THE PEDIATRIC SPINE PRINCIPLES AND PRACTICE

SECOND EDITION

THE PEDIATRIC SPINE
PRINCIPLES AND PRACTICE

SECOND EDITION

Editor

STUART L. WEINSTEIN, MD

Ignacio V. Ponseti Chair of Orthopaedic Surgery
Department of Orthopaedic Surgery
University of Iowa Hospitals
Iowa City, Iowa

LIPPINCOTT WILLIAMS & WILKINS
A **Wolters Kluwer** Company

Philadelphia · Baltimore · New York · London
Buenos Aires · Hong Kong · Sydney · Tokyo

Acquisitions Editor: Robert Hurley
Developmental Editor: Anne Snyder
Production Editor: Steven P. Martin
Manufacturing Manager: Colin J. Warnock
Cover Designer: Mark Lerner
Compositor: Maryland Composition
Printer: Edwards Brothers

© **2001 by LIPPINCOTT WILLIAMS & WILKINS**
530 Walnut Street
Philadelphia, PA 19106 USA
LWW.com

Printed in the USA

Library of Congress Cataloging-in-Publication Data
The pediatric spine : principles and practice / editor, Stuart L. Weinstein.—2nd ed.
     p. ; cm.
   Includes bibliographical references and index.
   ISBN 0-7817-1908-9 (casebound)
     1. Spine—Diseases. 2. Spinal cord—Diseases. 3. Pediatric orthopedics. I. Weinstein, Stuart L.
   [DNLM: 1. Spinal Diseases—Child. 2. Spinal Diseases—Infant. 3. Spinal
Diseases—surgery—Child. 4. Spinal Diseases—surgery—Infant. 5. Spinal Injuries—Child.
6. Spinal Injuries—Infant. 7. Spine—abnormalities. WE 725 P3713 2000]
   RD768.P363 2000
   618.92′73—dc21
                                                         00-042430

10 9 8 7 6 5 4 3 2 1

CONTENTS

CONTRIBUTING AUTHORS

Behrooz A. Akbarnia, MD Clinical Professor, Department of Orthopaedic Surgery, University of California, San Diego, Medical Director, San Diego Center for Spinal Disorders, 8010 Frost Street, Suite 401, San Diego, California 92123

Vincent Arlet, MD Associate Professor, Department of Orthopaedic Surgery, McGill University Health Center, Montreal Children's Hospital, 2300 Tupper Street, Montreal, Quebec, H3H 1P3 Canada

Elio Ascani, MD Ospedale Bambino Gesu, Centro Cura Delle Deformita, Della Colonna, Vertebrale, Via Torre de Palidoro, Passoscuro, Rome 1 00050, Italy

Gary M. Banks, MD Advanced Spine, Plymouth, Minnesota 55441

Michael J. Barnes, MB, ChB, FRACS Pediatric Spine Surgeon, Starship Children's Hospital, Eastwood Orthopaedic Clinic, 99 Remuera Road, Auckland 5, New Zealand

Randal R. Betz, MD Department of Orthopaedic Surgery, Temple University School of Medicine, Temple University Hospital, 3401 N. Broad Street; Chief of Staff, Shriners Hospitals for Children, 3551 North Broad Street, Philadelphia, Pennsylvania 19140

Stefano Boriani, MD Chief, Department of Orthopaedics and Traumatology, Ospedale Maggiore, Largo B. Nigrisoli, 2, Bologna, Italy 40133

J. Richard Bowen, MD Chairman, Department of Orthopaedics, duPont Hospital for Children, 1600 Rockland Road, PO Box 269, Wilmington, Delaware 19803

David S. Bradford, MD Professor and Chairman, Department of Orthopaedic Surgery, University of California, San Francisco, San Francisco, California 94143-0728

Keith H. Bridwell, MD Professor of Orthopaedic Surgery, Chief, Adult and Pediatric Spinal Surgery, Division of Orthopaedic Surgery, Washington University School of Medicine, One Barnes-Jewish Hospital Plaza, Suite 11300 West Pavilion, St. Louis, Missouri 63110

Wilton H. Bunch, PhD Beeson Divinity School, Samford University 800 Lakeshore Dr., Birmingham, Alabama 35339

Vincent J. Caiozzo, PhD Neuromuscular Research Laboratory, Department of Orthopaedics, University of California, Irvine College of Medicine, Irvine, California 92717

Laura Campanacci, MD Staff Orthopaedic Surgeon, Department of Skeletal Oncology, Ospedale Maggiore, Orthopaedics and Traumatology, Largo B. Nigrisoli, 2, Bologna, Italy 40133

Henry G. Chambers, MD Clinical Associate Professor, Department of Orthopaedic Surgery, University of California, San Diego, San Diego, California 92123; Chairman, Department of Orthopaedic Surgery, Children's Hospital and Health Center, 3030 Children's Way, Suite 410, San Diego, California 92123

Po-Quang Chen, MD, PhD Professor and Chief of Spine Section, Department of Orthopaedic Surgery, National Taiwan University Hospital, 7, Chung-Shan South Road, Taipei 100, Taiwan

Alvin H. Crawford, MD Professor, Department of Pediatric Orthopaedic Surgery, University of Cincinnati, Goodman Street, Cincinnati, Ohio 45229; Department Director, Department of Pediatric Orthopaedics, Children's Hospital Medical Center, 3333 Burnet Avenue, Cincinnati, Ohio 45229-3039

Mark S. Dias, MD Associate Professor, Department of Neurosurgery, State University of New York at Buffalo, Buffalo, New York 14222; Chief of Pediatric Neurosurgery, Departments of Pediatric Surgery and Neurosurgery, Children's Hospital of Buffalo, 219 Bryant Street, Buffalo, New York 14222

Robert A. Dickson, MA, ChM, FRCS, DSC Professor, University Department of Orthopaedic Surgery, Level 5, Room 5.8, Clinical Sciences Building, St. James University Hospital, Leeds, LS9 7TF, United Kingdom

Frederick Dietz, MD Professor, Department of Orthopaedic Surgery, University of Iowa, 200 Hawkins Drive, Iowa City, Iowa 52242

Carl DiRaimondo Department of Orthpaedic Surgery, Northwestern University, Chicago, Illinois 60611

Jean Dubousset, MD Professor of Pediatric Orthopaedics, Université René Descartes, Hôpital Saint Vincent de Paul, 82 avenue Denfert-Rochereau, 75674 Paris, France

Frank J. Eismont, MD   Department of Orthopaedics and Rehabilitation, University of Miami School of Medicine, Miami, Florida 33101

Georges Y. El-Khoury, MD   Department of Radiology University of Iowa, 200 Hawkins Drive, Iowa City, Iowa 52242-1077

François Fassier, MD   Department of Orthopaedic Surgery, McGill University Health Center, The Montreal Children's Hospital, 2300 Tupper Street, Montreal, Quebec H3H 1P3, Canada

Timothy M. Ganey, PhD   Director of Research, Atlanta Medical Center, Department of Orthopaedics, 303 Parkway Drive, NE, Director, co.don Tissue Engineering, Inc., 6104 River Terrace, Tampa, Florida 33604

Thomas M. Gavin, CO   Teaching Associate, Department of Orthopaedic Surgery, Loyola University Medical Center, 2160 First Avenue, Building 54, Maywood, Illinois 60153; President, Director of Clinical Services, Bio-Concepts, Inc., Orthotic-Prosthetic Centers, 100 Tower Drive, Suite 101, Burr Ridge, Illinois 60521

Teddy S. Govender, MD, FRCS   Professor and Chairman, Department of Orthopaedics, University of Natal Medical School, 719 Umbilo Road, Durban 4013, South Africa; Chief, Department of Spine Surgery, King George V Hospital, PO Box Domerton, Durban 4091, South Africa

Paul A. Grabb, MD   Department of Surgery, Division of Neurosurgery, University of Alabama at Birmingham, Children's Hospital of Alabama, Birmingham, Alabama 35233

Walter B. Greene, MD   Chairman and Professor, Department of Orthopaedic Surgery, University of Missouri Health Services Center, One Hospital Drive, MC213, Columbia, Missouri 65212

James T. Guille, MD   Chief Resident, Department of Orthopaedic Surgery, Hahnemann University Hospital, Broad & Vine Streets, Philadelphia, Pennsylvania 19120

Gregory V. Hahn, MD   Department of Orthopaedic Surgery, All Children's Hospital, 880 Sixth Street South, St. Petersburg, Florida 33701

Robert N. Hensinger, MD   Chairman and Professor, Section of Orthopaedic Surgery, University of Michigan Medical School, 1500 East Medical Center Drive, Ann Arbor, Michigan 48109

Eric K. W. Ho, FRCS (Glasg.), FRACS   Department of Orthopaedic Surgery, University of Hong Kong, Queen Mary Hospital, Hong Kong

Serena S. Hu, MD   Associate Professor and Staff Physician, Department of Orthopaedic Surgery, University of California, San Francisco, 500 Parnassus, Room MU 320W, San Francisco, California 94143-0728

Mark B. Kabins, MD   Department of Orthopaedics, University of Nevada Medical Center, 600 South Rancho Drive, #107, Las Vegas, Nevada 89106

Howard A. King, MD   St. Lukes Regional Medical Center, 190 E. Bannock Street, Boise, Idaho 83702

S. Jay Kumar, MD   Clinical Professor, Department of Orthopaedics Thomas Jefferson University Hospital, Philadelphia, Pennsylvania 19107; Senior Attending, Department of Orthopaedics, Alfred I. duPont Hospital for Children, 1600 Rockland Road, Wilmington, Delaware 19803

Hubert Labelle, MD   Clinical Professor, Department of Surgery, University of Montreal, C.P. 6128, Succursale Centre-Ville, Montreal, Quebec, Canada H3C 3J7; Staff Member, Division of Orthopaedics, Sainte-Justine Mother-Child University Hospital, 3175 Cote STE-Catherine Montreal, Quebec H3T 1C5, Canada

Guido La Rosa, MD   Ospedale Bambino Gesu, Centro Cura Delle Deformita, Della Colonna, Vertebrale, Via Torre de Palidoro, Passoscuro, Rome 1 00050, Italy

Nathan H. Lebwohl, MD   Associate Professor, Department of Orthopaedics and Rehabilitation, University of Miami School of Medicine, PO Box 016960 D-27, Miami, Florida 33101

John C. Y. Leong, FRCS, FRCSE, FRACS   Department of Orthopaedic Surgery, University of Hong Kong, Queen Mary Hospital, Hong Kong

Michael L. Levy, MD   Associate Professor, Department of Neurological Surgery, USC Keck School of Medicine, Division of Neurosurgery, Children's Hospital Los Angeles, 1300 North Vermont Ave #906, Los Angeles, California 90027

Mark A. Liker, MD   Clinical Instructor, Department of Neurological Surgery, USC Keck School of Medicine; Division of Neurosurgery, Children's Hospital Los Angeles, 1300 North Vermont Ave #906, Los Angeles, California 90027

Richard E. Lindseth, MD   Chairman and Professor, Department of Orthopaedic Surgery, Indiana University School of Medicine, 541 Clinical Drive, Room 600, Indianapolis, Indiana 46202-5111

Glenn E. Lipton   Temple University School of Medicine Philadelphia, Pennsylvania 19140,

Randall T. Loder, MD   Chief Surgeon, Shriners Hospitals for Children, Twin Cities Unit, 2025 East River Parkway, Minneapolis, Minnesota 55414

John E. Lonstein, MD   Clinical Professor, Department of Orthopaedic Surgery, University of Minnesota, Minneapolis, Minnesota 55455; Staff Physician, Twin Cities Spine Center, 913 East 26th Street, Minneapolis, Minnesota 55404

John P. Lubicky, MD, FAAOS, FAAP Professor, Department of Orthopaedic Surgery, Rush Medical College, 600 S. Paulina, Chicago, Illinois 60612; Chief of Staff, Shriners Hospitals for Children, 2211 North Oak Park Avenue, Chicago, Illinois 60707

Keith D. K. Luk, MCh, FRACS Department of Orthopaedic Surgery, University of Hong Kong, Queen Mary Hospital, Hong Kong

Aurelio G. Martinez-Lozano, MD Professor, Department of Orthopaedic Surgery, Universidad Autonoma de Nuevo Leon, Av. La Clinica, 2520 Number 214, Monterey, Mexico 64710

Richard E. McCarthy, MD Arkansas Spine Center, 500 South University, Suite 815, Little Rock, Arkansas 72205

J. Gordon McComb, MD Professor, Department of Neurological Surgery, USC Keck School of Medicine; Head, Division of Neurosurgery, Children's Hospital Los Angeles, 1300 North Vermont Avenue, Los Angeles, California 90027

David G. McLone, MD, PhD Professor of Neurosurgery, Northwestern University, 233 E. Erie, Chicago, Illinois 60611; Division Head, Pediatric Neurosurgery, Children's Memorial Hospital, 2300 Children's Plaza, Chicago, Illinois 60614

Michael J. McMaster, MD, FRCS Consultant Orthopaedic Spine Surgeon, Royal Hospital for Sick Children, Edinburgh EH10 7ED, Scotland

Kevin P. Meade, PhD Department of Mechanical, Materials and Aerospace Engineering, Illinois Institute of Technology, Chicago, Illinois 60616

Arnold H. Menezes, MD Professor and Vice Chairman, Division of Neurosurgery, University of Iowa, 200 Hawkins Drive, Iowa 52242

Nancy H. Miller, MS, MD Assistant Professor, Department of Orthopaedic Surgery, Johns Hopkins Hospital, 601 N. Caroline Street #5254, Baltimore, Maryland 21287-0882

Mary D. Moore, MD Department of Pediatrics, University of Iowa, 200 Hawkins Drive, Iowa City, Iowa 52242

Scott J. Mubarak, MD Clinical Professor, Department of Orthopaedics, University of California, San Diego, 200 W. Arbor Drive, San Diego, California 92123; Medical Director, Department of Orthopaedics, Children's Hospital, 3020 Children's Way, San Diego, California 92123

Mary Jane Mulcahey, MS, OTR/L Director, Department of Rehabilitation and Clinical Research, Shriners Hospitals for Children, 3551 North Broad Street, Philadelphia, Pennsylvania 19140

Virinder Nohria, MD, PhD Project Team Director, DevCo Pharmaceuticals Incorporated, 4825 Creekstone Drive—Suite 200, Research Triangle Park, Durham, NC 27703

Kenneth J. Noonan, MD Assistant Professor, Department of Orthopaedics, Indiana University School of Medicine, Riley Hospital for Children, 702 Barnhill Drive, Room 1134, Indianapolis, Indiana 46202

W. Jerry Oakes, MD Professor and Chief of Neurosurgery, Department of Surgery, University of Alabama, Birmingham, Children's Hospital of Alabama, 1600 7th Avenue, ACC 400, Birmingham, Alabama 35233

John A. Ogden, MD Atlanta Medical Center, 303 Parkway Drive, NE, Box 203, Atlanta, Georgia 30312

Avinash G. Patwardhan, PhD Department of Orthopaedic Surgery and Rehabilitation, Loyola University Medical Center, Maywood, Illinois 60143

Joseph H. Perra, MD Department of Orthopaedic Surgery, University of Minnesota, 420 Delaware Street SE, Box 492, Minneapolis, Minnesota 55455; Staff Surgeon, Twin Cities Spine Center, Piper Building, 913 East 26th, Suite 600, Minneapolis, Minnesota 55404-4515

William A. Phillips, MD Chief, Texas Children's Hospital, Professor, Orthopaedic Surgery and Pediatrics, Baylor College of Medicine, 6221 Fannin, Suite MC3-2295, Houston, Texas 77030

Thomas S. Renshaw, MD Professor of Orthopaedic Surgery, Department of Orthopaedics, Yale University School of Medicine, 800 Howard Avenue, YPB 133, New Haven, Connecticut 06510; Attending Physician, Department of Orthopaedic Surgery, Yale-New Haven Hospital, 20 York Street, New Haven, Connecticut 06510

David Ring, MD Instructor, Department of Orthopaedic Surgery, Harvard Medical School; Director of Research, Department of Orthopedic Surgery, Massachusetts General Hospital, Harvard Combined Orthopaedic Program, Boston, Massachusetts 02114

Timothy C. Ryken, MD Division of Neurosurgery, University of Iowa Hospitals and Clinics, University of Iowa, 200 Hawkins Drive, Iowa City, Iowa 52242-1061

John F. Sarwark, MD Associate Professor, Department of Orthpaedic Surgery, Northwestern University, Chicago, Illinois 60611; Interim Division Head, Division of Orthopaedic Surgery, Children's Memorial Hospital, 2300 Children's Plaza, No. 69, Chicago, IL 60614-3394

Yutaka Sato, MD Department of Radiology, University of Iowa, 200 Hawkins Drive, Iowa City, Iowa 52242-1077

Donald G. Schurr, CPO, PT American Prosthetics and Orthotics, Incorporated, The University of Iowa Hospitals and Clinics, Iowa City, Iowa 52242

James D. Schwender, MD Twin Cities Spine Center, 913 East 26th Street, Minneapolis, Minnesota 55404

Young-Shung Shen, MD Director, Po-Cheng Orthopaedic Institute, 100, Po-Ai 2nd Road, Kaohsiung 813, Taiwan

Russell D. Snyder, MD Professor, Department of Neurology and Pediatrics, University of New Mexico School of Medicine, 915 Camino de Salud, Albuquerque, New Mexico 87131-5281; Attending Physician, Department of Neurology, University of New Mexico Hospital, 2211 Lomas, NE, Albuquerque, New Mexico 87106

Paul D. Sponseller, MD Chief of Pediatric Orthopaedics and Professor, Department of Orthopaedic Surgery, Johns Hopkins University, 601 North Carolina Street #5253, Baltimore, Maryland 21287-0882

Ian A. F. Stokes, PhD Department of Orthopaedics and Rehabilitation, The University of Vermont, Stafford Hall 434, Burlington, Vermont 05405-0084

Ensor E. Transfeldt, MD University of Minnesota; Twin Cities Spine Center, 913 East 26th Street, Suite 600 Minneapolis, Minnesota 55404

William C. Warner, Jr., MD Associate Professor, University of Tennessee—Campbell Clinic, Department of Orthopaedic Surgery 910 Madison Avenue, Suite 500, Memphis, Tennessee 38103

James N. Weinstein, DO, MS Professor, Department of Community and Family Medicine, Dartmouth Medical School, 7251 Strasenburgh Hall, Hanover, New Hampshire 03755; Director, The Spine Center, Dartmouth-Hitchcock Medical Center, One Medical Center Drive, Lebanon, New Hampshire 03756

Stuart L. Weinstein, MD Ignacio V. Ponseti Chair of Orthopaedic Surgery, Department of Orthopaedic Surgery, University of Iowa, 200 Hawkins Drive, Iowa City, Iowa 52242

Dennis R. Wenger, MD Clinical Professor, Department of Orthopaedic Surgery, University of California, San Diego; Director of Pediatric Orthopaedics, Children's Hospital of San Diego, 3030 Children's Way, Suite 410, San Diego, California 92123

PREFACE

The practice of medicine is in an exciting era of change because of explosive advances in molecular genetics and biophysics, and the development of new biomaterials. The concepts and principles developed in the laboratory must be rapidly applied to the clinical setting. Pediatric patients with a disease or disorder of the spine often requires a multidisciplinary team of health care professionals. The effective management of these patients requires collaboration between basic scientists and clinicians of various disciplines to deal with these complex problems.

The Pediatric Spine brings together international experts from several disciplines to provide a definitive reference text for the health care professional interested in problems related to the pediatric spine. This book is the only comprehensive text devoted exclusively to this subject. It provides the reader with an in-depth study of disorders of the pediatric spine and related conditions. Strong emphasis is given to the basic sciences in the introductory chapters and throughout the text.

The authors of each chapter, with their considerable experience and expertise, provide complete and in-depth coverage of each subject. The chapters focusing on disease entities place strong emphasis on natural history, diagnosis, pathobiology of disease, and scope and breadth of operative and nonoperative management options.

The text also provides the reader with an in-depth look at related topics of imaging of the spine, and a detailed appendix of radiographic measurements, classifications, and definitions. Each chapter is accompanied by a comprehensive bibliography on the subject.

The Pediatric Spine is aimed at the senior resident and the practicing pediatric spine specialist. It should also be of interest to orthopaedic surgeons, pediatricians, neurosurgeons, bioengineers, therapists and orthotists, and anyone who has interest in patients with pediatric spinal disorders.

Stuart L. Weinstein, MD

ACKNOWLEDGMENTS

The completion of the first edition of The *Pediatric Spine: Principles and Practice* would not have been possible without the guidance, direction, encouragement, and hard work of Kathey Alexander of Lippincott Williams & Wilkins. Ms. Alexander's work ethic, dedication to purpose, and professional manner of dealing with the complex aspects of producing a high-quality textbook are greatly appreciated. Ms. Alexander was assisted by the equally capable and hardworking Beth Weiselberg. While their responsibilities and ongoing projects at Lippincott Williams & Wilkins are many, Ms. Alexander and Ms. Weiselberg always made me feel that *The Pediatric Spine: Principles and Practice* was their only concern. For this second edition, I would also like to thank Ms. Anne Snyder for her dedication to task and particularly for her perseverance.

I would also like to express my appreciation and gratitude to medical illustrators Tom Weinzeril of the University of Iowa and Paul Gross of Vanderbilt University, who worked very closely with each chapter author and the editor to bring the authors' words, principles, and techniques to life.

To Joyce Roller, my secretary and colleague over the last 22 years, I owe an extreme debt of gratitude for keeping me organized and on track. She never let being overworked interfere with her pleasant and professional manner in dealing with patients, families, and professional colleagues; she is an inspiration to all.

Finally, and most importantly, I am indebted to an outstanding group of experts who assembled their considerable knowledge and experience in the form of text chapters. Their spirit of cooperation and sense of common purpose was displayed time and time again during the production of this text in meeting editorial deadlines, revising and re-revising chapters, and sharing case photos and case materials. It is to these caring and talented health care providers that credit for this text is due.

Stuart L. Weinstein, M.D.

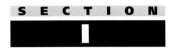

DEVELOPMENTAL ANATOMY

DEVELOPMENT AND MATURATION
OF THE AXIAL SKELETON

TIMOTHY M. GANEY
JOHN A. OGDEN

GENERAL DEVELOPMENTAL CONCEPTS

Developmental biology reflects the interactive dynamics of molecules and organisms guided by genetic and physical cues, including those external to the organism. These responses eventually bridge the distinction of genotype and phenotype, embryogenesis orchestrating a synthetic yet specific response to the workings of normal and modified mechanochemical controls (92,197).

The recognizable development of any specific axial skeletal structure begins with cellular proliferation (multiplication) to produce a critical cell mass, defined as the *anlage*, which may be affected by separate inductive biochemical and biophysical (mechanochemical) factors (245,249). Induction, coupled with permissive interactions, promotes further cell differentiation to form modified or additional anlagen (primordia) for the progressive development of intermediate and final overall vertebral structure.

Molecular, cellular, and tissue interactions; hierarchies; and increasing organ complexity are the fundamental features of embryonic development during axial embryogenesis (137,161). One of the most important aspects of the embryonic period is interactive induction, which is the evocative mechanochemical action of one cell or tissue type on another (252). Early cell or tissue forms may act on an adjacent type to elicit the origin of a third, usually different, cell or tissue. Specificity of such inductions not only resides in the inducing and responding cells but also is subject to the timing and duration of the interaction (126,137). Such interactions, which are molecularly based, are important to axial structuring of the vertebrate embryo, especially through progressive activation of homeoboxes (43).

Differentiation often is followed by a migration phase in which a committed cellular group moves to a more specific region within the embryo. During migration, animal cells release traces of material in the matrix as footprints of their locomotion and adhesion (116,378). Although the phenomenon is poorly understood, traces of integrin and other components of focal contacts in the tracks suggest that deposition and interactive recognition may extrude a patterned scaffold during elaboration of the anlage material (276). The group may either repeat the entire sequence (inductive cell change followed by further migra-

tion) or undergo revision in place to form the final structure through localized cell growth, matrix elaboration and modification, and, on occasion, programmed cell death (100,143–145). Changes to and virtual disappearance of the notochord typify such cellular alterations and disappearances (143,170,213,346).

Morphogenesis of the axial skeleton of vertebrates is characterized by mechanical and molecularly directed programmed movements of regions of embryonic cells to form and rearrange the three primary tissue groupings—ectoderm, endoderm, and mesoderm (51,53,70,102). These stages of reactive tissue pattern formation lead to progressive spatial biologic organization. Tabin (326) described such pattern formations as the "choreography of developmental processes in three dimensions." These cellular amalgamations, rearrangements, and migrations during embryogenesis play a critical role in organizing the basic physical structure that defines axial structure and orientation and in mediating those interactions between the various cell populations that regulate progressive patterns of gene expression, specification of cell fates, and the final definition of axial skeletal structures at the end of embryogenesis (45,90,91,102,146,161,186, 189,193,227).

Axial skeletogenesis is further characterized by the orderly, progressive appearance of mesenchymal, cartilaginous, and osseous cell types. These cellular "skeletal" changes are conferred as reactive modifications to the biosynthesis of extracellular matrix components. Matrix molecules such as hyaluronan may enhance a chondrogenic phase (endochondral bone formation), and fibronectin may inhibit cartilage differentiation (membranous bone formation) (375). Polarity of the cell may be instrumental in influencing differentiation of the cell. For instance, disrupting the actin cytoskeleton of mesenchymal cells causes them not only to round up but also to produce type II (versus type I) collagen (376). Wedging of one end of the neuroectodermal cells, due to the influence of the basement membrane, likewise facilitates progressive formation and deepening of the neural groove to form the neural tube (317,318).

ABNORMAL DEVELOPMENT

Alterations in a molecular or a macromolecular process may lead to structural defects involving the spine and spinal cord. Such defects may occur prenatally, manifest postnatally, or be combined over the course of both periods. The alterations can be divided into three basic categories from the standpoint of developmental pathogenesis.

T. M. Ganey and J. A. Ogden: Atlantic Medical Center, Atlanta, Georgia 30312.

Malformation

Malformation follows a failure of embryologic differentiation, development, or both of a specific anatomic structure, resulting in either absence or improper formation of the structure before the fetal period. An example in the axial skeleton is formation of a hemivertebra. Malformations involve a defect intrinsic to the developing embryo and thus occur during organogenesis. Once anatomically established, the defect may continue to adversely affect spinal development throughout subsequent fetal and postnatal periods. Malformations such as hemivertebrae or bars affect three-dimensional development and growth, contributing to both the rate of progression and severity of congenital scoliosis.

Ultimately, malformation and its severity depend on the stage of the developmental or maturation cycle affected (173). Inhibition of cellular proliferation before differentiation can cause either embryonic death or structural agenesis (e.g., failure to differentiate disc material, which may lead to fusion of adjacent vertebral bodies, although the posterior elements, which have a relatively independent origin, may remain separate). Failure of induction through a qualitative lack of an inducer substance or unresponsiveness of target cells also can lead to agenesis of a structure (e.g., lumbosacral agenesis), depending on when during embryogenesis the failure occurs (173). Because cell migration follows induction and differentiation, alterations at this stage in the cycle do not usually produce complete agenesis (222). In extreme cases, ineffective migration can cause adhesion of adjacent primordia and yield fused structures, as in Klippel-Feil syndrome. Failure in cell growth and maturation after migration may result in structural hypoplasia. Alterations at this stage may involve modification of an antecedent structure that had differentiated normally at first. Programmed cell death also is an important factor in the final shaping of structures.

Disruption

Disruption is a structural defect caused by destruction of a part that formed normally during the embryonic period. This mechanism involves the limbs (e.g., amniotic band syndrome with intrauterine autoamputation) more frequently than the spine during the fetal stage. Among children disruption is likely to have an acquired cause that involves alteration of growth patterns and destruction or distortion of basic morphologic features by trauma, infection, tumors, or metabolic alterations. Among children with discitis, for example, alteration of a structure, such as calcification of a disc, may cause fusion of the contiguous vertebrae and loss of the end plate contributions to longitudinal growth. Fractures of end plate growth mechanisms may cause kyphosis or scoliosis through altered growth patterns.

Deformation

Deformation embodies alteration in the shape or structure of an individual vertebra or the entire spine during the fetal or postnatal period. The involved region would have initially differentiated normally, as in infantile or adolescent scoliosis. The nature and severity of deformations are contingent not only on the magnitude and direction of the extrinsic deforming forces but also on the intrinsic properties of the structure or tissue on which they act. Relative resistance of each skeletal spinal tissue component to mechanical stress is important. However, inherent growth potential also is a factor in any final morphologic deformation (34). In general, compressive forces applied along a major growth axis such as the spine produce varying distortion in multiple planes as the tissues grow despite the imposed biomechanical restrictions.

Deformations may be divided between those intrinsically derived and those that are extrinsically acquired (173). *Intrinsic deformation* is caused by a reduction in the ability of the fetus or child to move away from normal imposed forces. It depends on the integrity of the neuromuscular system to respond effectively. Underlying abnormalities of the brain, spinal cord, peripheral nerves, neuromuscular junction, muscle, tendon, or bone may be responsible (340). Some of these are genetically derived and thus carry a latent risk of recurrence. Many deformations persist in their deleterious effects. The results are progressive spinal deformation and a reduction in the likelihood of normal function and response to treatments, which must often be directed at the deformation rather than at the specific underlying cause.

Extrinsic prenatal deformations are caused by a reduction in the space in which a developing fetus can move. Such reduction may be either physiologic or pathologic. Physiologic structural deformations usually are limited and relatively reversible once the constraining influences are removed. In contrast, pathologic structural deformation is permanent. In both physiologic and pathologic extrinsic deformation, the specific fetal part usually is genetically programmed to be normal. Because they usually are caused by extrinsic (epigenetic) factors, deformational and disruptive defects may occur or recur at variable periods throughout fetal and postnatal development.

Late gestational deformations have an excellent prognosis. Approximately 90% of deformations found at birth correct spontaneously. Of those that do not, most can be corrected by early means of postural intervention. This emphasizes the importance of early detection of infantile scoliosis (88). The earlier a deformation is recognized, the greater is the likelihood of correcting it or at least preventing progression, as with early bracing of idiopathic scoliosis.

BASIC PATTERNS OF BONE FORMATION

At birth the bones of the cranial vault consist of plates of resilient compact bone. After birth, the outer surface becomes a dense structure through rapid subperiosteal formation of new bone, cortical thickening, and mechanically induced remodeling. The inner surface, which undergoes both resorption and deposition, forms a less prominent inner table. This variable postnatal hardness of the outer and inner tables affects the ability to use halo fixation devices. Halo pins can easily penetrate this relatively soft bone of children, especially those younger than 10 years. Careful monitoring of pin sites is essential whenever pins are used to treat patients with immature skeletons.

A major method of cranial osseous expansion that is responsive to concomitant brain growth is *translation*. This is the tectonic displacement of the individual cranial plates relative to each other and the underlying neural tissue expansion. The sutures allow such expansion. When the sutures closure prematurely, as in Apert syndrome and other craniofacial abnormality syndromes, the brain continues to grow against a nonexpansile cranial vault. Early postnatal neurosurgical intervention to make pseudosutures may allow relatively adequate skull expansion and avert brain and intellectual impairment. Conversely, exaggerated expansion of the intracranial contents, as in hydrocephalus, can increase separation of the cranial plates and cause cranial enlargement. Early placement of a shunt usually prevents this complication for a patient with a myelomeningocele or any other predis-

posing neurologic condition. The expanding brain and uterine compression can cause microstructural failures and incomplete healing to form the multiple wormian bones of osteogenesis imperfecta.

The components of the axial skeletal are involved in membranous ossification. The cortex of the developing bone of the posterior elements is derived from specialized mesenchymal tissue known as *periosteum*, which surrounds the chondroosseous model (267,277). This periosteum-derived membranous bone eventually forms much of the cortical bone of the posterior elements of the mature axial skeleton of skeletal maturity (Fig. 1). Periosteal membranous bone contributes to the cortical shells of the vertebral bodies, but usually not until the primary ossifica-

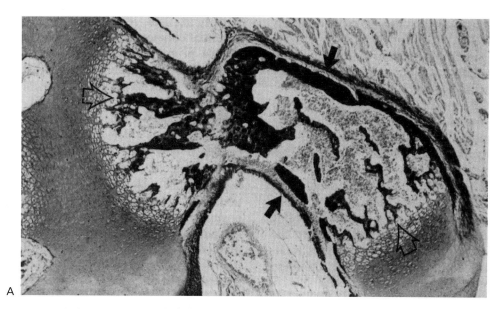

A

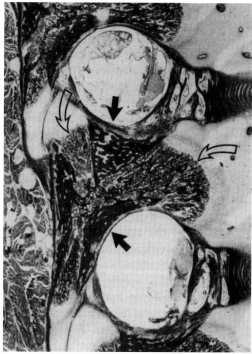

B

FIGURE 1. A: Combination of membranous cortical bone (*solid arrows*) and endochondral bone (*open arrows*) in the posterior segment (lamina and pedicle, as they extend from the vertebral centrum, *left*). A growth plate is present at each end of the expanding posterior primary ossification. Portions of the physis around the anterior primary ossification process are just visible at the *left*. **B:** More extensively remodeled posterior element membranous bone with thickened, mechanically defined trabecula (*solid arrows*) in contrast to the endochondral trabeculae associated with the physis adjacent to the facet joints (*open arrows*) and the junction with the vertebral centrum (*right*).

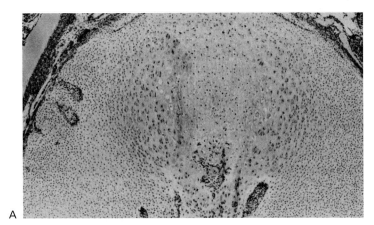
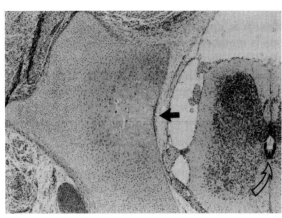

A   B

FIGURE 2. Early development of the primary ossification centers in the centrum **(A)** and posterior elements **(B)**. Definite osseous collars comparable with the long bones are not evident. Early vascular penetration is present anterolaterally and posteriorly. This eventually forms cartilage canals. Posteriorly **(B)** a condensation (*solid arrow*) indicates the first evidence of eccentric membranous bone formation. This condensation initially forms on the spinal canal surface. The closing neural canal is visible (*open arrow*).

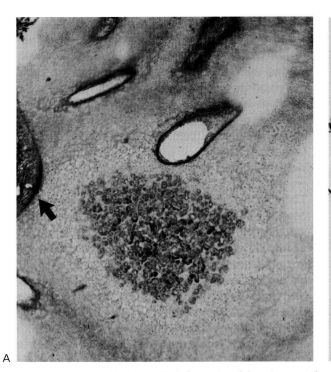
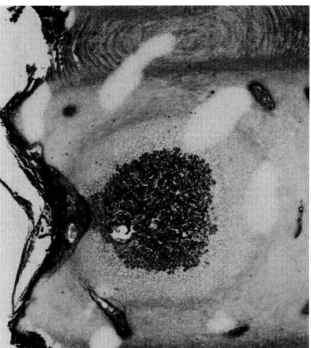

A   B

FIGURE 3. **A:** Early formation of the primary ossification center of a lumbar anterior segment (centrum). Large vessels are present within the cartilage. A very thin area of membranous bone is present anteriorly (*arrow*). This occurs in some vertebrae concomitant with ossification in the primary center. In other vertebrae it does not appear peripherally until after primary ossification begins. **B:** Ossification, more advanced than in **A**, within the primary center of a thoracic vertebra. This ossification has expanded eccentrically toward the anterior border. **A** and **B** are images of the same embryo, indicating the variable extent of ossification within the multiple spinal vertebrae. A forming intervertebral disc region is present in **B**.

tion center has expanded to the edges of the vertebral centrum and modified the perichondrium into periosteum. This modification varies with both postnatal age and spinal region.

Endochondral Bone Formation

Endochondral bone formation is the primary developmental process of the occipital bone and axial postcranial skeletal components in utero. Such bone formation is the result of synchronous replacement of the mesenchymal precursor first by a cartilaginous intermediate in the embryonic phase and then by osseous tissue, which prevails in the fetal phase. This overall process is a continuum that can be divided conceptually into a series of relatively discrete transformations (141).

Initial formation of a precartilaginous, cellular mesenchymal condensation—the basic anlage—elaborates extracellular matrix to form the hyaline cartilage model (41,138). Axial skeletal cartilage can be detected in the human embryo by the fifth week of gestation (140). Once they differentiate into chondroblasts, cells elaborate an appropriate extracellular matrix, the composition of which defines the basic cartilage types—hyaline cartilage, fibrocartilage, and elastic cartilage. The skeletal anlage of a given vertebra enlarges by means of cellular duplication, an increase in extracellular matrix, an appositional increase from the perichondrium, and subsequent selective hypertrophy of the chondrocytes in the central region of the anlage (211). The initial patterns of central and peripheral formation differ between the posterior and anterior elements (Fig. 2) The progressive chondroosseous transformation in each of the posterior elements is similar to, but not the same as, primary ossification of a typical longitudinal bone. In contrast, the anterior element (vertebral centrum) undergoes primary ossification in a manner analogous to secondary epiphyseal ossification in a long bone (Fig. 3).

In the long bones, concomitant with central cellular hypertrophy, peripheral primary membranous bone usually forms near the hypertrophic central chondrocytes. It is important to conceptualize that this initial bone is membrane-derived (woven) bone. Fibrovascular tissue then enters from the primary bone into the central region of hypertrophic cells, becoming the nutrient artery. The "directions" for the anlage to undergo hypertrophic changes, form membranous "outer" bone and then a primary ossification center are undoubtedly responses to biophysical (biomechanical) changes within the embryo (8,56,57, 60,129,139,187,257,275,371).

In the spine, however, the aforementioned processes are selectively modified in relation to the "classic" model of limb bone formation (108). A completely encircling periosteal "cortex" and shell are not significant early components of formation of either anterior or posterior elements. Instead, the vertebral centrum ossification center expands toward the periphery eventually to define the cortex in the fetal period. Vascular penetration is through a perichondrial sleeve rather than a periosteum and thin outer osseous shell. Vascular penetration is multiple in the anterior elements (Fig. 4) and more restricted in the posterior elements. True periosteum around the centrum is minimal until later fetal and postnatal stages. The posterior elements also differ. Peripheral membranous ossification begins eccentrically from the dural (inner) surface rather than centrally and symmetrically (see later).

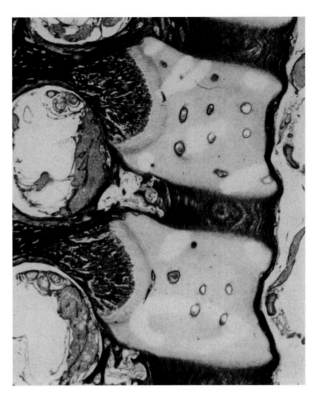

FIGURE 4. Numerous vascular channels in the thoracic vertebra, At this stage the channels have not begun primary ossification in the anterior elements. The posterior elements are well ossified. Physes extend toward the centrum, where they will contribute to the final vertebral body below, or anterior to the spinal canal.

The process of calcification in the hypertrophic regions of the developing vertebra involves ordered "remodeling" of the extracellular matrix (218). In the process calcified cartilage is modified and replaced with bone. This process extends toward each end of the centrum and posterior element anlagen. Reconstruction also entails integrated, concomitant development and extension of the periosteum and bone collar longitudinally toward the ends of the anlage. The periosteum and membranous bone collar, although incompletely encircling the pedicle, become well established in the posterior elements before there are any traces of such structures around the centrum. The combined processes form the primary ossification center, which enlarges to become the diaphyseal and metaphyseal equivalents of similar regions in the appendicular skeleton. As discussed later, these processes are variably modified in the chondroosseous transformation of the vertebral anlagen. Each of the three components of the final vertebra (one anterior, two posterior) form areas analogous to the diaphysis and metaphyses. The epiphyses become the neurocentral and spinous process synchondroses between anterior and posterior elements and the superior and inferior end plates of the centrum. An orderly arrangement of the cells is established adjacent to the expanding primary ossification centers and is equivalent in many respects to a long bone physis. This arrangement forms a site of active modeling and remodeling metaphyses more in the posterior elements than in the centrum (Fig. 5).

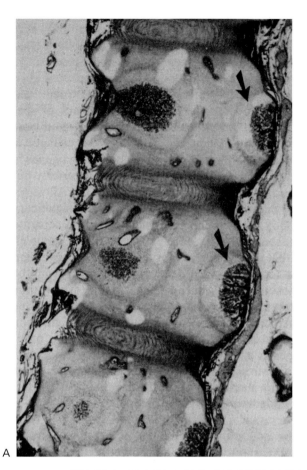

FIGURE 5. **A:** Formation of a primary ossification center in the anterior regions of the lumbar vertebrae (*left*). The presence of the anterior segment of peripheral membranous ossification is variable. A physis is evident around each anterior ossification center. Extension of the primary posterior ossification centers into the centrum is evident (*right, arrows*), a process also surrounded by a physeal region. **B:** More mature primary ossification in the centrum. The physeal region surrounds the ossification process, and the nonossified but vascularized ossification center extends to the membranous peripheral collar.

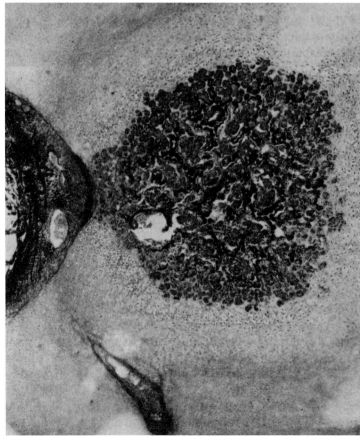

With the establishment of a primary ossification center within the centrum, endochondral bone formation progressively localizes to the ends and synchondroses of each vertebra. The central (diaphyseal) area models and remodels by means of peripheral membranous ossification that gradually replaces most, if not all, of the endochondral bone. The presence of growth regions like those of long bones helps explain the altered growth of vertebral height in the centrum in many types of skeletal dysplasia.

EMBRYOGENESIS

Molecular Embryology

Differentiation occurs through progressive, controlled division of cells. However, before most cells form specialized groupings, a master plan designating axial orientation and major body regions (e.g., head, trunk, tail) has been established at the molecular level. According to such a genetic blueprint, apparently identical combinations of cells and tissues (at least by current analytical methods) are arranged into distinctly different microanatomic regions and then recognizable macrostructures (76,77). Early establishment of the head-to-tail (craniocaudal) axis provides the orientation for subsequent structural development (236, 294–297,372).

Cellular regions that develop the potential for expression into a discrete structure are defined as *morphogenetic fields* (29, 77,370). Within each morphogenetic field, the potential for forming individual organs, such as specific bones, varies gradually. These areas of potential are called *gradient fields,* which correspond closely with the pattern of expression of certain more discrete sets of genes. *Craniocaudal, preaxial, postaxial,* and *proximodistal* are common terms that reflect such gradient-field expression.

The families of genes responsible for complex, early differentiation processes are called *homeobox genes* (77,119,157,233). They direct subdivision of the early embryo into progressively differentiated fields of cells with inherent potential for tissue and organ specificity. Homeobox genes specify the identities and fates of embryonic cells and gradually shape the body conformation into either a normal or an abnormal pattern (84,119, 124,125,127,166,179,185,186,189,193,197,282,289,298,319, 338,342,347,359,363–365,372,373).

According to homeobox gene expression patterns, embryo sequentially subdivides into fields of cells with different developmental capabilities. Such field subdivision precedes any histologic evidence of specific organs or structures (77). The identity and morphologic features of an individual vertebra can change if the domain of action of one of the homeobox genes is altered, as when it is normally expressed anteriorly but is instead expressed more posteriorly (179). All vertebrate organisms appear to have at least four important homeobox gene complexes, each located on separate chromosomes (86). These complex genes controlling early embryonic cellular expression are arranged sequentially (linearly) in the chromosomal DNA in the same order in which they are expressed along the craniocaudal body axis. This arrangement may have come about because homeobox genes must be sequentially activated in a specific order during early embryonic development (359). Homeobox genes are strongly expressed in sequential bands along the craniocaudal axis in early development. Later, when more specific tissues or organs are forming in discrete regions, the same homeobox genes may once again be intensely expressed (77).

An increased understanding of homeoboxes and diffuse growth factors has led to the embryologic concept of *morphoregulation,* in which the notion of biologic shape and intrinsic tissue patterns is linked to those of specific molecular regulatory loops, genetic controls, and cellular driving forces within both inductive and target tissues (92). The evocative forces that shepherd morphogenesis are cellular (biomechanical) in origin—division, movement, adhesion, cell death; they are extrinsic, often phenotypic, forces perceived by cells. Molecules, however, serve as the essential and regulating linkage between gene expression and mechanical driving forces (92,93).

The developmental patterns of disease expression often reflect a continuum of relatively discrete molecular processes. An abnormal developmental gene, initially active in embryogenesis, can be reactivated at various times throughout life in highly regular temporal and spatial patterns (87,123,174). Some of these genes and certain growth factors have the potential to become oncogenic when activated after birth (87,123).

Mesoderm Formation (Gastrulation)

In the spherical embryo of the clawed frog *Xenopus,* which is often used to understand the early phases of basic embryonic development, mesodermal formation is induced by growth factors released by cells within the ventral embryonic pole. The mesoderm forms at the "equator" between the ectodermal (animal) and endodermal (vegetal) hemispheres. Fibroblast growth factor may act as this ventrovegetalizing factor and induce mesoderm formation. Fibroblast growth factor may exert biologic effects on a wide variety of mesoderm- and neuroectoderm-derived cells. It also may act as a morphogen or mitogen in later phases of development (128).

The invagination process in the human embryo is analogous to gastrulation in spherical embryos (3,6,22,23,39,101,103,111, 147–149,184,243,301–303,344,360,368). At the caudal end of the bilaminar, flat mammalian embryo, circumscribed areas of tissue invaginate through a basement membrane between the ectoderm and the endoderm during the second week of gestation. This modified process first involves formation of a specialized cellular aggregation in the ectoderm, the *primitive streak* (22), which is located at the caudal end of the embryo. The area of invagination, the *primitive pit,* is surrounded by a cellular aggregation known as the *primitive knot.* These invaginating tissues elongate in a caudal to cranial direction. The mesenchymal tissues on either side of the primitive streak become mesoderm, establishing the trilaminar—ectoderm, mesoderm, endoderm—embryo.

In the midline the primitive knot produces the first important "skeletal" structure, the *notochord,* which intercalates between the ectoderm and the endoderm. Continuing elongation of both the notochord and the mesoderm takes place in a caudal to cranial sequence.

Notochord Formation and Induction

The initial notochord forms as the rostral extension of cells from the primitive streak that then fuses to the endoderm. A pit appears in the primitive node and extends in the caudal to cranial direction along the notochord as the *notochordal canal.* The canal floor undergoes degradation. The true notochord then forms from the dorsal portion associated with the ectoderm. Persistence of the canal has been implicated as a cause of diastematomyelia and the various rachischisis deformities (228,229). Abnormal ectoendodermal adhesion may cause split notochord syndrome, which consists of vertebral anomalies, a mediastinal cyst, and intestinal abnormalities. Several investigators have implicated this stage in the coexistence of spinal and enteric deformities (17,18,26).

When formation of the notochord is suppressed, as with lithium, several consequences may occur (337,349). The somites may fuse across the midline. The notochord normally acts as a barrier to prevent fusion of contralateral somites and block fusion of spinal ganglia across the midline until the appropriate stage of development. The neural tube may lack a floor plate. The notochord induces and localizes the floor plate of the neural tube. In regions lacking a notochord, cartilage develops variably or may not develop. Absence of the notochord may not uniformly suppress cartilage formation but certainly can lead to altered morphogenesis of the vertebral column (160,162). Instead of separate vertebrae, a continuous cartilage tube may develop that has openings for the segmented nerves. Neural arches and vertebral processes may form but may be fused. In various experiments investigators have concluded that the notochord is indispensable for development of the intervertebral regions (intervertebral discs) and individualization of somites to form vertebrae (337).

The notochord remains within the developing vertebral bodies but progressively constricts during the fetal period. It remains for a longer time between vertebrae in the presumptive disc region (Fig. 6). The retention of notochordal tissue is an inductive factor in further differentiation of the disc components.

Neurulation and Tube Closure

Critical developmental events usually are regulated by groups of genes that encode components of signal transduction pathways. One such group, the neurogenic loci, is required for normal segregation of epidermal from neural cell lineages (171). The neurogenic gene products are believed to function in cellular communication pathways that ultimately involve nuclear regulatory components (30,35,50,51). In neurulation, the final product is a group of cells (cell lineage) programmed to become the subsequent neural tube (306,320,345).

The basement membrane between the notochord and the ectoderm is necessary to induce the differentiation of the neuroectoderm (45,46,70). Cells must attach to this membrane to release the appropriate signal. Cells to be stimulated also must attach to the basement membrane. Attachment failures may be responsible for structural defects such as myelomeningocele (107,176,177,250).

Once the neural plate forms, the edges at the junction with the remaining surface ectoderm elevate and produce a neural groove that deepens until the apices of the folds approach and appose each other (Fig. 7A). Elevation of the neural fold is associ-

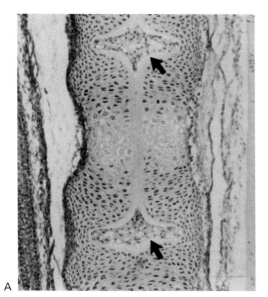

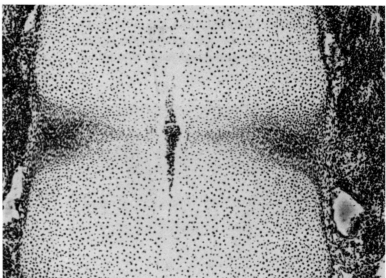

A   B

FIGURE 6.   A: Early developmental changes in hamster vertebrae. The notochord (*arrows*) is expanding between vertebrae to induce (form) the disc material, especially the nucleus pulposus. As in human embryonic vertebrae, there is notochordal continuity between the intervertebral discs. Central hypertrophy of cells on either side of the notochord traversing the vertebral body indicates the future site of the paired primary ossification centers that will coalesce around the notochord. **B:** Similar notochord presence in the center of the presumptive disc region of a human embryo. Condensation of disc material is more evident laterally than centrally, where the notochord is still evident but regressing.

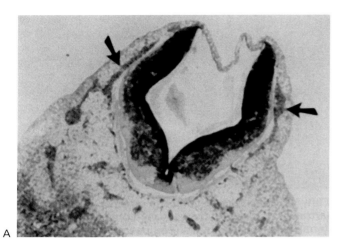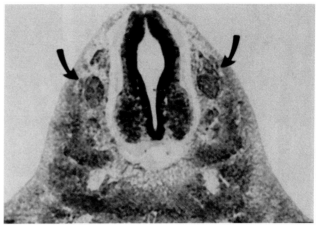

A

B

FIGURE 7. **A:** Closing neural tube. Although closure is incomplete, further cellular differentiation is evident within the lateral cord masses. The neural crest (*arrows*) is also starting to differentiate. **B:** Almost completed closure of the neural tube. The neuroectodermal cleft is still evident dorsally. Overlying nonneural ectoderm closure, however, is complete. Neural crest–derived spinal ganglia are forming (*arrows*). The differentiating vertebral anlagen (somites) and central notochord are evident below the neural tube. The presumptive somite has dorsal and ventral cellular regions separated by a relatively dense cellular zone.

ated with a change in cell shape from columnar to apically wedged (305,308,315–318). Cytoskeletal proteins likely stabilize this wedging process (168) as disassembly of microfilaments by cytochalasins results in the collapse of convex cranial neural folds (307).

The edges of the induced neural plate curve dorsally to progressively constitute the neural tube (248). This process begins centrally along the longitudinal axis and continues in both cranial and caudal directions, leaving the neural tube temporarily incomplete (open) at each end. Interruption of the tubularization process can lead to entities such as anencephaly or myelomeningocele. This bidirectional closure pattern also explains the frequent concomitant occurrence of abnormalities at each end of the neural system, such as hydrocephalus due to proximal ventricular abnormalities in association with distal myelomeningocele. If the notochord initially induces a defective neural plate or tube, either may induce defective differentiation of the paraxial mesoderm (spinal skeletal precursor) (96,133). The result may be abnormal vertebral development (congenital scoliosis) and abnormalities of the spinal cord (324).

The apposed folds fuse along the midline and lose continuity with the surface ectoderm, which then also fuses across the midline, internalizing the neural folds (Fig. 7B). As the neural folds contact each other, multiple cell surface projections interdigitate. The mechanics of neurulation appear to vary by level within the same embryo; this is particularly evident between cephalic and somitic levels in the chick (107). Convergence of the apposed folds is more important at cephalic and caudal regions than along the somites. Essential to convergence are isolation of the basal lamina from the nonneural ectoderm and formation of a new basal lamina associated with the nonneural ectoderm. At somitic levels this produces a cavity between the basal lamina through cellular adhesion. This process allows not only closure of the neural tube but also reestablishment of nonneural ectodermal

continuity over the closed tube. This concomitance of cellular fusion processes helps explain why dorsal skin does not form over a myelomeningocele.

Different mechanisms may underlie neurulation at different levels of the body axis (55,175,225,318). There appears to be a qualitative difference between de novo initiation of closure, bidirectional continuation of closure, and final closure at either end (36,225). Initial closure involves the embryo in establishing a new set of conditions, whereas continuation and final closure are the replication of a previously existing set of conditions to an adjacent portion of the body axis. Muller and O'Rahilly (244), who studied anencephalic fetuses, proposed independent development of the skull and the brain and suggested that certain disorders are related primarily to skeletal disturbance and only secondarily to the contiguous neural component.

Closure of the posterior neuropore appears to be the most susceptible to disturbance. The critical events are the coordinated growth of the various axially arranged tissue types and their mutual attachment by means of the extracellular matrices. Neural tube defects result when growth imbalances occur or when the axial components become dissociated from each other, as when the notochord becomes detached from the neural plate (242). Under such circumstances, axial elongation does not occur normally, or abnormal curvature is induced and neural tube defects result. Lack of adherence to the basement membrane and failure to transform cell shape (apical wedging) lead to failure to form a neural tube, leaving a relatively flat sheet of neuroectoderm that may differentiate further. Irregular neurologic development and subsequent attachment to the neural crest–derived ganglia may occur. Because the peripheral nerves are derived from neural crest ganglia, they may still develop normally, but these cellular groupings lack the appropriate completion of the neural loop as well as higher cortical connectivity.

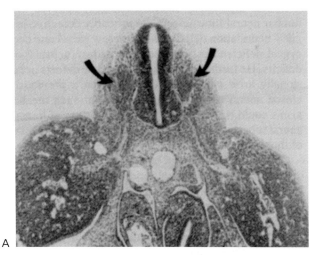
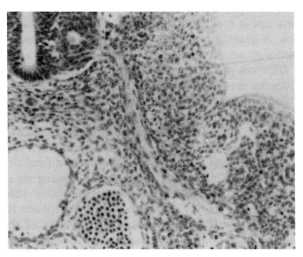

A   B

FIGURE 8. A: Section of embryo through upper limb bud level shows closed neural canal and neural crest condensations into ganglia (*arrows*). **B:** Higher-power view shows early formation of a peripheral nerve extending from the developing ganglion to the limb bud. Some communication with the developing spinal cord is evident. The regressing notochord is present just below the ventral cord cells.

Neural Crest Differentiation

As the neural tube is closing, another group of cells, the *neural crest* (Fig. 7), differentiates from the more lateralized neuroectoderm (1,232,350). The neural tube differentiates primarily into the various cellular components of the central nervous system. The neural crest cells give rise to the dorsal root ganglia and much of the peripheral nervous system, including the autonomic nervous system. They serve as the connecting link to the developing spinal cord and upper motor neurons (2,163,199,213).

Neural crest cell migration is the prime example of a system in which it was previously assumed that a population of precursor cells would migrate along different pathways and differentiate into specific cell types (13,353). It now appears that at a very early stage, the neural crest cells establish specific cell lineages. These "predetermined" cells then undergo differential migration (Fig. 8), particularly as they associate with limb morphogenetic fields for subsequent appendicular innervation (54, 206,223,234,253,254,352,377).

Neural crest cell migration, especially into the limb buds (Fig. 8), does not usually begin until neurulation is complete (231,243,285,311,312,336,361,362). Migration involves a change in intercellular adhesion. The notochord initially produces a molecular substance that inhibits neural crest cell migration while sclerotomal cells are attracted (74,251,279). There is a morphologic increase in extracellular space in the dorsal neuroepithelium immediately before migration of the neural crest (37,98,99). This is associated with decreased expression of cell adhesion molecules and expression of chondroitin sulfate proteoglycan, which is thought to decrease cell adhesion to fibronectin and collagen substrates. Changes in the basal lamina also may be necessary for crest migration. Abnormalities of the extracellular matrix may delay or prevent neural crest cell migration, as in the neural tube defect mutant splotch (230,231).

Neural Tube Maturation

The neural tube thins at both the roof and floor plates and the lateral walls thicken, effectively narrowing the central canal (Fig.

9). Lateral thickening leads to formation of distinct, chemically active cell masses—the alar (dorsal) plate and the basal (ventral) plate. These become, respectively, the afferent and efferent areas of the developing spinal cord and serve as the basis for the reflex loop (48). The alar plate cells form the dorsal roots, and the basal plates form the anterior root contributions to the spinal nerves. This process normally causes complete obliteration of the central canal. However, the canal may be retained as hydromyelia or may enlarge as a syrinx (syringomyelia), a phenomenon that may not become clinically evident until late adolescence or even adulthood. While the loops are forming, longitudinal pathways for interactive brain cell function also develop and

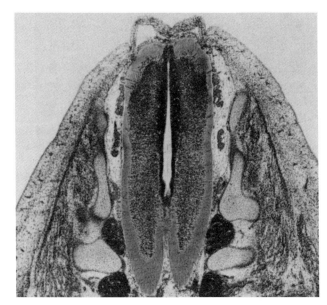

FIGURE 9. Further differentiation of the neural tube leads to formation of the intrinsic cellular structure necessary for progressive development of reflex loops and higher cortical communication.

integrate with appropriate spinal nerve levels (158,180). Fibroblast growth factor appears to be necessary for the development of the central nervous system neurons during these early stages (356).

Paraxial Mesoderm Formation

After differentiation of the notochord and neural tube, further mechanochemical induction produces the mesenchyma that forms the paraxial mesoderm (357,358). Additional proliferation of these two parallel cell masses results in elaboration of three distinct areas of the mesodermal plate—the medial paraxial columns, the intermediate columns, and the peripheral lateral plates. The lateral plates give rise to the layers of the thoracic and abdominal cavities; the intermediate columns differentiate into the urogenital system. Paraxial columns primarily form the axial musculoskeletal system. The early integration of neuromusculoskeletal anlagen and urogenital anlagen helps explain the frequent finding of urogenital abnormalities among patients with congenital scoliosis (88). The early morphologic developmental patterns of the neural, muscular, and axial skeletal elements are thus intimately coordinated and related to both the development of the notochord and the more generalized biologic process of metamerism (linear repetition of anatomically similar segments) (19,21,71,181,264).

Somite Formation

Cellular groupings along the notochord are evident in humans at 3 weeks of gestation. This serial segmentation depends on the presence of a normal notochord (182,194,220,221,270,271, 327,354,366), which conditions (patterns) the presomitic mesoderm. These mesodermal cells condense into paired segments, the *somites*. Although much emphasis is placed on the inductive role of the notochord in initial formation of the somites, further differentiation into vertebrae may be greatly affected by permissive interactions and interactive induction (mechanochemical) from the developing neural tube (65,80,113–115,159). As cellular proliferation and differentiation continue, the somites develop as distinct cell masses (274). The outer cell mass, which contributes to the tissue layers of the skin and subcutaneous tissue, is called the *dermatome*. The inner cell mass further differentiates into two components. A dorsal cellular aggregation becomes striated muscle (the *myotome*), and a ventral cell mass becomes skeletogenic tissue (the *sclerotome*) (5,20,121,255). The myotomal tissue may differentiate to some degree and independently of the contiguous sclerotomal tissue. Such differentiation may occur in the absence of somites (176).

Segmentation is a prevalent developmental feature that is not limited to mammals (117,118). The pair-rule gene family, shown to be involved in this process, is characterized by the presence of a paired-homeobox sequence (81,224). Mistakes during this segmentation and cellular rearrangement process, such as erroneous cellular boundary formation, may result in variable vertebral fusion or hemivertebra (segmented or unsegmented).

The cellular aggregation of each sclerotome follows a pattern of loosely packed cells in the cranial half and densely packed cells in the caudal half (Fig. 10) (272,310,328). These cellular groupings appear to be biochemically different (255). Theiler (337) stated that there is no resegmentation of the vertebral blastema, as originally proposed by Baur, Sensenig, Verbout, and others (16,310,348,349). What had been described as the *sclerotomic fissure* (16,337,349) was, in essence, the loosely packed cell population giving rise to the intervertebral disc material (278). Each sclerotome thus yields a single, centrally differentiating intervertebral disc that separates the cells that will become portions of adjoining vertebrae, as well as all the contiguous processes (rib, transverse, articular, and neural). Cells juxtaposed to the sclerotome (lateral mesenchymal condensations) give rise to vertebral processes; axial condensations independently form the perichordal ring (the precursor of the intervertebral disc) (195). The neural arch, the pedicle, and the ribs originate from one somite. The cellular structure of each mammalian vertebra is thus exclusively derived from a single somite rather than portions of adjacent somites. The sclerotomes of one pair of bilateral somites yield one single intervertebral disc, the adjoining vertebrae, and all the processes (rib, transverse, articular, and neural).

The somites acquire a craniocaudal polarity through aggregation of mesodermal cells. The segmental distribution of spinal nerves and ganglia is governed by the somites and their polarity. The notochord induces mesenchyma-cartilage transformation, induces the floor plate of the neural tube, and prevents the bilateral somites from premature fusion across the midline. It also promotes differentiation of the discs and yields cells to the nucleus pulposus. Somites may develop in the absence of the notochord. Theiler (337) presented a detailed array of genetic strains of mice with developing vertebral malformations that could have been caused by disturbances of somites, notochord, and sclerotome differentiation (alone or in combination).

Sclerotome differentiation, which primarily forms the anterior portion of the eventual vertebral body, appears to be mediated by the neural tube in conjunction with notochordal induction, whereas the neural crest may markedly and relatively independently affect or induce the neural arch (posterior) elements. Serial segmentation of the neural arches is integrated with (dependent on) the presence of developing spinal ganglia (neural crest derivation). Embryonic and fetal movement is essential for proper progressive development (198).

The vertebral bodies and neural arches thus are guided by separate inductive influences and retain a degree of independence in their initial developmental patterns. Congenital deformation of the spine may involve only posterior elements, only anterior elements, or respond to a variable combination of either. Fused vertebral bodies (centra) may not necessarily be associated with fused posterior (neural arch) elements, and vice versa. The extent of involvement affects the type and eventual rate of progression of congenital scoliosis. Aspects of such variable fusion are discussed in the section on congenital scoliosis.

When somite segmentation and initial vertebral condensation are completed, the notochord is surrounded by a series of vertebral centra derived from cells respective to somite determination (Fig. 11). Failure to adequately segment may be one mechanism that leads to formation of congenital scoliosis (Fig. 12). If the intervertebral sclerotomic cells do not occur bilaterally, fused vertebral bodies might result. Unilateral separation failure may produce a unilateral bar or hemivertebra. Unilateral develop-

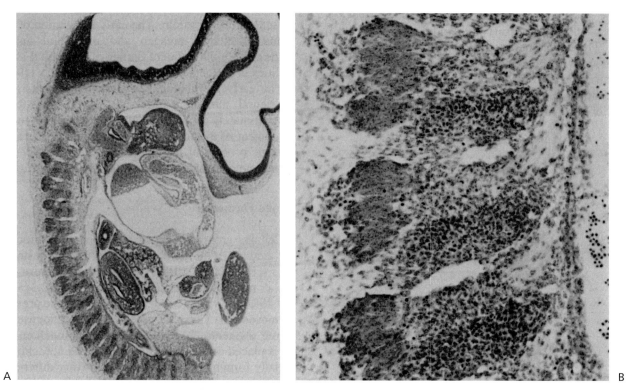

A   B

FIGURE 10. Early somite formation. Densely and loosely packed zones of cells are evident. Early muscle formation also is evident. **A:** Low-power midsagittal section of entire embryo. **B:** Higher-power image shows the division of each somite into a cell-loose cranial half and a cell-dense caudal half. A variably sized cell-free region separates each anlage (previously described as the sclerotomic fissure). Presumptive muscle paraxial muscle tissue (*left*) is associated principally with the loose cell zone. The muscle bridges the joint to associate with adjacent motion segments (vertebral bodies).

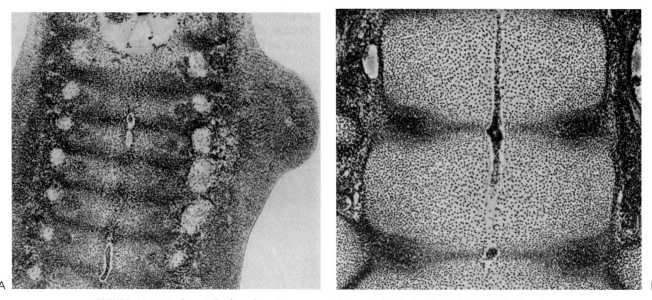

A   B

FIGURE 11. **A:** Early vertebral condensations around the central notochord. The intervertebral regions are beginning to demarcate from the vertebral bodies. **B:** Further development enlarges each vertebra and compresses the presumptive disc. Gradation typifies the disc region, even at this stage. The regressing notochord is slightly more retained in the disc regions.

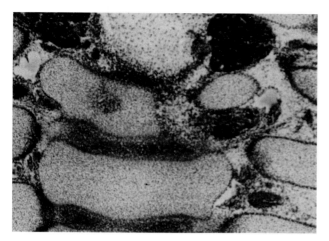

FIGURE 12. Partial condensation failure in an embryo. This probably would have resulted in a hemivertebra. The disc regions are well demarcated by a cellular vertebral boundary, the presumptive perichondrial tissue.

mental failure also may produce an unbalanced hemivertebra that is either fused or unfused to an adjacent vertebra (25).

Atlas and Axis Formation

Formation of the atlas (C1) and axis (C2) differs from the typical vertebral formation patterns. Cellular components from the fourth occipital somite may commingle with cellular material from the first cervical somite to form the proatlas. Although it is classically taught that the cranial bones are of membranous origin, the occipital bone exhibits considerable endochondral bone formation (Fig. 13). This differentiation facilitates extension of the ligaments from the skull to the odontoid process (dens) and to the cranial end of the odontoid process, the portion that eventually ossifies to become the os terminale. Failure of occipital and cervical somites to divide may cause variable fusion of C1 to the skull (occipitalization of C1).

The cell mass constituting the odontoid process (dens) appears to be derived from cellular components of the first and second cervical somites. This C1–2 somite amalgamation contributes to formation of the anterior arch (centrum) of C1 and some of the supporting ligaments connecting C1 to the odontoid process, at least in classic cellular embryology. Failure of the C1 centrum to separate into anterior arch and odontoid might be a cause of absence or hypoplasia of the odontoid process, especially in skeletal dysplasia. Trauma, however, is a more likely factor in the causation of os odontoideum among children with otherwise normal skeletons (109,152).

Neural Arch Formation

Cells of sclerotomal origin migrate dorsally (Fig. 14) juxtaposed to the neural tube to form the neural (vertebral) arch. The neural arch does not form until after anterior somite-centrum amalgamation is under way, another factor in the variable presentation of morphologic deformities of the spine. The neural arches alternate with the spinal ganglia and thus are situated intersegmentally with respect to the myotomes such that each neural arch is associated with two successive myotomal segments (59). An induced neural arch appears between successive ganglia. Absence of a ganglion may allow unilateral arch fusion (a congenital bar). The cellular components of each neural arch (in reality, paired arches per somite) progressively condense near the somite (basal region of the cord) toward the alar region, where the condensations must unite. Condensations continue farther dorsally to produce the anlagen of the spinous process or processes.

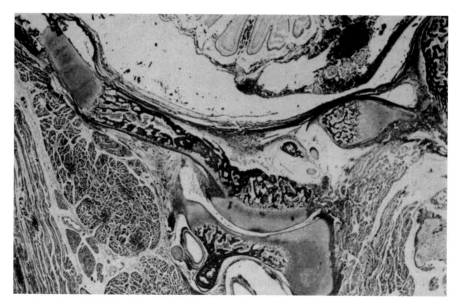

FIGURE 13. Occipital endochondral bone formation in a term woolly monkey fetus. Cartilage is evident where the occipital bone apposes other cranial bones in the anterior (*right*) and posterior (*left*) aspects. Inferiorly located occipital bone endochondral ossification is evident at the occiput-C1 joint.

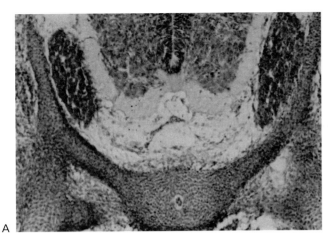 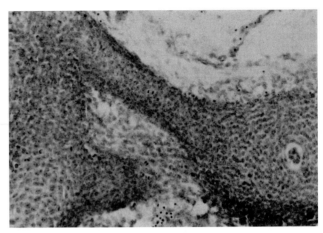

A   B

FIGURE 14. Mesenchymal vertebral anlage. Continuity of the differentiating posterior elements and ribs is evident. There is a centrally located notochord. **A:** Low power. **B:** High power.

Vertebral anomalies therefore can be caused by primary neurogenic defects that induce maldevelopment of the associated vertebral centrum, the neural arch, or both (330). The variable contributions of the neural arch to the centrum consequently progressively affect any specific pattern of congenital scoliosis.

Serious posterior chondroosseous defects may accompany major neural tissue defects (12,67,283). The various spinal cord membranes may be exposed (meningocele), or the neural tissue may be directly exposed (myelomeningocele). The flat structure of the exposed cord in myelomeningocele reflects early failure of neural tube closure, although the variable presence of spinal nerves indicates that failure of tubulation does not necessarily preclude further cellular differentiation within the spinal cord anlage. As such, scattered function below the level of a major osseous deformity is possible. Meningocele and myelomeningocele always coexist with posterior spina bifida. The suggestion is that a closed neural tube is a prerequisite for complete development of the neural arch anlagen.

Concomitant with developmental failure or hypoplasia of the neural arch is variable failure to bring portions of the myotome dorsally to form the dorsal paraxial musculature. As a result, this musculature may be shifted more anteriorly than is normal. Because of such positional changes, the developing (maturing) myotome may effectively function as a spinal flexor rather than an extensor, increasing the probability of progressive kyphosis.

Peripheral Innervation

The process of somite formation proceeds in conjunction with the formation of ganglia by the neural crest, such that a one nerve–one somite relation becomes established early, the dorsal root ganglion being situated opposite to the median surface of each myotome (24,40,63,73,79,122,132,204,212,214,215,313, 322). Thus any muscle derived from a particular somite, no matter how far it may subsequently migrate, retains its initial nerve relation (14,75,82,83,105,164,167,169,183,202,203,205, 207–209,237,238,256,314,322). However, there is a complex

relation between muscular and neural induction and interaction (104,200,201,269,339).

Notochord Regression

As the vertebral column differentiates, the notochord gradually regresses within the vertebral centra. This process allows cellular and matrix fusion across the midline to form the mesenchymal centrum. In contrast, notochordal cells between the vertebral bodies markedly affect formation of the nucleus pulposus and the anulus fibrosus. Remnants of the notochord may persist (Fig. 15), usually in either the basisphenoid region or the coccygeal region, where they may play a role in formation of a chordoma.

Chondrification

During the sixth embryonic week, the mesenchymal vertebral anlagen develop primary centers of chondrification (Fig. 16). As in bilateral somite differentiation, chondrifying centers appear on either side of the notochord and fuse to make a unified chondrified centrum (131). A center of chondrification also forms in each neural arch, fuses dorsally to establish a solid chondral neural arch, and begins chondrification within the spinous process (341). The final chondrification centers appear at the junctions of the centrum and neural arches and by means of lateral extension form the transverse processes. While vertebral chondrification is occurring, the perichordal tissue condenses into a dense anulus fibrosus around the differentiating nucleus pulposus. By means of expansion of the chondrification centers, the composite cartilaginous model of the vertebra becomes a solid unit, presenting variable demarcation between the body, neural arches, and transverse processes.

Ossification

After the cartilaginous axial skeleton forms, the next developmental stage is primary ossification (Figs. 17, 18). This process

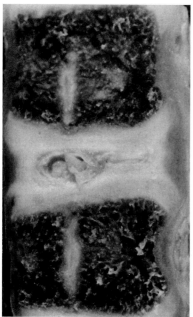
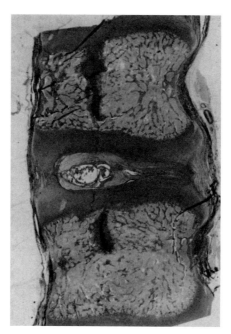
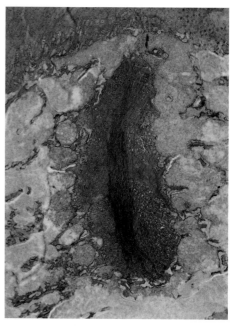

A,B

C

FIGURE 15. A: Segment of thoracic spine from a stillborn with congenital heart disease. Notochordal remnants are evident. **B:** Histologic features. **C:** Higher-power view shows cartilage around the notochordal remnants.

is enhanced with the onset of motion within the embryo (139,198,280). Within the centrum, this process is also highly dependent on the presence of a developing vascular system. Three primary centers of ossification are present within each vertebra, except for C1, C2, and the sacrum (270–273,290). According to most investigators, one ossification center appears in each body (centrum) and one in each of the neural arches (139,198). Chandraraj and Briggs (61) showed that in the neural arch, a single ossification center expands to effectively form three growth regions that become progressively independent. These

zones are for the pedicle, lamina, and transverse process. A few investigators have suggested that as many as six ossification centers may be present: two forming in the vertebral body; two forming the pedicles, lateral masses, and transverse processes; and two for the lamina and spinous processes (4,299).

Primary ossification in the centrum is similar to epiphyseal ossification in long bones but with minimal or no primary bone collar (Figs. 17, 18). Cartilage canals exist within the cartilage of the centrum (Fig. 19); however, no antecedent encircling ossification ring in the vertebra is evident, as in a long bone. In

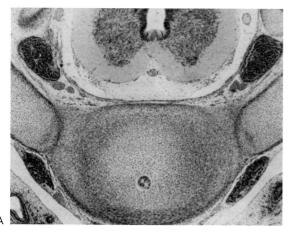
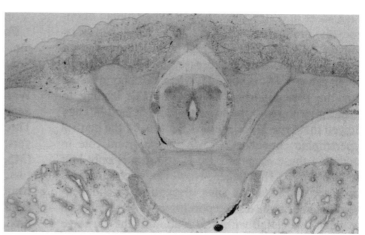

A

B

FIGURE 16. A: Thoracic vertebra during the early transition from mesenchymal to cartilaginous tissue. The change is initiated centrally, around the evident notochord. **B:** Further chondrification. The spinal cord is developing changes (gray and white matter). A demarcation is becoming evident between posterior and anterior elements and ribs. Chondrification is occurring throughout.

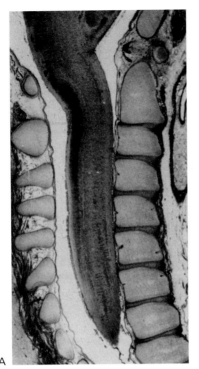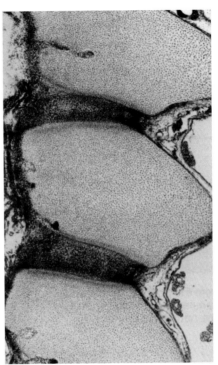

A   B

FIGURE 17. A: Low-power sagittal section of the chondrified cervical and upper thoracic spines. Early commencement of vascular ingrowth at multiple levels is evident. The dens of C2 appears to be below C1, but this finding is probably artifactual. An anterior slope on the dens is indicative of eventual flexion-extension between C1 and C2. **B:** Higher-power view of the vascular sprouts. Vascular establishment is essential for chondroosseous transformation.

contrast, formation of each primary ossification center in the posterior arches is similar to the diaphyseal ossification an eccentric bone collar forms and progressive vasoosseous transformation occurs (Figs. 20, 21).

Ossification of the vertebral body in humans begins in the

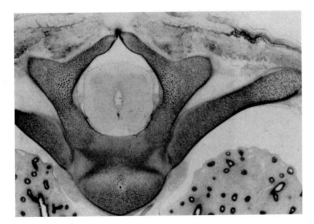

FIGURE 18. Localized hypertrophic cartilage changes preceding ossification within thoracic vertebral components. Relative demarcation of the anterior, posterior, and costal regions is evident. The posterior elements are incompletely fused (spina bifida occulta). Chondroosseous transformation apparently can occur even before the neural arch is fully fused into a spinal process anlage. Retention of this stage probably causes spina bifida occulta.

lower thoracic and upper lumbar regions and diverges craniad and caudad. In the cervical region, however, the primary ossification centers of the vertebral bodies appear sequentially after the primary centers appear in the vertebral arches (59). Within the cervical spine, centrum ossification begins in the lower region (C6, C7) before it starts in the upper region, an occurrence that may be fairly common throughout animal species (263). Again, disruption of the endochondral ossification process may adversely affect development of the spin as another causal mechanism of congenital scoliosis.

The ossification patterns of the atlas (C1) and axis (C2) differ from those of the other vertebrae (258,259). The atlas centrum has one primary center of ossification, and each of the two neural arches has a primary center. The two posterior centers are present prenatally, and the anterior center may not appear until several months postnatally—an important factor in assessing this region in neonates and infants. The axis develops five primary and two secondary centers of ossification. The centrum and neural arch centers form in the conventional manner, and the odontoid process forms two laterally situated centers. These two odontoid centers almost always fuse in the perinatal period, although a cleft may persist for several months after birth (259).

Posterior osseous defects in which the ossification centers of the neural arch fail to fuse are quite common, especially those involving the L5 and S1 vertebrae. In some studies the incidence of spina bifida occulta is estimated to be as high as 20% in the general population. This condition, however, is rarely accompa-

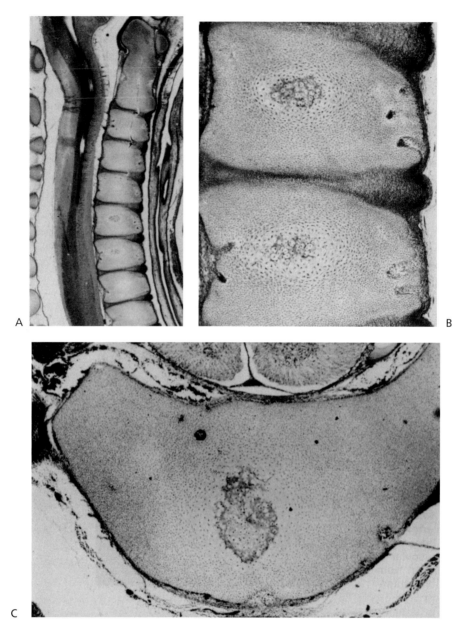

FIGURE 19. A: Early development of the cervical and thoracic spine. The continuity of the various component parts of C2 and the developing anterior portion of C1 is evident. The dens is now distinctly behind C1 (compare with Fig. 17A). Cartilage canals penetrate both anteriorly and posteriorly. The intervertebral discs, especially the nucleus pulposus, are minimally developed. The notochord is evident within C2 and C3. Ossification is beginning in C6 and C7. The incompletely closed neural canal extends from the brain to C4. **B, C:** Higher-power views demonstrate these hypertrophic preossification centers (**B,** sagittal; **C,** transverse). The ingrowing cartilage canals still do not reach these regions, and there is no peripheral bone collar, as in primary ossification of a long bone.

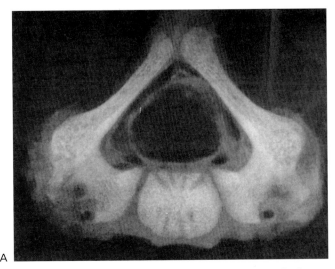
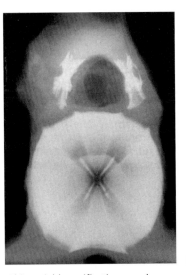

FIGURE 20. **A:** Irregular ossification of a cervical vertebral centrum. This variable ossification may be the basis for the concept of six ossification centers. **B:** Similar variable pattern of calcification in the thoracic vertebra of a shark seems to show four anterior regions and two posterior regions.

nied by serious primary neurologic defects. Larger areas of spina bifida may involve the sacrum and culminate in failure to form the spinous processes properly. The presence of large areas of spina bifida and may even predispose the child to a developmental form of spondylolisthesis in which there is progressive deformation of the normal angulation of the L5–S1 facet joints. Minor structural abnormalities in the neural arch, especially the facet joints, may be an overlooked cause of "idiopathic" scoliosis (172).

The intervertebral disc material becomes progressively defined in the embryonic period; more peripheral regions are characterized by greater cellularity (Fig. 22A). These peripheral regions differentiate and because of progressive motion develop a multilaminar appearance and an identity as the anulus fibrosus (Fig. 23A). Differentiating disc material is vascular and communicates with the contiguous vascular regions of the vertebral centrum and extraosseous circulations anterior and posterior to the vertebral body. The cells of the nucleus pulposus form a defined

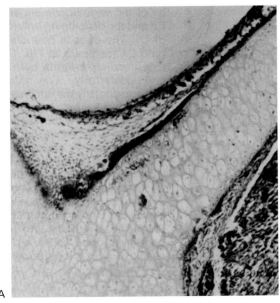
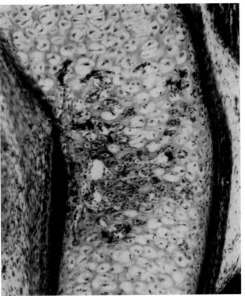

FIGURE 21. **A:** Early hypertrophy and eccentric bone collar formation in a posterior element. There is more definition of the bone collar on the canal side than on the muscle side. **B:** Subsequent vascular penetration from the canal side to form the ossification center.

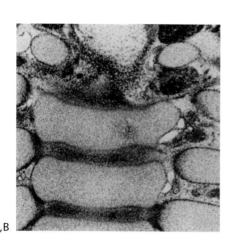
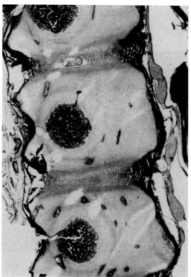
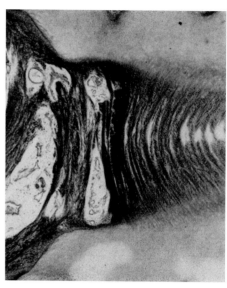

A,B

C

FIGURE 22. **A:** More defined condensation of disc tissue toward the end of the embryonic period. The cellular regions are more dense peripherally than centrally. **B:** As ossification begins in the fetal stage, the peripheral disc material assumes a multilaminar appearance. **C:** Maturation is associated with increased complexity of the laminations. This region also is extremely vascular.

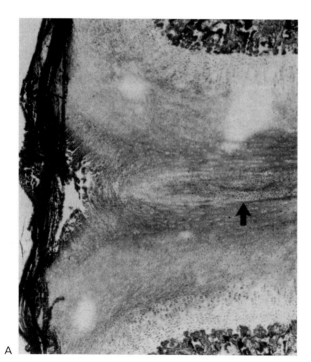
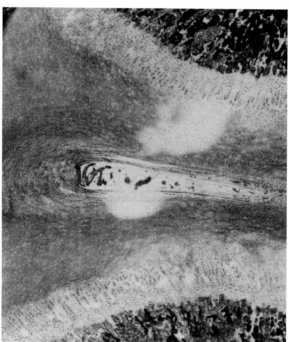

A

B

FIGURE 23. **A:** Central cellular condensation (*arrow*) in the region of the presumptive nucleus pulposus. The area is surrounded by hypertrophic cells that probably represent the developing epiphyseal analogue. **B:** This central disc region has considerable vascularity.

central cell grouping that is highly vascular in the fetus and child (Fig. 23B), a fact that may explain the concomitance of discitis, osteomyelitis, and eventual vertebral fusion among children.

POSTNATAL DEVELOPMENT

Normal postnatal development of the axial skeleton involves the progressive appearance of the characteristic curves (9,10), growth and expansion of the vertebral bodies (332), closure of the synchondroses, development of the ring apophysis, and changes in the longitudinal relations between the vertebrae and the spinal cord (262,349).

The diagnostic modalities used to examine the spines of adults must often be modified for children. On images of children, the presence of radiolucent cartilage produces large gaps between ossified parts, and ligamentous laxity allows greater motion during imaging, especially of the upper cervical spine (42,154,155,222,374).

Vertebral growth not only relies on genetic factors but also responds to epigenetic factors such as intrinsic tonicity in the paravertebral musculature, upright posture, and activity. Radiologic analysis of postnatal vertebral development among ambulatory and nonambulatory children supports a concept that vertebral body height in the midsagittal plane is relatively unaffected by mechanical factors and may even be primarily genetically determined (331). Latitudinal growth and peripheral vertebral growth are more dependent on upright posture. This differential growth response of the peripheral versus central portions may be a factor in the eccentric growth patterns that lead to development and progression of scoliosis and kyphosis.

Cord Growth

The spinal cord initially extends to the end of the vertebral canal, and the spinal nerves exit at or close to their respective levels of origin. Vettiveil (351) showed that there is rapid ascent of the conus medullaris relative to the vertebrae up to the 120-mm crown-rump length stage, when it reaches the fourth and sometimes the third lumbar vertebra. After that the ascent is fairly gradual; the cord terminates opposite the first or second lumbar vertebra in term neonates.

With postnatal growth, especially in the lumbar region during adolescence, the osteocartilaginous column elongates. Disparate rates of growth may occur between the vertebral bodies and the spinal cord. Positional changes cause the lumbosacral spinal roots to traverse more obliquely from the spinal cord to their respective neuroforamina and form an aggregate of nerve roots, the *cauda equina.* Some investigators believe that postnatal changes in cord level do not occur (15).

The filum terminale may attach as far as the first coccygeal vertebra and may cause progressive cord traction if elongation is not commensurate with the changing osseous-spinal cord relations (tethered cord syndrome). In diastematomyelia, differential growth may be a factor causing progressive development of neurologic abnormalities in a previously healthy child. The amount of disparate growth necessary to cause symptoms may be only a matter of millimeters.

Neurocentral Synchondroses

Progressive juxtaposition between the primary ossification centers of the anterior centrum and posterior arches occurs anteriorly to the anatomic pedicle, at the site of the neurocentral synchondrosis (Fig. 24). These regions are radiographically evident in the spines of infants and must not be interpreted as either congenital deformity or trauma (Fig. 25). It is also important to realize that as the most anterior portions of the neural arch contribute to vertebral body formation, a morphologic deformity such as fusion of adjacent posterior elements may affect the vertebral body to the margin of the neurocentral synchondrosis.

The cervical vertebrae, except for C1 and C2, and the thoracic

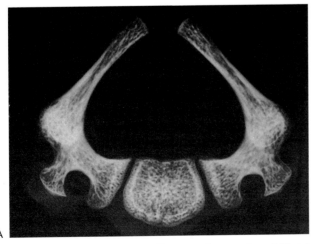
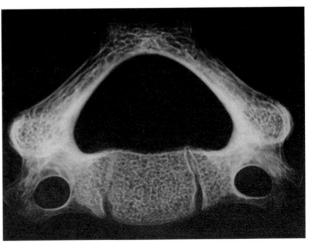

A   B

FIGURE 24. Differences of maturation of C3 at 1 year **(A)** and 6 years **(B)** of age. Posterior ossification is distinctly incomplete at 1 year of age. The neurocentral synchondroses are almost parallel and make up a large portion of the eventual vertebral body.

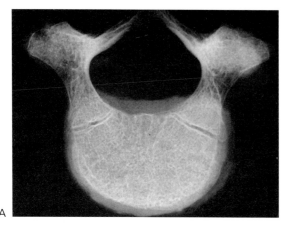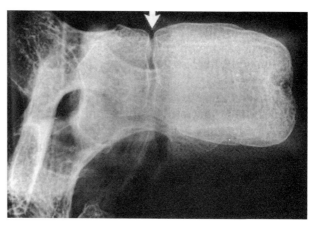

A   B

FIGURE 25. **A:** Radiograph of L3 at approximately 8 years. Compare the relative posterior contributions to the vertebral body with Figure 24. **B:** The neurocentral synchondrosis (*arrow*) is evident in this lateral view and should not be misconstrued as a fracture or congenital deformity.

and lumbar vertebrae follow this similar pattern of postnatal development with three ossification centers (two in the neural arches and one in the centrum) that meet within the vertebral body as the neurocentral synchondroses. Although the neurocentral synchondroses in the cervical vertebrae are almost parallel, such that the posterior centers contribute greatly to the lateral portions of each vertebral body, in the thoracic and lumbar vertebrae the posterior ossification centers contribute less and less to the final vertebral body (compare Figs. 25 and 26). The formation of unilateral bars in congenital scoliosis may include the variable anterior contribution. Thus an apparently posterior bar may extend anteriorly into a portion of the eventual vertebral body because of the segmental contribution of the posterior anlage. Such variable anterior extension of asymmetric fusions

(congenital bars) affects the rate of progression of congenital scoliosis. The symmetric or asymmetric contribution of the posterior elements to the eventual vertebral body also affects the risk of progression.

Because the neurocentral synchondroses are paired, growth in these regions must be equal if each vertebra is to develop normally. Experimental damage to one of the pair causes scoliosis (27,78,292). Subtle asymmetry of growth—one side versus the other—in these synchondroses may be a cause of scoliosis that affects the shape of the posterior elements and introduces asymmetric muscular function.

Canal Growth

The presence of three cartilaginous junctions within each composite vertebra allows progressive expansion of the spinal canal as the child grows. Conceptually these cartilaginous junctions are analogous to the triradiate cartilage in the acetabulum (347). Such multidimensional growth conglomerates are essential for enlarging three-dimensional morphologic features. Even if the posterior (spinous process) synchondrosis closes first, the paired neurocentral synchondroses still can grow longitudinally to allow further change in canal size.

Once the neurocentral synchondroses close (Figs. 26, 27), the spinal canal can no longer widen. Canal diameters throughout the spine appear to reach adult size by 6 to 8 years of age, after which little diametric canal growth occurs (112,154,155,374). Some remodeling and contour change in the spinal canal occurs through the periosteum on the inner and outer surfaces of the posterior elements. It is important to remember this early attainment of adult canal diameters.

A problem that may be caused by a decrease in the rate of growth or premature synchondrosis fusion is spinal stenosis. Either process, whether anterior or posterior, would lessen or preclude progressive canal widening. Because these are endochondral processes, failure to grow at a normal rate may impair proper diametric enlargement of the canal. Such growth impairment is a probable mechanism of spinal stenosis in skeletal dys-

FIGURE 26. Closing neurocentral synchondroses in a lumbar vertebra of a greater kudu (antelope). In the same way that is common among humans, a small area of spina bifida occulta is evident. The spinous process is from the adjacent vertebra.

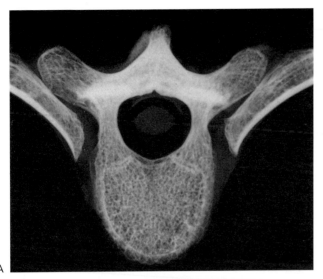

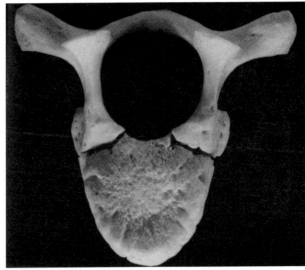

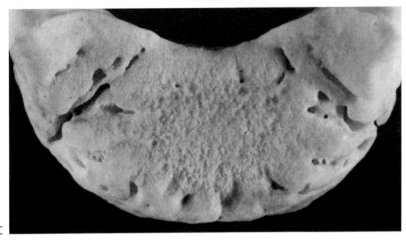

FIGURE 27. Closure stages of thoracic vertebra at 7 to 9 years. **A:** Radiograph of T6 at 9 years. **B:** Specimen of T5 at 7 years with open synchondroses. **C:** Closure of the synchondroses in T3 at 9 years. Anterior undulations counter shear stresses.

plasia such as achondroplasia. Eccentric or asymmetric growth or closure of the neurocentral synchondroses also may play a role in the development of scoliosis.

C1 (Atlas)

The anterior primary ossification center is present among fewer than 20% of neonates (Fig. 28). More commonly it appears 9 to 12 months after birth (range, 6 months to 2 years) (258). Usually this ossification center is unitary (Fig. 29). However, asymmetric, bifid, or multifocal ossification can occur (Fig. 29C) (258). The anterior center expands laterally toward each of the paired posterior ossification centers. The result is two cartilaginous gaps, which are defined as the *neurocentral synchondroses.* This anterior ossification center is called the *intercentraxium-1* (258). The anterior synchondroses are medial to the articular facets. In rare instances, the anterior center does not form, and the posterior centers progressively extend toward the centrum. By about 4 or 5 years of age, both the posterior synchondrosis and the anterior neurocentral synchondroses are fused. The spinal canal of C1 essentially reaches maximum (adult) size at a relatively early stage of postnatal development (5 to 6 years).

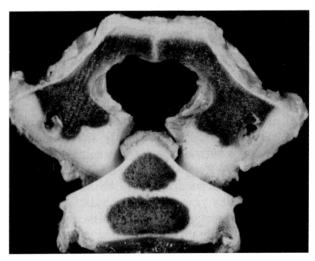

FIGURE 28. Development of C1 and C2 in a fetal Indian elephant. The anterior portion of C1, as in humans, is still cartilaginous. Only the posterior elements have ossified. Extensive confluence of cartilage of the dens and centrum of C2 is evident.

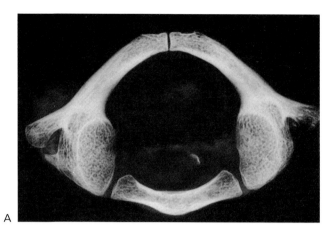

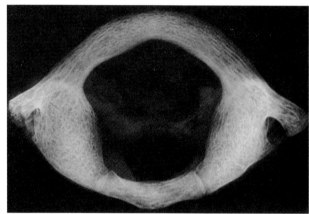

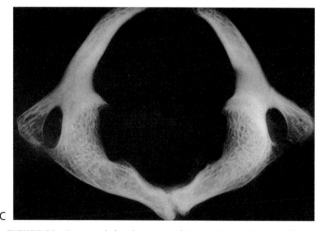

FIGURE 29. Postnatal development of C1. **A:** One and one half years. **B:** Five years. **C:** Anomalous development (8 years) with a single anterior synchondrosis (fusing) and spina bifida.

C2 (Axis)

The dens (odontoid process) develops two primary ossification centers that may not coalesce until 3 months after birth (Figs. 30, 31). This bifid nature is not the usual pattern in most mammals (259). The dens ossification is separated from the primary ossification center of the vertebral centrum by a cartilaginous region—the *dentocentral synchondrosis.* The dentocentral synchondrosis is below the level of the C1–2 articulations (Figs. 30,

31). The dentocentral synchondrosis normally closes between 5 and 7 years of age (Fig. 32). Remnants of the incompletely closed dentocentral synchondrosis may be evident on radiographs for many years after physiologic closure. The remnants must be differentiated from a fracture that can propagate along this structure as a physeal injury before skeletal maturity. The dens is a tubular bone analogue that forms a cartilaginous epiphysis at each end (chondrum terminale and dentocentral synchondrosis) and eventually forms a secondary ossification center in each end in most mammals (the os terminale and intercentraxium-2, respectively; Fig. 33). The centrum has superior and inferior epiphyses and secondary ossification centers. The inferior epiphysis of the dens and the superior epiphysis of the centrum fuse in embryos to form the dentocentral synchondrosis. The intercentraxium-2 is an analogue of secondary ossification in fused epiphyseal analogues. Humans appear unique in the absence of this secondary ossification in the dentocentral synchondrosis. There are no descriptions of this phenomenon in other higher primates.

Longitudinal growth of C2 occurs through three regions. First, the physis of the chondrum terminale contributes to the length of the dens. Failure of growth in this region may be a factor in the formation of a hypoplastic dens. Second, a small amount of longitudinal growth occurs within the dentocentral synchondrosis and contributes to both vertebral body height and dens length. Third, growth occurs inferiorly through the end plate physis.

The cartilaginous epiphysis at the tip of the dens may be transverse or form a cleft (*V* shape). This chondrum terminale at the superior end of the dens develops a secondary ossification center at 8 to 10 years of age—the os (ossiculum) terminale (Fig. 32B). Fusion of the os terminale with the rest of the dens occurs between 10 and 13 years of age (259). There is also an anterior acclivity, which is necessary to allow C1 to slide up and down during flexion and extension of the neck (325).

Mechanical Control of Growth

A factor involved in vertebral development is the exertion of physical forces on the tissues. Such forces are principally of two types. First, at the macromolecular level the developing musculature exert a force on the spinal column that increases as the tissue matures. Second, at the molecular level hydrodynamic forces are exerted on the cells as a result of retention of water within the extracellular matrix (129).

Carter and Wong and their coworkers (56,57,371) have shown that ossification centers appear in areas of high shear stresses, that the edge of the advancing ossification front is subject to high shear stresses, and that the intervertebral region is exposed to considerably hydrostatic compression. They believe that these observations support a general concept that shear stresses promote endochondral ossification and that intermittently applied hydrostatic compression inhibits or prevents cartilage degeneration and ossification.

Besides intrinsic limitations to cell division, there appears to be a mechanical restraint to elongation (275). This control factor is the periosteal sleeve, which is present to a limited degree in each vertebral body because of delayed development of the peri-

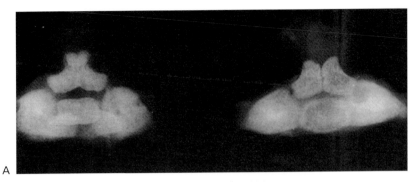

A

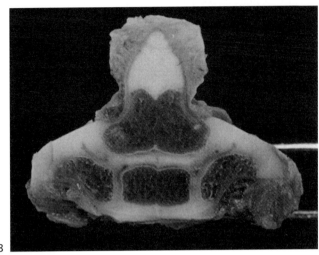

B

FIGURE 30. **A:** Radiographs of early development of C2 at term. The example on the *right* shows bifid ossification of the dens. **B:** Slab coronal section shows areas of cartilage and their continuities. **C:** Histologic appearance of C2. The dens ossification centers extend into the eventual vertebral body.

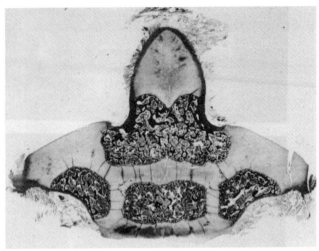

C

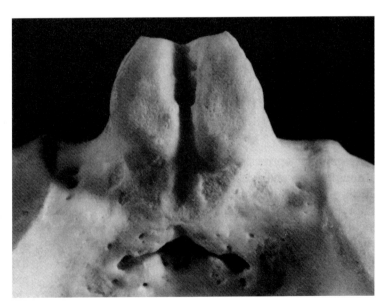

A

B

FIGURE 31. Specimen of C2 from a 10-year-old child with partial retention of the original bifid ossification process. **A:** Entire vertebra. **B:** Close-up view of dens. The underlying remnant of the dentocentral synchondrosis is also evident.

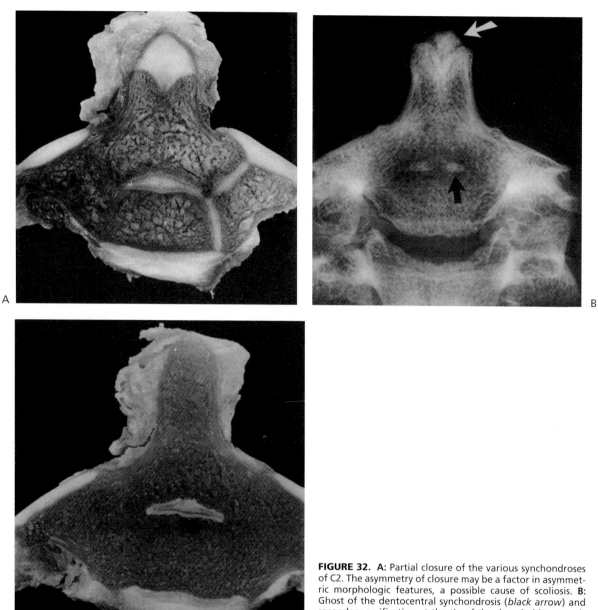

FIGURE 32. **A:** Partial closure of the various synchondroses of C2. The asymmetry of closure may be a factor in asymmetric morphologic features, a possible cause of scoliosis. **B:** Ghost of the dentocentral synchondrosis (*black arrow*) and secondary ossification at the tip of the dens (*white arrow*). **C:** Proximal maturation of ossification. A ghost of the dentocentral synchondrosis is still present.

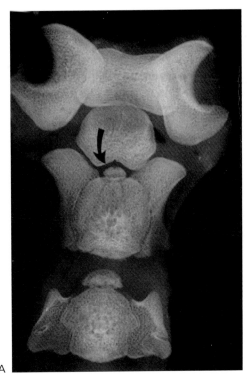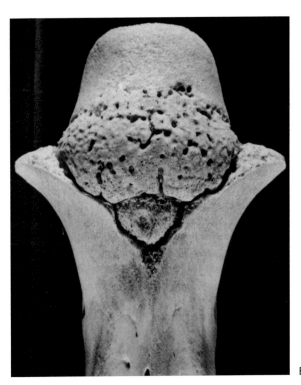

A   B

FIGURE 33. **A:** Radiograph shows upper cervical development in an addax (antelope). Secondary ossification (intercentraxium-2) is evident (*arrow*) within the dentocentral synchondrosis. **B:** Osseous specimen of C2 in a giraffe also contains the intercentraxium-2 and the multiple vascular penetrations of the lower dens. The more sclerotic cranial segment does not. A similar situation exists in humans and helps explain the problem of nonunion among adults with dens fractures.

osteum as a discrete tissue around the vertebra. In contrast, the posterior elements develop a more typical periosteal sleeve. The sleeve has an intrinsic elasticity affected by a varying collagenous composition. When this intrinsic tension is disrupted, as in a fracture, overgrowth of the bone in relation the contralateral bone is a recognized clinical phenomenon (260). Although not as dramatic in a vertebral fracture as in long bone, the overgrowth may be a factor in recovery of vertebral height after an anterior wedge fracture in a child.

GROWTH MECHANISMS

Vertebral Growth

The primary ossification center of each vertebral body is initially associated with a spherical physis, as in epiphyseal ossification (Fig. 5). However, this center is not associated with extensive cortical bone formation, as would be expected with a metaphyseal-diaphyseal analogue. Thus ossification within the centrum resembles epiphyseal ossification, and in essence the ring apophyses are more like tertiary ossifications. After birth, the ossification center enlarges toward the sides of the vertebral mass (centrum) and the intervertebral discs (Fig. 34). Gradually the spherical growth center expands to demarcate increasingly parallel growth plates located superiorly and inferiorly. The situation is similar to, but not exactly the same as, that involving the tubular limb

bones (95). Most animals have well-formed physes and epiphyses (epiphyseal ossification centers) in the superior and inferior aspects; humans and some other, but not all, large primates do not.

Longitudinal Growth

Physeal growth is the main mechanism by which each component of the axial skeleton enlarges (31–33). In the vertebral body, primary growth plates arise superiorly and inferiorly as a consequence of the formation of the enlarging primary ossification center (Fig. 34). These growth plates are characterized by an area of rapidly maturing cartilage that grades imperceptibly into the other cartilage of the chondroepiphysis. Although the primary function of the physis is to provide a mechanism for longitudinal growth, it also contributes greatly to circumferential expansion of the vertebral centrum. These physes change to variably undulated structures as the centrum increases in height and postnatal biomechanical demands change (260). Measurements of static diaphyseal regions such as the entrance of the nutrient artery suggest relatively equal contributions of each end plate physis to the height of the individual vertebrae.

Many species better exploit longitudinal vertebral growth through the end plate physes. A thicker end plate epiphysis is present in most mammals, and within this epiphysis a true epiphyseal ossification center forms and progressively enlarges rather than forming a thin, peripheral ring apophysis, as in ado-

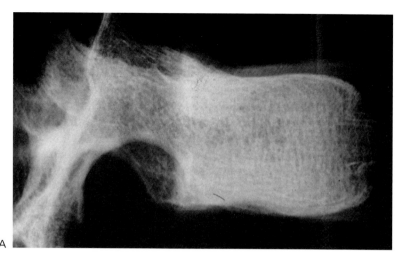
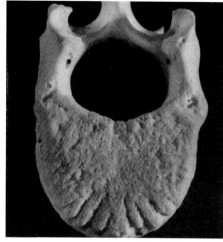

FIGURE 34. A: Characteristic lateral radiograph shows how the body often expands to the periphery in the central region first and then to the anterior and lateral "corners," leaving variable superior and inferior indentations where the remaining cartilage is present along the anterolateral margins. **B:** Osseous specimen shows how the cartilage of the end plate interdigitates with the expanding ossification center to counter shear forces as the trunk bends and twists. Anteriorly, these interdigitations have a radial (spokelike) appearance.

lescent humans. These structures reinforce the similarity of the increase in length (longitudinal growth) between vertebral bodies and limb bones and provide a coaptive stability for extension. The giraffe particularly exemplifies this process. Giraffes have seven cervical vertebrae that form a neck that can attain a length of more than 6 feet (1.8 m) (Fig. 35). An interesting finding was that among the large number of fetal to subadult giraffes we studied in detail, minor structural deformities, asymmetric growth, and mild cervical scoliosis appeared to be quite common (Ogden and Ganey, unpublished observations).

The contribution of the physes to longitudinal growth of the spine is important. Divided over approximately 20 to 25 vertebrae (40 to 50 growth plates), however, each physis makes a relatively small contribution to overall length. Longitudinal growth also occurs in each of the paired posterior elements. An anterior growth plate at each neurocentral synchondrosis and one posterior plate at the spinous process synchondrosis allow the laminar and pedicular regions to lengthen. As each posterior element elongates and grows away from the vertebral midline, the spinal canal enlarges. After the synchondroses close, usually at 5 to 8 years of age for most of the spine, the posterior elements are mature as far as longitudinal growth is concerned. In contrast, longitudinal growth of the anterior elements continues until 16 to 18 years of age. Asymmetric closure patterns of the neurocentral synchondroses (right versus left or longitudinally within a given synchondrosis) may be a subtle, yet predisposing factor in the eventual development of idiopathic scoliosis during adolescence.

Latitudinal Growth

Latitudinal growth of the vertebral body occurs in two ways. There is extensive latitudinal growth through the perichondrium, which surrounds most of the vertebral centrum during the first few years of development. There is also diametric growth in the physis and a thin, platelike epiphysis, both of which are responsive to physiologic stresses. As the spherical ossification center enlarges, there is an increase in appositional (membranous) bone along the sides where the ossification center extends to the periphery and induces discrete periosteum from the antecedent perichondrium (95,267,337). Individual vertebral bodies and even the posterior elements thus enlarge circumferentially by means of the combined processes of perichondral and periosteal apposition while they grow vertically (longitudinally) by means of endochondral ossification (Fig. 36). The vertebral physes enlarge in latitudinal directions by means of cell division and matrix expansion within the physis (interstitial growth). More important, they enlarge by means of cellular addition from the periphery. Interstitial growth in the transverse growth plate appears to be related to enlargement of the epiphyseal ossification center. When there is a chondroepiphysis, as there invariably is in a human vertebra, the cartilage of the epiphysis does not present a mechanical barrier to interstitial expansion within the juxtaposed growth plate.

While the physis is expanding latitudinally, the cortex of the vertebral centrum also must enlarge and serve as a peripheral structural support. This occurs through membranous bone formation, modeling, and remodeling (Fig. 37), all of which respond to biomechanical cues.

Histomorphology

The vertebral physis has a characteristic cytoarchitectural structure. The limited height of the vertebral physis after birth is a reflection of a relatively slow growth rate, especially in relation to the physis of a long bone.

In the zone of growth both longitudinal and diametric expansion of bone occurs. The reserve and dividing cells are associated

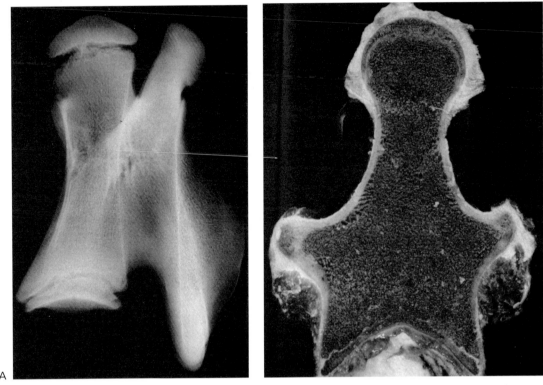

A   B

FIGURE 35. Development of a typical elongated cervical vertebra in a giraffe. In giraffes, the growth characteristics in the centrum are comparable with those of the long bones of a limb. A discrete physis and secondary epiphyseal ossification center are present at each end of the centrum. Such mechanisms are necessary to produce individual vertebrae that may attain heights of 6 to 10 inches (15 to 25 cm). **A:** Radiograph. **B:** Coronal slab section. Right-to-left asymmetry is evident. An interesting finding was that many cervical spines of giraffes studied had mild scoliosis.

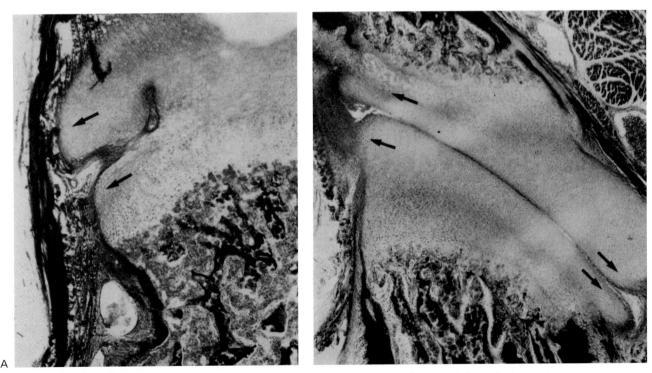

A   B

FIGURE 36.   A: Area of latitudinal expansion of the vertebral centrum (*arrows*). **B:** Latitudinal expansion (*arrows*) of the posterior elements at the facet joint. These are analogous to the zone of Ranvier of a long bone and allow circumferential expansion of the centrum and latitudinal enlargement of the facet joint. As in the long bones, the peripheral membranous bone extends into this zone.

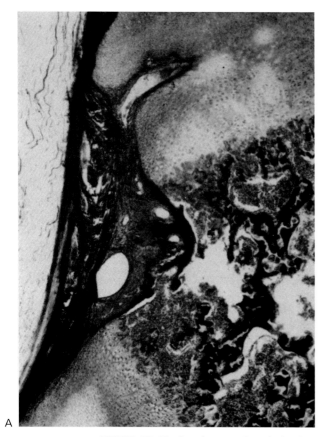 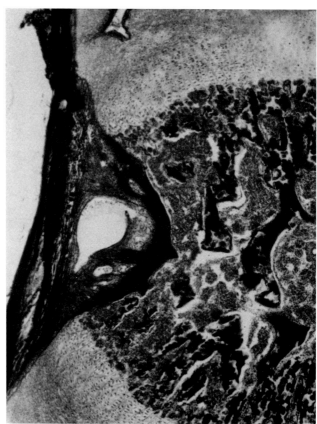

A

B

FIGURE 37. Varying degrees of cortical enlargement in thoracic **(A)** and lumbar **(B)** vertebrae. This process involves membranous bone formation, modeling, and remodeling, all of which are responsive to biomechanical demand.

with blood vessels less in vertebrae than they are in long bones (Fig. 38A). However, large transphyseal vessels are more frequent than in a long bone (Fig. 38). The zone of Ranvier is much less evident in a vertebra, in part because of the restricted advance of the peripheral perichondrial collar. In the zone of matrix formation, increased extracellular matrix is established and undergoes the several important biochemical changes necessary for eventual ossification. The matrix calcifies, and the chondrocytes become hypertrophic, a reflection of their changing metabolic activity.

In the last zone of cartilage transformation, the matrix (chondroid) is sufficiently calcified to allow vascular invasion by the metaphyseal sinusoidal loops. Endothelial cells and accompanying perivascular mesenchyme invade the space provided by hypertrophic cell apoptosis and provide cellular components for initial bone formation. Osteoblasts elaborate osteoid matrix directly on the preformed chondroid septa that are retained preferentially over the transverse septa that originally separated chondrocytes within hypertrophic columns.

This tissue is quickly mineralized to produce bone matrix, the primary spongiosa. By means of subsequent remodeling in the metaphyseal analogues, the initial bone is gradually removed and replaced by more mature secondary spongiosa that no longer contains remnants of the cartilaginous precursor. This process

is abbreviated in the area around the centrum but is more evident in posterior elements (Fig. 1). Remodeling occurs throughout the growth period and after skeletal maturation. Failure to remodel in response to biomechanical stress may be a predisposing factor for microinjury and may lead to increased kyphosis.

''Ring'' Apophysis

Because of ellipsoid enlargement of both the intervertebral disc and the primary ossification center in humans, the central epiphysis progressively thins and the lateral and anterior circumferential portions remain thick. The thickened periphery often is called *apophysis* (190,268), a term not completely appropriate. Most of the time these regions are subjected to compression and shear forces rather than pure tension, as befits the specific definition of an apophysis. On radiographs these regions may appear to be set in a groove extending around the upper and lower borders of the developing vertebral bodies. When this region is subjected to an increase in, if not pathologic, pressure, these indentations are accentuated, probably because of focal slowdown of endochondral ossification. The situation resembles formation of lateral irregularity and an increase in acetabular index in developmental dysplasia of the hip. This variation ossification may cause the vertebral changes usually called *Scheuer-*

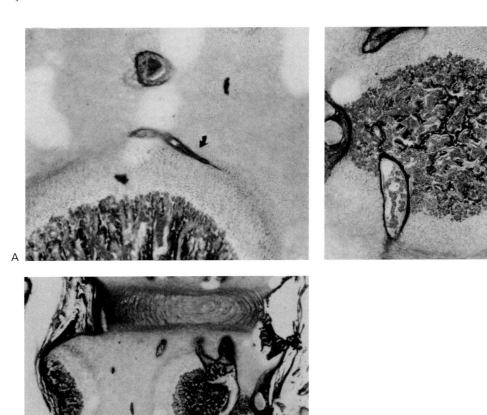

FIGURE 38. Vertebral vasculature. **A:** Epiphyseal (*E*) vessel (*arrow*) formation in the germinal zone comparable with that described for long bones. **B:** Large epiphyseal vessel (superiorly) and transphyseal vessel (inferiorly). The inferior vessel is surrounded by bone crossing the physis. However, in the absence of epiphyseal bone, impairment of growth does not occur. Such structures may be a defect that allows development of Schmorl nodules after skeletal maturation. **C:** Extensive vascular region extending across most of the vertebra and including both the superior and inferior physes.

mann disease. This is not a disease but is a biomechanical response to abnormal stress in an actively growing and remodeling segment of the axial skeleton.

Between 11 and 14 years of age, foci of ossification (Figs. 39–41) develop within the end plate epiphyses (31,33,156,190).

By 12 to 15 years of age, these ossific foci form the radiologic "ring" analogous to the secondary ossification center of the tubular bones. This ring extends to and usually beyond the neurocentral synchondrosis (Fig. 41). The ring does not involve the entire circumference of the vertebral body, and as a secondary ossifica-

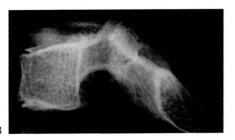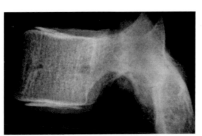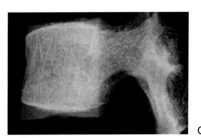

FIGURE 39. Variable stages of development of end plate and ring apophysis at T2 **(A)**, T8 **(B)**, and T12 **(C)** around 12 years of age. These form in the midthoracic region and extend cranially and caudally.

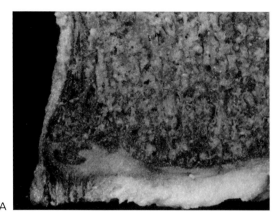
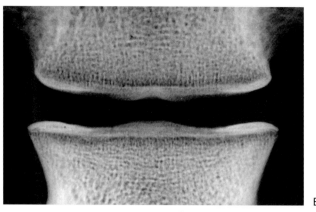

FIGURE 40. A: Appearance of a ring apophysis in L3 in a 16-year-old human. There is a very thin cartilage layer between the bone and the disc material. Impairment of growth and chondroosseous transformation in this region, comparable with impaired lateral acetabular development in hip dysplasia, is a likely cause of Scheuermann disease and thoracic kyphosis. **B:** Radiograph of fused ring apophyses in an adolescent baboon.

tion manifestation does not greatly contribute to growth of the vertebral body. Growth occurs, instead, through the contiguous, previously described physes. In humans rings develop primarily in the periphery. Most other mammals have a plate-like epiphyseal ossification center (Fig. 42). Because spinal flexibility is generally has a juncture at the disc articulations of opposing vertebral bodies, a complete epiphyseal plate buffers the physes from shear forces. When the cantilevered structure of the quadruped spine is taken into account, stress shielding offers a protective advantage in maintaining an aligned architecture and a balanced growth trajectory.

In deference to the prevalent morphologic features of mam-

mals, axial loading of the human spine in most instances neutralizes the value of a spanning epiphysis in the vertebral centrum. However, the susceptibility of the human spine to focal damage from shear forces is an important consideration. Both postural influence and sensitivity to acute injury are enhanced by the lack of a full epiphyseal plate. In some mammals, the ossification

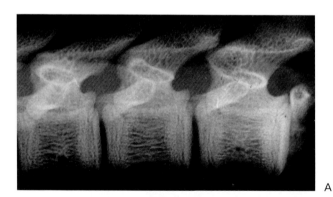

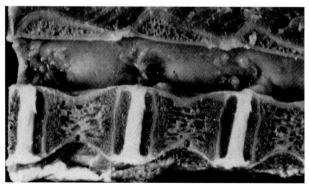

FIGURE 42. Most mammals have well-developed secondary ossification centers rather than ring apophyses. Radiograph **(A)** and midsagittal section **(B)** from an impala.

FIGURE 41. Transverse section of a cape water buffalo showing how the "ring" extends anterolaterally to the neurocentral synchondroses.

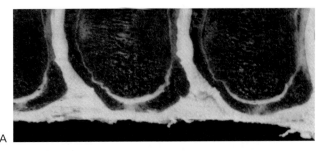

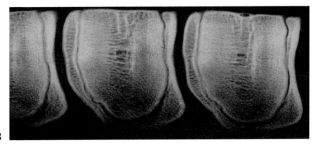

FIGURE 43. In some species, such as Grevy's zebra, the secondary centers grow toward each other anteriorly, producing a situation similar to the longitudinal epiphyseal bracket in humans. **A:** Midsagittal section. **B:** Radiograph. This process may direct the development of certain spinal curvatures in these animals. To our knowledge, this phenomenon has not been described for human vertebrae.

centers unite anteriorly, effectively limiting further longitudinal growth (Fig. 43). The analogous structure in humans, the longitudinal epiphyseal bracket, is distinctly abnormal (217).

Physeal Undulation

Throughout prenatal development, the physis vertebral centrum is usually a spheroid structure. With increasing biomechanical demands, especially shear stresses from walking and running (upright stance), the physis progressively changes contour (56,57,317,376). Biologic demands on a given species may be assessed by means of evaluation of these contour changes, which undoubtedly are affected by both genotypic and phenotypic factors. These undulations are not as prominent in a vertebra as in a long bone, but they can be visualized on prepared specimens (Figs. 27 and 34). In certain mammalian species, such as dolphins, these undulations are almost like the spokes of a bicycle wheel. They afford biomechanical structural modeling and adaptation to considerable rotatory shear forces during sinusoidal swimming motions (268).

Segments of the growth plate may be left behind as the physis continues to grow away from the central reference point (Fig. 44). This commonly occurs in the long bones and is evident in enchondromatosis. A similar phenomenon in the developing spine may be the precursor of Schmorl nodules. Disc tissue extends into these osseous defects after skeletal maturation.

Growth Slowdown Lines

Special radiographic lines reflect alterations in the rate of longitudinal growth from a given physis. These lines, called *Harris*

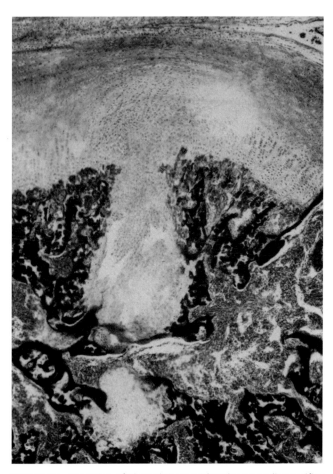

FIGURE 44. Retention of physeal tissue within the expanding ossification center. This may also be a precursor of a Schmorl nodule. Radiographically it would be of comparable appearance.

growth arrest or *slowdown lines,* are transversely oriented trabecular bands of increased radiodensity within the metaphyses and proximate diaphyses. Histologic examination shows these lines to be thickened, transversely interconnected trabecular networks with typical, longitudinally oriented trabecular bone on either side. The lines appear after a temporary slowdown of rapid longitudinal bone formation in the primary spongiosa and usually parallel the contours of the adjacent physis. At the interface of the advancing growth plate, bone formation yields a wake of longitudinally oriented trabeculae with interspersed marrow elements. When growth rates slow temporarily, trabeculae thicken in the hormonal milieu of differentiation and may fuse with each other transversely. When the abnormal process, such as a fracture or systemic illness, responsible for retarding growth subsides, rapid rates of endochondral growth and transformation resume, and the characteristic longitudinal trabecular orientation forms. As the bone elongates, these transverse lines are then progressively displaced from the physis. This phenomenon also occurs in the vertebral bodies (Fig. 45A), but it is not as easy to detect on clinical radiographs because of overlying tissue densities. As the metaphyseal bone remodels to diaphyseal bone, these trabecular lines gradually remodel and disappear com-

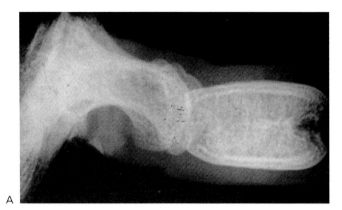

A

B

FIGURE 45. The spinal equivalent of Harris growth slowdown lines. **A:** Radiograph of T6 shows superior and inferior lines parallel to the end plate physes. **B:** Radiograph of a patient approximately 1 year of age shows vertebra-within-a-vertebra phenomenon. Patient had had severe sepsis in the neonatal period.

pletely by the time skeletal maturity is reached. This phenomenon may be present in a vertebra as a ghost or as a vertebra within a vertebra (Fig. 45B). No detailed studies of these lines in vertebrae have been undertaken.

Growth Cessation

Once physiologic stimulation of growth has stopped, the physes regressively cease to be a dynamic element in tissue modeling. In the vertebral body this is concomitant with fusion of the secondary (ring) ossification center to the contiguous metaphysis. This process begins earlier in girls than in boys and like the appearance of primary and secondary ossification centers follows a reasonably predictable sequence. The earlier closure in girls may be due to the presence of estrogenic compounds that accelerate cartilage replacement and osseous maturation. Although the time of onset and completion of fusion are influenced by the sex hormones, the chronologic relations between individual bones is similar for both sexes.

Fusion of the end plate ossification center with the primary ossification center of the vertebral body begins at 14 to 15 years of age but may not be completed until 20 to 22 years in the lumbar region, especially among men. Figure 42 illustrates the comparable process in an animal forming distinct epiphyseal ossification centers.

The closure pattern of the physes at the facet joints has not been studied despite its potential role in asymmetric growth in idiopathic scoliosis. However, continuing data from our skeletal development laboratory suggest that this region is progressively replaced by bone by direct invasion, not unlike the process that occurs in the nonepiphyseal ends of the phalanges, metacarpals, and metatarsals (266).

VASCULATURE

The developing vertebral chondroosseous skeleton has a complex blood supply within the anterior and posterior anlagen and at the perichondrial surface (68,69,106,134). These various macrocirculatory and microcirculatory systems flux constantly and are essential to initial bone formation and remodeling (Fig. 46), neither of which can occur in the absence of these systems (44,216).

The circulation varies structurally with the appearance and growth of the ossification center. Vessels initially enter and distribute throughout the centrum within specialized structures called *cartilage canals* (Figs. 1B, 17B, 19B, and 46A). These canals grow into the centrum from both the anterior and posterior aspects. Unlike the long bones, canals communicate frequently across the physes (Fig. 47) to supply germinal regions and the intervertebral tissues. They are a potential route for spread of infection or tumor from the metaphysis into the epiphysis and disc. Unlike the centrum, the posterior elements are not characterized by the presence of extensive cartilage canal. The posterior elements ossify by means of eccentric vascular penetration from the periosteum with a progressively enlarging eccentric ossification center that expands from the inner surface toward the outer surface as well as anteriorly and posteriorly.

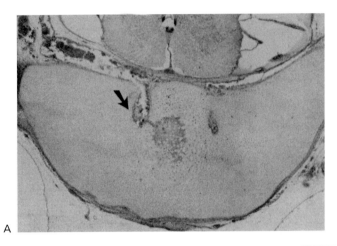

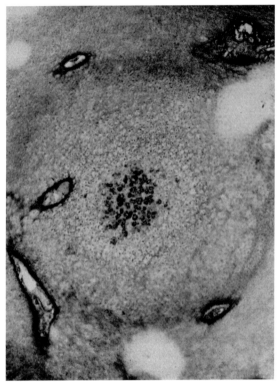

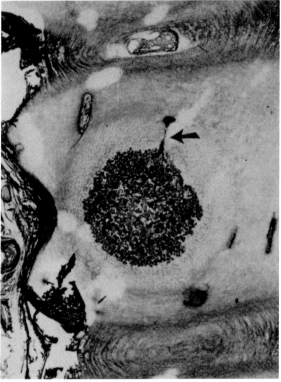

FIGURE 46. A: Extension of a cartilage canal (*arrow*) to reach the hypertrophic cells, a necessary step for ossification. **B:** Central hypertrophy and preossification surrounded by many cartilage canals. **C:** Further expansion ossification without peripheral bone collar. A contributing canal is evident (*arrow*).

Within the vertebral centrum, each cartilage canal contains a central artery and vein and a complex capillary network that surrounds the central vessels but stays within the confines of the canal and eventually forms a glomerular tuft as the end-arterial terminus of the canal system. Research has shown an absence of blood cells and, presumably, an absence of active circulation within these obvious anatomic structures before formation of the secondary ossification center (120). Calcification seems to enhance the activity of the circulation, as in the phenomenon of vascular invasion of the hypertrophic region of the calcified physis of a long bone. Such vascular invasion is impaired in calcium deficiency syndromes (rachitic disorders).

Cartilage canals serve several important functions. First, they supply discrete regions within the centrum with virtually no intraepiphyseal anastomoses between regions of the adjacent canalicular system. Second, the canals enter the centra at fairly regular intervals along each vertebra. Third, the canals serve as a cell conduit for additional chondroblastic and osteoblastic cells that facilitate continued chondroosseous maturation and enlargement of the ossification center.

The cartilage canals play a primary, essential role in the development of the ossification center of the centrum. The first sign of endochondral transformation is hypertrophy of the cartilage cells at the presumptive site of the ossification center (Fig. 46). This site, the preossification center, has both genetic and biomechanical determinants, a fact readily evident in the delayed secondary ossification of the capital femoral epiphysis of a subluxed or dislocated hip. The hypertrophic cells are brought into prox-

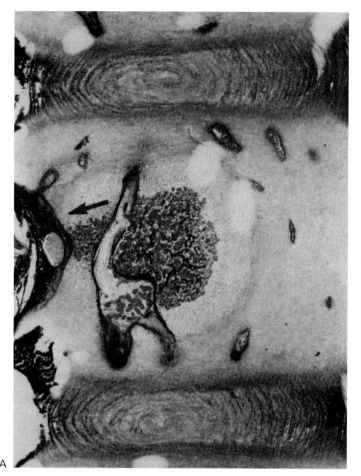

A

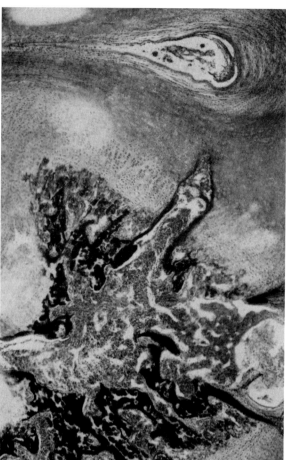

B

FIGURE 47. A: Anterior extension of the ossification center toward an early bone collar (*arrow*). A large vascular confluence is present. These appear to be relatively common in the developing centrum, unlike in the long bone epiphyseal-physeal vasculature. **B:** Extensions of vascularity and bone through the spherical physis toward the disc, which also has a large vascular region. This may be the anatomic explanation for combined osteomyelitis and discitis in childhood. The physis has well-demarcated regions similar to the physis of a long bone.

imity with a cartilage canal system by means of progressive in-growth. At first one and then multiple canals extend into this hypertrophic cell mass, but only after it has become analogous to the calcified, hypertrophic region of the physis. The ossification process enlarges, and a zone of hypertrophic and calcified carti-lage cells (a spherical physis) surrounds it. One or two vessels from the anterior and posterior surfaces usually develop as the predominant blood supply.

Guida et al. (134) studied the vascularization of the vertebral body at term. They demonstrated that each centrum has two anterolateral vessels stemming from the aorta and three or four posterior vessels that often originate from the same anterolateral vessels and transverse around the sides of the centrum and through the neuroforamen to reach the posterior centrum. Within the vertebral body there are multiple anastomoses.

Continued expansion of the centrum ossification center de-pend on the blood vessels (Figs. 47–50). When normal flow is disrupted, osteocytes die rapidly. After recovery, the damaged bone must be replaced with viable bone. The initial bone in the

secondary ossification center was biomechanically responsive in its trabecular orientation, but the rapidly formed new bone is not initially responsive and is thus susceptible to low-grade stress, especially at the interface of new and dead bone.

Within the vascularized chondroosseous epiphysis, the spher-ical growth plate expands centrifugally through rapid interstitial expansion and by means of radially directed longitudinal growth associated with metaphyseal ossification. Interstitial expansion of the spherical physis occurs almost throughout the existence of the ossification center. As the center expands toward the various surfaces of the vertebral body, the outer surface contains more and more platelike bone and fewer fenestrations. This delimits the amount of circulatory ingress, although, as demonstrated in Figs. 47 and 48, transphyseal circulation is frequent and may be an important source of epiphyseal circulation (germinal zone vascularity).

The enlargement of the centrum ossification center leads to juxtaposition of part of the spherical growth plate against the intervertebral tissues. The epiphyseal contribution is eventually

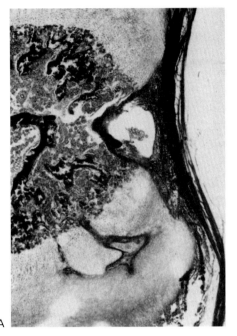
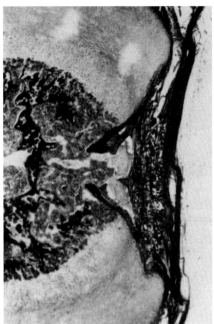
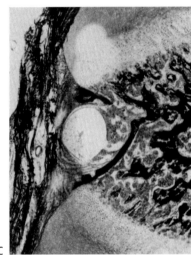

FIGURE 48. A–C: Variations in the posterior bone collar. This region is usually associated with a large vascular region (lakes). The vessels cross the physis in **A.**

replaced by a subchondral bone plate, but the remainder of the spherical growth plate may still be present at the interface of the epiphyseal margins and the peripheral boundary at the disc. This configuration allows continued osseous expansion commensurate with diametric expansion of the ossifying center. Actual latitudinal expansion of the centrum continues through the surrounding perichondrium and enlarges the cartilaginous antecedent model.

As the ossification center forms and enlarges, the epiphyseal circulatory pattern changes. When the subchondral (cribiform) plate forms, small vessels cross this osseous plate and form vascular expansions that supply discrete regions of the physis and extend toward the intervertebral tissues.

Ferguson (106) emphasized the concept of dorsal (posterior) and ventral (anterior) blood lakes. Evident in Fig. 48, these lakes are closely associated with the developing peripheral ossification processes, although the exact role they play in hemodynamics

is uncertain. These lakes can be disrupted with surgical exposure, and excessive bleeding can result.

Perichondrial Vessels

The perichondrial circulation shrouds each vertebral centrum, although with considerable anatomic variation, especially in relation to the vascular systems of the long bones. The most important derivation appears to be the system of small vessels within the zone of Ranvier (Fig. 48). The functional integrity of these vessels in the zone is essential to continued appositional growth at the periphery of the centrum and posterior element growth plates. Disruption of the perichondrial system may produce isolated areas of ischemia along the periphery and subsequent eccentric growth. Circulatory patterns in both the perichondrial circulation and its intraepiphyseal contributions change gradu-

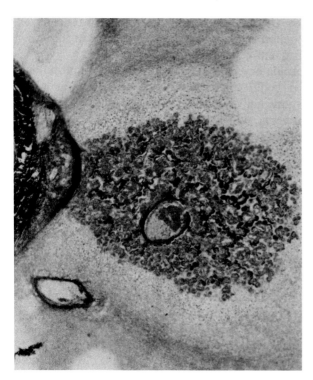

FIGURE 49. Vascular lake within the ossification center.

ally and affect the susceptibility of a region to ischemic damage. Impairment of this circulation in the anterolateral regions may seriously affect chondroosseous transition and may be a factor in irregular radiographic appearances.

Circulation in the Posterior Elements

The posterior elements derive their blood supply from branches of the same arteries that supply the centrum (93). These vessels

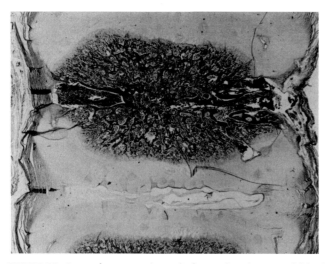

FIGURE 50. Image from near the end of gestation shows established fetal vertebral centrum and maturing anterior and posterior vascular contributions.

proceed dorsally to reach each of the paired posterior elements. As such, compromise of an anterior parent vessel can compromise posterior and anterior circulation and accentuate the progression of scoliosis because of asymmetric vascular insufficiency.

Vascular Disruption

When a region of the epiphyseal vasculature is either temporarily or permanently compromised, the zones of growth and transformation associated with these vessels cannot undergo appropriate cell division and maturation. Unaffected regions of the physis continue their longitudinal growth, and the affected region is left behind. The growth rate of the cells adjacent to the infarcted area is more mechanically compromised than that of cells farther away (277). If the involved area is peripheral, an angular deformity may occur. This may be a mechanism involved in Scheuermann disease.

Because vascular disruptions may be transient, the physis has a certain amount of recovery capacity. However, when circulation is restored, the cells most responsive are those that encircle the physis in and adjacent to the zone of Ranvier. DeSalis et al. (78) showed that circulatory disruption of one of the neurocentral synchondroses over several vertebrae caused scoliosis. Histologic studies showed that the neurocentral synchondroses on the convex side stayed open longer than those subject to vascular compromise. They also showed contiguous damage to the spinal cord preferentially on the side of the vascular damage rather than diffused throughout the spinal cord. Such cord changes may affect the segmented spinal musculature and further contribute to asymmetry of growth.

CLINICAL APPLICATION

It is extremely important to thoroughly assess all components of the spine and spinal cord and not to concentrate on only the radiologically obvious, that is, osseous, skeletal deformities when planning treatment, particularly when a patient has congenital spinal abnormalities. Deformities still in a cartilaginous phase may not be readily evident until sufficient postnatal growth and chondroosseous transformation have occurred to allow definition with routine radiography. Progression of deformity tends to be slower in the cartilaginous phase but becomes more evident with increasing ossification, not unlike the slow and later rapid progression of angular deformity in a limb bone from an osseous bridge after trauma or infection. The treating physician must be prepared to alter concepts of deformity and treatment, actual or intended, on the basis of the evolving anatomic deformity.

Arbitrary standards for values of various degrees of motion, distances, and so forth that are commonly applied to the evaluation of adult spines are not always applicable in the treatment of children. Nonossified cartilage can exaggerate a discrete measurement, placing it in the range that is pathologic for adults. It is important to base treatment decisions on the normal radiographic values for children rather than on those for adults (42,49,154,222).

The morphologic variations of congenital and acquired deformities, diseases, and trauma involving the spines of patients with immature skeletons are logically and clinically approached through an appreciation of prenatal and postnatal developmental biologic mechanisms at the molecular and cellular levels. Equally important is how the constantly changing microscopic and macroscopic anatomic differences of growing children compare with the relatively static skeletal components of adults (100). It is essential to realize the wide variation of basic steps in prenatal and postnatal skeletal development that may manifest in deformity despite initial radiographic similarity (286).

Congenital deformities invariably affect more than the evident osseous axial skeleton, especially among children younger than 5 years. Radiolucent cartilaginous, vascular, and neuromuscular structures may be altered or deficient and may thwart well-planned attempts at improvement if treatment is based only on radiologically evident changes (62). Acquired diseases and injuries can alter normal patterns of growth and necessitate modification of otherwise standard approaches, especially if the principles of adult surgery are applied. Deformities may recur among children because of inability to correct the causal (whether genetic or acquired) growth aberration. The biologically fluid (plastic), constantly remodeling skeleton does not always require the same types of prolonged immobilization and rigid fixation used for comparable treatment of adults.

Congenital spinal anomalies range from those so frequent that they should be considered normal variants, such as spina bifida occulta of L5, to major structural defects. Many major defects are related to somite malformations; these include block (unsegmented) vertebrae, wedge vertebrae (hemivertebrae and butterfly vertebrae), incomplete neural arch fusion, spina bifida, congenital bars, block vertebrae, absence of pedicle formation, and asymmetric pedicular enlargement. Limb abnormalities, such as radial hemimelia, often occur concomitantly with spinal

abnormalities. There also is a relatively high incidence of renal, genitourinary, and gastrointestinal deficits. The following sections briefly correlate developmental morphologic features with potential treatments and the usual course of the condition.

Hydromyelia and Syringomyelia

Hydromyelia occurs when the neural canal is retained (Fig. 19). This diagnosis is being made increasingly with the use of magnetic resonance imaging (324). Hydromyelia may be limited to only a few segments or extend for most of the cord. In most patients it is probably a structural variation rather than a definitive pathologic condition. Interpretation must be based on and correlated with the findings at clinical examination.

Syringomyelia can originate through slow dilation of the retained neural tube (canal). In children with spina bifida, syrinx enlargement may be caused by obstruction in the ventricular system. Syringes also may have posttraumatic or postischemic causes. Although most syringes appear stable, some may rapidly accumulate fluid, expand, and compress spinal cord tissue between the syrinx and the inner walls of the vertebral arch. Such a syrinx may be associated with the rapid onset and progression of scoliosis.

Cervical Hypermobility

The facet joints of the upper cervical spine are less oblique (more horizontal) than those of the lower cervical spine of young children (Fig. 51) (260). This allows considerable forward motion in flexion, especially at the C2–3 and C3–4 joints, and causes the phenomenon of pseudosubluxation (58,323). As the upper cervical spine matures, the facet angles become more oblique

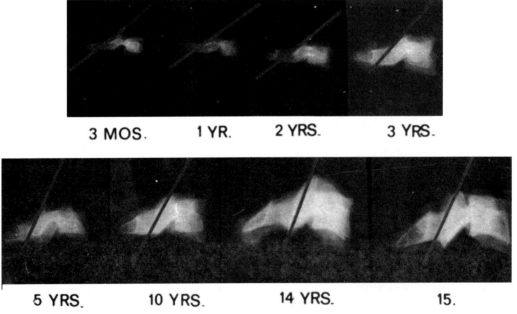

FIGURE 51. Changing pattern of angulation of the superior facet joint of C3 between 3 months and 15 years of age.

(more vertical) and subluxation becomes less accentuated (260). The thoracic and lumbar vertebrae follow similar developmental patterns of changes in facet orientation, but the phenomenon of pseudosubluxation is not as readily evident. Rotational changes in the orientation of the planes of the thoracolumbar facet joints also can occur. Asymmetric changes may be a subtle predisposing factor in idiopathic scoliosis. Such a predisposition to scoliosis with asymmetric development of the thoracic vertebrae has been found in rodents (172).

Congenital Scoliosis

Pathogenesis occurs very early in development, commonly before 6 weeks after ovulation (85,89,94,142,151,287,329). The deformity may occur by means of failure of formation. Typical patterns are unilateral hypoplasia (wedge vertebra) and aplasia (block vertebra or hemivertebra; Fig. 12). An alternative explanation is failure of segmentation that which leads to bar formation and affects anterior elements, posterior elements, or both. A combination of these deformities also may be present (Figs. 52, 53).

The anomalous vertebrae may or may not be radiographically

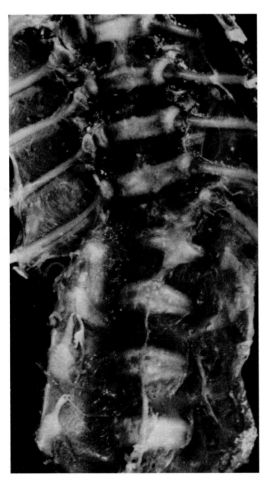

FIGURE 52. Congenital scoliosis in a greater kudu (antelope). The animal was stillborn.

evident at birth, depending on the extent of the abnormality and how much of the area has ossified (Fig. 53). For example, a hemivertebra may be represented by an asymmetric ossific center. Early definition of the exact structural defect may not be easy (Fig. 53). However, the earlier a specific deformity is properly classified, the sooner can appropriate treatment be instituted.

Longitudinal growth of the vertebral column occurs at each end plate anteriorly and by means of periosteal apposition posteriorly. If growth is tethered unilaterally by a bar, a deformity is likely because normal development occurs contralaterally. Conversely, absence of growth potential may lead to increasing deformity because of the present of normal posterior growth coupled with anterior deficiency. Congenital vertebral anomalies thus cause progressive curvature. The rate of progression, however, is highly variable.

Congenital Kyphosis

Congenital kyphosis often is caused by a hemivertebra located within the posterior aspect of the centrum. The size of the hemivertebra and whether it is attached by cartilage to an adjacent vertebra determine the rapidity of progression. A congenital kyphosis may not be clinically evident at birth, even with an evident hemivertebra. It manifests, however, as the vertebral column undergoes chondroosseous maturation and spinal elongation and particularly after the patient assumes an upright posture, whether sitting or standing.

The spinal cord appears to be much more susceptible to injury in congenital kyphosis than it is in congenital scoliosis. Any evidence of cord dysfunction necessitates urgent treatment to stop or reverse progression. Parents need to be warned of the risk of neurologic worsening, even with in situ, noninstrumented spinal fusions.

Klippel-Feil Syndrome

The Klippel-Feil syndrome involves variable portions of the cervical spine (Fig. 54), particularly fusions of several levels of the anterior and posterior components of the cervical and on occasion the upper thoracic spine (11,28,130,135,152,153,165, 188,192,239,265). Spina bifida and Sprengel deformity (omovertebral bone) are frequently present. The extent of deformity is not always evident in the first year or two of life. Many patients do not come to medical attention until adolescence, when they are being evaluated for neck pain after an evocative situation, such as football or wrestling (260).

Perhaps the most serious problem is the insidious impingement on the cord that occurs when limited motion segments begin to move excessively, especially during adolescence. For example, in cases of C1–3 and C4–7 fusion, there is only one important flexion-extension region, namely the C3-4 articulation. Forward motion (flexion) may chronically impinge on the cord and slowly lead to long-tract symptoms consequent to subtle, progressive spinal cord damage. Complete fusion of this "remaining motion" segment may be necessary to alleviate not only the symptoms but also cord damage.

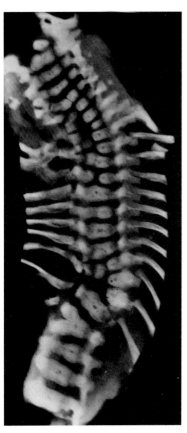

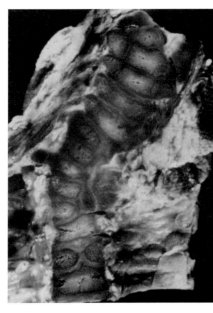

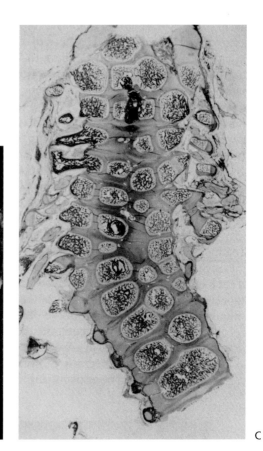

A,B

C

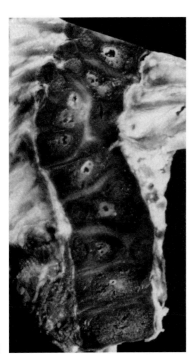

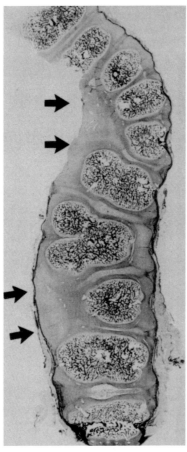

D,E

FIGURE 53. Multiple congenital vertebral anomalies in a human stillborn with congenital scoliosis. **A:** Radiograph of the entire spine. **B, C:** Morphologic and histologic sections of the cervical and upper thoracic regions. **D, E:** Morphologic and histologic sections of the lower thoracic and lumbar regions. Of particular importance is the cartilaginous continuity over several deformed segments (*arrows*). This would have been radiolucent at first, but it eventually formed a multilevel bar.

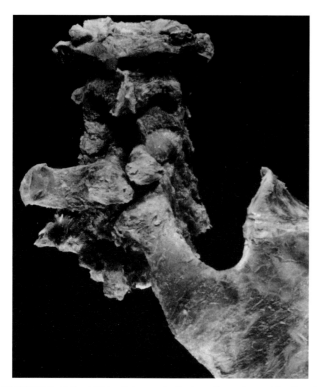

FIGURE 54. Spina bifida of the cervical spine of a patient with Klippel-Feil and Sprengel deformities.

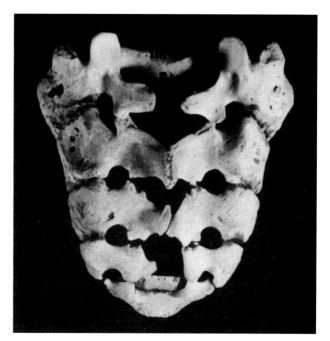

FIGURE 55. Spina bifida of the sacrum.

Spina Bifida and Dysraphism Complexes

Dysraphism is failure of fusion of posterior midline vertebral structures. In rare instances the anterior structures are affected. The spectrum of spina bifida, the most obvious form of spinal dysraphism, ranges from myeloschisis to myelomeningocele, meningocele, and spina bifida occulta (Fig. 55; see also Fig. 18). Myeloschisis and myelomeningocele probably occur during the embryonic period. Meningocele and spina bifida occulta more likely develop during the fetal period because of incomplete chondroosseous transformation. A minor defect in the spinal cord or meninges may prevent development of the normal amalgamation of the posterior element. However, the converse is not true. That is, an abnormal posterior arch can occur in the absence of a neurologic problem.

The posterior elements may be incompletely formed and oriented laterally (Fig. 56). This redirects the spinal extensor musculature anteriorly such that the muscles act as flexors and contribute to increased kyphosis at the level of the bifida defect. Failure of proper formation of the posterior elements contributes a great deal to the difficulty of instrumented spinal fusion. For example, pedicle screw placement is challenging if not impossible.

Lumbosacral Agenesis

The incidence of lumbosacral agenesis is high among prediabetic and diabetic mothers, yet the exact role of the metabolic abnormality as a causal factor has not been elucidated. The syndrome involves a spectrum of morphologic disorders ranging from mild dysplasia to complete absence of components of the lumbar or sacral spine or both. The most extreme manifestation is sirenomelia.

Diastematomyelia

Excessive width between pedicles may be associated with the presence of an osseous or cartilaginous mass extending from the vertebral body into the vertebral canal (62,91). The spinal cord or cauda equina is divided (cleft) around this fixed mass, which essentially transfixes the cord. Because of disparate longitudinal development of the spinal cord relative to the lengthening spine, children with this defect characteristically does not have neurologic symptoms until they are several years of age,

It had been assumed that the ascent of the spinal cord within the osseous vertebral canal has a progressive tethering effect. Barson (15) challenged this concept when showed in anatomic studies that the cord normally reaches the adult level (L1–2) within the canal by 2 months of age. Barson suggested that the normal ascent of the cord is unusually retarded in children with diastematomyelia or that the neurologic signs lack a simplistic mechanical explanation. In theory, one would expect a severe neurologic deficit at birth because most of the ascent, according to the usual concepts, occurs before this time.

Tethered Cord

Normally the filum terminale either elongates or detaches from its most distal (sacral) attachments during the fetal or early postnatal period to allow the aforementioned proximal migration. Failure to do so may produce progressive traction on the spinal

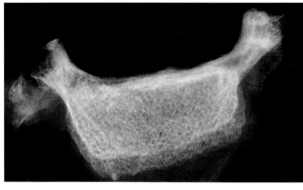
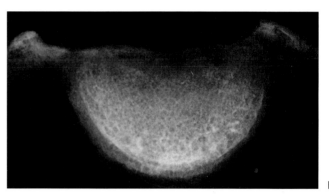

FIGURE 56. Representative myelomeningocele vertebra resected during kyphectomy. The amount of posterior element formation is limited in **A** and markedly lateralized in **B**.

cord or roots. The resulting change in neurologic function may necessitate intervention. The problem is fairly frequent among patients with spina bifida, either as a primary problem or as a secondary consequence (scarring) of primary closure of the defect in the neonatal period (235). The presence of tethered cord or another accompanying defect is not an indication for surgery; neurologic deterioration should be the basis for intervention.

Idiopathic Scoliosis

The origin of idiopathic scoliosis remains controversial (7, 191,247,300,333,335). Theories include neuromuscular imbalance, subtle growth abnormalities, and dysfunction at the cord or brain tissue level. Like slipped capital femoral epiphysis, three-dimensional alteration of the structure of the spine and curvature undoubtedly are outcomes that may have been derived from any one of several pathways.

Rönning and Kylämarkula (292) found that the potential of the neurocentral synchondroses to fuse at discrete times could be altered by changing biomechanical conditions. Altered muscular dynamics could feasibly allow asymmetric closure. Bequiristain and Cañadell et al. (27,52) showed that unilateral fusion with screws of several levels of the porcine thoracic spine produced scoliosis, They concluded that if symmetric growth of the neurocentral synchondroses was disturbed, rotation of the vertebral body would occur because of eccentric growth. Such eccentric development of the neurocentral synchondroses has been found in a large number of spines from cadavers of newborn infant (Ogden JA, unpublished observations). The asymmetric growth would produce three-dimensional change, as in Blount disease of a long bone or altered acetabular development in hip dysplasia.

The facet joint has a chondroosseous growth mechanism. In essence, each vertebra has four such facet physes (two superior, two inferior). Growth must be equal, right and left, to allow symmetric bone formation. Alteration of rates of growth can affect the shape of the posterior elements and secondarily affect muscle function, which can affect growth rates (loop effect).

Spinal Osteochondrosis and Scheuermann Disease

The cartilaginous plates appear to be relatively weaker mechanically where they are penetrated by vertebral vessels. These areas

conceptually have a decrease in resistance to the continuous pressure of the nucleus pulposus. Portions of the nucleus may be forced through the end plate into the vertebral body (Schmorl nodule). However, as shown in Fig. 44, the tissue in the radiolucent region may be unossified cartilage rather than disc material per se. During active growth this is a gradual process.

Multiple prolapse resulting in irregular end plates, associated with loss of anterior vertebral height in adolescents, is known as *Scheuermann kyphosis.* The specific cause of this sequence of events is not known. It is likely that some kyphosis occurs first, and then increased anterior pressure propagates the deformity (Hueter-Volkmann law) and allows uneven growth of the vertebral body, particularly with wedging. This produces a climate for variable growth similar to alteration of lateral acetabular growth in hip dysplasia. The narrowness of the intervertebral discs combined with the kyphosis contributes to abnormal biomechanical loading. This deformity can be corrected during further growth when these forces are mollified, as by bracing. The relatively dependable and rapid response to bracing supports a biomechanical cause rather than an intrinsic biologic (molecular) abnormality.

Chordoma

In normal development, notochordal cells progressively disappear from the vertebral centrum during the cartilaginous period of embryonic development. Persistence of the notochord, however, can form a mucoid streak (Fig. 15), a finding not uncommon among neonates. On radiographs these often appear as radiolucent depressions extending from the nucleus pulposus. Cohen et al. (66) described a number of patients with irregular radiolucencies in the vertebral centra due to retained segments of notochord that apparently impeded complete coalescence of ossific regions. During postmortem examinations, notochordal tissue remnants were found in 2% of cases. Notochordal cells may persist in the nucleus pulposus until term and may even be found in the nucleus as late as 10 years of age (331). Most are found in the region of the clivus (base of the skull) and in the sacrococcygeal region, where most chordomas occur. Chordomas are thought to arise from altered growth of these notochordal cells (331).

Canal Tumors

An excessively high sagittal diameter or excessive width between the pedicles during development suggests the presence of an expanding lesion within the spinal canal. A large vertebral foramen likewise should point to the possibility of the presence of a pathologic lesion (such as a neurofibroma). Many types of tumors affect the developing spine. Management is essentially the same as in other regions, but with an emphasis on preserving spinal stability and cord function. Tumors such as eosinophilic granuloma are associated with trabecular collapse (vertebra plana); recovery of vertebral height is variable.

The spine often is the initial site of malignant disease in children. Leukemia must be included in the differential diagnosis of back pain among children. Expansion of leukemia infiltrates within the trabecular bone may cause microstructural failure and painful symptoms. Wedging of the vertebrae may occur.

The spine may be the site of metastasis, especially of neuroblastoma. Radiation therapy for malignant tumors can alter growth if only a portion of the spine receives radiation exposure. The cord also is susceptible; radiation-induced fibrosis often develops. This may put the patient at risk of ischemic change if fusion is undertaken for the spinal deformity.

Os Odontoideum

The mechanism of formation of os odontoideum is reasonably well accepted (109,110,136,150,240,284,309,370). Fielding and Griffin (109) discovered that 17 of 35 cases of os odontoideum occurred an average of 3.5 years after initial trauma. In most cases, the radiograph obtained immediately after the trauma showed an intact dens.

Examination of radiographs that show antecedent os odontoideum clearly associated with C1 and some of the terminal ligaments allows easy postulation of a causal traumatic injury. Because of a lack of or minimal treatment, constant motion can contribute to the development of a pseudarthrosis that interferes with the blood supply to the distal part of the dens ossification center and causes progressive atrophy in the distal portion (290). The chondrum terminale, however, remains intact with all of its ligaments and vascularity attached (304). It then undergoes normal secondary ossification, which appears as a radiographically separate structure. Because the blood supply is cut off, there is minimal possibility of distal endochondral bone formation. However, the physis of the chondrum terminale, which has an intact circulation, enlarges, and if some blood gets into the proximal metaphysis, the ossiculum may enlarge.

End Plate Fractures

The expanding chondroosseous interface of the vertebral body, and possibly the posterior elements, presents a mechanically susceptible region analogous to the equivalent region of a long bone. The interface thus is susceptible to fractures that separate the physis and epiphysis from the ossification center of the centrum. These injuries may be subtle and often reduce spontaneously after the injury mechanism dissipates (260,261). Partial

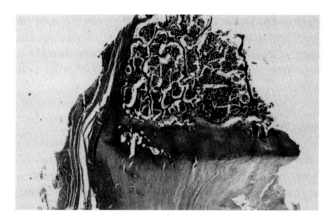

FIGURE 57. Avulsion of the corner lumbar fragment sustained through weight lifting.

fractures of the end plate (Figs. 57, 58) frequently involve the cervical spine anteriorly (210) and the lumbar spine posteriorly (260,262,291). In the latter instance, a lesion equivalent to a herniated disc develops. The cartilaginous cap may be avulsed as a physeal injury. The chondroosseous growth mechanism of the facet likewise may be disrupted and cause acute as well as long-term growth alteration.

Spondylolysis

No prenatal pattern of development of ossification centers in the lumbar neural arches suggests that the pars interarticularis defect in spondylolysis is the congenital result of failure of fusion of the posterior primary ossification centers. There is only one ossification center in each posterior element. The initial site of this onset of ossification also is the region involved in the spondylolytic defect. The normal site of ossific fusion of the centrum with the neural arches is well anterior to the pathologic defect, within the vertebral body. Any pars defect must be an acquired, traumatically incurred failure within the primary ossification center of the neural arch (214).

There are infrequent situations in which sacral spina bifida is associated with loss of the normal interspinous ligament support for the lumbar spine. Over a sufficient biomechanical time span, such an anatomic arrangement can lead to a more horizontal direction of the facets and attenuation of the developing pars interarticularis by plastic deformation of the bone (bone may be acutely stretched 3% to 7% of its length before fracturing). However, in most cases of spondylolysis, the pars is attenuated or broken by chronic, repetitive, often minimally or asymptomatic trauma, as in competitive gymnastics or figure skating. When both sides fail, biomechanical stability is affected, and spondylolisthesis may result.

Apparent spondylolytic defects can involve the upper cervical vertebra (66,260). These probably arise from variations in ossification of the region of the posterior element that contribute to the final vertebral body, which is more extensive in the cervical region than it is in other regions.

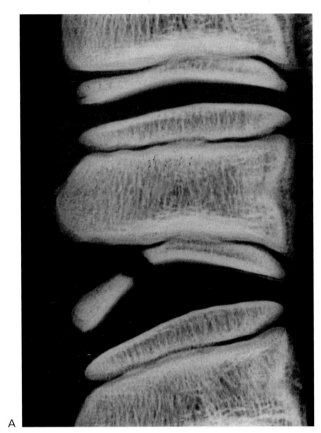
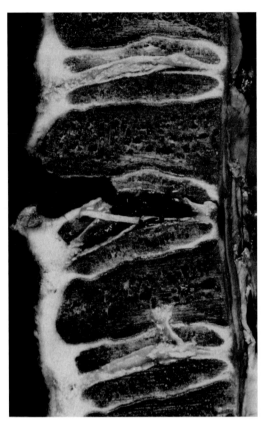

A   B

FIGURE 58. Spontaneously occurring end plate fracture in a zebra. **A:** Radiograph. **B:** Sagittal section.

Spondylolisthesis

Spondylolisthesis most often is an acquired disorder that requires antecedent bilateral spondylolysis (246,343,367). As mentioned earlier, a congenital deficiency also may allow the progressive forward slipping of one vertebral bone on another that typifies this lesion. In the most severe form, complete displacement occurs and the superior vertebra is located anterior to the inferior vertebra.

Dysplasia

The ossification center of the dens has both a proximal and a distal physis. In diseases that affect longitudinal growth, such as achondroplasia, the dens may not grow normally, leading to hypoplasia of the dens. This can occur with any skeletal dysplasia. *The shape and stability of this region always must be assessed for any child with dysplastic skeletal abnormalities* (293,355). Fusion, when necessary, should be performed with the patient's own bone because of the high risk of lysis of allografts among children (321).

In achondroplasia the vertebral canal may be narrowed throughout its length. Hence the normal spinal cord and cauda equina are housed in an inadequate bony canal. This abnormality is caused by a lack of growth in the pedicles and laminae. The sagittal width also is less than normal. The resultant spinal

stenosis can cause severe neurologic problems in adulthood (97). Kyphosis with or without wedging at the thoracolumbar junction is frequent (226).

Spondyloepiphyseal dysplasia affects the vertebral epiphyses of the spine as well as those of long bones (270). End plate ossification becomes irregular. Abnormalities of the vertebrae include irregular end plates, platyspondylia, and the appearance of a central tongue in the lumbar area. The end plates may manifest as multiple Schmorl nodules. However, these are more likely unossified dysplastic cartilage remnants similar to those shown in Fig. 44.

Several mucopolysaccharidosis syndromes include progressive abnormal development of the vertebral column (196,219). Ovoid vertebral bodies with wedging and kyphosis at the thoracolumbar junction are characteristic. The accumulation of abnormal molecular (metabolic) products in the trabecular spaces affects chondroosseous transformation and biomechanics. Thus the ability to grow normally is hindered by microstructural failure and variable collapse, especially in the anterior aspect. Platyspondylia is frequent in Morquio syndrome.

In Down syndrome, hypoplasia of the dens is common. However, a more difficult problem is increased joint laxity, which may particularly affect the atlantoaxial region (47,72,281,288). If instability persists, progressive myelopathy can damage the upper cord (Fig. 59) (355).

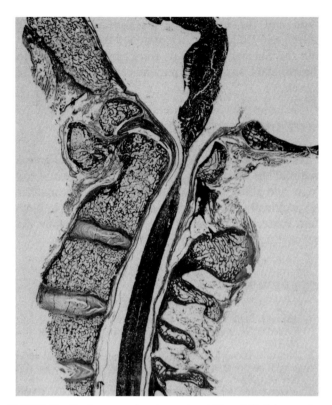

FIGURE 59. Cord compression due to instability of C1–2 in a patient with Down syndrome.

ACKNOWLEDGMENTS

The authors thank the Human Developmental Anatomy Center, National Museum of Health and Medicine, and the Armed Forces Institute of Pathology for making human embryonic and fetal material, especially that of the Carnegie collection, available for study; Busch Gardens Zoologic Park for providing a wide array of comparative animal material; and the Skeletal Educational Association for continued research support.

REFERENCES

1. Altman J, Bayer SA (1982): Development of the cranial nerve ganglia and related nuclei in the rat. *Adv Anat Embryol Cell Biol* 74:1–89.
2. Anderson DJ (1989): The neural crest cell lineage problem: neuropoiesis? *Neuron* 3:1–12.
3. Andries L, Harrisson F, Callebaut M (1987): Differential distribution of cell protrusions on the ventral surface of the deep layer in gastrulating quail and chick embryos. *Differentiation* 34:168–174.
4. Archer E, Batnitzky S, Franken EA, et al. (1977): Congenital dysplasia of C2–6. *Pediatr Radiol* 6:121–122.
5. Armstrong JB, Graveson AC (1988): Progressive patterning precedes somite segmentation in the Mexican axolotl (*Amblystoma mexicanum*). *Dev Biol* 126:1–6.
6. Azar Y, Eyal-Giladi H (1979): Marginal zone cells, the primitive streak-inducing component of the primary hypoblast in the chick. *J Embryol Exp Morphol* 52:79–88.
7. Badoux DM (1968): Some notes on the curvature of the spinal column of vertebrates with special reference to mammals. *Acta Morphol Neerl Scand* 7:29–40.
8. Bagi C, Burger EH (1989): Mechanical stimulation by intermittent compression stimulates sulfate incorporation and matrix mineralization in fetal mouse long-bone rudiments under serum-free conditions. *Calcif Tissue Int* 45:342–347.
9. Bagnall KM, Harris PF, Jones PRM (1977): A radiographic study of the human fetal spine, 1: the development of the secondary cervical curvature. *J Anat* 123:777–782.
10. Bailey DK (1962): The normal cervical spine in infants and children. *Radiology* 59:712–719.
11. Baird PA, Robinson GC, Buckler WSJ (1967): Klippel-Feil syndrome. *Am J Dis Child* 113:546–551.
12. Bale PM (1973): A congenital intraspinal gastroenterogenous cyst in diastematomyelia. *J Neurol Neurosurg Psychiatry* 36:1011–1017.
13. Barrofio A, Dupin E, LeDouarin NN (1988): Clone-forming ability and differentiation potential of migratory neural crest cells. *Proc Natl Acad Sci USA* 85:5325–5329.
14. Barry A (1956): A quantitative study of the prenatal changes in angulation of the spinal nerves. *Anat Rec* 126:97–110.
15. Barson AJ (1970): The vertebral level of termination of the spinal cord during normal and abnormal development. *J Anat* 106:489–497.
16. Baur R (1969): Zum Problem der Neugliederung der Wirbelsaule. *Acta Anat (Basel)* 72:321–356.
17. Beardmore HE, Wiglesworth FW (1958): Vertebral anomalies and alimentary duplications: clinical and embryological aspects. *Pediatr Clin North Am* 5:457–474.
18. Bellairs R (1953): Studies on the development of the foregut in the chick blastoderm, II: the morphogenetic movements. *J Embryol Exp Morphol* 1:369–385.
19. Bellairs R (1963): The development of somites in the chick embryo. *J Embryol Exp Morphol* 11:697–714.
20. Bellairs R (1979): The mechanism of somite segmentation in the chick embryo. *J Embryol Exp Morphol* 51:227–243.
21. Bellairs R (1984): Experimental analysis of control mechanisms in somite segmentation in avian embryos, II: reduction of material in the gastrula stages of the chick. *J Embryol Exp Morphol* 79:183–200.
22. Bellairs R (1986): The primitive streak. *Anat Embryol (Berlin)* 174: 1–14.
23. Bellairs R, Van Peteghem MC (1984): Gastrulation: is it analogous to malignant invasion? *Am Zool* 24:563–570.
24. Bennett MR, Davey DF, Uebel KE (1980): The growth of segmental nerves from the brachial myotomes into the proximal muscles of the chick forelimb during development. *J Comp Neurol* 189:335–357.
25. Benson DR, Muller F, O'Rahilly R (1982): A butterfly vertebra in a 63 millimeter human fetus. *Orthop Trans* 6:14–15.
26. Bentley JFR, Smith JR (1960): Developmental posterior enteric remnants and spinal malformation. *Arch Dis Child* 35:76–86.
27. Bequiristain JL, Gilli R, Cañadell J (1991): The role of the neurocentral cartilage. In: *Idiopathic scoliosis update.* Pamplona, Spain: University Press.
28. Bernini F, Elefante R, Smaltino F, et al. (1969): Angiographic study on the vertebral artery in cases of deformities of the occipitocervical joint. *Am J Roentgenol* 107:526–529.
29. Berrill NJ (1963): Morphogenetic fields, their growth and development. *Dev Biol* 7:342–347.
30. Bettler D, Schmid A, Yedvobnick B (1991): Early ventral expression of the *Drosophila* neurogenic locus *mastermind*. *Dev Biol* 144:436–439.
31. Bick EM (1952): The osteohistology of the human vertebra. *J Mt Sinai Hosp N Y* 19:490–527.
32. Bick EM, Copel JW (1950): Longitudinal growth of the human vertebra. *J Bone Joint Surg Am* 32:803–814.
33. Bick EM, Copel JW (1951): The ring apophysis of the human vertebra. *J Bone Joint Surg Am* 33:783–787.
34. Blechschmidt E, Gasser RF (1978): *Biokinetics and biodynamics of human differentiation.* Springfield, IL: Charles C Thomas.
35. Blum AS, Barnstable CJ (1987): O-acetylation of a cell-surface carbohydrate creates discrete molecular patterns during neural development. *Proc Natl Acad Sci USA* 84:8716–8720.
36. Bohmig R (1922): Ueber das primordialcranium eines menschlichen

embryos aus dem zweiten monat mit cranio-rachischisis. *Z Anat Entwicklungsgesch* 65:570–590.

37. Boisseau S, Simonneau M (1989): Mammalian neuronal differentiation: early expression of a neuronal phenotype from mouse neural crest cells in a chemically defined culture medium. *Development* 106: 665–674.

38. Bonewald LF, Mundy GR (1990): Role of transforming growth factor-beta in bone remodeling. *Clin Orthop* 250:261–276.

39. Bortier H, De Bruyne G, Espeel M, et al. (1989): Immunohistochemistry of laminin in early chicken and quail blastoderms. *Anat Embryol (Berlin)* 180:65–69.

40. Boss V, Wigston DJ (1989): Selective reinnervation of muscle basement membranes by their original motoneurons. *Soc Neurosci Abstr* 15:165.

41. Bradamante Z, Hall BK (1980): The role of epithelial collagen and proteoglycan in the initiation of osteogenesis by avian neural crest cells [abstract]. *Anat Rec* 197:305–315. Abstract 165.

42. Brandner ME (1970): Normal values of the vertebral body and intervertebral disk index during growth. *Am J Roentgenol* 110:618–627.

43. Brockes JP (1989): Retinoids, homeobox genes, and limb morphogenesis. *Neuron* 2:1285–1294.

44. Brookes M (1971): *The blood supply of bone: an approach to bone biology.* New York: Appleton.

45. Buck CA, Horwitz AF (1987): Cell surface receptors for extracellular matrix molecules. *Annu Rev Cell Biol* 3:179–205.

46. Buck CA, Shea E, Duggan K, et al. (1986): Integrin (the CSAT antigen): functionality requires oligomeric integrity. *J Cell Biol* 103: 2421–2428.

47. Burke SW, French HG, Roberts JM, et al. (1985): Chronic atlanto-axial instability in Down's syndrome. *J Bone Joint Surg Am* 67: 1356–1360.

48. Burt AM (1975): Choline acetyltransferase and acetylcholinesterase in the developing rat spinal cord. *Exp Neurol* 47:173–180.

49. Cacciarelli AA (1977): Posterior widening of the S1–S2 interspace in children: a normal variant of sacral development. *Am J Roentgenol* 129:305–307.

50. Campos-Ortega JA (1983): Topological specificity of phenotypic expression of neurogenic mutations of *Drosophila. Arch Dev Biol* 192: 317–326.

51. Campos-Ortega JA, Knust E (1990): Molecular analysis of a cellular decision during embryonic development of *Drosophila melanogaster:* epidermogenesis or neurogenesis. *Eur J Biochem* 190:1–10.

52. Canadell J, Bequiristain JL (1979): Experimental scoliosis by epiphysiodesis of the neurocentral cartilage in pigs. *J Bone Joint Surg Br* 61: 121.

53. Canning DR, Stern CD (1988): Changes in the expression of the carbohydrate epitope HNK-1 associated with mesoderm induction in the chick embryo. *Development* 104:643–655.

54. Carpenter EM, Hollyday M (1986): Defective innervation of chick limbs in the absence of presumptive Schwann cells. *Soc Neurosci Abstr* 12:1210.

55. Carter CO (1974): Clues to the aetiology of neural tube malformation [abstract]. *Dev Med Child Neurol* 16(Suppl 3):3–15. Abstract 1210.

56. Carter DR, Orr TE, Fyhrie DP, Schurman DJ (1987): Influences of mechanical stress on prenatal and postnatal skeletal development. *Clin Orthop* 219:237–250.

57. Carter DR, Wong M, Orr TE (1991): Musculoskeletal ontogeny, phylogeny, and functional adaptation. NASA symposium: Influence of gravity and activity on muscle and bone. *J Biomech* 24[Suppl 1]: 3–16.

58. Cattell JS, Filtzer DL (1965): Pseudosubluxation and other normal variations in the cervical spine in children. *J Bone Joint Surg Am* 47: 1295–1309.

59. Cave AJE (1975): The morphology of the mammalian cervical pleurapophysis. *J Zool* 177:377–393.

60. Chamay A, Tschantz P (1972): Mechanical influences in bone remodeling: experimental research on Wolff's law. *J Biomech* 5:173.

61. Chandraraj S, Briggs CA (1991): Multiple growth cartilages in the neural arch. *Anat Rec* 230:114–120.

62. Chernoff GF, Lyons KL (1983): Malformations in structural development. *Semin Perinatol* 7:244–246.

63. Chevallier A, Kieny M (1982): On the role of the connective tissue in the patterning of the chick limb musculature. *Arch Dev Biol* 191: 227–280.

64. Chevallier A, Kieny M, Mauger A (1977): Limb-somite relationships: origin of the limb musculature. *J Embryol Exp Morphol* 41:245–258.

65. Cohen AM, Hay ED (1971): Secretion of collagen by embryonic neuroepithelium at the time of spinal cord–somite interaction. *Dev Biol* 26:578–605.

66. Cohen J, Currarino G, Neuhauser EBD (1956): A significant variant in the ossification centers of the vertebral bodies. *Am J Roentgenol* 76: 469–475.

67. Cohen J, Sledge CB (1960): Diastematomyelia: an embryological interpretation with report of a case. *Am J Dis Child* 100:257–263.

68. Crock HV, Yoshizawa H (1977): *The blood supply of the vertebral column and spinal cord in man.* New York: Springer-Verlag.

69. Crock HV, Yoshizawa H, Karne SK (1973): Observation on the venous drainage of the human vertebral body. *J Bone Joint Surg Br* 55: 528–533.

70. Crossin KL, Prieto AL, Hoffman S, et al. (1990): Expression of adhesion molecules and the establishment of boundaries during embryonic and neural development. *Exp Neurol* 109:6–18.

71. Davidson D, Graham E, Sime C, et al. (1988): A gene with sequence similarity to *Drosophila engrailed* is expressed during the development of the neural tube and vertebrae in the mouse. *Development* 104: 305–316.

72. Davidson RG (1988): Atlantoaxial instability in individuals with Down's syndrome: a fresh look at the evidence. *Pediatrics* 81: 857–865.

73. Davies AM (1987): Molecular and cellular aspects of patterning sensory neuron connections in the vertebrate nervous system. *Development* 101:185–208.

74. Davies JA, Cook GMW, Stern CD, et al. (1990): Isolation from chick somites of a glycoprotein fraction that causes collapse of dorsal root ganglion growth cones. *Neuron* 4:11–20.

75. Decker C, Greggs R, Duggan K, et al. (1984): Adhesive multiplicity in the interaction of embryonic fibroblasts and myoblast with extracellular matrices. *J Cell Biol* 99:1398–1404.

76. DeRobertis EM, Gurdon JB (1979): Gene transplantation and the analysis of development. *Sci Am* 241:74–82.

77. DeRobertis EM, Oliver G, Wright CVE (1990): Homeobox genes and the vertebrate body plan. *Sci Am* 263:46–52.

78. DeSalis J, Beguiristain JL, Cañadell J (1991): Disorders of the vertebral blood supply. In: *Idiopathic scoliosis update.* Pamplona, Spain: University Press.

79. Detwiler SR (1934): An experimental study of spinal nerve segmentation in *Amblystoma* with reference to the plurisegmental contribution to the branchial plexus. *J Exp Zool* 67:395–441.

80. Detwiler SR, Holtzer H (1954): The inductive and formative influence of the spinal cord upon the vertebral column. *Bull Hosp Jt Dis* 15:114–123.

81. Deutsch U, Dressler GR, Gruss P (1988): *Pax 1,* a member of a paired box homologous murine gene family, is expressed in segmented structures during development. *Cell* 53:617–625.

82. Dias M, Lance-Jones C (1987): A possible role for somatopleural tissue in specific motoneuron guidance in the embryonic chick hindlimb [abstract]. *Soc Neurosci Abstr* 13:468. Abstract 468.

83. Dodd J, Jessell TM (1988): Axon guidance and the patterning of neuronal projections in vertebrates. *Science* 242:692–699.

84. Dolle P, Duboule D (1989): Two gene members of the murine HOX-5 complex show regional and cell-type specific expression in developing limbs and gonads. *EMBO J* 8:1507–1515.

85. Drvaric DM, Ruderman RJ, Conrad RW, et al. (1987): Congenital scoliosis and urinary tract abnormalities: are intravenous pyelograms necessary? *J Pediatr Orthop* 7:441–443.

86. Duboule D, Boncinelli E, DeRobertis E, et al. (1990): An update of mouse and human HOX gene nomenclature. *Genomics* 7:458–459.

87. Duboule D, Haenlin M, Galliot B, et al. (1987): DNA sequencing homologous to the Drosophila opa repeat are present in murine

mRNAs that are differentially expressed in fetuses and adult tissues. *Mol Cell Biol* 7:2003–2006.

88. Dunn LC, Gluecksohn-Schoenheimer S, Bryson V (1940): A new mutation in the mouse affecting spinal column and urogenital system. *J Hered* 31:343–348.

89. Dunn PM (1976): Congenital postural deformities. *Br Med Bull* 32:71–76.

90. Edelman GM (1976): Surface modulation in cell recognition and cell growth. *Science* 192:218–226.

91. Edelman GM (1986): Cell adhesion molecules in the regulation of animal form and tissue pattern. *Annu Rev Cell Biol* 2:81–116.

92. Edelman GM (1992): Morphoregulation. *Dev Dyn* 193:2–10.

93. Edelman GM, Thiery JP, eds. (1985): *The cell in contact: adhesions and junctions as morphogenetic determinants.* New York: John Wiley and Sons.

94. Ehrenhaft JL (1943): Development of the vertebral column as related to certain congenital and pathological changes. *Surg Gynecol Obstet* 76:282–292.

95. Ellender G, Feik SA, Carach BJ (1988): Periosteal structure and development in a rat caudal vertebra. *J Anat* 158:173–187.

96. Elliot GB, Tredwell SJ, Elliot KA (1970): The notochord as an abnormal organizer in production of congenital intestinal defect. *Am J Roentgenol* 110:628–634.

97. Epstein JA, Carras R, Epstein BS, et al. (1970): Myelopathy in cervical spondylosis with vertebral subluxation and hyperlordosis. *J Neurosurg* 32:421–426.

98. Erickson CA (1986): Morphogenesis of the neural crest. In: Browder L, ed. *Developmental biology: a comprehensive synthesis.* New York: Plenum Press, pp. 481–543.

99. Erickson CA (1987): Behavior of neural crest cells on embryonic basal lamina. *Dev Biol* 120:38–49.

100. Ettensohn CA (1990): The regulation of primary mesenchyme cell patterning. *Dev Biol* 140:261–271.

101. Everaert S, Espeel M, Bortier H, et al. (1988): Connecting cords and morphogenetic movements in the quail blastoderm. *Anat Embryol (Berlin)* 177:311–316.

102. Eyal-Giladi H (1984): The gradual establishment of cell commitments during the early stages of chick development. *Cell Differ* 14:245–255.

103. Eyal-Giladi H, Khaner O (1989): The chick's marginal zone and the primitive streak formation, II: quantification of the marginal zone's potencies—temporal and spatial aspects. *Dev Biol* 134:215–221.

104. Fallon JR, Nitkin RM, Reist NE, et al. (1985): Acetylcholine receptor aggregating factor is similar to molecules concentrated at neuromuscular junctions. *Nature* 315:571–574.

105. Ferguson BA (1983): Development of motor innervation of the chick following dorso-ventral limb bud rotations. *J Neurosci* 3:1760–1772.

106. Ferguson WR (1950): Some observations on the circulation in fetal and infant spines. *J Bone Joint Surg Am* 32:640–648.

107. Fernandez Caso M, DePaz P, Fernandez Alvarez JG, et al. (1992): Delamination of neuroepithelium and non-neural ectoderm and its relation to the convergence step in chick neuralization. *J Anat* 180:143–153.

108. Fielding JW (1965): Disappearance of the central portion of the odontoid process: a case report. *J Bone Joint Surg Am* 47:1228–1230.

109. Fielding JW, Griffin PO (1974): Os odontoideum: an acquired lesion. *J Bone Joint Surg Am* 56:187–190.

110. Fisher L, Neidhardt JH, Gerentes R, et al. (1969): Structure macroscopique de l'apophyse odontoide d'apres l'etude anatomoradiologique. *Lyon Med* 34:433–436.

111. Fontaine J, LeDouarin NM (1977): Analysis of endoderm formation in the avian blastoderm by the use of quail-chick chimaeras. *J Embryol Exp Morphol* 41:209–222.

112. Ford DM, McFadden KD, Bagnall KM (1982): Sequence of ossification in human vertebral neural arch centers. *Anat Rec* 203:175–178.

113. Fowler I, Watterson R (1953): The role of the neural tube in development of the axial skeleton of the chick. *Anat Rec* 117:555–556.

114. Fraser RC (1960): Somite genesis in the chick, III: the role of induction. *J Exp Zool* 145:151–167.

115. Fraser S, Keynes R, Lumsden A (1990): Segmentation in the chick embryo hindbrain is defined by cell lineage restrictions. *Nature* 344:431–435.

116. Fuhr G, Richter E, Zimmerman H, et al. (1998). Cell traces: footprints of individual cells during locomotion and adhesion. *Biol Chem* 379:1161–1173.

117. Gadow HF (1933): *The evolution of the vertebral column.* Cambridge, UK: University Press.

118. Gadow HF, Abott EC (1895): On the evolution of the vertebral column of fishes. *Philos Trans R Soc Lond Biol Sci* 186:163–221.

119. Galliott R, Dolle P, Vigneron M, et al. (1989): The mouse Hox-1.4 gene: primary structure, evidence for promoter activity and expression during development. *Development* 107:343–359.

120. Ganey TM, Love SM, Ogden JA, et al. (1992): Development of vascularization in the chondroepiphysis of the rabbit. *J Orthop Res* 10:496–510.

121. Gasser RF (1979): Evidence that sclerotomal cells do not migrate medially during embryonic development of the rat. *Am J Anat* 154:509–523.

122. Gatchalian CL, Schachner M, Sanes JR (1989): Fibroblasts that proliferate near denervated synaptic sites in skeletal muscle synthesize the adhesive molecules tenascin (J1), N-CAM, fibronectin, and heparan sulfate proteoglycan. *J Cell Biol* 108:1873–1890.

123. Gaunt SJ, Krumlauf R, Duboule D (1989): Mouse homeo-genes within a subfamily Hox-1.4, -2.6, and 5.1 display similar anteroposterior domains of expression in the embryo, but show stage- and tissue-dependent differences in their regulation. *Development* 107:131–141.

124. Gaunt SJ, Sharpe PT, Duboule D (1988): Spatially restricted domains of homeo-gene transcripts in mouse embryos: relation to a segmented body plan. *Development* 104:169–180.

125. Geduspan JS, MacCabe JA (1989): Transfer of dorsoventral information from mesoderm to ectoderm at the onset of limb development. *Anat Rec* 224:79–87.

126. Gehring WJ (1985): The molecular basis of development. *Sci Am* 253:153–162.

127. Gehring WJ (1987): Homeoboxes in the study of development. *Science* 236:1245–1252.

128. Gospodarowicz D (1990): Fibroblast growth factor: chemical structure and biologic function. *Clin Orthop* 257:231–248.

129. Gray ML, Pizzanelli AM, Grodzinsky AJ, et al. (1988): Mechanical and physicochemical determinants of the chondrocyte biosynthetic response. *J Orthop Res* 6:777–792.

130. Gray SW, Romaine CB, Skandalakis JE (1964): Congenital fusion of the cervical vertebrae. *Surg Gynecol Obstet* 118:373–385.

131. Grobstein, Holtzer C (1955): In vitro studies of cartilage induction in mouse somite mesoderm. *J Exp Zool* 128:333–357.

132. Grumet M, Hoffman S, Crossin KL, et al. (1985): Cytotactin, an extracellular matrix protein of neural and non-neural tissues that mediates glia-neuron interactions. *Proc Natl Acad Sci USA* 82:8075–8079.

133. Gruneberg H (1963): *The pathology of development: a study of inherited skeletal disorders in animals.* New York: John Wiley and Sons.

134. Guida G, Cigala F, Riccio V (1969): The vascularization of the vertebral body in the human fetus at term. *Clin Orthop* 65:229–234.

135. Gunderson CH, Greenspan RH, Glaser GH, et al. (1967): Klippel-Feil syndrome: genetic and clinical reevaluation of cervical fusion. *Medicine* 46:491–512.

136. Gwinn JL, Smith JL (1962): Acquired and congenital absence of the odontoid process. *Am J Roentgenol* 88:424–431.

137. Hall BK (1970): Cellular differentiation in skeletal tissue. *Biol Rev Camb Philos Soc* 45:455–484.

138. Hall BK (1971): Histogenesis and morphogenesis of bone. *Clin Orthop* 74:249–268.

139. Hall BK (1972): Immobilization and cartilage transformation into bone in the embryonic chick. *Anat Rec* 173:391–404.

140. Hall BK (1987): Earliest evidence of cartilage and bone development in embryonic life. *Clin Orthop* 225:255–272.

141. Hall BK (1988): The embryonic development of bone. *Am Sci* 76:174–181.

142. Hall JE (1985): Congenital scoliosis. In: Bradford DS, Hensinger RM, eds. *The pediatric spine.* New York: Thieme Medical Publishers. 181–195.

143. Ham RG, Veomett MJ (1980): Cell death and elimination of unneeded tissues. In: *Mechanisms of development.* St. Louis: Mosby.

144. Hamburger V, Oppenheim RW (1982): Naturally occurring neuronal death in vertebrates. *Neurosci Comment* 1:39–55.

145. Hamburger V, Yip JW (1984): Reduction of experimentally induced neuronal death in spinal ganglia of the chick embryo by nerve growth factor. *J Neurosci* 1:60–71.

146. Harrisson F (1990): The extracellular matrix and cell surface, mediators of cell interactions in chicken gastrulation. *Int J Dev Biol* 33: 407–428.

147. Harrisson F, Andries L, Vakaet L (1988): The chicken blastoderm: current views on cell biological events guiding intercellular communication. *Cell Differ* 22:83–106.

148. Harrisson F, Callebaut M, Vakaet L (1991): Features of polyingression and primitive streak ingression through the basal lamina in the chicken blastoderm. *Anat Rec* 229:369–383.

149. Harrisson F, Vanroelen C, Vakaet L (1985): Fibronectin and its relation to the basal lamina and to the cell surface in the chicken blastoderm. *Cell Tissue Res* 241:391–397.

150. Hawkins RJ, Fielding JW, Thompson WJ (1976): Os odontoideum: congenital or acquired—a case report. *J Bone Joint Surg Am* 58: 413–414.

151. Hensinger RN (1986): Osseous anomalies of the craniovertebral junction. *Spine* 11:323–333.

152. Hensinger RN (1991): Congenital anomalies of the cervical spine. *Clin Orthop* 264:16–38.

153. Hensinger RN, Lang JR, MacEwen GD (1974): The Klippel-Feil syndrome: a constellation of related anomalies. *J Bone Joint Surg Am* 56:1246–1253.

154. Hinck VC, Clark WM, Hopkins CE (1966): Normal interpediculate distances (minimum and maximum) in children and adults. *Am J Roentgenol* 97:141–153.

155. Hinck VC, Hopkins CE, Clark WM (1966): Sagittal diameter of the lumbar spinal canal in children and adults. *Radiology* 85:929–937.

156. Hindman BW, Poole CA (1970): Early appearance of the secondary vertebral ossification centers. *Radiology* 95:359–361.

157. Holland PWH (1989): Pursuing the functions of vertebrate homeobox genes: progress and aspects. *Trends Neurosci* 12:206–209.

158. Hollyday M (1980): Organization of motor pools in the chick lateral motor column. *J Comp Neurol* 194:143–170.

159. Holtzer H (1951): Morphogenetic influence of the spinal cord on the axial skeleton and musculature. *Anat Rec* 109:113–114.

160. Holtzer H (1952): An experimental study of the development of the spinal column, II: the dispensibility of the notochord. *J Exp Zool* 121: 573–592.

161. Holtzer H, Biehl J, Payette R, et al. (1982): TI cell diversification: differing roles of cell lineages and cell to cell interactions. *Prog Clin Biol Res* 110[Part B]:271–280.

162. Holtzer H, Detwiler S (1953): An experimental study of the development of the spinal cord, III: induction of skeletogenous cells. *J Exp Zool* 123:335–370.

163. Horstadius S (1950): *The neural crest.* London, UK: Oxford University Press.

164. Hunter DD, Shah V, Merlie JP, et al. (1989): A laminin-like adhesive protein concentrated in the synaptic cleft of the neuromuscular junction. *Nature* 33:229–234.

165. Illingworth RS (1956): Attacks of unconsciousness in association with fused cervical vertebrae. *Arch Dis Child* 31:8–11.

166. Ingham PW (1988): The molecular genetics of embryonic pattern formation in *Drosophila. Nature* 335:25–34.

167. Jacob M, Christ B, Jacob HJ (1979): The migration of myogenic cells from the somites into the leg region of avian embryos. *Anat Embryol (Berl)* 157:291–309.

168. Jacobson AJ, Oster GF, Odell GM, et al. (1986): Neurulation and the cortical tractor model for epithelial folding. *J Embryol Exp Morphol* 96:19–49.

169. Jaffredo T, Horwitz AF, Buck CA, et al. (1988): Myoblast migration specifically inhibited in the chick embryo by grafted CSAT hybridoma cells secreting an anti-integrin antibody. *Development* 103:431–446.

170. Jessell TM, Bovolenta P, Placzek M, et al. (1989): Polarity and patterning in the neural tube: the origin and function of the floor plate. *Ciba Found Symp* 144:255–276.

171. Johansen KM, Fehon RG, Artavanis-Tsakonas S (1989): The Notch gene product is a glycoprotein expressed on the cell surface of both epidermal and neuronal precursor cells during *Drosophila* development. *J Cell Biol* 109:2427–2440.

172. Johnson DR (1968): Reduced articular processes of thoracic vertebrae, a "minor skeletal variant" in the mouse. *J Anat* 102:311–320.

173. Jones MC (1983): Intrinsic versus extrinsically derived deformational defects: a clinical approach. *Semin Perinatol* 7:247–249.

174. Kaplan FS, Tabas JA, Zasloff MA (1990): Fibrodysplasia ossificans progressiva: a clue from the fly? *Calcif Tissue Int* 47:117–125.

175. Karfunkel P (1974): The mechanisms of neural tube formation. *Int Rev Cytol* 38:245–271.

176. Karfunkel P, Hoffman M, Phillips M, et al. (1978): Changes in cell adhesiveness in neurulation and optic cup formation. *Zoon* 6:23–31.

177. Keane RW, Mehta PP, Rose B, et al. (1988): Neural differentiation, NCAM-mediated adhesion, and gap junctional communication in neuroectoderm: a study in vitro. *J Cell Biol* 106:1307–1319.

178. Kenny Mobbs T (1985): Myogenic differentiation in early chick wing mesenchyme in the absence of the brachial somites. *J Embryol Exp Morphol* 90:415–436.

179. Kessel M, Balling R, Gruss P (1990): Variations of cervical vertebrae after expression of a Hox 1.1 transgene in mice. *Cell* 61:301–308.

180. Keynes RJ (1987): Schwann cells during neural development and regeneration: leaders or followers? *Trends Neurosci* 10:137–139.

181. Keynes RJ, Stern CD (1984): Segmentation in the vertebrate nervous systems. *Nature* 310:786–789.

182. Keynes RJ, Stern CD (1985): Segmentation and neural development in vertebrates. *Trends Neurosci* 8:220–223.

183. Keynes RJ, Stirling RV, Stern CD, et al. (1987): The specificity of motor innervation of the chick wing does not depend upon the segmental origin of muscles. *Development* 99:565–575.

184. Khaner O, Eyal-Giladi H (1989): The chick's marginal zone and primitive streak formation, I: coordinative effect of induction and inhibition. *Dev Biol* 134:206–214.

185. Kimelman D, Kirschner M (1987): Synergistic induction of mesoderm by FGF and TGF-beta and the early identification of an mRNA coding for FGF in the early *Xenopus* embryo. *Cell* 51:869–877.

186. Klambt C, Knust E, Tietze K, et al. (1989): Closely related transcripts encoded by the neurogenic gene complex: *Enhancer of split* of *Drosophila melanogaster. EMBO J* 8:203–210.

187. Klein-Nulend J, Veldhuijzen JP, Van de Stadt RJ, et al. (1987): Influence of intermittent compressive force on proteoglycan content of calcifying growth plate cartilage in vitro. *J Biol Chem* 262:15490–15495.

188. Klippel M, Feil A (1912): Un cas d'absence des vertebres cervicales avec cage thoracique remontant jusqu'a la base du crane. *Nouv Icon Salpetriere* 25:223–250.

189. Knust E, Tietze K, Campos-Ortega JA (1987): Molecular analysis of the neurogenic locus *Enhancer of split* of *Drosophila melanogaster. EMBO J* 6:4113–4123.

190. Knutsson F (1961): Growth and differentiation of the postnatal vertebrae. *Acta Radiol* 55:401–408.

191. Knutsson F (1963): A contribution to the discussion of the biological cause of ideopathic scoliosis. *Acta Orthop Scand* 33:98–104.

192. Koop SE, Winter RB, Lonstein JE (1984): The surgical treatment of instability of the upper part of the cervical spine in children and adolescents. *J Bone Joint Surg Am* 66:403–411.

193. Kopczynski CC, Muskavitch MAT (1989): Complex spatiotemporal accumulation of alternative transcripts from the neurogenic gene *Delta* during *Drosophila* embryogenesis. *Development* 107:623–636.

194. Kosher RA, Lash JW (1975): Notochordal stimulation of in vitro somite chondrogenesis before and after enzymatic removal of perinotochordal materials. *Dev Biol* 42:362–378.

195. Kucera P, Monnet-Tschudi F (1987): Early functional differentiation in the chick embryonic disc: interaction between mechanical activity and extracellular matrix. *J Cell Sci* 8:415–431.

196. Kulkarni MV, Williams JC, Yeakley JW, et al. (1987): Magnetic

resonance imaging in the diagnosis of the cranio-cervical manifestations of the mucopolysaccharidoses. *Magn Reson Imaging* 5:317–323.

197. LaBonne SG, Sunitha I, Mahowald AP (1989): Molecular genetics of *pecanex*, a maternal-effect neurogenic locus of *Drosophila melanogaster* that potentially encodes a large transmembrane protein. *Dev Biol* 136:1–16.

198. Laing NG (1982): Abnormal development of vertebrae in paralyzed chick embryos. *J Morphol* 173:179–184.

199. Lallier T, Bronner-Fraser M (1988): A spatial and temporal analysis of dorsal root and sympathetic ganglion formation in the avian embryo. *Dev Biol* 127:99–112.

200. Lance-Jones C (1988): The somitic level of origin of embryonic chick hind limb muscles. *Dev Biol* 126:394–407.

201. Lance-Jones C (1988): The effect of somite manipulation on the development of motoneuron projection patterns in the embryonic chick hindlimb. *Dev Biol* 126:408–419.

202. Lance-Jones C, Landmesser LT (1980): Motoneurone projection patterns in the chick hindlimb following early spinal cord deletions. *J Physiol (Lond)* 302:559–580.

203. Lance-Jones C, Landmesser LT (1980): Motoneurone projection patterns in the chick hind limb following early partial spinal cord reversals. *J Physiol (Lond)* 302:581–602.

204. Lance-Jones C, Landmesser LT (1981): Pathway selection by chick lumbosacral motoneurons during normal development. *Proc R Soc Lond B Biol Sci* 214:1–18.

205. Lance–Jones C, Landmesser LT (1981): Pathway selection by embryonic chick motoneurons in an experimentally altered environment. *Proc R Soc Lond B Biol Sci* 214:19–52.

206. Lance-Jones C, Yip JW (1988): The effect of neural crest deletions on the development of specific motoneuron projections in the embryonic chick [abstract]. *Soc Neurosci Abstr* 14:468.

207. Landmesser LT (1978): The distribution of motoneurons supplying chick hind limb muscles. *J Physiol (Lond)* 284:371–389.

208. Landmesser LT, Honig MG (1986): Altered sensory projections in the chick hindlimb following the early removal of motoneurons. *Dev Biol* 118:511–531.

209. Landmesser LT, O'Donovan MJ (1984): The activation patterns of embryonic chick motoneurones projecting to inappropriate muscles. *J Physiol (Lond)* 347:205–224.

210. Lash JW, Linask KK, Yamada KM (1987): Synthetic peptides that mimic the adhesive recognition signal of fibronectin: differential effects on cell-cell and cell-substatum adhesion in embryonic chick cells. *Dev Biol* 123:411–420.

211. Lawson JP, Ogden JA, Bucholz RW, et al. (1987): Physeal (end-plate) injuries of the cervical spine. *J Pediatr Orthop* 7:428–435.

212. Layer P, Alber R, Rathjen F (1988): Sequential activation of butyrylcholinesterase in rostral half somites and acetylcholinesterase in motoneurones and myotomes preceding growth of motor axons. *Development* 102:387–396.

213. LeDouarin NM (1982): *The neural crest.* New York: Cambridge University Press.

214. Lewis J, Al-Ghaith L, Swanson G, et al. (1983): The control of axon outgrowth in the developing chick wing. In: Fallon JF, Caplan AI, eds. *Limb development and regeneration.* New York: Alan R. Liss, pp. 195–205.

215. Lewis J, Chevallier A, Kieny M, et al. (1981): Muscle nerve branches do not develop in chick wings devoid of muscle. *J Embryol Exp Morphol* 64:211–232.

216. Light TR, McKinistry MP, Schnitzer J, et al. (1984): Bone blood flow: regional variation with skeletal maturation. In: Arlet J, Ficat RP, Hungerford DS, eds. *Bone circulation.* Baltimore: Williams & Wilkins pp. 178–185.

217. Light TR, Ogden JA (1981): The longitudinal epiphyseal bracket: implications for surgical correction. *J Pediatr Orthop* 1:299–305.

218. Linsenmayer TF, Gibney E, Schmid TM (1986): Segmental appearance of type X collagen in the developing avian notochord. *Dev Biol* 113:467–473.

219. Lipson SJ (1977): Dysplasia of the odontoid process in Morquio's syndrome causing quadraparesis. *J Bone Joint Surg Am* 59:340–344.

220. Lipton BH, Jacobson AG (1974): Analysis of normal somite development. *Dev Biol* 38:73–90.

221. Lipton BH, Jacobson AG (1974): Experimental analysis of the mechanisms of somite morphogenesis. *Dev Biol* 38:91–103.

222. Locke GR, Gardner JI, Van Epps EF (1966): Atlas-dens interval in children. *Am J Roentgenol* 97:135–140.

223. Loring JF, Erickson CA (1987): Neural crest cell migratory pathways in the trunk of the chick embryo. *Dev Biol* 121:220–236.

224. Love JM, Tuan RS (1992): Pair-rule genes are expressed during embryonic somite formation [abstract]. *Trans Orthop Res Soc* 17:640.

225. Lumsden A, Keynes R (1989): Segmental patterns of neuronal development in the chick hindbrain. *Nature* 337:424–429.

226. Lutter LD, Langer LO (1977): Neurological symptoms in achondroplastic dwarfs: surgical treatment. *J Bone Joint Surg Am* 59:87–92.

227. Mackie EJ, Tucker RP, Halfter W, et al. (1988): The distribution of tenascin coincides with pathways of neural crest cell migration. *Development* 102:237–250.

228. Marin-Padilla M (1966): Study of the vertebral column in human craniorhachischisis. *Acta Anat (Basel)* 63:32–48.

229. Marin-Padilla M (1979): Notochord-basichondrocranium relationships: abnormalities in experimental axial skeletal (dysraphic) disorders. *J Embryol Exp Morphol* 153:15–38.

230. Martins-Green M (1988): Origin of the dorsal surface of the neural tube by progressive delamination of epidermal ectoderm and neuropithelium: implications for neurulation and neural tube defects. *Development* 103:687–706.

231. Martins-Green M, Erickson CA (1986): Development of neural tube basal lamina during neurulation and neural cell crest migration in the trunk of the mouse embryo. *J Embryol Exp Morphol* 98:219–236.

232. Marusich MF, Weston JA (1992): Identification of early neurogenic cells in the neural crest lineage. *Dev Biol* 149:295–306.

233. Mavilio F, Simeone A, Giampaolo A, et al. (1986): Differential and stage-related expression in embryonic tissues of a new human homeobox gene. *Nature* 324:664–668.

234. Maxwell GD, Forbes ME, Christie DS (1988): Analysis of the development of cellular subsets present in the neural crest using cell sorting and cell cultures. *Neuron* 1:557–568.

235. McEnery G, Borzyskowski M, Cox TCS, et al. (1992): The spinal cord in neurologically stable spina bifida: a clinical and MRI study. *Dev Med Child Neurol* 34:342–347.

236. Melton DA, Ruii-Altaba A, Visraeli J, (1989): Localization of mRNA and axis formation during *Xenopus* embryogenesis. *Ciba Found Symp* 144:16–36,92–98.

237. Mendelson B, Frank E (1990): The time of origin of brachial sensory neurons is not correlated with neuronal phenotype. *J Comp Neurol* 300:1–11.

238. Mendez-Otero R, Schlosshauer B, Barnstable C, et al. (1988): A developmentally regulated antigen associated with neural cell and process migration. *J Neurosci* 8:564–579.

239. Michie I, Clark M (1968): Neurological syndromes associated with cervical and craniocervical anomalies. *Arch Neurol* 18:241–247.

240. Minderhoud JM, Braakman R, Penning L (1969): Os odontoidium: clinical, radiological, and therapeutic aspects. *J Neurol Sci* 8:521–544.

241. Mitrani E (1982): Primitive streak-forming cells of the chick invaginate through a basement membrane. *Rouxs Arch Dev Biol* 191:320–324.

242. Morriss GM, Solursh M (1978): The role of primary mesenchyme in normal and abnormal morphogenesis of mammalian neural folds. *Zoon* 6:33–38.

243. Morriss-Kay GM, Tan SS (1987): Mapping cranial neural crest cell migration pathways in mammalian embryos. *Trends Genet* 3:257–261.

244. Muller F, O'Rahilly R (1991): Development of anencephaly and its variants. *Am J Roentgenol* 190:193–218.

245. Murray JD, Maini PK, Tranquillo RT (1988): Mechanochemical models for generating biological pattern and form in development. *Phys Rep* 171:59–84.

246. Mutch J, Walmsley R (1956): The aetiology of cleft vertebral arch in spondylolisthesis. *Lancet* 1:74–77.

247. Nachemson AL, Sahlstrand T (1977): Etiologic factors in adolescent idiopathic scoliosis. *Spine* 2:176–184.

248. Nagele RG, Bush KT, Lynch FJ, et al. (1991): A morphometric and computer-assisted three-dimensional reconstruction study of neural tube formation in chick embryos. *Anat Rec* 231:425–436.

249. Nakamura H (1990): Do CNS anlagen have plasticity in differentiation? Analysis in quail-chick chimera. *Brain Res* 511:122–128.

250. Nardi JB (1981): Epithelial invagination: adhesive properties of cells can govern position and directionality of epithelial folding. *Differentiation* 20:97–103.

251. Newgreen DF, Scheel M, Kastner V (1986): Morphogenesis of sclerotome and neural crest in avian embryos: in vivo and in vitro studies on the role of notochordal extracellular matrix. *Cell Tissue Res* 244:299–313.

252. Nieuwkoop PD, Johnsen AG, Albers B (1985): *The epigenetic nature of early chordate development: inductive interaction and competence.* Cambridge, UK: Cambridge University Press.

253. Noakes PJ, Bennett MR (1987): Growth of axons into developing muscles of the chick forelimb is preceded by cells that stain with Schwann cell antibodies. *J Comp Neurol* 259:330–347.

254. Noakes PG, Bennett MR, Stratford J (1988): Migration of Schwann cells and axons into developing chick forelimb muscles following removal of either the neural tube or the neural crest. *J Comp Neurol* 277:214–233.

255. Norris WE, Stern CD, Keynes RJ (1989): Molecular differences between the rostral and caudal halves of the sclerotome in the chick embryo. *Development* 105:541–548.

256. O'Brien MK, Oppenheim RW (1990): Development and survival of thoracic motoneurons and hindlimb musculature following transplantation of the thoracic neural tube to the lumbar region in the chick embryo: anatomical aspects. *J Neurobiol* 21:313–340.

257. Ogden JA (1984): Radiology of postnatal skeletal development, IX: proximal tibia and fibula. *Skeletal Radiol* 11:169–292.

258. Ogden JA (1984): Radiology of postnatal skeletal development, XI: the first cervical vertebra. *Skeletal Radiol* 12:12–20.

259. Ogden JA (1984): Radiology of postnatal skeletal development, XII: the second cervical vertebra. *Skeletal Radiol* 12:169–177.

260. Ogden JA (1990): *Skeletal injury in the child,* 2nd ed. Philadelphia: WB Saunders.

261. Ogden JA (1990): Skeletal trauma. In: Grossman M, Dieckmann RA, eds. *Pediatric emergency medicine: a clinician's reference.* Philadelphia: WB Saunders, pp. 288–299.

262. Ogden JA (1991): The uniqueness of growing bones. In: Rockwood CA, Wilkins KE, King RE, eds. *Fractures,* 3rd ed., vol 3. Philadelphia: JB Lippincott.

263. Ogden JA, Conlogue GJ, Barnett JS (1981): Prenatal and postnatal development of the cervical portion of the spine in the short-finned pilot whale *Globicephala macrorhyncha. Anat Rec* 200:83–94.

264. Ogden JA, Conlogue G, Bronson M (1979): Radiology of postnatal skeletal development, II: the manubrium and sternum. *Skeletal Radiol* 4:189–195.

265. Ogden JA, Conlogue G, Phillips S, et al. (1979): Sprengel's deformity: radiology of the pathological deformation. *Skeletal Radiol* 4:204–211.

266. Ogden JA, Ganey TM, Light TR, et al. (1994): Nonepiphyseal ossification and pseudoepiphysis formation. *J Pediatr Orthop* 14:78–82.

267. Ogden JA, Grogan DP (1987): Prenatal skeletal development and growth of the musculoskeletal system. In: Albright JA, Brand RA, eds. *The scientific basis of orthopaedics,* 2nd ed. New York: Appleton & Lange, 47–89.

268. Ogden JA, Grogan DP, Light TR (1987): Postnatal skeletal development and growth of the musculoskeletal system. In: Albright JA, Brand RA, eds. *The scientific basis of orthopaedics,* 2nd ed. New York: Appleton & Lange, 47–89.

269. Oh TH, Markelonis GJ, Dion TL, et al. (1988): A muscle-derived substrate-bound factor that promotes neurite outgrowth from neurons of the central and peripheral nervous systems. *Dev Biol* 127:88–98.

270. O'Rahilly R, Benson DR (1985): The development of the vertebral column. In: Bradford DS, Hensinger RM, eds. *The pediatric spine.* New York: Thieme Medical Publishers.

271. O'Rahilly R, Meyer DB (1979): The timing and sequence of events in the development of the human vertebral column during the embryonic period proper. *Anat Embryol (Berl)* 157:167–176.

272. O'Rahilly R, Muller F, Meyer DB (1980): The human vertebral column at the end of the embryonic period proper, I: the column as a whole. *J Anat* 131:565–575.

273. O'Rahilly R, Muller F, Meyer DB (1983): The human vertebral column at the end of the embryonic period proper, II: the occipitocervical region. *J Anat* 136:181–195.

274. Ostrovsky D, Cheney CM, Seitz AW, et al. (1983): Fibronectin distribution during somitogenesis in the chick embryo. *Cell Differ* 13:217–223.

275. Oxnard CE (1976): Tensile forces in skeletal structures. *J Morphol* 134:425–435.

276. Palacek SP, Schmidt CE, Lauffenberger DA, et al. (1996). Integrin dynamics on the tail region of migrating fibroblasts. *J Cell Sci* 109:941–952.

277. Parkinson D (1991): Human spinal arachnoid septa, trabeculae, and "rogue strands." *Am J Anat* 192:498–509.

278. Peacock A (1951): Observations on the prenatal development of the intervertebral disc in man. *J Anat* 85:260–274.

279. Pettway Z, Guillory G, Bronner-Fraser M (1990): Absence of neural crest cells from the region surrounding implanted notochords in situ. *Dev Biol* 142:335–345.

280. Phelan KA, Hollyday M (1990): Axon guidance in muscleless chick wings: the role of muscle cells in motoneuronal pathway selection and muscle nerve formation. *J Neurosci* 10:2699–2716.

281. Pueschel SM, Scola FH (1987): Atlantoaxial instability in individuals with Down's syndrome: epidemiologic, radiographic, and clinical studies. *Pediatrics* 80:555–560.

282. Rao Y, Jan LY, Jan YN (1990): Similarity of the product of the *Drosophila* neurogenic gene *big brain* to transmembrane channel proteins. *Nature* 345:163–167.

283. Reichmann S, Lewin T (1969): Coronal cleft vertebrae in growing individuals. *Acta Orthop Scand* 40:3–22.

284. Ricciardi JE, Kaufer H, Lous DS (1976): Acquired os odontoideum following acute ligament injury: report of a case. *J Bone Joint Surg Am* 58:410–412.

285. Rickmann M, Fawcett JW, Keynes RJ (1985): The migration of neural crest cells and the growth of motor axons through the rostral half of the chick somite. *J Embryol Exp Morphol* 90:437–455.

286. Ridewood WA, MacBride EW (1921): On the calcification of the vertebral centra in sharks and rays. *Philos Trans R Soc Lond Biol Sci* 210:311–407.

287. Rivard CH, Narbaitz R, Uhthoff HK (1979): Congenital vertebral malformations: time of induction in human and mouse embryo. *Orthop Rev* 8:135–139.

288. Roach JW, Duncan D, Wenger DR, et al. (1984): Atlanto-axial instability and spinal cord compression in children: diagnosis by computerized tomography. *J Bone Joint Surg Am* 66:708–714.

289. Robert B, Sassoon D, Jacq B, et al. (1989): Hox-7, a mouse homeobox gene with a novel pattern of expression during embryogenesis. *EMBO J* 8:91–100.

290. Rockwell H, Evans FG, Pheasant HC, et al. (1938): The comparative morphology of the vertebrate spinal column: its forms as related to function. *J Morphol* 63:87–117.

291. Rolander SD, Blair WE (1975): Deformation and fracture of the lumbar vertebral end plate. *Orthop Clin North Am* 6:75–81.

292. Rönning O, Kylämarkula S (1979): Reactions of transplanted neurocentral synchondroses to different conditions of mechanical stress: a methodological study on the rat. *J Anat* 128:789–801.

293. Rowland LP, Shapiro JH, Jacobson HG (1958): Neurological syndromes associated with congenital absence of the odontoid process. *Arch Neurol Psychiatry* 80:286–291.

294. Ruiz-i-Altaba A, Melton DA (1989): Involvement of the *Xenopus* homeobox gene Xhox 3 in pattern formation along the anteroposterior axis. *Cell* 57:317–326.

295. Ruiz-i-Altaba A, Melton DA (1989): Binodal and graded expression of the *Xenopus* homeobox gene Xhox 3 during embryonic development. *Development* 106:173–183.

296. Ruiz-i-Altaba A, Melton DA (1989): Interaction between peptide growth factors and homeobox genes in the establishment of anteroposterior polarity in frog embryos. *Nature* 341:33–38.

297. Ruiz-i-Altaba A, Melton DA (1990): Axial patterning and the establishment of polarity in the frog embryo. *Trends Genet* 6:57–64.

298. Rushlow CA, Han K, Manley JL, et al. (1989): The graded distribution of the dorsal morphogen is initiated by selective nuclear transport in *Drosophila. Cell* 59:1165–1177.
299. Saidman J (1948): *Diagnostic et traitment des maladies de la collone vertebrate.* Paris: G Doin, pp. 1169–1177.
300. Samuelsson L, Lindell D, Kogler H (1991): Spinal cord and brain stem anomalies in scoliosis. *Acta Orthop Scand* 62:403–406.
301. Sanders EJ (1984): Labelling of basement membrane constituents in the living chick embryo during gastrulation. *J Embryol Exp Morphol* 79:113–123.
302. Sanders EJ, Prasad S (1986): Epithelial and basement membrane responses to chick embryo primitive streak grafts. *Cell Differ* 18: 233–242.
303. Sanders EJ, Prasad S (1989): Invasion of a basement membrane matrix by chick embryo primitive streak cells in vitro. *J Cell Sci* 92:497–504.
304. Schiff DCM, Parke WW (1973): The arterial supply of the odontoid process. *J Bone Joint Surg Am* 55:1450–1456.
305. Schoenwolf GC (1985): Shaping and bending of the avian neuroepithelium: morphometric analyses. *Dev Biol* 109:127–139.
306. Schoenwolf GC (1988): Microsurgical analyses of avian neurulation: separation of medial and lateral tissues. *J Comp Neurol* 276:498–507.
307. Schoenwolf GC (1991): Neurepithelial cell behavior during neurulation. In: Gerhart J, ed. *Cell-cell interactions in early development.* Forty-seventh Symposium of the Society for Developmental Biology. New York: Alan R. Liss.
308. Schoenwolf GC, Bortier H, Vakaet L (1989): Fate mapping the avian neural plate with quail/chick chimeras: origin of prospective median wedge cells. *J Exp Zool* 249:271–278.
309. Seimon LP (1977): Fracture of the odontoid process in young children. *J Bone Joint Surg Am* 59:943–948.
310. Sensenig E (1949): The early development of the human vertebral column. *Contrib Embryol* 33:21–49.
311. Serbedzija G, Bronner-Fraser M, Fraser SE (1989): Vital dye analysis of the timing and pathways of avian trunk neural crest cell migration. *Development* 106:806–816.
312. Smith CL (1990): The critical period for peripheral specification of dorsal root ganglion neurons is related to the period of sensory neurogenesis. *Dev Biol* 142:476–480.
313. Smith CL, Frank E (1987): Peripheral specification of sensory neurons transplanted to novel location along the neuraxis. *J Neurosci* 7: 1537–1549.
314. Smith CL, Frank E (1988): Peripheral specification of sensory connections in the spinal cord. *Brain Behav Evol* 31:227–242.
315. Smith JL, Schoenwolf GC (1987): Cell cycle and neuroepithelial cell shape during bending of the chick neural plate. *Anat Rec* 218: 196–206.
316. Smith JL, Schoenwolf GC (1988): Role of cell-cycle in regulating neuroepithelial cell shape during bending of the chick neural plate. *Cell Tissue Res* 252:491–500.
317. Smith JL, Schoenwolf GC (1989): Notochordal induction of cell wedging in the chick neural plate and its role in neural tube formation. *J Exp Zool* 250:49–62.
318. Smith J, Schoenwolf GC (1990): Mechanisms of neurulation: Traditional viewpoint and recent advances. *Development* 109:243–270.
319. Smoller D, Friedel C, Schmid A, et al. (1990): The *Drosophila* neurogenic locus *mastermind* encodes a nuclear protein unusually rich in amino acid homopolymers. *Genes Dev* 4:1688–1700.
320. Spratt NT Jr (1952): Localization of the prospective neural plate in the early chick blastoderm. *J Exp Zool* 120:109–130.
321. Stabler CL, Eismont FJ, Brown MD, et al. (1985): Failure of posterior cervical fusions using cadaveric bone graft in children. *J Bone Joint Surg Am* 67:370–375.
322. Stirling RV, Summerbell D (1988): Specific guidance of motor axons to duplicated muscles in the developing amniote limb. *Development* 103:97–110.
323. Sullivan RC, Bruwer AJ, Harris L (1958): Hypermobility of the cervical spine in children: a pitfall in the diagnosis of cervical dislocation. *Am J Surg* 95:636–640.
324. Sutterlin CE, Grogan DP, Ogden JA (1987): Diagnosis of developmental pathology of the neuraxis by magnetic resonance imaging. *J Pediatr Orthop* 7:291–297.
325. Swischuk LE, Hayden CK, Sarwar M (1979): The posteriorly tilted dens: a normal variation mimicking a fractured dens. *Pediatr Radiol* 8:27–28.
326. Tabin CJ (1991): Retinoids, homeoboxes, and growth factors: toward molecular models for limb development. *Cell* 66:199–217.
327. Tam PPL (1986): A study of the pattern of prospective somites in the presomitic mesoderm of mouse embryos. *J Embryol Exp Morphol* 92:269–285.
328. Tanaka T, Uhthoff HK (1981): Significance of resegmentation in the pathogenesis of vertebral body malformation. *Acta Orthop Scand* 52: 331–338.
329. Tanaka T, Uhthoff HK (1981): The pathogenesis of congenital vertebral malformations: a study based on observations made in 11 human embryos and fetuses. *Acta Orthop Scand* 52:413–425.
330. Tanaka T, Uhthoff HK (1983): Coronal cleft vertebrae, a variant of normal endochondral ossification. *Acta Orthop Scand* 54:389–395.
331. Taylor JR (1972): Persistence of the notochordal canal in vertebrae. *J Anat* 111:211–217.
332. Taylor JR (1975): Growth of human intervertebral discs and vertebral bodies. *J Anat* 120:49–68.
333. Taylor JR (1978): Genesis of scoliosis. *J Anat* 126:434–435.
334. Taylor JR (1980): Vertebral genesis of scoliosis. *J Anat* 130:197–198.
335. Taylor JR (1983): Scoliosis and growth: patterns of asymmetry in normal vertebral growth. *Acta Orthop Scand* 54:596–602.
336. Teillet MA, Kalcheim C, LeDouarin NM (1987): Formation of the dorsal root ganglia in the avian embryo: segmental origin and migratory behavior of the neural crest progenitor cells. *Dev Biol* 120: 329–347.
337. Theiler K (1988): Vertebral malformations. *Adv Anat Embryol Cell Biol* 112:1–99.
338. Thomas JB, Crews S, Goodman C (1988): Molecular genetics of the single-minded locus: a gene involved in the development of the Drosophila nervous system. *Cell* 52:133–141.
339. Tosney KW (1988): Proximal tissues and patterned neurite outgrowth at the lumbosacral level of the chick embryo: partial and complete deletion of the somite. *Dev Biol* 127:266–286.
340. Trauner DA (1983): Neuromuscular abnormalities as a cause of deformational defects. *Semin Perinatol* 7:250–252.
341. Trelstad RL (1977): Mesenchymal cell polarity and morphogenesis of chick cartilage. *Dev Biol* 59:153–163.
342. Tucker GC, Aoyama H, Lipinski M, et al. (1984): Identical reactivity of monoclonal antibodies HNK-1 and NC-1: conservation in vertebrates on cells derived from the neural primordium and on some leukocytes. *Cell Differ* 14:223–230.
343. Turing A (1952): The chemical basis of morphogenesis. *Philos Trans R Soc Lond Biol Sci* 237:37–72.
344. Vakaet L (1984): The initiation of gastrular ingression in the chick blastoderm. *Am Zool* 24:555–562.
345. Van Limborgh J (1956): The influence of adjacent mesodermal structures upon the shape of the neural tube and neural plate in bird embryos. *Acta Morphol Neerl Scand* 1:155–166.
346. Van Straaten HWM, Hekking JWM, Beursgens JPWM, et al. (1989): Effect of the notochord on proliferation and differentiation in the neural tube of the chick embryo. *Development* 107:793–803.
347. Vassin H, Bremer KA, Knust E, et al. (1987): The neurogenic gene *Delta* of *Drosophila melanogaster* is expressed in neurogenic territories and encodes a putative transmembrane protein with EGF-like repeats. *EMBO J* 6:3431–3440.
348. Verbout AJ (1976): A critical review of the "Neugliederung" concept in relation to the development of the vertebral column. *Acta Biotheor (Leiden)* 25:219–258.
349. Verbout AJ (1985): The development of the vertebral column. *Adv Anat Embryol Cell Biol* 90:1–122.
350. Verwoerd DCA, Van Oostrom CG (1979): Cephalic neural crest and placodes. *Adv Anat Embryol Cell Biol* 58:1–75.
351. Vettiveil S (1991): Vertebral level of the spinal cord in human fetuses. *J Anat* 179:149–161.
352. Vogel KS, Weston JA (1988): A subpopulation of cultured avian neural crest cells has transient neurogenic potential. *Neuron* 1: 569–577.
353. Vogel KS, Weston JA (1990): The sympathoadrenal lineage in avian

embryos, II: effects of glucocorticoids on cultured neural crest cells. *Dev Biol* 139:13–23.

354. Wachtler F, Christ B, Jacob HJ (1982): Grafting experiments on determination and migratory behavior of presomitic, somitic and so-matopleural cells in avian embryos. *Anat Embryol (Berl)* 164: 369–378.

355. Wadia NH (1967): Myelopathy complicating congenital atlantoaxial dislocation: a study of 28 cases. *Brain* 90:449–472.

356. Walicke PA (1988): Basic and acidic fibroblast growth factor have trophic effects on neurons from multiple CNS regions. *J Neurosci* 8: 2618–2626.

357. Watterson RL, Fowler I, Fowler BJ (1954): The role of the neural tube and notochord in development of the axial skeleton of the chick. *Am J Anat* 95:337–399.

358. Watterson RL, Goodheart CL, Lindberg G (1955): The influence of adjacent structures upon the shape of the neural tube and neural plate of chick embryos. *Anat Rec* 122:539–560.

359. Wedden SE, Pang K, Eichele G (1989): Expression pattern of homeo-box containing genes during chick embryogenesis. *Development* 105: 639–650.

360. Weinberger C, Penner PL, Brick I (1984): Polyingression, an impor-tant morphogenetic movement in chick gastrulation. *Am Zool* 24: 545–554.

361. Weston JA (1963): A radioautographic analysis of the migration and localization of trunk neural crest cells in the chick. *Dev Biol* 6: 279–310.

362. Weston JA (1970): The migration and differentiation of neural crest cells. *Adv Morphol* 8:41–114.

363. Wilkinson DG (1989): Homeobox genes and development of the vertebrate CNS. *Bioessays* 10:82–97.

364. Wilkinson DG, Bhatt S, Cook M, et al. (1989): Segmental expression of Hox-2 homeobox-containing genes in the developing mouse hind-brain. *Nature* 341:405–409.

365. Wilkinson DG, Peters G, Dickson C, et al. (1988): Expression of the FGF-related proto-oncogene int-2 during gastrulation and neuru-lation in the mouse. *EMBO J* 7:691–695.

366. Williams LW (1910): The somites of the chick. *Am J Anat* 11:55–100.

367. Willis TA (1931): The separate neural arch. *J Bone Joint Surg* 13: 709–721.

368. Winklbauer R, Nagel M (1991): Directional mesoderm cell migration in the *Xenopus* gastrula. *Dev Biol* 148:573–589.

369. Wollin DG (1963): The os odontoideum: separate odontoid process. *J Bone Joint Surg Am* 45:1459–1471.

370. Wolpert L (1978): Pattern formation in biological development. *Sci Am* 239:154–164.

371. Wong M, Carter DR (1988): Mechanical stress and morphogenetic endochondral ossification of the sternum. *J Bone Joint Surg Am* 70: 992–1000.

372. Wright CV, Cho KWY, Hardwicke J, et al. (1989): Interference with function of a homeobox gene in *Xenopus* embryos produces malforma-tions of the anterior spinal cord. *Cell* 59:81–93.

373. Wright CV, Cho KWY, Oliver G, et al. (1989): Vertebrate homeodo-main proteins: families of region-specific transcription factors. *Trends Biochem Sci* 14:52–56.

374. Yousefzadeh DK, El-Khoury GY, Smith WL (1982): Normal sagittal diameter and variation in the pediatric cervical spine. *Radiology* 144: 319–325.

375. Zanetti NC, Dress VM, Solursch M (1990): Comparison between ectoderm-conditioned medium and fibronectin in their effects on chondrogenesis by limb and mesenchymal cells. *Dev Biol* 139: 383–395.

376. Zanetti NC, Solursh M (1984): Induction of chondrogenesis in limb mesenchymal cultures by disruption of the actin cytoskeleton. *J Cell Biol* 99:115–123.

377. Ziller C, Dupin E, Brazeau P, et al. (1983): Early segregation of a neuronal precursor cell line in the neural crest as revealed by culture in a chemically defined medium. *Cell* 32:627–638.

378. Zimmermann H, Hagedorn R, Richter E, et al. (1999). Topography of cell traces studied by atomic force microscopy. *Eur Biophys J* 28: 516–525.

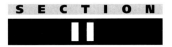

BIOMECHANICS

SPINAL BIOMECHANICS

IAN A. F. STOKES

This chapter surveys the biomechanics of the pediatric spine, especially the relation between forces and movements in the spine and the relation between forces and injury. These principles can be used to gain a better understanding of the spine from the point of view of growth and development, development of deformities, causes of injury to the spine, and the principles used in both conservative and surgical treatment. In describing the relation between forces and motion and between forces and tissue damage, properties of the spine must be described in mechanical terms. The spine can be considered a mechanical system that has geometric properties and tissue material properties. Together these characteristics determine the structural properties. First some basic mechanical concepts are reviewed.

The geometric characteristics of the spine—size, shape, motion, and the direction of forces applied to it—must be defined in three dimensions. This conventionally is done by means of a cartesian coordinate system. A cartesian coordinate system is uniquely defined according to the position of its origin and the direction of at least two of the three axes. The third axis by definition is perpendicular to the other two. Because the spine is flexible and moves, the definition of an axis system is not simple. Depending on the point of view, axes can be defined by reference to landmarks on an individual vertebra, by reference to the end vertebrae of the spine, or by reference to the position of the person's entire body (Fig. 1). The choice of axis system can be quite important, because measurements of spinal deformity and motion differ depending on whether a local, spinal, or global reference is used, if these axes systems are not coincident.

Once an axis system is selected, motion of the spine or motion of vertebrae can be considered as a combination of translations and rotations within this coordinate system. Forces, which produce primarily translation, and torques, which produce primarily rotations, can be considered to have components along and around the same set of axes. Because translations and rotations are fundamentally different, motion of the spine is considered to have six degrees of freedom (three translations and three rotations), and the force system acting on the spine has the same six degrees of freedom (91) (Fig. 2).

To simplify consideration of its biomechanics, the spine is often broken down into mechanical units called *motion segments*

or *functional spinal units.* Each motion segment consists of two vertebrae and all the passive structures (disc, ligaments, joint capsules, and so on) that link these two vertebrae (Fig. 2). The mechanical properties of the motion segment depend on its physical dimensions and proportions and the tissue material properties. Most investigations of properties of motion segments have been performed with aged specimens. How can these results be scaled or otherwise adapted to describe properties of the pediatric spine? During growth, the shape of vertebrae changes substantially. The dimensions of the neural canal approach adult size at an early age (109,143), but the vertebral bodies continue to grow (33). At the same time, there are probably age-related changes in tissue material properties. Because of the complex behavior of biologic tissues, numerous terms including those used in Fig. 3 must be used to describe the response.

STRESS AND STRAIN RELATIONS OF TISSUES

Deformation of tissue in response to applied load usually is displayed by means of a stress-strain graph (Fig. 3). Stress is a standardized measure of applied load in a particular direction (load divided by area of specimen), and strain is a standardized measure of the deformation in a specified direction (elongation divided by original length for direct strain, and shear deformation divided by specimen thickness for shear strain). In a stress-strain curve, numerous tissue characteristics are displayed and can be quantified. The elastic range is the range of deformation from which complete recovery is possible after unloading. Biologic tissues often have an initial region of laxity, an approximately linear elastic range, and a nonlinear elastic range. After the elastic limit, plastic deformation can occur. After a specimen that has been taken into the plastic range is unloaded, a permanent, plastic deformation remains. After the ultimate or maximum stress is passed, failure occurs. All these properties are illustrated in Fig. 3. Time-dependent properties are a function of the history of loading. These properties are illustrated in Fig. 4, which also shows how materials with time-dependent properties can be conveniently visualized and represented by equivalent structures consisting of springs and dampers. An example of time-dependent behavior is the decline in force magnitude in Harrington instrumentation that occurs over a period of hours after the operation (39,93).

I. A. F. Stokes: University of Vermont, Burlington, Vermont 05405.

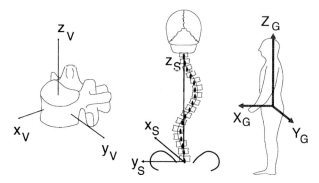

FIGURE 1. *Left to right,* Vertebral, spinal (spine with scoliosis), and global (body) axis systems. When making clinical measurements, such as from plain radiographs or computed tomographic sections, the axis systems should always be specified.

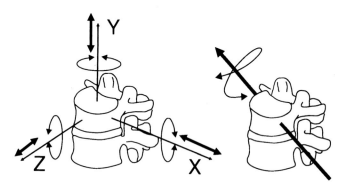

FIGURE 2. A motion segment, which consists of two vertebrae and the structures (disc and ligaments) that connect them, has six degrees of freedom. These produce six distinct components of motion (*left*)—three translations and three rotations. An alternative (*right*) is to express the six components of motion as motion along and around a helical axis. (Adapted from White AA, Panjabi MM (1978): *Clinical biomechanics of the spine.* Philadelphia: JB Lippincott, pp. 122–130, with permission.)

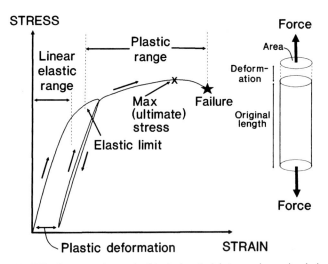

FIGURE 3. Stress-strain graph of typical material. A sample was loaded past its elastic limit, unloaded to demonstrate plastic deformation, and then loaded again to failure. Stress and strain are standardized measures of load and deformation. Representation of load and deformation as stress and strain allows comparison between tissue samples of different sizes.

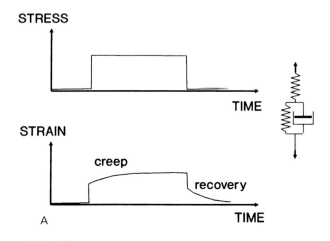

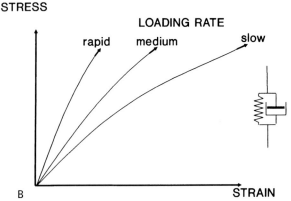

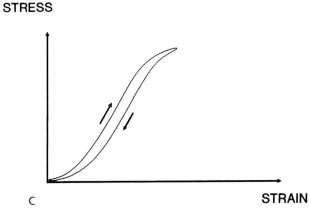

FIGURE 4. Three types of material behavior illustrated by stress and strain response and by equivalent spring and damper systems. **A:** Viscoelastic behavior. A step load produces a gradual increase in deformation, and unloading initiates slow recovery. **B:** Load-rate-dependent behavior. **C:** Hysteresis (unloading path different from loading path). Energy is absorbed in each load-unload cycle.

The acute and time-dependent behavior of the ligaments, vertebrae, discs, and other spinal structures during normal in vivo function, trauma, and treatment is a complex interaction between the tissue material properties and the sizes and shapes of these structures. In the same way as tissue properties can be displayed with a stress-strain graph, a load-deformation graph is used to display structural properties (Fig. 5).

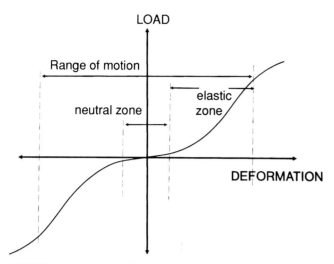

FIGURE 5. Idealized load-deformation behavior of a motion segment for loading along one axis, and the corresponding deformation along that axis. The motion segment displays nonlinear behavior that has been characterized by Panjabi (100) as having an initial region of minimal stiffness (neutral zone) followed by an elastic zone.

LOADING AND DEFORMATION OF THE SPINAL MOTION SEGMENT

The motion segment (Fig. 2) seldom moves in a single direction or even in a single plane. As described earlier, there are six degrees of freedom, but these normally occur in combination. In general, application of a single force or torque does not produce a single translation or rotation and may often produce all six translations and rotations in varying amounts. The tendency of certain degrees of freedom to be associated with each other, especially axial rotation and lateral bending, is called *coupling* (101). This complex mechanical behavior is difficult to visualize. One helpful concept is the instantaneous helical axis of rotation: for any instantaneous increment of motion, one vertebra can be considered rotating about and translating along an axis of rotation that is fixed relative to the other vertebra. If motion is considered planar, the point at which the axis of rotation cuts this plane is the center of rotation. However, the instantaneous axis of rotation is not fixed and depends on the direction of the applied forces and torques and on the position of the motion segment within its range of motion. The deformation of any tissue or structure depends on how far it is from the axis of rotation. Because the axis of rotation usually passes through the intervertebral disc, this minimizes the magnitudes of strains of tissues within the disc.

An experimental determination of the characteristics of the motion segment can be summarized in a load-deformation graph (Fig. 5). These graphs show a nonlinear relation between load and deformation. There typically is a region, called the *neutral zone,* of large deformation for small positive and negative loads (100). This region can be considered a region of laxity and is thought to place the spine at risk for instability. With increasing deformation, stiffness increases (elastic zone). With deformation beyond the elastic zone, damage can occur. Therefore the neutral

zone and the elastic zone together constitute the functional range of motion. Although these characteristics of the motion segment can be defined for cadaver spinal specimens, at present there is no way to determine their properties in vivo.

INJURIES TO THE MOTION SEGMENT

All the components of the motion segment contribute to flexibility and may contribute to ultimate strength, depending on the failure mechanism. This depends on the direction of loading. White and Panjabi (153) introduced the concept of major injuring vector to describe the predominant direction of loading during an injury. This leads to the idea that fractures and other injuries can be classified according to the magnitude and direction of forces acting at the time of injury. Fortunately, spinal injuries are somewhat rare in childhood and adolescence (18). Birney and Hanley (18) reviewed 84 injuries and found that the most common cause was falling from a height. Most of the others had recreational and athletic causes or were traffic and pedestrian injuries. Birney and Hanley drew attention to a problem that may be more common among children: spinal cord injury without radiologic evidence of injury or subluxation in the spinal column. In these cases it is difficult to establish the cause of injury or the necessary treatment.

Mechanisms of Injuries to the Spinal Cord

Each of the various tissues of the spine has a maximum strain beyond which injury occurs. Normal motion of the spine occurs around axes of motion that lie toward the posterior part of the intervertebral disc and maintaining acceptable ranges of deformation of the anterior disc and of the spinal cord and neural structures. It appears that direct trauma and sustained ischemia often combine to produce a neural deficit. Compression of short duration (71) and tension (95,96) on the spinal cord can produce irreversible ischemic damage. Sudden transverse deformation of the spinal cord produces a complex pattern of internal strain. For instance, anteroposterior compression tends to produce tension in the transverse direction (20,21). Standardized animal models for studying direct trauma to the spinal cord rely on dropping a standard weight from a standard height onto the exposed cord of an animal such as a rat (35,98,104). The effect of such trauma depends on many variables, including the shape of the dropped object, its mass, and the height from which it falls. The change of momentum of the dropped mass correlates better with the extent of the injury than does the kinetic energy of the mass before impact (98,104). Among patients the degree of spinal instability after injury indicates the probable degree of deformation of the cord at the time of the initial trauma but gives no indication of the duration of deformation. Thus the degree of spinal instability may not correlate with the degree of neurologic damage.

Contribution of the Intervertebral Disc to Flexibility and Strength

The intervertebral disc has a special mechanical role in transmitting large compressive forces and provides flexibility for rotations about all three axes. In compression loading, large pressures are generated in the nucleus pulposus, and these pressures are contained by tensile stresses in the anulus. Compression stiffness is relatively high initially, about 1 mm deflection per 1,000 N of compressive force, and it increases at greater forces. Disc compression (reduction in height) is accompanied by a similar amount of disc bulging (increase in disc radius). The high swelling pressure of the nucleus allows it to sustain high pressures without rapid loss of fluid. Although it has little effect on the compressive behavior of the disc (81), removal of the nucleus has a great effect on motion in other planes (102). Deformation causes a flow of fluid within the disc and causes changes in fluid content (volumetric changes). These are also apparent as diurnal changes in disc height. Whether these fluid fluxes augment the nutrition of intervertebral discs by means of a pumping mechanism is unclear (60,145), because diffusion may predominate. The vertebral end plates and the disc periphery are pathways for diffusion of nutrients and metabolites in and out of the avascular disc. The rates of diffusion of nutrients and metabolites along these pathways differ as a function of molecular weight (145).

Intervertebral discs can be subjected to quite large rotations without damage. Axial rotation allows the smallest range before damage occurs. Thus twisting has been considered a common source of injury to intervertebral discs (43), especially repetitive small injuries that cause disc degeneration in later life.

Contributions of the Vertebral Bodies to Flexibility and Strength

Vertebral bodies deform under compressive loading, and the end plates become more concave under the influence of intradiscal pressure (22). The end plate deformation at its center is of similar magnitude to the amount of radial bulging of the disc. Microscopic damage to the trabeculae (55) and herniation of the disc through the end plate (Schmorl nodule) apparently can occur at any age.

Contributions of the Posterior Elements and Ligaments to Flexibility and Strength

Depending on their orientation, which varies along the length of the spine, facet joints can contribute to resisting compressive loading, shear loading, and torsion loading (Fig. 6). However, probably because of flexibility in the neural arch, neither removing nor transfixing the facets has a great effect on the flexibility of the motion segment, except in torsion (132). Farfan (42) progressively cut away the posterior structures of lumbar motion segments and showed that the each facet joint contributes about 18% of the torsion stiffness. A large part of the remaining flexibility is provided by the intervertebral disc (Fig. 7). A similar experiment was conducted by Panjabi et al. (103) to investigate displacement in cervical motion segments in response to a posteriorly directed shear force (Fig. 8). When motion segment components were transected starting posteriorly (Fig. 2A), the largest increases in both rotational and translational displacements occurred with cutting of the disc and anterior ligament. When cutting was started anteriorly (Fig. 8B), sectioning of each structure produced a large increase in rotation and translation. Over-

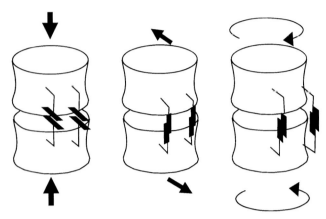

FIGURE 6. Orientation of facet joints that provide resistance to compression, forward shear, and axial rotation. (From Owen R, Goodfellow J, Bullough P, eds. (1980): *Orthopaedics and traumatology.* London: Heinemann, with permission.)

all it appears that the intervertebral disc is the most crucial structure for the mechanical integrity of the motion segment, but posterior structures help guide the motion segment and protect the disc from injury.

Special Considerations in the Immature Skeleton

Nearly all the information about mechanical properties of the motion segment and how they contribute to flexibility and strength of the spine comes from adult material tested in vitro. It is almost impossible to make measurements for living subjects, and very little material from young subjects has been tested. Ashton-Miller and Schultz (9) found that a child's spine is 5 to 10 times less stiff than the average adult spine. There is a loss of stiffness in both material (tissue) properties and mechanical (structural) properties of knee ligaments with age (158), which

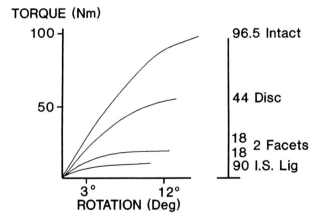

FIGURE 7. Results of torsion test of a motion segment of the lumbar spine with successive sectioning of components to show the relative contribution of each. (Redrawn from Farfan HF (1973): *Mechanical disorders of the low back.* Philadelphia: Lea & Febiger, with permission.)

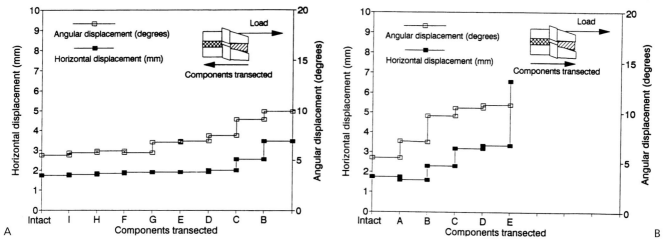

FIGURE 8. Results of an experiment in which a posteriorly directed force of 25% body weight was applied to the upper vertebra of a cervical spine motion segment and components of the joint were progressively transected. **A:** Components transected from posterior to anterior. **B:** Components transected from anterior to posterior. *A,* Anterior longitudinal ligament; *B,* anterior half of anulus; *C,* posterior half of anulus; *D,* posterior longitudinal ligament; *E,* intertransverse ligaments; *F,* capsular ligaments of facets; *G,* facets; *H,* ligamentum flavum; *I,* interspinous and supraspinous ligaments; *o,* angular displacement (degrees), *n,* horizontal displacement (mm). (Redrawn from Panjabi MM, White AA, Johnson RM (1975): Cervical spine mechanics as a function of transsection of components. *J Biomech* 8:327–336, with permission.)

probably is paralleled by similar changes in other soft tissues, including those of the spine.

IN VIVO LOADING OF THE SPINE: MOMENTS OF LIFTED OBJECTS AND MUSCLES

The spine is loaded by a combination of externally applied forces, body weight forces, and muscular forces. Because the moment arms of the muscles around the spine usually are smaller (73) than those of lifted weights and body weight contributions, the forces in muscles are correspondingly high. Figure 9 illustrates a case in which compressive load on the spine approaches 5,000

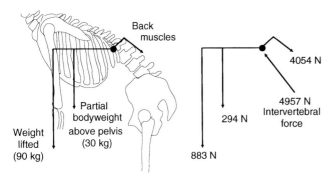

FIGURE 9. Simplified model of lifting mechanics. Deep muscles of the back provide extension moments to counteract flexion moments of the weight of the head, arms, and trunk and of the lifted weight. Possible effects of intraabdominal pressure are neglected in this model. (Adapted from Morris JM, Lucas DB, Bresler MS (1961): The role of the trunk in stability of the spine. *J Bone Joint Surg Am* 43:327–351, with permission.)

N (about one-half ton). This is close to the ultimate compressive strength of the adult spine. The weight being lifted together with the weights of body segments above the level of the spine being considered produce moments about the spine. The magnitude of each moment is the product of the force (weight) and its distance from the spine. These moments must be countered by moments generated by muscle and ligamentous forces. For any position of the body and for given external loading, the internal forces and moments acting on the spine can be estimated by means of considering the equilibrium between internal and external forces and torques around the spine with the help of a biomechanical model (4). When the trunk is at rest, all the forces and moments must balance to prevent motion. Free body analysis (Fig. 9) is an equilibrium analysis in which a system is split into real or imagined component parts (free bodies) to check that each part is in equilibrium. It can therefore be used to measure the internal stresses in joints and muscles when a body segment is subjected to external loads.

Biomechanical Models

Biomechanical analysis of spinal forces seldom has a unique solution because the redundant number of spinal muscles provides many combinations of synergistic and antagonistic muscle forces that can satisfy equilibrium. To resolve this redundancy in a model, the pattern of coactivation of muscles can be obtained from experimental electromyographic (EMG) recordings. However, the EMG-to-force conversion is always approximate, and the number of muscles that can be recorded is limited. Biomechanical models can be used to make assumptions about rules that govern muscle recruitment, that is, which muscles are active and which control strategies are used to activate them. This usually requires a presumed physiologic cost function, such as total muscle stress or intervertebral forces, that is considered to be minimized by the muscle control strategy. In simple sagittal-plane lifting tasks, it appears that both muscular activation levels and spinal compressive loadings are minimized but subject to increases in both muscle activation and spinal loading produced by antagonistic muscle forces. For example, in lifting tasks, antagonistic abdominal muscles are activated to produce a counterproductive flexion moment. This also produces intraabdominal pressure, which once was thought to augment the extension moments about the spine (92) and thus help to reduce compressive loading on the spine. This effect is now considered negligible (56,85,139), and it appears that abdominal muscle activation is important for maintaining the structural stability of the spine (4,47).

Another complicating factor in biomechanical models of the trunk is the contribution of ligamentous structures. These passive structures contribute to the forces acting on the spine only when they are in a tightened position. In lifting tasks performed with a flexed spine, the erector spinae muscles are electrically silent (120), and the ligaments provide a major contribution to the force. However, whether it is better to lift with the spine in a lordotic, kyphotic, or neutral position is unresolved (3,36).

Spinal Stability and Instability

Stability means that a system returns to equilibrium position after a perturbation. Buckling is a kind of instability in which a structure suddenly bends and collapses when a certain critical load is exceeded. The term *stability* unfortunately has been used in many different meanings in the context of the spine to refer to both clinical and biomechanical aspects. Biomechanical instability should not be confused with (a) large elastic deformation of the spine (high flexibility), (b) hypermobility of a spinal segment relative to its neighbors, (c) abnormal coupling of components of spinal motion, such as increased anterior shear motion accompanying flexion, (d) sudden and unpredictable changes in painful symptoms, or (e) slowly progressing posttraumatic or scoliotic deformity (9).

Equilibrium is a stable position of minimum potential energy. Because potential energy increases with deformation in an elastic structure, increased stiffness of a structure usually provides greater stability, but stiffness and stability are not equivalent. The spine consists of a column of vertebrae linked by relatively flexible articulations, so it is probably at risk of buckling when loaded by external forces and muscle forces. For equilibrium, all muscle tensions must be carefully balanced to prevent large deformations at individual articulations. Muscle stiffness is required to stabilize the spine. Because muscle stiffness increases with muscle activation, increased muscle coactivation can help to stabilize the spinal column. These ideas have been investigated analytically (16,31,47), and the results suggest a stabilizing role for antagonistic muscle activity, for muscles that cross several segments, and for the shorter muscles, such as the multifidus. Spinal instability is difficult to demonstrate in vivo. If it occurs, instability is most likely transient and unlikely to be recorded on an x-ray film.

BIOMECHANICS OF PAINFUL CONDITIONS OF THE SPINE

There is much disagreement about the role of biomechanical factors in the causation of low back pain among adults. When it occurs among children, low back pain should be taken seriously (116). The cause of low back pain in children is seldom mechanical (traumatic) or disc herniation or degeneration, and the underlying pathologic condition may be more ominous. An exception is spondylolysis, which is a risk among children who participate in certain sports (77). Although usually asymptomatic among children (124), spondylolysis may develop into spondylolisthesis during the adolescent growth spurt (157). Spondylolysis is more common among gymnasts (62) and football players (84,124) than it is among other children. Spondylolysis is reported to be present among 4.4% of the population at 6 years of age. The prevalence increases to 6% in adulthood (44). Important epidemiologic observations emerged from studies of skeletons removed from the graves of Alaskan natives (131). Four percent of the skeletons of 6-year-old children had this defect, which increased to 34% in adulthood. These observations led to the idea that spondylolysis is a fatigue fracture caused by repetitive loading. Cyron and Hutton (32) reproduced a spondylolysis fracture in cadaver vertebrae subjected to repetitive loading of the posterior elements. Their experiments were complemented by a simple mechanical model that showed how facet joint loading, combined with tension from the extensor muscles, produced bending moments in the neural arch. Rosenberg et al. (115) reported no instances of spondylolysis among persons with spinal paralysis. Their findings provide additional evidence of a mechanical cause of spondylolysis.

SPINAL DEFORMITIES

Simple mechanical consideration of the structural stability of the spine suggests that spinal deformities should be common. There are excellent controls over the growth and development of the spine in most persons, except when there is muscular weakness. The apparently spontaneous development of scoliosis and abnormal kyphosis is difficult to explain (113). Spinal growth and development are important factors in the progression of spinal deformities (19,150), but it is not clear whether abnormal growth initiates the deformity (135). Growth and maturation apparently are disturbed in idiopathic scoliosis. There are few indications why idiopathic scoliosis is more common among girls, except that their vertebrae might be slightly more slender (148) and there are differences in the development of the sagittal spinal curvatures (156). A set of subtle mechanical factors, including abnormal growth (13,38,51,76,127,141,144, 154,155), joint laxity (17), sagittal spinal curvature (156), and neurologic factors (57) may play a part (94).

Etiology and Progression of Scoliosis

The exact biomechanical mechanisms responsible for idiopathic scoliosis, especially the transverse plane rotations of the vertebrae, are not well understood. A number of biomechanical factors have been invoked to explain the biomechanics of scoliosis. These include intervertebral motion coupling, spinal tethering and buckling, and mechanical influences on growth.

It appears unlikely that coupling of rotational motion in intervertebral segments controls the development of vertebral rotation in scoliosis. Both lateral bending of the spine and scoliotic deformities show rotation in the transverse plane. However, the normal kinematic relations between lateral bending and axial rotation are different from those in scoliosis (133,151,152) and do not explain the pattern of deformity that develops in scoliosis with maximal vertebral rotation at the curve apex. Spinal tethering by posterior structures of the spine (33,63,130) also has been invoked to explain the spinal shape in scoliosis and its causation. There are several parts to this theory. Tethering is thought to prevent flexion of the spine and lead to a hypokyphotic or lordotic shape, which then has a greater tendency toward instability (34). Second, the tether is thought to maintain a straighter alignment of the posterior elements than of the vertebral bodies, thus rotating the vertebrae in the curve. That the sagittal plane of the spine is flattest in the early teen years (156) supports the idea that this shape places the spine at risk of development of scoliosis. The shape of the spine in scoliosis is reminiscent of that of a buckled beam, but buckling may not explain the development of lateral curvatures because buckling of the ligamentous spine first exaggerates the sagittal curvature.

It has been proposed that a small lateral curvature of the spine would load the vertebrae asymmetrically and cause asymmetric growth in the vertebral physes (106) and acceleration of the deformity in a vicious circle (111,136) after a certain threshold of spinal deformity has been reached. This theory of spinal growth sensitivity to loading asymmetry must explain why the normal spinal curvatures (kyphosis and lordosis) in the sagittal plane do not progress into hyperkyphosis and hyperlordosis by the same mechanism, although progressive deformity in Scheuermann kyphosis has been attributed to a similar mechanism (123). This concept of the mode of progression of deformity is attractive intuitively and is incorporated into the rationale for use of braces and other treatments. The concept cannot be quantified, however, without better knowledge of the normal spinal loading and of loading in the presence of scoliosis and knowledge of the sensitivity of growth to mechanical load magnitude and the time course of loading. Development of the rotational deformity in the spine complicates this process. The growth plates of long bones also are responsive to torsional loads (6,91), but the origin of such forces in the spine during progression of scoliosis is not clear. The clinical observation (79) that the risk of progression of scoliosis is a combination of both curve magnitude and amount of residual growth cannot be explained quantitatively with mechanical principles.

Spinal Biomechanics and Growth

Regulation of bone growth is complex. Genetic, vascular (66,129,142), hormonal (13,26,110), and biomechanical (24, 50,58,136) factors all play a role. Because the dimensions of the neural canal develop at such a young age, factors such as diet and health status in the perinatal period can influence spinal growth and subsequent health (29,108,109). Longitudinal

growth in the vertebral body occurs in the cartilage of the end plates (33) and is influenced by biomechanical loading (87,136). Roaf (112) developed a rationale for local epiphysiodesis in the treatment of patients with scoliosis with varying degrees of kyphosis and lordosis. It appears that the technique of vertebral growth arrest and stapling may be unsuccessful because it has been used when too little residual spinal growth has been present. The relation between mechanical factors and growth (modeling) is not well understood, and much of what is known about the interaction between mechanical forces and bone metabolism relates to remodeling of mature bone as opposed to the modeling of growing bone (24,78). The discs are implicated in scoliosis (106), and very little is known about the mechanical influences on the development and growth of the discs. Diaphyseal remodeling may not respond to mechanical loading in the same way as growth in physes. For example, the diaphyseal remodeling that straightens malunion of a long bone would require that the concave (compression) side experience apposition of bone and that the tension side experience resorption, the opposite of the growth modulation in physes.

Arkin and Katz (6) reported a sensitive response of long bone growth to compressive loading in rabbits. They found no evidence of a threshold level of load to produce growth modulation. They also found that limbs that were immobilized and relieved of weight bearing were elongated. Tension forces applied across the long-bone growth plates of sheep accelerated growth (107). Gooding and Neuhauser (49) found "tall vertebrae" in patients with paralysis and in younger patients who had been treated surgically with posterior fusion of the spine. Gooding and Neuhauser argued that the unloading of the spine increased longitudinal growth.

Clinical application of these principles of growth modulation implies direct application of loads to the skeleton or alteration of ambient loads with therapies such as exercises or brace wearing. Stapling of growth plates is thought to influence growth because of forces generated in the staples by growth of the underlying physis. Staples have been shown to have profound effects on growth (53) and the growth plate cells (41,59). However, other compensatory mechanisms may come into play. Hall-Craggs and Lawrence (52,53) found that rabbit tibia that had been stapled at one growth cartilage had accelerated growth at the growth cartilage at the other end of the bone.

Lack of understanding of the exact physiologic response of growing vertebrae to force has led to uncertainties about the efficacy of braces to manage idiopathic scoliosis. The relative timing of stimulus and response is unknown. Night bracing (overcorrection with a brace during the night) seemed intuitively attractive, because it is successful in orthodontic bracing. Clinical trials are showing, however, that night bracing is inferior to full-time use of a Boston brace for scoliosis (61,69). It may be that night bracing applies loading to the spine but in a way that does not influence growth. Bone metabolism also is known to have diurnal variations with greater mineralization activity at night but greater synthesis of collagen by day. The intuitively attractive idea of using electrical stimulation to treat scoliosis also failed, possibly because of insufficient understanding of the underlying physiologic mechanisms. Unknown factors include the muscle forces generated by the stimulation, the resulting adaptive changes in the muscles, the forces imposed on the spine by stimulation, and the growth response.

MECHANICAL CONSIDERATIONS IN THE MANAGEMENT OF SPINAL DEFORMITIES

In both conservative and surgical treatment of patients with spinal deformities, forces are applied to the spine. In the case of surgery, the desired forces usually can be applied more directly. Just as the motion segment has six degrees of freedom, there are, in general, six distinct components to any deformity of the spine, and forces can be applied to correct each of these components. Thus mechanical treatment of spinal deformities can involve horizontal forces in the frontal or sagittal planes, distraction forces, lateral bending or flexion-extension moments, or moments in the transverse plane (Fig. 10). In practice, precise control over the applied forces is difficult to achieve. However, both brace and surgical treatments are evolving in an attempt to address the three-dimensional components of spinal deformities.

Conservative Treatment

Brace treatment usually involves the principle of a three-point application of forces. The middle force is directed at the region of maximal deformity while equilibrium is provided by two additional forces at the extremes of the deformity (Fig. 10A). The present trend in bracing for scoliosis is to attempt to control both sagittal and frontal plane curvatures at the same time. The magnitude of scoliosis curves may be the best predictor of success of this treatment (89,90), but it is unclear why this treatment is not always successful. Changes in skeletal configuration (spine and rib cage) with the Boston brace among 40 patients with right thoracic idiopathic scoliosis were recorded with stereoradiography (75). It was found that both the frontal and the sagit-

tal plane curvatures were reduced, leaving the plane of maximum curvature almost unchanged. There was no significant improvement in vertebral rotation, but the ribs on the right (convex) side became angled more downward. Chase et al. (27) measured interface pressure between a Boston brace and 14 patients with adolescent scoliosis. The total force exerted through the brace averaged 58 $\pm$ 18 N and was associated with an initial curve correction of 37% $\pm$ 21%. The mean force level was maintained throughout the 6-month study, although the mean curve correction at 6 months had reduced to 15% $\pm$ 14%.

Braces apply forces directly to the trunk, and patients may be encouraged to recruit their own muscles in a beneficial way (passive and active theories of brace function). Wynarsky and Schultz (160) recorded muscular activity within a Boston brace and found little evidence of the second (active) mechanism.

Electrical stimulation of muscles for correction of scoliosis (11,12), although intuitively attractive as a way to load the growing skeleton, has not been successful (40). The treatment initially appeared promising and was used only at night, but the idea of night-brace treatment also has produced disappointing results (61,69). Night treatment raises the fundamental question about how a spinal deformity responds to the application of force. There are two possible modes of action. The brace or the electrical stimulation may apply forces directly that then modify the growth and development of the deformity. An alternative explanation is that the chronic stimulation or lengthening of muscles may change the resting length or tension of the muscles and prevent progression. Although the activity of bone cells has diurnal variation, it seems that providing a stimulus during the night is sufficient to produce marked differential growth. Unanswered questions remain about the biologic characteristics of bone and muscle.

Surgical Treatment

Instrumentation used in surgical treatment of spinal deformities has two separate mechanical roles. The first is to apply forces to correct or reduce the spinal deformity. The second is to produce the correct mechanical environment for spinal fusion by means of immobilizing the spine until fusion has occurred.

Control of the shape of the spine in three dimensions with instrumentation has proved to be challenging. The distraction forces applied to the spine with Harrington instrumentation were found to cause the flat-back complication (2,88,138). Curved rods were recommended to prevent this loss of curvature (25,67). Curving the rod can prevent its contacting intermediate vertebrae, but the forces at the end of the rod where the hook connects to the vertebrae are probably unchanged. Because of force equilibrium, the predominant forces at the instrumentation hooks must be equal and opposite along the line joining the saddles of the hooks in the absence of appreciable additional forces between the rod and the spine. With distraction instrumentation, there is a diminishing return with increasing distraction because the moment of the distraction force decreases as correction proceeds (Fig. 11). Distraction instrumentation can be augmented with segmental wires, which are attached to the posterior part of the vertebrae. In a scoliosis curve, they might be expected to pull the posterior parts of the vertebrae into

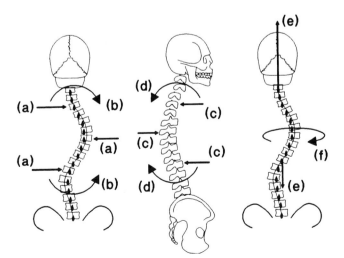

FIGURE 10. Forces that can be applied by means of instrumentation to correct scoliosis. *a*, lateral force; *b*, coronal moment; *c*, sagittal force; *d*, sagittal moment; *e*, distraction force; *f*, axial moment

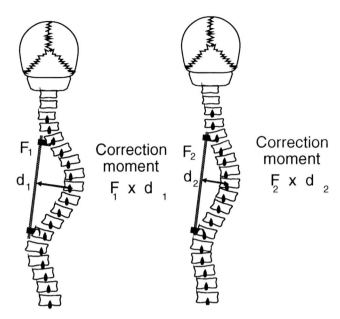

FIGURE 11. Distraction instrumentation produces decreasing increments of correction moment for increasing increments of force as correction proceeds.

the concavity of the curve and worsen the vertebral rotation. However, this does not appear to be an important effect (140).

There is little change in vertebral rotation after Harrington surgery (1,15,37,45,149), and there are small changes in the surface asymmetry of the back (65,149). This is not unexpected, considering that the distraction rod does not apply moments around the vertical axis. In contrast, the derotation maneuver used in the Cotrel-Dubousset procedure is intended to address the three-dimensional deformity of scoliosis by rotating the spine from a scoliosis curvature into kyphosis. However, the resulting derotation of the apical vertebrae and of the surface asymmetry of the back is quite small (14,159). The biomechanics of the Cotrel-Dubousset procedure are complicated because the operation can apply both distraction forces and lateral forces. The effects on the transverse plane should depend on the direction of the forces applied relative to the positions of the vertebrae in the deformed region of the spine (Fig. 12). This geometric configuration changes continually during the derotation maneuver (46). In theory, anterior instrumentation may be better placed to provide correction of both the lateral curvature and the vertebral rotation by means of pulling the spine toward the convexity of the curve (54). Anterior instrumentation also holds the promise of allowing shorter fusion while allowing fine surgical control over the fused part of the spine. The challenge of controlling the postoperative shape of unfused regions of the spine is even greater than that of manipulating the spinal shape within the bounds of the instrumentation. The control of posture and shape and balance of the spine is complex and is a poorly understood area of biomechanics of the spine and trunk.

Insights into the exact sequence of geometric changes in the spine during instrumentation are coming from intraoperative measurements. These measurements are technically demanding

and necessitate tracking the motion of landmarks on the spine by means of photogrammetry (118) or with sensors of magnetic fields (74). These measurements have shown that the proportion of curve correction of idiopathic scoliosis produced by distraction is almost equal to the proportion produced by the derotation maneuver of segmental instrumentation (36,94,97,101, 121). The curvature of the surgically exposed spine of a patient under anesthesia before instrumentation is substantially less than that present on preoperative radiographs.

After the operation, the process of graft incorporation and arthrodesis begins. More rigid fixation promotes more rapid fusion (68,82,83). There has been concern that extremely rigid fixation techniques would also produce stress shielding of bone and osteopenia. This was found among dogs (83,128) but not goats (68), and it does not appear to be important among humans.

In the spines of children, the question of graft placement is especially important in arthrodesis in the presence of continuing growth. The tethering effect of posterior fusion can produce continuing development of deformity of the vertebral column around the axis of the instrumentation. This is known as the *crankshaft phenomenon* (125). Very rigid fixation (anterior and posterior) may be able to arrest growth and prevent this from occurring (70). An alternative strategy is internal fixation without fusion, which allows continued growth while deformity is controlled. This method is associated with instrumentation problems because in the absence of fusion, the instrumentation is liable to fatigue failure due to the continued loading caused by patient activity.

It is suspected that the presence of a fused region results in greater everyday motion of the unfused motion segments, especially those adjacent to the fusion. This certainly appears to be true for the lumbosacral joints of patients with fusion that extends to L5 (30). Much of the clinical follow-up information about adjacent segments comes from patients who underwent fusion for degenerative conditions. It is not clear whether the adjacent segment degeneration is a result of natural history or whether the process is accelerated by the presence of the fusion.

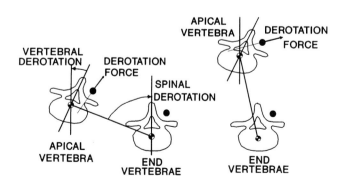

FIGURE 12. Transverse plane diagram of a spine with scoliosis before (*left*) and after (*right*) a derotation maneuver with a Cotrel-Dubousset rod on the concave side of the curve. The line of the force applied through the hook to the apical vertebra relative to its center of rotation determines the direction of the moment tending to reduce the axial rotation of the apical vertebra. These diagrams show that the derotation force tends first to derotate but then to rotate the apical vertebra.

Biomechanical Aspects of Surgical Planning

A surgeon planning surgical therapy for a spinal deformity has many variables to consider when using modern segmental instrumentation. These variables include the design of the instrumentation system, the number and location of vertebrae on which instrumentation is to be performed, rod shape (curvature), interconnections between instrumentation components, and the extent of the operative maneuvers. All of these factors can influence the correction of the deformity and the rigidity of the final construct. Surgical management of deformities must be viewed in three dimensions, which increases the challenges involved in surgical planning. There are four sources of information to help in decision making. First is empirical experience based on treatment of a large series of patients. Second, biomechanical studies in the laboratory provide information on the strength and flexibility of constructs applied to animal or human cadaveric spines. Third, animal experiments have been used to gain insight into the fate of both the instrumentation and the spinal fusion in vivo. Fourth, biomechanical analysis and biomechanical models can be used to predict the outcome of surgery on the basis of the underlying biomechanical principles.

Radiographic Assessment

Lateral bending radiographs may used in preoperative planning. The principle is that the amount of preoperative curve correction achieved by means of active of passive lateral bending or traction is predictive of the amount of change curvature during surgical treatment (28,147). Unfortunately, the amount of change in curvature with lateral bending is somewhat unrepeatable. It seems that fulcrum bending (side lying with a pad under the curve apex) produces the greatest change in curvature, which is quite predictive of surgical correction (80). In a study of the degree of vertebral rotational correction in lateral bending, spinal instrumentation markedly corrected the Cobb angle but minimally corrected apical vertebral rotation. In contrast, preoperative lateral bending produced a similar proportional correction of both (7).

Lateral bending radiographs also are used to help select the extent of fusion and the vertebrae for attachment of instrumentation (hook level selection). These rules are mostly empirical and based on qualitative concepts of spinal biomechanics, such as the neutral vertebra.

Mechanical Simulation of Surgical Maneuvers

In theory, if the mechanical properties of both the spine and the instrumentation were understood completely, biomechanical models can be used to predict the outcome of surgical therapy. There have been a number of attempts to develop and validate such models. Schultz and Hirsch (121,122) used a three-dimensional model adjusted to fit the frontal plane spinal deformity of six different patients to investigate the extent to which distraction forces from Harrington rods might alter the spinal deformity. These simulations demonstrated a nonlinear relation between the distraction force and correction, because the moment of the distraction force decreased as correction proceeded

(Fig. 11). These models also helped predict that distraction forces would produce very little derotation of vertebrae about the longitudinal axis. A similar model was used to study correction of deformity by means of electrical stimulation (119) and with braces (161).

One of the difficulties in using a mechanical model to predict the outcome of surgery for an individual patient is the unknown flexibility of each motion segment. Meade and Patwardhan et al. (86,105) developed a model that was used to estimate intervertebral stiffness by means of comparing predictions made with a two-dimensional model of the spine with the observed outcome of surgery. The results of these analyses indicated that motion segments near the apex have a flexibility similar to that of segments elsewhere in the curve (146). Subbaraj et al. (137) used a two-dimensional model of a patient's spine to simulate variations in surgical procedure. They estimated the flexibility of each motion segment based on radiographic measurements before and after application of traction. A three-dimensional model developed by Jayaraman et al. (64) was used for a similar purpose. Individualized simulation of six patients before and after Harrington rod surgery compared with the measured shape of each patient recorded with stereoradiography showed that model-predicted spinal curvature agreed better in the frontal plane than in the sagittal plane (134). The latter was sensitive to the properties of the intervertebral motion segments. Another problem in these simulations is incorporating nonlinear elastic and time-dependent material properties of the spine. These are known to be important in vivo, because the forces in instrumentation immediately postoperatively decay as much as one half in a few hours (39,93).

Segmental instrumentation offers surgeons many variables and multistep maneuvers to adapt to individual patients' needs. It also, however, produces many unknown inputs for the biomechanical analysis and difficulties in validation of predictions from models. To simulate these procedures, the surgical maneuvers for the concave-side rod of segmental instrumentation can be represented in four steps: (a) install the rod passively to the end hooks, then approximate the intermediate hooks to the rod; (b) displace the hooks along the rod to their final positions (hook distraction); (c) rotate the concave-side rod; (d) lock the hooks to the rod and relax the applied torque (spring-back). It has proved very difficult to quantify the required magnitude and direction of all these displacement inputs in the simulation.

Another possibility offered by analytical modeling is the ability to calculate stresses at selected sites in the spine and instrumentation. A finite element analyses were used to estimate stresses in internal fixation devices (48,126). These models have provided estimates of the change in bone stress for different vertebral injury situations with inclusion of plastic washers in the construct and after incorporation of bone graft. Biomechanical analyses also have been used to investigate the consequences of surgical variables, such as angulation of pedicle screws, on the rigidity of the construct (72,117).

Evaluation of Spinal Instrumentation

Much of the understanding about results of spinal fusion is empirical and based on results of follow-up studies. Biomechanical principles should provide additional information. The use of surgical instrumentation has a direct mechanical effect on the fused part of the spine and an indirect effect on the unfused region. It remains a challenge to biomechanics to further our understanding of the interactions between the spine, the instrumentation, and the muscular and other forces. The muscles and their control present the greatest difficulties, because central nervous system control of trunk balance is so poorly understood.

Mechanical Testing of Implants

There are three basic types of spinal implant construct testing—tests of individual implant components, such as hooks and rods; tests of the connections between an implant and the spine, such as hooks and pedicle screws; and tests of complete instrumentation assemblies. The performance of all constructs can all be evaluated tested in simulations of in vivo conditions. Laboratory testing of a spinal construct, which consists of test instrumentation applied to a standardized spinal specimen, can provide information about flexibility, strength, and fatigue life. Components such as pedicle screws can be tested in pull-out (72). The challenge in all these tests is to establish conditions that are representative of the in vivo situation. A test of strength (failure test) can be considered a test of instrumentation safety, and a test of stiffness can be considered a test of efficacy, because it is generally considered that stiffer fixation is more effective in achieving the goal of spinal arthrodesis. Thus strength and stiffness are desirable properties of instrumentation. Failure tests can be performed only once per specimen, whereas a stiffness or flexibility test can be repeated, provided that the installation of the instrumentation and the test itself do not greatly change the mechanical properties of the specimen. This may explain why there are a preponderance of reports of stiffness-flexibility tests over failure tests.

In a typical construct test, instrumentation is applied to a spine specimen, which is loaded. The resulting deformations are measured. A rare alternative is to test a construct by means of applying a displacement and measuring the necessary forces—a stiffness test. This test is the inverse of the flexibility test. In a typical flexibility test, a pure moment is applied with a coupling that consists of two equal parallel forces. The magnitude of the moment (torque) is the force magnitude multiplied by the distance between the parallel forces (Fig. 13A). As an alternative,

offset compression loading (Fig. 13B) is intended to be more physiologically realistic because the spine is compressed axially at the same time as a bending moment is produced. The latter kind of loading is more difficult to control, because it can cause buckling. Another problem is that as the specimen deforms, the loading position and direction can move relative to the specimen and alter the components of force and moments acting on it. Most reports give the resulting rotations about the same axis as the applied torque or collinear with the applied load. If additional rotations or displacements about other axes are recorded, these provide information about the coupled (as opposed to direct) stiffness. The motion typically is recorded by means of mechanical or optoelectronic methods or with magnetic sensors of position and orientation. For the motion measurements to be valid, it is important that the segments be firmly embedded at their ends.

If linear forces are used as applied loads, great care must be taken to define the axis system. Linear force can produce rotational moment that depends on the point at which it is applied and on the direction of force. Therefore an advantage of testing a construct by using applied couples and recording rotations is simplicity: the measured flexibility is sensitive only to the axis of testing, and this facilitates comparisons between tests of various construct designs. The disadvantage is that such testing ignores direct forces and linear displacement components, thus it may lose realism while gaining simplicity. This may explain why many reports give only the three rotational modes of testing and omit the other three (translational) degrees of freedom. The results for individual degrees of freedom usually are reported separately. Because these are referenced to an arbitrary axis system, it may be preferable to refer the resulting motion to a structure of anatomic interest, such as the motion occurring at the site of arthrodesis.

In the real in vivo biomechanical situation, the spine has six complex degrees of freedom that interact structurally. Because the stiffness of the lumbosacral spine increases with axial loading, testing under laboratory conditions without such preloading may lead to underestimation of the spinal contribution to stiffness. The spine is subject to complex muscular, ligamentous, and gravitational forces that we do not understand very well. Therefore, ideally we would first identify which combination of forces and moments is pertinent and then perform instrumentation tests that simulate this realistic combination of muscular, ligamentous, and gravitational forces with six degrees of freedom. Then we should record the resulting motion in a way that gives an indication of the probability of rapid fusion and the chances of failure of the metallic or biologic structures. The applicable loadings have not yet been determined, nor have the pertinent specimen deformations. Information about in vivo loading of internal fixators has been provided by means of telemetry of signals from force transducers built into the instrumentation (114). These show forces on the order of 250 N and moments on the order of 6 Nm transmitted through the instrumentation during walking, but this constitutes an unknown proportion of the total load carried by the spine and the instrumentation. For comparison, Cappozzo (23) calculated that the cyclic component of the compressive force in the spine during walking typically is 700 N, approximately body weight.

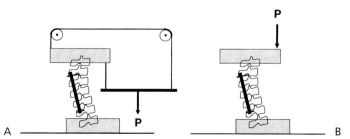

FIGURE 13. **A:** Mechanical test of an instrumentation construct with a pure moment that imposes flexion-extension by means of a coupling (equal parallel forces). **B:** Mechanical test with offset compression loading.

Fatigue testing is important to establish whether instrumentation will fail with repetitive loading. This kind of testing usually is conducted only on individual components of instrumentation or on constructs applied to inert fixtures, such as plastic blocks, because on the order of one million cycles of loading must be applied to ensure that failure would not occur under in vivo conditions. These tests provide values for the maximum safe loads under test conditions that must then be interpreted in terms of expected in vivo loading. Because this kind of test is time consuming, an alternative is to analyze expected loads in vivo to determine from a stress analysis whether the highest calculated stresses all are within the limits of those to which the instrumentation materials are resistant to fatigue. In this kind of analysis it is very important to ensure that small radii and features with other shapes that can produce stress concentrations (stress raisers) are taken into account.

Many instrumentation tests are performed on animal spines because human spines representative of the target population (persons who need implants) are difficult to obtain. Specimens of human spines also are more variable in their mechanical properties than are animal spines of similar ages taken from animals of the same breed. Bovine calf and pig spines have been shown to be a reasonable choice because they have vertebral dimensions and flexibility properties similar to those of humans.

Standardized protocols for testing of instrumentation should facilitate comparisons between tests performed in different laboratories (8,99). However, standardization is difficult. In addition to defining the exact conditions for the tests, standardization has to take into account the difficulty of obtaining suitable human cadaveric material or the appropriateness of using animal spines. Standardization has been elusive. To date only the testing of instrumentation systems attached to plastic blocks (corpectomy model) has been provisionally standardized by the American Society for Testing and Materials (5). If a greater degree of standardization could be achieved, there is no guarantee that the results of the tests would be predictive of clinical outcome.

It remains unclear how surgeons who operate on the spine should interpret the information in reports of stiffness and strength testing of spinal implants. Also unclear is what information is helpful in selecting an instrumentation system and adapting it to the needs of a particular patient. It appears that the stiffer instrumentation the better are the results, providing the size of the instrumentation components is not excessive. Given that there are six degrees of freedom possible in a stiffness test, it is not known which components of rotation and translational stiffness are most important. Biomechanical information can be used in conjunction with other information in making surgical decisions. Biomechanical testing ought to be used with the goal of reducing the need for empiricism in the development of knowledge about the outcomes of different surgical strategies.

CONCLUSIONS

The spine is a complex, flexible structure the biomechanics of which are difficult to understand. Each motion segment has six degrees of freedom that interact with one another. This interaction, combined with the inherent curvatures of the spine and the complex anatomic features of the muscles and ligaments, produces biomechanical behavior that is difficult to predict. The spines of children present additional challenges because the biomechanical behavior interacts with growth and continuing development. If, however, the underlying biologic characteristics that relate mechanical factors to biologic responses were better understood, new possibilities would emerge for effective treatments that are not possible on the spines adults, which no longer have growth potential. Because much of the pediatric management of spinal problems is based on biomechanical principles, biomechanical considerations are important in most clinical and surgical decisions.

ACKNOWLEDGMENTS

This work was supported by NIH grants R01 AR 40093 and R55 HD 34460 and by the Department of Orthopaedics and Rehabilitation, University of Vermont.

REFERENCES

1. Aaro S, Dahlborn M (1982): The effect of Harrington instrumentation on the longitudinal axis rotation of the apical vertebra and on the spinal and rib cage deformity in idiopathic scoliosis studied by computer tomography. *Spine* 7:456–462.
2. Aaro S, Öhlen G (1983): The effect of Harrington instrumentation on the sagittal configuration and mobility of the spine in scoliosis. *Spine* 8:570–574.
3. Adams MA, Hutton WC (1985): The effect of posture on the lumbar spine. *J Bone Joint Surg Br* 67:625–629.
4. Andersson GBJ, Winters JM (1990): Role of muscle in postural tasks: spinal loading and postural stability. In: Winters JM, Woo SLY, eds. *Multiple muscle systems: biomechanics and movement organization.* New York: Springer-Verlag 377–395.
5. Anonymous (1997): Standard test method for PS5–94 static and dynamic spinal implants assembly in a corpectomy model. West Conshohocken, PA: American Society for Testing and Materials.
6. Arkin AM, Katz JF (1956): The effects of pressure on epiphyseal growth: the mechanism of plasticity of growing bone. *J Bone Joint Surg Am* 38:1056–1076.
7. Aronsson DD, Stokes IA, Ronchetti PJ, et al. (1996): Surgical correction of vertebral axial rotation in adolescent idiopathic scoliosis: prediction by lateral bending films. *J Spinal Disord* 9:214–219.
8. Ashman RB, Bechtold JE, Edwards WT, et al. (1988): In vitro spinal implant mechanical testing protocols. *J Spinal Disord* 2:274–281.
9. Ashton-Miller JA, Schultz AB (1991): Spine instability and segmental hypermobility biomechanics: a call for the definition and standard use of terms. *Seminars in Spine Surgery* 3:136–148.
10. Aubin CE, Dansereau J, Petit Y, et al. (1998): Three-dimensional measurement of wedged scoliotic vertebrae and intervertebral disks. *Eur Spine J* 7:59–65.
11. Axelgaard J, Brown JC (1983): Lateral electrical surface stimulation for the treatment of progressive idiopathic scoliosis. *Spine* 8:242–260.
12. Axelgaard J, Nordwall A, Brown JC (1983): Correction of spinal curvatures by transcutaneous electrical muscle stimulation. *Spine* 8: 463–481.
13. Bagnall KM, Raso VJ, Hill DL, et al. (1996): Melatonin levels in idiopathic scoliosis: diurnal and nocturnal serum melatonin levels in girls with adolescent idiopathic scoliosis. *Spine* 21:1974–1978.
14. Beaumont SE, Burwell RG, Webb JK, et al. (1989): The effects of Cotrel-Dubousset operation on back shape and spinal movement: preliminary findings. (Abstract) *J Bone Joint Surg Br* 71:153.
15. Benson DR, DeWald RL, Schultz AB (1977): Harrington rod detrac-

tion instrumentation: its effect on vertebral rotation and thoracic compensation. *Clin Orthop* 125:40–44.

16. Bergmark A (1989): Stability of the lumbar spine: a study in mechanical engineering. *Acta Orthop Scand Suppl* 230:1–54.
17. Binns M (1988): Joint laxity in idiopathic adolescent scoliosis. *J Bone Joint Surg Br* 70:420–422.
18. Birney TJ, Hanley EN Jr (1989): Traumatic cervical spine injuries in childhood and adolescence. *Spine* 14:1277–1282.
19. Bjerkreim I, Hassan I (1982): Progression in untreated idiopathic scoliosis after end of growth. *Acta Orthop Scand* 53:897–900.
20. Brieg A, El-Nadi AF (1963): Biomechanics of the cervical spinal cord: relief of contact pressure on and overstretching of the spinal cord. *Acta Radiol [Diagn] (Stockh)* 1:1141–1160.
21. Brieg A, Turnbull I, Hassler O (1966): Effects of mechanical stresses on the spinal cord in cervical spondylosis: a study on fresh cadaver material. *J Neurosurg* 25:45–56.
22. Brinckmann P, Frobin W, Hierholzer E, et al. (1983): Deformation of the vertebral endplate under axial loading of the spine. *Spine* 8:851–856.
23. Cappozzo A (1984) Compressive loads in the lumbar vertebral column during normal level walking. *J Orthop Res* 1:292–301.
24. Carter DR (1987): Mechanical loading history and skeletal biology. *J Biomech* 20:1095–1109.
25. Casey MP, Asher MA, Jacobs RR, et al. (1987): The effect of Harrington rod contouring on lumbar lordosis. *Spine* 12:750–753.
26. Centrella M, Canalis E (1985): Local regulators of skeletal growth: a perspective. *Endocr Rev* 6:544–551.
27. Chase AP, Bader DL, Houghton GR (1989): The biomechanical effectiveness of the Boston brace in the management of adolescent idiopathic scoliosis. *Spine* 14:636–642.
28. Cheung KM, Luk KD (1997): Prediction of correction of scoliosis with use of the fulcrum bending radiograph. *J Bone Joint Surg Am* 79:1144–1150.
29. Clark GA, Hall NR, Armelagos GJ, et al. (1986): Poor growth prior to early childhood: decreased health and life-span in the adult. *Am J Phys Anthropol* 70:145–160.
30. Cochran T, Irstam L, Nachemson A (1983): Long-term anatomic and functional changes in patients with adolescent idiopathic scoliosis treated by Harrington rod fusion. *Spine* 8:576–584.
31. Crisco JJ III, Panjabi MM (1991): The intersegmental and multisegmental muscles of the lumbar spine: a biomechanical model comparing lateral stabilizing potential. *Spine* 16:793–799.
32. Cyron BM, Hutton WC (1978): The fatigue strength of the lumbar neural arch in spondylolysis. *J Bone Joint Surg Br* 60:234–238.
33. Dickson RA, Deacon P (1987): Annotation: spinal growth. *J Bone Joint Surg Br* 69:690–692.
34. Dickson RA, Lawton JO, Archer IA, et al. (1984): The pathogenesis of idiopathic scoliosis: biplanar spinal asymmetry. *J Bone Joint Surg Br* 66:8–15.
35. Dohrmann GJ, Panjabi MM, Banks D (1978): Biomechanics of experimental spinal cord trauma. *J Neurosurg* 48:993–1001.
36. Dolan P, Adams MA, Hutton WC (1988): Commonly adopted postures and their effect on the lumbar spine. *Spine* 13:197–201.
37. Dowell JK, Powell JM, Webb PJ, et al. (1990): Factors influencing the result of posterior spinal fusion in the treatment of adolescent idiopathic scoliosis. *Spine* 15:803–808.
38. Drummond DS, Rogala EJ (1980): Growth and maturation of adolescents with idiopathic scoliosis. *Spine* 5:507–511.
39. Dunn HK, Daniels AU, McBride GG (1982): Intraoperative force measurements during correction of scoliosis. *Spine* 7:448–455.
40. Durham JW, Moskowitz A, Whitney J (1990): Surface electrical stimulation versus brace in treatment of idiopathic scoliosis. *Spine* 15:888–892.
41. Ehrlich MG, Mankin HJ, Treadwell BV (1972): Biochemical and physiological events during closure of the stapled distal femoral epiphyseal plate in rats. *J Bone Joint Surg Am* 54:309–322.
42. Farfan HF (1973): *Mechanical disorders of the low back.* Philadelphia: Lea & Febiger.
43. Farfan HF, Cossette JW, Robertson GH, et al. (1970): The effects of torsion on the lumbar intervertebral joints: the role of torsion

in the production of disc degeneration. *J Bone Joint Surg Am* 52:468–497.
44. Fredrickson BE, Baker D, McHolick WJ, et al. (1984): The natural history of spondylolysis and spondylolisthesis. *J Bone Joint Surg Am* 66:699–707.
45. Gaines RW, McKinley CM, Leatherman KD (1981): Effect of the Harrington compression system on the correction of the rib hump in spinal instrumentation for idiopathic scoliosis. *Spine* 6:489–493.
46. Gardner-Morse M, Stokes IAF (1993): Three-dimensional simulations of scoliosis derotation by Cotrel-Dubousset instrumentation. *J Biomech* 27:177–181.
47. Gardner-Morse MG, Stokes IAF (1998): The effects of abdominal muscle co-activation on lumbar spine stability. *Spine* 23:86–92.
48. Goel VK, Pope MH (1995): Biomechanics of fusion and stabilization. *Spine* 15;20[24 Suppl]:85S–99S.
49. Gooding CA, Neuhauser EBD (1965): Growth and development of the vertebral body in the presence and absence of normal stress. *Am J Roentgenol Radium Ther Nucl Med* 93:388–394.
50. Greco F, de Palma L, Specchia N, et al. (1989): Growth-plate cartilage metabolic response to mechanical stress. *J Pediatr Orthop* 9:520–524.
51. Gross C, Graham J, Neuwirth M, et al. (1983): Scoliosis and growth. *Clin Orthop* 175:243–250.
52. Hall-Craggs ECB (1969): Influence of epiphyses on the regulation of bone growth. *Nature* 221:1245.
53. Hall-Craggs ECB, Lawrence CA (1969): The effect of epiphyseal stapling on growth in length of the rabbit's tibia and femur. *J Bone Joint Surg Br* 51:359–365.
54. Halm HF. Liljenqvist U, Niemeyer T, et al. (1998) Halm-Zielke instrumentation for primary stable anterior scoliosis surgery: operative technique and 2-year results in ten consecutive adolescent idiopathic scoliosis patients within a prospective clinical trial. *Eur Spine J* 7:429–434.
55. Hanssen T, Roos B (1981): Microcalluses of the trabeculae in lumbar vertebrae and their relation to the bone mineral content. *Spine* 6:375–380.
56. Hemborg B, Moritz U, Lowing H (1985): Intra-abdominal pressure and trunk muscle activity during lifting, IV: the causal factors of the intra-abdominal pressure rise. *Scand J Rehabil Med* 17:25–38.
57. Herman R, Mixon J, Fisher A, et al. (1985): Idiopathic scoliosis and the central nervous system: a motor control problem—1983 SRS Harrington lecture. *Spine* 10:1–14.
58. Hert J, Liskova M (1964): Regulation of the longitudinal growth of the long bone by mechanical influence. *Acta Univ Carol [Med] Praha* 20[Suppl]:32–34.
59. Herwig J, Schmidt A, Matthiab HH, et al. (1987): Biochemical events during stapling of the proximal tibial epiphyseal plate in pigs. *Clin Orthop* 218:283–289.
60. Holm S, Nachemson A (1983): Variations in the nutrition of the canine intervertebral disc induced by motion. *Spine* 8:866–874.
61. Howard A, Wright JG, Hedden D (1998): A comparative study of TLSO, Charleston, and Milwaukee braces for idiopathic scoliosis. *Spine* 23:2404–2411.
62. Jackson DW, Wiltse LL, Cirincione RJ (1976): Spondylolysis in the female gymnast. *Clin Orthop* 117:69–73.
63. Jarvis JG, Ashman RB, Johnston CE, et al. (1988): The posterior tether in scoliosis. *Clin Orthop* 227:126–134.
64. Jayaraman G, Zbib HM, Jacobs RR (1989): Biomechanical analyses of surgical correction techniques in idiopathic scoliosis: significance of biplanar characteristics of scoliotic spines. *J Biomech* 22:427–438.
65. Jefferson RJ, Weisz I, Turner-Smith AR, et al. (1988): Scoliosis surgery and its effect on back shape. *J Bone Joint Surg Br* 70:261–266.
66. Jenkins DHR, Cheng DHF, Hodgson AR (1975): Stimulation of bone growth by periosteal stripping: a clinical study. *J Bone Joint Surg Br* 57:482–484.
67. Johnston CE II, Ashman RB, Sherman MC, et al. (1987): Mechanical consequences of rod contouring and residual scoliosis in sublaminar segmental instrumentation. *J Orthop Res* 5:206–216.
68. Johnston CE II, Ashman RB, Baird AM, et al. (1990): Effect of spinal construct stiffness on early fusion mass incorporation: experimental study. *Spine* 15:908–912.

69. Katz DE, Richards BS, Browne RH, et al. (1997): A comparison between the Boston brace and the Charleston bending brace in adolescent idiopathic scoliosis. *Spine* 22:1302–1312.

70. Kioschos HC, Asher MA, Lark RG, et al. (1996): Overpowering the crankshaft mechanism: the effect of posterior spinal fusion with and without stiff transpedicular fixation on anterior spinal column growth in immature canines. *Spine* 21:1168–1173.

71. Kobrine AI, Evans DE, Rizzoli HV (1979): Experimental acute balloon compression of the spinal cord: factors affecting the disappearance and return of the spinal evoked response. *J Neurosurg* 51:841–845.

72. Krag MH (1991): Biomechanics of thoracolumbar spinal fixation: a review. *Spine* 16:S84–S99.

73. Kumar S (1988): Moment arms of spinal musculature determined from CT scans. *Clin Biomech (Bristol, Avon)* 3:137–144.

74. Labelle H, Dansereau J, Bellefleur C, et al. (1995): Peroperative three-dimensional correction of idiopathic scoliosis with the Cotrel-Dubousset procedure. *Spine* 20:1406.

75. Labelle H, Dansereau J, Bellefleur C, et al. (1996): Three-dimensional effect of the Boston brace on the thoracic spine and rib cage. *Spine* 21:59–64.

76. Leong JCY, Low WD, Mok CK, et al. (1982): Linear growth in southern Chinese female patients with adolescent idiopathic scoliosis. *Spine* 7:471–475.

77. Letts M, Smallman T, Afanasiev R, et al. (1986): Fracture of the pars interarticularis in adolescent athletes: a clinical-biomechanical analysis. *J Pediatr Orthop* 6:40–46.

78. LeVeau BF, Bernhardt DB (1984): Developmental biomechanics: effect of forces on the growth, development, and maintenance of the human body. *Phys Ther* 64:1874–1882.

79. Lonstein JE, Carlson JM (1984): The prediction of curve progression in untreated idiopathic scoliosis during growth. *J Bone Joint Surg Am* 66:1061–1071.

80. Luk KD, Cheung KM, Lu DS, et al. (1998): Assessment of scoliosis correction in relation to flexibility using the fulcrum bending correction index. *Spine* 23:2303–2307.

81. Markolf KL, Morris JM (1974): The structural components of the intervertebral disc. *J Bone Joint Surg Am* 56:675–687.

82. McAfee PC, Farey ID, Sutterlin CE, et al. (1989): Device-related osteoporosis with spinal instrumentation. *Spine* 14:919–926.

83. McAfee PC, Farey ID, Sutterlin CE, et al. (1991): The effect of spinal implant rigidity on vertebral bone density. *Spine* 16:S190–S197.

84. McCarroll JR, Miller JM, Ritter MA (1986): Lumbar spondylolysis and spondylolisthesis in college football players: a prospective study. *Am J Sports Med* 14:404–406.

85. McGill SM, Norman RW, Sharratt MT (1990): The effect of an abdominal belt on trunk muscle activity and intra-abdominal pressure during squat lifts. *Ergonomics* 33:147–160.

86. Meade KP, Bunch WH, Vanderby R Jr, et al. (1987): Progression of unsupported curves in adolescent idiopathic scoliosis. *Spine* 12:520–526.

87. Mente PL, Aronsson DD, Stokes IAF, et al. (1999): Mechanical modulation of growth for the correction of vertebral wedge deformities. *J Orthop Res* 17:518–524.

88. Mielke CH, Lonstein JE, Denis F, et al. (1989): Surgical treatment of adolescent idiopathic scoliosis: a comparative analysis. *J Bone Joint Surg Am* 71:1170–1177.

89. Montgomery F, Willner S (1989): Prognosis of brace-treated scoliosis: comparison of the Boston and Milwaukee methods in 244 girls. *Acta Orthop Scand* 60:383–385.

90. Montgomery F, Willner S, Appelgren G (1990): Long-term follow-up of patients with adolescent idiopathic scoliosis treated conservatively: an analysis of the clinical value of progression. *J Pediatr Orthop* 10:48–52.

91. Moreland MS (1980): Morphological effects of torsion applied to growing bone. *J Bone Joint Surg Br* 62:230–237.

92. Morris JM, Lucas DB, Bresler MS (1961): The role of the trunk in stability of the spine. *J Bone Joint Surg Am* 43:327–351.

93. Nachemson A, Elfström G (1971): Intravital wireless telemetry of axial forces in Harrington distraction rods in patients with idiopathic scoliosis. *J Bone Joint Surg Am* 53:445–465.

94. Nachemson A, Sahlstrand T (1977): Etiologic factors in adolescent idiopathic scoliosis. *Spine* 2:176–184.

95. Owen JH, Naito M, Bridwell KH (1990): Relationship among level of distraction, evoked potentials, spinal cord ischemia and integrity, and clinical status in animals. *Spine* 15:852–857.

96. Owen JH, Naito M, Bridwell KH, et al. (1990): Relationship between duration of spinal cord ischemia and postoperative neurologic deficits in animals. *Spine* 15:846–851.

97. Owen R, Goodfellow J, Bullough P, eds. (1980): *Orthopaedics and traumatology.* London: Heinemann, 92.

98. Panjabi MM (1987): Experimental spinal cord trauma: a biomechanical viewpoint. *Paraplegia* 25:217–220.

99. Panjabi MM (1988): Biomechanical evaluation of spinal fixation devices, I: conceptual framework. *Spine* 13:1129–1134.

100. Panjabi MM (1992): The stabilizing system of the spine, II: neural zone and instability hypothesis. *J Spinal Disord* 5:390–397.

101. Panjabi MM, Brand RM, White AA (1976): Three dimensional flexibility and stiffness properties of the human thoracic spine. *J Biomech* 9:185–192.

102. Panjabi MM, Krag MH, Chung TQ (1984): Effects of disc injury on mechanical behavior of the human spine. *Spine* 9:707–713.

103. Panjabi MM, White AA, Johnson RM (1975): Cervical spine mechanics as a function of transsection of components. *J Biomech* 8:327–336.

104. Panjabi MM, Wrathall JR (1988): Biomechanical analysis of experimental spinal cord injury and functional loss. *Spine* 13:1365–1370.

105. Patwardhan AG, Bunch WH, Meade KP, et al. (1986): A biomechanical analog of curve progression and orthotic stabilization in idiopathic scoliosis. *J Biomech* 19:103–117.

106. Perdriolle R, Becchetti S, Vidal J, et al. (1993): Mechanical process and growth cartilages: essential factors in the progression of scoliosis. *Spine* 18:343–349.

107. Porter RW (1978): The effect of tension across a growing epiphysis. *J Bone Joint Surg Br* 60:252–255.

108. Porter RW, Drinkall JN, Porter DE, et al. (1987): The vertebral canal, II: health and academic status, a clinical study. *Spine* 12:907–911.

109. Porter RW, Pavitt D (1987): The vertebral canal, I: nutrition and development, an archeological study. *Spine* 12:901–906.

110. Rappaport EB, Snoy P, Habig WH, et al. (1987): Effects of exogenous growth hormone on growth plate cartilage in rats. *Am J Dis Child* 141:497–501.

111. Roaf R (1960): Vertebral growth and its mechanical control. *J Bone Joint Surg Br* 42:40–59.

112. Roaf R (1963): The treatment of progressive scoliosis by unilateral growth-arrest. *J Bone Joint Surg Br* 45:637–651.

113. Robin GC (1990): *The aetiology of scoliosis: a review of a century of research.* Boca Raton, FL: CRC Press.

114. Rohlmann A, Bergmann G, Graichen F (1997): Loads on an internal spinal fixation device during walking. *J Biomech* 30:41–47.

115. Rosenberg NJ, Bargar WL, Friedman B (1981): The incidence of spondylolysis and spondylolisthesis in nonambulatory patients. *Spine* 6:35–38.

116. Rosenblum BR, Rothman AS (1991): Low back pain in children. *Mt Sinai J Med* 58:115–120.

117. Ruland CM, McAfee PC, Warden KE, et al. (1991): Triangulation of pedicular instrumentation: a biomechanical analysis. *Spine* 16:S270–S276.

118. Sawatzky BJ, Tredwell SJ, Jang SB, et al. (1998): Effects of three-dimensional assessment on surgical correction and on hook strategies in multi-hook instrumentation for adolescent idiopathic scoliosis. *Spine* 23:201–205.

119. Schultz A, Haderspeck K, Takashima S (1981): Correction of scoliosis by muscle stimulation. Biomechanical analyses. *Spine* 6:468–476.

120. Schultz AB, Haderspeck-Grib K, Sinkora G, et al. (1985): Quantitative studies of the flexion-relaxation phenomenon in the back muscles. *J Orthop Res* 3:189–197.

121. Schultz AB, Hirsch C (1973): Mechanical analysis of Harrington rod correction of scoliosis. *J Bone Joint Surg Am* 55:983–992.

122. Schultz AB, Hirsch C (1974): Mechanical analysis of techniques for improved correction of idiopathic scoliosis. *Clin Orthop* 100:66–73.
123. Scoles PV, Latimer BM, DiGiovanni BF, et al. (1991): Vertebral alterations in Scheuermann's kyphosis. *Spine* 16:509–515.
124. Semon RL, Spengler D (1981): Significance of lumbar spondylolysis in college football players. *Spine* 6:172–174.
125. Shufflebarger HL, Clark CE (1991): Prevention of the crankshaft phenomenon. *Spine* 16:S409–S411.
126. Skalli W, Lavaste F, Robin S, et al. (1993): A biomechanical analysis of short segment spinal fixation using a 3-D geometrical and mechanical model. *Spine* 18:536–545.
127. Skogland LB, Miller JAA (1980): Growth related hormones in idiopathic scoliosis. *Acta Orthop Scand* 51:779.
128. Smith KR, Hunt TR, Asher MA, et al. (1991): The effect of a stiff spinal implant on the bone-mineral content of the lumbar spine in dogs. *J Bone Joint Surg Am* 73:115–123.
129. Solá CK, Silberman FS, Cabrini RL (1963): Stimulation of the longitudinal growth of long bones by periosteal stripping: an experimental study on dogs and monkeys. *J Bone Joint Surg Am* 45:1679–1684.
130. Somerville EW (1952): Rotational lordosis: the development of the single curve. *J Bone Joint Surg Br* 34:421–427.
131. Stewart TD (1953): The age incidence of neural arch defects in Alaskan natives, considered from the standpoint of aetiology. *J Bone Joint Surg Am* 35:937–950.
132. Stokes IAF (1988): Mechanical function of facet joints in the lumbar spine. *Clin Biomech* 3:101–105.
133. Stokes IAF, Gardner-Morse M (1991): Analysis of the interaction between spinal lateral deviation and axial rotation in scoliosis. *J Biomech* 24:753–759.
134. Stokes IAF, Gardner-Morse M (1993): Three-dimensional simulation of Harrington distraction instrumentation for surgical correction of scoliosis. *Spine* 18:2457–2464.
135. Stokes IAF, Laible JP (1990): Three-dimensional osseo-ligamentous model of the thorax representing initiation of scoliosis by asymmetric growth. *J Biomech* 23:589–595.
136. Stokes IAF, Spence H, Aronsson DD, et al. (1996): Mechanical modulation of vertebral body growth: implications for scoliosis progression. *Spine* 21:1162–1167.
137. Subbaraj K, Ghista DN, Viviani GR (1989): Presurgical finite element simulation of scoliosis correction. *J Biomed Eng* 11:9–18.
138. Swank SM, Mauri TM, Brown JC (1990): The lumbar lordosis below Harrington instrumentation for scoliosis. *Spine* 15:181–186.
139. Tesh KM, Dunn JS, Evans JH (1987): The abdominal muscles and vertebral stability. *Spine* 12:501–508.
140. Thometz JG, Emans JB (1988): A comparison between spinous process and sublaminar wiring combined with Harrington distraction instrumentation in the management of adolescent idiopathic scoliosis. *J Pediatr Orthop* 8:129–132.
141. Torbjorn AHL, Albertsson-Wikland K, Kalén R (1988): Twenty-four-hour growth hormone profiles in pubertal girls with idiopathic scoliosis. *Spine* 13:139–142.
142. Trueta J, Amato VP (1960): The vascular contribution to osteogenesis, III: changes in the growth cartilages caused by experimentally induced ischaemia. *J Bone Joint Surg Br* 42:571–587.
143. Tulsi RS (1971): Growth of the human vertebral column: an osteological study. *Acta Anat (Basel)* 79:570–580.
144. Upadhyay SS, Hsu LCS, Ho EKW, et al. (1991): Disproportionate body growth in girls with adolescent idiopathic scoliosis: a longitudinal study. *Spine* 16:S343–S347.
145. Urban JPG, Holm S, Maroudas A, et al. (1982): Nutrition of the intervertebral disc: effect of fluid flow on solute transport. *Clin Orthop* 170:296–302.
146. Vanderby R Jr, Daniele M, Patwardhan A, et al. (1986): A method for the identification of in-vivo segmental stiffness properties of the spine. *J Biomech Eng* 108:312–316.
147. Vaughan JJ, Winter RB, Lonstein JE (1996): Comparison of the use of supine bending and traction radiographs in the selection of the fusion area in adolescent idiopathic scoliosis. *Spine* 21:2469–2473.
148. Veldhuizen AG, Baas P, Webb PJ (1986): Observations on the growth of the adolescent spine. *J Bone Joint Surg Br* 68:724–728.
149. Weatherley CR, Draycott V, O'Brien JF, et al. (1987): The rib deformity in adolescent idiopathic scoliosis: a prospective study to evaluate changes after Harrington distraction and posterior fusion. *J Bone Joint Surg Br* 69:179–182.
150. Weinstein SL, Ponseti IV (1983): Curve progression in idiopathic scoliosis. *J Bone Joint Surg Am* 65:447–455.
151. White AA (1971): Kinematics of the normal spine as related to scoliosis. *J Biomech* 4:405–411.
152. White A III, Hirsch C (1971): The significance of the vertebral posterior elements in the mechanics of the thoracic spine. *Clin Orthop* 81:2–14.
153. White AA, Panjabi MM (1978): Practical biomechanics of spine trauma. In: *Clinical biomechanics of the spine.* Philadelphia: JB Lippincott, pp. 115–190.
154. Willner S (1974): Growth in height of children with scoliosis. *Acta Orthop Scand* 45:854–866.
155. Willner S (1974): A study of growth in girls with adolescent idiopathic structural scoliosis. *Clin Orthop* 101:129–135.
156. Willner S, Johnson B (1983): Thoracic kyphosis and lumbar lordosis during the growth period in children. *Acta Pediatr Scand* 72:873–878.
157. Wiltse LL, Jackson DW (1976): Treatment of spondylolisthesis and spondylolysis in children. *Clin Orthop* 117:93–100.
158. Woo SLY, Hollis JM, Adams DJ, et al. (1991): Tensile properties of the human femur–anterior cruciate ligament–tibia complex: the effects of specimen age and orientation. *Am J Sports Med* 19:217–225.
159. Wood KB, Transfeldt EE, Ogilvie JW, et al. (1991): Rotational changes of the vertebral-pelvic axis following Cotrel-Dubousset instrumentation. *Spine* 16:S404–S408.
160. Wynarsky GT, Schultz AB (1989): Trunk muscle activities in braced scoliosis patients. *Spine* 14:1283–1286.
161. Wynarsky GT, Schultz AB (1991): Optimization of skeletal configuration: studies of scoliosis correction biomechanics. *J Biomech* 24:721–732.

CLINICAL APPLICATION OF BIOMECHANICS

GARY M. BANKS
JAMES D. SCHWENDER
ENSOR E. TRANSFELDT

The spine of a child is not simply a scaled-down version of the spine of an adult. Although axiomatic, this concept is frequently forgotten in the management of pediatric spinal disorders. Making treatment decisions without knowing the unique features of the pediatric spine is akin to prescribing a medication without knowing the mechanism of action of the drug or the side effects. A physician treating a child with a disorder of the spine usually has a general understanding of the structural features unique to the pediatric spine. It also, however, is incumbent on the physician to have a firm understanding of the unique functional features of a child's spine. This chapter is intended to bring the specific functional features of children's spines into clinical perspective.

Knowledge of the biomechanical characteristics of the pediatric spine and the changes with age is particularly important in dealing with pediatric spinal instability and deformity. An understanding of these unique biomechanical features is the cornerstone in the decisions about nonoperative or operative treatment. To achieve a successful outcome, it usually is necessary to address the biomechanical derangements present in the pediatric spinal column. An understanding of the biomechanical principles of the normal and altered pediatric spines with consideration of biologic factors leads to rational treatment decisions for individual patients. Although knowledge of the biomechanics of the pediatric spine remains incomplete, certain principles can be ascertained with our current knowledge.

Clinical error, including inaccurate diagnosis, suboptimal timing of treatment, and poor selection of treatment, may be the result of deviation from biomechanical principles. For example, physicians may diagnose pathologic C2-3 subluxation more often than it actually occurs if they are not aware that pseudosubluxation of C2 on C3 can be caused by the increase in ligamentous laxity and facet orientation that is normal in childhood (27). Conversely, true instability of C2 on C3 may be missed if the limits of physiologic ligamentous laxity are not realized.

The physician must select the procedure with the greatest likelihood of success in dealing with the primary pathologic con-

dition and the fewest potential complications. These two goals are not always met with a given surgical procedure. For example, cervical or thoracic laminectomy provides the most direct approach to spinal cord lesions. However, this procedure on a preadolescent patient is likely to cause progressive kyphosis at the level of the laminectomy (71). Knowledge of ligamentous laxity and the importance of the posterior tension band in these patients would lead to a decision to fuse the vertebrae at the level of the laminectomy. Knowledge of the plasticity of an immature posterior fusion mass in very young patients may lead to a decision to use localized instrumentation or a postoperative orthosis until the fusion consolidates. These examples highlight the clinical problems that can occur when there is no strong biomechanical or biologic rationale for treatment selection and implementation. The rest of this chapter describes basic biomechanical principles of the normal and pathologic pediatric spine and how these principles can be applied to clinical decision making.

BIOMECHANICAL PRINCIPLES SPECIFIC TO THE PEDIATRIC SPINE

One cannot understand specific pathologic conditions without understanding the biomechanical features that differentiate the normal spine of a child from the normal spine of an adult. These features are closely related to basic tissue differences and to capacity for growth and remodeling. The clinical utility of these principles also is discussed. Table 1 lists the basic biomechanical features typical of the pediatric spine. The following sections present a thesis for understanding the biomechanics of the pediatric spine.

Growth

A clear difference between the pediatric and the adult spine is that the pediatric spine is actively growing. Growth applies forces to the spine, the magnitude of which varies with the rate of growth. Because the growth velocity is highest in infant and adolescents, it is expected that the resulting forces applied to the spine are greatest at these ages. Even though they are not great, the forces that result from growth may change spinal structure because they are applied over long periods of time. In normal

J. D. Schwender and E. E. Transfeldt: Twin Cities Spine Center, Minneapolis, Minnesota 55404.

G. M. Banks: Advanced Spine, Plymouth, Minnesota 55441.

TABLE 1. BIOMECHANICAL FEATURES OF PEDIATRIC SPINES THAT DIFFERTIATE THEM FROM ADULT SPINES

Growth
Adaptability
Malleability
Hypermobility
Growth plate as weak link
Changes in mechanical properties with age
Development of structural sagittal contours with age
Changes in applied forces with age
Regenerative capability
Immature neuromuscular control

spinal growth, anterior and posterior growth and side to side growth are balanced. The result is lengthening of the spinal column with relatively small change in its gross contours. If, however, a pathologic condition causes asymmetric growth, the force vectors change and cause deformity. This is exemplified by anterior fusion, congenital or surgically induced, in a child. Because the anterior structures no longer grow but the posterior structures continue to grow, a progressive kyphotic deformity results (114).

The forces applied by asymmetric growth can be used to produce the progressive correction of congenital scoliotic curvature. This is the rationale for convex hemiepiphysiodesis for congenital scoliosis (115). Any correction obtained depends on the magnitude and rate of remaining growth on the concave side. Defects of segmentation lack concave growth, and convex hemiepiphysiodesis does not correct the deformity if the procedure is limited to the area of congenital anomaly. In contrast, a defect of formation can have considerable remaining growth potential, and the possibility exists that curve correction can be obtained with this technique. The often difficult to determine remaining spinal growth must be carefully considered in the management of pediatric spinal disorders. The ultimate goal should be to achieve a balanced spine.

The crankshaft phenomenon, which causes a progressive increase in curvature and rotational deformity, is an example of how spinal growth complicates the management of deformities of the pediatric spine. This phenomenon occurs in patients with immature skeletons who undergo isolated posterior fusion for the management of scoliosis. Despite solid fusion, progressive bending of the plastic posterior fusion mass can be caused by continued anterior growth of the spine at the fused levels (37). As expected, the risk of progression after posterior fusion is related to the amount of anterior growth remaining. Risk factors include being younger than 10 years of age at the time of fusion, Risser sign 0, or the presence of open triradiate cartilage (48,69,95,98). Progressive bending is common under these circumstances and can occur despite the presence of a thick fusion mass and rigid instrumentation. Anterior and posterior fusion often is recommended to prevent the crankshaft phenomenon among this population (68). Congenital scoliosis appears to carry lower risk of the crankshaft phenomenon than does idiopathic scoliosis, likely because of the limited growth potential remaining among many children with congenital scoliosis (37).

Adaptability

The pediatric spine can adapt to applied stresses much more readily than can the adult spine. This is related to growth potential, the lower modulus of elasticity, and prominent remodeling capability. The result of this adaptability is that a child often can maintain a functional level in the presence of a serious pathologic condition. For example, a large thoracic scoliosis curvature in a child is likely to be associated with a compensatory lumbar curve that causes net balance of the head over the pelvis. Despite this considerable spinal deformity, a child often continues to function well because of the compensatory mechanisms (63). Although immature musculoskeletal tissues have considerable capability to adapt and remodel, neural tissues do not have the same capability; this disparity can cause serious clinical problems (see later).

Malleability

In addition to being adaptable, which implies an active process, the pediatric spine also is substantially malleable. *Malleability,* a passive process, implies that the spine may be deformed with the application of a force external to the spinal column. One adverse outcome related to malleability is the scoliosis that often rapidly occurs after unilateral rib resection in a child (31). The same procedure is unlikely to cause progressive deformity in an adult. Malleability is a reflection of the intrinsic elasticity of ligamentous tissues and the modulus of bone. With maturation of these tissues, malleability decreases rapidly. This is one of the reasons the use of orthotic devices for the correction of deformities loses effectiveness with maturation (26). Malleability also is an important quality of the bony elements, as in spondylolisthesis, in which the pars interarticularis may undergo extensive elongation before fracture (57).

A corollary to malleability is that the pediatric spine is able to absorb considerable energy before failure. This partially accounts for the lower incidence of fractures of the spine among children than among adults (55). A spinal cord injury also can occur in a child without radiographic abnormality (*SCIWORA*) (62,65,89). In many cases, spinal cord injury is caused by over-distraction of the spinal cord, which is less elastic than young ligamentous tissues. Injury also may be caused by transient subluxation of vertebrae even though the ligamentous and bony elements are structurally intact.

Hypermobility

The physiologic range of motion of the pediatric spine is considerably greater than that of the adult spines. This is the result of differences in ligamentous restraints and orientation of the facet joint (110). In athletic activities such as gymnastics this hypermobility can be beneficial, but it generally is of questionable functional value. For example, among female gymnasts, spinal hypermobility can be accentuated to an extreme, as exemplified by the hyperextension used in back walkovers. This, however, exceeds the physiologic hypermobility of childhood, and the concentrated extension forces cause a high frequency of stress fractures of the susceptible pars interarticularis (58). Hypermobility must be appreciated in the assessment of patients with disorders such as pseudosubluxation of C2 on C3 (27). Physiologic hypermobility does not cause pathologic conditions when subjected to normal forces. Thus pseudosubluxation does not cause narrowing of the spinal canal. In general, physiologic hypermobility of the axial skeleton generally parallels that of the appendicular joints. These features can be used to assist in differentiating physiologic from pathologic hypermobility.

Weak Growth Plate

The growth plate is the weakest link in the axial skeleton when it is subjected to tensile forces. This has important implications for the types of injury most likely to occur in the pediatric spine. Odontoid injuries usually occur through the physeal plate, located near the base of the odontoid process (100). These are often in a position nearly equivalent to that of type II odontoid fractures in adults and are similarly unstable. However, because the pediatric injury occurs through the growth plate, the healing potential is high, and nonunion is infrequent. Because the spine does not have posterior column growth plates that can absorb traumatic force, injuries to the ligamentous and bony elements of the posterior column do occur. Physeal injuries frequently accompany disc protrusions among children. As an anular fragment protrudes from the disc space, traction through the ring apophysis avulses a fragment of bony end plate. This accounts for the present of extruded bony fragments on radiographs of the spines of these patients (8).

Changing Spinal Contours

The sagittal spinal contour begins as a gentle *C* arc. Secondary lordotic cervical and lumbar curves are added to this kyphotic curve with development. The development of these secondary curves has considerable biomechanical relevance, because the transitional regions between lordotic and kyphotic curvatures are regions of stress concentration and are susceptible to deformation. The predominance of burst fractures at the thoracolumbar junction is related to this stress concentration (110). It appears that the sagittal curve partially stabilizes the spine against the development of rotational and coronal plane deformity. With rapid spinal growth, as occurs during the adolescent growth spurt, anterior spinal growth appears to exceed posterior growth in many instances and to decrease thoracic lordosis. This may leave the spine susceptible to both rotational and coronal plane deformities, which cause scoliosis (103).

Changing Applied Forces

The forces to which the spine is subjected are important in the initiation, perpetuation, or exacerbation of various spinal diseases. These day-to-day forces change substantially during the process of growth and development. In infancy, the child is generally protected from large forces, partially as a result of a low level of activity. However, the head of an infant is large in relation to body mass; this is a potential source of considerable force during acceleration or deceleration. The force that this applies to the cervical spine can have devastating consequences (32,51). This vulnerability decreases with age with the decrease in the proportion of head to body mass, stabilization of the neck lever arm, and maturation of neuromusculoskeletal defenses against injury. The importance of lengthening spinal lever arms with growth is well known to physicians experienced in bracing. It is difficult to obtain adequate curve control with orthoses for very young patients with short spinal lever arms and abundant body fat (21).

The day-to-day forces to which a child is subjected usually increase through early childhood as play becomes more vigorous. Play is random at first, but as children become involved with organized sports they are more likely to be exposed to repetitive stress. It is at this time that the child becomes vulnerable to spinal disorders due to fatigue (34). These include spondylolisthesis, spondylolysis, disc protrusion, and muscle strain.

Immature Neuromuscular Control System

Myelination of the central nervous system is completed during the first 2 years of life. Balance and coordinated neuromuscular activities, however, continue to develop throughout childhood. The implications of this immaturity are, first, that the skeletal system, including the spine, is exposed to increased risk of injury. Second, immature motor control may predispose the child to conditions such as scoliosis (124). Postural equilibrium and balance require the complex integration of sensory stimuli from the proprioceptive, visual, and vestibular systems with control of the motor systems. Subtle abnormalities of this system may underlie at least some cases of idiopathic scoliosis (99,112).

Application of Biomechanical Principles to Clinical Practice

The importance of biomechanical principles depends on the specific clinical scenario. The rest of this chapter focuses on the application of basic biomechanical principles to the management of specific spinal disorders. Because biomechanical knowledge has its most profound effect on the management of spinal instabilities and deformities, the discussion is limited to these entities.

SCOLIOSIS

Three-dimensional Assessment of the Spine

The clinically important biomechanical features of scoliosis can be divided into those that are important in the initiation, progression, and management of curves. The three-dimensional nature of the deformity has been recognized because the original anatomic descriptions of scoliosis. Despite this, it is only in the last decade that the importance of the associated deformities in planes other than the coronal has come to light. The noncoronal plane components of the deformity appear to have both etiologic and therapeutic significance. Evidence suggests that decreased thoracic kyphosis and rotational deformity are important in the initiation of scoliotic curves. The importance of rotational deformity of the spine as a potential complication also has been

TABLE 2. BIOMECHANICAL FEATURES IMPORTANT IN EVALUATIONS FOR SCOLIOSIS

Spine
  Coronal curves
  Saqittal curves
  Rotational components
  Temporal analysis
Thoracic cage
  Paravertebral prominence
  Pulmonary function
Entire body
  Leg length
  Pelvic inclination
  Trunk shift
  Shoulder inclination
  C7 balance
  Occipital balance

stressed. It is essential that a physician managing scoliosis be adept at performing three-dimensional assessment of the spine, trunk, and entire body (Table 2). The findings must then be used in conjunction with biologic information and knowledge of the biomechanics of treatment modalities to arrive at the best therapeutic approach for a given patient.

A detailed clinical and radiographic assessment of a patient with scoliosis focuses not only on the various components of the spinal deformity but also on the resulting biomechanical alterations that occur in the trunk and the rest of the body. The spine must be evaluated to determine the magnitude and rigidity of the coronal, sagittal, and rotational deformities. This information must then be correlated with the effect of the spinal deformity on the function of the entire patient to assist in determining the best treatment.

The most obvious spinal deformity in scoliosis usually is curvature in the coronal plane. Radiographic evaluation of the magnitude of this curve has been standardized with the Cobb method. However, attempts to predict associated spinal and other deformities on the basis of the Cobb angle have met with little success (52). The magnitude of associated sagittal and rotational deformities does not correlate with the magnitude of the Cobb angle. This indicates that other factors are implicated in the development of the associated deformities. Despite poor correlation, there is excellent biomechanical evidence that spinal motions in different planes are coupled—deformity in the coronal plane affects the spinal configuration in the other planes (109). In the midthoracic spine, however, coupling is not entirely predictable. Ohlen et al. (87) showed that thoracic kyphosis among patients with idiopathic scoliosis was less than that among controls with normal spines. However, the degree of kyphosis or lordosis did not correlate with the Cobb angles.

Among most patients with thoracic scoliosis, rotation occurs and causes the spinous processes at the apex of the curve to rotate toward the concavity of the curve. However, nonstandard vertebral rotation is present in many patients with scoliosis. Most commonly this involves rotation that extends more than one segment beyond the end vertebra. Armstrong et al. (6) showed that rotation of the vertebral bodies to the side opposite the major curve occurred among 7% of the patients in their series.

As a result of this variability, the three-dimensional nature of curves must be assessed individually to determine optimal treatment regimens. These associated deformities may have a considerable functional effect on the patient. Rotation of the spine influences the perception of the sagittal and coronal plane deformities; this occurs because a lateral curvature is rotated out of the frontal plane. If there is substantial curve rotation, a spine that is lordotic may appear kyphotic on a standard lateral radiograph. For this reason, Stagnara et al. (104) described radiographs in the true plane of the deformity to assess scoliosis with a marked rotational component. These radiographs are not used frequently in scoliosis management in North America; however, the influence of rotational deformities on the assessment of coronal and frontal plane deformities should be kept in mind.

Assessment of spinal rotation with plain radiographs has been shown to be of limited accuracy. Both the Moe and Pedriolle methods have been shown to have measurement errors greater than 5 degrees. Assessment of vertebral rotation with plain radiographs is further complicated for curves greater than 50 degrees, with which deformities of the vertebral elements are common (3). For this reason, transverse computed tomographic sections with the vertebrae referenced to the thorax have been used for research. Accuracy within 0.3 degrees with vertebrae tilted up to 20 degrees in the sagittal and frontal planes has been reported with this technique (2). Aaro and Dhalborn (3) also found that vertebral rotation correlates roughly with the size of the lateral curve but not with the location or length of the curve.

Surgical improvement of vertebral rotation with instrumentation in idiopathic scoliosis is unpredictable at best (4). Wojcik et al. (119) found that the rotational correction obtained with Cotrel-Dubousset instrumentation is inconsistent. Wood et al. (120) pointed out that studies of rotational correction should reference vertebral correction to the pelvis, not to other vertebrae. These authors found that the entire vertebropelvic axis rotated around the frontal plane and that no selective derotation of the apical vertebrae occurred after Cotrel-Dubousset instrumentation. Wojcik et al. (119) also found no consistent rotational correction of the apical vertebrae of thoracic curves when segmental sublaminar wiring was used. These results were confirmed by Hullin et al. (56), who found that the rib hump often worsened with sublaminar wiring of thoracic curves. Hullin et al. found Luque wiring effective in achieving three-dimensional correction of thoracolumbar and lumbar curves. The reason for the difference in rotational correction according to curve location is unknown, but it may be related to the sequence of application of the Luque rods. Further therapeutic implications of spinal deformities outside the coronal plane are discussed later.

Static three-dimensional analysis of spinal deformity should be supplemented with an analysis of the flexibility of or ability to correct any deformities. General assessment of spinal flexibility can be made by means of clinical examination, but a more precise evaluation includes radiographic assessment. Supine side-bending radiographs have been used most frequently to assess spinal flexibility. The comparative value of standing, side-bending radiographs, manual pressure over curve apexes, and traction radiographs has not been scientifically assessed. These technical variations in the assessment of spinal flexibility may affect the magnitude of measured flexibility. Biomechanical data certainly indicate that longitudinal forces are more effective than transverse forces in achieving correction of curves greater than 55 degrees (110). This suggests the usefulness of traction in assessing large curves. The viscoelastic properties of the spine have not been accounted for in any of these assessments, so the bending time before radiography has not been standardized. Current methods for evaluating the flexibility of a curve are imprecise but are useful in patient care.

Bending radiographs contribute several factors to the biomechanical assessment of scoliosis, including assessment of the flexibility of major and compensatory curves, evaluation of the mobile disc spaces, and determination of which vertebrae become horizontal and come into the stable zone with side bending. Assessment of the flexibility of the curve provides a rough guide to the potential responsiveness to bracing and suggests the curve correction that can be obtained with surgery. The correlation between predicted preoperative correction based on bending radiographs and ultimate curve correction generally is good. However, the force generation that may be applied segmentally with Cotrel-Dubousset instrumentation and newer segmental devices often produces greater correction than predicted preoperatively. Overcorrection can cause postoperative decompensation and should be avoided (107). The lowest vertebra to become horizontal and stabilize with side bending and is adjacent to a mobile disc space determines the lowest level for Cotrel-Dubousset instrumentation. When a large and rigid lumbar curve is present, it is important that the distal end vertebra involved in instrumentation meet these criteria (10). This provides a stable and well-aligned caudal foundation for instrumentation and correction of the proximal curves and minimizes the risk of decompensation of the coronal plane with instrumentation.

In addition to the static and dynamic assessment of the three-dimensional spinal deformity, the clinical evaluation should define the chest wall deformity. This involves evaluation of the appearance of the paravertebral prominence and functional evaluation of thoracic capacity and pulmonary function. The paravertebral prominence in scoliosis is composed of the transverse processes, posterior aspects of the ribs, scapula, and overlying muscles on the convexity of the curve. The magnitude of the paravertebral prominence does not correlate well with the measured Cobb angle or with measured vertebral rotation at the curve apex. Aaro and Dahlborn (2) found that patients with early scoliosis often have clinically apparent posterior thoracic prominences, despite the absence of rotational deformity of the vertebrae. It appears that deformities of the ribs may play an important part in the development of rib humps (108). In addition, changes in the costovertebral joints may contribute to the rib prominence. The costovertebral joints allow motion, primarily in the coronal plane, as occurs with respiration. Because the cross-sectional contour of the ribs changes considerably depending on the cranial-caudal angulation of the ribs, minor changes in this angulation may have considerable effect on the perceived magnitude of the paravertebral prominence (3). Other factors that may contribute to the incomplete coupling between the convex paravertebral prominence and the severity of spinal deformity include asymmetric rib growth and accompanying deformities of the transverse processes and scapula.

Decrease in the paravertebral prominence can occur as a result

of coronal plane correction with minimal rotational correction of the spine, because the convex ribs may change from a horizontal to a more vertical pattern. This likely accounts for the often marked improvement in the paravertebral prominence with Cotrel-Dubousset instrumentation in the management of adolescent idiopathic scoliosis, despite only inconsistent rotational correction. However, clinical studies of instrumentation for scoliosis have shown that the posterior thoracic prominences may persist despite excellent correction of the spinal deformity (23,85,93). This has been demonstrated for Harrington, Harrington-Luque, and Cotrel-Dubousset instrumentation. Wojcik et al. (119) showed that the convex rib drooping present in idiopathic scoliosis usually is not corrected with segmental sublaminar wiring or Cotrel-Dubousset instrumentation. This may contribute to residual rib prominence. Persistent thoracic deformity may be caused by convex rib deformities (108), which may be managed best with spinal instrumentation and fusion combined with thoracoplasty. Although the main concern about the paravertebral prominence has been appearance, there is potential for biomechanical derangement of the scapulothoracic articulation. Some of our patients have had convex scapulothoracic pain or clicking with motion in association with a large convex paravertebral prominence. The functional importance of the paravertebral prominence to the scapulothoracic articulation remains unclear.

An important aspect of thoracic deformity is thoracic volume and, closely associated with this, dynamic pulmonary function. Thoracic volume is a complex measurement obtained with sophisticated techniques—either digitized radiography or computed tomography (86)—generally not performed in the clinic. Calculated thoracic volume is a reflection of the spinal deformities in the coronal and sagittal planes, the decrease in thoracic height, rib deformities, and elevation of the diaphragm. Ogilvie and Schendel (86) found that loss of thoracic kyphosis is the factor that correlates most closely with decreased thoracic volume in idiopathic scoliosis. Although actual thoracic volume is not measured, the sagittal plane alignment has considerable influence on thoracic volume and must be accounted for in clinical decision making. Dynamic measurements of pulmonary function in scoliosis obtained with spirometry must be interpreted with full knowledge that this measurement depends on patient effort and may have limited reproducibility. Despite the limitations, pulmonary function testing is frequently used (66). Pulmonary function is related to thoracic volume and thoracic muscle activity, both of which may be limited in scoliosis. Because the respiratory capacity of the thoracic musculature in scoliosis may be limited, particularly in neuromuscular scoliosis, improvement of thoracic volume may not produce similar improvement in pulmonary function. This appears to be particularly true with operative correction of curves greater than 90 degrees (66).

The final component of biomechanical assessment of the deformity in scoliosis involves determining how the spinal and thoracic deformities relate to the structure and balance of the entire patient. This often is the most functionally important portion of the assessment and requires knowledge of leg length discrepancy, pelvic inclination and rotation, lateral trunk shift, shoulder tilting, and C7 and occipital balance in both the coronal and sagittal planes. Understanding how the spinal deformity relates to the lower extremities, pelvic and shoulder girdles, and head position allows planning of treatment to address the most important components of the deformity for a given patient. Patients with large curves may be well balanced in the coronal and sagittal planes, and balance may be impaired with inadequately planned surgery (75). A patient's main concern may be related to shoulder obliquity or rotation of the shoulder girdle with respect to the pelvic girdle. If these concerns are not addressed with treatment, the patient may be dissatisfied despite excellent correction of the spinal deformity. The relations of structures at the cranial end of the spine to those at the caudal end often is more functionally important than the intervening scoliotic curves. The complex nature of the spinal deformity and the associated deformity of the body necessitates individualized assessment and management of scoliosis.

Leg length discrepancy may affect the pelvis and the spine. It appears that a leg length discrepancy greater than 2.5 cm is associated with a high incidence of scoliosis, often in the lumbar region, that usually is of small magnitude and is nonprogressive (90). A leg length discrepancy probably exerts its influence on the spine as a result of righting reflexes that act to maintain the patient's center of gravity in a stable position. Correction of the leg length discrepancy can resolve the curvature; however, Papaioannou et al. (90) showed that appreciable, although minor, lumbar scoliosis remains in many patients after neutralization of the discrepancy. Because leg length discrepancy causes pelvic obliquity that can be reversed initially with sitting, the patient's coronal plane balance may shift considerably between the standing and sitting positions. As the spine becomes more rigid with time, the ability to compensate for shifting balance becomes limited. As a result, it is important to attempt to account for the shifts in C7 or occipital balance that can occur with correction of a limb length discrepancy in a patient with scoliosis.

Pelvic obliquity can be caused by infrapelvic or suprapelvic problems (114). Infrapelvic problems include leg length discrepancy and iliotibial band contracture. Suprapelvic causes include neuromuscular imbalance and the fractional lumbosacral curve in scoliosis. The forces that contribute to the development of the pelvic obliquity also frequently cause an associated scoliotic deformity, particularly in the lumbar spine. Marked fixed pelvic obliquity in association with lumbar scoliosis may necessitate fusion to the pelvis with possible correction of the pelvic inclination with respect to the lumbar spine. If pelvic obliquity in this scenario is not addressed, the potential for producing an unbalanced spine is high.

Asymmetry of shoulder levels often is a problem among patients with scoliosis, particularly those with high thoracic curves. Most children without scoliosis have some normal shoulder asymmetry, mainly depression of the dominant shoulder. In any case, it is desirable to obtain reasonably level shoulders at the completion of treatment, because this is a potential source of patient dissatisfaction.

The combination of leg length discrepancy and pelvic inclination with the spinal curves determines whether the spine and the patient are balanced with the head centered over the pelvis. Although the relation of the occiput to the sacrum in the coronal and sagittal planes may be the most meaningful measurement, the relation of C7 to the sacrum is more commonly measured because this can be done readily measured on standing anteroposterior radiographs of the spine. It is important to realize that the occipital shift, which may be more important to the patient's perception of balance, may be substantially different from the C7 shift, particularly when curves extend into the cervical spine. In the frontal plane, the C7 plumb line should fall close to the midsacral line. Healthy children may show up to 2 cm of lateral shift from the midsacral line in neutral standing; this tends to decrease with age, possibly as a result of neural maturation (7). The mechanisms controlling spinal balance are poorly understood, as are the specific functional limitations caused by coronal imbalance.

In the sagittal plane, C7 is normally centered over the body of S2. Iatrogenic loss of lumbar lordosis (surgical flat back) often is associated with anterior displacement of C7 relative to S2 (67). The patient may be able to partially compensate and maintain C7 balance by means of extensor spinae contraction, hyperlordosis of the cervical spine, and knee flexion. Further implications of flat back syndrome are discussed later.

Initiation of Scoliosis

Numerous theories of the cause of idiopathic scoliosis have been presented in the literature over the past 50 years. Most of these have been disproved. Produced of melatonin by the pineal gland has been implicated as a possible etiologic factor. What is known is that melatonin deficiency caused by pinealectomy among chickens causes scoliosis. Machida (74) found lower melatonin levels among children with progressive curves than among children with normal spines. Hilibrand et al. (53), however, found no correlation when they compared children with and without scoliosis.

Subtle abnormalities of neuromuscular balance may be an important cause of idiopathic scoliosis. In much of the research in this area, it is difficult to differentiate primary from secondary abnormalities (124); however, abnormalities of postural control identified in the siblings without scoliosis of patients with scoliosis suggest that these may be of etiologic importance. Abnormal otolithic vestibular function has been found among children with scoliosis (112). Asymmetry of paraspinous muscle activity among patients with scoliosis also has been identified, but there is no evidence to suggest that this asymmetry is of primary importance in scoliosis.

Studies have emphasized biomechanical and structural changes early in the scoliotic process that may be of etiologic importance (Table 3). Experimental and clinical studies indicate that loss of normal thoracic kyphosis can cause a situation in which the spine is unstable during rotation and lateral bending (33). Using derotated views of the spine, Deacon et al. (29) showed with radiographs that patients with idiopathic scoliosis have less thoracic kyphosis than do children with normal spines. Although routine lateral views erroneously indicated a mean thoracic kyphosis of 41 degrees, derotated views showed actual lordosis of 14 degrees on average. Loss of thoracic kyphosis may occur if posterior spinal growth lags behind growth in the anterior spinal column. A linked column such as the spine loses

TABLE 3. BIOMECHANICAL FACTORS IN THE INITIATION AND PROGRESSION OF IDIOPATHIC SCOLIOSIS

Initiation
  Immature balance
  Hypokyphosis and rotational instability
  Nonstandard vertebral rotation
  Muscle imbalance
Progression
  Gravity effects
  Decrease in concave growth (Hueter-Volkmann law)

TABLE 4. BIOMECHANICAL PRINCIPLES OF MANAGEMENT OF SCOLIOSIS

Primary goals
  Prevent progression of deformity
  Correct spinal deformity
Secondary goals
  Balance spine, pelvis, and shoulders (coronal, sagittal, and rotational)
  Maintain mobile low lumbar segments
  Restore and maintain sagittal contours
Tertiary goals
  Increase truncal height
  Achieve cosmetic correction

stability when it is lengthened and straightened (110). This may allow rotational and coronal plane deformities to develop.

Another observation of potential etiologic importance in idiopathic scoliosis is that the direction of coupled rotation in the midthoracic spine is opposite that which occurs in other regions of the spine. With lateral bending in the midthoracic spine, the spinous processes rotate into the concavity of the curvature. Such nonstandard coupling of rotation and lateral bending may produce a rotationally unstable situation that may progress to the complete deformity of scoliosis (6). These theories must be described as interesting but speculative. They do not explain why certain persons and families are more prone to develop scoliosis than are others. Although the cause of idiopathic scoliosis remains unknown, it appears likely that biomechanical factors combine to produce a spine that lacks the stability to prevent axial rotation and bending in the coronal plane.

Progression of the Curve

The same factors that are involved in the initiation of scoliosis may be important in progression of the curve. Additional factors of probable importance in the progression of the deformity, particularly with larger curves, are the effects of gravity and asymmetric spinal growth. Biomechanical models have shown that the effects of gravity are more important than asymmetric functional capabilities of muscles in determining curve progression (45). As curves become larger, gravity applies an increasing bending force to the curvature in the upright posture. The deforming forces of gravity theoretically are more important in longer curves, in which there is a longer lever arm. Increasing deformity also is associated with increasing asymmetry of the force applied to the spinal growth plates. The increased concave pressure inhibits growth on this side of the spine, in accordance with the Hueter-Volkmann law. The result is progression of the deformity. Mente and Stokes et al. (80,105) applied the Hueter-Volkmann law experimentally in a rat tail model and found vertebrae loaded asymmetrically produced vertebral wedging due to asymmetric growth in the physis.

Biomechanics of the Management of Scoliosis

The primary goal in treating patients with scoliosis is to stabilize the curves to prevent further progression of the deformity (Table 4). Closely related to this is the goal of achieving correction of spinal deformity, although this is not part of the therapeutic regimen for every patient. The optimal treatment in a specific situation achieves the primary goal of prevention of curve progression and addresses as many secondary goals as possible. Treatment that neglects secondary goals can produce the unacceptable biomechanical situation of impaired function and possibly cause late pain.

The prevention of curve progression must counter the forces that tend to cause progression. The force causing progression is greatest in large curves in which gravity applies a bending force (45) and in young patients, among whom asymmetric spinal growth can accentuate the deformity. Methods for decreasing curve progression include decreasing the deforming force, applying a compensatory force, or a combination of these methods. Decreasing the deforming force can be achieved by means of decreasing the magnitude of curves with casting, bracing, or instrumentation. Decreasing the deforming force induced by asymmetric growth can be achieved by means of decreasing curve size or fusing the growing segments.

The compensatory force that can be applied by external devices usually is limited. External devices often are successful in neutralizing the deforming forces of small to moderate-sized curves (less than 40 degrees). In larger curves (40 to 50 degrees) the effectiveness of orthotic devices depends on achieving a substantial decrease in curve size and deforming forces (26).

Curve correction is not necessarily the primary goal in surgical treatment of patients with scoliosis. Correction of curves in the coronal plane may be useful for decreasing the deforming forces on the spine and for improving some aspects of appearance, but curve correction must be carefully coordinated with an overall plan to maintain the coronal, sagittal, and rotational balance of the patient. The issue of how much correction is appropriate for a patient is based on a risk to benefit analysis. With a rigid curve, correction may necessitate combined anterior and posterior procedures or may place undue stress on the instrumentation. In such cases, the benefits of curve correction may not be justified. The risk of traction on neural elements also must be accounted for in obtaining curve correction. There is no specific level of residual curvature that is best for all patients; this must be decided on an individual basis.

The biomechanics of obtaining curve correction have been studied extensively (110). The forces applied can include transverse loading, longitudinal traction on the curve concavity,

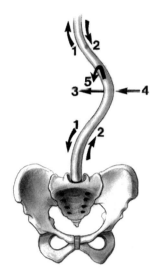

FIGURE 1. Schematic representation of force vectors that can affect correction of a spinal deformity. *1,* Concave distraction; *2,* convex compression; *3,* transverse force pulling the curve toward concavity; *4,* transverse force applied at curve apex; *5,* rotation of curve from coronal to sagittal plane.

compression on the curve convexity, and rotational forces (Fig. 1). With curves less than 55 degrees, transverse loading forces are the most effective in reducing the magnitude of the curve. For curves larger than 55 degrees, the force vectors change appreciably, making concave longitudinal distraction more effective than transverse loading. The usefulness of convex compression in correcting the deformity is substantially limited by the short lever arms provided by the transverse processes. Convex compression of large curves may actually apply a force that worsens the deformity, because the compressive force vector passes through the curve concavity. Rotational forces may improve the contours in both the coronal and the sagittal plane, but the actual rotational correction obtained with current instrumentation systems is limited. Correction with these systems may occur through a combination of transverse loading and longitudinal distraction.

Spinal deformities combine with the positions of the pelvis, shoulders, and head to determine whether the patient is balanced in the coronal and sagittal planes. A double curve in which there is a rigid and poorly aligned low lumbar curve often causes imbalance when the thoracic curve is corrected. This cause, at least in part, is inability of the rigid, caudal regions of the spine to compensate for changes induced in the midthoracic and thoracolumbar regions. Loss of spinal balance may produce an appearance that is worse than the initial deformity. Maintenance of sagittal contours also considerably improves the likelihood of a successful results of treatment.

An attempt must be made to preserve mobile motion segments in the lower lumbar spine. It is ideal that at least three healthy, mobile segments in the lower lumbar spine be preserved to avoid inordinate stresses on the remaining motion segments. Cochran and Nachemson (28) found that the incidence of serious low back pain increases from about 20% with fusion that

extends to L3 to 80% with fusion that extends down to L5. Maintenance of mobile distal lumbar segments is a problem with large lumbar curves in which instrumentation must be extended into the lower lumbar spine. The distal extent of fusion can be minimized with the use of anterior instrumentation or posterior segmental instrumentation supplemented with pedicle screws.

A basic component of many scoliosis curves is decreased thoracic kyphosis. One surgical goal in this population is to increase thoracic kyphosis. This may be achieved through the use of Luque instrumentation with sublaminar wiring that pulls the vertebrae posteriorly to contact the contoured rods (60). The use of segmental instrumentation devices may achieve increased thoracic kyphosis with less neurologic risk than that of sublaminar wiring. Kalen and Conklin (60) showed that correction of thoracic kyphosis does not increase lordosis in the lumbar spine on which instrumentation is not performed.

The importance of preventing iatrogenic flat-back deformity should be emphasized. As the name implies, flat-back deformity consists of loss of lumbar lordosis. Normal lumbar lordosis broadly ranges from 20 to 80 degrees (11). Iatrogenic flat-back syndrome is defined as a loss of lumbar lordosis that causes low back pain, upper and middle thoracic pain, cervical muscular strain, and knee pain (30). Lagrone et al. (67) found that the flat-back syndrome is most common when distraction instrumentation is extended into the lower lumbar spine or the sacrum. The next most common predisposing factor is preoperative thoracolumbar junctional kyphosis greater than 15 degrees. It appears that this complication can be minimized with knowledge of the sagittal plane contours and avoidance of the use of distraction instrumentation in the lower lumbar spine (106). Because surgical correction of flat-back deformity is a major procedure that necessitates an osteotomy such as a Smith-Peterson or pedicle subtraction osteotomy, avoidance of this complication is paramount.

Biomechanics of Orthotic Treatment

The effectiveness of orthotic treatment in preventing progression or achieving correction of a deformity is determined primarily on the basis of the factors in Table 5. The deforming force vectors interact with the orthotically applied force vectors to give a resultant or net force that determines the tendency of the spine to undergo correction or further deformation. This interaction can be represented as a balance with deforming forces on one side and applied or correcting forces on the other. The resistance

TABLE 5. FACTORS THAT DETERMINE THE EFFECTIVENESS OF ORTHOTICS

Deforming force, which depends on
  Spinal growth
  Severity of deformity
Applied force properties
  Magnitude
  Location
  Direction
  Temporal aspects
Spinal malleability or rigidity

to change represents spinal malleability or rigidity. This resistance decreases the effects of the resultant force on the spine. Greater forces are needed to effect changes in less malleable curves.

The primary factors determining the deforming forces are the rate of spinal growth (application of asymmetric forces to the spine) and the size of the curve (increasing the deforming effect of gravity). This biomechanical model is supported by results of clinical studies, which indicate that the remaining spinal growth and magnitude of the curve are most important in determining whether a curve progresses (72). The directional component of the applied force may be complex and three-dimensional, complicating this model.

There are several important aspects to the corrective forces applied by an orthotic device, including magnitude, location, direction, and temporal qualities. The magnitude of the corrective forces depends on the type and fit of the brace. These forces can be produced by passive correction by the brace or by the patient's active postural reaction to the brace. Passive correction is limited by patient tolerance of the direct pressure applied by the brace. Active correction is limited by the muscular forces that the patient can exert for prolonged periods. Studies have suggested that a patient's active postural reaction in the brace may be the most important force leading to correction (5,83). In either case, the applied forces usually are not large.

Traditional orthoses rely on the principle of three-point fixation to apply corrective forces to a deformity (21). Adequate force generation with this system depends on separation of the two end points from the central (apical) point of pressure application (Fig. 2). This creates adequate lever arms for force generation. The Milwaukee brace is a cervicothoracolumbosacral orthosis that is capable of producing adequate lever arms for the management of most curves, except those in the high thoracic region. Successful use of a thoracolumbosacral orthosis (TLSO) is restricted to curves with apexes below T7 (39); this is likely related to the shorter lever arm produced when cervical extension is not used.

It appears that bracing may provide some rotational correction of the scoliotic spine. Aaro et al. (1) showed that an average of 38% correction of rotation was achieved with the use of the Boston brace. However, the amount of correction varied dramatically among patients. Because it is unpredictable, rotational correction cannot be a prime goal of orthotic treatment. The ability of the Milwaukee brace to achieve correction of spinal decompensation was studied by Rudicel and Renshaw (97). The braces used were found to be inadequate for correction of spinal balance. It remains unclear whether adding trochanteric extensions to the brace improves decompensation correction.

The forces applied can be further limited if they are not directed in the appropriate plane for the deformation. Because it has a posterolateral apical pad, the Milwaukee brace produces lordosis in the thoracic spine; this effect can be minimized with optimal pad placement. Loss of thoracic kyphosis decreases thoracic volume and may impair pulmonary function (86). The presence of true lordosis of the thoracic spine is a contraindication to the use of a Milwaukee brace. Orthotic design also influences the location of maximal applied force, which should be at the curve apex to optimize the corrective force. The magnitude,

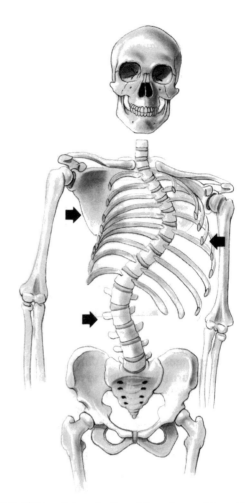

FIGURE 2. Three-point application of force (*arrows*) for orthotic correction of scoliosis. Correction of high thoracic curves is limited by the short lever arm achieved with an infraaxillary pad.

direction, and location of force must be optimized in the orthotic design for application of a suitable corrective, or counterprogressive, force.

The temporal characteristics of the force applied by an orthotic device also influence the ultimate magnitude of the curve. To have an optimal effect in countering the progressive forces, the force should be applied when the progressive forces are expected to be maximal. Maximal deforming forces generally occur when a patient is in an upright rather than prone or supine posture. For this reason, orthotic devices that are used only at night (92) probable function at a biomechanical disadvantage compared with braces that are prescribed for full-time use. Howard et al. (54) in a retrospective cohort study found the TLSO superior to the brace worn at night for preventing progression of the curve among adolescents with idiopathic scoliosis. Other investigators have found similar results with full-time brace wearing (41,61,96). Night bracing may be most useful during weaning from full-time brace wear.

The other important temporal characteristic of the applied force is its total duration of application. The application of force ideally should be continued until either the deforming force or spinal malleability decreases to a suitable level. Clinical experience has determined that both of these events generally occur around the time of skeletal maturity (26). Therefore it is biomechanically sound to continue orthotic treatment until skeletal maturity. Although the deforming force caused by spinal growth is no longer present in adults, the deforming force as a result of gravity is still present. This may cause continued curve progression after skeletal maturity, although such progression usually is slow because of decreased spinal malleability. The rate of progression may increase in later adult life with the increased overall spinal malleability that accompanies osteoporosis.

The decision to use an orthotic device for the management of a specific curve should be made when the applied forces can reasonably compensate for the deforming forces in a spine that is still malleable. Orthotic devices generally should not be used if the deforming forces are excessive (curves greater than 50 degrees), if the applied forces are minimal (because of skin problems or lack of patient compliance), or if the spine is rigid.

Biomechanics of Instrumentation and Fusion

The biomechanical goals for the surgical management of scoliosis include the general therapeutic goals for scoliosis described earlier and optimization of the biomechanical environment for fusion and minimization of complications related to instrumentation. The optimal biomechanical environment for fusion should place any bone graft under compressive stresses and minimize tensile stresses. Compression of an immature fusion mass promotes consolidation of bone. Conversely, tension promotes formation of fibrous tissue. The concave side of a scoliotic curve is the most desirable location for bone grafting, because this is the compressive side. Zagra et al. (125) used computed tomographic scans to follow consolidation of the fusion mass after posterior fusion for idiopathic scoliosis. Fusion consolidation was most pronounced on the concave side of the curve, as would be predicted with the Wolff law.

The importance of achieving relative immobilization of the spinal segments during fusion has been emphasized (79). Studies have shown that the rate of pseudarthrosis decreases from about 25% with a Risser cast to 15% with Harrington rods. This effect may be partially attributable to improved correction with Harrington rods. With current instrumentation systems, much of the compressive and tensile force is loaded through the instrumentation rather than through the spine. This appears to be particularly true of rigid pedicle-screw devices that may act in a load-bearing capacity. Use of such implants has the theoretical disadvantage of stress shielding of the immature fusion mass, possibly causing problems with fusion consolidation. However, these theoretical concerns have not been supported by either clinical or basic research. In an animal study, Johnston et al. (59) found that cross-linking and large diameter rods produce the stiffest fusion mass and no apparent stress shielding of the fusion. It does not appear that use of load-sharing devices has any substantial advantage over use of load-bearing devices in terms of fusion consolidation in the spine. Immobilization of the fused segments seems to be more important than cyclic loading to promote spinal fusion.

The anterior column of the spine is normally subjected to greater compressive forces than is the posterior column (110). This also is true of the scoliotic spine, particularly if residual thoracic kyphosis is present. Thus anterior fusion has a biomechanical advantage over posterior fusion. Anterior fusion also has the biologic advantage of a large, well-vascularized fusion bed. The advantages of anterior fusion are particularly useful when the anticipated pseudarthrosis rate with posterior fusion alone would be high, as in long fusions involving the thoracolumbar spine in which the transverse processes are relatively small and weak fusion often results. Anterior approaches in the management of spinal deformities should be used when needed to improve fusion rate, to improve correction of deformity, to allow anterior decompression of neural elements, or to prevent the crankshaft phenomenon.

Minimizing Complications of Instrumentation

Complications related to instrumentation include failure of instrumentation, iatrogenic fracture, decompensation, and neurologic complications. These problems can be minimized with knowledge of the biomechanical limitations of instrumentation systems. Because the spine has considerable viscoelasticity, the deformation that can be induced with a given applied force increases with the duration of application. This means that a given degree of correction of the curve can be achieved with small forces applied slowly. Minimizing the amount of force needed for curve correction is desirable, because this minimizes the risk of fracture of the posterior elements at the site of application of force. It is judicious to correct spinal deformities slowly and sequentially to take advantage of the viscoelastic properties of the spine during the correction process. Sequential correction with a minimum of 5 to 10 minutes between stages may be optimal (38). Stress relaxation occurs during this time, and little change occurs after this, if the force application is constant. With the advent of posterior instrumentation systems capable of applying large forces to the spine, the need to minimize the correcting force is even more important. The risk of iatrogenic spinal fracture can be decreased by respecting the inflection point of the spine. The inflection point is the point on the load deformation curve at which the amount of force needed for a given deformation increases dramatically. The inflection point may be palpably detected and should be interpreted as an indication that failure of the bony elements is imminent if the applied force is increased (110).

In a well-designed study, Nachemson and Elfstrom (84) used telemetrized Harrington rods to measure the forces to which the instrumentation was subjected in the postoperative period. These forces were found to vary considerably during routine daily activities. Forces during standing and walking were about 60% higher than those in the supine position. Axial forces were high when the patient lay on the convex side of the curve. The axial forces decreased considerably when a Milwaukee brace was used in the postoperative period. The investigators did not measure rotational and bending forces, which may be more important than axial forces as a predisposing factor for failure of instrumentation. Nevertheless, when Harrington rods were used, it was prudent to have patients avoid lying on the convex side, and care was taken to minimize the stress produced by Valsalva maneuvers (such as violent coughing and vomiting) during the immediately postoperative period. Segmentation fixation systems provide higher end-point fixation strength than the Harrington system; however, if there is uncertainty about the fixation, use of a postoperative brace and the aforementioned principles may decrease the risk of instrumentation failure.

Failure of the instrumentation used to manage idiopathic scoliosis most commonly occurs as the result of fatigue. Erwin et al. (40) found that fractures of Harrington rods occurred an average of 3.4 years postoperatively. As might be expected, larger curves had a higher rate of rod fracture and fractured earlier. These authors also identified rod fracture in the presence of a solid fusion; this is likely the result of repetitive elastic deformation of an immature fusion mass. Spinal fusion possesses considerable elasticity until 18 to 24 months after the operation. It is during this time that a rod is vulnerable to fracture, even though a bridging fusion is present. Segmental instrumentation has improved strength with fewer stress risers than has use of the Harrington system. As a result, fracture is less likely with the segmented systems.

Neurologic complications of the management of scoliosis are caused by cord compression, overdistraction, or purely vascular factors. Bridwell et al. (24) retrospectively identified 4 of 1,090 patients with intraoperative neurologic deficits; 3 of the 4 defects were purely vascular. Risk factors were anterior-posterior fusion and the presence of hyperkyphosis. Distraction of more rigid spinal segments causes rapid loss of spinal evoked potentials; this occurs more slowly in more flexible segments (88). Results of histologic studies suggest that actual structural damage to the cord occurs with distraction of stiff regions of the spine. It appears that ischemia rather than direct trauma is the cause of damage in more flexible regions. These important findings suggest the possibility of immediate onset of irreversible cord damage with distraction in rigid regions and must be carefully considered when correction of a severe and rigid spinal deformity is planned.

KYPHOSIS

Unlike the complex, multiplanar deformity of scoliosis, the deformity of kyphosis is confined to the sagittal plane. Because forward bending in pure kyphosis is symmetric relative to the facet joints, coupled deformities generally do not occur. To some extent, this simplifies the approach to the biomechanics of kyphosis. However, the biomechanical complications of neurologic compression and pseudarthrosis are of particular concern with kyphotic deformities.

Normal thoracic kyphosis tends to increase progressively with maturation until near the end of adolescence, but the normal range of kyphosis is large. Among older adolescents, the normal range of thoracic kyphosis is about 20 to 50 degrees (11,14). The presence of physiologic thoracic kyphosis allows for spinal balance, maximal thoracic volume, and spinal stability. Normal thoracic kyphosis combines with cervical and lumbar lordosis to keep the head centered over the sacrum in the sagittal plane. If the thoracic kyphosis increases in a child, there usually is

enough flexibility in the cervical and lumbar spines to maintain spinal balance. Among older adolescents and adults, loss of sagittal balance is more likely to be a clinical problem.

Initiation and Progression

Initiation of a kyphotic deformity can be caused by asymmetric growth, loss of the anterior buttress, loss of the posterior ligamentous tension band, or a combination of these factors (111). When posterior growth markedly exceeds anterior growth, the result is a tendency toward a kyphotic deformity. Congenital or acquired conditions can cause the loss of anterior growth potential in the vertebral column and progressive kyphotic deformity. As in any physis, the active cells are highly susceptible to damage (94); this biologic effect gradually is converted into the biomechanically significant deformity of kyphosis.

Loss of the posterior ligamentous restraints is of particular concern in the immature spine, because the remaining structural elements often are malleable enough to allow rapid progression of the deformity. In the thoracic spine, normal kyphosis produces a lever arm that tends toward progressive kyphosis. For this reason, laminectomy in the immature thoracic spine carries a particularly high risk of progressive kyphosis (71,122,123). With removal of several contiguous thoracic laminae, rounded kyphosis tends to develop with the addition of levels adjacent to those that were originally involved. When bilateral facetectomy is included with laminectomy, a more localized gibbus-type deformity tends to develop. The development of kyphotic deformities is predictable among patients younger than 10 years who are treated with these procedures.

Loss of the structural integrity of the anterior column of the spine causes loss of the ability of the spine to withstand anterior compressive loads; progressive kyphotic deformity often develops. Loss of the anterior buttress of the spine causes loss of the anterior pivot point for spinal motion and weakens the ability of the posterior ligamentous restraints to resist kyphotic forces. The combination of these factors causes loss of the anterior spinal buttress, which can lead to progressive kyphotic deformity. This situation can occur with burst fractures that cause greater than 50% loss of vertebral body height (78), neoplastic or infectious vertebral destruction, and congenital vertebral malformation involving anterior failure of formation of a vertebral body (type I). In the case of type I congenital kyphosis, the deficient anterior buttress combines with excessive posterior growth relative to anterior growth. The likely result is progressive kyphosis (46,81,114). When a kyphotic deformity has been initiated, the patient's center of gravity is displaced anteriorly, resulting in a larger lever arm for the body weight acting on the apex of the kyphosis (64). This tends to increase the kyphotic deformity.

Structural Features

The clinical distinction between flexible and rigid kyphosis has important implications for patient care. At the extreme of flexibility, a postural round-back deformity straightens completely with voluntary extension; the lack of any structural component of these curves makes treatment other than exercise superfluous (21). Flexible structural kyphosis gradually becomes more rigid.

This occurs as a result of thickening and lack of longitudinal growth of ligamentous structures, loss of disc height and mobility, and vertebral wedging (14). In the thoracic spine, loss of flexibility may be accentuated by severe deformities caused by shortening and deformity of the anterior chest wall, including the ribs, sternum, and intercostal muscles. The flexibility of the kyphosis determines whether bracing is likely to be successful. Curves that can be reduced to less than 50 degrees in the brace are much more likely to have a favorable outcome than curves that cannot be reduced to less than 60 degrees in the brace (22). Curves that can be corrected to less than 55 degrees likewise probably can be managed by means of posterior instrumentation alone (see later). Larger and less flexible curves usually are best managed with combined anterior release and posterior instrumentation and fusion to minimize instrumentation failure and pseudarthrosis.

Neurologic Impairment

Kyphotic deformities have a particular tendency toward neurologic impairment. The spinal cord is most susceptible to injury with direct transverse compression (43). For this reason, most cases of neurologic deterioration with kyphosis are the direct result of tethering of the cord over a large kyphotic deformity (73), particularly if a gibbus deformity is present. Because the cord has considerable inherent elasticity, isolated longitudinal distraction of the cord is less likely than is transverse compression to cause neurologic problems. However, longitudinal distraction of the cord in the presence of anterior compression increases the compressive effects on the cord (43). Thus the use of halo traction or instrumentation to distract the spine in the presence of a fixed kyphotic deformity without initial anterior decompression of the spinal cord poses considerable neurologic risk (117). If the spinal cord is already tented over a kyphotic deformity, a relatively small disc protrusion can have major effects on increasing spinal cord compression and neurologic deficit (18,121).

Orthotic Treatment

There is agreement that bracing can be effective for controlling and even correcting many cases of kyphosis. The uniplanar deformity of kyphosis is well suited to sagittal plane corrective forces applied through a Milwaukee brace. The principle of three-point fixation is used to apply posteriorly directed forces at the chin, sternum, and anterior pelvis and anteriorly directed forces at the apex of the kyphotic deformity. The success of bracing depends on reducing the deforming forces to an acceptably low magnitude. This necessitates that the kyphosis be flexible enough to achieve in-brace correction to less than 60 degrees and that the posterior growth potential not greatly exceed that in the anterior column (22). In the case of congenital kyphosis, particularly cases caused by failure of anterior vertebral formation, posterior growth continues in the brace, resulting in a high probability of progressive kyphosis (114). Results of clinical studies of the effectiveness of bracing in the management of Scheuermann kyphosis have indicated that this entity can be controlled or corrected in many cases. However, patients with kyphosis of greater than 70 degrees, vertebral wedging that averages more than 10 degrees, or skeletal maturity are unlikely to have a good result with bracing (22).

Biomechanics of Surgical Treatment

The goals of surgical management of kyphotic deformities are to obtain a solid arthrodesis over the length of the kyphosis, to attain some deformity correction, and to minimize risk to the neural elements. Correction of deformity is a goal only if it does not pose an inordinate risk to the patient. Correction of kyphotic deformity may be biomechanically desirable, because it may achieve improved balance in the sagittal plane and provide a biomechanical environment with increased compressive forces that favor fusion (17). However, the biomechanics of correction deformity always must be considered in conjunction with the previously discussed biomechanics and biologic characteristics of spinal cord compromise.

Achieving solid arthrodesis in kyphotic deformities is determined by several biomechanical factors. The entire length of the applicable segments optimally would be under compression to favor arthrodesis. This would require a direct line of weight transfer from each end of the segment. In the presence of substantial residual kyphosis, the posterior elements are in tension,

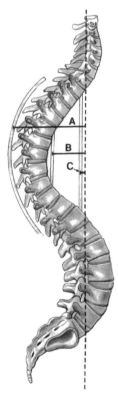

FIGURE 3. Limitations of posterior devices in stabilizing large kyphotic deformities. The moment arm *A* of force on a posterior implant is substantially greater than that on a short anterior strut *B*. The shortest moment arm is represented by a long strut graft *C*, which extends from vertebrae close to the weight-bearing axis (*dotted line*). Because the axis of rotation is anterior to the vertebral bodies, the strut grafts are under compression, and the posterior construct is subjected to biomechanically less favorable tensile forces.

tending toward formation of pseudarthroses (111). If the kyphosis is not flexible enough to correct to less than 55 degrees, anterior fusion should be added to achieve a graft in compression (17). Among a group of patients with congenital kyphosis greater than 50 degrees, Winter et al. (117) found a 55% rate of pseudarthrosis with posterior procedures alone. The rate of pseudarthrosis with combined anterior and posterior procedures was 15%.

If severe residual kyphosis is present, addition of anterior strut grafts across the length of the kyphosis can be used to achieve a more direct line of compressive force transfer and to relieve some of the posterior tensile forces (Fig. 3). The compressive strength of strut grafts depends on the type of graft selected. Fibular struts have the greatest strength followed by iliac crest; rib struts are weakest. Rib struts are highly susceptible to fracture if they are placed more than 4 cm anterior to the apex of the deformity. Graft fracture often occurs 6 to 12 months after the operation (17), presumably during the period of revascularization, in which the compressive strength is compromised. Vascularized rib grafts have been used successfully to reduce the fracture rate by avoiding the revascularization period (16). Regardless of the method of arthrodesis used, it is important to extend fusion over the length of the kyphosis (21). If fusion stops short of the end vertebra or a vertebra in the neutral weight-bearing axis, the kyphosing force is concentrated on the motion segment adjacent to the fusion. There is a considerable tendency for this segment to fall off and cause junctional kyphosis proximal or distal to the fusion.

SPONDYLOLYSIS AND SPONDYLOLISTHESIS

Solid biomechanical knowledge is important in the management of spondylolisthesis, because this condition is the combination of deformity and instability. The deformity of spondylolisthesis is forward displacement of one vertebra on another. The instability of spondylolisthesis is shown by the tendency for some cases to undergo progressive slipping. This section discusses the biomechanical features important in the causation of spondylolysis and those that are important in the progression and management of spondylolisthesis.

Etiology of Isthmic Spondylolysis

Spondylolysis has been rarely documented among persons younger than 6 years. The incidence increases between the ages of 6 and 14 years, when it approximates the 5% incidence among adults (9,49). It has been hypothesized that the involvement of children in organized athletic activities when they reach school age may account for the increased incidence during these years (113).

Isthmic spondylolysis is caused by repetitive stress, which produces a stress fracture of the pars interarticularis (113). The stresses to which the posterior elements are subjected are highest in the lumbosacral region. This large amount of stress is caused by the combination of lumbar lordosis that concentrates stress in the posterior elements, the long trunk lever arm in the lumbosacral region, and the transition between the mobile lumbar

segments and the immobile sacral segments (34). The concentration of stress at the L5 lamina largely accounts for the predominance of spondylolysis at L5 compared with other vertebral levels (57). Less commonly, L4 may be involved with a spondylolytic defect, particularly if L5 is a transitional vertebra (sacralized). The result is stress concentration in the posterior elements of L4. In anatomic studies, the pars interarticularis of children is thin and elongated. This relative weakness of the region may contribute to the development of stress fractures here (70).

In normal erect stance and gait, the posterior elements bear only about 20% of the weight transmitted through the spine. However, the force transmitted through the lumbar spine increases to about 50% when the spine is in a hyperlordotic position (111). When the lumbar spine is in a hyperextended position, the inferior facet of L4 impinges and levers on the posterior elements of L5 in the region of the pars interarticularis; this phenomenon has been disputed (57). This may cause direct transmission of force through this vulnerable region. Activities associated with accentuated lumbar lordosis place the pars interarticularis region of L5 at particularly high risk of spondylolysis. Activities that involve alternating flexion and extension produce large stress reversals in the pars and create the potential for stress failure (44). Participation in gymnastics, weight lifting, hockey, platform diving, and interior line football corresponds to a high incidence of spondylolysis (58,70).

The clinical importance of these biomechanical factors is that they provide the basis for ascertaining who is at risk of spondylolysis and appropriately minimizing that risk. Avoidance of repetitive, forceful lumbar hyperextension by children may greatly decrease the risk of development of spondylolysis; however, controlled studies have not been performed. In gymnastics, back walkovers should be avoided, because they place the L5 pars interarticularis at particularly high risk of stress fracture. Lumbar braces and corsets do not have an established role in minimizing the risk of spondylolysis in high-risk activities.

Biomechanics of Progression of Spondylolisthesis

Spondylolisthesis involves forward subluxation or slipping of a vertebra relative to its subjacent vertebra. The potential for progressive slipping is an important factor that may influence the decision to perform fusion. Progression of spondylolisthesis is a form of chronic instability and can be analyzed through the use of biomechanical principles. In normal spines, forces that tend to displace L5 anteriorly relative to the sacrum are balanced by forces that resist this translation. The deforming forces are those applied by body weight and muscle actions. The resistive forces are supplied by the posterior osteoligamentous tether and the anterior osseous buttress. Deficiencies of either of the columns that resist translation can produce a tendency toward progressive slipping and segmental kyphosis.

The posterior osseoligamentous tether is formed by the intact laminae, facet joints, spinous processes, and intervening ligamentous structures. When this column is anatomically intact, it can resist physiologic forces to prevent abnormal translation of the vertebral elements. Loss of the structural continuity of this column occurs with spondylolysis or with hypoplasia of

S1 facets (dysplastic spondylolisthesis). However, even in these situations, some resistance to displacement is provided by the posterior ligamentous structures and the anterior bony buttress to prevent immediate, catastrophic displacement of L5 on the sacrum. Laxity of ligamentous tissues may allow accelerated progression of spondylolisthesis. This may account for the considerably higher incidence of progression to severe spondylolisthesis among girls than boys and among younger than older children (9). Laminectomy and decompression of the neural elements in spondylolisthesis remove ligamentous and scar tissues that provide some residual resistance to the anterior translation of L5 on the sacrum. In the presence of this iatrogenic worsening of instability, it is advisable to perform fusion to decrease the risk of progression of the slip (20).

The intact anterior lip of the sacrum forms a buttress to prevent displacement and kyphotic angulation of L5. This buttress is deficient if the sacrum is substantially rounded, if L5 is wedged, if L5 has levered into kyphosis over the sacral promontory, or if L5 has translated more than 50% anteriorly relative to the sacrum. Natural history studies show that the combination of these features, which indicate a deficient anterior buttressing effect, increases the risk of progressive slipping (12,50).

For progression of spondylolisthesis to occur, the deforming forces must exceed the resisting forces supplied by the posterior tether and the anterior buttress. The force tending to displace the superior vertebra anteriorly increases when kyphosis is present at the spondylolisthetic level, resulting in an increased slip angle (Fig. 4). In this situation, the patient's center of gravity is displaced anteriorly relative to the level of the slip. This increases the moment arm for force transmission through the level of spondylolisthesis. The result is a net increase in the deforming force.

The presence of marked local kyphosis in spondylolisthesis is accompanied by compensatory changes in the rest of the spine that act to maintain balance in the sagittal plane. In the lumbar spine, this involves lumbar hyperlordosis; in the thoracic spine, hypokyphosis is commonly. It has been hypothesized that the decrease in thoracic kyphosis that accompanies spondylolisthesis may be associated with a tendency toward development of deformities in the coronal plane. This may account for the higher incidence of idiopathic-like scoliosis in association with spondylolisthesis than exists among the general population (101).

Mechanics of Neural Impairment

Although most neural deficits that occur with spondylolisthesis involve L5 radiculopathy, cauda equina compression can occur. Cauda equina syndromes most commonly are caused by a greater than 50% slip of dysplastic spondylolisthesis (76). Because the posterior elements of the slipping vertebra are intact, compression of the cauda between the lamina and vertebral body of S1 occurs. The biomechanics of cauda equina compression with spondylolytic spondylolisthesis are not well defined. One theory is that the cauda is stretched over the dome of the sacrum and that the stretching causes neural dysfunction; however, there is a poor correlation between the degree of the slip, radiographic cauda equina impingement, and a clinical cauda equina syndrome. It appears that in this scenario, other factors such as the rate of slip progression and presence of associated disc protrusions are important.

Biomechanics of Fusion for Spondylolisthesis

The surgical management of spondylolisthesis requires techniques that have a high likelihood of achieving solid arthrodesis while minimizing slip progression. By necessity, this means that the graft should be placed in a compressive mode and that the applicable levels should be immobilized. With less than 50% translation of one vertebra on the other, an intertransverse fusion between L5 and S1 is under acceptable compression. Slips greater than 50% cause anterior and inferior movement of the transverse processes of L5 toward the sacral ala. The result is inadequate area for posterior grafting that also is subjected to relative tensile forces (12). In this situation, including the transverse processes of L4 in the arthrodesis not only improves the graft bed available but also improves the compressive characteristics of the fusion (12,42). However, when there also is a substantial kyphotic deformity (slip angle greater than 45 degrees) at the spondylolisthetic level, even fusion to the transverse processes of L4 may not produce acceptable graft compression (Fig. 5). In this case, a more acceptable biomechanical environment for fusion can be obtained by means of using anterior-posterior arthrodesis, using a transsacral fibula, or reducing the slip angle (13,102). Anterior arthrodesis is anterior to the axis of rotation of the spondylolisthetic vertebra and therefore is under compression (15,19). Reduction of the slip angle can be achieved by means of casting,

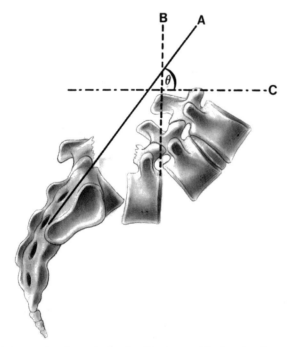

FIGURE 4. The slip angle (angle of lumbosacral kyphosis) is the angle formed by lines parallel to the posterior cortex of the sacrum *A* and the line perpendicular *C* to the superior end plate of L5 *B*. This measurement is biomechanically important because it is strongly related to the risk of progression of spondylolisthesis.

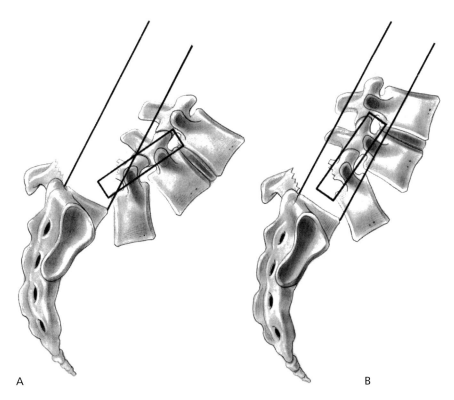

A

B

FIGURE 5. Effects of anterior translation and slip angle on intertransverse fusion biomechanics in spondylolisthesis. **A:** With greater than 50% slippage and a large slip angle, the fusion (*black box*) is not within the compressive zone over the ala of the sacrum (*black lines* projected parallel to the walls of the sacrum). This places the fusion under tensile forces that are predisposing factors for pseudarthrosis. **B:** With reduction of the slip angle, a transverse process fusion comes into the compressive zone despite greater than 50% residual translation.

instrumentation, or total excision of the spondylolisthetic vertebra. Reducing the slip angle causes a posterior change in the patient's center of gravity, so that a posterolateral graft is under increased compressive force. Reduction improves the contours of the sagittal plane and sagittal balance for many patients (13). Despite this, the surgeon's enthusiasm for reducing the slip angle and improving the biomechanical milieu for fusion must be tempered with the knowledge that reduction techniques, particularly those that involve instrumentation, carry considerable risk of iatrogenic neural deficits (15).

Among children, the posterior spinal fusion mass retains considerable plasticity, despite the presence of an apparently solid arthrodesis. Plasticity is most pronounced during the first 24 postoperative months but persists until maturity. Because of this plasticity, progression of the slip can occur despite the presence of a radiographically solid arthrodesis. Progression is most likely to occur with a large slip angle or extensive posterior decompression (13). In these situations, the potential for worsening of the spondylolisthesis should be recognized, and it may be prudent to institute use of an orthotic device.

As in fusion of joints in the extremities, achieving a high probability of successful arthrodesis in spondylolisthesis necessitates immobilization of the levels to be fused. To be effective in immobilizing the lumbosacral joint, an external device should incorporate at least one thigh in an extended position; this achieves relative immobilization of the pelvis and sacrum relative to the lumbar spine. Immobilization can be more rigidly obtained with internal fixation. The most rigid constructs are pedicle screw–rod devices with rigid cross linking. This rigid immobilization may reduce the rate of pseudarthrosis, but studies with

pediatric populations have not been performed. Except for older adolescents, the small pedicle size of these patients poses technical problems for the placement of pedicle screws.

CONCLUSIONS

Understanding the biomechanical characteristics of the pediatric spine provides a rational basis for the management of pediatric spinal disorders. Complete biomechanical analysis of this complicated, composite structure requires sophisticated inquiry. This chapter presents basic principles that can be applied to the normal and diseased spine to predict general biomechanical behavior. The analysis of scoliosis centers on the three-dimensional aspect of the deformity and how this influences treatment. In contrast, the deformity of kyphosis is confined to a single plane. This concentrates tensile forces on the posterior spine and predisposes the patient to pseudarthrosis and spinal cord injury. The combination of deformity and instability in spondylolisthesis makes biomechanical analysis essential to understanding the risk of progression and the basis for treatment.

REFERENCES

1. Aaro S, Burstrom R, Dahlborn M (1981): The derotating effect of the Boston brace. *Spine* 6:477–482.
2. Aaro S, Dahlborn M (1981): Estimation of vertebral rotation and the spinal and rib cage deformity in scoliosis by computer tomography. *Spine* 6:460–467.

3. Aaro S, Dahlborn M (1981): The longitudinal axis rotation of the apical vertebra, the vertebral, spinal, and rib cage deformity in idiopathic scoliosis studied by computer tomography. *Spine* 6:567–572.

4. Aaro S, Dahlborn M (1982): The effect of Harrington instrumentation on the longitudinal axis rotation of the apical vertebra and on the spinal and rib-cage deformity in idiopathic scoliosis studied by computer tomography. *Spine* 7:456–462.

5. Andriacchi TP, Schultz AB, Belytschko TB, et al. (1976): Milwaukee brace correction of idiopathic scoliosis: a biomechanical analysis. *J Bone Joint Surg Am* 58:806–815.

6. Armstrong GWD, Livermore NB, Suzuki N, et al. (1982): Nonstandard vertebral rotation in scoliosis screening patients. *Spine* 7:50–54.

7. Ashton-Miller JA, McGlashen KM, Schultz AB (1992): Trunk positioning accuracy in children 7–18 years old. *J Orthop Res* 10:217–225.

8. Aufdermaur M (1974): Spinal injuries in juveniles. *J Bone Joint Surg Br* 56:513–519.

9. Baker DR, McHolick W (1956): Spondylolysis and spondylolisthesis in children. *J Bone Joint Surg Am* 38:9–33.

10. Banks GM, Transfeldt EE, Hu SA, et al. (1992): Prognostic significance of decompensation occurring after Cotrel-Dubousset instrumentation. *Orthop Trans.*

11. Bernhardt M, Bridwell KH (1989): Segmental analysis of the sagittal plane alignment of the normal thoracic and lumbar spines and thoracolumbar junction. *Spine* 14:717–721.

12. Boxall D, Bradford DS, Winter RB, et al. (1979): Management of severe spondylolisthesis in children and adolescents. *J Bone Joint Surg Am* 61:479–496.

13. Bradford DS (1988): Closed reduction of spondylolisthesis: an experience in 22 patients. *Spine* 13:580–587.

14. Bradford DS, Ahmed KB, Moe JH, et al. (1980): The surgical management of patients with Scheuermann's disease: a review of twenty-four cases managed by combined anterior and posterior spine fusion. *J Bone Joint Surg Am* 62:705–712.

15. Bradford DS, Boachie-Adjei O (1990): Treatment of severe spondylolisthesis by anterior and posterior reduction and stabilization. *J Bone Joint Surg Am* 72:1060–1066.

16. Bradford DS, Daher YH (1986): Vascularized rib grafts for stabilization of kyphosis. *J Bone Joint Surg Br* 68:357–361.

17. Bradford DS, Ganjavian S, Antonious D, et al. (1982): Anterior strut-grafting for the treatment of kyphosis. *J Bone Joint Surg Am* 64:680–690.

18. Bradford DS, Garcia A (1969): Neurological complications in Scheuermann's disease. *J Bone Joint Surg Am* 51:567–572.

19. Bradford DS, Gotfried Y (1987): Staged salvage reconstruction of grade IV and V spondylolisthesis. *J Bone Joint Surg Am* 69:191–202.

20. Bradford DS, Hensinger RM (1985): *The pediatric spine.* New York: Thieme Medical Publishers.

21. Bradford DS, Lonstein JE, Moe JH, et al. (1987): *Moe's textbook of scoliosis and other spinal deformities.* Philadelphia: WB Saunders.

22. Bradford DS, Moe JH, Montalvo F, et al. (1974): Scheuermann's kyphosis and roundback deformity. *J Bone Joint Surg Am* 56:740–758.

23. Bridwell KH, Betz R, Capelli AM, et al. (1990): Sagittal plane analysis in idiopathic scoliosis patients treated with CD instrumentation. *Spine* 15:921–926.

24. Bridwell KH, Lenke LG, Baldus C, et al. (1998): Major intraoperative neurologic deficits in pediatric and adult spinal deformity patients: incidence and etiology at one institution. *Spine* 23:324–331.

25. Bunch WH, Smith D, Hakala M (1977): Kyphosis in the paralytic spine. *Clin Orthop* 128:107–112.

26. Carr WA, Moe JH, Winter RB, et al. (1980): Treatment of idiopathic scoliosis in the Milwaukee brace. *J Bone Joint Surg Am* 62:599–612.

27. Cattell HS, Filtzer DL (1965): Pseudosubluxation and other normal variations in the cervical spine in children. *J Bone Joint Surg Am* 47:1295–1309.

28. Cochran T, Nachemson A (1983): Long-term anatomic changes in patients with adolescent idiopathic scoliosis treated by Harrington rod fusion. *Spine* 8:576–584.

29. Deacon P, Flood BM, Dickson RA (1984): Idiopathic scoliosis in three dimensions. *J Bone Joint Surg Br* 66:509–512.

30. Denis F (1994): The iatrogenic loss of lumbar lordosis. *Spine State Art Rev* 8:659–672.

31. DeRosa GP (1985): Progressive scoliosis following chest wall resection in children. *Spine* 10:618–622.

32. Dickman CA, Zabramski JM, Hadley MN, et al. (1991): Pediatric spinal cord injury without radiographic abnormalities: report of 26 cases and review of the literature. *J Spinal Disord* 4:296–305.

33. Dickson RA, Lawton JO, Archer IA, et al. (1984): The pathogenesis of idiopathic scoliosis. *J Bone Joint Surg Br* 66:8–15.

34. Dietrich M, Kurowski P (1985): The importance of mechanical factors in the etiology of spondylolysis. *Spine* 10:532–542.

35. Drummond DS, Narechania RG, Rosenthal AN, et al. (1982): A study of pressure distributions measured during balanced and unbalanced sitting. *J Bone Joint Surg Am* 64:1034–1039.

36. Dubousset J, Gaf H, Miladi L, et al. (1986): Spinal and thoracic derotation with Cotrel-Dubousset instrumentation. *Orthop Trans* 10:36.

37. Dubousset J, Herring JA, Shufflebarger H (1989): The crankshaft phenomenon. *J Pediatr Orthop* 9:541–550.

38. Dunn HK, Daniels AU, McBride GG (1982): Intraoperative force measurements during correction of scoliosis. *Spine* 7:448–455.

39. Emans JB, Kaelin A, Bancel P, et al. (1986): The Boston bracing system for idiopathic scoliosis. *Spine* 11:792–801.

40. Erwin WD, Dickson JH, Harrington PR (1980): Clinical review of patients with broken Harrington rods. *J Bone Joint Surg Am* 62:1302–1307.

41. Fernandez-Feliberti R, Flynn J, Ramierz N, et al. (1995): Effectiveness of TLSO bracing in the conservative treatment of idiopathic scoliosis. *J Pediatr Orthop* 15:176–181.

42. Freeman BL, Donati NL (1989): Spinal arthrodesis for severe spondylolisthesis in children and adolescents: a long term follow-up study. *J Bone Joint Surg Am* 71:594–598.

43. Fujita Y, Yamamoto H (1989): An experimental study on spinal cord traction effect. *Spine* 14:698–705.

44. Green TP, Allvey JC, Adams MA (1994): Spondylolysis: bending of the inferior articular processes of lumbar vertebrae during simulated spinal movements. *Spine* 19:2683–2691.

45. Haderspeck K, Schultz A (1981): Progression of idiopathic scoliosis: an analysis of muscle actions and body weight influences. *Spine* 6:447–455.

46. Hall JE (1982): Congenital kyphosis. *Spine* 7:360–364.

47. Halsall AP, James DF, Kostuik JP, et al. (1983): An experimental evaluation of spinal flexibility with respect to scoliosis surgery. *Spine* 8:482–488.

48. Hamill CL, Bridwell KH, Lenke LG, et al. (1997): Posterior arthrodesis in the skeletally immature patient: assessing the risk for crankshaft—is an open triradiate cartilage the answer? *Spine* 22:1343–1351.

49. Hensinger RN (1983): Spondylolysis and spondylolisthesis in children. *Instr Course Lect* 32:132–151.

50. Hensinger RN, Lang JR, MacEwen GD (1976): Surgical management of spondylolisthesis in children. *Spine* 1:207.

51. Herzenberg JE, Hensinger RN, Dedrick DK, et al. (1989): Emergency transport and positioning of young children who have an injury of the cervical spine. *J Bone Joint Surg Am* 71:15–22.

52. Herzenberg JE, Waanders NA, Closkey RF, et al. (1990): Cobb angle versus spinous process angle in adolescent idiopathic scoliosis. *Spine* 15:874–879.

53. Hilibrand AS, Blakemore LC, Loder RT, et al. (1996): The role of melatonin in the pathogenesis of adolescent idiopathic scoliosis. *Spine* 21:1140–1146.

54. Howard A, Wright JG, Hedden D (1998): A comparative study of TLSO, Charleston, and Milwaukee braces for idiopathic scoliosis. *Spine* 23:2404–2411.

55. Hubbard DD (1974): Injuries of the spine in children and adolescents. *Clin Orthop* 100:56–65.

56. Hullin MG, McMaster MJ, Draper ERC, et al. (1991): The effect of luque segmental sublaminar instrumentation on the rib hump in idiopathic scoliosis. *Spine* 16:402–408.

57. Hutton WC, Stott JRR, Cyron BM (1977): Is spondylolysis a fatigue fracture? *Spine* 2:202–209.
58. Jackson DW, Wiltse LL, Cirincione RJ (1976): Spondylolysis in the female gymnast. *Clin Orthop* 117:68–73.
59. Johnston CE, Ashman RB, Baird AM, et al. (1990): Effect of spinal construct stiffness on fusion mass incorporation. *Spine* 15:908–912.
60. Kalen V, Conklin M (1990): Behavior of the unfused lumbar curve following selective thoracic fusion for idiopathic scoliosis. *Spine* 15:271–274.
61. Katz DE, Richards BS, Browne RH, et al. (1997): A comparison between the Boston brace and the Charleston bending brace in adolescent idiopathic scoliosis. *Spine* 22:1302–1312.
62. Kewalramani LS, Tori JA (1980): Spinal cord trauma in children. *Spine* 5:11–18.
63. King HA, Moe JH, Bradford DS, et al. (1983): The selection of fusion levels in thoracic idiopathic scoliosis. *J Bone Joint Surg Am* 65:1302–1313.
64. Kostuik JP, Maurais GR, Richardson WJ, et al. (1988): Combined single stage anterior and posterior osteotomy for correction of iatrogenic lumbar kyphosis. *Spine* 13:257–266.
65. Kriss VM, Kriss TC (1996): SCIWORA (Spinal Cord Injury Without Radiographic Abnormality) in infants and children. *Clin Pediatr (Phila)* 35:119–124.
66. Kumano K, Tsuyama N (1982): Pulmonary function before and after surgical correction of scoliosis. *J Bone Joint Surg Am* 64:243–248.
67. Lagrone MO, Bradford DS, Moe JH, et al. (1988): Treatment of symptomatic flatback. *J Bone Joint Surg Am* 76:569–580.
68. Lapinksy AS, Richards BS (1995): Preventing the crankshaft phenomenon by combining anterior fusion with posterior instrumentation: does it work? *Spine* 20:1392–1398.
69. Lee CS, Nachemson AL (1997): The crankshaft phenomenon after posterior Harrington fusion in skeletally immature patients with thoracic or thoracolumbar idiopathic scoliosis followed to maturity. *Spine* 22:58–67.
70. Letts M, Smallman T, Afansaciov R, et al. (1986): Fracture of the pars interarticularis in adolescent athletes: a clinical biomechanical analysis. *J Pediatr Orthop* 6:40–46.
71. Lonstein JE (1977): Post-laminectomy kyphosis. *Clin Orthop* 128:93–100.
72. Lonstein JE, Carlson JM (1984): The prediction of curve progression in untreated idiopathic scoliosis during growth. *J Bone Joint Surg Am* 66:1061–1071.
73. Lonstein JE, Winter RB, Moe JH, et al. (1980): Neurologic deficits secondary to spinal deformity. *Spine* 5:331–355.
74. Machida M (1996): Melatonin: a possible role in pathogenesis of adolescent idiopathic scoliosis. *Spine* 21:1147–1152.
75. Mason DE, Carango P (1991): Spinal decompensation in Cotrel Dubousset instrumentation. *Spine* 16:S394–S403.
76. Maurice HD, Morley TR (1989): Cauda equina lesions following fusion in situ and decompressive laminectomy for severe spondylolisthesis. *Spine* 14:214–216.
77. Mayfield JK, Erkkila JC, Winter RB (1981): *Spine* deformity subsequent to acquired childhood spinal cord injury. *J Bone Joint Surg Am* 63:1401–1411.
78. McAfee PC, Hansen AY, Lasda NA (1982): The unstable burst fracture. *Spine* 7:365–373.
79. McMaster MJ (1980): Stability of the scoliotic spine after fusion. *J Bone Joint Surg Br* 62:59–64.
80. Mente PL, Stokes IA, Spence H, et al. (1997): Progression of vertebral wedging in an asymmetrically loaded rat tail model. *Spine* 22:1292–1296.
81. Montgomery SP, Hall JE (1982): Congenital kyphosis. *Spine* 7:360–364.
82. Morris JM, Lucas DB, Bresler B (1961): Role of the trunk in stability of the spine. *J Bone Joint Surg Am* 43:327–340.
83. Mulcahy T, Galante J, DeWald R, et al. (1973): A follow-up study of forces acting on the Milwaukee brace on patients undergoing treatment for idiopathic scoliosis. *Clin Orthop* 93:53–68.
84. Nachemson A, Elfstrom G (1971): Intravital wireless telemetry of axial forces in Harrington distraction rods in patients with idiopathic scoliosis. *J Bone Joint Surg Am* 53:445–465.
85. Ogilvie JW, Millar EA (1983): Comparison of segmental instrumentation devices in the correction of scoliosis. *Spine* 8:416–419.
86. Ogilvie JW, Schendel MJ (1988): Calculated thoracic volume as related to parameters of scoliosis correction. *Spine* 13:39–42.
87. Ohlen G, Aaro S, Bylund P (1988): The sagittal configuration and mobility of the spine in idiopathic scoliosis. *Spine* 13:413–416.
88. Owen JH, Naito M, Bridwell KH (1990): Relationship among level of distraction, evoked potentials, spinal cord ischemia and integrity, and clinical status in animals. *Spine* 15:852–857.
89. Pang D, Wilgerger JE (1982): Spinal cord injury without radiographic abnormalities in children. *J Neurosurg* 57:114–129.
90. Papaioannou T, Stokes 1, Kenwright J (1982): Scoliosis associated with limb-length inequality. *J Bone Joint Surg Am* 64:59–62.
91. Pizzutillo PD, Mirenda W, MacEwen GD (1986): Posterolateral fusion for spondylolisthesis in adolescence. *J Pediatr Orthop* 6:311–316.
92. Price CT, Scott DS, Reed FE, et al. (1990): Nighttime bracing for adolescent idiopathic scoliosis with the Charleston bending brace. *Spine* 15:1294–1299.
93. Richards SB, Birch JG, Herring JA, et al. (1989): Frontal plane and sagittal plane balance following Cotrel-Dubousset instrumentation for idiopathic scoliosis. *Spine* 14:733–737.
94. Riseborough EJ (1977): Irradiation induced kyphosis. *Clin Orthop* 128:101–106.
95. Roberto RF, Lonstein JE, Winter RB, et al. (1997): Curve progression in Risser stage 0 or 1 patients after posterior spinal fusion for idiopathic scoliosis. *J Pediatr Orthop* 17:718–725.
96. Rowe DE, Bernstein SM, Riddick MF, et al. (1997): A meta-analysis of the efficacy of non-operative treatments for idiopathic scoliosis. *J Bone Joint Surg Am* 79:664–674,.
97. Rudicel S, Renshaw TS (1983): The effect of the Milwaukee brace on spinal decompensation in idiopathic scoliosis. *Spine* 8:385–387.
98. Sanders JO, Little DG, Richards BS (1997): Prediction of the crankshaft phenomenon by peak height velocity. *Spine* 22:1352–1356.
99. Schultz AB (1976): A biomechanical view of scoliosis. *Spine* 1:162–173.
100. Seimon LP (1977): Fracture of the odontoid process in young children. *J Bone Joint Surg Am* 59:943–948.
101. Seitsalo S, Osterman K, Poussa M (1988): Scoliosis associated with lumbar spondylolisthesis: a clinical survey of 190 young patients. *Spine* 13:889–904.
102. Smith MD, Bohlman HH (1990): Spondylolisthesis treated by a single-stage operation combining decompression with in situ posterolateral and anterior fusion: an analysis of eleven patients who had long-term follow-up. *J Bone Joint Surg Am* 72:415–421.
103. Somerville EW (1952): Rotational lordosis: the development of the single curve. *J Bone Joint Surg Br* 34:421–428.
104. Stagnara P, DeMauroy JC, Dran G, et al. (1982): Reciprocal angulation of vertebral bodies in a sagittal plane: approach to references for the evaluation of kyphosis and lordosis. *Spine* 7:335–342.
105. Stokes IA, Spence H, Aronsson DD, et al. (1996): Mechanical modulation of vertebral body growth: implications for scoliosis progression. *Spine* 21:1162–1167.
106. Swank SM, Mauri TM, Brown JC (1990): The lumbar lordosis below Harrington instrumentation for scoliosis. *Spine* 15:181–185.
107. Thompson JP, Transfeldt EE, Bradford DS, et al. (1990): Decompensation after Cotrel-Dubousset instrumentation of idiopathic scoliosis. *Spine* 15:927–931.
108. Thulbourne T, Gillespie R (1976): The rib hump in idiopathic scoliosis. *J Bone Joint Surg Br* 53:64–71.
109. White AA, Parjabi MM (1978): The basic kinematics of the human spine. *Spine* 3:12–29.
110. White AA, Panjabi MM (1990): *Clinical biomechanics of the spine*. Philadelphia: JB Lippincott.
111. White AA, Panjabi MM, Thomas CL (1977): The clinical biomechanics of kyphotic deformities. *Clin Orthop* 128:8–17 '
112. Wiener-Vacher SR, Mazda K (1998): Asymmetric otolith vestibulo-ocular responses in children with idiopathic scoliosis. *J Pediatr* 132:1028–1032.

113. Wiltse LL, Widell EH, Jackson DW (1975): Fatigue fracture: the basic lesion in isthmic spondylolisthesis. *J Bone Joint Surg Am* 57: 17–22.

114. Winter RB (1977): Congenital kyphosis. *Clin Orthop* 128:26–32.

115. Winter RB (1981): Convex anterior and posterior hemiarthrodesis and hemiepiphyseodesis in young children with progressive congenital scoliosis. *J Pediatr Orthop* 1:361–366.

116. Winter RB, Moe JH (1982): The results of spinal arthrodesis for congenital spinal deformity in patients younger than five years old. *J Bone Joint Surg Am* 64:419–433.

117. Winter RB, Moe JH, Lonstein JE (1985): The surgical treatment of congenital kyphosis. *Spine* 10:224–231.

118. Winter RB, Pinto WC (1986): Pelvic obliquity: its causes and treatment. *Spine* 11:225–233.

119. Wojcik AS, Webb JK, Burwell RG (1990): Harrington-Luque and Cotrel-Dubousset instrumentation for idiopathic thoracic scoliosis. *Spine* 15:424–431.

120. Wood KB, Transfeldt EE, Ogilvie JW, et al. (1991): Rotational changes of vertebral-pelvic axis following Cotrel-Dubousset instrumentation. *Spine* 16:S404–S409.

121. Yablon JS, Kasdon DL, Levine H (1988): Thoracic cord compression in Scheuermann's disease. *Spine* 13:896–898.

122. Yasuoka S, Peterson HA, Laws ER, et al. (1981): Pathogenesis and prophylaxis of post-laminectomy deformity of the spine after multiple level laminectomy: difference between children and adults. *Neurosurgery* 9:145–152.

123. Yasuoka S, Peterson HA, MacCarty CS (1982): Incidence of spinal column deformity after multilevel laminectomy in children and adults. *J Neurosurg* 57:441–445.

124. Yekutiel M, Robin GC, Yarom R (1981): Proprioceptive function in children with adolescent idiopathic scoliosis. *Spine* 6:560–566.

125. Zagra A, Lamartina C, Pace A, et al. (1988): Posterior spinal fusion in scoliosis: computer assisted tomography and biomechanics of the fusion mass. *Spine* 13:155–161.

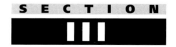

IMAGING TECHNIQUES

4

IMAGING MODALITIES

GEORGES Y. EL-KHOURY
YUTAKA SATO

RADIOGRAPHY

Wilhelm Conrad Roentgen discovered x-rays in 1895, for which he won the Nobel Prize for physics in 1901. Any physician can understand the basic physical principles of radiography, which are crucial for obtaining high-quality diagnostic examinations and protecting patients and medical staff from radiation exposure. Diagnostic imaging has recently advanced in giant leaps; nevertheless, radiography continues to be the mainstay of any diagnostic investigation. This fact is easily forgotten in the hospital environment, where physicians are surrounded by high-technology equipment. A radiographic examination should always precede any complex imaging procedure, and the interpretation of these complex studies should be undertaken only with the plain film examination at hand. Radiographs provide important information about the alignment of the vertebral bodies, disc space height, facet joint integrity, trabecular pattern, and cortical bone destruction.

Physical Principles

X-rays are a form of radiation belonging to the electromagnetic spectrum (Fig. 1) (40). Electromagnetic radiation consists of electric and magnetic fields that are perpendicular to each other. Electromagnetic radiation has a dual nature, behaving under some circumstances as waves and under different circumstances as particles or photons. The two concepts of wave and particle have been postulated to explain the variety of physical characteristics associated with electromagnetic radiation (9).

In diagnostic radiology, the most useful parts of the electromagnetic spectrum are x-rays and radio waves, both of which can travel through the human body (Fig. 1) (14). Under proper and predetermined conditions, x-rays and radio waves may carry useful diagnostic information that can be captured by appropriate receptors and recorded on films or displayed on television screens for viewing by physicians. X-rays can be either generated in x-ray tubes or emitted from radioactive nuclei. Those gener-

ated in x-ray tubes are generally used in radiography, fluoroscopy, conventional tomography, and computed tomography (CT). X-rays emitted from radioactive isotopes are used in nuclear medicine and radiation therapy. Radio waves are much less energetic than x-rays and are used extensively in magnetic resonance imaging (MRI) (14).

In diagnostic x-ray tubes (Fig. 2), x-rays are produced when a fast stream of electrons is suddenly stopped by the target or anode (positive terminal). The electrons originate on the negative terminal of the tube, which is also called the *cathode* or *filament* (9,40). On the cathode side, x-ray tubes are typically equipped with two filaments—one large and one small; the large filament is used for large exposures. The area of the target bombarded by electrons is referred to as the *focal spot*. Ideally, the focal spot should be as small as possible in order to produce a sharper image on the film (Fig. 3), although a large focal spot allows greater heat loading and therefore less damage to the target. The ability of the x-ray tube to achieve high x-ray outputs is limited by the heat generated at the target or anode. To overcome this problem, the rotating anode was developed, which allows the tube to withstand huge accumulations of heat generated during large exposures (Fig. 2) (9,26). In addition, both the filament and the target are made of tungsten, which has a very high melting point. To limit lack of image sharpness, the focal spot should not exceed 1.2 mm in size, and the spine should be placed as close as possible to the film. Patient motion during the exposure could also result in unsharp images; therefore, patients are instructed to remain perfectly still during the exposure.

With every exposure, an x-ray beam is emitted consisting of a wide spectrum of energies (7,26). The quantity of x-rays emitted from the x-ray tube is proportional to the number of electrons flowing from the filament (cathode) to the target (anode); this is measured in milliamperes. The milliampere setting on the control panel is preselected by the technologist. The quality, or penetrating power, of the x-rays is inversely related to the wavelengths of the x-rays emerging from the tube and is determined by the energy of the electrons striking the target (Fig. 1). More energetic electrons produce a preponderance of x-rays in the beam with shorter wavelengths (high-energy x-rays) and more penetrating qualities. The energy of the electrons bombarding the target is predetermined before the exposure by adjusting the kilovolt setting or potential difference between the

G. Y. El-Khoury: Department of Radiology, University of Iowa College of Medicine, Iowa City, Iowa 52242.

Y. Sato: Department of Radiology, University of Iowa College of Medicine, Iowa City, Iowa 52242.

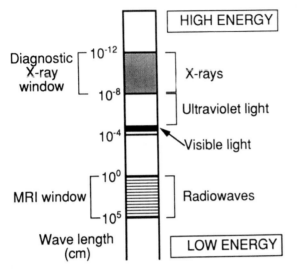

FIGURE 1. The electromagnetic spectrum. Radio waves with a long wavelength and low energy and x-rays with a relatively short wavelength and high energy are both useful in diagnostic imaging because they can travel through the human body.

FIGURE 3. The effect of the focal spot size on the sharpness of the image. **A:** A small focal spot, ideally a point source, produces sharp images. **B:** A large focal spot produces unsharp images with significant penumbra.

cathode and anode. Therefore, with any particular milliampere and kilovolt settings, a spectrum of x-rays of different wavelengths (polychromatic) and energies emerges from the x-ray tube (9,26). Very low-energy x-rays are not diagnostically useful and are actually harmful to the patient because most are absorbed by the first few centimeters of tissue; these low-energy x-rays fail to reach the film or detector with diagnostic information. X-ray tube casings are designed with filters to remove low-energy radiation. Filtration is extremely useful for changing the composition of x-rays in the beam. Aluminum (1 to 3 mm thickness)

is the most commonly used general-purpose filter. Filtration increases the ratio of x-rays in the beam that are useful for imaging to those that increase only the patient's dose of radiation. High-energy x-rays pass through the patient, carrying information, and are diagnostically useful (9).

A physical principle of practical importance in scoliosis examinations is called the heel effect, which becomes detectable when exposing long films (6 inches or longer). The intensity, or concentration, of x-rays within the beam is not uniform throughout all portions of the beam; it is less toward the anode side of the

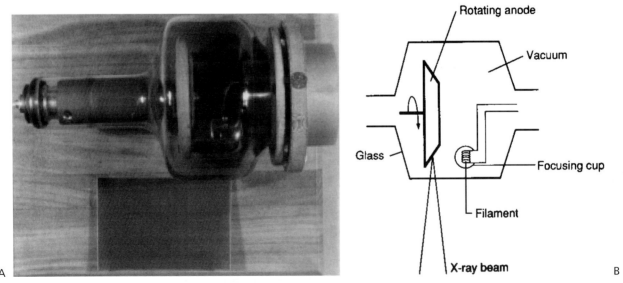

FIGURE 2. Photograph (**A**) and diagram (**B**) of an x-ray tube. The glass casing maintains a strict vacuum within the tube. All the components of the tube are designed to withstand high temperatures generated by changing the kinetic energy of the electrons into x-rays. This is not an efficient process; only 1% to 2% of the kinetic energy of the electrons is transformed into x-rays, and the rest changes to heat.

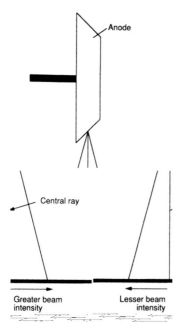

FIGURE 4. Beam intensity. The x-ray beam is more intense toward the anode side of the tube. This fact is put to practical use in the radiography of structures of uneven thickness.

tube (Fig. 4) (9,26). This fact is exploited to obtain balanced photographic densities on radiographs of body parts with different thicknesses. Ideally, when obtaining an anteroposterior view of the entire spine, the thicker body parts (abdomen) should be placed in the intense portion of the x-ray beam or toward the cathode side of the x-ray tube, and the thinner body parts (chest and neck) should be placed toward the anode side of the tube.

Principles governing the interaction of x-rays with matter are beyond the scope of this chapter. Generally, however, the interaction of x-rays with living or nonliving matter is dependent on the energy of the radiation. Low-energy diagnostic x-rays generate less scatter radiation and produce radiographs with good tissue contrast when compared with high-energy x-rays (20). Much of the low-energy radiation, however, is absorbed by thick body parts, and its clinical use is limited (40). High-energy diagnostic x-rays, produced by high kilovolt settings, are generally favored because less radiation is absorbed by the patient; however, they generate significant scatter, resulting in foggy images and diminished tissue contrast on radiographs. Without scatter control, the information content of x-ray images is severely compromised (Fig. 5). To control scatter and improve image quality, radiographic grids are used. The grid is the most common way of controlling scatter in medical radiography. Grids consist of lead strips separated by x-ray–transparent spacers. Primary x-rays travel in a straight line from the tube to the image receptor (Fig. 6A). X-rays that interact with the tissues and bounce off other atoms or electrons are deflected from a straight path and give rise to scattered radiation (Fig. 6B) (2). The amount of scatter is also proportional to the patient thickness and field size used. Thicker body parts produce much more scatter than thinner parts. Larger field size again results in more scatter and less tissue contrast on images (20). Limiting the field

size—in other words, restricting the size of the beam to the area of interest—achieves two very important objectives: It reduces scatter and cuts radiation to the patient by limiting radiation to body parts of clinical interest.

The grid is positioned between the patient and the image receptor; the x-rays traveling in a straight line carry useful information and, for the most part, pass through the lucent portion of the grid (Fig. 6). About 85% to 95% of the scattered x-rays are absorbed by the grid (2). Radiographic examinations of the thoracic and lumbar spine in older children cannot be performed without grids. One disadvantage of grids is that they absorb some of the primary radiation emerging from the patient as well as most of the scattered radiation; therefore, it becomes necessary to increase the radiation to the patient in order to maintain the proper photographic density on the film, which is the price paid to produce high-quality images when radiographing thick body parts (2). Controlling scatter therefore results in increasing patient dose and x-ray tube load. Equipment manufacturers and physicists continually strive to control scatter efficiently by trying to maximize image contrast and minimize radiation dose. Thin body parts, such as the cervical spine, produce little scattered radiation and can be radiographed without grids. One caution regarding the use of grids relates to the fact that grids are focused; therefore, proper alignment and proper distance from the x-ray tube should always be maintained, or the image quality will deteriorate quickly (2,9). This could become a serious problem in examinations performed in bed or in the operating room using portable x-ray machines.

Concepts controlling image formation are the key to the interpretation of radiographic examinations. Photons from the x-ray source interact with tissues and pass through the patient. Variations in tissue composition give rise to differences in attenuation and spatial variation in the x-ray beam exiting the patient. Most of the x-rays in a beam pass through air-containing tissues, such as the lung, with only minimal attenuation; however, most of the beam is absorbed or markedly attenuated as it passes through bone. Fat attenuates x-rays more than air, and water and soft tissues attenuate x-rays more than fat but less than bone. These alterations in the x-ray beam produce differences in the response and the light output of the intensifying screen in the film cassette (Fig. 7). As more x-rays pass through the patient and reach the intensifying screen, more visible light is generated by the screen, and the radiographic film becomes darker. Intensifying screens are used because the sensitivity of film to x-rays is low compared with its sensitivity to visible light. Intensifying screens are placed within x-ray cassettes to convert x-rays into visible light, which in turn exposes the film (Fig. 7). The efficiency of the intensifying screen in converting x-rays to visible light is important in reducing the radiation dose to the patient. State-of-the art radiography relies almost exclusively on the use of rare earth screen systems, which are more efficient than the old calcium tungstate screens (9,26,40).

The same physical principles of radiography apply to fluoroscopy except that the images are displayed on a television screen instead of films. Fluoroscopy plays a limited but important role in selected patients with spine problems. Needle biopsies of the vertebrae and discs are typically performed with biplane fluoroscopy.

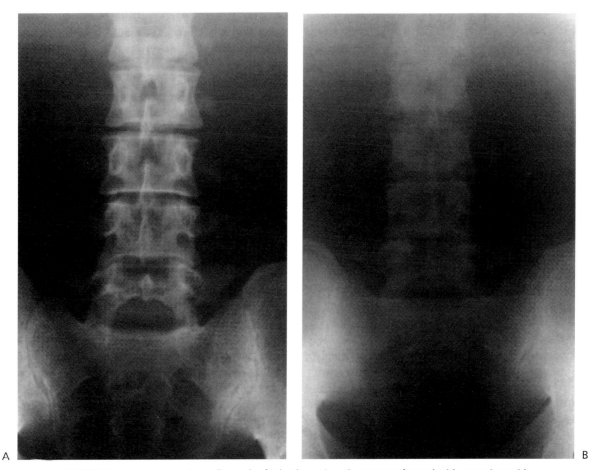

FIGURE 5. **A:** Anteroposterior radiograph of a lumbar spine phantom performed with a moving grid (Bucky) shows excellent trabecular detail and good contrast because most of the scattered radiation has been absorbed by the grid. **B:** The same spine phantom radiographed without a grid demonstrates inferior-quality image because of scatter.

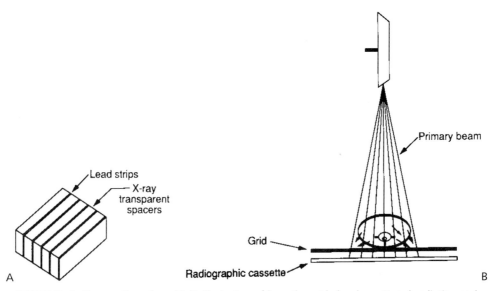

FIGURE 6. **A:** Cross section of a grid. **B:** Illustration of how the grid absorbs scattered radiation and allows the primary beam to pass through.

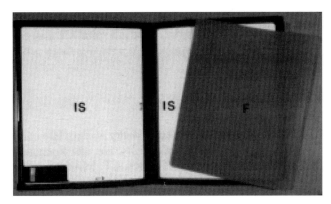

FIGURE 7. An opened cassette. On each side of the cassette, there is an intensifying screen (IS). When the cassette is closed, the film (F) is sandwiched between the two intensifying screens.

Technologic Advances

For more than 100 years, images have been captured on film. The era of filmless imaging is now here to stay. Digital radiography coupled with picture archiving and communications systems (PACS) is one of the fastest growing technologies in medicine. It is estimated that 66% of all hospitals in the United States will be using digital images that can be distributed to practitioners, both within and outside the hospital, using a PACS system by the year 2000. Factors promoting this change include faster and less expensive computers as well as memory storage devices with steadily increasing capacities. Another crucial component in this progress is the ease with which modern equipment manufactured by different companies can communicate digital information using standard protocols (e.g., Digital Imaging and Communication in Medicine [DICOM] standards).

Why do we need digital imaging? Digital imaging is more efficient to acquire and distribute than hard copies, and in the long run, digital images are less expensive to store and retrieve. Digital images can be made available to multiple physicians in different places at the same time. Digital images can be manipulated, that is, made darker or lighter, smaller or larger. Using Internet technologies, image distribution to distant locations can be easily accomplished at minimal cost.

Digital radiography is evolving. In the mid-1980s, indirect image capture was introduced and is still the dominant technology, although there is promise that direct electronic image capture may become the way of the future. With indirect image capture, the conventional screen-film system is replaced with a phosphor plate that can be stimulated, which stores a latent image (32). A laser image reader extracts the latent image from the phosphor plate, and data are handled by an image processor (20). Interactive workstations are connected to the image processor, replacing the light boxes for viewing the images. Direct electronic image capture was introduced in 1996. This technology used selenium or silicon detectors, which convert x-rays directly to electrons and subsequently to digital images.

The disadvantages of digital radiography include the high initial cost and complexity. The diagnostic quality of digital radiography is comparable to conventional screen-film radiography (28,32).

CONVENTIONAL TOMOGRAPHY

The radiograph is a two-dimensional image of three-dimensional structures superimposed over each other. Conventional tomography, also known as *body section radiography,* is an x-ray technique used to blur out superimposed structures and bring into focus structures of interest. The components of any tomographic unit are an x-ray tube and film cassette connected to a rigid arm. When the tube moves in one direction, the film moves in the opposite direction around a fulcrum or focal plane (Fig. 8). The amplitude (distance) of tube travel is measured in degrees and is referred to as the *tomographic angle.* The plane of interest within the patient is positioned at the level of the fulcrum and is the only plane that stays in sharp focus. Structures within the patient above or below the fulcrum are blurred (7,9).

There are several types of tube motions available, but the ones most commonly used in spine work are the circular motion and, to a lesser extent, the pluridirectional (or multidirectional) motion. Complex tube motions produce thorough blurring of structures outside the focal plane; however, complex motions expose the patient to more radiation and diminish image contrast (7).

Other factors to consider when planning tomographic examinations are section thickness and the interval between sections. The thickness of the section in sharp focus is inversely proportional to the amplitude (distance) of the tube travel measured in degrees. The more distance the tube travels, the thinner the section (7,9). The interval defines the distance between each tomographic section. The tube motion, travel, and interval are

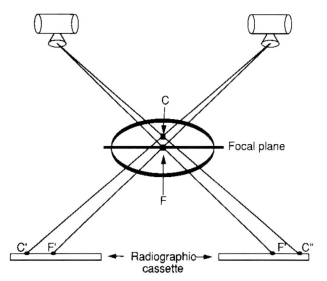

FIGURE 8. The basic principles of conventional tomography. During each exposure, the x-ray tube and radiographic cassette move in opposite directions. Structures above and below the fulcrum or focal plane become blurred, *C.* Only structures at the level of the focal plane stay in focus, *F.*

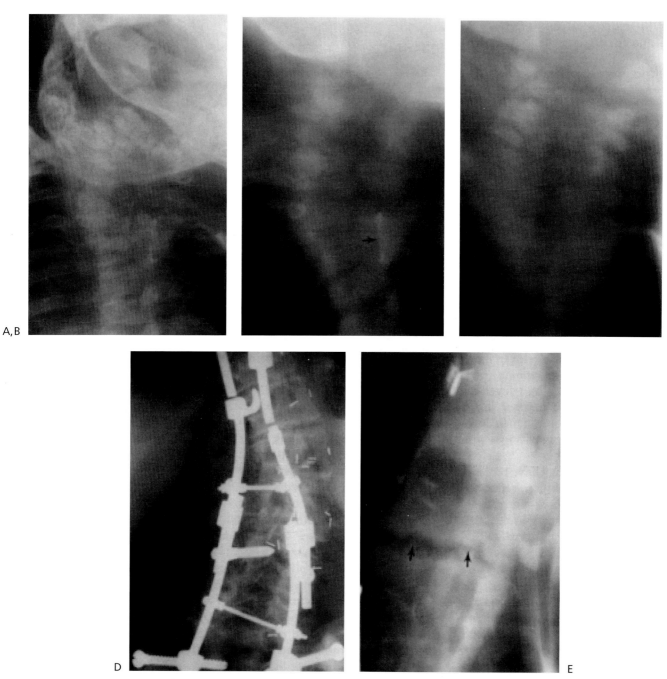

A,B

C

D

E

FIGURE 9. Three-month-old infant with congenital scoliosis. **A:** Anteroposterior radiograph demonstrates the scoliosis but fails to show in detail the multiple segmentation anomalies. **B:** Anteroposterior tomographic section at the level of the pedicles shows a pedicular bar on the left side (*arrow*). **C:** Another section through the vertebral bodies demonstrates multiple hemivertebrae. **D:** This 32-year-old woman presented with acute back pain, 3 years after posterior and anterior spine fusion. Plain films showed broken Cotrel-Dubousset rods. **E:** Conventional tomography demonstrates pseudarthrosis at the site of a previously fused disc (*arrow*).

predetermined for each examination depending on the size of the structure under evaluation. As an example, an osteoid osteoma within a pedicle is best studied with thin sections at intervals not exceeding 3 mm, whereas a large lytic or blastic lesion in the vertebral body can be studied with thicker sections at 5- to 10-mm intervals.

The numbers that appear on the films in a tomographic series indicate the distance between the plane in focus or fulcrum and the film. When reviewing a tomographic study, the films should be arranged in the proper sequence.

Although conventional tomography has been replaced, for the most part, by CT, it continues to be an effective tool in the evaluation of the spine. It is the modality of choice for mapping segmentation anomalies of the spine (Fig. 9). Failure of spinal fusion is still best studied with conventional tomography, although spiral CT may become the preferred modality to evaluate these problems in the future.

COMPUTED TOMOGRAPHY

The remarkable imaging modality of CT was put into clinical use in 1973 by Hounsfield (24). He, like Roentgen, won the Nobel Prize for physics. CT, however, is the end product of multiple discoveries by numerous investigators. The initial mathematical ideas were advanced as early as 1917 by the Austrian mathematician Radon. The basic principle behind CT is that the internal structure of an object can be reconstructed in the form of sections from multiple x-ray projections (9). CT, radiography, fluoroscopy, and conventional tomography use ionizing radiation to obtain images. The scanning gantry contains an x-ray tube, a series of detectors, and a couch with a precision positioning system. The x-ray beam is highly collimated, and the x-ray tube moves around the patient about 360 degrees during a single slice. The detectors capture the attenuated beam, and the resulting data are processed by a computer that displays the image on a matrix of 512 × 512 small squares, called *pixels*. Each pixel is given a CT number related to data obtained by the detectors. On the images, the CT numbers are displayed as various shades of gray, in which the lowest numbers appear black (e.g., air) and the highest numbers appear white (e.g., cortical bone) (7,41). The operator at the console can manipulate the window width (range of CT numbers in the gray scale) and the window level (center of the gray scale) to study either bone or soft tissue detail (Fig. 10) (40,41).

In planning a CT examination, the following parameters are selected: slice thickness, couch index or interval of slices (similar to conventional tomography), gantry angulation, proper window width and level for filming, and appropriate sagittal and coronal image reconstructions. For performing three-dimensional image reconstructions, a slice thickness of 3 mm with 1 mm of overlap is usually desirable.

Significant advances in CT technology have recently been made in the areas of image resolution, reduction of acquisition time, and software for three-dimensional reconstruction. Three-dimensional images do not add any new information that is not already available on axial images. CT actually displays complex anatomy and pathology in a more familiar and understandable fashion. In children, the complex problems of the craniovertebral junction have been appreciably simplified with the use of CT. Spiral or helical CT is a new technology that allows for faster image acquisition and for truly volumetric CT data. This has become possible because of technical refinements in the detector efficiency and greater tube cooling capability.

Three-Dimensional Computed Tomography

Traditionally, CT data have been presented in transaxial plane. With the advent of helical CT, volumetric data of a large area of interest, for example, the entire thoracolumbar spinal column, can be obtained in short period of time, about in 30 seconds. In helical CT, the volumetric data are obtained while the patient is translated continuously through a CT gantry in which the rotating x-ray tube is emitting x-ray without interruption. After the volumetric data are obtained, multiple overlapping axial images can be generated at arbitrary intervals, which provide superb source images for exquisite three-dimensional reconstruction (Fig. 11). These three-dimensional images can then be viewed

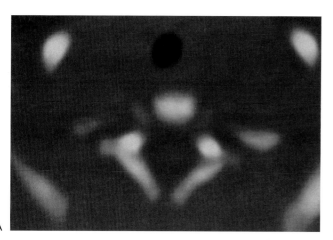
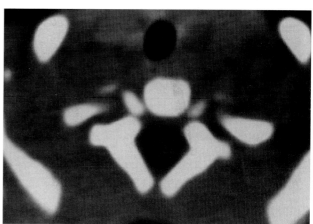

A B

FIGURE 10. CT examination of the upper thoracic spine in an infant. The same section is filmed with a bone window (**A**) and a soft tissue window (**B**).

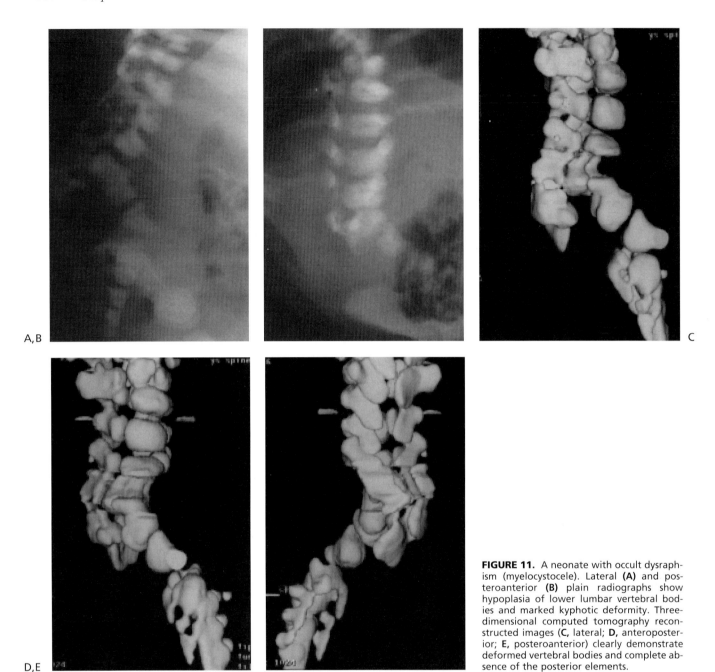

A, B

C

D, E

FIGURE 11. A neonate with occult dysraphism (myelocystocele). Lateral **(A)** and posteroanterior **(B)** plain radiographs show hypoplasia of lower lumbar vertebral bodies and marked kyphotic deformity. Three-dimensional computed tomography reconstructed images (**C**, lateral; **D**, anteroposterior; **E**, posteroanterior) clearly demonstrate deformed vertebral bodies and complete absence of the posterior elements.

from any direction without additional radiation to the patient. This is one of example of a postprocessing maneuver assisted by a graphic computer, which has become imminently important to present clinically pertinent information from vast amount of data obtained by newer CT and MRI technology.

BIOLOGIC EFFECTS OF RADIATION

The use of x-ray examinations continues to increase in both the United States and other countries (17). In the evaluation of spine problems, radiographic examinations are often crucial in

arriving at a specific diagnosis. Most physicians use ionizing radiation extensively in their diagnostic work; however, only a few are formally trained in handling ionizing radiation and radiation protection. Studies have shown that the lack of technical training results in excessive population exposure to ionizing radiation (10). The exposure of patients to medical x-rays continues to command increased attention by society and public health officials (22). If basic principles of radiation protection are followed, the same level of diagnostic information can be achieved with reduced risk to patients and health workers.

X-rays absorbed by tissues exert harmful effects on DNA by direct or indirect action. In direct action, dislodged electrons resulting from the absorption of x-rays interact with DNA to produce damage. In indirect action, the dislodged electrons interact with water molecules in the tissue, producing free radicals, which are highly reactive molecules. These, in turn, damage the DNA. With diagnostic x-rays, the dominant harmful effects on DNA are produced by indirect action. Whether the action of x-rays on DNA is direct or indirect, there are three principal biologic effects of ionizing radiation on humans: (a) genetic effects, in which radiation causes mutations in germ cells that will be expressed in some future generation; (b) carcinogenesis, in which radiation affects somatic cells, causing malignant mutations; and (c) cell killing, which affects embryogenesis because the resulting cell depletion can adversely affect the developing embryo and fetus (17).

In terms of the genetic effects of radiation, exposure to radiation does not produce bizarre or unique mutations, but it increases the frequency of mutations that occur naturally in the population (17,33). The radiation effects on a fetus depend on the stage of pregnancy. During preimplantation, or the first 10 days after conception, the main consequence is the death of the embryo. Radiation delivered during organogenesis, which occurs from 10 days to about 8 weeks after conception, leads to a broad spectrum of anomalies affecting organs and limbs. The natural prevalence of genetic disorders, however, is so high that small increments of fetal anomalies caused by radiation from diagnostic procedures are difficult to measure directly (17,33). There is evidence to suggest that irradiation of the fetus later in pregnancy can result in the future development of leukemia. Present data indicate that the risk for leukemia in a fetus exposed to more than 10 roentgens (R) increases from 1 in 3,000 to 1 in 2,000. To provide a basis for comparison, the average annual dose to the U.S. population from natural sources, or just from living in the United States, is 125 mR per year. The approximate fetal exposure from a chest x-ray to the mother is 1 mR, and an anteroposterior film of the lumbar spine is 50 mR (10,23). All estimates of the deleterious effects caused by radiologic procedures lead to the conclusion that the balance of risk versus benefit is heavily weighted in favor of benefits. If there is a valid medical indication to perform a diagnostic x-ray examination on a pregnant patient, the patient should not be denied the examination because of the pregnancy (43).

All health workers, including physicians, handling x-ray equipment should be familiar with the radiation protection guidelines at their institutions. The following are some general guidelines:

1. Appropriate personnel radiation-monitoring devices (PMDs) should be worn whenever there is a possibility of exposure to radiation.
2. PMDs should be worn only by the individual to whom they are assigned.
3. All exposure to the patient should be kept as low as reasonably possible by attempting to accomplish the following:
   a. Minimize the exposure time.
   b. Maximize the distance from the radiation source.
   c. Maximize filtration.
   d. Maximize film-screen speed (34).
   e. Use collimation.
   f. Use gonadal shielding.
   g. Eliminate unnecessary examination and views (36,37).

MAGNETIC RESONANCE IMAGING

MRI is a new technology that uses no ionizing radiation. It produces sectional images in any desirable plane revealing excellent anatomic detail with high tissue contrast (30). The demand for spinal MRI examinations continues to increase rapidly. The full potential of MRI has not been reached; nevertheless, its impact on the evaluation of spinal diseases has already altered our approach to many diagnostic problems.

In 1945, Bloch and Purcell independently discovered the phenomenon of nuclear magnetic resonance (NMR). They found that certain nuclei are capable of interacting with discrete frequencies of the electromagnetic spectrum—in this case, radio waves—when these nuclei are placed in a strong magnetic field. NMR became an important tool in chemistry for determining molecular structure. In 1952, Bloch and and Purcell shared the Nobel Prize in physics for their work with NMR. In 1972, Lauterbur was able to use the principles of NMR to produce images; this heralded the birth of clinical MRI as we know it today.

MRI is conceptually different from other diagnostic modalities, and a basic understanding of its physical principles is essential for practicing state-of-the-art spinal surgery.

Physical Principles

Nuclei with an odd number of protons or neutrons (^{1}H, ^{31}P, ^{23}Na) exhibit a spin, and because these nuclei are charged particles in motion, they create a magnetic field around them, behaving like small magnets. The nucleus most commonly used for medical imaging is hydrogen, because of its abundance in biologic tissues and its favorable magnetic characteristics. Normally, these small magnets (nuclei) are randomly oriented; when placed in a strong magnetic field, however, they orient themselves in the direction of the external magnetic field and are considered to be in a state of equilibrium. In this state, the nuclei not only spin but also precess around the axis of the external field, in a manner similar to the wobble of a spinning top (Fig. 12). The frequency of precession is directly proportional to the strength of the external field. If a specific radiofrequency (RF) pulse that is resonant with (i.e., has a frequency equal to) the frequency of precession is applied to these nuclei, they deflect from their alignment with the external magnet. When the strength of the RF pulse is chosen to cause a 90-degree deflection, the nuclei tip 90 degrees and precess perpendicular to the external magnetic field. Magnetic moments perpendicular to the external field are capable of producing an alternating current or signal in a receiver coil or antenna placed adjacent to the part being examined. After the RF pulse stops, the nuclei gradually return from the tipped position to their equilibrium state (realigning with the external field), and the emitted signals diminish. The signals captured by the receiver coil are electronically transformed into clinically useful images, or *spectra* (1,8,18).

Definitions

Resonance

The nuclei precess at a frequency that is directly proportional to the strength of the external magnet. The external magnetic

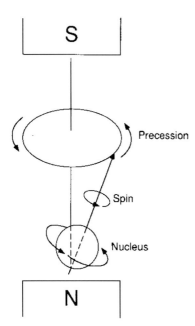

FIGURE 12. Nuclear spin and precession.

field is set at a gradient at which field strength gradually decreases across the scanned part, so that each slice or position is encoded with a known frequency of precession. In other words, the variation in the magnetic strength produces a corresponding variation in resonance frequencies across the sample volume. *Resonance* refers to the synchronization of the RF pulse with a specific precessing frequency of the nuclei in a particular slice (14,18).

T1 and T2 Relaxation Time

The T1 relaxation time (longitudinal relaxation or spin-lattice relaxation time) is a tissue-specific time constant. It is the time required for 63% of the deflected nuclei to realign with the external magnetic field or return to the equilibrium state after the termination of a 90-degree RF pulse (Fig. 13) (1,8,14,18).

The T2 relaxation time (transverse relaxation or spin-spin relaxation time) is also a tissue-specific time constant describing the rate at which nuclei get out of phase or out of precessing as one unit and start to process as individual nuclei. After the 90-degree RF pulse, all the deflected nuclei lying in the transverse plane precess in phase or as one unit. In a matter of milliseconds, they slip out of phase because of interactions with neighboring nuclei. As a result, transverse magnetization ceases, and the signal emitted from the scanned tissue diminishes. Maximum transverse magnetization is achieved immediately after the 90-degree RF pulse. Transverse magnetization decays exponentially at a time constant called T2. To put the nuclei back into phase or to make them spin as a unit, a 180-degree RF pulse is used (Fig. 14). This 90-degree RF pulse, followed by a 180-degree RF pulse, forms the basis for the commonly used spin-echo (SE) sequence, which is currently the workhorse for routine MRI (Fig. 14) (1,8,14,18).

T1 and T2 relaxation after the 90-degree RF pulse occur simultaneously. However, the T2 decay takes less time than T1 relaxation. For most soft tissues, the range of T1 is 220 to 3,000 msec; the range of T2 is 55 to 200 msec (35).

Pulse Sequence

A *pulse sequence* is a precisely defined pattern of RF pulses and listening times. The most commonly used pulse sequences in

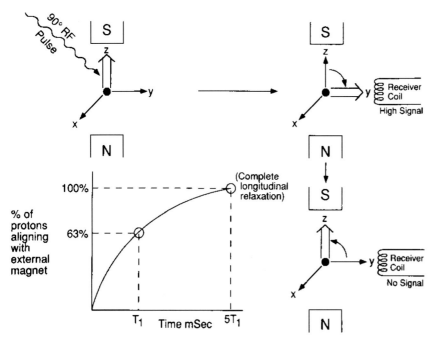

FIGURE 13. Sequence of events when a 90-degree radiofrequency pulse is applied. The magnetized hydrogen nuclei tip 90 degrees from the axis of the external magnet. The tipped nuclei then start to relax or realign with the external magnet at a rate defined by the T1 relaxation time of the tissue. By about five times the T1 relaxation time, all the tipped nuclei would have relaxed or realigned with the external magnetic field.

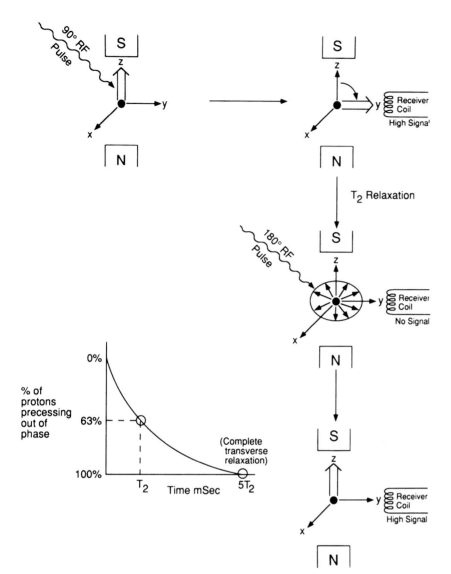

FIGURE 14. Sequence of events when a 90-degree radiofrequency pulse, followed by a 180-degree radiofrequency pulse, is applied. Note that the T2 relaxation time relates to the dephasing of the precessing nuclei, which occurs after they are tipped into the XY plane.

the study of the spine are the SE and gradient-refocused echo (GRE) or gradient echo sequences. A typical SE sequence consists of a 90-degree RF pulse, a pause, and then a 180-degree RF pulse. After an additional pause, the receiver coil is set to listen to a signal or echo emitted from the tissues; after a longer pause, the cycle of RF pulses and listening is repeated (Fig. 15). The SE sequence can be T1 weighted, accentuating the T1 properties of tissue, or T2 weighted, accentuating the T2 properties of tissue. T1-weighted sequences, sometimes called *partial saturation sequences,* have an echo time (TE) of less than 40 msec and a repetition time (TR) of less than 800 msec (Fig. 15). T2-weighted sequences have a TE of greater than 80 msec and a TR of greater than 1,500 msec (30,31,35). In general, T1-weighted images depict anatomy better, and T2-weighted images show pathology better. T2-weighted sequences tend to be lengthy and therefore costly. The other negative aspect of lengthy sequences has to do with patient motion because it is difficult for a patient to lie still for 30 minutes during image acquisition. Any motion during image acquisition results in

marked deterioration of the images. Infants and young children who cannot remain still during the entire course of the procedure have to be sedated or put under general anesthesia before a spinal examination. Recently, a fast SE sequence has been developed that can cut the scanning time to one third the conventional SE sequence without any loss in diagnostic quality.

Other imaging sequences have been devised to reduce the examination time. GRE sequences are rapid sequences commonly used in the evaluation of the spine. Two characteristics distinguish GRE sequences from traditional SE imaging: GRE uses a partial flip angle for excitation less than 90 degrees, and GRE techniques lack the 180-degree refocusing RF pulse. Instead, refocusing is achieved by the reversal of a magnetic field gradient. The short imaging time of GRE techniques does not replace the conventional SE; however, it allows for some unique applications. The most notable is three-dimensional volume acquisition, which is based on the collection of data from a block or slab of tissue rather than one slice of tissue at a time. The excited block of tissue is partitioned into individual sections or

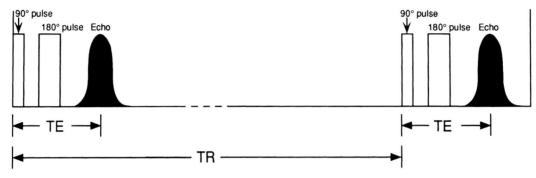

FIGURE 15. Typical T1-weighted spin-echo sequence.

images. With three-dimensional acquisition, structures can be studied with very thin sections, and data from the slab of tissue can be reconstructed in any desirable plane.

When using the GRE sequence, the flip angle is the most important factor in determining the type of tissue contrast produced. In general, small flip angles, in the range of 5 to 20 degrees, produce T2-weighted images. Mildly prolonged TE, in the range of 25 to 30 msec, also potentiates T2 contrast (16).

Echo Time and Repetition Time

The TE is defined as the time between the initial RF pulse and echo production (Fig. 15). The TR is defined as the time between the beginning of a pulse sequence and the beginning of the succeeding pulse sequence (Fig. 15). The TE and TR values are printed on the film with other data to inform the physician interpreting the scans which pulse sequences were used.

Tissue Contrast

Why do certain tissues appear bright or dark with particular pulse sequences? Contrast depends on the following inherent tissue properties: free hydrogen in the tissue (also known as *proton density*), T1 and T2 relaxation times, and flow (30). Most soft tissues in the body have similar proton densities; therefore, proton density alone is not a major contributor to tissue contrast. Flowing tissue, such as blood within arteries, does not persist in a fixed place for scanning and therefore appears dark on both T1- and T2-weighted images. This is caused by the migration of the excited (stimulated by RF pulse sequences) cylinder of blood from the scanning field and replacement by unexcited blood. These flow principles are employed in magnetic resonance angiography (MRA), which is a noninvasive technique used to demonstrate vessels. This leaves T1 and T2 relaxation times of tissues as the most important factors in determining tissue contrast in images. Most clinical protocols are designed with pulse sequences that exploit both the T1 and T2 characteristics of the tissue, so that a range of pathologic features may be identified and characterized. With SE sequences, the variables that are manipulated to produce image contrast are the TR and TE. Sequences with short TR and TE produce images dominated by T1 effect; in long TR and TE sequences, the influence of T2 on image contrast is maximized (Table 1) (30,31).

On T1-weighted sequences (35), tissues with short T1 relaxation times have high signal intensity (bright)—for example, fat. Tissues with long T1 relaxation times have low signal intensity (dark)—for example, cerebrospinal fluid. On T2-weighted sequences (35), tissues with short T2 relaxation times have low signal intensity (dark)—for example, tendon or ligament. Tissues with long T2 relaxation times have high signal intensity (bright)—for example, cerebrospinal fluid.

Because of prolonged T1 and T2 relaxation times, inflamed tissue appears dark on T1-weighted images and bright on T2-weighted images when compared with healthy neighboring tissue. The increased water in the form of edema is offered as an explanation. Neoplasms generally increase the T1 and T2 relaxation times relative to the host tissue; therefore, they appear dark or signal intense on T1-weighted sequences and bright on T2-weighted sequences. This is also thought to be caused by an increase in the free water content within tumors (Table 2).

Surface Coils

A high signal-to-noise ratio is a critical factor in producing high-quality MRI scans. One important source of noise is the patient; therefore, it is important to optimize the interface between the patient and the coil receiving the signals from the patient. The standard body coil is built into the MRI machine and is relatively distant from the patient. When a coil is applied directly to the

TABLE 1. RELATIVE RELAXATION TIMES OF PRACTICAL VALUE IN THE SPINE

Normal Tissue	T1	T2
Water	Long (dark)	Long (bright)
Cerebrospinal fluid	Long (dark)	Long (bright)
Fat	Short (bright)	Medium (gray, bright)
Fibrous connective tissue	Long (dark)	Very short (dark)
Tendons and ligaments	Very long (dark)	Very short (dark)
Bone	Very long (dark)	Very short (dark)
Muscle	Medium (gray)	Medium (gray)
Cartilage		
Hyaline cartilage	Medium (gray)	Medium (gray)
Fibrocartilage	Long (dark)	Very short (dark)

TABLE 2. RELATIVE RELAXATION TIMES OF SOME PATHOLOGIC PROCESSES

Abnormal Process	T1	T2
Infection/Inflammation	Long (dark)	Long (bright)
Neoplasm	Long (dark) or medium (isointense)	Long (bright)
Fibrosis	Long (dark)	Very short (dark)
Fatty infiltration	Short (bright)	Medium (bright)
Hemorrhage (acute)	Long (dark)	Long (bright)

body of the patient, it is called a *surface coil.* Surface coils are sophisticated antennae designed to receive radio waves generated by the precessing nuclei. These radio waves impinge on the coil and generate an alternating current within it. The efficiency of this process depends on how closely the wires are applied to the body part being examined. The anatomic region determines the design of the surface coil. Therefore, a surface coil for the cervical spine is different in design from a lumbar spine coil or a knee coil (Fig. 16). Surface coils greatly improve the quality of the

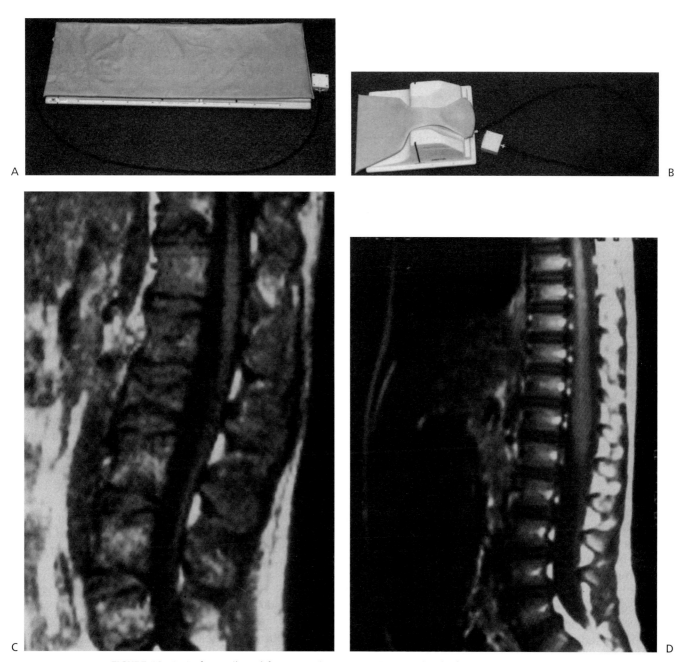

FIGURE 16. A: Surface coil used for magnetic resonance imaging (MRI) of the lumbar and thoracic spine. **B:** Surface coil for the cervical spine. **C:** A lumbar spine MRI study performed with a body coil that is built into the gantry and is not in direct contact with the patient. **D:** An MRI study performed with a surface coil shows significant improvement in the signal-to-noise ratio.

image by increasing the signal-to-noise ratio. Using surface coils, however, limits the field of view. When selecting surface coil, the region of sensitivity of the coil should match in size the region of interest and the field of view. The smallest possible coil should be used (13,27).

Phased-array coils (several surface coils combined to act as one) have the benefits of small surface coils (i.e., increased signal-to-noise ratio) yet provide a large field of view up to 48 cm in length. Both the thoracic and the lumbar spine can be imaged with this technique in about the same time as that required to image the lumbar spine alone (27).

Contrast Agents

The contrast agent presently approved by the U.S. Food and Drug Administration for clinical use is gadolinium diethylenetriamine pentaacetic acid (Gd-DTPA), which is a paramagnetic agent. Paramagnetic atoms possess unpaired electrons in their outer shells, thus creating their own small local magnetic field. Paramagnetic agents act in enhancing (shortening) the T1 and T2 relaxation times of surrounding hydrogen nuclei. T1 shortening produces higher (brighter) signals on T1-weighted images. Gd-DTPA displays pharmacokinetics similar to those of iodinated contrast media in that it penetrates highly vascularized areas and produces an increase in signal intensity in these areas on T1-weighted images. The paramagnetic properties of Gd-DTPA reduce the T1 relaxation time of penetrated tissues. In the musculoskeletal system, there is preliminary evidence that Gd-DTPA is useful in differentiating edema, cyst formation, and necrosis from the actual tumor and, therefore, helps in delineating the extent of a neoplastic process. It has also been used extensively in differentiating epidural scarring from recurrent disc herniation after disc surgery (3,45).

Nonionic gadolinium compounds with lower osmolality than that of Gd-DTPA are being developed. These newer compounds can be safely injected in larger doses than currently permitted with Gd-DTPA (3).

Safety and Contraindications

With the current clinical level of exposure, MRI is generally a safe technique. Recent studies indicate no interference with cardiac function or nerve conduction at 2 to 7 tesla magnet strength. The forceful attraction of ferromagnetic objects to the magnet is a definite risk. Caution must be exercised when there are ferromagnetic objects embedded in the patient, such as shrapnel, foreign bodies lodged within the eyes, or aneurysm clips in the brain. As a rule, MRI should not be performed on patients with cardiac pacemakers, aneurysm clips, or cochlear implants. Metallic orthopaedic appliances are generally not ferromagnetic, but they do create significant local artifacts that preclude scanning in the immediate vicinity of the appliance. MRI should be avoided during the first trimester of pregnancy (25,38).

MYELOGRAPHY

Myelography (5) has been replaced almost entirely by MRI, except on rare occasions, in the workup of pediatric spinal problems. When myelography is performed, low-osmolality, nonionic contrast material is used usually followed by a CT examination.

After adequate sedation and sterilization, the patient's back is anesthetized locally using 0.5% lidocaine (Xylocaine) at the L4–5 or L3–4 interspinous process. A 22-gauge spinal needle is inserted into the subarachnoid space, and contrast material is injected. If a complete block is suspected, a single drop of Pantopaque is injected. The table angle is changed so that the drop is moved to the level of the suspected block to identify it.

Indications for myelography include the following:

1. Identification of the exact anatomy of congenital anomalies, such as diastematomyelia, meningoceles, or other defects before corrective surgery
2. Documentation of drop metastases from such tumors as medulloblastomas, ependymomas, and pineal region tumors when the contrast-enhanced MRI study is negative
3. Confirmation of traumatic avulsion of the nerve sheath and posttraumatic pseudomeningocele

Major complications of myelography include death in association with anesthesia or sedation; respiratory arrest caused by tonsillar herniation or sedation; implantation epidermoid spinal abscess; chemical or infectious meningitis; and seizures.

ANGIOGRAPHY

The indication for spinal angiography (15,21,29) in the pediatric age group is primarily for the transcatheter treatment of vascular malformations and preoperative embolization of vascular tumors (Fig. 17) (21).

The cervical spinal cord is supplied by anterior spinal arteries branching off from the vertebral arteries and radiculomedullary arteries of the deep cervical and costocervical trunk. The upper thoracic segment (T1 to T7) of the spinal cord is perfused by radiculomedullary branches arising from the fourth to fifth intercostal arteries. In the thoracic region, the anterior spinal artery is smaller in diameter than the one in the cervical or thoracolumbar region. The artery of Adamkiewicz (arteria radicularis anterior magna) supplies the spinal cord from T8 through the conus. In 85% of cases, this artery arises from the intercostal or lumbar artery accompanying a nerve root between T9 and L2 (Fig. 17E). In the remaining cases, it arises between T5 and T8.

Liberal use of the digital subtraction technique is essential in the spinal angiogram for the identification of the lesion and arteries supplying the cord, particularly the artery of Adamkiewicz. Diversion of the flow in a radiculomedullary artery to the artery of Adamkiewicz by opening a potential communication during embolization is well known; thus, intermittent verification of the flow pattern during the process of embolization is necessary to prevent inadvertent complications.

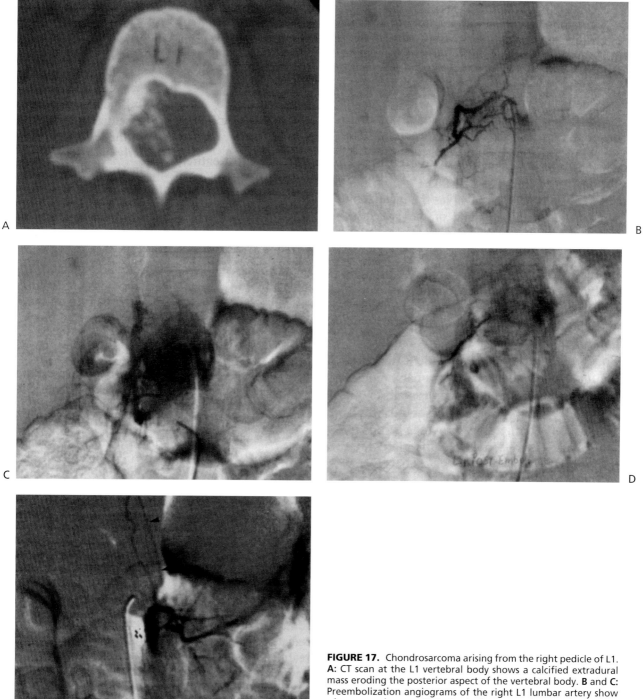

FIGURE 17. Chondrosarcoma arising from the right pedicle of L1. **A:** CT scan at the L1 vertebral body shows a calcified extradural mass eroding the posterior aspect of the vertebral body. **B** and **C:** Preembolization angiograms of the right L1 lumbar artery show a hypervascular mass. **D:** Postembolization angiogram shows obliteration of the tumor stain. **E:** Angiogram of the left L1 lumbar artery demonstrating the artery of Adamkiewicz (*arrowheads*).

RADIONUCLIDE BONE IMAGING

A common indication for radionuclide bone imaging in children is low back pain. Back pain in children is different from that in adults. Most radionuclide bone scanning in adults is performed to evaluate metastatic bone disease, but this is not the case in children.

Technetium-99m methylene diphosphonate (^{99m}Tc-MDP) is given 2 to 4 hours before scanning. The dose of radionuclide is calculated according to the body weight of the child. Two other agents are used for the detection of infection: gallium-67 citrate and indium-111–labeled white blood cells. The use of indium-111 is widely accepted and involves the incubation of the radionuclide with a sample of the patient's blood, which is reinjected into the patient; scanning is performed 24 hours later.

Single photon emission computed tomography (SPECT) is frequently used in the evaluation of low back pain (Fig. 18). SPECT is thought to improve the identification and localization of bone lesions, but no controlled studies comparing SPECT with planar scintigraphy are available for the spine. As with all

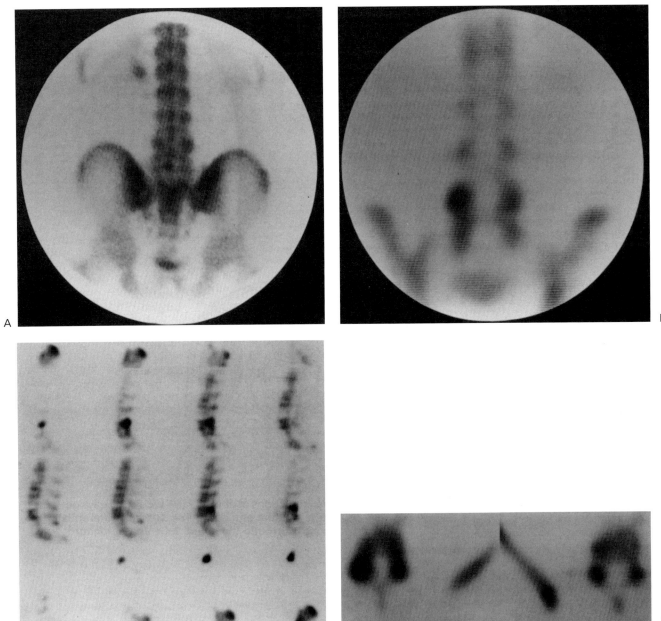

FIGURE 18. Nineteen-year-old athlete with low back pain. Radiographs were negative. Planar bone scintigraphy (**A**) is unremarkable. Coronal (**B**), sagittal (**C**), and axial (**D**) single photon emission computed tomography images show bilateral increased radiotracer uptake in the region of the pars interarticularis, more pronounced on the right side.

other imaging procedures, infants and young children must be adequately immobilized or sedated during image acquisition.

Bone scintigraphy is an excellent screening technique for young patients with low back pain. Because low back pain in children and adolescents is often associated with organic disease and should be vigorously pursued, bone scintigraphy provides a sensitive technique to exclude neoplasm, infection, fracture, or active spondylolysis (42).

UNIQUE FEATURES OF THE DEVELOPING SPINE

Embryology of the Spine

A brief review of the basic embryology of vertebral column formation may help in the analysis of the radiologic appearance of the pediatric spine (11,19,39).

Development of the bony spine evolves around the notochord, which acts as a framework for the developing spine and induces and controls the formation of vertebral bodies. The notochord forms from Hensen's node, a rapidly proliferating group of cells in the primitive streak, and develops into a chain of cells between the neural tube dorsally and the entoderm (developing gut) ventrally (Fig. 19).

There are three stages in the development of the vertebral column: formation of the membranous, cartilaginous, and osseous vertebral column.

Formation of the Membranous Vertebral Column

The fetal vertebral column begins to form toward the end of the third week, when the notochord separates from the primitive gut and the neural tube, and somites are formed from paraxial mesoderm on either side of the neural tube (Fig. 19). The ventral medial aspect of the somite further differentiates into the sclerotome, the precursor of the centra, neural arches, and ribs. The dorsal-lateral aspect of the somite forms the dermatome, the precursor of skin. The dorsal-medial aspect of the somite forms the myotome, the precursor of the paraspinous musculature. The sclerotomes surround the notochord in the ventral aspect

and the neural tube in the dorsal aspect, forming a continuous mesodermal sheath termed the *membranous vertebral column.* The sclerotome is then divided into cranial and caudal halves by an evanescent structure called the *sclerotomal fissure.* Adjacent halves of contiguous sclerotomes unite to form one vertebral body (Fig. 20). The intersegmental vessels that divided the sclerotomes now become incorporated within the center of the vertebral bodies, whereas segmental spinal nerves that originally related to the midpoint of the sclerotomal segment—site of the sclerotomal fissure—eventually relate to disc areas.

Formation of the Cartilaginous Vertebral Column

At about the fourth fetal week, chondrification of the vertebral column starts, and the membranous vertebral column is succeeded by the cartilaginous vertebral column. Two cartilaginous centers appear on either side of the notochord, forming the cartilaginous vertebral bodies (Fig. 19). A short time later, additional cartilaginous centers appear in the neural arches and in the costal processes to form pedicles, laminae, and costal processes of the cervical spine and ribs.

Formation of the Osseous Vertebral Column

At about the eighth fetal week, ossification of the vertebral column starts from the thoracolumbar junction and extends cranially and caudally. Ossification centers are formed dorsally and ventrally in the vertebral body, one for each neural arch (Fig. 21). Ossification centers start to appear in the bodies of the lower dorsal and lumbar regions at about the third month of gestation and, by the end of the fifth month, are present in all vertebral bodies. Ossification proceeds rapidly craniad and more slowly caudad. By the fourth month, all the centra are ossified.

The notochord, which remained as a solid cord during the membranous stage, is progressively squeezed from the vertebral body into the intervertebral discs by the increased pressure caused by the rapid enlargement of the vertebral bodies during chondrification and ossification. The notochord in the intervertebral discs forms the nucleus pulposus after some mucoid degeneration and proliferation.

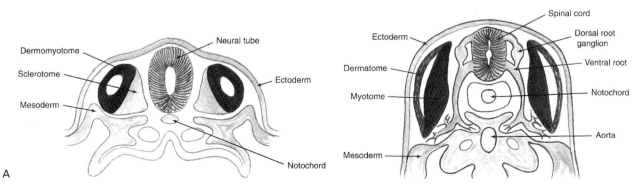

FIGURE 19. Early embryologic development. Axial sections at about 22 (**A**) and 30 (**B**) days' gestation. The notochord lies between the neural tube and the entoderm. The somites differentiate into sclerotomes, dermatomes, and myotomes and surround the neural tube and notochord.

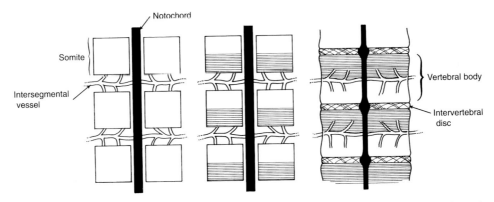

FIGURE 20. Development of the vertebral body and intervertebral disc. The vertebral bodies are formed by the fusion of the caudal segment with the cranial segment of the next somite. The intersegmental tissue containing intersegmental vessels becomes the center of the vertebral body. The intervertebral discs develop from the sclerotomes and remnants of the notochord.

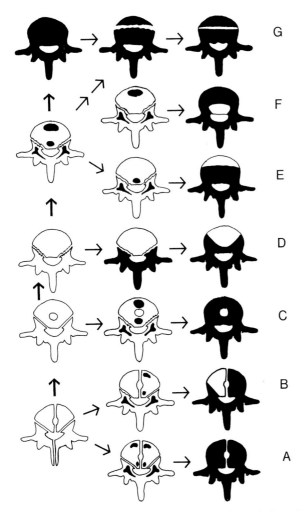

FIGURE 21. Development of the vertebral body and its variations. Cartilaginous formation is shown in white and osseous formation in black. Normal development is shown in the left row; variations and anomalies in the middle and right rows. *A,* sagittal cleft of body; *B,* hemivertebra; *C,* notochord remnant; *D,* absent vertebral body; *E,* hypoplastic vertebral body; *F, G,* coronal cleft (Adapted from Barnes GT (1991): Contrast and scatter in x-ray imaging. *Radiographics* 11:307–323, with permission.)

GENERAL DEVELOPMENT

The neonatal spine lacks the physiologic curvature of the adult spine (Fig. 22). At birth, the vertebral column is relatively straight and forms a single, long, shallow curve extending from the cervical to the lumbar segment with the convexity directed anteriorly. Cervical lordosis appears during the first year when the infant starts to have head control. Thoracic kyphosis and lumbar lordosis develop when the child starts to bear weight toward the latter half of the first year and gradually become more prominent during childhood. The complete loss of this physiologic curvature, however, may be pathologic even in neonates, suggesting conditions ranging from tumor to muscle spasms. In the neonatal period, the individual vertebral bodies are ovoid and wedge shaped when seen on lateral radiographs. They appear smaller in size relative to the intervertebral space, owing to the presence of nonossified cartilaginous zones on the superior and inferior surface. The "bone within a bone" appearance (Fig. 23) is normally seen, particularly in premature infants (4,19). The oval-shaped centrum has ventral and dorsal clefts, which are vascular channels (Fig. 22). The anterior notch is formed by a large sinusoidal blood space within the vertebral ossification center, whereas the posterior one is formed by a perforated indentation on the posterior wall of the vertebral body functioning as a conduit for basivertebral veins and nutrient arteries (39). Cartilaginous plates at the site of fusion of the sclerotome containing the intersegmental vessels can be observed routinely on MRI and occasionally on radiographs. The ventral channels gradually fade, but the dorsal channels may be seen even in adults (Fig. 24).

Neurocentral synchondroses, small nonossified parts of the attachment between ossification centers of the posterior neural arches and the vertebral body, are seen as radiolucent clefts in neonates and persist until the third to sixth years (Fig. 21). These should not be mistaken for fractures. The union of neurocentral synchondroses first occurs in the lumbar region shortly after birth, progresses cephalad, and reaches the cervical region by the second year. Clefts are also seen in the midline posteriorly between two ossification centers of the posterior neural arches and

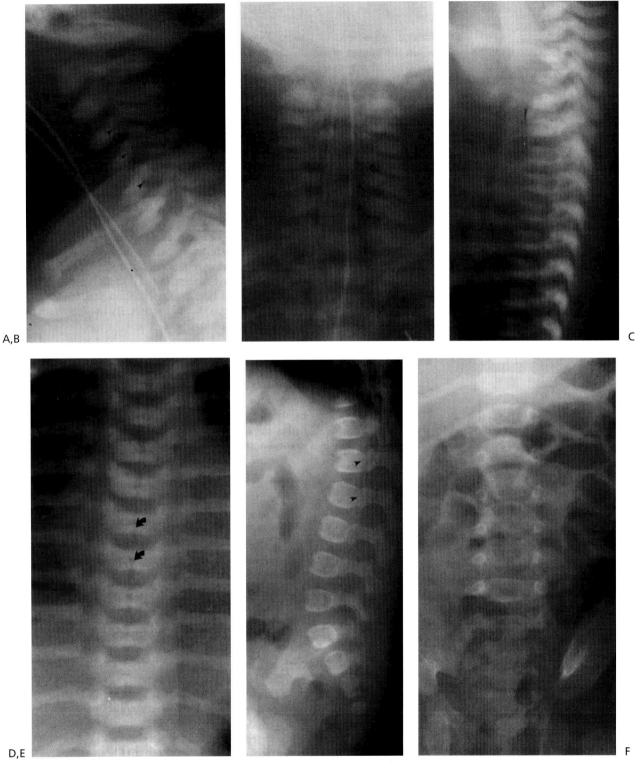

FIGURE 22. Neonatal spine. Cervical spine (**A and B**): Mid and lower cervical vertebral centra are round in shape and wedged anteriorly. Anterior arch of the atlas is not ossified and therefore cannot be seen. Physiologic kyphotic curvature is not developed. Neurocentral synchondrosis (*arrowheads*) between the centrum and neural arch is seen as a longitudinal radiolucency. The subdental synchondrosis (*curved arrow*) is not fused. Thoracic spine (**C and D**): Thoracic vertebral centra are more squared and show distinct anterior and posterior "notches." The midthoracic to upper lumbar region is the straightest segment. Central portions of the posterior arches, which are not ossified, are seen as a series of radiolucencies (*curved arrows*) in the midline. Lumbar spine (**E and F**): Mild kyphotic and lordotic curves are present in the upper lumbar and lumbosacral junction. Note the neurocentral synchondrosis (*arrowheads*).

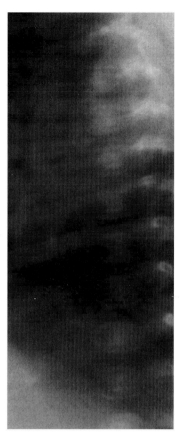

FIGURE 23. Neonatal spine. The "bone within a bone" appearance of the vertebrae is seen in the normal neonate.

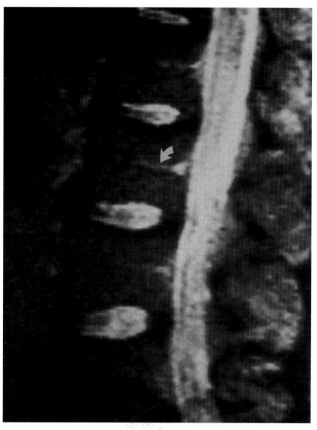

FIGURE 24. Dorsal vascular channel (*curved arrow*) is shown on a T2-weighted magnetic resonance image of a 25-year-old man.

appear as midsagittal radiolucencies on anteroposterior radiographs of the spine (Fig. 22D).

Coronal cleft vertebrae are normally present, most commonly in the lumbar region and predominantly in boys (12). This variation of the vertebral body is probably caused by the incomplete fusion of the anterior and posterior ossification centers of the centrum (Fig. 19). This defect usually disappears in a few weeks to months. This variation occurs more commonly in association with skeletal dysplasias such as chondrodysplasia punctata (Fig. 25) (6).

As the child grows, the spinal column attains a more adult configuration (Fig. 26). Physiologic lordosis of the cervical spine becomes more evident once head control is gained. Lumbar lordosis becomes prominent with walking. The vertebral bodies become more rectangular.

Secondary ossification centers appear at the tips of the several bony processes attached to the neural arch (39): transverse, articulating, and spinous processes (Fig. 27). These ossification centers do not participate in the longitudinal growth of the spinal column. They all appear at about puberty and fuse to the main mass of the neural arch at about 25 years of age. The annular ossification (Figs. 28 and 29) marginating the superior and inferior corners of the vertebral body appears as early as the seventh year and fuses with the vertebral body at about 25 years of age. The ossification of the ring apophyses may not occur simultaneously in the upper and lower surfaces of the same vertebral body and may easily be mistaken for a fracture. Complete ossification

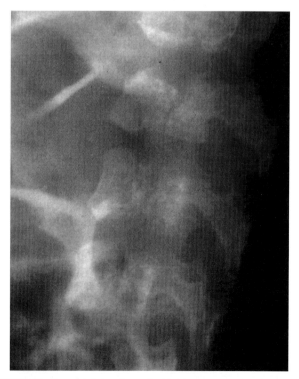

FIGURE 25. Coronal clefts of vertebral bodies. A coronal cleft is seen in multiple vertebral bodies in this infant with chondrodysplasia punctata. The cleft may be seen transiently in normal neonates.

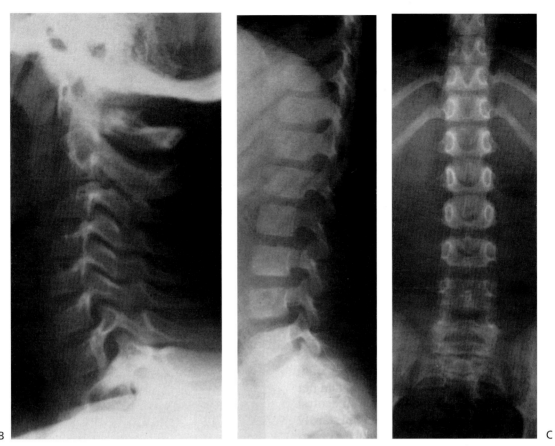

A,B   C

FIGURE 26. Normal 6-year-old cervical (**A**) and lumbar (**B and C**) vertebral column. Cervical and lumbar lordosis has developed, and the vertebral bodies have become more rectangular.

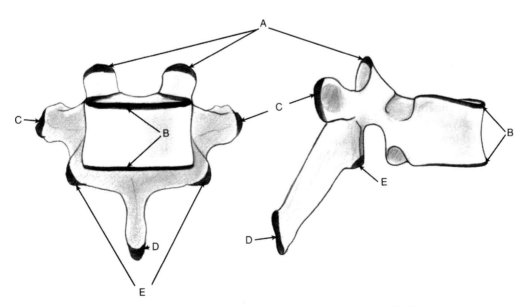

FIGURE 27. The secondary vertebral ossification centers. *A and E,* superior and inferior articular processes; *B,* annular ossification centers; *C,* transverse processes; *D,* spinous processes.

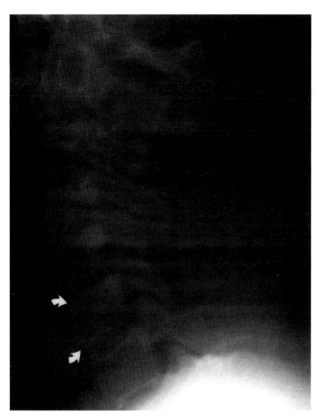

FIGURE 28. Annular ossification centers (*curved arrows*). Cervical spine in a 13-year-old boy.

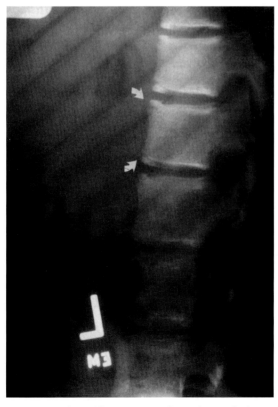

FIGURE 29. Annular ossification centers (*curved arrows*). Thoracolumbar junction in a 12-year-old girl.

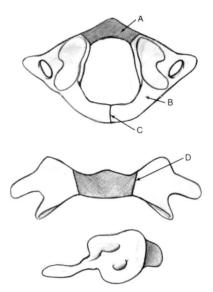

FIGURE 30. Development of the atlas. *A,* ossification center for the anterior arch; *B,* ossification center for the neural arch; *C,* the synchondrosis of the neural arches; *D,* the neurocentral synchondrosis.

and incorporation into the vertebral bodies usually occur by 18 years of age. Ring apophyses may be seen in the lumbar vertebrae of patients even in their twenties. When seen on lateral radiographs, ossifying ring apophyses appear as thin sclerotic lines along the end plates. The vertebral bodies are slightly beaked or notched, owing to the apophyseal edges of the anterior borders.

The development of the atlas and axis requires special attention (Figs. 30–33). At birth, the neural arches of the atlas are separated by cartilage in the midline dorsally. The arches fuse at about the fourth year. The anterior arch is cartilaginous at birth (Fig. 22A). Neurocentral synchondroses between the anterior arch and lateral masses fuse at about the eighth year of life. The failure of these fusions may cause confusion when evaluated in the context of trauma (Fig. 34). The transverse diameter of the atlas ring may be increased, causing lateral deviation of the lateral masses of the atlas in relation to the odontoid process, mimicking a Jefferson fracture.

The ossification of the axis is derived from five primary centers consisting of the centrum, neural arches, and dens; the latter two are paired (Fig. 31). The neural arches fuse dorsally at about the second year. The dens ossifies from two laterally placed cen-

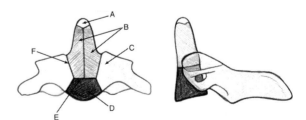

FIGURE 31. Development of the axis. *A,* ossification center for the os terminale; *B,* ossification centers for the odontoid process; *C,* ossification center for the neural arch; *D,* ossification center for the body of the axis; *E,* subdental synchondrosis; *F,* the neurocentral synchondrosis.

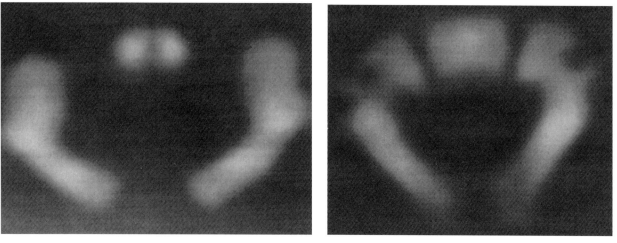

FIGURE 32. Computed tomography scans of the ossification centers of the atlas (**A**) and axis (**B**) in the neonate.

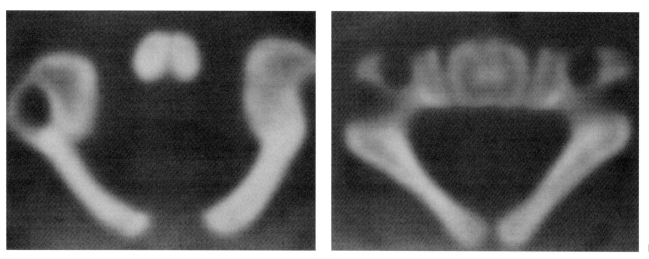

FIGURE 33. Computed tomography scan demonstrates the ossification centers of the atlas (**A**) and axis (**B**) in an 8-month-old infant.

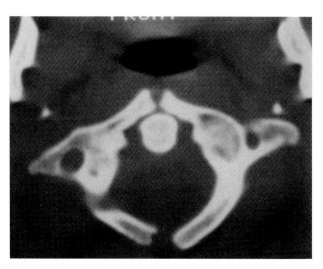

FIGURE 34. Nonfusion of anterior and posterior arches of the atlas in a 14-year-old boy. Open-mouth view (not shown) showed increased distance between the odontoid and lateral masses of the atlas. Jefferson fracture was suspected. Subsequent computed tomography scan revealed nonfusion (rachischisis) of both the anterior and posterior arches of the atlas.

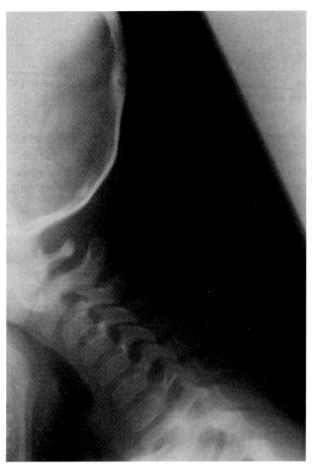
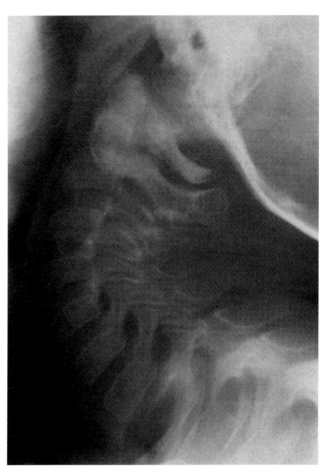

A   B

FIGURE 35. C2 to C3 pseudosubluxation. Lateral radiograph of a 6-year-old child in flexed neck position (**A**) shows prominent anterior movement of C2 to C3 and, to a lesser extent, C3 to C4, giving a subluxed appearance. On extension view (**B**), the alignment of the cervical spine is normal.

ters that fuse before birth. Neurocentral and subdental synchondroses ossify between 4 and 7 years of age. Remnants of these synchrondoses should not be mistaken for fractures. The terminal *ossicle,* or "summit" ossification center, in the tip of the odontoid process appears between the second and sixth years; it then fuses with the main mass of the odontoid at 11 to 12 years of age.

The upper cervical column has unique features in infants and young children. The upper cervical facet joints are oriented more horizontally, and vertebral bodies are wedged anteriorly. The fulcrum for maximal cervical flexion is higher, at the C2 to C3 level in this age group, as opposed to the C5 to C6 level in adults. This physiologic and anatomic uniqueness results in prominent anterior movement at the C2–3 and occasionally C3–4 spaces on flexed neck lateral radiographs, and it is often mistaken for a subluxation (Fig. 35).

MAGNETIC RESONANCE IMAGING SIGNAL CHANGES OF THE DEVELOPING SPINE

MRI signal characteristics in the normal pediatric spine evolve dramatically with age (5,44). The signal characteristics of the bone marrow of vertebral bodies, cartilaginous end plates, and intervertebral discs may be summarized as follows.

From birth to 6 months of age, the bone marrow of the vertebral body is ovoid in shape and shows hypointense signal intensity on both T1- and T2-weighted images. The cartilaginous end plates are hyperintense on T1-weighted images and hypointense on T2-weighted images. The discs remain hypointense on T1-weighted images and hyperintense on T2-weighted images throughout growth (Fig. 36).

By 6 to 12 months of age, the bone marrow of the vertebral body becomes more rectangular, and its signal intensity becomes more intense compared with that of the cartilage and disc on T1-weighted images. This reflects the infiltration of lipid into the marrow space. The cartilaginous end plates become ossified by this age and demonstrate no signal on T1- or T2-weighted images (Fig. 37).

By 2 years of age, each part of the vertebra is more distinct, and normal spinal curvature is established. The marrow shows a more marked hyperintense signal on T1-weighted images and a hypointense signal on T2-weighted images. The end plates are ossified and demonstrate no signal on T1- or T2-weighted images (Figs. 38–40).

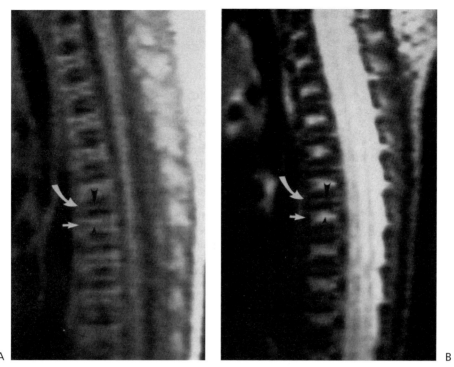

FIGURE 36. Magnetic resonance imaging of the spine in a newborn. The contour of the vertebral bodies is indistinct. **A:** T1-weighted image (SE 400/20) shows hypointensity of the bone marrow (*curved arrow*) with intersegmental vessels in the center (*arrowhead*), hyperintensity of the cartilaginous end plates (*arrow*), and hypointensity of the intervertebral discs (*small arrowhead*). **B:** T2-weighted image (SE 2,000/100) demonstrates hypointensity of the bone marrow (*curved arrow*) and the cartilaginous end plates (*arrow*) and hyperintensity of the discs (*small arrowhead*).

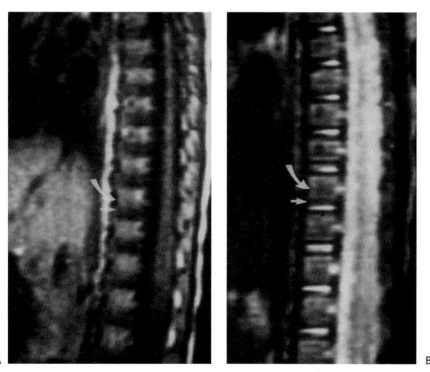

FIGURE 37. Magnetic resonance imaging of the spine in a 7-month-old infant. **A:** T1-weighted image (SE 400/20) shows slight hyperintensity of the bone marrow (*curved arrow*), hypointensity of the ossifying end plates (*arrow*), and hypointensity of the discs (*arrowhead*). **B:** T2-weighted (SE 2,000/100) image shows hypointensity of the bone marrow (*curved arrow*) and the cortical end plates (*arrow*) and hyperintensity of the discs (*arrowhead*).

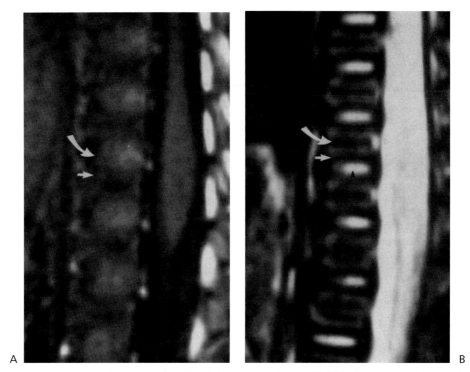

FIGURE 38. Magnetic resonance imaging of the spine in a 2-year-old child. The contour of the vertebral bodies is more distinct. **A:** T1-weighted (SE 400/10) image shows slight hyperintensity of the bone marrow (*curved arrow*) and hypointensity of the cortical end plates (*arrow*) and the discs (*arrowhead*). **B:** T2-weighted (SE 2,000/90) image shows slight hypointensity of the bone marrow (*curved arrow*), hypointensity of the cortical end plates (*arrow*), and hyperintensity of the discs (*arrowhead*).

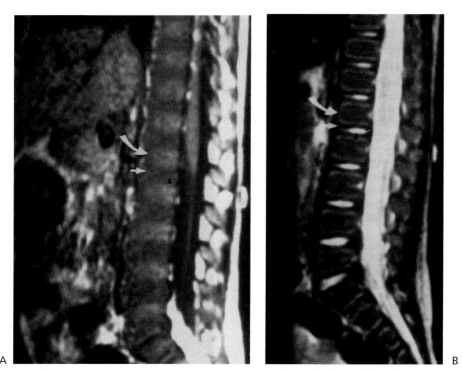

FIGURE 39. Magnetic resonance imaging of the spine in a 5-year-old child. **A:** T1-weighted image shows slight hyperintensity of the bone marrow (*curved arrow*), hypointensity of the cortical end plates (*arrow*), and isointensity of the discs (*arrowhead*). **B:** T2-weighted image shows slight hypointensity of the bone marrow (*curved arrow*), marked hypointensity of the cortical end plates (*arrow*), and marked hyperintensity of the discs (*arrowhead*).

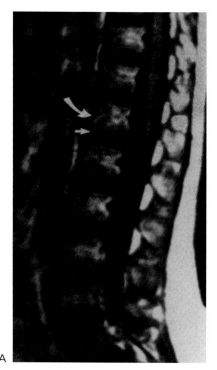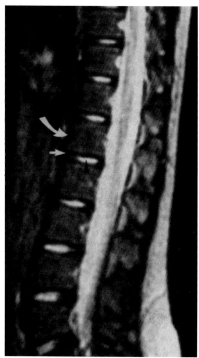

A　　　　　　　　　　　　　　　　　　　　　　B

FIGURE 40. Magnetic resonance imaging of the spine in a 9-year-old child. **A:** T1-weighted (SE 500/11) image shows marked hyperintensity of the bone marrow (*curved arrow*), marked hypointensity of the cortical end plates (*arrow*), and isointensity of the discs (*arrowhead*). **B:** T2-weighted (SE 2,000/90) image shows isointensity of the bone marrow (*curved arrow*), marked hypointensity of the cortical end plates (*arrow*), and marked hyperintensity of the discs (*arrowhead*).

SUMMARY

Familiarity with the developing spine, as well as the imaging modalities to evaluate it, is essential for diagnosing spinal disease. This chapter briefly discusses these issues and points out some of the technical developments that are looming on the horizon.

REFERENCES

1. Balter S (1987): An introduction to the physics of magnetic resonance imaging. *Radiographics* 7:371–383.
2. Barnes GT (1991): Contrast and scatter in x-ray imaging. *Radiographics* 11:307–323.
3. Beltran J, Chandnani V, McGhee RA Jr, et al. (1991): Gadopentetate dimeglumine-enhanced MR imaging of the musculoskeletal system. *Am J Roentgenol* 156:457–466.
4. Brill PW, Baker DH, Ewing ML (1973): "Bone-within-bone" in the neonatal spine. *Radiology* 108:363.
5. Byrd SE, Wilczynski MA (1991): Imaging modalities for the pediatric spine. *Curr Opin Radiol* 3:906–918.
6. Cohen J, Currarino G, Neuhauser EBD (1956): A significant variant in the ossification centers of the vertebral bodies. *Am J Roentgenol* 76:469–475.
7. Coulam CM, Erickson JJ (1981): Production of x-rays. In: Coulam CM, Erickson JJ, Rollo FD, et al., eds. *The physical basis of medical imaging.* New York: Appleton-Century-Crofts, p. 37.
8. Council on Scientific Affairs (1987). Fundamentals of magnetic resonance imaging. *JAMA* 258:3417–3423.
9. Curry TS III, Dowdey JE, Murry RC Jr (1990): *Christensen's physics of diagnostic radiology,* 4th ed. Philadelphia: Lea & Febiger, pp. 16–19, 222–225.
10. Doubilet PM, Judy PF (1981): Dosimetry of radiological procedures and dose reduction in diagnostic radiology. *Postgrad Radiol* 1:309–323.
11. Epstein BS (1976): *The spine: a radiological text and atlas,* 4th ed. Philadelphia: Lea & Febiger, 13–23.
12. Fielden P, Russel JGB (1970): Coronal cleft vertebra. *Clin Radiol* 21:327–328.
13. Fisher MR, Barker B, Amparo EG, et al. (1985): MR imaging using specialized coils. *Radiology* 157:443–447.
14. Fullerton GD (1987): Magnetic resonance imaging signal concepts. *Radiographics* 7:579–596.
15. Gellad FE, Sadato N, Numaguchi Y, et al. (1990): Vascular metastatic lesions of the spine: preoperative embolization. *Radiology* 176:683–686.
16. Haacke EM, Tkach JA (1990): Fast MR imaging: techniques and clinical applications. *Am J Roentgenol* 155:951–964.
17. Hall EJ (1991): Scientific view of low-level radiation risks. *Radiographics* 11:509–518.
18. Harms SE, Morgan TJ, Yamanashi WS, et al. (1984): Principles of nuclear magnetic resonance imaging. *Radiographics* 4:26–43.
19. Harwood-Nash D, Fitz CR (1976): *Neuroradiology in infants and children,* vol. 3. St. Louis: CV Mosby, pp. 1054–1071.
20. Hasegawa BH (1991): *The physics of medical x-ray imaging (or the photon and me: How I saw the light),* 2nd ed. Madison, WI: Medical Physics Publishing, pp. 36–37, 80–83.
21. Heinz ER (1984): Techniques in imaging of the spine. In: Rosenberg RN, ed. *The clinical neurosciences. Part 4: Angiography.* New York: Churchill Livingstone, pp. 818–825.
22. Hendee WR (1991): Personal and public perceptions of radiation risks. *Radiographics* 11:1109–1119.
23. Hogan MJ, ed (1987): X-rays and the pregnant woman. *Mayo Clin Update* 3:1–2.

24. Hounsfield GN (1973): Computerized transverse axial scanning (tomography): Part 1. Description of system. *Br J Radiol* 46:1016–1022.

25. Kanal E, Shellock FG, Talagala L (1990): Safety considerations in MR imaging. *Radiology* 176:593–606.

26. Kelsey CA (1985): *Essentials of radiology physics.* St. Louis· Warren H. Green, pp. 89–97.

27. Kneeland JB, Hyde JS (1989): High-resolution MR imaging with local coils. *Radiology* 171:1–7.

28. Lee KR, Siegel EL, Templeton AW, et al. (1991): State-of-the-art digital radiography. *Radiographics* 11:1013–1025.

29. McSweeney WJ, Benton C (1976): *Special procedures in infants and children. Practical approaches to pediatric radiology.* Chicago: Year Book Medical Publishers, pp. 363–419.

30. Merritt CRB (1987): Magnetic resonance imaging—a clinical perspective: image quality, safety and risk management. *Radiographics* 7:1001–1016.

31. Mitchell DG, Burk DL Jr, Vinitski S, et al. (1987): The biophysical basis of tissue contrast in extracranial MR imaging. *Am J Roentgenol* 149:831–837.

32. Murphey MD, Quale JL, Martin NL, et al. (1992): Computed radiography in musculoskeletal imaging: state of the art. *Am J Roentgenol* 158:19–27.

33. Murphy PH (1991): AAPM tutorial: acceptable risk as a basis for regulation. *Radiographics* 11:889–897.

34. Newlin N (1978): Reduction in radiation exposure: the rare earth screen. *Am J Roentgenol* 130:1195–1196.

35. Pavlicek W, Modic M, Weinstein M (1984): Pulse sequence and significance. *Radiographics* 4:49–65.

36. Roberts FF, Kishore PRS, Cunningham ME (1978): Routine oblique radiography of the pediatric lumbar spine: Is it necessary? *Am J Roentgenol* 131:297–298.

37. Scavone JG, Latshaw RF, Weidner WA (1981): Anteroposterior and lateral radiographs: an adequate lumbar spine examination. *Am J Roentgenol* 136:715–717.

38. Shellock FG, Curtis JS (1991): MR imaging and biomedical implants, materials, and devices: an updated review. *Radiology* 180:541–550.

39. Silverman FN. The spine. In: Silverman FN, ed. *Caffey's pediatric x-ray diagnosis: An integrated approach,* 8th ed., vol 1. Chicago: Year Book Medical Publishers.

40. Sprawls P Jr (1987): *Physical principles of medical imaging.* Rockville, MD: Aspen Publishers, 1987:25.

41. Sprawls P (1990): The principles of computed tomography image formation and quality. In: Gedgaudas-McClees RK, Torres WE, eds. *Essentials of body computed tomography.* Philadelphia: WB Saunders, pp. 1–9.

42. Summerville DA, Treves ST (1991): Radionuclide imaging of bone disease in children. In: Markisz JA, ed. *Musculoskeletal imaging: MRI, CT, nuclear medicine, and ultrasound in clinical practice.* Boston: Little, Brown, p. 129.

43. Swartz HM, Reichling BA (1978): Hazards of radiation exposure for pregnant women. *JAMA* 239:1907–1908.

44. Sze G, Baierl P, Bravo S (1991): Evolution of the infant spinal column: evaluation with MR imaging. *Radiology* 181:819–827.

45. Wolf GL (1989): Current status of MR imaging contrast agents: special report. *Radiology* 172:709–710.

The Pediatric Spine: Principles and Practice, 2nd ed., edited by Stuart L. Weinstein. Lippincott Williams & Wilkins, Philadelphia © 2001.

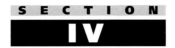

PATIENT EVALUATION

5

BACK PAIN IN CHILDREN

HOWARD A. KING

The problem of evaluating back pain in adults has been carefully studied, with numerous papers written that document the incidence of pain and symptoms. Treatment of the adult with back pain remains controversial, but the incidence and rate of pain have been well documented. In general, the literature suggests that in most adults with back pain, there is no definable cause of the symptoms, and symptoms resolve with time in most patients. The clinician generally has a grasp of those problems that will respond well to surgical treatment if the symptoms do not resolve with conservative management (e.g., spinal deformity, spinal stenosis, spondylolisthesis, disc herniation). We know far less about the incidence of back pain in children and the adolescent group. Reports suggest that the incidence of back pain in the younger age groups may be higher than once thought (1,8,15,19,25,26,29,33,36,40). Turner and colleagues (43) reported that less than 2% of patients younger than 15 years of age had been seen by a physician for an evaluation of back pain. Grantham (18), however, noted in a review of school children that 11.5% of adolescent boys were seen by a physician for low back pain. Fairbanks and associates (12) showed that 26% of students in English schools reported back pain on a questionnaire, and yet very few had sought medical attention for the symptoms. Olsen and coworkers (33) reported that complaints of back pain are rare before 10 years of age but increase between 12 and 15 years of age. Olsen and coworkers' data suggested that by 15 years of age, 36% of adolescents could be expected to have experienced back pain. Their data, however, showed that only 2% of their study group sought medical attention for their symptoms. Balague and colleagues (1) using a validated questionnaire found that 27% of Swiss schoolchildren had experienced back pain, but as in other studies, few of the study group had gone to see a physician. These investigators also noted that 23.6% of competitive and 15.8% of recreational athletes had low back pain.

Review of the current literature suggests that the incidence of back pain in children and adolescents is higher than earlier literature would suggest (1–33,35). Young patients, however, rarely have symptoms severe enough to warrant medical attention. Micheli and Wood (29) have shown that young athletes who present with back pain have a high incidence of spondylolysis as the cause of their symptoms. Turner and colleagues (43)

and I (21–23) have shown that children presenting to a physician with back pain frequently have a cause of their symptoms.

Physicians who see young people in their practices should be prepared to evaluate these patients if they present with symptoms of back pain. The physician should be prepared to take a detailed history, perform a thorough physical examination, and order appropriate radiographic examinations. If the physician is uncomfortable in performing this evaluation, an early referral to someone experienced is appropriate. It is ill advised to make the diagnosis of stress or psychosocial problems until all other organic causes have been excluded. Likewise, the diagnosis of "growing pains" should not be made; even when all other causes have been excluded, the diagnosis is more likely to be related to activity or overuse than growth.

The evaluation of the child with back pain requires a detailed history and physical examination. When appropriate, radiographs, laboratory tests, and special diagnostic imaging studies may be necessary to complete the workup. It is useful for the evaluating physician to have a good understanding of the differential diagnoses and studies that are appropriate to do a thoughtful and detailed evaluation.

MEDICAL HISTORY

The initial step in evaluating a child with back pain is a careful, detailed history. Both the child and the parent should be present to provide optimal information. Frequently, even adolescents are not good historians, and a parent can usually help fill in the details. A thorough history offers insight into the problem and how it affects the patient and family. The initial evaluation should take place in a well-lit and comfortable environment that is conducive to the development of a good rapport with the patient. It is also appropriate to study the interaction of the child with family members. Subtle comments and movements may hold keys to the underlying problem. Frequently, what is said is not as revealing as what is observed.

The history should start with general questions regarding the onset of symptoms, location, frequency, duration, and intensity. Acute traumatic symptoms must be distinguished from those with a slow insidious onset. It is important to inquire about sports and other specific activities. Spondylolysis is frequently seen in patients actively engaged in football, dance, or gymnastics (2,7,13,17,21–24,30,31,39,42,44). Inquiring about these ac-

H. A. King: St. Lukes Regional Medical Center, Boise, Idaho 83702.

tivities may help direct attention to possible "overuse" syndromes. It is also important to inquire about the frequency and intensity of these activities. Many young athletes may offer that they play a sport, but specific questions may reveal that they participate at a very high level and practice for many hours, supporting the diagnosis of stress fracture or overuse syndrome. Any abrupt changes or increase in activity may be associated with the onset of back symptoms. How the symptoms are interfering with the child's normal activities is a significant factor. Symptoms that are only occasionally present with home chores are not as worrisome as symptoms that cause a child to stop participating in a sport or pleasurable activity. Any child who has voluntarily given up a pleasurable activity because of back pain is by definition disabled and has severe symptoms. These complaints alone are adequate to proceed with an aggressive workup regardless of initial findings.

It is appropriate to inquire about frequency, duration, location, and intensity of the symptoms. Movements or activities that aggravate or relieve the symptoms should be identified. It is also important to inquire about night pain. Night pain is a worrisome symptom that can be associated with tumors, infections, and inflammatory conditions. Generally, problems such as spondylolysis, spondylolisthesis, Scheuermann disease, muscle pulls, or overuse are improved by bed rest. If a family or child reports night symptoms, the physician's level of concern should be heightened. Nighttime back pain mandates a complete and meticulous workup.

The nature of the pain is frequently difficult to determine. It is, however, helpful to inquire about localized, diffuse, or radiating pain. Localized pain may be seen with spondylolysis and tumors. Generalized pain or pain over a fairly wide anatomic region is frequently seen with overuse problems, Scheuermann disease, or inflammatory conditions. Radiating pain into the upper or lower extremities or complaints of numbness, tingling, or weakness suggest neurocompression and warrant the appropriate studies.

The patient and family should be questioned about alterations in neurologic function. It is important to inquire about changes in bowel and bladder habits. Families are frequently embarrassed to discuss issues of bed-wetting or incontinence; hence, the information may not be volunteered unless specifically addressed. These symptoms may be subtle and should therefore be thoroughly discussed. Inquiries about changes in balance and coordination must also be made. Families may not place any significance on the fact that a child falls or stumbles more frequently than other children, unless the right questions are asked. Mild changes in gain and coordination suggest subtle neurologic changes and warrant the appropriate evaluation.

Finally, inquiries must be made about similar symptoms in other family members or role models. Even though the diagnosis of conversion reaction is a diagnosis of exclusion, children do mimic complaints they see and hear from others, including parents, grandparents, siblings, or friends. These symptoms may not seem to correlate with the child's problems, and many families will not associate the two problems unless specifically asked. Even if the symptoms and complaints appear to mimic a role model, a detailed workup should be performed before the diagnosis of a conversion reaction can be made.

A general systems review should be included in the evaluation. Other medical problems can present with a chief complaint of back pain. Weight loss, fever, lethargy, skin rashes, and joint pain and swelling should be noted. Any family history of genetic conditions should also be reviewed. Lymphomas, infections, and rheumatologic conditions have presented with the primary complaint of back pain. The clinician must be aware of the myriad diagnoses that may present as back pain.

PHYSICAL EXAMINATION

The physical examination should be carried out in comfortable, well-lit surroundings. The examination must be thorough, and the patient should wear only underpants and a hospital gown. Boys frequently prefer the use of gym trunks. Modesty should be maintained but not at the cost of being able to see the patient. Observation of the torso and limbs is basic to a thorough back evaluation.

The initial step is a general screening examination, which should include a review of the head, neck, upper and lower limbs, and gait pattern. This allows the physician to watch the patient move and observe the torso and limbs for symmetry; abnormalities in the patient's gait might suggest a neurologic problem.

The spinal examination should start with a general review of posture, alignment, and skin patterns. It is important to look for obvious spinal deformities, trunk decompensation, and evidence of muscle spasm. Midline skin defects, café-au-lait spots, and cysts can indicate serious underlying problems and should be carefully reviewed. Midline cysts, hemangiomas, and lipomas frequently communicate with the underlying nerve structures; therefore, any evidence of midline skin defect should be noted and worked up aggressively to exclude a neural defect or lesion.

The forward-bending test is a crucial part of the examination (Fig. 1A, B). Things to look for include thoracic and lumbar asymmetry and evidence of limited or asymmetric movement of the spine. The amount of movement is a sensitive sign of possible problems. When the child has listing and dysrhythmia or a rigid lumbar lordosis on forward bending, a cause of the back pain is frequently found. An abnormal positive forward-bending test is nearly always a sign of underlying pathology. A positive examination is not pathognomonic of a specific condition but is almost always associated with a documentable diagnosis (Fig. 1A–1B).

The neurologic examination should be thorough. Careful study of the gait provides valuable information, especially when spinal cord or cauda equina pathology is suspected. Motor, sensory, and reflex testing should also be performed and recorded. A sensory examination may not be reliable in young children, however. It is important to look for clonus and the Babinski sign. Evaluation of the abdominal reflexes should also routinely be performed. An abnormal abdominal reflex is a subtle sign of spinal cord pathology. Asymmetry or absence of the reflex has been associated with syringomyelia and spinal cord tumors. Straight-leg raising and crossed straight-leg raising may indicate the presence of radiculopathy. If positive neurologic findings are noted, pediatric neurologic consultation may be indicated.

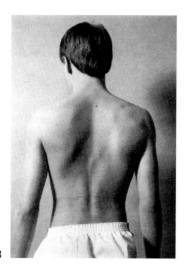
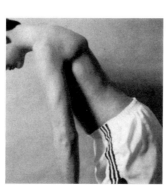

A,B

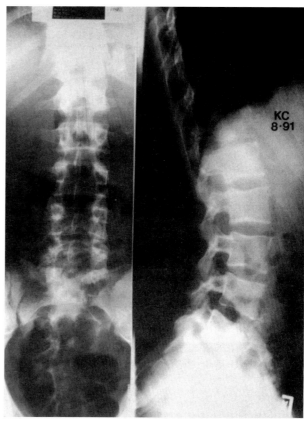

FIGURE 1. **A and B:** This 15-year-old boy presented with a 4-month history of midthoracolumbar back pain and stiffness. This forward-bending test demonstrates severe limitation of motion on forward bending. Note that the patient's lumbar lordosis does not flatten with forward bending. These findings invariably occur when a patient has a true organic cause for back pain. **C:** Anteroposterior and lateral radiographs in the same patient. There is some early narrowing of the T12–L1 disc space. These films were, however, interpreted as normal. **D to F:** Radiographs obtained 4 months after the initial onset of back symptoms. The T12-L1 disc space shows marked narrowing and erosive changes of the end plates, suggesting the diagnosis of hematogenous discitis. *(Figure continues.)*

C

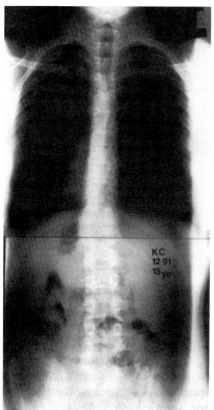
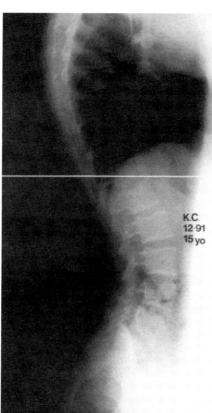
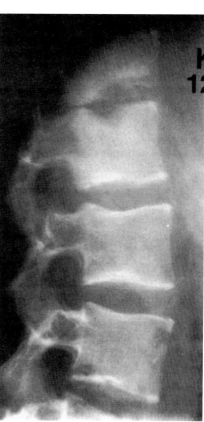

,E

F

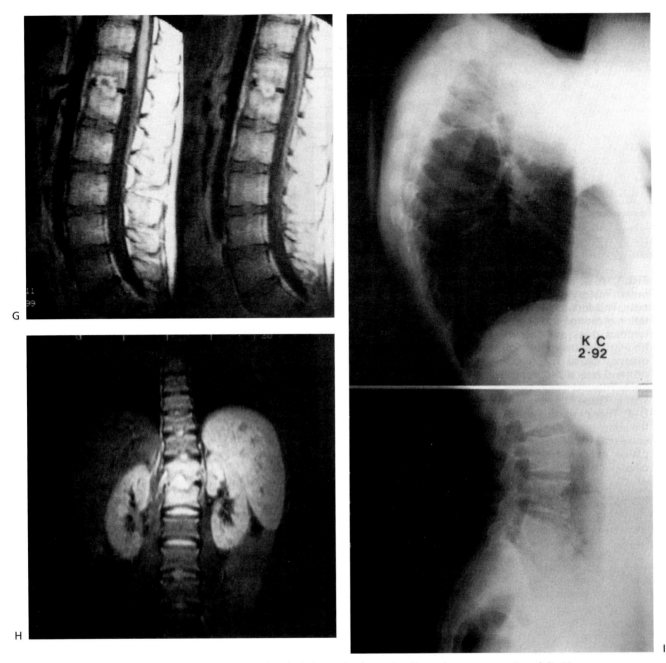

FIGURE 1. *Continued.* **G** and **H:** The physical examination and radiographs were suggestive of discitis. Because of the severe symptoms, a magnetic resonance imaging scan was obtained, which confirmed the diagnosis of discitis. The patient's sedimentation rate was elevated. He was treated with thoracolumbosacral orthoses and intravenous antibiotics. **I:** This radiograph was obtained after 6 weeks of brace and intravenous antibiotic therapy. The patient was completely free of symptoms and had regained normal back motion. The film demonstrates residual changes at the T12-L1 disc space.

RADIOGRAPHIC EVALUATION

Every child who presents with back pain should have at least an anteroposterior and lateral radiograph of the spine (Fig. 1C, D). Oblique radiographs are not necessary on a routine basis but can be useful if the initial films are negative or equivocal. Good-quality films are important, especially when looking for tumors and stress fractures. If the findings are subtle, they may be missed on a poor-quality study. It is also important to visualize fully the area of maximal symptoms. Communicating with the radiology technologist regarding location of symptoms and maximal area of interest will ensure adequate visualization. Experience suggests that spondylolisthesis and spondylolysis are the most common causes of low back pain. Generally, the pars interarticularis defect can be seen on the lateral film. In addition, oblique views and caudocephalic views may be useful in better defining the pathology if the anteroposterior and lateral views are equivocal or non-diagnostic.

IMAGING STUDIES

Bone Scan

If a child is having significant symptoms and the plain radiographs are not diagnostic, a bone scan using technetium-99m should be done (Fig. 2D). If the symptoms have lasted less than 1 month and the physical examination is unremarkable, the decision to do a scan may be delayed. In a patient with severe symptoms or a highly suspicious examination, however, a bone scan should be done promptly. The scan has been useful in finding tumors, discitis, and stress fractures. The radioactive material is more readily absorbed in areas with increased vascularity.

It is important to outline the specific information hoped to be obtained from the scan. The nuclear medicine team can do various views to help define a suspicious area. For example, pinhole images may be useful to give better detail around a tumor nidus or pars interarticularis stress fracture. Generally, the scan is performed 2 to 3 hours after injection of a radioactive tracer. If the vascularity of the lesion is a concern, a three-phase scan can be performed, consisting of an initial-phase dynamic flow study (nuclear angiography), an immediate postflow image, and then the usual delayed blood pool image (28). Generally, however, the standard delayed study is of most benefit.

The bone scan studies should include the entire spine and pelvis. A total-body scan is generally not necessary unless a tumor or a suspicious lesion has been identified. Under these circumstances, a total-body scan is performed to exclude metastatic or multifocal disease. It is most important to include the pelvis because lesions in the pelvis can present as and mimic lumbar symptoms. Lesions around the ischium and greater sciatic notch may even cause the patient to present with radicular-type symptoms. Even though there is no neural compression, the symptoms may closely resemble sciatica. Lesions or a stress reaction around the sacroiliac joints may cause symptoms similar to those of spondylolisthesis and spondylolysis. It is important to realize that a positive scan may be a nonspecific finding and must be correlated with symptoms, plain radiographs, and other studies, such as computed tomography (CT) and magnetic resonance imaging (MRI) scans.

Occasionally, the bone scan does not show focal increased activity, yet the symptoms and plain radiographs may suggest a suspicious lesion. Lowe and associates (27), in a prospective study of 53 military recruits with low back pain and spondylolysis, confirmed an increased incidence of positive bone scan and active symptoms. Papanicolaou and colleagues (34) found that although bone scans were useful in evaluating patients with spondylolysis, plain radiographs were better for making the diagnosis; bone scans may be more useful in determining the activity level of a pars fracture.

Single photon emission computed tomography (SPECT) is a technique that links the bone scan with CT techniques. This technology dates back to the early 1980s but has only recently been integrated into routine scanning studies (3,14). The technique is basically CT of a conventional scan. Collier and cowork-ers (9) and Bellah and associates (2) have shown that SPECT imaging is more sensitive in looking for stress fractures than plain scanning techniques (Fig. 2D, E). Bodner and colleagues (3) have shown that SPECT scans are more sensitive in identifying stress fractures in the lumbar spine and have more precision in locating lesions. They believe that by using axial images, they can be more precise in locating the exact anatomic area involved. SPECT studies can be useful when the plain bone scan is negative or equivocal. The SPECT image can help locate stress fractures and differentiate unilateral from bilateral pars fractures when the plain bone scan shows only a unilateral lesion (Fig. 2D, E).

Computed Tomography Scan

CT scans can be useful in evaluating low back pain. CT can be used as an adjunct in the evaluation of suspicious bony lesions seen on x-ray or bone scan. Although CT is not much help as a screening study, it is useful in evaluating tumors, fractures, and disc herniations. CT may also be used to evaluate spondylitic lesions in the lumbar spine. If brace or cast immobilization has been used, CT scans may be used to determine whether healing has occurred in the pars area.

CT scans are also used to evaluate neural compression after myelography. Although MRI has decreased the number of myelograms performed, CT can be effective in enhancing a myelographic study, especially in adolescent patients with difficult-to-evaluate disc herniation. Using CT-enhanced myelograms is an effective way of outlining the pathology. CT is an accurate tool when MRI shows multiple levels of disc pathology or when there are equivocal studies that do not match the symptoms.

Magnetic Resonance Imaging

MRI scanning techniques have revolutionized the evaluation of children's spines. MRI techniques are extremely useful in evaluating the spinal cord and neural elements, and tumors and syringomyelia have been much more accurately evaluated with MRI.

One caution, however, involves the tendency to overread MRI scans positive for disc pathology as the cause of low back pain. Tertti and associates (42) studied two groups of young adolescents—one with back pain and the other free of symptoms. They found that 38% of the patients with back pain and 26% of the symptom-free patients had disc degeneration by 15 years of age. They were unable to find any statistical significance in their data. They concluded that by 15 years of age, disc degeneration is already a common finding on MRI scans and may not correlate with back symptoms.

Although MRI studies are excellent diagnostic tools, they should not be used as a "shotgun" screening examination and should not be performed before a thorough examination and plain radiographs are obtained. Because of their cost and inconvenience, MRI studies must be reserved for those cases in which clinical signs and symptoms deem them appropriate. Specifically, MRI has been extremely useful in evaluating the spine when neurologic findings or symptoms are present. It is invaluable in diagnosing spinal cord tumors, syringomyelia, bone tumors, discitis, and other conditions. However, it does not seem

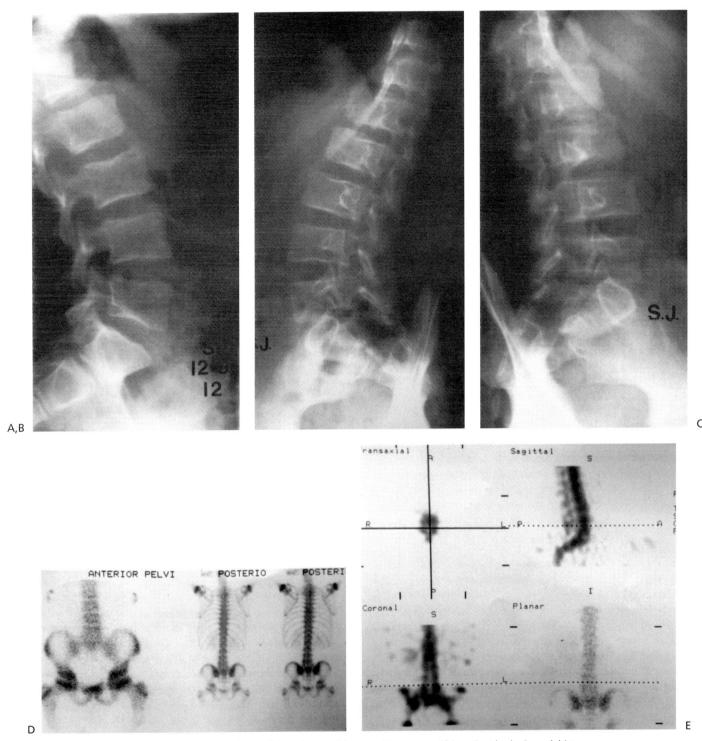

A,B

C

D

E

FIGURE 2. **A:** Lateral radiograph in a 12-year-old competitive runner. This patient had a 3-week history of low back pain localized to the left side at the lumbosacral junction. A high index of suspicion for spondylolysis was noted because of the patient's high level of sports activity. The anteroposterior and lateral radiographs were interpreted as normal. **B and C:** These oblique radiographs were used to evaluate the sacs interarticularis. They were interpreted as showing no evidence of fracture. **D:** A bone scan was obtained. The initial planar study did not demonstrate uptake in the spine or pelvis. **E:** This image, using single photon emission computed tomography techniques, demonstrates an area of increased activity at the L5–S1 pars interarticularis on the left. This area was compatible with the patient's symptoms, which subsided with brace immobilization.

as effective as some other diagnostic modalities for diagnosing stress fractures and should not replace a careful history and physical examination.

When using MRI, physicians must communicate their suspicions to the radiologists. Because many radiologists are more familiar with adult conditions, some extra prescan planning can be useful in getting maximal value from the studies, especially in young children for whom sedation or general anesthesia is necessary to obtain an optimal study.

LABORATORY EVALUATION

A careful laboratory evaluation may be indicated based on the complaints and clinical findings. In cases in which infection, rheumatologic disease, lymphoma, or leukemia are included in the differential diagnosis, laboratory studies are useful. A complete blood count, sedimentation rate, urinalysis, electrolytes, and enzymes can be used to screen for general medical conditions. HLA-B27, rheumatoid factor, antinuclear antibody, and Lyme titers can be obtained if a rheumatologic condition is suspected.

Because numerous medical conditions can present with back pain as one of the early symptoms, physicians must never forget the importance of evaluating the entire patient. Diagnostic tests and imaging cannot replace a thoughtful physician who understand the many conditions that might bring a child with back pain in for evaluation.

DIFFERENTIAL DIAGNOSIS

The differential diagnosis can generally be established after a careful history and physical examination. The imaging and laboratory studies may be diagnostic or add to the clinical information to help establish a diagnosis.

Bunnell (7) has divided back pain in children into four categories (Table 1):

1. Mechanical disorders
2. Developmental disorders
3. Inflammatory disorders
4. Neoplastic disorders

I have suggested a fifth category, conversion reaction, be added to the list (21,22). The categories outlined by Bunnell are an invaluable guide in helping the physician's thinking process as the evaluation of the child with back pain begins.

After the initial history and physical examination, a working differential diagnosis can be established. Radiographs and laboratory studies can be added to complete the workup and help confirm a diagnosis. The child should not be compared with the adult, and the diagnosis of overuse and lumbar strain can be included after all other possible causes of the symptoms have been excluded. If the diagnosis is not obvious despite a thorough evaluation, it is appropriate to repeat periodic examinations until the symptoms resolve or the diagnosis becomes apparent. It is fair to assume that serious problems do not resolve spontaneously.

TABLE 1. CATEGORIES OF CAUSES OF BACK PAIN

Mechanical disorders
  Postural problems
  Muscular disorders
    Overuse syndromes
  Herniated nucleus pulposus
Developmental disorders
  Spondylolysis/spondylolisthesis
  Scheuermann disease
Inflammatory disorders
  Discitis
  Disc space calcification
  Osteomyelitis
  Rheumatologic conditions
    Juvenile rheumatoid arthritis
    Ankylosing spondylitis
Neoplastic disorders
  Vertebral column
  Spinal cord/canal
  Muscle
  Metastatic tumors
Conversion reaction
  Psychosomatic back pain

Turner and coworkers (43) have shown that more than half of children 15 years of age or younger with nontraumatic back complaints were diagnosed with a problem thought to be compatible with the presenting symptoms. Tufel and I (23) reported on a prospective study of 54 children presenting to a spine clinic at a regional children's hospital. None of the patients presented with a confirmed diagnosis. This study demonstrated that 34 of 54 patients were found to have a diagnosis that was thought to be the cause of the presenting symptoms. It is important to keep in mind that both of these studies were done in a specialty clinic at tertiary referral centers. The incidence of positive findings may be less in a primary care setting, but in specialized centers, back pain is frequently associated with physical problems. It is also important to realize that our study was a prospective study done on patients who were referred and had no diagnosis at the time of initial evaluation. The most alarming finding in our study was the high incidence of tumors found in the study patients. In our series (23), 6 of 54 (11%) patients, and in Turner's series (43), 4 of 61 (6%) patients were found to have tumors around the spine.

The age at presentation can frequently be helpful in developing a differential diagnosis. In my experience, patients younger than 10 years of age at presentation are more likely to have discitis or a tumor, and patients older than 10 years of age at presentation are more likely to have spondylolysis, spondylolisthesis, or Scheuermann disease as a causes of symptoms.

Spondylolysis and Spondylolisthesis

Both Turner and colleagues (43) and I (21–23) showed that spondylolysis and spondylolisthesis were the most common causes of back pain in the study groups in children 10 years of age or older. Spondylolysis appears to be uncommon in children 5 years of age or younger. The fracture of the pars interarticularis appears to occur in activities that accentuate lumbar lordosis and with repeated movement create the stress fracture. Jackson and coworkers (20) have demonstrated an 11% incidence of spondylolysis in young gymnasts. Kono and associates (24) reported a 10.9% incidence of spondylolysis in athletic Japanese boys. Ferguson and coauthors (13) have shown an increased incidence of spondylolysis in college football linemen. Teitz (41) reported a 5% to 20% incidence of spondylolysis in dancers who presented with symptoms of back pain. These studies would suggest that certain activities appear to have an increased incidence of stress fracture in the lumbar spine. Numerous studies have suggested that there is a definite heritable association with spondylolysis (31,32,45).

Patients with symptomatic spondylolysis usually complain of pain with strenuous activity that is usually relieved with rest. The symptoms may be acute or, more frequently, insidious in onset. Some patients present with lumbosacral pain only. The symptoms may vary from mild without limitations in activity to more severe, causing the elimination of all strenuous activities.

The diagnosis can frequently be made on radiographs by obtaining anteroposterior, lateral, and oblique views. When the radiographs are inconclusive, a bone scan with SPECT imaging can be done. If the x-rays and bone scan are equivocal, fine-cut 1-mm CT scans can be done. In my experience, MRI scans have not been useful in establishing the diagnosis of spondylolysis.

The initial treatment of symptomatic patients with spondylolysis is usually modification of activities and the use nonsteroidal antiinflammatory drugs. In patients who persist in having symptoms despite a conservative treatment program, the use of thoracolumbosacral orthosis may be helpful. I generally immobilize the spine for 6 to 12 weeks. Morita and colleagues (30) have shown that about 73% of patients with early defects heal with brace immobilization. In patients with more chronic defects, healing was much less likely. My experience has shown that healing is not as common, but brace immobilization has led to relief of symptoms with subsequent return to normal activities.

Surgical treatment for spondylolysis has been reserved for patients whose symptoms do not respond to nonoperative therapies. In L5- to S1-level spondylolysis, a posterolateral fusion would be recommended. For pars defects at L4 to L5 or above, a pars defect repair can be considered. In my experience, surgical treatment is rarely needed because most patients respond well to conservative programs.

Wiltse (45) has categorized spondylolisthesis into five types: (1) isthmic, which is the most common cause seen in adolescents; (2) dysplastic; (3) traumatic; (4) degenerative; and (5) pathologic. The degree of slip has been categorized by the amount of displacement of one vertebral body on the other: grade 1, 0 to 25% slip; grade 2, 25% to 50% slip; grade 3, 50% to 75% slip; grade 4, 75% to 100% slip. In mild grade 1 to 2 slips, conservative treatment is generally all that is necessary to allow these children to resume their sports and activities. In those with progressive slips and in growing children with grade 3 and above slips, a posterolateral fusion is probably indicated. Controversy exists about the need for instrumentation and reduction in the management of spondylolisthesis.

Scheuermann Disease

In the series reported by Turner and colleagues (43) and myself (21–23), Scheuermann disease was the second most common cause of back pain. Patients generally present with pain that starts later in the day or after strenuous activity. Frequently, these patients also complain of poor posture, with the development of thoracic kyphosis. Rarely are the symptoms so severe that the patients have voluntarily halted activities. The symptoms are usually described as aggravating but not limiting. The physical examination is generally nonspecific unless a deformity is present. The forward-bending test may reveal an obvious kyphosis, with sloping of the ribs and an increase in the anteroposterior dimensions of the chest. A lateral radiograph of the spine shows the typical findings of end plate irregularities and wedging of three or more vertebral bodies. Generally, the diagnosis can be established by physical examination and radiographs. If the symptoms and history do not match the radiographic findings, bone scans can be done to exclude other concomitant causes of symptoms. Bone scans are generally not useful in diagnosing Scheuermann disease unless a fracture has recently occurred. A fracture or avulsion of the end plate may occur in addition to the typical Scheuermann findings.

Osteomyelitis and Discitis

Vertebral osteomyelitis and discitis tend to occur in patients between 1 and 12 years of age, with the mean age of presentation being 6 years (5,38,44). These conditions can occur at any age, however. These patients usually have had symptoms of a fairly long duration. They may or may not be febrile, but they generally appear ill. They may present with back pain, but it is not uncommon for a young child to present with refusal to walk. It is possible to confuse this condition with a septic hip or pelvic osteomyelitis.

Radiographs can frequently confirm the diagnosis, but early in the course of the disease, a bone scan may be more useful, especially if disc narrowing has not yet occurred. Sedimentation rates and white blood cell counts are frequently elevated and can help establish the diagnosis. MRI studies may also be useful in localizing the lesion and defining the extent of bone and soft tissue involvement. Even though tuberculosis of the spine is rare in the United States, there are several new cases each year. It is important to consider this condition when a child presents with back pain and radiographs show vertebral collapse and soft tissue mass. In addition, a careful neurologic evaluation should be done to document the possibility of cord compression.

In the early stages of discitis, the white blood cell count may not be elevated. Wenger and associates (44) have shown that blood cultures were positive in 9 of 32 patients and were more useful in the acute period. Disc space biopsy has been shown to have 25% accuracy factor and, when positive, usually shows *Staphylococcus aureus* as the organism. Because of the low yield of disc space biopsy, blood cultures are obtained, and the patients are treated as though they have *S. aureus* infection. Treatment includes brace or cast immobilization and parenteral antibiotics, especially in patients who present with fever and systemic symptoms. Most patients respond to brace and antibiotic treatment. Rarely is surgery indicated in these patients.

Disc Herniation

Although disc herniation is not a common cause of back and leg pain in children, it does occur (4–6,11,16). Children and adolescents account for about 1% to 2% of all patients who present with disc herniations (9). These patients generally tend to present with a paucity of neurologic signs, yet most have positive straight-leg raising signs. DeLuca and colleagues (10) noted that 98% of children with disc herniation presented with back pain, some with and some without sciatica. Epstein and associates (11) reported on 25 patients with disc herniation and noted trauma as a precipitating cause in more than half. All patients had straight-leg raising signs, and 17 patients had positive crossed straight-leg raising signs. Epstein and others (11) have noted a high incidence of other anomalies along the spine in addition to the herniated disc. Such anomalies as transitional vertebra, spondylolisthesis, congenital spinal stenosis, and lateral recess narrowing have been noted.

The evaluation should include imaging studies. MRI and CT-enhanced myelograms are the two best means for confirming the diagnosis. The MRI scan, however, can be overly sensitive and may lead to false-positive results. DeLuca and colleagues (10) have shown that most herniations occur at L4–5 or L5–S1 levels.

A displacement of the posterior growth apophysis can occur in young patients. These patients frequently present acutely after trauma. Clinical symptoms and presentation can otherwise mimic disc herniation. CT scans and MRI studies do a good job of demonstrating the displacement of the vertebral apophysis and frequently a piece of adjacent bone. The history and physical examination can be suggestive of the problem, but radiographs and imaging studies are necessary to confirm the diagnosis and differentiate the condition from a more typical disc herniation. Differentiation of a disc herniation from apophyseal separation is useful because surgical treatment may vary, depending on the location and size of the fragments.

Tumor

Studies have shown that children with back pain can and do present with tumors (21,22,43). These lesions can occur in the bone or along the spinal cord and soft tissues, and they may be difficult to identify and diagnose. Tachdjian and Matson (39) showed that the diagnosis of cord tumors may take a long time because of the unusual presentation. When these lesions present with marked neurologic deficits, it is easy to proceed with a prompt diagnostic workup. Frequently, however, these patients present with nonspecific complaints of back pain or a constellation of unusual symptoms. They may present with complaints of night pain or pain unrelated to any activity. Although the history may be specific for changes in coordination and bowel and bladder habits, the children frequently have no neurologic signs or changes. On occasion, patients with cord lesions have presented with such unusual complaints that their symptoms have been attributed to hysteria. As mentioned previously, the diagnosis of psychosomatic back pain can be made only when all organic causes have been excluded.

The clinical examination may reveal back listing or atypical scoliosis. Left thoracic scoliosis or scoliosis extending into the cervical spine has been associated with tumors. A careful neurologic examination should be done, paying careful attention to reflexes, especially the abdominal reflexes. Reflex changes of clonus, Babinski sign, or asymmetry of the abdominal reflex may indicate a subtle myelopathy. Any hard neurologic finding demands a prompt evaluation, including sophisticated spinal imag-

ing. MRI scans with and without gadolinium appear to be the best techniques for evaluating spinal cord and soft tissue tumors.

Psychosomatic Pain

Throughout this chapter, it has been stressed that psychosomatic back pain in children should be a diagnosis of exclusion. There are times, however, when careful diagnostic evaluations are done and no firm diagnosis can be made. In patients whose symptoms appear to exceed the findings and who may be subject to other home or school factors, psychosomatic reactions must be considered. These patients often present after relatively minor trauma. They generally report severe incapacitating symptoms but rarely have positive physical findings. During the initial evaluation, it is important to learn about the patient's social and family situations. Children are under great pressure to do well at school, be model citizens, and compete in athletics. When these stresses are masked outwardly, they may result in a myriad of symptoms, including back pain. It is also not uncommon to find that another family member has similar problems and that the child has subconsciously taken on those symptoms. The clinician must be aware of these potential problems and inquire about them.

One study analyzed the experience of managing 17 patients who presented to a clinic with symptoms and findings compatible with the diagnosis of reflex neurovascular dystrophy (37). The clinic program included a careful medical evaluation to exclude organic causes of symptoms. If the symptoms seemed to exceed those related to normal overuse, the patients underwent a careful psychological evaluation, which generally revealed other symptoms or predisposing problems. In that series, role modeling was noted in 71%, hyperesthesias in 59%, parental marital discord in 47%, headache in 41%, abdominal pain in 41%, and conversion symptoms in 41%. Half the patients complained of minor preceding trauma. These patients and their parents viewed themselves as quite ill. In fact, these patients viewed themselves as more ill than did a group of patients newly diagnosed with juvenile rheumatoid arthritis.

The diagnostic studies included a Family Environment Scale, Brief Symptoms Inventory, and Childhood Depressive Inventory. These are standardized tests that can be useful in adding objective data toward the establishment of a diagnosis. Family environment scales demonstrated two family types: one with a highly cohesive, low conflict, high intellectual and recreational orientation; the other with high levels of conflict and low intellectual orientation. Brief Symptoms Inventory studies showed a high level of conflict in 41% of families, especially in the cohesive family type. Only one patient was noted to be depressed based on the Childhood Depressive Inventory. The common denominator for most of these patients was a stressful environment with a fairly high level of family conflict. As a general rule, these patients were not clinically depressed.

Treatment in these patients included aggressive psychological and physical therapy. In patients with severe incapacitating symptoms or a chaotic home situation, hospital admission may be appropriate. Aggressive management has achieved a 94% recovery rate.

Psychosocial elements can play a large role in children's back pain; however, only when a detailed medical evaluation is negative for physical causes should one consider the possibility of psychosocial problems as the cause of symptoms. It is useful to consult colleagues who are familiar with childhood psychosocial problems to aid in the workup and evaluation of these patients. A team approach appears to give optimal long-term results.

SUMMARY

Back pain in children is a fascinating area of pediatric orthopedics. The incidence of back pain in children is fairly high when a large group is screened by questionnaire. Most of these patients never seek medical advice or present for consultation. In patients who do seek medical attention, however, the incidence of a definable cause of symptoms is high. Careful, detailed medical and radiographic evaluations must be performed. Imaging studies should be used when indicated. With diligent workup and evaluation, one can expect to find a cause of the symptoms in more than half of patients. Psychosocial problems may also be masked as low back pain in children and cannot be overlooked when doing an initial evaluation. Even with all our modern technology, nothing replaces the watchful eye of a caring and knowledgeable physician.

REFERENCES

1. Balague F, Dutoit G, Waldburger M (1988): Low back pain in school children: an epidemiological study. *Scand J Rehabil Med* 20:175–179.
2. Bellah RD, Summerville DA, Treves ST, et al. (1991): Low back pain in adolescent athletes: detection of stress injury to the pars interarticularis with SPECT. *Radiology* 180:509–512.
3. Bodner RJ, Heyman S, Drummond DS, et al. (1988): The use of single photon emission computed tomography (SPECT) in the diagnosis of low-back pain in young patients. *Spine* 13:1155–1160.
4. Borgesen SE, Vang PS (1974): Herniation of the lumbar disc in children and adolescents. *Acta Orthop Scand* 45:540–549.
5. Boston HC Jr, Bianco AL Jr, Rhodes KH (1975): Disc space infections in children. *Orthop Clin North Am* 6:953–964.
6. Bradford DS, Garcia A (1969): Herniations of the lumbar intervertebral disc in children and adolescents. *JAMA* 210:2045–2051.
7. Bunnell WA (1982): Back pain in children. *Orthop Clin North Am* 13:587–604.
8. Burton AK, Clarke RD, McClune TD, et al. (1996): The natural history of low back pain in adolescents. *Spine* 21:2323.
9. Collier BD, Johnson RP, Carrera GF, et al. (1985): Painful spondylolisthesis studied by radiography and single photon emission computed tomography. *Radiology* 154:207.
10. DeLuca PF, Mason DE, Weiand R, et al. (1994): Excision of herniated nucleus pulposus in children and adolescents. *J Pediatr Orthop* 14:318–322.
11. Epstein JA, Epstein NE, Marc J, et al. (1984): Lumbar intervertebral disc herniation in teenage children: recognition and management of associated anomalies. *Spine* 9:427.
12. Fairbanks JCT, Pynsent PB, Van Poortvliet JA, et al. (1984): Influence of anthropometric factors and joint laxity in the incidence of adolescent back pain. *Spine* 9:461.
13. Ferguson RJ, McMasters MC, Stanitski CL (1974): Low back pain in college football linemen. *J Bone Joint Surg Am* 56:1300.
14. Fidler MW, Hoefnagel CA (1984): Lateral and computerized transverse 99m Tc-Mdp bone scintigrams to supplement the anteroposterior bone scintigram for spinal hot spot localization. *Spine* 6:655–657.
15. Flato B, Aasland A, Vandvik IH, et al. (1997): Outcome and predictive factors in children with chronic musculoskeletal pain. *Clin Exp Rheumatol* 15:569.
16. Garrido E, Humphreys RP, Hendrick EB, et al. (1978): Lumbar disc disease in children. *Neurosurgery* 2:22–26.
17. Gerbino PG, Micheli LJ (1995): Back injuries in the young athlete. *Clin Sports Med* 14:571–590.
18. Grantham VA (1977): Backache in boys: a new problem? *Practitioner* 218:226–229.
19. Hollingsworth P. (1996): Back pain in children. *Br J Rheumatol* 35:1022.
20. Jackson DW, Wiltse LL, Cirinicione RJ (1976): Spondylolysis in the female gymnast. *Clin Orthop* 117:68–73.
21. King HA (1984): Back pain in children. *Pediatr Clin North Am* 31:1083–1095.
22. King HA (1986): Evaluating the child with back pain. *Pediatr Clin North Am* 33:1489–1493.
23. King HA, Tufel D (1986): Prospective study of back pain in children. *Orthop Trans* 10:9–10.
24. Kono S, Hayashi N, Kashahara G, et al. (1975): A study on the etiology of spondylolysis with reference to athletic activities. *J Jpn Orthop Assoc* 49:125.
25. Kristjansdottir G (1996): Prevalence of self-reported back pain in school children: a study of sociodemographic difference. *Eur J Pediatr* 155:984.
26. Leboeuf-Yde, Kyvik KO (1998): At what age does low back pain become a common problem? *Spine* 23:228.
27. Lowe J, Schachner E, Hirschberg E, et al. (1984): Significance of bone scintigraphy in symptomatic spondylolysis. *Spine* 9:653–655.
28. Maymont JV, Bergfeld JA (1991): Nuclear scintigraphy in the diagnosis of sports related injuries. *Med Orthop* 10:1–5.
29. Micheli LJ, Wood R (1995): Back pain in the young athlete: significant differences from adults. Causes and patterns. *Arch Pediatr Adolesc Med* 149:15–18.
30. Morita T, Ikata T, Katoh S, et al. (1995): Lumbar spondylolysis in children and adolescents. *J Bone Joint Surg Br* 77:620–625.
31. Newman PH (1956): The etiology of spondylolisthesis. *J Bone Joint Surg Br* 45:933.
32. Ota H (1967): Spondylolysis: familial occurrence and its genetic implications. *J Jpn Orthoped Assoc* 41:931–939.
33. Olsen TL, Anderson RL, Dearwater SR, et al. (1992): The epidemiology of low back pain in the adolescent population. *Am J Public Health* 82:606–609.
34. Papanicolaou N, Wilkinson RH, Treves S, et al. (1985): Bone scintigraphy and radiography in young athletes with low back pain. *Am J Radiol* 145:1039–1044.
35. Payne WK III, Ogilvie JW (1996): Back pain in children and adolescents. *Pediatr Clin North Am* 43:899–917.
36. Salminen JJ (1984): The adolescent back: a field study of 310 Finnish schoolchildren. *Acta Orthop Scand Suppl* 315:1–22.
37. Sherry SD, King HA, Wallace C (1991): Analysis of psychosomatic back pain in seventeen children. *Orthop Trans* 15:120–121.
38. Spiegel PG, Kergla KW, Issacson AS, et al: Intervertebral disc space inflammation in children. *J Bone Joint Surg Am* 1972;54:284–296.
39. Tachdjian MO, Matson DD (1965): Orthopaedic aspects of intraspinal tumors in infants and children. *J Bone Joint Surg Am* 1965;17:223–248.
40. Taimela S, Kujala UM, Salminen JJ, et al. (1997): The prevalence of low back pain among children and adolescents. *Spine* 22:1132.
41. Teitz CC (1982): Sports medicine concern in dance and gymnastics. *Pediatr Clin North Am* 29:1399–1421.
42. Tertti MO, Salminen JJ, Paajanen HE, et al. (1991): Low back pain and disc degeneration in children: a control MR imaging study. *Radiology* 180:503–507.
43. Turner PG, Hancock PG, Green JH, et al. (1989): Back pain in childhood. *Spine* 14:812–814.
44. Wenger DR, Bobechko WP, Gilda DL: The spectrum of intervertebral disc space infections in children. *J Bone Joint Surg Am* 60:100–108.
45. Wiltse LL (1969): Spondylolisthesis: classification and etiology. In: American Academy of Orthopaedic Surgeons: *Symposium on the spine*. St. Louis, CV Mosby, pp. 143–168.

6

EVALUATION OF THE PATIENT WITH DEFORMITY

RICHARD E. MCCARTHY

SCREENING

Concept of Screening

Screening has been defined as the presumptive identification of unrecognized disease or a defect by the application of tests, examinations, or other procedures that can be applied rapidly to sort out apparently well people who have the disease from those who probably do not. A screening test is not intended to be diagnostic; rather, physicians can establish a diagnosis after appropriate referrals are made (13). Screening can be undertaken to determine the frequency or natural history of a condition or, as in the case of scoliosis, can be directed toward the early detection of the disease process or its precursors as a guide to the management of individuals (42). Certain presumptions regarding the disease are made regarding the risk or occurrence of the disease and the management of that disease. Some have debated the value of screening for scoliosis based on these presumptions.

The detection of spinal deformities for most patients begins soon after birth. There are, however, cases in which prenatal ultrasounds have detected the presence of spinal deformities, as in the case of spina bifida. The benefit of prenatal detection with myelodysplasia is realized at birth when preparations may be necessary for a cesarean birth or the availability of specialists such as pediatric neurosurgeons for prenatal sac closure. Certainly, there is a benefit derived from the early anticipation of that birth and the emotional adjustment of the parents.

Initial inspection of the newborn in the nursery may identify early signs of spinal dysraphism associated with cutaneous sinuses, midline hairy patches, or other cutaneous lesions. Truncal asymmetries can be detected within the first few years of life, with some congenital deformities, such as a hemivertebra, causing scoliosis or kyphosis. It is important that pediatricians keep this in mind during their routine physical examinations of newborns and toddlers. Developmental changes marked by a delay in reaching milestones or an abnormal gait may reflect early signs of neuromuscular diseases that, late in the course of the disease, may be associated with spinal deformities.

An examination for spinal deformities during the juvenile years should be part of the routine physical in the pediatrician's office. This may elicit early signs of coronal or sagittal plane deformities associated with congenital or idiopathic causes. Children with known congenital or acquired diseases associated with known higher incidence of spinal deformities should be examined and, in some cases, radiographs taken on a yearly basis in an effort to detect those deformities early. Children with myelodysplasia and high neurologic levels should be reviewed with a radiograph yearly to look for scoliosis. The purpose of early detection of any spinal deformity is to institute a timely plan of care and intervention for treatment. For juveniles, this may mean observation, for some bracing, and for others surgery. Surgery may mean the insertion of "growing rods," in situ fusions, excision of hemivertebra, or merely a diagnostic test such as a muscle biopsy. For most, after documentation of the magnitude of the deformity is established, close observation is the mainstay of treatment.

Early detection of spinal deformities during adolescence has been shown to affect the ultimate outcome of this disorder significantly by decreasing the number of cases detected late and allowing for better treatment plans (23,26,32,48).

School Screening

Population

Most school screening in North America has been performed in grades 5 to 9, that is, in the 10- to 14-year-old age group, as recommended by the Scoliosis Research Society (35). The differential prevalence of this disease in girls has prompted some locations to recommend that boys be screened less frequently (2).

Screening Technique

Before the initiation of the screening process, training programs have been established in most locales for the proper training and education of the primary screeners. The primary screeners often consist of nurses, interested teachers, educated laity, physical therapists, and occasionally physicians. Letters are sent out to the parents before the screening day advising them of the process to take place. Schools have traditionally cooperated with preventive care programs for screening of other medical problems (hearing and vision). Examining the students in the school setting

R. E. McCarthy: Arkansas Spine Center, Little Rock, Arkansas 72205.

generally allows for an efficient use of the students' and the examiners' time with a minimal amount of actual on-site cost. The support of the school administration is essential, as is the proper training of the screeners. Medical advisors have often served as consultants to screening programs in the United States. At times, slide shows and movies have helped to educate both students and parents by increasing their awareness of scoliosis (22,32). The screening should take place in the school nurse's office, a physical education class, or some other suitable location, to provide a reasonable degree of privacy. Boys and girls should be examined separately, and girls should be screened by or in the presence of a female examiner. Boys should take their shirts off; girls should be encouraged to wear a bathing suit or bra to preserve modesty.

The actual examination begins with the student standing in a straight but relaxed posture while the examiner observes from behind (Fig. 1). Asymmetries of the neck, shoulder, rib margins, waist, flank, or hips can be noted. Defects in postural balance may be noted as poor positioning of the head and shoulders over the center of the pelvis. A prominence of the scapula on the side of a convex curve or elevation of the shoulder on that side may reflect a thoracic scoliosis. Unequal distances between

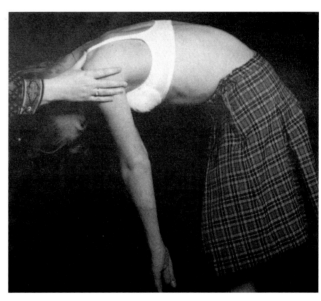

FIGURE 2. The Adams forward-bending test for school screening.

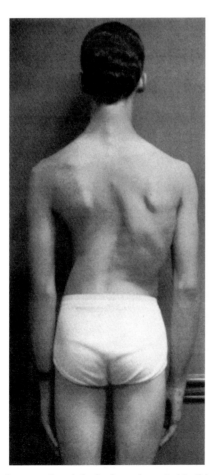

FIGURE 1. Asymmetries of the back can be noted in this 15-year-old boy, distinguished by elevation of the left shoulder area, lateral trunk shift to the right, and prominence of the right-sided rib hump.

the torso and the hanging arms may reflect a truncal shift, whereas an unequal waistline or a high hip may reflect a pelvic obliquity in addition to truncal shift. The limb length inequality may be noted in the standing position by an asymmetry of the top of the underwear or in the forward-bending position with an elevation in the hemipelvis on the long side. The child is then asked to bend forward with the arms hanging freely rather than joined exactly together (37). The feet are together and the knees straight; the child is asked to bend at the hip to nearly 90 degrees (Fig. 2). If hamstring tightness does not allow for full forward flexion, a slight symmetric bend to the knee will allow for further hip flexion. The child can be then observed from the head or back looking for truncal asymmetries. These are seen as a prominence in the rib height (hump) associated with a thoracic scoliosis or a prominence of the paraspinal muscle mass associated with rotation of a lumbar curve (Fig. 3). These deformities are caused by vertebral rotations associated with scoliosis. Not uncommonly, ipsilateral prominences are be noted. The right thoracic idiopathic curve is often noted as a right-sided rib hump with a left-sided lumbar prominence. Any asymmetries in this position can be measured with the use of an inclinometer device such as recommended by Bunnell (5) to better establish the angle of truncal rotation (ATR) (Fig. 4). Readings can be taken with this device on those areas of the spine that are horizontal to the ground, fixing the center of the scoliometer over the spinous process. Further forward flexion of the hips is necessary to place the lumbar prominence in a horizontal position, and then less flexion for measurement of the high thoracic curves. Wherever asymmetries of truncal rotation are noted, measurements should be taken and recorded.

The child should be viewed from the side in both the forward-bending and standing positions. The long sloping curve of postural kyphosis will be noted differently from the acute gibbous deformity of a congenital kyphosis (Fig. 5), or the abnormal

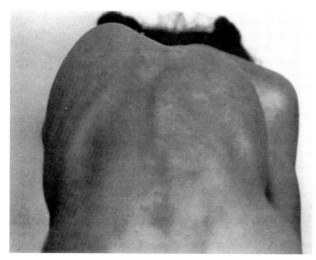

FIGURE 3. The forward-bending test gives the best visualization of truncal asymmetries.

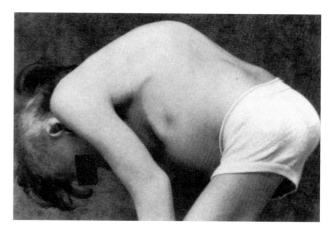

FIGURE 5. Congenital kyphosis on forward-bending test in an 11-year-old boy.

kyphosis of Scheuermann disease (Fig. 6). The findings should be recorded for each student and kept in his or her school health record. Most screening programs across the United States have reported carrying out their screening with the aid of an inclinometer (2). These have been found by many to be helpful in establishing specific criteria for referral of patients. The scoliometer is inexpensive, portable, and allows for a number to be recorded for those youngsters thought to be at risk for scoliosis. The criteria for referral in many centers has been based heavily on

the ATR. It has been suggested that an ATR of 5 degrees should be referred for further follow-up (5–7). Ashworth has pointed out that an ATR of 5 degrees supplies 100% sensitivity but only 47% of specificity, whereas an ATR of 7 degrees has a sensitivity of 83% but a specificity of 86%, thereby minimizing referrals based on false-positive test results (3). Based on those recommendations adopted in each of the screening programs, appropriate referrals are made.

It is generally thought that a second screening should be carried out to confirm the findings for those students considered at risk for spinal deformities. Many centers have found the use of

A
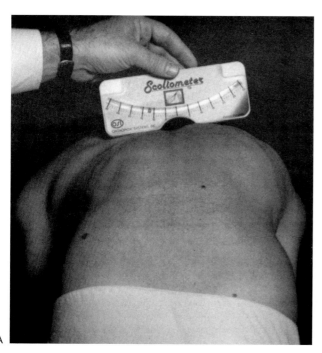

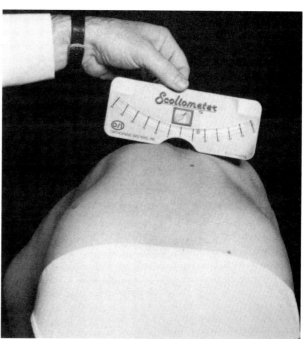
B

FIGURE 4. Measurement of angle of truncal rotation with scoliometer in forward-bending position with measurements of both thoracic (**A**) and lumbar (**B**) curves in the same patient. The maximal reading for each curve is recorded.

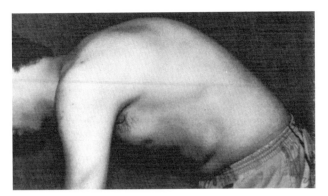

FIGURE 6. Scheuermann kyphosis on forward-bending test in a 17-year-old boy.

the inclinometer especially helpful during this second screening session. Usually, this second screening is carried out by a more experienced screener or a physician to confirm the presence of criteria for referral and keep low the incidence of false positive referrals. After the criteria have been met, the child's parents should be informed of the results and a recommendation made for a timely follow-up examination by the child's physician. Those youngsters at greater risk with large degrees of truncal rotation (ATR of 8 degrees or greater) should be referred directly to an orthopaedist. A follow-up telephone call can insure that the family is aware of the recommendation and the importance of compliance.

Upon referral to the primary care physician, the child is carefully assessed to confirm the asymmetry, to eliminate other causes of scoliosis, and to evaluate maturity. At times, referrals are made to a physician's offices for an elevation of the scapula not associated with any truncal rotation. Elevations of the scapula can occur with mild forms of Sprengel deformity. Leg length inequality may produce a truncal rotation in the standing position, but with examination in the sitting position, the asymmetry is eliminated (8). Referral to an orthopaedist may or may not be in order depending on the magnitude of limb length inequality. Painful scoliosis may or may not be associated with an abnormal neurologic examination, but painful scoliosis should raise a "red flag" for further assessment to exclude intraspinal pathology (24). Signs of other medical problems may also be elicited by the primary care physician, such as café-au-lait skin pigmentations (possible neurofibromatosis), midline hairy patches (possible spinal dysraphism), abnormalities in height indicative of dwarfism or Marfan disease, or other possible illnesses. An assessment of skeletal maturity at the time of that visit would be most helpful in determining both the risk of progression and the urgency of referral. The Tanner grading system offers signs of secondary sex characteristics with which pediatricians are the most familiar (38). These are based on the presence or absence of breast tissue, pubic hair, and development of the genitalia in assessing maturity.

For many physicians, the confirmation of a curvature merely confirms the need to refer the child to an orthopaedist who cares for scoliosis. If that is the case, then a radiograph is not necessary. If the primary physician wishes to participate in the decision

making and assessment, then a standing radiograph of the spine on either a 36-inch film or a 14- × 17-inch film may be appropriate. This may be helpful for the early identification of congenital curves that cannot be differentiated from idiopathic curves on physical examination alone. The importance of this lies in the increased incidence of renal anomalies that accompany this defect. Workup with renal ultrasound or intravenous pyelogram (IVP) may be indicated (32). The film should be positioned so that the entire spine appears on the one film with the lower end of the cassette positioned at the level of the anterosuperior iliac spine and with the child in the erect position. Posteroanterior projections minimize breast radiation dosages. Based on his examination, the primary care physician will then make a further referral, continue to observe the patient himself, or discharge the patient (29). Some record of that evaluation should then be returned to the school, where data can be collected and an analysis carried out by the screening program, to keep records of the prevalence of the disease and the results of the screening program.

One of the dilemmas facing physicians specializing in the care of patients with scoliosis and spinal deformities is the question of how to minimize the delay in transfer of appropriate patients to them. This should be done to minimize the involvement in the medical care system of those patients who need observation only or no form of treatment at all. Hopefully, as each branch of the decision making tree learns the importance of its role in either holding onto or expediting the referral of those patients, the dilemma faced by the patient in the accompanying figure will not be repeated (Fig. 7).

Scoliometer

Since 1948, a number of diagnostic techniques have been used to describe the rib hump deformity characteristic of scoliosis. The level and ruler described by Cobb (10) have the time-honored tradition of being used by all the spine surgeons trained at the Twin Cities Scoliosis Center (4) (Fig. 8). Other contour-describing devices have been introduced by Willner, Rogala, Burwell, and Thulbourne (8,34,39,43,44,45,46). None of these devices has gained widespread use, and compared with the scoliometer, they are somewhat inconvenient. Bunnell (6) introduced an inclinometer in 1984 that has become known as the *scoliometer*. The idea for this device came from his experiences as a sailor with a similar on-board device used to measure inclination of the sailboat in a strong wind.

An inclinometer is designed to measure the rotational deformity by better defining the angle of thoracic inclination. That angle is the construct between the horizontal and a plane across the posterior rib cage at the greatest prominence of the rib (5). Bunnell chose to apply this device to rotational deformity occurring throughout the spine as it describes the angle of trunk rotation. He defined this angle as that which occurs between the horizontal plane and the plane across the posterior aspect of the trunk at the point of maximal deformity, when that section of the spine is observed in the horizontal plane. Patients are placed in the forward-bending position (Adams test), and the degree of hip flexion is adjusted to place either the thoracic or the lumbar spine in the horizontal position (Fig. 4). The

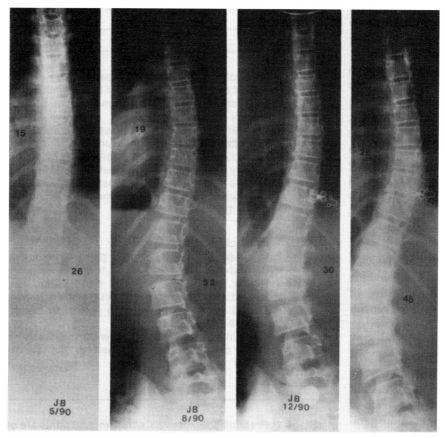

FIGURE 7. Scoliosis noted at age 11 years and followed without intervention until age 13 years, at which time the patient was referred for evaluation and treatment.

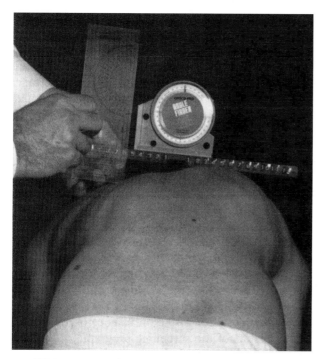

FIGURE 8. Truncal rotation measured by the spirit ruler.

scoliometer has a false-negative result rate of 0.1% and a high degree of sensitivity (6). It has been reported as an effective screening tool in the identification of children at risk for significant scoliosis (more than 10 degrees) (1,3,19,25,41). Ashworth (3) found that adding the scoliometer to the Adams test increased the specificity of that test from 56% to 86%. Bunnell (6) found that the mean Cobb angle in patients with 5 degrees of truncal rotation was 11 degrees of scoliosis, and for a truncal rotation of 7 degrees, the mean Cobb angle was 20 degrees. The recommendation was made, therefore, to refer all patients with an ATR of 5 degrees or greater because they are in the at-risk population for spinal deformity. Some authors have recommended increasing this cutoff to 7 degrees, but at the same time, concern has been expressed that some patients with curves greater than 20 degrees will not be picked up on initial screening (3,19). Others believe that the scoliometer is insufficient to use as the sole method of patient diagnosis and management. It remains a worthwhile tool for school screening, however (1,7,28).

GENERAL EVALUATION FOR DEFORMITY

History

Disorders of the renal or nervous system may reflect scoliosis associated with a number of possible syndromes (47).

It is important to establish developmental milestones, especially any delays during the first 2 years of life or the presence of any protracted hospitalizations or illnesses. Abnormalities in gait, difficulties in learning, hearing abnormalities, visual problems, cleft lips, cardiac murmurs, extremity disorders, genitourinary problems, and certainly neurologic disorders all may be pieces of the puzzle to establish the diagnosis. For many children, scoliosis is merely one piece of a syndrome, all of which must be considered when any correction of the deformities is contemplated. General questions regarding previous operations or illnesses may elicit a history of disorders in other organ systems.

It is a good discipline to force oneself to ask all the questions regarding other organ systems before the obvious history of the spinal deformity. In this manner, the possibility of missing an associated disorder is minimized. Questions regarding the spinal deformity itself can then be directed toward how the deformity was detected, whether it was known from many years before and forgotten, picked up on a recent visit to the pediatrician's office, or identified in school screening. At times, the patients themselves have noticed asymmetries in their clothing but have delayed the referral until a friend or parent brings it to their attention. At times, the parents notice asymmetries in the torso while making clothing for their children. The question of who detected the deformity is an important one, and feedback should be provided to the school screening program, if that is the source of the referral, so that the school screening programs can improve their screening techniques.

The presence or absence of pain is an important piece of the history and has been discussed previously. Has there been any previous treatment of this disorder? If so, what type of bracing or surgery was carried out? How reliably was the brace worn? Or exactly what kind of surgery was done? Records of those procedures are very helpful in the proper evaluation of these patients. All of the details related to the previous course of treatment, and the patient's interpretation of that course, are important in assessing both the physical and psychological situation.

An assessment of maturity can be carried out by questions related to the onset of menarche in girls, which generally signals the beginning of slowdown of growth. The amount of growth remaining after menarche is generally 2 years. For boys, the appearance of axillary hair and the initiation of shaving are generally signs that are equivalent to menarche and, therefore, growth slowdown. It is well known that the general range of maturity is varied for different adolescents, and boys may continue growing into their late teens. The 6 months before and immediately after these peak markers form the period of most rapid growth. It is during these times that youngsters with spinal deformities are at greatest risk for progression of curvature.

Physical Examination

It has been stated that "more mistakes are made from want of proper examination than for any other reason" (27). In the area of spinal disorders, the physical examination and an excellent history are essentials to proper diagnosis (27). Patients should be examined without clothing in a hospital gown that opens in the back.

The examiner begins his observations upon entering the room, first noting the posture of the child and the ability and manner of interactions with the parent or care provider. Then he notices the ability or inability of the child to interact with the examiner. These first impressions may have important consequences not only for diagnosis but also for the outcome of any treatment recommendations. Adolescents who are able to confront the reality of their spinal disorder and deal with it directly in a mature manner are more likely to have a successful outcome, both physically and psychologically, from whatever treatment modalities are recommended. Wherever possible, adolescents and children should be directly involved in the history taking and questions, in order to set the stage for a comfortable physical examination.

The physical examination of the spine begins with a general inspection in the standing position (Fig. 1). Boys can leave off the hospital gown, and girls can have the back of the gown moved aside for proper examination while maintaining modesty. At some time during the evaluation, however, the chest should be examined. Body habitus should be noted. The presence of obesity can mask the early signs of spinal deformities, and these patients present later in the course with a larger curve. Extremely tall, thin individuals may manifest the body habitus of Marfan disease; if this is suspected, examination of the oropharynx may reveal a high-arched palate. Increased arm span may also be noted. Patients with dwarfism should be checked for corneal clouding characteristic of mucopolysaccharidosis or limb deformities (40). Obvious asymmetries should then be noted along the contours of the back, especially elevation of the shoulder, prominence of the scapula, an uneven waistline, and the presence of rib humps. Cutaneous lesions may be noted across the back with midline hairy patches, sinuses, or clefts indicative of spinal dysraphism (Fig. 9). Café-au-lait spots can masquerade as simple birth marks, but when they occur as large blotches or are greater

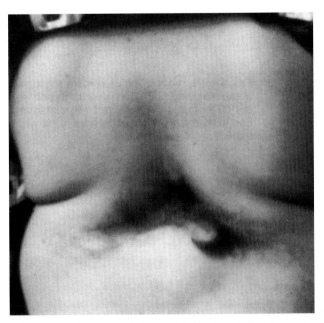

FIGURE 9. Lumbar midline hairy patch indicative of spinal dysraphism. (Courtesy of Tom Dempsey, M.D.)

than five in number, they are thought to represent early signs of neurofibromatosis (14). A characteristic area for café-au-lait spots to appear is the axilla.

The head should be directly aligned over the sacrum, and any deviation from midline may reflect a spinal deformity. This can be demonstrated by dropping a plumb line from the spinous process of C7 down to and beyond the gluteal crease. The distance of that plumb line from the gluteal crease can be recorded in centimeters for future reference (Fig. 10). If a leg length discrepancy is suspected, small wooden blocks underneath the shortened extremity will eliminate the contribution of the leg length discrepancy to any pelvic obliquity (Fig. 11). Performing the forward-bending test in the sitting position eliminates the effect of the leg length discrepancy on the spine (Fig. 12). By viewing the patient from the side, the sagittal curves can be noted between the occiput and the sacrum, including a normal cervical lordosis, thoracic kyphosis, and lumbar lordosis, which generally maintain a proper balance of the head and trunk over the pelvic girdle (20) (Fig. 13).

In this same position, the range of motion of the spine can be tested in flexion, extension, and the side-bending position. Passive side bending is often necessary to visualize the maximal

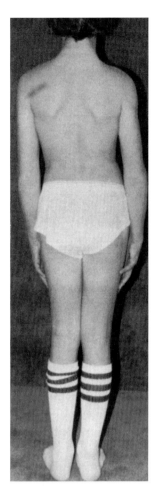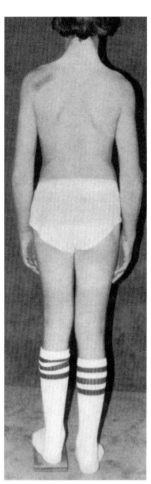

A,B

FIGURE 11. Scoliosis can occur secondary to leg length discrepancy (**A**) and is corrected by a ¾-inch block beneath the short extremity (**B**).

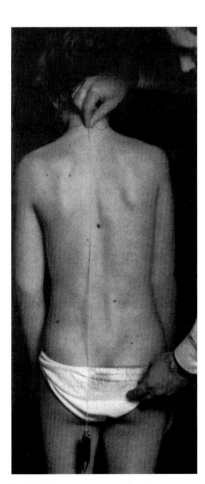

FIGURE 10. Plumb-line measurement for truncal asymmetry in the standing position. The plumb bob is dropped from the C7 spinous process, and the distance of the plumb line from the gluteal cleft is measured with a ruler as an indication of balance.

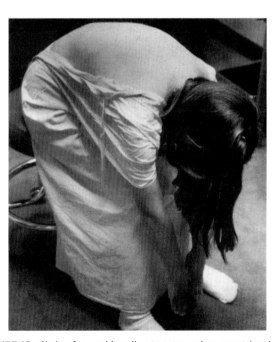

FIGURE 12. Sitting forward-bending test: truncal asymmetries viewed from the sitting position eliminate the effect of leg length discrepancies.

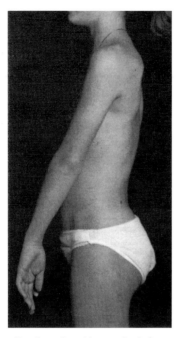

FIGURE 13. Standing lateral position to check for presence of abnormal sagittal curves noted here as the hypokyphosis often seen in idiopathic scoliosis.

amount of flexibility in a curve (Fig. 14). Clinical bending tests may be necessary in the supine position with three-point bending using a hand over the apex of the curve to be tested and contralateral forces over the shoulder and iliac crest during forced correction (Fig. 15). Flexibility can also be tested by grasping the head in the area of the mastoid processes and lifting the patient from the standing or sitting posture (4) (Fig. 16). Tests of clinical and radiographic flexibility supply important information for the planning of surgical instrumentation in order to balance thoracic curves properly over the flexible lumbar spine and pelvis. In severe curves, deformities are exaggerated and should be noted. For instance, if a large lumbar curve is present, it can produce a protrusion of the lower rib cage that abuts the pelvis. This usually accompanies a markedly shortened torso out of proportion to arm length.

While in the standing position, palpation of the lower lumbar spine posteriorly may reveal a palpable step-off felt at the level of the slip in spondylolisthesis (Fig. 17). In its exaggerated forms, the characteristic lumbosacral kyphotic deformity can be seen in the standing position, but this is not common. Careful palpation of the spinous processes may be the only finding on physical examination besides tight hamstrings.

The forward-bending test is carried out with the patient's feet placed together, the knees straight, and flexion through the hips. The patient is instructed to touch the toes with the hands thrust forward at the same level (Fig. 18). Some authors have

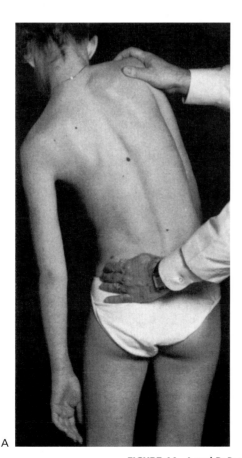

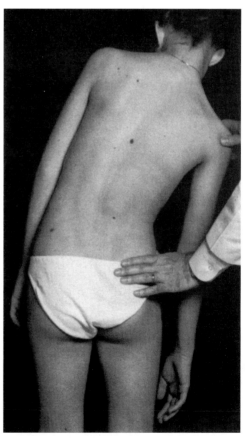

A   B

FIGURE 14. **A and B:** Passive standing side-bend test.

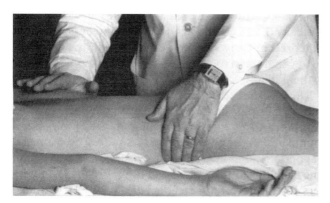

FIGURE 15. Prone three-point flexibility testing.

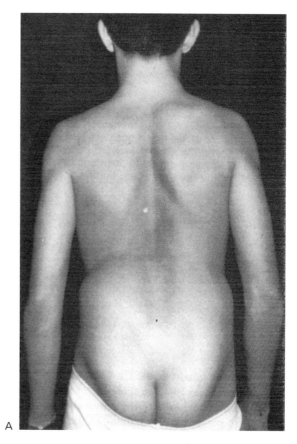

A

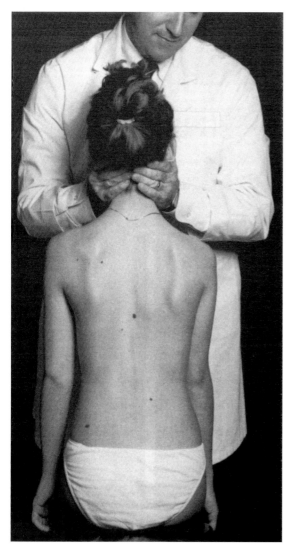

FIGURE 16. Sitting passive traction test for flexibility.

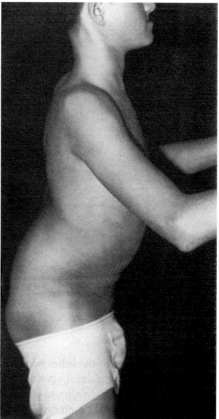

B

FIGURE 17. **A and B:** Clinical appearance of 16-year-old boy with isthmic spondylolisthesis, grade IV.

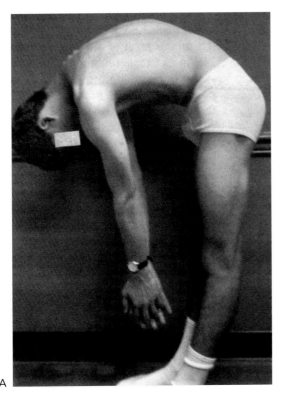

A

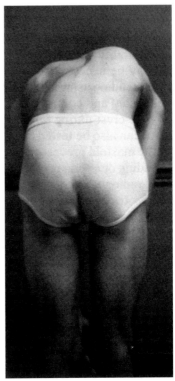

B

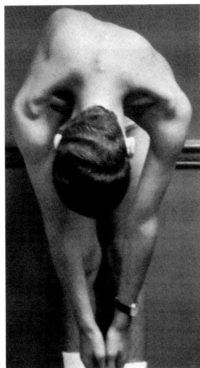

C

FIGURE 18. A–C: Adams forward-bending test. Asymmetries of the back are best viewed with the Adams forward-bending test as viewed from three positions to best outline the truncal asymmetries.

pointed out that asymmetries in arm lengths may lead to some confusion when the hands are joined together during the Adams test. The back should be viewed both from the head and the bottom end to maximize visualization of the truncal rotation, especially in cases in which the youngster is unable to bend fully forward because of tight hamstrings. When visualized from the bottom end, deviations to one side or the other on forward bending may be indicative of a painful scoliosis (Fig. 19). Asymmetries in truncal rotation should be defined in some manner (6,39). The most commonly used devices are the scoliometer to

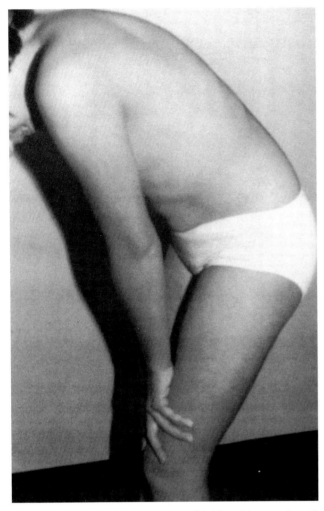

FIGURE 19. Painful scoliosis in a 9-year-old girl unable to perform the forward-bending test because of discitis.

determine the ATR and the spirit level to measure in centimeters the height of the rib hump or lumbar prominence (Figs. 4 and 8). The scoliometer should be placed over the maximal area of the paraspinal prominence where it is positioned horizontal to the floor. The maximal reading of the scoliometer is recorded after multiple readings are taken both superiorly and inferiorly to the side of the apex; this number represents the ATR. The ATR for each curve identified should be recorded (6).

The forward-bending test for small children can be done over the examiner's leg or over the parent's legs while keeping the child's feet on the floor. If there is difficulty in performing the forward-bending test because of tightness of the hamstrings, such as that seen in spondylolisthesis, an equal flexion in the knees allows for increased flexion at the waist and a better examination. Also during the forward-bending test, the spine should be viewed from the side (Fig. 18) to determine whether there are any signs of kyphosis either of a gradual or acute nature, such as might be seen in a congenital deformity secondary to an acute type 1 kyphosis. If there is a rigid lordosis, the spinous processes through the lumbar spine will not reverse on the forward-

bending test as they usually do; this can be indicative of an intrathecal mass and warrants a full workup with possible need for a magnetic resonance imaging (MRI) scan.

After the forward-bending test, the patient is asked to stand up and walk across the room so that any abnormalities in gait or balance can be elicited. These may be reflective of problems of a neurologic nature or of lower extremity abnormalities, which may lead to the underlying diagnosis. The abnormalities in the lower extremities associated with spondyloepiphyseal dysplasia may not be identified until the time of the referral for spinal deformities.

The patient is asked to walk toward the examiner, first on the toes and then on the heels to check for muscle functioning. While still in the standing position, a Romberg test can be carried out. An abnormal Romberg test with ataxia during gait may be the initial signs leading to a diagnosis of Friedreich ataxia (9,21). Examination of the chest and rib cage, axillary areas, and pubic areas can elicit signs of chest wall deformities, such as pectus carinatum or excavatum, and also supply information for the Tanner rating.

The patient is then asked to sit on the examination table for a neurologic examination of the upper extremities, when indicated, and a full examination of the lower extremities, including reflex testing, sensory testing, and further motor testing. Muscle atrophy can be noted by the measurement of the calf or quadriceps area associated with polio or other neurologic abnormalities (Fig. 20). Straight-leg raising should be carried out in both the sitting and lying positions (29). In the supine position, leg lengths can be evaluated by pulling the legs into full extension and placing one's thumbs beneath the medial malleoli. Unequal leg lengths can be confirmed with a tape measure from the anterosuperior iliac spine to the distal limit of the medial malleolus. An active attempt at situps can give some indication of abdominal musculature and spinal flexibility. Abdominal reflexes should be elicited by stroking the abdomen toward the umbilicus to watch for appropriate deviation of the umbilicus (Fig. 21). In the prone position, palpation of the spinal deformity and any possible areas of tenderness can be examined. An active prone hyperextension test may elicit painful areas in the spine or give some idea of flexibility and muscle strength. The examination of the lower extremities should also include any abnormalities of the feet, remembering that cavus deformities may be indicative of diastematomyelia or neuromuscular disorders. Generalized hyperlaxity (Fig. 22) and flat feet may be consistent with collagen diseases, such as Ehler-Danlos and Down syndromes. Joint contractures of the lower extremities may be noted around the hip, with flexion contractures in achondroplastic and spina bifida patients contributing to excessive lumbar lordotic posturing. Flexion contractures around the knee are consistent with a multiplicity of disorders, including arthrogryposis. Full examination of the child should include a height and weight and placement on a growth chart if there is any indication or suspicion of abnormality in height.

Laboratory Studies

Occasionally, the child presenting with spinal deformities requires further laboratory workup to exclude infectious or inflam-

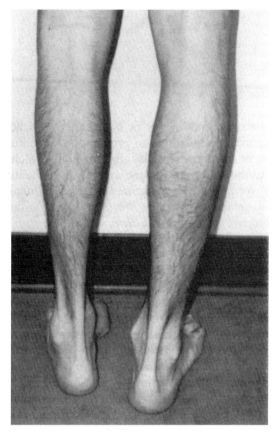

FIGURE 20. Cavus foot and calf atrophy associated with an intrathecal lipoma in a 16-year-old boy.

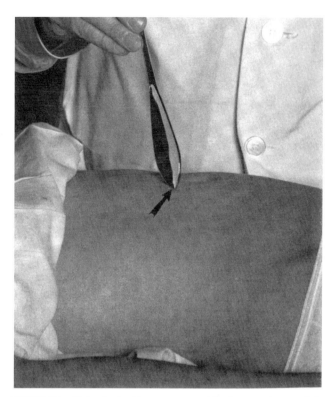

FIGURE 21. Abdominal reflexes are tested in four quadrants of the abdomen, with the skin stroked lightly toward the umbilicus with the handle of a reflex hammer (*arrow*). The lack of umbilical deviation toward the tested quadrant reflects an upper motor neuron lesion.

matory causes. A complete blood count and sedimentation rate may show an elevation in white blood cells, with an elevation in the sedimentation rate indicative of infection. Sedimentation rates can be elevated for many causes, including some spinal tumors, such as Hodgkin disease and histiocytosis X. Older adolescents may show signs of ankylosing spondylitis, necessitating a rheumatologic workup, including an HLA-B27 evaluation.

In patients undergoing surgical correction for spinal deformities, preoperative pulmonary function studies may be indicated. In the presence of severe curvature or neuromuscular diseases, a preoperative workup should also include arterial or capillary blood gases.

Radiographic Studies

On presentation to the orthopaedist's office, any previously done radiographs irrespective of quality or position should be brought with the patient and examined by the orthopaedist. Information from these radiographs may shed light on the type of deformity, the stage of maturity, and the location of the deformity. If the radiographs are recent, no further radiographs may be necessary. The purpose of radiographs is to establish the diagnosis suspected on physical examination. Ideally, radiographs should be taken on 36-inch film. A 17- × 14-inch radiograph can be used but must be positioned so that the entire spine appears on one

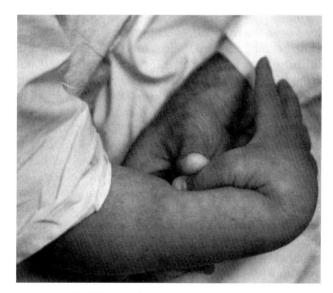

FIGURE 22. Flexibility test for generalized hyperlaxity.

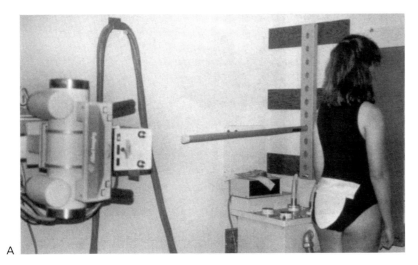

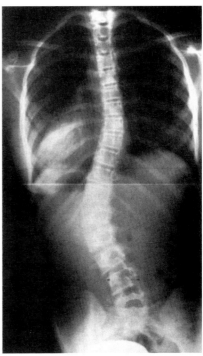

FIGURE 23. **A:** Positioning for posteroanterior radiographs for scoliosis. **B:** Erect 36-inch anteroposterior spine radiograph with scoliosis placed on illuminator with right side on the right as seen anatomically from the back.

radiograph with the lower end of the cassette positioned at the level of the anterosuperior iliac spine. This is done to include the top of the iliac apophysis. Some authors are of the opinion that all patients referred for evaluation of spinal deformities warrant a radiograph (32), whereas others believe that adolescents with mild curves do not need radiographic examination provided that the examiner is experienced and the parents understand that clinical follow-up is necessary (16).

If a radiograph is to be taken, a single upright anteroposterior or posteroanterior view is sufficient for diagnosis and for observational treatment of most patients with curves of less than 20 degrees (Fig. 23). If, however, there is indication of back pain or suspicion of other causes of the scoliosis, a more extensive examination is necessary. Lateral and oblique radiographs of the spine are not indicated for the routine screening referral. Lateral radiographs are indicated for pain or sagittal plane deformities, such as hyperkyphosis or hyperlordosis (Fig. 24). Oblique radiographs of the lower lumbar spine are indicated for the assessment of pars defects associated with spondylolysis (Fig. 25). All these views other than the obliques should be taken in the functional upright position. For wheelchair patients, this is a sitting position. For ambulatory patients, it is a standing positions. For infants, the functional position is supine. Special plane views, such as Stagnara views, bend radiographs, and stretch radiographs, are rarely indicated and are usually taken only before instituting some form of treatment, such as bracing or surgery. Supine radiographs may be indicated for improved definition of bony structures, as in congenital deformities such as scoliosis or kyphosis. Upright radiographs best represent the actual effect on the development of compensatory curves to achieve spinal balance.

Thought must be given to why the radiograph is being taken. "Routine" sets of scoliosis radiographs are unwarranted and unnecessarily expose adolescents to irradiation during a critical stage in their development. Attempts should be made whenever possible to minimize the number of radiographs used to make the diagnosis, and the same effort should be made on subsequent visits. Not uncommonly, surface topography devices, such as the scoliometer, can be used to follow smaller curves as indicators of whether an increase in truncal rotation has occurred, warranting a radiograph. It is well known that increased gonadal radiation increases the mutation rate of reproductive cells, and if pregnancy were to occur within 6 months, the effects of the irradiation might be seen. Certain organs in the body, however, are sensitive in a cumulative fashion to irradiation. The developing breasts, bone marrow, and thyroid gland are vulnerable; therefore radiographic techniques should minimize irradiation to keep organ dosage to a minimum (4,15).

Most patients being evaluated by orthopaedists for spinal deformities are girls first seen during early adolescence at a critical time for breast tissue development. The best way to minimize irradiation of these youngsters is to avoid taking a radiograph unless truly indicated. Attempts have been made to decrease the dose of irradiation by improving the quality of the radiograph, using rare earth screens and aluminum screens to filter out a portion of the radiograph beam (15,18). Standing radiographs can be taken with a shield over the pelvis to shield the gonads. On anteroposterior view radiographs, some centers have found the use of breast shields useful and unencumbering, whereas others have thought that any device hung around the neck and draped across the chest will cause further spinal deformity. Positioning the patient for a posteroanterior view with the chest

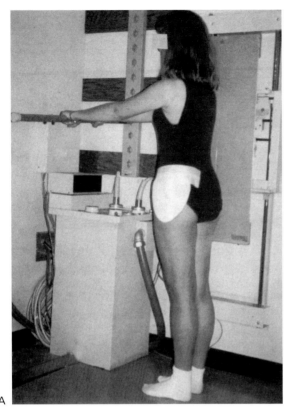
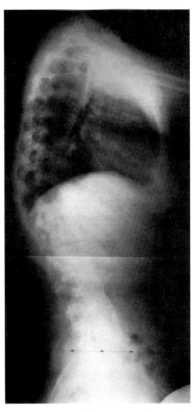

FIGURE 24. **A:** Positioning for lateral 36-inch scoliosis radiograph. **B:** Lateral 36-inch scoliosis radiograph.

positioned against the screen decreases the amount of direct irradiation to the breast tissue without the need for shields. This radiograph can extend from the occiput to the midpelvic region, where a gonadal shield is placed on a free stand in front of the patient or taped to the patient. At least one initial radiograph should be taken with no shielding to look for other possible associated anomalies.

Technique

For erect radiographs, the patient is instructed to stand straight in his functional position (Fig. 23). In the standing position, the feet are together, with arms out to the side and the shoulders pressed against the radiograph plate. For the neuromuscular child, sitting on a stool in front of the plate with an anteroposterior view works adequately. Accessory supports or people may be required to hold the patient upright in an attempt to mimic his usual functional posture. Occasionally, radiographs taken of the patient in the wheelchair may best represent the functional position. For these patients, it is important to visualize the pelvis on the radiograph.

For the lateral projection, most centers have positioned the patient with the right side against the radiograph plate and with the patient looking forward and arms raised at 60 degrees (Fig. 24). It has been pointed out by Stagnara (36) that moving the humeri forward 45 degrees from the vertical line does not

modify kyphosis or lordosis. He found that raising the arms straight out in front or above the head considerably changed kyphosis and lordosis. Gonadal shields can be used for this radiograph, but as noted, judgment must be exercised in deciding when to order this radiograph because it does require a higher radiation dose than the standard anteroposterior or posteroanterior views.

Special Views

Evaluation of the patient with low back pain may warrant the use of supine oblique views to better visualize the pars area (Fig. 25). These are generally taken at an angle of 45 degrees off the vertical, visualizing the right and left sides on different radiographs with the beam centered on the L4 to L5 area. Further evaluation of the low lumbar spine for spondylolisthesis frequently requires the use of a standing spot view of the L5 to S1 region to assess the percentage of slip of L5 on S1 (Fig. 26). Occasionally, a Ferguson view taken at a 30-degree angle and tilting the beam cephalad allows for better visualization in patients with low lumbar deformities because this view eliminates the lordosis (Fig. 27). This view has a high irradiation exposure dosage to the gonads. Bending radiographs can be done in the supine or standing position. These are used to assess the flexibility of a particular curve (11). A bending radiograph is generally done with active side bending in the supine position using a 14-

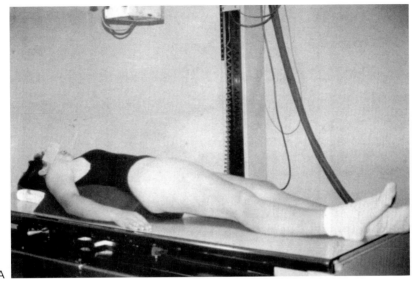

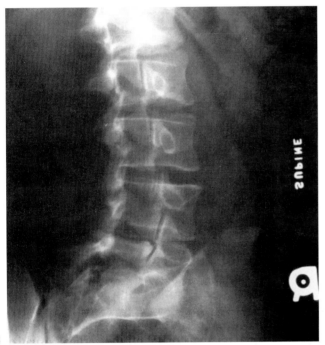

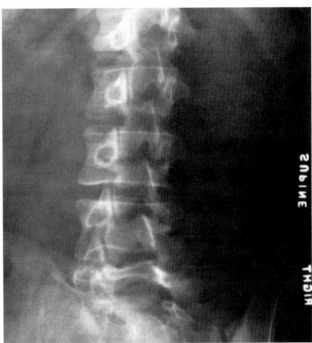

FIGURE 25. A: Positioning for lumbar supine oblique radiograph. **B and C:** Supine oblique radiograph demonstrating bilateral isthmic spondylolysis.

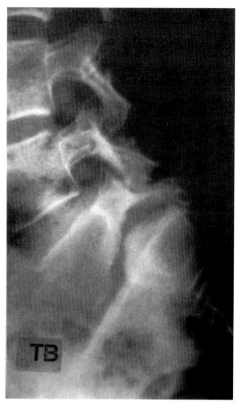

FIGURE 26. Standing lateral radiograph of L5 to S1 demonstrating congenital spondylolisthesis.

× 17-inch radiograph (Fig. 28). Separate exposures are required for each side bend. Occasionally, forceful bending with a gloved hand is required, especially in assessment of neuromuscular curves (Fig. 28). The traction radiograph, taken on a Risser table with pelvic straps and a cervical halter, can substitute for bend radiographs by supplying similar information especially helpful in the case of neuromuscular patients.

Hyperextension views over a bolster are frequently helpful in assessing the flexibility of kyphotic curvatures when the patient is laid supine over the foam bolster and a shoot-through lateral radiograph is taken (Fig. 29). The flexibility of lumbar lordosis can be assessed with the patient similarly aligned on the radiograph table without the bolster, drawing the hips into a fully flexed position, clasping the knees across the chest in a knee-chest position (Fig. 30). This can be coupled with thoracic flexion when the patient is placed in a side-lying position for the same view.

In severe curves, the Stagnara view helps to assess the true magnitude of the deformity in extreme positions of rotation (Fig. 31). The radiograph is taken in such a way as to eliminate rotation and look at a true lateral view and the apex of the curve. This is, therefore, actually an oblique radiograph of the apex. An oblique view is taken with the cassette positioned parallel to the medial aspect of the rotational rib prominence, with the x-ray beam positioned at right angle to the cassette. This gives a true coronal view of the apical vertebra.

Curve Assessment

Curves are measured by the Cobb method where the top of the vertebra that best delineates the curve pattern is chosen, and a

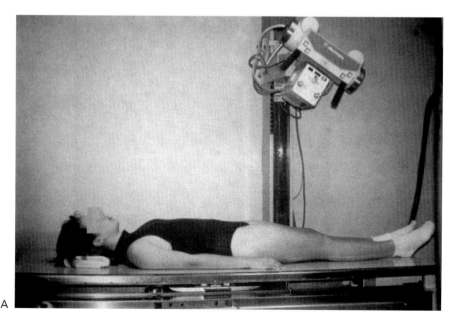

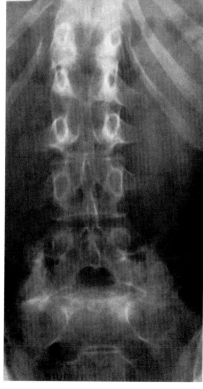

FIGURE 27. A: Positioning for Ferguson view. **B:** This view is most helpful in visualizing low lumbar fusions, such as this posterior intertransverse fusion between L5 and S1.

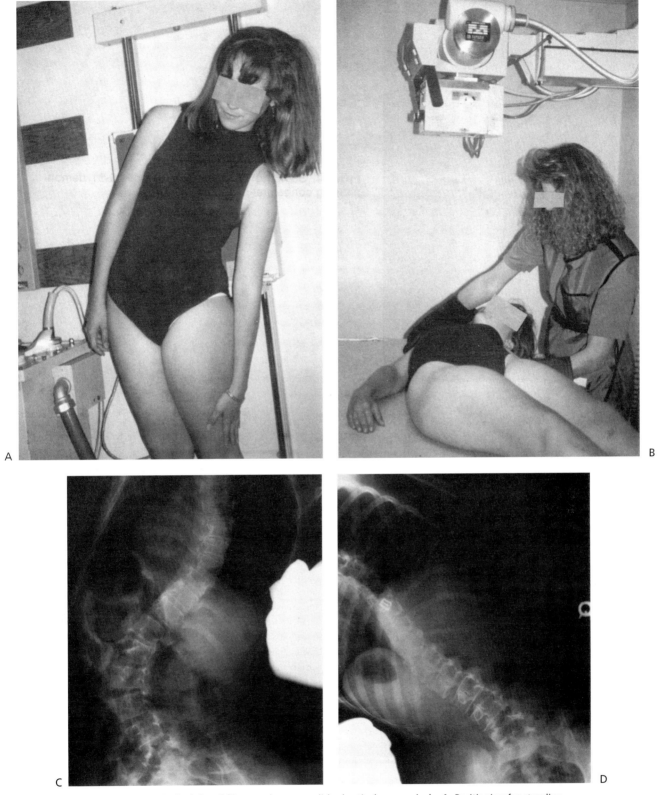

FIGURE 28. Scoliosis bend films can be accomplished actively or passively. **A:** Positioning for standing active-bend radiographs. **B:** Positioning for passive supine radiographs with technologist using a gloved fist over the apex of the spinal curve and pressure exerted with three-point resistance. **C and D:** Supine passive-bend films to determine the maximal degree of flexibility of a scoliotic curvature.

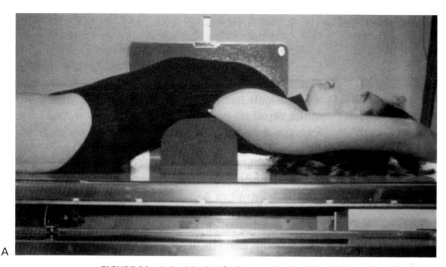
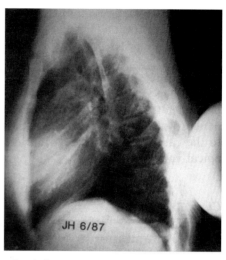

JH 6/87

A   B

FIGURE 29. **A:** Positioning for hyperextension lateral thoracic radiograph over a firm bolster positioned at the apex of kyphosis. **B:** Hyperextension cross-table lateral radiograph of a 15-year-old girl with Scheuermann disease demonstrating maximal flexibility of the curvature.

line perpendicular to the top of that vertebral body is drawn. A similar perpendicular line is drawn across the bottom of the vertebral body that best delineates the maximal curve in its lower aspect. The intersection of these two perpendicular lines is the Cobb angle, which is calibrated with the goniometer on the Cobb ruler (Fig. 32). It is occasionally difficult to determine the location of the bottom of the vertebral body in the immature spine; therefore, the ovoid of the apophysis is outlined, and the limits of the ovoid are marked at their extremes and joined with a line that is then drawn across the bottom of the vertebral body. Occasionally, in the thoracic spine with severe deformities, it is difficult to visualize the top of the vertebral bodies, and in this situation, the top of the corresponding facet joints can be chosen above which to draw the line. In assessment of congenital curves, the best-

guess method should be used, but it must be used consistently on subsequent comparison radiographs. For assessment of kyphotic curves, the end vertebra that is T3 and T12 is thought to represent true kyphosis (10). Curve magnitudes are recorded on the radiograph, and subsequent radiographs are measured in a similar manner.

Vertebral rotation as demonstrated by rotation of the pedicles has been graded using the system of Nash and Moe (30) (Fig. 33). Grades 0 through 4 have designated increased degrees of rotation. Perdriolle and Vidal (31), Coestier and colleagues (12), and Bunnell (6) have also described methods for description of curve rotation. Both erect radiographs and flexibility radiographs can be assessed with the Cobb method to assess the changes in the curve with motion. The vertebral levels are numbered in a standard fashion with 7 cervical levels, 12 thoracic levels, and 5 lumbar levels. Occasionally, extra levels or fewer levels are identified, and judgment must be used to determine whether to number the extra levels as additional or deficient thoracic or lumbar levels. Generally, each thoracic vertebra has ribs attached to it, except in the case of congenital deformities. The Risser sign appears across the top of the iliac crest, progressing from a small area of ossification laterally and growing medially (Fig. 34). When it first appears, it is designated Risser 1; when halfway across, Risser 2; when three quarters way, Risser 3; and when completely to the medial side (capped), Risser 4. Risser 5 describes a fused apophysis and complete maturity. Risser 4 represents completion of spinal growth (33). Additional radiographs may be required for the proper assessment of bone age, with the use of a left wrist and hand radiograph to be compared with the Gruelich and Pyle atlas (17). This atlas has an accuracy of plus or minus 6 months at best. The iliac crest is generally visible on radiographs and readily available for assessment of skeletal maturity in most cases. Occasionally, this fails to appear when expected based on physical maturity, and the wrist for bone age radiograph is helpful. The vertebral apophyses also give some indication of skeletal maturity, and they can appear as a second-

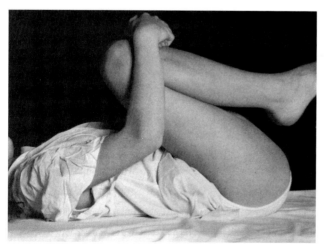

FIGURE 30. Position for lateral shoot-through radiograph of the lumbar spine to assess flexibility.

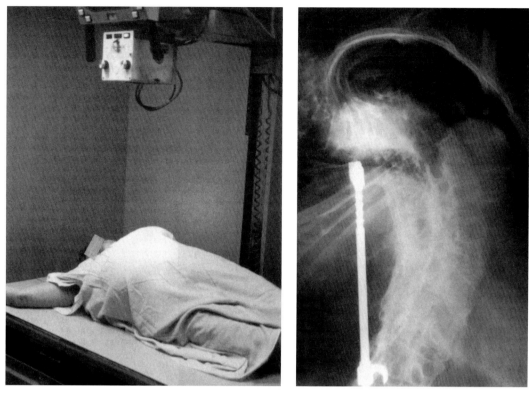

FIGURE 31. **A:** Positioning for Stagnara view in severe scoliosis to visualize a true lateral of the apical vertebral bodies. The degree of thoracic obliquity depends on the severity of the curve. **B:** Stagnara view showing a lateral view of the apical vertebral bodies in this severe scoliotic treated previously.

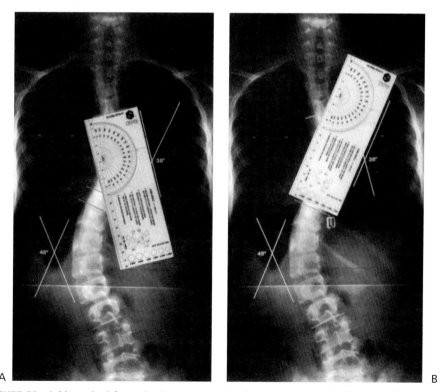

FIGURE 32. Cobb method for scoliosis measurement using transparent ruler. Lines are drawn across the top of the vertebral body that best represents the curve and the bottom of the lowest vertebral body in the curve; perpendiculars to these lines intersect, and that angle is the Cobb angle. **A and B:** Measurement of the thoracic curve. *(Figure continued.)*

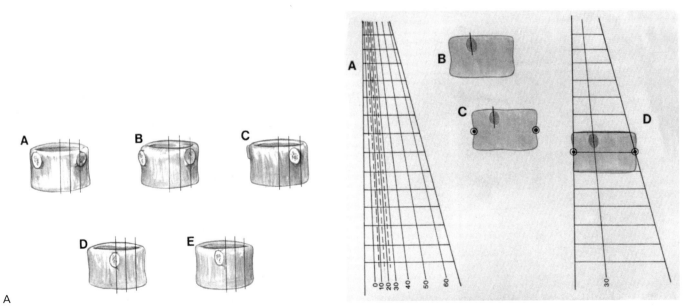

C,D   E

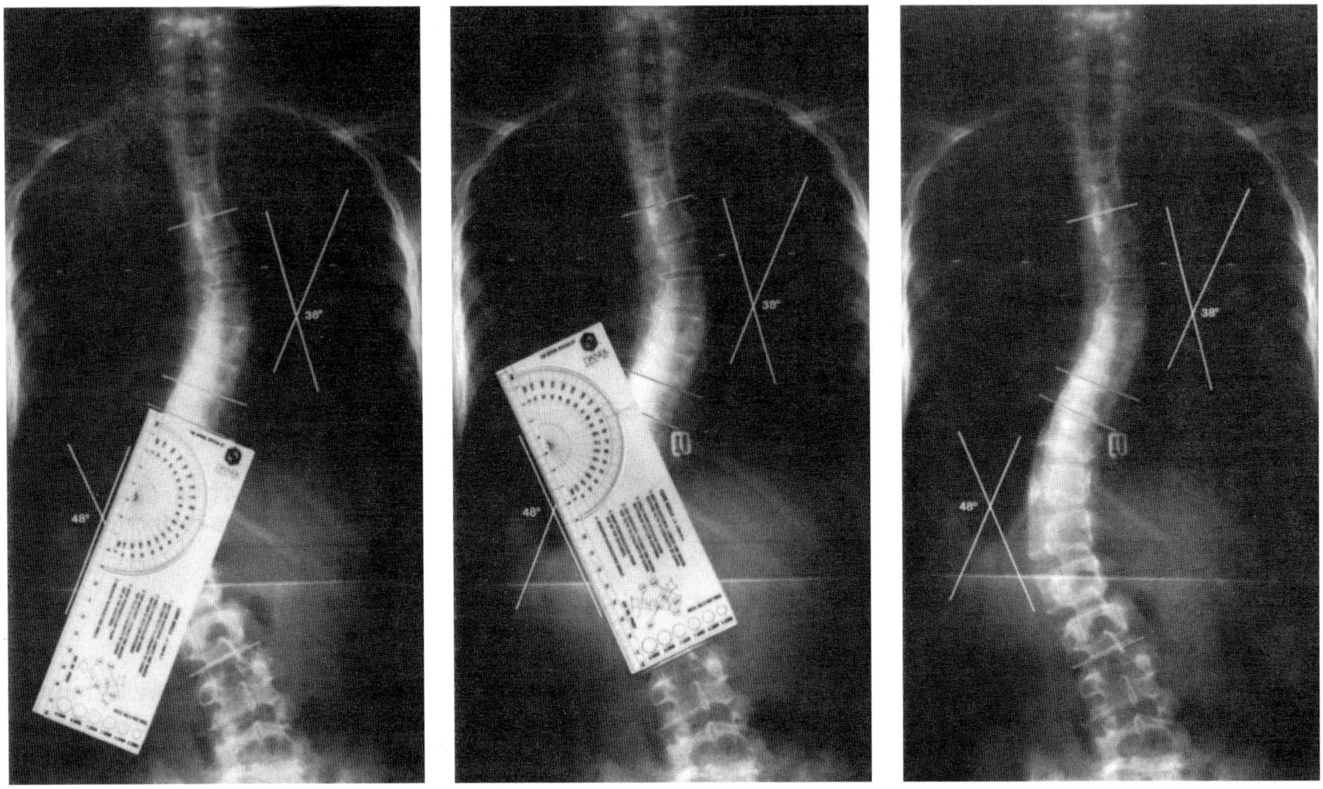

FIGURE 32. *Continued.* **C and D:** Measurement of the lumbar curve. **E:** Completed curve measurements.

FIGURE 33. A: The Nash-Moe method for determining vertebral rotation on an anteroposterior radiograph. **B:** Pedicle method of measurement of vertebral rotation.

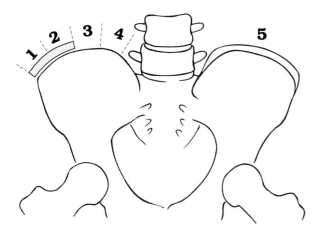

FIGURE 34. Risser sign. The Risser sign is a reflection of skeletal maturity. Risser *1*, initial appearance of lateral ossification of iliac apophysis; Risser *2*, migration halfway across the top of the iliac wing; Risser *3*, migration across three fourths of the distance; Risser *4*, ossification crossing the iliac wing; Risser *5*, complete ossification of the iliac apophysis.

ary density on both the anteroposterior and lateral views. The lumbar spine apophyses mature before the thoracic levels in a sequential fashion.

Ancillary Studies

Myelogram

Myelograms are rarely indicated by present-day standards except in cases of gross deformity, in which MRI and computed tomography (CT) scans have too much variability in the planes visualized. In that case, the use of a myelogram with a follow-up CT scan can be most helpful. Water-soluble dye is desirable and adequately visualizes the spinal canal to demonstrate any pathology therein (Fig. 35).

Myelograms have been found useful in situations in which hardware is in place, preventing the use of MRI for intrathecal assessment.

Computed Tomography

CT scanning of the spine has proved to be extremely useful in many spinal anomalies (Fig. 36). CT scanning has allowed for better visualization of the bone, and with improved techniques, the amount of diffraction from adjacent metal rods can be minimized.

Of late, CT scanning has been coupled with three-dimensional reconstruction to better visualize congenital anomalies, especially those that have been poorly understood and are best seen with three-dimensional scanning (Fig. 37). Postmyelography CT scan is extremely useful for visualization of spinal cord or nerve root compression and after discograms to better visualize in a coronal plane extravasation of dye from a torn annulus.

Magnetic Resonance Imaging

MRI has proved to be an extremely valuable tool that has provided a great deal of information in the field of spinal deformi-

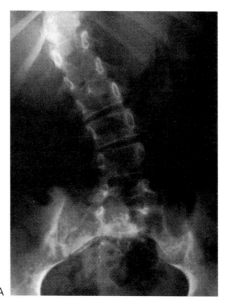

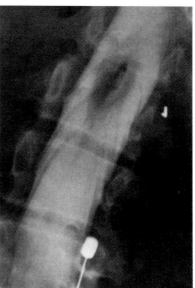

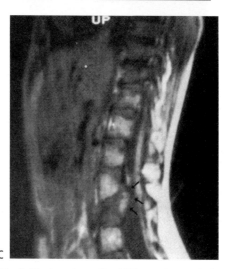

FIGURE 35. **A:** Diastematomyelia at L2 on anteroposterior lumbar radiograph with central calcification best seen on **(B)** water-soluble myelogram outlining the diastematomyelia. **C:** Magnetic resonance imaging view.

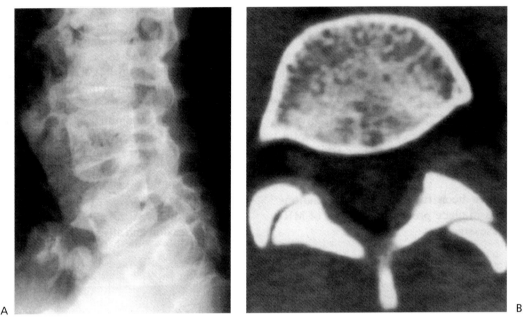

FIGURE 36. **A:** Plain lateral radiographs of a 14-year-old motorcyclist with a unilateral facet dislocation at L5 to S1. **B:** This is best visualized on computed tomography scan, coronal view.

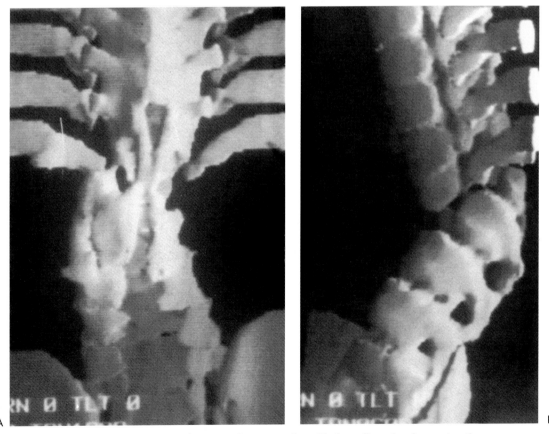

FIGURE 37. **A and B:** Computed tomography scan studies with three-dimensional reconstruction may be helpful in delineating congenital bony deformities as in this 2-year-old boy with segmental spinal dysgenesis.

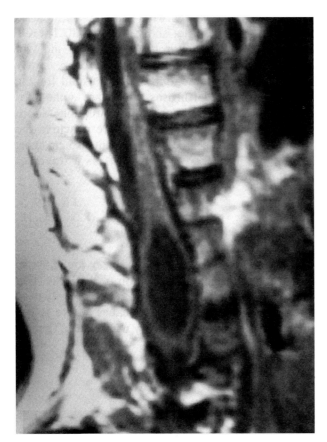

FIGURE 38. Preoperative magnetic resonance imaging in a 12-year-old boy with congenital scoliosis. A large syringomyelia was noted in the cervical canal.

ties. Children who had otherwise not been diagnosed as so have been found to have a high incidence of intrathecal anomalies. Lewonowski and associates (22) have identified a high incidence of syringomyelia and other anomalies in a population of juvenile "idiopathic" scoliotic patients (Fig. 38). Numerous youngsters who had previously been watched as they developed severe curvatures have now been identified as having associated intrathecal pathology causing the spinal deformities. The MRI is readily able to identify a thickened filum and other anomalies, such as lipomas, not previously diagnosed easily (Fig. 39). The CT scan remains the best technique for visualization of bony deformities.

Tomograms

Traditionally, laminagrams have been used in cases in which radiographs did not show good detail. The CT scanning has shown better visualization of most of those cases in which laminagrams were previously used. Tomograms remain useful, however, for the delineation of pseudarthroses, which are sometimes poorly visualized on CT scans and in situations in which the diffraction from adjacent hardware obscures the bony outline. In those situations, fine cuts 0.5 cm apart can show the line of a pseudarthrosis as it traverses across the spine.

Ultrasound

The Doppler ultrasound study has been found useful not only in the prenatal evaluation of the fetus but also in the postnatal situation, in which it has been widely used for the assessment of renal anomalies, where it has gained wide acceptance as a useful tool. The use of intraoperative ultrasound for assessment of the spinal cord is also gaining wider acceptance in the hands of neurosurgeons.

Intravenous Pyelogram

IVPs and retrograde pyelograms have been used for the assessment of the renal deformities seen with congenital scoliosis. In large part, these have been replaced by renograms and ultrasound studies, which better visualize the renal collection system without the potential for allergic reactions to iodine in the IVP dye.

Bone Scan

Bone scans have been useful especially in the assessment of the patient with painful spinal deformity (Fig. 40) or in situations in

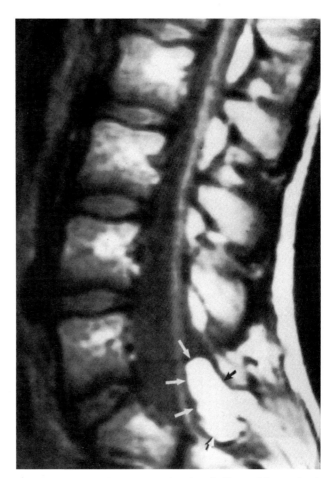

FIGURE 39. Magnetic resonance imaging findings of lipoma in the distal spinal canal with sinus tract and thickening of the filum terminale causing a tethered spinal cord in a 17-year-old boy.

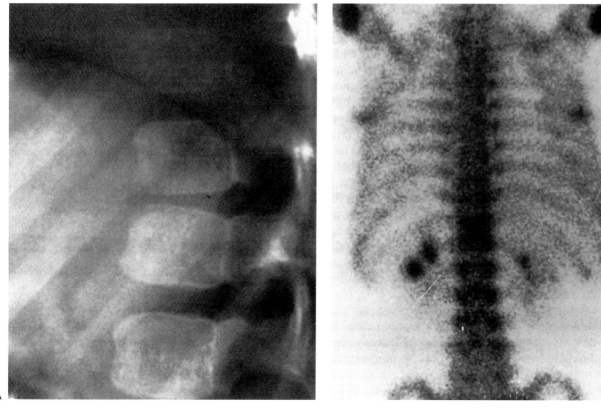

FIGURE 40. A: Lateral radiograph of a 4-year-old with discitis demonstrating disc space narrowing. **B:** A positive bone scan with increased uptake at T11 and T12 confirms inflammatory involvement on both sides of the disc.

which the acuteness of a spondylolysis needs assessment. Indium scans can be useful for identification of spinal and paraspinal infections. The use of single photon emission computed tomography (SPECT) bone scanning has also been an adjunct to the localization of tumors and infections in an anteroposterior plane.

SUMMARY

The early diagnosis of the patient with a spinal deformity is dependent on screening examinations that begin from early life extending through the school years into adolescence. School screening programs carried out between the fifth and ninth grades have been carried out in many states to detect truncal asymmetries indicative of spinal deformities. About 2% to 3% of school children have been identified as having spinal deformities and then referred for further evaluation. To minimize inappropriate referrals and maximize on the topographic signs of deformity, certain techniques have been developed to aid in the screening process. Inclinometers have found a place in many screening programs.

The examination of the patient in the physician's office should include a careful physical examination, the use of devices to describe the topographic asymmetry, and judicious use of radiographs. To minimize the dose of radiation to the growing child, only those radiographs necessary for the appropriate diag-

nosis should be acquired. Further evaluation with special views are often indicated for patients with excessive deformities. Occasionally, ancillary radiographic studies are also indicated, such as MRI and CT of the spine, to exclude soft tissue problems in or around the spinal canal or to better delineate bony deformities. The proper assessment needs to be individualized for each patient and should be appropriate for the specific deformity.

REFERENCES

1. Amendt L, Ause-Ellias K, Eybers J, et al. (1990): Validity and reliability testing of the scoliometer. *Phys Ther* 70:108–117.
2. Asher M, Beringer G, Orrick J, et al. (1989): The current status of scoliosis in North America, 1986. *Spine* 14:652–662.
3. Ashworth M, Hancock J, Ashworth L, et al. (1988): Scoliosis screening: an approach to cost/benefit analysis. *Spine* 13:1187–1188.
4. Bradford D, Lonstein J, Moe J, et al. (1987): *Moe's textbook of scoliosis and other spinal deformities.* Philadelphia: WB Saunders.
5. Bunnell W (1984): *Vertebral rotation: a simple method of measurement on routing radiographs.* Presented at 19th annual meeting of the Scoliosis Research Society, Sept. 19–22, 1984, Orlando, FL.
6. Bunnell W (1984): An objective criterion for scoliosis screening. *J Bone Joint Surg Am* 66:1381–1387.
7. Bunnell W (1987): When does scoliosis need referral? *Patient Care* 15: 53–60.
8. Burwell R, James N, Johnson F, et al. (1983): Standardised trunk asymmetry scores. *J Bone Joint Surg Br* 65:452–463.
9. Cady R, Bobechko W (1984): Incidence, natural history, and treatment of scoliosis in Friedreich's ataxia. *J Pediatr Orthop* 4:673–767.

10. Cobb J (1948): Outline for the study of scoliosis. *Instr Course Lec* 5: 261–275.
11. Cobb J (1960): The problem of the primary curve. *J Bone Joint Surg Am* 42:1413–1425.
12. Coestler M, Vercauteren M, Moerman P (1977): A new radiographic method for measuring vertebral rotation in scoliosis. *Acta Orthop Belg* 43:598–605.
13. Commission on Chronic Illness (1957): *Chronic illness in the United States,* vol. 1. Cambridge, MA: Harvard University Press.
14. Crawford A (1989): Pitfalls of spinal deformities associated with neurofibromatosis in children. *Clin Orthop* 245:29–42.
15. Desmet A, Cook L, Tarlton M (1981): Assessment of scoliosis using three-dimensional radiographic measurements. *Automedica* 4:25–36.
16. Emans J (1985): Scoliosis: detecting the curves that mandate treatment. *J Musculoskel Med* March: 11–27.
17. Gruelich W, Pyle S (1959): *Radiographic atlas of skeletal development of the hand and wrist.* Stanford, CA: Stanford University Press.
18. Harcke H, Mandell G, Grissom L, et al (1991): *Digital radiology: musculoskeletal application.* Presented at American Roentgen Ray Society, Annual Meeting.
19. Hopkins R, Grundy M, Sherr-Mehl M (1984): X-ray filters in scoliosis x-rays. *Orthop Trans* 8:148.
20. Hughes L, McCarthy R, Glasier C (1998): Segmental spinal dysgenesis: a case report. *J Pediatr Orthop* 18:227–232.
21. Keppler L, Wenger D, Speck G, et al. (1984): Curve progression in mild scoliosis. *Orthop Trans* 9:111.
22. Lewonowski K, King J, Nelson M (1992): Routine use of magnetic resonance imaging in idiopathic scoliosis patients less than eleven years of age. *Spine* 17:S109–S116.
23. Lonstein J (1977): Scoliosis screening in Minnesota schools. *Clin Orthop* 126:33–42.
24. Lonstein J (1988): Why school screening for scoliosis should be continued. *Spine* 13:1198–1199.
25. Lonstein J (1989): Scoliosis update: managing school screening referrals. *J Musculoskel Med* July: 37–54.
26. Lonstein J, Morrissy R (1989): Scoliosis school screening: is it of value? *Orthopedics* 12:1589–1593.
27. McCarthy R (1987): Prevention of the complications of scoliosis by early detection. *Clin Orthop* 222:73–78.
28. McNab I, McCulloch J (1990): *Backache.* Baltimore: Williams & Wilkins.
29. Moreland M, Cobb L, Pope M, et al. (1983): Pattern recognition topograms. *J Pediatr Orthop* 3:120.
30. Nash C, Moe J (1969): A study of vertebral rotation. *J Bone Joint Surg Am* 51:223–229.
31. Perdriolle R, Vidal J (1981): Etude de la courbure scoliotique. *Revue De Chir Orthop* 67:25–34.
32. Renshaw T (1988): Screening school children for scoliosis. *Clin Orthop* 229:26–33.
33. Risser J (1958): The iliac apophysis: an invaluable sign in the management of scoliosis. *Clin Orthop* 11:111–119.
34. Rogala E, Drummond D, Gurr J (1978): Scoliosis: incidence and natural history. *J Bone Joint Surg Am* 60:173–176.
35. Scoliosis Research Society (1986): *Scoliosis: a handbook for patients.* Park Ridge, IL: Scoliosis Research Society.
36. Stagnara P, DeMauroy J, Dran G, et al. (1982): Reciprocal angulation of vertebral bodies in a sagittal plane: an approach to references for the evaluation of kyphosis and lordosis. *Spine* 7:335–342.
37. Stirling A, Smith R, Dickson R (1986): Screening for scoliosis: the problem of arm length. *Br Med J* 292:1305–1306.
38. Tanner J (1975): Growth and endocrinology of the adolescent. In: Gardner L, ed. *Endocrine and genetic disease of childhood.* Philadelphia: WB Saunders, p. 4.
39. Thulbourne R, Gillespie R (1976): The rib hump in idiopathic scoliosis. *J Bone Joint Surg Br* 58:64–71.
40. Tolo V (1985): Spinal deformity in dwarfs. In: Hensinger R, Bradford D, eds. *The pediatric spine.* New York: Thieme, pp. 38–349.
41. Tolo V (1988): Treatment, follow-up, or discharge. *Spine* 13:1189–1190.
42. Williams J (1988): Criteria for screening: are the effects predictable? *Spine* 13:1178–1186.
43. Willner S (1979): Moire topography for the diagnosis and documentation of scoliosis. *Acta Orthop Scand* 50:295–305.
44. Willner S (1979): Moire topography: a method for school screening of scoliosis. *Arch Orthop Trauma Surg* 95:181–185.
45. Willner S (1982): A comparative study of the efficiency of different types of school screening for scoliosis. *Acta Orthop Scand* 53:769–774.
46. Willner S (1984): Prevalence study of trunk asymmetries and structural scoliosis in 10-year-old school children. *Spine* 9:644–647.
47. Winter R (1983): *Congenital deformities of the spine.* New York: Thieme-Stratton.
48. Winter R, Moe J (1974): A plea for the routine school examination of children for spinal deformity. *Minn Med* May: 419–424.

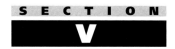

CONGENITAL ABNORMALITIES

CONGENITAL SCOLIOSIS

MICHAEL J. MCMASTER

Congenital scoliosis is a lateral curvature of the spine caused by developmental vertebral anomalies that produce a lateral longitudinal imbalance in the growth of the spine. The term *congenital scoliosis* is slightly misleading because it implies that the curvature is present at birth, but this is not necessarily so. The vertebral anomalies are present at birth, but the clinical deformity may not become evident until later childhood, when scoliosis develops and the diagnosis is made radiographically. This type of scoliosis must not be confused with *infantile idiopathic scoliosis,* which can also present as a deformity in early childhood. In these patients, however, the spinal radiograph shows that there are no vertebral anomalies.

Congenital scoliosis is relatively uncommon, but the true incidence in the general population remains unknown because some vertebral anomalies produce so little deformity that they remain undetected.

The radiographic appearance of vertebral anomalies varies considerably. As a result, congenital scoliosis was for many years thought to be unpredictable in its behavior, and some thought that it seldom required treatment (2,6). In 1952, Kuhns and Hormell (35) reviewed 165 children with congenital scoliosis and concluded that this was usually a relatively benign condition that progressed slowly. It was not until 1968 that Winter and associates (68), in a major study involving 234 children, firmly established the much more serious prognosis for certain types of congenital scoliosis and described a radiographic classification based on the types of vertebral anomalies that cause it.

Ohtsuka and I studied the natural history of 251 patients with congenital scoliosis and found that all degrees of severity of curvature were seen at all ages (44). Some patients presented in their late teens with small curves that did not deteriorate significantly, whereas others presented in the first few years of life with curves that deteriorated rapidly, becoming severe deformities before the child reached the age of 10 years. These severe curves were often rigid, and surgical correction was difficult and dangerous. It is therefore important to be able to anticipate when a congenital scoliosis is at risk for rapid deterioration so that treatment can be initiated when the curve is small, rather than having to attempt dangerous surgical salvage procedures after the curve has become severe. Planning, such prophylactic treatment, requires a thorough knowledge of the pathogenesis

and natural history of all types of congenital scoliosis and the various methods of treatment that are available.

ETIOLOGY

A family history of congenital scoliosis is unusual. Wynne-Davies (73) found that an isolated single anomaly, such as a hemivertebra, was usually sporadic, and there was no hereditary risk. Multiple vertebral anomalies and spina bifida cystica were etiologically related, however, and there was a 5% to 10% risk of either of these anomalies occurring in siblings or subsequent children. In contrast, Winter (64), found no significant relationship between multiple vertebral anomalies and relatives with spina bifida cystica. In addition, he found that an isolated single vertebral anomaly had about a 1 in 100 chance of occurring in a first-degree relative.

There are two rare hereditary conditions associated with congenital scoliosis in which most of the vertebrae in the thoracic and lumbar regions are malformed (55). In spondylothoracic dysostosis (Jarcho-Levin syndrome) (30), there are, in addition to the vertebral anomalies, also multiple posterior rib fusions that constrict the thorax and result in death from respiratory failure in early infancy. In spondylocostal dysostosis, the ribs are not so severely affected, and there is a normal life expectancy but with marked stunting of the trunk because of the vertebral anomalies.

Reports of congenital scoliosis in monozygotic twins have shown that if one twin has a vertebral anomaly, the other twin usually has a normal spine or less frequently an anomaly at a different level (23,51,52). Monozygotic twins have the same genetic material, and any difference in their vertebral development is likely to be due to an environmental insult rather than genetic factors. Mice embryos subjected to hypobaric hypoxia or carbon monoxide at an age equivalent to a 6-week-old human embryo also develop vertebral anomalies similar to those seen in congenital scoliosis (38,54). It can therefore be postulated that other environmental factors may have a similar effect on the human embryo vertebral column at this stage of its development.

PATHOGENESIS

To understand the natural history of congenital scoliosis and the great disparity in prognosis, it is necessary to correlate the

---

M. J. McMaster: Royal Hospital for Sick Children, Edinburgh, Scotland.

principles of normal growth of the spine with the pathologic anatomy of the various types of congenital vertebral anomalies that may cause scoliosis. The embryologic development of the vertebral column is a complex and rapid process. The complete anatomic pattern is formed in mesenchyma during the first 6 weeks of intrauterine life (see Chapter 1). Defects of formation or segmentation of the primitive vertebrae occur during this period. After the abnormal mesenchymal mold is established, the cartilaginous and bony stages follow that pattern, and the vertebral anomalies are fully established at birth.

Normal longitudinal growth of the spine is the sum total of growth occurring at the end plates on the upper and lower surfaces of the vertebral bodies (5). This growth occurs symmetrically; as a result, the spine grows in a balanced manner without a pathologic curvature. In the presence of a congenital vertebral anomaly, however, there is an asymmetric deficiency in either the number of growth plates or their rate of growth, resulting in a longitudinal growth imbalance and an increasing spinal deformity as the child grows.

Congenital scoliosis, kyphoscoliosis, and kyphosis are part of a gradually blending spectrum of spinal deformities due to developmental anomalies that produce a localized imbalance in the longitudinal growth of the spine. The type of deformity that develops depends on whether the impaired growth occurs unilaterally producing a pure scoliosis or lies anterior or anterolateral to the transverse axis of vertebral rotation in the sagittal plane, producing kyphosis or kyphoscoliosis. Lordosis, caused by impaired posterior growth of the spine, is uncommon by itself and is usually associated with scoliosis. In a study of 584 consecutive patients with closed congenital spine deformities, I found that 472 patients had pure congenital scoliosis, 76 had kyphoscoliosis, and 36 had a pure kyphosis (48). Care was taken to distinguish between scoliosis with marked rotation, which could mimic kyphosis in the sagittal plane, and true kyphoscoliosis. This chapter deals only with those patients whose major deformity is scoliosis.

The rate of deterioration and final severity of congenital scoliosis are proportional to the degree of growth imbalance produced by the vertebral anomalies. This deterioration continues until skeletal maturity, when the growth plates fuse. However, the rate of spinal growth is not uniform. There are two periods of accelerated growth during which the scoliosis deteriorates more rapidly. The first occurs during the first 2 years of life, and the second occurs later during the adolescent growth spurt, which usually occurs in girls between the ages of 10 and 13 years and in boys about 2 years later. It is during these two periods that congenital scoliosis is most frequently diagnosed. On average, 25% of curves are nonprogressive, 25% progress slowly, and 50% progress more rapidly.

The neural axis and the vertebral column develop at the same time. It is therefore not surprising that neural and vertebral malformations often coexist and are termed *spinal dysraphism*. Abnormalities of the spinal cord are often associated with a failure of development of the posterior vertebral arches and overlying soft tissues, resulting in an "open" spinal defect, such as a myelomeningocele. This type of malformation often presents with major neurologic deficits in the lower limbs and paralysis of the trunk muscles, which contribute to the development of scoliosis.

This chapter deals only with "closed" congenital scoliosis in which the skin overlying the spine remains intact, although there may be mild neurologic abnormalities in the lower limbs as a result of occult intraspinal anomalies.

CLASSIFICATION AND NATURAL HISTORY

The major advances in the management of congenital scoliosis have been not in devising new methods of correcting severe deformities but rather in achieving a better understanding of the natural history of the condition and knowing when to apply prophylactic surgical treatment to balance the abnormal growth of the spine before there is a significant deformity.

The classification of the developmental vertebral anomalies that produce congenital scoliosis is based on the embryologic development of the spine. There are two basic groups of anomalies: those caused by a defect of formation and those caused by a defect of segmentation of one or more vertebrae (Table 1). About 80% of vertebral anomalies can be classified in this manner (Fig. 1). The remaining 20% are unclassifiable because there is a jumble of anomalies or the anomaly cannot be accurately identified, or because the scoliosis is so severe that it obscures the radiographic characteristics of the anomaly.

Vertebral anomalies may also be present in other areas of the spine outside the scoliotic curve, but these are ignored for the purposes of classification of the scoliosis if they do not contribute to the development of the deformity. Anomalies of the ribs are also common in association with congenital scoliosis, but these are not included in the classification because they do not cause scoliosis by themselves.

Defects of Vertebral Segmentation

Defects of vertebral segmentation may be either unilateral or bilateral and occur most frequently in the thoracic or thoracolumbar region.

Unilateral Failure of Segmentation

A unilateral failure of segmentation of two or more vertebrae results in a unilateral unsegmented bar, which is one of the most

TABLE 1. TYPES OF DEVELOPMENTAL VERTEBRAL ANOMALIES CAUSING CONGENITAL SCOLIOSIS

Defects of segmentation
  Unilateral
    Unsegmented bar
    Unsegmented bar with contralateral hemivertebrae
  Bilateral
    Block vertebra
Defects of formation
  Complete unilateral
    Hemivertebra: fully segmented, semisegmented, nonsegmented, incarcerated
  Partial unilateral
    Wedge vertebra
Mixed or unclassifiable anomalies

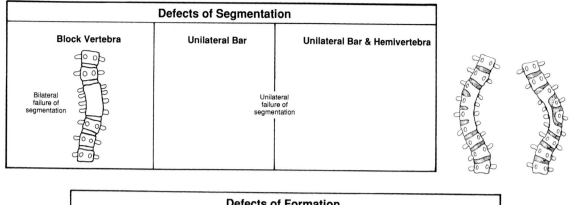

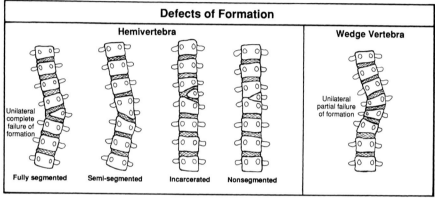

FIGURE 1. Congenital scoliosis.

common causes of congenital scoliosis (8,41,44,68). This type of anomaly consists of a bar of bone fusing the disc spaces and facet joints on one side of the spine while leaving the other side relatively unaffected. The unsegmented bar does not contain growth plates and therefore does not grow longitudinally. Some degree of growth continues on the opposite side of the spine, resulting in the development of scoliosis (Fig. 2). Rib fusions and other abnormalities of the ribs are often seen adjacent to the unsegmented bar, but they do not by themselves contribute to the development of the scoliosis. The rate of deterioration and the final severity of the scoliosis depend not only on the extent of the unsegmented bar but also on the growth potential on the convexity of the spine opposite the unsegmented bar. If the disc spaces on the convexity are well formed, it is more likely that the growth will be relatively normal, resulting in the development of a severe curvature. However, if the disc spaces are narrow and indistinct, there is likely to be impaired growth, resulting in a lesser curvature. On average, these curves deteriorate at a rate of 5 degrees a year, and most exceed 50 degrees by 10 years of age, resulting in a severe deformity.

There is also a small but important subgroup of patients who, in addition to the unsegmented bar, have one or more hemivertebrae on the convexity of the curve at the same level as the bar. Radiographically, this type of anomaly is seen most clearly in the first few years of life, but as the curve deteriorates and rotates, the hemivertebrae often become obscured by the deformity (Fig. 3). It is most important to recognize a unilateral unsegmented bar with contralateral hemivertebrae at an early

stage because this type of anomaly produces the most severe and rapidly progressive of all types of congenital scoliosis (47,50). Although there is no longitudinal growth on the side of the bar, the hemivertebrae produce a greater growth potential on the convexity than in patients with an unsegmented bar alone. On

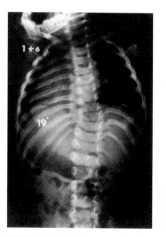 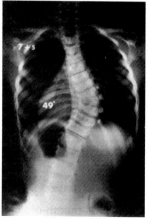

A,B

FIGURE 2. A: A boy aged 1 year, 6 months with a unilateral unsegmented bar on the left extending from T8 to T10 and producing a right thoracic scoliosis measuring 19 degrees. The disc spaces on the convexity opposite the bar are clearly seen, indicating a relatively normal growth potential; no growth is occurring in the unsegmented bar. No treatment was given. **B:** By the age of 7 years, 5 months, the thoracic curve had deteriorated to 49 degrees.

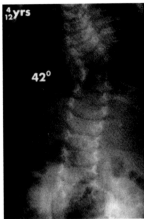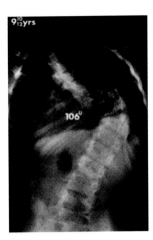

A,B

FIGURE 3. A: A 4-month-old girl with a 42-degree right thoracic scoliosis due to a unilateral unsegmented bar on the right extending from T7 to T10, with three adjacent contralateral hemivertebrae at the eighth to the tenth thoracic levels. No treatment was given. **B:** By the age of 9 years, 10 months, the scoliosis had increased to 106 degrees, and the contralateral hemivertebrae were no longer visible. There was marked malalignment of the trunk and distortion of the rib cage, reducing the vital capacity.

average, these curves deteriorate 6 degrees or more a year, and most exceed 60 degrees by 4 years of age. In addition, there is usually severe vertebral rotation and distortion of the rib cage due to the crankshaft effect produced by continuing growth of the hemivertebrae anterolaterally combined with the tethering effect of the unsegmented bar on the concavity of the curve. If untreated, these children become extremely deformed at an early age, and there is often significant respiratory impairment, which can lead to cor pulmonale.

In treating patients with an unsegmented bar with or without contralateral hemivertebrae, it is important to remember that it is not possible to create growth on the concave side of the spine where none exists. The only way to stop deterioration of the deformity is to prevent further growth on the convex side of the curve opposite the unsegmented bar, and this can only be accomplished by a spinal fusion.

Bilateral Failure of Segmentation

A bilateral failure of segmentation of a number of adjacent vertebrae results in a block vertebra. The disc spaces between the affected vertebrae are very narrow or fused. As a result, longitudinal growth is impaired on both sides of the spine, producing a shortened segment. When this occurs in the neck, it is part of the Klippel-Feil syndrome (25,70) and is usually diagnosed because of the short neck, low hairline, and restricted movement. A block vertebra occurring elsewhere in the spine is diagnosed less frequently because it produces little if any deformity. Occasionally, the longitudinal growth impairment is not symmetric, which can result in the development of lesser scoliosis that rarely exceeds 20 degrees and never requires treatment. Most commonly, the block vertebra is diagnosed as part of a complex of other congenital vertebral anomalies that may produce a more severe deformity.

Defects of Vertebral Formation

A lateral defect of vertebral formation can vary from mild wedging to the complete absence of half of the vertebra (i.e., a hemivertebra). These anomalies may affect one or more vertebrae and can occur in any part of the spine.

Unilateral Complete Failure of Formation

A hemivertebra is one of the most common causes of congenital scoliosis. It is caused by the complete failure of a vertebra to form on one side, resulting in a laterally based wedge of bone consisting of half a vertebral body, a single pedicle, and hemilamina. If the hemivertebra is in the thoracic region, there is usually an attached rib, resulting in an unequal number of ribs.

There are four different types of hemivertebrae, depending on the pathologic anatomy and relationship to the adjacent vertebrae (Fig 1). The hemivertebra may be fully segmented (nonincarcerated), which is most common; semisegmented, which is less common; nonsegmented; or incarcerated, which is the least common. It is important to distinguish among these different types. Each has a different growth potential, and the severity of the resultant scoliosis is related to the degree of segmentation (46).

Fully Segmented Hemivertebra

A fully segmented (nonincarcerated) hemivertebra has a normal disc space above and below and is completely separate from its adjacent vertebrae. Longitudinal growth occurs on the upper and lower surfaces of the hemivertebra, whereas there is an absence of two growth plates on the unformed side. As the hemivertebra grows, it acts as an enlarging wedge, producing scoliosis that usually deteriorates relatively slowly at a rate of 1 to 2 degrees a year.

A single fully segmented hemivertebra lies at the apex of the scoliosis, and as the curve deteriorates, the body of the hemivertebra tends to protrude slightly from the lateral margin of the spine. There may also be slight secondary wedging of the adjacent normal vertebrae (Fig. 4A, B). Lower thoracic and thoracolumbar curves deteriorate most rapidly and can exceed 45 degrees at skeletal maturity. However, there is often only a moderate cosmetic deformity because the hemivertebra does not have the same tethering effect on the concavity of the curve as a unilateral unsegmented bar and there is much less vertebral rotation (Fig. 4C).

A fully segmented hemivertebra at the lumbosacral junction is a particularly pernicious anomaly because it causes the lumbar spine to take off obliquely from the sacrum. This results in the development of long compensatory scoliosis in the thoracolumbar region. The secondary thoracolumbar curve, which does not contain any congenital anomalies, is initially mobile, but it later becomes fixed and rotated, with the upper body listing to the side opposite the hemivertebra (Fig. 5). This can produce a major cosmetic deformity and is best treated by prophylactic surgery at an early stage before the compensatory curve becomes fixed.

Two fully segmented hemivertebrae on the same side of the spine are less common but cause a much greater growth imbal-

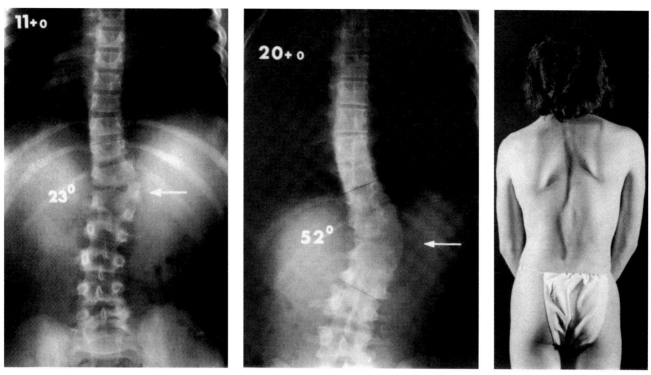

FIGURE 4. **A:** A boy aged 11 years with a 23-degree right thoracolumbar scoliosis due to a fully segmented (nonincarcerated) hemivertebra at L1. No treatment was given. **B:** By the age of 20 years, the patient was skeletally mature, and the curve had deteriorated to 52 degrees. **C:** Despite the severity of the curve, the cosmetic deformity was relatively mild.

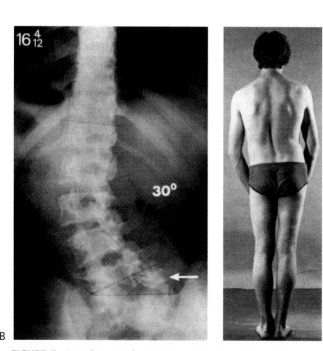

FIGURE 5. **A:** A boy aged 16 years, 4 months with a single unsegmented (nonincarcerated) hemivertebra at the lumbosacral junction, causing the lumbar spine to take off obliquely from the sacrum. A long secondary lumbar curve has developed, which measures 30 degrees and does not contain any congenital anomalies. **B:** The main cosmetic deformity is caused by the secondary lumbar curve and the tendency of the upper body to list to the left.

ance because there is an absence of four growth plates on the concavity of the curve. These curves deteriorate much more rapidly than those caused by a single hemivertebra. They deteriorate by about 3 degrees a year, and all exceed 50 degrees by 10 years of age (Fig. 6A, B). Without treatment, these curves could reach 70 degrees by skeletal maturity. Therefore, early prophylactic surgical treatment should be given as soon as they are diagnosed.

Two opposing fully segmented hemivertebrae are thought to be caused by an embryologic hemimetameric shift. The severity of the deformity depends on whether the hemivertebrae are close together or in different regions of the spine. If they are close together, separated by only one or two normal vertebrae, they tend to balance each other, causing only two small kinks in the spine. This produces minimal cosmetic deformity, and no treatment is required. If the hemivertebrae are in different regions of the spine, they produce separate curves that may be unbalanced, causing spinal decompensation and a significant cosmetic deformity (Fig. 7).

Semisegmented Hemivertebra
A semisegmented hemivertebra is synostosed to its neighboring vertebra and has only one disc space either above or below. As a result, two growth plates are obliterated on the convexity of the curve, which tends to balance the absence of the two growth plates on the unformed side of the hemivertebra. Although growth of the spine is theoretically balanced, the hemivertebra causes a tilting of the spine, which can induce slowly progressive scoliosis (Fig. 8). These curves usually do not exceed 40 degrees

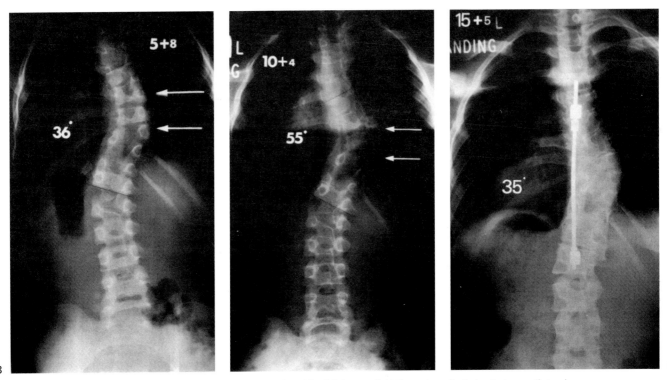

A,B   C

FIGURE 6. **A:** A girl aged 5 years, 8 months with a 36-degree right thoracic scoliosis due to two unilateral fully segmented (nonincarcerated) hemivertebrae at T7 and T9. No treatment was given. **B:** By the age of 10 years, 4 months, the thoracic curve had deteriorated to 55 degrees. At this time, the patient was treated by means of a posterior spinal fusion with instrumentation, which corrected the curve to 35 degrees. **C:** At 15 years, 5 months, there had been no deterioration.

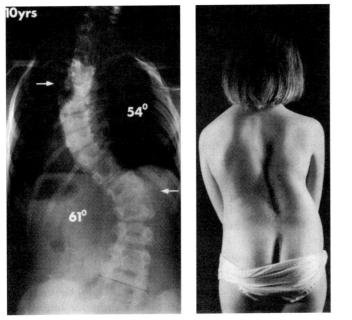

A,B

FIGURE 7. **A:** A girl aged 10 years with two opposing hemivertebrae occurring in different regions of the spine at T5 and L2. These hemiver-tebrae have produced two curves that are unbalanced. **B:** The patient lists to the left, and there is a significant cosmetic deformity.

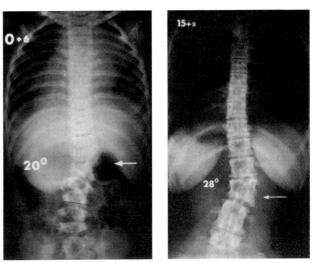

A,B

FIGURE 8. **A:** A girl aged 6 months with a 20-degree right lumbar scoliosis due to a semisegmented hemivertebra at L2. The hemivertebra is synostosed with L3. No treatment was given. **B:** The curve deterio-rated very slowly to measure 28 degrees at 15 years, 8 months, when the patient was skeletally mature.

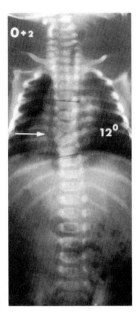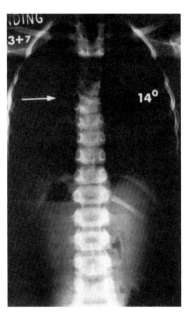

A,B

FIGURE 9. A: An infant aged 2 months with a minimal 12-degree left thoracic scoliosis due to an incarcerated hemivertebra at T6. No treatment was given. **B:** There was virtually no deterioration at 13 years, 7 months.

at skeletal maturity. Treatment is not usually required, except possibly when the semisegmented hemivertebra occurs at the lumbosacral junction.

Nonsegmented Hemivertebra

A nonsegmented hemivertebra is synostosed to both of its adjacent vertebrae and has no disc spaces either above or below. This type of hemivertebra, which usually occurs in the thoracic region, has no growth potential and therefore does not cause progressive scoliosis. There is no cosmetic deformity, and no treatment is required.

Incarcerated Hemivertebra

An incarcerated hemivertebra is more ovoid in shape and smaller than a fully segmented (nonincarcerated) hemivertebra. This type of hemivertebra is tucked into the side of the spine and set into a niche scalloped out of the adjacent vertebrae. The vertebrae above and below are shaped in such a way that they tend to compensate for the hemivertebra. As a result, the alignment of the pedicles on that side of the spine remains straight, and there is minimal scoliosis (Fig. 9). The disc spaces above and below the incarcerated hemivertebra are usually narrow and poorly formed, indicating a poor growth potential. The resulting scoliosis deteriorates very slowly if at all. Occasionally, the disc spaces become even narrower with growth and may fuse with the adjacent vertebrae. An incarcerated hemivertebra rarely produces scoliosis exceeding 20 degrees at skeletal maturity and never requires treatment.

Unilateral Partial Failure of Formation

A wedge vertebra is an uncommon cause of congenital scoliosis and is due to partial failure of a vertebra to form on one side.

The malformed vertebra contains two pedicles and is slightly wedged toward one side of the spine. There is retarded longitudinal growth on the hypoplastic side, which causes scoliosis that deteriorates relatively slowly. Surgical treatment may occasionally be necessary, especially if there are more than one wedged hemivertebra situated close together on the same side of the spine.

ASSOCIATED DEFORMING FEATURES

Apart from the severity of the congenital scoliosis, there are also a number of important secondary deforming features related to the site of the vertebral anomalies. These features contribute significantly to the overall disability and deformity of the patient and must be taken into consideration when planning treatment.

Upper thoracic curves are relatively common in congenital scoliosis. Although most never become very large, they can cause a significant cosmetic deformity because of elevation of the shoulder line and, less frequently, tilting of the head (Fig. 10). The higher the apex of the curve, the more severe the deformity. A 30-degree curve is probably at the upper limit of acceptability, especially in girls.

Midthoracic curves with their apex at T5, T6, or T7, especially those caused by a unilateral unsegmented bar with or without contralateral hemivertebrae, are frequently associated with the development of a long secondary structural curve in the lower thoracic or thoracolumbar region (Fig. 11). As the congenital scoliosis deteriorates, it produces a rotational effect that is transmitted further down the spine into the lower thoracic and thoracolumbar region, resulting in secondary scoliosis on the opposite side. This curve, which does not contain any congenital anomalies, is initially compensatory and correctable. Later, it becomes fixed and may deteriorate even more rapidly than the primary

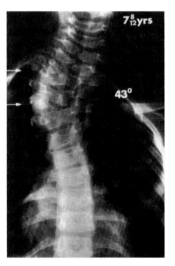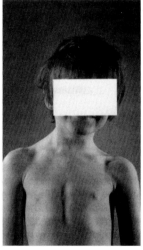

A,B

FIGURE 10. A: A girl aged 7 years, 8 months with a 43-degree right upper thoracic scoliosis due to two unilateral fully segmented (nonincarcerated) hemivertebrae at T2 and T4. **B:** Her main cosmetic deformity is the elevation of the right shoulder and slight tilting of the head to the left.

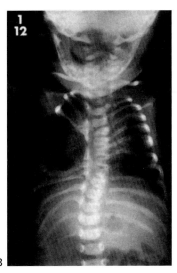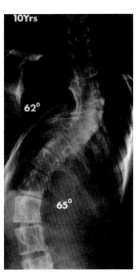

A,B

FIGURE 11. A: An infant aged 1 month who had a radiograph because of asymmetry of the thoracic cage. This showed that the spine was relatively straight, but there were absent ribs and a unilateral unsegmented bar extending from T3 to T7 on the left. No treatment was given. **B:** By the age of 10 years, the unilateral unsegmented bar had produced a 62-degree right upper thoracic scoliosis. However, the main deformity was caused by the secondary development of a severe left structural thoracolumbar scoliosis, which contained no congenital anomalies.

congenital curve. The congenital thoracic curve is often only moderately rotated, but the lower secondary curve is frequently severely rotated, producing the major cosmetic deformity of a large rib hump. In these circumstances, a severe, apparently "idiopathic" curve can develop below a congenital anomaly whose significance may not be fully appreciated.

Lower thoracic, thoracolumbar, and lumbar curves, especially those caused by a long unilateral unsegmented bar with or without contralateral hemivertebrae, often fail to develop compensatory curves either above or below that are sufficient to balance the congenital curve (Fig. 3). There are too few normal mobile vertebrae between the rigid anomalous segment and either the upper end of the spine or the sacrum. This results in a severe cosmetic deformity because, in addition to the spinal curvature, there is severe malalignment of the body, often associated with pelvic obliquity and an apparent leg length discrepancy.

Severe distortion of the rib cage frequently occurs secondary to the development of significant thoracic scoliosis. When this occurs before the child is 8 years of age, it interfere with the normal development of the lungs (13). Increasing deformity is associated with a steady decrease in vital capacity and may lead to cor pulmonale and possibly death in early adult life. Surgical treatment of the spine is associated with a further reduction in vital capacity, especially in patients with multiple thoracic anomalies (14).

ASSOCIATED OCCULT INTRASPINAL ANOMALIES

The development of the spinal cord is closely associated with that of the vertebral column. It is therefore not surprising that

neural and vertebral malformations often coexist. The spinal deformity may be obvious, but the intraspinal anomaly may not be recognized because the skin overlying the spine is intact and any associated neural deficit in the lower limbs may be mild or absent. It is important to detect these intraspinal anomalies because they may restrict movement of the spinal cord within the spinal canal and attempts to correct the spinal deformity could result in stretching of the neural tissues and serious complications.

A diastematomyelia is found in 5% to 21% of patients with congenital scoliosis (7,18,27,45,65). This is a sagittal split in a localized segment of either the spinal cord or cauda equina. Lying within the split is an osseous or fibrocartilaginous spur that projects backward from one or more adjacent vertebral bodies. The term *diastematomyelia* refers to the split in the neural structures and not to the spur or septum. It should not be confused with diplomyelia or true division of the spinal cord. Other types of congenital neural abnormalities—epidermoid cysts, dermoid cysts, neurenteric cysts, lipomas, and teratomas—may be found either alone or in association with diastematomyelia. The spinal cord or cauda equina may also be tethered by fibrous bands, a tight filum terminale, ectopic posterior nerve roots, or arachnoid adhesions to the dura or vertebral column.

In the past, myelography was used to diagnose these intraspinal anomalies. However, magnetic resonance imaging (MRI) is a much better method because it is noninvasive and more sensitive in the visualization of soft tissue abnormalities of the spinal cord. Using MRI, Bradford and coworkers (11) found a 38% prevalence of intraspinal anomalies in 42 patients with congenital spinal deformities; of these, 16 had a tethered cord, 4 had a diastematomyelia, 3 had a diplomyelia, 3 had a low-lying conus, 1 had a teratoma of the sacrum, and, surprisingly, 4 had an unsuspected syringomyelia. Winter and colleagues (72) found a similar prevalence of 41% in 48 patients.

Intraspinal abnormalities may be found in association with all sites and types of congenital scoliosis. However, the most common association (50%) is with a unilateral unsegmented bar with contralateral hemivertebra, producing scoliosis in the lower thoracic or thoracolumbar region (11,45).

An intraspinal anomaly may not be immediately obvious, but there are a number of clues to its presence. An abnormality of the skin overlying the spine, such as a dimple, nevus, hairy patch, or lipoma, is present in about 70% of affected patients. These stigmata, however, may also occur without an accompanying intraspinal anomaly (45). Neurologic abnormalities affecting the lower limbs may also be present, but they are often very mild and easily missed. Frequently, only one leg is affected. The leg may be slightly short with a small foot that may have a mild cavus deformity and slight clawing of the toes (29). In addition, the spinal radiograph may show a spina bifida occulta affecting one or more adjacent vertebrae associated with widening of the interpedicular distance and narrowing of the disc spaces. Occasionally, the bony spur associated with a diastematomyelia may be visible on the plain spinal radiograph, but an MRI is necessary to confirm its presence and reveal other possible neural abnormalities.

It is widely accepted that an intraspinal anomaly that tethers the spinal cord should be surgically released if there is a progressive neurologic deficit or before attempting to correct a spinal deformity (49). Excision or release of the intraspinal anomaly will not improve the neurologic status, but it will prevent further deterioration and decrease the risk for complications after correction of the scoliosis. MRI is not necessary for all patients with congenital scoliosis, but it should be used in those with suspicious clinical or radiologic findings and in those who are about to undergo surgery to correct the spinal deformity. If the intraspinal anomaly is diagnosed during the routine assessment of children younger than 5 years of age, it should probably be removed as a prophylactic measure to prevent the possible development of neurologic deterioration. In older children, however, the presence of an intraspinal anomaly is not necessarily an indication for its removal unless there are symptoms or corrective surgery is planned.

OTHER CONGENITAL ANOMALIES

Congenital scoliosis is frequently associated with congenital anomalies in other systems, especially those formed from mesenchyma. These anomalies are often asymptomatic and may remain undetected until the patient is fully assessed after diagnosis of a congenital scoliosis. Beals and associates (3) found that up to 60% of patients with vertebral anomalies have one or more associated anomalies in other systems and that many of these are medically important. The prognosis for these patients is excellent if the associated anomalies are detected and, if necessary, treated.

The genitourinary system may be affected in up to 25% of patients. The most common anomalies diagnosed by means of an intravenous pyelogram (IVP) or ultrasound scan are a unilateral kidney, duplication of the kidney, or ureteric obstruction (15,43). The Klippel-Feil syndrome may be found in 25% (25,70) and congenital heart disease in 10% of patients (53).

Sprengel deformity (congenital elevation of the scapula) is often found in association with congenital scoliosis in the upper thoracic or cervicothoracic region. When it is present on the convexity of the curve, the combination of these two anomalies causes a significant deformity because of elevation of the shoulder line. In these circumstances, the elevated scapula should also be reduced when the scoliosis is treated surgically. If the elevated scapula is on the concavity of the curve, however, it may partially compensate for the scoliotic deformity by leveling the shoulders. In these circumstances, it should not be reduced.

Goldenhar syndrome (oculoauricular vertebral dysplasia) is uncommon (19,20). Its main features are unilateral malformation of the ear and facial hypoplasia, and it is associated with congenital scoliosis, usually in the upper thoracic region.

PROGNOSIS

The prognosis for congenital scoliosis with regard to its rate of deterioration and final severity depends on three factors (Table 2):

1. *The type of vertebral anomaly and the degree of growth imbalance it produces.* The type of anomaly that causes the most severe scoliosis is a unilateral unsegmented bar with contralateral hemivertebrae at the same level. Next in severity is a scoliosis caused by a unilateral unsegmented bar alone, followed by two unilateral fully segmented hemivertebrae, a single fully segmented hemivertebra, and a wedge vertebra. The least severe deformity is caused by a block vertebra. Congenital scoliosis caused by a jumble of unclassifiable anomalies can be difficult to predict and requires careful monitoring. The poor prognosis associated with a unilateral unsegmented bar with or without contralateral hemivertebrae is so predictable that these curves should be treated immediately without any period of observation.

2. *The site of the anomaly.* For any type of vertebral anomaly, the rate of deterioration of the resulting scoliosis are most severe in the thoracic and thoracolumbar regions and are usually less severe in the upper thoracic and lumbar regions.

TABLE 2. MEDIAN YEARLY RATE OF DETERIORATION (IN DEGREES) WITHOUT TREATMENT FOR EACH TYPE OF SINGLE CONGENITAL SCOLIOSIS IN EACH REGION OF THE SPINE

Site of Curvature	Type of Congenital Anomaly					
	Block Vertebra	Wedge Vertebra	Hemivertebra		Unilateral Unsegmented Bar	Unilateral Unsegmented Bar and Contralateral Hemivertebrae
			Single	Double		
Upper thoracic	<1°–1°	★–2°	1°–2°	2°–2.5°	2°–4°	5°–6°
Lower thoracic	<1°–1°	2°–2°	2°–2.5°	2°–3°	5°–6.5°	5°–8°
Thoracolumbar	<1°–1°	1.5°–2°	2°–3.5°	5°–★	6°–9°	7°–14°
Lumbar	<1°–★	<1°–★	<1°–1°	★	>5°–★	★
Lumbosacral	★	★	<1°–1.5°	★	★	★

◙ No treatment required ▢ May require spinal surgery ▢ Requires spinal fusion ★ Too few or no curves
Ranges represent the degree of deterioration before and after 10 years of age.
Modified from McMaster MJ, Ohtsuka K (1982): The natural history of congenital scoliosis: a study of 251 patients. *J Bone Joint Surg Am* 66: 588–601 and McMaster MJ (1998): Congenital scoliosis caused by a unilateral failure of vertebrae segmentation with contralateral hemivertebrae. *Spine* 23: 998–1005.

The site of the congenital scoliosis is also an important factor in the degree of cosmetic deformity produced, which can be tilting of the head, elevation of the shoulder line, decompensation of the trunk, and pelvic obliquity.

3. *The age of the patient at the time of diagnosis.* Congenital curves generally stabilize at skeletal maturity. A scoliosis presenting as a clinical deformity in the first few years of life has a particularly bad prognosis because this indicates a marked growth imbalance that will continue throughout the period of growth, resulting in a severe deformity. In addition, the rate of deterioration is not constant; it becomes much more severe after the age of 10 years, during the adolescent growth spurt. Even after skeletal maturity, severe curves may continue to deteriorate slowly as a result of plastic deformation of the spine.

TREATMENT

The objective of treatment in congenital scoliosis is to produce a spine that will be as straight as possible at the end of growth. It is not possible, however, to create growth on the concavity of the scoliosis, where it is either retarded or nonexistent. For patients with a marked spinal growth imbalance, there is no perfect treatment. The best that can be achieved is to balance spinal growth by retarding the growth on the convexity. In these circumstances, the optimal result is a short, relatively straight spine rather than the severely crooked spine that would have developed without treatment. There are three key factors in achieving an optimal result in patients with congenital scoliosis:

1. *Early diagnosis.* If the diagnosis is made early, while the curvature is still small, there is an opportunity for prophylactic surgery to balance the growth of the spine. Congenital vertebral anomalies are frequently diagnosed in infants on radiographs taken for other reasons, before there is an obvious clinical deformity (Fig. 11A). These radiographic findings should not be ignored. They may provide an opportunity for early prophylactic treatment before a deformity develops (Fig. 11B).
2. *Anticipation.* The prognosis for deterioration of congenital scoliosis can be anticipated based on the amount of spinal growth remaining, the type and site of the vertebral anomaly, and the degree of growth imbalance it produces. This requires careful study of good-quality spinal radiographs and a thorough knowledge of the natural history of the condition. Often, the most helpful radiographs are those taken at an early stage before the vertebral anomalies are obscured by the developing deformity (Fig. 3).
3. *Prevention of deterioration.* It is easier to prevent a severe deformity than to correct one. Some types of congenital scoliosis, such as those caused by a unilateral unsegmented bar with or without contralateral hemivertebrae, have such a bad prognosis that no observation is necessary; they require immediate surgical treatment no matter how young the patient. Other types of congenital scoliosis may be observed, but one of the most common errors is to fail to recognize slow and relentless progression until it is too late for prophylactic treat-

ment. All patients require careful radiologic assessment at 4- to 6-month intervals. After progression is established, immediate treatment is necessary to prevent further deterioration. A simple operation to balance the growth of the spine and prevent increasing curvature is preferable to a hazardous multistage surgical procedure to correct a severe and rigid deformity at a later stage.

Radiographic Assessment

Spinal radiographs are necessary to identify the type of vertebral anomaly that is causing the congenital scoliosis and to monitor any deterioration of the deformity.

Identification of the vertebral anomalies requires good-quality supine anteroposterior and lateral spinal radiographs centered on the abnormal levels. The diagnosis of a congenital scoliosis is made on the anteroposterior spine radiograph. It is also important to examine carefully the lateral radiograph to detect any associated kyphosis because this will affect the treatment. If only the anteroposterior radiograph is viewed, a patient with a posterolateral quadrant vertebra producing kyphoscoliosis may be misdiagnosed as having a lateral hemivertebra producing scoliosis. Treatment by means of a combined anterior and posterior convex epiphysiodesis, which may be appropriate for a lateral hemivertebra, would be contraindicated for kyphoscoliosis because it would increase the deformity in the sagittal plane. A misdiagnosis is also possible in infants with a short unilateral unsegmented bar, which may not appear radiographically until it is fully ossified. A coned-down oblique radiograph of the apex of the curve gives a true anteroposterior view of the more severely rotated spine and may detect hidden vertebral anomalies. An anteroposterior view aligned through the lumbosacral junction shows whether a lumbosacral hemivertebra is fully segmented or semisegmented. An MRI scan may also help define the type of vertebral anomaly.

After the vertebral anomalies have been clearly identified on the anteroposterior radiograph, it should be possible to count the number of vertebral growth plates on both sides of the spine and estimate the potential growth imbalance. Allowance should be made for any disc space that is narrowed or ill defined because this indicates an impaired growth potential. It may be difficult to assess the prognosis in young infants with mixed vertebral anomalies; they require careful radiologic follow-up to detect deterioration of the scoliosis.

Follow-up radiographic assessment of congenital scoliosis does not require detailed visualization of the vertebral anomalies after they have been fully identified. Serial full-length standing anteroposterior spinal radiographs are best for assessing deterioration. The Cobb angle of the scoliosis is always measured at exactly the same vertebral levels with reference to the standing radiograph taken when the patient was first seen (39). These radiographs show any deterioration of the scoliosis as well as any change in shoulder symmetry, decompensation of the trunk, or pelvic obliquity.

Nonoperative Treatment

Certain types of congenital scoliosis can occasionally be managed by the application of an orthosis, but this is never an alternative to appropriate surgical treatment. The problem being treated is one of spinal growth imbalance, and an orthosis should never be applied if there is a severe growth imbalance or a rigid curve such as that produced by a unilateral failure of segmentation.

In young children with congenital scoliosis, the application of a plaster jacket or underarm brace in an attempt to prevent deterioration of the deformity constricts the chest and may have an adverse effect on the developing respiratory system. Winter and colleagues (67) found that the Milwaukee brace does not have the same adverse effects on pulmonary function. It has the advantage of being a nonconstricting device yet is able to apply corrective forces to selected areas of the trunk. This type of brace works best on long flexible thoracic or thoracolumbar curves with a short anomalous segment, such as a hemivertebra at the apex of the curve. A Milwaukee brace is unlikely to be effective if the scoliosis is greater than 40 degrees or if there is less than 50% flexibility assessed on side-bending or distraction radiographs.

If the brace does not control the congenital curve, it is pointless to continue its use. The patient requires immediate surgery. After surgery, a brace may be helpful in controlling spinal alignment and the development of compensatory curves that were not included in the fusion. These secondary structural curves are easier to control than primary congenital curves because they occur in areas of the spine where the vertebrae are relatively normal and therefore much more mobile than the anomalous segment, which is often rigid. Tilting of the head may be controlled in a Milwaukee brace with a head extension. An underarm brace may be sufficient for an adolescent with a secondary thoracolumbar or lumbar curve.

Surgical Treatment

Surgical treatment is frequently necessary for congenital scoliosis and is indicated at any age if the deformity is severe or the curve is increasing and cannot be controlled. There is no one operative procedure that can be applied to all types of deformities. The method of surgery selected depends on the age of the patient, the site and type of vertebral anomaly, and the size of the curvature. Successful surgical treatment depends on selecting the right procedure and applying it at the right time.

Prophylactic surgical procedures are applied to young patients presenting with small curves that have a bad prognosis. The objective of treatment is to prevent further deterioration by balancing the growth of the spine. After prophylactic surgery, these curves must be carefully followed to skeletal maturity because further surgical treatment may be required later.

Salvage surgical procedures are necessary for patients who present at a later stage with larger deformities that require correction. The primary objective is still to prevent further deterioration, and correction is attempted only if it can be safely achieved.

Prophylactic Convex Growth Arrest (Hemiepiphysiodesis)

A convex growth arrest procedure (combined anterior and posterior convex hemiepiphysiodesis) is the optimum form of early prophylactic surgical treatment for patients with a small progres-

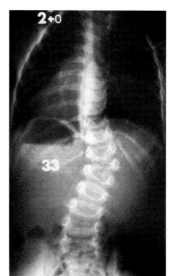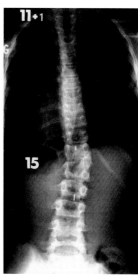

A,B

FIGURE 12. **A:** An infant aged 2 years with a 33-degree right thoracolumbar scoliosis due to a single fully segmented (nonincarcerated) hemivertebra at L1. A combined anterior and posterior convex growth arrest procedure was performed. **B:** By the age of 11 years, 1 month, the curve had improved to 15 degrees.

sive scoliosis due to a unilateral failure of vertebral formation in which there is some growth potential on the concavity at the site of the vertebral anomaly. This procedure is best applied to patients younger than 5 years of age with a short curve caused by a fully segmented hemivertebra that corrects to less than 40 degrees, with the patient supine (1,9,59,61,63,71) (Fig. 12). The objective of the surgery is to balance the growth of the spine by preventing further unbalanced growth on the convexity at the site of the hemivertebra. Theoretically, this should allow the scoliosis to correct slowly by means of the continuing growth on the concavity. This is a relatively safe procedure; the only disadvantage is the slow and often uncertain correction because of the unpredictable growth potential on the concavity of the curve. Even if there is no correction of the deformity, however, a convex growth arrest is often sufficient to stabilize the deformity.

This procedure does not result in correction of the scoliosis in patients with a unilateral failure of vertebral segmentation because there is no potential for growth on the concavity of the curve. The presence of any degree of kyphosis is also a contraindication to the procedure because the anterior convex growth arrest aggravates the deformity.

The surgery is performed in two stages that are usually carried out under the same anesthetic. The spine is first approached anteriorly on the convexity of the scoliosis through a thoracotomy, a thoracoabdominal retroperitoneal exposure, or a purely retroperitoneal approach beneath the diaphragm, depending on the site of the hemivertebra. The lateral half of the discs and their adjacent end plates are removed not only at the site of the hemivertebra but also at one intervertebral level above and below. This removes the anterior growth plates at the site of the anomaly, which are the main cause of the increasing scoliosis. To create an anterior convex fusion, the excised disc spaces are packed with chips of bone taken from an excised rib. The second stage of the procedure is performed through a separate posterior exposure of the convexity of the curve at the site of the hemivertebra. Care is taken not to strip the paraspinal muscles on the concavity of the curve and possibly interfere with the growth potential on this side of the spine. A posterior convex fusion is performed by excising the facet joints and decorticating the posterior elements not only at the site of the hemivertebra but also to one intervertebral level above and below. Strips of excised rib are applied to the fusion area. Several days after surgery, partial correction may be attempted by means of manual traction and the application of a plaster jacket, which is maintained for 6 months until the convex growth arrest has soundly healed.

A transpedicular anterior convex epiphysiodesis, which can be performed at the same time as the posterior convex epiphysiodesis, has been described as an alternative that obviates the need for a separate anterior approach (31,34). The pedicle of the hemivertebra and the pedicles of the vertebrae above and below are entered on the convexity. Using a curette, the hemivertebra is decancellated along with the convex half of the vertebrae above and below. Curved curettes are used to perforate the end plates of the vertebrae to be included in the hemiepiphysiodesis. Strips of autogenous iliac crest bone graft are then placed through the pedicles and into the decancellated portion of the vertebral bodies and packed across the disc spaces. This technique has the potential advantage of reducing the morbidity associated with a separate thoracotomy or thoracoabdominal retroperitoneal approach. There are as yet no long-term follow-up reports of this procedure, however, and the results can only be fully assessed at skeletal maturity.

Minimally invasive thoracoscopic and laparoscopic procedures have recently gained considerable clinical interest and can also be used to perform an anterior convex epiphysiodesis or arthrodesis as well as excise the body of a hemivertebra. These procedures have the potential to reduce postoperative pain and recovery time, and they produce a more cosmetically pleasing result because of small incisional scars. There is a considerable learning curve associated with these techniques, however, and as yet, there are no long-term results.

Excision of a Hemivertebra

Excision of a fully segmented hemivertebra is theoretically attractive as a prophylactic procedure because it removes the primary cause of the scoliosis, which is the enlarging wedge on the convexity at the apex of the curve (12,56,62). This also creates a wedge osteotomy of the spine, which, when closed, produces correction.

The major advantage of resecting a hemivertebra is that it allows maximal correction of the deformity and realignment of the spine. Most single hemivertebrae, however, do not cause significant spinal imbalance when seen at an early stage. Most surgeons, therefore, use the simpler combined anterior and posterior convex growth arrest procedure, which is a less risky operation, but it has the relative disadvantage of less predictable correction that depends on continuing growth on the concavity of the curve. If there is a more severe deformity, excision of the hemivertebra and realignment of the spine can be a more beneficial, although more hazardous, procedure.

The hemivertebra is excised in two stages. The spine is approached both anteriorly and posteriorly in a manner similar to that for a convex growth arrest procedure. In the first stage, the body of the hemivertebra and the anterior part of the pedicle are removed along with the adjacent discs and vertebral end plates, and the dura is visualized. In the second stage of the procedure, the spine is exposed posteriorly, and the posterior elements of the hemivertebra are removed, along with the transverse process and posterior part of the pedicle. This is a technically demanding procedure with a risk for direct injury to the spinal cord and bleeding from the epidural veins (26). It has also been suggested that the dissection necessary to resect the hemivertebra may interfere with the segmental blood supply to the spinal cord (32). To prevent possible ischemic neurologic complications, some surgeons have advocated that the two stages be separated by 10 days to allow time for the vasculature to recover (33,36,64). However, it has now been established that successful results can be achieved when both procedures are performed under the same anesthetic (4,10).

After the hemivertebra has been excised, the scoliosis can be corrected by closing the wedge osteotomy. During this procedure, the spine remains relatively stable because the ligaments have been maintained on the concavity and act as a stabilizing hinge as the wedge is closed. However, correction may be difficult to obtain in the thoracic region because of the supporting rib cage. Correction is easier and safer in the more mobile lumbar spine, where the cauda equina is also more resilient. Spinal compression instrumentation applied to the convexity of the curve above and below the excised hemivertebra may be used posteriorly to close the wedge osteotomy (4,26). This requires strong bone to seat the hooks. Care must be taken not to compress the emerging nerve root as the osteotomy is closed, especially at the lumbosacral junction. It may be difficult or dangerous to apply this type of instrumentation to very small children. In these situations, correction may be easier and safer to obtain by the postoperative application of a double-pantaloon spica cast; this may be wedged at a later stage to obtain further correction (10). Regardless of the method of correction, the patient must wear a spica cast for 3 months after the surgery. This should be followed by 3 months in a brace until the osteotomy is soundly healed.

The objective of excising the hemivertebra is to achieve a balanced spine and prevent curve progression. The operation should be performed early while the scoliosis is still relatively mobile and before the development of secondary structural changes in the curve. The best long-term results after resection of a hemivertebra are achieved if the scoliosis can be nearly completely corrected. It is usually possible to obtain up to 30 degrees of correction of lumbar curves. Larger curves, especially those that have already developed secondary structural changes or fixed compensatory curves, do not fully correct and often continue to deteriorate. This may be partially prevented by extending the surgery to include an anterior and posterior convex growth arrest of the disc spaces one level above and below the excised hemivertebra. Failure to fuse the whole length of the scoliosis often leads to a slow progressive loss of correction, which necessitates further posterior surgery to extend the fusion when the child is older.

In my opinion, the best indication for hemivertebra excision is its occurrence at the lumbosacral junction, where it causes an oblique take-off of the lumbar spine and a major spinal imbalance. The only way of realigning the trunk is by excising the hemivertebra and closing the osteotomy (57). This is successful only at a relatively early stage before the secondary thoracolumbar compensatory curve becomes fixed.

Prophylactic Early Spine Arthrodesis In Situ

Arthrodesis in situ is the optimal form of early prophylactic surgical treatment for a congenital scoliosis caused by a unilateral failure of vertebral segmentation when seen at an early stage before there is significant deformity. A convex growth arrest procedure would not correct this type of deformity because there is no growth potential in the unsegmented bar on the concavity of the curve. These anomalies produce very rigid deformities with a known potential for severe progression. After significant scoliosis has developed, it can be corrected only by a spinal osteotomy, which can be a difficult and hazardous procedure. The object of an early spine arthrodesis is to stabilize the curve at an early stage by creating a solid thick fusion that will stop the unbalanced growth of the spine. The arthrodesis should be performed as soon as the anomaly is recognized, and the best results are achieved when this is carried out before the age of 2 years (47,66). The argument that an early spine fusion will stunt the growth of the spine is of no relevance with this type of congenital scoliosis. The abnormal segment is not contributing to vertical height, and it is only making the spine more crooked. It is much better to achieve a short, relatively straight spine that is balanced than a spine that is even shorter because of the severe curvature.

The congenital scoliosis contains not only the unilateral unsegmented segment but also a number of relatively normal vertebrae at the upper and lower ends that are also tilted into the curve. Failure to include all of these vertebrae in the fusion results in continued progression of the deformity (47). With this type of congenital scoliosis, the surgeon is unlikely to regret operating too early or fusing too many vertebrae but will always regret delaying surgery or having fused too few vertebrae.

Loss of correction after an early posterior spinal fusion in infantile and juvenile idiopathic scoliosis has been attributed to either a weak fusion mass or increasing rotation of the spine resulting from the crankshaft effect produced by continuing unbalanced anterior growth of the spine in the presence of the posterior tether caused by the fusion (16,24). This phenomenon, however, does not usually occur to a great extent in congenital scoliosis because the anterior growth plates in the anomalous segment are also frequently abnormal. A posterior arthrodesis alone can produce an acceptable result in congenital scoliosis, provided it results in a strong, thick fusion capable of overcoming the anterior growth of the spine (58). The crankshaft effect is seen only in those patients who already have marked vertebral rotation as part of the deformity (40).

In my experience, it is usually advisable to perform a single-stage combined anterior and posterior spine arthrodesis if there is a severe growth imbalance, such as that produced by a unilateral unsegmented bar with contralateral hemivertebra (47). This pro-

cedure has the advantage of directly overcoming any possible crankshaft effect and producing a more solid stable fusion. The rib excised at the time of the thoracotomy provides a good source of autogenous bone graft, which may not be available from the iliac crest in these very young children. Postoperatively, a spinal jacket is applied for 6 months to allow the fusion to heal.

The secondary structural thoracolumbar scoliosis, which can develop below congenital thoracic scoliosis with its apex at T5, T6, or T7, also requires prophylactic treatment. This secondary deformity is not controlled by an early fusion of the primary congenital scoliosis. Bracing may control the secondary curve and postpone extending the fusion to the lower lumbar region, especially if many years of further growth are anticipated. Alternatively, it is possible at the time of the posterior arthrodesis of the congenital curve to apply pediatric spine instrumentation across both curves without fusing the secondary curve. Subsequent serial extension of the instrumentation allows additional longitudinal growth in the unfused thoracolumbar curve before extending the fusion when the child is older.

Correction and Posterior Spinal Arthrodesis

Attempted correction of the deformity and posterior spinal arthrodesis is the usual surgical procedure for an older child with a moderately severe congenital curve that is still relatively flexible (Fig. 13). The object of surgery is to achieve overall balance of the spine rather than excessive correction of the congenital curve. The posterior arthrodesis is performed over the whole length of the deformity from the upper to the lower neutral vertebrae and not just at the anomalous segment. Although it is not usually possible to obtain correction at the site of the anomalous vertebrae, moderate correction may be achieved at the relatively normal vertebral levels that lie above and below this area and are still within the scoliosis. Correction may be attempted either intraoperatively by the insertion of instrumentation at the time of the posterior spinal arthrodesis or postoperatively by the application of a spinal jacket.

An MRI scan is essential in all patients before intraoperative correction of the deformity is attempted. This may reveal the presence of an intraspinal anomaly, such as a diastematomyelia, that could be tethering the cord. If this is not removed, the patient could develop serious neurologic complications if a distraction force is applied to the spine to correct the deformity (Fig. 13C). Because of the complexity of the two operative procedures, it is best to have the intraspinal anomaly removed during a separate neurosurgical procedure performed several weeks before the attempted correction of the spinal deformity and posterior arthrodesis.

The safest method of correcting the deformity is to apply a spinal jacket 5 days after the posterior spinal arthrodesis. The patient is awake during this procedure, and the jacket is applied on a traction frame. With this technique, there is negligible risk for neurologic complications. The disadvantages are that it produces relatively little correction, and the patient has to wear a cumbersome spinal jacket extending from the neck to the pelvis for 6 months until the fusion is solid. This method is best applied to young children whose bones are too soft or underdeveloped to allow the effective application of internal fixation.

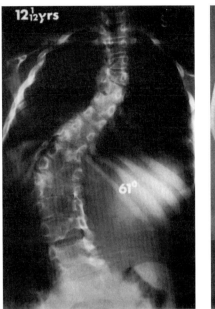
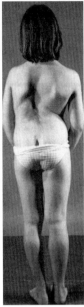
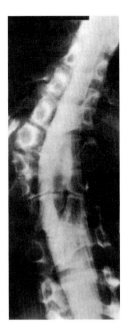
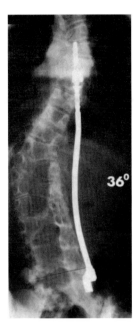
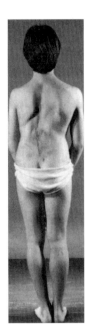

A,B,C

D,E

FIGURE 13. A: A girl aged 12 years, 1 month with a 61-degree thoracolumbar scoliosis due to complex multiple vertebral anomalies. The spinal radiograph also shows a spina bifida occulta affecting a number of adjacent vertebrae in the thoracolumbar region, associated with widening of the interpedicular distance and narrowing of the disc spaces. **B:** The patient had a hairy patch at the thoracolumbar junction, and there was slight shortening and hypoplasia of the left leg. **C:** A myelogram shows a diastematomyelia at the thoracolumbar junction. **D:** The diastematomyelia was excised, and the scoliosis was corrected to 36 degrees with Harrington instrumentation. **E:** At the age of 15 years, there is a solid fusion with no loss in correction and a good cosmetic result.

The use of posterior spinal instrumentation to correct a congenital scoliosis at the time of the spinal arthrodesis has several advantages: It achieves moderately better correction and reduces the incidence of pseudarthrosis when compared with a posterior spinal fusion in a spinal jacket alone (21,69). Spinal instrumentation does, however, carry a greater risk for neurologic complications because of the effect of distraction on the spinal cord while the patient is anesthetized. Of the various types of scoliosis, the congenital variety carries the highest risk for neurologic complications after intraoperative correction. Arthrodesis and instrumentation without correction, other than that achieved passively while the patient is lying on the operating table, should be used if there is any suspicion of an intraspinal anomaly, even if it has been removed before the surgery. The instrumentation should be used only as an internal strut to support the spine and aid the development of a solid fusion (42).

Despite the risks, spinal instrumentation is frequently used to obtain moderate correction in patients with congenital scoliosis, but specific measures must be taken during the surgery to detect the possible development of neurologic complications. Spinal cord monitoring using evoked potentials is essential, but unfortunately it is not completely reliable (17). The wake-up test (60) or the ankle clonus test (28) should be performed immediately after correction of the deformity. These tests, however, monitor only the current neurologic status, and it is possible for neurologic abnormalities to develop at a later stage in the operative procedure (22,37).

In the past, Harrington instrumentation has been used most frequently in the treatment of congenital scoliosis (21,69). Newer forms of segmental spinal instrumentation using multiple hooks, pedicle screws, or sublaminar wires are more controversial in their application. Congenital abnormalities of the laminae may make it difficult to apply these types of instrumentation. It may also be dangerous to pass wires or hooks into the spinal canal at the site of the anomalous segment, which could be congenitally narrowed or contain an abnormal spinal cord. Regardless of the method of instrumentation, it is important to remember that the main objective is to achieve trunk balance rather than excessive correction of the scoliosis, which may be dangerous. If there is any suspicion that a neurologic deficit may have developed during the surgery, the spinal instrumentation should be removed immediately and the patient treated postoperatively in a plaster jacket.

Anterior and Posterior Spinal Osteotomy, Vertebrectomy, Correction, and Arthrodesis

A spinal osteotomy is a major salvage procedure that theoretically should never be necessary in congenital scoliosis. Its use is indicative of a failure to apply the basic principles of early diagnosis, anticipation, and prevention of increasing deformity. Patients who require a spinal osteotomy would have been much better treated at an earlier stage by simpler surgical procedures.

The indication for a spinal osteotomy is a severe rigid deformity with either fixed pelvic obliquity or marked decompensation of the upper trunk relative to the pelvis (Fig. 14). These

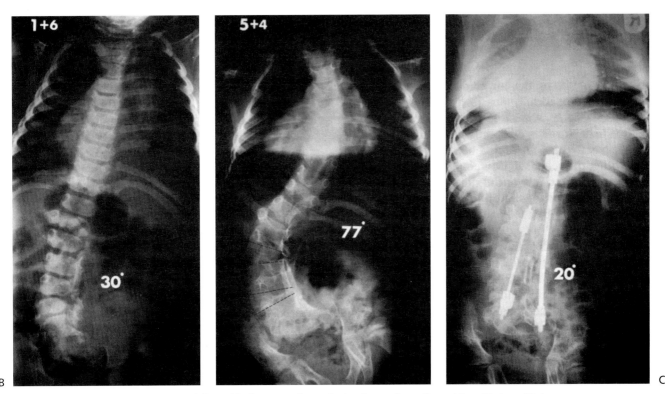

A,B   C

FIGURE 14. **A:** An infant girl who was radiographed at 1 year, 6 months and found to have 30-degree left lumbar scoliosis due to a unilateral unsegmented bar on the right extending from L4 to the sacrum, with a contralateral hemivertebra at L6. No treatment was given. **B:** By the age of 5 years, 4 months, the scoliosis had increased to 77 degrees, resulting in a severe rigid deformity with translocation of the trunk and marked pelvic obliquity. **C:** Two-stage anterior and posterior spinal osteotomies were performed at two levels in the lumbar region, and the scoliosis was corrected to 20 degrees with posterior spinal instrumentation.

severe spinal deformities are usually caused by a unilateral unsegmented bar with or without contralateral hemivertebrae.

The object of the surgery is to osteotomize the spine both anteriorly and posteriorly to create mobility, which will allow correction and enable the head and upper trunk to be balanced over a level pelvis. This is a technically demanding procedure with a significant neurologic risk and should be performed only by an experienced spinal surgeon after full consultation with the patient or parents and only if there are no alternatives.

The surgery can be performed as a single combined procedure or in two stages separated by 5 to 7 days. In the first stage, the spine is exposed anteriorly through a thoracotomy or a thoracoabdominal retroperitoneal approach, depending on the site of the vertebral anomalies. The intervertebral discs and their associated end plates are excised over the whole length of the deformity. The unsegmented bar on the concavity is then osteotomized through the sites of the excised discs. Simply osteotomizing the unsegmented bar will not allow the spine to grow straight because there is no growth potential on that side of the curve. To obtain significant correction, it may also be necessary to perform a wedge resection of a vertebral body at the apex of the curve, with the base of the wedge on the convexity and tapered toward the concavity. This is a difficult and dangerous procedure that is often associated with significant blood loss from the raw bony surfaces and epidural veins.

In the second stage of the procedure, the whole length of the congenital scoliosis is exposed posteriorly. The sites of the anterior osteotomies are identified, and posterior osteotomies are performed at the same levels by removing part of the lamina and facet joints on the convexity and dividing the unsegmented bar on the concavity. If an anterior vertebrectomy has been performed at the apex of the curve, it will be necessary to carry out a posterior wedge osteotomy at the same level by excising the lamina and removing the pedicle and transverse process on the convexity. The safest and best site for a vertebrectomy is in the lumbar region, where it is easier to close the wedge because there is no interference from the rib cage and the cauda equina is more resilient than the spinal cord.

After the anterior and posterior osteotomies have been performed, correction is obtained by applying posterior compression instrumentation to the convexity to close the wedge osteotomies. This shortens the spinal column and relaxes the neural structures, decreasing the risk for complications as well as straightening the scoliosis and balancing the spine (36). Only after this has been achieved is it safe to apply instrumentation to the concavity—not to achieve further correction but to act as a supporting strut and to maintain correction over the whole length of the deformity. A posterior spinal arthrodesis is performed over the entire length of the scoliosis extending from the upper to the lower neutral vertebrae and not just at the site of the osteotomy. Postoperatively, a plaster jacket or spica is applied to help stabilize the spine until the fusion is solid.

SUMMARY

Congenital scoliosis is a potentially serious condition that can result in an extreme deformity with malalignment of the body. Ideally, this type of scoliosis should be diagnosed at an early stage when it is possible to anticipate the prognosis based on the amount of spinal growth remaining, the type and site of the vertebral anomalies, and the degree of growth imbalance they produce. Deterioration of the deformity must always be prevented. Scoliosis that is at risk for progression requires immediate prophylactic surgical treatment, no matter how young the patient. It is much better to carry out a relatively simple operation to balance the growth of the spine at an early stage than to wait and perform a dangerous surgical salvage procedure when the deformity is severe.

REFERENCES

1. Andrew T, Piggott H (1985): Growth arrest for progressive scoliosis: combined anterior and posterior fusion of the convexity. *J Bone Joint Surg Br* 67:193–197.
2. Arkin AM (1953): Conservative management of scoliosis. *Clin Orthop* 1:99–108.
3. Beals RK, Robbins JR, Rolfe B (1993): Anomalies associated with vertebral malformations. *Spine* 18:1329–1332.
4. Bergoin M, Bollini G, Taibi L, et al. (1986): Excision of hemivertebrae in children with congenital scoliosis. *Ital J Orthop Traumatol* 12:179–184.
5. Bick EM, Copel JW (1950): Longitudinal growth of the human vertebra: a contribution to human osteogeny. *J Bone Joint Surg Am* 32:803–814.
6. Billing EL (1955): Congenital scoliosis: an analytical study of its natural history. *J Bone Joint Surg Am* 37:404–405.
7. Blake NS, Lynch AS, Dowling FE (1986): Spinal cord abnormalities in congenital scoliosis. *Ann Radiol* 29:377–379.
8. Blount WP (1960): *Congenital scoliosis transactions.* 8th Congres International Societe de Chirurgia Orthopedique et Traumatologic, New York, Sept. 4–9. Bruscelles Impremerre des Sciences, pp. 748–762.
9. Bradford DS (1982): Partial epiphyseal arrest and supplemental fixation for progressive correction of congenital spine deformity. *J Bone Joint Surg Am* 64:610–614.
10. Bradford DS, Boachie-Adjei O (1990): One-stage anterior and posterior hemivertebral resection and arthrodesis. *J Bone Joint Surg Am* 72:536–540.
11. Bradford DS, Heithoff KB, Cohen M (1991): Intraspinal abnormalities and congenital spine deformities: a radiographic and MRI study. *J Pediatr Orthop* 11:36–41.
12. Compere EL (1932): Excision of hemivertebrae for correction of congenital scoliosis: report of 2 cases. *J Bone Joint Surg* 14:555–562.
13. Davies G, Reid L (1971): Effect of scoliosis on growth of alveoli and pulmonary arteries and right ventricle. *Arch Dis Child* 46:623–632.
14. Day GA, Upadhyay SS, No EKW, et al. (1994): Pulmonary functions in congenital scoliosis. *Spine* 19:1027–1031.
15. Drvac DM, Ruderman RJ, Coonrad RW, et al. (1987): Congenital scoliosis and urinary tract abnormalities. *J Pediatr Orthop* 7:441–443.
16. Dubousset J, Herring JA, Shufflebarger H (1989): The crankshaft phenomenon. *J Pediatr Orthop* 9:541–550.
17. Forbes HJ, Allen PW, Waller CS, et al. (1991): Spinal cord monitoring in scoliosis surgery: experience with 1168 cases. *J Bone Joint Surg Br* 73:487–491.
18. Goldberg C, Fenton G, Blake NS (1984): Diastematomyelia: a critical review of the natural history of treatment. *Spine* 9:367–372.
19. Goldenhar M (1952): Associations malformations de L'oeil et de L'oreille, en particuliar le syndrome dermoide epibullaire: appendices auriculaires-fistula auris congenita et ses relations avex la dysostose mandibulo faciale. *J Genet Hum* 1:243–282.
20. Gorlin RJ, Kenneth LJ, Jacobsen U, et al. (1973): Oculo auricular vertebral dysplasia. *J Pediatr* 63:991–999.
21. Hall JE, Herndon WA, Levine CR (1981): Surgical treatment of congenital scoliosis with or without Harrington instrumentation. *J Bone Joint Surg Am* 63:608–619.
22. Hall JE, Levine CR, Sudhir KG (1978): Intraoperative awakening to monitor spinal cord function during Harrington instrumentation and spine fusion. *J Bone Joint Surg Am* 60:533–536.
23. Hattaway GL (1977): Congenital scoliosis in one of monozygotic twins: a case report. *J Bone Joint Surg Am* 59:837–838.
24. Hefti FL, McMaster MJ (1983). The effect of the adolescent growth spurt on early posterior fusion in infantile and juvenile idiopathic scoliosis. *J Bone Joint Surg Br* 65:247–254.
25. Hensinger R, Lang JE, MacEwen GD (1974): Klippel-Feil syndrome: a constellation of associated anomalies. *J Bone Joint Surg Am* 56:1246–1253.
26. Holte DC, Winter RB, Lonstein JE, et al. (1995): Excision of hemivertebrae and wedge resection in the treatment of congenital scoliosis. *J Bone Joint Surg Am* 77:159–171.
27. Hood RW, Riseborough E, Hehme A, et al. (1980): Diastematomyelia and structural spinal deformities. *J Bone Joint Surg Am* 62:520–528.
28. Hoppenfield S, Gross A, Andrews C, et al. (1997): The ankle clonus test for assessment of the integrity of the spinal cord during operations for scoliosis. *J Bone Joint Surg Am* 79:208–212.
29. James CCM, Lassman LP (1970): Diastematomyelia and the tight filum terminale. *J Neurol Sci* 10:193–196.
30. Jarcho S, Levin PM (1938): Hereditary malformations of the vertebral bodies. *Bull Johns Hopkins Hosp* 62:216–226.
31. Keller PM, Lindseth RE, De Rosa GP (1994): Progressive congenital scoliosis treatment using a transpedicular anterior and posterior convex hemiepiphysiodesis and hemiarthrodesis: a preliminary report. *Spine* 19:1933–1939.
32. Keim HA, Hilal SK (1971): Spinal angiography in scoliosis patients. *J Bone Joint Surg Am* 53:904–912.
33. King JD, Lowery MD (1991): Results of lumbar hemivertebral excision for congenital scoliosis. *Spine* 16:7, 778–782.
34. King AG, MacEwen GD, Bose WJ (1992): Transpedicular convex anterior hemiepiphysiodesis and posterior arthrodesis for progressive congenital scoliosis. *Spine* 17:291–294.
35. Kuhns JG, Hormell RS (1952): Management of congenital scoliosis. *Arch Surg* 65:250–263.
36. Leatherman KD, Dickson RA (1979): Two-stage corrective surgery for congenital deformities of the spine. *J Bone Joint Surg Br* 61:324–328.
37. Letts RM, Hollenberg C (1977): Delayed paresis following spinal fusion with Harrington instrumentation. *Clin Orthop* 125:45–48.
38. Loder RT, Hernandez MJ, Lerner AL, et al. (1998): The induction of congenital spinal deformities in mice by maternal carbon monoxide exposure. Paper presented at Scoliosis Research Society Meeting, New York, September 1998.
39. Loder RT, Urquhart A, Steen H, et al. (1995): Variability in Cobb angle measurements in children with congenital scoliosis. *J Bone Joint Surg Br* 77:768–770.
40. Lopez-Sosa FH, Guille JT, Bowen JR (1993): Curve progression and spinal rotation in congenital scoliosis. *Orthop Trans* 17:382.
41. MacEwen GD, Conway JT, Miller WT (1968): Congenital scoliosis with a unilateral bar. *Radiology* 90:711–715.
42. MacEwen GD, Bunnell WP, Sriram K (1975): Acute neurological complications in the treatment of scoliosis: a report of the Scoliosis Research Society. *J Bone Joint Surg Am* 57:404–408.
43. MacEwen GD, Winter RB, Hardy JH (1972): Evaluation of kidney anomalies in congenital scoliosis. *J Bone Joint Surg Am* 54:1341–1454.
44. McMaster MJ, Ohtsuka K (1982): The natural history of congenital scoliosis: a study of 251 patients. *J Bone Joint Surg Am* 64:1128–1147.

45. McMaster MJ (1984): Occult intraspinal anomalies and congenital scoliosis. *J Bone Joint Surg Am* 66:588–601.
46. McMaster MJ, David CV (1986): Hemivertebra as a cause of scoliosis. *J Bone Joint Surg Br* 68:588–595.
47. McMaster MJ (1998): Congenital scoliosis caused by a unilateral failure of vertebral segmentation with contralateral hemivertebrae. *Spine* 23:998–1005.
48. McMaster MJ, Singh H (1999): The natural history of congenital kyphosis and kyphoscoliosis. A study of one hundred and twelve patients. *J Bone Joint Surg Am* 81:1367–1383.
49. Miller A, Guille JT, Bowen JR (1993): Evaluation and treatment of diastematomyelia. *J Bone Joint Surg Am* 75:1308–1317.
50. Nasca RJ, Stelling FH, Steel HH (1975): Progression of congenital scoliosis due to hemivertebrae and hemivertebrae with bars. *J Bone Joint Surg Am* 57:456–466.
51. Peterson HA, Peterson LF (1967): Hemivertebrae in identical twins with dissimilar spinal columns. *J Bone Joint Surg Am* 49:938–942.
52. Pool RD (1986): Congenital scoliosis in monozygotic twins. Genetically determined or acquired in utero? *J Bone Joint Surg Br* 68:194–196.
53. Reckles LH, Peterson HA, Bianco AJ, et al. (1975): The association of scoliosis and congenital heart defects. *J Bone Joint Surg Am* 57:449–455.
54. Rivard CH, Duhaime M, Labelle P, et al. (1982): Perturbation of cell proliferation in mouse embryo after treatment of the mouse mother with hypobaric hypoxia as teratogenic agent producing congenital vertebral malformations. *Orthop Trans* 6:14.
55. Roberts AP, Connor AN, Tolmie JL, et al. (1988): Spondylothoracic and spondylocostal dysostosis: hereditary forms of spinal deformity. *J Bone Joint Surg Br* 70:123–126.
56. Royle ND (1928): Operative removal of an accessory vertebra. *Med J Aust* 1:467–468.
57. Slabaugh P, Winter R, Lonstein J, et al. (1980): Lumbosacral hemivertebrae: a review of 24 patients with resection in eight. *Spine* 5:234–244.
58. Terek RM, Wehner J, Lubicky JP (1991): Crankshaft phenomenon and congenital scoliosis: a preliminary report. *J Pediatr Orthop* 11:527–532.
59. Thompson AG, Marks DS, Sayampanathan SRE, et al. (1995): Long-term results of combined anterior and posterior convex epiphysiodesis for congenital scoliosis due to hemivertebrae. *Spine* 20:1380–1385.
60. Vauzelle C, Stragnara P, Jouvinroux P (1973): Functional monitoring of spinal cord activity during spinal surgery. *Clin Orthop* 93:173–178.
61. Von Lackum WH, Smith A de F, Wylie R (1954): Stapling vertebral bodies in congenital scoliosis. *J Bone Joint Surg Am* 36:342–347.
62. Wiles P (1951): Resection of dorsal vertebrae in congenital scoliosis. *J Bone Joint Surg Am* 33:151–154.
63. Winter RB (1981): Convex anterior and posterior hemi-arthrodesis and epiphyseodesis in young children with progressive congenital scoliosis. *J Pediatr Orthop* 1:361–366.
64. Winter RB (1983): Congenital deformities of the spine. New York: Thieme-Stratton.
65. Winter RB, Haven JJ, Moe JH, et al. (1974): Diastematomyelia and congenital spine deformities. *J Bone Joint Surg Am* 56:27–39.
66. Winter RB, Moe JH (1982): The results of spinal arthrodesis for congenital spine deformity in patients younger than 5 years old. *J Bone Joint Surg Am* 64:419–432.
67. Winter RB, Moe JH, MacEwen GD, et al. (1976): The Milwaukee brace in the non-operative treatment of congenital scoliosis. *Spine* 1:85–96.
68. Winter RB, Moe JH, Eilers VE (1968): Congenital scoliosis: a study of 234 patients treated and untreated. *J Bone Joint Surg Am* 50:1–47.
69. Winter RB, Moe JH, Lonstein JE (1984): Posterior spinal arthrodesis for congenital scoliosis: an analysis of 290 patients 5 to 19 years old. *J Bone Joint Surg Am* 66:1188–1197.
70. Winter RB, Moe JH, Lonstein JE (1984): The incidence of Klippel-Feil syndrome in patients with congenital scoliosis and kyphosis. *Spine* 9:363–366.
71. Winter RB, Lonstein JE, Davis F, et al. (1988): Convex growth arrest for progressive congenital scoliosis due to hemivertebrae. *J Pediatr Orthop* 8:633–638.
72. Winter RB, Lonstein JE, Denis F, et al. (1992): Prevalence of spinal canal or cord abnormalities in idiopathic, congenital and neuromuscular scoliosis. *Orthop Trans* 16:135.
73. Wynne-Davies R (1975): Congenital vertebral anomalies: etiology and relationship to spina bifida cystica. *J Med Genet* 12:280–288.

CONGENITAL KYPHOSIS AND LORDOSIS

JEAN DUBOUSSET

Congenital deformities in the sagittal plane result from congenital vertebral anomalies, leading to immediate deformities (e.g., when one element is missing) or progressive deformities (e.g., when the normal balance of growth potential of the various segments of the spine is more or less altered depending on the nature of congenital defect).

A sagittal plane abnormality means that the major deformity will be either an increase of the normal sagittal alignment of the affected segment of the spine or a decrease. Most of the time the deformity is not purely sagittal but also involves the coronal plane to some degree; thus, in kyphoscoliosis or lordoscoliosis the major deformity is in the sagittal plane. The deformity must be viewed in a spacial fashion for pure congenital kyphosis or lordosis as well as for the scoliosis group (kyphoscoliosis or lordoscoliosis). This is logical from the anatomical, mechanical, clinical, and surgical viewpoints because all treatment will be directed to the prevention and alleviation of any spinal cord and spinal canal compromise.

PATHOLOGIC ANATOMY, MECHANISM, AND SPONTANEOUS EVOLUTION

The embryologic (9–11) and anatomical relationships for congenital anomalies of the spine indicate that there is a permanent association between osteoarticular elements that are more or less abnormal at the various levels of the vertebra (e.g., disc, pedicles, ligaments, bodies) and the nervous elements (e.g., spinal cord, meninges). The nervous system may be absolutely normal or congenitally disordered (e.g., dysraphism, lipoma).

CARTILAGINOUS, BONY, JOINT, AND LIGAMENT ANOMALIES

Bone and joint anomalies result from an embryologic defect at the time of vertebral formation or segmentation or both. Tondury (10), Rivard et al. (9), and Watanabe (11) demonstrated

J. Dubousset: Hôpital Saint Vincent de Paul, Université René Descartes, Paris, France.

(either in experimental work or correlation with human embryonic studies) that vertebral malformations are acquired at the mesenchymal phase of development between the twentieth and thirtieth day of embryonic life, most of the time secondary to dysfunction of notochord cells. Most nervous system malformation also develops during this time frame of embryonic life, in addition to other anomalies, such as cardiac or urinary. After birth, the analysis of these bone and joint defects can be done in conjunction with an analysis of the central nervous system anomalies (2).

Computed tomography (CT) and magnetic resonance imaging (MRI), in addition to the clinical examination and plain frontal and sagittal radiography, allow one to study the deformity in three dimensions, establishing the balance for stability, spinal growth potential, and potential danger to the nervous structures so well seen on MRI.

However, even today (Fig. 1) we cannot predict the growth potential of an area based on the clear space (on radiograph) or dark space (on MRI sequences). In fact, we may be viewing stable or unstable fibrous tissue without the potential to form bone, or ossifying fibrocartilage without growth potential, or growing cartilage. Most of the time it is necessary to observe and follow the patient over time to determine if an anomaly is getting worse.

CONGENITAL KYPHOSIS

Congenital kyphosis may be attributed to three causes: failure of formation, failure of segmentation, and rotatory dislocation of the spine.

Failure of Formation

Failure of formation leads to a total or partial absence of one or more vertebral bodies, and the abnormalities of the posterior arch determine the degree of stability of the spine (Fig. 2).

The analysis must consider two mains points:

1. *Location of the malformation.* Bodies, pedicles, and posterior arch may each be absent, totally or partially and symmetrically or asymmetrically.
2. *Alignment of the canal,* particularly at the level of the posterior

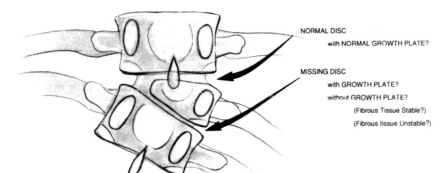

NORMAL DISC
with NORMAL GROWTH PLATE?

MISSING DISC
with GROWTH PLATE?
without GROWTH PLATE?
(Fibrous Tissue Stable?)
(Fibrous tissue Unstable?)

FIGURE 1. Congenital kyphosis or kyphoscoliosis factor for progression. Prognostic value of the "clear space."

wall of the bodies in the sagittal plane. A well-aligned canal may exist with an acute kyphosis or a dislocated canal may exist when the alignment of vertebral bodies results in an offset or sudden loss of continuity.

Three types of failure of formation can be found:

1. *Partial failure of formation with a well-aligned canal.* Pure anterior and symmetrical failure is rare and results in an angular kyphosis. The posterior arch is strong, and normal kyphosis in such a condition progresses slowly. It is difficult to determine the exact value and histologic nature of this anterior "empty space." Is it cartilaginous, nuclear, or fibrous tissue?

The differential growth potential results in a progressive kyphosis and spinal cord tethering. This type of deformity may

also be seen in the case of binuclear or butterfly symmetrical bodies. These cases may progress 5 degrees to 7 degrees per year.

If the failure of formation is anterolateral, as in the posterolateral hemivertebra, the bending of the canal occurs at only one level. This leads to kyphoscoliosis, with a more or less normal posterior arch. The more acute the kyphosis, the greater the risk to the spinal cord even if the cord is always located on the concave side. If there is a fused hemivertebra, there is little or no progression of the kyphoscoliosis; but if the hemivertebra is "free," meaning movement of the half vertebral plateau on each side above and below the normal half disc space, a progression of 3 degrees to 5 degrees per year is anticipated in the sagittal as well as the coronal plane (1).

This abnormality progresses at an increased rate once the pubertal growth spurt starts. If the defect is an asymmetrical binuclear vertebra, the pedicles may be absent, and more than 10 degrees progression may occur in a year. This condition exists mostly in the thoracic or thoracolumbar region and frequently leads to a progressively increasing neurologic deficit.

2. *Partial failure of formation with a dislocated canal* (Fig. 3B). This condition was described in 1973 using the term "congenital

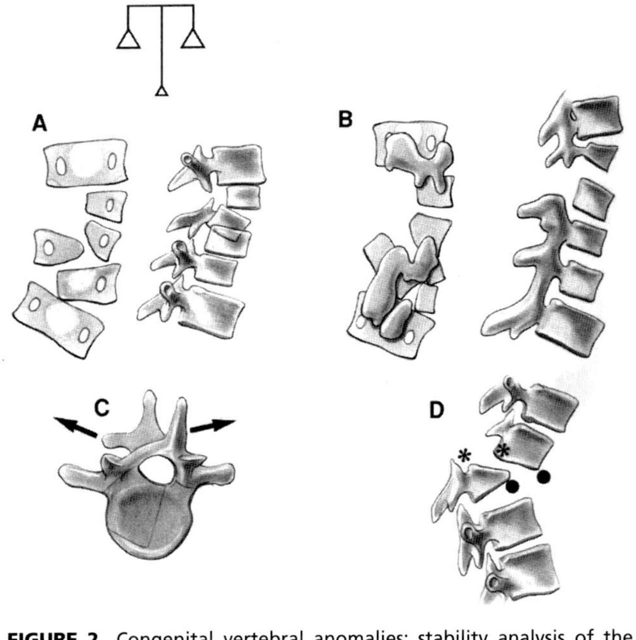

FIGURE 2. Congenital vertebral anomalies: stability analysis of the three-dimensional studies in the coronal, sagittal, and horizontal planes. *A,* Anterior column disc space and bodies. *B,* Posterior bolt elements—pedicles; joints; lamina; transverse and spinous processes; ligaments. *C,* Instability on the horizontal plane. *D,* An example of a congenitally dislocated spine.

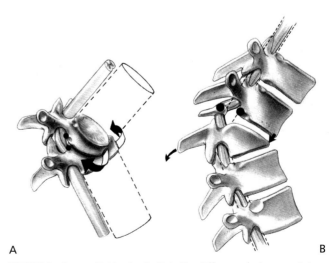

FIGURE 3. Congenital kyphosis. Note the difference between rotatory dislocation of the spine with a continuous canal **(A)** and congenital dislocated spine **(B).**

dislocation of the spine" (5). Here the offset is clear, and the neurologic risk for the spinal cord is greater. It is also more dramatic because the condition (neurologic injury) can occur suddenly (e.g., as the result of a minor trauma). If the offset is clear on the sagittal radiograph, it can also frequently be seen in the coronal plane and almost always has a bayonet-type appearance. Frequently there is a narrowing of the right and left pedicles and some coronal and horizontal stenosis of the spinal canal.

With this malformation there is always a defect of the posterior arch, which explains the often considerable instability, but the defect is not always demonstrated by the dynamic radiographs. This is why we call the instability "potential," that is, because the defect is revealed only as the result of a minor or major trauma. Progression of such an unstable kyphotic spine is always observed (e.g., 45 degrees at age 1 year to 135 degrees at age 15 years). During anterior surgery we have sometimes seen "neojoints" with fluid between the anterior part of the two adjacent bodies, demonstrating real mobility. The normal or dysplastic spinal cord often escapes from the normal spinal canal above and courses directly under the skin to enter the spinal canal below the offset. The cord can be severed accidentally by too vigorous a posterior approach because the skin covering it may be completely normal or may have a mild "angioma aspect," which might be indicative of dysraphism or a mild lipoma.

But the big danger is instability where a minor trauma to a normal spinal cord can lead to a nonreversible, acute paraplegia, in contrast to those cases in which the spinal cord is progressively stretched.

Frequently, in this condition of "dislocated congenital spine" there is an associated dysraphic cord. Therefore, it is important to know the neurologic status at birth. We have seen completely normal patients as well as a patient in whom the only manifestation of a dysraphic condition was a paralytic club foot and a neurogenic bladder. We also have a patient manifesting complete congenital paraplegia, as is seen in some cases of lumbar agenesis. Generally, the location of the dislocated spine is thoracolumbar. That is why we describe this type of congenital kyphosis as a partial form of suspended lumbar agenesis.

The prenatal diagnosis can be made with ultrasonography, but the prognosis for normal or automatic motion of the lower limbs is guarded.

3. *Total failure of formation of the vertebral bodies* (1) results in the agenesis of one, two, three, or more vertebral bodies, with or without agenesis of their posterior arches. This occurs more frequently at the lumbar spine level. In such patients, there is almost always a congenital paraplegia and very often an increased motion at the kyphosis between the two parts of the spine. The hips may be normal, or subluxated, or dislocated and stiff in extension, in such cases, all mobility of the trunk and flexion-extension of the lower limbs occurs at the site of agenesis.

There is often a complete motor spastic or flaccid paraplegia, with urinary problems and generally with normal sensation of the skin at the level of the lower limbs. We have observed a wide variety of findings, from dislocated spine, to spinal canal stenosis, to partial or total lumbar agenesis with sacrum, to partial or total agenesis of the sacrum and caudal regression syndrome.

Failure of Segmentation

Anterior or Anterolateral Typical Bar

The defect of anterior or anterolateral typical bar involves one or multiple levels (Fig. 4). When strictly anteriorly located, a pure kyphosis results. When anterolaterally located, a kyphoscoliosis results from the posterior elements that continue to grow in the face of the anterior elements having no growth potential. The resulting kyphosis generally has a smooth contour with no sharp angles and thus imposes minimal neurologic risk.

Delayed Fusion Anterior Bar

There is a special type of defect of segmentation that may not be evident at first glance but in which a progressive ossification of a part of or of a complete disc space develops slowly (7). It is often necessary to distinguish this type of defect from Scheuermann kyphosis, which has a similar appearance clinically and radiographically; however, with growth and maturation the spontaneous anterior fusion becomes evident. The fusion generally begins at age 8 to 10 years, but it is unpredictable and sometimes ossification is completed only when growth is completed. A histologic specimen of such a defect looks like bipolar cartilage progressively ossifying without any nucleus pulposus disc material in between. The angulation may be considerable, and we have one patient progressing from 20 degrees at age 3 years to 135 degrees at the end of puberty. The hereditary factor in these cases is evident because among the 10 cases of this progressive defect that we have reported, 7 cases involved only two families (one family in four generations and one family with three cases in two generations).

Rotatory Dislocation of the Spine

Rotatory dislocation of the spine (6) (Fig. 3A) is a mechanical deformity caused by the sudden presence of a kyphotic zone between two areas of scoliosis, each of them often in lordosis and rotating in opposite directions. In the first report (1973) of this deformity, we described three patients (one with neurofibromatosis, one with chondrodystrophy, and one with congenital vertebral anomalies). The deformity may be anywhere in the spine but generally is located in the upper thoracic or thoracolumbar region. The sudden kyphosis is angular, with a scissoring effect at the apex with often considerable collapse of the spine. Because this apex is abrupt and because of the twist of the spinal cord inside the spine, neurologic complications are common. The progression of this type of kyphosis is variable and depends on the progression of each scoliotic curve above and below. When an early diagnosis of neurologic impairment is made, traction may be beneficial and often allows complete neurologic recovery. This is followed by anterior and posterior fusion, which can stabilize the spine without the need for neurologic decompression.

CONGENITAL LORDOSIS

Congenital lordosis or lordosciolosis is the result of three factors (Fig. 4):

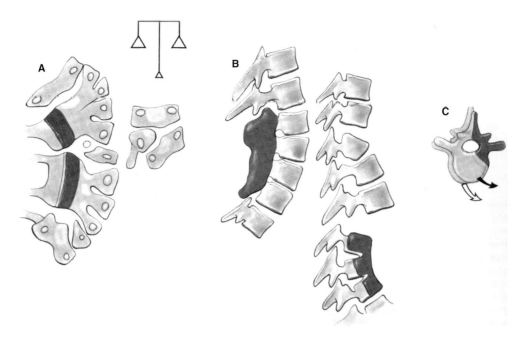

FIGURE 4. Congenital vertebral anomalies: analysis of the three-dimensional local growth potential asymmetry. *A,* Right–left coronal view showing scoliosis. *B,* Front–back sagittal view showing lordosis. *C,* Horizontal view showing rotation.

1. The most important factor is *posterior defects of segmentation* associated with a normal anterior growth. A symmetrical posterior bar leads to pure lordosis. If asymmetrical this lead to lordoscoliosis, which is sometimes very severe, especially when it involves almost the entire thoracic area. The consequence is a severe impairment of pulmonary function; the worse the lordosis, the worse the pulmonary function. In some cases, the resulting intrathoracic vertebral protrusion gives compression of the main bronchi with temporary or permanent atelectasia, leading to frequent pulmonary infection and sometimes lung abscess (Fig. 9). Sometimes several ribs are missing, which makes surgical treatment very difficult. In a few cases, the lordosis involves the cervical area with secondary esophageal compression. When it occurs in the thoracolumbar area there is usually only postural impairment (12).

2. The second factor is *posterior failure of formation* or absence of the posterior elements in the face of normal anterior elements. This occurs in patients with myelomeningocele as well as in those with dysraphism. The lordosis is more or less pure according to the mixture with partial posterolateral congenital bars.

3. The third factor that must be taken into consideration is the *postural factor* whereby lordosis can be increased by the evolution or progression of a congenital kyphosis below.

Prognosis

Because of associated anomalies, mainly skeletal (ribs fusion), nervous (dysraphism), cardiopulmonary, and urinary, the prognosis (Fig. 5) of congenital sagittal anomalies must be studied from three major perspectives: mechanical, neurologic, and respiratory.

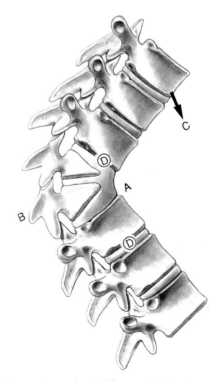

FIGURE 5. Prognosis, mechanical factors. *A,* Anterior empty space (fibrous and soft, fibrous and strong, or cartilaginous?). *B,* Quality and stability of the posterior bold. *C,* Effect of gravity (angular deformity, value of the angulation). *D,* Growth factors—growth imbalance at the level of the malformation and bad orientation of the growth plates on normal elements.

Mechanical

From the mechanical perspective, two factors must be analyzed:

1. *Stability and instability* (4). Particularly for a kyphotic deformity, when an anterior empty space is filled with nonosseous tissue, a potential instability exists, where even with good posterior "bolts" created by normal posterior elements the progression of deformity is inevitable.

From time to time, where posterior anomalies exist, there is great risk for sudden neural injury even by minor trauma.

Evidently, when there is a congenital absence of anterior and posterior elements, maximum instability is apparent. Very often this is associated with congenital spinal cord defects detected not only by skin anomalies on the back but by problems such as a unilateral paralytic foot, or urinary or bladder dysfunction. For all these congenital anomalies, MRI is mandatory from skull to coccyx.

Once an existing instability (on dynamic imaging) or a potential instability is detected, it is necessary to stabilize and fuse the spine both anteriorly and posteriorly. Lordotic deformities are much less prone to produce such instability.

2. *Growth imbalance.* Regardless of the defect (hemivertebra, asymmetrical binuclear vertebra, unsegmented bar, or a mixture of all these basic defects), growth imbalance must be studied in three dimensions. The spatial location of the defect of segmentation, for example, will determine the orientation of the deformity: defects of the bodies cause pure kyphosis, whereas defects solely of the posterior elements that develop in a symmetrical fashion induce pure lordosis. However, if the defect is slightly lateralized, it will induce the scoliotic component, with either a lordotic or kyphotic deformity depending on whether there is an posterolateral or anterolateral congenital bar. The bar's extent will determine the degree of deformity. Finally, the importance of the pubertal growth spurt must be stressed because it is at this time when suddenly an previously undetected deformity may quickly progress. Once such progression is documented, the best treatment is epiphysiodesis of the opposite side to balance the entire spine, if there is growth remaining.

Neurological Aspect

Instability or a progressive deformity will lead to neurologic complications, suddenly or gradually. However, as previously noted, often the neural structures are also congenitally abnormal. This is best documented with MRI. In specific patients, the existing dysraphism requires neurosurgical treatment (e.g., lipoma removal or release of an attached filum, or removal of a dermoid cyst). This treatment is often combined with definitive orthopedic treatment. The prognosis for the neurologic deficits occurring with such anomalies depends on three factors: clinical, pathoanatomical, and the "rest test."

1. *Clinical factor.* The longer the neurologic deficit has been present and the more severe the neurologic deficit from cord compression is, the less chance of recovery one can expect. Some deficits may have been present before birth; some are secondary to malformation of the cord; and some are secondary to the evolution of the spinal deformity itself. Only the last type can be expected to recover following treatment; the first two cannot. The prognosis is better if the neurologic compromise occurs progressively rather than suddenly, as in trauma to the cord. Complete paraplegia has a worse prognosis than incomplete but progressive paraplegia with persistent sensation on the skin below the level of the lesion or if some small voluntary motion persists. Recovery from a progressive neurologic deficit is better for younger patients (infants and children) than it is for older patients. Cord compression in the upper thoracic spine has a worse prognosis than other areas of the spine because of the precarious cord blood supply at this level.

2. *Pathoanatomy of the deformity.* If the apex of the deformity is acutely kyphotic and stiff during a hyperextension test, there is danger in applying traction for reduction. On the other hand, if the apex is flexible, traction is often recommended and generally leads to recovery, especially in a "rotatory dislocation" pattern.

3. *Rest test.* Very often it is sufficient to place the recently compromised spinal cord at rest—for example, with a cast or halo cast—to see if improvement occurs; sometimes complete recovery occurs. If recovery occurs, then surgical stabilization both anteriorly and posteriorly without opening the canal can prevent any further problems. If recovery does not occur, then direct surgical decompression is mandatory.

Respiratory Aspect

Progressive lordosis or lordoscoliosis, as in an unsegmented thoracic posterior or posterolateral bar, can have associated severe respiratory compromise. The increased transverse rib orientation decreases the rib excursion and motion. Often multiple rib fusions increase chest rigidity. The diaphragm may not function normally. The bronchi may be stretched on the vertebral "billot" and create atelectasia and lung collapse. The respiratory compromise in such a cases may be dramatic. These problems must be detected early and treatment by appropriate epiphysiodesis implemented promptly.

Multiple absent ribs on one side in the absence of lung and cardiac anomalies is a less dangerous anomaly than multiple fused ribs.

Sometimes kyphosis and kyphoscoliosis may also induce respiratory compromise, but much less so than lordotic deformities.

Treatment: General Principles

The treatment of congenital kyphosis and lordosis is exclusively surgical. Nonoperative treatment alone has no value in halting the progression of these congenital anomalies; however, it may have some role in controlling compensatory deformities above or below the congenital defect, but only when the level of the congenital anomaly is stabilized or stopped from progressing.

Before any surgical treatment is undertaken, it is necessary to make some general and specific assessments, with emphasis on cardiopulmonary anomalies, associated visceral or urinary anomalies, and neurologic problems (e.g., filum terminal, lipoma, Arnold-Chiari syndrome, various dysraphism considerations). These findings will sometimes change the timing of and the approach to treatment. The limits of the fusion both posteriorly and anteriorly must be established prior to surgery. For the very young patient, a fusion should be as short as possible to allow the normal spine to balance as best it can naturally, but it should be sufficiently long to achieve some correction using the growth potential of the normal levels involved in the fusion area to balance the defect. For the older patient close to puberty or at adolescence, the entire deformity must sometimes be fused front and back, as is done for an adult patient. The fusion must be as close as possible to the gravity line. This can be determined preoperatively by the sagittal bending radiographs either in flexion for lordotics or hyperextension for kyphotics to achieve good balance and to keep one or two disc levels free below the fusion.

EMERGENCY SITUATIONS NEEDING TREATMENT TO PROTECT LIFE ITSELF AND ITS QUALITY

1. *When instability is diagnosed,* there is the risk of sudden damage to the spinal cord. For the very young child (a few weeks to a few months old) with an unstable congenital kyphosis, external immobilization by a cast with posterior and anterior fusion of the unstable levels as early as a few weeks of age is the recommended treatment. In the author's experience, the youngest patient to receive this treatment for a dislocated spine with normal nervous function was 3 weeks old. The child was successfully casted and a posterior fusion was performed leaving intact the midline structures extending the fusion to the laminae and the transverse process. The facets were left intact (their destruction would increase the instability). The fusion extended two levels above and below the pathologic one, with a second reinforcement fusion 4 months after the initial fusion. In a similar case, a pseudarthrosis was found at the second reinforcement fusion; in this case, an anterior interbody fusion was also done at the same time.

Of course, when such an emergency situation is encountered in an older patient, one has to adapt the techniques (with or without instrumentation). In general, anterior fusion is done in conjunction with a protein fusion as soon as the child is older than 3 or 4 years.

2. *When progressive neural deficits are demonstrated,* the condition must be considered an emergency and treated immediately. This would apply whatever the age of the patient, with the same basic principle that we will use for the older child. These include, for example, the rotatory dislocation phenomena, or where growth increases the neural deficit of a spinal dysraphism, or when progressive deformity stretches the spinal cord and causes neural impairment.

3. *When respiratory function is clearly involved* and worsened by a spinal deformity (mainly congenital lordoscoliosis) and/or lung abnormalities, this must be considered an emergency that requires immediate treatment in conjunction with the cardiopulmonary team. For the orthopedic team in such a case, the immediate partial correction of the lordosis can be attempted, as can airway decompression if necessary, but generally the correction

is achieved progressively by epiphysiodesis and in some cases by thoracic rib distraction.

PROGRESSIVE DEFORMITIES DURING INFANCY AND CHILDHOOD AS BEST INDICATIONS FOR EPIPHYSIODESIS OR HEMIVERTEBRA EXCISION

Preoperative Planning

The preoperative planning of an epiphysiodesis (Fig. 6) of the spine, with or without hemivertebra excision, requires knowledge of the normal growth of a vertebral unit and its growing

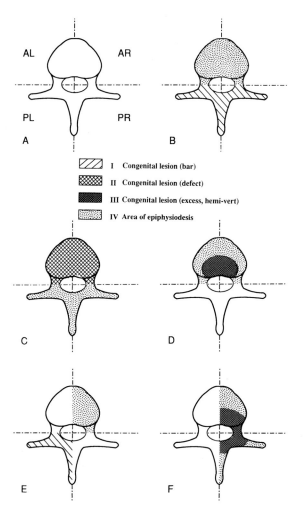

FIGURE 6. Planning for epiphysiodesis of the spine. *A,* Schematic division of the vertebral element into four quadrants in the horizontal plane. *B,* Symmetrical posterior bar and the required area of the epiphysiodesis. *C,* Symmetrical absence or failure of formation of the body—posterior symmetrical epiphysiodesis required. *D,* Pure anterior hemivertebra. An increase in the relative anterior length results in lordosis. Epiphysiodesis is required along with anterior fusion. *E,* Posterolateral congenital bar. An anterior convex hemiepiphysiodesis is required. *F,* Anterolateral hemivertebra requires simultaneous anterior and posterior homolateral hemiepiphysiodesis.

cartilages in three dimensions. Consider the entire vertebra to be a cube divided into four quadrants, with all vertebrae growing equally around the spinal canal.

When an imbalance in the growth potential exists, it is necessary to plan preoperatively the exact zones to be fused to reestablish good balance. We use a schematic axial drawing divided into four quadrants and a schematic sagittal drawing where all of the vertebrae belonging to the lesion are included. This gives a mental three-dimensional reconstruction and plan of exactly what has to be done (Fig. 7). By doing this we can treat any

kind of deformity by adapting the three-dimensional defect to the three-dimensional area of epiphysiodesis.

When a single posterolateral hemivertebra leads to a kyphoscoliosis at the lower thoracic, thoracolumbar, or lumbar area, the author favors hemivertebra excision and short fusion.

Technique of Epiphysiodesis (3)

Outcomes are classified according in three ways: *improvement effect,* when clinical and radiologic improvement can be mea-

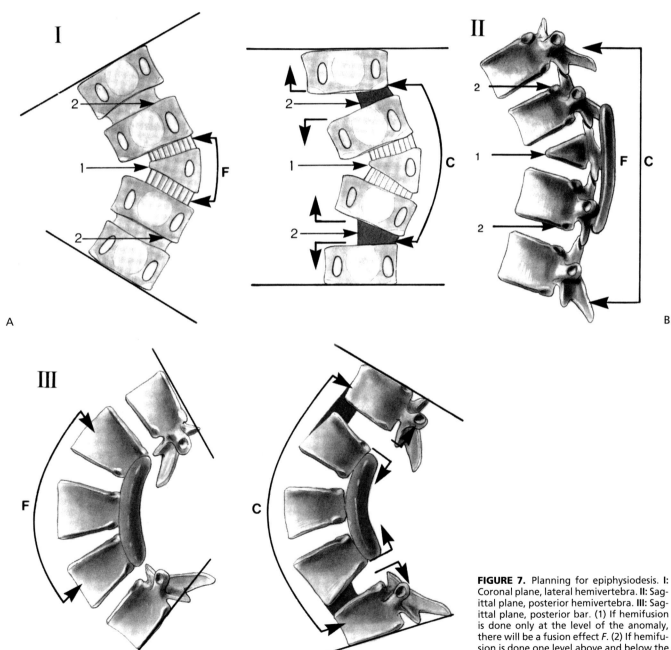

FIGURE 7. Planning for epiphysiodesis. **I:** Coronal plane, lateral hemivertebra. **II:** Sagittal plane, posterior hemivertebra. **III:** Sagittal plane, posterior bar. (1) If hemifusion is done only at the level of the anomaly, there will be a fusion effect *F.* (2) If hemifusion is done one level above and below the anomaly, there will be a correcting effect *C.*

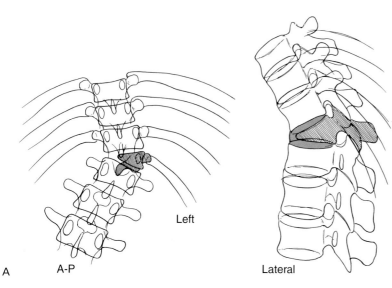

FIGURE 8. Kyphosing hemivertebra of the thoracolumbar junction (T12), posterolateral hemivertebra excision. **A:** What we see on a regular radiograph anteroposteriorly and laterally. Anteroposterior: it is important to know where the hemiposterior arch is located. Lateral: Note that the posterior hemivertebral body shadow overlaps the upper and lower adjacent bodies. **B:** Technique:

(a) What has to be removed on the front?
• The hemibody of T12, including more than half the length of the pedicle inside the canal.
• The adjacent growth plates of T11 and L1.

We always start with the anterior approach. After removal, we secure the canal lateral to the dura with a piece of Surgicel tape and place between the two vertebral plateaux T11 and L1 mashed cancellous bone.

(b) What has to be removed on the back, the hemilamina, facets, and remaining pedicle?

What do we see on the back and the hemilamina to be removed? Note: Do not strip the periosteum of vertebrae T10 and L2 because of risk of extending the fusion.

(c) After removing the hemiarch, we see the dura, the root, and the piece of Surgicel tape placed in front.

(d) Compression is done posteriorly by any device between T11 and L1 (we use Baby CD) to close the gap unilaterally until both posterior arches of T11 and L1 have been approximated.

Posterior fusion is achieved with cancellous bone coming from the body excised and chips of the rib used for the approach.

The postoperative cast is realized 3 or 4 days after with general anesthesia.

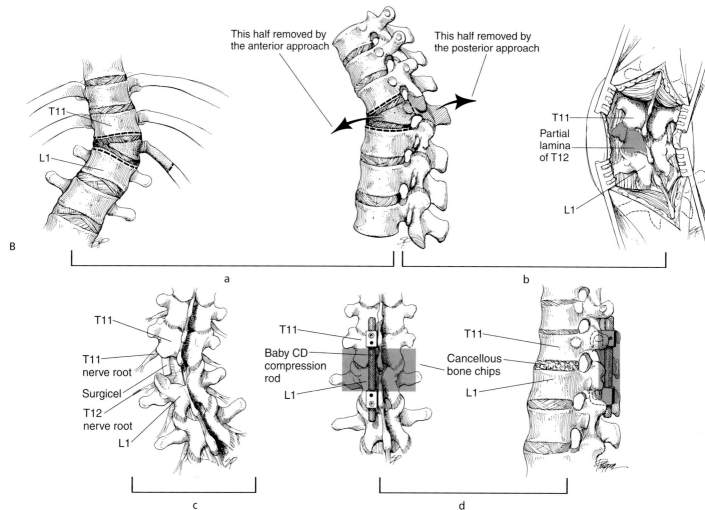

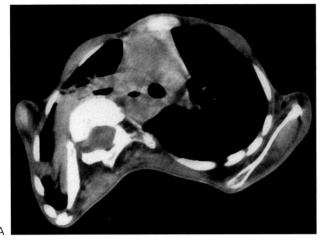

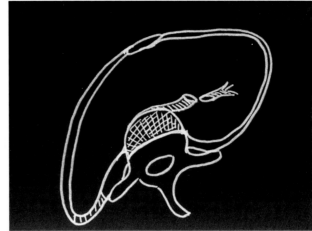

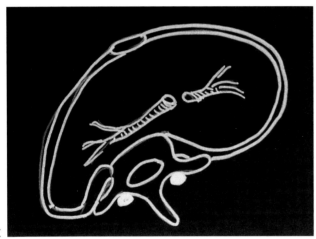

FIGURE 9. Decompression of the airway. **A:** Congenital lordoscoliosis with CT scan atelectasia of the inferior main bronchi of the right lung. **B:** Drawing of the planned resection of vertebral body "billot." **C:** After anterior resection and proper kyphosing posterior instrumentation, the airway is free.

sured by more than a 5-degree Cobb angle; *fusion effect,* when even with a considerable cosmetic improvement there is no change above or below 5 degrees from the angle from the postoperative cast; and *worsening effect,* where the curve has been exacerbated by more than 5 degrees.

For example, for *kyphosis* secondary to pure symmetrical posterior hemivertebra, symmetrical posterior epiphysiodesis on both sides is required.

For *kyphoscoliosis* caused by a posterolateral hemivertebra, an anterior and posterior convex hemiepiphysiodesis on the same side as the hemivertebra is required. In fact, if we start first with a posterior convex hemiepiphysiodesis, we achieve correction of the kyphotic component but not for the coronal plane component, and we observe a crankshaft phenomenon that is avoided by the simultaneous anterior fusion. For this reason, particularly in the thoracolumbar or lumbar spine, we prefer to perform a *unilateral hemivertebra excision* with closure of the posterior elements with a small compressive device, correcting at the same time the anteroposterior and sagittal plane and simultaneous fusion and postoperative cast (Fig. 8).

For *lordoscoliosis* caused by posterolateral bar, we need to perform an anterior and posterior convex hemiepiphysiodesis, which is located at the opposite side of the bar. Sometimes

compression of the airway exists due to protrusion of the vertebral bodies at the same time that epiphysiodesis anterior hemivertebral body resection is being performed (Fig. 9).

Finally, in some patients with lordoscoliosis associated with asymmetrical defect of segmentation and absence of ribs, the use of a progressive rib distractor (see Chapter 7 on congenital scoliosis), in young children gives surprising good results both pulmonary and spinal without any direct vertebral epiphysiodesis.

ESTABLISHED DEFORMITIES IN OLDER, ADOLESCENT, OR END-OF-GROWTH CHILDREN

Patients without Neurologic Deficits

1. *For kyphosis and kyphoscoliosis,* the plan of treatment will depend on the stiffness or flexibility of the curve, particularly the mobility at the apex. For a *flexible apex,* preoperative traction with hyperextension with careful close neurologic evaluation is useful. This should be followed by anterior and posterior fusion. It is recommended that one start with the anterior approach and release of fibrous tissue, with the disc spaces remaining. This improves the reduction either with a temporary anterior dis-

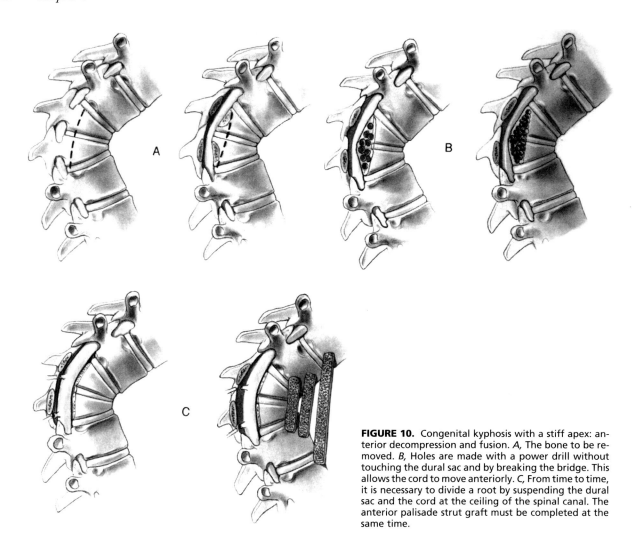

FIGURE 10. Congenital kyphosis with a stiff apex: anterior decompression and fusion. *A,* The bone to be removed. *B,* Holes are made with a power drill without touching the dural sac and by breaking the bridge. This allows the cord to move anteriorly. *C,* From time to time, it is necessary to divide a root by suspending the dural sac and the cord at the ceiling of the spinal canal. The anterior palisade strut graft must be completed at the same time.

tractor or, more often, with posteroanterior pressure directly on the apex to open the anterior gap, where struts of tibial graft are inserted in a palisade fashion from the bottom of the apex as symmetrically as possible above and below this apex until the gravity line is approached (Fig. 10 for palisade graft example). This results in segmental anterior multilevel bridges. We favor the concave approach when we treat a kyphoscoliosis in order to be well aligned in the gravity line. We do not like to start with the posterior approach because it can increase a previously unrecognized instability that may result in neurological compromise.

One can do the posterior fusion first only if there is certainty regarding stability and if the hyperextension test demonstrates mobility.

With time this palisade graft consolidates. Only in very few cases have we used vascularized rib because generally this type of anterior material does not give immediate stability. We never use it alone, only in association with rigid struts.

For a *rigid apex,* in the case of a congenital cause, we do not favor osteotomy, cord decompression, and fusion because these may result in only partial improvement of the cosmetic aspect

and from time to time may cause a neurologic deficit. We prefer to do the anterior approach first to keep the apex intact and to have partial correction through the disc spaces above and below, followed by a posterior fusion. This approach, while not giving cosmetic correction, does preserve spinal cord function.

2. *For lordosis,* flexibility of the congenital lordosis deformity is very uncommon, existing mainly in cases where the absence of the posterior elements explains the reducibility. In such cases, the best treatment is anterior release with shortening and anterior instrumentation with any compressive system (if located in a safe area for the great vessels), followed by posterior instrumentation and fusion, with a kyphosing distraction effect on the mobile levels.

More often, the lordotic curve is rigid. Correction is generally achieved with the anterior approach first and sometimes anterior body resection when airway compromise exists, followed by posterior osteotomies with posterior instrumentation and fusion, or in a reverse order, with posterior osteotomies first, followed by anterior multiple wedging and anterior compressive instrumentation when possible. For younger children, in the thoracolumbar area, we have used this technique without instrumentation.

The closure of the anterior wedge was achieved with 4 weeks of traction with the hips and knees flexed 90 degrees and vertical suspension of the inferior part of the body. Then a body cast extending down to the hips and knees for another 2 months is used.

The advantage of not using metallic implants is that safe neurologic control can be achieved afterward with CT or MRI. Generally, for lordoscoliosis, it is always better to shorten the anterior convexity without lengthening the posterior concavity.

Patients with Neurologic Deficits

A clear difference must be established between neurologic signs that are secondary to the progressive deformity and those existing from birth because of malformation of nervous tissues (8).

Congenital kyphosis and kyphoscoliosis are the most common cause of neurologic complication secondary to an angular kyphosis, sometimes occurring in young children but usually appearing only at puberty, especially when the congenital defect is in the upper thoracic spine (T3-5) and thoracolumbar junction (T12-L1). If *the apex is flexible* the deformity can be partially reduced, especially if the patient has previous radiographs that show a less pronounced deformity—either angular or of the rotatory dislocation type. If the neurologic signs were definitely acquired recently, the deformity may be progressively reduced using a distraction cast, very often combined with halo traction independent of the cast. The patient must be monitored very closely for the evolution of neurologic signs. The author prefers the distraction cast to the direct halo traction because the cast adds spatial stabilization to the spine, which is not the case with a simple halo traction in the bed.

Once recovery occurs, the same strategy can be used as described for patients without neurologic deficit. Both anterior and posterior fusion must be accomplished to ensure a good outcome.

If *the apex is stiff and not reducible,* then rest and immobilization are the first line of therapy. If improvement occurs, one can wait 1 or 2 months or more; in some cases there is complete recovery, and an in situ anterior and posterior fusion is performed. If there is no change in neurologic status or progression, decompression of the spinal cord must be accomplished. However, in patients with long-term neurologic deficit (over 3 years or from birth, i.e., congenital), decompression of the cord in our experience gives no improvement and runs the risk of loss of one or two additional roots.

In all other cases (major neurologic compromise relatively recent—3 years or less—or worsening seen during the short rest period), decompression of the cord is combined with an anterior and posterior fusion.

If the anatomy demonstrates pure kyphosis (Fig. 10), decompression is achieved with the anterior approach. This involves removing the bony apex but never starting at the apex, instead creating a big hole from one or more levels above and below the apex, in the bodies, and creating a bridge. The bridge is then removed without touching the dural sac at any time. Anterior strut interbody fusion is done under direct visualization of the sac. Posterior fusion is performed the same day or a few days later, with internal fixation done whenever possible. Of course, in young children, external immobilization by halo cast is recommended and the surgery is performed inside the cast on a relatively stable spine. With *kyphoscoliosis,* decompression is done through the costal transversectomy approach on the concave side using the technique described by Guiot. The dural sac and the cord are moved gently outside the canal and are often close to the rib heads or stumps (Fig. 11).

It is mandatory to perform the anterior fusion at the same time. Not doing this renders it dangerous to approach the spine with a dural sac "inside" the chest but outside the canal!

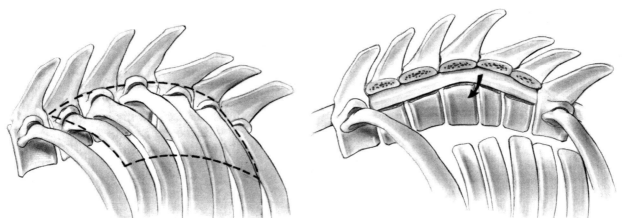

A   B

FIGURE 11. Anterolateral decompression for kyphoscoliosis using the Guiot-Capener approach. **A:** Approach is done on the concave side from the spinous processes to the ribs. The route of the canal follows one root through a foramen that is distant from the apex with a costal transversectomy. *(Figure continues.)*

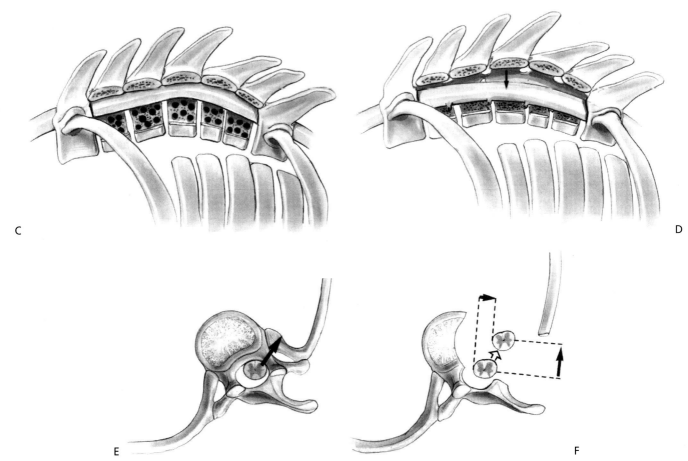

C

D

E

F

FIGURE 11. *Continued* **B, C:** Once the canal and bodies are exposed, a power drill is used to create a bridge under the cord. One must break the bridge in the direction from the cord to the hole (and not the reverse) to avoid touching the cord at the apex. **D:** The cord is transposed more or less on the heads and strump of the ribs. **E, F:** Horizontal view of the surgery showing anterior and lateral transposition of the dural and cord elements.

In the French experience with approximately 40 patients having congenital anomalies with acquired progressive neurologic signs, we used the preoperative traction strategy. Improvement occurred in about 60% of the cases, and this without having to perform decompression but only anterior and posterior fusion. We have never seen recurrence of neurologic signs after this circumferential fusion in such patients. In patients on whom we performed decompression and circumferential fusion, significant improvement or recovery of the neurologic signs was observed only in 50%, while 20% showed a worsening of signs.

So far, we have not seen any patient with congenital spinal anomaly without neurologic signs who was appropriately treated by fusion (circumferential if necessary) during infancy and childhood who later developed neurologic impairment.

CONCLUSION

Persons with sagittal plane congenital anomalies require the earliest possible diagnosis and proper evaluation of the pathoana-tomy, including stability, growth potential imbalance, associated anomalies, and consequences on the vital functions (primarily cardiopulmonary and neurologic). Early treatment should be provided to correct the deformity—if possible. But treatment should mainly be directed at *preventing* any worsening of the deformity and any onset of progression of the consequences of the deformity on vital functions.

REFERENCES

1. Bradford DS, Hensinger RM, eds. (1985): *The pediatric spine,* vol. 1. Stuttgart: Thieme Verlag, pp. 196–217.
2. Cruveilhier E (1845): *Anatomie pathologique descriptive,* vol. 1. Paris.
3. Dubousset J (1993): Epiphysiodesis of the spine; indications, techniques, results. *J Pediatr Orthop B* 1:123–130.
4. Dubousset J, Gonon G (1983): Cyphoses et cyphoscolioses angulaires. *Rev Chir Orthop* 69 [Suppl II]:1.
5. Dubousset J, Duval-Beaupere G, Anquez L (1973): In: Rougerie J, ed. *Deformations vertébrales congénitales compliquées de troubles neurologiques. Compressions médullaires chez l'enfant,* vol. 1. Paris: Masson, pp. 193–207.
6. Duval-Beaupere G, Dubousset J (1972): La dislocation rotatoire progressive du rachis. *Rev Chir Orthop* 58:323–334.

7. Kharrat K, Dubousset J (1980): Bloc vertebral anterieur progressif chez l'enfant. *Rev Chir Orthop* 66:485–492.
8. Lonstein JE, Winter RB, Moe JH, et al. (1980): Neurologic deficits secondary to spinal deformity; a review of the literature and report of 43 cases. *Spine* 5:331–335.
9. Rivard C, Nairbait Z, Vithoff HK (1979): Congenital vertebral malformation. *Orthop Rev* 8:135–139.
10. Tondury G (1958): *Entwick lungs geschilte Fehlbidddren der wirbelsaüle.* Stuttgart: Hypokates.
11. Watanabe H (1983): Pathological anatomy of congenital kyphosis and kyphoscoliosis. Presented at ESDS, Dubrovnik, 1983.
12. Winter RB (1983): *Congenital deformities of the spine.* New York: Thieme Stratton.

SACRAL AGENESIS

WILLIAM A. PHILLIPS

Sacral agenesis is the term commonly applied to a group of disorders characterized by absence of a variable portion of the caudal portion of the spine. Individuals with sacral agenesis lack motor function below the level of the remaining normal spine, similar to those with myelomeningocele. In myelomeningocele, however, sensory nerve function is impaired below the level of affected vertebrae. In sacral agenesis, sensation tends to be present at much more caudal levels. In more severe cases of sacral agenesis, part or all of the lumbar spine and even the lower thoracic spine may be absent. By convention, even these severely affected individuals are referred to as having sacral agenesis, despite attempts by some to use the more descriptive term *lumbosacral agenesis* (14,25,27,35,38,42).

Individuals with sacral agenesis frequently have other abnormalities of the musculoskeletal system. Of greatest interest to the spinal surgeon is the abnormal articulation between the pelvis and the remaining normal spine that characterizes children with agenesis of the lumbar spine. With increasing severity of vertebral agenesis (i.e., more proximal involvement), the articulation between the spine and pelvis becomes more abnormal and the lower extremities present with more severe deformities. Abnormalities of the renal system are commonly reported, and other viscera can also be affected.

In this chapter, management of the lower-extremity deformities and of the articulation of the spine and pelvis unique to this condition are discussed. This approach is necessary because these problems and their management are often interdependent.

NOMENCLATURE

Sacral agenesis has been referred to by a variety of terms, including congenital absence of the sacrum (15,22,51), congenital anomaly of the sacrum (6), sacrococcygeal agenesis (18), vertebral agenesis (10), caudal regression (5,23,38,39), caudal dysplasia (29,56), and sacral aplasia. Williams and Nixon (57) in 1957 appear to have been the first to use the term sacral agenesis. As the absence of the coccyx is not known to cause any problems (22), mention of its absence seems unnecessary.

The level of involvement in sacral agenesis is best described by the most caudal normal vertebral body (42,47). Although there may be a more caudal nubbin of malformed bone, the last vertebral body usually corresponds well to the degree of motor impairment seen in affected children.

Renshaw (47) classified patients by the amount of sacrum remaining and the characteristics of the articulation between the spine and the pelvis (Fig. 1):

Type I has either total or partial unilateral agenesis of the sacrum.

Type II has partial sacral agenesis with a bilaterally symmetrical defect, a normal or hypoplastic first sacral vertebra, and a stable articulation between the ilia and the first sacral vertebra.

Type III has variable lumbar and total sacral agenesis, with the ilia articulating with the sides of the lowest vertebra present.

Type IV has variable lumbar and total sacral agenesis, with the caudal end plate of the lowest vertebra resting above either fused ilia or an iliac amphiarthrosis.

Sacral agenesis is considered by some to be a form of caudal regression or caudal dysplasia syndrome (16,23,39).

EPIDEMIOLOGY FACTORS

Sacral agenesis is an uncommon congenital affliction of the spine occurring in approximately 1 of 25,000 live births (50). The actual incidence may be higher because minor defects of the sacrum without other external manifestations may not be obvious at birth. The first reported case of sacral agenesis is attributed to Hohl (27) in 1852.

The majority of reported cases involve absence of the sacrum and perhaps some lumbar vertebrae. Complete absence of the lumbar spine is uncommon. Based on a cumulative review of the literature (more than 500 cases of sacral agenesis), there appears to be little difference in the incidence of sacral agenesis between males and females.

ETIOLOGIC FACTORS

The exact cause of sacral agenesis is unknown. In 1959, Blumel et al. (6) first called attention to the increased incidence of diabetes in mothers of affected children. The incidence of maternal diabetes is about 16% (29). Rusnak and Driscoll (50) reviewed the cases of 1,150 infants born to diabetic mothers. Three had

W. A. Phillips: Texas Children's Hospital and Baylor College of Medicine, Houston, Texas 77030.

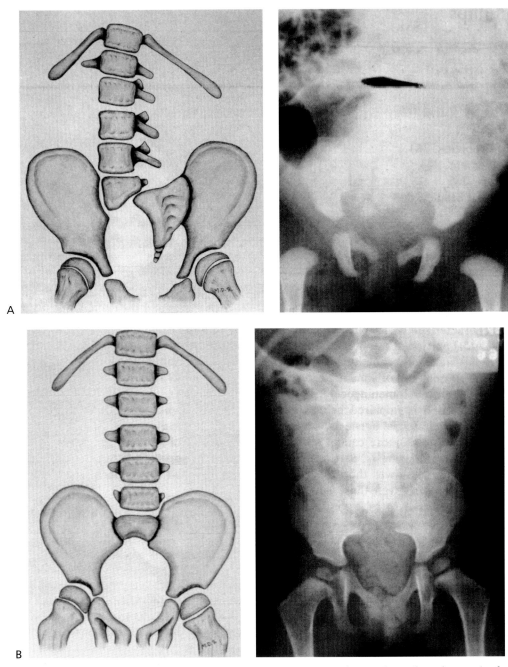

FIGURE 1. Renshaw classification of sacral agenesis. **A:** Type I sacral agenesis—unilateral agenesis of the sacrum. **B:** Type II sacral agenesis—partial sacral agenesis with a bilaterally symmetrical defect, a normal or hypoplastic first sacral vertebra, and a stable articulation between the ilia and the first sacral vertebra. *(Figure continues.)*

sacral agenesis, making the incidence 1 of every 350 births to diabetic mothers. Passarge (39) estimated that no more than 1% of infants born to diabetic mothers have sacral anomalies. The degree of sacral agenesis does not appear to be related to the severity of the maternal diabetes, and severe defects have been noted in children whose mothers had no evidence of diabetes or were in a prediabetic state (42). Kalter (30) suggested the association of maternal diabetes and specific malformations cannot be established from case reports due to selection bias. He

notes that the incidence of these malformations is too low for the incidence of diabetes in women of childbearing age.

Several kindreds have been described in which a sacral defect is inherited and there is no association with maternal diabetes (43). Welch and Aterman (56) described three forms of familial sacral dysgenesis: familial hemisacrum type I (Cohn-Bay-Nielsen syndrome), familial hemisacrum type II (Ashcraft syndrome), and familial partial sacral agenesis. Chromosomal studies have been normal (4,8,40), with a few exceptions (5,53).

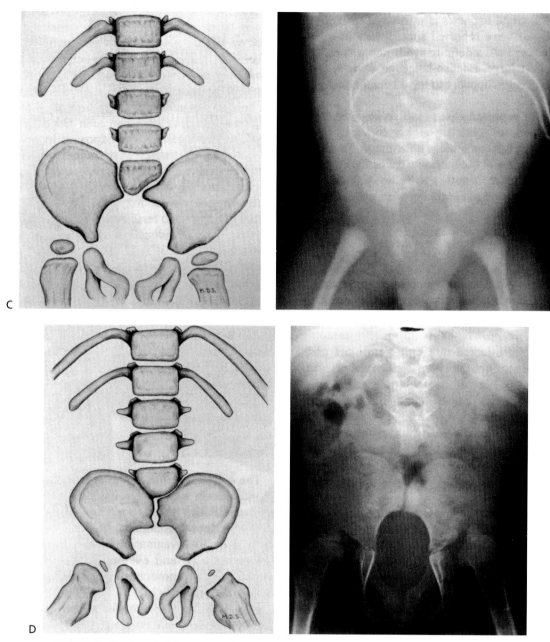

FIGURE 1. *Continued.* **C:** Type III sacral agenesis—variable lumbar and total sacral agenesis with the ilia articulating with the sides of the lowest vertebra present. **D:** Type IV sacral agenesis—variable lumbar and total sacral agenesis with the caudal end plate of the lowest vertebra resting above either fused ilia or an iliac amphiarthrosis. (From Renshaw TS (1978): Sacral agenesis: a classification and review of twenty-three cases. *J Bone Joint Surg Am* 60:373–383, with permission.)

CLINICAL FEATURES

Just as the degree of agenesis of the spine can vary greatly in children with sacral agenesis, so can the number and severity of associated problems. Renshaw (47) and others (42) have noted that higher levels of agenesis seem to be associated with more anomalies of greater severity (Fig. 2). Certain problems are associated with specific patterns of agenesis.

The Renshaw type I pattern of unilateral sacral agenesis (the so-called scimitar sacrum) is often inherited in either an autoso-mal or a sex-linked dominant pattern (7,59). In familial hemisa-crum type I (Cohn-Bay-Nielsen syndrome), anterior meningo-cele is often seen (13). In familial hemisacrum type II (Ashcraft syndrome), there is a high incidence of presacral teratoma (31).

Musculoskeletal Problems

Musculoskeletal problems related to sacral agenesis can be di-vided into those that are dependent on the level of agenesis of the spine and neural elements and those that are independent

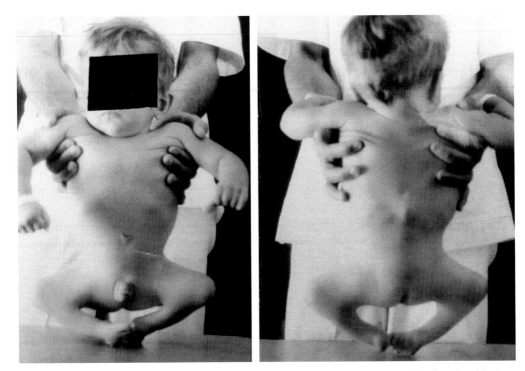

FIGURE 2. A child with agenesis of the spine below T12. Note the small pelvis, the flexed webbed knees, and clubfeet in the posterior view. Note the prominent nubbin at the end of the thoracic spine, which represents the end of the spine in this child. (From Phillips WA, Cooperman DR, Lindquist TC, et al. (1982): Orthopaedic management of lumbosacral agenesis. *J Bone Joint Surg Am* 64:1282–1294, with permission.)

of the level. Orthopedic problems not related to the level of agenesis include foot deformities, such as clubfoot, and other anomalies of the spine, such as congenital scoliosis, myelomeningocele, and Klippel-Feil syndrome. Problems dependent on the level of involvement include spinal-pelvic instability, dislocation of the hips, and knee flexion contractures, sometimes with popliteal webbing. These tend to be seen most frequently in children with Renshaw III or IV sacral agenesis. Involvement of the upper extremities is rare (6,47).

Spine

In the more severe forms of sacral agenesis (Renshaw types III and IV), the articulation between the spine and pelvis is rudimentary (type III) or nonexistent (type IV). This results in a kyphosis at the end of the spine as well as an abnormal amount of motion between spine and pelvis. Affected individuals sit in the so-called Buddha position with knees flexed and legs crossed, leaning forward because of their kyphosis (51). This motion has been commonly referred to as spinal-pelvic instability (3,14, 41,42,58) (Fig. 3).

A variety of other spinal abnormalities have been reported in children with sacral agenesis. In several series, few of the children had normal spines above the level of agenesis (4,47). Congenital scoliosis due to hemivertebra and duplicated or fused ribs has been reported (26). Developmental scoliosis (i.e., with no obvious bony defect in the spine above the level of agenesis) is also

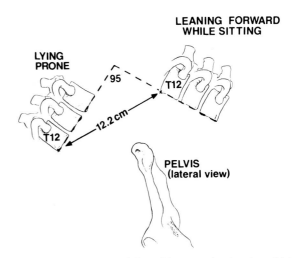

FIGURE 3. Spinal pelvic instability. This composite drawing of lateral radiographs of the spinal-pelvic junction of a 35-year-old woman with lumbosacral agenesis at the twelfth thoracic level was made while she was lying prone and while she was sitting leaning forward. The iliac wings appear flattened due to absence of the sacrum. Note the large translation as well as rotation possible. This patient was asymptomatic. (From Phillips WA, Cooperman DR, Lindquist TC, et al. (1982): Orthopaedic management of lumbosacral agenesis. *J Bone Joint Surg Am* 64: 1282–1294, with permission.)

common (42). Klippel-Feil syndrome has also been reported occasionally in children with sacral agenesis (4,21,42,44,47).

Hips

The possible inclusion of children with myelomeningocele in some reports makes it difficult to determine the exact incidence of hip problems occurring in sacral agenesis. Hip dislocation in sacral agenesis usually occurs in cases of relatively severe involvement. Hip dislocation in higher level sacral agenesis appears to be a consequence of muscle imbalance (42). The situation is similar to myelomeningocele, in which preservation of hip flexor and adductor power with loss of hip abduction and extension is associated with a high incidence of hip problems.

Knees

One of the most striking features in children with high-level sacral agenesis (L1 and above) is the presence of severe knee flexion contractures, often with popliteal webbing. The contractures, which can be greater than 120 degrees, preclude the use of a brace and attempts at ambulation (14). Lack of active quadriceps power appears to correlate with the severity of the knee flexion contracture. Children with L1 and above sacral agenesis tend to have the most severe contractures. Children with sacral agenesis below the L1 level tend to have less severe contractures that rarely need intervention.

Feet

Foot deformities in sacral agenesis tend to be stiff and similar to those seen in arthrogryposis. Clubfoot, vertical talus, and cavus foot deformities have been reported (1,4,22,23).

Neurologic Involvement

The degree of neurologic involvement varies and is usually related to the amount of spine remaining. In most individuals, the level of motor function is usually within one level of the last normal-appearing vertebral body. Because the absence of the sacral vertebrae suggests absence of the corresponding sacral motor nerves, virtually all individuals with sacral agenesis above S2 (i.e., missing two or more sacral segments) will have a neurogenic bladder (24,57). Sensation tends to be spared more distally, and even high-level children tend to have at least protective sensation in their feet. Most also have at least some sensation in the perianal region. Pressure sores have been reported only rarely, and it is unclear whether these children had sacral agenesis alone or myelomeningocele as well (4). Pathologic fractures appear to be uncommon and are not mentioned in most reports.

In most cases of sacral agenesis, the neurologic level does not change. There have been occasional reports of children with sacral agenesis who developed progressive neurologic deficits that improved with surgical intervention. Tethered cord (11,37), lipomas (25), and dural sac stenosis (12) have been described. In most cases, the child presented with a progressive neurologic deficit. Several recent reports in the neurosurgical literature have

suggested taking a more aggressive approach to asymptomatic anomalies. Muthukumar (34) reported improved urinary continence after tethered-cord releases in several patients with stable deficits.

Myelomeningocele is often associated with sacral agenesis. In these individuals, the neurologic deficits correspond to the level of involvement, with both motor and sensory loss. Spinal lipomas and tethering of the spinal cord have been noted in conjunction with myelomeningocele, and a child may occasionally present with a progressive neurologic deficit due to one of these conditions. Intelligence seems normal in individuals with sacral agenesis who do not have the hydrocephalus associated with myelomeningocele (10,42).

IMAGING AND FUNCTIONAL STUDIES

The pathognomonic finding on radiographs is the absence of part or all of the sacrum and possibly the lumbar spine. In more severe cases, the ilia tend to be rotated back almost parallel to each other in the coronal plane rather than forming the typical 90-degree angle. This is a result of the absence of the sacrum.

Imaging studies beyond plain radiography that are helpful in evaluating patients with sacral agenesis include myelography, computed tomography (CT), magnetic resonance imaging (MRI), ultrasonography, and intravenous pyelography. Both CT and MRI have been used to delineate the spinal cord pathology and to detect the occasional tethered spinal cord (5,9, 25,38,55.36). Ultrasonography has been used to detect anterior meningocele and presacral teratomata in individuals with the hereditary forms of sacral agenesis as well as to screen for renal and collecting system abnormalities.

PATHOANATOMY

Observations on sacral agenesis have been based on autopsy studies, surgical dissections, and amputation specimens. The extremities tend to have muscle replaced with fibrofatty tissue with irregular nerve structures, similar to that seen in arthrogryposis (21,50). In severely involved individuals with popliteal webbing, the neurovascular bundle tends to take the shortest course and is often just below the skin at the apex of the webbing. This can hinder attempts at correcting the severe knee flexion contractures.

Examination of the spine at autopsy or during attempts at spinal-pelvic fusion has found irregular threads of nerves coming from the end of the vertebral column and extending down through the pelvis (21,82). In some cases, no distal extension of the spinal cord was found, even in patients who had distal sensation (41,58). The spinal cord and dural sac often terminate at the same level as the vertebral column (2,21,25,28,50,55–57).

NATURAL HISTORY

Most reported cases of sacral agenesis are in children. Reported causes of death in infancy have included cardiac anomalies (2,10) and other severe congenital anomalies. Deaths in childhood have been due to sepsis or renal failure (42). The highest known level of spinal agenesis in which the patient is known to have survived is at the T7 level (54). Information on adults with sacral agenesis is sparse, with no longitudinal studies (4,13,20,22,32,35,42, 45,49,59).

Most higher level patients become wheelchair users as adults despite attempts at orthotic or prosthetic management of their lower extremity deformities. Virtually all the adults reported in the literature received no special treatment for their spinal-pelvic instability, and few had problems that could be attributed to spinal-pelvic instability. Many were dependent on others for assistance with activities of daily living. Urinary and fecal incontinence seems to become less of a problem for adults with sacral agenesis. Satisfactory sexual function is possible. The lack of education and society's indifference to the handicapped appear to have contributed to these individuals' dependent states.

ORTHOPEDIC MANAGEMENT

High-level sacral agenesis presents the orthopedic surgeon with two unique problems—spinal-pelvic instability and severe knee flexion contractures with popliteal webbing—whose solutions are often interrelated. Before planning a surgical procedure on a child for one of these two problems, one must plan for the other. Otherwise, the options for management may be unnecessarily restricted.

Spine

Several problems have been attributed to spinal-pelvic instability and have been offered as justification for attempts to fuse the shortened spine to the abnormal pelvis. Perry et al. (41) were the first to report in English on results of spinal-pelvic fusion in children with sacral agenesis. Their justification for performing spinal-pelvic fusion was threefold:

1. To free the upper extremities from the necessity of supporting an unstable collapsing back
2. To protect the viscera from unphysiologic compression and angulation
3. To establish a stable vertebral-pelvic complex about which lower-extremity contractures can be stretched or surgically released.

Few reports have been published on the technique and results of fusions for spinal-pelvic instability (33,41,52,58,46,17).

Winter (58) reported a case of T10 level agenesis that he successfully fused when the patient was 5 years 11 months old. He used Harrington compression rods in a claw configuration on the top and bottom of the pelvis linked to the upper thoracic spine (Fig. 4). Simultaneous knee disarticulation provided bone graft. When the patient was aged 10 years 6 months and 12 years 6 months, Winter osteotomized the fusion mass and lengthened it each time by an inch in an attempt to prevent crowding of the patient's internal organs.

Satisfactory results of spinal-pelvic fusion have been reported.

No neurologic complications (e.g., loss of sensation) and few pseudarthroses have been reported, although several authors reported exploring the fusion mass in the first 6 months and adding more bone. Hand-free sitting and gastrointestinal function have been reported to be improved after surgery.

Although the reported attempts at spinal-pelvic fusion have generally been successful, a solid fusion may not solve all problems. Phillips et al. (42) reported an 18-year-old who was fused at age 5 but had daily back pain despite a solid fusion. Andrish et al. (3) noted that "multiple problems have been related to spinal-pelvic stabilization, primarily related to the hips. Several patients had minimal hip motion discovered postoperatively. In some, resection of the proximal femur was necessary to improve sitting balance, but made them non-ambulating."

The three reasons advanced to justify spinal-pelvic fusion—to allow hand-free sitting, to prevent visceral compression, and to stretch hip flexion contractures—are at best relative indications. The natural history of untreated spinal-pelvic instability should also be considered.

Andrish et al. (3) noted that as patients get older, the degree of instability (i.e., the excessive motion of the spinal-pelvic junction) decreases. In another series (42), 17 of 19 patients with unfused spines (both children and adults) could sit with their hands free.

The risk of visceral compression due to spinal-pelvic instability is difficult to assess. Instances of documented problems are uncommon (19).

Given the risk of obstructive uropathy resulting from anomalous urinary tracts and an abnormally innervated bladder and sphincter mechanism, it may be difficult to determine the cause of an obstructive uropathy in patients with sacral agenesis. In reports of adults with sacral agenesis, problems with visceral compression have seldom been noted. Further investigation of this problem is needed. Adults with severe sacral agenesis tend to be barrel-chested, suggesting that they compensate for lack of trunk height by increased trunk width (42,49).

Stabilization of the spinal-pelvic junction may allow stretching of severe hip flexion contractures (41). The children with the most severe spinal-pelvic instability have the least functioning musculature in the lower extremities and will probably become wheelchair users as adults. The necessity of correcting hip flexion contractures in such patients has not been established.

Currently, spinal-pelvic fusion does not seem justified for asymptomatic spinal-pelvic instability. The risk of visceral compression remains largely unsubstantiated, and the functional benefits seem few. If spinal-pelvic fusion is to be performed, the technique of Dumont et al. (17) of segmental instrumentation with claws on the pelvis and spine is recommended. If amputation of the legs is not performed, large segments of allograft bone can be used to maintain a more normal trunk height, although the long-term results of this are unknown. A limited amount of autocraft can be obtained by harvesting the lower ribs. Use of allograft cortical bone would require prolonged postoperative immobilization to protect the graft during its slow incorporation. Regardless of the type of graft used, prolonged postoperative immobilization in the recumbent position is often necessary. Subsequent lengthening of the fusion mass to gain trunk height may be possible, but the impact on the child and

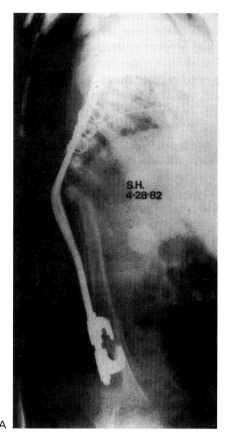 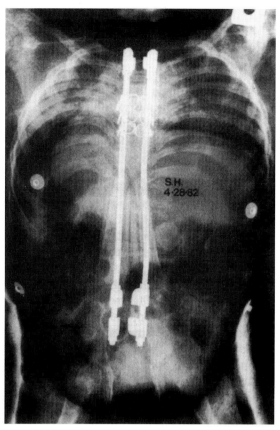

FIGURE 4. Postoperative radiographs of a child with T10 level lumbosacral agenesis who underwent posterior spinal pelvic stabilization using amputated tibiae for bone graft and large Harrington compression rods, sublaminar wires, and Harrington hooks for internal fixation. (From Winter RB (1991): Congenital absence of the lumbar spine and sacrum: one-stage reconstruction with subsequent two-stage spine lengthening. *J Pediatr Orthop* 11:666–670, with permission.)

family of repeated operations with prolonged recovery times should be carefully weighed against the potential benefits.

Knees

To assist these children in standing with braces, attempts have been made to straighten knee flexion contractures, with mixed success.

Most recently, the Ilizarov device has been used to correct these contractures. Even with this device, the contractures can recur and the long-term outcome is unknown.

Even if the knee flexion contracture is straightened, how useful are the limbs? It is unclear how much passive knee motion can be obtained.

Faced with severe hip and knee flexion contractures in paralyzed limbs (frequently accompanied by foot deformities), some surgeons have elected amputation and prosthetic fitting for these children.

There is general agreement that the severe knee flexion contractures seen in some children with sacral agenesis can interfere not only with brace wear and standing but also with sitting and hand walking (14). Such severely affected children will probably not be functional ambulators as adults. The parents must be informed that the alternative to amputation is a *series* of procedures to maintain correction as the child grows. The aesthetics of preserving limbs of limited function should be weighed against the physical and emotional costs of repeated hospitalization and surgery. The "best" treatment may depend on the degree of deformity, the presence of other anomalies, the parents' concerns, and the medical resources available.

A combination of soft-tissue releases, supracondylar extension osteotomies, and serial casting will probably result in satisfactory correction of some knee contractures. Prolonged nighttime splinting is also needed (4). Recurrence with growth should be anticipated. If amputation is chosen, disarticulation at the knee is the recommended level of amputation. There is little need for subtrochanteric amputation as long as any hip flexion contracture is compensated for by increased motion at the spinal-pelvic junction. As the tibiae are a commonly used source of bone graft for spinal-pelvic fusion, arrangements to preserve the bones for later use should be considered.

Feet

The feet in children with sacral agenesis are often deformed. Clubfeet have been reported in up to 50% (22). Both equinovarus and calcaneocavus foot deformities have been reported.

The decision to correct foot deformities depends on what other lower-extremity anomalies are present and the ambulatory potential of the child. Conventional methods of managing paralytic foot deformities seem satisfactory. The presence of protective sensation makes both serial casting and orthotics less of a problem than in a similarly deformed child with myelomeningocele.

Hips

The decision to treat hip dislocation in sacral agenesis depends on the type of dislocation and the ambulatory potential of the child. Bilateral, paralytic hip dislocations in children with high-level sacral agenesis (Renshaw III and IV) probably do not need reduction. The occasional unilateral dislocation seen in lower level (Renshaw I and II) sacral agenesis can be managed much like a developmental dislocation in normal children. Richards's (48) caution about the Salter osteotomy and the potential for excessive motion at an abnormal sacroiliac joint should be kept in mind.

Other Problems

Occasionally, a child with sacral agenesis may present with a progressive neurologic deficit. In some but not all cases, the deficit has improved following surgical exploration and correction of an anatomical problem. Despite sporadic reports of neurologic improvement following surgical exploration of the spinal cord in sacral agenesis, routine exploration is probably not indicated. Most of these patients had developed symptoms of a progressive neurologic deficit, such as a limp, weakness, incontinence, or pain. Pang and Hoffman (37) recommended serial neurologic examinations with imaging of the spinal cord at the first sign of deterioration.

SUMMARY

Orthopedic management of a child with sacral agenesis will never be routine. The clinical picture can vary tremendously. Although intervention will alter the child, will it allow him or her to be a more functional person? Given what is currently known about the natural history of untreated adults with sacral agenesis, it is important to set realistic goals for each child, allowing him or her to lead as normal a life as possible.

REFERENCES

1. Abraham E (1979): Sacral agenesis with associated anomalies (caudal regression syndrome): autopsy case report. *Clin Orthop Rel Res* 145: 168–171.
2. Anderton JM, Owen R (1983): Absence of the pituitary gland in a case of congenital sacral agenesis. *J Bone Joint Surg Br* 65:182–183.
3. Andrish J, Kalamchi A, MacEwen GD (1979): Sacral agenesis: a clinical evaluation of its management, heredity, and associated anomalies. *Clin Orthop Rel Res* 139:52–57.
4. Banta JV, Nichols O (1969): Sacral agenesis. *J Bone Joint Surg Am* 51: 693–703.
5. Barkovich AJ, Raghavan N, Chuang S, et al. (1989): The wedge-shaped cord terminus: a radiographic sign of caudal regression. *Am J Neuroradiol* 10:1223–1231.
6. Blumel J, Evans EB, Eggers GWN (1959): Partial and complete agenesis or malformation of the sacrum with associated anomalies. *J Bone Joint Surg Am* 41:497–518.
7. Brem H, Beaver BL, Colombani PM, et al. (1989): Neonatal diagnosis of a presacral mass in the presence of congenital anal stenosis and partial sacral agenesis. *J Pediatr Surg* 24:1076–1078.
8. Bronsteen RA, Wolfe HM, Zador IE, et al. (1987): Topics in perinatal ultrasonography. *J Perinatol* 7:264–266.
9. Brooks BS, Gammal TE, Hartlage P, et al. (1981): Myelography of sacral agenesis. *Am J Neuroradiol* 2:319–323.
10. Carlo WA, Kliegman RM, Dixon MS, et al. (1982): Vertebral agenesis. *Am J Dis Child* 136:533–537.
11. Carson JA, Barnes PD, Tunell WP, et al. (1984): Imperforate anus: the neurologic implication of sacral abnormalities. *J Pediatr Surg* 19: 838–842.
12. Cerisoli M, Davidovits P, Giulioni M (1983): Sacral agenesis: usefulness of CT study. *J Neurosurg Sci* 27:261–264.
13. Cohn J, Bay-Nielsen E (1969): Hereditary defect of the sacrum and coccyx with anterior sacral meningocele. *Acta Paediatr Scand* 58: 268–274.
14. Dal Monte A, Andrisano A, Capanna R (1979): The surgical treatment of lumbosacral coccygeal agenesis. *Ital J Orthop Traumatol* 5:259–266.
15. Del Duca V, Davis V, Barroway JN (1951): Congenital absence of the sacrum and coccyx. *J Bone Joint Surg Am* 33:248–253.
16. Duhamel B (1961): From the mermaid to anal imperforation: the syndrome of caudal regression. *Arch Dis Child* 36:152–155.
17. Dumont C, Damsin J, Forin V, et al. (1993): Lumbosacral agenesis: three cases of reconstruction using Cotrel-Dubousset or L-rod instrumentation. *Spine* 18:1229–1235.
18. Duncan PA, Shapiro LR, Klein RM (1991): Sacrococcygeal dysgenesis association. *Am J Med Genet* 41:153–161.
19. Elting J, Allen JC (1972): Management of the young child with bilateral anomalous and functionless lower extremities. *J Bone Joint Surg Am* 54:1523–1530.
20. Fellous M, Boue J, Malbrunot C, et al. (1982): A five-generation family with sacral agenesis and spina bifida: possible similarities with the mouse T-locus. *Am J Med Genet* 12:465–487.
21. Frantz CH, Aitken GT (1967): Complete absence of the lumbar spine and sacrum. *J Bone Joint Surg Am* 49:1531–1540.
22. Freedman B (1950): Congenital absence of the sacrum and coccyx: report of a case and review of the literature. *Br J Surg* 37:299–303.
23. Guidera KJ, Raney E, Ogden JA, et al. (1991): Caudal regression: a review of seven cases, including the mermaid syndrome. *J Pediatr Orthop* 11:743–747.
24. Guzman L, Khoshbin S, Bauer SB, et al. (1983): Evaluation and management of children with sacral agenesis. *Urology* 12:506–510.
25. Hafeez M, Tihansky DP (1984): Intraspinal tumor with lumbosacral agenesis. *Am J Neuroradiol* 5:481–482.
26. Helin I, Pettersson H, Alton D (1983): Extensive spinal dysraphism and sacral agenesis without urologic disturbances. *Acta Radiol Diagn* 24:209–212.
27. Hohl AF (1852): *Zur Pathologie des Beckens. I. Das schrag-ovale Becken.* Leipzig: Wilhelm Engelmann, p. 61.
28. Hudson LP, Ramsay, DA (1993): Malformation of the lumbosacral spinal cord in a case of sacral agenesis. *Pediatr Pathol* 13:421–429.
29. Jones KL (1988): Caudal dysplasia sequence (caudal regression syndrome) and sirenomelia sequence. In: *Smith's recognizable patterns of human malformation.* Philadelphia: WB Saunders, pp. 574–575.
30. Kalter H (1993): Case reports of malformations associated with maternal diabetes: history and critique. *Clin Genet* 43:174–179.
31. Kenefick JS (1973): Hereditary sacral agenesis associated with presacral tumours. *Br J Surg* 60:271–274.
32. Lotan D, Hertz M, Aladjem M, et al. (1981): Sacral agenesis. *Isr J Med Sci* 17:437–440.
33. Mayfield JK (1981): Severe spinal deformity in myelodysplasia and sacral agenesis: an aggressive surgical approach. *Spine* 6:498–509.
34. Muthukumar N (1996): Surgical treatment of nonprogressive neuro-

logic deficits in children with sacral agenesis. *Neurosurgery* 38: 1133–1138.

35. Nichol WJ (1972): Lumbosacral agenesis in a 60-year-old man. *Br J Surg* 59:577–579.

36. O'Neill OR, Piatt JH, Mitchell P, et al. (1995): Agenesis and dysgenesis of the sacrum: neurosurgical implications. *Pediatr Neurosurg* 22:20–28.

37. Pang D, Hoffman HJ (1980): Sacral agenesis with progressive neurological deficit. *Neurosurgery* 7:118–126.

38. Pappas CTE, Seaver L, Carrion C, et al. (1989): Anatomical evaluation of the caudal regression syndrome (lumbosacral agenesis) with magnetic resonance imaging. *Neurosurgery* 25:462–465.

39. Passarge E (1966): Syndrome of caudal regression in infants of diabetic mothers: observations of further cases. *Pediatrics* 37:672–675.

40. Perrot LJ, Williamson S, Jimenez JF (1987): The caudal regression syndrome in infants of diabetic mothers. *Ann Clin Lab Sci* 17:211–220.

41. Perry J, Bonnett CA, Hoffer MM (1970): Vertebral pelvic fusions in the rehabilitation of patients with sacral agenesis. *J Bone Joint Surg Am* 52:288–294.

42. Phillips WA, Cooperman DR, Lindquist TC, et al. (1982): Orthopaedic management of lumbosacral agenesis. *J Bone Joint Surg Am* 64: 1282–1294.

43. Pierson PM, Faulon M, Vigneron J, et al. (1985): Conseil genetique et syndrome de regression caudale. *J Genet Hum* 33:405–418.

44. Raas-Rothschild A, Goodman RM, Grunbaum M, et al. (1988): Klippel-Feil anomaly with sacral agenesis: an additional subtype, Type IV. *J Craniofac Genet Dev Biol* 8:297–301.

45. Redhead RG, Vitali M, Trapnell DH (1968): Congenital absence of the lumbar spine. *BMJ* 3:595–596.

46. Reiger MA, Hall JE, Dalury DF (1990): Spinal fusion in a patient with lumbosacral agenesis. *Spine* 15:1382–1384.

47. Renshaw TS (1978): Sacral agenesis: a classification and review of twenty-three cases. *J Bone Joint Surg Am* 60:373–383.

48. Richards BS (1988): Partial sacral agenesis with congenital hip dislocation. *Orthopedics* 11:973–977.

49. Ruderman RJ, Keats P, Goldner JL (1977): Congenital absence of the lumbo-sacral spine: a report of an unusual case. *Clin Orthop Rel Res* 124:177–180.

50. Rusnak SL, Driscoll SG (1965): Congenital spinal anomalies in infants of diabetic mothers. *Pediatrics* 35:989–995.

51. Russell HE, Aitken GT (1963): Congenital absence of the sacrum and lumbar vertebrae with prosthetic management. *J Bone Joint Surg Am* 45:501–508.

52. Saint-Supery G, Wallon P, Bucco P, et al. (1985): A propos de 3 observations d'agenesie lombosacree, place de la greffe lombo-iliaque. *Chir Pediatr* 26:181–186.

53. Schrander-Stumpel C, Schrander J, Fryns J-P, et al. (1988): Caudal deficiency sequence in 7q terminal deletion. *Am J Med Genet* 30: 757–761.

54. Sonek JD, Gabbe SG, Landon MB, et al. (1990): Antenatal diagnosis of sacral agenesis syndrome in a pregnancy complicated by diabetes mellitus. *Am J Obstet Gynecol* 162:806–808.

55. Tihansky DP, Hafeez M (1984): Case report: CT findings in lumbosacral agenesis. *J Comput Tomogr* 8:325–329.

56. Welch JP, Aterman K (1984): The syndrome of caudal dysplasia: a review, including etiologic considerations and evidence of heterogeneity. *Pediatr Pathol* 2:313–327.

57. Williams DI, Nixon HH (1957): Agenesis of the sacrum. *Surg Gynecol Obstet* 105:84–88.

58. Winter RB (1991): Congenital absence of the lumbar spine and sacrum: one-stage reconstruction with subsequent two-stage spine lengthening. *J Pediatr Orthop* 11:666–670.

59. Yates VD, Wilroy RS, Whitington GL (1983): Anterior sacral defects: an autosomal dominantly inherited condition. *J Pediatr* 102:239–242.

CONGENITAL AND DEVELOPMENTAL SPINAL STENOSIS

MARK B. KABINS

Stenosis is defined as "the narrowing or stricture of a passage, duct or opening" (90). The effects of stenosis on any inner contents are caused by compression by two or more directly opposed forces (47). The term *spinal stenosis* has been elegantly demonstrated by Verbiest (164) to be ambiguous in that it does not identify the location, nature, or cause of the process. For general purposes, this chapter uses the definition of spinal stenosis established by Arnoldi et al. (4): any type of narrowing of the spinal canal, nerve root canals, or intervertebral foramina.

Spinal stenosis may occur locally or segmentally, or it may be generalized. It may be caused by bone or soft tissue, and the narrowing may involve the bony canal, the dural sac, or both. Furthermore, spinal stenosis may be absolute or relative, static or dynamic. Verbiest (162–167) stated that those with absolute stenosis may be symptomatic in the absence of additional stimuli or compressive forces. In other words, there is no remaining reserve capacity, which implies a noninterfered, physiologic space between the thecal sac and the surrounding bone and soft tissue (172). With relative stenosis, the reserve capacity is so small that minor additional compressive forces, such as a herniated disc, spondylosis, or disc space narrowing, may produce symptomatic stenosis. In fact, it has been suggested that individuals with reduced functional spinal reserve capacities may be potential occupational hazards (171). Clinically significant stenosis does not always occur as a static phenomenon but frequently occurs as part of a dynamic process (80).

Congenital stenosis, which occurs as a result of a congenital malformation, constitutes only a small subset of patients with spinal stenosis. Sarpyener (133,134) was one of the first to recognize and describe this entity in the thoracolumbar spine. He identified a "congenital stricture of the spinal canal" in patients with spina bifida occulta, spastic diplegia, clubfeet, enuresis, and/ or spastic or flaccid paralysis. He stated: "The narrowing of the bony canal compresses the cord, and, by the law of Delpech, prevents it from normal development." Our understanding of congenital stenosis has grown since then, but it remains limited.

Developmental stenosis, as described by Verbiest (159–161,164,166), is caused by a growth disturbance of the bony walls of the vertebral canal during the pre- and postnatal periods. Vertebral stenosis in patients with achondroplasia is an example of developmental stenosis.

CLASSIFICATION AND DEFINITIONS

In the past, the distinction between congenital and developmental stenosis was vague. In fact, some authors considered the terms to be synonymous. In 1976, Verbiest (164) limited the term *congenital stenosis* to cases of abnormally narrow spinal canals resulting from congenital malformation. Congenital stenosis of the thoracolumbar spine typically is identified in young children and infants, although it can be first identified in adults. It is often associated with spina bifida, failure of vertebral segmentation, congenital tumors in the lumbosacral region (most commonly, lipoma), diastematomyelia, gait abnormalities, enuresis, and developmental abnormalities of the hips, knees, and feet.

Developmental stenosis refers to a genetic disturbance of both fetal and postnatal development that usually continues until maturity. Periosteal apposition of bone that may occur after maturity is also included in the category of developmental stenosis.

Developmental stenosis may be idiopathic or part of a generalized growth disturbance, which is most frequently found in achondroplasia. *Idiopathic* implies that the cause of the condition is not known. Generalized growth disturbances typically occur as a result of an inherited chromosomal abnormality or a mutation.

Nightingale (99) has identified an association between cervical spine developmental canal stenosis and somatotype. Specifically, those with developmentally narrow cervical canals are more likely to have relatively shorter long-bones (particularly in the upper arms) and longer trunks.

Idiopathic developmental stenosis of the lumbar spine is typically identified later in life than congenital stenosis. Verbiest (164) reported that his youngest patient with idiopathic developmental stenosis was 22 years old, and that the average age at onset of symptoms was between 45 and 50 years. Associated musculoskeletal anomalies are rare, with the exception of coinciding idiopathic cervical stenosis.

Acquired spinal stenosis implies a process that occurs following birth that is caused by degenerative changes, trauma, or bone diseases or is iatrogenic in nature. Most cases of clinically

M. B. Kabins: Department of Orthopedics, University of Nevada Medical Center, Las Vegas, Nevada 89106.

significant stenosis that involve an acquired process likely have underlying idiopathic developmental stenosis. Verbiest (164, 167,168) and Schatzker and Pennal (135) suggested that spondylotic, traumatic, and iatrogenic stenoses likely represent processes occurring within a developmentally ("relative") stenotic canal, and that acquired processes alone seldom lead to clinically significant stenosis.

Porter et al. (121,124), Heliovaara et al. (55), and others (41,128,173) demonstrated that patients who present with symptomatic herniated discs generally have significantly smaller than normal spinal canals. Porter et al. (121,124), Ramani (128), and Winston et al. (173) reported significant differences in the midsagittal diameters in this group of patients. Surgical failures of patients with herniated discs frequently occur because of the presence of underlying developmental stenosis that has not been recognized. These patients frequently require a more extensive decompression rather than a nucleotomy or disc excision alone.

Porter et al. (118,121) stated that the risk of developing disabling symptoms from disc protrusion is inversely related to the size of the spinal canal, and that prophylactic measures in childhood may ultimately reduce morbidity in adulthood.

DEVELOPMENT OF THE VERTEBRAL CANAL

Vertebral bodies enlarge circumferentially through perichondral and periosteal apposition and grow vertically through endochondral ossification (103,104,109,174). The spine consists of anterior primary centers of ossification located within the vertebral body and posterior primary centers of ossification located within the posterior elements. The anterior ossification centers enlarge toward the posterior ossification centers, creating two obliquely oriented cartilaginous gaps, which are referred to as *neurocentral junctions.* Upon closure of the neurocentral junctions, canal expansion for the most part ceases. Thus, canal diameters tend to approximate adult size by 3 to 6 years of age, which is when the neurocentral junctions close.

Ogden (103,104) noted that some remodeling of the canal may occur later through the periosteum on the inner and outer surfaces of the posterior elements. Spinal stenosis may result from premature fusion of the synchondroses or from premature osseous fusion anteriorly or posteriorly. Disorders of endochondral ossification, such as that seen in achondroplasia and other forms of dwarfism, affect canal diameter and may ultimately lead to stenosis.

After studying 155 pediatric and 839 adult vertebrae, Porter (118) reported that individuals younger than 4 years had mean midsagittal diameters in the lumbar spine that were approximately 10% greater than those found in adults. This reduction in size with age is likely a reflection of the remodeling witnessed within the posterior portion of the vertebral body. The mean interpedicular diameter in pediatric vertebrae was reported to be approximately 85% of the adult size. This additional increase in interpedicular distance from early childhood to adulthood occurs through membranous bone formation with internal resorption and external deposition. Vertebrae located in the cephalad portion of the lumbar spine were found to mature earlier than the more caudal vertebrae. Radiographic studies (79,81)

have independently shown similar findings: interpedicular diameters increase until puberty, and growth in the lower lumbar spine continues after cessation of growth in the upper lumbar spine.

The shape of the lumbar spinal canal has also been shown to change with age. Porter et al. (118,120,123) demonstrated that the anterior vertebral borders of the lumbar canal—in particular those of L4 and L5—were generally concave in infancy and convex in adulthood. When convexity of the vertebral body occurred with continued widening of the interpedicular distance, the canal was molded into a trefoil configuration. Eisenstein (31,32) identified 15% of negroid and caucasoid skeletons as being trefoil in shape at L5. None of these changes was seen before puberty. However, the canal at L2 was shown to become dome-shaped with maturity.

The association between smaller vertebral canals and impairment of health and certain intellectual abilities has been demonstrated (122). Individuals with smaller vertebral canals have been found by association to have more cardiovascular and gastrointestinal symptoms along with fewer post-school qualifications. This may arise, in part, from adverse environmental factors that affect several growing systems prior to the age of 4 years. The smaller canal can be considered a marker of a more generalized developmental disturbance.

Porter et al. (121) also demonstrated that the lumbar canal in women was larger than that of men in age-matched individuals in a South Yorkshire population. They speculated that a larger canal would be advantageous during pregnancy, when the spine is subjected to altered mechanical forces and increased ligamentous laxity. They also showed that the canals of women contained more extradural fat than those of men.

Interpedicular distance typically widens as one proceeds down the lumbar spine. An unusual relative increase in interpedicular distance at a particular level should be considered a warning sign and may reflect the presence of an underlying neoplasm, dural ectasia, or dysraphism (60,109). In the cervical or thoracic spine, an unusually enlarged area of the canal may occur as a result of syringomyelia, hydromyelia, or Arnold-Chiari malformation (62).

In utero, the spinal canal develops partially in response to the underlying spinal cord. The spinal cord spans the length of the spinal canal in neonates. During childhood, particularly during the adolescent growth spurt, the vertebral bodies and their accompanying discs elongate at a faster rate than the spinal cord (103). The cord ultimately terminates in adults at the T12–L1 level. Unlike the midsagittal diameter of the spinal canal, the midsagittal diameter of the spinal cord varies little among individuals (20,33,100), depending on sex (15) and age, and is not dependent on body habitus.

RADIOGRAPHIC ANALYSIS

Determination of spinal canal size to identify stenosis can be accomplished through various imaging techniques.

Plain radiography is used most frequently to screen for spinal abnormalities and stenosis. Interpretation of plain films is highly dependent on the radiographic and measurement techniques.

Plain radiographic measurements are affected by gantry-to-patient distance, patient-to-grid distance, angulation, and patient position. Standardization of technique and knowledge of the technique used when interpreting such films are critical in maximizing the reliability and validity of measurements. In the cervical spine, the most commonly used focus-grid distance measures 183 cm (72 in.) (17,33,112,177); in the lumbar spine, the standard focus-grid distance measures 101.6 cm (40 in) (61,83).

When assessing for stenosis by plain radiography, it is important to first recognize the normal values (means and ranges) of various measurements. Many authors have studied and published their findings (Table 1) (53,54,57,60–62,88,96,138). This information is helpful as a reference when screening patients, but only when using radiographic measuring techniques and focus-grid distances identical to those used for comparison.

Many techniques for measuring canal size and determining the presence of stenosis through the use of lateral radiographs have been described. Kessler (72) believes that the lateral view of the cervical spine is the most critical for measurement and identification of stenosis. In the cervical spine, canal size is usually measured from the posterior aspect of the vertebral body at the midpoint between the superior and inferior end plates to the nearest point of the radiopaque line marking the inner aspect of the lamina directly under the spinous process (developmental segmental sagittal diameter) (28,29,62,88). The spondylotic segmental sagittal diameter is also directly measured from the lateral radiograph (Fig. 1A). The adult developmental sagittal canal diameter between C2 and C7, with a target distance of 183 cm, has been shown to average 17 ± 5 mm. Using the same target distance and measuring techniques, Epstein et al. (36,37) and Countee and Vijayanathan (17) reported severe spinal stenosis at less than 13 and 14 mm, respectively. According to Kessler (72), subaxial values under 14 mm were below the standard deviation for any cervical segment and were associated with myelopathy and neurapraxic symptoms. The cervical spinal cord is widest at the midcervical level (C4–C5), with a maximum sagit-

tal diameter in the adult of 10 mm (10,20,130,177). Unfortunately, the spinal canal is narrowest at C4, followed by C5 (67).

Pavlov's ratio (111,148–150) (Fig. 1B) compensates for variations in radiographic technique because the sagittal diameters of the canal and the vertebral body are similarly affected by magnification. Generally, this ratio is a more reliable indicator of cervical stenosis than absolute measurements made by plain lateral radiographs. There is normally a 1:1 relationship between the sagittal diameter of the spinal canal and that of the vertebral body. Using a cutoff ratio of 0.82, Pavlov et al. (111) showed that this method was more than 2.5 times more sensitive than direct measuring techniques and that the ratio method was a more specific indicator of spinal stenosis. A Pavlov ratio of 0.80 or less has been shown to have a high sensitivity (93%) for transient neurapraxia (151). However, the low positive predictive value of the ratio (0.2%) precludes its use as a screening mechanism for determining the suitability of an athlete for participation in contact sports.

Odor et al. (102) found contrast-enhanced computed tomography (CT) to be more accurate in the detection of cervical stenosis than the Pavlov ratio method. They evaluated 34 adult cervical spines (139 levels) from symptomatic patients using both methods. At all levels where the ratio method was less than or equal to 0.80, contrast-enhanced CT measured midsagittal diameters to be 10 mm or less. Although the ratio method proved highly specific, it demonstrated a 19% false-negative rate in detecting cervical spinal stenosis.

Using myelography, Nurick (101) and others have studied the measurements of intrathecal contrast in the cervical spine and have defined critical stenosis as a measurement equal to or less than 10 to 12 mm. Nakstad (97) reported that a quotient of less than 0.9 between the sagittal diameter of the spinal canal, as determined through myelography, and the midsagittal diameter of the vertebral body was indicative of stenosis in the cervical spine.

Plain lateral radiographs are not as helpful in the lumbar

TABLE 1. SAGITTAL DIAMETER OF THE BONY CERVICAL SPINAL CANAL IN 120 NORMAL CHILDREN: RELATION TO AGE

Age group Sex n	3–6 years			7–10 years			11–14 years		
	Boys 20 Mean mm	Girls 20 Mean mm	Total 40 Mean/SD mm	Boys 20 Mean mm	Girls 20 Mean mm	Total 40 Mean/SD mm	Boys 20 Mean mm	Girls 20 Mean mm	Total 40 Mean/SD mm
C1	20.2	19.6	19.9 ± 1.3	20.5	20.6	20.6 ± 1.3	21.2	21.4	21.3 ± 1.4
C2	18.2	17.6	17.9 ± 1.3	18.8	18.9	18.8 ± 1.0	19.3	19.5	19.4 ± 1.1
C3	16.3	15.8	16.0 ± 1.3	17.3	17.2	17.2 ± 1.0	17.8	17.7	17.8 ± 1.0
C4	16.0	15.6	15.8 ± 1.3	17.0	16.9	16.9 ± 0.9	17.3	17.2	17.3 ± 0.9
C5	15.9	15.5	15.7 ± 1.3	16.7	16.6	16.7 ± 0.9	17.1	16.9	17.0 ± 0.9
C6	15.8	15.3	15.6 ± 1.2	16.5	16.3	16.4 ± 0.9	16.8	16.6	16.7 ± 0.9
C7	15.6	15.0	15.3 ± 1.1	16.1	15.9	16.0 ± 0.9	16.3	16.2	16.2 ± 0.9

These data are based on studies of lateral radiographs of the cervical spine measured from the middle of the posterior surface of the vertebral body to the nearest point on the ventral line of the cortex seen at the junction of the spinous process and lamina. The radiographs were taken with patients standing erect and their necks in the neutral position. The focus-film distance was 150 cm (59.05 in.). (Data from Hensinger RN, ed. *Standards in pediatric orthopedics. Tables, charts, and graphs illustrating growth.* New York: Raven Press, 1986; and Markuske H, ed. Sagittal diameter measurement of the bony cervical spinal canal in children. *Pediatr Radiol* 1927;6:129–131.)

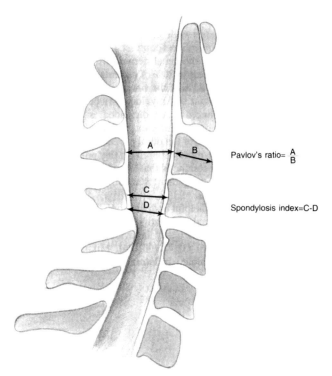

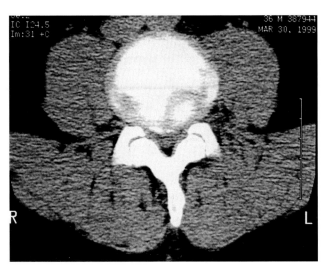

FIGURE 2. Axial lumbar CT scan of a symptomatic 36-year-old man with underlying developmental stenosis and small disc protrusion.

FIGURE 1. **(a)** The cervical developmental segmental sagittal diameter (DSSD) *C,* and the spondylotic segmental sagittal diameter (SSSD) *D,* are illustrated. Using standard lateral radiographic techniques and a focal-grid distance of 72 in., perpendicular lines are drawn to the posterior margin of the spinal canal at the level of the pedicular-vertebral body junction and at the level of the disc space. The difference between the two measurements is the spondylosis index and represents stenosis due to degenerative disease. (From Epstein JA, Carras R, Hyman RA (1979): Cervical myelopathy caused by developmental stenosis of the spinal canal. *J Neurosurg* 15:489–496; Epstein JA, Carras R, Rerrar J, et al. (1982): Conjoined lumbosacral nerve roots. Management of herniated discs and lateral recess stenosis in patients with this anomaly. *J Neurosurg* 55:585–589. Redrawn with permission.) **(b)** The ratio of the spinal canal *A,* to the vertebral body *B,* equals Pavlov's ratio. The vertebral body is measured from the midpoint of the anterior and posterior vertebral body, and the canal is measured from the midpoint of the posterior aspect of the vertebral body to the nearest point on the spinolaminar line. A ratio of less than 0.80 is indicative of stenosis. (From Torg JS, Pavlov H, Warren R, et al. (1991): The relationship of cervical spinal canal narrowing (stenosis) to permanent neurological injury to the athlete: an epidemiological survey. *Proceedings of the sixth annual meeting of the Federation of Spine Association.* Redrawn with permission.)

spine in the screening for stenosis (108). Myelography is the radiologist's gold standard in the diagnosis of spinal stenosis. Bolender et al. (9) reported better accuracy in the diagnosis of lumbar stenosis with myelography, in comparison to CT without intrathecal contrast. They reported that the dimensions of the canal derived from CT provided a correct diagnosis in 20% of patients, and myelography was accurate 83% of the time.

It is important that myelography be performed with the subarachnoid space distended, such as with the patient standing. Since extension of the spine decreases the size of the dural sac, milder degrees of stenosis may be more apparent in this position (142).

CT is most helpful in delineating the bony shape and size

of the canal (24,33,82,166) (Fig. 2). Mikhael et al. (91) used CT to evaluate the lateral recesses in symptomatic and asymptomatic patients. They reported that normal lateral recesses decreased in size from L2 to S1. Symptomatic lateral recess stenosis occurred most often at the L5–S1 level. Lateral recess depth of 3 mm or less was likely to be associated with symptoms.

Magnetic resonance imaging (MRI) (52,132) is helpful in identifying thecal sac and nerve root impingement, cord abnormalities (e.g., hydromyelia, Arnold-Chiari malformation, syringomyelia, tethered cord), degenerative changes, and disc herniations, but it does not demonstrate the surrounding bony structures as well as CT does.

Ultrasonography is a noninvasive, safe, and relatively inexpensive and accurate way for evaluating canal dimensions (34). Intraoperative sonography can be valuable in assessing the degree of neural compression in up to 90% of patients. (112) Intraoperative sonography may be used to diagnose calcified posterior longitudinal ligaments, spinal cord atrophy, myelomalacia, herniated discs, and osteophytes at all levels in the spine.

CONGENITAL AND DEVELOPMENTAL STENOSIS BY LOCATION AND TYPE

Cervicomedullary Junction and Rostral Cervical Spine

Brain stem and upper cord stenosis can occur as a result of congenital abnormalities. This may occur due to static forces, such as basilar impression, narrowing of the foramen magnum, elevation of the dens, shortening of the clivus, invagination of the occipital condyles, and elevation of the petrous pyramids, or dynamic forces, such as instability associated with os odontoideum and absence of the dens. Developmental atlantoaxial instability may also be found in patients with Down syndrome, spinal epiphyseal dysplasia, Larson syndrome, Morquio syndrome, osteogenesis imperfecta, and neurofibromatosis.

Congenital basilar impression occurs as a result of the failure of formation (or fusion) of the occipital somites. It is often associated with other vertebral defects, including unilateral or bilateral atlantooccipital fusion (181), hypoplasia of the atlas, bifid posterior arch of the atlas, odontoid abnormalities, and Klippel-Feil syndrome (58). Occipital hypoplasia is frequently associated with other congenital malformations of the base of the skull, cervical spine, and brain stem. Narrowing of the foramen magnum is also associated with the presence of accessory occipital vertebrae, which have been found to occur unilaterally and bilaterally.

Bony anomalies of the cervicomedullary junction are not necessarily associated with anomalies of the nervous system. However, Arnold-Chiari malformation, syringomyelia, and hydromyelia are often associated with these bony anomalies (181).

Developmental stenosis of the foramen magnum has been shown to occur in patients with achondroplasia. The foramen magnum is narrowed through hypertrophy of its bony rim. This is frequently accompanied by hypoplasia of the clivus and basilar impression and occasionally by stenosis of the remaining cervical spine. Together these findings produce kinking at the junction of the brain stem and the cord. Although patients with achondroplasia and thoracolumbar stenosis typically present in adulthood, those with significant stenosis of the foramen magnum usually present in infancy. Yamada et al. (179) reported respiratory insufficiency, quadriparesis, and a high rate of mortality in patients with achondroplasia and stenosis of the foramen magnum. Patients typically respond to foramen magnum decompression.

Hypoplasia of the completed posterior arch of C1 (114) has been identified in Asians. It creates congenital stenosis that becomes increasingly symptomatic with age and advancement of degenerative disease. Effective surgical intervention consists of removal of the shortened posterior C1 arch and surrounding degenerative ligaments.

Prakash et al. (126) first identified localized spinal stenosis as a cause of myelopathy due to developmental hypertrophy of the posterior neural arch of C2. The cause was likely premature fusion of the posterior cartilaginous neurocentral synchondrosis. Decompression with laminectomy alleviated symptoms.

Congenital malformations of the dens may also lead to stenosis (140). Duplication of the dens occurs secondary to an abnormality in segmentation and frequently presents with torticollis. Condylicus tertius syndrome may be diagnosed when a large abnormal dens is found to articulate with the third occipital condyle on the anterior rim of the foramen magnum. Cord compression occurs at the level of the narrowed foramen magnum.

Idiopathic Developmental Cervical Stenosis

Heightened awareness of idiopathic developmental cervical stenosis, particularly among adolescents and young adults, arose in the mid-1980s following the historic publications of Torg et al. (152) and Ladd and Scranton (78), in which they described the presence of neurapraxia of the spinal cord with transient quadriplegia in football players with developmental cervical stenosis.

Prior to this, Payne and Spillane (112) reported the association of myelopathy in patients with developmental cervical stenosis and recognized that spondylosis and degenerative disc disease were confounding factors. Symptomatic idiopathic stenosis was recognized to occur primarily in older boys. In 1970, Moiel et al. (92) reported a case of an 18-year-old individual with developmental stenosis (without spondylosis) who developed a central cord syndrome following a hyperextension injury. Grant and Puffer (49) subsequently reported a case of quadriparesis in an 18-year-old with developmental stenosis. This patient's canal reportedly measured 13 mm from C4 to C6. In 1979, Countee and Vijayanathan (17) described an association between quadriplegia following traumatic events and underlying idiopathic developmental stenosis. This was found to occur primarily in black males with cervical canal diameters of 14 mm or less. The association of developmental cervical stenosis with an increased risk of spinal cord injury was also reported by Epstein et al. (42) in 1980 and Eismont et al. (33) in 1984.

In a retrospective review, Epstein et al. (42) reported 23 patients with cervical spinal stenosis and traumatic myelopathy without evidence of fracture or dislocation. Plain radiographs and myelography demonstrated 7 patients to have "absolute" developmental stenosis without evidence of degenerative changes. The remaining 16 patients had degenerative changes along with "relative" stenosis. Absolute stenosis was defined as a canal diameter of less than 10 mm, measured on lateral films from the posterior aspect of the vertebral body to the posterior laminar line. Relative stenosis measured less than 13 mm, using the prominent vertebral osteophytes as the anterior landmark. Patients with narrower canals presented with more severe myelopathies. When stenosis is severe, any additional pressure, swelling, and/or edema from trauma may cause neurologic catastrophe (46). The neurologic level of injury most frequently occurs between C4 and C6.

Eismont et al. (33) examined 98 patients with fracture dislocations of the cervical spine. Forty-five patients demonstrated no neurologic deficit, 39 had incomplete quadriplegia, and 14 had complete quadriplegia. The greatest percentage of neurologic deficits occurred between C4 and C6. Patients with small sagittal diameters, as evaluated by plain lateral radiographs, were significantly more likely to have neurologic deficits (Fig. 3); patients with larger canals were more likely to be spared neurologic injury. This finding was not surprising because the midsagittal diameter of the canal varies between individuals (15,33, 112,177), unlike that of the spinal cord, which does not vary significantly (20,100).

Later, Torg et al. (152) and Ladd and Scranton (78) described 19 (17 and 2, respectively) patients with developmental cervical stenosis who sustained spinal cord neurapraxia and transient quadriplegia. Torg also reported similar presentations in patients with failure of segmentation of the cervical spine, diffuse idiopathic skeletal hyperostosis, instability, and intervertebral disc disease. They theorized that spinal cord neurapraxia occurred because of narrowing of the anteroposterior diameter of the spinal canal with or without concomitant degenerative changes, herniated discs, posttraumatic instability, or congenital anomalies. All but three of the patients sustained their injuries while playing football. All patients were male and ranged in age from

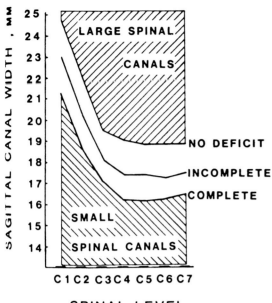

FIGURE 3. Ninety-eight patients suffered cervical spine fracture-dislocations. The area labeled "large spinal canals" represents patients with midsagittal canal diameters larger than the mean and without neurologic injury. The area labeled "small cervical canals" represents patients with midsagittal diameters less than the mean and with complete neurologic deficit. (From Eismont FJ, Clifford S, Goldberg M, et al. (1984): Cervical sagittal canal size in spine injury. *Spine* 9:663–666, with permission.)

15 to 32 years. The mechanism of injury was thought to be hyperextension in eight cases, hyperflexion in six cases, and axial loading in five cases.

It has been shown that patients with cervical stenosis are particularly at risk during hyperextension (113,152). Hyperextension leads to infolding and thickening of the ligamentum flavum and posterior longitudinal ligament, resulting in further canal compromise (1,14,147). Hyperextension in addition to hyperflexion may lead to further canal compromise by as a result of "pinching" of the cord between the vertebral body and the lamina of the adjacent level. Penning (113) demonstrated this through measurement of plain lateral radiographs in varying degrees of flexion and extension. He described the "pincer mechanism," whereby the cord is pinched between the inferior portion of the superior vertebral body and the closest point on the spinolaminar line of the inferior vertebra in hyperextension, and between the superior portion of the inferior vertebral body and the closest point on the spinolaminar line of the superior vertebra in hyperflexion. He stated that pinching was dependent on underlying (developmental) stenosis, the extent of flexion and extension, and the size of underlying degenerative osteophytes. Sagittal diameters of less than 11 mm in extreme ranges of motion represented an increased risk for spinal cord compression. The cord in the spondylitic spine has also been shown to move in the rostral and caudal direction by as much as 3 mm at the C7 level during flexion and extension, thus angulating the nerve roots at their foramina (14).

Patients with neurapraxia of the spinal cord can experience burning pain, paresthesias, numbness, anesthesia, motor weakness, or even complete quadriplegia (78,148,152). Symptoms may be present in the upper extremities, lower extremities, or all four extremities. Except for burning paresthesias, pain in the neck is not usually present at the time of injury. These episodes are temporary, and recovery usually occurs in 10 to 15 minutes; sometimes there may be gradual resolution of symptoms over 36 to 48 hours. Motor function returns completely, and full, pain-free motion of the cervical spine usually ensues. Motor and sensory function at times returns in a cephalad to caudad direction. Routine radiographs usually show no evidence of fracture or dislocation.

The incidence of transient paresthesias in all four extremities with quadriplegia has been reported to be 1.3 per 10,000 athletes in a survey of 503 schools (39,377 participants) in the National Collegiate Athletic Association. Six per 10,000 reported transient paresthesias in all four extremities (152).

Because of anthropomorphic differences, asymptomatic football players demonstrate somewhat smaller Pavlov ratios, and players who experience cervical cord neurapraxia demonstrate significantly ($P < .001$) smaller Pavlov ratios than their asymptomatic controls (153).

Individuals with cervical canal narrowing, defined as a Pavlov ratio of less than 0.8, are no more susceptible to permanent neurologic injury than individuals in the general population and should not be precluded from participating in contact sports if symptoms of spinal cord neurapraxia are absent (152). According to Torg et al. (148–150), even neurapraxia of the spinal cord does not predispose individuals to permanent neurologic injury, and patients with developmental stenosis or failure of segmentation should be managed on an individual basis. None of the original 17 patients with transient quadriplegia and developmental stenosis later developed permanent neurologic injury. Nine abandoned football after one episode; three resumed playing temporarily and later gave it up after experiencing a second episode. One patient returned to football and, despite a second episode, went on to play for 3 years without additional difficulties; three returned without any problems at 2 years follow-up. A professional boxer received a laminectomy following two episodes of transient quadriplegia and continued to box without problems at 5 years follow-up.

One hundred seventeen football players with permanent quadriplegia were studied separately to determine the occurrence of antecedent cord symptoms (153). None had experienced a previous motor event, and only one had experienced a previous sensory event before the catastrophic injury.

Torg et al. (150) recently reviewed 110 cases of transient cervical cord neurapraxia. They concluded that in uncomplicated cases, patients may return to their previous activities without increased risk of permanent neurologic injury; congenital or developmental narrowing of the sagittal diameter was a causative factor; the recurrence rate after return to play was 56%; and the risk of recurrence was strongly and inversely correlated with sagittal canal diameter and was predictive of future episodes of cervical cord neurapraxia.

Torg et al. (148,152,149,154) specifically recommend that patients with developmental stenosis and concomitant instability, intervertebral disc disease with cord compression, MRI evidence of cord defect or swelling, symptoms of positive neurologic findings lasting more than 36 hours, more than one recurrence, and/or acute or chronic degenerative changes not be allowed to participate in contact sports. He later described a clinical entity called the "spear tacklers spine" (155). This constituted an absolute contraindication to participation in football. These individuals had developmental cervical stenosis, persistent straightening or curve reversal of the cervical spine, preexisting posttraumatic radiographic abnormalities, and employment of the spear tackler's technique.

In contrast, Ladd and Scranton (78) believe that a potentially dangerous situation may arise if any individual with developmental cervical stenosis is permitted to participate in contact sports. They found that stenosis was present in a large percentage of athletes with neck injuries that resulted in permanent neurologic deficit, including quadriplegia and death (personal communication).

Edwards and LaRocca (28,29) demonstrated that clinical symptoms in patients with degenerative spondylosis of the cervical spine were related to the underlying (developmental) size of the canal. They measured the cervical developmental sagittal diameter and the spondylotic segmental sagittal diameter from C4 to C7 in 63 symptomatic patients and calculated the spondylosis index (Fig. 1A). Patients were labeled as having narrow (C5 < 17 mm) or wide (C5 ≥ 17 mm) cervical canals. Symptomatic patients with narrow canals had a spondylosis index averaging 2.08 mm per segment, and those with wide canals had a spondylosis index averaging 3.29 mm. Myelopathic patients presented with average midcervical (developmental) canal diameters of 11.7 mm per segment, with 2.43 mm of additional degenerative (spondylosis index) narrowing per segment. Premyelopathic patients had developmental midcervical canal diameters from 10 to 13 mm, with a spondylosis index of 2 to 4 mm. Patients with canals measuring 13 to 17 mm were reported to be less likely to present with myelopathy but may be prone to symptomatic cervical spondylosis. Patients with canal (developmental) diameters greater than 17 mm were believed to be less likely to develop symptomatic cervical spondylosis. They concluded that larger midcervical (developmental) diameters may enable a patient to better tolerate degenerative disease with fewer or no symptoms.

Ogino et al. (105) studied spinal cord destruction in nine cadaveric specimens with cervical spondylotic myelopathy. The degree of spinal cord destruction correlated well with the ratio of anteroposterior diameter to transverse diameter. Of the factors responsible for a decrease in the ratio, developmental narrowing of the spinal canal was the most significant; multiplicity of spondylotic protrusion was less so. Developmental narrowing resulted in extensive demyelination of the posterolateral funiculus and infarction of the gray matter. Recurrent trauma also caused distinct manifestations and cord pathology.

Combined Developmental Cervicolumbar Stenosis

Combined cervical and lumbar developmental stenosis (without spondylosis or disc injury) has been reported (156) in young, symptomatic patients. Clinical manifestations include back pain,

intermittent claudication, polyradiculopathy, and myelopathy. The additive effects of irritation to both the spinothalamic tract at the cervical level and the nerve roots at the lumbar level probably lead to the early onset of symptoms. Cervical cord compression alone has been reported to cause symptoms in the lumbar region (18,43). Surgical decompression for symptomatic combined cervical and lumbar stenosis can be performed under a single anesthetic (156) or staged.

Klippel-Feil Syndrome

Although most patients with Klippel-Feil syndrome have normal or enlarged canals, several authors have described patients with Klippel-Feil syndrome and congenitally narrow canals (35,37, 42,112,116,127,132) (Fig. 4). Patients with congenital cervical fusions are also at increased risk of developing spondylosis and hypermobility at adjacent segments (50,58,115,127,132). These conditions alone or in combination may lead to the development of radiculopathy, myelopathy, or sudden quadriplegia.

Patients may not reveal their symptoms until directly questioned (50,132). They may experience episodic weakness, paresthesias, pain in the upper or lower extremities, or bowel or bladder dysfunction. Case reports of sudden quadriplegia after minor trauma have also been described. For example, Strax and Baran

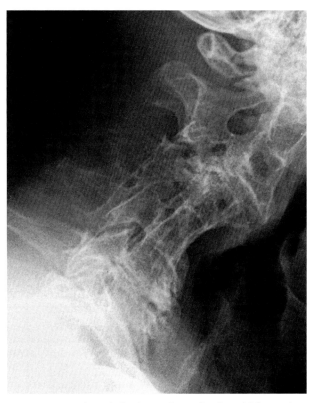

FIGURE 4. Lateral cervical spine radiograph of a middle-aged man with Klippel-Feil syndrome. The second cervical vertebra is dysplastic and C3–C4–C5 are nonsegmented. Note the instability at the C2–3 level and the spondylosis adjacent to the fused segments. This patient presented with radiculopathy and myelopathy due to underlying congenital and developmental stenosis.

(146) described a 13-year-old boy with Klippel-Feil syndrome who fell out of bed attempting to silence an alarm clock and became quadriplegic. A male with Klippel-Feil syndrome who became quadriplegic following a whiplash injury in an automobile accident was also described. Elster (35) described a patient with Klippel-Feil syndrome who became quadriplegic following a fall onto the back of his head. The coexistence of congenital stenosis with hypermobility (instability) in patients with Klippel-Feil syndrome is potentially hazardous and may predispose them to quadriplegia following minor trauma (127).

Congenital stenosis may occur at one or more segments. It may occur at, above, or, more typically, below the level of the congenital fusion (132). Patients may have "absolute" (midsagittal diameter ≤ 10 mm) or "relative" (midsagittal diameter between 10 and 13 mm) stenosis (42,127). The unlikely coexistence of spinal cord neoplasms [e.g., multiple intradural meningiomas (65)] should also be considered when evaluating symptomatic patients with Klippel-Feil syndrome.

Pizzutillo et al. (116) examined lateral cervical spine radiographs of 81 patients between 3 and 14 years of age with Klippel-Feil syndrome. Sagittal diameters were measured and compared with both control groups and previously published norms. Significant narrowing was detected at unfused levels, which included C1, C3, and C4.

Prusick et al. (127) described a 23-year-old patient with Klippel-Feil syndrome and failure of segmentation at C2–C3. This patient demonstrated an elliptically shaped and eccentrically positioned stenotic canal from C3 to the upper thoracic spine on myelography and CT. Following laminoplasty from C4 to C7, the patient's neck and back pain improved, and her radiculopathy resolved.

Dynamic MRI studies in flexion and extension may also be helpful in delineating the site of pathology and identifying the mechanism by which neurologic compression occurs. Ritterbusch et al. (132) examined 20 pediatric Klippel-Feil patients ranging in age from 3 to 20 using MRI. They identified five (25%) with instability and five (25%) with stenosis (canal diameter of 9 mm or less below C1). Three (12%) cord abnormalities were identified, including hydromyelia with Arnold-Chiari malformation in one and diplomyelia in two.

The above reports clearly document that stenosis occurs in pediatric patients with Klippel-Feil syndrome. Previous notions that the diameters of the spinal canal were normal, and that stenosis and subluxation were events of adult life secondary to degenerative changes and hypermobility, are incorrect (35).

It is the author's opinion that patients with Klippel-Feil syndrome should be screened for underlying stenosis and instability through plain radiographic examinations that include lateral flexion and extension views. Disastrous complications can occur if these findings go unrecognized. Patients with congenital scoliosis and kyphosis are at increased risk (25%) of having associated segmentation defects of the cervical spine (58,115,174). They should also be screened with lateral radiographs of the cervical spine.

Segmental Spinal Dysgenesis

Segmental spinal dysgenesis is a localized congenital defect in which severe stenosis occurs with malalignment and focal agenesis or dysgenesis in the thoracolumbar or lumbar spine (139,175,176). Patients may be neurologically intact or they may have complete paraplegia. Generally, neurologic deficits occur at the cord or root level and are usually present at birth. Patients may have congenital absence of roots or segments of the spinal cord. However, patients with associated instability due to progressive kyphosis and/or scoliosis can develop additional neurologic deficits in childhood and adulthood. Lower limb deformities, such as congenital talipes equinovarus, occasionally accompany this syndrome. The canal above and below the involved segment is usually normal. The sacrum is also well formed, differentiating this syndrome from sacral agenesis. Additional congenital deformities, including heart disease, may be present.

Several authors have described patients with this syndrome using various names, including "congenital stricture of the spinal canal" (133,134), "congenital kyphosis" (26,94), "congenital kyphosis and subluxation" (84), and "congenital duplication of the spinal canal" (89).

Sarpyener (133,134) was one of the first to describe patients with this syndrome. Strictures occurred with and without concomitant spina bifida. He classified patients in four categories. The first group consisted of patients with "ring constriction" of the cord at one or more levels. These patients typically had neurogenic bladders (enuresis). Laminectomy readily improved symptoms within a few hours after surgery. The second group consisted of patients with more extensive regional strictures, which were usually associated with spastic paralysis. The third group consisted of those with localized strictures causing paralysis of certain groups of muscles. This was associated with and thought to be responsible for clubfoot formation. The fourth group consisted of atypical cases with clefts in the cord and occasionally in the dura.

Initially, Winter et al. (175) referred to this syndrome as "congenital spinal stenosis," because nine patients presented with focal narrowing of the spinal canal in both the sagittal and frontal diameters. This localized area of canal stenosis occurred at the lower thoracic and upper lumbar spine. It was commonly, but not always, part of a congenital scoliosis or kyphosis. Congenital absence of one or more vertebral segments was typical. They reported that CT scans and myelography were helpful in diagnosis.

In 1988, Scott et al. (139) named this entity "segmental spinal dysgenesis." They described three children with this syndrome, all of whom demonstrated failure of formation, spinal dysraphism, and spinal cord tethering. In neonatal cases, ultrasonography was extremely helpful in demonstrating the absence of the dorsal bony elements, the anatomy of the thecal sac at and adjacent to the area of maximal involvement, and the presence of a low-lying conus.

Winter et al. (175) later described 20 additional patients with this syndrome. Localized spinal stenosis was a universal finding, thus explaining their original name for this syndrome. The stenotic area typically extended three vertebral segments but could be as long as six. Patients presented from birth to 19 years of age, with the majority between 1 and 4 years old. Most deformities were at the thoracolumbar junction, but two patients had deformities in the upper thoracic spine, and one had a deformity that extended as far caudad as L4. Kyphosis at the level of stenosis was seen in 12 patients (60%) and ranged from 10 degrees to 87 degrees. Five (25%) had concomitant sagittal plane subluxation, and three (15%) had frontal plane subluxation. Scoliosis ranging from 10 degrees to 71 degrees was identified in eight patients (40%). Three patients were reported to have ribs at the level of the lesion that crossed in front of the vertebral bodies from one hemithorax to the other. The neurologic status was normal in four patients, neurogenic bladders were present in two, and the remainder had varying degrees of motor weakness. The spinal cord itself was usually much smaller than normal, especially in those with neurologic deficits.

The cause of this process is unknown. No genetic explanations, history of exposure to toxic agents, or maternal illnesses (such as diabetes) have been identified. Scott et al. (139) stated that the cause of these anomalies appears to be "embryological segmental maldevelopment."

Surgical decompression may be helpful in patients with partially functioning nerve roots and spinal cords. According to Scott et al. (139), surgical decompression may be indicated in children when neurologic function is preserved below the level of the anomaly and when significant compression of the spinal cord can be demonstrated by myelography. However, stability would be further compromised with decompression alone, and fusion and bracing would also be required.

Clearly, patient management must be individualized. Fusion should be performed whenever conservative measures, such as bracing, fail to prevent progression of instability at the dysgenic site. Progressive neurologic deficit caused by tethering of the spinal cord or instability requires immediate attention. An appropriately performed release, decompression, and/or combined anterior and posterior fusion is advised.

Winter et al. (176) reported that they could not bring about improvement in children born with neurologic deficit by decompression of the canal. They were, however, able to reverse worsening paraparesis in an adolescent with progressive spinal deformity through a posterolateral spinal cord transposition as well as an anterior and posterior spinal fusion.

Other Forms of Congenital Stenosis of the Lumbar Spine

Congenital stenosis of the lumbar spine without accompanying malformations is rare (19). Symptoms may present at any time. Verbiest (164,165) described four patients whose first symptoms appeared between ages 45 and 50. Two patients had block vertebrae (failure of segmentation) with hypoplastic articulations, and the remainder had occult dysraphism with upward-directed lamina, paramedial clefts, and narrowed interpedicular diameters.

Verbiest (168) also described an unusual form of congenital intermittent stenosis in which the S1 lamina is absent and the posterior spinous process of L5 is enlarged, hooked downward, and possibly connected to a rudimentary spinous process of S1. Patients were symptomatic in the upright standing position as lordosis increased and the spinous process of L5 and the rudimentary process of S1 compressed the canal through the sacral cleft at S1. Symptoms were relieved with flexion of the lumbar

spine. Symptoms resolved following resection of the spinous process.

Borkow and Kleiger (11) reported a case of spondylolisthesis at the L4–L5 level in a newborn. This patient likely had congenital stenosis, as the vertebral body and canal at L5 were smaller than the vertebrae cephalad to L4. This neurologically intact patient developed a lumbar kyphotic deformity. Fusion was performed posteriorly from L3 to S1, and the patient did well postoperatively without a decompression.

Conjoined nerve roots have been reported to occur in 1% to 2% of the population (38). These patients are predisposed to symptoms of stenosis and suffer a greater risk of becoming symptomatic due to small disc protrusions, subarticular narrowing, and disc space narrowing (38,56).

Idiopathic Developmental Lumbar Stenosis

Developmental stenosis is usually uniform and involves the entire lumbar spine. However, it also may be isolated, involving the L2–L3 or L4–L5 segments (12), or it may be associated with developmental stenosis of the cervical spine (29,43). The sagittal canal diameter is frequently narrowed, yet the interpedicular diameter is usually not significantly affected (12,22,31,32,119,123,135,161,163,166,167).

Verbiest (168) reported similarities between patients with idiopathic developmental stenosis and those with stenosis associated with achondroplasia, in that scalloping (posterior lipping) of the vertebral bodies occurs above the L4 level, disc herniations are common, and hypertrophy of the vertebral arches can occur. Hypertrophy is usually limited to the posterior bony column of the spine (163,166). Prior to the onset of degenerative changes, the ligamentum flavum does not typically increase in thickness or hypertrophy (161). The laminae may be enlarged, which results in a decrease of the interlaminar space. In fact, the laminae may become so large that they begin to overlap. Bowen et al. (12) termed this "shingling of the laminae." This usually occurs at L4–L5 and/or L5–S1 and can also be seen with spondylolisthesis. The facets are also frequently hypertrophied. Verbiest (163,166) showed that the medial borders of the inferior articular processes may extend close to midline and can encroach upon the canal.

Porter and Pavitt (123) reported that stenosis resulted not only from narrowing of the midsagittal diameter but also from the trefoiled shape of the canal seen in individuals following puberty. This was most prominent at L5, but it also occurred at L4. They reported that trefoiling was associated with smaller midsagittal diameters. With continued interpedicular growth, the canal was hypothesized to become trefoiled in shape.

Verbiest (168) used a stenosimeter to examine 195 patients with developmental stenosis. Intraoperative measurements demonstrated that midsagittal diameters of 10 mm or less appeared to produce symptomatic stenosis. He defined "absolute," "relative," and "mixed" stenosis through measurement of the midsagittal diameter (162). Absolute stenosis was defined as a midsagittal diameter of 10 mm or less. Midsagittal diameters between 10 and 13 mm were termed relative stenosis. Mixed stenosis represented patients with midsagittal diameters less than or equal to 10 mm in some locations and between 10 and 13 mm in other locations. Most patients had absolute stenosis (42%), as compared with mixed (30%) or relative (28%) stenosis.

Overall, men present more often than women with signs, symptoms, and radiographic features of developmental stenosis (110,121,160,161,168). Newman (98) reported that the normal spinal canal varied in volume at different levels and according to sex. It was characteristic for males to have narrow canals at the L3–L4 and L4–L5 levels, whereas females had narrow canals at the lumbosacral level. He related this narrowing at the mid-lumbar region in males with the greater incidence and prevalence of developmental stenosis in men.

Verbiest (162,168) reported that in absolute and mixed stenoses, males were afflicted more frequently than females. However, females and males had an equal incidence of relative stenosis. This substantiated Verbiest's belief that relative stenosis was a variant of an otherwise normal vertebral canal and did not represent a pathologic condition.

Patients with absolute stenosis were generally symptomatic due to compression of the cauda equina and/or nerve roots. Patients with relative stenosis alone were not symptomatic but were predisposed to developing symptoms later in life due to trauma, disc pathology, and/or osteophyte formation.

The cause of developmental lumbar stenosis is unknown. Familial cases have been described in the literature (125, 158,162), lending credence to the notion that the dimensions of the canal may be regulated by genetic factors. In further support of genetic regulation, Eisenstein (31,32) showed that the shape of the vertebral canal is markedly consistent across race and sex. The trefoil configuration of the canal, which almost invariably occurs at the L5 level, was considered by Eisenstein to be a variation of normal anatomy. The low average age (46 years) and the low incidence of associated degenerative changes support a developmental etiologic process over a degenerative process. Eisenstein also showed that the negroid canal was marginally smaller than the caucasoid canal in skeletons of both sexes. However, caucasoids predominated in symptoms, which was theorized to be due to "soft-tissue structures bordering the canal."

Eisenstein (32) reported that developmental lumbar stenosis was found in 27 of 433 (6.3%) adult negroid and caucasoid skeletons—4.3% in the midsagittal plane and 2% in the frontal (interpedicular) plane. He stated that this incidence of stenosis was high for any population and that a large number of these patients were "very slightly subnormal." The shortest midsagittal diameter was 11 mm; he had defined the low limit of normal to be 13 mm. The narrowest interpedicular distance was reported to be 16 mm; his low-normal limit was 18 mm. Eisenstein reported that bony degenerative changes were more likely to cause neurologic compression in the nerve root tunnel than in the spinal canal.

Adverse environmental factors in the first years of life have also been shown to be associated with developmental stenosis. Porter and Pavitt (121) theorized that a narrow canal in an adult may be a marker of impaired development in early life. Narrowing of the midsagittal diameter—the primary marker of developmental stenosis—was believed to be highly influenced by the environment, both prenatally and postnatally (first 4 years of life). They examined the lumbar canals in adult spines from two archaeological populations and demonstrated an association between small midsagittal diameters, small interpedicular diameters, and trefoiling of the canal at L4 and L5 and physiologic indicators of stress (cribra orbitalia, porotic hyperostosis, dental hypoplasia, Harris lines).

Porter et al. (119) retrospectively and prospectively demonstrated a crude association between canal size, as measured ultrasonographically, and health and academic status during childhood. Patients with smaller canals tended to have a greater incidence ($P < .1$) of childhood illnesses and infections.

Clark et al. (16) presented evidence to suggest that infant malnutrition may be related to developmental vertebral stenosis. Lumbar and thoracic vertebrae were measured from a prehistoric Native American population. Over time (950 to 1300 AD), their diet reportedly changed from a hunting-gathering, protein-rich diet to a maize agriculture, protein-deficient diet. Multivariate analysis was used to control for age, sex, and culture. Canal size was shown to be significantly smaller in the population that consumed the protein-deficient diet. The sagittal diameters and the lumbar segments were shown to be more affected by growth disruption than the frontal (interpedicular) diameters and the thoracic segments, respectively. Canal size was shown to be independent of stature and was ultimately determined to be the most powerful index for the assessment of infant malnutrition. Platt and Stewart's (117) laboratory findings in neonatal pig malnutrition substantiate these findings. They found that the vertebral canal was approximately 20% smaller in malnourished pigs than in their well-fed littermates.

Patients with developmental stenosis may be continuously or intermittently symptomatic (110). Bowen et al. (12) stated that patients with developmental stenosis usually become symptomatic when their condition is complicated by a herniated nucleus pulposus, degenerative stenosis, or both. Young adults usually present because of a herniation in the lower lumbar spine. Patients aged 30 through 50 years frequently relate a history of many years of low back pain, often following a traumatic episode. These patients present with low back pain and pain in one or both legs. Symptoms in this age group are produced by mild to moderate degenerative changes and/or disc herniations superimposed on an already developmentally stenotic canal. Older individuals between 40 and 70 present with a clinical picture of degenerative stenosis.

Achondroplasia

Spinal deformities are most common among those with achondroplastic dwarfism. Stenosis arises from two processes: kyphosis at the thoracolumbar junction and concentric narrowing of the vertebral canal (5,23,24,27,40,168). Thoracolumbar kyphosis is most common in almost all patients prior to walking (59). It resolves spontaneously in most patients (5,75,178), but approximately 15% to 20% have clinically significant kyphosis in adulthood (5,69,178). Narrowing of the canal and foramina continues through childhood and adulthood, in part through excessive periosteal bone formation, which causes the bone to thicken (40,168). All regions of the spinal canal may be affected. Stenosis may occur at the level of the foramen magnum, and potentially devastating consequences can arise should this go unrecognized or untreated (87,95,145,179).

One hallmark of stenosis in persons with achondroplasia is progressive narrowing of the interpedicular distance in the caudal direction of the midthoracic and lumbar spine (69,86,178). This is not found in every patient, however, and is not always a reliable indicator of the extent of stenosis (23,85). Stenosis occurs at the canal and foramina level by means of narrowing of the interpedicular and midsagittal diameters, shortening and thickening of the pedicles, thickening of the lamina and inferior facets, concomitant disc pathology (e.g., bulging, protrusion, herniation), spondylosis (e.g., scalloping of the vertebral body and osteophyte formation), excessive lordosis (in part due to hip flexion contractures), and thoracolumbar kyphosis (69,86, 168,178). Stenosis may increase in severity from the midthoracic level toward the lower lumbar spine, or it may be localized at the thoracolumbar junction or upper lumbar spine.

Symptoms of stenosis in persons with achondroplasia include back pain (present in over 50%), leg pain, neurogenic claudication, neurogenic bowel and bladder, paresthesias, anesthesia, weakness, and paraplegia (3,5,69,75,85,95,137,178). Stenosis in the lower thoracic spine may lead to bowel and bladder difficulties, spasticity, and weakness. Intermittent neurogenic claudication may result from compression at the thoracic or lumbar spine. When neurogenic claudication occurs as a result of cord compression, the patient may complain of weakness, loss of sensation, or incontinence that occurs during or shortly after activity and dissipates with rest. Generally, symptoms are slowly progressive. They may tentatively improve with changes of position, including forward bending or squatting. Onset of symptoms typically occurs from 20 to 40 years of age but may occur in childhood (5,40,85,178).

Wynne-Davies et al. (178) reported that neurologic complications (e.g., severe back or leg pain with weakness, paralysis) are rare in patients with simple narrowing of the spinal canal or persistence of a thoracolumbar kyphosis. However, when these two are combined, the risk of neurologic complications is high. Specifically, when the ratio of the interpedicular distance at L1 to that at L4 is greater than 1.3 and there is persistent thoracolumbar kyphosis, serious neurologic sequelae are likely. Kahanovitz et al. (69) reported similar findings. They also reported that interpedicular distances less than 20 mm at L1 or less than 16 mm at L5 were associated with symptoms of stenosis.

Neurogenic claudication without accompanying neurologic deficit has been reported to improve with rest alone (85). Conservative treatment may be worthwhile in the absence of progressive neurologic deficit (85).

Patients with symptoms unamenable to conservative treatment and those with progressive neurologic deficit or cauda equina syndrome require surgical decompression. Decompressions may extend from the lower aspect of the thoracic spine throughout the lumbar spine. In fact, Grabias (48) stated that decompressions in achondroplastic patients should include laminectomies and partial facetectomies from the first sacral vertebra through at least the tenth thoracic vertebra, as either a single or a staged procedure.

Disc herniations are a common cause of radiculopathy and tension signs in persons with achondroplasia (27,85,95,144).

Appropriate treatment in this case entails discectomy along with a generous posterior decompression.

Results following decompression for thoracolumbar and lumbar stenosis have varied (40,85,95,137). The earlier surgical intervention is performed in the symptomatic adult, the better the outlook for improvement (48). For example, Bethem et al. (8) reported that six patients with paraparesis lasting from 6 weeks to 2 years who were treated by laminectomy did not improve neurologically. Verbiest (168) stated that neural complications are often not detected during early stages of this developmental process, which may contribute to the mixed results following decompression. In a considerable number of patients, operative treatment does not result in noticeable improvement and may fail to arrest progressive neurologic deficits, even in cases of symptomatic stenosis thought to be limited to the lumbar spine. Verbiest emphasized the importance of early detection. He suggested that profile radiographs of the cervicooccipital region be taken soon after birth to identify potential life-threatening malformations. Frequent histories and examinations must be performed because neural disturbances, including neurogenic claudication, may not be recognized by the patient or family.

Surgical failures can occur because of the surgeon's failure to perform a complete decompression or to recognize additional pathology (69,85,95).

Postlaminectomy instability may also arise following a wide multilevel decompression. For this reason, Bethem et al. (8) recommend fusion following decompression. However, Kopits (75) believes that this is not necessary, provided the facets are not significantly damaged following decompression. The transverse processes are frequently small, which sometimes makes posterolateral fusion more difficult. Under these conditions, an anterior interbody fusion should be considered to maximize the possibility of obtaining a solid fusion.

If thoracolumbar kyphosis is associated with stenosis and neurologic deficit, an anterior decompression and strut grafting should be performed (8,59), along with a posterior decompression and fusion. Posterior decompression alone produces poor results.

Hypochondroplasia

Hypochondroplasia was first described in the English literature in 1969 by Beals (6). As reported by Wynne-Davies et al. (178) and others (5,168), its features are similar to those of achondroplasia but are less severe and usually do not involve the skull. Hands and feet also tend to exhibit more normal proportions. Hypochondroplasia in its most severe form is indistinguishable from achondroplasia. Like achondroplasia, this disorder is inherited as autosomal dominant, though most patients in the community present as new mutations. The foramen magnum and spinal canal are concentrically reduced in size, but usually not of the magnitude seen in achondroplasia. Symptoms, diagnosis, prognosis, and treatment are similar to those of achondroplasia.

Miscellaneous Forms of Developmental Stenosis

Developmental stenosis is seen in other forms of dwarfism, including diastrophic dwarfism (7,8), thanatophoric dwarfism, and Morquio syndrome (7,13). In Morquio syndrome, bony stenosis can occur at any level but is most common in the lumbar spine (168). Developmental stenosis can occur in association with many congenital anomalies, including, but not limited to, brachydactyly, syndactyly, and hyperopia (66).

Adults with Down syndrome (106) appear to have an increased prevalence of spondylosis with associated stenosis in the lower cervical spine. This seems to occur at an earlier age than in the normal population, predisposing these individuals to myelopathy.

Patients with hereditary multiple exostoses (68,168) are also at risk for developmental stenosis. This occurs through bony exostoses that can extend from any location into the canal.

Wackenheim (169,170) described a developmental entity called cheirolumbar dysostosis (168) in which patients presented with lumbar spinal stenosis along with acromelic disturbances, such as brachyphalangia. Approximately 25% demonstrated a circular, symmetrical type of stenosis, with the remaining patients showing shortening of the midsagittal diameter as typically seen in idiopathic developmental stenosis.

Diffuse developmental stenosis has been identified in patients with acrodysostosis (52). Findings associated with this rare skeletal dysplasia include peripheral dysostosis, nasal hypoplasia, and mental retardation. Loss of normal caudad widening of the coronal and sagittal diameters is frequently observed.

Narrowing of the spinal canal has been reported in patients with acromegaly (24,30,44) and is related to generalized bony overgrowth. Pseudogout (24,71) (calcium pyrophosphate dihydrate deposition) may also cause stenosis through crystal deposition and accumulation in the ligamentum flavum. Degenerative disc disease and facet joint disease can also occur in these patients. Spinal stenosis in patients with Paget disease (24,25, 45,136) most commonly results from bony overgrowth at a single lumbar vertebra and paraspinal masses of incompletely ossified osteoid. Neurologic complications are unusual, and partial or complete relief following medical therapy has been described.

Developmental stenosis is rare, but it does occur in patients with ankylosing spondylitis (21,24,76,141). Outpouching of the dural sac (arachnoid diverticula) most commonly occurs dorsally, which can cause back and leg pain. Symptoms may occur as long as 10 to 40 years after the primary disease has become quiescent. Destructive lesion of the disc spaces (inflammatory and noninflammatory) and vertebral bodies can also cause stenosis.

Other diseases in which developmental stenosis can occur include calcification and ossification of the posterior longitudinal ligament (24,39,63,64,73,74,131,157,180), diffuse idiopathic skeletal hyperostosis (2,131), and calcification and ossification of the ligamenta flavum (70,77,107).

TREATMENT

Treatment of patients with congenital and developmental stenosis of the spine should be determined on an individual basis. A general knowledge of the pathophysiologic factors, natural history, and prognosis of a given disease is helpful for making appropriate treatment recommendations.

In general, surgical decompressions are recommended for patients who have progressive functional and/or neurologic deficits without sustained remission (48,129,144,165). Once severe symptoms of spinal stenosis develop, it is unlikely that improvement will occur without surgical treatment (48). (This is in contrast to younger patients with disc herniations, who frequently improve over time.) Fusions and reconstructive surgery are also recommended for patients with instability or progressive deformity (e.g., kyphotic gibbus) with natural or iatrogenic causes. The goals of treatment are the relief of pain and the preservation or restoration of neurologic function and spinal stability.

REFERENCES

1. Adams CBT, Logue V (1971): Studies in cervical spondylotic myelopathy. I. Movement of the cervical roots, dura and cord, and their relations to the course of the extrathecal roots. *Brain* 94:557–568.
2. Alenghat JP, Hallett M, Kido DK (1982): Spinal cord compression in diffuse idiopathic skeletal hyperostosis. *Radiology* 142:119–120.
3. Alexander E (1969): Significance of the small lumbar spinal canal: cauda equina compression syndromes due to spondylosis. 5. Achondroplasia. *J Neurosurg* 31:513–519.
4. Arnoldi CC, Brodsky AE, Cauchoix J, et al. (1976): Lumbar spinal stenosis and nerve root entrapment syndromes. Definition and classification. *Clin Orthop Rel Res* 115:4–5.
5. Bailey JA (1970): Orthopaedic aspects of achondroplasia. *J Bone Joint Surg Am* 52:1285–1301.
6. Beals RK (1969): Hypochondroplasia: report of 5 kindreds. *J Bone Joint Surg Am* 51:728–736.
7. Bethem D, Winter R, Lutter L (1980): Spinal disorders of the spine in diastrophic dwarfism. *J Bone Joint Surg Am* 62:529–536.
8. Bethem D, Winter R, Lutter L, et al. (1981): Spinal disorders of dwarfism. *J Bone Joint Surg Am* 63:1412–1425.
9. Bolender N-F, Schonstrom NSR, Spengler DM (1985): Role of computed tomography and myelography in the diagnosis of central spinal stenosis. *J Bone Joint Surg Am* 67:240–246.
10. Boltshauer E, Hoare RD (1976): Radiographic measurements of the normal cord in childhood. *Neuroradiology* 10:235–237.
11. Borkow SE, Kleiger B (1971): Spondylolisthesis in the newborn: a case report. *Clin Orthop* 81:73–76.
12. Bowen V, Shannon R, Kirkaldy-Willis (1978): Lumbar spinal stenosis. A review article. *Child's Brain* 4:257–277.
13. Brailsford JF (1952): Chondro-osteo-dystrophy. *J Bone Joint Surg Br* 34:53–63.
14. Breig A, Turnbull I, Hassler O (1966): Effects of mechanical stresses on the spinal cord in cervical spondylosis: a study of fresh cadaver material. *J Neurosurg* 25:45–56.
15. Burrows EH (1963): The sagittal diameter of the spinal canal in cervical spondylosis. *Clin Radiol* 14:77–86.
16. Clark GA, Panjabi MM, Wetzel FT (1985): Can infant malnutrition cause adult vertebral stenosis? *Spine* 10:165–170.
17. Countee RW, Vijayanathan T (1979): Congenital stenosis of the cervical spine: diagnosis and management. *J Natl Med Assoc* 71:257–264.
18. Dagi TF, Tarkington MA, Leech JA. (1987): Lumbar and cervical spinal stenosis: natural history prognostic indices and results after surgical decompression. *J Neurosurg* 66:842–849
19. Dauser RC, Chandler WF (1982): Symptomatic congenital spinal stenosis in a child. *Neurosurgery* 11:61–63.
20. Devkota J, El Gammal T, Lucke JF (1982): Measurement of the normal cervical cord by metrizamide myelography. *South Med J* 79: 1363–1365.

21. Dihlmann W, Delling G (1978): Discovertebral destructive lesions (so-called Andersson lesions) associated with ankylosing spondylitis. *Skel Radiol* 3:10–16.

22. Dommisse GF (1975): Morphological aspects of the lumbar spine and lumbosacral region. *Orthop Clin N Am* 6:163–175.

23. Donaldson DH, Brown CW, Moore MR (1991): Dysplastic conditions of the spine. In: Bridwell KH, Dewald RL, eds. *The textbook of spinal surgery.* Philadelphia: JB Lippincott, pp. 445–498.

24. Dorwart RH, Vogler JB, Helms CA (1983): Spinal stenosis. *Radiol Clin N Am* 21:301–325.

25. Douglas DL, Duckworth T, Kanis JA, et al. (1981): Spinal cord dysfunction in Paget's disease of bone. Has medical treatment a vascular basis? *J Bone Joint Surg Br* 63:495–503.

26. Dubousset J (1985): Congenital kyphosis. In: Stuttgart, ed. *The pediatric spine.* Stuttgart: Thieme Verlag, pp. 196–217.

27. Duvoisin RC, Yahr MD (1962): Compressive spinal cord and root syndromes in achondroplastic dwarfs. *Neurology* 12:202–207.

28. Edwards WC, LaRocca H (1983): The developmental segmental sagittal diameter of the cervical spinal canal in patients with cervical spondylosis. *Spine* 8:20–27.

29. Edwards WC, LaRocca SH (1985): The developmental segmental sagittal diameter in combined cervical and lumbar spondylosis. *Spine* 10:42–49.

30. Efird TA, Genant HK, Wilson CB (1980): Pituitary gigantism with cervical spinal stenosis. *Am J Radiol* 134:171–173.

31. Eisenstein S (1976): Measurements of the lumbar spinal canal in 2 racial groups. *Clin Orthop Rel Res* 115:42–46.

32. Eisenstein S (1977): The morphometry and pathological anatomy of the lumbar spine in South African negroes and caucasoids with specific reference to spinal stenosis. *J Bone Joint Surg Br* 59:173–180.

33. Eismont FJ, Clifford S, Goldberg M, et al. (1984): Cervical sagittal canal size in spine injury. *Spine* 9:663–666.

34. Eismont FJ, Green BA, Berkowitz BM, et al. (1984): The role of intraoperative ultrasonography in the treatment of thoracic and lumbar spine fractures. *Spine* 9:782–787.

35. Elster AD (1984): Quadriplegia after minor trauma in the Klippel-Feil syndrome. A case report and review of the literature. *J Bone Joint Surg Am* 66:1473–1474.

36. Epstein JA, Carras R, Epstein BS, et al. (1970): Myelopathy in cervical spondylosis with vertebral subluxation and hyperlordosis. *J Neurosurg* 32:421–426.

37. Epstein JA, Carras R, Hyman RA (1979): Cervical myelopathy caused by developmental stenosis of the spinal canal. *J Neurosurg* 15:489–496.

38. Epstein JA, Carras R, Rerrar J, et al. (1982): Conjoined lumbosacral nerve roots. Management of herniated discs and lateral recess stenosis in patients with this anomaly. *J Neurosurg* 55:585–589.

39. Epstein JA, Epstein NE (1989): The surgical management of cervical spinal stenosis, spondylosis, and myeloradiculopathy by means of the posterior approach. In: Cervical Spine Research Society Editorial Committee, ed. *The cervical spine,* 2nd ed. Philadelphia: JB Lippincott, pp. 625–643.

40. Epstein JA, Malis LI (1955): Compression of spinal cord and cauda equina in achondroplastic dwarfs. *Neurology* 5:875–881.

41. Epstein NE, Epstein JA, Carras R (1988): Spinal stenosis and disc herniation in a 14-year-old male. *Spine* 13:938–941.

42. Epstein N, Epstein JA, Benjamin V, et al. (1980): Traumatic myelopathy in patients with cervical spinal stenosis without fracture dislocation. Methods of diagnosis, management, and prognosis. *Spine* 5:489–496.

43. Epstein NE, Epstein JA, Carras R, et al. (1984): Coexisting cervical and lumbar spinal stenosis: diagnosis and management. *Neurosurgery* 15:489–496.

44. Epstein N, Whelan M, Benjamin V (1982): Acromegaly and spinal stenosis. Case report. *J Neurosurg* 56:145–147.

45. Feldman F, Seaman WB (1969): The neurologic complications of Paget's disease in the cervical spine. *Am J Roentgenol* 105:375–382.

46. Firooznia H, Ahn JH, Rafic M, et al. (1985): Sudden quadriplegia after minor trauma. The role of pre-existing spinal stenosis. *Surg Neurol* 23:165–168.

47. Garfin SR, Herkowitz HN, Mirkovic S (1999): Spinal stenosis. *J Bone Joint Surg Am* 81:572–586.

48. Grabias S (1980): Current concepts review: the treatment of spinal stenosis. *J Bone Joint Surg Am* 62:308–313.

49. Grant TT, Puffer J (1976): Cervical stenosis: a developmental anomaly with quadriparesis during football. *Am J Sports Med* 4:219–221.

50. Hall JE, Simmons ED, Danylchuk K, et al. (1990): Instability of the cervical spine and neurologic involvement in Klippel-Feil syndrome. A case report. *J Bone Joint Surg Am* 72:460–462.

51. Hamanishi C, Matukura N, Fujita M, et al. (1994): Cross-sectional area of the stenotic lumbar dural tube measured from transverse views of magnetic resonance imaging. *J Spinal Dis* (F): 388–393.

52. Hamanishi C, Nagata Y, Nagao Y, et al. (1993): Acrodysostosis associated with spinal canal stenosis. *Spine* 18:1922–1925.

53. Hanley EN Jr, Matteri RE, Frymoyer JW (1976): Accurate roentgenographic determination of lumbar flexion-extension. *Clin Orthop Rel Res* 115:145–148.

54. Haworth JB, Keillor GW (1962): Use of transparencies in evaluating the width of the spinal canal in infants, children, and adults. *Radiology* 79:109–114.

55. Heliovaara M, Vanharanta H, Korpi J, et al. (1989): Herniated lumbar disc syndrome and vertebral canals. *Spine* 11:433–435.

56. Helms CA, Dorwart RH, Gray M (1982): The CT appearance of conjoined nerve roots and differentiation from a herniated nucleus pulposus. *Radiology* 144:803–807.

57. Hensinger RN, ed. (1986): *Standards in pediatric orthopaedics. Tables, charts, and graphs illustrating growth.* New York: Raven Press.

58. Hensinger RN, Fielding JW (1990): The cervical spine. In: Morrissy RT, ed. *Pediatric orthopaedics,* 3rd ed. Philadelphia: JB Lippincott, pp. 703–737.

59. Herring JA (1983): Kyphosis in an achondroplastic dwarf. *J Pediatr Orthop* 3:250–252.

60. Hink VC, Clark WM, Hopkins CE (1966): Normal interpediculate distances (minimum and maximum) in children and adults. *Am J Roentgenol Radium Ther Nucl Med* 97:141–153.

61. Hinck VC, Hopkins CE, Clark WM (1965): Sagittal diameter of the lumbar spinal canal in children and adults. *Radiology* 89:929–937.

62. Hinck VC, Hopkins CE, Savara BS (1962): Sagittal diameter of the cervical spinal canal in children. *Radiology* 79:97–108.

63. Hirabayashi K, Watanabe K, Wakano K, et al. (1983): Expansive open-door laminoplasty for cervical spinal stenotic myelopathy. *Spine* 8:693–699.

64. Hiramatsu Y, Nobechi T (1971): Calcification of the posterior longitudinal ligament of the spine among Japanese. *Radiology* 100:307–312.

65. Holliday PO III, Davis C Jr, Angelo J (1984): Multiple meningiomas of the cervical spinal cord associated with Klippel-Feil malformation and atlantooccipital assimilation. *Neurosurgery* 14:353–357.

66. Iida H, Shikata J, Yamamuro T, et al. (1988): A pedigree of cervical stenosis, brachydactyly, syndactyly, and hyperopia. *Clin Orthop Rel Res* 80–86.

67. Inoue H, Ohmoir K, Takatsu T, et al. (1996): Morphological analysis of the cervical spinal canal, dural tube and spinal cord in normal individuals using CT myelography. *Diag Neuroradiol* 38:1148–1151.

68. Johnson CE (1988): Multiple hereditary exostoses with spinal cord compression. *Orthopedics* 11:1213–1216.

69. Kahanovitz N, Rimoin D, Sillence DO (1982): The clinical spectrum of lumbar spine disease in achondroplasia. *Spine* 7:137–140.

70. Kamakura K, Namko S, Furokawa T, et al. (1979): Cervical radiculomyelopathy due to calcified ligameta flava. *Ann Neurol* 5:193–195.

71. Kawano N, Yoshida S, Ohwada T, et al. (1980): Cervical radiculomyelopathy caused by deposition of calcium pyrophosphate dihydrate crystals in the ligamenta flava. Case report. *J Neurosurg* 52:279–323.

72. Kessler JT (1975): Congenital narrowing of the cervical spinal canal. *J Neurol Neurosurg Psychiatry* 38:1218–1224.

73. Kimura I, Oh-Hama M, Shingu H (1984): Cervical myelopathy treated by canal-expansive laminaplasty. *J Bone Joint Surg Am* 66: 914–920.

74. Kimura I, Shingu H, Yamasake G (1980): Operative treatment for cervical myelopathy. *J West Jpn Res Spine* 6:10–16.

75. Kopits SE (1976): Orthopaedic complications of dwarfism. *Clin Orthop Rel Res* 114:153.

76. Kramer LD, Kruth GJ (1978): Computerized tomography. An adjunct to early diagnosis in the cauda equina syndrome of ankylosing spondylitis. *Arch Neurol* 35:116–118.

77. Kubota M, Baba I, Sumida T (1981): Myelopathy due to ossification of the ligamentum flavum of the cervical spine. A report of two cases. *Spine* 6:553–559.

78. Ladd A, Scranton PE (1986): Congenital cervical stenosis presenting as transient quadriplegia in athletes. Report of two cases. *J Bone Joint Surg Am* 68:1371–1374.

79. Larsen JL (1981): The lumbar spinal canal in children. II. *Eur J Radiol* 2:312–327.

80. Larsen JL, Smith D (1980): Size of the subarachnoid space in stenosis of the lumbar canal. *Acta Radiol Diagn* 21:627–632.

81. Larsen JL, Smith D (1981): The lumbar spinal canal in children. *Eur J Radiol* 1:163–170.

82. Lee BCP, Kazam E, Newman AD (1978): Computed tomography of the spine and spinal cord. *Radiology* 128:95–102.

83. Lehmann TR, Spratt KF, Tozzi JE, et al. (1987): Long-term follow-up of lower lumbar fusion patients. *Spine* 12:97–104.

84. Lorenzo RL, Hungerford GD, Blumenthal BI, et al. (1983): Congenital kyphosis and subluxation of the thoraco-lumbar spine due to vertebral aplasia. *Skel Radiol* 10:255–257.

85. Lutter LD, Langer LO (1977): Neurological symptoms in achondroplastic dwarfs—surgical treatment. *J Bone Joint Surg Am* 59:87–92.

86. Lutter LD, Lonstein JE, Winter RB, et al. (1977): Anatomy of the achondroplastic lumbar canal. *Clin Orthop Rel Res* 126:139.

87. Luyendyk W, Matricale B, Thomeer R (1978): Basilar impression in an achondroplastic dwarf: causative role in tetraparesis. *Acta Neurochir* 41:243–253.

88. Markuske H (1977): Sagittal diameter measurement of the bony cervical spinal canal in children. *Pediatr Radiol* 6:129–131.

89. McKay DW (1980): Congenital duplication of the spinal canal. *Spine* 5:390–391.

90. McKechnie JL (1983): *Webster's new universal unabridged dictionary.* New York: New World Dictionaries/Simon and Schuster.

91. Mikhael MA, Ciric I, Tarkington JA, et al. (1981): Neuroradiological evaluation of lateral recess syndrome. *Neuroradiology* 140:97–107.

92. Moiel RH, Raso E, Waltz TA (1970): Central cord syndrome resulting from congenital narrowness of the cervical spinal canal. *J Trauma* 10:502–510.

93. Montalvo BM, Quencer RM (1986): Intraoperative sonography in spinal surgery: current state of the art. *Neuroradiology* 28:551–590.

94. Montgomery SP, Hall JE (1982): Congenital kyphosis. *Spine* 7: 3350–3364.

95. Morgan DF, Young RF (1980): Spinal neurological complications of achondroplasia. Results of surgical treatment. *J Neurosurg* 52: 463–472.

96. Naik DR (1970): Cervical spinal canal in normal infants. *Clin Radiol* 21:323–326.

97. Nakstad P (1987): Myelographic findings in cervical spines without degenerative changes. Special reference to sagittal diameter of the dural sac. *Neuroradiology* 29:256–258.

98. Newman PH (1976): Stenosis of the lumbar spine in spondylolisthesis. *Clin Orthop Rel Res* 115:116–121.

99. Nightingale S (1989): Developmental spinal canal stenosis and somatotype. *J Neurol Neurosurg Psychiatry* 52:887–890.

100. Nordquist L (1964): The sagittal diameter of the spinal cord and subarachnoid space in different age groups. *Acta Radiol* [Suppl] 227: 1–96.

101. Nurick S (1972): The pathogenesis of the spinal cord disorder associated with cervical spondylosis. *Brain* 95:87–100.

102. Odor J, Watkins RG, Dillin W, et al. (1991): Cervical spinal stenosis: Torg ratios versus contrast CT canal diameters. *Proceedings of the Sixth Annual Meeting of the Federation of Spine Associations.*

103. Ogden JA (1990): Development and maturation of the neuromusculoskeletal system. In: Morrissy RT, ed. *Lovell and Winter's pediatric orthopaedics,* 3rd ed. Philadelphia. JB Lippincott, pp. 1–33.

104. Ogden JA, Grogan DP (1987): Prenatal skeletal development and growth of the musculoskeletal system. In: Albright JA, Brand RA, eds. *The scientific basis of orthopaedics,* 2nd ed. New York: Appleton & Lange.

105. Ogino H, Tada K, Okada K, et al. (1983): Canal diameter, anteroposterior compression ratio, and spondylotic myelopathy of the cervical spine. *Spine* 8:1–15.

106. Olive PM, Whitecloud TS, Bennett JT (1988): Lower cervical spondylosis and myelopathy in adults with Down's syndrome. *Spine* 13(7): 781–784.

107. Omojola MF, Cardoso ER, Fox AJ, et al. (1982): Thoracic myelopathy secondary to ossified ligamentum flavum. *J Neurosurg* 56: 448–450.

108. Omojola MF, Wenzel V, Banna M (1981): Plain film assessment of spinal canal stenosis. *J Can Assoc Radiol* 32:95–96.

109. O'Rahilly R, Benson DR (1985): The development of the vertebral column. In: Bradford DS, Hensinger RM, eds. *The pediatric spine.* Stuttgart: Thieme Verlag, pp. 3–17.

110. Paine KWE (1976): Clinical features of lumbar spinal stenosis. *Clin Orthop Rel Res* 115:77–82.

111. Pavlov H, Torg JS, Robie B, et al. (1987): Cervical spinal stenosis: determination with vertebral body ratio method. *Radiology* 771–775.

112. Payne EE, Spillane JD (1957): The cervical spine: an anatomico-pathological study of 70 specimens (using a special technique) with particular reference to the problem of cervical spondylosis. *Brain* 80: 571–596.

113. Penning L (1962): Some aspects of plain radiography of the cervical spine in chronic myelopathy. *Neurology* 12:513–519.

114. Phan N, Marras C, Midha R, et al. (1998): Cervical Myelopathy caused by Hypoplasia of the Atlas: two case reports and review of the literature. *Neurosurgery* 43:629–633.

115. Pizzutillo PD (1989): Klippel-Feil syndrome. In: Cervical Spine Research Society Editorial Committee, ed. *The cervical spine,* 2nd ed. Philadelphia: JB Lippincott; 258–271.

116. Pizzutillo PD, Mandell GA, Schoedler S (1991): Spinal stenosis and the Klippel-Feil syndrome. *Proceedings of the 58th Meeting of the American Academy of Orthopaedic Surgeons.*

117. Platt BS, Stewart RJC (1962): Transverse trabeculae and osteoporosis in bones in experimental protein-calorie count. *Br J Nutr* 16: 483–494.

118. Porter R (1990): Lumbar spinal stenosis. Development of the vertebral canal. In: Weinstein JN, Wiesel SW, eds. *The lumbar spine.* Philadelphia: WB Saunders, pp. 589–594.

119. Porter RW, Drinkall JN, Porter DE, et al. (1987): The vertebral canal. II. Health and academic status: a clinical study. *Spine* 12:907–911.

120. Porter RW, Hibbert C (1981): Relationship between the spinal canal and other skeletal measurements in a Romano-British population. *Ann R Coll Surg Engl* 63:47.

121. Porter RW, Hibbert C, Wellman P (1980): Backache and the lumbar spinal canal. *Spine* 5:99–105.

122. Porter RW, Oakshot G (1994): Spinal stenosis and health status. *Spine* 19:901–903.

123. Porter RW, Pavitt D (1987): The vertebral canal. I. Nutrition and development: an archaeological study. *Spine* 12:901–906.

124. Porter RW, Wicks M, Hibbert C (1978): The size of the lumbar spinal canal in the symptomatology of disc lesion. *J Bone Joint Surg Br* 60:485–487.

125. Postacchini F, Massobrio M, Ferro L (1985): Familial lumbar stenosis. Case report of three siblings. *J Bone Joint Surg Am* 67:321–323.

126. Prakash SG, Chandy MJ, Abraham J (1992): Stenosis of the axis and cervical myelopathy. *J Neurosurg* 76:296–297.

127. Prusick VR, Samberg LC, Wesolowski DP (1985): Klippel-Feil syndrome associated with spinal stenosis. A case report. *J Bone Joint Surg Am* 67:161–164.

128. Ramani PS (1976): The spinal canal in symptomatic lumbar disc lesions. *Clin Radiol* 27:301–307.

129. Reale F, Delfini R, Gambacorta D, et al. (1978): Congenital stenosis of lumbar spinal canal: comparison of results of surgical treatment for this and other causes of lumbar syndrome. *Acta Neurochir* 42:199–207.

130. Resjo IM, Harwood-Nash DC, Fitz CR, et al. (1979): Normal cord in infants and children examined with computed tomographic metrizamide myelography. *Radiology* 130:691–696.

131. Resnick D, Guerra J, Robinson CA, et al. (1978): Association of diffuse idiopathic skeletal hyperostosis (DISH) and calcification and ossification of the posterior longitudinal ligament. *Am J Roentgenol* 131:1049–1053.

132. Ritterbusch JF, McGinty LD, Spar J, et al. (1991): Magnetic resonance imaging for stenosis and subluxation in Klippel-Feil syndrome. *Spine* 16:S539–S541.

133. Sarpyener MA (1945): Congenital stricture of the spinal canal. *J Bone Joint Surg* 27:70–79.

134. Sarpyener MA (1947): Spina bifida aperta and congenital stricture of the spinal canal. *J Bone Joint Surg* 29:817–821.

135. Schatzker J, Pennal GF (1968): Spinal stenosis, a cause of cauda equina compression. *J Bone Joint Surg Br* 50:606–618.

136. Schmidek HH (1977): Neurologic and neurosurgical sequelae of Paget's disease of bone. *Clin Orthop Rel Res* 127:70–77.

137. Schreiber F, Rosenthal H (1952): Paraplegia from ruptured discs in achondroplastic dwarfs. *J Neurosurg* 9:648–651.

138. Schwarz GS (1956): The width of the spinal canal in growing vertebra with special reference to the sacrum, maximum interpediculate distances in adults and children. *Am J Radiol* 76:476–481.

139. Scott RM, Wolpert SM, Bartoshesky LE, et al. (1988): Segmental spinal dysgenesis. *Neurosurgery* 22:739–744.

140. Sherk HH, Uppal GS (1991): Congenital bony anomalies of the cervical spine. In: Frymoyer JW, ed. *The adult spine: principles and practice.* New York: Raven Press, pp. 1015–1037.

141. Soeur M, Monseu G, Baleriaux-Waha D, et al. (1981): Cauda equina syndrome in ankylosing spondylitis. Anatomical, diagnostic, and therapeutic considerations. *Acta Neurochir (Wien)* 55:303–315.

142. Sortland O, Magnaes B, Hauge T (1977): Functional myelography with metrizamide in the diagnosis of lumbar spinal stenosis. *Acta Radiol* S355:42–54.

143. Spengler DM (1987): Current concepts review: Degenerative stenosis of the lumbar spine. *J Bone Joint Surg Am* 69:305–308.

144. Spillane JD (1952): Three cases of achondroplasia with neurological complications. *J Neurol Neurosurg Psychiatry* 15:246–252.

145. Spillane JD, Pallis C, Jones AM (1957): Developmental abnormalities in the region of the foramen magnum. *Brain* 80:11–48.

146. Strax TE, Baran E (1975): Traumatic quadriplegia associated with Klippel-Feil syndrome: discussion and case reports. *Arch Phys Med Rehab* 56:363–365.

147. Taylor AR (1951): The mechanism of injury to the spinal cord in the neck without damage to the vertebral column. *J Bone Joint Surg Br* 33:543–547.

148. Torg JS (1989): Risk factors in congenital stenosis of the cervical spinal canal. In: Cervical Spine Research Society Editorial Committee, ed. *The cervical spine*, 2nd ed. Philadelphia: JB Lippincott, pp. 272–285.

149. Torg JS (1995): Cervical spinal stenosis with cord neuropraxia and transient quadriplegia. *Sports Med* 20:429–434.

150. Torg JS, Corcoran TA, Thibault LE, et al. (1997): Cervical cord neuropraxia classification pathomechanics, morbidity, and management guidelines. *J Neurosurg* 87: 843–850.

151. Torg JS, Naranja RJ, Pavlov H, et al. (1996): The relationship of developmental narrowing of the cervical spinal canal to reversible and irreversible injury of the cervical spinal cord in football players. *J Bone Joint Surg Am* 78(9):1308–1314.

152. Torg JS, Pavlov H, Genuario SE, et al. (1986): Neurapraxia of the cervical spinal cord with transient quadriplegia. *J Bone Joint Surg Am* 68:1354–1370.

153. Torg JS, Pavlov H, Warren R, et al. (1991): The relationship of cervical spinal canal narrowing (stenosis) to permanent neurological injury to the athlete: an epidemiological survey. In: *Proceedings of the Sixth Annual Meeting of the Federation of Spine Association.*

154. Torg JS, Ramsey-Emrhein JA (1997): Suggested managment guidelines for participation in collision activities with congenital developmental or post injury lesoins involving the cervical spine. *Med Sci Sports Exerc* 29[7 Suppl]:256–272.

155. Torg JS, Sennett B, Pavlov H, et al. (1993): Spear tackler's spine. An entity precluding participation in tackle football and collision activities that expose the cervical spine to axial energy inputs. *Am J Sports Med* 21:640–649.

156. Tseng S-H (1993) Combined form of developmental cervical-lumbar stenosis of the spinal canal in two young patients. *J Formosan Med Assoc* 92:388–391.

157. Tsuji H (1982): Laminoplasty for patients with compressive myelopathy due to so-called spinal canal stenosis in cervical and thoracic regions. *Spine* 7:28–34.

158. Varughese G, Quartey GRC (1979): Familial lumbar spinal stenosis with acute disc herniations. Case reports of four brothers. *J Neurosurg* 51:234–236.

159. Verbiest H (1949): Sur certaines formes rares de compression de la queue de cheval. I. Les stenoses osseuses du canal vertebral. In: *Hommage a Clovis Vincent.* Paris: Maloine, pp. 161–174.

160. Verbiest H (1954): A radicular syndrome from developmental narrowing of the lumbar vertebral canal. *J Bone Joint Surg Br* 36:230–237.

161. Verbiest H (1955): Further experiences on the pathological influence of a developmental narrowness of the bony lumbar vertebral canal. *J Bone Joint Surg Br* 37:576–583.

162. Verbiest H (1973): Neurogenic intermittent claudication in cases with absolute and relative stenosis of the lumbar vertebral canal (ASLC and RSLC), in cases with narrow lumbar intervertebral foramina, and in cases with both entities. *Clin Neurosurg* 20:204–214.

163. Verbiest H (1975): Pathomorphologic aspects of developmental lumbar stenosis. *Orthop Clin N Am* 6:177–196.

164. Verbiest H (1976): Fallacies of the present definition, nomenclature, and classification of the stenoses of the lumbar vertebral canal. *Spine* 1:217–225.

165. Verbiest H (1977): Results of surgical treatment of idiopathic developmental stenosis of the lumbar vertebral canal. A review of twenty-seven years' experience. *J Bone Joint Surg Br* 59:181–188.

166. Verbiest H (1979): The significance and principles of computerized axial tomography in idiopathic developmental stenosis of the bony lumbar vertebral canal. *Spine* 4:369–378.

167. Verbiest H (1990): Lumbar spinal stenosis. Morphology, classification and long-term results. In: Weinstein JN, Wiesel SW, eds. *The lumbar spine.* Philadelphia: WB Saunders, pp. 546–589.

168. Verbiest H (1990): Lumbar spine stenosis. In: Youmans JR, ed. *Neurological surgery,* 3rd ed. Philadelphia: WB Saunders, pp. 2805–2855.

169. Wackenheim A (1980): Cheirolumbar dysostosis: Developmental brachycheiry and narrowness of the lumbar canal. In: Wackenheim A, Babin E, eds. *The narrow lumbar canal.* New York: Springer-Verlag, pp. 147–155.

170. Wackenheim A (1981): Cheirolumbar dysostosis. *Eur J Radiol* 1:189–194.

171. Weisz G (1986): Lumbar canal stenosis an occupational hazard. *Int Surg* 71(3):199–201.

172. Weisz GM, Lee P (1983): Spinal canal reserve capacity: radiologic measurements and clinical applications. *Clin Orthop Rel Res* 179:134–140.

173. Winston K, Rumbaugh C, Colucci V (1984): The vertebral canals in lumbar disc disease. *Spine* 9:414–417.

174. Winter RB, Erickson DL, Lonstein JE, et al. (1991): Segmental spinal dysgenesis: a report of 20 cases. *Proceedings of the 58th Meeting of the American Academy of Orthopaedic Surgeons.*

175. Winter RB, Lonstein JE, Erickson D, et al. (1985): Congenital spinal stenosis. *Orthop Trans* 9:131.

176. Winter RB, Moe JH, Lonstein JE (1984): The incidence of Klippel-Feil syndrome in patients with congenital scoliosis and kyphosis. *Spine* 9:363–366.

177. Wolf BS, Khilnani M, Malis L (1956): The sagittal diameter of the bony cervical spinal canal and its significance in cervical spondylosis. *J Mt Sinai Hosp* 23:283–292.

178. Wynne-Davies R, Walsh WK, Gormley B (1981): Achondroplasia and hypochondroplasia: clinical variations and spinal stenosis. *J Bone Joint Surg Br* 63:508–515.

179. Yamada H, Nakamura S, Tajima M (1981): Neurological manifestations of pediatric achondroplasia. *J Neurosurg* 54:49–57.

180. Yamamoto I, Kageyama N, Nakamura K, et al. (1979): Computed tomography in ossification of the posterior longitudinal ligament in the cervical spine. *Surg Neurol* 12:414–418.

181. Zingesser LH (1972): Radiological aspects of anomalies of the upper cervical spine and craniocervical junction. *Clin Neurosurg* 20:220–231.

11

CRANIOVERTEBRAL JUNCTION ABNORMALITIES IN THE PEDIATRIC SPINE

ARNOLD H. MENEZES AND TIMOTHY C. RYKEN

EMBRYOLOGY AND DEVELOPMENT OF THE CRANIOVERTEBRAL JUNCTION

The cranial aspect of the craniovertebral junction (CVJ) is composed of the squamous occipital bones posteriorly, the exoccipital bones laterally, and the basioccipital bones anteriorly (9). They coalesce to form the foramen magnum in their center. The atlas vertebra acts as a washer between the cranium and the axis (32). The funnel-shaped bony enclosure encompasses the medulla oblongata and the cervical spinal cord. Bony abnormalities affecting this complex result in dysfunction of the neural structures by compression along the entire circumference, by alteration in the arterial supply as well as the venous drainage, and by alteration in the cerebrospinal fluid dynamics (34,52,57,65). Thus, a vast array of congenital, developmental, and acquired lesions that arise or are located at the CVJ produce changes that ultimately affect the neural structures.

Their clinical significance was appreciated only after the classic radiographic studies on basilar invagination by Chamberlain in 1939 (15) and the recognition of the neurologic syndromes by List in 1941 (52). Early classification of the limited atlantoaxial abnormalities was attempted by Greenberg (34). Until then, the treatment of bony lesions at the CVJ consisted of posterior decompression with enlargement of the foramen magnum and removal of the posterior arch of the atlas (6,102). Greenberg recognized that anteriorly placed lesions at the foramen magnum that were treated in such a manner had a very high mortality and morbidity, especially when an irreducible ventral lesion of the CVJ caused cervicomedullary compression (34).

In 1977, we proposed a physiologic approach to treatment of abnormalities of the CVJ based on an understanding of the stability of the craniovertebral region, the dynamics, the associated neural abnormalities, and the site of encroachment (65). Since then, 3,500 patients with neurologic symptoms and signs secondary to an abnormality of the craniovertebral region have been evaluated. Advances in imaging and instrumentation have

led to treatment of such lesions. Although these abnormalities may appear complex, they are easily understood, and their treatment is simplified with knowledge of the bony anatomy, biomechanics, and embryology (64,99,100).

Anomalies of the CVJ appear to be the result of faulty development of the cartilaginous neural cranium and adjacent vertebral skeleton during the early embryonic weeks. Congenital anomalies at the base of the skull in the atlantooccipital region involve both the osseous structures and the nervous system (30,54,79,99). The frequent occurrence of patterns with various combinations suggests an interrelationship if not a common cause of the origin and development (43,47,86).

LYMPHATIC DRAINAGE OF THE CRANIOVERTEBRAL JUNCTION

The lymphatics of the synovial bursa that line the occipitoatlantoaxial joint complex drain primarily into the retropharyngeal lymph nodes and up the cervical chain (9,71,72). This set of nodes also receives drainage from the paranasal sinuses, the nasopharynx, and the retropharyngeal areas. It is important to keep in mind that a retrograde infection from any of these areas may affect the synovial lining of the craniovertebral joint complex, resulting in effusion and instability as an inflammatory response (64,71). This may result in neurologic deficit and is what contributes to Grisel syndrome (36).

BIOMECHANICS OF THE OCCIPITOATLANTOAXIAL COMPLEX

The occipitoatlantoaxial complex serves as a transition between the skull and the completely different vertebral joint structures (99,100,106). This functions as a single unit and is the most mobile part of the axial skeleton (32).

Cadaveric studies of infants have shown that during hyperflexion at the CVJ, the odontoid process invaginates into the foramen magnum in 25% of individuals (99). Likewise, extreme hyperextension may cause the posterior arch of the atlas to in-

A. H. Menezes and T. C. Ryken: University of Iowa Hospitals and Clinics; Division of Neurosurgery, University of Iowa College of Medicine, Iowa City, Iowa 52242.

trude into the spinal canal and into the foramen magnum, causing compromise of the cervicomedullary junction. Extreme hyperflexion or hyperextension may occur as a result of the positions in which infants are extracted during breech delivery. A similar situation may arise during general anesthesia (64).

Injury to the craniovertebral region is more common in infants and young children than in the older pediatric population due to the large infantile head and small body, resulting in high torques being applied to the neck with acceleration and deceleration (50,64). The cervical musculature does not become supportive until puberty (43,46,48). In addition, the ligaments and joint capsules are lax in small children, allowing for mobility at the cost of stability (99,105). The facets in the first three cervical vertebrae have a horizontal orientation to the articular surfaces, permitting increased translation motion. These facets never become as oblique as the lower cervical spine. There is an incomplete development and flattening of the uncinate processes in children younger than 10 years, making them ineffective in withstanding flexion-rotation forces. Finally, the fulcrum of cervical motion may be higher in young children than in adolescents and adults (99).

Both the occipitoatlantal and the atlantoaxial articulations are involved with flexion-extension (99,105). In a child, the amount of anterior-posterior translation that occurs between the dens and the anterior ring of the atlas can be up to 5 mm (25,53,64). When the transverse component of the cruciate ligament has been disrupted, the alar ligaments are still intact; hence, the amount of displacement stays between 5 and 6 mm until the alar ligaments become incompetent (25,48,78).

The anatomical design of the occipitoatlantal articulation precludes rotation (85,86). The largest degree of rotation occurs at the atlantoaxial joint and is explained by the geometry of the articular surfaces, which is meant to allow maximum mobility. When rotation exceeds 40 to 45 degrees, an interlocking of the facets takes place (64,85,105,106). More importantly, rotation of more than 35 degrees produces an angulation of the contralateral vertebral artery. With greater rotation, there is stretching of the vertebral artery, and at 45 degrees the ipsilateral artery may demonstrate angulation or occlusion. This phenomenon has implications in sudden rotation of the head as may occur with general anesthesia, chiropractic manipulations, and wrestling and football injuries (64). Usually, a large part of the rotation that takes place in the neck is shared by the atlantoaxial joint as well as the remainder of the cervical spine (32).

It has been recognized that muscular action is principally responsible for holding the head firmly to the neck and preventing abnormal excursions. When the protective muscles are relaxed or inadequately developed, as in the case of a child under general anesthesia, the CVJ becomes inherently less stable than in an adult.

Between 1977 and 1999, 3,500 symptomatic patients with abnormalities of the CVJ were evaluated. A wide variety of congenital, developmental, and acquired abnormalities of the CVJ exists and may occur as single or multiple anomalies in the same individual. These entities have been categorized as congenital, developmental, and acquired disorders for the purposes of understanding and discussing CVJ abnormalities (Table 1).

TABLE 1. CLASSIFICATION OF CRANIOCERVICAL JUNCTION ABNORMALITIES

I. Congenital malformations
  A. Malformations of occipital bone (e.g., bifid clivus, remnants around foramen magnum, dens anomalies, atlas anomalies, assimilation of atlas, condylar hypoplasia, basilar invagination)
  B. Malformations of atlas (e.g., assimilation of atlas, atlantoaxial fusion, hypoplasia of arches)
  C. Malformations of axis [e.g., segmentation defects of C1-2, C2-3); dens dysplasia (os terminale, os odontoideum, hypoplasia)]
II. Developmental abnormalities
  A. Abnormalities at the foramen magnum
    1. Foraminal stenosis (e.g., achondroplasia, rickets)
    2. Secondary basilar invagination (e.g., Paget disease, Hajdu-Cheney disease, osteogenesis imperfecta)
  B. Atlantoaxial instability
    1. Errors of metabolism (e.g., mucopolysaccharidosis, types II and IV)
    2. Bone dysplasia (e.g., spondyloepiphyseal dysplasia)
    3. Miscellaneous (e.g., Conradi syndrome, fetal warfarin syndrome, Scott syndrome, Goldenhar syndrome)

CLINICAL PRESENTATION OF CRANIOVERTEBRAL JUNCTION ABNORMALITIES

The most interesting feature of the region's pathology is the diverse presentation. Frequently, there is an antecedent history of minor trauma, which sets off a pattern of symptoms and signs that may progress at a rapid pace. Alternatively, neurologic progression may be insidious and gradual but may suddenly precipitate death (18,22,43,57,60,66,86,91).

The symptoms of craniovertebral dysfunction may be insidious; at times, it may present with false localizing signs (64, 85,105,106). A constellation of symptoms and signs may occur as a result of compromise of the brain stem, cervicomedullary junction, cranial nerves, cervical roots, and their vascular supply as well as alterations in cerebrospinal fluid dynamics. Varied pictures exist with hindbrain herniation syndromes, hydromyelia, foramen magnum constriction, and hydrocephalus. This list of pathologic states that affect the CVJ is extensive (64). Each of these abnormalities may vary in the magnitude of neurologic dysfunction and abnormal findings, exclusive of involvement of the central nervous system.

Congenital abnormalities of the CVJ are often associated with an abnormal general physical appearance (2,5,7,18,33,50, 88,101). This may involve a short stature and an abnormally short neck; at times, the head may be cocked to one side or the other, as with patients with rotary luxation of the atlas on the axis vertebra. An abnormally low hairline may be present posteriorly, with limitation of neck motion—part of the classical triad of Klippel-Feil syndrome (49). In addition, there may be facial asymmetry and webbing of the neck. Scoliosis is present in a significant number of these individuals. Sprengel shoulder deformity and abnormal stature also fall within the spectrum of Klippel-Feil syndrome. It is not uncommon to see children with a small dysmorphic stature. There is an increased incidence of associated defects involving the genitourinary and cardiopulmonary systems, as well as defects of the skeletal and nervous systems in Klippel-Feil syndrome (4,37,55,69).

The skeletal dysplasias have a peculiar propensity for developmental abnormalities involving the CVJ. Disease states, such as achondroplasia, spondyloepiphyseal dysplasia, and the related diseases of dwarfism, are well represented in this region (2,3, 7,10,21,33,38,50,77,80,88,90,108).

The most common deficit in the author's series of children with abnormalities of the CVJ is myelopathy. The most common symptom is neck pain, present in 85% (64). This originates in the suboccipital area with radiation to the cranial vertex. False localizing signs associated with abnormalities of the foramen magnum are usually motor and may present with hemiparesis, monoparesis, paraparesis, and quadriplegia. The "central cord syndrome" was often seen in children with basilar invagination in whom the myelopathy mimicked a lower cervical disturbance (64,66). In 1974, in a classical experimental study, Taylor and Byrnes (96) investigated this phenomenon and proved that the venous drainage of the central gray matter in the lower portion of the cervical cord occurs in an upward direction. A separate venous drainage exists for the white and gray matter of the spinal cord. Thus, in compressive lesions of the cervicomedullary junction, there is venous stagnation in the lower cervical spinal cord, leading to hypoxia and dysfunction in the anterior horn cells. This may present as a lower cervical myelopathy between the C6 and C8 levels.

The sensory abnormalities are related to posterior column dysfunction. Brain stem and cranial nerve deficits were exhibited by abnormalities such as sleep apnea, dysphagia, and aspiration pneumonia. Not uncommonly, internuclear ophthalmoplegia was present and led to a misdiagnosis of upper brain stem dysfunction. Downbeat nystagmus was present in compressive lesions of the craniovertebral border, whether they were associated with Chiari malformations or not.

The most common cranial nerve dysfunction was hearing loss in 25% of children (64). This had an increased incidence in Klippel-Feil syndrome. A bilateral or unilateral paralysis of the soft palate and pharynx led to repeated bouts of aspiration pneumonia as well as poor feeding and inability to gain weight. Vascular symptoms, such as intermittent attacks of altered consciousness, confusion, and transient loss of visual fields, as well as vertigo occurred in 15% to 20% of children. At times, this was provoked by extension of the head or rotation, as with manipulation of the head and neck.

The syndrome of "basilar migraine" was frequently encountered in children with basilar invagination with atlas assimilation and compression of the medulla as well as the vertebrobasilar tree (22,35). In these individuals, the symptoms completely regressed upon surgical decompression of the area. The excessive mobility of an unstable occipitoatlantoaxial joint may cause repeated trauma to the anterior spinal artery and the perforating vessels of the medulla and upper cervical cord, leading to occlusion or spasm and the attendant neurologic deficits.

Children with nasopharyngeal infections and neck spasm or torticollis must be suspected of harboring CVJ abnormalities, which may be caused by an osseous abnormality secondary to effusion into the CVJ joints or rotary luxation.

NEURORADIOLOGIC INVESTIGATIONS

The diagnosis of CVJ abnormalities should be suspected when symptoms and signs referable to the brain stem, high cervical cord, and cerebellum are present. The factors that influence treatment are as follows (62):

1. Reducibility
2. Mechanics of compression
3. Cause of the associated neurologic abnormalities, such as Chiari malformation, syringohydromyelia, or associated vascular abnormalities
4. Presence of abnormal ossification centers and epiphyseal growth plates with anomalous development

The primary treatment for reducible craniovertebral lesions is stabilization. Surgical decompression is performed in patients with irreducible pathology. When irreducible lesions are encountered, the decompression is performed in the manner in which encroachment occurs (60). If a ventral encroachment is present, a transpalatopharyngeal decompression or LeForte I drop-down maxillotomy is made; alternatively, a lateral extrapharyngeal approach may be performed if decompression is possible by this route. When dorsal compression is present, a posterior decompression is mandated. In either circumstance, if instability follows, posterior fixation is required.

The above factors regarding treatment are determined by plain radiographs and dynamic studies that include the flexed and extended positions (Fig. 1A, B), computed tomography (CT) of the craniovertebral area, and magnetic resonance imaging (MRI). The effects of cervical traction must be documented. Magnetic resonance angiography and CT angiography is supplemented by direct visualization with selective vertebral angiography, when necessary. Each of these techniques has important features and provides complementary information about the CVJ and the presence of any incidental and pathologic changes in normal as well as abnormal relationships (19,35,47,57,68).

There has been a gradual trend toward the use of MRI as the only neurodiagnostic procedure other than plain radiography of the craniovertebral border. MRI cannot completely visualize the osseous pathology and cannot delineate the true extent of congenital and developmental lesions in this region. The authors rely on three-dimensional CT for identifying the osseous pathology (Fig. 1C, D). Dynamic imaging is performed in the flexed and extended positions and, subsequently, with cervical traction. This defines the bony pathology and acts as a preoperative assessment of the stability in both the anterior-posterior and vertical dimensions. Cervical traction with an MRI-compatible halo is used to determine the stability and reducibility of the lesion.

The predental space, also called the atlas-dens interval, is the space seen on the lateral radiograph between the anterior aspect of the dens and the posterior aspect of the anterior arch of the atlas vertebra. Locke et al. (53), in a radiographic study performed at the University of Iowa in 1966, reviewed 160 patients and observed the lateral radiographs in normal individuals. The

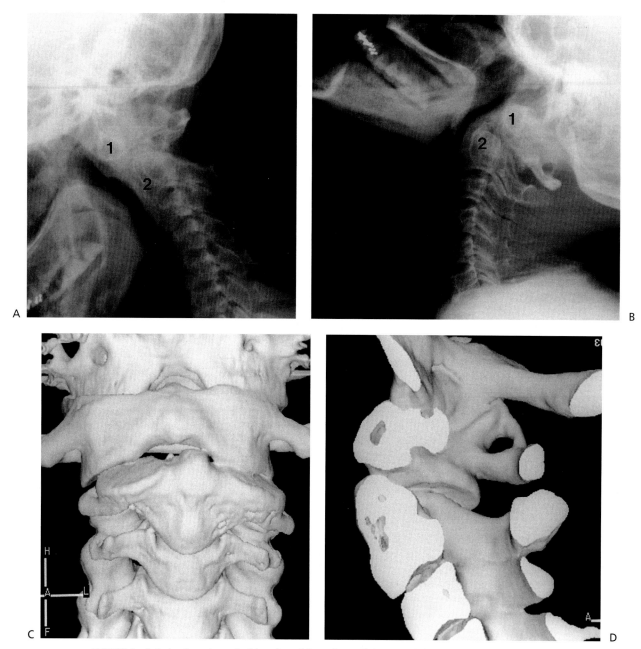

FIGURE 1. A: Lateral craniocervical junction plain radiograph in a 14-year-old boy with severe spastic quadriparesis in the flexed position. Note the os odontoideum, the anterior position of the anterior atlantal arch, and the marked widening of the interspinous distance between the atlas and the axis vertebrae. **B:** Lateral craniocervical radiograph of patient in **A** in the extended position. There is significant dorsal displacement of the anterior atlantal arch together with the dystopic os odontoideum. **C:** Three-dimensional computed tomographic construction of the craniocervical junction and upper cervical spine. Note the lateral atlantoaxial displacement and the hypoplastic dens. **D:** Midsagittal view of the craniocervical junction from within the spinal canal. There is a dystopic os odontoideum with an offset of the lateral atlantal mass on the superior articular facet of the axis vertebra.

TABLE 2. CRANIOMETRIC RELATIONSHIP OF THE CRANIOVERTEBRAL JUNCTION AS SEEN ON PLAIN LATERAL RADIOGRAPHS

Synonym	Definition	Normal Measurements	Implications
Chamberlains palatooccipital line	Joins posterior tip of hard palate to posterior tip of foramen magnum	Tip of dens below this line ± 4 mm	In basilar invagination, the odontoid process bisects the line
McRae's foramen magnum line	Joins anterior and posterior edges of foramen magnum	Tip of odontoid is below foramen magnum	When effective sagittal diameter of canal is less than 20 mm, neurologic symptoms occur
Wackenheims clivus–canal line	Line drawn along clivus into cervical spinal canal	Odontoid is ventral to this line	Odontoid transects the line in basilar invagination
Bulls angle	Angle between Chamberlains line and central plane of atlas	13 degrees or less	If the angle is more than 13 degrees, basilar impression is present due to either hypoplastic clivus or occipital condyles

maximum amount of flexion-permitted motion is between 3 and 4 mm; in very rare instances, there was up to 5 mm of predental space. The upper limit of normal in adults is 3 mm (26,48), and in children below age 8 years it is 5 mm. The atlantodental interval is of limited value in evaluating chronic atlantoaxial instability resulting from congenital anomalies. In these situations, the odontoid process may be small and hypermobile. List (52) and subsequently McRae (56) called attention to the relationship between neurologic symptoms and the effective sagittal diameter of the spinal canal at the foramen magnum. They noted that when the effective diameter of the spinal canal at the foramen magnum (the space available for the cervicomedullary junction) was less than 19 mm, neurologic deficits ensued. In our own series this held true. However, with the availability of MRI, this measurement can be more specifically defined.

A general consensus is that the space behind the anterior arch of the atlas and the spinous interlaminar line is divided into thirds. The first third is occupied by the odontoid process and the second third by the spinal cord; the last third is a free safe "space" that is roughly equal to the transverse diameter of the odontoid process. The craniometric lines of reference are enumerated in Table 2 and illustrated in Figure 2 (15,16,47,64, 86,95).

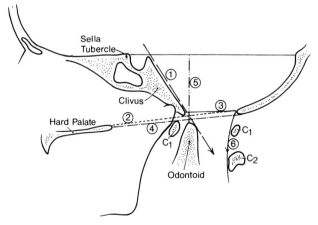

FIGURE 2. Lateral craniometry of the craniocervical junction with points of reference. *1,* Wackenheim clivus-canal line; *2,* Chamberlain line; *3,* McRae line; *4,* McGregor line; *5,* Height index of Klaus; *6,* Spinous interlaminar line (posterior canal line).

SPECIFIC CONDITIONS

Griesel Syndrome

Griesel syndrome is defined as a spontaneous subluxation of the atlantoaxial joint following parapharyngeal infection (36). This inflammatory subluxation has been ascribed to metastatic inflammation causing ligamentous stretching, subluxation, muscle spasm, and regional hyperemia with decalcification of the ligamentous attachments (64). These children present with a stiff neck with neck pain, torticollis, and neurologic deficit. This may occur with tonsillitis, mastoiditis, retropharyngeal abscess, and otitis media. Most children affected are younger than 12 years. This may be explained by the greater ligamentous laxity and vascularity of the region in the pediatric population (72).

In 1987, Wilson et al. reviewed 62 cases of nontraumatic subluxation of the atlantoaxial articulation that fulfilled the otolaryngologic criteria of Griesel syndrome (107). In 14 children this occurred following surgical procedures for tonsillectomy, adenoid removal, mastoiditis, and resection of a pharyngeal rhabdomyosarcoma. Twelve children had symptoms of pharyngitis or cervical adenitis, several had tonsillitis, and seven harbored a cervical abscess. There were five children who had acute rheumatic fever and four with acute mastoiditis. Several patients were assigned the diagnosis of non-specific parapharyngeal infection. In children with Griesel syndrome, the neurologic deficit may range from paresthesias to quadriparesis, suggesting compression of the cervicomedullary junction or arterial compromise. In our own experience with 29 children, the causes were similar. Unilateral or bilateral rotary subluxation of the atlantoaxial complex was evident (64).

Treatment of such lesions consists of precise visualization of the region by means of MRI and CT. It is paramount that the source of infection be eliminated. Stabilization is achieved with a sterno-occipitomandibular immobilizing brace or a halo vest. In the acute phase, a Philadelphia collar may be applied to allow careful monitoring of the respiratory function. Once the infection is under control it is important that further diagnostic procedures be obtained to define the instability and possible rotational abnormalities. These are corrected by traction, derotation, and immobilization for 10 to 12 weeks. It is rare that a fusion procedure is necessary. We have not had to do this in any of our 29 children.

Malformations of Occipital Vertebrae

Anomalies and malformations of the most caudal of the occipital sclerotomes are collectively called manifestations of occipital vertebrae (31,51,57,86,88). An occipital vertebra occurs when there is failure of the third occipital sclerotome to be incorporated into the more rostral two occipital sclerotomes (64,100). The occipital condyles are then attached to the vertebra, and if the occipital vertebra has a transverse process, it does not have a foramen for the vertebral artery (100). In contrast, in occipitoatlantal fusion or assimilation of the atlas, the transverse process of the atlas maintains the bony foramina of the vertebral arteries. This latter condition is the most commonly recognized anomaly of the craniovertebral joint. It is frequently associated with Klippel-Feil syndrome.

A significant abnormality representing malformation of the occipital vertebra is a pseudojoint formed by an abnormal articulation between the clivus, anterior arch of the atlas, and apical segment of the dens (50,54,86). Even though the bony abnormality is situated extracranially at the anterior margin of the foramen magnum, an abnormal angulation of the CVJ occurs, with ventral compression of the cervicomedullary junction. The normal clivus canal angle should not be less than 130 degrees in flexion (99). This particular abnormality is often associated with Chiari malformation and syringohydromyelia (23,35, 61,67). When the hypochordal bow assumes a large knobby configuration, it has been called the third condyle and may in itself form an abnormal articulation.

Abnormal segmentation of the clivus is not uncommon and should not be mistaken for the sphenooccipital suture line (61,99).

There are many anomalies that involve the proatlas. For example, in a 12-year-old boy with severe spastic quadriparesis, the proatlas component of the dens failed to separate from the portion that forms the basiocciput of the clivus (Fig. 3). The anterior arch of the atlas thus rests above the axis body, and the neurocentral synchondrosis of the axis itself is well visualized. The abnormality moves in unison with the clivus, grossly distorting the cervicomedullary junction ventrally, especially in flexion. This anomaly is similar to the reptilian spine in lower vertebrates. An anterior decompression is essential. In the author's experience with such individuals, a dorsal occipitocervical fusion is mandatory following anterior decompression.

Assimilation of the Atlas

Occipitalization, or assimilation, of the atlas implies bony union between the skull and first cervical vertebra. This anomaly occurs in 0.25% of the population (56,64,100). It is defined as failure of segmentation between the fourth occipital sclerotome and the first spinal sclerotome. It involves the skull and the anterior arch of the atlas, or the lateral atlantal masses, causing a disappearance of the joint space (14). This anomaly may be bilateral, unilateral, segmental, or focal (64). In most instances, it occurs in conjunction with other abnormalities, such as basilar invagination and Klippel-Feil syndrome (5,12,42,69). Fusion between the second

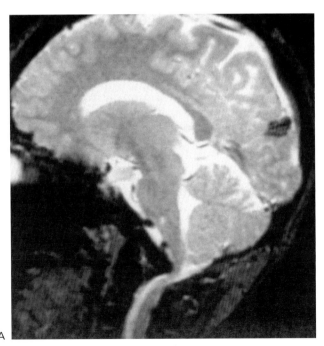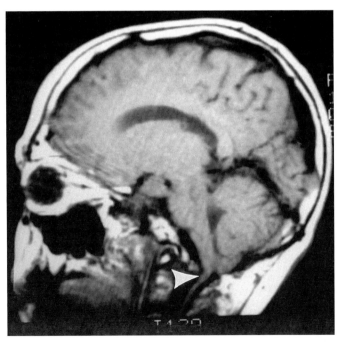

A B

FIGURE 3. A: Midsagittal T1-weighted magnetic resonance image of head and upper cervical region in a 12-year-old boy. The proatlas component of the odontoid is attached to the clivus and projects into the spinal canal with severe ventral compression of the lower medulla oblongata. **B:** T2-weighted magnetic resonance image of head and craniocervical region. Note the extension of the clivus into the ventral spinal canal with severe compression of the cervicomedullary junction.

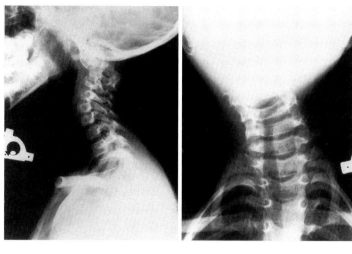

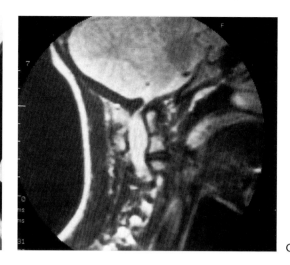

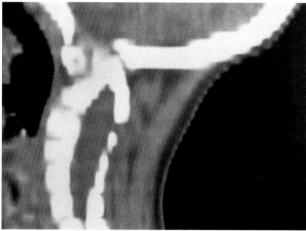

FIGURE 4. A: Composite of lateral and frontal cervical spine radiographs in a 5-year-old girl. She had torticollis and was unable to walk. There is segmentation failure of C2–3 and atlantoaxial dislocation. **B:** Reformatted computed tomogram of the craniovertebral junction in the midsagittal plane. There is atlas assimilation with marked odontoid invagination and dorsal displacement of the odontoid process. **C:** Midsagittal T2-weighted magnetic resonance image of the craniovertebral junction. The subarachnoid sac of the cervicomedullary junction is grossly deformed and compressed by the abnormal odontoid process.

and third cervical vertebrae was present in 18 of 25 patients with occipitalization of the atlas reported by McRae and Barnum (56). In the senior author's own series reviewed in 1988 (64), 96 such patients were detected among 890 patients with CVJ abnormalities. There were 32 segmentation failures between the second and third cervical vertebrae (Fig. 4). In all of these patients a Chiari malformation existed. In addition, Chiari malformation was seen in 42 of 96 patients with assimilation of the atlas. Paramesial invagination was present in 12 of 42 individuals with Chiari malformation (Fig. 5). Reducible atlantoaxial instability, or reducible basilar invagination, was detected in 15 of 18 children younger than 14 years (61). As age progressed, the lesion became irreducible. In partially reducible lesions there was prolific granulation tissue around the dislocation. In those individuals in whom an irreducible lesion was present, the granulation tissue was tough and fibrotic. An irreducible basilar invagination was more often than not associated with a horizontally oriented clivus and abnormal grooving behind the occipital condyles, articulating with the lateral masses of the axis vertebra (61). There is an inability to move in a rostral-caudal dimension or in a sagittal plane.

In keeping with these findings, the authors believe that the combination of assimilation of the atlas and segmentation failures between the second and third cervical vertebrae results in progressive laxity of the atlantodental joint, with development of luxation between the dens and the atlas in childhood (64). As a result of this instability, progressive proliferation of granulation tissue occurs. During this time, there is remodeling of the inferior surfaces of the foramen magnum, involving the occipital condyles as well as the unsegmented atlas vertebra. This then leads to an irreducible state, with the newly formed "socket" attended to by the ball-like configuration of the superior facet of the axis vertebra placed in an abnormal position behind the occipital condyle and within the socket formed by the structures of the assimilated atlas. The odontoid invagination then combines with the abnormal clivus, leading to progressive neural compromise. These children become symptomatic during adolescence.

Acute trauma and infections of the upper respiratory tract have been implicated in precipitating symptoms of atlantoaxial instability. In developing countries, the carrying of heavy loads on the head constitutes a chronic trauma that results in flexion-extension injuries and further instability. Unfortunately, this has been termed congenital atlantoaxial subluxation; however, the

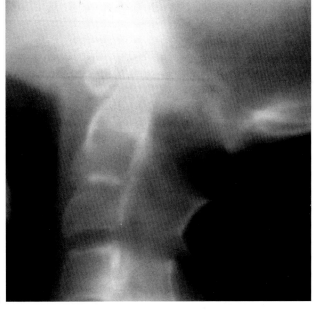

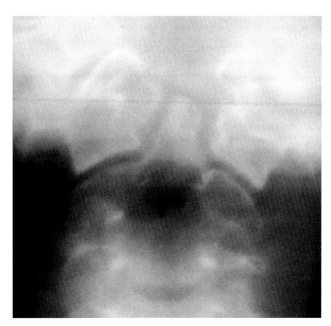

A

B

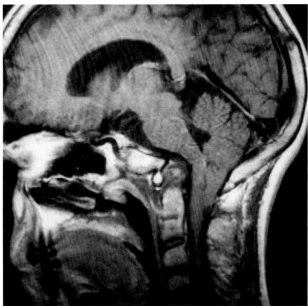

C

FIGURE 5. A: Midline lateral pluridirectional tomogram of the craniovertebral junction. Note the atlas assimilation and odontoid invagination. **B:** Frontal tomogram through the plane of the odontoid process. There is assimilation of the atlas lateral masses (C1) with an abnormally angulated and elongated odontoid process. The skull base is elevated. **C:** Midsagittal T1-weighted magnetic resonance image of the head and cervical spine. There is near-horizontal position of the clivus (platybasia) and a 100-degree clivus-odontoid angle. This indents into the ventral pontomedullary junction. There is a hindbrain herniation into the cervical canal. The vertical height of the posterior fossa has been markedly reduced.

phenomenon should be considered developmental rather than congenital (6). Irregular segmentation of the atlas and the axis may be associated with assimilation and unilateral fusion between the axis and the atlas vertebra. These fusions are not common and may be associated with other anomalies.

The initial treatment is traction. If reduction is not adequate, as documented by MRI, a ventral decompression of the clivus-odontoid complex with the associated granulation tissue is essential, and subsequent stabilization is needed.

Basilar Invagination and Basilar Impression

The terms *basilar invagination, basilar impression,* and *platybasia* are often used erroneously (15). Basilar invagination applies to

the primary form of basilar impression consisting of a distinct developmental defect of the chondrocranium, which is often associated with anomalies in the region of the CVJ, such as occipitalization of the atlas and Klippel-Feil syndrome (Fig. 5B, C) (64). It is also associated with anomalies of development in the epichordal neural axis, such as Chiari malformation, syringobulbia, and syringomyelia (5,22,55,59,65,79).

Basilar impression refers to the secondary, acquired form of basilar invagination that is caused by softening of the bone (100). This is characterized by invagination at the base of the skull as a consequence of such abnormalities as osteomalacia, hyperparathyroidism, osteogenesis imperfecta, Paget disease, Hurler syndrome, rickets, tumors or infections with local bone destruction, and ligamentous injury (Fig. 6) (7,10,38,39,73–75,92,104).

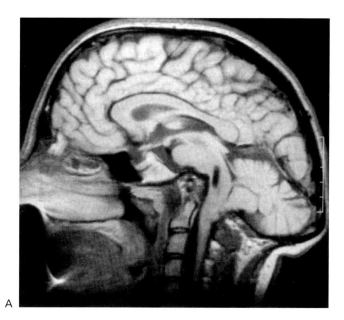

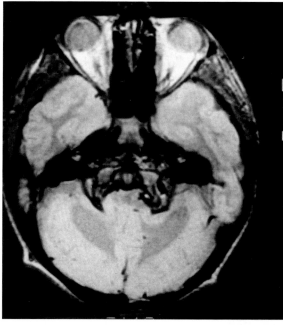

FIGURE 6. A: Midsagittal T1-weighted magnetic resonance image of the head and upper cervical spine. This 16-year-old with Paget disease presented with headaches, arm weakness, and lower cranial nerve palsies. Note the horizontal clivus. There is severe secondary skull base upward invagination, and compression of the cerebellum and brain stem. There is a 90-degree angle at the pontomedullary junction. **B:** Axial T2-weighted magnetic resonance image through the plane of the clivus. Note the invaginated atlas and odontoid process.

Platybasia, on the other hand, refers only to an abnormally obtuse basal angle formed when the plane of the clivus joins with the plane of the anterior fossa of the skull. This angle is of anthropologic significance only (100). There are no symptoms or signs that can be attributed to platybasia. It is not a measure of basilar invagination, although it may be associated with invagination. Confusion between platybasia and basilar impression

dates to Chamberlain's 1939 paper (15). Although the title of Chamberlain's paper implies that the terms platybasia and basilar impression are synonymous, they do not refer to the same anomaly.

In basilar invagination, all three parts of the occipital bone are deformed. Two types are distinguished: anterior and paramedian (64,100). In anterior basilar invagination, there is shortening of the basiocciput and an associated platybasia, which raises the plane of the foramen magnum. In paramedian basilar invagination, hypoplasia of the exoccipital bone is present. There is a medial elevation of this portion of the occipital bone; on anteroposterior skull views, this can be seen as the rise of the skull base toward the foramen magnum. The distinction between these two forms is not important clinically, and an admixture does occur (Fig. 7).

The radiographic diagnosis of basilar invagination is based on a pathologic alteration in craniometric relationships made visible by plain radiographs, pleuridirectional tomography, CT, and MRI (19,64,99). Basilar invagination should be suspected when the lateral atlantoaxial articulations cannot be clearly visualized in the open-mouth anteroposterior view of the upper cervical spine (100). The tip of the dens should normally not exceed the bimastoid line by more than 10 mm. The digastric or biventral line is approximately 10 mm rostral to the bimastoid line. This should not be crossed by the normal dens. There are multiple reference lines to identify basilar invagination on the lateral projection. The tip of the odontoid process should usually lie below Chamberlain's line and not more than 2.5 mm above it (99). McRae's line represents the plane of the foramen magnum and should not be encroached on by the dens under normal circumstances (57). When the sagittal diameter at the foramen magnum is less than 19 mm, neurologic deficits have been recognized.

In basilar invagination, there is elevation of the floor of the posterior fossa (35,99,100). This may be simulated by an abnormally short clivus, resulting in upward elevation of the anterior aspect of the foramen magnum. The elevation of the floor of the posterior fossa is most prominent around the foramen magnum, so the margins may curve upward; the lateral portions of the posterior fossa may curve downward. Thus, the space within the posterior fossa is compromised (35,38,64,79).

When chronic instability is present, as with occipitalization of the atlas, an excess of granulation tissue may build up around the odontoid process. This in itself acts as a space-occupying mass in the anterior portion of the foramen magnum. In addition, fibrous bands and dural adhesions are common in the posterior cervicomedullary junction and around the cerebellar tonsils in both primary and secondary basilar invagination.

A severe form of secondary basilar invagination may occur following childhood diseases of bone, such as renal rickets. Although the patient shows no manifestations of the problem at a later age, the invagination has occurred and persists. In this situation, it is very difficult to differentiate this form of invagination from the other varieties.

Condylar hypoplasia is often a feature of malformations of the CVJ and leads to the paramedian type of basilar invagination (99,100). The occipital condyles are flattened, leading to an elevated position of the atlas and the axis. There are transitional

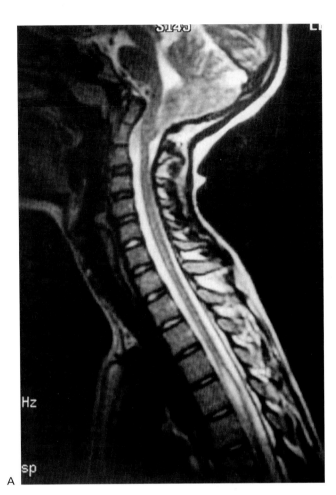

A

FIGURE 7. **A:** Midsagittal T2-weighted midsagittal magnetic resonance image of posterior fossa, cervical and upper thoracic spine. There is atlas assimilation with foreshortened clivus and a 90-degree angle between the clivus and odontoid process. This invaginates into the pontomedullary junction. A hind-brain herniation is also present with upper thoracic syringohydromyelia. This 13-year-old boy presented with difficulty swallowing, basilar migraines, and spastic quadriparesis with thoracic scoliosis. **B:** Three-dimensional computed tomogram of craniocervical junction viewed from within the cranium and posterior fossa. Note the orientation such that the odontoid process is to the right. Thus, there is atlas assimilation seen better on the left. There is gross atlantoaxial dislocation with severe canal compromise at foramen magnum. **C:** Axial T2-weighted magnetic resonance image through the plane of the atlas vertebra. The odontoid process is now visible to the left of the midline, and atlantoaxial dislocation is evident with significant compression of the medulla.

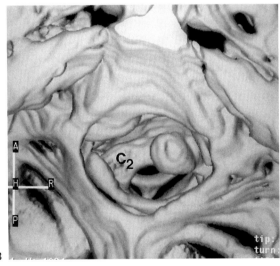

B

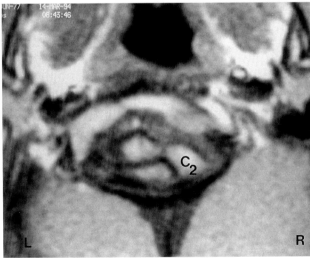

C

stages between condylar hypoplasia and basilar invagination. Condylar hypoplasia limits movement of the atlantooccipital joint and at times may lead to vertebral artery compression as a result of the backward glide of the occiput. An asymmetrical flattening of the occipital condyle may produce scoliotic changes in the cervical spine. In some instances, medial placement of the occipital condyles causes a marked reduction in the transverse diameter of the foramen magnum, resulting in lateral medullary compression that is compounded by an existing Chiari malformation. A secondary form of this is seen in children with osteogenesis imperfecta, where there is paramesial invagination due to the side-to-side intrusion of the occipital condyles into the foramen magnum (2,3,7,39,73,75,77).

Symptomatic patients with basilar invagination require cervical traction using an MRI-compatible halo ring. Basilar invagination associated with Chiari malformations is not uncommon (22,61). When this is the case and there is ventral compression of the cervicomedullary junction by a bony abnormality, a ventral decompression must be performed before the posterior surgical procedure. The ability to reduce the invagination is age-related. The presence of a syringohydromyelia does not mean that a posterior operative procedure is indicated (Fig. 7A). The majority of the syringohydromyelia will disappear once the ventral abnormality has been corrected (59). This occurs because of an equalization of the abnormal cerebrospinal fluid dynamics such that the cerebrospinal fluid flow is restored to its normal values. In addition, the bony compression is reduced, leading to an improved neurologic state. If a posterior decompression is performed first, a significant number of patients will show no improvement or experience a progressive deterioration of brain stem and high cervical cord function (6,34,64,99,102). Posterior decompression and rerouting of the cerebrospinal fluid pathway should be performed before a cervical fusion, after the ventral pathology has been corrected. The secondary basilar invagination that is seen with osteogenesis imperfecta and the Hajdu-Cheney syndrome with acroosteolysis requires bracing as early as possible (17,38,45,81), preferably with a Minerva brace or a custom-fitted one. The youngest child seen by the authors was fitted with a brace shortly after birth.

Anomalies of the Odontoid Process

Aplasia-Hypoplasia of the Dens

Aplasia-hypoplasia of the dens may be expressed in several degrees; a rudimentary dens may be present or it may be completely absent (13). In this entity, the cruciate ligament is incompetent, leading to atlantoaxial instability. Extensive hypoplasia may be combined with developmental forms of os odontoideum (28,29,34,43,62). A significant vascular compromise—the result of stretching and distortion of the vertebral arteries—has been seen in such lesions. Chronic atlantoaxial dislocation in this situation may result in the formation of granulation tissue at the site of the luxation, with compression of the cervicomedullary junction.

Os Odontoideum

The term *os odontoideum* was first coined by Giacomini in 1886 (62). It refers to an independent bone seen cranial to the axis, in the place of the dens. It is not an isolated dens but exists apart from a small hypoplastic dens. Radiographically, the os odontoideum has rounded, smooth cortical borders that are separated by a variable gap from a small odontoid process (100). It is usually located in the position of the normal odontoid tip or near the basiocciput in the area of the foramen magnum, where it may fuse with the clivus. The gap between the free ossicle and the axis usually extends above the level of the axis superior facets. This leads to incompetence of the cruciate ligament and subsequent atlantoaxial instability.

Fielding has described two types of os odontoideum: the orthotopic variety wherein the ossicle lies in the position of the normal dens and moves in unison with the atlas and the axis vertebrae, and the dystropic variety wherein the ossicle lies near the inferior end of the clivus and fuses with the occipital bone and moves in unison with the clivus (27) (Fig. 8).

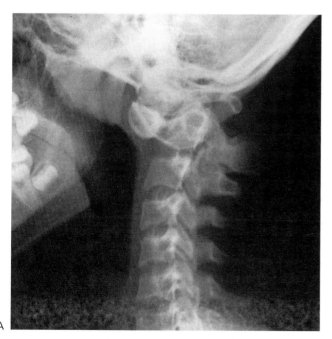 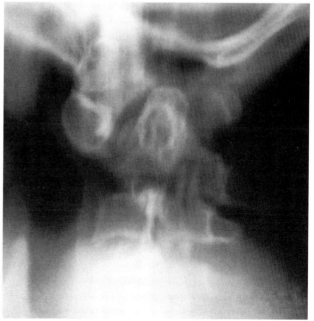

FIGURE 8. A: Lateral cervical radiograph of a 12-year-old girl who presented with hemiparesis after gymnastics. There is gross atlantoaxial instability, with the anterior atlas arch descending toward the C2–3 interspace. **B:** Midline polytomograms of the craniovertebral junction reveal a large dystopic os attached to the inferior clivus, with sclerotic borders. The anterior C1 arch is enlarged. The hypoplastic odontoid process and the axis body have ascended and moved dorsally.

Radiographically it may be difficult to differentiate an os odontoideum from an old odontoid fracture. In the traumatic nonunion, the gap between the fracture fragments is characteristically irregular and narrow and extends into the body of the axis below the level of the superior facets of the axis vertebra (62). The bone fragments appear to have no cortical margin or rounded appearance, and the fragments "match."

Evidence favors an unrecognized fracture in the region of the base of the odontoid as the most common cause of os odontoideum (27). It has been seen in patients who have had a recognized complete odontoid process in early childhood and subsequently progressed to have an os odontoideum in one of identical twins who had cervical trauma and in patients with gross ligamentous laxity, such as that associated with Down syndrome and Morquio syndrome (3,28,40,44,62,78,92). Following fracture of the odontoid in early childhood or acute ligamentous injury, a separation may take place. With time and contracture of the alar ligaments, a distraction force pulls the odontoid fragments away from the centrum of the axis toward the occipital bone. The blood supply of the odontoid is easily traumatized and may contribute to poor healing or callus formation that would now retard closure of the gap (1,27,64,71,83,91). The ossicle is then supplied through the proximal arterial arcade, accounting for the hypertrophy of the anterior atlantal arch that

shares the same blood supply. There is now increasing evidence that os odontoideum is more commonly associated with trauma, upper respiratory infections, bony abnormalities such as spondyloepiphyseal dysplasia, and previously mentioned Morquio syndrome and Down syndrome (28,62,91) (Fig. 9).

The biomechanics of os odontoideum must be carefully studied because it is varied. The movement of os odontoideum is individual with each patient and cannot be extrapolated to another. In the dystropic variety, a dorsal compromise of the spinal cord may occur by the forward position of the posterior arch of the atlas in the flexed position, as well as ventral compromise by the odontoid ossicles. At times the axis may be displaced dorsally in extension and increase the ventral compromise (Fig. 10A–C). Thus, each patient should be carefully assessed by dynamic studies in the flexed and extended and the lateral positions. Lateral displacement of the atlantoaxial complex is a common finding at the time of operative fixation in such individuals (27,62) (Fig. 1).

Direct pathologic examination of the area at the time of ventral decompressive surgery has shown that an irreducible state may be caused by slippage of the transverse portion of the cruciate ligament beneath the ossicle and at times even in front of it (58). In addition, intense granulation proliferation may occur ventral to the bone defect owing to repeated luxations. In severe

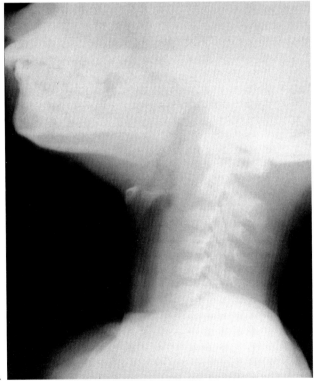

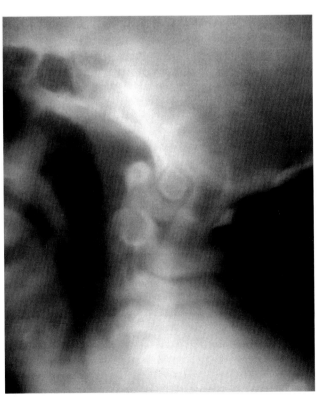

A   B

FIGURE 9. A: Lateral cervical radiograph made in a 4-year-old with traumatic atlantoaxial dislocation. She was treated with cervical traction and a pediatric Minerva cast (1967). **B:** Midline pluridirectional myelotomogram of craniocervical junction. Iohexol outlines the cerebrospinal fluid spaces. This study was made in 1980, when the patient was 17 years old. The patient had acute quadriparesis following a minor accident. Note the dystopic os odontoideum with ventral compression of the cervicomedullary junction. The odontoid process was intact at age 4, as seen in **A.**

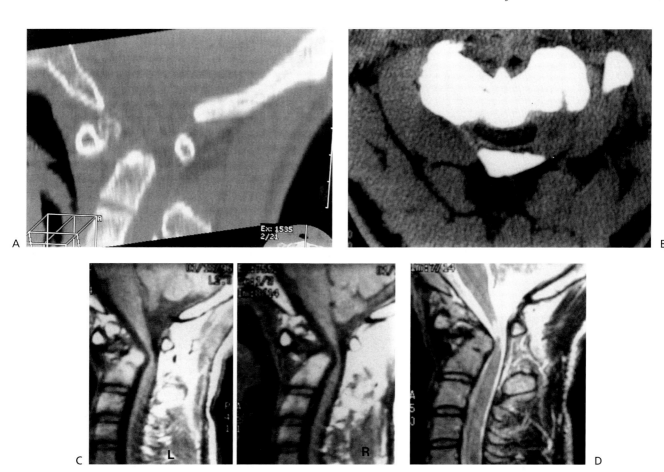

FIGURE 10. A: Midsagittal two-dimensional computed tomographic reconstruction of craniocervical region. This 15-year-old presented with spastic quadriparesis and ninth and tenth nerve cranial palsies. There is a dystopic os odontoideum with a dorsal and upward migration of the axis body, causing severe canal compromise. **B:** Axial computed tomogram through the plane of the superior axis body. Note the dorsally displaced axis with marked compromise of the cervicomedullary junction between the axis body and the posterior atlantal arch. **C:** Composite of T1-weighted magnetic resonance image of craniocervical junction in the sagittal and parasagittal location. There is significant ventral compression of the cervicomedullary junction by the displaced axis body. **D:** T2-weighted midsagittal magnetic resonance image through the craniocervical region. There is atlantoaxial dislocation with a dystopic os odontoideum. The compression of the ventral cervicomedullary junction is caused by the dorsal aspect of the superior axis body. Note the contusion within the cervicomedullary junction at the level of the axis compression.

chronic dislocation, this may become fixed over several years, accompanied by severe basilar invagination. At its worst, os odontoideum has significant implications concerning the compression of the cervicomedullary junction. There is no argument that in unstable situations, as well as in cases involving neurologic deficits, therapy is mandated. However, the most difficult question to answer is whether an asymptomatic child, recognized as having an os odontoideum on a routine cervical spine radiographic after head trauma, should undergo treatment. It is not uncommon for children who are asymptomatic with os odontoideum to have severe neurologic deficits following minor trauma, as with dental work, sports activities, and gymnastics. We believe that all patients with recognizable instability at the craniocervical junction and associated os odontoideum should undergo stabilization. If a fixed irreducible abnormality exists, decompression should be done first.

Down Syndrome (Fig. 11)

The incidence of craniovertebral anomalies related to Down syndrome warrants special comment. The treatment of instability at the CVJ in patients with Down syndrome has become somewhat controversial because some authors have reported high fusion-related complication rates and suggested that the incidence of neurologic abnormality associated with this abnormal motion may be low. This has led to neurologic disasters with minor neck manipulations, as with tonsillectomy under general anesthesia. The authors have reported on the clinical and radiographic findings in 33 patients treated at their institution (63,94). Common presenting symptoms included neck pain (14 patients), torticollis (12 patients), myelopathy manifesting as hyperreflexia (21 patients), or varying degrees of quadriparesis (11 patients). Four patients suffered acute neurologic insults,

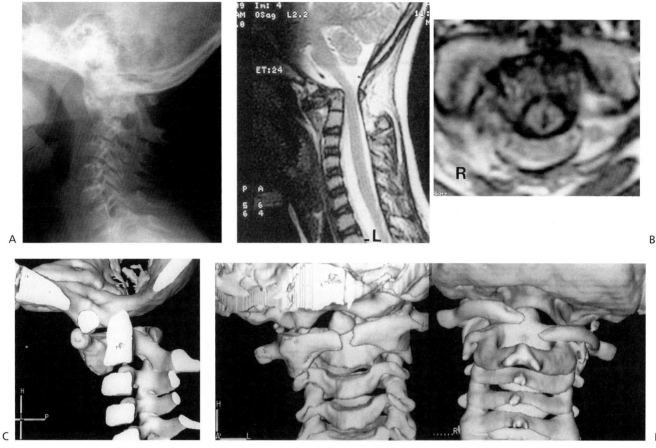

FIGURE 11. **A:** Lateral cervical radiograph in a 9-year-old girl with Down syndrome. She presented with head tilt, arm weakness, and inability to walk. Note the gross atlantoaxial dislocation. **B:** Composite of T2-weighted midsagittal magnetic resonance image of craniocervical junction on the left and axial view through the plane of the axis body. A dystopic os odontoideum is seen. However, the cervicomedullary compression is caused ventrally by the superior aspect of the axis body and dorsally by the posterior arch of C1. **C:** Midsagittal view of three-dimensional computed tomogram of craniocervical junction viewed from within. Note the os odontoideum, the bifid posterior and anterior arch of C1, the atlantoaxial dislocation, and the upward migration of the axis body. **D:** Composite of three-dimensional craniocervical images viewed from in front *(left)* and behind *(right)*. The atlas is bifid anteriorly and posteriorly in the midline. There is a lateral displacement of the lateral atlantal masses with a rotary luxation of the right lateral mass being displaced forward and downward. This is a grossly unstable craniocervical junction.

two after receiving routine general anesthetics for minor surgical procedures and two other patients following minor falls. Atlantoaxial instability was the most common abnormality documented on radiography (22 patients). Atlantooccipital instability (15 patients) was also frequently observed and was coexistent with the presence of atlantoaxial luxations in 14 patients. A rotary component of the atlantoaxial luxation was present in 13 cases. In 17 patients, bony anomalies were present, the most frequent of which was os odontoideum (10 patients). Twenty-four patients underwent operative intervention, and successful fusion was achieved in 23. In 6 of 9 patients with basilar invagination, reduction was achieved with preoperative traction, avoiding the need for ventral decompressive procedures. There were no incidents of postoperative deterioration, and 22 patients made excellent or good recoveries. The results of this series highlight the clinicopathologic phenomena of craniovertebral insta-

bility in patients with Down syndrome and suggest that satisfactory outcomes can be achieved with a low rate of surgical morbidity.

The most common chromosomal abnormality in humans, trisomy 21, occurs approximately once in every 700 births. The clinical syndrome associated with this genetic aberration was originally described in 1866 by John Langdon Down and subsequently bore his name (76,89,96). Down syndrome is well recognized by its phenotypic features, which include characteristic facies, hypotonia, ligamentous laxity, mental retardation, and transverse palmar creases. This disorder can variably affect nearly every organ system, resulting in numerous potential complications. Manifestations of the disease affecting the CVJ were first described in 1961 by Spitzer et al., who reported on 9 of 29 patients with atlantooccipital dislocations (89).

The generalized ligamentous laxity associated with Down

syndrome, as well as incidence of bony anomalies, predisposes the CVJ to instability because of the complex interaction of ligamentous and bony anatomy required to maintain stability. In 7% to 40% of patients with Down syndrome there is radiographic evidence of atlantoaxial instability, although the incidence of symptomatic instability may be less than 1%. Atlantooccipital instability and rotary luxation of the atlas are well described in patients with Down syndrome and should not be overlooked. Parfenchuck et al. have suggested that the incidence of posterior atlantooccipital hypermobility in Down syndrome is 8.5% (70). Bony anomalies, such as os odontoideum and hypoplasia of various craniovertebral elements, including the atlantal ring and condyles, likely increase the risk for instability at the CVJ. This evidence in part prompted the American Academy of Pediatrics Committee on Sports Medicine and Fitness to mandate that participants with Down syndrome undergo physical examination and radiographic screening of the cervical spine prior to competition in the Special Olympics (63).

Evidence regarding the natural history of atlantoaxial instability suggests that it may be a progressive disease. In follow-up of 33 patients over a 13-year period, 7 were found to have developed instability (predental space of more than 5 mm), as compared with only one patient in whom this instability was present at the start of the study (13). Two patients underwent arthrodesis and one died of the pathologic process. Pueschel et al. evaluated 95 patients over a 3- to 10-year period and found that in 7 a predental space greater than 5 mm had developed (77). These authors claimed that no patient became symptomatic. Ferguson et al. recently called into question the relationship of neurologic abnormality and atlantoaxial instability (25). Eighty-four patients with Down syndrome were evaluated for a predental space of 4 mm or greater or 2 mm of translation in flexion and extension. In 20% (17 patients), instability at the atlantoaxial joint was demonstrated. In a comparison of results of neurologic examinations with patients in whom subluxation was present with those in whom it was not, no significant difference could be found relative to incidence (29% and 27%, respectively) or type of positive neurologic finding. Results of our series demonstrate not only that children with this phenomenon are predisposed to neural compromise but also that a high rate of neurologic recovery can be expected (94).

Atlantooccipital and occipitoatlantoaxial instability are expected findings in the Down syndrome population (97). Clinical correlations were not made in the first description of atlantooccipital luxation by Spitzer et al. (89). Neurologic abnormalities have been found in up to 66% of patients with atlantooccipital instability. In a prospective review of 64 patients with atlantooccipital instability, 61% of the patients were shown to have a posterior occipital subluxation greater than 4 mm and 21% to have a predental space greater than 5 mm. Uno et al. reviewed flexion and extension cervical radiographs obtained in 75 patients with Down syndrome. Comparing their findings with those of 30 age-matched controls, they found a significant number of patients in whom atlantooccipital hypermobility was demonstrated (98). Furthermore, they found occipitoaxial instability coexistent with atlantoaxial instability in all cases. In 11 of the 14 patients in our series, atlantoaxial instability along with atlantooccipital instability was found, which supports their finding,

although correlation is not absolute. In this light, both Brooke et al. and El-Khoury et al. have reported two patients with Down syndrome in whom atlantooccipital instability was present without atlantoaxial abnormality (11,24).

Rotary luxations of the atlantooccipital and atlantoaxial joint were initially described in a Down syndrome patient in 1969 by Sherk and Nicholson (87). Surgical intervention was not undertaken, and 9 years after the diagnosis was made this female patient developed acute quadriplegia and died of respiratory failure. Other investigators have recognized a rotary component of instability in some patients with Down syndrome (20). In more than one third of the patients in our series a component of rotary luxation at C1–2 was found, and in one patient rotary luxation at *occiput -C-C2* was demonstrated. It is important to recognize this phenomenon because the ipsilateral vertebral artery can kink and the contralateral vessel put on stretch as the rotation at C1 exceeds 35 degrees (85). Subsequently, the facets may lock, resulting in a fixed luxation, and can only be disengaged if traction and derotation are performed. One must recognize that this rotary component can worsen the canal compromise and increase the stress placed on the cruciate ligament; thus, it can worsen the stability of an already compromised CVJ in a patient with Down syndrome.

The bony anomalies associated with Down syndrome, particularly os odontoideum, deserve emphasis. Unsuspected fractures of the odontoid, with secondary pull of the alar and apical ligaments, may result from repeated minor traumatic events in these patients. Over time, the cruciate ligament becomes incompetent, resulting in atlantoaxial dislocation and possibly allowing for decompression at the ventral cervicomedullary junction because the odontoid ascends into the foramen magnum. In 1985, Burke described 20 patients in whom myelopathy had developed secondary to atlantoaxial instability; in nine of these patients, either an os odontoideum or odontoid hypoplasia was present (8). Pueschel and Scola have provided evidence that a higher rate of cervical bony anomalies exists in the subgroup of Down syndrome patients in whom atlantoaxial instability is present (31 of 39) (76). In this report, the authors also reviewed the bony anomalies in Down syndrome patients, and os odontoideum and ossiculum terminale were shown to be common. This evidence supports the findings in our series that in nearly half of patients with bony anomalies, the particular anomaly was os odontoideum, followed by posterior atlantal arch hypoplasia (Fig. 11).

In the clinical setting, achieving consistent, successful outcomes in this patient population is challenging. Incomplete evaluation or understanding of the complex interactions at the CVJ has resulted in poor pre- and perioperative planning and treatment, including failure to recognize simultaneous instability at the different segments of the CVJ, failure to obtain proper reduction prior to the decompression and fusion procedure, and performance of intraoperative reduction without application of traction. In our own clinical experience, we have seen fusion failure as a result of inappropriate postoperative immobilization, failure to recognize and appropriately treat ventral pathologic processes, and inadequate bone grafting. Segal et al. have reported successful initial fusion in only 2 of 10 patients and bone graft absorption in 6 patients (84). More recently, in 7 of 15 patients with

Down syndrome, a nonunion occurred after attempted posterior arthrodesis (20). In this series, reported by Doyle et al. (20), 4 of the 7 patients achieved solid bony fusion after reoperation; in 3 of these 4 patients, fusion was preceded by loss of reduction and neurologic deterioration, and successful fusion was achieved only after the occiput was incorporated on the second attempt.

Abnormal physiologic processes in the Down patient may also contribute to poor outcome (8). The T-cell-dependent processes of the immune system in patients with Down syndrome are deficient as measured both quantitatively and qualitatively. The overall number of T lymphocytes is decreased as is the synthesis of lymphokines and the secretory products of these cells. These products may affect the initial inflammatory stages of bone graft incorporation. Other authors have implicated a collagen defect intrinsic to Down syndrome patients as responsible for bone graft resorption and poor graft maturation (84). The sequential forms of collagen required for successful graft incorporation may be deficient and thus contribute to nonunion or graft absorption.

Based on our own series and our interpretation of the literature, we find that occipitocervical fusion is required to address cranial settling, reducible basilar invagination, and anterior, posterior or lateral cranial dislocation within the CVJ. This is performed in as far lateral an interlaminar fashion as possible between the axis and atlas. Although iliac crest may be harvested, we favor the use of autologous full-thickness rib as the donor bone. Sawin et al. have shown that posterior rib harvesting was not associated with significant pulmonary morbidity when compared with autologous iliac crest harvesting in patients undergoing cervical fusion procedures (82). Furthermore, rib grafting was associated with an excellent fusion rate in their series. Titanium cable is used to purchase the exoccipital bone to improve the stiffness of the construct. Generally, patients are immobilized in a halo vest for 3 to 4 months for atlantoaxial fusion and up to 6 months for atlantooccipital fusion. Inadequate immobilization invites nonunion, resorption of the graft, and progressive instability.

Skeletal Dysplasias

The practical approach to skeletal dysplasias in infancy was formulated by Dutton based on the international nomenclature of constitutional disease of the bone (21). Many authors have attempted to clarify the older well-known titles of dysplasias, which now fall into the category of skeletal dysplasias. Skeletal dysplasias are divided into five large categories: (a) osteochondral dysplasia; (b) dysostosis; (c) idiopathic osteolysis; (d) chromosomal aberrations; and (e) primary metabolic abnormalities.

Osteochondral dysplasias and dysostosis account for the largest and most complex entities. Each category is further subdivided into numerous subcategories and individual diagnoses. Osteochondral dysplasias are defined as abnormalities of cartilage or bone growth in development. This category includes achondrogenesis, thanatophoric dysplasia, chondrodysplasia punctata (Conradi-Hünermann syndrome), achondroplasia, dystrophic dysplasia, metatrophic dysplasia, spondyloepiphyseal dysplasia, Kniest dysplasia, cleidocranial dysplasia, and multiple epiphyseal dysplasias (33,41,43,77,81,90,94,108,109).

The dysostoses are defined as malformations of individual bones manifested singly or in combination. The category may include Crouzon, Apert, and Carpenter syndromes with vertebral defects. This category also includes Sprengel deformity and Klippel-Feil syndrome.

The subcategory of idiopathic osteolysis includes the diagnosis of spondyloepiphyseal dysplasia tarda, fibrous dysplasia, neurofibromatosis, osteogenesis imperfecta, and multicentric forms such as the Hajdu-Cheney form (17,38,90).

The primary metabolic and chromosomal abnormalities are numerous. The metabolic abnormalities include problems with calcium or phosphorus metabolism, such as rickets and pseudohypoparathyroidism. Abnormalities of calcium and phosphorous metabolism will lead to bone softening and a secondary form of invagination. This may be paramesial, which is common with achondroplasia, in which case the sagittal diameter of the foramen magnum is preserved whereas the transverse diameter is markedly reduced. In addition, an inward bending of the exoccipital bone results in further invagination and creation of a dural shelf, which compresses the dorsal cervicomedullary junction (80) (Fig. 12). Thus, in these syndromes, posterior decompression is necessary with a duraplasty. Upper cervical and spinal stenosis is a well-known entity with such syndromes as achondroplasia and Morquio syndrome (50,93,103).

Atlantoaxial instability occurs with increasing incidence in the skeletal dysplasias. In patients with achondroplasia, we have noted cervicomedullary compromise most frequently in those younger than 3 years (80). Sleep apnea has been a major symptom, as has progressive spastic quadriparesis. In this situation,

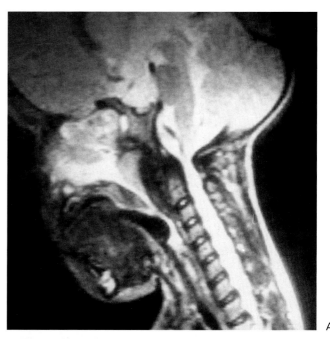

A

FIGURE 12. A: Midsagittal T2-weighted magnetic resonance image of craniocervical region in a 4-year-old girl with achondroplasia. She presented with weakness in the arms and gait difficulty. Note the constriction of the subarachnoid sac at the foramen magnum and C1 level. The brain stem is abnormally "vertical," with the pons above the sella turcica. *(Figure continues.)*

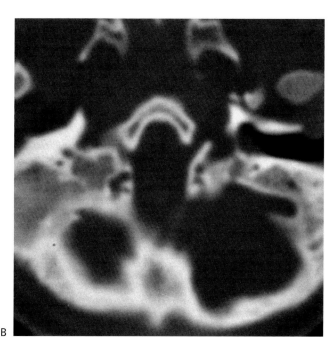

B

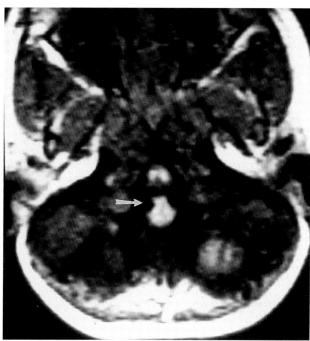

C

FIGURE 12. *(continued)* **B:** Axial computed tomogram through plane of foramen magnum. The bone formatted windows demonstrate a narrowing of the transverse diameter of the foramen magnum with paramesial invagination. **C:** T1-weighted magnetic resonance image at foramen magnum illustrates a paramesial invagination with compromise of the cervicomedullary junction.

CT myelography with iohexol has permitted visualization of the compression at the foramen magnum as well as at C1 and C2. There is an inward bending of the posterior arch of the atlas, further compromising the stenosis. Prior to embarking on therapy, one must confirm that prior attention has been given to hydrocephalus, if present.

Spondyloepiphyseal dysplasia is a complex disorder with atlantoaxial instability seen in infancy. Our approach has been to brace the infant with a custom-built orthosis until definitive surgical treatment can be performed between ages 2 and 4 years (59). In individuals in whom this occurs at a later age, the treatment would be as previously outlined.

REFERENCES

1. Althoff B, Goldie IF (1977): The arterial supply of the odontoid process of the axis. *Acta Orthop Scand* 48:622–626.
2. Aryanpur J, Hurko O, Francomano C, et al. (1990): Craniocervical decompression for cervicomedullary compression in pediatric patients with achondroplasia. *J Neurosurg* 73:375–382.
3. Ashraf J, Crockard HA, Ransford AO, et al. (1991): Transoral decompression and posterior stabilization in Morquio's disease. *Arch Dis Child* 66:1318–1321.
4. Baga N, Chusid EL, Miller A (1969): Pulmonary disability in the Klippel-Feil syndrome. *Clin Orthop* 67:105–110.
5. Baird PA, Robinson GC, Buckler WSTJ (1962): Klippel-Feil syndrome. A study of mirror movements detected by electromyelography. *Am J Dis Child* 113:546–661.
6. Barucha EP, Dastur HM (1964): Craniovertebral anomalies. *Brain* 87:469–480.
7. Berger FE, Tew JM Jr (1982): Basilar impression and platybasia in osteogenesis imperfecta tarda. *Surg Neurol* 17:116–119.
8. Braakhekke JP (1988): Symptomatic atlantoaxial dislocation in Down's syndrome. *Ann Neurol* 23:421.
9. Brasch JC (1958): *Cunningham's manual of practical anatomy.* Oxford: Oxford University Press, pp. 258–295.
10. Brill CB, Rose JS, Godmilow L, et al. (1978): Spastic quadriparesis due to C1–C2 subluxation in Hurler's syndrome. *J Pediatr* 92: 441–443.
11. Brooke DC, Burkus JK, Benson DR (1987): Asymptomatic occipitoatlantal instability in Down syndrome (trisomy 21). Report of two cases in children. *J Bone Joint Surg Am* 69:293–295.
12. Bull JWD, Nixon WLB, Pratt RTC (1955): The radiological criteria and familial occurrence of primary basilar impression. *Brain* 78: 229–247.
13. Burke SW, French HA, Robert S, et al. (1985): Chronic atlantoaxial instability in Down's syndrome. *J Bone Joint Surg Am* 67:1356–1360.
14. Bystrow A (1931): Assimilation des atlas und manifestation des proatlas. *Z Anat* 95:210–242.
15. Chamberlain WE (1938–1939): Basilar impression (platybasia). *Yale J Biol Med* 11:487–496.
16. de Oliveira E, Rhoton AL Jr, Peace D (1985): Micro-surgical anatomy of the region of the foramen magnum. *Surg Neurol* 24:293–352.
17. Cheney WD (1965): Acro-osteolysis. *Am J Roentgenol* 94:595–607.
18. Cohen ME, Rosenthal AD, Matson DD (1967): Neurological abnormalities in achondroplastic children. *J Pediatr* 71:367–372.
19. Daffner RH (1996): CT of the craniovertebral junction. *Am J Roentgenol* 167(2):365–366.
20. Doyle JS, Lauerman WC, Wood KB, et al (1996): Complications and long-term outcome of upper cervical spine arthrodesis in patients with Down syndrome. *Spine* 21:1223–1231.
21. Dutton RV (1987): A practical radiologic approach to skeletal dysplasias in infancy. *Radiol Clin N Am* 25:1211–1233.
22. Dyck P (1978): Os odontoideum in children: neurological manifestations and surgical management. *Neurosurgery* 2:93–99.
23. Dyste GN, Menezes AH (1988): Presentation and management of pediatric Chiari malformations without myelodysplasia. *Neurosurgery* 23:589–597.

24. El-Khoury GY, Clark CR, Dietz FR, et al (1986): Posterior atlanto-occipital subluxation in Down syndrome. *Radiology* 159:507–509.

25. Ferguson RL, Putney ME, Allen BL Jr (1997): Comparison of neurologic deficits with atlanto-dens intervals in patients with Down syndrome. *J Spinal Disord* 10:246–252.

26. Fielding JW, Cochran GB, Lawsing JR III, et al (1974): Tears of the transverse ligament of the atlas. A clinical and biomechanical study. *J Bone Joint Surg Am* 56:1683–1691.

27. Fielding JW, Hensinger RN, Hawkins RJ (1980): Os odontoideum. *J Bone Joint Surg Am* 62:376–383.

28. Freiberger RH, Wilson PD Jr, Nicholas JA (1965): Acquired absence of the odontoid process: a case report. *J Bone Joint Surg Am* 47:1231–123.

29. Fromm GH, Pitner SE (1963): Late progressive quadriparesis due to odontoid agenesis. *Arch Neurol* 9:291–296.

30. Ganguly DN, Roy KK (1964): A study on the craniovertebral joint in the man. *Anat Anz* 114:433–452.

31. Gladstone J, Erickson-Powell W (1915): Manifestations of occipital vertebra and fusion of atlas with occipital bone. *J Anat Physiol* 49:190–199.

32. Goel VK, Clark CR, Gallaes K, et al. (1988): Movement-rotation relationships of the ligamentous occipito-atlanto-axial complex. *J Biomech* 21:678–680.

33. Goldberg MJ (1976): Orthopedic aspects of bone dysplasias. *Orthop Clin N Am* 7:445–456.

34. Greenberg AD (1968): Atlanto-axial dislocations. *Brain* 91:655–684.

35. Greenlee J, Garell PC, Stence P, et al. (1999): Comprehensive approach to Chiari malformation in pediatric patients. *Neurosurg Focus* 6(6):4.

36. Grisel P (1930): Enucleation des l'atlas et torticollis nasopharyngien. *Presse Med* 38:50–53.

37. Guillo JT, Miller A, Bowen R, et al. (1995): The natural history of Klippel-Feil Syndrome: clinical, roentgenographic, and magnetic resonance imaging findings at adulthood. *J Pediatr Orthop* 15:617–625.

38. Hajdu N, Kauntze R (1948): Cranioskeletal dysplasia. *Br J Radiol* 21:42–48.

39. Harkey HL, Crockard HA, Stevens JM, et al. (1990): The operative management of basilar impression in osteogenesis imperfecta. *Neurosurgery* 27:782–786.

40. Hawkins RJ, Fielding JW, Thompson WJ (1976): Os odontoideum: congenital or acquired. *J Bone Joint Surg Am* 58:413–414.

41. Hecht JT, Horton WA, Butler IJ, et al. (1986): Foramen magnum stenosis in homozygous achondroplasia. *Eur J Pediatr* 145:545–547.

42. Hensinger RN, Lang JE, MacEwen D (1976): Klippel-Feil syndrome. A constellation of associated anomalies. *J Bone Joint Surg Am* 6:1246–1253.

43. Hensinger RN (1986): Osseous anomalies of the craniovertebral junction. *Spine* 11:323–333.

44. Hukuda S, Ota H, Norikazu O, et al. (1980): Traumatic atlantoaxial dislocation causing os odontoideum in infants. *Spine* 5:207–210.

45. Hunt TE, Dekaban AS (1982): Modified head-neck support for basilar invagination with brain stem compression. *Can Med Assoc J* 126:947–948.

46. Jirout J (1973): Changes in the atlas-axis relations on lateral flexion of the head and neck. *Neuroradiology* 6:215–218.

47. Johnson MH, Smoker WR (1994): Lesions of the craniovertebral junction. *Neuroimag Clin N Am* 4(3):599–617.

48. Jones MD (1960): Cineradiographic studies of the normal cervical spine. *Calif Med* 93:293–296.

49. Klippel M, Feil A (1912): Un cas D'absence des vertebres cervicales avec cage thoracique remontant jusqu'a base du cranie. *Nouv Icon Selpetriere* 25:223–250.

50. Kopits SE, Perovic MN, McKusick V, et al. (1972): Congenital atlanto-axial dislocations in various forms of dwarfism. *J Bone Joint Surg Am* 54:1349–1350.

51. Lanier RR Jr (1939): Anomalous cervico-occipital skeleton in man. *Anat Rec* 73:189–207.

52. List CF (1941): Neurologic syndromes accompanying developmental anomalies of occipital bone, atlas and axis. *Arch Neurol Psychiatry* 45:577–616.

53. Locke GR, Gardner JI, VanEpps EF (1966): Atlas-dens interval (ADI) in children: A survey based on 200 normal cervical spines. *Am J Roentgenol* 97:135–150.

54. Macalister A (1892–1893): Notes on the development and variations of the atlas. *J Anat Physiol* 27:519–542.

55. MacEwen D (1975): The Klippel-Feil syndrome. *J Bone Joint Surg Br* 57:261–267.

56. McRae DL, Barnum AS (1953): Occipitalization of the atlas. *Am J Roentgenol* 70:23–46.

57. McRae DL (1960): The significance of abnormalities of the cervical spine. *Am J Roentgenol* 84:3–25.

58. Menezes AH (1988): Os odontoideum—pathogenesis, dynamics and management. In: Marlin AE, ed. *Concepts in pediatric neurosurgery*, vol 8. Basel: Karger, pp. 133–145.

59. Menezes AH (1991): Surgical approaches to the craniocervical junction. In: Frymoyer J, ed. *The adult spine: principles and practice*, vol 2. New York: Raven Press, pp. 967–986.

60. Menezes AH (1992): The anterior midline approach to the craniocervical region in children. In: McLone DG, ed. *Concepts in pediatric neurosurgery*. Basel: Karger.

61. Menezes AH (1995): Primary craniovertebral anomalies and the hindbrain herniation syndrome (Chiari I): data base analysis. *Pediatr Neurosurg* 23(5):260–269.

62. Menezes AH (1999): Pathogenesis, dynamics and management of os odontoideum. *Neurosurg Focus* 6(6):2.

63. Menezes AH, Ryken TC (1992): Craniovertebral abnormalities in Down's syndrome. *Pediatr Neurosurg* 18:24–33.

64. Menezes AH, VanGilder JC (1990): Anomalies of the craniovertebral junction. In: Youman J, ed. *Neurological surgery*, 3rd ed., vol 2. Philadelphia: WB Saunders, pp. 1359–1420.

65. Menezes AH, Graf CJ, Hibri N (1980): Abnormalities of the craniovertebral junction with cervicomedullary compression. A rational approach to surgical treatment in children. *Chil's Brain* 7:15–30.

66. Mitchie I, Clark M (1968): Neurological syndromes associated with cervical and craniocervical anomalies. *Arch Neurol* 18:241–247.

67. Muhonen MG, Menezes AH, Sawin PD, et al. (1992): Scoliosis in pediatric Chiari malformations without myelodysplasia. *J Neurosurg* 77:69–77.

68. Nicholson JT, Sherk HH (1968): Anomalies of the occipitocervical articulation. *J Bone Joint Surg Am* 50:295–304.

69. Palant DI, Carter BL (1972): Klippel-Feil syndrome and deafness. *Am J Dis Child* 123:218–221.

70. Parfenchuck TA, Bertrand SL, Powers MJ, et al (1994): Posterior occipitoatlantal hypermobility in Down syndrome: an analysis of 199 patients. *J Pediatr Orthop* 14:304–308.

71. Parke WW (1978): The vascular relationships of the upper cervical vertebrae. *Orthop Clin N Am* 9:879–889.

72. Parke WW, Rothman RH, Brown MD (1984): The pharyngovertebral veins. An anatomical rationale for Grisel's syndrome. *J Bone Joint Surg Am* 66:568–574.

73. Pauli RM, Gilbert EF (1986): Upper cervical cord compression as a cause of death in osteogenesis imperfecta type II. *J Pediatr* 108:579–581.

74. Poppel MH, Jacobson HG, Duff BK (1953): Basilar impression and platybasia in Paget's disease. *Radiology* 61:639–644.

75. Pozo JL, Crockard HA, Ransford AO (1984): Basilar impression in osteogenesis imperfecta. A report of three cases in one family. *J Bone Joint Surg Br* 66:233–238.

76. Pueschel SM, Scola F (1987): Atlantoaxial instability in individuals with Down's syndrome: epidemiologic, radiographic and clinical studies. *Pediatrics* 80:555–560.

77. Reid CS, Pyeritz RE, Kopits SE, et al (1987): Cervicomedullary compression in young patients with achondroplasia: value of comprehensive neurologic and respiratory evaluation. *J Pediatr* 110:522–530.

78. Riccardi JE, Kaufer H, Louis DS (1976): Acquired os odontoideum following acute ligament injury. *J Bone Joint Surg Am* 58:410–412.

79. Roth M (1986): Craniocervical growth collision: another explanation

of the Arnold-Chiari malformation and of basilar impression. *Neuroradiology* 28:187–194.

80. Ryken TC, Menezes AH (1994): Cervicomedullary compression in achondroplasia. *J Neurosurg* 81:43–48.

81. Sawin PD, Menezes AH (1997): Basilar invagination in osteogenesis imperfecta and related osteochondrodysplasias: medical and surgical management. *J Neurosurg* 86:950–960.

82. Sawin PD, Traynelis VC, Menezes AH (1998): A comparative analysis of fusion rates and donor site morbidity for autogeneic rib and iliac crest bone grafts in posterior cervical fusions. *J Neurosurg* 88:255–265.

83. Schiff DCM, Parke WW (1972): The arterial blood supply of the odontoid process (dens). *Anat Rec* 72:339–400.

84. Segal LS, Drummond DS, Zanotti RM, et al (1991): Complications of posterior arthrodesis of the cervical spine in patients who have Down's syndrome. *J Bone Joint Surg Am* 73:1547–1554.

85. Selecki BR (1969): The effects of rotation of the atlas on the axis: experimental work. *Med J Aust* 1:1012–1015.

86. Shapiro R, Robinson F (1976): Anomalies of the craniovertebral border. *Am J Roentgenol* 127:281–287.

87. Sherk HH, Nicholson JT (1969): Rotary atlanto-axial dislocation associated with ossiculum terminale and mongolism. A case report. *J Bone Joint Surg Am* 51:957–964.

88. Spillane JD, Pallis C, Jones AM (1957): Developmental abnormalities in the region of the foramen magnum. *Brain* 80:11–48.

89. Spitzer R, Rabinowitch JY, Wybar KC (1961): A study of the abnormalities of the skull, teeth and lenses in mongolism. *Can Med Assoc J* 84:567–572.

90. Spranger JW, Langer LO (1970): Spondyloepiphyseal dysplasia congenita. *Radiology* 94:313–322.

91. Steinbok P, Hall J, Flodmark O (1989): Hydrocephalus in achondroplasia: the possible role of intracranial venous hypertension. *J Neurosurg* 71:42–48.

92. Stevens JM, Chong WK, Barber C, et al. (1994): A new appraisal of abnormalities of the odontoid process associated with atlantoaxial subluxation and neurological disability. *Brain* 117:133–148.

93. Stevens JM, Kendall BE, Crockard HA (1991): The odontoid process in Morquio-Brailsford's disease; the effects of occipitocervical fusion. *J Bone Joint Surg Br* 73:851–858.

94. Taggard DA, Menezes AM, Ryken TC (1999): Instability of the crani-

overtebral junction and treatment outcomes in patients with Down's syndrome. *Neurosurg Focus* 6(6):1–7.

95. Tanzer A (1956): Die basilare impression. *Radiol Clin* 25:135–142.

96. Taylor AR, Byrnes DP (1974): Foramen magnum and high cervical cord compression. *Brain* 97:473–480.

97. Tishler J, Martel W (1965): Dislocation of the atlas in mongolism: preliminary report. *Radiology* 84:904–906.

98. Uno K, Kataoka O, Shiba R (1996): Occipitoatlantal and occipitoaxial hypermobility in Down's syndrome. *Spine* 21:1430–1434.

99. VanGilder JC, Menezes AH, Dolan K, eds. (1987). *Craniovertebral junction abnormalities.* Mount Kisco, NY: Futura Publishing.

100. VonTorklus D, Gehle W (1972): The upper cervical spine. Regional anatomy, pathology and traumatology. In: Georg Thieme Verlag, ed. *A systemic radiological atlas and textbook.* New York: Grune & Stratton, pp. 2–77.

101. Wackenheim A (1969): A radiologic diagnosis of congenital forms, intermittent forms and progressive forms of stenosis of the spinal canal of the level of the atlas. *Acta Radiol Diagn (Stockh)* 9:481–486.

102. Wadia NH (1967): Myelopathy complicating congenital atlanto-axial dislocation (a study of 28 cases). *Brain* 90:449–474.

103. Wald SL, Schmidek HH (1984): Compressive myelopathy associated with type VI mucopolysaccharidosis (Maroteaux-Lamy syndrome). *Neurosurgery* 14:83–88.

104. Weil VH (1981): Osteogenesis imperfecta: historical background. *Clin Orthop Rel Res* 159:6–10.

105. Werne S (1957): Studies in spontaneous atlas dislocation. *Acta Orthop Scand* 23[Suppl]:1–50.

106. White AA III, Punjabi MM (1978): The clinical biomechanics of the occipito-atlanto-axial complex. *Orthop Clin N Am* 9:867–878.

107. Wilson BC, Jarvis BL, Handon BC (1987): Nontraumatic subluxation of the atlantoaxial joint. Grisel's syndrome. *Ann Otol Rhinol Laryngol* 96:703–708.

108. Wong VC (1991): Basilar impression in a child with hypochondroplasia. *Pediatr Neurol* 7:62–64.

109. Wynne-Davies R, Hall CM, Young ID (1986): Pseudoachondroplasia: clinical diagnosis at different ages and comparison of autosomal dominant and recessive types. A review of 32 patients (26 kindreds). *J Med Genet* 23:425–434.

12

CONGENITAL ABNORMALITIES OF THE CERVICAL SPINE

FREDERICK DIETZ

Development of the cervical vertebral column begins with the process of gastrulation, during which the embryonic mesoderm and the notochordal plate are formed. This process is completed by the third week of embryonic life. The notochord induces formation of the neural groove, which gradually closes from cranial to caudad to form the neural tube. By the twenty-third day of fetal life, the neural groove is closed except for the most cranial and caudal ends, which are called the neuropores. These usually close by the end of the fourth week.

With the formation of the neural tube, the mesoderm on each side of the notochord develops lateral, intermediate, and paraxial proliferations. The lateral plate mesoderm gives rise to the pleural pericardium, peritoneum, and mesentery, blood vessels, and limb-bud mesoderm. The intermediate mesoderm gives rise to the urogenital system. The paraxial mesoderm becomes the vertebrae and ribs as well as the dermis and musculature. At the end of the third week of development, the paraxial mesoderm segments into paired masses, called somites. The somites are formed craniad and extend caudally, with each somite differentiating into three portions: the dermatome laterally, the sclerotome ventromedially, and the myotome in between. The dermatome differentiates into the dermis of the skin; the myotome into muscles, tendons, and fascia; and the sclerotome into the vertebral discs and ligaments of the vertebral column and ribs.

At the fourth week, the sclerotomic cells from each pair of somites migrate medially, meeting around the notochord and separating it from the dorsal neural tube and the ventral gut. Between adjacent somitic segments is a transverse intersegmental artery. The segmental spinal nerves originally lie at the midportion of the somitic sclerotomal mass. A process of resegmentation of sclerotomic tissues occurs at about $4\frac{1}{2}$ weeks. Each somitic sclerotome thins out cranially and condenses caudally by variable-rate mitosis. Part of the condensed portion migrates cranially to the center of the sclerotome, and this central condensed portion differentiates into the intervertebral disc. The rest of the dense caudal portion of each sclerotome unites with the less condensed cranial part of the next sclerotome to form the primordium of the vertebra. Thus, the skeletal portions of the somites no longer correspond to the original segmentation. The segmental spinal nerves, which were originally in midsomite, now lie at the level of the disc. The intersegmental artery, initially located between somites, comes to lie at the midportion of the vertebral bodies, and the myotomes now bridge the vertebrae. Although somites form from craniad to caudad, the resegmentation process with intervertebral disc formation progresses caudally to cranially in the cervical spine. Cartilage appears in the primordia of the bodies of the cervical vertebrae during the fifth week and in the posterior arches slightly later. Ossification, like segmentation, begins in the thoracic region and progresses both cranially and caudally. Segmentation of the cartilaginous anlagen of the vertebrae occurs in the sixth to eighth weeks and is generally completed by the end of the eighth week.

A physical and temporal proximity of the developing urogenital ridge to the developing spinal column explains the high association of anomalies in these two systems. Furthermore, the physical proximity of the brachial arches, which arise from the intermediate mesoderm, helps explain the high incidence of malformations of the ear and facial bones associated with congenital cervical spine fusions.

KLIPPEL-FEIL SYNDROME

The appellation *Klippel-Feil syndrome* has been used in two different ways. Some authors use Klippel-Feil syndrome to denote only those patients with the clinical triad of a short neck, a low posterior hairline, and marked limitations of neck range of motion. This usage stems from Maurice Klippel and André Feil's 1912 description of a single patient who manifested these signs as a result of massive fusion of the cervical spine (52).

Feil reported additional cases and developed a classification system in 1919. The common element in the patients he described was a congenital fusion of at least two vertebrae, resulting in use of the term Klippel-Feil syndrome to denote any congenital cervical spinal fusion. Feil described three patterns of congenital cervical fusions that are still used for classification today. Type I lesions consist of a massive fusion of the cervical vertebrae, sometimes extending to the upper thoracic spine. Type II lesions consist of only one or two fused vertebral segments. Type III lesions are type I or II lesions with distant anomalies in the thoracic or lumbar spine.

F. Dietz: Department of Orthopaedic Surgery, University of Iowa, Iowa City, Iowa 52242.

Klippel-Feil syndrome refers to any congenital fusion of the cervical spine, with or without the originally described clinical triad. Therefore, Klippel-Feil syndrome can denote a wider range of disorders representing different etiologic processes with varying associated anomalies and differing clinical implications. Nonetheless, the implications for the mechanics of the spine and the occurrence of embryologically related anomalies are sufficiently similar to warrant considering all cervical vertebral fusions as a single group, at least for clinical convenience. Often, it is more important to treat the associated anomalies of the central nervous system, genitourinary system, cardiovascular system, gastrointestinal system, and musculoskeletal system than it is to diagnose and treat the cervical spine anomaly.

Incidence

The incidence and prevalence of Klippel-Feil syndrome are unknown. No population screening studies have been done. Only sketchy information about prevalence can be obtained from cases that have come to medical attention in reasonably closed populations. The best of these studies is that of Gjorup and Gjorup (38). They reviewed the radiographic files of all of the hospitals in Copenhagen and determined the incidence of congenital spine fusions by comparing the number of spine fusions found to the population of Copenhagen. This is a minimal estimate of the incidence because asymptomatic cases could not be ascertained and some of the hospitals had not maintained radiographs from the entire study period. They found a prevalence of 0.2 symptomatic congenital fusion per 1,000 in their population.

A little more illumination is gained from a study by Brown et al. (14), who reviewed 1,400 skeletal specimens in a collection at Washington University School of Medicine in St. Louis. They found that 0.71% of the skeletons had congenital fusions. The selection criteria for inclusion in the collection are not stated, and this number may be artificially high if pathologic specimens were selectively preserved. However, if one assumes that many single-level fusions are asymptomatic throughout life, this prevalence seems reasonable when compared with the 0.2 clinically evident congenital fusion per 1,000 found in the Copenhagen study. In a related investigation, Brown et al. (14) reviewed all of the radiographic examinations of the cervical spine made for 1 year at their institution and found 7 congenital cervical fusions among 1,158 patients, yielding an incidence of 0.6% congenital fusion in patients radiographed for symptoms of cervical spine problems.

Because the incidence and prevalence of Klippel-Feil syndrome are not known, counseling patients is difficult. For those who are found to have a congenital fusion after minor trauma or after a radiograph is taken for unrelated reasons, the chance of their developing problems is unknown (Fig. 1).

Etiologic Factors

The cause of Klippel-Feil syndrome is unknown. Conflicting hypotheses include those proposing a primary vascular disruption, a global fetal insult, a primary neural tube abnormality, a primary genetic causation, or failure of facet joint segmentation.

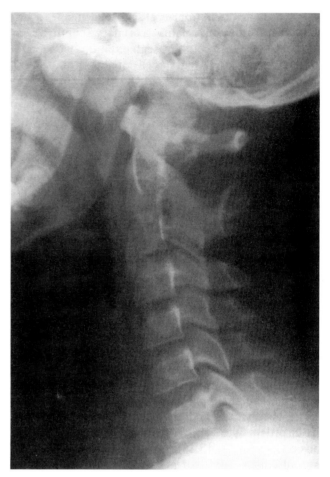

FIGURE 1. This 12-year-old boy was found to have a C2–3 block vertebra during evaluation for a depressed skull fracture. Flexion and extension radiographs revealed no instability. He was entirely asymptomatic and neurologically intact. Appropriate couseling of this patient about the natural history of this lesion is difficult because of the uncertainties about its prevalence.

Congenital cervical fusion also occurs occasionally in other well-recognized syndromes.

Primary Vascular Disruption

A prominent hypothesis to explain the causes not only of Klippel-Feil syndrome but also of Poland anomaly, Möbus syndrome, absence of the pectoralis major, isolated terminal transverse limb defects, and Sprengel deformity is the subclavian artery disruption sequence (10). Disruption occurs when a normal embryo suffers a destructive process with cascading consequences. As all the tissues affected in these various disorders receive their major blood supply from the subclavian artery, it is hypothesized that a defect of arterial formation or an injury to existing arteries causes these various congenital defects. The location and extent of tissue abnormality is determined by the extent, location, and timing of the interruption of normal blood supply.

The observation underlying this hypothesis is that the disorders listed above often occur together in various combinations

(10,12). According to this scheme, Klippel-Feil syndrome results from an interruption of flow in the vertebral arteries or their branches, causing arrest of the normal segmentation process if it occurs at the appropriate embryologic time (about 6 to 7 weeks). Ischemia at this time might interrupt the normal vertebral segmentation process, resulting in the congenital fusions.

If a single longitudinal anastomosis between two intersegmental arteries is blocked, fails to develop, or is delayed in forming past the critical developmental stage, then a single level of fusion occurs. If many longitudinal anastomoses are blocked or fail to form, a more extensive fusion occurs. A disruption of the vertebral artery near its origin or a disruption of the subclavian artery proximal to the vertebral artery takeoff, resulting in reversal of flow in the vertebral artery, would result in a massive fusion, often with associated anomalies. Because the vertebral artery gives rise to the basilar and labyrinthine arteries supplying the cochlea and vestibular structures, disruption of this vessel could explain the sensorineural hearing defects often found in patients with Klippel-Feil syndrome.

The hypothesis of vascular disruption is attractive because it can explain the varying severity of cervical anomalies seen in Klippel-Feil syndrome as well as many of the associated anomalies. Furthermore, this hypothesis easily explains the generally sporadic occurrence of this disorder. There are limitations to this hypothesis, however. It fails to explain the many anomalies unrelated to the subclavian artery that are often associated with Klippel-Feil syndrome. It does not easily account for the hereditary occurrence of Klippel-Feil syndrome, although a genetic propensity toward vascular disruption or abnormal vessel formation can certainly be hypothesized. The major difficulty with the hypothesis, however, is whether the vascular anomalies cause the embryologic abnormalities, or the vascular abnormalities are the effect of a more primary cause or a reflection of the distorted tissues supplied.

Global Fetal Insult

Beals and Rolfe (9) pointed out that, in addition to the major components of the VATER association (i.e., vertebral defects, imperforate anus, tracheoesophageal fistula, and radial and renal dysplasia), another group of anomalies, including Klippel-Feil syndrome, was associated in a nonrandom fashion. They argued that these anomalies are not embryologically related either spacially or temporally and that no single insult could reasonably explain the wide range of associated anomalies. They suggested that a global insult with variable effects on different tissues or multiple separate insults might best explain the associated anomalies. That 34% of rabbits whose mothers were subjected to decreased oxygen between the ninth and eleventh days of gestation developed vertebral anomalies, including fusion, supports the concept of global insult causing vertebral anomalies (25).

Genetic Causation

Evidence for a genetic cause of Klippel-Feil syndrome comes from the work of Gunderson et al. (43). Eleven probands with Klippel-Feil syndrome were identified. All were symptomatic, most because of neck pain. Of these 11 probands, seven had type II lesions with only one or two interspaces fused; four had type I with a more massive fusion. Eleven of 52 radiographs of type II patients' relatives showed a type II fusion. In six of the seven families of probands with type II lesions, multiple family members were radiographed; in four of these six families, the affected family members had the same vertebral fusion at either C2–3 or C5–6, as did the probands. In two of these six families, relatives and probands had different vertebrae fused. Gunderson's interpretation was that congenital C2–3 fusion is an autosomal dominant condition with variable expressivity and penetrance; congenital C5–6 fusion is an autosomal recessive condition. These conclusions are weakened by incomplete ascertainment of relatives of probands and by simple segregation analysis. Nonetheless, this study strongly suggests a hereditary component in isolated fusions of C2–3. The four patients with type I fusions (massive fusions) had no affected family members with similar fusions.

Clark et al. studied a family with four generations of vocal impairment and two generations in which cervical vertebral fusions were associated with vocal impairment and inherited in an autosomal dominant manner. In affected individuals C2–3 were always fused, with C4–5 or C6–7 fusions occurring as well in some individuals. A gene locus on chromosome 8 has been identified based on an incision in 8q that segregates with the anomaly (17).

In Gray's (41) review of 418 cases of Klippel-Feil syndrome reported in the literature, there were 168 family histories, 136 of which were negative. Of the 32 positive family histories, 15 came from 10 families; the other 17 were cases in which another family member was believed to be affected. This suggests a much lower incidence of inheritance than that reported by Gunderson.

Syndromic Associations

Klippel-Feil syndrome is associated with other well-identified syndromes. One of these, fetal alcohol syndrome, has a known cause, although the mechanism remains obscure (57,101). Fetal alcohol syndrome results from heavy maternal alcohol use and is characterized by developmental delay, poor growth, and characteristic facies. Tredwell et al. (101) radiographed the cervical spines of 38 patients with fetal alcohol syndrome and found that 19 (50%) had congenital fusion. Ten of these 19 patients had fusion of C2–3 alone, six more had a C2–3 fusion plus one or more other levels, and three had more than two levels that did not include C2–3. Only two patients were found to have clinically abnormal necks on physical examination. The result causing fetal alcohol syndrome is believed to occur between the twenty-fourth and twenty-eighth day of fetal life, which is a little earlier than most hypotheses place the timing of failure of segmentation of the cervical spine. Reports of multiple-level fusions in siblings affected with fetal alcohol syndrome support maternal alcohol abuse and a hereditary predisposition as etiologic factors (57).

Congenital cervical fusion is also seen in Goldenhar syndrome slightly less than 10% of the time (7). This is a sporadic disorder of unknown cause characterized by hemifacial microsomia with ocular dermoid cysts, ear appendages, and fistulae. It is associated with other musculoskeletal anomalies, including clubfoot, Sprengel deformity, developmental dysplasia of the hip, and radial limb defects.

Clinical Features

The best available data on the clinical features of Klippel-Feil syndrome come from several medical centers' experience with this disorder (38,47,58,103). Articles that review the available literature are obviously biased by the unusual findings that warranted case reports (41,46,90). Surveys of Klippel-Feil patients seen at single medical institutions are uniform in showing a gender predominance of females over males of 1.5:1 (38,47, 58,103). The age at presentation is extremely variable, extending throughout the entire life span. Massive fusions are often noted in infancy or early childhood because of the cosmetic deformity. Less extensive fusions may come to light because of associated anomalies detected in infancy or childhood. Neurologic problems in infancy are usually related to craniovertebral junction abnormalities, although cervical-vertebral fusions may also be present in this age group. In general, higher fusions near the craniovertebral junction present earlier; C1–2 fusions often present in childhood, usually with pain (28). Lower cervical fusions, if not massive, often do not present until the third decade or even later in life, when degenerative changes or instability of adjacent segments develops (41,55). Overall, about 20% of the patients destined to develop neural symptoms do so in the first 5 years. Sixty-five percent of patients who eventually develop neurologic symptoms will do so before age 30 (41). One clue to finding a congenital cervical vertebral anomaly in the newborn is asymmetrical crying facies due to a partial seventh nerve palsy (75). Many of these children will have a hemivertebra; occasionally, a congenital fusion will also be found. This clinical finding should prompt a radiographic search for vertebral anomalies.

The clinical triad of short neck, decreased range of motion, and low posterior hairline is seen in 40% to 50% of patients. In single-institution surveys, decreased range of motion is the most common finding, occurring in 50% to 76% of patients (47,58,103). The decrease in motion is most commonly in lateral bending and rotation; flexion and extension are relatively well preserved, except in the most massive fusions. In general, if fewer than two motion segments are fused or if the fusion is confined to the lower cervical spine, minimal or no detectable diminution in range of motion may be evident clinically. A normal range of motion due to excessive motion at motion segments adjacent to the fused vertebra is common. Definite shortening of the neck is evident in less than half of patients, and a low posterior hairline seems to reflect this shortening of the neck rather than being a separate entity (Fig. 2).

Patients with Klippel-Feil syndrome present with a wide range of chief complaints, including cosmesis (either of the neck or due to associated anomalies such as Sprengel deformity), neck pain alone, radicular pain with or without weakness, slowly progressive or acute paraparesis or quadriparesis, and complications caused by associated anomalies of the genitourinary, cardiovascular, or gastrointestinal systems.

Radiographic Features

One-level fusions are the most common pattern. Gjorup and Gjorup (38), in a review of 76 patients with Klippel-Feil syn-

drome, found 44 patients with one-level fusions, 19 patients with two to five fused vertebrae, and 13 patients with six or more levels fused. Similarly, in a review of skeletal specimens, Brown et al. (14) found 69 with one-level fusions and three with two separate one-level fusions. Van Kerckhoven and Fabry (103), in their population in Copenhagen, found 14 patients with one- or two-level fusions, 1 with a massive fusion, and 3 with either a limited or a massive fusion and associated lower spine anomalies. In a review of reported cases by Gray et al. (41), 20% of patients had one joint affected and 50% had three or fewer joints affected. Variable patterns of fusion may be seen, with anterior, lateral, and posterior fusion occurring in about half of patients. Anterior fusion alone occurs in about 20% of patients. Isolated posterior or lateral fusions make up the remainder. Generally, the involved vertebrae have flat wide bodies (32). The disc spaces are absent or hypoplastic (28,47,103). Spinal stenosis at the level of the segmentation defect has been reported (67,79), but this is not uniform, and a decrease in canal size is not thought to be common in children (28,47). Two brief reports suggest a higher incidence of stenosis in children than generally accepted (77,78). Pizzutillo et al. (77) reported a high incidence of decreased spinal canal width at unfused C1, C3, and C4 segments in children and adolescents with Klippel-Feil syndrome as compared with controls. Spinal stenosis often develops with aging due to degenerative changes from adjacent segment hypermobility (55). The C1–2 articulation is generally spared, as is the C7–T1 motion segment. Massive fusions beginning at the C4–5 level often extend into the upper thoracic spine and include the cervicothoracic segment.

The diagnosis of congenital cervical fusion in infants and young children can be difficult because the lack of vertebral ossification makes the hypoplastic or absent disc spaces difficult to appreciate. Flexion and extension radiographs can demonstrate a lack of motion between fused segments, and flexion and extension laminograms may be needed to confirm the diagnosis. In massive fusions, overlap of the mandible often makes the upper cervical spine anatomy difficult to appreciate on plain radiographs. Laminograms are most helpful in defining the bony architecture, but computed tomography (CT) can also be used. Care must be taken in the radiographic diagnosis to assess the craniovertebral junction, as anomalies are common and an abnormal cranial-cervical junction coupled with a lower cervical fusion may increase the risk of neurologic injury (67,68). Occipitalization of the atlas, basilar impression, os terminale, os odontoideum, hypoplastic dens, and other less common anomalies of the craniovertebral junction may be found (60,67,68,93,103).

Clinically unapparent vertebral abnormalities of the thoracic, lumbar, and sacral spines are associated with Klippel-Feil syndrome (47,82). Radiographic evaluation of the entire spine is appropriate. Conversely, 15% to 25% of children presenting with congenital scoliosis will be found to have Klippel-Feil syndrome, suggesting a need for routine cervical spine films in any child with a congenital scoliosis (109). If plain radiographs, flexion-extension laminograms, or CT scans are suggestive of instability, magnetic resonance imaging (MRI) is indicated to assess the space available for the spinal cord. Obviously, in patients with neurologic symptoms, a combination of CT, lami-

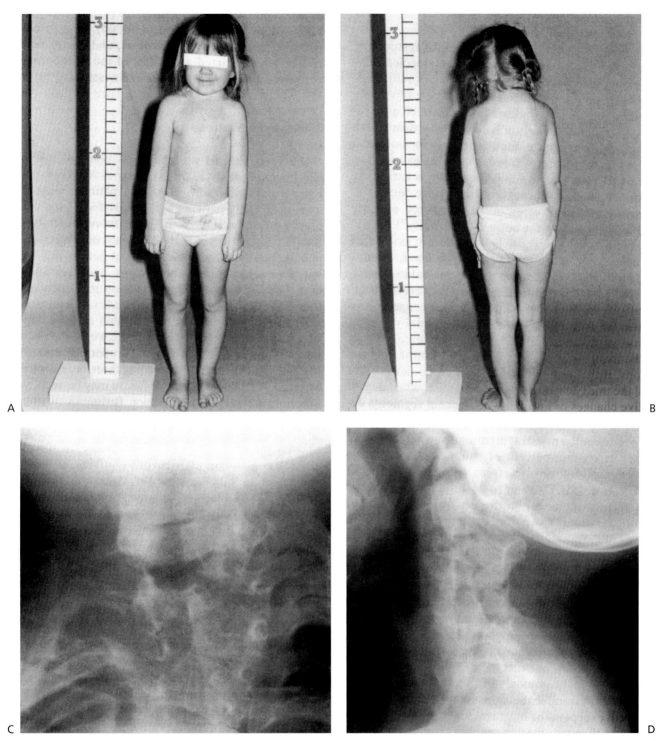

FIGURE 2. Photographs **(A, B)** and radiographs **(C, D)** of a 4-year-old girl with multiple segmentation defects of the cervical spine, congenital scoliosis, and Sprengel deformity. She also had a moderate sensorineural hearing loss in the right ear and a cleft palate.

nography, and MRI may be necessary to define the pathoanatomy and guide appropriate treatment.

The majority of patients with massive cervical fusion have spina bifida occulta, and somewhat less than half have cleft vertebral bodies and cervical hemivertebra in addition to the congenital fusions (6,38,41,58,109).

Associated Anomalies

Multiple anomalies associated with Klippel-Feil syndrome have been reported. Some of these are common, whereas others have been reported in so few case reports that their occurrence may be coincidental. Nonetheless, the search for associated anomalies is warranted with the finding of Klippel-Feil syndrome, as these anomalies may threaten the patient's life, health, or development. Therapeutic interventions may be necessary.

Musculoskeletal Anomalies

The most common associated musculoskeletal anomaly is scoliosis (usually congenital), occurring in up to 60% of patients with Klippel-Feil syndrome (38,41,47,99,103). Compensatory curves containing apparently normal vertebrae below primary congenital curves have a strong propensity to progress and may create significant deformities (46,47). These should be carefully monitored and appropriate treatment of bracing or fusion undertaken. The high incidence of congenital scoliosis reflects the high associated occurrence of hemivertebra (58,103). Unilateral bars may occur, and reports of combined failures of formation and segmentation in the cervical spine and in other areas of the spine are common in this syndrome (88).

Sprengel deformity is commonly reported in 20% to 30% of patients but was found in 50% of patients in one series (38,41,47,58,103). Therefore, screening of the cervical spine for congenital fusions is appropriate in patients with Sprengel deformity. An omovertebral bone may be associated with Sprengel deformity; this has been reported to contribute to cord compression in association with instability resulting from a congenital C4–C5 fusion (93).

Cervical ribs occur in 12% to 15% of patients with Klippel-Feil syndrome, which is much higher than the 1% prevalence in the general population (38,41,90). When evaluating the cause of neurologic symptoms in patients with Klippel-Feil syndrome, the possibility of thoracic outlet syndrome should be kept in mind, even though there are no reported cases associated with Klippel-Feil syndrome. The known association of cervical ribs with thoracic outlet syndrome suggests that this may occur (2,18,23,24,89). If degenerative changes and/or instability have resulted from congenital fusion, the possibility of a thoracic outlet syndrome based on a cervical rib might be overlooked.

Rib anomalies are common and occur in about one third of patients with Klippel-Feil syndrome (41,58,103). Absence of ribs occurs with appropriately equal frequency. Less common associated musculoskeletal anomalies include hypoplastic pectoralis major, radial clubhand, syndactyly of the fingers, hypoplastic thumb, supernumerary digits, clubfoot, and sacral agenesis (41, 47,103).

Torticollis, neck webbing, and facial symmetry are often combined in reviews, and one or more of these findings occur in 21% to 50% of the patients (41,47,103). Torticollis stems largely from congenital spinal anomalies, but muscular torticollis does occur (13). Neck webbing may be severe, and other joints webbings are occasionally seen. Treatment of the associated musculoskeletal anomalies is generally standard for the individual deformity. Treatment of Sprengel deformity in patients with Klippel-Feil syndrome is the same as and produces similar results to treatment of patients without congenital fusions of the cervical spine (46,58). If muscular torticollis is present, release is appropriate (13). Severe pterygium colli may be treated with Z-plasty of the soft tissues, which occasionally improves cosmesis with or without resection of underlying muscle (41,58,90). Resection of cervical ribs may be indicated for symptoms or cosmesis. Bonola (11) reported that resection of the cervical ribs plus the posterior portions of the first, second, and third thoracic ribs increased the apparent length of the neck. He reports no complications and good cosmetic results from this procedure.

Craniofacial Anomalies

Hearing loss is one of the most common anomalies associated with Klippel-Feil syndrome. Institutional surveys report a 15% to 36% incidence of hearing loss or congenital deafness (47,58,103). The majority of the hearing loss is sensorineural due to abnormalities of the inner ear. However, at least one third appears to be conductive hearing loss associated with abnormalities of the ossicular chain, particularly fixation of the stapes foot plate (50,59,74,85). Mixed conductive and sensorineural hearing loss also occurs in some patients (71,95,96). Early recognition of an auditory defect is important so that patients can be rehabilitated for deafness and not miss crucial developmental milestones in language skills and speech. Audiologic tests should be performed on all children with Klippel-Feil syndrome (62,74). Malformations of the middle and external ear are also reported, including absence of the external auditory meatus (71).

Klippel-Feil syndrome and congenital hearing loss have been associated with a third finding, called Duane syndrome. Duane syndrome, or retraction bulbi, results from an abducens nerve palsy in which the adducting eye becomes retracted, causing narrowing of the palpebral fissure and enophthalmus (20,56). This combination of anomalies was called cervicooculoacoustic syndrome by Wildervanck, who initially described the association in 1960 (19,22,91,98,105). It is now more commonly referred to as Wildervanck syndrome. There is a marked female predominance of this syndrome of about 10:1, and the family history is almost always negative for similar defects. A review of 126 patients with Duane syndrome showed that 5 had Klippel-Feil syndrome and 12 had congenital hearing loss (51). Of the 3 patients who had all three components in this series, 2 also had pseudopapilledema.

Approximately 10% of patients with maxillonasal dysplasia, also called Binder syndrome, have congenital fusions of the cervical spine (73,81). Other anomalies of the cervical spine, especially defects at the craniovertebral junction and scoliosis, are even more common with Binder syndrome (73,81). Binder syndrome is characterized by premaxillary agenesis.

Although cleft lip and palate are not commonly associated

with Klippel-Feil syndrome, Klippel-Feil syndrome is dispropor-tionately represented among those with cleft lip and palate, oc-curring in about 4% of patients (94). Less common oral facial abnormalities reported with Klippel-Feil syndrome include fron-tal nasal dysplasia, mandibular duplication, and velopharyngeal insufficiency (26,37,54).

Central Nervous System Anomalies

The most commonly associated central nervous system anomaly is the occurrence of mirror movements (synkinesia), which are involuntary paired movements of the hands and arms. Fifteen to twenty percent of patients with Klippel-Feil syndrome show clinically evident mirror movements (46,103). Mirror move-ments are not always abnormal; they are common in preschool children and may occur as a familial trait. If mirror movements are persistent or severe, occupational therapy can often help a child disassociate the movements and improve upper extremity function.

Other congenital central nervous system anomalies have been reported less commonly. Syringomyelia, neuroschisis (failure of closure of the neural tube), fibrous diastematomyelia with cervi-cal spinal cord duplication, posterior fossa dermoid cysts, and an isolated aberrant bony fragment embedded in the cord have all been reported (27,41,66,107). These unusual problems can give rise to confusing neurologic symptoms. One must consider underlying central nervous system pathology as a possible cause of a patient's neurologic problems in addition to possible neuro-logic injury from instability or stenosis due to the congenital cervical fusions.

Genital and Urinary Anomalies

Significant renal abnormalities are present in 25% to 35% of patients with Klippel-Feil syndrome (47,58,63,80,103). The most common renal anomaly is unilateral renal agenesis, with other structural abnormalities, such as malrotation, ectopic kid-ney, horseshoe kidney, and pelvic and ureteral duplication, oc-curring less often (63). Ultrasonography is an effective noninva-sive screening tool without the small risk associated with intravenous pyelography (29). If a structural anomaly is found by ultrasonography, intravenous pyelography should be done to identify other problems, such as ureteral vesicular reflux, which, if untreated, could result in permanent damage to an abnormal or singular kidney. All patients with Klippel-Feil syndrome should have a renal ultrasonography as a screening precaution.

Genital anomalies have been infrequently reported. Ten to twenty percent of patients with Mayer-Rokitansky-Küster-Hauser syndrome, consisting of congenital absence of the uterus and upper vagina, have congenital skeletal abnormalities, includ-ing congenital cervical fusion (108). Gonadal dysplasia has also been reported with congenital cervical fusion, as well as hypospa-dias and cryptorchidism (44).

Cardiovascular Anomalies

The incidence of cardiac anomalies in patients with Klippel-Feil syndrome is difficult to define. From a review of the literature,

Morrison et al. (64) believed that a minimum of 4.2% of those with Klippel-Feil syndrome had cardiovascular anomalies. Nora et al. (70) reported that five of eight patients admitted to their hospital with Klippel-Feil syndrome had significant cardiac dis-ease. All of these patients had a ventricular septal defect as a component of their anomalies. Two surveys of patients seen at single institutions where cardiovascular anomalies were sought found an incidence of 14% and 29%, respectively (47,103). The anomalies noted were ventricular septal defect, atrial septal defect, bicuspid aortic valve, mitral insufficiency, pulmonary ste-nosis, and patent ductus arteriosus. Most of the cardiac condi-tions that are commonly associated with Klippel-Feil syndrome involve a murmur. Forney et al. (36) reported on three members of a family, all of whom had congenital cervical spine fusions, conductive deafness due to a malformed stapes, and mitral insuf-ficiency.

Gastrointestinal Anomalies

Rarely, anomalies of the gastrointestinal tract are associated with Klippel-Feil syndrome (41). These include intrathoracic gastro-genic cysts and mediastinal cysts of foregut origin (1,35,104). These may result from a failure of the notochord to separate completely from the primitive gut. There have been several re-ports of recurrent meningitis in patients with Klippel-Feil syn-drome, usually due to defects of or fistulae from the inner ear.

Pulmonary Problems

Pulmonary disease associated with Klippel-Feil syndrome is gen-erally related to scoliosis or chest wall deformities (47). Restric-tive lung disease has been reported from multiple rib fusions. Deformity and shortening of the thoracic spine have also been associated with restrictive lung disease and should be sought in the appropriate setting (8).

Miscellaneous Associations

Case reports of Klippel-Feil syndrome associated with meningio-mas, dural hemangiolipomas, and lipomas of the spinal cord have been published (16,49,110). The presence of craniocervical dermoid cysts presenting as aseptic meningitis in a patient with Klippel-Feil syndrome has been reported (27).

Natural History and Treatment

Congenital cervical fusions can cause serious neurologic compro-mise. The lesions can cause anything from persistent pain with radiculopathy to sudden death from minor traumas (31,34,41, 60,65,67,68,79,82,92,97,106). The risk of significant disability or injury from these lesions is not known. If the incidence figures quoted at the beginning of this chapter are within an order of magnitude of being correct, the risk of death or serious disability is small. However, because the accuracy of these figures is un-known, the physician's task of counseling families and patients is difficult.

Pain can result from stress on motion segments above or

below fused segments, and the articulations above and below fixed segments often are not entirely normal (61,65,76). Instability can develop, resulting in pain and spinal cord injury, including complete quadriplegia. The excess stress on motion segments adjacent to fused areas can cause degenerative changes with osteophyte formation, resulting in acquired spinal stenosis that can cause cord compromise or foraminal stenosis with radiculopathy. Both instability and the lever arm of a congenital fusion can put an individual at risk for spinal cord injury from relatively minor trauma. The combination of fusion and spinal stenosis puts the cord at risk as well.

If a neurologic lesion is present, significant pain persists despite conservative measures, or instability is documented, then spinal fusion must be considered. Similarly, if neurologic injury is present and stenosis is documented, decompression with or without fusion is indicated. One must be cautious, especially with congenital fusions associated with craniovertebral anomalies, to rule out intrinsic cord anomalies, such as syringomyelia and diastematomyelia (65,82). In an asymptomatic patient, it is difficult to decide whether prophylactic treatment is appropriate because the natural history of Klippel-Feil syndrome is not known. For this reason, attempts to identify high-risk patients are warranted.

Gray et al. (41), in their review of all reported cases up to 1964, found that 34% of patients exhibited spasticity or hyperreflexia. Pain was present in 38%. Flaccid paralysis, weakness, anesthesia, or paresthesia was found in 10% to 15% of the reported cases. This is obviously a highly selected group; neurologic injury in association with the bony abnormality would tend to warrant a case report, whereas less dramatic sequelae would not.

Nagib et al. (67,68) attempted to identify high-risk patients with Klippel-Feil syndrome and described three patterns of deformity that they believe put patients at particular risk for neurologic injury. Pattern 1 consists of two sets of block vertebrae with open intervening disc spaces. This puts the patient at risk for gradual subluxation or acute subluxation with minor trauma at the open disc space. The second pattern consists of craniocervical anomalies (most commonly occipitalization of the atlas and basilar invagination) with a congenital fusion below C2. This lesion may cause increased mobility at the craniocervical junction and risks foramen magnum encroachment. An Arnold-Chiari malformation, syringobulbia, or syringomyelia may occur with this pattern. Pattern 3 consists of fusion at one or more levels associated with spinal canal stenosis. Stenosis may occur above, below, or at the level of the fusion. This classification scheme was based on only 21 patients with Klippel-Feil syndrome seen over a 20-year period. Of this group, 12 had no neurologic symptoms; nine of these asymptomatic patients had only two vertebrae fused, and two more had a single massive fusion. Of the nine patients with neurologic symptoms, three had the unstable fusion pattern (pattern 1), four had craniovertebral abnormalities and a lower fusion (pattern 2), and two had congenital fusion with associated spinal stenosis (pattern 3). Support for the potential problems of these three patterns is present in the literature. Two sets of fused vertebrae separated by an open interspace have caused quadriplegia, according to several authors reporting single cases (31,61,65). The association

of craniovertebral anomalies with cervical fusions is the most commonly reported cause of cord injury (48,60,61,65,84,92) (Fig. 3). Spinal cord damage in patients with spinal stenosis and congenital fusions has also been reported by other authors (34,45,79). In a study of 25 cases of occipitalization of the atlas by McRae and Barnum (60), there was significant cord involvement with long-tract signs of spasticity or weakness in 16 patients. Eleven of these had a congenital fusion of C2–3 in addition to the craniovertebral anomaly (Fig. 4). Klippel-Feil syndrome associated with spinal stenosis is not commonly reported in the literature, but the combination certainly does predispose the patient to significant cord injury with minor trauma. Of 32 patients described by Torg et al. (100) with neurapraxia of the cervical cord causing transient quadriplegia, four had Klippel-Feil syndrome in addition to congenital stenosis. Other reports of transient or permanent quadriplegia after trauma with this combination of anomalies exist (31,34).

Fusions that do not fit Nagib's at-risk groups have also been reported to cause neurologic damage ranging from radiculopathy to quadriplegia to death from minor trauma (33,55). Graaff (40) evaluated 145 patients with cervical myelopathy and purposely excluded those with craniocervical abnormalities and severe Klippel-Feil syndrome. Nonetheless, eight of these 145 patients had an isolated C2–3 fusion, and one also had a C5–6 fusion. These patients all had quadriparesis and upper extremity dysfunction.

Pizzutillo et al. (76) reviewed 111 patients with Klippel-Feil syndrome and found five patients with neurologic deficits, four of whom had instability of the upper cervical spine. Twelve other patients had degenerative changes or instability of the lower cervical spine that generally resulted in pain but not neurologic deficit.

It may be that Gray's (41) 1964 assessment of patients at risk for neurologic injury remains correct: "The level of fusion does not greatly affect the incidence of neurologic symptoms. The most frequent defect—occiput to first cervical vertebra and second and third cervical vertebra—also produced the most symptoms. Lesions beginning below the third and fourth cervical vertebra were slightly less likely to be accompanied by symptoms as lesions starting higher."

All patients with congenital cervical fusion should be treated as being at increased risk of pain, instability, or neurologic injury. Some evidence and common sense suggest that certain patterns, such as occipitalization of the atlas with C2–3 fusion, would stress the C1–2 articulation and cause a high incidence of instability and potential cord injury. One should be especially cautious about the potential for damage in these patients.

Certain principles are apparent. If a congenital fusion is identified, stability must be assessed. Flexion and extension radiographs may be sufficient if the patient is asymptomatic, but flexion and extension laminography or CT may be needed if the anatomy is obscured. Plain radiographs must be scrutinized for evidence of either congenital or acquired spinal stenosis and for evidence of degenerative changes that would compromise the neural foramina. If none of these abnormalities is present in an asymptomatic patient, it is unwise to recommend prophylactic fusion or decompression. In cases in which the anomalies are such that there is concern about the space available for the cord, MRI in flexion and extension should be performed. If it

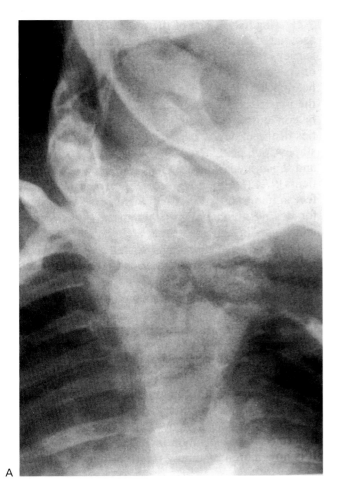

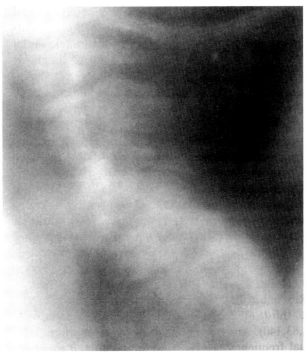

B

FIGURE 3. This 3-month-old girl had multiple segmentation defects as well as a unilateral bar on the left, resulting in congenital scoliosis. She had a bifid thumb but no other congenital anomalies. She eventually underwent posterior in situ fusion on the left from T2 to T5 and on the right from T1 to T7 for progressive deformity. **A:** Anteroposterior radiograph. **B:** Midline lateral tomogram.

A

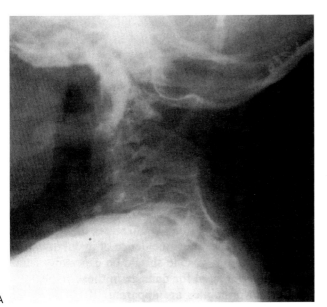

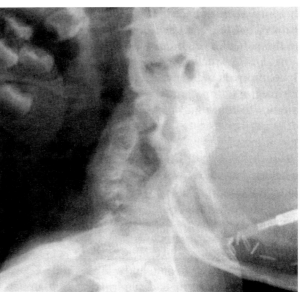

A

B

FIGURE 4. This 3-year-old boy with massive fusion but no instability had an associated posterior fossa dermoid cyst that was resected. With occipitalization of C1 and fusion of C2–3 and C4–5, this cervical spine would seem to be at risk for developing instability. Flexion **(A)** and extension **(B)** tomograms in early childhood did not reveal any instability, but continued follow-up would be appropriate.

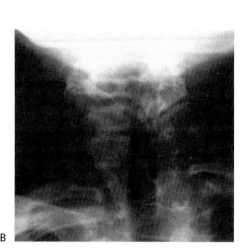
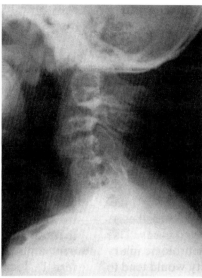
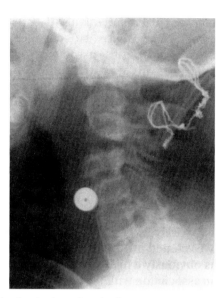

A,B

C

FIGURE 5. This 10-year-old boy with chronic severe neck pain was recognized as having Klippel-Feil syndrome at age 6 years. Over the years, he developed progressively increasing neck pain that was unresponsive to conservative therapy. He had occipitalization of C1 with basilar invagination and segmentation defect from C2 to C7, sparing only the C3-4 articulation **(A,B)**. Magnetic resonance imaging (MRI) revealed impingement of the ventral cervicomedullary junction by an abnormal odontoid process in an invaginated position from the foramen magnum. In spite of halo ring traction, he had persistent compression of the cervicomedullary junction as revealed by MRI. The patient underwent a transoral transphalangeal decompression of the cervicomedullary junction followed by a posterior occipital cervical fusion with rib graft **(C)**.

demonstrates a significantly small space available for the spinal cord, prophylactic decompression and/or fusion might be considered. It instability is demonstrated prior to the onset of significant symptoms, it is difficult to decide when prophylactic fusion should be done. Koop et al. (53) reported several asymptomatic patients who developed cervical instability of 6 to 18 mm who underwent posterior fusion with excellent results.

It is prudent to obtain flexion and extension radiographs periodically to seek developing instability in patients with Klippel-Feil syndrome. Patients may become symptomatic at any time, and it is a matter of philosophy whether lifelong assessments are made or the patient is simply counseled about the warning signs of neurologic compromise so that these can be detected and treated soon after the onset of symptoms (Fig. 5). All patients with congenital cervical fusion should avoid contact sports as well as occupations and recreational activities that put them at risk for head trauma. Patients who do develop symptoms of nerve root injury, irritation, or cord injury need a careful workup to identify the source of the neurologic symptoms because more than one anomaly with the potential to cause symptoms might be present. This is especially critical with anomalies of the craniovertebral junction. Therapy must be tailored to the pathology and often involves the combined services of a neurosurgeon and an orthopaedic surgeon.

Summary

Klippel-Feil syndrome encompasses a wide range of cervical anomalies, all characterized by a failure of segmentation of at least one motion segment. Several causes of this disorder may exist. A high index of suspicion for Klippel-Feil syndrome should be maintained in the presence of other congenital anomalies; conversely, if congenital cervical fusions are found, a diligent search for associated anomalies should be done. Management of this disorder requires recognition of the limitation of our knowledge concerning its general incidence so that overtreatment is avoided. However, the potential for catastrophic outcomes with this lesion must be kept in mind. Long-term follow-up and careful counseling of patients and families should be undertaken.

CERVICAL RIBS

Cervical ribs are a common anatomical variation that is rarely symptomatic in childhood. The prevalence of cervical ribs in the general population is estimated at between 0.5% and 1% (21). More than 90% of these apparently cause no problems. The remaining 10% are most commonly associated with thoracic outlet syndrome, which usually develops in the third to fifth decade (21). Cervical ribs are generally considered to be of two types: complete or incomplete. The complete cervical rib arises from the transverse process and is continuous with the first thoracic rib. The incomplete cervical rib does not have bony continuity with the first thoracic rib, although it usually does have a fibrous connection; the remaining cervical ribs end in the soft tissues without a fibrous or bony connection to the thoracic cage. A nonrib bony connection between the cervical spine and rib cage has been reported (39). The diagnosis of a cervical rib is generally made on plain radiographs and is an incidental finding, although unsuspected cervical ribs have been found with other imaging techniques (69). If the transverse process of the cervical vertebra is larger than the transverse process of the first thoracic vertebra, a rudimentary cervical rib is felt to be present. Although cervical ribs are most common at the seventh cervical level, they do occur at the sixth level and rarely at the fifth level.

Cervical ribs seem to be inherited in an autosomal dominant fashion, although extensive population studies have not been done to confirm this. A carefully pedigreed family showed a high degree of dominance and complete penetrance (86). There was variable expressivity, with some affected members showing bilateral complete cervical ribs and others showing only rudimentary unilateral cervical ribs. Cervical ribs occur approximately twice as commonly in females as males, and they are bilateral twice as often as unilateral.

The most common problem with cervical ribs is irritation of the brachial plexus, causing the neural symptoms of thoracic outlet syndrome. There is an extensive literature addressing the appropriate treatment, and disagreement still exists whether anterior scalenotomy is sufficient or cervical rib resection is necessary for relief of symptoms (15). This is largely a problem of adults, although thoracic outlet-like symptoms relieved by cervical rib resection in a child as young as 6 years have been reported (3). Vascular compromise from cervical ribs can cause vague symptoms of the thoracic outlet syndrome type, but it may also cause arterial stenosis with aneurysm development, thrombosis, and embolism (87). If a cervical rib causes direct compression resulting in stenosis or aneurysm, resection of the rib is obviously indicated, along with all other soft tissues compressing the vessel (87). A subclavian artery aneurysm due to a cervical rib was reported in a 9-year-old child (102). This presented as a mass with a bruit that had probably been present since infancy. Cervical ribs have also been implicated in axillary vein thrombosis occurring in young athletes without other risk factors or with risk factors such as the taking of oral contraceptives (5). In this setting, the decision of whether to excise the cervical ribs largely depends on whether a return to the activities that precipitated the thrombosis is desired and anticipated. A rare complication of cervical ribs was reported by Grimer et al. (42) in which a brachial plexus injury occurred after correction of a right thoracic scoliosis in a patient with cervical ribs. Isolated cervical rib fracture after blunt trauma has been reported (30).

MISCELLANEOUS DISORDERS

Cervical meningocele is an uncommon disorder (26). Meningoceles are distinctly less common than myelomeningoceles; only 4% to 20% of spinal bifida cysticas have no neural elements and qualify as meningoceles. Less than 10% of these meningoceles are in the cervical spine. Meningocele is far more common in the lumbosacral spine. Cervical meningoceles warrant special attention because of the high incidence of associated central nervous system anomalies. Hydrocephalus, Arnold-Chiari malformations, hydromyelia, lipomyelocele, tethered cord, Klippel-

Feil syndrome, and diastematomyelia have all been found in association with cervical meningocele (26). Therefore, in spite of the generally benign nature of this lesion, a careful evaluation and probably MRI of the entire spinal cord should be done when this condition is found.

Cervical diastematomyelia is also quite rare (4,72). Thoracic and lumbar diastematomyelia are far more common. Vertebral abnormalities occur in 85% to 90% of patients with cervical diastematomyelia and provide a clue to the presence of this disorder. Cervical diastematomyelia may present with primary upper extremity signs and symptoms. Although this condition usually manifests itself in childhood, adult presentation has rarely been reported (72).

REFERENCES

1. Al-Rajeh S, Chowdhary UM, Al-Freihi H, et al. (1990): Thoracic disc protrusion and situs inversus in Klippel-Feil syndrome. *Spine* 15:1379–1381.
2. Adson AW (1986): The classic. Surgical treatment for symptoms produced by cervical ribs and the scalenus anticus muscle. *Clin Orthop Rel Res* 207:3–12.
3. Alp M, Urdakul Y, Gürses A, et al. (1982): Symptomatic cervical rib in childhood. *Turk J Pediatr* 24:121–125.
4. Anand AK, Kuchner E, James R (1985): Cervical diastematomyelia: uncommon presentation of a rare congenital disorder. *Comput Radiol* 9:45–49.
5. Aquino BC, Barone E (1989): "Effort" thrombosis of the axillary and subclavian vein associated with cervical rib and oral contraceptives in a young woman athlete. *J Am Board Fam Pract* 2:208–211.
6. Avery LW, Rentfro CC (1936): The Klippel-Feil syndrome. *Arch Neurol Psychiatry* 3:1068–1076.
7. Avon SW, Shively JL (1988): Orthopaedic manifestations of Goldenhar syndrome. *J Pediatr Orthop* 8:682–686.
8. Baga N, Chusid EL, Miller A (1969): Pulmonary disability in the Klippel-Feil syndrome. A study of two siblings. *Clin Orthop Rel Res* 67:105–110.
9. Beals RK, Rolfe B (1989): Current concepts review. VATER association. *J Bone Joint Surg Am* 71:948–950.
10. Bouwes Bavinck JN, Weaver DD (1986): Subclavian artery supply disruption sequence: hypothesis of a vascular etiology for Poland, Klippel-Feil and Mobius anomalies. *Am J Med Genet* 23:903–918.
11. Bonola A (1956): Surgical treatment of the Klippel-Feil syndrome. *J Bone Joint Surg Br* 38:440–449.
12. Brill CB, Peyster RG, Keller MS, et al. (1987): Isolation of the right subclavian artery with subclavian steal in a child with Klippel-Feil anomaly: an example of the subclavian artery supply disruption sequence. *Am J Med Genet* 26:933–940.
13. Brougham DI, Cole WC, Dickens RV, et al. (1989): Torticollis due to a combination of sternomastoid contracture and congenital vertebral anomalies. *J Bone Joint Surg Br* 71:404–407.
14. Brown MW, Templeton AW, Hodges FJ (1964): The incidence of acquired and congenital fusions in the cervical spine. *Am J Roentgenol* 92:1255–1259.
15. Brown SCW, Charlesworth D (1988): Results of excision of a cervical rib in patients with the thoracic outlet syndrome. *Br J Surg* 75:431–433.
16. Bucy PC, Ritchey H (1947): Klippel-Feil's syndrome associated with compression of the spinal cord by an extradural hemangiolipoma. *J Neurosurg* 4:476–481.
17. Clark RA, Singh S, McKenzie H, et al. (1995): Familial Klippel-Feil syndrome and paracentric inversion inv(8)(q22.2q23.3). *Am J Hum Genet* 57:1364–1370.
18. Cormier JM, Amrane M, Ward A, et al. (1989): Arterial complications of the thoracic outlet syndrome: fifty-five operative cases. *J Vasc Surg* 9:778–787.

19. Cremers WRJ, Hoogland GA, Kuypers W (1984): Hearing loss in the cervico-oculo-acoustic (Wildervanck) syndrome. *Arch Otolaryngol* 110:54–57.

20. Cross HE, Pfaffenbach DD (1972): Duane's retraction syndrome and associated congenital malformations. *Am J Ophthalmol* 73:442–450.

21. Dale WA, Lewis MR (1975): Management of thoracic outlet syndrome. *Ann Surg* 181:575–578.

22. Daniilidis J, Demetriadis A, Triaridis C, et al. (1980): Otological findings in cervico-oculo-auditory dysplasia. *J Laryngol Otol* 94: 533–544.

23. Daskalakis MK (1983): Thoracic outlet syndrome: current concepts and surgical experience. *Int Surg* 68:337–344.

24. Davies AH, Walton J, Stuart E, et al. (1991): Surgical management of the thoracic outlet compression syndrome. *Br J Surg* 78:1193–1995.

25. Degnehardt KH, Klodetzky L (1956): Malfmoraciones de la columna vertebrale y del esbozo de la corda dorsalis. *Actua Pediatr Barcelona* 7:1.

26. Delashaw JB, Park TS, Cail WM, et al. (1987): Cervical meningocele and associated spinal anomalies. *Child's Nerv Syst* 3:165–169.

27. Guiroy-Diekmann B. Huang PS (1989): Klippel-Feil syndrome in association with a craniocervical dermoid cyst presenting as aseptic meningitis in an adult: case report. *Neurosurgery* 25:652–655.

28. Dolan KD (1977): Developmental abnormalities of the cervical spine below the axis. *Radiol Clin North Am* 15:167–175.

29. Drvaric DM, Ruderman RJ, Conrad RW, et al. (1987). Congenital scoliosis and urinary tract abnormalities: are intravenous pyelograms necessary? *J Pediatr Orthop* 7:441–443.

30. Du Poit JGA, De Muelenaere PFRG (1982): Isolated fracture of a cervical rib. *South Afr Med J* 62:454–456.

31. Elster AD (1984): Quadriplegia after minor trauma in the Klippel-Feil syndrome. *J Bone Joint Surg Am* 66:1473–1474.

32. Erskine CA (1946): An analysis of the Klippel-Feil syndrome. *Arch Pathol* 41:269–281.

33. Epstein JA, Carras R, Epstein BS, et al. (1970): Myelopathy in cervical spondylosis with vertebral subluxation and hyperlordosis. *J Neurosurg* 32:421–426.

34. Epstein NE, Epstein JA, Zilkha A (1984): Traumatic myelopathy in a seventeen-year-old child with cervical spine stenosis (without fracture or dislocation) and a C2–C3 Klippel-Feil fusion. *Spine* 9: 344–346.

35. Fallon M, Gordon ARG, Lendrum AC (1954): Mediastinal cysts of fore-gut origin associated with vertebral abnormalities. *Br J Surg* 41: 520–533.

36. Forney WR, Robinson SJ, Pascoe DJ (1966): Congenital heart disease, deafness, and skeletal malformations: a new syndrome? *J Pediatr* 68: 14–26.

37. Fragoso R, Cid-Garcia A, Hernandez A, et al. (1982): Frontonasal dysplasia in the Klippel-Feil syndrome: a new associated malformation. *Clin Genet* 22:270–273.

38. Gjorup PA, Gjorup L (1964): Klippel-Feil's syndrome. *Dan Med Bull* 11:50–53.

39. Goodwin CB, Simmons EH, Taylor I (1984): Cervical vertebral-costal process (costovertebral bone)—a previously unreported anomaly. *J Bone Joint Surg Am* 69:1477–1479.

40. Graaff R de (1982): Congenital block vertebrae C2–C3 in patients with cervical myelopathy. *Acta Neurochir* 61:111–126.

41. Gray SW, Romaine CB, Skandalakis JE (1964): Congenital fusion of the cervical vertebrae. *Surg Gynecol Obstet* 118:373–385.

42. Grimer RJ, Mulligan PJ, Thompson AG (1983): Thoracic outlet syndrome following correction of scoliosis in a patient with cervical ribs. *J Bone Joint Surg Am* 65:1172–1173.

43. Gunderson CH, Greenspan RH, Glaser GH, et al. (1967): The Klippel-Feil syndrome: genetic and clinical reevaluation of cervical fusion. *Medicine* 46:491–512.

44. Haddad HM, Wilkins L (1959): Congenital anomalies associated with gonadal aplasia. *Pediatrics* 23:885–902.

45. Hall JE, Simmons ED, Danylchuk K, et al. (1990): Instability of the cervical spine and neurological involvement in Klippel-Feil syndrome. *J Bone Joint Surg Am* 72:460–462.

46. Hensinger RN (1991): Congenital anomalies of the cervical spine. *Clin Orthop Rel Res* 264:16–38.

47. Hensinger RN, Lang JE, MacEwen GD (1974): Klippel-Feil syndrome. *J Bone Joint Surg Am* 56:1246–1253.

48. Herring JA, Bunnel WP (1989): Instructional case. Klippel-Feil syndrome with neck pain. *J Pediatr Orthop* 9:343–346.

49. Holliday PO III, Davis C Jr, Angelo J (1984): Multiple meningiomas of the cervical spinal cord associated with Klippel-Feil malformation and atlantoccipital assimilation. *Neurosurgery* 14:353–357.

50. Jarvis JF, Sellars SL (1974): Klippel-Feil deformity associated with congenital conductive deafness. *J Laryngol Otol* 88:285–289.

51. Kirkham TH (1969): Cervico-oculo-acusticus syndrome with pseudo-papilloedema. *Arch Dis Child* 44:504–508.

52. Klippel M, Feil A (1975): The classic. A case of absence of cervical vertebrae with the thoracic cage rising to the base of the cranium (cervical thoracic cage). *Clin Orthop Rel Res* 109:3–8.

53. Koop SE, Winter RB, Lonstein JE (1984): The surgical treatment of instability of the upper part of the cervical spine in children and adolescents. *J Bone Joint Surg Am* 66:403–411.

54. Lawrence TM, McClatchey KD, Fonseca RJ (1985): Congenital duplication of mandibular rami in Klippel-Feil syndrome. *J Oral Med* 40:120–122.

55. Lee CK, Weiss AB (1981): Isolated congenital cervical block vertebrae below the axis with neurological symptoms. *Spine* 6:118–124.

56. Livingstone G, Delahunty JE (1968): Malformation of the ear associated with congenital ophthalmic and other condition. *J Laryngol Otol* 82:495–504.

57. Lowry RR (1977): The Klippel-Feil anomalad as part of the fetal alcohol syndrome. *Teratology* 16:53–56.

58. McElfresh E, Winter R (1973): Klippel-Feil syndrome. *Minn Med* 56:353–357.

59. McLay K, Maran AGD (1969): Deafness and the Klippel-Feil syndrome. *J Laryngol Otol* 83:175–184.

60. McRae DL, Barnum AS (1953): Occipitalization of the atlas. *Am J Roentgenol* 70:23–46.

61. Michie I, Clark M (1968): Neurological syndromes associated with cervical and craniocervical anomalies. *Arch Neurol* 18:241–247.

62. Miyamoto RT, Yune HY, Rosevear WH (1983): Klippel-Feil syndrome and associated ear deformities. *Am J Otol* 5:113–119.

63. Moore WB, Matthews TJ, Rabinowitz R (1975): Genitourinary anomalies associated with Klippel-Feil syndrome. *J Bone Joint Surg Am* 57:355–357.

64. Morrison SG, Perry LW, Scott LP (1968): Congenital brevicollis (Klippel-Feil syndrome). *Am J Dis Child* 115:614–620.

65. Mosberg WH Jr (1953): The Klippel-Feil syndrome. Etiology and treatment of neurologic signs. *J Nerv Ment Dis* 117:479–491.

66. Nagib MG, Larson DA, Maxwell RE, et al. (1987): Neuroschisis of the cervical spinal cord in a patient with Klippel-Feil syndrome. *Neurosurgery* 20:629–631.

67. Nagib MG, Maxwell RE, Chou SN (1984): Identification and management of high-risk patients with Klippel-Feil syndrome. *J Neurosurg* 61:523–530.

68. Nagib MG, Maxwell RE, Chou SN (1985): Klippel-Feil syndrome in children: clinical features and management. *Child's Nerv Syst* 1: 255–263.

69. Newmark H III, Cassidy TD (1986): Cervical rib diagnosis by computerized tomography. *Comput Radiol* 10:171–173.

70. Nora JJ, Cohen M, Maxwell GM (1961): Klippel Feil syndrome with congenital heart disease. *Am J Dis Child* 102:110–116.

71. Ohtani I, Dubois-Northrop C (1985): Aural abnormalities in Klippel-Feil syndroem. *Am J Otol* 6:468–471.

72. Okada K, Fuji T, Yonenobu K, et al. (1986): Cervical Diastematomyelia with a stable neurological deficit. *J Bone Joint Surg Am* 68: 934–937.

73. Olow-Nordenram MAK, Radberg CT (1984): Maxillo-nasal dysplasia (Binder syndrome) and associated malformations of the cervical spine. *Acta Radiol* 25:353–360.

74. Palant DL, Carter BL (1972): Klippel-Feil syndrome and deafness. *Am J Dis Child* 123:218–221.

75. Pape KE, Pickering D (1972): Asymmetric crying facies: an index of other congenital anomalies. *J Pediatr* 81:21–30.
76. Pizzutillo PD, Woods MW, Nicholson L (1987): Risk factors in Klippel-Feil syndrome. *Orthop Trans* 11:473.
77. Pizzutillo PD, Woods MW, Nicholson L (1987): Risk factors in Klippel-Feil syndrome. *Orthop Trans* 15:759–760.
78. Pollock M, Carpenter D, Trinkle J, et al. (1991): Quantitative assessment of full range of motion cervical rotation strength. *Orthop Trans* 15:694–695.
79. Prusick VR, Samberg LC, Wesolowski DP (1985): Klippel-Feil syndrome associated with spinal stenosis. *J Bone Joint Surg Am* 67: 161–164.
80. Ramsey J. Bliznak J (1971): Klippel-Feil syndrome with renal agenesis and other anomalies. *Am J Roentgenol* 113:460–463.
81. Resche F, Tessier P, Delaire J (1980): Craniospinal and cervicospinal malformations associated with maxillonasal dysostosis (Binder syndrome). *Head Neck Surg* 3:123–131.
82. Rish BL (1982): Klippel-Feil syndrome: case report: *Va Med* 109: 520–521.
83. Raas-Rothschild A, Goodman RM, Grunbaum M, et al. (1988): Klippel-Feil anomaly with sacral agenesis: an additional subtype, type IV. *Craniofac Genet* 8(4):297–301.
84. Rouvreau MD, Glorion C, Langlais J, et al. (1998): Assessment and neurologic involvement of patients with cervical spine congenital synostosis as in Klippel-Feil syndrome: study of 19 cases. *J Pediatr Orthop B* 7:179–185.
85. Sakai M. Shinkawa A, Miyake H, et al. (1983): Klippel-Feil syndrome with conductive deafness and histological findings of removed stapes. *Ann Otol Rhinol Laryngol* 92:202–206.
86. Schapera J (1987): Autosomal dominant inheritance of cervical ribs. *Clin Genet* 31:386–388.
87. Scher LA, Veith FJ, Haimovici H, et al. (1984): Staging of arterial complications of cervical rib: guidelines for surgical management. *Surgery* 95:644–649.
88. Schlitt M, Depsey PJ, Robinson RK (1989): Cervical butterfly-block vertebra. A case report. *Clin Imaging* 13:167–170.
89. Sellke FW, Kelley TR (1988): Thoracic outlet syndrome. *Am J Surg* 156:54–57.
90. Sherk HH, Uppal GS (1991): Congenital bony anomalies of the cervical spine. In: Frymoyer JW, ed. *The adult spine: principles and practice.* New York: Raven Press, pp. 1015–1037.
91. Scolapurkar SL, Dhall GI (1991): Cervico-oculo-acousticus syndrome with pregnancy. *Gynecol Obstet Invest* 31:116–118.
92. Shoul MI, Ritvo M (1952): Clinical and roentgenological manifestations of the Klippel-Feil syndrome (congenital fusion of the cervical vertebrae, brevicollis). *Am J Roentgenol* 68:369–385.
93. Southwell RB, Reynolds AF, Badger VM, et al. (1980): Klippel-Feil syndrome with cervical cord compression resulting from cervical subluxation in association with an omo-vertebral bone. *Spine* 5:480–482.
94. Stadnicki G, Rassumowski D (1972): The association of cleft palate with the Klippel-Feil syndrome. *Oral Surg* 33:335–340.
95. Stark EW, Borton TE (1973): Klippel-Feil syndrome and associated hearing loss. *Arch Otol* 97:415–419.
96. Steward EJ, O'Reilly BF (1989): Klippel-Feil syndrome and conductive deafness. *J Laryngol Otol* 103:947–949.
97. Strax TE, Baran E (1975): Traumatic quadriplegia associated with Klippel-Feil syndrome: discussion and case reports. *Arch Phys Med Rehabil* 56:363–365.
98. Strisciuglio P, Raia V, Di Meo A, et al. (1982): Wildervanck's syndrome with bilateral subluxation of lens and facial paralysis. *J Med Genet* 20:72–73.
99. Thomsen MN, Schneider U, Weber M, et al. (1997): Scoliosis and congenital anomalies associated with Klippel-Feil syndrome types I–III. *Spine* 22(4):396–401.
100. Torg JS, Pavlov H, Genuario SE, et al. (1986): Neurapraxia of the cervical spinal cord with transient quadriplegia. *J Bone Joint Surg Am* 68:1354–1370.
101. Tredwell SJ, Smith DF, Macleod PJ, et al. (1982): Cervical spine anomalies in fetal alcohol syndrome. *Spine* 7:331–334.
102. Vaksmann G, Noblet D, Dupuis C (1987): Subclavian artery aneurysm secondary to a cervical supernumerary rib in a child. *Eur J Pediatr* 146:209–210.
103. Van Kerckhoven MF, Fabry G (1989): The Klippel-Feil syndrome: a constellation of deformities. *Acta Orthop Belg* 55:107–118.
104. Veeneklaas GMH (1952): Pathogenesis of intrathoracic gastrogenic cysts. *Am J Dis Child* 83:500–507.
105. West PDB, Gholkar A, Ramsden RT (1989): Wildervanck's syndrome—unilateral mondini dysplasia identified by computed tomography. *J Laryngol Otol* 103:408–411.
106. Whitehouse GH, Harrison RJ (1970); Klippel-Feil syndrome. *Proc R Soc Med* 63:287–288.
107. Whittle IR, Besser M (1983): Congenital neural abnormalities presenting with mirror movements in a patient with Klippel-Feil syndrome. *J Neurosurg* 59:891–894.
108. Willemsen WMP (1982): Combination of the Mayer-Rokitansky-Kuster and Klippel-Feil syndrome—a case report and literature review. *Eur J Obstet Gynecol Reprod Biol* 13:229–235.
109. Winter RB, Moe JH, Lonstein JE (1984): The incidence of Klippel-Feil syndrome in patients with congenital scoliosis and kyphosis. *Spine* 9:363–366.
110. Wycis HT (1953): Lipoma of the spinal cord associated with Klippel-Feil syndrome. *J Neurosurg* 10:625–678.

NEUROSURGICAL MANAGEMENT OF SPINAL DYSRAPHISM

MARK S. DIAS
DAVID G. MCLONE

Spinal dysraphism encompasses several spinal malformations. All have in common a disorder of dorsal midline development that involves any or all of the dorsal midline structures—skin, dorsal muscles, vertebrae, and the neural tube and its coverings. Dysraphic malformations can be conveniently classified according to type of skin covering into open malformations (spina bifida aperta) and closed malformations (spina bifida occulta). Open dysraphic malformations lack an intact skin covering over the neural malformation, and the neural lesion is readily visible on the back of the infant. Occult dysraphic malformations are covered by an intact, although often abnormally formed, skin covering. Myelomeningocele is the most common open malformation. The frequency is approximately 1 in 1,400 live births (16,69,134). Other, less common open dysraphic malformations include meningocele and combined anterior and posterior spina bifida (12,22,25,27,31,135). The most commonly encountered occult dysraphic lesions is lipomyelomeningocele (spinal lipoma). Other occult dysraphic lesions include split-cord malformation (diastematomyelia), dermal sinus tract and dermoid tumor, thickened filum terminale, and myelocystocele. More complex malformations may have combinations of the foregoing anomalies and are not as readily classified (23). A working knowledge of normal and abnormal neuroembryology helps in understanding the anatomy, presentation, and management of these lesions.

NORMAL NEURAL DEVELOPMENT

The human embryo at the end of the first week is composed of two layers—the epiblast adjacent to the amnionic cavity and the hypoblast adjacent to the yolk sac (Fig. 1A). During the second week, a midline structure, the primitive streak, forms in the midline in the caudal half of the embryo; the cranial end of the primitive streak is called *Hensen's node* (Fig. 1B). Cells of

the epiblast migrate toward the primitive streak and enter between the epiblast and hypoblast in a process known as *gastrulation*. This gives the embryo three layers—ectoderm, mesoderm, and endoderm. The ectodermal cells give rise to the surface ectoderm and neuroepithelium; the mesodermal cells give rise to the somites and mesenchyme of the embryo; and the endodermal cells give rise to the gut.

During gastrulation, the primitive streak first elongates toward the cranial end of the embryo then regresses back toward the caudal end of the embryo. During regression, cells within Hensen's node are laid down to form the midline notochordal process between the overlying neuroepithelium and the underlying endoderm. These prospective notochordal cells enter through the primitive pit within the center of Hensen's node and enter between the ectoderm and endoderm rostral to the retreating Hensen's node (Fig. 1C). The notochordal process initially is rod shaped and has a central lumen, the notochordal canal, which is contiguous with the amnionic cavity through the primitive pit (Fig. 2A). Later, the notochordal process fuses, or intercalates, with the underlying endoderm to form the notochordal plate (Fig. 2B). The fusion of the notochordal process with the endoderm places the amnionic cavity and yolk sacs in direct communication through the primitive neurenteric canal. This canal lasts approximately 3 days, after which the notochordal plate detaches, or excalates, from the endoderm (Fig. 2C), and the primitive neurenteric canal is closed. With regression of the primitive streak and Hensen's node during gastrulation, the primitive pit ultimately occupies a caudal position at the coccyx; benign coccygeal dimples are thought by many to represent a remnant of the primitive pit. Abnormal development of the notochord during gastrulation has been implicated as a cause of split-cord malformations and other complex dysraphic malformations (25).

The nervous system and the skin are both derived from ectoderm. The development of the neuroectoderm to form the neural tube is called *primary neurulation*. By gestational day 16, the neuroectoderm is visible as pseudostratified columnar epithelium in the midline of the dorsal surface of the embryo. It overlies the notochord and is contiguous laterally with the cutaneous ectoderm. By day 18, the neural groove (median hinge point)

M.S. Dias: Departments of Pediatric Surgery and Neurosurgery, Children's Hospital of Buffalo, State University of New York at Buffalo, Buffalo, New York 14222.

D.G. McLone: Department of Neurosurgery, Children's Memorial Hospital, Northwestern University, Chicago, Illinois 60614.

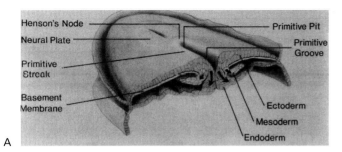

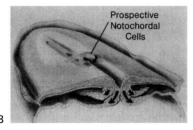

FIGURE 1. Illustrations show early human development. **A:** Human embryo at the time of gastrulation is composed of two layers—the epiblast adjacent to the amnionic cavity and the hypoblast adjacent to the yolk sac. During gastrulation, cells of the epiblast migrate toward and enter the primitive streak to form the endoderm and mesoderm. **B:** Presumptive notochordal cells in Hensen's node enter the primitive pit during the latter half of gastrulation (during regression of the primitive streak) to form the notochordal process.

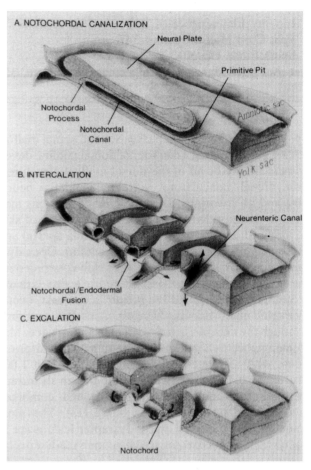

FIGURE 2. Formation of the notochord. *A,* The notochordal process contains a central lumen (the notochordal canal), which is continuous with the amnionic cavity through the primitive pit. *B,* During intercalation, the canalized notochordal process fuses with the underlying endoderm. The communication of the amnion with the yolk sac forms the primitive neurenteric canal. *C,* During excalation, the notochord rolls up and separates from the endoderm to become the definitive notochord. The primitive neurenteric canal is obliterated.

forms in the midline of the neuroectoderm, and the two adjacent neural folds begin to elevate (Fig. 3A). This is the beginning of primary neurulation, the process whereby the neural plate undergoes several morphogenetic movements to form the neural tube (129).

As primary neurulation continues, the neural groove deepens, and the adjacent neural folds continue to elevate dorsally (Fig. 3B). Later, two dorsolateral hinge points form on both sides of the developing neural tube, bringing the neural folds together in the midline (Fig. 3C). The apposition and fusion of the neural folds completes the neural tube; simultaneously, the cutaneous ectoderm separates from the neural folds to form the skin of the back. Mesenchymal tissues intercalating between the newly formed neural tube and the overlying cutaneous ectoderm form the paraspinous muscles and dorsal vertebral arch.

Closure of the neural tube in human embryos usually begins in the midcervical region and proceeds both cranially and caudally from this point. Whereas neurulation was previously thought to occur in a simple linear manner, as the closing of a zipper, from the point of initial closure, it is now known that there are multiple points of closure (42,43,95). The last areas to close are the cranial neuropore, located near the optic chiasm at the lamina terminalis, and the caudal neuropore, located at the second sacral level of the spinal cord. The cranial neuropore closes at about gestational day 24, and the caudal neuropore at about day 26 (96,97). More caudal regions of the neural tube (the spinal cord caudal to the S2 segment and the filum terminale) are formed thereafter through a process known as *secondary*

neurulation. This secondary neural tube develops from the caudal cell mass, a pluripotent group of cells that additionally gives rise to the caudal vertebrae and mesenchyme through a process of canalization and fusion of adjacent tubules (Fig. 4). The secondary neural tube eventually becomes contiguous with the neural tube formed by means of primary neurulation (71,97, 126–128).

Beginning during the sixth embryonic week and continuing into postnatal life, the neural tube undergoes several morphogenetic changes collectively called the *ascent of the conus medullaris.* Before embryonic day 54, the caudal neural tube undergoes morphogenetic changes known as *retrogressive differentiation.* The result is formation of the filum terminale and an apparent ascent of the conus medullaris. After day 54, differential growth of the vertebral column relative to the neural tube causes a progressive length discrepancy so that the conus medullaris undergoes a true

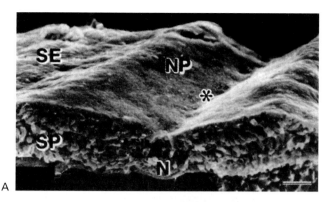

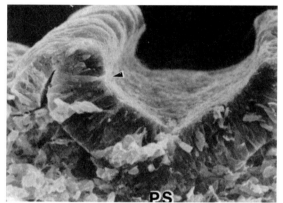

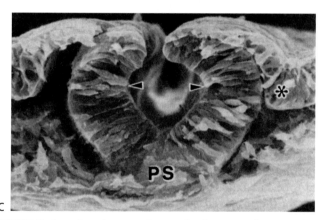

FIGURE 3. Scanning electron micrographs show neurulation in the chick embryo. **A:** Midline bending of the neural plate (*NP*) over the notochord (*N*) to form the neural groove, or median hinge point (*asterisk*). *SE,* Surface epithelium; *SP,* segmental plate mesoderm. **B:** Further elevation of the neural folds about paired dorsolateral hinge points (*arrowhead*). *PS,* Primitive streak. **C:** Apposition of neural folds in preparation for fusion to form the neural tube. *Asterisk,* Surface epithelium; *arrowheads,* dorsolateral hinge points; *PS,* primitive streak. (From Shoenwolf GC [1986]: On the morphogenesis of the early rudiments of the developing central nervous system. In: Schoenwolf GC. ed. *Scanning electron microscopy studies of embryogenesis.* O'Hare, IL: SEM, Inc., pp. 289–308, with permission.)

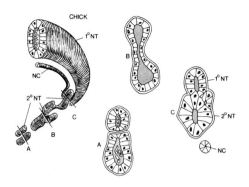

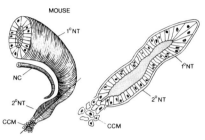

FIGURE 4. Secondary neurulation in chick and mouse. *A,* In the chick (*top*), cells of the caudal cell mass located caudal to the primary neural tube (*1°NT*) form multiple independent vesicles. *B,* These vesicles fuse to form a secondary neural tube (*2°NT*). *C,* The secondary neural tube then fuses with the primary neural tube. *NC,* Notochord. In the mouse (*bottom*), cells of the caudal cell mass (*CCM*) fuse directly with the caudal end of the primary neural tube to form the secondary neural tube. Among humans, it is unclear whether secondary neurulation more closely resembles that of the chick or the mouse.

ascent (Fig. 5). The conus by 1 to 2 months after birth normally lies opposite or craniad to the L1–2 disc space (4,26,149,151). A more caudally positioned conus suggests spinal cord tethering (see later).

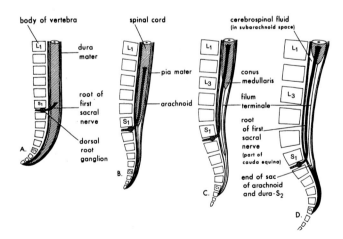

FIGURE 5. *A, B, C, D:* Ascent of the conus medullaris. The conus ascends by means of a combination of morphologic changes in the terminal neural tube and by means of differential growth of the vertebral column relative to the developing spinal cord. *A:* 8 weeks. *B:* 24 weeks. *C:* Newborn. *D:* Adult. (From Moore KL [1982]: *The Developing Human,* 3rd ed. Philadelphia: WB Saunders, p. 383, with permission.) *(Figure continues.)*

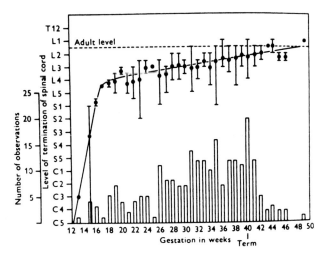

FIGURE 5. *Continued. E,* Level of the conus medullaris in humans during gestation and postnatal development (From Barson AJ [1970]: The vertebral level of termination of the spinal cord during normal and abnormal development. *J Anat* 106:489–497, with permission.)

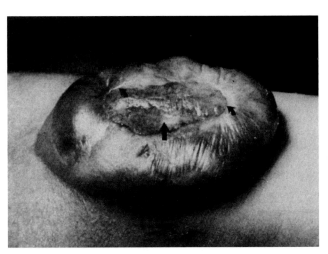

FIGURE 6. Myelomeningocele in a newborn infant. *Straight arrow* points to the neural placode on the dorsal aspect in the center of the sac. *Curved arrows* denote the junction of the neural placode with the surrounding skin (cutaneous ectoderm).

EMBRYOGENESIS OF SPINAL DYSRAPHISM

Dysraphic spinal cord malformations are the result of abnormalities of early neural development during the first 4 through 6 weeks of embryogenesis. Myelomeningocele involves either primarily or secondarily a failure of the neural tube to close properly over a portion of its length. Occult dysraphic lesions are thought to arise through a variety of mechanisms involving several key processes in early neural development. The embryogenesis of all of these malformations is beyond the scope of this chapter, and the interested reader is referred to more extensive discussions of this topic (24,25,84). This chapter concentrates on four disorders of the spinal neural tube: (a) myelomeningocele, (b) meningocele, (c) lipomyelomeningocele, and (d) split-cord malformations. Also included is a review of the embryogenesis of spina bifida occulta.

Myelomeningocele

Myelomeningocele arises through a localized failure of neural tube closure. The nonclosure theory (146) suggests that these malformations arise through a primary failure of neural tube closure, whereas the reopening or overdistention theory (37–40,93) suggests that the neural tube reopens after an initial period of normal closure. In most cases, myelomeningocele arises by means of the former mechanism. Myelomeningocele is likely the end product of a variety of environmental, teratogenic, and genetic abnormalities and has a heterogeneous and multifactorial origin. Neither the contributing etiologic factors nor the molecular events that underlie human neural tube defects are known with certainty (15).

Use of the terms *myelomeningocele* and *myeloschisis* is confusing, in part because various authors have used these terms to refer to what they have considered to be two distinct disorders. *Myeloschisis* has traditionally referred to a malformation in which

the neural tube has failed to close over a large portion of its length. The involved neural tissue is flat, lies open on the back, and has no investing meninges (59). In contrast, the term *myelomeningocele* refers to an open neural tube that sits atop a spinal-fluid-containing sac (Fig. 6). These terms are confusing and misleading. In both disorders, a portion of the neural tube has failed to close, the neural folds remain attached to the adjacent cutaneous ectoderm, and a portion of the neural plate—the placode—is therefore exposed on the dorsal embryonic surface. Because the exposed placode remains attached to the cutaneous ectoderm, cerebrospinal fluid (CSF) can form only in the subarachnoid space beneath the placode. The extent to which the underlying CSF elevates the placode determines the type of malformation. If CSF accumulates beneath the placode and displaces it to the top of a fluid-filled sac, a myelomeningocele results (Fig. 6). If CSF is vented, perhaps through the central canal or through a tear in the attenuated surrounding tissues, it does not accumulate, the placode lies flat on the dorsal surface, and myeloschisis results. These two malformations therefore differ not in origin but in subsequent development. The term *myeloschisis* should be discarded, and all such lesions called myelomeningocele.

Another point of confusion is the use of the term *closed myelomeningocele* to refer to a fluid-filled lumbosacral mass covered with full-thickness skin. When neurulation fails to occur, the neuroectoderm remains attached to the skin laterally, and myelomeningocele is by definition an open lesion. "Closed myelomeningocele" is not a myelomeningocele at all. Most often it is a myelocystocele, a terminal dilation of the spinal cord contained within a dilated, fluid-filled, thecal sac (88,106).

Meningocele

Meningocele is a skin- or membrane-covered sac, usually in the lumbar region, that contains no demonstrable neural tissue. The sac, which contains CSF, comprises the spinal dura mater and

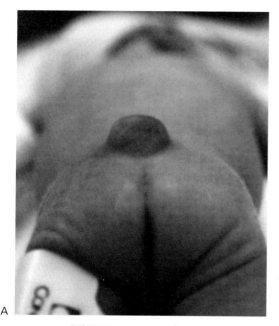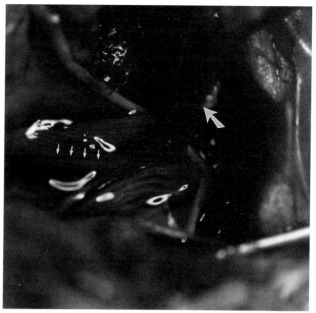

FIGURE 7. Meningocele in a newborn infant. **A:** The malformation consists of a fully skin-covered lesion with no spinal fluid leakage. **B:** Operative photograph shows the distal spinal cord terminating in a filum terminale (*small arrows*). A track of mesenchymal tissue (*large arrow*) is attached to the dorsal portion of the distal spinal cord just cranial to the tip of the conus and separate from the filum terminale. This projects into and ends within the skin-covered sac.

underlying arachnoid, which balloon dorsally from the spinal thecal sac. The spinal cord is normal and within the spinal canal. True meningocele, which has no element of neural tissue, is extraordinarily rare. In many cases, the sac contains strands of mesenchymal or central or peripheral neural tissue that connects with the dorsal surface of a low-lying (tethered) spinal cord (Fig. 7). The neural-tissue-containing lesions probably are a form of myelomeningocele. Meningocele likely is caused by either a postneurulation disorder of cutaneous ectodermal or dorsal mesenchymal development or by abnormal separation of cutaneous ectoderm from neuroectoderm. Despite the presence of small amounts of neural tissue in some of the malformations, these patients usually have normal neurologic findings, and their prognosis is excellent if the spinal cord is properly untethered. Hydrocephalus and Chiari malformation are unusual.

Lipomyelomeningocele

Lipomyelomeningocele (spinal lipoma) is a malformation that contains an element of fat (lipoma) contiguous with a low lying, or tethered, spinal cord. Lipoma usually is an isolated malformation, although it can occur in combination with myelomeningocele and other dysraphic malformations. Most lipomyelomeningoceles involve the lumbosacral spinal cord, filum terminale, or both. Cervical or thoracic lesions are rare. Two general types of lipomyelomeningocele have been described. In the first and more frequent type, a subcutaneous fatty mass of variable size is contiguous with the spinal cord through a dorsal vertebral

and dural defect (Fig. 8A). In the second type, the dura and posterior vertebral elements are intact, and the fat is located solely within the thecal sac (Fig. 8B). In both cases, the spinal cord has failed to close properly at the level of the lipomyelomeningocele, and the fat arises from the dorsal spinal cord through the defect (Fig. 9). The dorsal nerve roots, which are derived from neural crest and normally arise from the neural folds just lateral to the site of dorsal midline fusion, are located immediately lateral to the junction between the fat and the dorsal cord. Lipomyelomeningocele is thought to arise from disordered neural tube closure in which the cutaneous ectoderm separates prematurely from the approximating neural folds before neural tube closure is complete (Fig. 9). The surrounding mesenchyme enters the central lumen of the neural tube and is induced to form fat (78).

Split-cord Malformations (Diastematomyelia)

Split-cord malformation is an anomaly whereby the spinal cord is clefted over a portion of its length to form a double neural tube. The two hemicords both may be contained within a single dural sheath, or each may be contained within its own, separate dural sheath. Split-cord malformations can occur in isolation or in association with myelomeningocele or other closed dysraphic malformations. Early classification schemes were confusing and misleading. The term *diastematomyelia* (from the Greek "diastema" meaning *cleft* and "melos" meaning *medulla*) was used to describe malformations in which the spinal cord was "split" into two half-cords, each with a single, lateral set of dorsal and

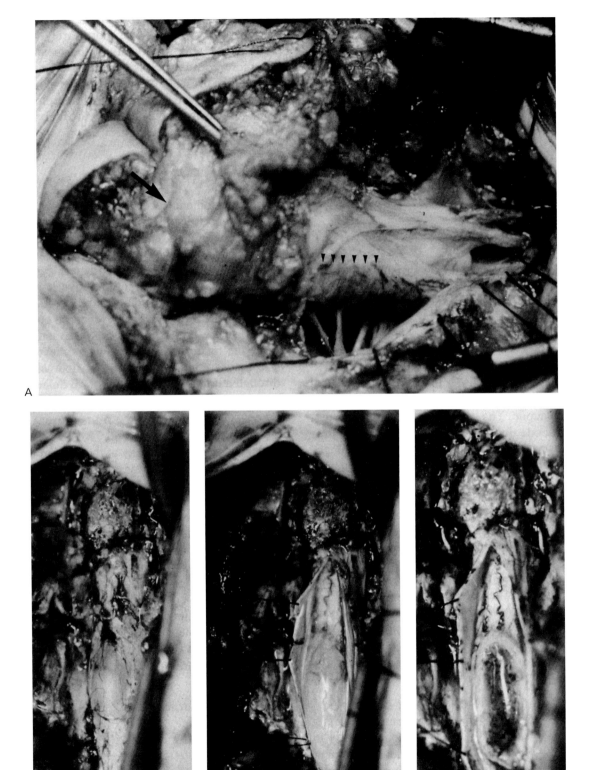

FIGURE 8. Lipomyelomeningocele. **A:** Lipoma with subcutaneous extension (*arrow*). The subcutaneous mass enters the spinal cord through a dorsal dural defect and infiltrates the central canal of the cord. The nerve roots exit immediately lateral to the lateral edge of the lipoma (*arrowheads*). **B:** Intradural lipoma. The lipoma is located entirely within the dural sac. *Left,* Before dural opening, the lipoma is visible through the thinned dura. *Center,* After dural opening but before resection. *Right,* After resection.

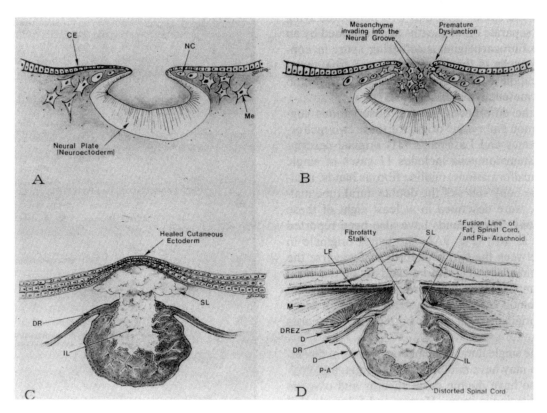

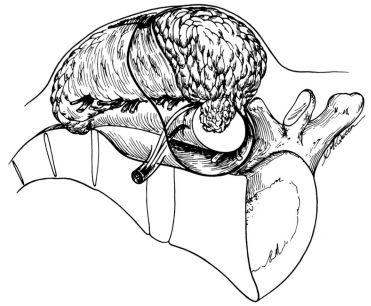

FIGURE 9. A, B, C, D: Embryogenesis of lipomyelomeningocele. *A,B,* Premature dysjunction of the cutaneous ectoderm (*CE*) from the neuroepithelium allows mesenchymal cells (*Me*) to gain access to the central canal of the neural tube. *C,D,* These cells form a fibrofatty subcutaneous lipoma (*SL*) beneath the surface ectoderm and extending into the central canal. The dorsal roots (*DR*) arise immediately lateral to the lipoma. *NC,* Neural crest; *LF,* lumbodorsal fascia; *DREZ,* dorsal root entry zone; *D,* dura; *P-A,* pia and arachnoid; *IL,* intracanalicular lipoma. (From Pang D: Tethered cord syndrome. In: Hoffman HJ, ed [1986]: *Advances in Pediatric Neurosurgery. Neurosurgery: State of the Art Reviews,* vol. 1, no. 1: Philadelphia, Hanley and Belfus, with permission.) **E:** Anatomic features of lipomyelomeningocele. The subcutaneous mass extends through the dorsal aspect of the spinal cord to end within the central canal. The dorsal roots arise immediately lateral to the lipoma at the dorsal root entry zone (From Oakes WJ [1991]: Management of spinal cord lipomas and lipomyelomeningoceles. In Wilkins RH, Rengachary SS, eds. *Neurosurgery Update II.* New York: McGraw-Hill, pp. 345–352 with permission.)

E

ventral nerve roots. The term *diplomyelia* was used to describe complete duplication of the spinal cord, each cord containing both medial and lateral sets of ventral and dorsal nerve roots (20,52,53,64,98).

The confusion has been compounded by classification of these malformations according to the composition of their dural coverings or by the presence or absence of tethering midline structures. In diastematomyelia, each of the hemicords lies within its own dural sheath, whereas in diplomyelia, both duplicated cords lie within a common dural sheath. In diastematomy-

elia, midline bony, cartilaginous, or fibrous tethering bands are present between the two hemicords. In diplomyelia, no such midline structures are thought to be present. Thus the widespread belief has been that diastematomyelia involves a splitting of the spinal cord into two half-cords lying within two separate dural sheaths and separated by an osseous or fibrocartilaginous tethering spur. Diplomyelia, however, is thought to be a true spinal cord duplication within a common dural tube with no interposed tethering elements (20,52).

Several more recent observations suggest that diastematomye-

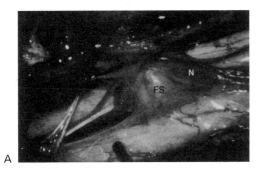

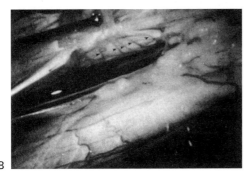

FIGURE 10. Intraoperative photographs of a split-cord malformation with a single dural sac. **A:** A thick, fibrous band (*FS*) arises from between the two hemicords and tethers them to the dorsal dura. Median dorsal nerve roots (*N*) are visible in the cranial margin of the band. **B:** After the fibrous band and dorsal roots are removed, median ventral nerve roots (*arrowheads*) course up from the ventral aspect of the left hemicord and end in the median septum. (From Pang D, Dias, MS, Ahab-Barmada M [1992]: Split-cord malformation, I: a unified theory of embryogenesis for double spinal cord malformations. *Neurosurgery* 31: 451–480, with permission.)

lia and diplomyelia represent different variations of the same malformation and share a common embryonic origin. James and Lassman's (64) original description of diastematomyelia included 11 cases of "single dural tube" malformations, eight of which contained midline intradural fibrous "bands" analogous to the osseocartilaginous spurs of the double dural tube malformations. These tethering bands also have been described by Pang et al. (Fig. 10A). The intradural bands originate in the cleft between the two hemicords and traverse the subarachnoid space to end more caudally on the dura. They are composed of tough, fibrous connective tissue, prominent blood vessels, and dystrophic median nerve roots that originate from one or both of the hemicords (103). Similar midline intradural fibrous bands were described by Herren and Edwards (52) in several cases of "diplomyelia"; cases of double and single dural tube malformations occurred with equal frequency in the series.

Dystrophic median nerve roots projecting from one or both hemicords have been associated with both diastematomyelia and diplomyelia (Fig. 10B) (52,64,102,103,120). These dystrophic roots originate from one or both hemicords and insert onto the midline osseocartilaginous spurs or fibrous bands. Both dorsal and ventral roots and ganglion cells have been described (102,103,120). The presence of both lateral and median sets of nerve roots strongly suggests the presence of at least partial spinal cord duplication in both malformations. Autopsies of persons

who died with diastematomyelia or diplomyelia have shown neither absolute splitting nor complete duplication of the cord in any instance. Rather, the hemicords are incomplete duplications with relatively well preserved lateral halves and dystrophic medial halves (20,52,72,119,120).

All these observations suggest that diastematomyelia and diplomyelia represent a spectrum of split-cord malformations that have a common embryonic mechanism. The exact nature of the resultant malformation depends in part on the severity of the initial embryologic insult and the success of subsequent embryonic repair. Pang et al. (102,103) has classified split-cord malformations into types I and II. Type I malformations contain two hemicords, each within its own dural sheath, with an intervening extradural tethering osseocartilaginous spur (Fig. 11). Type II malformations contain the two hemicords within a single dural tube and a midline intradural fibrous tethering band (Fig. 12).

Split-cord malformations can be isolated or associated with

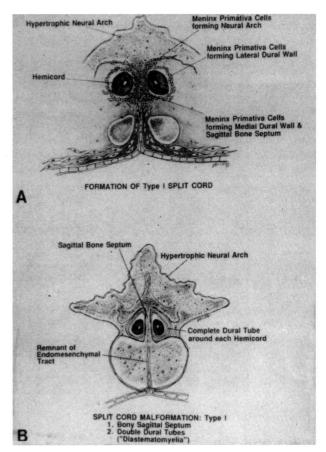

FIGURE 11. Embryogenesis of double dural tube malformation, classified as split-cord malformation type I by Pang et al. **A:** Cells of the meninx primitiva form two separate dural sheaths that surround each of the two hemicords. The midline cells of the malformation form an osseous or fibrocartilaginous spur that bisects the two hemicords. The midline cells also contribute to hypertrophy of the neural arch. **B:** Fully formed malformation. The remnant of the endomesenchymal tract of the malformation is visible. (From Pang D, Dias, MS, Ahab-Barmada M [1992]: Split-cord malformation, I: a unified theory of embryogenesis for double spinal cord malformations. *Neurosurgery* 31:451–480, with permission.)

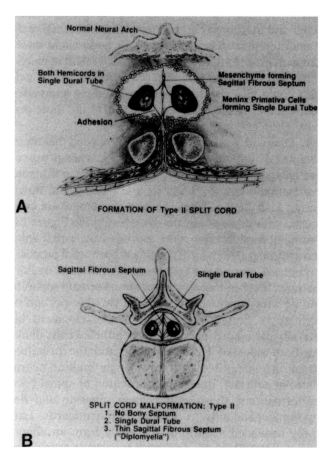

FIGURE 12. Formation of a single dural sac malformation, classified as split-cord malformation type II by Pang et al. **A:** The meninx primitiva forms a single dural sheath that surrounds both hemicords. The cells of the endomesenchymal tract form a midline fibrous band or septum, which bisects the two hemicords and tethers them to the surrounding dura. **B:** Fully formed single dural sac malformation. (From Pang D, Dias MS, Ahab-Barmada M [1992]: Split-cord malformation, I: a unified theory of embryogenesis for double spinal cord malformations. *Neurosurgery* 31:451–480, with permission.)

a wide variety of malformations, including combined anterior and posterior) spina bifida, also called *split notochord syndrome*; hemimyelomeningocele; myelomeningocele, (in which SCMs are found in as many as one-third of autopsies); cervical myelomeningocele; neurenteric cyst; some instances of Klippel-Feil syndrome, iniencephaly, and caudal agenesis; and certain intestinal duplications and diverticula. All these complex dysraphic malformations have in common stereotypical anomalies that involve tissues derived from all three primary germ layers and are thought to share an embryonic origin (25,39). The following four putative embryonic mechanisms have been proposed (25).

Ectodermal-Endodermal Adhesion Theory

Beardmore and Wigglesworth (5) proposed that adhesion between the epiblast and hypoblast before or during the outgrowth of the notochordal process could split the notochord around the adhesion. The result would be a split notochord and independent development of paired neural tubes to form two hemicords.

Remnants of this endodermal-ectodermal adhesion could give rise to endodermal remnants anywhere between the gut and the cutaneous ectoderm. This mechanism would work only if the notochord extended cranially from the Hensen node. If, on the other hand, the notochord is laid down as the node regresses, as has been demonstrated in the chick embryo (139), one would have to postulate an adhesion within the primitive streak caudal to the Hensen node, around which the notochord might be split during node regression (113).

Accessory Neurenteric Canal Theory

Bremer (9) studied combined spina bifida (split notochord syndrome), which is characterized by an open neural tube defect and widespread underlying vertebral anomalies. Midsagittal splitting of the involved vertebrae forms two hemivertebral columns around a central cleft. Through this cleft passes a variable amount of endodermal tissue, ranging from a neurenteric cyst to entire loops of intestine, that arises from the abdominal cavity and projects onto the dorsum of the child. The intraabdominal intestine also may contain variable duplications or diverticula. An associated split-cord malformation is invariably present; the two hemicords surround the central cleft. Visceral malformations are exceedingly common (5,12).

Both the central cleft in combined spina bifida and the neurenteric canal of normal embryos connect the embryonic endoderm and ectoderm. However, the dorsal opening of the neurenteric canal—the primitive pit—ultimately descends to the level of the coccyx, whereas combined spina bifida (and other variants of split-cord malformations) arise at more cranial levels of the neuraxis. Bremer proposed that the endoderm herniates dorsally in these malformations and splits the notochord and neural plate to produce an accessory neurenteric canal. However, the impetus for such a dorsal herniation is unknown.

Notochordal Duplication Theory

McLetchie et al. (76) and Saunders (125) suggested that the initial abnormality is a duplication of the notochord that allows a secondary endodermal-ectodermal interaction between the paired notochords. Dodds (27) suggested that during normal embryogenesis, bilaterally paired prospective notochordal cell anlagen might be integrated into a single midline structure during primitive streak regression. Feller and Sternberg (32) proposed that abnormal rests of undifferentiated cells in Hensen's node might interfere with proper midline integration and result in paired notochords. Subsequent differentiation of these cell rests might give rise to a variety of midline anomalies composed of tissues derived from any of the three primary germ cell layers.

Abnormal Gastrulation Theory

Dias and Walker (25) proposed that all these malformations arise during a time when prospective anlagen from the three germ layers are in intimate association during gastrulation. The events of this model are contrasted to those of normal develop-

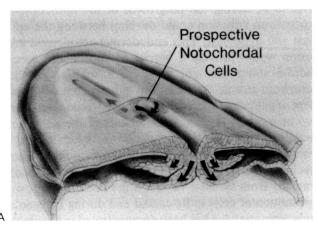
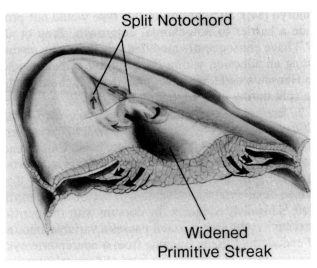

FIGURE 13. Embryogenesis of split-cord malformations. **A:** Normal gastrulation. **B:** Formation of split-cord malformation. During gastrulation, presumptive notochordal cells in Hensen's node, rather than forming a single notochordal process, become functionally separate and begin to form two separate notochordal processes. The overlying and adjacent neuroectoderm also forms two separate hemineural tubes, each of which overlies a heminotochord. Intervening cells of Hensen's node between the two hemicords have pluripotent potential and can develop into a variety of normal or abnormal tissues derived from any of the three primary germ layers (From Dias MS, Walker M [1992]: The embryogenesis of complex dysraphic malformations: a disorder of gastrulation? *Pediatr Neurosurg* 18:229–253, with permission.)

ment in Fig. 13. During normal development, paired notochordal anlagen are integrated to form a single notochordal process. In contrast, during the formation of split-cord malformations, these notochordal precursors remain separate and develop independently over a variable portion of their length. During normal development, bilaterally paired prospective neuroepithelial cells likewise flank both sides of Hensen's node, and the primitive streak are integrated to form a single midline neural plate. In contrast, during the formation of split-cord malformations, these cells remain separate and develop independently to produce two hemicords. Laterally displaced somitic tissue would form an abnormally widened spinal canal with numerous associated vertebral segmentation anomalies, including sagittally clefted (butterfly) vertebrae, fused vertebrae (single or multiple, as in Klippel-Feil syndrome), hemivertebrae, absent vertebrae (single or multiple, as in caudal agenesis syndrome), or if displaced widely enough, incompletely duplicated vertebrae (as in combined spina bifida).

The space between the paired hemicords comprises pluripotent primitive streak cells and could give rise to a variety of tissue types from any of the three primary germ layers, including enteric structures (neurenteric cysts, loops of intestine), mesenchymal tissues (bony or fibrous midline structures, blood vessels, muscle, and fat encountered in split-cord malformations; anomalous vertebrae; immature renal tissues) and ectodermal tissue (dermoid and epidermoid tumors), and even pathologic tissues such as teratomas and Wilms tumors (14,33,144). All of these clinical variations have been described. Both the clinical spectrum and embryologic theory have been reviewed by Dias and Walker (25).

Spina Bifida Occulta

Spina bifida occulta is an isolated disorder of posterior vertebral development in which a failure of posterior vertebral fusion results in absence or dysplasia of spinous processes and laminae. The malformation most commonly affects the S1 vertebral level, and is estimated to occur among as many as 30% of the population (8). The underlying spinal cord is normally formed and the findings of the neurologic examination are normal, suggesting a disorder that arises after neurulation is complete and which involves only the dorsal vertebral arch. Spina bifida occulta is therefore almost certainly unrelated pathogenetically to myelomeningocele.

Because it is an isolated anomaly, spina bifida occulta is usually of no clinical consequence. However, posterior vertebral malformations can occur in association with underlying occult spinal dysraphism. Posterior vertebral malformations usually are more extensive, and there are either cutaneous manifestations of underlying spinal dysraphism or signs and symptoms of spinal cord tethering. Isolated spina bifida occulta of the S1 lamina without other signs or symptoms of spinal dysraphism need not be investigated further; however, complex bony malformations or those that accompany signs or symptoms of spinal cord tethering should be investigated further.

NEUROSURGICAL MANAGEMENT OF SPINAL DYSRAPHISM

Children with spinal dysraphism comprise one of the largest groups of patients for whom pediatric neurosurgeons care. Their care is often extraordinarily complex and may require the integrated efforts of caregivers from many disciplines, including neurosurgeons, orthopaedists, urologists, physiatrists, physical and occupational therapists, orthotists, gastroenterologists, endocrinologists, speech and swallowing experts, pulmonologists, and intensive care specialists. The concept of the spina bifida team, in which a core of dedicated clinicians and staff provide coordinated, multidisciplinary care, provides the best opportunity to minister comprehensively to a child with spinal dysraphism. The medical care rendered is both higher in quality and ultimately less expensive (66) than uncoordinated care. Herein are reviewed management issues for the neurosurgical treatment of a child with myelomeningocele, lipomyelomeningocele, or split-cord malformation.

Treatment of Children with Myelomeningocele

Treatment of a child with a myelomeningocele has undergone a striking evolution over the past several decades. From the early 1900s, improvements in surgical techniques have allowed early closure of the back wound without infection. The introduction of effective CSF shunting systems in the 1950s led to dramatic improvements in the management of hydrocephalus. The introduction in 1975 of clean intermittent catheterization for the management of associated neurogenic bladder dysfunction dramatically reduced the mortality from chronic renal failure. Therapy for symptomatic Chiari malformation with posterior fossa and cervical decompression; therapy for progressive spinal cord dysfunction by means of spinal cord untethering and shunting of syringomyelia; and aggressive orthopaedic management of spinal and lower extremity deformities all have led to improved long-term function among many of these children.

Perhaps the greatest change has been in attitude. In the past, many physicians considered treatment of these children to be cruel, thinking it more merciful to allow them to die. In 1971, in an effort to better decide which patients should be treated, the Lorber criteria were developed to allow withholding of treatment from certain infants with myelomeningocele. The Lorber criteria included (a) the presence of severe hydrocephalus at birth, (b) total paraplegia, (c) spinal kyphosis at birth, and (d) any additional birth defect (73).

None of these criteria, either in isolation or in combination, is an entirely accurate predictor of outcome (79). Moreover, the outcome among children treated without regard to selection criteria (nonselective treatment) (77) compares favorably with the outcomes in Lorber's and others' series (17,45,74), in which selection was performed. In a comparison between the unselected series of McLone (77) and the selected series of Lorber and Salfield (74), the mortality for the unselected group was comparable with that for the highest-ranking infants in the selected group. The overall mortality for the unselected group was 15%, and that for the selected group, including infants thought to be at poor risk and therefore allowed to die, was nearly 70%. The IQs of the highest-ranking infants from the selected group were slightly higher than those of infants in the unselected group (15% more children had normal IQs). The higher IQs, however, were more than offset by the tremendous increase in mortality.

From another perspective, 60% of the children from the selected group who were allowed to die would have been "competitive" had they been allowed to survive (80). Finally, parents rarely regret a decision to treat their child. Only 13 of 300 parents expressed regret over their decision to treat their child; remarkably, 9 of the 13 regretted an initial decision not to treat their child (79).

This is not to say that every child with a myelomeningocele should be treated. Children with multiple severe or potentially fatal associated malformations and those with severe chromosomal abnormalities may not be chosen for treatment. However, the decision to withhold treatment from any child should be individualized and made only after a frank and realistic discussion with the parents about the chances for meaningful survival. In our experience, these children are fewer than 1% of infants born with myelomeningocele.

The parents of children with myelomeningocele are initially overwhelmed with the complexity of the disorder. Confused and often frightened, they most often follow the suggestions of the treating physician. It is incumbent upon physicians, then, to present accurately the nature of myelomeningocele, the likely sequelae of the malformation, and the outlook for intellectual, sensorimotor, urinary, sexual, and societal function. Although each has a bias based on personal, ethical, or religious principles, physicians must refrain from transmitting this bias to parents. It is they rather than physicians who will ultimately care for the child.

It is important that certain facts be transmitted accurately to parents. First, almost all children with myelomeningocele survive initially with proper treatment (80,116), although a few children die each year. The most common causes of death are Chiari malformation in infancy and unrecognized shunt obstruction in later life. Among 100 unselected children with myelomeningocele consecutively treated at the Children's Memorial Hospital in Chicago for whom 8- to 12-year follow-up information was available, the overall mortality was 15%. The neonatal mortality was 2%, mortality during the first 3 years was 10%, and mortality during the first 5 years of life was 14%. Hindbrain dysfunction was the most frequent cause of death in this series because of associated stridor, apnea, and aspiration pneumonitis (85). The long-term mortality in other series has been as high as 35% to 50% by adulthood (60,62).

Between 80% and 90% of children need a shunt for control of hydrocephalus (80,81,85); 30% to 40% of these need at least one shunt revision during the subsequent year, 60% within 5 years, and 85% within 10 years (85,140). Approximately 75% of children with myelomeningocele have IQs greater than 80, and this figure is not affected appreciably by the presence of hydrocephalus (61,82,85,132,137). However, among the children with normal intelligence, 60% have learning disabilities (35,81,132).

Approximately 60% to 70% of children who survive are community ambulators (34,81,141). Ability to walk depends on and is directly correlated with sensorimotor level (34). Excluding children with severe developmental delay and hypotonia, who account for about 13% of patients, approximately 89% of preadolescent children can be community ambulators with aggressive multidisciplinary orthopaedic and neurosurgical management. This percentage includes all of those with low lumbar and sacral lesions and 63% of those with higher-level lesions (81). After adolescence, however, the proportion of children who achieve community ambulation decreases to about 50% as it becomes more energy efficient to use a wheelchair (85).

Social continence (being free of urinary incontinence in social situations, with or without clean intermittent catheterization) is achieved by about 85% of school-age children (80,110, 122,138). Most have chronic constipation. Although almost all patients with myelomeningocele have abnormal genital sensation, about two thirds of boys report at least some genital sensation, and 70% to 75% report the ability to achieve erections. In an objective assessment of 15 selected male patients by Sandler et al.(123), 60% had objective evidence of at least some nocturnal erections.

Orthopaedic procedures are extremely common (10,141). In one study of 206 unselected children with 6-month to 18 year follow-up results, 64% underwent at least one orthopaedic procedure, and an average of 5.4 procedures were performed per patient (141).

Despite their disabilities, many children with myelomeningocele mature to become contributing members of society. Eighty-two percent of adults with myelomeningocele are independent in activities of daily living. Thirty percent are in, or have finished, college, but only 32% are employed (89).

The neurosurgical treatment of children with myelomeningocele is divided into three phases: (a) stabilization of the infant's condition and closure of the myelomeningocele, (b) assessment and management of hydrocephalus, when present, and (c) management of associated problems, including signs and symptoms of hindbrain (Chiari II) malformation, tethered spinal cord, and syringomyelia.

Stabilization of the Infant and Closure of the Myelomeningocele

The myelomeningocele should be protected from external mechanical trauma and desiccation, and should be kept as clean as possible, because the malformation may contain functional neural tissue and frequently leaks spinal fluid. The malformation is best covered with gauze dressings soaked in sterile saline solution. Iodine-containing compounds such as povidone-iodine (Betadine) should be avoided, because they may further injure the exposed tissues. Plastic wrap may be placed atop the gauze to keep the dressings moist.

Initial sensorimotor level can be be assessed readily by means of observation of the spontaneous movements of the lower limbs and of the response to pinprick stimulation (Table 1). Muscle

imbalance produces characteristic postures of the lower limbs and is a good indicator of sensorimotor level. For example, imbalance between iliopsoas and quadriceps muscles of an infant with an upper lumbar lesion causes a flexed-hip deformity. Imbalance between quadriceps and hamstrings muscles of an infant with a midlumbar lesion produces a characteristic knee extension deformity. Imbalance between the foot dorsiflexors and plantar flexors of an infant with a low lumbar lesion produces a dorsiflexed ankle deformity.

An open malformation should be closed in a timely manner to avoid the development of meningitis. The lesion ideally should be repaired on the first day of life; however, studies have suggested that closure can be delayed up to 48 hours without an appreciable increase in neurologic morbidity or infectious complications (17). The techniques for closure of myelomeningocele are detailed elsewhere (83) and are summarized here (Fig. 14). The neural placode is sharply dissected from the surrounding skin at the perimeter of the malformation. No cutaneous

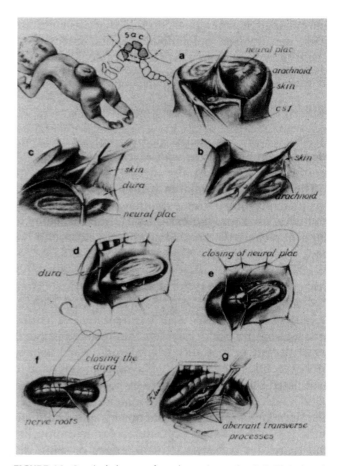

FIGURE 14. Surgical closure of myelomeningocele. *A, B,* The placode is dissected away from the surrounding skin at the arachnoid-skin interface. Care is taken not to include skin in the placode. *C, D,* The dura is dissected from the lateral aspects of the sac in preparation for closure. *E,* The neural placode is closed dorsally to reapproximate a neural tube. *F,* The dura is closed over the closed placode. The remaining fascia and skin are closed over the malformation with a vertical closure if possible. (From Reigel DH [1979]: Kyphectomy and myelomeningocele repair. In: Ransohoff J, ed: *Neurosurgery. Modern techniques in surgery,* vol 13. Mt Kisco, NY: Futura, pp. 1–9, with permission.)

TABLE 1. ASSESSMENT OF NEUROLOGIC LEVEL OF PATIENTS WITH MYELOMENINGOCELE

Level	Motor	Sensory
T10	Rectus abdominus	Umbilicus
L1–2	Hip flexion	Anterolateral thigh
L2–3	Hip adduction	Anteromedial thigh
L3–4	Knee extension	Knee, anterior shin
L4–5	Foot dorsiflexion	Dorsum of foot
L5	Extensor hallucis longus	First, second interspace
S1	Plantar flexion	Plantar aspect of foot

tissue should be left with the placode, or an inclusion dermoid may form (83,115). The lateral edges of the placode and its associated pial coverings are brought together in the midline to reapproximate a tubular structure. This makes subsequent untethering procedures much less difficult should they become necessary. Once the placode is repaired, the surrounding dura is dissected from the underlying fascia and reapproximated. The dural sac should be kept as capacious as possible to minimize the risk of later tethering.

The lumbodorsal fascia can be closed to provide an additional layer. However, the benefits of this technique are unclear. Reigel and McLone (116) suggested that there is no additional benefit to closing the lumbodorsal musculature and fascia as a separate layer. Troup et al. (143), however, suggested that wound leakage of CSF is less frequent and that shunting is required less often after myofascial closure. If myofascial closure is performed, care must be taken not to strangle the underlying neural tissue. The overlying skin is trimmed and closed. Vertical closure is preferred because it simplifies later procedures, such as untethering and spinal fusion, should they become necessary.

Initial Treatment of Hydrocephalus

Associated hydrocephalus is present among 80% to 90% of children with myelomeningocele (85,141). Among some infants, hydrocephalus is apparent at birth. The infant has an enlarged head (greater than 2 standard deviations above the mean for age), a bulging fontanel, and split sutures. Sunsetting eyes, poor feeding, vomiting, irritability, or lethargy occasionally is present when hydrocephalus is severe. Hydrocephalus can promote or exacerbate symptoms of Chiari malformation, including lower cranial nerve dysfunction (weak or high-pitched cry, choking during feeding, poor swallowing, vocal cord palsy, aspiration pneumonitis, or facial palsy), and arm or hand weakness (see later). Cranial ultrasonography, computed tomography (CT), or magnetic resonance imaging (MRI) shows enlarged ventricles (Fig. 15). Under these circumstances, hydrocephalus should be managed when the myelomeningocele is closed, because the risk of infectious or other complications does not increase when permanent insertion of a ventriculoperitoneal shunt (VPS) is performed at myelomeningocele closure. An alternative is temporary diversion of CSF to a bedside bag by means of external ventricular drainage for several days followed by insertion of a VPS.

Hydrocephalus often is not obvious immediately after birth, because CSF is being vented from the back wound, but develops within days or weeks after closure of the myelomeningocele. In addition to the signs described earlier, CSF under increased pressure may dissect beneath, and eventually leak from, the healing wound. Any collection or leakage of CSF from the back wound should alert the clinician to the presence of hydrocephalus. When hydrocephalus develops, it should be managed promptly with a VPS.

One may reasonably ask, "Why not insert shunts in all children from the outset?" Although most children with myelomeningocele ultimately need a shunt, a VPS commits both the patient and physician to a lifelong struggle to maintain the patency of the shunt. Even a functioning shunt wreaks havoc on the

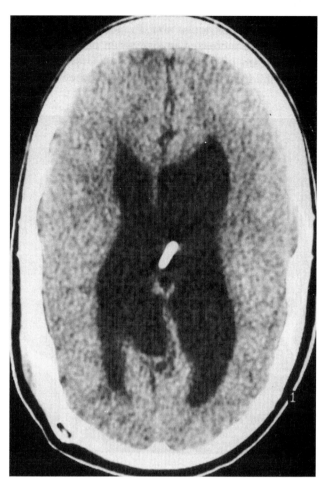

FIGURE 15. Computed tomographic scan shows hydrocephalus in a patient with myelomeningocele. The ventricles are misshapen because of developmental changes in the surrounding cerebral hemispheres from Chiari II malformation. The shunt catheter is visible within the right lateral ventricle.

patient and family. Because signs of shunt malfunction include headache, nausea, vomiting, and listlessness, every viral syndrome prompts another trip to the hospital to exclude shunt malfunction. Finally, although it is a controversial issue, some authors consider every child with a myelomeningocele and shunted hydrocephalus shunt dependent for life (118). We place shunts only in patients with demonstrated hydrocephalus.

A bewildering variety of shunt systems exist to manage hydrocephalus (114). The typical shunt system has three basic components—a ventricular catheter, a valve mechanism, and a variable length of distal tubing (Fig. 16). The valve can be proximally located under the skin on the scalp or distally located as simple slits in the distal catheter within the abdomen. Whatever the shape or configuration, almost all valves serve two purposes: they retard retrograde flow of spinal fluid back into the brain, and they regulate the amount of CSF that can be drained as a function of the pressure differential across the valve. Many shunts also contain a subcutaneous reservoir from which to tap the shunt if necessary to assess shunt function or to sample CSF.

The peritoneum is the overwhelming choice as the site for

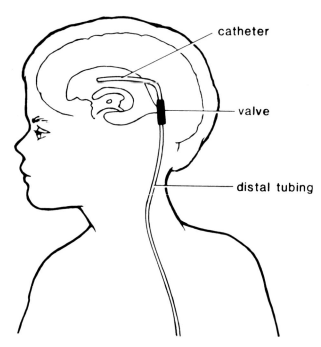

catheter

valve

distal tubing

FIGURE 16. Shunt components.

the distal shunt catheter. If the catheter cannot be placed within the peritoneum, children older than 5 years can undergo shunting to the pleural space, a ventriculopleural shunt, through a small incision beneath a rib and insertion through a trocar. Children much younger than 5 years do not usually tolerate a ventriculopleural shunt because they do not adequately reabsorb CSF from the pleural space. Ventriculoatrial shunts implanted into the common facial or jugular veins and threaded into the right atrium were preferable years ago. A number of serious complications, however, including sepsis, endocarditis, pulmonary emboli with pulmonary hypertension (30,36), and renal failure from shunt nephropathy, in which a chronically infected shunt incites immune complex deposition within the renal glomeruli (147),have limited their use. We reserve ventriculoatrial shunts for children younger than 5 years who cannot tolerate a VPS. In rare instances the gallbladder can be used for a shunt if the other sites are unavailable.

The signs and symptoms of shunt malfunction in a child with myelomeningocele are legion and often can confuse even the most experienced clinician. The oft-quoted signs and symptoms of intracranial hypertension, including headache, nausea and vomiting, poor feeding, listlessness or lethargy, and sunsetting eyes or extraocular abduction palsy, although indicative of a shunt malfunction, may be absent among a large number of children. For many of these patients, a shunt malfunction may become manifest through any of the following symptoms: (a) cognitive changes such as a decline in school performance or worsening behavior, (b) the onset of or a change in the frequency of seizures without another demonstrable cause, (c) a change in motor performance such as a decrease in muscle strength, loss of previously acquired motor skills, or increase in spasticity of either upper or lower extremities, (d) a change in

ambulation without another definable cause, (e) a change in urinary or bowel function, such as more frequent accidents or urinary tract infections or an increase in frequency of catheterization, (f) a change in lower cranial nerve function suggestive of hindbrain dysfunction, (g) pain in the back or legs, particularly that which occurs at the myelomeningocele closure site, and (h) worsening scoliosis or orthopaedic deformities of the lower extremity. Viewed another way, a shunt malfunction can mimic the signs and symptoms of tethered spinal cord, syringomyelia, or hindbrain dysfunction from the Chiari malformation. It is our firm belief that once a shunt is placed, any deterioration in neurologic, orthopaedic, or urologic function always should prompt an investigation of the shunt to exclude a malfunction before any other treatment is initiated. Some children with a shunt malfunction may be completely free of symptoms yet have florid papilledema on physical examination. The papilledema improves after shunt revision. A good fundoscopic examination therefore is essential to properly evaluate a child with a shunt.

The evaluation of a child with a suspected shunt malfunction includes CT or MRI to evaluate ventricular size. In many children, the ventricles are larger than they appeared on baseline scans. In some children, fortunately a minority, the ventricles may be slitlike or may not change appreciably, and the diagnosis of shunt malfunction is made solely on clinical grounds. A child with unrecognized shunt malfunction may progress to herniation and death even though a CT scan shows no change in ventricular size. Any patient whose condition is rapidly deteriorating should be assumed to have a shunt malfunction, even in the absence of a change in ventricular size, and should be examined immediately by a neurosurgeon. Patients with signs of herniation (stupor or coma, motor posturing, signs of brain stem compromise) should undergo an immediate shunt tap from the reservoir, if present, to withdraw CSF and relieve intracranial pressure. Urgent shunt exploration and either revision or external drainage are warranted immediately thereafter.

In summary, the need to keep the ventricular shunt foremost in one's mind when assessing a child with myelomeningocele cannot be overemphasized. Shunt malfunction can mimic any symptom complex in these children and can occur without any visible symptoms or demonstrable changes in the radiologic studies. Nowhere else in pediatric neurosurgery is clinical judgment so important and misjudgment so treacherous. The watchwords in evaluating any neurologic change are *always evaluate the shunt first*.

Management of the Chiari II Malformation

Almost all children with myelomeningocele have an associated hindbrain malformation that consists of caudal displacement of the cerebellar tonsils and vermis, the caudal medulla, and variably the fourth ventricle into the cervical spinal canal (Fig. 17). The malformation has been called *Chiari II malformation* to differentiate it from the Chiari I malformation, in which only the cerebellar tonsils are displaced. Chiari II malformation actually consists of a number of brain abnormalities. It is a pancerebral malformation (Table 2) that involves almost all areas of the brain. A unifying theory has been proposed to explain the origin of Chiari II malformation. Venting of CSF during the period

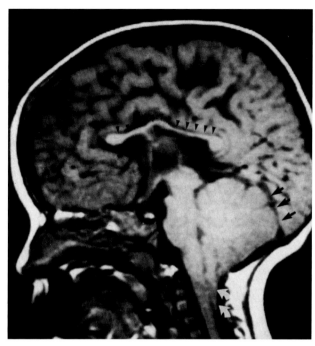

FIGURE 17. Magnetic resonance image of a child with myelomeningocele and Chiari II malformation. The tentorium is low lying (*black arrows*), and the posterior fossa is small. The cerebellar tonsils and caudal brain stem (*white arrows*) have descended through the foramen magnum at the skull base. The corpus callosum is malformed (*arrowheads*), and the cerebral cortex has several areas of abnormality.

of mesenchymal condensation to form the skull produces inadequate stimulus to skull growth, particularly for the posterior fossa surrounding the cerebellum and brain stem. Subsequent growth of the cerebellum occurs within a compartment that is too small. The result is downward displacement of the inferior cerebellum and brain stem and upward displacement of the supe-

TABLE 2. CHIARI-ASSOCIATED MALFORMATIONS OF THE CENTRAL NERVOUS SYSTEM

Disorders of the skull
  Lückenschädel of the skull
  Small posterior fossa
  Low-lying tentorium cerebelli with large incisura
  Scalloping of the petrous bone
  Shortening of the clivus
  Enlargement of the foramen magnum
Disorders of the cerebral hemispheres
  Polymicrogyria
  Cortical heterotopia
  Dysgenesis of the corpus callosum
  Large massa intermedia
Disorders of the posterior fossa
  Descent of the cerebellar vermis through the foramen magnum
  Caudal displacement of the pons and medulla
  Rostral displacement of the superior cerebellum through tentorium
  Kinking of brain stem
  Loss of pontine flexure
  Aqueductal stenosis or forking
  Beaking of tectum

rior cerebellum, beaking of the midbrain, and enlargement of the tentorial notch. Secondary disorders of neuronal histogenesis cause many of the other associated malformations, such as callosal dysgenesis, cortical heterotopia, and stenogyria (87,91).

Although Chiari II malformation is anatomically present in nearly every child with a myelomeningocele and many have occasional mild symptoms referable to the malformation, between 29% and 76% have grave problems (19,29,56,57,77,85,104, 112). About one third need surgical treatment. Treatment should be reserved for children with symptoms and signs that suggest substantial brain stem compromise. Symptoms may develop at any age but are most common during infancy. Swallowing dysfunction is the most frequent sign. Disorders of swallowing represent injury to the lower cranial nerves or their associated brain stem nuclei. They occur more frequently during infancy and may become manifest as choking or coughing on food, nasal regurgitation during drinking, frequent vomiting, or gastroesophageal reflux (112). Other signs of lower brain stem dysfunction include frequent episodes of aspiration pneumonitis, apnea and cyanotic spells, dysarthria, inspiratory stridor, and a hoarse or high-pitched cry. Often these babies have soft, feeble cries and are therefore described as ''good babies'' (99). Other signs and symptoms of Chiari II malformation include weakness or spasticity of the upper extremities, headache or neck pain, cerebellar dysfunction, oculomotor problems, and scoliosis.

Chiari II malformation is best evaluated with MRI (Fig. 17). Associated hydrocephalus, syringomyelia, and spinal cord tethering can be evaluated simultaneously. Treatment includes cervical or foramen magnum (posterior fossa) decompression with dural opening and patch grafting (duraplasty). The foramen magnum in these patients usually is quite large and usually does not require substantial decompression. In our series of 43 patients, posterior fossa decompression offered no additional benefit over cervical decompression alone. Moreover, opening the posterior fossa dura entails great risk of bleeding from intradural venous sinuses. Other procedures, such as opening or stenting the fourth ventricle (105) or plugging the obex (3,37,148) have not proved to be of additional benefit. We therefore recommend simple bony decompression and duraplasty for most patients. Cervical laminectomy is performed to below the inferiormost level of the cerebellar tonsils, and a generous patch graft of periosteum, cadaver dura, or bovine pericardium is sewn to the dural edges.

Outcome depends on the age of the patient and the mode of presentation. Patients with symptoms present at birth generally fare poorly. Only 1 of 7 (14%) such patients in our series improved postoperatively. Postmortem studies of these infants often show a disorganized and chaotic brain stem architecture (41). Many infants undergo tracheostomy, Nissen fundoplication, and insertion of gastrostomy feeding tubes because of persistent swallowing difficulties, vocal cord palsy, repeated bouts of aspiration pneumonitis, and gastroesophageal reflux. Older children, however, often improve after decompression, particularly if the operation is performed before severe and irreparable damage to the brain stem has occurred (111). In our series, upper extremity weakness, cerebellar dysfunction, and pain improved in more than 80% of patients. Swallowing dysfunction, apnea, and vocal cord palsy improved in only 50%.

Postlaminectomy kyphosis can occur after cervical decompression. We do not recall treating any patient with myelodysplasia who had this complication, although an incidence as high as 40% has been reported (1). Treatment involves occipital-cervical lateral mass fusion that spans the laminectomy defect and at a minimum includes the most cranially located intact vertebral segment.

Management of the Tethered Spinal Cord

Spinal cord tethering is a well-recognized cause of neurologic deterioration. It is responsible for delayed and progressive neurologic deficits, urologic dysfunction, and orthopaedic deformities among patients with myelomeningocele (6,51,65,86,117,121, 142,145). Symptoms referable to spinal cord tethering necessitate treatment of about 30% of patients with myelomeningocele (145). The pathophysiologic basis for neurologic decline among patients with spinal cord tethering was well illustrated by Yamada et al., who demonstrated changes in mitochondrial oxidative metabolism in response to spinal cord tethering both in cats during experimental spinal cord stretching and in humans during operations for untethering (152,153). In humans, growth and development of the vertebral column may progressively stretch the tethered spinal cord. The increased incidence of the tethered cord syndrome during periods of rapid growth (50,55,94,142) supports this concept. In addition, intermittent and transient traction on the tethered spinal cord may increase with flexion movements of the pelvis and spine (90) and contribute to repetitive neurologic injury. Several studies have documented improvement or stabilization of neurologic function (2,18,50,51,130,142) urologic disorders (65), and orthopaedic deformities (86,117,121) after untethering.

The importance of spinal cord tethering as a potential cause of neurologic deterioration is perhaps most evident in comparisons between the long-term neurologic outcome among patients with sacral-level myelomeningocele in two programs, one that offered untethering for patients with deterioration and another that did not. In a program offering spinal cord untethering to patients with deterioration, 62 consecutively registered patients with sacral-level lesions who underwent closure of the lesions at Children's Memorial Hospital and were observed for 18 years, no patient lost the ability to walk, and all but one (who had a severe balance deficit) were community ambulators (141). In contrast, among 36 patients with sacral-level myelomeningocele observed for an average age of 25 years (range 19 to 51 years) in a program in which spinal cord untethering was not routinely offered for deterioration, one third had a deterioration in gait, and only 24 of 35 patients (69%) who started as community ambulators remained so. Eleven patients became wheelchair users. Spinal deformities and soft tissue contractures of the hip or knee, developed in 16 patients each (44%) (10). Although these two studies are not strictly comparable in many respects, the differences in outcome suggest that untethering can prevent what appears to be otherwise inevitable deterioration for many patients with myelomeningocele. It has become increasingly evident to us that the neurologic deterioration so prevalent among patients with myelomeningocele does not represent the natural

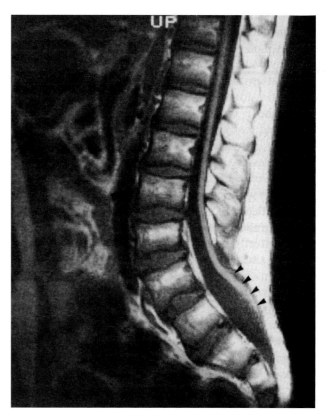

FIGURE 18. Magnetic resonance image of a child with myelomeningocele shows radiographic evidence of tethered spinal cord. The conus medullaris is low lying. The placode is displaced posteriorly and is adherent to the dorsal dura (*arrowheads*).

course of the disorder but reflects progressive injury from spinal cord tethering.

The diagnosis of tethered-cord syndrome in a patient with myelomeningocele is made on clinical not radiologic grounds. Almost every patient with myelomeningocele has a low-lying conus medullaris on radiographic images (Fig. 18), yet relatively few have clinical signs of tethering. Moreover, the position of the conus on MR images does not change appreciably after spinal cord untethering, yet the clinical condition of many patients improves (11). The clinical features of tethering in some cases are initially subtle and advance so slowly that parents, child, and physician do not recognize the inexorable decline. It is only after untethering and subsequent improvement that everyone recognizes, in retrospect, the extent to which the child had deteriorated. A vigilant eye, keen clinical judgment, and objective, accurate, and reproducible means of evaluating patients, such as serial manual muscle testing, urodynamic studies, and scoliosis radiographs, are necessary to properly evaluate and observe a child with a tethered spinal cord. Signs and symptoms of spinal cord tethering can be conveniently divided into six broad categories, as follows: (a) pain, either in the back or legs, (b) motor deterioration, manifested as a decrease in muscle strength or an increase in tone (spasticity), (c) a change in sensory level, (d) a change in bowel or bladder function, (e) a deterioration in gait, and (f) progressive orthopaedic deformities, either in the lower extremities (hip dislocation, pes cavus, equinovarus) or spine (scoliosis).

Pain is a relatively common presenting symptom of spinal cord tethering in our experience but is usually minor and seldom the predominant symptom. When present, pain usually accompanies other objective changes in neurologic function. The pain may be present in the back or legs and even extend even into areas that have no sensation. The pain usually is ill defined, dull, or achy in character and is often, although not invariably, exacerbated by exercise or effort. Leg pain may have a dysesthetic or neuropathic quality. We have found that pain is almost universally relieved with untethering.

A change in motor function is the most frequent manifestation of tethering. Changes in motor performance include a decrease in muscle strength or an increase in tone (spasticity). In our clinics, manual muscle testing of individual muscles performed by physical therapists at least one a year and more frequently if clinically indicated provides a quantifiable assessment of motor function. We consider a consistent decrease of at least one grade in several muscles significant. In some cases, muscles innervated by the last intact root are lost, and motor paralysis ascends to a higher level. More commonly, a more diffuse pattern of muscle weakness develops in muscles innervated by more rostral spinal levels.

In addition to weakness, muscle tone may be increased and become manifest as classic spasticity (a velocity-dependent resistance to movement that is greatest at the initiation of movement and declines thereafter—the so-called clasp-knife phenomenon), a progressive increase in muscle contractures, or a change in gait (see later). Muscle tone may reliably be assessed with the modified Ashworth scale (Table 3) (7), and contractures by means of measurement of various joint angles. We have found that untethering improves muscle strength and decreases spasticity among affected children and leads to improved ambulation and a decrease in the frequency of soft-tissue releases.

Subjective changes in sensation are common. They consist of numbness or dysesthesia in areas previously sensate. However, objective deterioration in sensation is seldom found at physical examination and when present is usually evanescent and unreliable. We therefore do not rely solely on changes in sensation to determine the need for untethering. Fortunately, changes in sensation usually are associated with other objective signs of neurologic deterioration.

Urologic dysfunction is present among many children with myelomeningocele. Clinical signs of progressive neurourologic deterioration suggest tethering. They include increasingly frequent accidents or urinary dribbling between catheterizations of a child previously dry, an increase in the frequency of catheterizations or decrease in the volumes of urine obtained with each catheterization, and increasingly frequent urinary tract infections without another cause. Serial urodynamic testing provides objective evidence of changes in bladder function, including a smaller bladder capacity or increased bladder pressures, reduced threshold for the initiation of bladder contraction (uninhibited bladder contraction), and worsening coordination of bladder contraction with urethral sphincter relaxation (detrusor-sphincter dyssynergia). All of these urodynamic changes can suggest progressive bladder spasticity. High-pressure bladders with uninhibited contractions are of particular concern. Improvement can be expected among approximately 60% of patients after untethering (65). Although less common, abnormalities of defecation can accompany tethering. These include increasing problems with constipation and intermittent stool soilage. Most patients improve after untethering (65).

Gait abnormalities are present among almost all children with myelomeningocele. However, excluding patients with severe retardation or hypotonia, about 89% of preteens with myelomeningocele are community ambulators (89). Many continue to walk into adulthood; the exception, in our experience, is the teen-ager or adult with an upper lumbar or thoracic lesion who, although initially an ambulator, finds a wheelchair to be a more efficient means of transportation. Although they may abandon their braces for a wheelchair, these patients generally do not have accompanying changes in muscle strength or tone or any of the other changes of tethering. The change in ambulation is a personal decision rather than a change in neurologic function per se. With this single exception, ambulation among all children with myelomeningocele generally improves with advancing age. Ambulation never should regress without a good reason. Suggestions that a deterioration in gait reflects the natural course of myelomeningocele, is the result of an inevitable and therefore irreparable degeneration of the placode, or is the result of increasing weight gain are simply untrue. We have found that any deterioration in gait usually is caused by progressive muscle weakness, increasing spasticity, or orthopaedic deformities. Among many patients, these problems can be attributed to spinal cord tethering and often improve or stabilize after an untethering procedure.

Orthopaedic deformities are common among children with myelomeningocele; however, the presence of progressive deformities, especially those associated with progressive increases in muscle tone, such as progressive or recurrent hip subluxation, pes cavus, or equinovarus deformities, should prompt a thorough search for other clinical evidence of tethered cord. In most instances the presence of associated muscle weakness or spasticity, urologic abnormalities, and pain corroborates the diagnosis and makes the decision to untether easier. Some children, however, have progressive foot deformities for which no other explanation

TABLE 3. MODIFIED ASHWORTH SCALE OF MUSCLE TONE

Score	Definition
0	Hypotonic; less-than-normal muscle tone; floppy
1	Normal; no Increase in muscle tone
2	Mild; slight increase in tone or minimal resistance to movement through less than half of range
3	Moderate; more marked increase in tone through most of range, but affected part is easily moved
4	Severe; considerable increase in tone; passive movement difficult
5	Extreme; affected part rigid in flexion or extension

Adapted from Peacock WJ, Staudt L (1991): Functional outcomes following selective posterior rhizotomy in children with cerebral palsy. *J Neurosurg* 74:380–385, with permission.

is evident. Under these circumstances, we perform untethering, and many patients improve (unpublished observations).

Spinal cord tethering can cause progressive scoliosis. Scoliosis is present among as many as 90% of patients with myelomeningocele (109,133) and is more frequent with upper lumbar and thoracic lesions (117). The cause of scoliosis is likely multifactorial. In any patient scoliosis can be caused by (a) paravertebral muscle weakness and sensorimotor imbalance, (b) structural deformities from vertebral malformations such as hemivertebrae and segmental bars, (c) pelvic obliquity or hip contracture, and (d) neurosurgical problems such as Chiari malformation, syringomyelia, and spinal cord tethering (109,117). Progressive scoliosis above a low-lying placode in a patient without underlying vertebral anomalies is most likely caused by spinal cord tethering and less frequently by Chiari malformation or hydrosyringomyelia. In a study involving 30 patients with progressive scoliosis and radiographic evidence of tethering without symptoms of Chiari malformation or hydromyelia, scoliosis improved after untethering among 21% and stabilized among 42%. Considering only children with curves of less than 50 degrees, scoliosis improved among 8 of 24 (33%) and stabilized among 15 of 24 (63%) patients. In contrast, scoliosis continued to progress and ultimately necessitated spinal fusion in 5 of 6 patients with preoperative curves greater than 50 degrees (86). In another study of 216 patients with myelomeningocele, untethering improved or stabilized scoliosis in patients with sacral and lumbar level lesions but did not halt the progression of scoliosis among patients with thoracic-level lesions (117). In a study involving children with low-level (L3 and below) lesions treated with untethering for progressive scoliosis, first-year results showed stable (60%) or improving (15%) curves. Long-term (3 to 10 years) follow-up studies showed stable (57%) or improving (7%) curves but late progression among 36% of the patients (124). The results of these studies suggest that spinal cord tethering is an important cause of scoliosis and that untethering performed early reverses or stabilizes scoliosis for selected patients.

Once tethering is suspected because of clinical evidence, manual muscle testing, urodynamic studies, and scoliosis radiographs are obtained to document associated changes that may not be evident clinically. Radiologic evaluation includes MRI to confirm tethering and to identify associated lesions such as lipoma, split-cord malformations, and hydromyelia (see later), which may contribute to neurologic deterioration. CT or MRI of the head is performed to evaluate ventricular size. Changes in ventricular size or symptoms that suggest shunt malfunction should prompt shunt revision, and untethering is deferred for 8 to 12 weeks. If signs or symptoms improve or stabilize after the shunt revision, nothing further is done; if the child's condition continues to deteriorate, untethering is performed.

Untethering is accomplished by means of reopening the wound, exposing the dural sac, and dissecting the placode from the overlying dural closure. During dissection of the placode, care is taken to remain outside the arachnoid plane to minimize injury to the nerve roots. The spinal cord cranial to the placode is freed from any bony impingement or surrounding scar. The caudal end is inspected for tethering lesions. A surprising number of patients have an unrecognized filum terminale which can also tether the placode. Any associated tethering lesions identi-

fied at preoperative MRI are repaired. The dural sac is reapproximated primarily, and the is wound closed in several layers to prevent CSF leakage. A dural graft usually is not necessary, because the thecal sac is already quite capacious in most patients, and a graft is of no demonstrated benefit in preventing retethering.

Although the situation is uncommon, some patients initially improve or stabilize after untethering only to have delayed (usually several years) signs and symptoms of retethering. These patients may benefit from a second, or even a third or fourth, untethering procedure.

Management of Hydrosyringomyelia

Hydromyelia is CSF-containing dilatation of the central canal of the spinal cord. Syringomyelia is a similar cavity of CSF that develops within the substance of the spinal cord but is still in communication with the central canal. Among patients with myelomeningocele, hydromyelia and syringomyelia occur in combination. It is impossible to differentiate one from the other with clinical or radiographic evidence (Fig. 19). Therefore the term *hydrosyringomyelia* is more appropriate. Hydrosyringomyelia is present in 50% to 80% of patients with myelomeningocele (13,75,81) and can cause progressive neurologic deterioration due to spinal cord deformation and injury. The most common presenting features include upper extremity weakness or loss of function, back pain, scoliosis, and worsening spasticity and ascending motor loss in the lower extremities. Dissociated sensory loss (loss of pain or thermal sensation with preservation of proprioception) occasionally is discerned and may follow a cape distribution (99). We have found that the latter finding though classic is uncommon. Extension of hydrosyringomyelia into the brain stem can cause lower cranial neuropathy and brain stem dysfunction. Changes in urinary function are rare and should suggest spinal cord tethering as a cause of the incontinence (99). Scoliosis caused by hydrosyringomyelia often is rapidly progressive and is thought to be caused by asymmetric anterior motor column damage (47,48,63).

Because hydrosyringomyelia is present among so many patients with myelomeningocele, one must rely on clinical judgment to determine which patients require treatment. Some patients have only a small cavity and are unlikely to have symptoms. Moreover, the risks of surgical therapy for a small cavity probably outweigh any potential benefit. We would pursue other avenues of therapy in this instance. Among other patients, symptomatic hydrosyringomyelia may be the consequence of incipient malfunction of a ventricular shunt (47,49), and symptoms resolve after shunt revision. In the absence of shunt malfunction, the initial management of symptomatic hydrosyringomyelia for these patients is controversial. One option is posterior fossa–cervical decompression if Chiari malformation is documented. This option is based on the premise that abnormal CSF dynamics at the foramen magnum (documented best among patients with Chiari I malformation) caused by the Chiari malformation allow expansion of the central spinal canal (100). An alternative is to place a shunt directly from the syrinx cavity to the peritoneum (syringoperitoneal shunt) or to the pleural cavity (syringopleural shunt). Some surgeons prefer to

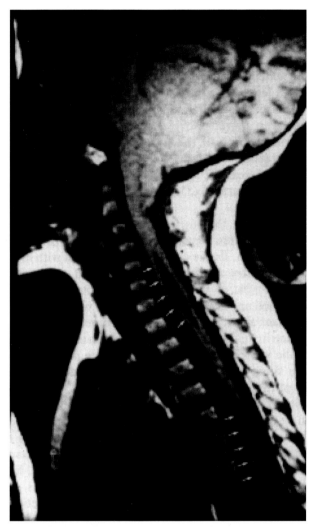

FIGURE 19. Magnetic resonance image of a child with myelomeningocele, Chiari II malformation (caudally displaced cerebellar tonsils and medulla are visible), and extensive hydrosyringomyelia (*arrows*).

place a stent locally from the syrinx cavity to the spinal subarachnoid space (syringosubarachnoid shunt). In an analysis of various therapies for symptomatic hydrosyringomyelia among 50 patients with myelomeningocele, posterior fossa decompression alone was successful (syrinx unchanged or enlarging) among only 14%, whereas syringosubarachnoid shunting alone was successful among 70%. A combination of posterior fossa decompression and syringosubarachnoid shunting was successful for two patients on whom it was performed (136). These data suggest that the ideal initial therapy for symptomatic hydrosyringomyelia among children with myelomeningocele and a functioning shunt is placement of a syringosubarachnoid shunt.

In summary, the single greatest long-term neurosurgical problem among these children is maintenance of proper shunt function. Every year, several children with myelomeningocele die of unrecognized shunt malfunction. Most of these deaths can be prevented with prompt recognition of the malfunction and treatment. If we can educate other physicians about the signs

and symptoms of shunt malfunction among this population and impart an understanding that the size of the ventricle on CT scans may not change in the face of acute shunt malfunction, we have advanced the care of these children considerably.

We reject the concept that delayed deterioration among these children is simply the natural course of this disorder. We emphasize that neurologic decline can be controlled in many cases. Aggressive management of associated neurosurgical disorders such as Chiari malformation, hydrosyringomyelia, and spinal cord tethering have improved ambulation and urinary function, prevented a large number of orthopaedic deformities, and in many cases eliminated the need for spinal fusion for scoliosis and soft-tissue release for lower limb spasticity. With further advances, the outlook for these children remains ever more hopeful.

Treatment of Children with Lipomyelomeningocele

Lipomyelomeningocele (LMC; also called spinal lipoma) is the most common occult dysraphic malformation. It accounts for 20% to 50% of cases of occult spinal dysraphism and for 35% of skin-covered lumbosacral masses (90). Most of these lesions involve the conus medullaris and the caudal end of the spinal cord. In rare instances LMC involves the thoracic or cervical region, where they arise from the dorsal aspect of the underlying spinal cord.

Because lipoma is a disorder of premature dysjunction with the lipoma that arises from the central canal of the neural tube (Fig. 9), the stalk of the lipoma therefore lies between the entrance of the dorsal roots (which arise from neural crest cells at the edges of the closing neural folds) to the spinal cord and extends into the central canal of the spinal cord through this dorsal dysraphic defect. Knowledge of this anatomic arrangement is crucial to the safe removal of a LMC.

For LMCs that extend beyond the dura and have a large subcutaneous portion, a subcutaneous mass often is obvious at birth. The mass is sometimes eccentric and may reflect an embryologic origin from only one neural fold. Other associated cutaneous abnormalities include cutaneous dimples, dermal sinuses, hemangiomas, hairy patches, and skin tags. These skin lesions may appear with or without an associated subcutaneous fatty mass. For a purely intradural LMC that lacks a subcutaneous component, these skin lesions may be the only clue to the presence of an underlying dysraphic abnormality. Finally, cutaneous markers may be absent in as many as 15% of patients with lipoma, and the first manifestation of the problem may be the development of neurologic abnormalities, urologic dysfunction, or orthopaedic deformities from tethering.

Neurologic abnormalities usually are lacking among neonates with LMC, but progressive neurologic deficits and associated urologic and orthopaedic abnormalities develop regularly with advancing age. In one surgical series, only 3% of children had no symptoms after the first year of life, and none did so after the second year. Among 87 children with symptomatic LMC, 54% had weakness as the initial symptoms, 7% had spasticity, 13% had gait abnormalities, 18% had pain, 10% had numbness, 38% had incontinence, 9% had urinary retention, 15% had foot deformities, and 12% had scoliosis (some patients had more than one symptom) (70).

Among 197 children with LMC treated at Children's Memorial Hospital, sensorimotor function was preserved among nearly two thirds of patients younger than 9 months when they came to medical attention. Function was intact among only 12% of children 9 months or older. By the age of 2 years, more than 50% of children have marked sensorimotor loss. A similar trend of increasing dysfunction with advancing age was observed for both urologic abnormalities and orthopaedic deformities. More than 50% of children had marked bladder dysfunction by 4 years of age, and 50% had orthopaedic deformities (small or asymmetric feet, pes cavus, claw toe deformity, and equinovarus being the most common) by 7 years of age (unpublished observations). It therefore appears that with advancing age untreated children with LMC most often have, in chronologic order, neurologic deficits, urologic abnormalities, and orthopaedic deformities.

Lipoma is best imaged with MRI. The lipoma is readily visible on T1-weighted images as a hyperintense mass in continuity with the distal spinal cord (Fig. 20). The lipoma usually is dorsal to the conus and often extends caudad to the conus as well. The finding of a low-lying conus medullaris confirms spinal cord tethering. The conus occasionally is rotated 90 degrees with the lipoma oriented dorsolaterally rather than immediately dorsally to the rotated spinal cord. The lipoma in these rare cases often drapes asymmetrically over the spinal cord into the lateral gutters of the thecal sac, and the nerve roots may run through the fatty mass. This configuration makes complete untethering difficult or even impossible. Neurologic deficits in children with laterally

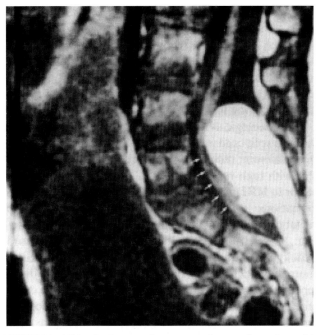

FIGURE 20. Midsagittal magnetic resonance image of a patient with a spinal lipoma. The spinal cord (*arrows*) is low-lying at the sacral level, indicating tethering. The lipoma, which is *white* on this T1-weighted image, is dorsal to the spinal cord.

situated lipoma, if present, usually are asymmetric and are worse on the side to which the lipoma is attached.

Additional preoperative tests include manual muscle testing, urodynamic evaluation, and comprehensive orthopaedic assessment of both the spine and lower extremities. Manual muscle testing confirms the presence of individual muscle weakness or change in function. Urodynamic studies may show a small- or large-capacity bladder, uninhibited bladder contraction, detrusor-sphincter dyssynergia, or other evidence of a neurogenic bladder. Orthopedic deformities of the lower extremities and scoliosis may be evident at physical examination or on radiographs.

Repair of LMC usually is straightforward. The subcutaneous portion of the lipoma, if present, often can be readily differentiated from the surrounding subcutaneous fat and is dissected down to the lumbodorsal fascial defect. The lumbodorsal fascia is opened, and the laminae and spinous processes are exposed. Dysraphic posterior elements are common. The stalk of the lipoma enters the dura through a dorsal dural defect (duraschisis). The dura is opened around the stalk, and the stalk is followed to its attachment to the spinal cord, where it inserts between the more laterally situated dorsal roots as they enter the spinal cord. Dissection of the fibrofatty stalk is limited laterally by these roots (Fig. 8). The lipoma is gently dissected from within, from dorsal to ventral with bipolar cautery and scissors, ultrasonic aspirator, or carbon dioxide laser (78). Dissection continues from within the lipoma as it approaches the central canal of the spinal cord. Dissection of the more laterally situated lipoma can be more difficult and dangerous. As the anatomic features become distorted by the rotated spinal cord and the root sleeves are misplaced, the fat extends laterally or even ventrolaterally to the cord and obscures the roots. The roots may even run within the fat itself.

Spinal lipoma is essentially an intramedullary spinal cord tumor, although not a neoplasm, with a dorsal exophytic component. Untethering usually involves incomplete removal of the fat as it arises from the spinal cord substance. If a carbon dioxide laser is being used, one can see a distinct change in the response of the tissues as the interface between the fat and the normal spinal cord substance is approached. The bubbling of the vaporized fat ceases as normal spinal cord tissues are approached. Once most of the lipoma has been removed, the normal tubular contour of the spinal cord is reconstructed by means of reapproximation of the exposed pial surfaces. The dura is closed either primarily or with a dural patch graft.

The results of untethering depend on whether dysfunction has evolved before intervention. In a series of 213 children with lipoma (55 children with lipoma of the filum and 158 with LMC), no patient who had normal neurologic function preoperatively was permanently worsened by the operation. For the 158 children with LMC and preexisting deficits, 29% had marked improvement in all symptoms after surgical treatment (12% returned to normal condition), and 69% had improvement in at least one symptom or remained in stable condition. Two patients with preexisting deficits were in worse condition after the operation (70).

Patients with sensorimotor deficits and pain were most likely to improve—66% of those with preoperative weakness, 83% of those with spasticity, 79% of those with pain, and 100% of those with gait disturbances improved postoperatively. Patients with preexisting urologic dysfunction improved less frequently; 38% of those with preoperative urinary retention and 29% of those with incontinence improved postoperatively. Patients with orthopaedic deformities were least likely to improve; 22% of patients with preoperative foot deformities and none of those with scoliosis improved postoperatively. However, 72% of patients with foot deformities and 95% of those with scoliosis were in stable condition postoperatively (70). These results emphasize the importance of early detection and therapy for LMC, before neurologic, urologic, or orthopaedic dysfunction intervenes.

Clinical deterioration due to spinal cord retethering continues to be a problem, occurring among 10% to 47% of patients (21,70,107,108). Because essentially all patients with lipoma have radiographic signs of tethering at follow-up MRI, the diagnosis of recurrent tethering is not made on the basis of MRI findings alone. All patients with lipoma should ideally be observed carefully in a multidisciplinary setting with serial neurologic examinations, urodynamic studies, and orthopaedic evaluations to detect early evidence of clinical deterioration.

Treatment of Children with Split-cord Malformations

Like those with occult dysraphic malformations, many children with split-cord malformations are born with normal or nearly normal neurologic function. When examined carefully, however, many are found to have subtle neurologic abnormalities that suggest spinal cord dysfunction. More important, with growth and development, almost all patients have insidious and progressive neurologic deficits, urologic dysfunction, and orthopedic deformities of the legs or spine or both (46,102). It is very rare to encounter an adult who is truly free of symptoms. Children younger than 2 years often look healthy or have only subtle abnormalities. More than one half of those older than 2 years, however, and nearly all adults have developed considerable neurologic dysfunction that can be attributed to spinal cord tethering (102). Once they occur, neurologic deficits often do not improve even after resection of the tethering malformation (46,102). For this reason, we and most pediatric neurosurgeons recommend early repair of the malformation, before deficits occur. In particular, patients in being considered for an operation to correct scoliosis should absolutely be evaluated by a neurosurgeon familiar with developmental anomalies. The underlying split-cord malformation should be addressed before orthopaedic intervention. Without prior untethering, corrective spinal surgery may cause sudden and disastrous neurologic loss.

Most children with split-cord malformations (88% in the series of Pang et al. [101–103]) have associated visible cutaneous signs that suggest the diagnosis before neurologic deficits occur. Cutaneous and mesenchymal lesions include hypertrichosis (hairy patch) among 20% to 55% of patients, capillary hemangioma, dermal sinus (approximately half of which have an associated intraspinal dermoid tumor), and obvious bony malformations of the dorsal arch (46,68,101,102). Hypertrichosis is the most common, and the most specific, indicator of an underlying split-cord malformation (102).

Neurologic abnormalities include motor dysfunction, sensory loss, and pain. Muscle weakness usually is insidious and progressive but can be acutely precipitated by means of sudden stretching of the spinal cord, as occurs, for example, with a jackknife posture during a sporting event or auto accident or during the lithotomy position for surgery or obstetric delivery (67,92). Weakness can be symmetric or predominantly or even exclusively unilateral. Asymmetric motor deficits are observed in two groups: (a) patients in whom the two hemicords are asymmetrically divided resulting in one larger and one smaller hemicord (102) and (b) patients with hemimyelomeningocele, in which one hemicord fails to properly close, manifests as an open neural placode, and causes ipsilateral sensorimotor deficits while the other hemicord remains within the spinal canal and provides more normal innervation to the contralateral leg (28).

Associated changes in motor tone and vegetative sensorimotor functions are common and include spasticity, muscle atrophy, and even sympathetic dystrophy with hairlessness, anhidrosis, dependent rubor, thickened toenails, nonhealing ulcers, and recurrent osteomyelitis. Muscle imbalances can cause progressive secondary orthopaedic difficulties, such as pes cavus, claw toe, and equinovarus deformities (68,102).

Sensory disturbances occur most frequently in combination with motor weakness. Both altered sensation and sensory loss may be apparent. Sensory symptoms include paresthesia (spontaneously occurring disagreeable sensations such as pins and needles or burning), dysesthesia (unpleasant sensory responses to innocuous sensory stimuli), and hyperpathia (heightened painful responses to painful sensory stimuli). Pain is more common among adults than children. It characteristically involves the legs, perineum, or perianal region and usually has an unpleasant paresthetic or dysesthetic quality (102).

Urinary dysfunction is more frequent with advancing age (102). Symptoms of progressive bladder disturbance include intermittent accidents or urinary dribbling, frequent urinary tract infections, and difficulty with toilet training. Among toddlers who have not yet mastered toilet training, progressive loss of bladder function may become apparent only in retrospect, when the child later does not achieve urinary control. Urodynamic testing (see earlier) may provide important information regarding preoperative urinary function and should be a part of every evaluation.

Scoliosis is a common presenting feature of split-cord malformations and its cause is likely multifactorial. Underlying causes of scoliosis include associated underlying vertebral anomalies such as unbalanced hemivertebrae and segmental bars (58), underlying static muscle imbalance or tonal asymmetry, and asymmetric neurologic dysfunction. In particular, spinal cord tethering, either from the split-cord malformation or an associated foreshortened filum terminale, has been proposed as a potential cause of scoliosis. There remains considerable and lively debate about the degree to which spinal cord tethering contributes to progressive scoliosis. Several authors have suggested that scoliosis among patients with split-cord malformations is most commonly the result of underlying vertebral malformations and that untethering is unlikely to change the progression of the curve (44,54,58,67,92,150). In a series of 27 patients referred to Winter et al. (150) because of scoliosis and split-cord malformations, all but one patient had multiple underlying vertebral abnormalities. Most curves were congenital (10 were present at birth, and the average age at presentation was 3 years), and the scoliosis was most commonly at the level of the underlying vertebral malformations (150). In a study of 34 patients conducted by Hilal et al. (54), scoliosis among untreated patients progressed gradually and was most severe among those with multiple underlying vertebral malformations. Among 20 patients described by Keim and Greene (67), most of whom had malformations of the vertebral bodies, 14 came to medical attention with scoliosis. Twelve of these underwent resection of the bony spur, and 6 of the 12 needed subsequent surgery to correct the scoliosis. In a series of 30 patients described by Gower (44), 7 came to medical attention with scoliosis. Surgery for correction of the split-cord malformation stabilized progressive scoliosis for 1 patient, did not halt progression for 2, and had no effect on stable scoliosis for 4 (44). In Keim and Greene's series, however, scoliosis in 6 of 12 patients remained stable after untethering. Among 39 patients described by Pang (102), 5 of whom had progressive and 16 nonprogressive scoliosis, 4 of 5 children with progressive scoliosis achieved stability, and 1 of 5 had progression. Fourteen of 16 patients with stable scoliosis remained stable postoperatively, whereas 2 of 16 eventually needed corrective surgery for scoliosis.

These studies all had a variety of problems. First, the reported correlation between malformations of the vertebral bodies and scoliosis among patients with split-cord malformations does not necessarily imply a causal relation. Second, details regarding the following factors and a host of other variables were neither adequately described nor systematically examined in any of the studies: level and extent of the malformation; severity and progression (if any) of the curves at diagnosis; ages of the patients at diagnosis; presence or absence of additional presenting features, such as neurologic deterioration, urologic worsening, or orthopaedic deformities of the lower limbs; the nature, severity, and extent of underlying vertebral malformations; and the extent of untethering surgery and associated spinal cord malformations. Third, some patients underwent untethering and some did not, introducing a potential element of bias. Fourth, as Pang (101,102) pointed out, there are often multiple sites of tethering in these patients. For example, many split-cord malformations have an associated thickened filum terminale, 10% to 15% have tandem lesions at other levels of the neuraxis, others have hidden ventral tethering elements in addition to the obvious dorsal elements, and still others may have other malformative tethering elements, such as median nerve roots that attach to or pass through the dura (so-called myelomeningocele manqué), lipoma, dermal sinus, neurenteric cyst, teratoma, and a variety of other malformations. The conditions of patients with type II malformations, who previously have been thought to harbor no tethering element, do indeed deteriorate, and the deterioration would complicate surgical results. Earlier surgical series are much more likely to have missed these associated elements. The result is partially controlled malformations and ongoing deterioration.

Scoliosis among patients with split-cord malformations no doubt is multifactorial and probably most often is related to underlying vertebral malformations. However, in a child with a split-cord malformation and progressive scoliosis but without underlying vertebral malformations, tethering should be strongly considered a potential cause of the scoliosis. No comprehensive, systematic studies have examined either the contribution of tethering to scoliosis or the effect of spinal cord untethering on

stabilizing or improving scoliosis among these patients. Nevertheless, there appears to be agreement among most authors that (a) nearly all patients with split-cord malformations eventually have neurologic deterioration, (b) untethering in patients without symptoms will likely avert the development of neurologic deterioration and improve some and stabilize almost all patients with symptoms, and (c) therapy for scoliosis without first untethering the malformation can cause abrupt neurologic deterioration. For these reasons, we and others recommend that the split-cord malformation be untethered before patients undergo corrective scoliosis surgery, even if the scoliosis is thought to be unrelated to the underlying spinal cord malformation.

The radiologic evaluation of a child with a suspected split-cord malformation should include both MRI and CT through the entire area. The CT scan shows any bone spurs to better advantage. Myelography with high-resolution CT (CT myelography) may be superior to MRI in demonstrating some of the details of these malformations (102). Whether this provides practical information that would justify the additional discomfort and risk is debatable. Vertebral malformations such as hemivertebrae, sagittally clefted (butterfly) vertebrae, fused (block) vertebrae, and missing vertebrae are more frequent in type I (double dural tube) than the type II (single dural tube) malformations (102). The midline osseous spur in type I malformation is almost always evident at MRI or CT myelography, whereas the midline fibrous bands of type II malformations are present among fewer than one third of patients (102). Median nerve roots occasionally are visible projecting from the hemicords to the intervening fibrous band (102) (Fig. 10).

For a patient with a type II malformation, both the dura surrounding the hemicords and the intervening osseous or fibrocartilaginous spur tether the spinal cord (Fig. 21). Both the spur and the surrounding dural cuff must be removed. As would be predicted, the tethering spur in these patients usually transfixes the spinal cord at the caudal end of the malformation, where the two hemicords reunite to form a single caudal spinal cord, although they may be present anywhere within the split segment. The spur may be attached either ventrally to the underlying ventral dura and vertebral body, dorsally to the lamina, or at both ends. The spur is removed with rongeurs before the dura is opened. Vigorous bleeding may occur from vessels within the spur, and the surgeon should be prepared to control this with bone wax and bipolar cautery. After the spur is removed, the cuff of dura is excised. Adherent, nonfunctional median nerve roots that project from the hemicords to the dural sleeve are carefully sectioned. The ventral dura is difficult to close and usually is left open, and the dorsal dura is closed in a watertight manner.

Type II malformations lack a visible extradural osseous spur and traditionally have not been thought to contain tethering lesions (20,52,131). However, the intradural midline fibrous bands in single dural sheath malformations can tether the spinal cord in a manner analogous to that of the osseous spurs of double dural tube malformations (102,103). Like the osseous spurs of type I malformations, the intradural fibrous bands in type II malformations (Fig. 10) often are located at the caudal end where the hemicords reunite, although they may be found anywhere within the split segment. The bands pass from the cleft between the hemicords to the adjacent dorsal and ventral dura. They are

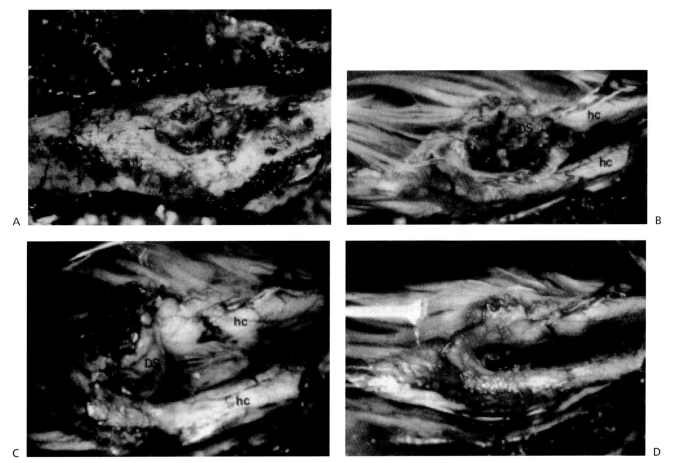

FIGURE 21. Surgical management of a double dural sac malformation. **A:** Partial resection of the osseous spur (*arrows*). **B:** The dura has been opened. The median cuff of the dural sheath (*DS*) is visible adherent to the two hemicords (*hc*). **C:** The dural sleeve (*DS*) is retracted caudally to show its cranial base. **D:** After complete removal of both the osseous spur and surrounding dural sheath, the two hemicords lie freely within a common dural sac. (From Pang D [1992]: Split-cord malformation, II: the clinical syndrome. *Neurosurgery* 31:481–500, with permission.)

resected to untether the hemicords. A thickened filum terminale also is frequently present and must also be sectioned. Among 11 patients with single dural sheath malformations, all had fibrous bands at surgery that were thought to be tethering the hemicords. Therefore, all split-cord malformations, regardless of type, should be explored operatively (102).

The results of treatment depend largely on whether untethering is performed before or after neurologic deficits have intervened. Surgical morbidity is acceptable (7% in one series) when untethering is performed on patients without symptoms and is lower for type II than type I malformations (102). For patients with symptoms, pain is relieved by means of untethering in almost all cases. However, once they develop, neurologic, urologic, and orthopaedic deficits are frequently stabilized but less frequently are improved by means of surgery. Preoperative sensorimotor deficits in one series improved in 38%, stabilized in 59%, and worsened in 3% of cases. Progressive deficits of recent onset were much more likely to improve than were static, longstanding deficits. For example, progressive sensorimotor deficits improved in 58% and stabilized in 42% cases, whereas static deficits improved in no cases, stabilized in 82%, and worsened

in 9%. Progressive bowel and bladder dysfunction likewise improved in 45%, stabilized in 45%, and worsened in 10% of cases, whereas static urologic abnormalities improved in none, stabilized in 90%, and worsened in 10%. Scoliosis improved in no cases, stabilized in 86%, and progressed (requiring spinal fusion) in 14% (102).

SUMMARY

It is increasingly apparent that neurologic and related urologic and orthopaedic dysfunction among children with both myelomeningocele and occult dysraphic lesions such as lipomyelomeningocele and split-cord malformations are the result of progressive and in some cases irreversible injury due to spinal cord tethering. Animal studies have implicated progressive spinal cord ischemia as the pathophysiologic mechanism underlying progressive injury from cord tethering in humans. The improvements that follow untethering for all types of dysraphic malformations strongly support a vigilant and aggressive neurosurgical approach to dysraphic malformations. For children with myelomeningocele, untethering should be considered whenever objective clinical evidence of neurologic dysfunction becomes evident, provided that incipient shunt malfunction has been excluded. For children with an occult dysraphic malformation, the mere presence of a potentially tethering lesion is reason for neurosurgical intervention. Untethering is best performed before dysfunction becomes evident and sensorimotor changes, urologic dysfunction, and orthopaedic deformities intervene. The operation should be performed by a neurosurgeon experienced with such malformations.

REFERENCES

1. Aronson DD, Kahn RH, Canady A, et al. (1991): Instability of the cervical spine after decompression in patients who have Arnold-Chiari malformation. *J Bone Joint Surg Am* 73:898–906.
2. Bakker-Niezen SH, Walder HAD, Merx JL (1984):The tethered spinal cord syndrome. *Z Kinderchir* 39[Suppl 2]:100–103.
3. Barnett HJM, Foster JB, Hudgson P (1973): *Syringomyelia*. Philadelphia: Saunders.
4. Barson AJ (1970): The vertebral level of termination of the spinal cord during normal and abnormal development. *J Anat* 106:489–497.
5. Beardmore HE, Wigglesworth FW (1958): Vertebral anomalies and alimentary duplications. *Pediatr Clin North Am* 5:457–474.
6. Begeer JH, Meihuizen de Regt MJ, HogenEsch I, et al. (1986): Progressive neurological deficit in children with spina bifida aperta. *Z Kinderchir* 41[Suppl 1]:13–15.
7. Bohannon RW, Smith MB (1987): Interrater reliability of a modified Ashworth scale of muscle spasticity. *Phys Ther* 67:206–207.
8. Boone D, Pansons D, Lachman SM, et al. (1985): Spina bifida occulta: lesion or anomaly? *Clin Radiol* 36:159–161.
9. Bremer JL (1952): Dorsal intestinal fistula; accessory neurenteric canal: diastematomyelia. *Arch Pathol* 54:132–138.
10. Brinker MR, Rosenfeld SR, Feiwell E, et al. (1994): Myelomeningocele at the sacral level. *J Bone Joint Surg Am* 76:1293–1300.
11. Brophy JD, Sutton LN, Zimmerman RA (1989): Magnetic resonance imaging of lipomyelomeningocele and tethered cord. *Neurosurgery* 25:336–340.
12. Burrows FGO, Sutcliffe J (1968): The split notochord syndrome. *Br J Radiol* 41:844–847.
13. Cameron AH (1957): The Arnold-Chiari and other neuro-anatomical malformations associated with spina bifida. *J Pathol Bacteriol* 73:195–211.
14. Cameron AH (1957): Malformations of the neuro-spinal axis, urogenital tract and foregut in spina bifida attributable to disturbances of the blastopore. *J Pathol Bacteriol* 73:213–221.
15. Campbell LR, Dayton DH, Sohal GS (1986): Neural tube defects: a review of human and animal studies on the etiology of neural tube defects. *Teratology* 34:171–187.
16. Centers for Disease Control and Prevention (1992): Spina bifida incidence at birth—United States. *MMWR* 41:497.
17. Charney EB, Weller SC, Sutton LN, et al. (1985): Management of the newborn with myelomeningocele: time for a decision-making process. *Pediatrics* 75:58–64.
18. Chaseling RW, Johnston IH, Besser M (1985): Meningoceles and the tethered cord syndrome. *Childs Nerv Syst* 1:105–108.
19. Cochrane DD, Adderley R, White CP, et al. (1990–91): Apnea in patients with myelomeningocele. *Pediatr Neurosurg* 16:232–239.
20. Cohen J, Sledge CB (1960): Diastematomyelia: an embryological interpretation with report of a case. *Am J Dis Child* 100:127–133.
21. Colak A, Pollack IF, Albright AL (1998): Recurrent tethering: a common long-term problem after lipomyelomeningocele repair. *Pediatr Neurosurg* 29:184–190.
22. Dénes J, Honti J, Léb J (1967): Dorsal herniation of the gut: a rare manifestation of the split notochord syndrome. *J Pediatr Surg* 2:359–363.
23. Dias MS, Klein DM (1996): Occipital plagiocephaly: deformation or lambdoid synostosis? II: a unifying theory regarding pathogenesis. *Pediatr Neurosurg* 24:69–73.
24. Dias MS, Pang D (1995): split-cord malformations. *Neurosurg Clin N Am* 6:339–358.
25. Dias MS, Walker ML (1992): The embryogenesis of complex dysraphic malformations: a disorder of gastrulation? *Pediatr Neurosurg* 18.229–253.
26. DiPietro MA (1993): The conus medullaris: normal US findings throughout childhood. *Radiology* 188:149–153.
27. Dodds GS (1941): Anterior and posterior rhachischisis. *Am J Pathol* 17:861–872.
28. Duckworth T, Sharrard WJ, Lister J, et al. (1968): Hemimyelocele. *Dev Med Child Neurol* 16:69–75.
29. Dyste GN, Menezes AH, Vangilder JC (1989): Symptomatic Chiari II malformations: an analysis of presentation, management, and long-term outcome. *J Neurosurg* 71:159–168.
30. Emery JL, Hilton HB (1961): Lung and heart complications of the treatment of hydrocephalus by ventriculoauriculostomy. *Surgery* 50:309–314.
31. Faris JC, Crowe JE (1975): The split notochord syndrome. *J Pediatr Surg* 10:467–472.
32. Feller A, Sternberg H (1929): Zur kenntnis der fehlbildungen der wirbelsäule, I: die wirbelkörperspalte und ihre formale genese. *Virchows Arch Pathol Anat* 272:613–640.
33. Fernbach SK, Naidich TP, McLone DG, et al. (1984): Computed tomography of primary intrathecal Wilms tumor with diastematomyelia. *J Comput Assist Tomogr* 8:523–528.
34. Findley TW, Agre JC, Habeck RV, et al. (1987): Ambulation in the adolescent with myelomeningocele, I: early childhood predictors. *Arch Phys Med Rehabil* 68:518–522.
35. Fletcher JM, Francis DJ, Thompson NM, et al. (1992): Verbal and non-verbal skill discrepancies in hydrocephalic children. *J Clin Exp Neuropsychol* 14:593–609.
36. Friedman S, Zita-Gozum C, Chatten J (1964): Pulmonary vascular changes complicating ventriculovascular shunting for hydrocephalus. *J Pediatr* 64:305–314.
37. Gardner WJ (1965): Hydrodynamic mechanism of syringomyelia: its relationship to myelocele. *J Neurol Neurosurg Psychiatry* 28:247–259.
38. Gardner WJ (1966): Embryologic origin of spinal malformations. *Acta Radiol [Diagn] (Scand)* 5:1013–1023.
39. Gardner WJ (1973): *The dysraphic states from syringomyelia to anencephaly*. Amsterdam: Excerpta Medica.
40. Gardner WJ (1980): Hypothesis: overdistention of the neural tube may cause anomalies of non-neural organs. *Teratology* 22:229–238.
41. Gilbert JN, Rorke LB, James HE, et al. (1988): The pathological basis for the failure of surgery to relieve the symptomatic Arnold-Chiari malformation. *Concepts in Pediatric Neurosurgery* 8:70–75.
42. Golden JA, Chernoff GF (1993): Intermittent pattern of neural tube closure in two strains of mice. *Teratology* 47:73–80.
43. Golden JA, Chernoff GF (1995): Multiple sites of anterior neural tube closure in humans: evidence from anterior neural tube defects (anencephaly). *Pediatrics* 95:506–510.
44. Gower DJ (1988): Diastematomyelia: a forty year experience. *Pediatr Neurosci* 14:90–96.
45. Gross RH, Cox A, Tatyrek R, et al. (1983): Early management and decision making for the treatment of myelomeningocele. *Pediatrics* 72:450–457.
46. Guthkelch AN (1974): Diastematomyelia with median septum. *Brain* 97:729–742.
47. Hall PV, Campbell RL, Kalsbeck JE (1975): Meningomyelocele and progressive hydromyelia: progressive paresis in myelodysplasia. *J Neurosurg* 43:457–463.
48. Hall PV, Lindseth RE, Campbell RL, et al. (1976): Myelodysplasia and developmental scoliosis: a manifestation of syringomyelia. *Spine* 1:48–56.
49. Hall P, Lindseth R, Campbell R, et al. (1979): Scoliosis and hydrocephalus in myelocele patients: the effects of ventricular shunting. *J Neurosurg* 50:174–178.
50. Hendrick EB, Hoffman HJ, Humphreys RP (1982): The tethered spinal cord. *Clin Neurosurg* 30:457–463.
51. Herman JM, McLone DG, Storrs BB, et al. (1993): Analysis of 153 patients with myelomeningocele or spinal lipoma reoperated upon for a tethered cord. *Pediatr Neurosurg* 19:243–249.

52. Herren RY, Edwards JE (1940): Diplomyelia (duplication of the spinal cord). *Arch Pathol* 30:1203–1214.

53. Hertwig O (1892): Urmund und spina bifida. *Arkh Mikr Anat* 39:353–503.

54. Hilal SK, Marton D, Pollack E (1974): Diastematomyelia in children: radiographic study in 34 cases. *Radiology* 112:609–621.

55. Hoffman HJ (1985): The tethered spinal cord. In: Holtzman R, Stein BM, eds. *The tethered spinal cord.* New York: Thieme-Stratton, pp. 91–98.

56. Hoffman HJ, Hendrick EB, Humphreys RP (1975): Manifestations and management of Arnold Chiari malformation in patients with myelomeningocele. *Childs Brain* 1:255–259.

57. Holinger PC, Holinger LD, Reichert TJ, et al. (1978): Respiratory obstruction and apnea in infants with bilateral abductor vocal cord paralysis, meningomyelocele, hydrocephalus, and Arnold-Chiari malformation. *J Pediatr* 92:368–373.

58. Hood RW, Riseborough EJ, Nehme AM, et al. (1980): Diastematomyelia and structural spinal deformities. *J Bone Joint Surg Am* 62:520–528.

59. Humphreys RP (1985): Spinal dysraphism. In: Wilkins RH, Rengachary SS, eds. *Neurosurgery,* vol. 3. New York: McGraw-Hill pp. 2041–2052.

60. Hunt GM (1990): Open spina bifida: outcome for a complete cohort treated unselectively and followed into adulthood. *Dev Med Child Neurol* 32:108–118.

61. Hunt GM, Holmes AE (1974): Some factors relating to intelligence in treated children with spina bifida cystica. *Dev Med Child Neurol Suppl* 35:65–70.

62. Hunt GM, Poulton A (1995): Open spina bifida: a complete cohort reviewed 25 years after closure. *Dev Med Child Neurol* 37:19–29.

63. Isu T, Chono Y, Iwaski Y, et al. (1992): Scoliosis associated with syringomyelia presenting in children. *Childs Nerv Syst* 8:97–100.

64. James CCM, Lassman JP (1964): Diastematomyelia: a critical survey of 24 cases submitted to laminectomy. *Arch Dis Child* 39:125–130.

65. Kaplan WE, McLone DG, Richards I (1988): The urological manifestations of the tethered spinal cord. *J Urol* 140:1285–1288.

66. Kaufman BA, Terbrock A, Winters N, et al. (1994): Disbanding a multidisciplinary clinic: effects on the health care of myelomeningocele patients. *Pediatr Neurosurg* 21:36–44.

67. Keim HA, Greene AF (1973): Diastematomyelia and scoliosis. *J Bone Joint Surg Am* 55:1425–1435.

68. Kennedy PR (1979): New data on diastematomyelia. *J Neurosurg* 51:355–361.

69. Khoury MJ, Erickson JD, James LM (1982): Etiologic heterogeneity of neural tube defects: clues from epidemiology. *Am J Epidemiol* 115:538–548.

70. LaMarca F, Grant JA, Tomita T, et al. (1997): Spinal lipomas in children: outcome of 270 procedures. *Pediatr Neurosurg* 26:8–16.

71. Lemire RJ (1975): Secondary caudal neural tube formation. In: Lemire RJ, Loeser JD, Leech RW, et al., eds. *Normal and abnormal development of the human nervous system.* Hagerstown, MD: Harper & Row, pp. 71–83.

72. Lichtenstein BW (1940): "Spinal dysraphism": spina bifida and myelodysplasia. *Arch Neurol* 44:792–810.

73. Lorber J (1971): Results of treatment of myelomeningocele: an analysis of 524 unselected cases, with special reference to possible selection for treatment. *Dev Med Child Neurol* 13:279–303.

74. Lorber J, Salfield S (1981): Results of selective treatment of spina bifida cystica. *Arch Dis Child* 56:822–830.

75. Mackenzie NG, Emery JL (1971): Deformities of the cervical cord in children with neurospinal dysraphism. *Dev Med Child Neurol* 13:59–67.

76. McLetchie NGB, Purves JK, Saunders RL (1954): The genesis of gastric and certain intestinal diverticula and enterogenous cysts. *Surg Gynecol Obstet* 99:135–141.

77. McLone DG (1983): Results of treatment of children born with a myelomeningocele. *Clin Neurosurg* 30:407–412.

78. McLone DG (1986): Laser resection of fifty spinal lipomas. *Neurosurgery* 18:611–615.

79. McLone DG (1986): Treatment of myelomeningocele: arguments against selection. In: Little JR, ed. *Clinical neurosurgery,* vol. 33. Baltimore: Williams & Wilkins, pp. 359–370.

80. McLone DG (1992): Continuing concepts in the management of spina bifida. *Pediatr Neurosurg* 18:254–256.

81. McLone DG (1996): Myelomeningocele. In: Youmans JR, ed. *Neurological surgery,* 4th ed, vol. 2. Philadelphia: WB Saunders, pp. 843–860.

82. McLone DG, Czyzewski D, Raimondi AJ, et al. (1982): Central nervous system infections as a limiting factor in the intelligence of children born with myelomeningocele. *Pediatrics* 70:338–342.

83. McLone DG, Dias MS (1991–92): Complications of myelomeningocele closure. *Pediatr Neurosurg* 17:267–273.

84. McLone DG, Dias MS (1994): Normal and abnormal early development of the nervous system. In: Cheek WR, ed. *Pediatric neurosurgery: Surgery of the developing nervous system.* Philadelphia: WB Saunders, pp. 3–39.

85. McLone DG, Dias L, Kaplan WE, et al. (1985): Concepts in the management of spina bifida. *Concepts in Pediatric Neurosurgery* 5:14–28.

86. McLone DG, Herman JM, Gabrieli AP, et al. (1990–91): Tethered cord as a cause of scoliosis in children with a myelomeningocele. *Pediatr Neurosurg* 16:8–13.

87. McLone DG, Knepper PA (1989): The cause of Chiari II malformation: a unified theory. *Pediatr Neurosurg* 15:1–12.

88. McLone DG, Naidich TP (1985): Terminal myelocystocele. *Neurosurgery* 16:36–43.

89. McLone DG, Naidich TP (1989): Myelomeningocele: outcome and late complications. In: McLaurin RL, Schut L, Venes JL, et al., eds. *Pediatric neurosurgery: surgery of the developing nervous system.* Philadelphia: WB Saunders, pp. 53–70.

90. McLone DG, Naidich TP (1989): The tethered spinal cord. In: McLaurin RL, Venes JL, Schut L, et al., eds. *Pediatric neurosurgery. Surgery of the developing nervous system.* Philadelphia: WB Saunders, pp. 71–96.

91. McLone DG, Nakahara S, Knepper PA (1991): Chiari II malformation: pathogenesis and dynamics. *Concepts Pediatr Neurosurg* 11:1–17.

92. Miller A, Guille JT, Bowen R (1993): Evaluation and treatment of diastematomyelia. *J Bone Joint Surg Am* 75:1308–1317.

93. Morgagni JB (1769): *The seats and causes of disease investigated by anatomy.* London: A. Millar and T. Cadell.

94. Moufarrij NA, Palmer JM, Hahn JF, et al. (1989): Correlation between magnetic resonance imaging and surgical findings in the tethered spinal cord. *Neurosurgery* 25:341–346.

95. Müller F, O'Rahilly R (1985): The first appearance of the neural tube and optic primordium in the human embryo at stage 10. *Anat Embryol (Berl)* 172:157–169.

96. Müller F, O'Rahilly R (1986): The development of the human brain and the closure of the rostral neuropore at stage 11. *Anat Embryol (Berl)* 175:205–222.

97. Müller F, O'Rahilly R (1987): The development of the human brain, the closure of the caudal neuropore, and the beginning of secondary neurulation at stage 12. *Anat Embryol (Berl)* 176:413–430.

98. Naidich TP, Harwood-Nash DC (1983): Diastematomyelia: hemicord and meningeal sheaths—single and double arachnoid and dural tubes. *Am J Neuroradiol* 4:633–636.

99. Oakes WJ (1985): Chiari malformations, hydromyelia, syringomyelia. In: Wilkins RH, Rengachary SS, eds. *Neurosurgery,* vol. 3. New York: McGraw-Hill, pp. 2102–2124.

100. Oldfield EH, Muraszko K, Shawker TH, et al. (1994): Pathophysiology of syringomyelia associated with Chiari I malformation of the cerebellar tonsils: implications for diagnosis and treatment. *J Neurosurg* 80:3–15.

101. Pang D (1995): split-cord malformation. In: Pang D, ed. *Disorders of the Pediatric Spine.* New York: Raven Press, pp. 203–251.

102. Pang D (1992): split-cord malformation, II: the clinical syndrome. *Neurosurgery* 31:481–500.

103. Pang D, Dias MS, Ahab-Barmada M (1992): split-cord malformation, I: a unified theory of embryogenesis for double spinal cord malformations. *Neurosurgery* 31:451–480.

104. Park TS, Hoffman HJ, Hendrick EB, et al. (1983): Experience with surgical decompression of the Arnold-Chiari malformation in young infants with myelomeningocele. *Neurosurgery* 13:147–152.

105. Paul KS, Lye RH, Strang FA, et al. (1983): Arnold Chiari malformation: review of 71 cases. *J Neurosurg* 58:183–187.

106. Peacock WJ, Murovic JA (1989): Magnetic resonance imaging in myelocystoceles: report of two cases. *J Neurosurg* 70:804–807.

107. Pierre-Kahn A, Lacombe J, Pinchon J, et al. (1986): Intraspinal lipomas with spina bifida: prognosis and treatment in 73 cases. *J Neurosurg* 65:756–761.

108. Pierre-Kahn A, Zerah M, Renier D, et al. (1997): Congenital lumbosacral lipomas. *Childs Nerv Syst* 13:298–334.

109. Piggott H (1980): The natural history of scoliosis in myelodysplasia. *J Bone Joint Surg Br* 62:54–58.

110. Pike JG, Berardinucci G, Hamburger B, et al. (1991): The surgical management of urinary incontinence in myelodysplastic children. *J Pediatr Surg* 26:466–470.

111. Pollack IF, Pang D, Albright AL, et al. (1992): Outcome following hindbrain decompression of symptomatic Chiari malformations in children previously treated with myelomeningocele closure and shunts. *J Neurosurg* 77:881–888.

112. Pollack IF, Pang D, Kocoshis S, et al. (1992): Neurogenic dysphagia resulting from Chiari malformations. *Neurosurgery* 30:709–719.

113. Prop N, Frensdorf EL, van de Stadt FR (1967): A postvertebral entodermal cyst associated with axial deformities: a case showing the "entodermal-ectodermal adhesion syndrome." *Pediatrics* 39:555–562.

114. Pudenz RH (1981): The surgical treatment of hydrocephalus: an historical view. *Surg Neurol* 15:15–26.

115. Reigel DH (1983): Tethered spinal cord. *Concepts Pediatr Neurosurg* 4:142–164.

116. Reigel DH, McLone DG (1988): Myelomeningocele: operative treatment and results. *Concepts Pediatr Neurosurg* 8:41–50.

117. Reigel DH, Tchernoukha K, Bazmi B, et al. (1994): Change in spinal curvature following release of tethered spinal cord associated with spina bifida. *Pediatr Neurosurg* 20:30–42.

118. Rekate HL (1984): To shunt or not to shunt: hydrocephalus and dysraphism. *Clin Neurosurg* 32:593–607.

119. Rokos J (1975): Pathogenesis of diastematomyelia and spina bifida. *J Pathol* 117:155–161.

120. Ross GW, Swanson SA, Perentes E, et al. (1988): Ectopic midline spinal ganglion in diastematomyelia: a study of its connections. *J Neurol Neurosurg Psychiatry* 51:1231–1234.

121. Rotenstein D, Reigel DH, Lucke JF (1996): Growth of growth hormone-treated and nontreated children before and after tethered spinal cord release. *Pediatr Neurosurg* 24:237–241.

122. Rudy DC, Woodside JR (1991): The incontinent myelodysplastic patient. *Urol Clin North Am* 18:295–308.

123. Sandler AD, Worley G, Leroy EC, et al. (1996): Sexual function and erection capability among young men with spina bifida. *Dev Med Child Neurol* 38:823–829.

124. Sarwark JF, Weber DT, Gabrieli AP, et al. (1996): Tethered cord syndrome in low motor level children with myelomeningocele. *Pediatr Neurosurg* 25:295–301.

125. Saunders RL (1943): Combined anterior and posterior spina bifida in a living neonatal human female. *Anat Rec* 87:255–278.

126. Schoenwolf GC (1977): Tail (end) bud contributions to the posterior region of the chick embryo. *J Exp Zool* 201:227–246.

127. Schoenwolf GC (1984): Histological and ultrastructural studies of secondary neurulation in mouse embryos. *Am J Anat* 169:361–376.

128. Schoenwolf GC, DeLongo J (1980): Ultrastructure of secondary neurulation in the chick embryo. *Am J Anat* 158:43–63.

129. Schoenwolf GC, Smith JL (1990): Mechanisms of neurulation: traditional viewpoint and recent advances. *Development* 109:243–270.

130. Scott RM (1985): Delayed deterioration in patients with spinal tethering syndromes. In: Holtzman R, Stein BM, eds. *The tethered spinal cord*. New York: Thieme-Stratton, pp. 116–120.

131. Scotti G, Musgrave MA, Harwood-Nash DC, et al. (1980): Diastematomyelia in children: metrizamide and CT metrizamide myelography. *Am J Roentgenol* 135:1225–1232.

132. Shaffer J, Wolfe L, Freidrich W, et al. (1986): Developmental expectations; intelligence and fine motor skills. In: Shurtleff DB, ed. *Myelodysplasias and extrophies: significance, prevention, and treatment*. New York: Grune and Stratton, pp. 359–372.

133. Shurtleff DB, Goiney R, Gordon LH, et al. (1976): Myelodysplasia: the natural history of kyphosis and scoliosis—a preliminary report. *Dev Med Child Neurol Suppl* 37:126–133.

134. Shurtleff DB, Lemire RJ (1995): Epidemiology, etiologic factors, and prenatal diagnosis of open spinal dysraphism. *Neurosurg Clin N Am* 6:183–193.

135. Singh A, Singh R (1982): Split notochord syndrome with dorsal enteric fistula. *J Pediatr Surg* 17:412–413.

136. Sklar F, Shapiro K (1998): Surgical management of hydromyelia: a retrospective review. Presented at the 21st Annual Meeting of the American Society for Pediatric Neurosurgens, January 25–31 1998, Lana'i, Hawaii.

137. Soare PL, Raimondi AJ (1977): Intellectual and perceptual motor characteristics of treated myelomeningocele children. *Am J Dis Child* 131:199–204.

138. Spindel MR, Bauer SB, Dyro FM, et al. (1987): The changing neurologic lesion in myelodysplasia. *JAMA* 258:1630–1633.

139. Spratt NT (1947): Regression and shortening of the primitive streak in the explanted chick blastoderm. *J Exp Zool* 104:69–100.

140. Steinbok P, Irvine B, Cochrane DD, et al. (1992): Long-term outcome and complications of children born with meningomyelocele. *Childs Nerv Syst* 8:92–96.

141. Swank M, Dias L (1992): Myelomeningocele: a review of the orthpaedic aspects of 206 patients treated from birth with no selection criteria. *Dev Med Child Neurol* 34:1047–1052.

142. Tamaki N, Shirataki K, Kojima N, et al. (1988): Tethered cord syndrome of delayed onset following repair of myelomeningocele. *J Neurosurg* 69:393–398.

143. Troup EC, Sanford RA, Muhlbauer MS, et al. (1998): Myofascial closure for myelomeningocele: a 20-year experience. Presented at the Annual Meeting of the American Association of Neurological Surgeons, April 1998, Philadelphia.

144. Ugarte N, Gonzalez-Crussi F, Sotelo-Avila C (1980): Diastematomyelia associated with teratoma. *J Neurosurg* 53:720–725.

145. Vernet O, Farmer JP, Houle AM, et al. (1996): Impact of urodynamic studies on the surgical management of spinal cord tethering. *J Neurosurg* 85:555–559.

146. von Recklinghausen E (1886): Untersuchungen über die spina bifida. *Arch Pathol Anat* 105:243–373.

147. Wald SL, McLaurin RL (1978): Shunt-associated glomerulonephritis. *Neurosurgery* 3:146–150.

148. Williams B (1978): A critical appraisal of posterior fossa surgery for syringomyelia. *Brain* 101:223–250.

149. Wilson DA, Prince JR (1989): MR imaging determination of the location of the normal conus medullaris throughout childhood. *Am J Roentgenol* 152:1029–1032.

150. Winter RB, Haven JJ, Moe JH, et al. (1974): Diastematomyelia and congenital spine deformities. *J Bone Joint Surg Am* 56:27–39.

151. Wolfe S, Schneble F, Tröger J (1992): The conus medullaris: time of ascendence to normal level. *Pediatr Radiol* 22:590–592.

152. Yamada S, Iacono RP, Yamada BS (1996): Pathophysiology of the tethered spinal cord. In: Yamada S, ed. *Tethered cord syndrome*. Park Ridge, IL: American Association of Neurological Surgeons, pp. 29–48.

153. Yamada S, Zinke D, Sanders D (1981): Pathophysiology of "tethered cord syndrome." *J Neurosurg* 54:494–503.

14

THE SPINE IN SKELETAL DYSPLASIAS

PAUL D. SPONSELLER

Skeletal dysplasia is a group of disorders caused by a systemic defect in the formation of the skeleton. The mutations and the mechanisms by which they cause dysplasia have been greatly elucidated in the past few years (3). Almost all affect either the matrix of cartilage or the process of endochondral ossification. There are several ways of classifying dysplasia. The more traditional method, the International Classification of Skeletal Dysplasias (1), is summarized in Table 1. The more recent method of grouping dysplasia according to families of similar mutation is summarized in Table 2 (37). The group of skeletal types of dysplasia merges with other types of disorders such as connective tissue disorders and metabolic disorders. For instance, disorders that affect cartilage oligomeric matrix protein affect not only cartilage but also ligament, and mucopolysaccharidosis is both metabolic derangement and skeletal dysplasia. Therefore it is somewhat debatable which conditions should be included. This chapter emphasizes principles common to all types of skeletal dysplasia and discusses unique features of each of the most common disorders. These are summarized in Table 3.

For persons treating patients with skeletal dysplasia, it is not uncommon to be faced with syndromes that are rare or even new to the practitioner. This is unavoidable. However, certain patterns of problems occur that are common to many types of skeletal dysplasia. These are instability, deformity, and stenosis. They may occur in different planes and at different levels of the spine, but it is helpful to think of these classes of problems when approaching the care of a patient with a skeletal dysplasia. Almost every type of dysplasia may manifest any or several of these problems, with the following exceptions: cervical kyphosis occurs only in diastrophic dysplasia and Larsen syndrome, and symptomatic stenosis is by far most common in achondroplasia. Another phenomenon that confounds the practitioner is the phenotypic variability of genetic disease. Some patients with achondroplasia have severe thoracolumbar kyphosis, whereas others do not have any at all despite the presence of a reasonably constant mutation. That makes it all the more important to be open-minded when evaluating these patients for the first time. However, some useful generalizations are as follows.

Instability most commonly occurs at the atlantoaxial level. It may be caused by os odontoideum, odontoid hypoplasia or aplasia, or laxity of the transverse ligament. This is most common in mucopolysaccharidosis (7), spondyloepiphyseal dysplasia (11), and metatropic dysplasia. It is helpful for the novice to recognize that this problem is quite rare in that most common of all dysplasia, achondroplasia. Plain radiographs should be obtained of the cervical spines of most patients with dysplasia, especially if an intervention is to be performed. The odontoid process should be clearly visualized. Not all patients with a radiographic anomaly have clinical instability, however. If an anomaly is found, active flexion-extension lateral radiographs of the cervical spine should be obtained. If it is not clear whether cord compression or impingement is developing, magnetic resonance imaging (MRI) in neutral, flexion, and extension is the next step. During MRI any pathologic changes are likely to be underestimated because imaging is performed in a confined space in a lateral position. Sometimes the images show an additive compressive effect from cervical stenosis at the same levels. If translation between the most caudal portion of the arch of C1 and the anterior-superior cortex of C2 is more than 8 mm, atlantoaxial fusion usually is recommended. If the translation is between 5 and 8 mm, observation may be justified unless the patient is very small, is at higher-than-average risk of trauma, has neurologic signs indicating cord compression, or is poorly compliant.

Among patients who need atlantoaxial fusion, it is desirable to preserve atlantooccipital motion, unless this level is already fused or ankylosed or is stenotic and in need of decompression. Computed tomography (CT) can be helpful in assessing the shape of the posterior ring of the atlas, because this structure often is bifid and may even be missing. If the bone size and quality are of adequate condition for internal fixation, there are many techniques of stabilization to choose from. These are left to the surgeon's discretion. However, it is wise to have several options available because the anatomic features may not appear as expected. If internal fixation is not feasible, graft and fusion with halo-vest immobilization are quite successful in the care of young children (45). Graft sources may include one or both iliac crests and the proximal tibial metaphysis if needed. Reliance on allograft is inadvisable, because there is a high risk of pseudarthrosis (88). The upper cervical spine is best stabilized in a halo

P.D. Sponseller: Pediatric Medicine, Johns Hopkins University, Baltimore, Maryland 21287.

TABLE 1. INTERNATIONAL CLASSIFICATION OF SKELETAL DYSPLASIAS (1992 PARTIAL LIST)

A. Defects of the tubular and flat bones of the axial skeleton
   Achondroplasia group
      Achondroplasia
      Hypochondroplasia
      Thanatophoric dysplasia
   Metatropic dysplasia
   Atelosteogenesis and diastrophic dysplasia group
   Osteogenesis imperfecta
   Kneist-Stickler group
   Spondyloepiphyseal dysplasia congenita group
   Other spondyloepi (metaphyseal) dysplasia groups
   Storage disorders
      Mucopolysaccharidosis
      Mucolipidosis
   Multiple epiphyseal dysplasia
   Metaphyseal dysplasia
   Dysplasia with defective mineralization
      Hypophosphatasia
      Hypophosphatemic rickets
      Neonatal hypoparathyroidism
   Dysplasia with increased bone density
B. Disorganized development of cartilaginous and fibrous components of the skeleton
   Multiple cartilaginous exostosis
   Dysplasia epiphysealis hemimelica
   Enchondromatosis
   Fibrous dysplasia
C. Idiopathic osteolysis

TABLE 2. ETIOLOGIC CLASSIFICATION OF DYSPLASIA

FGFR3 group (Fibroblast Growth Factor Receptor 3, a local regulator of cartilage growth)
   Achondroplasia
      Hypochondroplasia
      Thanatophoric dysplasia
COL1A group (collagen 1, structural osseous protein)
   Osteogenesis imperfecta
COL2A 1 group (collagen 2, structural cartilage protein)
   Spondyloepiphyseal dysplasia (SED) congenita
   Kneist dysplasia
   Stickler dysplasia
   Strudwick dysplasia
   SED tarda
DDST group (Diastrophic Dysplasia Sulfate Transport, defective sulfate transport enzyme)
   Diastrophic dysplasia
   Achondrogenesis
COMP group (cartilage oligomeric matrix protein, structural cartilage protein)
   Multiple epiphyseal dysplasia (MED)
   Pseudoachondroplasia
Storage disorders
   Mucopolysaccharidosis
   Mucolipidosis

TABLE 3. SPINAL DISORDERS IN SKELETAL DYSPLASIA

Condition	Instability	Cervical Deformity	Scoliosis	Kyphosis	Stenosis	Comments
Achondroplasia	None	None	None	Thoracolumbar	Foramen magnum Lumbosacral greater than thoracic or cervical	Brace if not resolved at 2–3 years of age
Hypochondroplasia	Rare	None	None	Rare	Rare	
Metatropic	Yes	None	Yes	Yes	None	
Diastrophic	Rare	Kyphosis	Yes	Yes	Yes	Cervical kyphosis may resolve; spina bifida may affect other levels
Kneist	Yes	No	Yes	Yes	No	Scoliosis usually mild
Spondyloepiphyseal dysplasia	Yes	No	Yes	Yes	No	
Pseudoachondroplasia	Yes	No	Yes	No	No	Cervical instability rare
Chondrodysplasia punctata	Yes	No	Yes, congenital	No	Cervical (rhizomelic)	
Metaphyseal dysplasia	Rare	No	Rare	No	No	
Cleidocranial dysplasia	No	No	Yes	No	No	Scoliosis may be associated with syrinx
Larsen Syndrome	Rare	Kyphosis	Yes	Yes	No	Spina bifida occulta Lumbar spondylolysis possible
Stickler Syndrome	Rare	No	Yes	Yes	No	

device. Postoperative immobilization in a halo vest should take into account the patient's age as well as any cranial anomalies. Patients younger than 6 years should have the halo pins tightened to 2 to 4 inch-pounds, and more than four pins are recommended for patients younger than 4 years (17).

Rotatory instability, such as spondyloepiphyseal dysplasia and metatropic dysplasia can occur with skeletal dysplasia. Subaxial instability can occur in Larsen syndrome or more rarely in other conditions. Evaluation and treatment should proceed according to the principles described earlier.

Deformity in the cervical spine takes the form of cervical kyphosis. This is most common in Larsen syndrome and diastrophic dysplasia (36,41,74). In both conditions, deformity arises in conjunction with cervical spina bifida and hypoplasia of the midcervical vertebrae. One contrast between the two conditions is that in diastrophic dysplasia, kyphosis can reverse spontaneously (36). In Larsen syndrome this has not been reported. Bracing does not have a clear-cut role in the management of this deformity. In either case, if the deformity becomes severe, myelopathy can occur (41,49,60). Anterior and posterior decompression is indicated if this complication develops.

The most common deformity in dysplasia is thoracic or thoracolumbar kyphosis. This is most severe when it is focal and not associated with scoliosis. The value of brace treatment has not been proved with clinical research. The rarity and variability of these conditions makes a controlled trial difficult. If a patient is young and there is flexibility in the curve, a Milwaukee brace can be corrective (7,68). Surgical treatment depends on the magnitude of the curve and the associated scoliosis. If kyphosis is greater than 60 to 70 degrees, anterior and posterior fusion may be necessary (7).

Scoliosis is most common in diastrophic, spondyloepiphyseal, Kneist, and metatropic dysplasia. Bracing remains an option, although the rate of successful stabilization is unknown. When the curve exceeds 50 to 69 degrees, bracing does not have much value. Surgery is indicated if a curve is unbalanced or associated with severe kyphosis. Low-profile instrumentation is indicated, and the hooks must be carefully placed. If pedicle screws are used, preoperative CT of the pedicles is recommended to evaluate size.

Stenosis most commonly involves achondroplasia. It can occur from the foramen magnum to the sacrum (see later). If frequent claudication or neurologic deficit is present, decompression must extend to the sacrum. If stenosis extends proximally across a kyphosis, this area also must be fused. Stenosis also occurs among diastrophic persons and in rare instances is clinically symptomatic (43,72). Stenosis at the ring of the atlas can complicate spondlyoepiphyseal dysplasia.

The surgical treatment of a patient with skeletal dysplasia poses problems for the anesthesiologist (90,91), who should be experienced in this area and extra time should be allowed for induction. Intravenous access may be difficult, especially central access. Intubation is complex because of abnormal oropharyngeal anatomic features, mandible or neck stiffness, and, in some cases, cervical instability. Intraoperative positioning must be geared to the patient's size and unique anatomic features. Postoperative management is complicated because the patient often has coexisting disabilities. Inpatient rehabilitation sometimes is necessary after spinal surgery. These considerations should be taken into account in surgical planning.

SPECIFIC DISORDERS

Achondroplasia

Achondroplasia is the most common skeletal dysplasia. The incidence is about 1 case per 30,000 livebirths (28). Although the most noticeable involvement is rhizomelic shortening of the extremities, the length of the spine is at the lower limits of normal. This disorder is autosomal dominant, but for 70% of affected persons this disorder is a spontaneous mutation. The genetic defect is a specific mutation in fibroblast growth factor receptor protein 3 (62,80). This protein has an inhibitory effect on cells in the proliferative zone of the growth plate. The mutation increases the inhibitory effect. The growth of the vertebrae normally occurs from the two neurocentral synchondroses (growth plates) in the vertebral body near the bases of the pedicles (53,63) (Fig. 1). They are obliquely oriented and provide growth in width of the spinal canal as well as length of the pedicles. Growth does not occur in these regions of persons with achondroplasia, and a canal develops that is narrow in all dimensions.

Radiographic Findings

The cervical spine rarely displays deformity or instability in achondroplasia, in contrast to the features of many of types of skeletal dysplasia. However, in the spine of a person with achondroplasia the posterior vertebral body cortex is close to the lamina, indicating stenosis. Anteroposterior radiographs show nar-

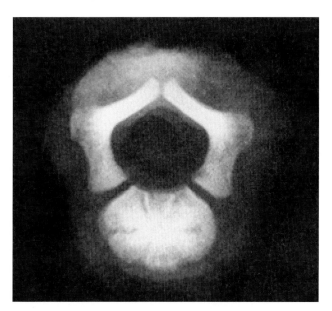

FIGURE 1. Pedicles in a person with achondroplasia come closer together in the more distal parts of the spine. This is in contrast to the usual pattern, in which there is greater interpediculate distance in the distal portions of the spine.

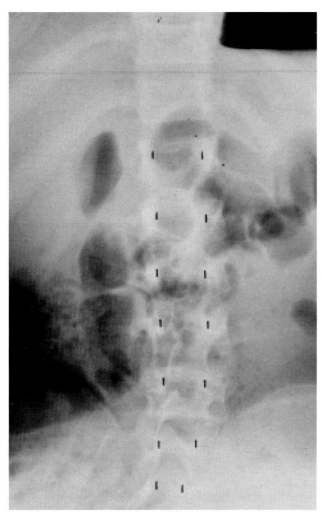

FIGURE 2. Growth of each vertebra and the pedicular separation is determined by the growth plates labeled *neurocentral synchondroses*. These grow by means of endochondral ossification and are therefore impaired in achondroplasia.

rowing of the pedicles from the upper lumbar spine to the sacrum in contrast to the normal widening (70) (Fig. 2). All areas of the spine from skull base to sacrum are prone to stenosis. The lumbar spine is more lordotic than normal, an alignment that worsens the stenosis. The vertebral bodies are taller than they are wide in the mediolateral or anteroposterior dimension, and the posterior margins are scalloped. There is often mild, residual thoracolumbar kyphosis, which persists into adulthood.

Clinical Problems

Foramen Magnum Stenosis

The base of the skull around the foramen magnum, being formed from endochondral bone, is congenitally stenotic in almost all infants with achondroplasia but usually improves with age (33,35). In some infants this stenosis becomes critical and causes symptoms of sleep apnea, hypotonia, aspiration, or gener-

alized developmental delay. If a child does not meet milestones or displays respiratory problems, a sleep study may confirm brain stem compression (66,104,112). Foramen magnum decompression by an experienced neurosurgeon usually improves the symptoms noticeably. This is necessary in the care of fewer than 10% of persons with achondroplasia. Along with the posterior edge of the foramen magnum, usually only the ring of the atlas is removed during this procedure. No postoperative immobilization is needed. Late sequelae have not been seen. However, if two or more laminae are removed, it is necessary to monitor for upper cervical kyphosis.

Thoracolumbar Kyphosis

Mild to moderate thoracolumbar kyphosis occurs among 80% of infants in the sitting position. Contributory factors most likely include hypotonia of the trunk extensors, ligamentous laxity, the largeness of head in relation to the rest of the body, and delayed standing. Most instances of kyphosis resolve spontaneously at about the time the child begins to stand (65). Those that do not resolve tend to occur among children with greater hypotonia, often those who needed foramen magnum decompression. The vertebrae, usually the T12 and L1, tend to become progressively wedged (Fig. 3). There are several reasons why this kyphosis should be corrected. First, it causes mild pressure on the conus, which may add to other factors in causing symptoms. Second, it necessitates an increase in compensatory lower lumbar lordosis, which increases stenosis there (82). Third, because adolescents or adults with achondroplasia often need decompressive laminectomy of the entire lumbar spine, any kyphosis present may markedly increase after posterior decompression (Fig. 4).

Pauli et al. (65) recommend prohibition of sitting at an angle greater than 69 degrees. I believe this leads to greater flexion force at the thoracolumbar junction, because patients try to sit up anyway. We recommend observing kyphosis until 2 years of age or walking age, whichever comes first. Patients who do not improve or who have neurologic signs and symptoms should be treated with a brace. I recommend a modified Knight double-upright thoracolumbosacral orthosis (TLSO) with a movable posterior pad to be placed at the apex and to be raised as the patient grows (Fig. 5). If this treatment fails or the patient is noncompliant, serial hyperextension casts can be applied over the course of a few months. The extension moment is gradually increased while the patient is allowed to stand and walk. This therapy has the advantage that the cast must be worn full time, and constant correction is applied. If a satisfactory response has been obtained (correction of more than 50% after 3 to 4 months), the patient can be placed in a TLSO for additional correction and transition to active spinal support (Fig. 6). For patients with thoracolumbar kyphosis greater than 30 to 40 degrees that persists beyond 5 years of age, consideration should be given to posterior fusion in situ over this region to stabilize the spine or allow it to grow straighter (96) (Fig. 7).

Spinal Stenosis

Stenosis is common among persons with achondroplasia; the prevalence is 80% to 90% (110). Symptoms usually develop in late teens to early adult years but may begin even in early adolescence. The most common symptoms is cramping or fa-

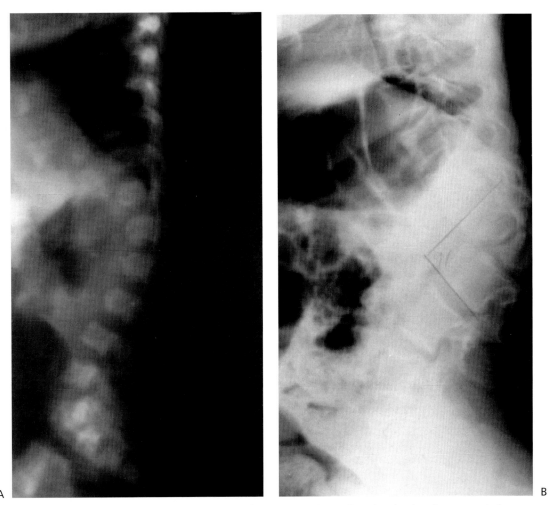

FIGURE 3. Thoracolumbar kyphosis in achondroplasia is mechanically induced rather than congenital. **A:** This patient had moderate thoracolumbar kyphosis at 6 months of age. The typical flaring of the vertebral body at the apex is evident. No treatment was given. **B:** At 12 years of age, severe kyphosis with marked vertebral wedging has developed.

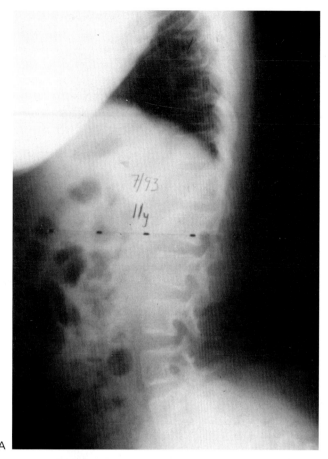

A

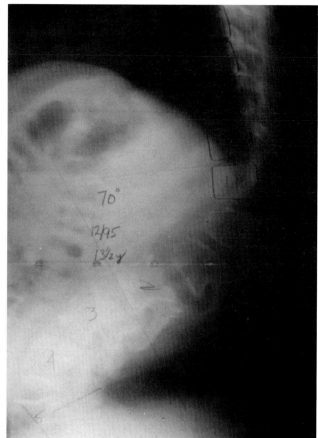

B

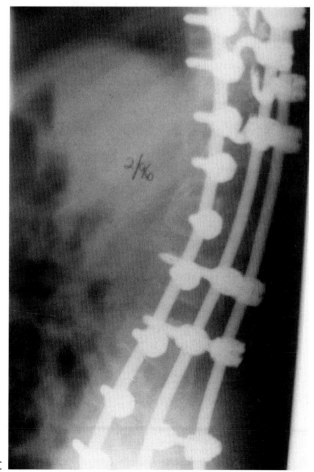

C

FIGURE 4. Images of a patient with achondroplasia and spinal stenosis that necessitated laminectomy of T10–S1 during adolescence. **A:** At the time of decompression, no stabilization had been performed. **B:** Ten months later, kyphosis of the thoracolumbar junction had progressed and was painful. **C:** Anterior and posterior stabilization was chosen because of the extreme kyphosis and limited size of posterior elements.

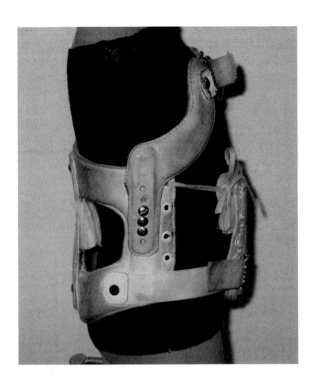

FIGURE 5. A chair-back brace is especially suitable for achondroplastic kyphosis because it does not impair abdominal movement and can be adjusted with growth. The posterior pad over the apex of the curve can be adjusted under direct vision.

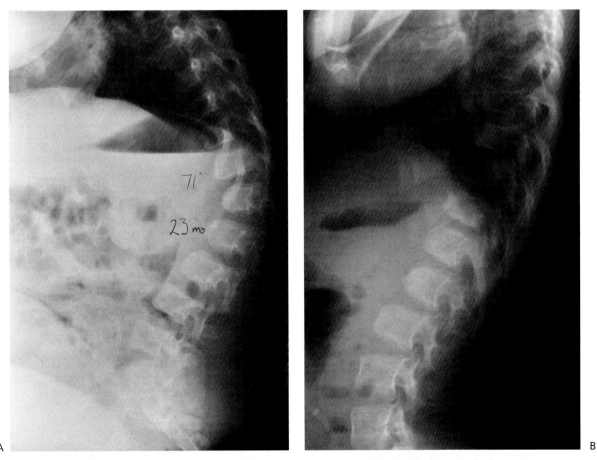

A

B

FIGURE 6. A: Image of a 5-year-old child who had a 71-degree curve that had not resolved. Severe thoracolumbar kyphosis improved with bracing. **B:** A hyperextension cast was used for 3 months and a brace for 1 year. The curve decreased to less than 20 degrees.

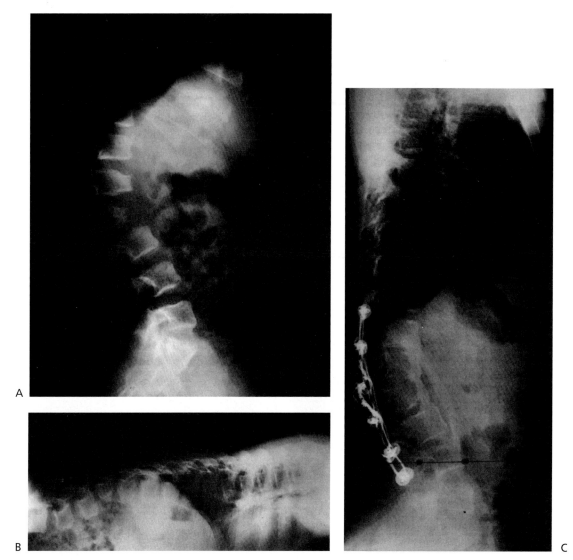

FIGURE 7. Lateral spinal radiograph of an 8-year-old child with achondroplasia shows residual 50-degree kyphosis with wedging of the apical vertebrae at L1 and L2. Resolution of kyphosis after this age is not expected. **B:** Prone lateral radiograph of the child in **A** shows partial correction of kyphosis. **C:** Lateral radiograph of the spine obtained immediately after anterior and posterior spinal fusion. Postoperative casting was used for 6 months. The patient could walk in the cast. *(Figure continues.)*

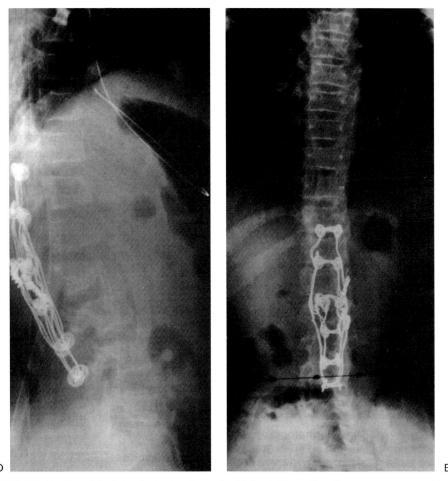

D   E

FIGURE 7. *Continued.* **D:** Lateral spinal radiograph obtained 19 months after surgery shows residual 30-degree kyphosis and solid bony fusion. The child was free of symptoms. **E:** Anteroposterior radiograph of the spine 19 months after anterior and posterior spinal fusion shows method of wiring used posteriorly between the spinous processes to act as a tension band and provide partial correction.

tigue in the thighs, knees, or legs after walking that is relieved by leaning forward and resting hands on the knees in a crouched position (52). Not being able to walk more than a block or two indicates considerable stenosis. Numbness or partial foot drop may complicate more serious cases. A thorough neurologic examination should be performed to evaluate hyperreflexia, weakness, hypoesthesia, and bowel and bladder function. If a deficit is found, or symptoms limit daily activities, posterior decompression probably is indicated. The level of the block is best determined with myelography and CT myelography, because MRI shows stenosis over such a wide region that the level of critical impingement is difficult to determine. The myelographic contrast agent is best introduced from the cervical region. CT usually shows that the canal is reduced to barely more than a slit at the lumbosacral level (Fig. 8). The decompression should be performed carefully. A burr is used to develop a trough on each side near the facets, and the laminae are carefully removed with a fine rongeur (98). Partial facetectomy is performed if needed, but most of the pathologic changes are central. Laminectomy should extend from one to two levels above the block, all the way to the sacrum. The lumbosacral area is difficult to expose for two reasons. First, lumbosacral lordosis is often greater than

normal (Fig. 9). Second, the ilia are very prominent posteriorly, and this configuration increases the distance to the laminae (Fig. 10). The dura is thin and often is adherent to the laminae, and dural tears are common. If a tear occurs, the lumbar nerve roots often protrude through it and are difficult to replace.

The degree of difficulty increases markedly if there is kyphosis along with the stenosis. If kyphosis is more than 20 to 30 degrees, fusion and instrumentation should be added to treatment. Pedicle screws should be used whenever possible; 5-mm screws may be necessary. Hooks should not be placed inside the canal wherever there is stenosis (Fig. 11). Correction should be minimal, if any; stabilization is the goal. Spinal cord monitoring should be conducted. The distal extent of fusion is a matter of controversy. Some surgeons believe fusion should extend to the sacrum to prevent junctional stenosis. Others believe it should extend to L4. Sacral screws are difficult to insert because of the narrowness of the sacrum and the prominence of the ilia. Iliac screws are another option. The historical incidence of postoperative neurologic deficits with this combined decompression and fusion is among the highest reported in spinal surgery, but it can be minimized by experience. The course of untreated stenosis is one of further worsening (73).

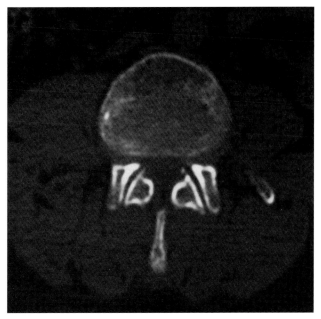

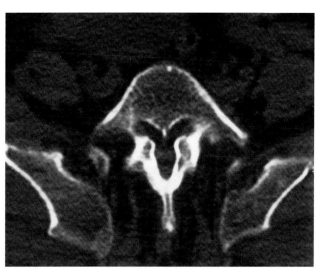

FIGURE 10. The posterior iliac crests in achondroplasia often project far posteriorly, and this configuration produces a deep space. Stenosis of the sacral canal is evident.

FIGURE 8. Computed tomographic scan of the lumbar spine of a patient with achondroplasia shows both central and foraminal stenosis.

Hypochondroplasia

Hypochondroplasia is a disorder distinct from but related to achondroplasia. Like achondroplasia, hypochondroplasia is caused by a mutation in fibroblast growth factor receptor protein 3, but the mutation occurs in a different domain (57). Stature is not as diminished as in achondroplasia and may reach the low

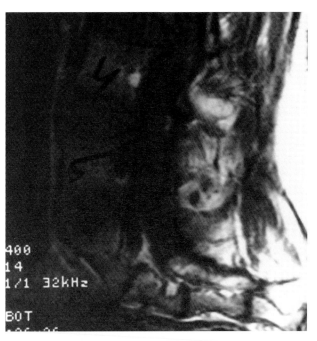

FIGURE 9. Lordosis of the lumbosacral junction in achondroplasia can be severe.

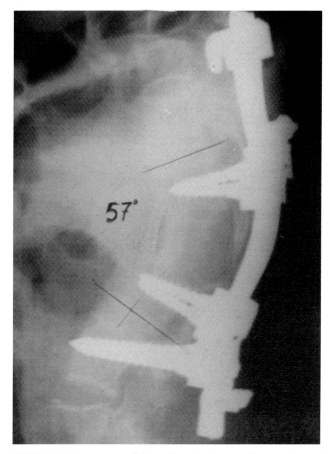

FIGURE 11. Appearance of the patient in Figure 3 after anterior and posterior decompression for symptomatic stenosis. Myelopathy had developed when the spine was corrected to a greater degree. The instrumentation was removed with complete neurologic recovery. One week later correction had occurred to the degree shown here.

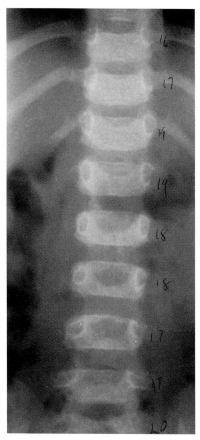

FIGURE 12. The spine of a 2-year-old with hypochondroplasia lacks the caudal narrowing of the pedicles typical of achondroplasia. However, the pedicles do not widen normally either. Mild platyspondyly is present.

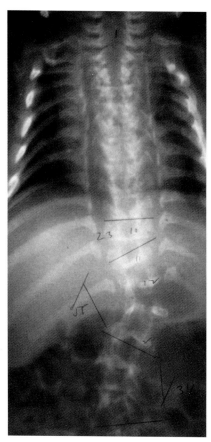

FIGURE 13. Radiograph of a patient with metatropic dysplasia shows early scoliosis, delayed vertebral mineralization, and hypoplasia of the thorax.

normal range (3,19). Midfacial hypoplasia is not noticeable. Spinal involvement is rare; only a small number of patients have caudal narrowing of the pedicles or kyphosis (24,26,78) (Fig. 12). Spinal decompression rarely is indicated, but when it becomes necessary, the principles of management of achondroplasia should be followed (see earlier).

Metatropic Dysplasia

Metatropic dysplasia is a rare disorder with a high infant mortality due to thoracic hypoplasia. It also is characterized by enlarged metaphyses, joint contractures, and a long, skin-covered coccygeal "tail." Spinal involvement is prominent with radiographic findings of flattening of all vertebrae. Some patients have odontoid hypoplasia with cervical instability. Scoliosis, often with kyphosis at the junction between curves, develops early among most patients (Fig. 13).

Treatment Implications

The cervical spine should be imaged in a neutral position when the patient is first examined to rule out subluxation (4,77,81), although lack of ossification may make it difficult to see detail

at an early age. The radiographs should be obtained in flexion and extension when the patient is older to rule out odontoid hypoplasia. If atlantoaxial translation is more than 5 mm on these radiographs, clinical signs of myelopathy should be sought or MRI performed in flexion. If clinical or radiographic evidence of cord compression is present, posterior fusion is indicated. Posterior fixation is not always possible if the patient is young or the bone quality is poor. Halo cast or halo vest immobilization is indicated until the fusion is solid. For young patients, halo pin torque has to be decreased to 2 to 4 inch-pounds (17).

Scoliosis has often been reported to exceed 90 degrees and to become quite rigid in adulthood. Paraparesis caused by the kyphotic component has been reported (7). Because these curves often arise in quite young children, it would be useful to know the efficacy of brace treatment. Unfortunately, no studies on this topic have been conducted. It is probably futile to brace curves greater than 45 degrees because of rigidity and lack of mechanical effectiveness. Larger curves should be managed surgically when they exceed this magnitude to prevent worsening of kyphosis. Indications for anterior release in addition to posterior fusion include skeletal immaturity or the presence of a rigid curve. Correction has been achieved by a period of carefully monitored halo traction between the two steps (7). Correction is nevertheless limited by the rigidity of the spine.

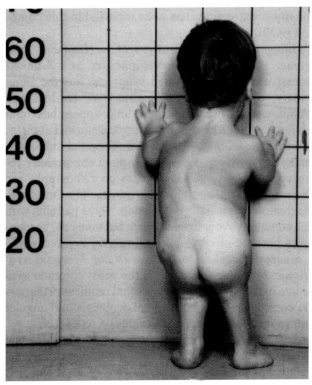

FIGURE 14. Image of a 2-year-old boy with diastrophic dysplasia and progressive severe thoracolumbar kyphosis. (Courtesy of Vernon T. Tolo, MD.)

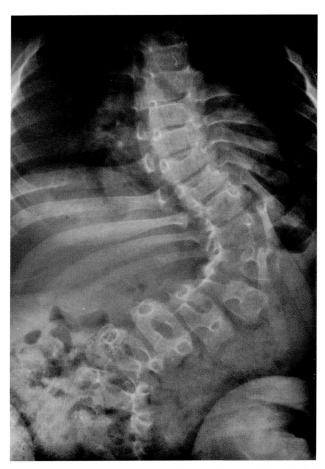

FIGURE 15. Image of a 6-year-old child with diastrophic dysplasia is advanced but resembles idiopathic scoliosis.

Diastrophic Dysplasia

Diastrophic dysplasia has possibly the most widespread and unique manifestations throughout the skeleton of any dysplasia (39,102). Patients show abducted (hitchhiker) thumbs, cauliflower ears, equinovarus feet, and multiple joint contractures with epiphyseal dysplasia (48,54) (Fig. 14). Possible spinal problems include cervical kyphosis, thoracolumbar scoliosis, and kyphosis. The genetic defect has been shown to be a defect in sulfate transport through all cartilage; the result is undersulfation of proteoglycans (31,32). The defect is transmitted in an autosomal recessive condition. The highest concentration of patients with this condition occurs in Finland, as do most clinical reports.

Clinical and Radiographic Findings

Throughout the spine, the vertebrae of persons with diastrophic dysplasia are relatively flat. The foramen magnum is abnormally wide. In the cervical spine, there is relative stenosis (6,102), but it rarely becomes clinically significant as it does in achondroplasia. Spina bifida may be present at any region of the spine, but it is usually in the form of occult clefts in the lamina. The discs appear underhydrated throughout life on MR images (75), most likely because of decreased sulfation of proteoglycans and a resultant decrease in water binding. Stiffness and degenerative changes begin relatively early. Trunk height remains very short throughout life.

The cervical spine of persons with diastrophic dysplasia usu-

ally does not have atlantoaxial instability, although a case has been reported (76). The most common neck problem is kyphosis in the midcervical spine. This occurs among about 15% of persons with diastrophic dysplasia (74,75). It is associated with spina bifida occulta of the same region. The vertebral bodies at the apex are hypoplastic. It is not clear whether the hypoplasia is primary or whether the bodies become underossified because of kyphosis. Amazingly, some cases have been reported to improve spontaneously, even with curves as large as 85 degrees (6,36). Some cases, however, do progress; they may exceed 100 degrees and can cause myelopathy (43).

The prevalence of scoliosis varies from 50% in some series (72) to 100% in others (6). The latter cases may be influenced by referral bias. Two types have been described—a gradual, idiopathic type of curve (Fig. 15) and a sharper, dystrophic curve, which is more difficult to manage (97).

Orthopaedic Treatment

Cervical Kyphosis

Frequent neurologic examinations should be performed. Cervical kyphosis initially should be followed to see whether it resolves spontaneously. Many cases do (6,36) (Fig. 16). The risk of ky-

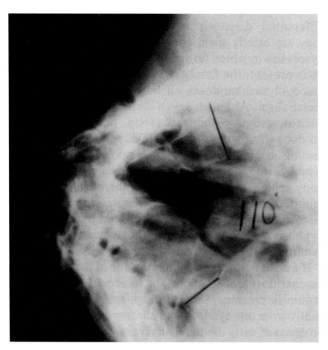

FIGURE 16. Kyphosis in diastrophic dysplasia can be focal. (Courtesy of Vernon T. Tolo, MD.)

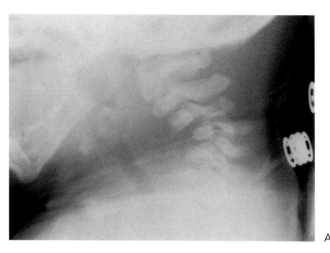

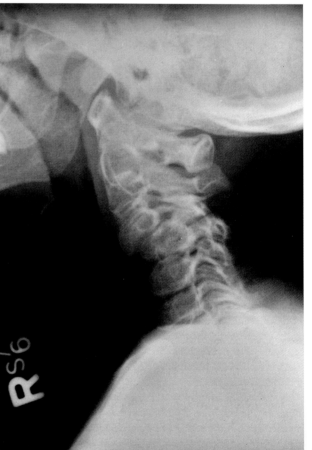

FIGURE 17. Images of a child with diastrophic dysplasia at 9 months **(A)** and 5 years **(B)** of age. Cervical kyphosis improved over time without treatment. At no time did the patient have evidence of myelopathy.

phosis is greater if the curve exceeds 50 degrees (74). If progression is observed, treatment with a Milwaukee brace has been associated with improvement. If the brace is not tolerated or treatment is not successful, surgical fusion may be necessary. Posterior fusion may allow spontaneous correction through anterior growth. Care should be exercised during the surgical approach because of the bifid posterior elements. Postoperative immobilization should be in a halo cast or halo vest. The best position achieved by means of careful passive stretching can be maintained with gentle distraction and use of a posterior pad behind the apex and suspended from the halo uprights. Immobilization should be continued until fusion can be documented radiographically, usually about 4 months. Additional protection in an orthosis can be carried out until the surgeon is confident of solid fusion. If the patient has myelopathy, anterior decompression may be indicated along with strut grafting and posterior fusion (6). This operation can be difficult, however, because of the small size of the patient and of the vertebrae at the time this problem develops. If postoperative pseudarthrosis at the apex develops, it should be corrected when it is detected, or recurrent deformity may develop.

Kyphosis

Kyphosis can develop in isolation or at the junction between two scoliotic curves. Improvement in the former type has been reported, usually with use of a Milwaukee brace. Because of the compact size of the patient, the brace must be carefully fitted and must be adjusted with age to maintain the corrective potential. If the kyphosis is severe and focal, surgery may be indicated to prevent neurologic compromise (Fig. 17).

Scoliosis

Scoliosis can be managed with a Milwaukee brace if it is not too great. Posterior fusion with instrumentation usually is indicated for larger curves. This procedure usually is combined with instrumentation. Sublaminar hook fixation can be used with care (97). For patients who are too small, halo cast immobiliza-

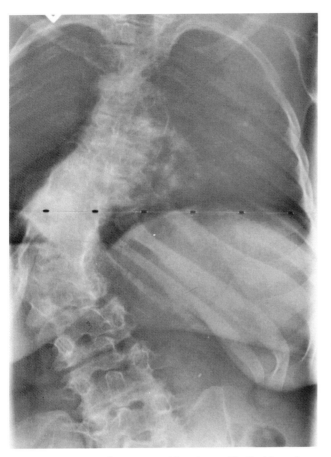

FIGURE 18. Image of a 35-year-old patient with Kneist syndrome shows scoliosis that has been stable at 46 degrees since the patient reached maturity.

tion can provide correction and stabilization. Spinal stenosis has not been reported to become a surgical problem (72).

Kneist Dysplasia

Kneist dysplasia is a disorder of type II collagen (12,71,105). It commonly results in enlarged, stiff joints (23,44,87). Many patients are disabled by retinal detachment (83,85). Radiographic changes include odontoid hypoplasia and severe platyspondyly with irregular end points as well as scoliosis, which usually is mild to moderate.

Orthopaedic Treatment

Patients should be observed with neurologic examinations and periodic lateral radiographs of the cervical spine (59). If marked instability is detected with either method, posterior fusion is indicated to prevent neurologic damage. Internal fixation may not be possible because of small bone size or young age, so halo cast immobilization may be indicated. Scoliosis rarely necessitates surgical treatment, possibly because the stiffness of the spine prevents curves from becoming too large (Fig. 18).

Spondyloepiphyseal Dysplasia Congenita, Tarda

Spondyloepiphyseal dysplasia is caused by a defect in type II collagen resulting from a mutation in COL2A1 at a location different from that of Kneist dysplasia (30,94,111). Spondyloepiphyseal dysplasia congenita causes more pronounced skeletal involvement and is inherited in an autosomal dominant pattern. The tarda form usually is X linked and therefore more common among boys and men (42,106,108). Severely short stature often results because of altered growth in both the spine and epiphyses.

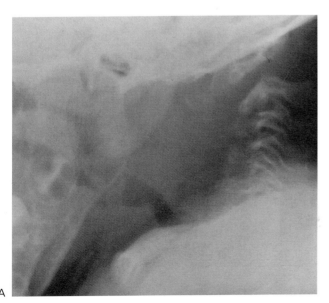

A

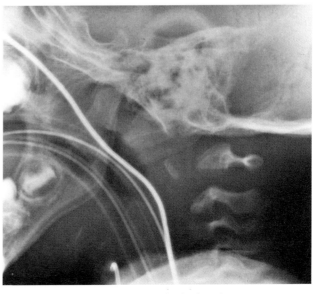

B

FIGURE 19. Images of a 3-year-old child with spondyloepiphyseal dysplasia congenita who had markedly delayed milestones and clonus show odontoid aplasia with atlantoaxial instability and stenosis at C1. **A:** Neutral upright showing subluxation. **B:** Repositioned in operating room. *(Figure continues.)*

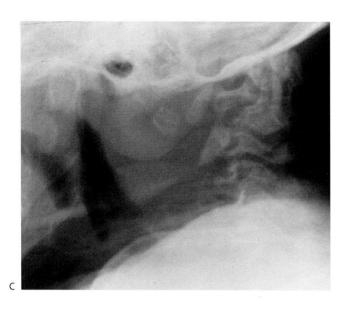

C

FIGURE 19. *Continued.* **C:** Solid fusion after C1 decompression and occipital-C2 fusion. Standing and walking improved gradually, although they remained limited by hip and knee contractures.

Several different spinal problems can develop, as can degenerative arthritis of the major joints. Retinal detachment can occur with spondyloepiphyseal dysplasia congenita. Radiographic findings include decreased vertebral and intervertebral height and posterior flattening of the vertebrae to form a pattern called *pear shaped* (86). The end plates are irregular. The second cervical vertebra may show os odontoideum, hypoplasia, or aplasia, although in many patients it is not unstable. The ring of C1 is stenotic in some patients. Kyphosis or scoliosis each develops in about one half of patients (7).

Orthopaedic Treatment

Approximately one third of children with spondyloepiphyseal dysplasia congenita have atlantoaxial instability. Cervical radiographs should be obtained at the initial evaluation. Flexion-extension lateral radiographs should be obtained if no static abnormality is present or if the shape of the odontoid cannot be determined from the plain radiographs. If an abnormality is present but is stable, radiographs still should be obtained periodically during follow-up care. If more than 5 mm of translation of the most cranial portion of the anterior arch of C1 with respect to the cranial portion of the body of C2 is seen on flexion-extension views and the findings of the neurologic examination are normal, the patient should be examined especially frequently. If the examination findings are abnormal or the translation is greater than 8 mm, the atlantoaxial interval should be fused in a reduced position (Fig. 19). If it cannot be reduced or if there is severe stenosis, the posterior arch of the atlas should be decompressed and the fusion extended to the occiput.

Thoracolumbar Spine

Kyphosis, which occurs among about one half of patients, responds to treatment with a Milwaukee brace among some patients during the growing years (7). If fusion is performed, the surgeon should consider anterior and posterior fusion or verify the solidity of the fusion mass, because considerable loss of cor-

rection has been reported after pseudarthrosis (7). The most common pattern of scoliosis is a double curve, which may become quite severe (Fig. 20). It is not as responsive to brace treatment as kyphosis is. Surgery may be indicated for large or progressive curves near adulthood (Fig. 21). Low-profile, segmental instrumentation should be used. Because of the rigidity of the curves, permanent correction is not impressive; it averaged only 17% success at follow-up evaluation in one series (7). Spon-

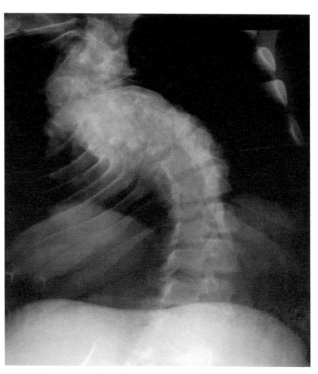

FIGURE 20. Image of a patient with spondyloepiphyseal dysplasia congenita shows severe, focal scoliosis.

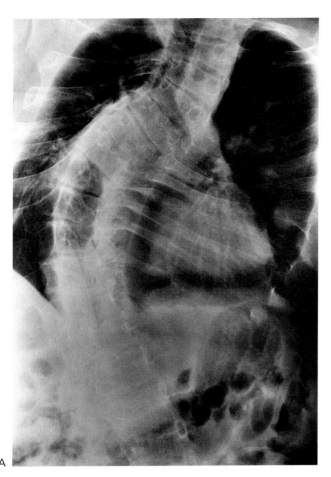

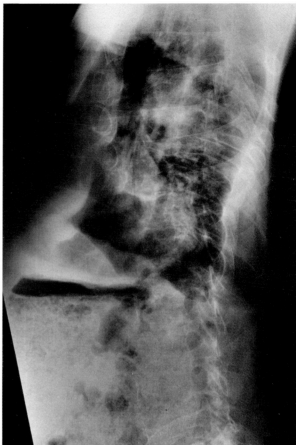

A

B

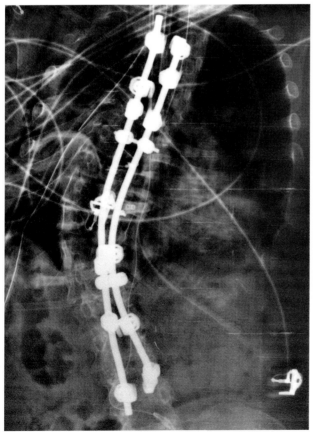

C

FIGURE 21. A, B: Images of a patient with spondyloepiphyseal dysplasia congenita who had progression of scoliosis during adulthood. **C:** After anterior release and posterior instrumented fusion, correction was achieved to the limit of the stiffness of the curve. (Courtesy of Michael C. Ain, MD).

dyloepiphyseal dysplasia tarda involves mild flattening of the thoracolumbar vertebrae and their disc spaces but rarely produces marked spinal deformity (42,69). If kyphosis or scoliosis develops, however, it should be managed as described earlier (Fig. 22).

Pseudoachondroplasia

Pseudoachondroplasia is caused by a defect in cartilage oligomeric matrix protein, an extracellular protein that is present in the territorial matrix of chondrocytes (13,15,34,67,89). Patients have nearly normal stature at birth, but stature lags with growth as abnormal matrix products accumulate (38,57,58,109). The patients have characteristic deformities, especially of the knees, which may become windswept (20,27,29,46).

The atlantoaxial segment can become unstable, although this is not common. Nevertheless, patients should be checked for this instability before undergoing surgery on the knees or hips. Treatment guidelines are the same as for spondyloepiphyseal dysplasia. Scoliosis of a mild degree may develop (Fig. 23). It should be managed with a brace if it exceeds 25 to 30 degrees (7). Surgery is not commonly needed.

Chondrodysplasia Punctata

Chondrodysplasia punctata refers to a series of disorders that produce punctate epiphyseal calcifications and generalized skeletal dysplasia (2,14,56,61). The most common forms are the Conradi-Hünermann type (18,84) and the rhizomelic type (22). The cause of the former is not known; the latter is an enzyme defect (79,107). The latter type is more severe and is most commonly fatal in infancy (103). It may be characterized by os odontoideum or odontoid hypoplasia (5). Cervical stenosis has been found in the recessive type, but whether to do anything to manage the stenosis depends on the patient's medical condition. We are not aware of any patients who undergone treatment of this disorder. The Conradi-Hünermann form may be associated with congenital vertebral malformations such as congenital scoliosis or congenital kyphosis. Patients with this disorder should be observed with periodic radiographs and undergo fusion if the condition is progressive.

Metaphyseal Chondrodysplasia

There are several types of metaphyseal chondrodysplasia (47). They are characterized by metaphyseal irregularities and bowing of the long bones. These conditions resemble rickets. The two most common types are Schmid type and McKusick type (55,92,99). The latter may also be associated with gastrointestinal and immune disturbances in childhood and with malignant disease in adulthood. Both types have been reported (7) to cause atlantoaxial instability in rare instances, so it is probably worth obtaining a cervical spinal radiograph to screen for this disorder.

Cleidocranial Dysplasia

Cleidocranial dysplasia is a condition characterized by complete or partial absence of the clavicles and a widened cranium

(8,25,40). The genetic defect is in the CBFA1 gene, which induces osteoblast differentiation (21,51,64). The stature usually is at the lower end of normal. A small proportion of these patients have been reported to have scoliosis associated with syringomyelia (16,93,100). Therefore they should be screened for scoliosis, and MRI should be performed if a marked curve develops.

Larsen Syndrome

Larsen syndrome is a condition best known for dislocation of multiple joints, including the elbows, hips, and knees, and the presence of equinovarus feet (49,50,101). Bifid posterior elements may occur at any level of the spine (9). Facial features include hypertelorism and a depressed nasal bridge (95). There usually is an accessory ossification center of the calcaneus. Because of the profound deformities of the skeleton, any developmental delay often is ascribed to them, and serious problems in the spine often are overlooked. This problem is severe cervical kyphosis that may develop along with cervical spina bifida; it may worsen to cause paraparesis (41). Spina bifida occulta is present in most patients, and the kyphosis is present in 12% to 50% of patients. The fourth and fifth cervical vertebral bodies may be extremely hypoplastic, either primarily or perhaps as a result of the pressure of kyphosis. Spontaneous improvement has not been reported to occur in this condition as it has in kyphosis occurring with diastrophic dysplasia (9,41). Symptoms include hypotonia, delay in motor milestones, or apnea. Sudden death has been reported among children with this syndrome. The deaths probably are caused by kyphosis (49,60). Other findings in the spine include atlantoaxial instability, spondylolysis of the lumbar spine, and scoliosis.

Orthopaedic Treatment

All patients with Larsen syndrome should have a cervical spinal radiograph obtained at the first orthopaedic visit. If the cervical kyphosis is greater than approximately 40 degrees, strong consideration should be given to posterior fusion in situ, so that correction can occur by means of anterior growth. Often this decision must be made when the patient is very young (less than 2 years) (41). If fusion is not performed at this time, the patient should be observed very closely so that any worsening can be detected and controlled. The fusion should extend from the neutral vertebrae above to those below the kyphosis. Care should be exercised in exposing the vertebrae because of the presence of bifid laminae. Postoperative immobilization should be performed with a halo cast or vest or with a Minerva cast. The solidity of the fusion mass should be visualized radiographically because pseudarthrosis can cause loss of correction (41). If the kyphosis is allowed to progress to more than 60 degrees, the likelihood of a successful posterior fusion diminishes.

Patients with myelopathic findings should undergo MRI. If marked cord compression is present, anterior decompression and anterior and posterior fusion should be performed (41).

Patients should be observed for atlantoaxial instability and scoliosis. Fewer than 5% to 10% of patients need surgical treat-

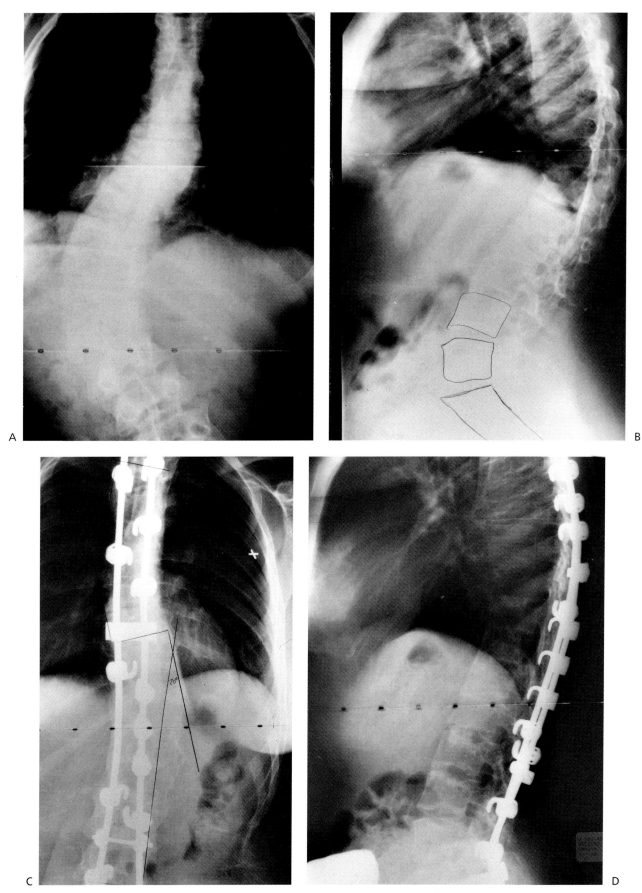

FIGURE 22. A to D: Spondyloepiphyseal dysplasia tarda can be associated with marked curvature of the spine, such as this painful, progressive kyphoscoliosis in a 15-year-old patient. Fusion was carried down to the sacrum because of painful degenerative changes in this area.

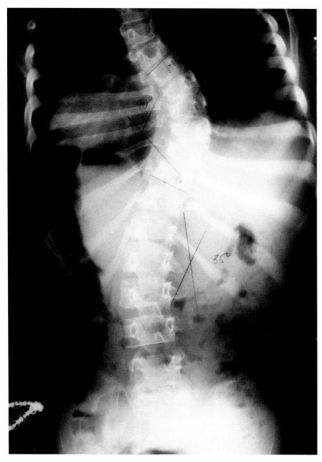

FIGURE 23. Scoliosis with pseudoachondroplasia.

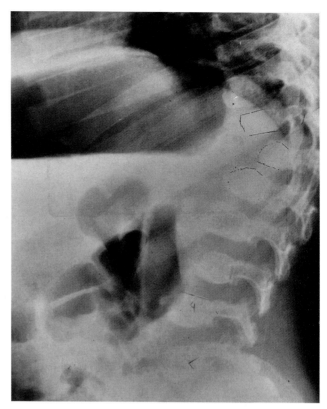

FIGURE 24. Thoracolumbar kyphosis with apical translation is common at the thoracolumbar junction in Hurler syndrome.

ment of either of these conditions (9). Painful lumbar kyphosis also has occurred (9).

Mucopolysaccharidosis

In mucopolysaccharidosis, a group of almost a dozen conditions, enzyme defects lead to intracellular buildup of metabolites. The skeletal effects may not become apparent until later in childhood, by which time other children may have been born into the family. Although specifics vary from subtype to subtype, the general pattern is short stature, organomegaly, epiphyseal abnormality, and risk of odontoid hypoplasia or upper cervical instability. The most common of these is the Hurler syndrome (mucopolysaccharidosis type I, which produces mental retardation and often death by the end of the first decade. With the advent of bone marrow transplantation, many patients live longer than this. In this condition, besides the upper cervical instability, marked kyphosis with vertebral translation may develop at the thoracolumbar junction and may necessitate treatment with a brace or surgery (Fig. 24). If the kyphosis is flexible, posterior reduction and stabilization are an option for treatment. Morquio syndrome (mucopolysaccharidosis type IV) is another disorder that usually involves spinal problems. The vertebrae are flattened, often with a characteristic flame-shaped pattern of

ossification. There patients have not only scoliosis and kyphosis of the thoracolumbar spine but also atlantoaxial instability. These patients often are limited by cardiopulmonary compromise, and evaluation should proceed if surgery is necessary.

Stickler Syndrome

Also known as *hereditary arthroophthalmopathy,* Stickler syndrome is characterized by myopia, risk of retinal detachment, tall stature, and premature degenerative joint disease. Inheritance is autosomal dominant. A defect in type II collagen is the basis of the disorder. A number of spinal abnormalities have been described, including block vertebrae, scoliosis, kyphosis, and narrowing of the intervertebral disc space. Some success with bracing has been reported. The main value of recognizing the syndrome is to encourage routine ophthalmologic follow-up evaluation.

Jarcho-Levin Syndrome

In 1938, Jarcho and Levin described a patient with numerous thoracic vertebral malformations, including hemivertebrae and bars, fused and absent ribs, a short trunk, and respiratory distress. A more common term for these conditions is *spondylothoracic* or *spondylocostal dysplasia.* Although many cases are sporadic, both autosomal recessive and dominant transmission have been

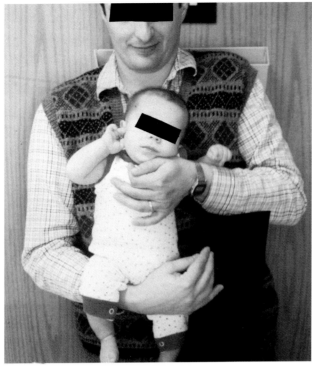

A

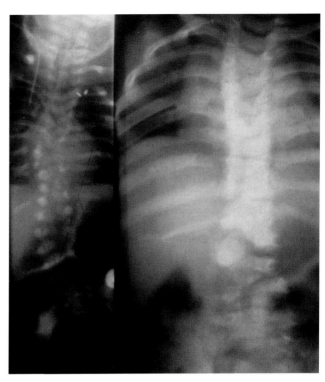

B

FIGURE 25. Spondylocostal dysplasia often is familial, as shown in this father-son **(A)** pair. A radiograph of the father at the same age is shown next to that of the son **(B)**.

observed (Fig. 25). The congenital spinal curve may be progressive, although there are many instances in which the vertebral malformations balance each other out, causing no net curvature. If net progression of considerable degree is observed, localized fusion over the progressive area is indicated, according to the guidelines for congenital scoliosis. The role of the fused ribs in progression of the deformity has not been conclusively shown. Do they act as a tether, or do they grow en masse with the spine? Does managing the bony rib dysplasia help either the curve or the patient's respiratory status? A clinical trial is ongoing to explore the effect of titanium rib expanders in the care of patients with infantile thoracic hypoplasia. The investigators' hypothesis is that both areas can be helped (10).

CONCLUSION

The subject of spinal disorders in skeletal dysplasia has become much better understood in the past two decades. This understanding has been fueled by the development of the specialty of medical genetics, which has improved diagnosis and centralized care. Nevertheless, gaps in our knowledge remain. In many disorders, we still do not know which thoracolumbar curves respond well to bracing and which may not. For many disorders there have been no outcome studies to show that surgery improves patients' health status, although in many cases it is reasonable to expect improvement. Research into these questions is hampered by the rarity of the conditions and by the substantial variation in expression of many of these disorders. For these

reasons, it is important that care of persons with skeletal dysplasia be provided in centers experienced and interested in these conditions. Continued research into the clinical care and basic science of skeletal dysplasia is critical and should yield more answers to these questions.

REFERENCES

1. Aldigheri R, et al. (1988): Lengthening of the lower limbs in achondroplastic patients. *J Bone Joint Surg Br* 70:69–73.
2. Andersen PE, Justesen P. (1987): Chondrodysplasia punctata: report of two cases. *Skeletal Radiol* 16:223.
3. Beals RK (1969): Hypochondroplasia: a report of five kindreds. *J Bone Joint Surg Am* 51:728–736.
4. Beck M, et al. (1983): Heterogeneity of metatropic dysplasia. *Eur J Pediatr* 140:231.
5. Bethem D (1982): Os odontoideum in chondrodystrophia calcificans congenita: a case report. *J Bone Joint Surg Am* 64:1385.
6. Bethem D, Winter RB, Lutter L (1981): Disorders of the spine in diastrophic dwarfism. *J Bone Joint Surg Am* 62:529–539.
7. Bethem D, Winter RB, Lutter L, et al. (1981): Spinal disorders of dwarfism: review of the literature and report of eighty cases. *J Bone Joint Surg Am* 63:1412–1425.
8. Bick EM, Marie P, Saiton P (1968): The classic: on hereditary cleidocranial dysostosis. *Clin Orthop* 58:5.
9. Bowen JR, et al. (1985): Spinal deformities in Larsen's syndrome. *Clin Orthop* 197:159–163.
10. Carey JC (1994): Titanium expandable rib implant. *Trans AAOS* 77: 1225–1225.
11. Carroll KL, et al. (1999): Clinical correlation to genetic variations of hereditary multiple exostosis. *J Pediatr Orthop* 19:785–791.
12. Cole WG (1997): Abnormal skeletal growth in Kneist dysplasia caused by type II collagen mutations. *Clin Orthop* 341:162–169.

13. Cooper RR, Ponseti IV, Maynard JA (1973): Pseudoachondroplastic dwarfism: a rough-surfaced endoplasmic reticulum storage disorder. *J Bone Joint Surg Am* 55:475.
14. Curry CJR, et al. (1984): Inherited chondrodysplasia punctata due to deletion of the terminal short arm of X-chromosome. *N Engl J Med* 311:1010.
15. Deere M, et al. (1999): Identification of nine novel mutations in COMP in patients with pseudoachondroplasia and multiple epiphyseal dysplasia. *Am J Med Genet* 85:486–490.
16. Dore DD, MacEwen GD, Boulos MI (1987): Cleidocranial dysostosis and syringomyelia: case report and review of the literature. *Clin Orthop* 214:231–234.
17. Dormans JP, et al. (1995): Complications in children managed with immobilization in a halo vest. *J Bone Joint Surg Am* 77:1370–1373.
18. Fairbank HAT (1949): Dysplasia epiphysealis punctata: symptoms—stippled epiphyses, chondrodystrophia calcificans congenita (Hunermann). *J Bone Joint Surg Br* 31:114.
19. Fasanelli S. (1999): Hypochondroplasia: radiological diagnosis and differential diagnosis. In: Nicoletti B, ed. *Human achondroplasia: a multidisciplinary approach.* New York: Plenum Press, pp. 163–166.
20. Ferguson HL, Deere M, Evans R, et al. (1999): Mosaicism in pseudoachondroplasia. *Am J Med Genet* 85:486–490.
21. Geoffroy V, et al. (1999): Genomic organization, expression of the human CBFA1 gene, and evidence for an alternative splicing event affecting protein function. *Mamm Genome* 9:54–57.
22. Gilbert EF, et al. (1976): Chondrodysplasia punctata: rhizomelic form, pathologic and radiographic studies of three infants. *Eur J Pediatr* 123:89.
23. Gilbert-Barnes E, Langer LO (1996): Kneist dysplasia: radiologic histopathologic and scanning em findings. *Am J Med Genet* 63:34–45.
24. Glass L, et al. (1981): Audiological findings of patients with achondroplasia. *J Pediatr Otorhinolaryngol* 129–135.
25. Gupta SK, et al. (1992): Cleidocranial dysostosis-skeletal abnormalities. *Australas Radiol* 36:238–242.
26. Hall BD, Spranger J (1979): Hypochondroplasia: clinical and radiological aspects in 39 cases. *Radiology* 133:95.
27. Hall JG (1975): Pseudoachondroplasia. *Birth Defects* 1:187.
28. Hall JG (1988): The natural history of achondroplasia. *Basic Life Sci* 48:3–9.
29. Hall JG, et al. (1969): Pseudoachondroplastic SED, recessive Maroteaux-Lamy type. *Birth Defects* 5:254.
30. Harrod MJ, et al. (1984): Genetic heterogeneity in spondyloepiphyseal dysplasia congenita. *Am J Med Genet* 18:311.
31. Hastbacka J, de la Chappelle A, Mahtani MM, et al. (1994): The diastrophic dysplasia gene encodes a novel sulfate transporter: positional cloning by fine-structure linkage disequilibrium mapping. *Cell* 78:1073–1087.
32. Hastbacka J, Sistonen P, Kaitila I, et al. (1991): A linkage map spanning the locus for diastrophic dysplasia (DTD). *Genomics* 11:968–973.
33. Hecht JT, Horton WA, Reid CS, et al. (1989): Growth of the foramen magnum in achondroplasia. *Am J Med Genet* 32:528–535.
34. Hecht JT, Montufar-Solis D, Decker G, et al. (1998): Retention of cartilage oligometric membrane protein (COMP) and cell death in dedifferentiated pseudoachondroplasia chondrocytes. *Matrix Biol* 17:625–633.
35. Hecht JT, Nelson FW, Butler IJ, et al. (1985): Computerized tomography of the foramen magnum: achondroplastic values compared to normal standards. *Am J Med Genet* 20:355–360.
36. Herring JA (1978): The spinal disorders in diastrophic dwarfism. *J Bone Joint Surg Am* 60:177.
37. Horton WA (1996): Evolution of the bone dysplasia family. *Am J Med Genet* 63:4–10.
38. Horton WA, Hall JG, Scott CI, et al. (1982): Growth curves for height for diastrophic dysplasia, spondyloepiphyseal dysplasia congenita and pseudoachondroplasia. *Am J Dis Child* 136:316–319.
39. Horton WA, Rimoin DL, Lachman RS, et al. (1978): The phenotypic variability of diastrophic dysplasia. *J Pediatr* 93:609–613.
40. Jarvis JL, Keats TE (1974): Cleidocranial dysostosis: a review of 40 new cases. *Am J Roentgenol Radium Ther Nucl Med* 121:5–16.
41. Johnston CE, Birch JG, Daniels JL (1996): Cervical kyphosis in patients who have Larsen syndrome. *J Bone Joint Surg Am* 78:538–548.
42. Kaibara N, Takagishi K, Katsuki I (1983): Spondyloepiphyseal dysplasia tarda with progressive arthropathy. *Skeletal Radiol* 10:10–13.
43. Kash IJ, Sane SM, Samaha FJ (1974): Cervical cord compression in diastrophic dwarfism. *J Pediatr* 78:862.
44. Kneist W (1952): Zur Abgrenzung der Dysostoses endochondralis von der Chondrodystrophie. *Z Kinder* 70:633.
45. Koop SE, Winter RB, Lonstein JE (1984): The surgical treatment of instability of the upper part of the cervical spine in children and adolescents. *J Bone Joint Surg Am* 66:403–502.
46. Kopits SE, Lindstrom JA, McKusick VA (1974): Pseudoachondroplastic dysplasia: pathodynamics and management. *Birth Defects* 10:341.
47. Kozlowski K (1976): Metaphyseal and spondylometaphyseal chondrodysplasia. *Clin Orthop* 114:83–93.
48. Lamy M, Maroteaux P (1960): Le nanisme diastrophicque. *Presse Med* 68:1977.
49. Larsen LJ, Schottstaedt ER, Bost FC (1950): Multiple congenital dislocations associated with characteristic facial abnormality. *J Pediatr* 37:574.
50. Laville JM, Lakermore P, Limouzy F (1994): Larsen's syndrome: review of the literature and analysis of thirty-eight cases. *J Pediatr Orthop* 14:63–73.
51. Lee B, et al. (1997): Missense mutations abolishing DNA binding of the osteoblast-specific transcription factor OSF2/CBFA1 in cleidocranial dysplasia. *Nat Genet* 16:307–310.
52. Lutter LD, Langer LO (1977): Neurological symptoms in achondroplastic. *J Bone Joint Surg Am* 59:87–92.
53. Lutter LD, Longestein JE, Winter RB, et al. (1977): Anatomy of the achondroplastic lumbar canal. *Clin Orthop* 126:139–142.
54. Makitie O, Kaitila I (1991): Growth in diastrophic dysplasia. *J Pediatr* 130:641–646.
55. Makitie O, Kaitila I (1993): Cartilage-hair hypoplasia: clinical manifestations in 108 Finnish patients. *Eur J Pediatr* 152:211–217.
56. Manzke H, Christophers E, Wiedmann HR (1980): Dominant sex-linked inherited chondrodysplasia punctata. *Clin Genet* 17:97.
57. Maroteaux P, Lamy M (1959): Les formes pseudoachondroplastique des dysplasies spondyloepisaires. *Presse Med* 67:383.
58. McKeand J, Rotta J, Hecht JT (1996): Natural history study of pseudoachondroplasia. *Am J Med Genet* 63:406–410.
59. Merrill KD (1990): Occipitoatlantal instability in a child with Kneist syndrome. *J Pediatr* 116:596.
60. Micheli LJ, Hall JE, Watts HG (1976): Spinal instability in Larsen syndrome: report of three cases. *J Bone Joint Surg Am* 58:562.
61. Mueller RF, et al. (1985): X-linked dominant chondrodysplasia punctata. *Am J Med Genet* 20:137.
62. Muenke M, Schell U (1981): Fibroblast growth factor receptor mutations in human skeletal disorders. *Trends Genet* 11:308–313.
63. Nehme AME, Riseborough EJ, Tredwell SJ (1976): Skeletal growth and development of the achondroplastic dwarf. *Clin Orthop* 116:88–23.
64. Otto F, Thornell AP, Crompton T (1997): cfba1, a candidate gene for cleidocranial dysplasia syndrome, is essential for osteoblast differentiation and bone development. *Cell* 89:765–771.
65. Pauli RM, Breed A, Horton VK, et al. (1997): Prevention of fixed, angular kyphosis in achondroplasia. *J Pediatr Orthop* 17:726–733.
66. Pauli RM, Horton VK, Glinski LP, et al. (1995): Prospective assessment of risks for cervicomedullary-junction compression in infants with achondroplasia. *Am J Hum Genet* 56:732–744.
67. Pedrini-Mille A, Maynard JA, Pedrini VA (1984): Pseudoachondroplasia: biochemical and histochemical studies of cartilage. *J Bone Joint Surg Am* 66:1408.
68. Pierre-Kahn A, Hirsch JF, Renier D (1980): Hydrocephalus and achondroplasia: a study of 25 observations. *Childs Brain* 7:205.
69. Pinelli G, Cottefava F, Senes FM (1988): Spondyloepiphyseal dysplasia tarda: linkage with genetic markers from the distal short arm of the X chromosome. *Hum Genet* 81:61.
70. Ponseti IV (1970): Skeletal growth in achondroplasia. *J Bone Joint Surg Am* 52:701–716.

71. Poole AR, et al. (1988): Kneist dysplasia is characterized by an apparent abnormal processing of the C-propeptide of type II collagen resulting in imperfect fibril assembly. *J Clin Invest* 81:579.

72. Poussa M, et al. (1991): The spine in diastrophic dysplasia. *Spine* 16:881.

73. Pyeritz RE, Sack G.H, Udvarhelyi GB (1987): Thoracolumbosacral laminectomy in achondroplasia: long-term results in 22 patients. *Am J Med Genet* 28:433–444.

74. Remes V, Marttinen E, Poussa M, et al. (1999): Cervical kyphosis in diastrophic dysplasia. *Spine* 24:1990–1995.

75. Remes V, Tervahartiala P, Poussa M, et al. (2000): Cervical spine in diastrophic dysplasia: an MRI analysis. *J Pediatr Orthop* 20:48–53.

76. Richards BS (1991): Atlanto-axial instability in diastrophic dysplasia: a case report. *J Bone Joint Surg Am* 73:614.

77. Rimoin DW, et al. (1982): Metatropic dwarfism, the Kneist syndrome and the pseudoachondroplastic dysplasias. *Clin Orthop* 176:70.

78. Rousseau F, et al. (1996): Clinical and genetic heterogeneity of hypochondroplasia. *J Med Genet* 33:749–752.

79. Sheffield LJ, et al. (1989): Clinical, radiologic, and biochemical classification of chondrodysplasia punctata. *Am J Med Genet* 1989; 45[Suppl]:A64.

80. Shiang R, et al. (1994): Mutations in the transmembrane domain of fgfr3 cause the most common genetic form of dwarfism, achondroplasia. *Cell* 78:335–342.

81. Shohat M, Lachman R, Rimoin DL (1989): Odontoid hypoplasia with vertebral subluxation and ventriculomegaly in metatropic dysplasia. *J Pediatr* 114:239.

82. Siebens AA, Hungerford DS, Kirby NA (1978): Curves of the achondroplastic spine: a new hypothesis. *Johns Hopkins Med J* 142:205–210.

83. Siggers DC, et al. (1974): The Kneist syndrome. *Birth Defects* 10:193.

84. Silengo MC, Luzzatti L, Silverman FN (1980): Clinical and genetic aspects of Conradi-Hunermann disease: a report of three familial cases and review of the literature. *J Pediatr* 97:911.

85. Spranger J, Winterpracht A, Zabel B (1997): Kneist dysplasia: Dr. W. Kneist, his patient, the molecular defect. *Am J Med Genet* 69:79–84.

86. Spranger JW, Langer LO JR (1970): Spondyloepiphyseal dysplasia congenita. *Radiology* 94:313.

87. Spranger JW, Maroteaux P (1974): Kneist disease. *Birth Defects* 10:50.

88. Stabler CL, et al. (1985): Failure of posterior cervical fusions using cadaveric bone graft in children. *J Bone Joint Surg Am* 67:370–375.

89. Stevens JW (1999): Pseudoachondroplastic dysplasia: an Iowa review from human to mouse. *Iowa Orthop J* 19:53–57.

90. Stokes DC, Pyeritz RE, Wise RA, et al. (1988): Spirometry and chest wall dimensions in achondroplasia. *Chest* 1988 93:34.

91. Stokes DC, Wohl ME, Wise RA, et al. (1990): The lungs and airways in achondroplasia: do little people have little lungs? *Chest* 98:145–152.

92. Sulisalo T, et al. (1995): Genetic homogeneity of cartilage-hair hypoplasia. *Hum Genet* 95:157–160.

93. Taglialavoro G, Fabris D, Agostini S (1999): A case of progressive scoliosis in a patient with craniocleidopelvic dysostosis. *Ital J Orthop Traumatol* 9:507–513.

94. Tiller GE, et al. (1995): An RNA-splicing mutation in the type II collagen gene in a family with spondyloepiphyseal dysplasia congenita. *Am J Hum Genet* 56:388–395.

95. Tobias JD (1996): Anesthetic implications of Larsen syndrome. *J Clin Anesth* 8:255–257.

96. Tolo VT (1986): Surgical treatment of kyphosis. In: Nicoletti B, ed. *Human achondroplasia: a multidisciplinary approach.* New York, Plenum Press, pp. 257–263.

97. Tolo VT, Kopits SE (1983): Spinal deformity in diastrophic dysplasia. *Orthop Trans* 7:31.

98. Uematsu S, Hurko O (1986): The subarachnoid fluid space in achondroplastic spinal stenosis: the surgical implications. In: Nicoletti B, ed. *Human achondroplasia: a multidisciplinary approach.* New York: Plenum Press, pp. 275–283.

99. van der Burgt I, et al. (1991): Cartilage hair hypoplasia. description of seven patients and review of the literature. *Am J Med Genet* 41:371–380.

100. Vari R, Puca A, Meglio M (1996): Cleidocranial dysplasia and syringomyelia. *J Neurol Sci* 49:125–128.

101. Vujic M, et al. (1999): Localization of a gene for autosomal dominant Larsen syndrome to chromosome region 3p21.1–14.1 in the proximity of, but distinct from, the COL7A1 locus. *Am J Hum Genet* 57:1104–1113.

102. Walker BA, et al. (1972): Diastrophic dwarfism. *Medicine (Baltimore)* 51:41.

103. Wardinsky TD, et al. (1990): Rhizomelic chondrodysplasia punctata and survival beyond one year: a review of the literature and five case reports. *Clin Genet* 38:84.

104. Waters KA, et al. (1995): Treatment of obstructive sleep apnea in achondroplasia: evaluation of sleep, breathing and somatosensory-evoked potentials. *Am J Med Genet* 59:460–466.

105. Wilkin DJ, et al. (1999): Small deletions in the type II collagen triple helix produce Kneist dysplasia. *Am J Med Genet* 85:105–112.

106. Williams B, Cranley RE (1974): Morphologic observations on four cases of SED congenita. *Birth Defects* 10:75.

107. Wulfsberg EA, Curtis J, Jayne CH (1992): Chondrodysplasia punctata: a boy linked with X-linked recessive chondrodysplasia punctata due to an inherited X-Y translocation with a current classification of these disorders. *Am J Med Genet* 43:823.

108. Wynne-Davies R, Hall C (1982): Two clinical variants of spondyloepiphyseal dysplasia congenita. *J Bone Joint Surg Br* 64:435.

109. Wynne-Davies R, Hall CM, Young ID (1986): Pseudoachondroplasia: clinical diagnosis at different ages and comparison of autosomal dominant and recessive types: a review of 32 patients. *J Med Genet* 23:425–434.

110. Wynn-Davies R, Walsh WK, Gormley J (1981): Achondroplasia and hypochondroplasia: clinical variation and spinal stenosis. *J Bone Joint Surg Br* 63:508–515,.

111. Yang SS, et al. (1980): Spondyloepiphyseal dysplasia congenita: a comparative study of chondrocyte inclusions. *Arch Pathol Lab Med* 104–208.

112. Zucconi M, et al. (1996): Sleep and upper airway obstruction in children with achondroplasia. *J Pediatr* 129:743–749.

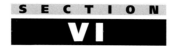

SECTION VI

DEVELOPMENTAL ABNORMALITIES

DEVELOPMENTAL ABNORMALITIES OF THE CERVICAL SPINE

RANDALL T. LODER
ROBERT N. HENSINGER

TORTICOLLIS

Torticollis is a combined head tilt and rotatory deformity. Pure torticollis indicates a problem at C1–2, whereas a head tilt alone indicates a more generalized problem in the cervical spine. The differential diagnosis of torticollis (Table 1) is large.

Nonosseous Types

Congenital Muscular Torticollis

Congenital muscular torticollis is the most common cause of torticollis among infants and young children. A disproportionate number of these children have a history of primiparous birth or breech or difficult delivery. The deformity is caused by contracture of the sternocleidomastoid muscle. The head tilts toward the involved side, and the chin rotates toward the opposite shoulder (Fig. 1). If the child is examined during the first 4 weeks of life, a mass or "tumor" may be palpable in the neck (43). This mass usually is a nontender, soft enlargement beneath the skin and attached to or located within the belly of the sternocleidomastoid muscle. This tumor reaches its maximum size within the first 4 weeks of life and gradually regresses. After 4 to 6 months of life, only the contracture and the torticollis remain. Because there is an association with developmental dysplasia of the hip (43), a careful hip examination should be performed. If the deformity is progressive, deformities of the skull and face (plagiocephaly) can develop, often within the first year of life. The facial flattening occurs on the side of the contracted muscle. If a child is untreated for many years, the levels of the eyes and ears become unequal and there is considerable cosmetic deformity.

The cause of congenital muscular torticollis is unknown. One theory is that it is a compartment syndrome caused by compression on the soft tissues of the neck during delivery. The histopathologic features of resected surgical specimens suggest that the lesion may be caused by occlusion of the venous outflow of the sternocleidomastoid muscle (8) with edema, degeneration of muscle fibers, and fibrosis of the muscle body. The amount of fibrosis is variable. It has been suggested that the clinical deformity is related to the ratio of fibrosis to remaining functional muscle. If ample muscle remains, the sternocleidomastoid will probably stretch with growth, and the child will not have torticollis. If fibrosis predominates, there is little elastic potential, and torticollis will develop. With the passage of time, the fibrosis of the sternal head may entrap the branch of the spinal accessory nerve to the clavicular head of the muscle; the result can be a later progressive deformity (63). Another theory is in utero crowding, because three of four children have the lesion on the right side and there is an association with developmental hip dysplasia. The final theory concerns remnant mesenchymal cells in the sternocleidomastoid from its embryogenesis (73). After birth, environmental changes stimulate these cells to differentiate, and the sternocleidomastoid tumor develops. If the myoblasts undergo normal development and differentiation, no persistent torticollis occurs and conservative treatment will likely succeed. If the myoblasts mainly undergo degeneration, the remaining fibroblasts produce large amounts of collagen with sternocleidomastoid contracture and typical torticollis.

Radiographs of the cervical spine should be obtained to rule out congenital vertebral anomalies. These are always normal among children with muscular torticollis, aside from the head tilt and rotation. If there is any concern about the hips, appropriate imaging should be performed.

Treatment consists of nonoperative measures first and surgical measures when those fail. A success rate as high as 90% success can be expected with stretching exercises alone (5). The exercises are performed by the caregivers and guided by a physiotherapist. The ear opposite the contracted muscle should be positioned to the shoulder, and the chin should be positioned to touch the shoulder on the same side as the contracted muscle. When adequate stretching has occurred in the neutral position, the exercises should be graduated up to the extended position, which will achieve maximum stretching and prevent residual contractures. Other treatment consists of modifying the child's toys and crib so that the infant will extend his or her neck when reaching for or looking at objects of interest.

Surgery is recommended after 1 year of age, because stretch-

R.T. Loder: Shriners Hospital for Children, Minneapolis, Minnesota 55414.
R.N. Hensinger: Section of Orthopaedic Surgery, University of Michigan Medical School, Ann Arbor, Michigan 48109.

TABLE 1. DIFFERENTIAL DIAGNOSIS OF TORTICOLLIS

Congenital
  Occipitocervical anomalies
  Basilar impression–primary
  Atlanto-occipital anomalies
  Asymmetry of occipital condyles
  Unilateral absence of C1 facet
  Odontoid anomalies (aplasia, hypoplasia, os odontoideum)
  Klippel-Feil syndrome
  Familial cervical dysplasia
  Pterygium colli
  Congenital muscular torticollis
Acquired
  Basilar impression–secondary
  Idiopathic/inflammatory
  Atlantoaxial rotary displacement, subluxation, fixation
  Neurogenic
  Spinal cord tumors
Cerebellar tumors, posterior fossa tumors
  Syringomyelia
  Ocular dysfunction
Bulbar palsy
  Arnold-Chiari malformation
Inflammatory
  Cervical adenitis, Grisel syndrome, retropharyngeal abscess
  Juvenile rheumatoid arthritis, rheumatoid arthritis
Disc space calcification
Tuberculosis
Neoplasm
  Osteoid osteoma
  Aneurysmal bone cyst
Sandifer syndrome

ing measures are then usually unsuccessful (17). Established facial deformity or a loss of more than 30 degrees of motion usually precludes a good result with stretching alone, and surgery is needed to prevent further facial flattening and cosmetic deterioration. Asymmetry of the face and skull can improve as long as adequate growth potential remains after the deforming pull of the sternocleidomastoid is removed.

Surgical options include a unipolar release at either the sternoclavicular or mastoid pole, bipolar release, and even complete resection. Bipolar release (Fig. 2) combined with Z-plasty of the sternal attachment yielded 92% satisfactory results in one series, whereas only 15% satisfactory results were obtained with other procedures (17). The Z-plasty maintains the *V* contour of the neck for improved appearance. Care must be taken during surgery not to transect the spinal accessory nerve, the anterior and external jugular veins, the carotid vessels and sheath, or the facial nerve. Skin incisions should never be located directly over the clavicle because of unacceptable scar spreading. The incisions should be made one finger breadth proximal to the medial end of the clavicle and sternal notch and in line with the cervical skin creases. The postoperative protocol can vary from simple stretching exercises to cast immobilization, depending on the severity of the torticollis, the ease and amount of correction achieved intraoperatively, and the cooperation of the child with stretching exercises.

Sandifer Syndrome

Sandifer syndrome involves gastroesophageal reflux with abnormal posturing of the neck and trunk, usually torticollis (58). It

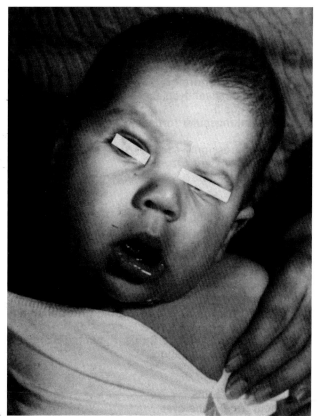

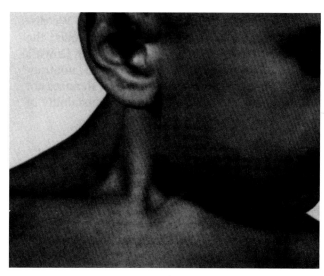

FIGURE 1. A: A 6-month-old infant with right-sided congenital muscular torticollis. Rotation of the skull and asymmetry and flattening of the face on the side of the contracted sternocleidomastoid are evident. **B:** An older child with a right-sided congenital muscular torticollis. Prominence of the sternal and clavicular heads and the tight and shortened belly of the sternocleidomastoid muscle are evident.

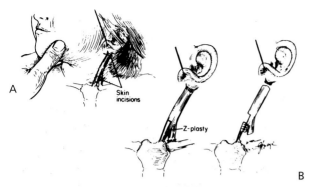

FIGURE 2. Z-plasty for torticollis. **A:** Location of the skin incisions. **B:** The clavicular and mastoid attachments of the sternocleidomastoid muscle are cut, and Z-plasty is performed. The medial aspect of the sternal attachment is preserved. (From Ferkel RD, Westin GW, Dawson EG, et al. [1983]: Muscular torticollis: a modified surgical approach. *J Bone Joint Surg Am* 65:894–900, with permission.)

is common among infants or children with cerebral palsy. The torticollis is the child's attempt to decrease the discomfort of gastroesophageal reflux. The incidence of gastroesophageal reflux among infants is as high as 40% (7). The principal symptoms are vomiting, failure to thrive, recurrent respiratory disease, dysphagia, various neural signs, torticollis, and even respiratory arrest. In careful examination of these infants, the tight and short sternocleidomastoid muscle or its tumor is not seen, eliminating congenital muscular torticollis. If further evaluation excludes dysplasia and congenital anomalies of the cervical spine, postinfectious causes, central nervous system and ocular disorders, Sandifer syndrome should be considered.

Radiographs of the cervical spine, which are normal in Sandifer syndrome, should be obtained to rule out congenital anomalies or dysplasia. Contrast studies of the upper gastrointestinal tract demonstrate hiatal hernia or gastroesophageal reflux. An esophageal pH study also may be necessary (32). Treatment, once the diagnosis has been made, starts with medical therapy. When this fails, fundoplication can be considered.

Neurogenic Causes

Although neurogenic causes are rare, they should be considered in the differential diagnosis of any torticollis that is unusual, especially when it is unresponsive or progressive in the face of appropriate therapy. The major neurogenic causes are central nervous system tumors, syringomyelia, Arnold-Chiari malformation, ocular dysfunction, and paroxysmal torticollis of infancy.

Posterior fossa tumors can manifest as torticollis (72) and may mimic a local ocular inflammatory condition (37). Tumors of the cervical spinal cord also can manifest as torticollis, often early in their course. Signs of such tumors that often are overlooked are spinal rigidity, early spinal deformity, and spontaneous or induced vertebral pain (24). Among young children the pain may be expressed as irritability and restlessness. Imaging of a child with a potential central nervous system tumor should consist of plain radiography of the skull and cervical spine followed by magnetic resonance imaging (MRI). Vertebral angiography also may be needed for neurosurgical planning.

The Arnold-Chiari malformation is downward displacement of the medulla oblongata with extrusion of the cerebellar tonsils through the foramen magnum. It is encountered among older children (12) and often is associated with headaches and paracervical muscle spasm. The evaluation of a child with a potential Chiari malformation consists of plain radiography of the skull and cervical spine followed by MRI. Treatment is neurosurgical.

Ocular dysfunction can cause atypical torticollis (61,80). The face may be simply turned about a vertical axis; the head may be tilted to one shoulder with the frontal plane of the face remaining coronal; or the chin may be elevated or depressed. The abnormal head position is assumed to optimize visual acuity or maintain binocularity. A detailed ophthalmologic examination established the diagnosis. Therapy for ocular torticollis usually is surgical.

Paroxysmal torticollis of infancy is a rare, episodic type of torticollis that lasts for minutes to days with spontaneous recovery (53). The attacks usually occur in the morning, last from 10 minutes to 14 days (variable within and between individuals), and have a frequency of less than one per month to three or four per month. The attacks can be associated with lateral trunk curvature, eye movements or deviations, and alternating sides of torticollis. The children are more commonly girls (71%). The average age at onset is 3 months (range 1 week to 30 months), and the average time of recovery is 24 months (range 6 months to 5 years). Paroxysmal torticollis of infancy may be an equivalent of a migraine headache—29% of patients have a family history of migraine—or a forerunner of benign paroxysmal vertigo of childhood. Whatever the cause, paroxysmal torticollis usually is self-limiting and does not necessitate therapy.

Inflammatory Causes

Juvenile Rheumatoid Arthritis

The subtypes of juvenile rheumatoid arthritis that usually involve the cervical spine are those of polyarticular or systemic onset; the pauciarticular type rarely affects the cervical spine (27). These children come to medical attention with neck stiffness, usually in the first 1 to 2 years after onset of the disease. Pain and torticollis are rare; when they occur, causes other than arthritis, such as fracture, infection, or tumor, should be suspected (27). Neurologic findings are infrequent.

The radiographic features (27) consist of the following seven types (Fig. 3): anterior erosion of the odontoid process, anterior-posterior erosion of the odontoid process (apple-core lesion), subluxation of C1 on C2, focal soft-tissue calcification anterior to the ring of C1, apophyseal joint ankylosis, growth abnormalities, and subaxial subluxations between C2 and C7. Although mild hypermobility at C1–2 may exist, true instability or myelopathy is rare. Basilar invagination, common in adult rheumatoid arthritis, is rare in juvenile rheumatoid arthritis. The radiographic findings of juvenile rheumatoid arthritis that are most different from those of adult rheumatoid arthritis are late destruction of articular cartilage and bone, growth disturbances, spondylitis with associated vertebral subluxation, apophyseal joint ankylosis, and micrognathia (27). Other imaging studies are occasionally needed in the evaluation of a child with juvenile

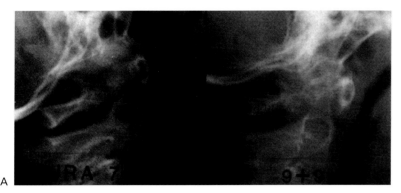

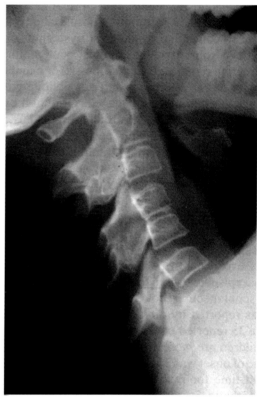

FIGURE 3. **A:** Images of a boy with polyarticular juvenile rheumatoid arthritis who at age 7 years shows only slight erosion in the anterior portion of the odontoid process. By 9 years of age there is anterior and posterior erosion of the odontoid process, called the *apple-core lesion.* **B:** Image of a 13-year-old girl with polyarticular juvenile rheumatoid arthritis. Posterior ankylosis is present at C2–3 and C3–4. The vertebral bodies are small, and the disc space between the involved segments is of minimal height. (From Hensinger RN, DeVito PD, Ragsdale CG [1986]: Changes in the cervical spine in juvenile rheumatoid arthritis. *J Bone Joint Surg Am* 68:189–198, with permission.)

rheumatoid arthritis and pain to look for occult fractures, infections, and bony tumors. Bone scans can pinpoint the exact anatomic location of activity, and computed tomography (CT) can be used to study the anatomic features in detail.

The presence of inflammatory synovitis and pannus of the synovial ring around the odontoid process causes odontoid erosion. This pannus erodes both anteriorly and posteriorly but leaves the apical and alar ligament attachments free, producing an apple-core lesion. This apple-core lesion is susceptible to fracture. Ankylosis of the apophyseal joints often affects young children. This posterior ankylosis of the immature cervical spine acts as a tether to prevent further anterior growth; the result is a decrease in disc space height and the size of the vertebral bodies (both longitudinally and circumferentially).

Treatment generally is nonsurgical in conjunction with good rheumatologic care. A cervical collar is recommended for patients those with involvement of the odontoid process or subaxial subluxation whenever they are in an automobile or other vehicle. If these patients need surgery for any reason, intubation can be difficult because of micrognathia, flexion deformity, and neck stiffness. Cervical fusion should be reserved for the rare child with documented instability and progressive neurologic deterioration.

Intervertebral Disc Calcification

More than 100 cases of intervertebral disc calcification have been reported in the literature (70). The cause is unclear. Theories include antecedent trauma and recent upper respiratory infection. There is no evidence to suggest a metabolic disorder or an accelerated aging process. This disorder is slightly more common among boys than among girls (7:5 ratio). The average age at presentation is 8 years (range 8 days to 13 years). Calcification is most common in the cervical spine, where it is especially symptomatic. About one half of children have neck pain (70) as the initial symptoms; torticollis occurs among approximately one fourth of patients. The onset of symptoms is abrupt, 12 to 48 hours, and 23% of patients have a fever when they come to medical attention. Decreased cervical motion and spinal tenderness also can occur. Radicular signs and symptoms are rare but never without local symptoms. Myelopathy is very rare.

Calcified deposits delineate the nucleus pulposus (Fig. 4A). The number of calcified discs averages 1.7 per child (70). Children without symptoms do not have protrusions, but children with symptoms frequently have detectable protrusions. MRI may show involvement of the vertebral body (29) (Fig. 4B).

Two thirds of children are symptom free within 3 weeks, and 95% by 6 months. Regression or disappearance of the calcific deposits occurs among 90% of patients; about one half of this improvement occurs within 6 months. Children without symptoms may not have radiographic regression even when observed for long periods. Children with multiple lesions have different rates of regression at the different disc levels.

Because of the course of the disorder, treatment is symptomatic in the absence of spinal cord compression. Analgesics, sedation, and cervical traction can be used, depending on the severity of symptoms. A short trial of a soft cervical collar also may be helpful. Surgical intervention is needed only for myelopathy or severe radiculopathy (49,69).

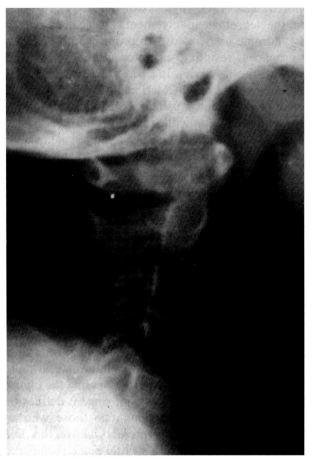

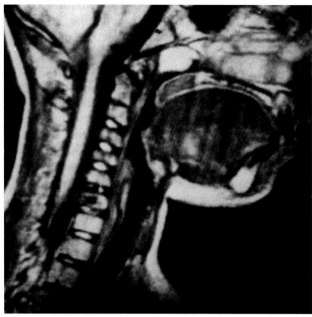

FIGURE 4. A: Lateral radiograph of a child with cervical disc calcification at the C3–4 interspace. **B:** Lateral magnetic resonance image of a child 1 month after onset of pain from cervical disc calcification. Disc abnormalities and decreased signal of the body of C6 are present. (From Herring JA, Hensinger RN [1988]: Cervical disc calcification: instructional case. *J Pediatr Orthop* 8:613–616, with permission.)

Tuberculosis

Mycobacterium tuberculosis infection of the cervical spine is rare compared with that of the thoracolumbar spine. Because of an increase in immigration from countries where tuberculosis is prevalent, the rise of HIV infection, and the emergence of drug-resistant strains, North America will most likely see an increase in the number of cases of tuberculosis. There have been two thorough reviews of this subject (15,30).

Children with tubercular involvement of the upper cervical spine have neck pain and stiffness. Torticollis also may be present along with headaches and constitutional symptoms. Neurologic symptoms vary from none to severe tetraparesis. Children with involvement of the lower cervical spine also may have dysphagia, asphyxia, inspiratory stridor, and kyphosis. Among children younger than 10 years, more diffuse and extensive involvement occurs with large abscesses but with a decreased incidence of paraplegia and quadriplegia. The neurologic symptoms have a gradual onset over a period of 4 to 8 weeks. Sinus formation is not a prominent feature because of the thickness of the cervical prevertebral fascia, which contains the abscess.

Radiographs show osteolytic erosions and an increase in the width of the retropharyngeal soft-tissue space. Instability at C1–2 can occur; rarely is there fixed C1–2 rotatory subluxation. One fourth of patients with lower cervical spine involvement have kyphosis. Cord compression is caused by the abscess or the

kyphosis. Because the infection is anterior, most patients with spinal tuberculosis have spinal cord compression or paralysis if left untreated.

All children receive antituberculous chemotherapy. Chemotherapy alone is the established method of controlling tuberculosis in the thoracic and lumbar spine (14). Surgery is recommended for patients with tuberculosis of the cervical spine, because the pain, upper respiratory obstruction, and spinal cord compression resolve rapidly. Débridement is performed with or without grafting. Most children need halo traction with reduction before drainage, if possible. Children younger than 2 years usually do not need grafting. Anterior transoral drainage and fusion across the lateral facet joints can be considered in the care of children with upper cervical spine involvement.

Osseous Types

Occipitocervical synostosis, basilar impression, and odontoid anomalies are the most common developmental malformations of the occipitovertebral junction. These lesions arise from faulty development of the neocranium and adjacent vertebral skeleton during formation of the mesenchymal anlage. The basilar portion of the occiput, along with lateral masses and posterior arches of the atlas, is derived from the mesenchyma of the most caudal occipital sclerotome, also known as the *proatlas* (66). The ossiculum terminale also arises from this sclerotome. These areas of primitive mesenchyma separate from each other during fetal growth and then undergo chondrification and subsequent ossification as distinct units. An abnormality in formation of the mesenchymal anlage can thus produce malformation of the occipitovertebral junction.

Basilar Impression

Basilar impression is an osseous deformity at the margin of the foramen magnum. The skull floor is indented by the upper cervical spine; the odontoid tip may even protrude into the opening of the foramen magnum. This may encroach on the brain stem, with potential for neurologic damage from injury, vascular compromise, or alteration of flow of cerebrospinal fluid (74).

There are two types of basilar impression: primary, which is by far the most common, and secondary. Primary basilar impression is a congenital abnormality often associated with other vertebral defects, such as Klippel-Feil syndrome, odontoid abnormalities, atlantooccipital fusion, and atlas hypoplasia. Secondary basilar impression is a developmental condition attributed to softening of the bone at the base of the skull. The primary type has been discussed in other chapters and is not addressed here.

Secondary basilar impression (9) can occur with any osseous softening disorder. This includes metabolic bone diseases such as Paget disease, renal osteodystrophy, rickets, and osteomalacia; bone dysplasia and mesenchymal syndromes such as osteogenesis imperfecta, achondroplasia, hypochondroplasia, and neurofibromatosis; and rheumatologic disorders such as rheumatoid arthritis and ankylosing spondylitis.

Patients with secondary basilar impression have a short neck (9), but it is only an apparent shortness because of the basilar impression. They also may show asymmetry of the skull or face, a painful range of cervical motion, and torticollis. Neurologic signs and symptoms often are present (42). Many children have acute onset of symptoms precipitated by minor trauma (75). In cases of pure basilar impression, the neurologic involvement is a pyramidal syndrome that causes motor weakness or limb paresthesia. In cases of basilar impression associated with Arnold-Chiari malformation, the neurologic involvement usually is cerebellar and causes motor incoordination with ataxia, dizziness, or nystagmus. There may be cranial nerve involvement, particularly of nerves that emerge from the medulla oblongata—trigeminal (V), glossopharyngeal (IX), vagus (X), and hypoglossal (XII). Ataxia is a common finding among children (75). Hydrocephalus may develop from obstruction of flow of cerebrospinal fluid by the odontoid process at the foramen magnum.

Basilar impression is difficult to assess radiographically. The most commonly used lines are the Chamberlain, McRae, and McGregor (Fig. 5). The McGregor line is best for screening, because the landmarks can be clearly defined at all ages on a routine lateral radiograph. The McRae line is helpful in assessing the clinical significance of basilar impression, because it defines the opening of the foramen magnum. Among patients without symptoms, the odontoid process projects above this line. CT with sagittal plane reconstructions can show the osseous relations at the occipitocervical junction more clearly, and MRI can show impingement on the neural structures.

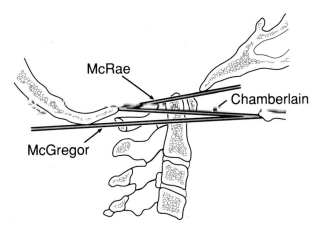

FIGURE 5. Lateral craniometry. These are the three lines commonly used to determine basilar impression. The Chamberlain line is drawn from the posterior lip of the foramen magnum to the dorsal margin of the hard palate. The McGregor line is drawn from the upper surface of the posterior edge of the hard palate to the most caudal point of the occipital curve of the skull. The McRae line defines the opening of the foramen magnum. The McGregor line is best used for screening, because the bony landmarks can be defined clearly at all ages on a routine lateral radiograph. (From Hensinger RN, Fielding JW [1990]: The cervical spine. In: Morrissy RT, ed. *Lovell and Winter's Pediatric Orthopaedics.* Philadelphia: JB Lippincott, pp. 703–739, with permission.) (28)

Management of basilar impression is difficult and requires a multidisciplinary approach (orthopedics, neurosurgery, neuroradiology) (77). In rare instances the symptoms can be relieved with custom-made orthotic devices (31), but the primary treatment is surgical. If the symptoms are caused by hypermobility of the odontoid process, surgical stabilization in extension at the occipitocervical junction is needed. Anterior excision of the odontoid process is needed if the hypermobility cannot be reduced (41), but this step should be preceded by posterior stabilization and fusion. If the symptoms are caused by posterior impingement, suboccipital decompression and often upper cervical laminectomy are needed. The dura often has to be opened in a search for a tight posterior band (9,77). Posterior stabilization should be performed. These are general statements, and each case should be considered individually.

Atlantooccipital Anomalies

The appearance of these children is similar to that of those with Klippel-Feil syndrome. They have short, broad necks and restricted neck movement, a low hairline, high scapulae, and torticollis (2). The skull may be deformed. These children may have associated anomalies, including dwarfism, funnel chest, jaw anomalies, cleft palate, congenital ear deformities, hypospadias, genitourinary tract defects, and syndactyly. Neurologic symptoms can occur during childhood but more often occur at 40 to 50 years of age. The most common signs and symptoms, in decreasing order of frequency, are neck and occipital pain, vertigo, ataxia, limb paresis, paresthesia, speech disturbances, hoarseness, diplopia, syncope, auditory malfunction, and dysphagia (25). These symptoms can be initiated by traumatic or inflammatory processes and progress slowly and relentlessly.

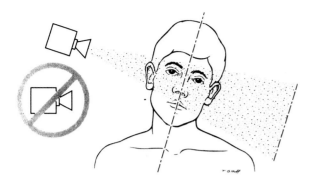

FIGURE 6. A lateral radiograph of the skull gives a satisfactory view of the occipitocervical junction, even in the presence of fixed bony deformity or a patient's inability to cooperate, because the ring of C1 stays with the occiput. (From Hensinger RN, Fielding JW [1990]: The cervical spine. In: Morrissy RT, ed. *Lovell and Winter's Pediatric Orthopaedics.* Philadelphia: JB Lippincott, pp. 703–739, with permission.)

Plain radiographs are difficult to interpret because of fixed bony deformities and overlapping shadows from the mandible, occiput, and foramen magnum. If the x-ray beam is perpendicular to the skull rather than to the cervical spine, a satisfactory view of the occipitocervical junction usually can be obtained (Fig 6). CT is used to further study the bony anatomy. The anterior arch of C1 is commonly assimilated to the occiput, usually in association with a hypoplastic posterior ring. The variable decrease in height of C1 allows the odontoid process to project upward into the foramen magnum (primary basilar impression). The position of the odontoid relative to the opening of the foramen magnum was described by McRae. The distance measured is that from the posterior aspect of the odontoid to the posterior ring of C1 or the posterior lip of the foramen magnum, whichever is closer (40). This distance should be determined with the patient in flexion, because this position maximizes the reduction in the space available for the cord. If this distance is less than 19 mm, a neurologic deficit usually is present. Associated C1–2 instability has been reported to develop among 50% of these patients. Lateral flexion-extension radiographs of the upper cervical spine often show as much as 12 mm of space between the odontoid process and the C1 ring anteriorly. This instability is determined when the distance is greater than the normal 4 mm between the anterior aspect of the odontoid and the posterior aspect of the anterior ring of C1 in children, compared with the 3-mm value used for adults. The 1-mm difference in normal values is a result of the considerably more cartilaginous nature of both structures (incomplete ossification) and of the greater laxity among children. The odontoid process also may be misshapen or maldirected posteriorly. As many as 70% of these children have congenital fusion between C2 and C3. Occipital vertebrae and condylar hypoplasia also may be present.

MRI is used to examine the neural structures. The upper spinal cord or medulla often is encroached posteriorly by a dural constricting band. Cerebellar tonsil herniation also can occur. Anterior compression of the brain stem or upper cervical cord occurs from a backward projecting odontoid process. Pyramidal tract signs and symptoms (spasticity, hyperreflexia, muscle weakness, gait disturbances) are most common, although cranial nerve involvement (diplopia, tinnitus, dysphagia, auditory disturbances) may be seen. Compression from the posterior lip of the foramen magnum or dural constricting band can disturb the posterior columns with a loss of proprioception, vibration, and tactile senses. The commonly occurring nystagmus also is probably caused by posterior cerebellar compression. Vertebral artery disturbances can cause syncope, seizures, vertigo, and unsteady gait. The altered mechanics of the cervical spine may cause dull, aching pain in the posterior occiput and neck with intermittent stiffness and torticollis.

Treatment of patients with atlantooccipital anomalies is difficult, and surgery carries a higher morbidity and mortality than does surgery for anomalies of the odontoid process (2,46). Nonoperative methods should be attempted initially, such as cervical collars, braces, and traction. These often help those with persistent head and neck pain that occurs after minor trauma or infection. Immobilization may achieve only temporary relief if neurologic deficits are present.

When symptoms or signs of instability of the C1–2 complex are present, posterior C1–2 fusion is indicated. Preliminary traction to attempt reduction is used if necessary. If reduction is possible and there are no neurologic signs, surgery has an improved prognosis (2,25). The role of concomitant posterior fusion has not yet been determined, but if decompression, whether anterior or posterior, could destabilize the spine, concomitant posterior fusion should be considered. Results vary from complete resolution to increased deficits and death (2,25).

Unilateral Absence of C1

This congenital malformation is hemiatlas, or congenital scoliosis of C1. It often is associated with other anomalies common with congenital spine deformities, such as tracheoesophageal fistula. Dubousset (11) described a series of 17 patients who did not have a C1 facet.

Two thirds of cases of unilateral absence of C1 are present at birth. In the other one third torticollis develops, and the anomaly is noticed later. A lateral shift of the head on the trunk with variable degrees of lateral tilt and rotation is the most striking finding. It is best appreciated from the back. Instead of sternocleidomastoid muscle tightness, aplasia of the muscles in the nuchal concavity of the tilted side is noticed. Neck flexibility is variable and decreases with age. Plagiocephaly can occur and increases as the deformity increases. About one fourth of patients have neurologic signs (headaches, vertigo, myelopathy).

Standard anteroposterior and lateral radiographs rarely give enough information for a diagnosis, although the open-mouth odontoid view may provide a clue. Tomograms or CT scans provide the information necessary to see the anomaly (Fig. 7). There are three types. Type I is an isolated hemiatlas. Type II is partial or complete aplasia of one hemiatlas with other associated anomalies of the cervical spine, such as fusion of the third and fourth vertebrae or congenital bars in the lower cervical vertebrae. Type III is partial or complete atlantooccipital fusion and symmetric or asymmetric hemiatlas aplasia with or without anomalies of the odontoid process or lower cervical vertebrae.

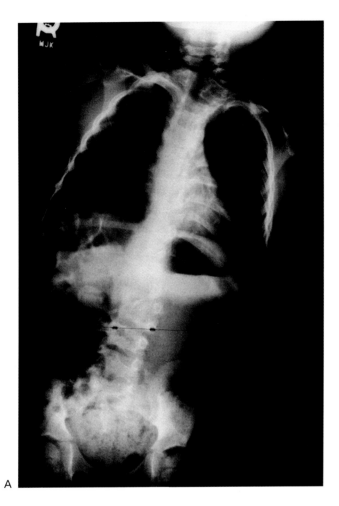

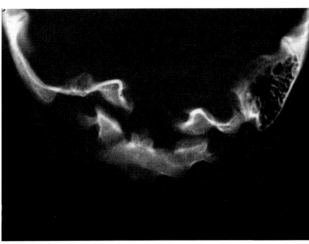

FIGURE 7. Images of a boy with VATER syndrome who was born with imperforate anus, absent right kidney, ventricular septal defect, and spinal anomalies. Physical examination showed mild scoliosis and right head tilt. **A:** Standing posteroanterior radiograph of the spine shows congenital vertebral anomalies at the cervicothoracic junction and the lower thoracic and upper lumbar spine. Head tilt to the right is apparent. **B:** Computed tomographic scan of the cervical spine. The right occipital condyle is superiorly located because of hypoplasia of the left lateral mass of C1 (*arrow*).

Radiographs of the entire spine should be obtained to rule out other congenital vertebral anomalies.

Vertebral angiography should be performed if operative intervention is undertaken. Arterial anomalies, such as multiple loops and abnormal routes between C1 and C2, often are found on the aplastic side. MRI should also be performed before surgery, because these children may have stenosis of the foramen magnum or Arnold-Chiari malformation.

The deformity should be followed for progression. Bracing does not halt progression of the deformity. Surgical intervention is recommended for children with progression or severe deformities. Preoperative halo cast correction is used until correction has been achieved. It is followed by posterior fusion from the occiput to C2 or C3, depending on the extent of the anomaly. Decompression of the spinal canal is performed if the canal size is inadequate or if it is projected to be inadequate in the future. The ideal age for posterior fusion is 5 to 8 years.

Familial Cervical Dysplasia

The clinical presentation of familial cervical dysplasia (62) varies. It can be an incidental finding, a passively correctable head tilt, suboccipital pain, or decreased cervical motion. In rare instances clunking of the upper cervical spine is noticed. Plain radiographs

are often difficult to interpret. The anatomic features are best seen with CT and three-dimensional reconstruction (Fig. 8). Partial absence of the posterior ring of C1 is most common. Various anomalies of C2 also exist, usually a shallow hypoplastic left facet. Other forms of dysplasia of the lateral masses, facets, and posterior elements and occasionally spondylolisthesis can occur. Occiput-C1 instability is common; C1–2 instability is rare. When symptoms of instability are present, MRI in flexion and extension is recommended to assess the presence and magnitude of neural compression.

Nonsurgical treatment is close observation for the development of instability. Surgical intervention is recommended for persistent pain, torticollis, and especially neurologic symptoms. Posterior fusion from the occiput to C2 typically is required after gradual preoperative reduction with an adjustable halo cast.

Atlantoaxial Rotary Displacement

Atlantoaxial rotary displacement is one of the most common causes of childhood torticollis. It has several causes. Rotary displacement is a characteristic pediatric problem but also can occur among adults. Because they are the same for all pediatric causes, the radiographic findings and treatment regimens are discussed as a unit. Individual exceptions are mentioned when necessary.

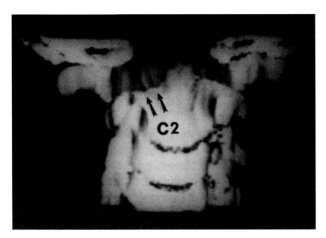

FIGURE 8. Three-dimensional CT scan of the upper cervical spinal cord of a child with familial cervical dysplasia. The left superior facet of C2 is shallow and hypoplastic (*arrows*). (From Saltzman CL, Hensinger RN, Blane CE, et al. [1991]: Familial cervical dysplasia. *J Bone Joint Surg Am* 73:163–171, with permission.)

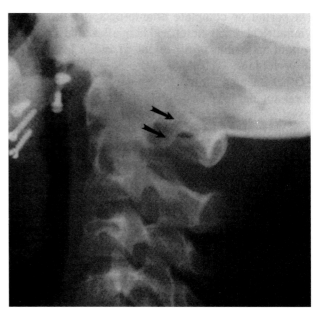

FIGURE 9. Lateral cervical spine radiograph of the child in Figure 10. The posterior arches do not superimpose because of the head tilt (*arrows*).

The terminology is confusing. It includes *rotary dislocation, rotary deformity, rotational subluxation, rotary fixation,* and *spontaneous hyperemic dislocation* (20). These multiple terms indicate a lack of understanding of the pathophysiologic and pathoanatomic aspects of the anomaly. *Atlantoaxial rotary subluxation* is probably the most accepted term. *Subluxation* can be misleading, however, because cases of subluxation usually occur within the normal range of motion of the atlantoaxial joint. *Rotary displacement* is a more appropriate and descriptive term. If the deformity persists, the children have resistant and unresolving torticollis, and it is best termed *atlantoaxial rotary fixation* or *fixed atlantoaxial displacement.* Gradations exist between mild, easily correctable rotary displacement and rigid fixation.

Atlantoaxial rotary displacement can occur spontaneously after minor or major trauma, upper respiratory infection, or head and neck surgery. The child has cocked robin torticollis and resists attempts to move the head because of pain. The associated muscle spasm is noticed on the side of the long sternocleidomastoid muscle because the muscle is attempting to correct the deformity. This is opposite the situation with congenital muscular torticollis. When the deformity becomes fixed, the pain subsides and the torticollis persists along with reduced neck motion. In long-standing cases, plagiocephaly and facial flattening may develop on the side of the tilt.

The radiographic findings of rotary displacement sometimes are difficult to see because positioning for the study is painful. With rotary displacement torticollis, the lateral mass of C1 that has rotated forward appears wider and closer to the midline (medial offset). The opposite lateral mass is narrower and away from the midline (lateral offset). The facet joints may be obscured because of apparent overlapping. The lateral view shows the wedge-shaped lateral mass of the atlas lying anteriorly where the oval arch of the atlas normally lies, and the posterior arches fail to superimpose because of the head tilt (Fig. 9). These findings may suggest occipitalization of C1 because with the neck tilt the skull may obscure C1. The normal relation between the

occiput and C1 is believed to be maintained among children with atlantoaxial rotary displacement. Thus a lateral radiograph of the skull may show the relative position of C1 and C2 more clearly than a lateral radiograph of the cervical spine.

The dilemma is differentiating the position of C1 and C2 of a child with subluxation from that of a healthy child whose head is rotated; both give the same picture. Open-mouth views are difficult to obtain and interpret. Cineradiography has been recommended, but the radiation dose is high, and patient cooperation can be difficult because of muscle spasms (18). Dynamic rotational CT is helpful in this situation (22). Views with the head maximally rotated to the right and then to the left show atlantoaxial rotary fixation when there is a loss of normal rotation (Fig. 10).

The four types of rotary displacement (20) are as follows (Fig. 11). Type I is simple rotary displacement without an anterior shift. Type II is rotary displacement with an anterior shift of 5 mm or less. Type III is rotary displacement with an anterior shift greater than 5 mm. Type IV is rotary displacement with a posterior shift. The amount of anterior displacement considered to be pathologic is greater than 3 mm among older children and adults and greater than 4 mm among younger children (19,36). Type I is the most common type among children. It usually is benign and commonly resolves on its own. Type II is potentially more dangerous and must be approached carefully. Types III and IV are rare, but because of the potential for neurologic involvement and even instant death, management must be approached with great caution.

The cause of atlantoaxial rotary displacement is multifactorial and still not totally known (38,52). Rotary displacement can occur spontaneously after minor or major trauma, upper respiratory infection (Grisel syndrome), or after operations on the oral

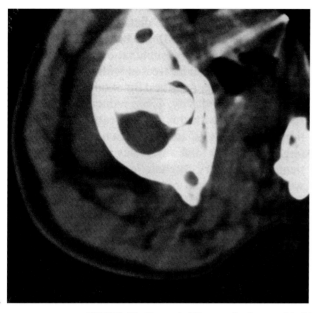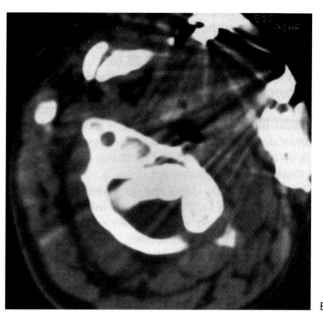

A   B

FIGURE 10. Dynamic CT scan of a 9-year-old girl with fixed atlantoaxial rotary displacement. **A:** The head maximally rotated to the left. **B:** The head maximally rotated to the right, which in this case is not even to the midline. The ring of C1 is still in the same relation to the odontoid as in **A**, indicating fixed rotary subluxation.

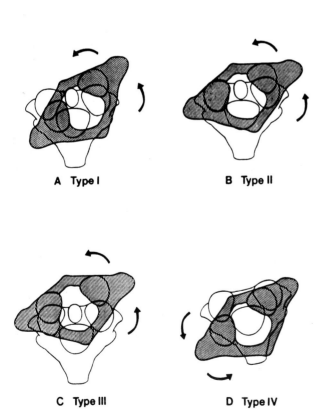

FIGURE 11. The four types of atlantoaxial rotary displacement. (From Fielding JW, Hawkins RJ [1977]: Atlanto-axial rotatory fixation. *J Bone Joint Surg Am* 59:37–44, with permission.)

pharynx, mostly tonsillectomy and adenoidectomy. A direct connection exists between the pharyngovertebral veins and the periodontal venous plexus and suboccipital epidural sinuses (52). This provides a route for hematogenous transport of pharyngeal septic exudates or postsurgical inflammatory products to the upper cervical spine, which causes atlantoaxial hyperemia. Regional lymphadenitis causes spastic contracture of the cervical muscles. This muscle spasm, combined with ligamentous laxity caused by hyperemia due to pharyngovertebral venous drainage can lock the overlapping edges of the articular facets. This prevents easy repositioning and causes atlantoaxial rotary displacement. Highly vascular meniscus-like synovial folds occur in the atlantooccipital and lateral atlantoaxial joints of children but not those of adults, and the dens-facet angle of the axis is steeper in children than in adults (34). Excessive C1–2 rotation due to this steeper angle, compounded by ligament laxity from underlying hyperemia, allows the meniscus-like synovial folds to become impinged in the lateral atlantoaxial joint, leading to rotary fixation.

Most atlantoaxial rotary displacements resolve spontaneously. If the deformity becomes fixed, the pain subsides but torticollis remains. The duration of symptoms and deformity dictates the recommended treatment (54). Patients with displacement of less than 1 week's duration can be treated with immobilization in a soft cervical collar and rest for about 1 week. Close follow-up evaluation is mandatory. If reduction does not occur spontaneously with this initial treatment, hospitalization and the use of halter traction, muscle relaxants, such as diazepam, and analgesics is the next step. Patients with rotary subluxation of greater than 1 week's but less than 1 month's duration should be imme-

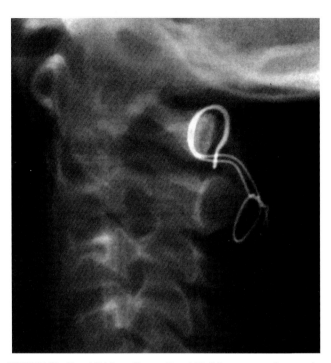

FIGURE 12. The child from Figures 9 and 10 did not respond to traction treatment, including halo traction, because the deformity had been fixed for 6 months after maxillofacial surgical reconstruction for deformities associated with Goldenhar syndrome. She underwent posterior C1–2 Gallie-type fusion. Nine months after the operation she had 80-degree rotation to the left, 45-degree rotation to the right, and a solid arthrodesis.

diately hospitalized for therapy with cervical traction, muscle relaxants, and analgesics. Halo traction occasionally is needed to achieve reduction. After reduction is documented clinically and confirmed with dynamic CT, cervical support is continued until symptoms have subsided. If there is anterior displacement, immobilization is continued for 6 weeks to allow ligamentous healing. Patients with rotary subluxation that lasts longer than 1 month need cervical traction, usually halo skeletal, for up to 3 weeks, but the prognosis is guarded. These children usually fall into two groups. The first is children with rotary subluxation that can be reduced with halo traction but who despite a prolonged period of immobilization have a reoccurrence of the resubluxation when immobilization is stopped. The second is children with subluxation that cannot be reduced and is fixed.

When the deformity is fixed, especially when anterior C1 displacement is present, the transverse atlantal ligament is compromised and there is potential for catastrophe. In this situation, posterior C1–2 fusion should be performed. The indications for fusion are neurologic involvement, anterior displacement, failure to achieve and maintain correction, presence of the deformity for more than 3 months, and recurrence of the deformity after an adequate trial of conservative management, at least 6 weeks of immobilization after reduction. Forceful or manipulative reduction should not be performed. Simple positioning in a halo cast or vest should be done after fusion and can be expected to provide satisfactory alignment. We prefer Gallie-type fusion (21) with sublaminar wiring at the ring of C1 and through the spinous process of C2 (Fig. 12) to Brooks-type fusion, in which the wire is sublaminar at both C1 and C2. Brooks fusion carries a higher risk of neurologic injury.

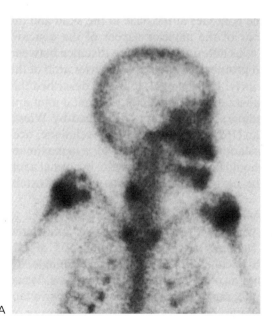

A

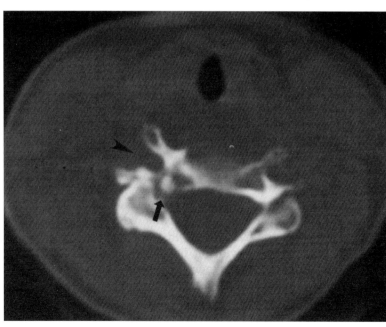

B

FIGURE 13. **A:** Bone scan of a 9-year-old girl with a 3-month history of neck pain, which was worse at night, and torticollis. The pain responded to aspirin. The scan shows markedly increased uptake on the right side of C5. **B:** Computed tomographic scan of the same patient shows a nidus with surrounding lucency (*arrow*). The nidus is close to the vertebral artery (*arrowhead*). It was successfully excised through a posterior approach.

Neoplasms

The most common neoplasm that causes childhood torticollis is osteoid osteoma. The incidence of torticollis among children with cervical osteoid osteoma ranges from 10% to 100% (1,35,45). The pain classically responds to aspirin or other non-steroidal antiinflammatory medications. The intense inflammatory nature of these lesions and their proximity to the neural elements likely causes nerve root irritation with pain and muscle spasm; the result is torticollis.

Osteoid osteoma is not easily seen on plain radiographs. A radionuclide bone scan is intensely hot with an osteoid osteoma. This study can be followed with CT to localize the lesion (Fig. 13). Osteoid osteoma causes a sclerotic reaction in the surrounding bone but usually does not invade the epidural space. This tumor is most commonly located in the laminae.

Osteoid osteoma does not undergo malignant transformation. However, continued torticollis and pain can cause fixed spinal deformities. For this reason, we advocate surgical resection. Prophylactic fusion should be performed if resection renders the spine unstable. Pain relief with complete resection is dramatic. Reports of postoperative pain as severe as the preoperative pain indicate either incomplete resection or recurrence.

DOWN SYNDROME

Because of underlying collagen defects among children with Down syndrome, cervical instabilities can develop at both the occiput-C1 and C1–2 levels. The instability may occur at more than one level and in more than one plane, such as the sagittal and rotary planes.

Atlantoaxial instability among children with Down syndrome was first reported in 1961. Sine then there have been many reports on this instability. None, however, documents the true incidence of atlantoaxial dislocation in contrast to instability, and no long-term studies have been conducted on the course of this problem. Organizers of the Special Olympics have concerns about the participation of children with Down syndrome. The appropriate approach to the problem of upper cervical instability among these children is unclear.

The incidence of atlantoaxial instability among children with Down syndrome varies from 9% to 22% (6,56,76). It is a gradually progressive lesion (3). The incidence of symptomatic atlantoaxial instability has been reported to be much lower, 2.6% among a series of 236 patients with Down syndrome (56). Progressive instability and neurologic deficits are more likely to develop among male patients older than 10 years (3). Children with Down syndrome have a high incidence of cervical skeletal anomalies, especially persistent synchondrosis and spina bifida occulta of C1, than do other children (57). These spinal anomalies may be a contributing factor in the cause of atlantoaxial instability among these children. Children with Down syndrome who have atlantoaxial instability have a higher frequency of cervical spinal anomalies than do children with Down syndrome who do not have these anomalies (57).

The incidence of occiput-C1 instability has been reported to be as high as 60% among children with Down syndrome (76). Measurement reproducibility is poor (33), but a Power ratio less than 0.55 is likely to be associated with neurologic symptoms (51). No guidelines exist regarding the frequency of periodic screening or indications for atlantooccipital fusion except when symptoms are present. Treatment of these children depends on the amount of room available for the cord rather than absolute values of displacement for both atlantoaxial and atlantooccipital instability (76). This area requires further investigation.

Most cases of atlantoaxial or occipitoatlantal hypermobility are asymptomatic (6,39). When symptoms occur, they usually are pyramidal tract symptoms, such as gait abnormalities, hyperreflexia, easy fatigability, and tetraparesis. Local symptoms, such as head tilt, torticollis, neck pain, or limited neck mobility, occasionally exist. The neurologic deficit is not necessarily caused by hypermobility of the atlantoaxial or occipitoatlantal joint. Neurologic symptoms in one series of adult patients with Down syndrome were equally as common among those with an large atlantodens interval as among those with a normal atlantodens interval (16). Further evaluation with flexion-extension CT or MRI to assess for cord compression is needed in this situation.

In the past, screening of patients with Down syndrome by means of lateral flexion-extension radiographs had been recommended. However, symptomatic atlantoaxial instability is extremely rare, and the chances of a sports-related catastrophic injury are even rarer. The reproducibility of radiographic screening for atlantoaxial and occipitoatlantal mobility is poor (33,65). The radiologic signs also can change gradually, most frequently from abnormal to normal. Because of all these factors, and the absence of any evidence that a screening program is effective in preventing symptomatic atlantoaxial and occipitoatlantal mobility, lateral cervical radiographs are of unproven value. The American Academy of Pediatrics has retired its recommendation that screening radiographs be obtained.

Sudden catastrophic death rarely occurs. Nearly all of the patients who have sustained catastrophic injury to the spinal cord have had weeks to years of preceding, less severe neurologic abnormalities. In a recent review by the American Academy of Pediatrics, 41 cases of symptomatic atlantoaxial instability were compiled. In only three of these 41 children did the initial symptoms or worsening of symptoms of atlantoaxial instability occur after trauma during organized sports (6).

Ascertaining which patients have symptoms or signs of symptomatic spinal cord injury is more important than obtaining radiographs. Neurologic examination often is difficult to perform and interpret for these children (76). Parental education about the early signs of myelopathy is extremely important. A thorough history and neurologic examination are more important before participation in sports than are screening radiographs. However, further research is needed into this confusing matter. Because of persistent concerns, the Special Olympics does not plan to remove its requirement that all athletes with Down syndrome undergo radiography of the cervical spine before participating.

Spinal radiographs often are obtained without neurologic symptoms. When these radiographs are available, they should be reviewed to determine whether there are associated anomalies,

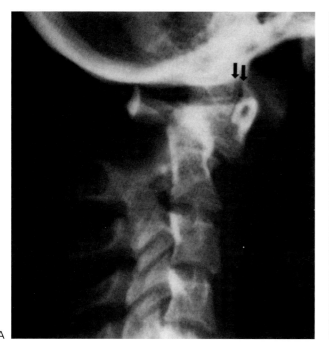 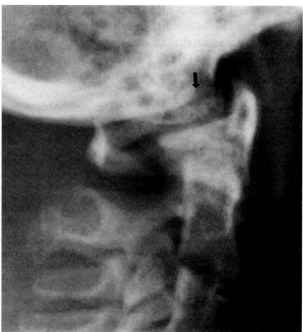

A   B

FIGURE 14. A: Lateral flexion radiograph of the cervical spine of a 20-year-old woman with Down syndrome who had no symptoms. The atlantooccipital distance measured 2 mm (*arrows*). According to the method described by Tredwell et al. (76), the relation is measured as the distance between the anterior margin of the condyles at the base of the skull and the sharp contour of the anterior aspect of the concave joint of the atlas. The atlantodens distance measures 8 mm. **B:** Lateral extension radiograph shows posterior subluxation at the atlantooccipital joint. The distance measures 9 mm (*arrows*), greater than the 4-mm upper limit of normal according to Tredwell (76). The atlantodens distance is reduced to 1 mm. This patient has both atlantooccipital and atlantodens hypermobility.

such as persistent synchondrosis of C2, spina bifida occulta of C1, ossiculum terminale, os odontoideum, or other less common anomalies. When the plain radiographs indicate atlantoaxial or atlantooccipital instability of 6 mm or more in a patient who does not have symptoms (Figs. 14, 15), CT and MRI in flexion and extension can help determine the extent of neural encroachment and cord compression.

Once a patient with Down syndrome has radiographic instability, what treatment should be instituted? Patients with asymptomatic atlantoaxial or occipitoatlantal hypermobility probably should undergo repeated neurologic examinations. The role of repeated radiographs is unclear. Because the risk of catastrophic spinal cord injury is extremely low among children with Down syndrome who do not have neurologic findings and participate in organized sports, avoidance of high-risk activities must be individualized. For children with sudden onset or recent progression of neurologic symptoms, immediate fusion should be undertaken if appropriate imaging confirms cord compromise. The most difficult question concerns patients with upper cervical hypermobility who have minimal or nonprogressive chronic symptoms. Before arthrodesis is undertaken, imaging with flexion-extension MRI (78) or CT scans should be performed to confirm the presence of cord compression from the hypermobility and to eliminate other central nervous system causes of neurologic symptoms. Even if stabilization is successful, patients with chronic symptoms often have little symptomatic improvement after arthrodesis (55).

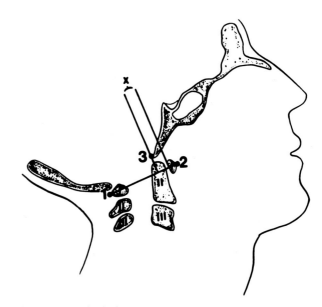

FIGURE 15. Method of measuring atlantooccipital instability according to Wiesel and Rothman (79). The atlantal line joins points 1 and 2. A perpendicular line to the atlantal line is made at the posterior margin of the anterior arch of the atlas. The distance from point 3, which is the basion, to the perpendicular line is measured in flexion and extension. The difference represents the anteroposterior translation at the atlantooccipital joint. For a healthy adult, this translation should be no more than 1 mm. (From Gabriel KR, Mason DE, Carango P [1990]: Occipito-atlantal translation in Down's syndrome. *Spine* 15:996–1002, with permission.) (23)

Posterior cervical fusion at the levels involved is the recommended surgical treatment. The classic technique for posterior C1–2 fusion entails autogenous iliac crest bone grafting with wiring and postoperative halo immobilization. Internal fixation with wiring provides protection against displacement, shortens the time of postoperative immobilization, allows the consideration of using less rigid forms of external immobilization, and is reported to aid in obtaining fusion. However, internal fixation with sublaminar wiring poses added risk. If the instability does not decrease on routine extension radiographs, the patient is at high risk of development of iatrogenic quadriplegia during sublaminar wiring and acute manipulative reduction (48). Satisfactory results can be obtained with onlay bone grafts and rigid external immobilization without internal fixation (60). For this reason it has been recommended that preoperative traction be used to effect the reduction. If reduction does not occur with traction, only an onlay bone grafting should be performed without sublaminar wiring (48). Sublaminar wiring at C2 is not recommended regardless of the success of reduction—sublaminar wiring at C2 was associated with the only death at our institution (67,68). If wiring is to be performed, pliable, small-caliber wires should be used.

In a study of the results of surgical fusion among 35 children with Down syndrome who had symptoms, eight made complete recoveries, 14 showed improvement, seven did not improve, four died, and the outcome for two is unknown (56). Patients with long-standing symptoms and marked neural damage had no or little postoperative improvement, whereas patients with more recent onset of symptoms usually had an excellent recovery. Patients with Down syndrome are at higher risk of postoperative complications, neurologic and otherwise, after fusion (10, 64,68). Neurologic complications can range from complete quadriplegia and death to Brown-Séquard syndrome (68). Other complications are loss of reduction despite halo immobilization and resorption of the bone graft with a stable fibrous union or unstable nonunion (60,64). Persons with Down syndrome who

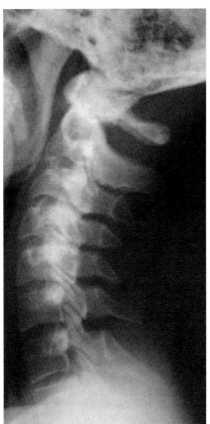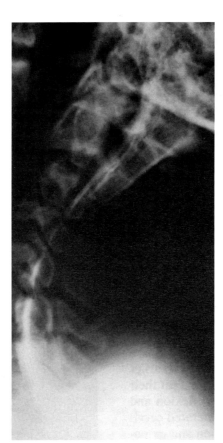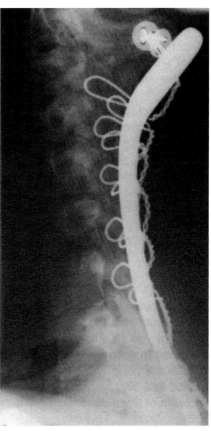

A,B

C

FIGURE 16. Images of a girl 14 years, 6 months of age with spastic tetraparesis and progressive loss of upper-extremity function, which affected her ability to feed herself and control her wheelchair. She also had mild neck pain. **A:** Lateral radiograph shows marked stenosis at C3–6 with decreased space available for the cord. **B:** Myelogram shows near-complete block of the column of contrast material from C3 to C5. The patient underwent posterior laminectomy from C3 to C7, posterior cervical fusion from C2 to T1, and Luque rectangle fixation with wiring spinous processes and facet joints. **C:** Lateral radiograph obtained 8 months after the surgical procedure shows stable fixation and facet joint fusion. By this time the patient had a marked increase in upper-extremity strength and was able to feed herself.

undergo short cervical fusion are at risk of development of instability above the level of fusion, such as occiput-C1 after C1–2 fusion or C1–2 after lower-level fusion (44).

DEVELOPMENTAL CERVICAL STENOSIS: CEREBRAL PALSY

Cervical radiculopathy and myelopathy in cerebral palsy (13,59) were first described in the athetoid types and now has been described in the spastic types. Patients with athetoid cerebral palsy experience cervical disc degeneration at a younger age than do otherwise healthy persons. This degeneration progresses rapidly and involves several levels. Angular and spondylolisthetic instability also are more frequent and appear at a younger age (26) than they do among otherwise healthy persons. The combination of disc degeneration and spondylolisthetic instability predisposes these patients to a relatively rapid, progressive neurologic deficit.

The symptoms of cervical spondylotic myelopathy in cerebral palsy are brachialgia and weakness of the upper extremity with limited functional use or an increase in paraparesis or tetraparesis. Among persons with cerebral palsy who can walk, loss of ambulatory ability often is the initial symptom. Occasional loss of bowel and bladder control also occurs.

Radiographic findings (Fig. 16) are narrowing of the spinal canal and premature development of cervical spondylosis; malalignment of the cervical spine with localized kyphosis, increased lordosis, or both; and instability of the cervical spine manifested as spondylolisthesis. Flattening of the anterosuperior margins of the vertebral bodies and beak-like projections of the anteroinferior margins are radiographic findings of spondylosis. Myelography shows stenosis, disc protrusion, osteophyte projection, and blocks in dye flow, most commonly at the C3–4 and C4–5 levels.

The kyphosis, herniated discs, and osteophytes compress the nerve roots and cord. It is believed that these young adults with cerebral palsy have degenerative cervical stenosis at an earlier age than persons without cerebral palsy. Among the latter whom stenosis develops in the late fourth and fifth decades of life because of exaggerated flexion and extension of the neck, which accelerate cervical degeneration. Exaggerated flexion and extension occur among patients with athetosis and writhing movements. Difficulty with head control also can cause exaggerated flexion and extension among patients with spastic cerebral palsy.

Treatment is primarily surgical. Anterior discectomy, resection of osteophytes, and interbody fusion have been the most effective methods. Posterior spinal fusion also may be needed. Postoperative immobilization can be a problem, but a halo seems to be best and is well tolerated by patients with athetosis (47). For this reason, some authors recommend adding posterior fusion and wiring to minimize the duration of postoperative immobilization is needed. Posterior laminectomy alone (47) is contraindicated because this increases instability.

PSEUDOINSTABILITY AND SUBLUXATION OF THE CERVICAL SPINE

It is known that the C2–3 and, to a lesser extent, C3–4 interspaces of children have a normal physiologic displacement. In a study involving 161 children, Cattell and Filtzer (4) documented that marked anterior displacement of C2 on C3 occurred among in 9% of children between 1 and 7 years of age. In some children, the anterior physiologic displacement of C2 on C3 is so pronounced that it appears pathologic. To differentiate this from true pathologic subluxation, Swischuk described a differentiating line drawn from the anterior cortex of the posterior arch of C1 to the anterior cortex of the posterior arch of C3, called the *posterior cervical line* (Fig. 17) (71). In pathologic dislocation of C2 on C3, the posterior cervical line misses the posterior arch of C2 by 2 mm or more.

During growth, the facets of the lower cervical spine change from 55 to 70 degrees, whereas the upper cervical spine facets

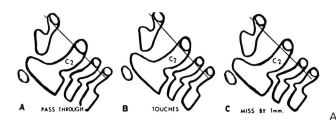

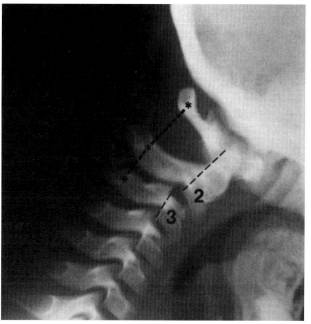

FIGURE 17. A: The posterior cervical line of Swischuk shows the normal limits. *A,* Passing through or just behind the anterior cortex of C2. *B,* Touching the anterior aspect of the cortex of C2. *C,* Coming within 1 mm of the anterior aspect of the cortex of C2. (From Swischuk LE [1977]: Anterior displacement of C2 in children: physiologic or pathologic—a helpful differentiating line. *Radiology* 122:759–763, with permission.) **B:** Lateral cervical radiograph of a child with pseudosubluxation at C2–3. The step-off at C2–3 is present, but the posterior cervical line of Swischuk is normal.

(C2–4) may have initial angles as low as 30 degrees that gradually change to 60 to 70 degrees (50). This variation in facet orientation is an important factor in pseudosubluxation among infants and young children, as are normal looseness of the soft tissues and intervertebral discs and the greater size and weight of the skull in relation to the trunk. No therapy is needed for this normal physiologic pseudosubluxation.

REFERENCES

1. Azouzi EM, Kozlowski K, Marton D, et al. (1986): Osteoid osteoma and osteoblastomas of the spine in children: report of 22 cases with brief literature review. *Pediatr Radiol* 16:25–31.
2. Bharucha EP, Dastur HM (1964): Craniovertebral anomalies (a report on 40 cases). *Brain* 87:469–480.
3. Burke SW, French HG, Roberts JM, et al. (1985): Chronic atlanto-axial instability in Down syndrome. *J Bone Joint Surg Am* 67: 1356–1360.
4. Cattell HS, Filtzer DL (1965): Pseudosubluxation and other normal variations in the cervical spine in children. *J Bone Joint Surg Am* 47: 1295–1309.
5. Cheng JCY, Au AWY (1994): Infantile torticollis: a review of 624 cases. *J Pediatr Orthop* 14:802–808.
6. Committee on Sports Medicine and Fitness of the American Academy of Pediatrics (1995):. Atlantoaxial instability in Down syndrome: subject review. *Pediatrics* 96:151–154.
7. Darling DB, Fisher JH, Gellis SS (1974): Hiatal hernia and gastroesophageal reflux in infants and children: analysis of the incidence in North American children. *Pediatrics* 54:450–455.
8. Davids JR, Wenger DR, Mubarak SJ (1993): Congenital muscular torticollis: sequela of intrauterine or perinatal compartment syndrome. *J Pediatr Orthop* 13:141–147.
9. de Barros MC, Farias W, Ataide L, et al (1968):. Basilar impression and Arnold-Chiari malformation. *J Neurol Neurosurg Psychiatry* 31: 596–605.
10. Doyle JS, Lauerman WC, Wood KB, et al. (1996): Complications and long-term outcome of upper cervical spine arthrodesis in patients with Down syndrome. *Spine* 21:1223–1231.
11. Dubousset J (1986): Torticollis in children caused by congenital anomalies of the axis. *J Bone Joint Surg Am* 68–A:178–188.
12. Dure LS, Percy AK, Cheek WR, et al. (1989): Chiari type I malformation in children. *J Pediatrics* 115:573–576.
13. Ebara S, Harada T, Yamazaki Y, et al. (1989): Unstable cervical spine in athetoid cerebral palsy. *Spine* 14:1154–1159.
14. Eighth report of the Medical Research Council Working Party on Tuberculosis of the Spine (1982): A 10-year assessment of a controlled trial comparing debridement and anterior spinal fusion in the management of tuberculosis of the spine in patients on standard chemotherapy in Hong Kong. *J Bone Joint Surg Br* 64:393–398.
15. Fang D, Leong JCY, Fang HSY (1983): Tuberculosis of the upper cervical spine. *J Bone Joint Surg Br* 65:47–50.
16. Ferguson RL, Putney ME Jr (1997): Comparison of neurologic deficits with atlanto-dens intervals in patients with Down syndrome. *J Spinal Disord* 10:246–252.
17. Ferkel RD, Westin GW, Dawson EG, et al. (1983): Muscular torticollis: a modified surgical approach. *J Bone Joint Surg Am* 65:894–900.
18. Fielding JW (1964): Normal and selected abnormal motion of the cervical spine from the second cervical vertebra to the seventh cervical vertebra based on cineroentgenography. *J Bone Joint Surg Am* 46: 1779–1781.
19. Fielding JW, Cochran GVB, Lawsing III JF, et al. (1974): Tears of the transverse ligament of the atlas: a clinical and biomechanical study. *J Bone Joint Surg Am* 56:1683–1691.
20. Fielding JW, Hawkins RJ (1977): Atlanto-axial rotatory fixation. *J Bone Joint Surg Am* 59:37–44.
21. Fielding JW, Hawkins RJ, Ratzan SA (1976): Spine fusion for atlanto-axial instability. *J Bone Joint Surg Am* 58:400–407.

22. Fielding JW, Stillwell WT, Chynn KY, et al. (1978): Use of computed tomography for the diagnosis of atlanto-axial rotatory fixation. *J Bone Joint Surg Am* 60:1102–1104.
23. Gabriel KR, Mason DE, Carango P (1990): Occipito-atlantal translation in Down's syndrome. *Spine* 15:996–1002.
24. Giuffrè R, di Lorenzo N, Fortuna A (1981): Cervical tumors of infancy and childhood. *J Neurosurg Sci* 25:259–264.
25. Greenberg AD (1968): Atlantoaxial dislocation. *Brain* 91:655–684.
26. Harada T, Ebara S, Anwar MM, et al. (1996): The cervical spine in athetoid cerebral palsy. *J Bone Joint Surg Br* 78:613–619.
27. Hensinger RN, DeVito PD, Ragsdale CG (1986): Changes in the cervical spine in juvenile rheumatoid arthritis. *J Bone Joint Surg Am* 68:189–198.
28. Hensinger RN, Fielding JW (1990): The cervical spine. In: Morrissy RT, ed. *Lovell and Winter's Pediatric Orthopaedics*. Philadelphia: JB Lippincott, pp. 703–739.
29. Herring JA, Hensinger RN (1988): Cervical disc calcification. Instructional case. *J Pediatr Orthop* 8:613–616.
30. Hsu LCS, Leong JCY (1984): Tuberculosis of the lower cervical spine (C2–C7). *J Bone Joint Surg Br* 66B:1–5.
31. Hunt TE, Dekaban AS (1982): Modified head-neck support for basilar impression with brain-stem compression. *Can Med Assoc J* 126: 947–948.
32. Jolley SG, Johnson DG, Herbst JJ, et al. (1978): An assessment of gastroesophageal reflux in children by extended pH monitoring of the distal esophagus. *Surgery* 84:16–24.
33. Karol LA, Sheffield EG, Crawford K, et al. (1996): Reproducibility in the measurement of atlanto-occipital instability in children with Down syndrome. *Spine* 21:2463–2468.
34. Kawabe N, Hirotani H, Tanaka O (1989): Pathomechanism of atlantoaxial rotatory fixation in children. *J Pediatr Orthop* 9:569–574.
35. Kirwan EOG, Hutton PAN, Pozo JL, et al. (1984): Osteoid osteoma and benign osteoblastoma of the spine: clinical presentation and treatment. *J Bone Joint Surg Br* 66:159–167.
36. Locke GR, Gardner JI, van Epps EF (1966): Atlas-dens interval (ADI) in children: a survey based on 200 normal cervical spines. *Am J Roentgenol* 97:135–140.
37. Marmor MA, Beauchamp GR, Maddox SF (1990): Photophobia, epiphora, and torticollis: a masquerade syndrome. *J Pediatr Ophthalmol Strabismus* 27:202–204.
38. Mathern GW, Batzdorf U (1989): Grisel's syndrome: cervical spine clinical, pathologic, and neurologic manifestations. *Clin Orthop* 244: 131–146.
39. Matsuda Y, Sano N, Watanabe S, et al. (1995): Atlanto-occipital hypermobility in subjects with Down's syndrome. *Spine* 20:2283–2286.
40. McRae DL (1960): The significance of abnormalities of the cervical spine. *Am J Roentgenol* 84:3–25.
41. Menezes AH, VanGilder JC (1988): Transoral-transpharyngeal approach to the anterior craniocervical junction. *J Neurosurg* 69:895–903.
42. Michie I, Clark M (1968): Neurological syndromes associated with cervical and craniocervical anomalies. *Arch Neurol* 18:241–247.
43. Morrison DL, MacEwen GD (1982): Congenital muscular torticollis: observations regarding clinical findings, associated conditions, and results of treatment. *J Pediatr Orthop* 2:500–505.
44. Msall M, Rogers B, DiGaudio K, et al. (1991): Long-term complications of segmental cervical fusion in Down syndrome. *Dev Med Child Neurol Suppl* 33:5.
45. Nemoto O, Moser RP, van Dam BE, et al. (1990): Osteoblastoma of the spine: a review of 75 cases. *Spine* 15:1272–1280.
46. Nicholson JT, Sherk HH (1968): Anomalies of the occipitocervical articulation. *J Bone Joint Surg Am* 50:295–304.
47. Nishihara N, Tnabe G, Nakahara S, et al. (1984): Surgical treatment of cervical spondylotic myelopathy complicating athetoid cerebral palsy. *J Bone Joint Surg Br* 66:504–508.
48. Nordt JC, Stauffer ES (1981): Sequelae of atlantoaxial stabilization in two patients with Down's syndrome. *Spine* 6:437–440.
49. Oga M, Terada K, Kikuchi N, et al. (1993): Herniation of calcified cervical intervertebral disc causes dissociated motor loss in a child. *Spine* 18:2347–2350.

50. Ogden JA (1990): *Skeletal injury in the child,* 2nd ed. Philadelphia: WB Saunders,
51. Parfenchuck TA, Bertrand SL, Powers MJ, et al. (1994): Posterior occipitoatlantal hypermobility in Down syndrome: an analysis of 199 patients. *J Pediatr Orthop* 14:304–308.
52. Parke WW, Rothman RH, Brown MD (1984): The pharyngovertebral veins: an anatomical rationale for Grisel's syndrome. *J Bone Joint Surg Am* 66:568–574.
53. Parker W (1989): Migraine and the vestibular system in childhood and adolescence. *Am J Otol* 10:364–371.
54. Phillips WA, Hensinger RN (1989): The management of rotatory atlanto-axial subluxation in children. *J Bone Joint Surg Am* 71:664–668.
55. Pueschel SM, Findley TW, Furia J, et al. (1987): Atlantoaxial instability in Down syndrome: roentgenographic, neurologic, and somatosensory evoked potential studies. *J Pediatr* 110:515–521.
56. Pueschel SM, Herndon JH, Gelch MM, et al. (1984): Symptomatic atlantoaxial subluxation in persons with Down syndrome. *J Pediatr Orthop* 4:682–688.
57. Pueschel SM, Scola FH, Perry CD, et al. (1981): Atlanto-axial instability in children with Down syndrome. *Pediatr Radiol* 10:129–132.
58. Ramenofsky ML, Buyse M, Goldberg MJ, et al. (1978): Gastroesophageal reflux and torticollis. *J Bone Joint Surg Am* 60:1140–1141.
59. Reese ME, Msall ME, Owen S, et al. (1991): Acquired cervical impairment in young adults with cerebral palsy. *Dev Med Child Neurol* 33:153–166.
60. Rizzolo S, Lemos MJ, Mason DE (1995): Posterior spinal arthrodesis for atlanto-axial instability in Down syndrome. *J Pediatr Orthop* 15:543–548.
61. Rubin SE, Wagner RS (1986): Ocular torticollis. *Surv Ophthalmol* 30:366–376.
62. Saltzman CL, Hensinger RN, Blane CE, et al. (1991): Familial cervical dysplasia. *J Bone Joint Surg Am* 73:163–171.
63. Sarnat HB, Morrissy RT (1981): Idiopathic torticollis: sternocleidomastoid myopathy and accessory neuropathy. *Muscle Nerve* 4:374–380.
64. Segal LS, Drummond DS, Zanotti RM, et al. (1991): Complications of posterior arthrodesis of the cervical spine in patients with have Down syndrome. *J Bone Joint Surg Am* 73:1547–1554.
65. Selby KA, Newton RW, Gupta S, et al. (1991): Clinical predictors and radiological reliability in atlantoaxial subluxation in Down's syndrome. *Arch Dis Child* 66:876–878.
66. Sensenig EC (1957): The development of the occipital and cervical segments and their associated structures in human embryos. *Contrib Embryol Carnegie Inst* 36:141–156.
67. Smith MD, Phillips WA, Hensinger RN (1990): Fusion of the upper cervical spine in children and adolescents: an analysis of 17 patients. *Spine* 16:695–701.
68. Smith MD, Phillips WA, Hensinger RN (1991): Complications of fusion to the upper cervical spine. *Spine* 16:702–705.
69. Smith RA, Vohman MD, Dimon JH III, et al. (1977): Calcified cervical intervertebral discs in children. *J Neurosurg* 46:233–238.
70. Sonnabend DH, Taylor TKF, Chapman GK (1982): Intervertebral disc calcification syndromes in children. *J Bone Joint Surg Br* 64:25–31.
71. Swischuk LE (1977): Anterior displacement of C2 in children: physiologic or pathologic—a helpful differentiating line. *Radiology* 122:759–763.
72. Taboas-Perez RA, Rivera-Reyes L (1984): Head tilt: a revisit to an old sign of posterior fossa tumors. *Bol Assoc Med P R* 76:62–65.
73. Tang S, Liu Z, Quan X, et al. (1998): Sternocleidomastoid pseudotumor of infants and congenital muscular torticollis: fine structure research. *J Pediatr Orthop* 18:214–218.
74. Taylor AR, Chakravorty BC (1964): Clinical syndromes associated with basilar impression. *Arch Neurol* 10:475–484.
75. Teodori JB, Painter MJ (1984): Basilar impression in children. *Pediatrics* 74:1097–1099.
76. Tredwell SJ, Newman DE, Lockitch G (1990): Instability of the upper cervical spine in Down syndrome. *J Pediatr Orthop* 10:602–606.
77. VanGilder JC, Menezes AH (1985): Craniovertebral junction anomalies. In: Wilkins RH, Rengachary SS, eds. *Neurosurgery.* New York: McGraw–Hill, pp. 2097–2102.
78. Weng MS, Haynes RJ (1996): Flexion and extension cervical MRI in a pediatric population. *J Pediatr Orthop* 16:359–363.
79. Wiesel SW, Rothman RH (1979): Occipitoatlantal hypermobility. *Spine* 4:187–191.
80. Williams CRP, O'Flynn E, Clarke NMP, et al. (1996): Torticollis secondary to ocular pathology. *J Bone Joint Surg Br* 78:620–624.

EARLY-ONSET IDIOPATHIC SCOLIOSIS

ROBERT A. DICKSON

Idiopathic scoliosis traditionally has been divided into three categories according to age of onset: infantile (0 to 3 years), juvenile (4 to 9 years), and adolescent (10 years to maturity) (19). These three ages of onset were supposed to mirror the three phases of increased growth velocity during childhood and adolescence. Although growth velocity increases during infancy and adolescence, it is steady during the juvenile period. Accordingly, juvenile-onset scoliosis is uncommon and does not merit a category of its own. What is crucial about age of onset is whether a substantial thoracic deformity is present before the age of 5 years, in which case there is a real risk of cardiopulmonary compromise (4). Therefore idiopathic scoliosis should be divided into two subgroups: early onset (0 to 5 years) and late onset (after the age of 5 years). Late-onset idiopathic scoliosis is solely a question of appearance and deformity, although patients with large deformities can be socially and psychologically disadvantaged. Patients with early-onset scoliosis not only have the deformity but also can have serious organic health problems.

UNTREATED IDIOPATHIC SCOLIOSIS

In the 1960s, several reports of patients with untreated scoliosis appeared to attribute to adolescent idiopathic scoliosis a high morbidity and mortality from cardiopulmonary problems. However, these investigations were confusing and open to misinterpretation. The 102 patients traced by Nilsonne and Lundgren (33) had a curve magnitude greatly in excess of that normally associated with late-onset idiopathic scoliosis. The proper interpretation of this important investigation is that a large number of these patients had early-onset scoliosis. The finding of increased cardiac and pulmonary disease, which accounted for 60% of deaths, therefore is not surprising. In Nachemson's (32) oft-quoted study, some of the patients did not have idiopathic scoliosis but had congenital and miscellaneous etiologic factors. Nevertheless, a small subset with late-onset idiopathic scoliosis was identified, and the organic health of these patients was no different from that of their straight-backed counterparts.

The study by Collis and Ponseti (7) was retrospective, and had a recall rate of only 30%. However, the finding that two thirds of patients with thoracic curves greater than 60 degrees had diminished vital capacity appeared to support the notion of intervening surgically in idiopathic scoliosis once that curve magnitude has been reached. An alternative interpretation of these data is that many of Collis and Ponseti's patients had early-onset idiopathic scoliosis with marked curves. The theory that early-onset deformities threaten cardiopulmonary function was entirely, although accidentally, supported in a study of scoliosis and cor pulmonale (41). Twenty patients with cor pulmonale and an average Cobb angle of 135 degrees participated in the study. Six had paralytic scoliosis, seven had congenital scoliosis, and five had early-onset idiopathic scoliosis. Meanwhile, several long-term studies involving patients with late-onset idiopathic scoliosis clearly demonstrated that pulmonary function remains normal even if curve magnitude exceeds 100 degrees (14,21,34).

The chest abnormalities of scoliosis among patients with cardiopulmonary compromise has been thoroughly investigated. The studies showed that if the deformity was of considerable magnitude at the time of development of the pulmonary parenchyma, evidence of cardiopulmonary dysfunction could be expected (10,35). If severe deformities developed after this time, the tendency toward cardiopulmonary compromise was mitigated. Therefore the old-fashioned figure of 60 degrees as a threshold to proceed with surgical intervention is of real relevance only when age of onset also is taken into consideration. The old view that the lungs at birth are a smaller but fully developed version of the adult organs is wrong. At birth, the development of all the conductive airways is complete, but only a small number of the respiratory bronchioles and alveoli exist. Branching of these final orders of the respiratory tree continues until the age of 8 years, when the full 23 generations of airways of adults are present (15,16,35). It is estimated that at birth there are 20 million alveoli. This number increases rapidly, reaching 250 million by the age of 4 years. The full adult complement is reached by the age of 8 years.

Restriction of the available space in the thoracic cavity has a variable effect on lung development, depending on the time of onset of considerable restriction. If onset is before birth, development of the major airways is limited; the earlier this occurs, the more serious is the problem. The best example is the pulmonary

R.A. Dickson: University Department of Orthopaedic Surgery, St. James University Hospital, Leeds LS9 7TF, United Kingdom.

hypoplasia that occurs in the presence of a major congenital diaphragmatic hernia, in which respiratory failure can cause death. Pathologic studies of these lungs have shown the lack of airway development (3). Even congenital spinal deformities do not reach such a degree at birth to cause major pulmonary hypoplasia. From birth until the age of 8 years, the effect is on the number of alveoli rather than the airways, and this number has been shown to be considerably reduced among children with early-onset scoliosis. In this situation, the alveoli are of normal size and outline. This finding suggests reduced formation rather than secondary atrophy or simple compression (10).

Pulmonary arterial hypertension accompanies respiratory failure among persons with scoliosis, so it is appropriate to consider the development of the pulmonary vascular tree. Development and remodeling of this vasculature appears to by secondary to development of the alveoli. The arteries develop to a size appropriate to the size of the lung rather than to the patient's age. There also is evidence of abnormal distribution of muscle in the walls of these vessels. This is probably caused by the initial restriction in growth of the arteries. Subsequent development of hypoxemia leads to secondary arterial muscle hypertrophy and extension into the acinus itself (10). Right heart hypertrophy and failure (cor pulmonale) are the inevitable complications of pulmonary hypertension.

In a long-term study of uncontrolled idiopathic scoliosis, Branthwaite (4) conducted a follow-up study with several hundred of the late Dr. Phillip Zorab's patients with particular reference to heart and lung function. Branthwaite showed quite clearly that only if the onset of scoliosis was before the age of

5 years was there any risk of subsequent cardiopulmonary compromise. The occasional case of cardiopulmonary compromise encountered among patients with late-onset scoliosis was attributable not to the deformity but to another serious heart or lung problem, such as congenital heart disease or excessive smoking. The belief that surgery is indicated because of a risk of lung dysfunction in an adolescent whose curve reaches 60 degrees is erroneous. The real risk of death of idiopathic scoliosis concerns thoracic deformity that develops in the first year of life and progresses relentlessly (Fig. 1).

CLINICAL FEATURES

Although early-onset idiopathic scoliosis is clearly not a new condition, it was described for the first time only 60 years ago (17). Since then the course of the condition has changed dramatically, particularly regarding the percentage of cases that resolve or progress. In 1951, James (18) found that only 4 cases among his 33 patients resolved. He later reported 52 cases (19) and then a total of 212 (20); in the latter group, 64% of cases progressed and 36% resolved. Scott and Morgan's (39) figures from Oxford indicated that four times as many cases progressed as resolved.

Then, for no apparent reason, things changed for the better. In the 1960s, published series showed that a convincing majority of cases resolving spontaneously (26,43), 92 of 100 cases in the London series resolving (25). Since then, not only has the resolving proportion remained very high, but also the incidence rate of the condition has rapidly declined.

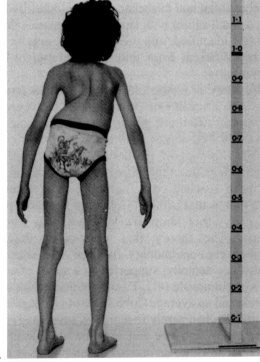
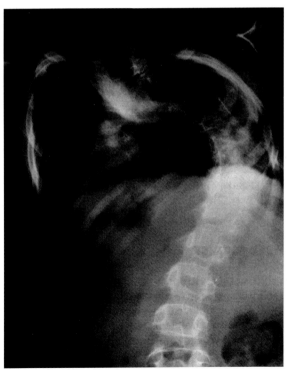

FIGURE 1. A: Clinical photograph. **B:** Posteroanterior radiograph of the spine of a 4-year-old boy with a severe early-onset thoracic curve. Just over a year earlier the deformity measured only 30 degrees.

There are two main notions as to how the deformity develops—intrauterine molding and postnatal pressure due to a constant oblique supine position. Browne (5,6) first put forward the intrauterine molding view and also thought that this might cause the associated deformities of plagiocephaly, plagiopelvy, and limited hip abduction. This view was supported by Mehta (29). The problem with this hypothesis is that the scoliosis and associated deformities are not present until after birth. This led Mau (26) to the belief that it was the infant's position in the crib that provided pressure molding. He suggested that the oblique supine position favored in Europe, as opposed to the prone position favored in North America, was responsible for the marked difference in incidence between these two continents. That the side of the plagiocephaly was related to the convex side of the scoliosis, the side of the hip dysplasia, the side of the bat ear, and the side of the sternomastoid tightness supported the pressure-molding theory (44), as did Wynne-Davies's (45) observation that 97 of her 134 cases developed curves during the first 6 months of life. In contrast, only just over one fourth of healthy children were found to have an asymmetric skull.

Mehta (29) found that a floppy hypotonic baby was much less able to resist deformation than was a normal–birth-weight normotonic baby going through its milestones at the usual rate. Added congenital malformations (8), such as hiatal hernia, and mental retardation (45) are risk factors for progression. Wynne-Davies (45) also observed a higher prevalence of congenital heart disease, breech delivery, inguinal hernia, older mothers, and developmental dysplasia of the hip. She also found the prevalence of scoliosis among the parents and siblings of affected infants was 30 times greater than expected, suggesting that there is no great difference genetically between early- and late-onset idiopathic scoliosis.

Boys are affected more commonly than girls. Unlike the situation in late-onset idiopathic scoliosis, three fourths of thoracic curves are convex to the left. Thoracic and thoracolumbar curves tend to resolve, but double structural curves with a thoracic component have a definite progression potential. Not surprisingly, initial curve size and the amount of associated rotation are prognostic factors. Girls with right-sided thoracic curves have a worse prognosis (42).

Mehta (28) found that by looking at the inclination of the ribs on each side of the apical vertebra, progressive curves could be differentiated from resolving ones (Fig. 2). She measured the apical rib-vertebra angles as the angles subtended by the neck of the rib on each side of the apical vertebra with reference to its vertical axis. On the convex side of the curve, the angle is more acute; on the concave side, it is more obtuse. If the difference between the angles—the rib-vertebra angle difference (RVAD)—exceeds 20 degrees, the curve is likely to be progressive. It is important in trying to determine the prognosis that serial radiographs be obtained and the RVAD calculated on more than one occasion (29).

For practical purposes, an infant referred to a scoliosis clinic with a suspected spinal deformity should be carefully examined for the presence of a scoliosis and the other associated abnormalities of the head, neck, pelvis, and hips. A history should be obtained regarding birth weight and milestone development. If possible, a neurologic examination should be performed, but

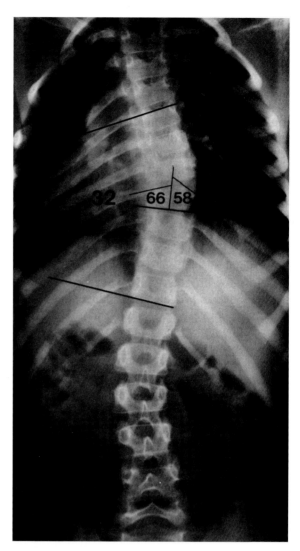

FIGURE 2. Posteroanterior radiograph of a 32-degree early-onset right thoracic curve. The rib-vertebra angle difference at the apex is only 8 degrees, strongly suggesting that the deformity is of the spontaneously resolving variety.

plain radiographs should help differentiate idiopathic from congenital scoliosis. Another important prognostic determinant is the degree of curve rigidity. The child should be suspended to assess flexibility and laid horizontally over the examiner's knee with the convex side downward to assess whether the curve will correct with lateral pressure. Then the RVAD should be calculated. In the double structural thoracic and lumbar curve pattern, the RVAD at the apex of the upper curve often is minimal; the presence of the lower curve may not always be perceptible as a lateral curvature on a posteroanterior radiograph. The presence of a negative RVAD at the level of T12 confirms the presence of a double structural curve. A negative RVAD means that the rib-vertebra angle is smaller on the side of the concavity of the thoracic curve when measured at the level of T12 (Fig. 3).

Over the past 18 years, more than 150 cases of early-onset idiopathic scoliosis have been referred to my center. The sex ratio was 3.5 boys to 1 girl. Seventy percent of curves were

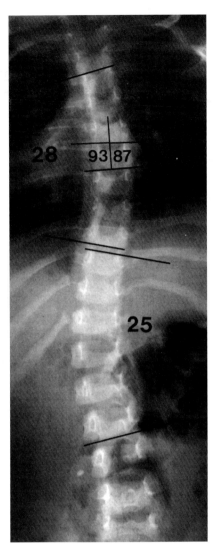

FIGURE 3. Posteroanterior radiograph of an early-onset double structural curve. Although the rib-vertebra angle difference (RVAD) of the upper curve is minimal, the twelfth rib on the left side is directed very obliquely downward, indicating a large negative RVAD and the presence of a double structural curve.

single thoracic and three fourths of these were left sided. Age at presentation ranged from 2 months to 5 years. Evidence of body molding, such as plagiocephaly or bat ear, was equally distributed by curve site, side, and sex. There was no appreciable association between Cobb angle and sex, side, site, presence of molding, or even age at presentation. Curves with an RVAD greater than 20 degrees were considerably larger than curves with smaller RVADs. An RVAD greater than 20 degrees was the single most important factor predicting progression. Fifty percent of patients with an RVAD greater than 20 degrees had an increase in Cobb angle of 10 degrees or more compared with less than 15% when the RVAD was less than 20 degrees. Fifty percent of single right thoracic curves progressed, and only 15% of left thoracic curves did so. The presence of molding features and the absence of psychomotor retardation were more common in resolving

curves. It would certainly appear that early-onset idiopathic scoliosis is pursuing a more benign course with the passage of time.

Increasing attention is being paid to the appearance of the spinal cord at magnetic resonance imaging (MRI) of patients with idiopathic scoliosis, at least younger patients. However, the need or value of this particular investigation in routine cases is by no means certain, no matter what the age of onset. Experienced scoliosis surgeons readily recognize suspicious cases as being unusual curve patterns (e.g., right lumbar or left thoracic), unusual patients (e.g., a boy with a progressive curve), or unusual symptoms (e.g., serious spinal pain, night pain, or headache). These suspicious cases alert the surgeon. At physical examination, a slight but objective neurologic abnormality often confirms the initial suspicion. These patients *must* undergo appropriate spinal cord imaging—usually MRI. Although patients with suspect findings certainly should undergo appropriate spinal cord imaging to rule out a syrinx or neoplasm, the need to perform MRI on all idiopathic scoliosis patients has not been validated.

Just as with late-onset idiopathic scoliosis, these deformities are lordoscoliosis (1,11,13,37,40) (rotated lordosis). What happens in the future is to a large extent determined by whether normal thoracic kyphosis redevelops.

MANAGEMENT

Until relatively recently, therapy for early-onset idiopathic scoliosis was disappointing. Milwaukee bracing, or a look-alike, was empirically prescribed, although there has been no convincing evidence that the course of scoliosis was favorably affected. Posterior spinal fusion was prescribed for larger curves or those "not responding" to brace treatment (24,27). Performing posterior spinal fusion for early-onset scoliosis when the principal deformity is lordosis is about as logical as performing posteromedial fusion for clubfoot (Fig. 4). Not surprisingly, the back of the spine is further tethered, and there is more rapid progression of the three-dimensional deformity. Fortunately, both conservative and operative treatments are now more logical and effective.

Serial elongation derotation flexion (EDF) casting is the conservative treatment of choice. Even deformities with all the hallmarks of progression can be made to resolve or at least remain static (30). Clearly not all cases require casting, but if a low birth-weight, floppy child has evidence of other associated deformities, a large curve and RVAD, and relative curve rigidity, an EDF cast should be applied without delay. This is best done in the operating room with a standard Cotrel EDF casting frame under light general anesthesia on an outpatient basis. Manual pressure over the convex rotational prominence while the cast is drying facilitates derotation, as does a window cutout on the concave side posteriorly and the convex side anteriorly. The cast is generally well tolerated, and it is surprising how easy the inner stockinette can be changed to maintain hygiene. A cast can generally be tolerated for 3 or 4 months before it must be changed. Skin care is essential while the cast is in place, but it may be necessary to remove the cast a week or so before it is due to be changed to allow adequate skin cleansing. Casting is repeated until the deformity has been seen to improve or even resolve completely, which may take 3 or 4 years (Fig. 5).

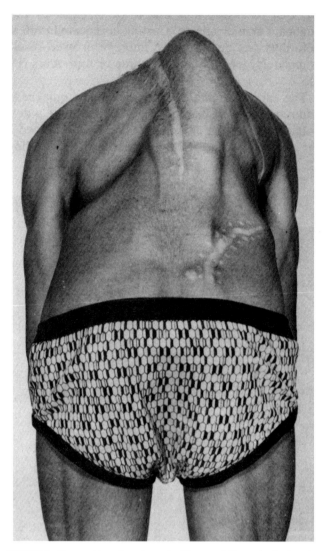

FIGURE 4. Forward bending view of a 16-year-old boy who had undergone posterior fusion for an early-onset progressive curve 10 years previously. The lordosis has been further tethered in bone, which has increased the progression potential of the curve. It is difficult to conceive of a more deleterious procedure than posterior fusion for early-onset scoliosis.

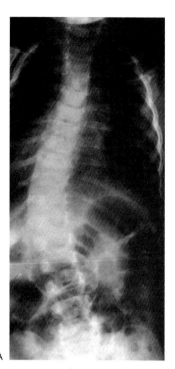 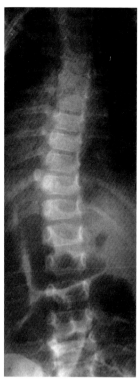

A   B

FIGURE 5. Posteroanterior radiographs of an early-onset progressive curve before **(A)** and after **(B)** serial EDF casting show the benefits of conservative treatment when the cast is applied promptly.

The earlier casting is commenced, the quicker the results. Unfortunately, there often is quite a delay between the parents' first noticing the spinal asymmetry and their bringing the child to a scoliosis surgeon. In this respect, physicians can be worse than parents, often reassuring the parents that the "rib asymmetry" will go away with growth when the reverse can occur (9).

There is little point in continuing cast treatment after the age of 4 or 5 years. By then infantile growth velocity has reached a plateau. Beyond the age of 5 years, children should be examined regularly as outpatients. Radiographs should be obtained sparingly; any change is better perceived by means of inspection or measurement of surface shape. With curves that resolve either spontaneously or with treatment, the rotational component often takes several years to disappear when the spine has become straight in the frontal plane.

If the curve is deemed clinically and radiographically of the resolving variety, casting is not required. Should there be any uncertainty, the child should be examined again in 3 months, radiography should be repeated, and the RVAD should be further assessed. Even if the RVAD was more than 20 degrees initially, improvement at the second visit indicates the possibility of spontaneous resolution. The child should be examined again in 3 months and radiography repeated. In this manner, those who really need EDF cast treatment can be identified.

At my center more than 50 young children have had a series of EDF casts. The ability of casting to greatly reduce curve size has been impressive, even when the cast is applied at somewhat older than optimum age (Fig. 6).

OPERATIVE TREATMENT

Should serial EDF casting be unsuccessful in preventing progression, surgical treatment is necessary. Surgery can, however, make matters worse, and posterior fusion alone is contraindicated. The essence of treatment should be to reduce anterior spinal growth, and there is relatively little time available (vertebrae are half the adult size by the age of 2 years) (Fig. 7). Both Somerville (40) and Roaf (37), who understood perfectly well that lordosis was the driving force in the production of structural scoliosis, recommended that anteroposterior spinal growth imbalance be addressed surgically. Roaf (36) had the idea of anteroconvex epiphysiodesis—stopping the growth of the leading edge of the spine—but unfortunately, by the time epiphysiodesis had actu-

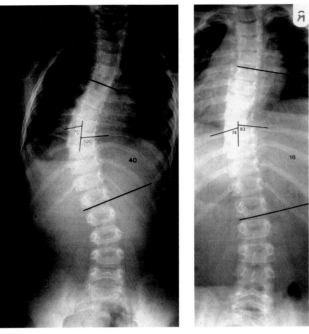

A   B

FIGURE 6. A: Early onset progressive curve at age three with a big Cobb angle and RVAD. Four EDF casts were prescribed. **B:** Eight years later—satisfactory resolution is occurring.

ally occurred, the unfavorable biomechanics of buckling lordosis had overcome his biologic intentions. Andrew and Piggott (2) clearly demonstrated that such a technique was ineffective in the management of either congenital or idiopathic lordoscoliosis but was effective for hemivertebrae, which exist principally in the coronal plane with little or no associated rotation.

To reduce anterior spinal growth, the discs and growth plates must be excised completely over the four or five apical segments (24) (Fig. 8). Although these children are small and much of the spine is cartilaginous, this procedure through a standard thoracotomy is simple and straightforward. In a second-stage posterior procedure, "growing instrumentation" can be inserted to allow the back of a spine to continue to grow and, it is hoped, catch up with the front. The subcutaneous Harrington rod is no more effective than an ordinary Harrington rod, because it does not affect rotation (38). Luque trolley-type instrumentation as recommended by Leatherman, who spent a lifetime trying to alter the forces of the young deforming spine, and Dickson (23) is one possible procedure. Standard sublaminar wiring to two Luque L rods is performed. With growth, the rods separate on the vertical axis, because subperiosteal exposure does not necessarily lead to bony fusion (Fig. 9). A similar effect can be achieved with a single distraction rod and concave sublaminar wiring to a

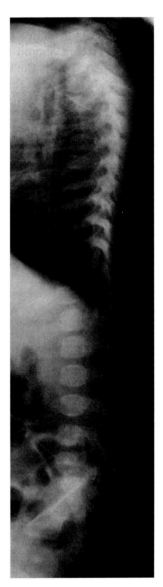

FIGURE 7. Lateral radiograph of a patient with early-onset progressive thoracic scoliosis shows apical lordosis. If the patient is to be treated successfully, this anterior leading edge must be shortened.

kyphotic Harrington rod configuration (Leeds procedure) (12). Fusion is withheld at this young age, although it may have to be added later if spontaneous fusion does not eventually occur (Fig. 10). It is, however, worthwhile to try another round of EDF casting after the anterior growth-arresting multiple-discectomy procedure. The possible tethering effect of posterior surgery can then be obviated or at least delayed.

FIGURE 10. Nine-year follow-up results for a boy treated with growing instrumentation. **A:** Posteroanterior radiograph obtained at 5 years of age shows early-onset right thoracic idiopathic curve with a great deal of apical rotation and a large rib-vertebra angle difference. **B:** Lateral radiograph obtained after one-stage posterior reproduction of thoracic kyphosis without fusion. **C:** Postoperative posteroanterior radiograph shows curve correction in three planes. **D:** Lateral radiograph obtained 2 years after C shows migration of the rod from the lower hook. **E:** Lateral follow-up radiograph shows considerable distance between the lower end of the rod and the lower hook. The thoracic kyphosis has been maintained. No deformity was discernible at clinical examination.

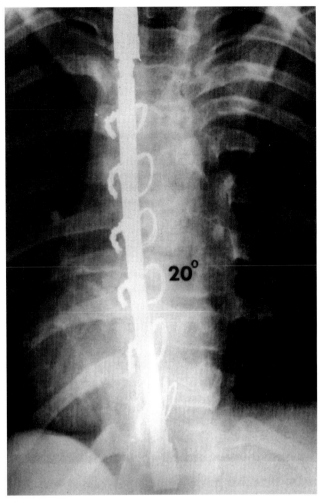

FIGURE 8. Posteroanterior radiograph of a patient with an early-onset idiopathic thoracic scoliosis managed by means of of thoracotomy and excision of the five apical discs and growth plates. In the second posterior stage, thoracic kyphosis was reproduced with a single kyphotic Harrington rod and concave sublaminar wires (Leeds procedure).

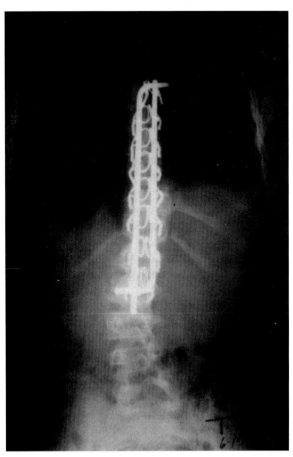

FIGURE 9. Posteroanterior radiograph of a patient with early-onset progressive thoracic curve managed in the second stage by means of Luque trolley instrumentation without fusion. Leatherman was the first to perform this procedure (23).

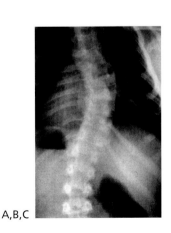
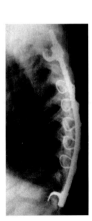
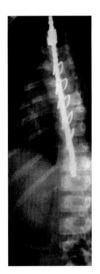
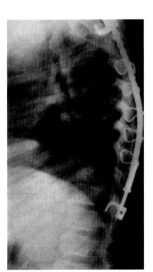
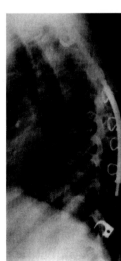

A,B,C   D,E

For children with inexorable progression to considerable severity, even a growth-equalizing attempt is insufficient. In addition to multiple discectomy with removal of growth plates over the apical segments, closing-wedge removal of the apical vertebra should be performed (22). This is the keystone vertebra, and its removal leads to appreciable three-dimensional correction when the bony surfaces above and below are coapted.

Tackling progressive early-onset scoliosis surgically by means of both anterior and posterior surgical approaches may appear to be a daunting prospect, but it is far better to perform an operation that addresses the three-dimensional lordoscoliotic deformity than to see considerable disfigurement and morbidity result from less aggressive approaches.

REFERENCES

1. Adams W (1865): *Lectures on the pathology and treatment of lateral and other forms of curvature of the spine.* London: Churchill and Sons.
2. Andrew T, Piggott H (1985): Growth arrest for progressive scoliosis: combined anterior and posterior fusion of the convexity. *J Bone Joint Surg Br* 67:193–197.
3. Areechon W, Reid L (1963): Hypoplasia of the lung associated with congenital diaphragmatic hernia. *Br Med J* 1:230–233.
4. Branthwaite MA (1986): Cardiorespiratory consequences of unfused idiopathic scoliosis. *Br J Dis Chest* 80:360–369.
5. Browne D (1936): Congenital deformities of mechanical origin. *Proc R Soc Med* 29:1409–1431.
6. Browne D (1956): Congenital postural scoliosis. *Proc R Soc Med* 49:395–398.
7. Collis DK, Ponseti IV (1969): Long term follow up of patients with idiopathic scoliosis not treated surgically. *J Bone Joint Surg Am* 51:425–445.
8. Conner AN (1969): Developmental anomalies and prognosis in infantile idiopathic scoliosis. *J Bone Joint Surg Br* 51:711–713.
9. Conner AN (1984): Early onset idiopathic scoliosis: call for awareness. *Br Med J* 289:962–963.
10. Davies G, Reid L (1971): Effect of scoliosis on growth of alveoli and pulmonary arteries and on right ventricle. *Arch Dis Child* 46:623–632.
11. Dickson RA (1988): Dogma disputed: the aetiology of spinal deformities. *Lancet* 1:1151–1155.
12. Dickson RA, Archer IA (1987): Surgical treatment of late-onset idiopathic thoracic scoliosis: the Leeds procedure. *J Bone Joint Surg Br* 69:709–714.
13. Dickson RA, Lawton JO, Archer IA, et al. (1984): The pathogenesis of idiopathic scoliosis: bi-planar spinal asymmetry. *J Bone Joint Surg Br* 66:8–15.
14. Dickson RA, Leatherman KD (1976): Spinal deformity in adults: changing concepts. *J Bone Joint Surg Am* 58:729.
15. Dunnill MS (1962): Postnatal growth of the lung. *Thorax* 17:329–333.
16. Emery JL, Mithal A (1960): The number of alveoli in the terminal respiratory unit of man during late intrauterine life and childhood. *Arch Dis Child* 35:544–547.
17. Harrenstein RJ (1930): Die skoliose bei saueglingen und ihre behandlung. *Z Orthop Chir* 52:1–40.
18. James JIP (1951): Two curve patterns in idiopathic structural scoliosis. *J Bone Joint Surg Br* 33:399–406.
19. James JIP (1954): Idiopathic scoliosis: the prognosis, diagnosis, and operative indications related to curve patterns and the age at onset. *J Bone Joint Surg Br* 36:36–49.
20. James JIP, Lloyd-Roberts GC, Pilcher MF (1959): Infantile structural scoliosis. *J Bone Joint Surg Br* 41:719–735.
21. Kostuik JP, Israel J, Hall JE (1973): Scoliosis surgery in adults. *Clin Orthop* 93:225–234.
22. Leatherman KD, Dickson RA (1979): Two-stage corrective surgery for congenital deformities of the spine. *J Bone Joint Surg Br* 61:324–328.
23. Leatherman KD, Dickson RA (1988): *The management of spinal deformities.* London: John Wright.
24. Letts RM, Bobechko WP (1974): Fusion of the scoliotic spine in young children. *Clin Orthop* 101:136–145.
25. Lloyd-Roberts GC, Pilcher MF (1965): Structural idiopathic scoliosis in infancy. *J Bone Joint Surg Br* 47:520–523.
26. Mau H (1968): Does infantile scoliosis require treatment? *J Bone Joint Surg Br* 50:881.
27. McMaster MJ, MacNicol MF (1979): The management of progressive infantile idiopathic scoliosis. *J Bone Joint Surg Br* 61:36–42.
28. Mehta MH (1972): The rib vertebra angle in the early diagnosis between resolving and progressive infantile scoliosis. *J Bone Joint Surg Br* 54:230–243.
29. Mehta MH (1984): Infantile idiopathic scoliosis. In: Dickson RA, Bradford DS, eds. *Management of spinal deformities.* London: Butterworths International Medical Reviews, pp. 101–120.
30. Mehta MH, Morel G (1979): The non-operative treatment of infantile idiopathic scoliosis. In: Zorab PA, Siegler D, eds. *Scoliosis: Proceedings of the Sixth Symposium 1979.* London: Academic, 71–84.
31. Millner PA, Helm RH, Dickson RA (1992): Early onset idiopathic scoliosis: natural history and outcome. *J Bone Joint Surg Br* 74[Suppl II]:154–155.
32. Nachemson A (1968): A long term follow-up study of non-treated scoliosis. *Acta Orthop Scand* 39:466–476.
33. Nilsonne U, Lundgren KD (1968): Long term prognosis in idiopathic scoliosis. *Acta Orthop Scand* 39:456–465.
34. Ponder RC, Dickson JH, Harrington PR, et al. (1975): Results of Harrington instrumentation and fusion in the adult idiopathic scoliosis patient. *J Bone Joint Surg Am* 57:797–801.
35. Reid L (1965): Autopsy study of the lungs in kyphoscoliosis. In: Zorab PA, ed. *Proceedings of a symposium on scoliosis: action for the crippled child monograph.* London, pp. 71–77.
36. Roaf R (1963): The treatment of progressive scoliosis by unilateral growth arrest. *J Bone Joint Surg Br* 45:637–651.
37. Roaf R (1966): The basic anatomy of scoliosis. *J Bone Joint Surg Br* 786–792.
38. Schultz AB, Hirsch C (1973): Mechanical analysis of Harrington rod correction in idiopathic scoliosis. *J Bone Joint Surg Am* 55:983–992.
39. Scott JC, Morgan TH (1955): The natural history and prognosis of infantile idiopathic scoliosis. *J Bone Joint Surg Br* 37:400–413.
40. Somerville EW (1952): Rotational lordosis: the development of the single curve. *J Bone Joint Surg Br* 34:421–427.
41. Swank SM, Winter RB, Moe JH (1982): Scoliosis and cor pulmonale. *Spine* 7:343–354.
42. Thompson SK, Bentley G (1980): Prognosis in infantile idiopathic scoliosis. *J Bone Joint Surg Br* 62:151–154.
43. Walker GF (1965): An evaluation of an external splint for idiopathic structural scoliosis in infancy. *J Bone Joint Surg Br* 47:524–525.
44. Watson GH (1971): Relation between side of plagiocephaly, dislocation of the hip, scoliosis, bat ears and sternomastoid tumours. *Arch Dis Child* 46:203–210.
45. Wynne-Davies R (1975): Infantile idiopathic scoliosis. *J Bone Joint Surg Br* 57:138–141.

17

JUVENILE IDIOPATHIC SCOLIOSIS

WILLIAM C. WARNER, JR.

Idiopathic scoliosis is divided into three distinct age-related types: infantile, juvenile, and adolescent (6,45). Infantile scoliosis occurs between birth and 3 years of age, juvenile scoliosis occurs between the ages of 4 and 10 years (39), and adolescent scoliosis occurs among children older than 10 years. Idiopathic scoliosis has been divided into these three age-related types because of distinct differences in the course of the condition, although some overlap may occur between infantile and early juvenile types and between the late juvenile form and adolescent form. Mehta (63) suggested that any classification based on the age of the child at detection is only a statement of the level of awareness and skill of the person who detects the scoliosis, the circumstances of detection, and the magnitude of the deformity when it is discovered. This may explain some of the overlap among the three types. These age-based divisions of juvenile idiopathic scoliosis still are useful because they allow generalizations about risk of progression and response to both nonoperative and operative treatment.

Because of the overlap of infantile and adolescent idiopathic scoliosis, juvenile idiopathic scoliosis may manifest as a spontaneously resolving curve, similar to that in infantile scoliosis, as a slowly progressive curve that responds to nonoperative treatment, or as a progressive curve that does not respond to nonoperative treatment, similar to that of adolescent scoliosis.

Many articles in the orthopaedic literature have delineated the course and management of adolescent idiopathic scoliosis. Infantile idiopathic scoliosis also has received much attention, especially in the British literature. Although it has not received as much attention, juvenile idiopathic scoliosis has a distinct course that provides a basis for treatment recommendations. The same questions that are asked about other types of scoliosis apply to juvenile idiopathic scoliosis: Which curves will progress? Which will require treatment? What will occur with no treatment? What effect can be expected from treatment? A knowledge of the usual course of this condition is essential to answer these questions.

The effect of spinal growth on scoliosis has been well documented. Adolescent idiopathic scoliosis progresses most rapidly during a peak growth spurt of the spine. Because patients with

juvenile scoliosis already have a marked curve before this growth spurt, they are at high risk of curve progression.

Dimeglio (18) identified two periods of rapid spinal growth: between birth and 5 years of age and the onset of puberty during the adolescent growth spurt. Between these two periods of rapid growth, there is a relative plateau of spinal growth, during which the spine continues to grow but not at the rapid rate it does during the first several years of life and during the adolescent growth spurt. Treatment of patients with juvenile idiopathic scoliosis must consider the remaining spinal growth of these children.

EPIDEMIOLOGY

Juvenile idiopathic scoliosis is reported to occur among 12% to 21% of patients with idiopathic scoliosis (11,39,45,56,61). Several authors have reported an increased familial occurrence of juvenile idiopathic scoliosis (101) similar to that of adolescent idiopathic scoliosis (14,15,51,80,82). Figueiredo and James (27) found that 13% of their patients had family histories of scoliosis. The only report of conditions associated with juvenile idiopathic scoliosis was by the same authors (27), who found that 12% of their patients had mental deficiencies and 2% had epilepsy. Magnetic resonance imaging (MRI) has shown an association between juvenile scoliosis and intraspinal pathologic changes, most commonly Arnold-Chiari malformation and syringomyelia (3,34,47,85,89,93).

Juvenile idiopathic scoliosis differs from adolescent and infantile forms not only in age at onset but also in its varied presentation. Adolescent scoliosis occurs most often among girls and most frequently manifests as a right thoracic curve that progresses during the adolescent growth spurt. Brace treatment arrests progression for many patients with adolescent scoliosis (10,23,43,49,64). Infantile scoliosis occurs most frequently among boys and is most often a left thoracic curve; most curves resolve spontaneously (45,61,63).

In contrast to the clear differences between adolescent and infantile idiopathic scoliosis, the juvenile form may resemble either of these two forms. There is a gradual transition from the characteristics of infantile curvature to those of adolescent curvature. The reported overall female to male ratio for juvenile idiopathic scoliosis ranges from 2:1 to 4:1 (27,56,92). However, a more detailed analysis by age belies this predominance

W. C. Warner, Jr.: Department of Orthopaedic Surgery, University of Tennessee—Campbell Clinic, Memphis, Tennessee 38103.

329

of female patients. Among children between the ages of 3 and 6 years, the female to male ratio is almost 1:1. The higher frequency among boys in this age group may represent infantile curves that have progressed and have been detected after 3 years of age. This is supported by the findings that left thoracic curves are more frequent among this younger group (less than 6 years of age) and that curves that are resolving are diagnosed at a younger age (61,65). Mannherz et al. (56) also found that these resolving curves tended to be left thoracic and left lumbar curves. Among children between the ages of 6 and 10 years, girls are more frequently affected, with a ratio ranging from 8:1 to 10:1 (27,56), which is similar to that for adolescent scoliosis. McMaster (61) found that the average age of boys at diagnosis of juvenile scoliosis was 5 ± 8 years and of girls 7 ± 2 years. That girls usually mature earlier than boys adds to the evidence that juvenile idiopathic scoliosis among boys tends to resemble more closely the infantile type and among girls the adolescent type.

The curve patterns of juvenile idiopathic scoliosis usually resemble those of adolescent scoliosis, with right thoracic and double major curve patterns predominating. The ratio of right thoracic curves to left thoracic curves is about 3:1 (16,27,56,61), although McMaster (61) found that among patients younger than 6 years, left and right curves occurred with equal frequency. Among their patients with juvenile scoliosis, Figueiredo and James (27) found that thoracic curves were most frequent (62%), followed by double thoracic (22%), thoracolumbar (15%), and lumbar (1%) curves (15). Mannherz et al. (56) found similar percentages of thoracic, double major, thoracolumbar, and lumbar curves.

Identifying the curve type can be difficult. As the child grows, the primary curve may extend, the end vertebra in the curve changes. McMaster (61) found that even though the end vertebra may change over time, the apical vertebra remains the same. Single thoracic curves have been reported to change to double major curves over time despite active brace treatment (27,56).

ETIOLOGY

The cause of juvenile idiopathic scoliosis is unknown. Excluding the increased incidence of syringomyelia and Arnold-Chiari malformation among patients with juvenile scoliosis, the proposed causes of juvenile scoliosis are the same as those of adolescent idiopathic scoliosis. It is possible that scoliosis is a symptom of several distinct processes.

The most popular etiologic theories have entailed mechanical (17,77–79), neuromuscular (4,42,97), central nervous system (55), or neurohormonal abnormalities (52–54). Mechanical causes of scoliosis are believed to be a discrepancy between anterior and posterior spinal growth that produces a relatively lordotic spinal segment. As it rotates laterally, this lordotic segment causes scoliotic deformity. Neuromuscular and central nervous system causes have been suggested by the findings of proprioceptive and vibratory abnormalities, which may indicate posterior spinal column dysfunction (4,42,97). Changes in somatosensory evoked potentials and the findings of brain stem asymmetry during MRI suggest a central nervous system cause of scoliosis

(55). A deficiency in the hormone melatonin has been proposed as a neurohormonal cause of scoliosis (52–54), and abnormalities in development of bone (13) and collagen (22,26) have been implicated. At present the exact cause of scoliosis is unknown. Because the cause of juvenile idiopathic scoliosis is unknown and scoliosis therefore cannot be prevented, a knowledge of the course of the condition is essential for making treatment recommendations and giving the family and patient reasonable expectations about how treatment will affect the scoliosis and what to expect if no treatment is instituted.

HISTORY AND CLINICAL EXAMINATION

The history and clinical examination are extremely important in the evaluation of a patient with juvenile idiopathic scoliosis. Because of the increased frequency of spinal cord disorders among children with scoliosis, any underlying causes of the curvature must be eliminated before the diagnosis of juvenile idiopathic scoliosis is made. Several important questions should be answered. How was the curve discovered? Is the condition painful? Does it interfere with the child's activities? Is there numbness? Are there bowel or bladder changes? Has the curve progressed rapidly? A positive response to any of these questions requires the physician to make a more thorough evaluation for intraspinal pathologic changes. Has the child undergone any surgical procedure? Some surgical procedures, such as thoracotomy and other operations on the chest, cause curves to be more progressive and less responsive to nonoperative treatment (24). Is the child's development normal? A developmental abnormality can be an early clue to an underlying neurologic condition.

The clinical examination starts with evaluation of the back for spinal deformity. Any midline dimples or hairy patches should be documented and should prompt further investigation of the spinal cord. A complete neurologic evaluation is performed to find any subtle neurologic changes or signs. Special attention is paid to the sensory and motor examinations. A cavus foot deformity can be an early sign of a neurologic cause of the scoliosis (71). Hugus et al. (38) reported that the loss of abdominal reflexes was sometimes the only clinical finding besides scoliosis for a patient with a syrinx (Fig. 1).

The initial radiographic examination should include unshielded posteroanterior and lateral views of the spine, but subsequent radiographs should be obtained with a shield because of the linear nature of accumulated radiation exposure (71). Supine bending views are not necessary unless surgery is being considered or the distinction between a compensatory and a structural curve is essential to treatment decisions. Bone-age radiographs can be obtained to correlate bone age with chronologic age but generally are needed only when there is a discrepancy between the patient's size and his or her chronologic age. The Risser sign is generally 0, and other signs of maturity, such as Tanner stages, are absent (Fig. 2).

Serial Cobb angle measurements (12) are used to measure progression, which is usually considered to be a change of 5 degrees or more. Morrissy et al. (72) and Carman et al. (9) emphasized the importance of using the same end vertebra and

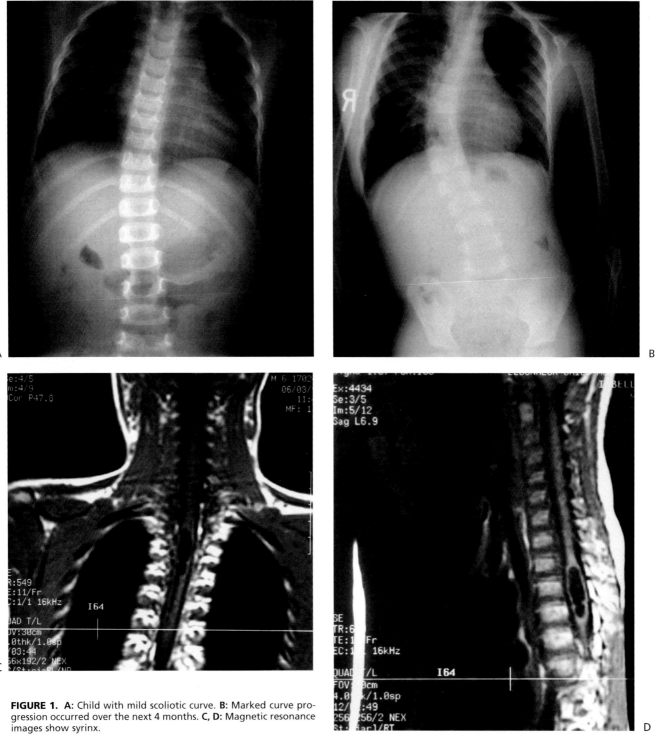

FIGURE 1. **A:** Child with mild scoliotic curve. **B:** Marked curve progression occurred over the next 4 months. **C, D:** Magnetic resonance images show syrinx.

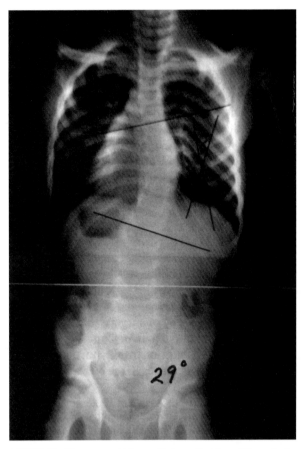

FIGURE 2. Nine-year-old boy with juvenile idiopathic scoliosis.

having the same person make the measurement at each examination.

Mehta (62) divided the stages of the curvature into two phases. The first phase is characterized by separation of the head of the rib from the vertebral body at the apex on both sides. As the curve progresses into phase 2, the rib head overlaps the vertebral body on the convex side. The measurement of the rib-vertebra angle is made in phase 1. A line perpendicular to the

apical vertebral end plate is drawn, and another line is drawn from the midneck to the midhead of the corresponding rib. The angle formed by the intersection of these two lines is the rib-vertebra angle. The rib-vertebra angle difference (RVAD) is the difference between the values of the rib-vertebra angles on the concave and convex sides of the curve (Fig. 3). Although the Mehta RVAD (34) has been used to predict progression of infantile scoliosis, it has not proved as useful for predicting progression of juvenile scoliosis. Serial RVAD measurements, however, have been useful in predicting response to brace treatment of children in this age group (56,92). McMaster (61) found that a progressive RVAD was indicative of a progressive curve and that resolving curves had improved RVADs. This may actually reflect the nature of the curve, because increasing vertebral rotation causes an increase in the RVAD.

Other authors have described other indicators of progression. Mannherz et al. (56) found kyphosis of less than 20 degrees on the initial lateral radiograph to be a strong risk factor for progression. Kahanovitz et al. (41) found that all patients with curves of more than 45 degrees at the beginning of brace treatment ultimately needed surgery, as did one half of those with curves of more than 35 degrees.

Further evaluation, which may include MRI examination, is indicated when there are abnormal findings in the history or physical examination, such as back pain that interferes with sleep or the child's normal activities, rapid curve progression (more than 2 to 3 degrees per month), left thoracic curves, focal neurologic abnormalities, cavus feet, abnormal abdominal reflexes, and any changes in bowel or bladder function. Because of the frequency of neural axis abnormalities among children with scoliosis (4% to 30%), Lewonowski et al. (47) recommended routine MRI examination of all children with scoliosis who are younger than 11 years. Gupta et al. (34) also recommended MRI examination of patients with juvenile idiopathic scoliosis who have curves of more than 20 degrees. Other authors have recommended performing MRI only if abnormalities are found in the history or physical examination, in particular any abnormal neurologic findings. Because of the increased incidence of abnormalities in this age group, I usually obtain an MRI in patients younger than 10 years of age.

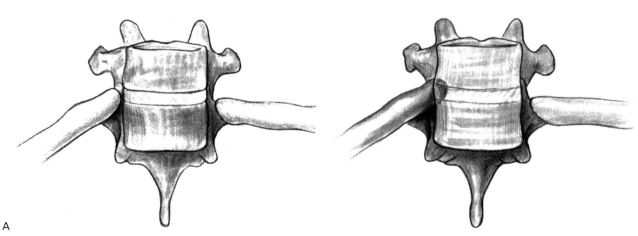

A

B

FIGURE 3. Mehta phase 1 **(A)** and phase 2 **(B)**. *(Figure continues.)*

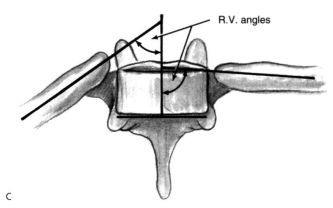

FIGURE 3. *Continued.* **C:** Measurement of rib-vertebra angles.

DIFFERENTIAL DIAGNOSIS

Juvenile idiopathic scoliosis is a diagnosis of exclusion. Before the diagnosis of juvenile idiopathic scoliosis is made, other conditions that cause scoliosis among young patients must be considered. Differential diagnoses should include neurofibromatosis (16,88), benign bone tumors (such as osteoid osteoma) (98), malignant or benign intraspinal tumors (16,88), spinal infection (66,98), connective tissue disease (such as Marfan syndrome and Ehlers-Danlos syndrome), chromosomal abnormalities (such as Down syndrome), congenital scoliosis, syringomyelia, tethered cord syndrome, metabolic bone disease, degenerative neurologic conditions (such as Friedreich ataxia) (16,27), primary muscle disease, and intervertebral disc abnormalities (31). Once these other possible causes of scoliosis in a young patient have been excluded and the diagnosis of idiopathic juvenile scoliosis is made, the parents can be informed of the distinct course of this condition, and treatment recommendations can be made.

COURSE OF DISEASE

A relative plateau in the growth of the spine occurs between the ages of 5 and 10 years. Periods of rapid spinal growth occur between 0 and 5 years and during the adolescent growth spurt (6). A unique characteristic of juvenile idiopathic scoliosis is the tendency toward progression during the growth plateau and rapid progression during the growth spurt. Because of this tendency toward progression, the course of juvenile idiopathic scoliosis is much more aggressive than that of adolescent idiopathic scoliosis. Approximately 70% of curves among patients with juvenile scoliosis progress and necessitate treatment; about one half of patients with curve progression need surgery (27,50, 56,61,92).

Curve progression is not surprising, considering the considerable amount of spinal growth remaining in these patients. According to the probabilities of progression described by Lonstein and Carlson (48), almost all juvenile scoliotic curves should progress; however, a small number do not. In the study by Mannherz et al. (56), 6 of 12 uncontrolled curves resolved spontaneously. Tolo and Gillespie (92) reported that 6 of 59 curves did not progress, even without treatment. McMaster (61) re-

ported 5 resolving curves among 109 patients. All five were younger patients (less than 6 years) with little vertebral rotation and RVADs less than 20 degrees. These resolving curves may represent a variant of infantile idiopathic scoliosis.

Knowing that most juvenile curves progress, what is the expected rate of progression? Tolo and Gillespie (92) found that uncontrolled curves progressed about 6 degrees a year during the juvenile growth period. McMaster (61) reported that among juvenile curves managed with a brace, the rate of progression decreased to 1 to 3 degrees a year during the juvenile period and increased to 4.5 to 11 degrees a year during the adolescent growth spurt.

How does this progression affect patients with juvenile scoliosis? Pehrsson et al. (76), in a study of mortality and its causes among 115 patients with uncontrolled scoliosis, found that mortality was significantly higher among patients with infantile and juvenile scoliosis than it was among those with adolescent scoliosis. The higher risk was apparent when patients became 40 to 50 years of age and was related to respiratory and cardiovascular disease. Weinstein and Ponseti (96) also documented that curves greater than 50 to 60 degrees will continue to progress even after skeletal maturity.

CLASSIFICATION

Robinson and McMaster (83) classified juvenile curves into four types according to the apical vertebra (Fig. 4). The apical vertebra was used because the tendency toward extension of the primary curve can change the end vertebra, and compensatory secondary curves tend to become fixed primary curves or double major curves. Group I curves were progressive thoracic curves with an apex at T8. This group was divided into IA and IB subtypes. Group IA was a single midthoracic curve, and group IB was a midthoracic curve and a secondary minor lumbar curve. Group II curves had the apical vertebra at T8, T9, or T10. Unlike vertebrae in group I curves, the lumbar vertebrae were rotated in the same direction as in the primary curve and a compensatory lumbar curve did not develop. Patients with this type of curve had a severe list and unsightly deformity. Group III curves were long thoracolumbar curves with the apex at T12. Group IV curves were primary lumbar curves and secondary thoracic curves. The importance of this classification is that 73 (97%) of 75 of Robinson and McMaster's patients classified as having group I or II curves needed operative treatment. The 20 patients with group III or IV curves had much slower curve progression, and only 3 (15%) needed surgery.

TREATMENT
Nonoperative Treatment

As with other forms of scoliosis, treatment depends on the severity of the curve and the rate of its progression. In general, the indications for nonoperative management of juvenile scoliosis are more liberal than those for management of adolescent scoliosis. Curves of more than 25 degrees that are first detected in the juvenile years and curves with documented progression are

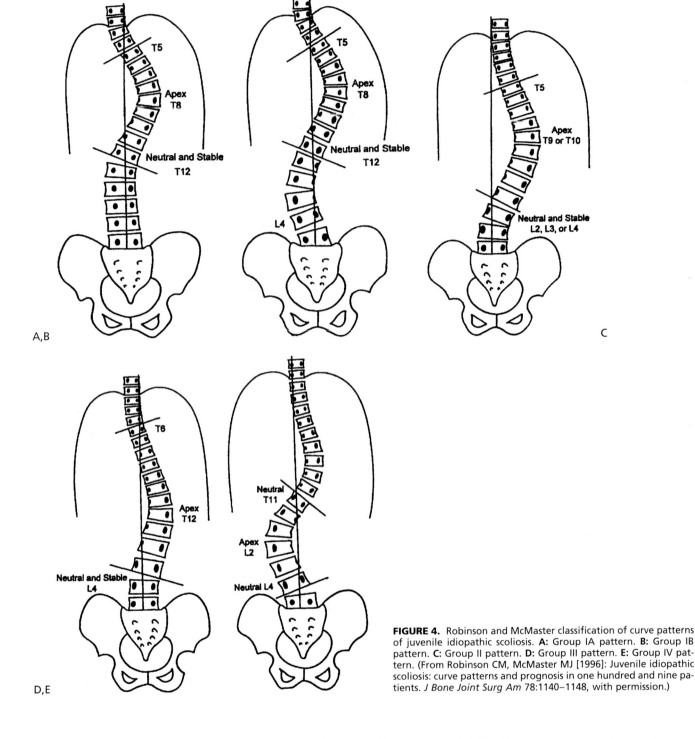

FIGURE 4. Robinson and McMaster classification of curve patterns of juvenile idiopathic scoliosis. **A:** Group IA pattern. **B:** Group IB pattern. **C:** Group II pattern. **D:** Group III pattern. **E:** Group IV pattern. (From Robinson CM, McMaster MJ [1996]: Juvenile idiopathic scoliosis: curve patterns and prognosis in one hundred and nine patients. *J Bone Joint Surg Am* 78:1140–1148, with permission.)

indications for instituting a brace treatment program. Brace treatment also may be indicated for some patients with thoracic curves of 20 degrees or more when they come to medical attention because of the high rate of progression of these curves. A Milwaukee brace or a modified Boston brace is generally preferred for children with juvenile idiopathic scoliosis because these braces do not cause chest wall compression. Rib cage distortion is possible with the use of a total-contact thoracolumbosacral orthosis (TLSO) because the child must wear the brace

for a long time (6). Bending braces worn at night, such as the Charlestown brace, have been reported to be effective in the management of some adolescent idiopathic curves (25), but the effectiveness in juvenile idiopathic scoliosis has not been proved.

General principles of bracing are as described by Tolo and Gillespie (92). The brace is worn full time at first, except for 2 hours each day, for at least 1 year. Radiographs are obtained every 4 to 6 months. If stabilization of the curve is apparent, brace wear becomes part time; the brace can be removed for 4 hours each day. If the curve does not progress, brace wear is decreased in 2- to 4-hour increments until the device is worn only during sleep. Tolo and Gillespie used serial measurements of the RVAD to evaluate the success of brace treatment. If RVAD values declined as treatment continued, part-time brace wear was deemed adequate. Patients with RVAD values near or less than zero at the time of diagnosis progressed from full-time to part-time wear in a relatively short time. If the RVAD did not decrease to less than 10 degrees, progression could be expected and full-time brace wear was continued. An increase in RVAD was sometimes seen before any change occurred in the Cobb angle. If the curve responded to brace treatment, part-time wear was continued until maturity.

The reported success of bracing programs in the management of juvenile scoliosis has been variable. Kahanovitz et al. (41) reported an excellent prognosis with part-time bracing for curves of less than 35 degrees and RVADs of less than 20 degrees. Patients with curves of more than 45 degrees and RVADs of more than 20 degrees had a poorer prognosis for successful brace treatment. Among patients with curves between 35 and 45 degrees, the response to brace treatment was unpredictable. Tolo and Gillespie (92) found that only 19% of their patients needed surgery, but other authors have reported much higher percentages of patients who needed surgery despite bracing: Figueiredo and James (27), 62%; Dabney and Bowen (16), 33%; Mannherz et al. (56), 80%; and McMaster (61), 86%.

If the curve progresses despite brace treatment, the goal of bracing changes. Bracing is then used to slow progression of a curve of 45 to 50 degrees so that surgery can be delayed until more growth has been completed. The hope is to avoid the crankshaft phenomenon, which often occurs when posterior spinal fusion with instrumentation is performed on an immature spine. Bracing should be used only if the patient and parents understand that the goal is to delay—not prevent—surgery. Close follow-up care and patient compliance are necessary.

Reported problems with brace wear include skin pressure problems, rib cage deformity with the use of a total-contact TLSO, and change of a single thoracic curve to a double curve.

Electrical stimulation has been recommended as an alternative to brace treatment. Several authors have reported favorable results with electrical stimulation (7,28,60), but others have found this modality less effective than bracing (8,21,32,74,90). At present, electrical stimulation is not a recommended therapeutic alternative for juvenile idiopathic scoliosis.

Operative Treatment

The indications for surgical management of juvenile scoliosis are generally the same as for other forms of scoliosis (5,6). Surgery is recommended for progressive curves of more than 40 to 45 degrees, although some surgeons may continue bracing until the curve reaches 50 degrees in younger patients.

When surgical management of a curve that has not been controlled by bracing is being considered for a young patient, the amount of spinal growth remaining is of prime importance. How spinal fusion affects spinal growth is a controversial topic. Many authors initially believed the immature posterior fusion mass possessed biologic plasticity and had potential for longitu-

dinal growth (91), but several studies have demonstrated that the posterior fusion mass does not grow longitudinally (40,46, 70,81). Anterior growth of the spine continues despite solid posterior fusion, which explains some of the findings among young patients who have undergone posterior fusion. Anterior growth of the vertebral body initially causes loss of disc space height. If the disc space height does not decrease at one or more levels after posterior fusion, pseudarthrosis is likely present. Marjedtoko (58) found a gradual deterioration of clinical results with continued anterior vertebral body growth, including progressive apical rotation and apical deviation, increased prominences of the ribs or paraspinal muscles, and increased Cobb angles. This was initially reported as "bending of the fusion mass." It was found that the younger the child, the more likely were these clinical findings. The period of highest risk was during the adolescent growth spurt.

Hefti and McMaster (36) also described this phenomenon of anterior spinal growth and subsequent clinical deterioration. Dubousset et al. (19) called this process the *crankshaft phenomenon*. Sanders et al. (86) found that patients with a Risser 0 sign and open triradiate cartilages are at high risk of crankshaft phenomenon if a posterior fusion alone is performed. The crankshaft phenomenon occurred among 45% of patients who had open triradiate cartilages and only 5% who had closed triradiate cartilages. The description of the crankshaft phenomenon has changed the recommendations for posterior spinal fusion among juvenile and young adolescent patients with progressive scoliosis. To prevent the crankshaft phenomenon, anterior growth arrest and fusion have been recommended in addition to posterior fusion.

When operative management of juvenile scoliosis is chosen, an important consideration is the expected loss of growth caused by the fusion. Dimeglio (18) described two periods of rapid spinal growth: from birth to 5 years and from 10 to 16 years of age. From 5 to 10 years of age the spine grows at a steady rate but not at the rapid rate that is does during the other two periods of growth. Dimeglio found that during the 5- to 10-year period of growth, each spinal segment averages 0.05 cm of growth each year. After the age of 10 years, growth increases to 0.11 cm per segment per year. As emphasized by Anderson et al. (2), the growth remaining in sitting height is determined by contributions from the head; the cervical, thoracic, and lumbar portions of the spine; and the pelvis. Fifty percent of the sitting height is from T1 to S1, the thoracic spine contributing two thirds and the lumbar spine one third. At 5 years of age the T1-S1 segment has reached about 66% of its definitive size among boys and 69% among girls. At this point there should be about 15 cm of growth remaining, including an average of 10 cm in the thoracic spine and 5 cm in the lumbar spine. The deficit in sitting height caused by spinal fusion can be calculated with this information (Fig. 5).

Winter (79) used the calculations of Anderson et al. (2) to devise a formula for determining potential shortening after spinal fusion: Amount of shortening in centimeters equals 0.07 multiplied by the number of segments fused multiplied by the number of years of remaining growth. This formula allows the surgeon to inform the family of the estimated shortening to be expected after spinal fusion. The family should understand that even with-

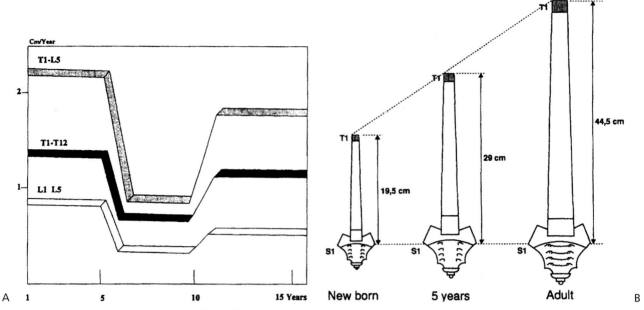

FIGURE 5. **A:** Growth velocity of T1–L5 segment, thoracic segment T1–12, and lumbar segment L1–5. **B:** Evolution of the T1–S1 segment. The figures are average values to indicate extent of the phenomenon. (From Dimeglio A [1992]: Growth of the spine before age 5 years. *J Pediatr Orthop B* 1:102–107, with permission.)

out fusion, some height will be lost because of the scoliotic deformity (Fig. 6).

The goal of surgery is to halt progression of the scoliotic curve. This may be obtained by any of several methods: (a) posterior instrumentation with fusion, (b) anterior instrumentation with or without fusion, (c) posterior instrumentation with both anterior and posterior fusion, (d) posterior instrumentation without fusion, (e) anterior fusion without instrumentation, and (f) posterior fusion in situ.

Posterior Fusion with Instrumentation

The smaller the child, the more difficult it is to insert a spinal instrumentation system safely. The current hook and rod systems may be too large to be safely used in the care of a young patient, but several spinal instrumentation systems come in pediatric sizes that are better suited for young patients. Because these rods are more flexible than the adult instrumentation systems and the hooks may not give as secure a purchase for correction of the deformity, postoperative immobilization may be necessary. If posterior fusion and instrumentation are considered, several questions must be answered. How flexible is the curve, and how much correction can be expected with the instrumentation? How much anterior growth is expected after surgery? What amount of crankshaft deformity will occur after surgery? Is the curve a single curve or a double curve? Is there a marked compensatory curve that might require postoperative bracing?

Posterior fusion and instrumentation alone cause some loss of correction among young patients because of continued anterior growth of the vertebral bodies. With the loss of correction, there will be an associated increase in rotation of the apical vertebra and an increase in the rib prominence. Dubousset et al. (19) reported that curves progressed after posterior spinal fusion in

all their patients younger than 10 years, including those with idiopathic and neuromuscular curves. Among those with idiopathic curves, average progression in Cobb angle was 13 degrees; the increase in rotation, as measured by means of the Perdriolle method (77,78), was 11 degrees. At final follow-up examinations, some patients still had Risser 0, so further progression could be expected. Hefti and McMaster (36) reported that after posterior fusion the disc spaces initially bulge before decompensation of the curve, so there may be a period during which continued anterior growth is absorbed by the disc spaces and no correction is lost. If posterior fusion alone is performed for a patient with juvenile scoliosis, some increase in deformity should be expected. The younger the patient, the greater is the increase in deformity. At present the exact amount of postoperative progression cannot be predicted preoperatively, but some degree of progression should be expected after posterior instrumentation and fusion (Figs. 7, 8).

Anterior Fusion with or without Instrumentation

Good results have been reported after anterior fusion and instrumentation of the thoracic spine in certain types of adolescent idiopathic scoliosis, but whether this technique can be used in the care of patients with juvenile scoliosis is unknown. Because the vertebral bodies are smaller, safe insertion of anterior vertebral body screws may be more difficult in operations on younger children. This approach is attractive because it solves the problem of continued anterior growth and may help improve the associated thoracic hypokyphosis usually present in this condition. In thoracolumbar and lumbar curves, anterior instrumentation may be possible if the vertebrae are large enough. Anterior fusion and instrumentation in management of these curves have the advantage of saving mobile lumbar segments while correcting

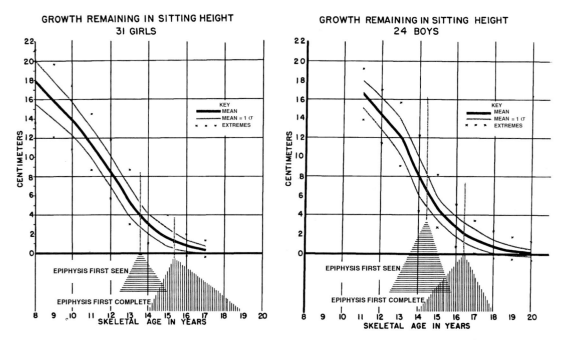

FIGURE 6. Growth remaining in trunk for different skeletal ages in girls and boys. (From Anderson M, Hwang SC, Green WT [1965]: Growth of the normal trunk in boys and girls during the second decade of life, related to age maturity, and ossification of the iliac epiphyses. *J Bone Joint Surg Am* 47:1554–1564, with permission.)

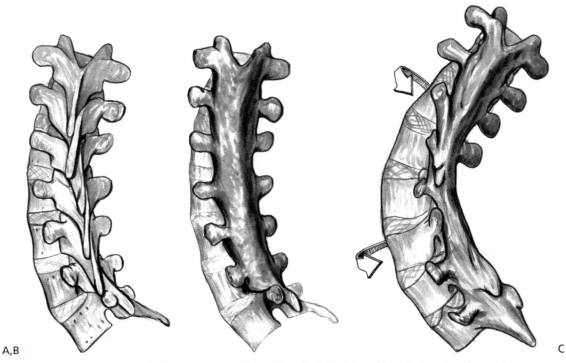

FIGURE 7. Crankshaft phenomenon. **A:** Spine with scoliosis. **B:** Spine with scoliosis and solid posterior fusion mass. **C:** Despite solid posterior fusion, continued anterior growth causes increase in deformity.

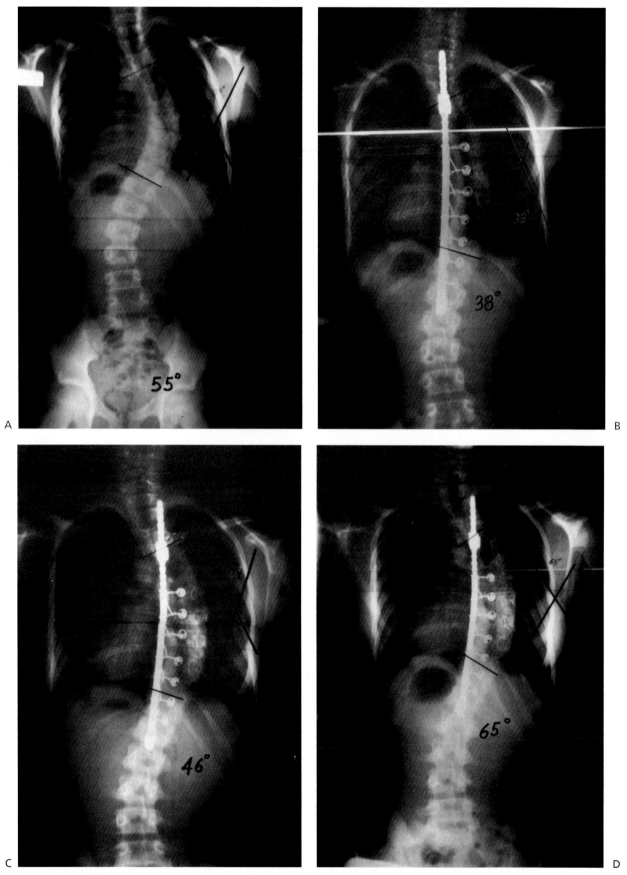

FIGURE 8. Clinical example of crankshaft phenomenon. **A:** Nine-year-old patient with a 55-degree curve. **B:** One year after posterior spinal fusion and instrumentation, curve is 38 degrees. **C:** At 2.5 years after fusion, curve is 46 degrees. **D:** Five years after fusion, curve is 65 degrees despite solid posterior fusion.

the scoliotic deformity. One disadvantage is that kyphosis can be produced in the thoracolumbar or lumbar area. This problem can be lessened with the use of a rigid rod construct anteriorly.

Combined Anterior and Posterior Fusion

Anterior fusion followed by posterior instrumentation and fusion is currently recommended for patients with progressive juvenile scoliosis. Although performing two procedures increases morbidity, the possibility of the occurrence of the crankshaft phenomenon is eliminated, and better correction of the primary curve is obtained. Shufflebarger and Clark (87) reported no loss of correction or progression of rotational deformity after combined fusions among patients who were at high risk of development of the crankshaft phenomenon after posterior fusion alone. Anterior fusion can be done through a thoracoscopic approach, which allows good exposure of the anterior vertebrae and disc spaces. Reported fusion rates after use of the thoracoscopic approach are equal to those with open methods (33,37,73,84,95), and a thoracoscopic approach has the advantages of less morbidity and smaller incisional scars than open techniques. Disadvantages are that there is a learning curve with this technique and that the assistance of a general surgeon trained in this technique is required. If such assistance is not available, a standard thoracotomy can be used.

Instrumentation without Fusion or with Limited Fusion

Another alternative for control of curves during growth is instrumentation without fusion of the curve or with fusion of only the end vertebra into which the hooks are inserted (20,29,30,75). Harrington (35) first described this technique in the 1960s. Moe (67,68), who used it specifically on growing children, called it the subcutaneous Harrington rod technique. Moe (67,68) designed a rod for this purpose, and Moe et al. (69) reported using a Harrington rod in this manner. Several companies have developed so-called growth rods that can be lengthened periodically to maintain curve correction, and the technique has been modified to replace subcutaneous placement of the rods with subfascial insertion. Problems with the use of growth rods include the necessity for a surgical procedure every 6 to 12 months to lengthen or exchange the rod. Most surgeons recommend postoperative full-time brace wear to prevent rod breakage or hook dislodgment. Despite these problems, this method is an alternative for controlling curves until the child is mature enough for definitive posterior fusion (Fig. 9).

Another alternative is to combine subcutaneous or subfascial posterior rod fixation with localized anterior fusion of the apical vertebrae (1,44,94). This technique has the advantage of provid-

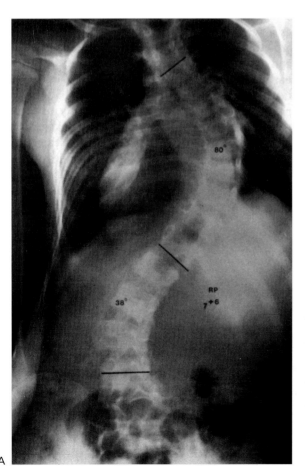
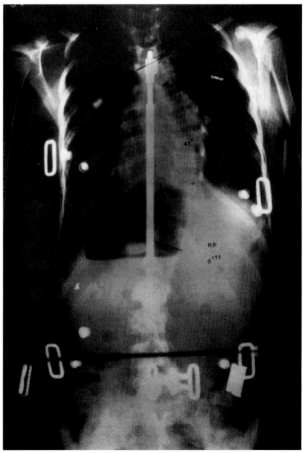

A   B

FIGURE 9. A: Boy 7 years 6 months of age with an 80-degree curve. **B:** One year 5 months after insertion of a Moe subcutaneous rod with fusion at hook sites. (Courtesy of Stuart L. Weinstein, MD.)

ing partial correction with instrumentation. Localized anterior fusion stops progression of the curve and growth of the apical vertebra, which may help lessen any increase in deformity caused by continued vertebral rotation. This combined approach helps control progression of scoliosis while the child continues to grow in the unfused segments. Several authors have reported good results with this technique because it allows some spinal growth and control of the progressive curve before definitive fusion is performed. Vanlommel et al. (94) reported that the initial intraoperative correction averaged 25 degrees, but this decreased to only 8 degrees of correction at final lengthening. The authors suggested that the spine became stiffer with each lengthening and that the stiffness made subsequent correction more difficult. Klemme et al. (44) also found that the curve response tended to decline with consecutive lengthenings. Among their patients the growth of the unfused spinal segments averaged 3.1 cm over a treatment period of 3.1 years.

A technique with Luque rods and wires without fusion (the so-called Luque trolley) has been described as a way to correct the curve and still allow spinal growth (46,59). Extraperiosteal spinal dissection and segmental fixation with Luque rods and sublaminar wires are performed. Although extraperiosteal dissection is used, the incidence of spontaneous fusion is high. Mardjetko et al. (59) reported that nine patients treated with the Luque trolley without fusion all had spontaneous fusion. This method has the advantage of providing segmental fixation, but the risk of passing sublaminar wires, the difficulty of removing the wires, the possibility of wire breakage, and the high incidence of spontaneous fusion preclude recommendation of this technique.

Technique of Insertion of Subfascial Rods

After induction of general anesthesia, the patient is placed prone on a four-poster frame (1). The back is prepared and draped in the usual sterile manner. The proper level for exposure is identified on a radiograph before the incision is made. A radiograph must be obtained to mark both the upper and lower vertebrae that are to be instrumented. The neutral vertebrae at each end of the curve are selected, and after infiltration of 1:500,000 epinephrine solution, a 3- to 4-cm incision is made over the lamina at each level to be instrumented. An alternative method is to make the skin incision the length of the curve but to expose only the fascia overlying the spine that is to be instrumented with hooks (Fig. 10). Moe et al. (69) initially described subcutaneous placement of the rod, but now the rod is placed beneath the dorsal fascia to improve stability and to reduce the potential for skin problems (1).

Dissection is carried down to the lamina and spinous process of the end vertebra on the concave side. A Cobb elevator is used to expose the lamina on the concave side, and care is taken not to cut the interspinous ligament or to extend the dissection past the midline. The facet joints at the sites selected for hook insertion are exposed. The ligamentum flavum is stripped from the underside of the selected lamina at each end.

A claw-type construct can be used at the upper and lower

levels. If the Harrington rod system is used, a special pediatric hook is used; otherwise, a 1254 hook without a sharp edge is preferred. A rod of the appropriate length is contoured to accommodate thoracic kyphosis and lumbar lordosis. If a Harrington rod is used, the ratchet end of the rod is placed at the lower hook site to prevent prominence of the unused portion of the rod. The rod is placed in the hook sites, and distraction is applied to correct the deformity. Somatosensory evoked potentials or a wake-up test is used for neurologic evaluation.

With the newer growth rod system, two rods are used. One rod is attached to the upper hooks and one to the lower hooks. These two rods are allowed to overlap and are connected with a growth connector. Distraction is achieved by means of lengthening the two rods at the connector site. In addition, so called end fusions, as described by Marchetti and Faldini (57), are performed at the initial instrumentation in most patients. Akbarnia and McCarthy (1) place a subfascial distraction rod on the concave side and an additional subfascial compression rod on the convex side of the curve (Fig. 11).

After the operation, a Milwaukee brace is worn full time for external support. Ambulation is begun within 48 hours, and the patient is discharged from the hospital. Winter and Lonstein (99,100) recommended repetition of lengthening 3 months after the initial rod insertion rather than waiting for curve deterioration before lengthening. After the second lengthening, subsequent rod lengthening should be done every 3 to 6 months. Posteroanterior and lateral radiographs are obtained to evaluate the status of the rod and correction of the deformity. Only the area over the growth connectors has to be exposed for the lengthening. This technique is a method of temporarily managing the curve. Definitive spinal fusion is required when the patient is more mature.

Complications

Complications of management of juvenile scoliosis are similar to those of management of adolescent scoliosis: pseudarthrosis, wound infection, paralysis, and malalignment after fusion with instrumentation. Complications that are more frequent among patients with juvenile scoliosis include trunk shortening, the crankshaft phenomenon, and progression of unfused curves.

The amount of trunk shortening can be accurately predicted with growth charts and growth-remaining tables or Winter's (99) formula (see earlier). Although trunk shortening is a consideration when with surgical treatment, the family should understand that even without surgery the trunk will be short and deformed because the spine is not growing straight. After correction of a single curve, careful follow-up evaluation is necessary to determine whether bracing is necessary for secondary curves. What were believed to be compensatory curves during brace treatment can progress after surgery (for example, a primary single curve can become a primary double major curve).

The crankshaft phenomenon remains a major problem after operations for juvenile scoliosis. Although the loss of correction in the coronal plane and the increase in vertebral rotation cannot be accurately predicted at this time, it is known that this will

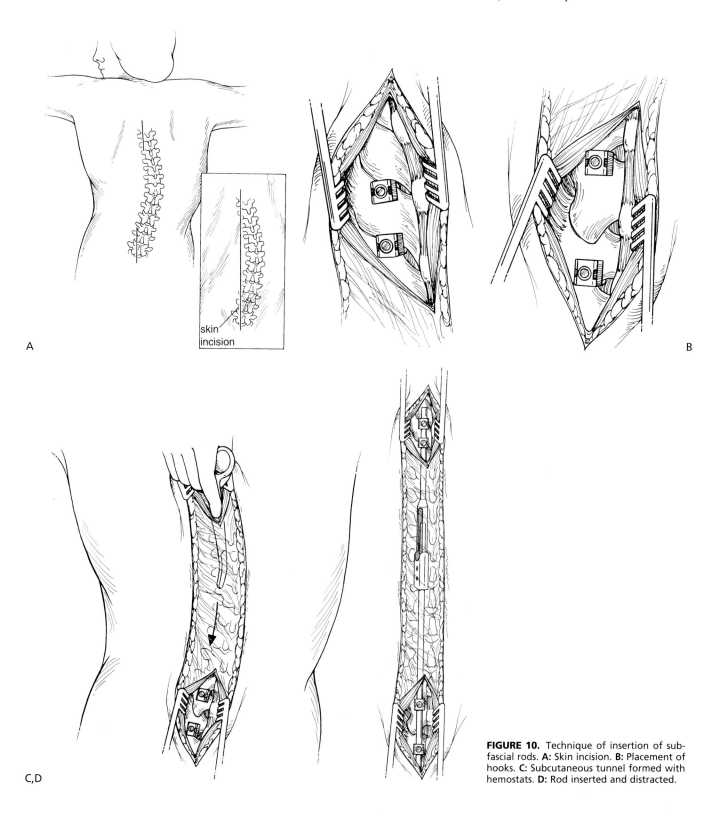

A

B

C,D

FIGURE 10. Technique of insertion of sub-fascial rods. **A:** Skin incision. **B:** Placement of hooks. **C:** Subcutaneous tunnel formed with hemostats. **D:** Rod inserted and distracted.

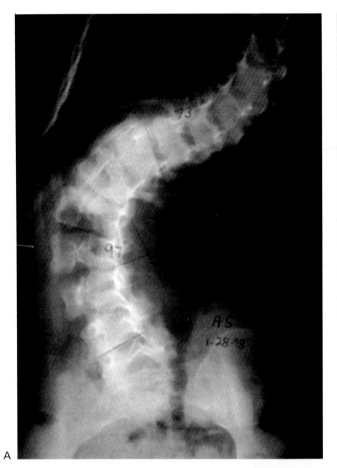

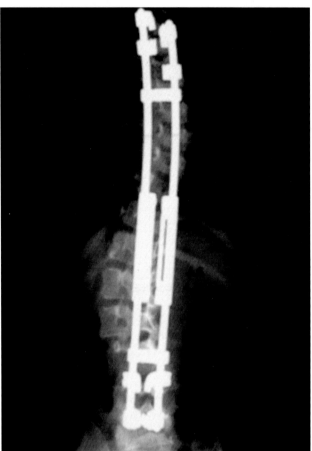

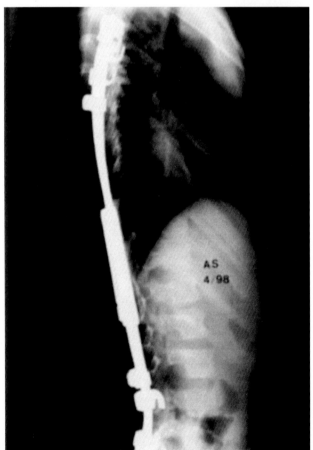

FIGURE 11. **A:** Juvenile idiopathic scoliosis with 73-degree thoracic curve and 97-degree lumbar curve. **B, C:** After insertion of dual subfascial growth rods. Distraction rod on concave side and compression rod on convex side of curve. (Courtesy of Behrooz A. Akbarnia, MD.)

occur after almost all posterior fusions among patients who have a Risser sign of 0 (19) and an open triradiate cartilage. To avoid this problem, clinical judgment must be exercised to determine whether brace treatment should be continued for a longer time and for a larger curve, for example curves of 50 to 55 degrees. If brace treatment cannot control the curvature, instrumentation without fusion should be considered to allow continued growth of the spine before definitive fusion. If fusion is planned for a patient with juvenile scoliosis, circumferential fusion is recommended to avoid the crankshaft phenomenon.

SUMMARY

Juvenile idiopathic scoliosis occurs between the ages of 4 and 10 years without any known cause of the curvature. A detailed history and examination are required to exclude other known causes of scoliosis among this age group. Curves less than 20 to 25 degrees are simply observed. If the curve progresses, brace treatment is begun. The RVAD is used to help follow the response of the curve to brace treatment. If the curve continues to progress in the brace, bracing can be continued in an attempt to delay surgery. If surgery is needed, instrumentation without fusion can be used to control the curve until the spine is more mature. If surgical fusion of the immature spine is needed, anterior fusion and posterior fusion with instrumentation are recommended to prevent loss of correction and deterioration of appearance caused by the crankshaft phenomenon.

REFERENCES

1. Akbarnia BA, McCarthy RE (1998): Basics: Pediatric Isola instrumentation without fusion for the treatment of progressive early onset scoliosis. In: *Instrumentation for growth. Spinal instrumentation techniques,* vol. 2. Rosemont IL: Scoliosis Research Society.
2. Anderson M, Hwang SC, Green WT (1965): Growth of the normal trunk in boys and girls during the second decade of life, related to age maturity, and ossification of the iliac epiphyses. *J Bone Joint Surg Am* 47:1554–1564.
3. Arai S, Ohtsuka Y, Moriya H, et al (1993): Scoliosis associated with syringomyelia. *Spine* 18:1591–1592.
4. Barrack RL, Wyatt MP, Whitecloud TS III, et al. (1988): Vibratory hypersensitivity in idiopathic scoliosis. *J Pediatr Orthop* 8:389–395.
5. Birdwell K, DeWald R, eds (1991): *The textbook of spinal surgery.* Philadelphia: JB Lippincott.
6. Bradford DS, Lonstein E, Moe JH, et al., eds (1978): *Moe's textbook of scoliosis and other spinal deformities,* 2nd ed. Philadelphia, WB Saunders.
7. Brown JC, Axelgaard J, Howson DC (1984): Multicenter trial of a noninvasive stimulation method for idiopathic scoliosis. *Spine* 9: 382–387.
8. Bylund P, Aaro S, Gottfries B, et al.: Is lateral electric surface stimulation an effective treatment for scoliosis? *J Pediatr Orthop* 7:298–300.
9. Carman DL, Browne RH, Birch JG (1990): Measurement of scoliosis and kyphosis radiographs: intraobserver and interobserver variation. *J Bone Joint Surg Am* 72:328–333.
10. Carr WA, Moe JH, Winter RB, et al. (1980): Treatment of idiopathic scoliosis in the Milwaukee brace. *J Bone Joint Surg Am* 62:599–612.
11. Chen PQ (1990): Spinal deformities among children under 10 years old: a clinical analysis of 41 cases. *J Formos Med Assoc* 89:772–776.
12. Cobb J (1948): Outline for the study of scoliosis. *Instr Course Lect* 5:261–275.
13. Cook SD, Harding AF, Morgan EL, et al. (1987): Trabecular bone mineral density in idiopathic scoliosis. *J Pediatr Orthop* 7:168–174.
14. Cowell HR, Hall JN, MacEwen GD (1972): Genetic aspects of idiopathic scoliosis. *Clin Orthop* 86:121–131.
15. Czeizel A, Bellyei A, Barta O, et al. (1978): Genetics of adolescent idiopathic scoliosis. *J Med Genet* 15:424–427.
16. Dabney KW, Bowen JR (1991): Juvenile idiopathic scoliosis. *Semin Spine Surg* 3:524–530.
17. Dickson RA, Lawton JO, Archer IA, et al. (1984): The pathogenesis of idiopathic scoliosis: biplanar spinal asymmetry. *J Bone Joint Surg Br* 66:8–15.
18. Dimeglio A (1992): Growth of the spine before age 5 years. *J Pediatr Orthop B* 1:102–107.
19. Dubousset J, Herring JA, Shufflebarger H (1989): The crankshaft phenomenon. *J Pediatr Orthop* 9:541–550.
20. Dubousset J, Katti E, Seringe R (1992): Epiphysiodesis of the spine in young children for congenital spinal deformations. *J Pediatr Orthop B* 1:123–130.
21. Durham JW, Moskowitz A, Whitney J (1990): Surface electrical stimulation versus brace in treatment of idiopathic scoliosis. *Spine* 15: 888–892.
22. Echenne B, Barneon G, Pages M, et al. (1988): Skin elastic fiber pathology and idiopathic scoliosis. *J Pediatr Orthop* 8:522–528.
23. Edmonson AS, Morris JT (1977): Follow-up study of Milwaukee brace treatment in patients with idiopathic scoliosis. *Clin Orthop* 126: 58–61.
24. Farley FA, Phillips WA, Herzenberg JE, et al. (1991): Natural history of scoliosis in congenital heart disease. *J Pediatr Orthop* 11:42–47.
25. Federico DJ, Renshaw TS (1990): Results of treatment of idiopathic scoliosis with the Charleston bending orthosis. *Spine* 15:886–887.
26. Fernandez-Bermejo E, Garcia-Jimeniez MA, Fernandez-Pafomeque C, et al. (1993): Adolescent idiopathic scoliosis and joint laxity. *Spine* 18:918–922.
27. Figueiredo UM, James JI (1981): Juvenile idiopathic scoliosis. *J Bone Joint Surg Br* 63:61–66.
28. Fisher DA, Rapp GF, Emkes M (1987): Idiopathic scoliosis: transcutaneous muscle stimulation versus the Milwaukee brace. *Spine* 12: 987–991.
29. Fisk JR, Peterson HA, Laughlin R, et al. (1995): Spontaneous fusion in scoliosis after instrumentation without arthrodesis. *J Pediatr Orthop* 15:183–186.
30. Gillespie R, O'Brien J (1981): Harrington instrumentation without fusion. *J Bone Joint Surg Br* 63:461.
31. Grass JP, Dockendorff IB, Soto VA, et al. (1993): Progressive scoliosis with vertebral rotation after lumbar intervertebral disc herniation in a 10-year-old girl. *Spine* 18:336–338.
32. Goldberg C, Dowling FE, Fogarty EE, et al. (1988): Electro-spinal stimulation in children with adolescent and juvenile scoliosis. *Spine* 13:482–484.
33. Gonzalez Barrios I, Fuentes Caparros S, Avila Jurado MM (1995): Anterior thoracoscopic epiphysiodesis in the treatment of a crankshaft phenomenon. *Eur Spine J* 4:343–346.
34. Gupta P, Lenke LG, Bridwell KH (1998): Incidence of neural axis abnormalities in infantile and juvenile patients with spinal deformity: is a magnetic resonance imaging screening necessary? *Spine* 23: 206–210.
35. Harrington PR (1962): Treatment of scoliosis: correction and internal fixation by spine instrumentation. *J Bone Joint Surg Am* 44:591–610.
36. Hefti FL, McMaster MJ (1983): The effect of the adolescent growth spurt on early posterior spinal fusion in infantile and juvenile idiopathic scoliosis. *J Bone Joint Surg Br* 65:247–254.
37. Holcomb GW III, Mencio GA, Green NE (1997): Video-assisted thoracoscpic diskectomy and fusion. *J Pediatr Surg* 32:1120–1127.
38. Hugus JJ, Taylor TKF, McGee-Callett M, et al. (1990): Syringomyelia and scoliosis: a new view. Presented at the 25th Annual Meeting of the Scoliosis Research Society, Honolulu, Hawaii, September 27.
39. James JIP (1954): Idiopathic scoliosis: the prognosis, diagnosis, and operative indications related to curve patterns and the age at onset. *J Bone Joint Surg Br* 36:35–49.

40. Johnson JTH, Southwick WO (1960): Bone growth after spine fusion: a clinical survey. *J Bone Joint Surg Am* 42:1396–1412.

41. Kahanovitz N, Levine DB, Landone J (1982): The part-time Milwaukee brace treatment of juvenile idiopathic scoliosis: long-term follow-up. *Clin Orthop* 167:145–151.

42. Keessen W, Crowe A, Hern M (1992): Proprioceptive accuracy in idiopathic scoliosis. *Spine* 17:149–155.

43. Keiser RP, Shufflebarger HL (1976): The Milwaukee brace in idiopathic scoliosis: evaluation of 123 completed cases. *Clin Orthop* 118:19–24.

44. Klemme W, Denis F, Winter RB, et al (1997): Spinal instrumentation without fusion for progressive scoliosis in young children. *J Pediatr Orthop* 17:734–742.

45. Koop SE (1988): Infantile and juvenile idiopathic scoliosis. *Orthop Clin North Am* 19:331–337.

46. Letts RM, Bobechko WP (1974): Fusion of the scoliotic spine in young children. *Clin Orthop* 101:136–145.

47. Lewonowski K, King JD, Nelson MD (1992): Routine use of magnetic resonance imaging in idiopathic scoliosis in patients less than eleven years of age. *Spine* 17[Suppl 6]:S109–S116.

48. Lonstein JE, Carlson JM (1984): The prediction of curve progression in untreated idiopathic scoliosis during growth. *J Bone Joint Surg Am* 66:1061–1071.

49. Lonstein JE, Winter RB (1988): Adolescent idiopathic scoliosis: non-operative treatment. *Orthop Clin North Am* 19:239–246.

50. Lonstein JE, Winter RB (1988): Milwaukee brace treatment of juvenile idiopathic scoliosis. Presented at the 23rd Annual Meeting of the Scoliosis Research Society, Baltimore, Maryland, October 1.

51. MacEwen GD, Cowell HR (1970): Familial incidence of idiopathic scoliosis and its implications in patient treatment. *J Bone Joint Surg Am* 52:405.

52. Machida M, Dubousset J, Imamura Y (1993): An experimental study in chickens for pathogenesis of idiopathic scoliosis. *Spine* 18:1609–1615.

53. Machida M, Dubousset J, Imamura Y, et al. (1992): Melatonin: a possible role in pathogenesis of adolescent idiopathic scoliosis. *Spine* 21:1147–1152.

54. Machida M, Miyashita Y, Murai I, et al. J (1997): Role of serotonin for scoliotic deformity in pinealectomized chicken. *Spine* 22:1297–1301.

55. Maguire J, Madigan R, Wallace S, et al. (1993): Intraoperative long-latency reflex activity in idiopathic scoliosis demonstrates abnormal central processing. *Spine* 18:1621–1626.

56. Mannherz RE, Betz RR, Clancy M, et al. (1988): Juvenile idiopathic scoliosis followed to skeletal maturity. *Spine* 13:1087–1090.

57. Marchetti PG, Feldini A (1978): "End fusions" in the treatment of progressing or severe scoliosis in childhood or early adolescence. *Orthop Trans* 2:271.

58. Mardjetko SM (1997): Infantile and juvenile scoliosis. In: Bridwell KH, DeWald RL, eds. *The textbook of spinal surgery.* Philadelphia: Lippincott-Raven, pp. 401–422.

59. Mardjetko S, Hammerberg K, Lubicky JP (1990): The Luque trolley revisited: review of 9 cases requiring revision. Presented at the 25th Annual Meeting of the Scoliosis Research Society, Honolulu, Hawaii, September 26.

60. McCollough NC III (1986): Nonperative treatment of idiopathic scoliosis using surface electrical stimulation. *Spine* 11:802–804.

61. McMaster MJ (1983): Infantile idiopathic scoliosis: can it be prevented? *J Bone Joint Surg Br* 65:612–617.

62. Mehta MH (1972): The rib-vertebra angle in the early diagnosis between resolving and progressive infantile scoliosis. *J Bone Joint Surg Br* 54:230–243.

63. Mehta MH (1992): The conservative management of juvenile idiopathic scoliosis. *Acta Orthop Belg* 58[Suppl 1]:91–97.

64. Mellencamp DD, Blount WP, Anderson AJ (1977): Milwaukee brace treatment of idiopathic scoliosis: late results. *Clin Orthop* 126:47–57.

65. Mellin G, Poussa M (1992): Spinal mobility and posture in 8- to 16-year-old children. *J Orthop Res* 10:211–216.

66. Millner PA, Dickson RA (1992): Scoliosis secondary to subphrenic abscess. *Spine* 17:116–117.

67. Moe JH (1958): A critical analysis of methods of fusion for scoliosis: an evaluation in 266 patients. *J Bone Joint Surg Am* 40:529–554.

68. Moe JH (1980): Modern concepts of treatment of spinal deformities in children and adults. *Clin Orthop* 150:137–153.

69. Moe JH, Kharrat K, Winter RB, et al. (1984): Harrington instrumentation without fusion plus external orthotic support for the treatment of difficult curvature problems in young children. *Clin Orthop* 185:35–45.

70. Moe JH, Sundberg B, Gustilo R (1964): A clinical study of spine fusion in the growing child. *J Bone Joint Surg Br* 46:784.

71. Morrissy RT (1985): Clinical and radiologic evaluation of spinal disease. In: Bradford D, Hensinger R, eds. *The pediatric spine.* New York: Thieme Medical Publishers, pp. 24–40.

72. Morrissy RT, Goldsmith GS, Hall EC, et al. (1990): Measurement of the Cobb angle on radiographs of patients who have scoliosis: evaluation of intrinsic error. *J Bone Joint Surg Am* 72:320–327.

73. Newton PO, Wenger DR, Mubarak SJ, et al. (1997): Anterior release and fusion in pediatric spinal deformity: a comparison of early outcome and cost of thoracoscopic and open thoracotomy approaches. *Spine* 22:1398–1406.

74. O'Donnell CS, Bunnell WP, Betz RR, et al. (1988): Electrical stimulation in the treatment of idiopathic scoliosis. *Clin Orthop* 229:107–113.

75. Patterson JF, Webb JK, Burwell RG (1990): The operative treatment of progressive early-onset scoliosis. *Spine* 15:809–815.

76. Pehrsson K, Larsson S, Oden A, et al. (1992): Long-term follow-up of patients with untreated scoliosis: a study of mortality, causes of death, and symptoms. *Spine* 17:1091–1096.

77. Perdriolle R (1979): *La scoliose.* Paris: Maloine.

78. Perdriolle R, Vidal J (1985): Thoracic idiopathic scoliosis curve evaluation and prognosis. *Spine* 10:785–791.

79. Raso VJ, Russell GG, Hill DL, et al. (1991): Thoracic lordosis in idiopathic scoliosis. *J Pediatr Orthop* 11:599–602.

80. Riseborough EJ, Wynne-Davies R (1973): A genetic survey of idiopathic scoliosis in Boston, Massachusetts. *J Bone Joint Surg Am* 55:974–982.

81. Risser JC, Norquist DM, Cockrell BR Jr, et al. (1966): The effect of posterior spine fusion on the growing spine. *Clin Orthop* 46:127–136.

82. Robin GC, Cohen T (1975): Familial scoliosis: a clinical report. *J Bone Joint Surg Br* 57:146–147.

83. Robinson CM, McMaster MJ (1996): Juvenile idiopathic scoliosis: curve patterns and prognosis in one hundred and nine patients. *J Bone Joint Surg Am* 78:1140–1148.

84. Rothenberg S, Erickson M, Eilert R, et al. (1998): Thoracoscopic anterior spinal procedures in children. *J Pediatr Surg* 33:1168–1170.

85. Samuelsson L, Lindell D (1995): Scoliosis as the first sign of a cystic spinal cord lesion. *Eur Spine J* 4:284–290.

86. Sanders JO, Herring JA, Browne RH (1995): Posterior arthrodesis and instrumentation in the immature (Risser grade 0) spine in idiopathic scoliosis. *J Bone Joint Surg Am* 77:39–45.

87. Shufflebarger HL, Clark CE (1990): Prevention of the crankshaft phenomenon. Presented at the 25th Annual Meeting of the Scoliosis Research Society, Honolulu, Hawaii, September 26.

88. Skages DL, Roye DP (1994): Idiopathic and juvenile scoliosis. *Spine State Art Rev* 8:605–615.

89. Sponseller PD (1992): Syringomyelia and Chiari I malformation presented with juvenile scoliosis as sole manifestation [Clinical Conference] [published correction appears in *J Spinal Disord* 5:382, 1992] *J Spinal Disord* 5:237–239.

90. Sullivan JA, Davidson R, Renshaw TS, et al. (1986): Further evaluation of the Scolitron treatment of idiopathic adolescent scoliosis. *Spine* 11:903–906.

91. Terek RM, Wehner J, Lubicky JP (1991): Crankshaft phenomenon in congenital scoliosis: a preliminary report. *J Pediatr Orthop* 11:527–532.

92. Tolo VT, Gillespie R (1987): The characteristics of juvenile idiopathic scoliosis and results of its treatment. *J Bone Joint Surg Br* 60:181–188.

93. Tomilson RJ Jr, Wolfe MW, Nadall JM, et al. (1994): Syringomyelia and developmental scoliosis. *J Pediatr Orthop* 14:580–585.

94. Vanlommel E, Fabry G, Urlus M, et al. (1992): Harrington instru-

mentation without fusion for the treatment of scoliosis in young children. *J Pediatr Orthop* Part B 1:116–118.

95. Waisman M, Saute M (1997): Thoracoscopic spine release before posterior instrumentation in scoliosis. *Clin Orthop* 336:130–136.

96. Weinstein SL, Ponseti IV (1983): Curve progression in idiopathic scoliosis. *J Bone Joint Surg Am* 65:447–451.

97. Whitecloud TS III, Brinker MR, Barrack RL, et al. (1989): Vibratory response in congenital scoliosis. *J Pediatr Orthop* 9:422–426.

98. Wimpee MW, Moale GE, Hudkins PG, et al. (1986): Scoliosis secondary to osteoblastoma of the rib. *J Pediatr Orthop* 7:589–593.

99. Winter R (1997): Scoliosis and spinal growth. *Orthop Rev* 6:17–20.

100. Winter R, Lonstein J (1992): Juvenile and adolescent scoliosis. In: Rothman R, Simeone F, eds. *The spine,* 3rd ed. Philadelphia: WB Saunders, pp. 373–430.

101. Wynne-Davies R (1968): Familial (idiopathic) scoliosis: a family survey. *J Bone Joint Surg Br* 50:24–30.

ADOLESCENT IDIOPATHIC SCOLIOSIS: ETIOLOGY

NANCY H. MILLER

DEFINITION

Adolescent idiopathic scoliosis is a structural lateral curvature of the spine evident in the late juvenile or adolescent period in otherwise normal children (63). The diagnosis is frequently suspected through screening examinations for the presence of back asymmetry. Confirmation of a positive diagnosis can only be obtained through evidence of a 10-degree lateral curvature with vertebral rotation on a standing upright radiograph of the spine (63). The definition of a 10-degree lateral curvature is based on the fact that a graph of scoliosis prevalence among the general population is a smooth exponential function in which the sharpest change in slope occurs at 10 degrees (63). Multiple topographic methods have been used to study back asymmetry; however, there is no definitive correlation with underlying bony structure (5,21). Radiographic analysis is the definitive methodology for documentation of the true idiopathic nature of the scoliosis from one of alternative origins and for measurement of curve magnitude (5,112). Finally, careful history and clinical examination must eliminate features of alternative disorders that are known to have an increased incidence of scoliosis (i.e., Marfan syndrome, osteogenesis imperfecta) to maintain the true idiopathic nature of the diagnosis (18,32,69,113).

Prevalence studies indicate that 2% to 3% of children have idiopathic scoliosis (20,24,64). Curves of small magnitude are of equal prevalence in both males and females. As curve size increases, however, the female-to-male incidence ratio is about 4:1. Additionally, the overall prevalence of the disorder decreases to 0.2% for curves of a magnitude of more than 30 degrees and to less than 0.1% for curves greater than 40 degrees (20,63,71,127,131,136). Despite the overwhelming prevalence of idiopathic scoliosis diagnosed through screening, studies of the natural history of this disorder indicate that less than 10% of the positively screened patients require active treatment (20,71,83,102,136).

In 1984, Lonstein and Carlson (71) correlated the Risser sign, a sign of skeletal maturation, with curve progression. They found that immature patients (Risser grades 0 and 1) with a spinal

curvature measuring less than 20 degrees had a 22% probability of progression, whereas small curves in mature patients had only a 1.6% chance of progression. As curve magnitude increased to 20 to 29 degrees, immature patients had a 68% probability of progression, whereas patients closer to maturity (Risser grades 2 to 4) had a 23% probability of progression. A second long-term follow-up of 102 patients with idiopathic scoliosis demonstrated that 68% of all diagnosed curves progressed after spinal maturity (130). Curves measuring less than 30 degrees at maturity were least likely to progress, whereas curves measuring 30 to 50 degrees progressed an average of 10 to 15 degrees over a normal lifetime. Those measuring 50 to 75 degrees at maturity progressed steadily at a rate of about 1 degree per year. A report from the Scoliosis Research Society confirmed that a younger age at detection and a larger curve magnitude correlate with a higher probability of progression (85). Multiple studies have shown, however, that girls maintain 10 times the risk for curve progression as compared with boys (6,22,71,102,127,129).

RESEARCH DIRECTED TO ETIOLOGY

Despite significant research efforts directed to the etiology of adolescent idiopathic scoliosis, the cause of this disorder remains elusive. Multiple hypotheses have been proposed, with no one model supported by significant convincing evidence. Different observations, such as connective tissue abnormalities, differing growth patterns, neuromuscular aberrations, central nervous system asymmetries, and hormonal variations, have been noted in select patient populations. Studies have failed, however, to establish conclusively any one factor as the causative agent of the scoliotic condition (10,25,42,44,47,66,79,96,106,141,147). The primary disadvantage of the past work is the difficulty of differentiating an observation as the primary etiologic factor of a disorder from secondary changes that may result from the deformity. Despite this disadvantage, this research is important not only in potentially revealing the etiologic factors of scoliosis but also in adding to our knowledge of the effects of the scoliotic deformity on the immature skeleton.

Genetics

Although the specific cause of idiopathic scoliosis has not been determined, the role of hereditary or genetic factors in the devel-

N. H. Miller, M.D.: Johns Hopkins University, Baltimore, MD 21287-9553.

opment of this condition is widely accepted (12,16,37,43,59, 134,137,143). Clinical observations and formalized population studies have documented scoliosis within families, with a higher incidence of the condition within relatives as opposed to the general population (41,49,51,55,72,100,101,143). Harrington (59) studied women whose scoliotic curves exceeded 15 degrees and found a 27% incidence of scoliosis among their daughters. Population studies involving index patients and their families indicate that 11% of first-degree relatives are affected, as are 2.4% and 1.4% of second- and third-degree relatives, respectively (100).

Twin studies have consistently shown monozygous twins to maintain a high concordance rate of about 73% for the condition. Dizygous twins may or may not be concordant in the expression of the disease and have a concordance rate of 36% (27,41,54,62,65,78,84,110). This value is consistently higher than that reported of a first-degree relative from more global population studies (100,143). This may be related to the high rate of radiographic confirmation of affectation status within twin studies as compared with that of large population studies of families. Radiographic confirmation of disease potentially lowers the false-negative rate because small scoliotic curves undetectable by clinical examination would then be ascertained as positive.

Despite the documentation of the familial nature of this condition, the mode of inheritance has been debated within the literature. Studies based on a wide variety of populations have suggested an autosomal dominant, X-linked, or multifactorial inheritance pattern (9,14,19,28,39,48,53,55,69,80,82). Wynne-Davies and Riseborough (100,143) published studies of 2,000 and 2,869 individuals, respectively. The first work suggested a dominant mode of inheritance; however, a major percentage of individuals lacked radiographic confirmation of disease. The second series performed with a more rigidly defined population was more consistent with a multifactorial inheritance pattern.

In 1972, Cowell and colleagues (37), noting the paucity of male to male transmissions in the literature, selected 17 families (192 individuals) for examination and radiographs and reported a pattern consistent with X-linked inheritance. With the advent of statistical analysis directed to the potential linkage of genes to known disorders (genetic linkage analysis), Miller and associates (80) investigated X-linkage in 14 families (136 individuals). Overall results did not support X-linkage within the population as a whole.

An alternative statistical method directed to the clarification of a genetic model and penetrance of a familial disease is complex segregation analysis. This methodology is applied to an unscreened population and can confirm clinical observations that a genetic determination exists for a specific disorder. Aksenovich and associates (3,7) used complex segregation analysis (as implemented in S.A.G.E. (103) to study a population of 101 families (788 individuals). The initial results supported a genetic model; however, the best-fitting genetic model was equivocal. When the authors excluded 27 families with probands with mild scoliosis, a mendelian model with sex-dependent penetrance could not be rejected when compared with a general model ($P < .1$), whereas an environmental model was strongly rejected ($P < .001$). These results are similar to those reported by Bonaiti and coauthors

(19), suggesting either an autosomal mode of inheritance with incomplete penetrance (higher in girls than in boys) or a genetic model with a mixture of dominant and multifactorial modes of inheritance.

Advances in the mapping of the human genome and current genetic methodology now allow screening of the entire genome of an individual with known genetic markers evenly spaced along the chromosomes. This type of analysis can be performed on individuals or populations in an effort to associate a genomic area with a disease trait. Wise and associates (139) in a genomic scan of a single extended family with idiopathic scoliosis (seven affected individuals) reported suggestive evidence for linkage of the disease state on chromosomes 6, 10, 12, and 18. When these candidate genomic regions were studied in four additional families, one family showed supporting evidence again of genetic linkage on chromosome 10. An additional family showed a suggestive linkage on chromosome 2.

The above studies collectively attempt to indicate that scoliosis is a single gene disorder that follows the simple patterns of mendelian genetics. This is dependent on specific features characteristic to the study population. The simple patterns of mendelian inheritance, however, are known to be susceptible to the genetic principles of variable penetrance and heterogeneity. The wide prevalence of scoliosis associated with high clinical variability is potentially a result of significant locus or intrafamilial heterogeneity. This would confound interpretation of data and possibly conflicting results. As a result of these principles, the genetic mode of inheritance of a disorder may not be clearly evident within a smaller family or group but rather may demand the study of an extensive, well-characterized population through genomic wide-scanning methodology.

Connective Tissue

As a functional biomechanical unit, spinal stability relies on the structural integrity of its various constituents (bone, disc, and ligamentous elements), all of which are composed of the viscoelastic connective tissue elements of collagen, proteoglycan, elastic fibers and additional extracellular matrix components. Because scoliosis is a phenotypic characteristic of multiple connective tissue disorders, such as the Marfan syndrome and osteogenesis imperfecta, the hypothesis that a defect within the connective tissue is the etiologic factor of adolescent idiopathic scoliosis is plausible (18,58,113). Investigators have addressed the issue from two different approaches, that is, a localized defect within one tissue element, or a generalized extracellular matrix abnormality.

Enneking and Harrington in 1969 (47) studied the histology and ultrastructure of the vertebral elements of the scoliotic spine and found no abnormalities as compared with those of controls. This, in conjunction with the fact that long-term studies of idiopathic scoliosis show increasing deformity after completion of vertebral growth (33,43), suggests that the deformity may be secondary to an extraosseous cause and that the change in the vertebral bone and cartilage may be secondary adaptations.

Work focusing on the proteoglycan and collagen of the intervertebral discs has conflicting results. Beard and colleagues in 1981 (13) identified a decrease in type III collagen but no significant differences in type I and II collagen within scoliotic discs. Pedrini and coauthors (96) reported a 25% decrease in the glycosaminoglycan content and a 25% increase in collagen in the nucleus pulposus of scoliosis patients. This finding was supported in 1980 by Taylor and Slinger (126) and Zaleske and colleagues (150). An increase in lysosomal activity of the discs of patients with scoliosis was also documented. In contrast to these reports, Oegema and coauthors (94) did not find any difference in absolute concentrations of proteoglycans in discs of patients with scoliosis from those of controls.

In an effort to view a potential connective tissue abnormality as a more global etiologic factor in adolescent idiopathic scoliosis, Francis and associates studied collagen cross-linking within the skin of patients with scoliosis (52). They found a decrease in the stability of extracted skin polymeric collagen from patients with scoliosis as compared with controls; however, in more mature affected patients, the collagen appeared to be normal. Echenne and colleagues (46) studied the role of an elastic fiber abnormality in the skin of patients with idiopathic scoliosis. A significant number of patients maintained abnormalities in the middle and deep dermis; however, muscle fiber type I abnormalities were also observed in half of patients. Hadley-Miller and coauthors in 1994 (58) focused on the elastic fiber system within the ligamentous structures of patients with idiopathic scoliosis and found a significant number of patients exhibiting elastic fiber abnormalities as compared with controls. Further study in vitro of harvested fibroblasts indicated a potential failure of matrix incorporation of elastic fiber components in a select number of scoliotic patients.

Two works by Carr and colleagues (28) and Miller and associates (80) are directed to the genes responsible for the structural components of the extracellular matrix system. Both groups selected families in which scoliosis was expressed in an autosomal dominant pattern. Through a candidate gene approach the structural genes of collagen types I and II, fibrillin (FBN1) and elastin were excluded as potential causative factors of idiopathic scoliosis within the studied populations.

Muscle and Platelet

Multiple authors have postulated a generalized growth or functional defect within the skeletal muscle as a factor in the etiology of adolescent idiopathic scoliosis (26,50,68,104,119,122,147, 148). Documented changes in the morphology, ultrastructure, and biochemistry have been described; however, many appear to be localized to specific areas, that is, the convexity or concavity of the spinal curvature.

Morphologically, Spencer and Eccles (122) were the first to record a decrease in type II (fast-twitch) muscle fibers as compared with type I (slow-twitch) fibers in patients with idiopathic scoliosis. They postulated a denervation or myopathic process as a causative factor. Other investigators have found abnormalities in fiber size and fiber type distribution in the paraspinous muscle areas of affected patients as compared with controls; however, they differ in their observations (26,50,104,119,147,148). Fidler and Jowett (50) noted atrophy of type II fibers on the concave aspect of the scoliotic deformity and a greater number of type I fibers on the convexity. Bylund and colleagues (26), in a comparative study including patients with idiopathic scoliosis and healthy age-matched controls, did not observe any difference in fiber type on the convex side of the curve but did note a relative decrease in type I fibers on the concave side of the curve. In an effort to support a global myopathy, Yarom and Robin (147,148) and Sahgal (104) studied skeletal muscle from alternative sites (gluteus medius, deltoid, and trapezius muscles). Both groups reported myopathic changes or a fiber-type disproportion at these more distant sites. These myopathic changes were further documented through histologic work to include myofilament disarray, central core formation, and fiber splitting at both the light and electron microscopy levels.

Biochemical analyses of the muscle in patients with idiopathic scoliosis have focused on tissue enzyme activity and protein synthesis. Activity of multiple enzymes, including aspartic and thiol proteinase and adenosine triphosphatase, were found to be decreased on the concave aspect of the curve, in addition to increased levels of calcium (17,36). Investigators postulate a potential defect in the calcium pump across the cellular membrane as a contributing factor of the scoliotic deformity.

Muscle protein synthesis as detected by the uptake of radioactive L-leucine was noted to be higher at the apex of the curve on the convex side than on the concave side of the curve in nine patients with idiopathic scoliosis (57). These changes are potentially consistent with a simple increase in muscle contractile activity and muscle immobilization, which occurs on the concave aspect of the curve.

Because of the physiologic relationship of the muscular contractile proteins and that of the thrombocyte, the thrombocyte or platelet has been a focus of etiologic research of scoliosis. The platelet is also not localized to the skeleton but found systemically, which intuitively suggests that any abnormalities may be primary, not secondary, in nature.

Wong and associates in 1977 (140) and Yarom and Robin in 1979 (148) reported elevations in platelet intracellular calcium and phosphorous concentrations in patients with idiopathic scoliosis as compared with age-matched controls. This elevation is believed to be localized to the "dense bodies," a platelet intracellular histologic finding. In a second study, Yarom and colleagues (146) compared histologic findings of patients with mild scoliosis (less than 15 degrees) and those with more severe scoliosis (greater than 20 degrees). The number of dense bodies was found to be increased in patients with scoliosis in direct proportion to the degree of curvature. These findings collectively have led to a hypothesis of a calcium transport defect of the cellular membrane or contractile complex as a factor. More recently, investigators have reported abnormalities in levels of platelet calmodulin, a calcium-binding protein, among patients with scoliosis as compared with age-matched controls (31,67). Calmodulin interacts with actin and myosin and mediates calcium flux through the sarcoplasmic reticulum. Thus, it is a known regulator of the contractile properties of muscles and platelets. In a comparison of patients with idiopathic scoliosis and matched controls, Kindsfater and coauthors (67) found that skeletally immature patients with progressive curves maintained significantly higher levels of platelet calmodulin than did controls and those patients with stable curves. The significance of this finding and its relationship to parallel research related to melatonin, a hormone known to bind and enhance the action of calmodulin, is unknown.

Neuromotor Mechanisms

Immature patients with known neuromotor disorders are subject to the development of scoliosis; therefore, a subclinical dysfunction or anatomic abnormality of the neurologic system has been hypothesized as an etiologic factor related to adolescent idiopathic scoliosis. In clinical studies, authors have tested a wide range of functions, including proprioception, postural equilibrium, the oculovestibular complex, and vibratory sensation. Multiple techniques have been used, including electronystomography, electroencephalography, and electromyography in select affected patient populations in an effort to distinguish any potential neuromotor differences from those of controls (11,70,106,141,142,144). Abnormal findings are hampered by the inability to determine whether they are a cause or an effect of the scoliosis. Through intuitive scientific deduction, many reports are, rightfully or wrongfully, considered to be a secondary phenomenon of the scoliotic deformity.

Wyatt and colleagues (142) and Barrack and associates (10) evaluated vibratory sensation with a BioThesiometer in patients who had scoliosis and suggested a lesion of the dorsal columns. The reliability of the BioThesiometer used, however, is now considered questionable. Yekutiel and associates in 1981 (149) tested proprioception in scoliotic patients through a wide range of tests and concluded that no abnormality could be consistently demonstrated in patients with scoliosis as compared with age-matched controls.

Early studies by Yamamoto (1982) (145) suggested postural equilibrium dysfunction among scoliotic patients. Further work by Lidstrom and colleagues (1988) (70) demonstrated that the abnormalities parallel the deterioration of the curve, and, further, that as a patient matures, the postural sway corrects itself. In conclusion, the observed equilibrium abnormality is now believed to be secondary to the curve and indicates a compensatory phenomenon of a normal immature neurologic system.

Multiple spinal and central monitoring techniques have been used to localize a defect within the brain stem or higher cortical function within patients with scoliosis (29,77,105–107). One of interest is that of oculovestibular function. Work by Sahlstrand and colleagues (105,106) showed an abnormal nystagmus response through calorific testing among patients with idiopathic scoliosis, indicating an oculovestibular abnormality. Herman and MacEwen (60) showed consistent oculovestibular dysfunction present in affected patients and proposed a defect in the sensory input involved in the visual and vestibular areas of the hindbrain. Conversely, children with vestibular dysfunction have been shown to have a lower incidence of idiopathic scoliosis than is seen in age-matched control populations (141).

The advent of neuromotor and sensory monitoring during the surgical intervention of patients with severe scoliosis has led investigators to question whether the cerebral cortex may be a source of the scoliotic deformity (29,77). Asymmetric latency potentials have been correlated with the direction of the scoliotic

deformity and, to some degree, with the progression of the curvature in some patients.

Research related to the neuroanatomy of scoliosis is focused in two areas: first, clinical work related to the identification of a central asymmetry or abnormality related to the scoliotic condition, and, second, experimental work related to the development of an animal model for scoliosis. Geissele and colleagues in 1991 (56) and Stevens in 1992 (124) reported asymmetries of the midbrain and hindbrain in patients with scoliosis as compared with controls. Because of the limited number of controls and the relatively new application of magnetic resonance imaging to illustrate subtle size differences within areas of the central nervous system, this work needs further investigation.

Animal studies have focused on the development of a bipedal animal model for the experimental study of scoliosis. The production of localized and asymmetric lesions of the spinal cord through selective posterior rhizotomies can lead to a scoliotic deformity; however, its features are that of a neuropathic etiology (125). A well-publicized series of works by Machida and colleagues (73–75) reported a chicken animal model that, after pinealectomy, developed a significant scoliotic deformity paralleling that of an idiopathic type. The pineal gland is the primary source of melatonin, a neurohormone whose function is not clearly understood. The authors additionally observed abnormal cortical evoked somatosensory potentials within the pinealectomized animals and hypothesized an abnormality of somatosensory conduction as a primary etiologic factor in the development of the scoliotic condition.

Growth and Hormonal System

The relationship of growth and idiopathic scoliosis has been well recognized (129,130). Growth is essential to the development and progression of a structural scoliosis, and small scoliotic curves stabilize after maturity. However, growth as a primary or a secondary factor in the etiology of scoliosis remains undetermined. Multiple longitudinal and cross-sectional studies from Scandinavia documented an increased standing height in girls with idiopathic scoliosis both before and after correction for the loss of height due to the scoliotic deformity (89,118,132) This finding was confirmed by other authors in differing ethnic populations (40,45). Further study by Willner (134) indicated that in those children who developed scoliosis, the growth rate the year before the onset of curvature was markedly elevated as compared with those children who did not develop scoliosis. However, this difference did not seem to persist, and the initial difference in height between the two groups decreased at the end of the growth period. Although multiple anthropometric studies have found that scoliotic patients are taller than nonscoliotic controls, other authors have found no association with height or rate of growth between children with or without scoliosis (40,45,126). These variable results may reflect differences in study methodology because some studies do not correct for the loss of height resulting from the spinal curvature.

The possibility that a disproportionate relationship exists between the length of the trunk and that of the lower extremities has been studied in scoliotic patients in comparison with controls (87,133). No difference in the proportion of legs to trunk, sitting height, suprapelvic height, or weight has been found in female patients with idiopathic scoliosis as compared with controls.

The accelerated growth in the prepubertal growth period observed in girls with idiopathic scoliosis as compared with age-matched controls indicates a potential deviation in the normal growth pattern. This observation has led to the study of growth-stimulating hormones within scoliotic patients (2,117,135). Skogland and Miller (117) noted an increase in release of growth hormone in scoliotic patients between the ages of 7 and 12 years. Similar findings have been found by other groups (2,135). Misol and colleagues (81) and Yamada and coauthors (144) report no difference in growth hormone levels between scoliotic and nonscoliotic girls; however, the ages of the study groups either was not reported or the study population was mature at the time of study. The fact that growth hormone secretion after experimental stimuli and in relation to pubertal maturation is episodic in nature significantly limits the comparison of the studies. Evidence exists that a differential growth pattern secondary to growth hormone stimulation may be present within the scoliotic population and requires additional investigation.

A second hormonal system under investigation within the scoliotic population is that of melatonin (76). As discussed previously, the pinealectomized chicken has been used as an experimental animal model for idiopathic scoliosis (73,74). Melatonin is the primary hormonal product of the pineal gland and is known to have an effect on the control of circadian rhythms (35). In this role, it has been available to the general public as a solution to jet lag. A second interaction of melatonin is on calcium regulation through an interaction with the calmodulins (15). As mentioned previously, peripheral calmodulin levels are under investigation as a potential marker for patients with progressive scoliosis.

Patients with scoliosis do produce melatonin. Machida and coauthors (74,76) have reported that patients with severe and progressive scoliosis maintain significantly decreased nighttime levels of melatonin levels as compared with controls and patients individuals with stable scoliosis. These findings, however, have not been confirmed by other authors (8,61). Although the association between melatonin and the etiology of idiopathic scoliosis is speculative, the given ubiquitous nature of this hormone and its involvement in multiple cellular regulatory processes warrants further investigative efforts.

Biomechanics

As a functional biomechanical unit, spinal alignment and stability rely on the integrity of the tissue elements, the functional load applied to the spinal column, and the growth pattern of the immature vertebrae. The fact that the loss of structural integrity of the supporting elements, as seen in known connective tissue disorders, leads to scoliosis indicates that specific biomechanical factors are essential for normal spinal development (18,113). The potential that biomechanical factors initiate the development of idiopathic scoliosis has been suggested.

Individual elements of the spine (i.e., the vertebral bodies, the rib and trunk muscles, the ligaments and intervertebral discs) have been investigated for an alteration in their intrinsic mechanical properties that would lead to an abnormal response to bio-

mechanical loading. A subtle alteration in the laxity or stiffness of the tissues would cause the column to buckle when load is applied to the spinal column in the bipedal state. As reviewed previously, multiple authors have identified changes within the musculature or within the extracellular matrix of the spinal ligaments or intervertebral discs (25,38,58,59,88,94,97—99). Most concluded, however, that the observed differences were most likely secondary to the scoliotic deformity rather than a primary etiologic factor (59,97,114). Decreased bone density in patients with idiopathic scoliosis has been documented in several studies (30,34,108,128). Although poor bone quality (osteoporosis) is known to contribute to some existing scoliotic deformities, the role of decreased bone density in the development of idiopathic scoliosis in the immature skeleton is unknown.

Clinical observation has shown that with the loss of normal thoracic kyphosis, a structural scoliosis may develop. In 1952, Somerville (121) suggested that a growth differential between the anterior and posterior columns of the spine or vertebrae could lead to hypokyphosis. This, in turn, would cause a biomechanical rotational abnormality of the spine producing the scoliosis. This theory has been furthered by marked circumstantial evidence (23,43,44,120,138). However, the technical inability to study differential growth patterns of immature vertebrae in children and the lack of a good animal model make this theory difficult to test.

A fundamental mechanism for the development of scoliosis is potentially the asymmetric application of loading forces as one assumes the bipedal state. A series of work by Normelli and colleagues (90–93) focus on the asymmetry of the rib structure, anterior thoracic wall, and vascular supply to the chest within patients with right thoracic scoliosis as compared with controls. Their results indicate significant differences between the left and right sides, particularly within the size of the ribs and breasts. They hypothesized that the increased vasculature to the left could lead to increased growth potential and result in asymmetric loading of the spine. In turn, collapse of the right side and a scoliotic condition develop. Sevastik and coauthors (111) reported asymmetric growth of the pedicle elements within spines with vertebral rotation. Further support for the theory of growth asymmetry has been generated by the successful production of scoliosis in a rabbit animal model through the unilateral stimulation of rib overgrowth (1).

Although spinal stability is primarily considered a static configuration, the biomechanics of spinal stability, particularly in relationship to the immature skeleton, is a dynamic process. As a person moves and grows, spinal stability is a continuous realignment of the head over the pelvis. This mechanical process is dependent on the integration of static and dynamic elements in both a localized area and on a more unified structural level. Although the dynamic process of the spinal stability is recognized, research within this area is now directed to the innovative application of computerized technology to develop mathematical models of the spine (4,86,95,109,115,116,123).

SUMMARY

Adolescent idiopathic scoliosis is a prevalent disorder that is known to occur within families for unknown reasons. Knowledge of the natural history of this disease process has shown us that through clinical assessment, specific patient groups maintain certain risks and patterns of progression. The role of genetic factors is widely documented; however, the genetic mode of inheritance of familial idiopathic scoliosis is undetermined. Multiple areas have been investigated for the potential etiology of this disorder, with no one element showing definitive evidence as the primary etiologic factor. Abnormalities have been documented in the skeleton, neuromotor system, connective tissue, biomechanics, and hormonal system. The primary difficulty of most investigations is whether the observed abnormalities are primary or secondary features in the pathogenesis of this disorder. Genetic studies directed to a wide population may aid in the delineation of a primary etiologic factors through modern genotyping techniques. A better understanding of the etiology of idiopathic scoliosis and factors related to the clinical variability of this disorder should improve the ability to assign a more specific prognosis and modify current treatment regimens.

REFERENCES

1. Agadir M (1988): Induction of scoliosis in the growing rabbit. *Spine* 13:1065–1069.
2. Ahl T, Albertsson-Wikland K, Kalen R (1988): Twenty-four-hour growth hormone profiles in pubertal girls with idiopathic scoliosis. *Spine* 13:139–142.
3. Aksenovich TI, Semenov IR, Ginzburg EK, et al. (1988): Preliminary analysis of inheritance of scoliosis [Russian]. *Genetika* 24:2056–2063.
4. Andriacchi T, Schultz AB, Belytschko T, et al. (1974): A model for studies of mechanical interactions between the human spine and rib cage. *J Biomech* 7:497–507.
5. Armstrong GW, Livermore NB, Suzuki N, et al. (1982): Nonstandard vertebral rotation in scoliosis screening patients: its prevalence and relation to the clinical deformity. *Spine* 7:50–54.
6. Ascani E, Bartolozzi P, Logroscino CA, et al. (1986): Natural history of untreated idiopathic scoliosis after skeletal maturity. *Spine* 11:784–789.
7. Axenovich TI, Zaidman AM, Zorkoltseva IV, et al. (1988): *Segregation analysis of idiopathic scoliosis: evidence for a major-gene effect*. Abstract of the 10th International Philip Zorab Symposium, Oxford, UK, March 30–April 1, 1998, pp. 19–21.
8. Bagnall KM, Raso VJ, Hill DL, et al. (1996): Melatonin levels in idiopathic scoliosis: diurnal and nocturnal serum melatonin levels in girls with adolescent idiopathic scoliosis. *Spine* 21:1974–1978.
9. Ballesteros S, Grove HM, Campusano C, et al. (1977): Genetic study in a family affected of idiopathic scoliosis [Author's translation]. *Rev Med Chile* 105:224–226.
10. Barrack RL, Whitecloud TS, Burke SW, et al. (1984): Proprioception in idiopathic scoliosis. *Spine* 9:681–685.
11. Barrack RL, Wyatt MP, Whitecloud TS, et al. (1988): Vibratory hypersensitivity in idiopathic scoliosis. *J Pediatr Orthop* 8:389–395.
12. Beals RK (1973): Nosologic and genetic aspects of scoliosis. *Clin Orthop* 93:23–32.
13. Beard HK, Roberts S, O'Brien JP (1981): Immunofluorescent staining for collagen and proteoglycan in normal and scoliotic intervertebral discs. *J Bone Joint Surg Br* 63:529–534.
14. Bell M, Teebi AS (1995): Autosomal dominant idiopathic scoliosis? *Am J Hum Genet* 55:112.
15. Benitez-King G, Rios A, Martinez A, et al. (1996): In vitro inhibition of Ca2 + /calmodulin-dependent kinase II activity by melatonin. *Biochim Biophys Acta* 1290:191–196.
16. Berquet KH (1996): Considerations on heredity in idiopathic scoliosis [German]. *Z Orthop Ihre Grezgeb* 101:197–209.
17. Blatt JM, Rubin E, Botin GC, et al. (1984): Impaired calcium pump activity in idiopathic scoliosis: possible etiological role of a membrane defect. *Orthop Trans* 8:143.
18. Boileau C, Jondeau G, Babron MC, et al. (1993): Autosomal dominant Marfan-like connective-tissue disorder with aortic dilation and skeletal anomalies not linked to the fibrillin genes. *Am J Hum Genet* 53:46–54.
19. Bonaiti C, Feingold J, Briard ML, et al. (1976): Genetics of idiopathic scoliosis. *Helv Pediatr Acta* 31:229–240.
20. Brooks HL, Azen SP, Gerberg E, et al. (1975): Scoliosis: a prospective epidemiological study. *J Bone Joint Surg Am* 57:968–972.
21. Bunnell WP (1984): An objective criterion for scoliosis screening. *J Bone Joint Surg Am* 66:1381–1387.
22. Bunnell WP (1986): The natural history of idiopathic scoliosis before skeletal maturity. *Spine* 11:773–776.
23. Burwell RG, Cole AA, Cook TA, et al. (1992): Pathogenesis of idiopathic scoliosis: the Nottingham concept. *Acta Orthop Belg* 58:33–58.
24. Burwell RG, James NJ, Johnson F, et al. (1983): Standardised trunk asymmetry scores: a study of back contour in healthy school children. *J Bone Joint Surg Br* 65:452–463.
25. Bushell GR, Ghosh P, Taylor TK, et al. (1979): The collagen of the intervertebral disc in adolescent idiopathic scoliosis. *J Bone Joint Surg Br* 61:501–508.
26. Bylund P, Jansson E, Dahlberg E, et al. (1987): Muscle fiber types in thoracic erector spinae muscles: fiber types in idiopathic and other forms of scoliosis. *Clin Orthop* 214:222–228.
27. Carr AJ (1990): Adolescent idiopathic scoliosis in identical twins. *J Bone Joint Surg Br* 72:1077.
28. Carr AJ, Ogilvie DJ, Wordsworth BP, et al. (1992): Segregation of structural collagen genes in adolescent idiopathic scoliosis. *Clin Orthop* 274:305–310.
29. Cheng JCY (1998): *Adolescent idioapthic scoliosis: the correlation of curve severity, SEP, and MRI findings*. Aetiology of Adolescent Idiopathic Scoliosis. 10th Annual International Philip Zorab Symposium. March 30–April 1, 1998.
30. Cheng JCY, Guo X (1997): Osteopenia in adolescent idiopathic scoliosis: a primary problem or secondary to the spinal deformity? *Spine* 22:1716–1721.
31. Cheung WY (1982): Calmodulin. *Sci Am* 246:62–70.
32. Codorniu AH-R (1958): "Idiopathic" scoliosis of congenital origin. *J Bone Joint Surg Br* 40:94.
33. Collis DK, Ponseti IV (1969): Long-term follow-up of patients with idiopathic scoliosis not treated surgically. *J Bone Joint Surg Am* 51:425–445.
34. Cook SD, Harding AF, Morgan EL, et al. (1987): Trabecular bone mineral density in idiopathic scoliosis. *J Pediatr Orthop* 7:168–174.
35. Copinschi G, Van CE (1995): Effects of ageing on modulation of hormonal secretions by sleep and circadian rhythmicity. *Horm Res* 43:20–24.
36. Cotic V, Bizjak F, Turk V (1983): The activity of proteinases of the paravertebral muscles in idiopathic scoliosis. In: Pecina M, ed. *Scoliosis and kyphosis*. Dubrovnik, p. 250.
37. Cowell HR, Hall JN, MacEwen GD (1972): Genetic aspects of idiopathic scoliosis: a Nicholas Andry Award essay, 1970. *Clin Orthop* 86:121–131.
38. Cutler AD, Riggins RS, Lin HJ, et al. (1981): Stress relaxation in tendons of chickens with scoliosis. *J Biomech* 14:439–441.
39. Czeizel A, Bellyei A, Barta O, et al. (1978): Genetics of adolescent idiopathic scoliosis. *J Med Genet* 15:424–427.
40. Dangerfield PH, Roaf R (1974): Anthrophotometry and scoliosis. *J Bone Joint Surg Br* 56:382.
41. DeGeorge FV, Fisher RL (1967): Idiopathic scoliosis: genetic and environmental aspects. *J Med Genet* 4:251–257.
42. Dickson RA (1988): The aetiology of spinal deformities. *Lancet* 1:1151–1155.
43. Dickson RA (1992): The etiology and pathogenesis of idiopathic scoliosis. *Acta Orthop Belg* 58:21–25.
44. Dickson RA, Lawton JO, Archer IA, et al. (1984): The pathogenesis of idiopathic scoliosis: biplanar spinal asymmetry. *J Bone Joint Surg Br* 66:8–15.
45. Drummond DS, Rogala EJ (1988): Growth and maturation of adolescents with idiopathic scoliosis. *Spine* 5:507–511.

46. Echenne B, Barneon G, Pages M, et al. (1988): Skin elastic fiber pathology and idiopathic scoliosis. *J Pediatr Orthop* 8:522–528.
47. Enneking WF, Harrington P (1969): Pathological changes in scoliosis. *J Bone Joint Surg Am* 51:165–184.
48. Faber A (1935): Skoliose bei eineiigen zwillingen. *Der Erbartz* 2:102.
49. Faber A (1936): Untersuchungen uber die erblichkeit der skoliose. *Arch Orthop Unfallchir* 36:247–249.
50. Fidler MW, Jowett RL (1976): Muscle imbalance in the aetiology of scoliosis. *J Bone Joint Surg Br* 58:200–201.
51. Filho NA, Thompson MW (1971): Genetic studies in scoliosis. *J Bone Joint Surg Am* 53:199.
52. Francis MJ, Sanderson MC, Smith R (1976): Skin collagen in idiopathic adolescent scoliosis and Marfan's syndrome. *Clin Sci Molec Med* 51:467–474.
53. Funatsu K (1980): Familial incidence in idiopathic scoliosis *Nippon Seikeigeka Gakkai Zasshi* 54:633–649.
54. Gaertner RL (1979): Idiopathic scoliosis in identical (monozygotic) twins. *South Med J* 72:231–234.
55. Garland HG (1934): Hereditary scoliosis. *Br Med J* 1:328.
56. Geissele AE, Kransdorf MJ, Geyer CA, et al. (1991): Magnetic resonance imaging of the brain stem in adolescent idiopathic scoliosis. *Spine* 16:761–763.
57. Gibson JNA, McMaster MJ, Scrimgeour CM, et al. (1984): Rates of muscle protein synthesis in paraspinal muscles: literal disparity in children with idiopathic scoliosis. *Spine* 9:373–376.
58. Hadley-Miller N, Mims B, Milewicz DM (1994): The potential role of the elastic fiber system in adolescent idiopathic scoliosis. *J Bone Joint Surg Am* 76:1193–1206.
59. Harrington PR (1977): The etiology of idiopathic scoliosis. *Clin Orthop* 126:17–25.
60. Herman R, MacEwen GD (1979): Idiopathic scoliosis: a visuo-vestibular disorder? Proceedings of the 6th Zorab Scoliosis Symposium, March 30–April 1, 1998, pp. 61–69.
61. Hilibrand AS, Blakemore LC, Loder RT, et al. (1996): The role of melatonin in the pathogenesis of adolescent idiopathic scoliosis. *Spine* 21:1140–1146.
62. Hull BL (1961): Scoliosis in biovular twins. *J Bone Joint Surg Br* 43:285.
63. Kane WJ (1977): Scoliosis prevalence: a call for a statement of terms. *Clin Orthop* 126:43–46.
64. Kane WJ, Moe JH (1970): A scoliosis-prevalence survey in Minnesota. *Clin Orthop* 69:216–218.
65. Kesling KL, Reinker KΛ (1997): Scoliosis in twins: a meta-analysis of the literature and report of six cases. *Spine* 22:2009–2015.
66. Khosla S, Tredwell SJ, Day B, et al. (1980): An ultrastructural study of multifidus muscle in progressive idiopathic scoliosis: changes resulting from a sarcolemmal defect at the myotendinous junction. *J Neurol Sci* 46:13–31.
67. Kindsfater K, Lowe T, Lawellin D, et al. (1994): Levels of platelet calmodulin for the prediction of progression and severity of adolescent idiopathic scoliosis. *J Bone Joint Surg Am* 76:1186–1192.
68. Langenskiold A, Michelsson JE (1961): Experimental progressive scoliosis in the rabbit. *J Bone Joint Surg Br* 43:116–120.
69. Levaia NV (1981): Genetic aspect of dysplastic (idiopathic) scoliosis. *Ortop Travmatol Protez* 2:23–29.
70. Lidstrom J, Friberg S, Lindstrom L, et al. (1988): Postural control in siblings to scoliosis patients and scoliosis patients. *Spine* 13:1070–1074.
71. Lonstein JE, Carlson JM (1984): The prediction of curve progression in untreated idiopathic scoliosis during growth. *J Bone Joint Surg Am* 66:1061–1071.
72. MacEwen GD (1969): *Familial incidence of idiopathic scoliosis and experimental scoliosis.* New York: Columbia Presbyterian Medical Center, New York Orthopaedic Hospital, p. 78.
73. Machida M, Dubousset J, Imamura Y, et al. (1993): An experimental study in chickens for the pathogenesis of idiopathic scoliosis. *Spine* 18:1609–1615.
74. Machida M, Dubousset J, Imamura Y, et al. (1995): Role of melatonin deficiency in the development of scoliosis in pinealectomised chickens. *J Bone Joint Surg Br* 77:134–138.
75. Machida M, Dubousset J, Imamura Y, et al. (1994): Pathogenesis of idiopathic scoliosis: SEPs in chicken with experimentally induced scoliosis and in patients with idiopathic scoliosis. *J Pediatr Orthop* 14:329–335.
76. Machida M, Dubousset J, Imamura Y, et al. (1996): Melatonin: a possible role in pathogenesis of adolescent idiopathic scoliosis. *Spine* 21:1147–1152.
77. Maguire J, Madigan R, Wallace S, et al. (1993): Intraoperative long-latency reflex activity in idiopathic scoliosis demonstrates abnormal central processing: a possible cause of idiopathic scoliosis. *Spine* 18:1621–1626.
78. McKinley LM, Leatherman KD (1978): Idiopathic and congenital scoliosis in twins. *Spine* 3:227–229.
79. Miller NH, Mims B, Child A, et al. (1996): Genetic analysis of structural elastic fiber and collagen genes in familial adolescent idiopathic scoliosis. *J Orthop Res* 14:994–999.
80. Miller NH, Sponseller PD, Bell J, et al. (1998): Genomic search for X-linkage in familial AIS. In: Stokes IAF, ed. *Research into spinal deformities,* vol. 2. Amsterdam: IOF Press, pp. 209–213.
81. Misol S, Ponseti IV, Samaan N, et al. (1971): Growth hormone blood levels in patients with idiopathic scoliosis. *Clin Orthop* 81:122–125.
82. Mongird-Nakonieczna J, Kozlowski B. (1976): Familial occurrence of idiopathic scoliosis. *Chir Narzadow Ruch Ortop Pol* 41:161–165.
83. Montgomery F, Willner S (1997): The natural history of idiopathic scoliosis: incidence of treatment in 15 cohorts of children born between 1963 and 1977. *Spine* 22:772–774.
84. Murdoch G (1959): Scoliosis in twins. *J Bone Joint Surg Br* 41:736.
85. Nachemson A, Lonstein J, Weinstein S. *Report of the SRS prevalence and natural history committee 1982;* Denver, Colorado; Scoliosis Research Society.
86. Nachemson A, Pope MH (1991): Concepts in mathematical modeling. *Spine* 16:675–676.
87. Nicolopoulos KS, Burwell RG, Webb JK (1985): Stature and its components in adolescent idiopathic scoliosis. *J Bone Joint Surg Br* 67:594–601.
88. Nordwall A (1973): Studies in idiopathic scoliosis relevant to etiology, conservative, and operative treatment. *Acta Orthop Scand* 44:150.
89. Nordwall A, Willner S (1975): A study of skeletal age and height in girls with idiopathic scoliosis. *Clin Orthop* 110:6–10.
90. Normelli H, Sevastik J, Ljung G, et al. (1985): Anthropometric data relating to normal and scoliotic Scandinavian girls. *Spine* 10:123–126.
91. Normelli H, Sevastik JA, Akrivos J (1985): The length and ash weight of the ribs of normal and scoliotic persons. *Spine* 10:590–592.
92. Normelli H, Sevastik JA, Ljung G, et al. (1986): The symmetry of the breasts in normal and scoliotic girls. *Spine* 11:749–752.
93. Normelli H, Sevastik JA, Wallberg H (1986): The thermal emission from the skin and vascularity of the breasts in normal and scoliotic girls. *Spine* 11:405–408.
94. Oegema TRJ, Bradford DS, Cooper KM, et al. (1983): Comparison of the biochemistry of proteoglycans isolated from normal, idiopathic scoliotic and cerebral palsy spines. *Spine* 8:378–384.
95. Panjabi MM (1973): Three-dimensional mathematical model of the human spine structure. *J Biomech* 6:671–680.
96. Pedrini VA, Ponseti IV, Dohrman SC (1973): Glycosaminoglycans of intervertebral disc in idiopathic scoliosis. *J Lab Clin Med* 82:938–950.
97. Ponseti IV, Pedrini V, Wynne-Davies R, et al. (1976): Pathogenesis of scoliosis. *Clin Orthop* 120:268–280.
98. Riggins RT, Abbott UK, Ashmore CR, et al. (1977): Scoliosis in chickens. *J Bone Joint Surg Am* 59:1020–1026.
99. Riggins RT, Lewis DA, Benson DR, et al. Mechanical properties of the tibia from chickens with idiopathic scoliosis. *J Biomech* 16:59–67.
100. Riseborough EJ, Wynne-Davies R (1973): A genetic survey of idiopathic scoliosis in Boston, Massachusetts. *J Bone Joint Surg Am* 55:974–982.
101. Robin GC, Cohen T (1975): Familial scoliosis: a clinical report. *J Bone Joint Surg Br* 57:146–148.
102. Rogala EJ, Drummond DS, Gurr J (1978): Scoliosis: incidence and natural history. A prospective epidemiological study. *J Bone Joint Surg Am* 60:173–176.
103. S.A.G.E. (1999): *Statistical analysis for genetic epidemiology.* Cleveland,

OH: Case Western University, Department of Epidemiology and Bio-statistics.

104. Sahgal V, Shah A, Flanagan N, et al. (1983): Morphologic and morphometric studies of muscle in idiopathic scoliosis. *Acta Orthop Scand* 54:242–251.

105. Sahlstrand T, Ortengren R, Nachemson, A (1978): Postural equilibrium in adolescent idiopathic scoliosis. *Acta Orthop Scand* 49(4): 354–365.

106. Sahlstrand T, Petruson B, Ortengren R (1979): Vestibulospinal reflex activity in patients with adolescent idiopathic scoliosis: postural effects during caloric labyrinthine stimulation recorded by stabilometry. *Acta Orthop Scand* 50:275–281.

107. Sahlstrand T, Sellden U (1980): Nerve conduction velocity in patients with adolescent idiopathic scoliosis. *Scand J Rehabil Med* 12:25–26.

108. Saji MJ, Upadhyay SS, Leong JCY (1995): Increased femoral neck-shaft angles in adolescent idiopathic scoliosis. *Spine* 20:303–311.

109. Schultz AB (1991): The use of mathematical models for studies of scoliosis biomechanics. *Spine* 16:1211–1216.

110. Scott TF, Bailey RW (1963): Idiopathic scoliosis in fraternal twins. *J Mich Med Soc* 62:283.

111. Sevastik B, Xiong B, Sevastik JA, et al. (1995): Vertebral rotation and pedicle length asymmetry in the normal adult spine. *Eur Spine J* 4: 95–97.

112. Shands AR Jr, Eisberg HB (1955): The incidence of scoliosis in the State of Delaware: a study of 50,000 films of the chest made during a survey for tuberculosis. *J Bone Joint Surg Am* 37:1243.

113. Shapiro JR, Burn VE, Chipman SD, et al. (1989): Osteoporosis and familial idiopathic scoliosis: association with an abnormal alpha 2(I) collagen. *Connect Tissue Res* 21:117–123.

114. Skaggs DL, Bassett GS (1996): Adolescent idiopathic scoliosis: an update [see Comments]. *Am Fam Physician* 53:2327–2335.

115. Skalli W, Lavaste F, Descrimes E (1995): Quantification of three-dimensional vertebral rotations in scoliosis: what are the true values? *Spine* 20:546–553.

116. Skalli W, Robin S, Lavaste F, et al. (1993): A biomechanical analysis of short segment spinal fixation using 3-D geometrical and mechanical model. *Spine* 18:545.

117. Skogland LB, Miller JA (1980): Growth related hormones in idiopathic scoliosis: an endocrine basis for accelerated growth. *Acta Orthop Scand* 51:779–780.

118. Skogland LB, Miller JA (1981): The length and proportions of the thoracolumbar spine in children with idiopathic scoliosis. *Acta Orthop Scand* 52:177–185.

119. Slager UT, Hsu JD (1986): Morphometry and pathology of the paraspinous muscles in idiopathic scoliosis. *Dev Med Child Neurol* 28: 749–756.

120. Smith RM, Dickson RA (1987): Experimental structural scoliosis. *J Bone Joint Surg Br* 69:576–581.

121. Somerville EW (1952): Rotational lordosis: the development of the single curve. *J Bone Joint Surg Br* 34:421–427.

122. Spencer GS, Eccles MJ (1976): Spinal muscles in scoliosis. Part V. The proportion and size of type I and type II skeletal fibers measured using a computer controlled microscope. *J Neurol Sci* 30:143–154.

123. Stambough J, Geraidy A, Guo L (1995): A mathematical lifting model of the lumbar spine. *J Spinal Disord* 8:264–277.

124. Stevens WR (1992): MRI of the posterior fossa and evoked potential analysis in adolescent idiopathic scoliosis. Abstract of the 27th SRS Annual Meeting, Kansas City, MO, p. 89.

125. Suk SI, Song HS, Lee CK (1989): Scoliosis induced by anterior and posterior rhizotomy. *Spine* 14:692–697.

126. Taylor JR, Slinger BS (1980): Scoliosis screening and growth. *Med J Aust* 1:475–478.

127. Torell G, Nordwall A, Nachemson A (1981): The changing pattern of scoliosis treatment due to effective screening. *J Bone Joint Surg Am* 63:337–341.

128. Warren MP, Brooks-Gunn J, Hamilton LH, et al. (1986): Scoliosis and fractures in young ballet dancers: relation to delayed menarche and secondary amenorrhea. *N Engl J Med* 314:1348–1353.

129. Weinstein SL (1986): Idiopathic scoliosis: natural history. *Spine* 11: 780–783.

130. Weinstein SL, Ponseti IV (1983): Curve progression in idiopathic scoliosis. *J Bone Joint Surg Am* 65:447–455.

131. Weinstein SL, Zavala DC, Ponseti IV (1981): Idiopathic scoliosis: long-term follow-up and prognosis in untreated patients. *J Bone Joint Surg Am* 63:702–712.

132. Willner S (1975): A study of height, weight and menarche in girls with idiopathic structural scoliosis. *Acta Orthop Scand* 46:71–83.

133. Willner S (1975): The proportion of legs to trunk in girls with idiopathic structural scoliosis. *Acta Orthop Scand* 46:84–89.

134. Willner S (1994): Adolescent idiopathic scoliosis: etiology. In: Weinstein SL, ed. *The pediatric spine: principles and practices.* New York: Raven, pp. 445–462.

135. Willner S, Nilsson KO, Kastrup K, et al. (1976): Growth hormone and somatomedin A in girls with adolescent idiopathic scoliosis. *Acta Paediatr Scand* 65:547–552.

136. Willner S, Uden A (1982): A prospective prevalence study of scoliosis in Southern Sweden. *Acta Orthop Scand* 53:233–237.

137. Winter RB (1982): Evolution in the treatment of idiopathic scoliosis in Minnesota: a family report. *Minn Med,* 65:627–629.

138. Winter RB, Lovell WW, Moe JH (1975): Excessive thoracic lordosis and loss of pulmonary function in patients with idiopathic scoliosis. *J Bone Joint Surg Am* 57:972–977.

139. Wise CA, Caudle DL, Barnes R, et al. (1998): Genome wide scan for susceptibility to familial idiopathic scoliosis. *Am J Hum Genet* 63: A315.

140. Wong YC, Yau AC, Low WD, et al. (1977): Ultrastructural changes in the back muscles of idiopathic scoliosis. *Spine* 2:251–260.

141. Woods LA, Haller RJ, Hansen PD, et al. (1995): Decreased incidence of scoliosis in hearing-impaired children: implications for a neurologic basis for idiopathic scoliosis. *Spine* 20:776–780.

142. Wyatt MP, Barrack RL, Mubarak SJ, et al. (1986): Vibratory response in idiopathic scoliosis. *J Bone Joint Surg Br* 68:714–718.

143. Wynne-Davies R (1968): Familial (idiopathic) scoliosis: a family survey. *J Bone Joint Surg Br* 50:24–30.

144. Yamada K, Yamamoto H, Nakagawa Y, et al. (1984): Etiology of idiopathic scoliosis. *Clin Orthop* 184:50–57.

145. Yamamoto H (1982): *A postural dysequilibrium as an etiological factor in idiopathic scoliosis.* Presented at the 17th annual meeting of the Scoliosis Research Society. Denver, Colorado.

146. Yarom R, Meyer S, More R, et al. (1982): Metal impregnation abnormalities in platelets of patients with idiopathic scoliosis. *Haemostasis* 12:282–289.

147. Yarom R, Robin GC (1979): Muscle pathology in idiopathic scoliosis. *Isr J Med Sci* 15:917–924.

148. Yarom R, Robin GC (1979): Studies of spinal and peripheral muscles from patients with scoliosis. *Spine* 4:12–21.

149. Yekutiel M, Robin GC, Yarom R (1981): Proprioceptive function in children with adolescent idiopathic scoliosis. *Spine* 6:560–566.

150. Zaleske DJ, Ehrlich MG, Hall JE (1980): Association of glycosaminoglycan depletion and degradative enzyme activity in scoliosis. *Clin Orthop* 148:177–181.

19

ADOLESCENT IDIOPATHIC SCOLIOSIS: NATURAL HISTORY

STUART L. WEINSTEIN

All treatment decisions about disease entities are ideally made in light of a thorough knowledge of the natural history of the condition. These treatment decisions must be critically and continually assessed in light of outcome studies on patients treated with various nonsurgical and surgical methods. All treatments must alter natural history in a positive way. This chapter is concerned only with those patients who carry the diagnosis of late-onset scoliosis or what is more commonly referred to in North America as *adolescent idiopathic scoliosis* (AIS). Understanding the natural history enables physicians to make thoughtful and appropriate management decisions that will alter the course of the disease in a positive way.

The literature on the natural history of idiopathic scoliosis has many shortcomings. First and foremost among these is the paucity of information on the topic (7,37,41,42,54,55,63, 69,78,84,91,97,101,124,129,130). Most long-term follow-up studies are retrospective in nature and suffer the faults of all retrospective studies, particularly lost patients. Most studies include small numbers of patients, and thus "significant" findings may not be statistically significant. Patients with other etiologies for their spinal deformity and patients with early-onset idiopathic scoliosis are often included. Patients with scoliosis of varying etiologies and those with idiopathic scoliosis of early onset cannot be compared with the specific group of patients with adolescent onset of their spinal deformity. The effects of spinal deformity can be profound on the growth of the spine as well as on adjacent structures and internal organs, such as the ribs and pulmonary parenchyma. Curve patterns, gender, magnitude, and other factors affect outcome, and this information is often lacking in the literature. Other variables include whether the patient was actually seen and examined and the variability and reliability of questionnaires used to assess outcome parameters.

By definition, AIS is a structural lateral curvature of the spine that occurs at or near the onset of puberty for which no cause can be established (65,123). The diagnosis of AIS is generally suspected by the presence of body asymmetries in the standing position. These asymmetries may include variance in shoulder height (acromioclavicular [AC] joint level), scapular prominences, chest prominences, or decompensation by a plumb line from C7 (121,132,134). The rotational asymmetries are best detected by the Adams forward-bending test (2). Unfortunately, all the screening tests used to make the diagnosis of AIS (e.g., moiré topography, Integrated Shape Imaging System (ISIS) scanning, forward-bending test) are sensitive for detecting body asymmetries but are not specific for scoliosis or curve magnitude (6). Hence, the diagnosis can be confirmed only by the presence of a curvature of at least 10 degrees, measured by the Cobb method, on a standing upright radiograph of the spine (65). By this criterion, the prevalence of AIS in the at-risk population (children 10 to 16 years of age) is about 2% to 3% (8,16–18, 21,22,50,51,65,66,81,82,92,94,95,105,107,109,110,114, 115,129). As curve magnitude increases, the overall prevalence of the condition decreases (Table 1). There is an overall female predominance of 3.6:1. The male-to-female ratio of patients with small curves in the range of 10 degrees is about equal. In curves of larger magnitude, however, there is an overwhelming female predominance (8,16,17,21,22,36,66,73,74,110,117, 133,134,138,140) (Table 1). There had been some question about whether the incidence and hence natural history of AIS had changed in recent years. Montgomery and Willner (82), however, demonstrated in a longitudinal cross-sectional analysis that in a cohort of children followed over a 15-year period, there was no support for a change in the natural history of scoliosis.

Epidemiologic and natural history studies indicate that less than 1% of the screened population and less than 10% (range 3% to 9%) of positively screened patients (curve greater than 10 degrees) require active treatment (8,16,17,74,81,107,134). This small group of patients with curves greater than 10 degrees is the focus of the remainder of this chapter.

It is well known that the prognosis of scoliosis varies according to the etiology. The natural history of patients with untreated AIS does not necessarily apply to the natural history of scoliosis with known etiologies. The various natural histories of curves with different etiologies, as well as their associated problems, may have a significant bearing on the ability of patients to meet the demands of daily life and work.

Curve patterns must be taken into consideration when reviewing the natural history. The four main curve patterns in AIS are thoracic, lumbar, thoracolumbar, and double major

S. L. Weinstein: Department of Orthopaedics, University of Iowa Hospitals, Iowa City, IA.

TABLE 1. ADOLESCENT IDIOPATHIC SCOLIOSIS PREVALENCE

Cobb Angle (degrees)	Female-to-Male Ratio	Prevalence (%)
>10	1.4–2:1	2–3
>20	5.4:1	0.3–0.5
>30	10:1	0.1–0.3
>40		<0.1

(Figs. 1–4). There may be some confusion in the literature when differentiating curve patterns; many authors put some thoracolumbar curves in the lumbar group, and vice versa. The definitions used here specifically refer to the location of the apical vertebrae. Each curve has its own particular characteristics, predicted course, and outcomes (12,23,24,28,29,40,62,72,84,96, 97,100,102,124,126,128,129). Other, less common curve patterns include the cervicothoracic, double thoracic, and thoracic thoracolumbar (102).

Patients with AIS and their families are often upset by misinformation about the condition and its ultimate effect on their lives. There are few natural history studies available on AIS. Most that do exist are retrospective and are open to criticism on various points (7,41,42,63,69,84,91,97,103,124,129).

In 1968, Nachemson (84) and Nilsonne and Lundgren (91) published long-term follow-up studies that expressed a grim

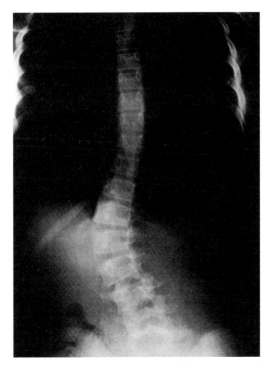

FIGURE 2. Lumbar curve. Seventy percent left convexity involving an average of six vertebrae: apex L1, L2; upper end vertebrae T11, T12; lower end vertebrae L3, L4.

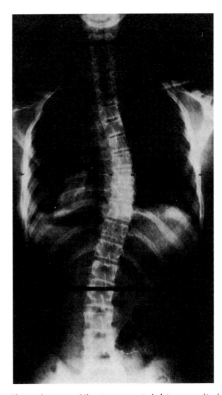

FIGURE 1. Thoracic curve. Ninety percent right convexity involving an average of six vertebrae: apex T8, T9; upper end vertebrae T5, T6; lower end vertebrae T11, T12.

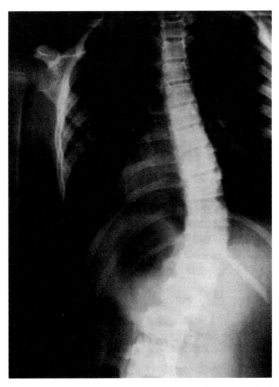

FIGURE 3. Thoracolumbar curve. Eighty percent right convexity involving an average of six to eight vertebrae: apex T11, T12; upper end vertebrae T6, T7; lower end vertebrae L1, L2.

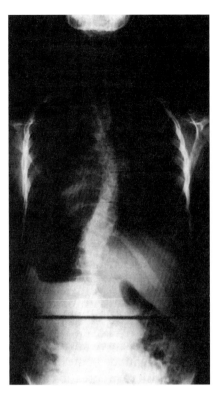

FIGURE 4. Double curve. Ninety percent right thoracic convexity and left lumbar convexity. Thoracic component averages four vertebrae: apex T7, upper end vertebrae T5, T6; lower end vertebrae T10. Lumbar component averages three vertebrae: apex L2, upper end vertebrae T11; lower end vertebra L4.

prognosis for patients with untreated scoliosis. Nachemson reported a 38-year follow-up of 130 patients with untreated scoliosis. Thirty percent claimed disability because of their deformity. There was a 100% increase in the mortality rate compared with that of the general population, and 16 of the 20 deaths were due to cor pulmonale. Thirty-seven percent of the patients had constant backache, and 14% complained of cardiopulmonary symptoms. Only 59 patients (45%) in this study, however, had idiopathic scoliosis; the remainder included patients with congenital scoliosis, paralytic scoliosis, and scoliosis secondary to tuberculosis, neurofibromatosis, and other miscellaneous diseases. Only 12 patients were actually seen in that particular follow-up study. Of the 16 deaths due to cor pulmonale, only three occurred in patients with idiopathic scoliosis, and it is uncertain whether these patients had adolescent-, juvenile-, or infantile-onset idiopathic scoliosis. Although no radiographs were available, Nachemson postulated that the constant backache in these patients was probably caused by osteoarthritis (84).

In a more recent and further follow-up study, Pehrsson and associates (97) reported on 115 patients with scoliosis born between 1902 and 1937: 30 patients had infantile-onset scoliosis, 31 juvenile-onset, and 52 adolescent-onset; 26 had polio, 19 had rickets, and in 69, the etiology was unknown. The average age at death was 54 years (range, 16 to 75 years). Sixty patients were alive at follow-up. All patients were younger than 30 years of age at their first visit, with a mean age of 14 years (0 to 30

years). Of the 55 patients who died, 21 died of respiratory failure and 17 of cardiovascular disease. The study confirmed an increased mortality rate in untreated scoliosis if one considers all the etiologies together. However, no patient with adolescent-onset scoliosis of unknown etiology (AIS) died from respiratory failure. Therefore, respiratory failure and premature death may develop in idiopathic scoliosis, but there is no indication from this study that this will occur in patients who have adolescent- or late-onset idiopathic scoliosis.

Nilsonne and Lundgren (91) reported a 50-year follow-up of 113 patients. This group had a mortality rate that was twice the rate in the general population. Sixty percent of the deaths were attributed to cardiopulmonary disease. Of the living patients, half were unable to work, 76% were unmarried, 90% had back symptoms, 30% were on disability pensions for back pain or scoliosis, and 17% were disabled but not on pensions. The major shortcoming of this study was that Nilsonne and Lundgren had no radiographs to ascertain the etiology of scoliosis in their patients. In addition, it is uncertain whether any of the patients were actually examined on follow-up.

A study by Fowles and associates (51) was based on 65 patients who were followed for an average of 23 years. Ten patients had died; of the rest, 22% were unemployed, 40% had intermittent backache, 22% had frequent backache, 9% were on disability pensions, and 63% of the women were unmarried. This study included patients with scoliosis of mixed etiologies, including idiopathic scoliosis, paralytic scoliosis (secondary to poliomyelitis), congenital scoliosis, and kyphosis. Only 24 (44%) of the 55 living patients had idiopathic scoliosis.

In a recent four-part follow-up of a scoliosis cohort from Ste. Justine in Montreal (54,55,78,101), the authors reported on a 14-year follow up survey on surgically and nonsurgically treated patients. Seventy-one percent of the cohort returned the questionnaire. In the nontreated patient group, there was a 45% incidence of current back pain. The authors concluded that patients with scoliosis perceived themselves as less healthy than other people of the same age, and they experienced limitations in certain activities, such as lifting, walking long distances, standing and sitting for periods of time, and being able to travel and socialize outside of the home. The scoliosis patients also reported more current back pain and pain that was more intense than did controls. Among the shortcomings of this study was that most of the information was obtained by a telephone survey and questionnaire. Although the authors used many validated questionnaire instruments, the patients were not reevaluated personally or radiographed at follow-up. More important, the population-based control group was made up of patients randomly selected from the telephone directory but not actually seen and screened to exclude the presence of spinal deformity.

A study by Dickson and colleagues (37) following a group of 81 surgically treated adults with AIS for an average of 5 years after surgery also included a group of 30 patients who declined surgery. These two groups were then compared with a group of nonscoliotic patients. At 5-year follow-up, the surgically treated patients reported significantly more improvement in self-image and ability to perform physical functional and positional tasks than did untreated patients. It is questionable, however, whether this small group, who presented as adults for evaluation, who refused surgical treatment for progression or pain, and who were followed for only 5 years, would constitute a natural history study or could be compared with untreated patients followed longitudinally.

The remainder of this chapter synthesizes what is currently known about the natural history of AIS in patients not treated surgically. We examine outcomes referable to curve progression, pulmonary function, mortality, back pain and disability, psychosocial effects, and effects of and on pregnancy.

CURVE PROGRESSION

The main concern in the skeletally immature patient relates to curve progression. In this group, nonsurgical and operative treatment decisions are generally made on the basis of curve progression or the probability thereof. It is often assumed by treating physicians that progressive curves will eventually lead to pain,

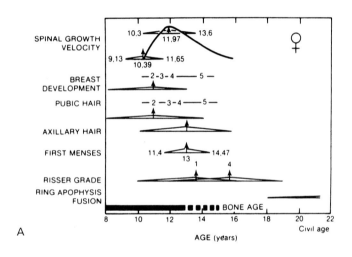

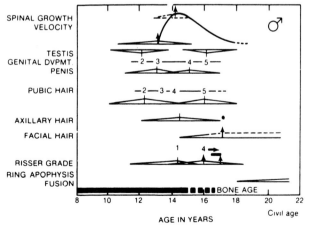

FIGURE 5. The relationship of spinal growth velocity to maturity landmarks and the events of puberty in girls (**A**) and boys (**B**). Numbers above breast development, pubic hair, axillary hair, and genital development refer to Tanner stages. (Modified from Trevor S, Kleinman R, Bleck EE [1980]: Growth landmarks and the evolution of scoliosis: a review of pertinent studies on their usefulness. *Dev Med Child Neurol* 22:675, with permission.)

diminution of pulmonary function, and psychosocial problems. The long-term sequelae related to these topics are discussed later in the chapter.

In the immature patient, the risk for progression is related primarily to specific curve factors and growth potential. Assessment of growth potential is essential for prognostication regarding curve progression. The relationship of spinal growth to the events of puberty (Fig. 5) must be evaluated in the skeletally immature patient (118).

Most information available on curve progression is from studies of girls, particularly those with thoracic curves. From these studies, six factors have been determined to influence the probability of progression in the skeletally immature patient. Four of these factors are related to growth potential; the remaining two are related to the particular curve. The curve factors include the following:

1. Double-curve patterns have a greater tendency to progress than single-curve patterns.
2. The larger the magnitude of the curve at detection, the greater the risk for progression (19,20,24,34,40,67,74,87,108, 134,139).

The growth factors are as follows:

1. The younger the patient at the time of diagnosis, the greater the risk for progression.
2. There is a greater risk for progression before the onset of menarche in girls.
3. The lower the Risser grade at curve detection, the greater the risk for progression.
4. Boys with comparable curves have about one tenth the risk for progression as girls (7,8,19,24,39,74,87,89,107,123–125, 128,129,134,140). A recent study (57) refutes this point.

In 1982, Nachemson and colleagues (87) calculated the probability of curve progression before skeletal maturity based on all known prognostic factors available at the time (Table 2).

TABLE 2. PROBABILITY OF PROGRESSION: MAGNITUDE OF CURVE AT INITIAL DETECTION VERSUS AGE

Curve Magnitude at Detection (degrees)	Age at Detection (ys)		
	10–12	13–15	16
<19			
20–29			
30–59			
>60	25%		
60			
90			
100		10%	
40			
70			
90		0%	
10			
30			
70			

From Nachemson A, Lonstein J, Weinstein S (1992): *Report of the SRS Prevalence and Natural History Committee 1982*. Presented at the SRS meeting, Denver, with permission.

TABLE 3. PROBABILITY OF PROGRESSION BASED ON RISSER GRADE AND CURVE MAGNITUDE AT DETECTION

Risser Grade	Curve Magnitude (degrees)	
	5–19	20–29
0–1		
2–4	22%	
1.6	68%	
23		

From Lonstein JE, Carlson JM (1984): The prediction of curve progression in untreated idiopathic scoliosis during growth. *J Bone Joint Surg Am* 66: 1061, with permission.

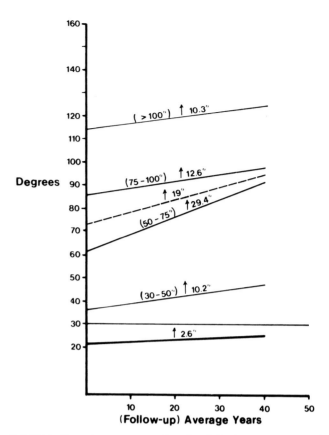

FIGURE 6. Thoracic curve progression after skeletal maturity. The *thick black line* represents average curve progression for all curves less than 30 degrees at skeletal maturity. The *thick dashed line* represents average curve progression for all curves of more than 30 degrees at skeletal maturity. The *thin black lines* represent average curve progression for each range in parentheses. Progression is not necessarily linear. Lines connect average values at maturity and at average 40-year follow-up. (Adapted from Weinstein SL, Ponseti IV [1983]: Curve progression in idiopathic scoliosis: long-term follow-up. *J Bone Joint Surg Am* 65:447, with permission.)

Lonstein and Carlson (74) evaluated the probability of progression based on Risser grade (Table 3). These studies show that risk for curve progression decreases with increasing skeletal maturity. With larger-magnitude curvatures, however, there may be a considerable risk for progression despite maturity.

Another factor that no doubt has some influence on the likelihood of curve progression is the loss of thoracic kyphosis. The importance of loss of thoracic kyphosis has been demonstrated by Dickson and others (33,35,99,113). How the loss of thoracic kyphosis affects curve progression is yet to be determined. Thoracic hypokyphosis also causes diminution of pulmonary function and may affect nonoperative as well as operative treatment decisions (43,45,135–137).

It was once thought that when the patient reached skeletal maturity, there would be no further curve progression (27,104). The study by Duriez (39) and several subsequent studies (7,41,102,124,128–130) demonstrated, however, that curves may continue to progress throughout life.

In a review of 102 patients followed for an average of 40 years at the University of Iowa, 68% of the curves progressed after maturity (124,125,128,129). This trend has continued in a 50-year longitudinal study (130). From this group of patients, multiple factors that lead to curve progression after maturity were identified (Table 4). In the thoracic curve pattern, patients with curves of less than 30 degrees at maturity tended to have

TABLE 4. PROGRESSION FACTORS IN CURVES GREATER THAN 30 DEGREES AT SKELETAL MATURITY

Thoracic	Lumbar	Thoracolumbar	Combined
Cobb angle	>50°		
Apical vertebral rotation	>30%		
Mehta angle	>30°		
Cobb angle	>30°		
Apical vertebral rotation	>30%		
Curve direction			
Relation of L5 to intercrest line			
Translatory shifts		Cobb angle	>30°
Apical vertebral rotation	>30%		
Translatory shifts		Cobb angle	>50°

From Weinstein SL (1986): Idiopathic scoliosis: natural history. *Spine* 11: 780, with permission.

apical vertebral rotation of less than 20 degrees (89) and Mehta angles (79) of less than 20 degrees; these curves did not progress. Thoracic curves of more than 30 degrees at maturity progressed an average of 19 degrees during the 40-year follow-up period. The most marked progression was noted in curves between 50 and 75 degrees at maturity. These continued to progress at 0.75 to 1 degree per year during the follow-up period (Fig. 6). All these patients had Mehta angles of greater than 20 degrees and apical vertebral rotation of more than 30% (125,128) (Fig. 7). The Mehta angle appears to be influenced by extreme degrees of vertebral rotation (98,99).

The importance of the rib cage to spinal stability has been demonstrated by Langenskiold and Michelsson in a study of rabbits in which resection of the costovertebral ligaments or the dorsal rib ends reliably produced scoliosis (71,80). Farkas (49,103) indicated that intrasegmental movement of the vertebral body in scoliosis is caused by relaxation of the costovertebral joints. Andriacchi and colleagues (4) demonstrated that the rib cage markedly increases the axial stability of the spine.

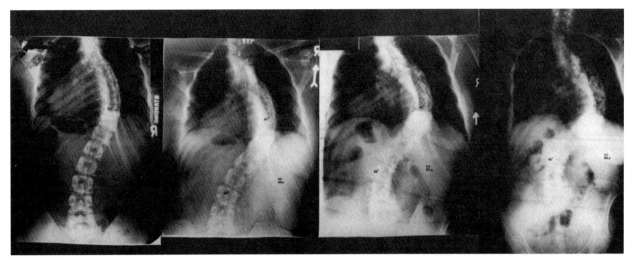

FIGURE 7. Natural history scenario of a thoracic curve. At maturity (21 years of age), the patient's curve measured 53 degrees. Note the slow steady progression of about 1 degree per year (age 43 years, 67 degrees; age 53 years, 86 degrees) to her current curve of 94 degrees at age 66 years.

In the lumbar curve pattern, curves of less than 30 degrees did not progress after skeletal maturity (Fig. 8). In our series (75), only one patient with a lumbar curve of less than 30 degrees progressed from 24 degrees at 18 years of age to 45 degrees at 54 years of age. This patient had an apical vertebral rotation of more than 33% and a high-riding fifth lumbar vertebra (the intercrest line passed through the body of the fifth lumbar vertebra). A translatory shift of the third lumbar vertebra on the fourth developed, with lateral tilting of the fourth lumbar vertebra on the fifth (Fig. 9).

All lumbar curves of more than 30 degrees at maturity had apical vertebral rotation of more than 33%. All but four of these curves progressed; no progression was seen in two patients in whom the fifth lumbar vertebra was deeply seated and in two other patients in whom the fifth lumbar vertebra was sacralized. These four curves were the only ones that did not develop translatory shifts at follow-up. Thus, in lumbar curves, the factor leading to progression is a curve greater than 30 degrees at maturity, particularly one with apical vertebral rotation of more than 33%. If the fifth lumbar vertebra is high riding, translatory shifts develop at the third lumbar vertebra on the fourth, with lateral tilting of the fourth lumbar vertebra on the fifth. Right lumbar curves tend to progress twice as often as left lumbar curves. The reasons for this could not be determined (125,128).

Farfan and colleagues (47,48) demonstrated that annular tears are the result of torsional rather than compressive failures. MacGibbon and Farfan (75) demonstrated in 554 patients that a high intercrest line (an interiliac crest line falling at or above the fourth or fifth lumbar disc space; in this situation, L5 is said to be well seated) is an antitorsional device, which reduces the risk for annular tears and disc degeneration. A low intercrest line provides no antitorsional protection to the discs between the fourth and fifth lumbar vertebrae and the fifth lumbar and the first sacral vertebrae (75). When the fifth lumbar vertebra is not well seated and there is a high percentage of vertebral

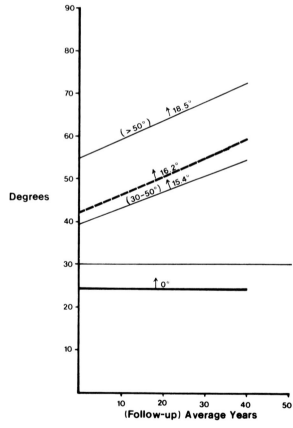

FIGURE 8. Lumbar curve progression after skeletal maturity. The *thick black line* represents average curve progression for all curves of less than 30 degrees at skeletal maturity. The *thick dashed line* represents average curve progression for all curves of more than 30 degrees at skeletal maturity. The *thin black lines* represent average curve progression for each range in parentheses. Progression is not necessarily linear. Lines connect average values at maturity and at average 40-year follow-up. (Adapted from Weinstein SL [1987]: The natural history of scoliosis in the skeletally mature patient. In: Dickson JH, ed. *Spinal deformities,* vol. 1, no. 2: *Spine, state of the art reviews.* Philadelphia: Hanley and Belfus, pp. 195–212, with permission.)

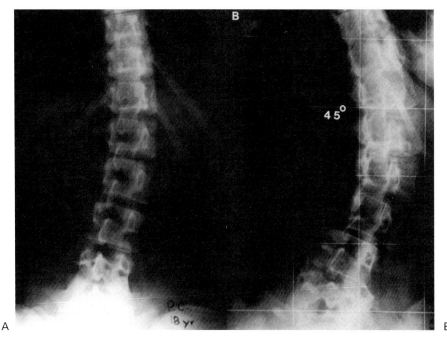

FIGURE 9. Progressive right lumbar curve. **A:** At 18 years of age, the right lumbar curve measures 24 degrees. The apical vertebral rotation is 33%, and the fifth lumbar vertebra is riding high in relation to the intercrest line. **B:** At 53 years of age, the curve measures 45 degrees, vertebral rotation has increased to 41%, and there is a translatory shift of the third lumbar vertebra on the fourth.

rotation, the curve tends to progress; significant translatory shifts (lateral listhesis) occur at the lower end of the curve, often accompanied by tilting of the fourth and fifth lumbar vertebrae toward the convexity of the curve (128) (Fig. 10). The roles of torsional rotation were investigated by Perdriolle and Vidal (98–100) and were found to be prognostic factors in progression of the thoracic curves.

The thoracolumbar curve pattern manifested the most significant amounts of apical vertebral rotation (40% to 65%) of any curve pattern (Fig. 11). This rotation increased with increasing curve severity. As with lumbar curves, patients with thoracolum-

bar curve patterns develop translatory shifts at the lower end of the curves. The marked vertebral rotation, in combination with translatory shifts at the lower end of the curve, leads to significant curve progression.

In our recent 50-year follow-up of untreated patients, the number of translatory shifts increased dramatically over time, with 20% having at least one translatory shift at maturity, increasing to 71% having at least one translatory shift at 50-year follow up (130).

In double (combined) curves, there were no correlative factors for curve progression after maturity. The apical vertebral rotation

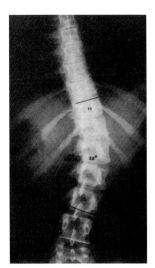
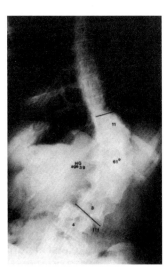

FIGURE 10. Sixteen-year-old girl with 38-degree right lumbar curve from T11 to L3 *(left)*. Her skeletal maturity is assessed as grade 5 on the Risser scale. At 39 years of age, her right lumbar curve has increased to 61 degrees *(right)*. Note the translatory shift of L3 on L4 *(arrows)*. (From Weinstein SL, Ponseti IV [1983]: Curve progression in idiopathic scoliosis: long-term follow-up. *J Bone Joint Surg Am* 65:447, with permission.)

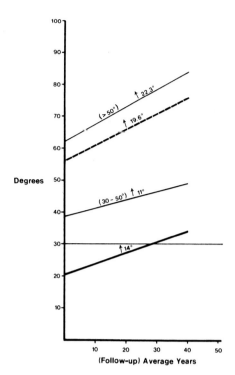

FIGURE 11. Thoracolumbar curve progression after skeletal maturity. The *thick black line* represents average curve progression for all curves of less than 30 degrees at skeletal maturity. The *thick dashed line* represents average curve progression for all curves of more than 30 degrees at skeletal maturity. The *thin black lines* represent average curve progression for each range in parentheses. Progression is not necessarily linear. Lines connect average values at maturity and at average 40-year follow-up. (Adapted from Weinstein SL [1987]: The natural history of scoliosis in the skeletally mature patient. In: Dickson JH, ed. *Spinal deformities*, vol. 1, no. 2: *Spine, state of the art reviews*. Philadelphia: Hanley and Belfus, pp. 195–212, with permission.)

tended to be less than that in thoracolumbar curves. The ribs remain level in the thoracic component; therefore, the Mehta angles were usually low. There was no prognostic value in the relationship of the fifth lumbar vertebra to the intercrest line in combined curves (125,128) (Fig. 12). Of note is the fact that at maturity, the magnitude of the thoracic component of the double major curve pattern tends to be larger than the lumbar component; with time, however, there are selectively greater increases in the lumbar curve magnitude as compared with the thoracic curve to balance the patient better. In addition, all patients tend to compensate better with time by increases in their secondary curvatures (125,128).

Ascani and coauthors (7) published the results of a multicenter Italian study of 187 patients followed for 34 years. The results of this study and the Iowa study (118,120) are similar concerning the amount of progression during the follow-up period for each specific curve pattern. Thus, in considering postmaturity curve progression, curves of less than 30 degrees at skeletal maturity regardless of curve pattern tend not to progress in adult life. Many curves, however, do continue to progress throughout adult life, in particular thoracic curves between 50 and 80 degrees.

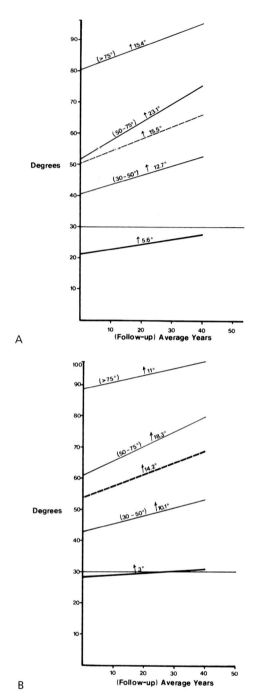

FIGURE 12. A: Thoracic component of double (combined) curve progression after skeletal maturity. The *thick dashed line* represents average curve progression for all curves of more than 30 degrees at skeletal maturity. The *thin black lines* represent average curve progression for each range in parentheses. Progression is not necessarily linear. Lines connect average values at maturity and at average 40-year follow-up. (Adapted from Trevor S, Kleinman R, Bleck EE [1980]: Growth landmarks and the evolution of scoliosis: a review of pertinent studies on their usefulness. *Dev Med Child Neurol* 22:675, with permission.) **B:** Lumbar component of double (combined) curve progression after skeletal maturity. The *thick dashed line* represents average curve progression for all curves of more than 30 degrees at skeletal maturity. The *thin black lines* represent average curve progression for each range in parentheses. Progression is not necessarily linear. Lines connect average values at maturity and at average 40-year follow-up. (Adapted from Weinstein SL, Ponseti IV [1983]: Curve progression in idiopathic scoliosis: long-term follow-up. *J Bone Joint Surg Am* 65:447, with permission.)

BACK PAIN

The incidence of back pain in the general population is varied and is questionnaire dependent (52). Howe and Frymoyer (60) evaluated 207 patients who were followed a minimum of 10 years after a single lumbar disc operation. They used 14 different questionnaires measuring surgical outcomes and demonstrated that outcome depends on the questionnaire design. In their review, satisfactory outcomes for the procedure ranged from 97% to 60%, depending on the questionnaire (statistically significant). The authors concluded that the reported outcomes for lumbar spinal surgery are significantly manipulated by the criteria selected for the assessment of end results.

The incidence of back pain in the general population is reported to range from 60% to 80% (13,30,52,58,61,70,85, 88,129). Jackson and colleagues (61) reported the incidence of back pain in the general population to be 80%; Kostuik and Bentivoglio (70) reported a 60% incidence. Horal (58), in an epidemiologic study of back pain in Gothenburg, Sweden, found that 81% of the population had some spinal pain, with 66% complaining of lumbar pain. Bjure and Nachemson (13) reported a 66% incidence of back pain in the general population, and Frymoyer and coauthors (52) reported a 67% incidence in 292 subjects in a randomly selected group of 1,221 men, with 20% of these subjects having severe pain.

The incidence of back pain in patients with scoliosis is comparable to the incidence of back pain in the general population. In the Iowa long-term follow-up study of 161 living patients with AIS (average follow-up, 40 years), 80% complained of some backache (127,129). In a control group of 100 patients who were age and sex matched and did not have scoliosis, 86% reported backache. Twenty-four percent of the patients with scoliosis had been to a doctor because of back pain, and 6% had been hospitalized for backache. In the control group, 30% had been to a doctor for backache, and 16% required hospitalization (Table 5). The incidence of frequent or daily backache was slightly higher in the scoliosis group (37%) compared with the control group (25%). Patients with lumbar or thoracolumbar curves, particularly those with translatory shifts at the lower end of their curves, tended to have a slightly greater incidence of backache than did patients with other curve patterns. The presence of translatory shifts on radiographs is associated with backache (129).

In a recent 50-year follow up of these same patients, patients filled out the same questionnaire they filled out at 30- and 40-year follow-up, in addition to filling out a more detailed questionnaire using validated instruments (130). This allowed us to make solid inferences over time and compare the group against an age- and gender-matched group of controls who were all screened physically to make certain they had no evidence of spinal deformity. Our study demonstrated an incidence of current back pain in 77% of scoliotic patients compared with 37% of controls. The incidence of chronic back pain was 61% in scoliotic patients compared with 35% in controls. The ability of these patients to perform activities of daily living and work was similar to that of controls. When patients rated their pain at 30, 40 and 50 years on a scale of 1 (none) to 5 (daily), the frequency of back pain was rated as 3 (occasional) during each study period.

An estimated 1% of patients with scoliosis eventually require surgery specifically for backache, an incidence similar to that for the general population (30,85). Horal (58), in his epidemiologic study, showed that scoliosis cases did not represent a disproportionate number of disability pensions. Furthermore, the three Swedish long-term follow-up studies of AIS, all with follow-up periods of longer than 30 years and all with more than 90% of the patients traced, demonstrated that low back pain is not a significant problem in these patients (69,84,91). The most common complaints of patients with scoliosis include backache at the end of a strenuous day or after unusual activities, with pain generally relieved by rest. The location of the pain is variable and generally unrelated to the location or magnitude of the curve (Fig. 13).

In the Iowa long-term series, at skeletal maturity, only 2% of the patients had any evidence of osteoarthritis. At 40-year follow-up, 38% of the patients had radiographic evidence of degenerative joint disease of the spine (129), and at 50-year follow-up, osteoarthritic changes were seen in 91% of patients (130). The history of back pain in this scoliotic group was generally unrelated to the severity of the radiographic osteoarthritic changes, except in areas of translatory shifts in thoracolumbar and lumbar curves. These changes ranged from minimal osteo-

TABLE 5. BACK PAIN IN SCOLIOTIC PATIENTS

Clinical findings	Scoliotic Patients[a] (Percentage at 40-year follow-up; N=161)	Scoliotic Patients[b] (Percentage at 50-year follow-up; N=106)	Controls[a] (Percentage; N=100)
Never have pain	20	13	14
Rare pain (one to five times in life)	19	13	25
Occasional pain (few days per year)	24	33	36
Frequent pain (few days per month)	20	22	19
Daily pain	17	19	6

[a] Data adapted from Weinstein SL, Zarala DC, Ponseti IV (1981): Idiopathic Scoliosis: Long-term follow-up and prognosis in untreated patients. *J Bone Joint Surg Am* 63: 702–712.
[b] Data adapted from Weinstein SL, Dolan LA, Spratt KF, et al. (1998): Natural history of adolescent idiopathic scoliosis: back pain at 50 years. Presented at the SRS meeting, New York City, September 17, 1998.

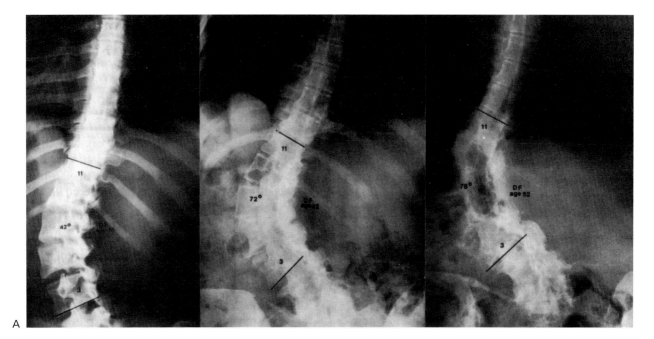

A

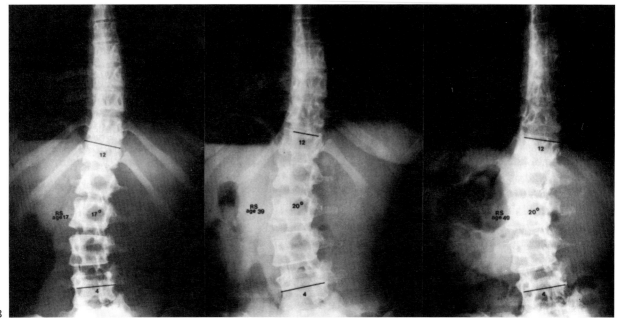

B

FIGURE 13. A: Fifteen-year-old girl (Risser grade 4) with a 42-degree left lumbar curve from T11 to L3 *(left)*. At 42 years of age *(center)*, the patient's curve has increased 30 degrees to 72 degrees. At 52 years of age *(right)*, the patient's curve has increased 6 degrees, to 78 degrees. Patient never had backache. (From Willner S [1984]: Prevalence study of trunk asymmetries and structural scoliosis in 10 year old school children. *Spine* 9:644–647, with permission.) **B:** Seventeen-year-old girl (Risser grade 5) with a 17-degree left lumbar curve from T12 to L4 *(left)*. At 39 years of age *(center)*, the patient's curve has increased 3 degrees, to 20 degrees. At 49 years of age *(right)*, the patient's curve remains stable at 20 degrees. The patient reports daily low backache for as long as she can remember. (From Weinstein SL [1987]: The natural history of scoliosis in the skeletally mature patient. In: Dickson JH, ed. *Spinal deformities*, vol. 1, no. 2: *Spine, state of the art reviews*. Philadelphia: Hanley and Belfus, pp. 195–212, with permission.)

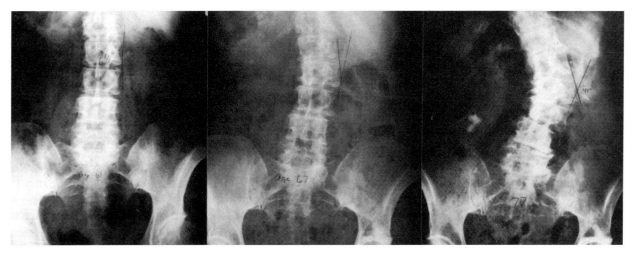

FIGURE 14. Degenerative scoliosis (supine radiographs) at 61 years of age *(left)*, 67 years of age *(center)*, and 77 years of age *(right)*. Note the development of a severe lumbar curve with marked degenerative changes. Clinically, the patient reported increasing back pain. (From Weinstein SL [1987]: The natural history of scoliosis in the skeletally mature patient. In: Dickson JH, ed. *Spinal deformities*, vol. 1, no. 2: *Spine, state of the art reviews.* Philadelphia: Hanley and Belfus, pp. 195–212, with permission.)

phyte formation and mild narrowing at the intervertebral disc space to moderate facet joint sclerosis and rarely to spontaneous fusion on the curve concavity. At 50-year follow-up, more than 90% of the patients had osteoarthritic changes in the spine. Radiographs continued to be unrelated to the duration or intensity of pain (130).

Back pain may develop in the compensatory curves below lumbar and thoracolumbar curves (30,38,61,85). It must not be assumed that a scoliotic patient's back pain is related to the curve. It is incumbent on the physician to determine whether the cause of pain is curve related or not before treatment decisions are made.

Kostuik and Bentivoglio (70) and Robin and associates (106) demonstrated that lumbar and thoracolumbar curves may arise de novo in adult life. This "degenerative" scoliosis may cause severe pain and discomfort requiring treatment. This type of scoliosis and its related problems should not be confused with the natural history of untreated AIS (Fig. 14). The cause of back pain in the adult scoliotic patient is unknown, but it may be spondylogenic or discogenic in origin.

PULMONARY FUNCTION

Only in thoracic curves is there a direct correlation between curve magnitude and effects on pulmonary function (1,9,15,31, 32,53,56,59,64,72,76,77,83,93,96,111,112,120,129,131,137, 141). Pulmonary function studies in patients with untreated AIS demonstrate that only in patients with thoracic curves is there a direct correlation between decreased pulmonary function and increasing curve severity. Vital capacity and forced expiratory volume in 1 second decreased as the severity of thoracic curves

increased (Fig. 15). The same correlation applies to PaO₂ (Fig. 16). In all other curve patterns, there was no correlation between curve severity and loss of pulmonary function.

The pattern of pulmonary disease in affected patients is uniformly that of restrictive lung disease (129). Smokers are generally affected much more severely than nonsmokers. Most studies show that significant limitations of forced vital capacity in nonsmokers do not occur until the curve approaches 100 to 120 degrees. The presence of thoracic hypokyphosis, however, increases the loss of pulmonary function associated with curve severity (137). Thus, curves of lesser magnitude with significant

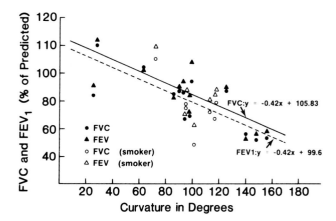

FIGURE 15. Relationship between forced vital capacity (FVC), forced expiratory volume in 1 second (FEV₁), and size of the curve in 20 patients with thoracic scoliosis, using a line of regression. (From Weinstein SL, Zavala DC, Ponseti IV [1981]: Idiopathic scoliosis: long-term follow-up and prognosis in untreated patients. *J Bone Joint Surg Am* 63:702–712, with permission.)

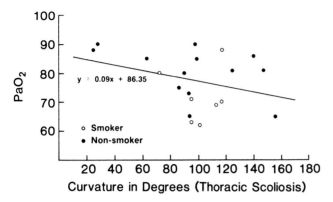

FIGURE 16. Relationship between PaO₂ and size of curve in 20 patients with thoracic scoliosis using a line of regression. (From Weinstein SL, Zavala DC, Ponseti IV [1981]: Idiopathic scoliosis: long-term follow-up and prognosis in untreated patients. *J Bone Joint Surg Am* 63:702–712, with permission.)

hypokyphosis may cause significant diminution of pulmonary function.

MORTALITY

Mortality rates in patients with AIS are comparable to those in the general population (129). Previous natural history studies of scoliosis (84,91) claimed an exaggerated mortality rate for patients with idiopathic scoliosis.

In the aforementioned study by Pehrsson and coauthors (97) on 115 patients with scoliosis of mixed etiology, the average age at death was 54 years (range, 16 to 75 years). Sixty patients were alive at follow-up. All patients were less than 30 years of age at their first visit, with a mean age of 14 years (0 to 30 years). Of the 55 patients who died, 21 died of respiratory failure and 17 of cardiovascular disease. The study confirmed an increased mortality rate in untreated scoliosis if one considers all the etiologies together. No patient with adolescent-onset scoliosis of unknown etiology (AIS), however, died from respiratory failure. Therefore, respiratory failure and premature death may develop in idiopathic scoliosis, but there is no indication from this study that this will occur in patients who have AIS (15,32,97).

In AIS, only patients with high-angle thoracic curves of more than 100 degrees are at increased risk for death from cor pulmonale and right ventricular failure. In the Iowa 40-year long-term study, the mortality rate was 15%, and in only one case was cor pulmonale secondary to scoliosis implicated as the cause of death. Actuarial data for patients born in the same years as the study patients coincided (119,129). At 50-year follow-up, the number of deaths increased as expected but was no different than actuarial predicted rates for patients born in the same years. In only two additional cases could scoliosis be implicated as a contributing cause of death.

PSYCHOSOCIAL EFFECTS

Scoliosis causes varying degrees of cosmetic deformity secondary to spinal rotation. Psychological effects of scoliosis do not appear to manifest in childhood unless curve magnitude is severe. Unhappiness with the rib prominence is often a concern of young patients with severe rotation and rib prominence of more than 3 cm. The same concerns are often expressed by patients treated surgically with large residual rib prominences. The psychological effects of scoliosis have been widely studied (3,5,25,26,46,90), particularly with reference to attitudes toward operative and nonoperative treatment (44). Psychological effects of scoliosis appear to be better tolerated by middle-aged patients than by teenagers (129). Some adults, however, with moderate to severe deformity may become mentally disabled by the deformity (12,129). There is no correlation between the location or degree of the curvature and the extent of the psychosocial effect (129).

Many patients with minimal curvatures have severe limitations psychosocially. These limitations are often expressed as buying clothing to try to hide the deformity. Other patients with severe deformities express little psychosocial limitation and are more accepting of their conditions. There are many studies on the psychological effects, but most conclusions are based on clinical judgment rather than empirical data (12,44). Significant radiographic changes of curvature may not occur over the course of time in many untreated patients. Increase in rotation, however, as manifested by increased rib or paraspinous muscle prominence may develop in the absence of significant changes of the Cobb angle on radiographs (7,130), causing changes in the patient's appearance. In adult patients with untreated AIS, the main concerns are often cosmetic; this is often the major reason these patients seek surgical consultation (68,116). The cosmetic aspects of the disorder should not be underplayed.

PREGNANCY

There has been great controversy about whether curves progress during pregnancy and whether scoliotic women can have normal reproductive experiences. With respect to the effects of pregnancy on scoliosis, Nachemson and colleagues (86) demonstrated a statistically significant effect on curve progression in patients who had multiple pregnancies before 23 years of age. They recommended avoidance of pregnancy in the early 20s, particularly in brace-treated patients. Blount and Mellencamp (14) and Berman and coauthors (10) also demonstrated that scoliosis progressed as a result of pregnancy. Blount and Mellencamp related this effect to the curve stability. Bunnell (19), however, was unable to detect any deleterious effect of pregnancy on scoliosis in his natural history study group. In the Iowa series (129), there were only two women who required cesarean sections. Significant complications during pregnancy or delivery were subjectively attributed to the women's spinal deformities (129).

Betz and associates (11) examined the charts and radiographs on 355 affected patients who had reached skeletal maturity (Risser grade 4). These patients were divided into two groups: 175 patients who had had at least one pregnancy (group A), and 180 who had never been pregnant (group B). The groups were comparable with regard to treatment. Curve progression of more than 5 degrees was seen in 25% and progression of more than 10 degrees in 10% of patients in each group. The age of the patient at the time of her first pregnancy did not influence the risk for progression, and the stability of the curve before pregnancy did not decrease the risk for progression during pregnancy.

The authors concluded that pregnancy does not increase the risk for progression of a scoliotic curve in a patient whose curve is not severe. The risk for progression was unaffected by the age of the patient at the time of first pregnancy, the number of pregnancies, or curve stability.

From the obstetric point of view, a recent study by Visscher and associates (122) demonstrated that reproductive experiences of scoliotic women do not differ from those of nonscoliotic women. In addition, in the Betz series (11), the effect of pregnancy and delivery was evaluated in 175 women who had had at least one pregnancy. No specific problems were directly related to the scoliosis, except in four patients in whom delivery posed difficulties. The incidence of cesarean section was half of the national average, and no cesarean sections were directly related to the mother's scoliosis. The authors concluded that mild to moderate scoliosis does not have a deleterious effect on pregnancy or delivery. The incidence of delivery by cesarean section and health problems in children of women who have scoliosis is no greater than that for the nonscoliotic population. These findings mirror the results of the Iowa long-term follow-up study (129).

SUMMARY

Increased public awareness about scoliosis, national scoliosis associations, and screening clinics have resulted in an increased number of children being referred for orthopaedic opinion, less severe curves at initial detection, and early institution of treatment. The natural history data presented in this chapter, particularly with reference to curve progression, are based on limited numbers of patients and are generally based on information from female patients with thoracic curves. Even in patients with progressive curves, we do not know, for example, whether the natural history of a progressive 30-degree curve would be to progress to 38 degrees or to 78 degrees.

Therefore, the conclusions presented in this chapter represent generalities. Decisions for each patient must be individualized, taking into consideration the probabilities of curve progression based on curve magnitude, skeletal maturity, sexual maturity, and age. Appropriate decisions for AIS require a thorough knowledge of natural history. Long-term results of various treatments, surgical or nonsurgical, for AIS must be viewed in light of the natural history of the disorder.

REFERENCES

1. Aaro S, Ohlund C (1984): Scoliosis and pulmonary function. *Spine* 9:220–222.
2. Adams W (1865): *Lecture on the pathology and treatment of lateral and other forms of curvature of the spine.* London: Churchill and Sons.
3. Anderson JD, D'Amba P (1976): The adolescent patient with scoliosis: a nursing care standard. *Nurs Clin North Am* 11:699.
4. Andriacchi T, Schultz A, Belytschko T, et al. (1974): A model for studies of mechanical interactions between the human spine and rib cage. *J Biomech* 7:497–507.
5. Apter A, Morein G, Munitz H, et al. (1978): The psychosocial sequelae of the Milwaukee brace in adolescent girls. *Clin Orthop* 131:156.
6. Armstrong GWD, Livermore NB, Suzuki N, et al. (1982): Nonstandard vertebral rotation in scoliosis screening patients. *Spine* 7:50.
7. Ascani E, Bartolozzi P, Logroscino CA, et al. (1986): Natural history of untreated idiopathic scoliosis after skeletal maturity. *Spine* 11:784.
8. Ascani E, Giglio GC, Salsano V (1980): Scoliosis screening in Rome. In: Zorab PA, Siegler D, eds. *Scoliosis.* London: Academic Press, pp. 39–44.
9. Bergofsky GH, Turino GM, Fishman AP (1959): Cardiorespiratory failure in kyphoscoliosis. *Medicine* 38:263–317.
10. Berman AT, Cohen DL, Schwentker EP (1982): The effects of pregnancy on idiopathic scoliosis: a preliminary report on eight cases and review of the literature. *Spine* 7:76.
11. Betz R, Bunnell WP, Lambrecht-Mulier E, et al. (1987): Scoliosis and pregnancy. *J Bone Joint Surg Am* 69:90–96.
12. Bjerkreim I, Hassan I (1982): Progression in untreated idiopathic scoliosis after end of growth. *Acta Orthop Scand* 53:897–900.
13. Bjure J, Nachemson A (1973): Nontreated scoliosis. *Clin Orthop* 93:44.
14. Blount WP, Mellencamp DD (1980): The effect of pregnancy on idiopathic scoliosis. *J Bone Joint Surg Am* 62:1083.
15. Branthwaite MA (1986): Cardiorespiratory consequences of unfused idiopathic scoliosis patients. *Br J Dis Chest* 80:360–369.
16. Brooks HL (1980): Current incidence of scoliosis in California. In: Zorab PA, Siegler D, eds. *Scoliosis.* London: Academic Press, pp. 7–12.
17. Brooks HL, Azen SP, Gerberg E, et al. (1975): Scoliosis: a prospective epidemiological study. *J Bone Joint Surg Am* 57:968.
18. Bruszewski J, Kamza A (1957): Czestosc wystepowania skolioz na podstawie anaciizy zdec maxoobrakowych. *Chir Narzadow Ruchu Ortop Pol* 22:115.
19. Bunnell WP (1986): A study of the natural history of idiopathic scoliosis before skeletal maturity. *Spine* 11:773.
20. Bunnell WP (1988): The natural history of idiopathic scoliosis. *Clin Orthop* 229:20–25.
21. Burwell RG, James JN, Johnson F, et al. (1982): The rib hump score: a guide to referral and prognosis? *J Bone Joint Surg Br* 64:248.
22. Burwell RG, James NH, Johnson F, et al. (1983): Standardized trunk asymmetry scores: a study of back contours in healthy school children. *J Bone Joint Surg Br* 65:453.
23. Chapman EM, Dill DB, Graybill A (1939): The decrease in functional capacity of the lungs and heart resulting from deformity of the chest: pulmonocardiac failure. *Medicine* 18:167–202.
24. Clarisse P (1974): Pronostic evolutif des scolioses idiopathiques mineures de 10° á 29°, en Période de Croissance. Thesis, Lyon.
25. Clayson D, Levine DB (1967): Adolescent scoliosis patients: personality patterns and effects of corrective surgery. *Clin Orthop* 116:99.
26. Clayson D, Luz-Alterman S, Cataletto MM, et al. (1987): Long term psychological sequelae of surgically versus non surgically treated scoliosis. *Spine* 12:983–986.
27. Cobb JR (1948): Outline for the study of scoliosis. In: *American Academy of Orthopaedic Surgeons: instructional course,* vol 5. Ann Arbor, MI: JW Edwards.
28. Collis DK, Ponseti IV (1969): Long-term follow-up of patients with idiopathic scoliosis not treated surgically. *J Bone Joint Surg Am* 51:425.
29. Cruickshank JL, Koike M, Dickson RA (1989): Curve patterns in idiopathic scoliosis. *J Bone Joint Surg Br* 71:259–263.
30. Dahlberg L, Nachemson A (1977): The economic aspects of scoliosis treatment. In: Zorab PA, ed. *Proceedings of the 5th symposium on scoliosis.* London: Academic Press.
31. Daruwalla JS, Tan WC (1985): Spirometric pulmonary function tests before and after surgical correction of idiopathic scoliosis in adolescents. *Ann Acad Med Singapore* 14:475–478.
32. Davies G, Reid L (1971): Effect of scoliosis on growth of alveoli and pulmonary arteries and on right ventricle. *Arch Dis Child* 46:623–632.
33. Deacon P, Flood BM, Dickson RA (1984): Idiopathic scoliosis in three dimensions: a radiographic and morphometric analysis. *J Bone Joint Surg Br* 66:509–512.
34. Dickson R, Deacon P (1987): Spinal growth. *J Bone Joint Surg Br* 69:690–692.
35. Dickson RA, Lawton JO, Archer IA, et al. (1983): Combined median

and coronal plane asymmetry: the essential lesion of progressive idiopathic scoliosis. *J Bone Joint Surg Br* 65:368.

36. Dickson RA, Stirling AJ, Whitaker IA, et al. (1988): Prognostic factors derived from screening studies: prognosis in scoliosis. In: *Proceedings of the 8th Phillip Zorab scoliosis symposium,* London; October 26–28, 1988; pp. 1–4.

37. Dickson JH, Mirkovic S, Noble MS, et al. (1995): Results of operative treatment of idiopathic scoliosis in adults. *J Bone Joint Surg Am* 77: 513–523.

38. Dove J (1988): The fate of unfused thoracolumbar curves: a specific pain pattern. In: *Proceedings of the 8th Phillip Zorab scoliosis symposium,* London; October 26–28, 1988; pp. 79–82.

39. Duriez J (1969): Evolution de la scoliose idiopathique chex: adulte. *Acta Orthop Belg* 33:547–550.

40. Duval-Beaupere G, Lamireau TH (1985): Scoliosis of less than 30 degrees: properties of the evolutivity (risk of progression). *Spine* 10: 421–424.

41. Edgar MA (1987): The natural history of unfused scoliosis. *Orthopaedics* 10:931–939.

42. Edgar MA, Mehta M (1988): Long term followup of fused and unfused idiopathic scoliosis. *J Bone Joint Surg Br* 70:712–716.

43. Edmonson AS, Morris JT (1977): Follow-up study of Milwaukee brace treatment in patients with idiopathic scoliosis. *Clin Orthop* 126:48.

44. Eliason JM, Richman LC (1984): Psychological effects of idiopathic adolescent scoliosis. *Dev Behav Pediatr* 5:169.

45. Emans J, Kaelin A, Bancel P, et al. (1986): Boston brace treatment of idiopathic scoliosis. *Spine* 11:792.

46. Fallstrom K, Nachemson AL, Cochran TP (1984): Psychologic effect of treatment for adolescent idiopathic scoliosis. *Orthop Trans* 8:150.

47. Farfan HF, Cossette J, Robertson GH, et al. (1970): The effects of torsion on lumbar intervertebral joints: the role of the torsion in disc degeneration. *J Bone Joint Surg Am* 52:468.

48. Farfan HF, Huberdeau RM, DuBow HI (1972): Lumbar intervertebral disc degeneration: the influence of geometrical features on the pattern of disc degeneration—a post mortem study. *J Bone Joint Surg Am* 54:492–510.

49. Farkas A, cited in Ogilvie JW, Schendel MJ (1988): Calculated thoracic volume as related to parameters of scoliosis correction. *Spine* 13: 39–42.

50. Floman Y, Span Y, Makin M, et al. (1980): The prevalence of scoliosis in the Jerusalem school population. *Orthop Rev* 9:73.

51. Fowles JV, Drummond DS, L'Ecuyer S, et al. (1978): Untreated scoliosis in the adult. *Clin Orthop* 134:212–217.

52. Frymoyer JW, Newberg A, Pope MH, et al. (1984): Spine radiographs in patients with low back pain: an epidemiologic study in men. *J Bone Joint Surg Am* 66:1048–1055.

53. Gazioglu K, Goldstine LA, Femi-Pearse D, et al. (1968): Pulmonary function in idiopathic scoliosis: comparative evaluation before and after orthopaedic correction. *J Bone Joint Surg Am* 50:1391–1399.

54. Goldberg MS, Mayo NE, Poitras B, et al. (1994): The Ste-Justine Adolescent Idiopathic Scoliosis Cohart Study. I. Description of the study. *Spine* 19:1551–1561.

55. Goldberg MS, Mayo NE, Poitras B, et al. The Ste-Justine Adolescent Idiopathic Scoliosis Cohart Study. II. Perception of health, self and body image, and participation in physical activities. *Spine* 19: 1562–1572.

56. Gucker T (1962): Changes in vital capacity in scoliosis: preliminary report on effect of treatment. *J Bone Joint Surg Am* 44:469–481.

57. Hassan I, Bjerkreim I. (1983): Progression in idiopathic scoliosis after conservative treatment. *Acta Orthop Scand* 54:88–90.

58. Horal J (1969): The clinical appearance of low back disorders in the city of Göteberg, Sweden. *Acta Orthop Scand* 118[Suppl].

59. Hornstein S, Inman S, Ledsome JR (1987): Ventilatory muscle training in kyphoscoliosis. *Spine* 12:859–863.

60. Howe J, Frymoyer JW (1985): The effects of questionnaire design on the determination of end results in lumbar spine surgery. *Spine* 10:804–805.

61. Jackson RP, Simmons EH, Stripinis D (1983): The incidence and severity of back pain in adult idiopathic scoliosis. *Spine* 8:749.

62. James JIP (1954): Idiopathic scoliosis: the prognosis, diagnosis and operative indications related to curve pattern and age at onset. *J Bone Joint Surg Br* 36:36–49.

63. Johnson M (1988): Long term follow-up of fusion versus no fusion. In: *Proceedings of the 8th Phillip Zorab scoliosis symposium.* London; October 26–28, 1988; pp. 135–139.

64. Kafer ER (1977): Respiratory and cardiovascular functions in scoliosis. *Bull Eur Physiopathol Respir* 13:299–321.

65. Kane WJ (1977): Scoliosis prevalence: a call for a statement of terms. *Clin Orthop* 126:43–46.

66. Kane WJ, Moe JH (1970): A scoliosis prevalence survey in Minnesota. *Clin Orthop* 69:216.

67. Karol LA, Browne RH, Johnston CE (1991): *Incidence of curve progression in male idiopathic scoliosis.* Presented at the SRS Annual Meeting; September; Minneapolis, MN.

68. Kitahara H, Inoue S, Minami S, et al. (1989): Long term results of spinal instrumentation surgery for scoliosis, five or more after surgery, in patients over twenty-three years of age. *Spine* 14:744–749.

69. Kolind-Sörensen V (1973): A follow-up study of patients with idiopathic scoliosis. *Acta Orthop Scand* 44:98.

70. Kostuik JP, Bentivoglio J (1981): The incidence of low-back pain in adult scoliosis. *Spine* 6:268–273.

71. Langenskiöld A, Michelsson JE (1961): Experimental progressive scoliosis in the rabbit. *J Bone Joint Surg Br* 43:116–120.

72. Lindh M, Bjure J (1975): Lung volumes in scoliosis before and after correction by Harrington instrumentation method. *Acta Orthop Scand* 46:934–948.

73. Lonstein JE, Bjoklund S, Wanninger MH, et al. (1982): Voluntary school screening for scoliosis in Minnesota. *J Bone Joint Surg Am* 64: 481–488.

74. Lonstein JE, Carlson JM (1984): The prediction of curve progression in untreated idiopathic scoliosis during growth. *J Bone Joint Surg Am* 66:1061.

75. MacGibbon B, Farfan HF (1979): A radiologic survey of various configurations of the lumbar spine. *Spine* 4:258–266.

76. Makley JT, Herndon CH, Inkley S, et al. (1968): Pulmonary function in paralytic and nonparalytic scoliosis before and after treatment: a study of sixty-three cases. *J Bone Joint Surg Am* 50:1379–1390.

77. Mankin HJ, Graham JJ, Schack J (1964): Cardiopulmonary function in mild and moderate idiopathic scoliosis. *J Bone Joint Surg Am* 46: 53–62.

78. Mayo NE, Goldberg MS, Poitras B, et al. (1994): The Ste-Justine Adolescent Idiopathic Scoliosis Cohart Study. III. Back pain. *Spine* 19:1573–1581.

79. Mehta MH (1972): The rib vertebral angle in the early diagnosis between resolving and progressive infantile scoliosis. *J Bone Joint Surg Br* 543:230–243.

80. Michelsson JE (1965): The development of spinal deformity in experimental scoliosis. *Acta Orthop Scand* 81[Suppl].

81. Montgomery F, Willner S (1988): The natural history of idiopathic scoliosis: a study of the incidence of treatment. *Spine* 13:401–404.

82. Montgomery F, Willner S (1997): The natural history of idiopathic scoliosis: incidence of treatment in 15 cohorts of children born between 1963 and 1977. *Spine* 22:772–774.

83. Muirhead A, Conner AN (1985): The assessment of lung function in children with scoliosis. *J Bone Joint Surg Br* 67:699–702.

84. Nachemson A (1968): A long-term follow-up study of nontreated scoliosis. *Acta Orthop Scand* 39:446.

85. Nachemson A (1979): Adult scoliosis and back pain. *Spine* 4: 513–517.

86. Nachemson A, Cochran TP, Irstam L, et al. (1981): *Pregnancy after scoliosis treatment.* Presented at SRS annual meeting; September 1981; Montreal.

87. Nachemson A, Lonstein J, Weinstein S (1982): Report of the SRS Prevalence and Natural History Committee 1982. *Presented at SRS meeting;* September 1982; Denver.

88. Nagi SJ, Riley LE, Newby LG (1973): Social epidemiology of back pain in general population. *J Chronic Dis* 26:769.

89. Nash CL Jr, Moe JH (1969): A study of vertebral rotation. *J Bone Joint Surg Am* 51:223–229.

90. Nathan SW (1977): Body image of scoliotic female adolescents before and after surgery. *Matern Child Nurs J* 6:139.

91. Nilsonne U, Lundgren KD (1968): Long-term prognosis in idiopathic scoliosis. *Acta Orthop Scand* 39:456.

92. O'Brien JP (1980): The incidence of scoliosis in Oswestry. In: Zorab PA, Siegler D, eds. *Scoliosis.* London: Academic Press.

93. Ogilvie JW, Schendel MJ (1988): Calculated thoracic volume as related to parameters of scoliosis correction. *Spine* 13:39–42.

94. Owen R, Taylor JF, McKendrick O, et al. (1980): Current incidence of scoliosis in school children in the city of Liverpool. In: Zorab PA, Siegler D, eds. *Scoliosis.* London: Academic Press, pp. 31–34.

95. Patynski J, Szczekot J, Szwaluk F (1957): Boczne skrywienie kregosyupa w awietle statystyki. *Chir Narzadow Ruchu Ortop Pol* 22:111.

96. Pehrsson K, Bake B, Larsson S, et al (1991): Lung function in adult idiopathic scoliosis: a 20 year follow-up. *Thorax* 46:474–478.

97. Pehrsson K, Larsson S, Nachemson A, et al. (1991): A long term follow-up of patients with untreated scoliosis: a study of mortality, causes of death, and symptoms. *Spine* 17:1091–1096.

98. Perdriolle R (1979): *La scoliose: son etude tridimensionnelle.* Paris: Maloine.

99. Perdriolle R, Vidal J (1981): Etude de lat cour bure scoliotique, importance de l'extension et de la rotation vertebral. *Rev Chir Orthop* 67:25–34.

100. Perdriolle R, Vidal J (1985): Thoracic idiopathic scoliosis curve evolution and prognosis. *Spine* 10:785–791.

101. Poitras B, Mayo NE, Goldberg MS, et al. (1994): The Ste-Justine Adolescent Idiopathic Scoliosis Cohart Study. IV. Surgical correction and back pain. *Spine* 19:1582–1588.

102. Ponseti IV, Friedman B (1950): Prognosis in idiopathic scoliosis. *J Bone Joint Surg Am* 32:381.

103. Ponseti IV, Pedrini V, Wynne-Davies R, et al. (1976): Pathogenesis of scoliosis. *Clin Orthop* 120:268–280.

104. Risser JC, Ferguson AB (1936): Scoliosis, its prognosis. *J Bone Joint Surg Am* 18:667–670.

105. Robin GC, Meyer V, Meyer S (1988): A follow-up study of 1000 children referred from school survey programs. In: *Proceedings of the 8th Phillip Zorab scoliosis symposium;* October 26–28, 1988; London, pp. 9–13.

106. Robin GC, Span Y, Steinberg R, et al. (1982): Scoliosis in the elderly: a follow-up study. *Spine* 7:355.

107. Rogala EJ, Drummond DS, Gurr J (1978): Scoliosis: incidence and natural history. A prospective epidemiological study. *J Bone Joint Surg Am* 60:173–176.

108. Scott MM, Piggott H (1981): A short-term follow-up of patients with mild scoliosis. *J Bone Joint Surg Br* 63:523.

109. Segil CM (1974): The incidence of idiopathic scoliosis in the Bantu and white population groups of Johannesburg. *J Bone Joint Surg Br* 56:393.

110. Shands AR, Eisberg HB (1955): The incidence of scoliosis in the state of Delaware: a study of 50,000 minifilms of the chest made during a survey for tuberculosis. *J Bone Joint Surg Am* 37:1243.

111. Shannon DC, Roseborough EJ, Valenca LM, et al. (1970): The distribution of abnormal lung function in kyphoscoliosis. *J Bone Joint Surg Am* 52:131–144.

112. Shneerson J (1988): Respiratory consequences of spinal fusion. In: *Proceedings of the 8th Phillip Zorab scoliosis symposium;* October 26–28, 1988; London, pp. 139–141.

113. Shufflebarger HL, King WF (1987): Composite measurements of scoliosis: a new method of analysis of the deformity. *Spine* 12:228.

114. Skogland LB, Miller JAA (1978): The incidence of scoliosis in northern Norway: a preliminary report. *Acta Orthop Scand* 49:635.

115. Smyrnis PM, Valanis J, Voutsinas S, et al. (1980): Incidence of scoliosis in the Greek Islands. In: Zorab PA, Siegler D, eds. *Scoliosis.* London: Academic Press, pp. 13–18.

116. Sponseller PD, Cohen MS, Nachemson AL, et al. (1987): Results of surgical treatment of adults with scoliosis. *J Bone Joint Surg Am* 69:667–675.

117. Torell G, Nordwall A, Nachemson A (1981): The changing pattern of scoliosis treatment due to effective screening. *J Bone Joint Surg Am* 63:337–341.

118. Trevor S, Kleinman R, Bleck EE (1980): Growth landmarks and the evolution of scoliosis: a review of pertinent studies on their usefulness. *Dev Med Child Neurol* 22:675.

119. U.S. Department of Health, Education and Welfare, (1978): *Vital Statistics of the United States,* vol II, sec 5: *life tables.* Hyattsville, MD: Public Health Service National Center for Health Statistics.

120. Veraart BEEMJ, Jansen BJ (1990): Changes in lung function associated with idiopathic thoracic scoliosis. *Acta Orthop Scand* 61[Suppl 235]:1.

121. Vercauteren M, Van Beneden M, Verplaetse, et al. (1982): Trunk asymmetries in a Belgian school population. *Spine* 7:555.

122. Visscher W, Lonstein JE, Hoffman DA, et al. (1988): Reproductive outcomes in scoliosis patients. *Spine* 13:1096–1098.

123. Weinstein SL (1985): Adolescent idiopathic scoliosis: prevalence, natural history, treatment indications. Iowa City: University of Iowa Printing Service.

124. Weinstein SL (1986): Idiopathic scoliosis: natural history. *Spine* 11:780.

125. Weinstein SL (1987): The natural history of scoliosis in the skeletally mature patient. In: Dickson JH, ed. *Spinal deformities,* vol. 1, no. 2: *spine, state of the art reviews.* Philadelphia: Hanley and Belfus, pp. 195–212.

126. Weinstein SL (1988): Adolescent idiopathic scoliosis, morbidity in unfused adults. In: *Proceedings of the 8th Phillip Zorab scoliosis symposium;* October 26–28, 1988; London, pp. 83–91.

127. Weinstein SL (1988): In view of the long term results in untreated patients, can surgery be justified? In: *Proceedings of the 8th Phillip Zorab scoliosis symposium;* October 26–28, 1988; London, pp. 142–146.

128. Weinstein SL, Ponseti IV (1983): Curve progression in idiopathic scoliosis: long-term follow-up. *J Bone Joint Surg Am* 65:447.

129. Weinstein SL, Zavala DC, Ponseti IV (1981): Idiopathic scoliosis: long-term follow-up and prognosis in untreated patients. *J Bone Joint Surg Am* 63:702–712.

130. Weinstein SL, Dolan LA, Spratt KF, et al. (1998): *Natural history of adolescent idiopathic scoliosis: back pain at 50 years.* Presented at the SRS meeting, New York City, September 17, 1998.

131. Westgate HD, Moe JH (1967): Pulmonary function in kyphoscoliosis before and after correction by Harrington instrumentation method. *J Bone Joint Surg Am* 51:935–946.

132. Willner S (1984): Prevalence study of trunk asymmetries and structural scoliosis in 10 year old school children. *Spine* 9:644–647.

133. Willner S (1988): Natural history of early curves: prognosis in scoliosis. In: *Proceedings of the 8th Phillip Zorab scoliosis symposium;* October 26–28, 1988; London, pp. 4–8.

134. Willner S, Uden A (1982): A prospective prevalence study of scoliosis in southern Sweden. *Acta Orthop Scand* 53:233–237.

135. Winter RB, Carlson JM (1977): Modern orthotics for spinal deformities. *Clin Orthop* 126:74.

136. Winter RB, Lonstein JE, Droght J, et al. (1986): The effectiveness of bracing in the non-operative treatment of idiopathic scoliosis. *Spine* 11:790.

137. Winter RB, Lovell WW, Moe JH (1975): Excessive thoracic lordosis and loss of pulmonary function in patients with idiopathic scoliosis. *J Bone Joint Surg Am* 57:972–977.

138. Wynne-Davies R (1968): Familial scoliosis: a family survey. *J Bone Joint Surg Br* 50:24.

139. Yamauchi Y, Yamaguchi T, Asaka Y (1988): Prediction of curve progression in idiopathic scoliosis based on initial roentgenograms: a proposal of an equation. *Spine* 13:1258–1261.

140. Zaoussis AL, James JIP (1958): The iliac apophysis and the evolution of curves in scoliosis. *J Bone Joint Surg Br* 40:442–453.

141. Zorab PA, Prime FJ, Harrison A (1978): Lung function in young persons after spinal fusions for scoliosis. *Spine* 4:22–28.

ADOLESCENT IDIOPATHIC SCOLIOSIS: NONSURGICAL TECHNIQUES

KENNETH J. NOONAN

This chapter outlines the different methods of nonoperative treatment in immature patients with adolescent idiopathic scoliosis (AIS). Most of this chapter focuses on bracing because this is the main nonoperative treatment used today. Emphasis is placed on commonly used braces and their pertinent biomechanics, brace manufacture, indications, and brace use. Compliance and complications are discussed. Review of the results of previous studies using nonoperative therapy centers on the effectiveness of treatment in meeting objectives and altering the natural history of AIS.

PHYSICAL THERAPY

Most would agree that isolated physical therapy has no role in the treatment of AIS. In a controlled study of patients with mild scoliosis, Stone and associates (92) found that progression of scoliosis was not affected by an exercise protocol consisting of pelvic tilts, situps, leg lifts, and trunk strengthening. Only half of their patients were found to be compliant with the protocol. Others have also noted poor compliance with exercises in combination with bracing (64).

It is controversial whether physical therapy in conjunction with bracing has an important effect on halting curve progression. Originally, exercises (pelvic tilts, back extensions, lateral shifts, and chest expansion) were performed in and out of the Milwaukee brace and were considered integral in maximizing treatment. Subsequently, Carman and colleagues (22) evaluated 24 compliant patients treated with bracing—12 who performed exercises as described by Blount and Moe with 12 who performed no exercises. Both groups were similar in age and curve magnitude, yet no difference in outcome was documented. Based on these findings, specific exercises are no longer routinely prescribed to prevent curve progression. Currently, however, patients are encouraged to participate in athletic activities even in the brace. Removal of the orthosis during extreme or contact

sports is allowed so that the patient can enjoy the obvious physical and psychological benefits of these activities. Some authors promote specific exercises to avoid atrophy of the paraspinal and abdominal muscles (20) and to prevent possible hip flexion contractures resulting from prolonged brace treatment (33).

ELECTRICAL STIMULATION

Experimental studies in laboratory animals demonstrated that electrical stimulation could produce scoliotic deformities (9). Extrapolation to human subjects showed that electrical stimulation along the convexity of a curve produces variable initial correction. Because of this, several centers started to use electrical stimulation as an alternative to orthotic treatment in the nonoperative management of immature patients with AIS. Proponents of these systems have theorized better patient acceptance and therefore greater compliance than braced patients (30,54). Immature patients are stimulated for 8 to 12 hours per night in the prone position. This is continued until maturity or failure to halt curve progression.

Originally, some investigators used electrodes that were surgically implanted and controlled by means of external transmitters (15,51). The potential cost and morbidity (including need for removal, infection, or pneumothorax [51]) of implantable systems paved the way for transcutaneous stimulator units. Single (single-curve) or double (double-curve) channeled devices are placed laterally along paraspinal muscles in the convexity of the scoliosis. Greater initial correction of curves is noted with lateral placement of electrodes compared with paraspinal placement. Worsening of curves is possible by placing an electrode in the concavity of a compensatory curve (9).

Several studies reported good results by halting curve progression in 72% to 84% of cases (6,8,15,17,37,51,66). Many were preliminary reports, had poor follow-up, or included patients at low risk for curve progression (6,8,17,37,51,66). Those studies that published results of patients at higher risk for progression or with longer follow-up demonstrated curve progression in up to 56% (21,42,94). O'Donnell and coauthors (80) reported 62 fully compliant patients and noted progression of 8 to 18 degrees in 83% of patients. Similar to natural history studies, greater

K. J. Noonan, M.D.: Indiana University, Department of Orthopaedic Surgery, Riley Children's Hospital, Indianapolis, IN.

rates of failure were noted in thoracic and double major curves and in curves with greater magnitude. Other authors have also reported poor results (progression in 50% to 86% of patients), suggesting that electrical stimulation does not alter the natural history of AIS (3,28,76). In addition, with further follow-up, the potential benefit of increased compliance in comparison to bracing has not held true, with rates of noncompliance of 24% to 50% (21,42,54). Decreased compliance is secondary to poor patient tolerance as a result of back pain, difficulty sleeping, and skin irritation because of electrode placement (6,16,21,30,37, 51,54). There are currently no indications for electrical stimulation in the treatment of AIS.

BRACING

History of Bracing

The modern history of orthotic treatment in AIS began in the 1940s when external devices were used in the postoperative stabilization of in situ fusion of spinal deformities. In 1946, Blount and Schmidt introduced the Milwaukee brace to be used as alternative to casting after such procedures. In 1958, they sug-

gested that the Milwaukee brace may be useful in the nonoperative treatment of AIS provided the existing deformity would be acceptable at skeletal maturity (14). The Milwaukee brace was the first orthosis to be widely used in AIS; and although many physicians still use this brace, many other types of orthoses have been designed and are currently in widespread use.

Types of Braces

One type of orthosis used in AIS can be classified as a CTLSO (cervical-thoracic-lumbar-sacral orthosis), for which the Milwaukee brace is the standard. Lower-profile braces that do not immobilize the cervical spine were later developed and are considered thoracic-lumbar-sacral orthoses (TLSOs). TLSOs were primarily designed to circumvent the objectionable appearance of the cervical extension present with the Milwaukee brace, which is associated with poor compliance (20,98). TLSOs can also be classified as *high profile* (higher trim lines) or *low profile* according to their potential for holding curves with apices higher in the thoracic region. Examples of common TLSOs include the Boston brace, the Wilmington brace, and the Miami brace. Other TLSOs have been developed but are not discussed in this

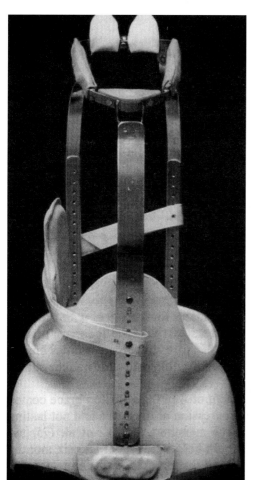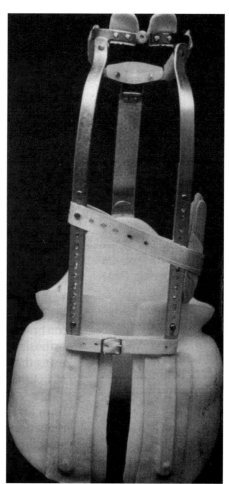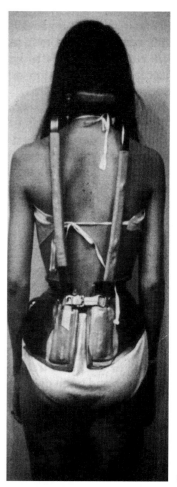

A,B

C

FIGURE 1. The Milwaukee brace. **A:** Front view of the Milwaukee brace, showing the pelvic girdle and lateral rib pad. **B:** Posterior view of the Milwaukee brace. **C:** A patient wearing the Milwaukee brace.

chapter (see Chap. 52). Although the Charleston bending brace is technically a TLSO, it is designed to unbend the structural curves and must be worn at night only.

Theoretically, bracing works by applying external forces to the trunk, which imparts corrective force to the spine. Resultant decreases in deformity, as measured by the Cobb method, are thought to alter the growth in some unknown manner, preventing significant progression. Forces that have been used include longitudinal traction and lateral pressure from pads, straps, or the brace itself.

Milwaukee Brace

The original Milwaukee brace consisted of a molded pelvic leather girdle with an attached metal superstructure positioned in slight lumbar flexion (Fig. 1). Over time, the leather pelvic module was replaced by custom-made or prefabricated thermoplastic pelvic modules that are easier and less expensive to construct. To correct lumbar scoliosis, pads are often incorporated into the pelvic portion. Pressure pads (thoracic curves) and trapezius pads and axillary slings (for high thoracic curves) can be attached to the superstructure with leather straps and are adjusted in relationship to curve location. Axillary slings provide a point of counterpressure for thoracic curves with apices from the fifth to the eighth thoracic vertebra (T5 to T8); in addition, they prevent increased pressure at the throat mold. Pad placement is critically analyzed and expected to be below the apical rib with posterolateral pressure.

The superstructure consisting of three metal uprights was chosen to minimize thoracic pressure, possibly leading to pulmonary problems in postoperative polio patients. Attached to the superstructure was a fixed mandibular and occipital assembly used to stabilize the head. Because of potential orthodontic deformity, the mandibular component was later replaced by a throat mold, which serves to position the head over the thorax and the occipital pads. A lower profile design of the Milwaukee brace has been developed for use in patients with lower apical vertebrae.

The patient is thought to produce traction and improve spine correction by actively extending against the occipital pads with movement and prescribed exercises. This theory has not been supported by Galante and colleagues (40), who demonstrated maintenance of corrective forces even during sleep. Forces produced by traction have been estimated to be 10 to 20 Newton, with twice that seen with lateral pads. Subsequent biomechanical studies have demonstrated that correction generated through traction in the occipital and mandibular support or throat mold is possible for minor or moderate curves (40,74). Most of the corrective forces are due to direct pressure from the lateral pads (particularly in larger curves) (5) or backward tilt of the pelvis.

Boston Brace System

The Boston brace system was developed at Boston Children's Hospital in the 1970s and consisted of six standardized prefabricated polypropylene pelvic and thoracolumbar modules lined with soft foam polyethylene. With time, a total of 16 to 20 prefabricated modules became available. It is estimated that 95%

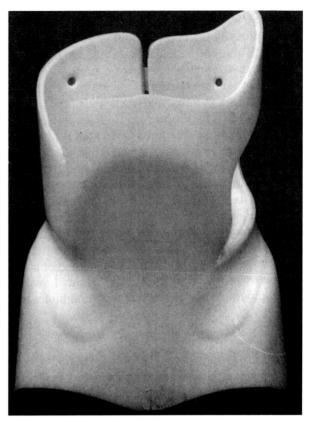

FIGURE 2. The Boston brace.

of children can be braced with the entire prefabricated inventory, and most children (80%) can be fitted with one of the six original modules. Originally, a cervical superstructure (Boston-Milwaukee brace) was added for curves with an apex above T10 (98).

A brace blueprint is constructed from the radiographs for correct pad placement and trim-line planning. The prefabricated pelvic girdle is trimmed, and pressure pads for derotation are inserted according to the location of the apex on radiographs (Fig. 2). Areas of relief or voids are present opposite pads, allowing passive and possibly active curve movement away from the pads. Lumbar lordosis is purposefully reduced by flexing the spine in the brace with an abdominal concavity and flattening the posterior lumbar contours with low posterior trim lines. Trim lines can be further altered to control the curves with posterosuperior extension (for hypokyphosis) or trochanteric extension (for lower lumbar curves).

The Boston brace system consists of variations according to the curve to be braced and include Boston-thoracic, Boston-thoracolumbar, and Boston-lumbar braces. The Boston-thoracic brace was developed to control thoracic curves with a higher apex (up to T7) without using a superstructure. This was accomplished by adding an axillary support on the concave side with lateral pressure from a convex pad (53,61,96). The main difference in the Boston-thoracolumbar and Boston-lumbar types is due to pad placement and trim lines designed to control each of these curve patterns.

Advantages of the Boston brace include decreased construction time of 2 to 3 hours (98); uniform initial curve correction in the brace greater than 50% (47,98); and better patient acceptance than with the Milwaukee brace (47). The Boston brace diminishes curve magnitude through the use of decreased lumbar lordosis and direct pressure from lateral pads and from the brace itself, which was originally molded on children without scoliosis. Several reports have documented a decrease in the initial Cobb angle measurement of 33% to 50% resulting from a decrease in lumbar lordosis alone (2,62,95,96). In the early 1990s, the original brace design with no lumbar lordosis was modified by incorporating 15 degrees of lordosis into the pelvic module. In a preliminary study, Olafsson and associates (81) documented no difference in initial Cobb angle correction (62% to 65%) between the two different brace designs. However, better derotation of the curves were noted with the later design. Addition of lateral pads with pressure on ribs or the transverse processes in the lumbar spine also contributes to the correction of the curves, with greater effects in minor or moderate curves of less than 50 degrees (24,95).

Wilmington Brace

In the early 1970s, the Wilmington brace was independently developed at Wilmington Children's Hospital in Delaware as an alternative to the Milwaukee brace (Fig. 3). This brace is fabricated from Orthoplast after making a mold of the patient, whose curvature is reduced on a Cotrel or Risser table with transverse forces and longitudinal traction. Transverse reduction forces are produced during the molding at the apices of the curves. After molding the brace, trim lines are cut high in the axilla and low to capture the pelvis yet are trimmed in a manner to allow hip flexion while sitting. The brace is designed as a body jacket with an anterior opening secured with Velcro straps; a cotton undergarment is worn because of its intimate fit. Advantages to this system include greater patient acceptance and relatively inexpensive and rapid production as compared with the Milwaukee brace. The fact that the Orthoplast jacket tended to break down and that there is little room for growth can be counted as relative disadvantages to this system. Commonly, patients would require manufacture of at least two braces during the treatment time period (20). Other centers have used the same brace design principles but have increased durability with polypropylene (48).

Miami Brace

Originally designed in 1975, the Miami brace is a custom-made TLSO constructed of polypropylene with built-in Plastizote pads (Fig. 4). The brace is designed to allow lateral motion away from the curve concavity and promote some hip flexion but limit hip extension. Advantages of this system include a relatively rigid nature and areas of concave pressure relief that stimulate active correction and assist with ventilation in warmer climates. The brace is not adaptable for curves with apices higher than T7 or for kyphotic deformities (67). Preliminary results in 20 patients who have completed treatment have been favorable, but no large studies with longer follow-up have been published to date (67).

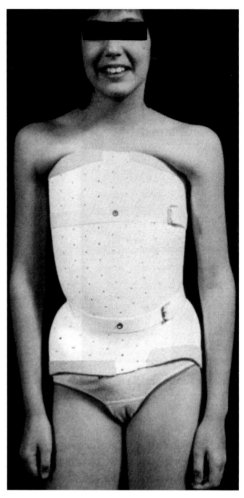

FIGURE 3. The Wilmington jacket.

Charleston Bending Brace

The Charleston bending brace is a custom-made orthosis that was originally developed as an alternative to full-time brace wear (86). During brace production, the orthotist maintains pressure at the apex while applying an unbending force above the curve. A positive mold is made with soft foam padding in areas of maximal pressure. The brace is constructed from two lateral halves riveted in the back to allow anterior opening only. Because of the awkward positioning, this brace is designed for nighttime use only.

Single curves are the easiest to brace, and trim lines are carefully cut to produce maximal unbending of the primary curves without increasing the compensatory curves. In patients with double major curves, it is crucial to determine whether the pattern is consistent with King type I or II curves. In King type I curves, the trim line should be below the rib of the apex of the thoracic curve. If one prescribes a brace with a higher trim line into the axilla (King type II), the thoracic curve is exaggerated. The importance of adequate brace fitting cannot be underestimated, and the manufacturers currently arrange educational seminars for physicians who are unfamiliar with its design and

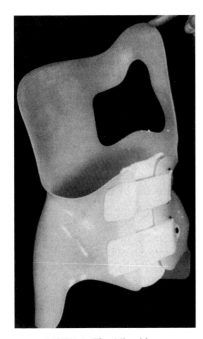

FIGURE 4. The Miami brace.

use. At brace fitting, a supine anteroposterior radiograph is obtained in the brace with the Velcro straps sufficiently tightened. Initial correction is considered adequate if there is greater than 75% correction of the primary curve and 20% correction of compensatory curves (Fig. 5). For very stiff curves, it is reasonable to accept the amount of correction seen on side-bending films.

Indications for Bracing

Before bracing, several key variables must be assessed and determined to be appropriate before recommending treatment in patients with AIS. These variables include maturity, curve magnitude by Cobb measurement, and curve pattern. Bracing is designed to prevent curve progression during the adolescent growth spurt and therefore is not indicated in patients who are skeletally mature. Mature patients are those who have complete capping of the iliac apophysis, have had menses for at least 1 year, and have had no increase in height for at least 6 months.

Bracing is recommended for curves in immature patients (Risser grade 1 or less) with a minimal magnitude of 25 degrees at bracing onset. Curves of less than 25 degrees should be braced only after there is documented progression of 5 degrees or more in patients who are Risser grade 1 or less. Scoliosis greater than

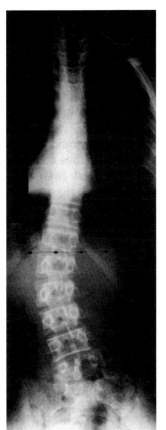
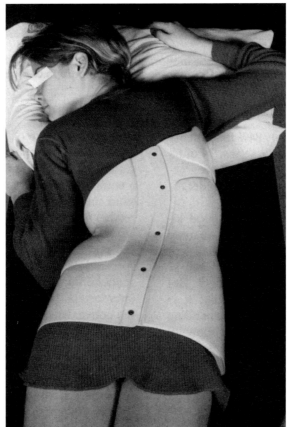
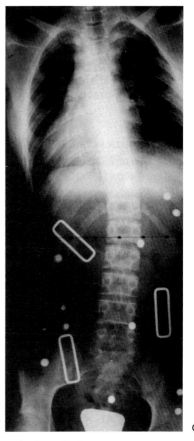

A,B

C

FIGURE 5. An example of the Charleston bending brace. **A:** Anteroposterior radiograph of a patient with a left lumbar scoliosis. **B:** The same patient wearing the brace. **C:** Radiograph of the same patient showing in-brace correction.

40 to 45 degrees usually continues to progress despite adequate bracing, especially if the patient is relatively immature (Risser grade 1 or less or premenarchal). In patients with well-balanced curve patterns (40 to 45 degrees) (33), it is reasonable to recommend bracing to the patient and family, yet they should be made aware of the increased chance of failure and the possible need for surgery. Curves in immature patients with AIS of greater than 45 to 50 degrees meet indications for surgery and should not be braced.

The use of bracing in more mature patients (greater than Risser grade 2 or who have begun menses within the last 6 months) should be individualized for each patient. Curves that are 35 to 40 degrees should probably be braced. Continued observation in these "more mature" patients with curves of less than 35 degrees is reasonable. In this instance, families should be educated on the diminished likelihood of progression into a surgical range compared with the cost and transient psychosocial effects of bracing. After this discussion, the choice of bracing versus observation is made and is usually more palatable to the patient and family. Additionally, it is important to realize that rates of noncompliance tend to be higher in the more mature patient as opposed to the younger patient (27). Clearly, a brace should not be prescribed to a patient with a social situation that precludes compliant brace wear. Other relative contraindications include severe thoracic lordosis, massive obesity, or insensate or fragile skin.

Finally, the type of curve pattern affects bracing indications. Most believe that curves with an apex at or above the seventh thoracic (T7) vertebra are not amenable to braces without a superstructure, such as that seen with a Milwaukee brace or one of the TLSOs with an attached superstructure. Because the results of bracing with CTLSOs improve in curves with more caudal apices (below T7), some authors question whether any orthosis can alter the natural history of more proximal curves (23,33,64). Additional evidence suggests that not all braces are equally efficacious for all curve patterns. Katz and coauthors (56) compared the results of the Charleston bending brace with the Boston brace in 319 patients. They found the Boston brace system to be more effective in larger curves and in thoracic or double major curve patterns (56). As such, the remaining indication for the Charleston bending brace may be isolated lumbar or thoracolumbar curves of moderate magnitude, for which both braces were found to be equally effective. Double curves may not be as amenable (as compared with single major curves) to bracing because maximal correction of one curve necessarily decreases the correctability of the adjacent curve.

Full-time Bracing Protocol

After the patient has received a brace, he or she should be examined to ensure that the orthosis fits reasonably well with minimal gaps (less than 1 finger), that the pelvis is adequately captured, and that there are no significant pressure points. Patients are allowed an initial adjustment period of 5 to 10 days, during which the straps can be incrementally tightened, and to increase brace wear up to 22 hours per day. After 1 month of progressive brace wear, the patient should have a standing radiograph in the brace after it is appropriately tightened. This radiograph documents accurate pad placement as well as initial curve correction of the primary and compensatory curves. Most orthopaedists do not prescribe a detailed exercise program, and the brace may be removed for 1 to 2 hours per day for athletic activities, bathing, and swimming. The brace is not designed to be socially restrictive, and the patient should be allowed the opportunity to abstain from brace wear during the occasional special event.

The patient should return every 4 to 6 months for an interview and assessment of problems and compliance. The trunk is examined for signs of skin irritation and pressure points. Most authors recommend follow-up radiographs out of the brace, and some have recommended removal of the brace for a standard time period before radiographs (45). Regardless of preference, radiographs should be done in a standard fashion at each clinic appointment. Full-time bracing is continued until skeletal maturity if the patient remains compliant and there is no significant progression. Some orthopaedists allow decreasing brace wear if there is at least 50% correction after 9 months of full-time brace wear (33).

The typical course of bracing can be summarized in Figure 6. After bracing is started, the structural curve decreases to a variable magnitude dictated by several factors. These include curve flexibility, presenting curve magnitude, and the unique ability of each brace to correct the curve initially. Greater initial correction is routinely documented with more modern TLSOs (30% to more than 60%) (10,33,53,56,67,96,98,101) as opposed to the Milwaukee brace (less than 30% to 40%) (65,69, 78,79,96). In addition, greater initial correction may be expected in younger patients as opposed to older patients (18). It appears from follow-up reports of bracing that better initial correction correlates with improved long-term outcome and decreased risk for progression (23,78,81,82).

With continued bracing, the curve continues to progress from maximal initial correction until the brace is stopped. In the successfully braced patient, the curve magnitude at brace cessation is less than or equal to curve magnitude at presentation. Brace weaning is begun based on certain radiographic or chronologic features. Most authors recommend full-time bracing until Risser grade 4 in girls. In boys, continued curve progression has been noted until Risser grade 5; therefore, boys should be braced until full healing of the iliac apophysis (55). Other indicators of maturity can be used when the Risser status is difficult to evaluate or is discordant with other features. Full-time bracing is recommended until there is cessation of longitudinal growth for at least 6 months, the vertebral ring apophyses have fused, female patients have had menses for at least 1 year, or a skeletal age of 15 to 16 years has been reached according to the Gruelich and Pyle atlas. After skeletal maturity is documented, the patient is started on gradual daytime weaning to nighttime brace wear over 8 to 12 months. Brace wear is encouraged during the night until the brace breaks or no longer fits.

After skeletal maturity and complete stoppage of brace wear, the patient should have radiographs at increasing intervals to assess for curve progression. The degree of curve progression after bracing varies between each study and depends on curve magnitude when the brace is stopped. Postbrace progression may average up to 3 degrees a year (49), yet most reports document

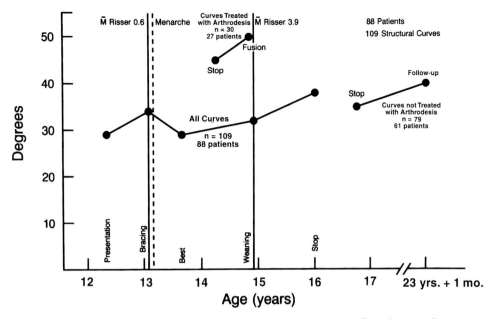

FIGURE 6. Graph of the results of Milwaukee bracing for all structural curves from the report by Noonan and colleagues (78). After brace initiation, there is progression from the time of the best correction in the brace *(Best)* to the time when bracing was stopped *(Stop)*. There is also continued progression of the curves that were not treated with an arthrodesis from the time when bracing was stopped to the time of follow-up. In successfully managed patients, the initial curve is equal to that at the time of brace cessation.

progression to be less than 1 to 3 degrees per year (10,23, 65,69,73,78,79,84,93).

The total magnitude of progression obviously depends on the available length of follow-up in the literature. Most practitioners follow patients for several years after brace cessation to determine whether the curve progresses to a surgical magnitude. Montgomery and colleagues (73) studied the degree of progression in 168 patients for an average of 6.9 years after successfully brace management. The average progression was 5.1 degrees, and they concluded that progression of the curve may continue into the 20s. They determined, however, that follow-up of 2 years is sufficient to detect and treat malignant progression in 97% of cases.

Compliance With Full-time Brace Wear

It is difficult to assess the degree of treatment compliance resulting from uniform patient dissatisfaction with bracing. The disparity of actual and reported brace wear remains unknown because no compliance meter is widely used. Each patient is caught in a conflict of trying to please parents and physicians with the unpleasantness of bracing; especially during school hours (27). Patients are at higher risk for adjustment and compliance problems if they have lower overall intelligence or if they are not adequately educated to the benefits of bracing versus the implications of further curve progression (33,99). Other risk factors include concurrent personal or family strife (50); older versus younger adolescence at treatment onset (27,46); treatment with a CTLSO versus a TLSO (98); and longer duration of treatment (27,75). Authors report some noncompliance in 10% to 85% of

patients (20,23,26,27,31,36,46,57,67,71,75,78,81). The wide disparity is due to variable ways of defining complete compliance, partial compliance, and noncompliance. Compliance is probably increased with supportive families and a medical team that fully educates each patient to the benefits of bracing. Scheduling clinic appointments with other patients who are similarly treated decreases the sense of isolation and stimulates patient acceptance and understanding.

Another approach to brace wear is to assume a certain degree of noncompliance and to make the brace more acceptable by decreasing the number of prescribed hours. DiRaimondo and Green (27) compared 38 patients who were prescribed full-time brace wear with 38 patients who were prescribed part-time brace wear. After 2 years of treatment, all patients were wearing the brace only 8 to 9 hours per day irrespective of their bracing schedule. Whether decreasing the number of hours of prescribed brace wear effects outcome is subject to some debate. From a practical standpoint, however, noncompliance with full-time bracing is probably underestimated, and it is unclear how many hours of actual brace wear are required to alter the natural history of immature patients with AIS.

Results of Bracing

Postural Changes With Bracing

In addition to the main goal of preventing curve progression, braces have been reported to improve spinal decompensation, posture, and cosmetic appearance (57,79). Moe and Kettleson (71) had noticed in some patients with double curves that bracing had improved cosmesis with less rib prominence and better balance despite little improvement in Cobb angle measurement. Further studies with the Milwaukee brace have documented variable short-term and long-term improvements in spinal decompensation (90) or truncopelvic alignment (4). Rudicel and associates (90) examined 22 patients with lumbar or thoracolumbar curves treated with the Milwaukee brace and found no predictable improvement in this small study. In a larger study by Andrews and coauthors (4), an improvement in "truncopelvic alignment" (lateral trunk shift) was documented in 14.6% at brace cessation. Although 49% of patients demonstrated an improved alignment at follow-up, the correction was considered unpredictable and the actual correction in centimeters was small. In a thesis from the Netherlands, Styblo (93) failed to demonstrate any significant predictable improvement in rib hump after treatment with the Milwaukee brace. On the other hand, he recorded some improvement in spinal dysbalance at follow-up; most improvement was noted in patients with imbalance greater than 1 centimeter at treatment.

Two studies of the Wilmington brace have documented improvements in lateral trunk shift and spinal decompensation. Bassett and colleagues (11) defined lateral trunk shift as the radiographic distance from the center of the trunk to a line connecting C7 to the center of the sacrum. Before bracing, trunk shift averaged 1.9 to 2.2 cm, with slightly more shift noted in lumbar or thoracolumbar curves. At an average follow-up of less than 2 years, these authors documented an average improvement of trunk shift to 0.9 to 1.2 cm. In 61% of patients, there was an improvement in lateral trunk shift that was independent of curve progression. A later study from the same institution (12) documented improvement in spinal decompensation (defined as the distance of C7 to the center sacral line) in 71 patients treated with the Wilmington brace. In this study, all patients had decompensation greater than 1 cm, with an average prebracing decompensation of 1.9 to 2.5 cm. At follow-up, the average distance improved to 1 to 1.4 cm, depending on curve pattern. Of 18 patients with decompensation greater than 3 cm, all had an average of 2.1 cm improvement. Based on these two well-documented studies, the authors suggest some cosmetic benefits to bracing that may be independent of the effect on Cobb angle measurements. On the other hand, two studies using stereoradiographic techniques or CT scans in patients treated with the Boston brace failed to demonstrate changes in rib hump, rotation, or spinal balance (60,100).

In summary, it is controversial whether bracing results in significant long-term improvements in posture as quantified by rib hump, spinal balance, or trunk shift. Although several well-documented studies have suggested improvement in spinal balance or trunk shift, it is likely that the effects are small. Additionally, one should keep in mind that reliability and variability testing for measurement error have not been performed and that the natural history of these parameters in untreated patients is unknown.

Results of Bracing on Curve Progression

To determine the effectiveness of bracing, it is important to have an abbreviated understanding of the fate of untreated curves in immature patients with AIS. Key factors that affect the natural history are curve magnitude and maturity. Lonstein and Carlson (63) documented progression of greater than 5 degrees in 68% of patients who have curves from 20 to 30 degrees and who are Risser grade 0 or 1. Others have documented progression of 52% to 79% in immature patients whose curves measured 20 to 30 degrees at presentation (19,39,85,89). Peterson and Nachemson (83) recently reported progression of 6 degrees in 50% of patients with curves from 25 to 35 degrees treated with electrical stimulation or observation. Higher rates of progression have been noted in curves with greater curve magnitude (19,39, 76,83). In addition to these factors, differences in curve pattern are likely to affect different rates of progression in untreated patients. In general, lumbar or thoracolumbar curves are less likely to progress than are double or thoracic curves (19,29,63).

Part-time Brace Wear

Some physicians have recommended part-time brace wear to make bracing less invasive to normal adolescent life. The prescribed time for part-time brace wear may vary from nighttime-only wear (Charleston bending brace) to less than 22 hours per day (usually without having to wear the brace during school). In 1986, Green (45) reported 44 patients treated with either a Milwaukee or Boston brace for 16 hours per day. In this report, the average curve at bracing was 31 degrees; at a minimum follow-up of 5 months, the authors noted that 89% of their patients had no progression of their curves and that compliance was greater than 90% in patients. They concluded that part-time brace wear does decrease the risk for progression. Two other reports of patients treated with the full-time Boston brace were also unable to determine differences in results between compliant patients (full-time brace wear) and partially compliant patients (part-time brace wear) (33,82).

The Wilmington brace has also been prescribed on a part-time basis with good results (3,48). Allington and Bowen (3) compared the effectiveness of full-time versus part-time (12 to 16 hours/day) bracing and patients treated with electrical stimulation. All patients met contemporary indications for bracing and were followed to maturity. The rates of progression greater than 5 degrees were 36%, 41%, and 70% of patients treated with full-time bracing, part-time bracing, and electrical stimulation, respectively. No significant differences between full-time and part-time wear were detected.

As mentioned previously, the Charleston bending brace was designed for nighttime-only wear. After presentation of favorable preliminary results (35,86), longer-term follow-up on patients treated exclusively with the Charleston bending brace is available. Price and associates (87) presented results of a prospective multicenter trial of 98 patients treated for curves between 25 to 49 degrees who were Risser grade 2 or less at treatment onset. At minimal follow-up of 1 year, they reported no curve progression in 66% of patients, with acceptable results in 79% of patients who did not require surgery or change to a different orthosis. Similar to Katz and colleagues (56), better results were noted in single lumbar or thoracolumbar curves as opposed to double curves.

In summary, from these papers, it appears that part-time brace wear is at least as effective as full-time brace wear in the management of AIS. If this is true, patients who are prescribed full-time brace wear may not be fully compliant and are actually wearing the brace in a part-time manner (27). Alternatively, both protocols are meeting a minimal number of hours required to alter the natural history of AIS.

Full-time Brace Wear

Milwaukee Brace

The earliest and largest experience of bracing has been reported over the years from physicians in Minneapolis and St. Paul, Minnesota. In 1970, Moe and Kettleson (71) reported the results of 169 juvenile and adolescent scoliosis patients treated with the Milwaukee brace. With mean correction ranging from 10% to 23%, the authors conclude that the Milwaukee brace was effective in controlling mild to moderate scoliosis. In 1980, Carr and colleagues (23) continued studying 74 of 133 patients with greater than 5 years of follow-up. In this series, the overall correction in thoracic, lumbar, and high thoracic curves was 2, 4, and − 1 degrees, respectively. Greater progression was noted in larger curves or curves that did not have substantial correction in the brace. A later separate review of 95 patients with only thoracic curves of 30 to 39 degrees also demonstrated effective control of curve progression in 84% of patients (102). In 1994, Lonstein and Winter (64) presented the cumulative experience of Milwaukee bracing in 1020 patients treated from 1954 to 1979. Twenty-two percent of patients required surgical intervention; in the remaining patients, the authors noted an average improvement of 1 to 4 degrees. The authors selected a subgroup of patients who would meet contemporary brace indications for comparison with natural history data. They concluded that the Milwaukee brace is effective in preventing curve progression in 20- to 29-degree curves at the time of brace cessation. However, significant differences could not be found at the time of follow-up; nor could significant differences be found in braced curves from 30 to 39 degrees at brace cessation or follow-up.

Other centers have also published good results of Milwaukee bracing, with average corrections at the time of follow-up from 1 to 6 degrees, depending on curve location (4,31,57,69,70,79). These authors concluded that the Milwaukee brace is effective in preventing curve progression. When looked at objectively, these studies have some shortcomings because of short or incomplete follow-up, exclusion of noncompliant or surgical patients, or inclusion of patients at low risk for progression. In 1991, Styblo (93) presented a well documented thesis of 290 patients treated with Milwaukee bracing. In a selected subgroup of 128 patients, he recorded no progression in 72% of patients. The patients who required surgery or had progression tended to be younger and skeletally immature with less correction in the brace. Cochran and Nachemson (26) reviewed 85 of 95 compliant patients treated with the Milwaukee brace. The average curve at bracing was 30 degrees, with 4 degrees of progression at follow-up. Based on their findings and the shortcomings of previously published papers, they concluded that the true effectiveness of bracing had yet to be determined.

In 1996, we reported our results in 111 patients treated with Milwaukee bracing (78). In an effort to eliminate some of the bias present in previous publications, we restricted our study to 88 patients who were considered at high risk for progression. At an average follow-up of 6.3 years, we documented progression of 5 degrees in 48% of patients. Forty-two percent of patients had or met radiographic indications for surgery. Patients who failed treatment tended to be younger and to have decreased maximal correction in the brace. Based on these findings, we questioned whether the Milwaukee brace significantly alters the natural history of progressive AIS.

Wilmington Brace

In 1980, Bunnell and coauthors (20) presented initial results of the Wilmington brace in 48 patients. After initial correction of 74% in the brace, progression of more than 5 degrees was noted in only 10%. Later follow-up in 79 patients with curves from 20 to 39 degrees in patients who were Risser grade 1 or less was published by Bassett and colleagues (10). In this paper, the mean initial correction was 50%; at an average follow-up of 2.5 years, only 28% had progression greater than 5 degrees. Thoracic and double major curve patterns were noted to have greater rates of progression. In 1990, the group was reexamined at an average follow-up of 8.1 years (84). Only 12% of patients required surgery, and 21% had progression after the brace was discontinued. This series of papers from Wilmington suggests a positive effect on the natural history and corroborates similar results on two later papers comparing full-time and part-time treatment with the Wilmington brace (3,48).

Boston Brace

After the Boston brace was introduced, several authors presented preliminary results of initial curve correction ranging from 40% to 65% (41,61,81,96,98,101). Greater initial correction with the Boston system has been appreciated with lumbar and thoracolumbar curves as opposed to double, thoracic, or high thoracic curves. In 1984, Jonasson-Rajala and associates (53) examined the efficacy of the Boston-Milwaukee, original Boston, and Boston-thoracic braces. In their study and in comparison with the literature, they found that the Boston-thoracic brace gave better initial correction than the other types. The only exception is in the lumbar region, where initial correction is better with the original Boston brace. This paper and that by Laurnen and coauthors (61) have examined the Boston-thoracic brace and documented potential success with apices up to T7.

In 1986, Emans and colleagues (33) presented follow-up data on 295 patients treated with the Boston or Boston-Milwaukee braces. At an average follow-up of 1.4 years, only 11% of patients required surgery, and progression of 5 degrees or more was documented in 7% of cases. Progression and need for surgery were more likely in patients younger than 13 years of age with curves greater than 30 degrees. The authors found no difference in results between the Boston and the Boston-Milwaukee brace in curves with apices at T7 or below. Katz and colleagues (56) recently published a comparative study between the Charleston bending brace and the Boston brace. In this study, the Boston brace significantly outperformed the Charleston bending brace. Thirty-four percent of patients treated with the Boston brace had progression greater than 5 degrees; surgery was required in

16% of patients. Both studies are limited because of short follow-up, although the report from Boston also includes some patients at lower risk for progression.

Despite the good results published, one study questioned the ability of the Boston brace to affect the natural history (43). In this study from two centers, 32 patients treated with bracing were compared with 32 patients matched by curve size, location, and age, and all were noted to be Risser grade 0. The authors did note a nonstatistical improvement in braced patients; however, there was no significant difference in regard to curve progression greater than 10 degrees or progression beyond 45 degrees. Although provocative, the results should be viewed in light of possible selection bias.

Other publications have compared the results of the Boston brace or similar TLSOs with those of the Milwaukee brace. In these studies, the Milwaukee brace has been inferior in regard to initial correction and final outcome (72,97). In 1998, Howard and coauthors (52) compared 35 patients treated with the Milwaukee brace with 45 and 95 patients treated with a TLSO and the Charleston bending brace, respectively. In this study, no differences in presenting age, curve magnitude, or Risser grade was noted. At follow-up, the TLSO demonstrated significantly decreased rates of progression of 6 and 10 degrees in comparison to the other two braces. Although these studies are convincing, one must keep in mind that selection bias may exist whereby patients with higher apical curves (and worse prognosis) are preferentially treated with a Milwaukee brace.

Scoliosis Research Society Study

In 1995, Nachemson and Peterson (76) presented the results of a prospective multicenter trial of 286 female patients with thoracic or thoracolumbar curves from 25 to 35 degrees at presentation. Three treatment protocols included a TLSO, electrical stimulation, and observation. In this landmark article, the percentages of curve progression greater than 5 degrees were 26%, 66%, and 67%, respectively. These findings demonstrate a statistically significant effect of bracing in this population over observation and electrical stimulation—both correlating closely with previous published natural history studies. These patients, however, were followed to the end of bracing only, and it remains to be seen whether differences in curve magnitude will continue to exist between the groups after 5 years of follow-up.

Complications of Brace Wear

Although bracing is considered nonoperative treatment, it should not be considered conservative treatment because complications are possible and have been reported. Potential complications include pain, alterations in renal and pulmonary function, skin irritation or pressure sores (up to 16% [71]), nerve irritation (meralgia paresthetica [45] or axillary nerve pressure [86]), and psychosocial impairment.

Renal testing of patients treated with the Boston brace has demonstrated that transient changes in the glomerular filtration rate, renal plasma flow, and urinary excretion of sodium return to normal after prolonged brace wear (1,13). Pulmonary function testing has also been performed by multiple investigators. Various parameters in pulmonary function testing have been

altered by up to 80% of normal values after immediate bracing with both the Milwaukee brace and various TLSOs (20,88,91). It is theorized that these changes may be due to cephalad displacement of abdominal contents (58) or restriction of the chest wall. With time, however, most parameters return to normal, and no significantly deleterious effects of bracing on lung function have been recorded (59,88,91).

Normally, significant stresses are already present in adolescents because of rapid physical change and emerging concept of self and secondary sexual characteristics. In patients to be braced, it is important to recognize these issues because compliance and possible family and personal stress are directly related. Clayson and associates (25) compared 23 braced and 23 surgically treated patients with 23 age-matched controls. The scoliosis patients were found to have lower self-esteem and body image than controls; the surgical patients had slightly higher self-esteem than braced patients. In a detailed retrospective review by Fallstrom and colleagues (34), 157 treated patients (92 with arthrodesis; 65 with Milwaukee bracing) were evaluated at a minimal 5-year follow-up. In this study, surgical patients had less anxiety, were more satisfied with their treatment, and had higher body image. The authors concluded that although braced patients were getting on fairly well, they felt that the brace led to a lesser body image that may complicate identity development.

In 1997, we examined the psychosocial characteristics of 95 patients treated for scoliosis with bracing or with both bracing and surgery (77). Although there were no significant long-term signs of depression, the scoliosis patients who were between 13 and 21 years of age felt that they were more frequently discriminated against than did a group of age-matched controls. Fortunately, as they aged, this difference became insignificant. The results of this study are encouraging in that we found relatively few differences between the patient and control samples. These findings correlate with previous literature on the psychosocial effects of bracing. In such patients, a fairly standard initial psychological effect is present and includes anxiety, fear, and withdrawal. Fortunately, these problems usually improve with time (7,32,34,44,50,68,75).

FUTURE DIRECTIONS FOR NONOPERATIVE TREATMENT

At this time, it appears that bracing is the only nonoperative modality that has been shown to affect progression in the immature patient with AIS. Further efforts need to be continued in the areas of optimizing brace design and to develop ways to improve the assessment of compliance. After an accurate means of documenting compliance is in place, we will be able to determine how much time is needed to alter the natural history. It is hard to evaluate the current literature when we are not sure how often and how well the treatment is applied.

Bracing as a treatment in AIS is still a controversial topic. Some physicians who treat AIS are convinced that bracing either is or is not effective. Most physicians who continue to prescribe braces may not be completely convinced of their practical effectiveness. This situation stems from differences and flaws in the older literature in comparison to more recent articles. Historically, older reports of bracing often included patients at low risk for progression because of small curve magnitude or increased skeletal maturity. Additionally, some publications exclude surgical patients from their follow-up analysis, which biases results in a favorable manner. Other studies exclude noncompliant patients, and one should also question the practicality of a treatment that cannot be effectively used because of poor patient acceptance. Further hindrances include grouping of adolescent and juvenile patients; poor documentation of risk factors; short-term or inadequate follow-up; and a failure to compare results with natural history controls.

It is true that bracing alters the natural history in smaller curves (20 to 35 degrees) by significantly lowering the rate of progression of 5 to 6 degrees in selected curves (76). However, it is not known whether similar effects are present in larger curves (35 to 45 degrees). It is well known that the risk for progression is much greater in this group (38,73). If one assumes a minimal magnitude (45 to 50 degrees) to be an indication for surgery in immature patients, perhaps we should reexamine the natural history and the results of bracing in more practical terms.

In the recent Scoliosis Research Society study, significant improvements in rates of curve progression are noted with bracing, yet it is unknown whether differences in surgical treatment also exist (76). In other words, a 30-degree curve that is braced would currently be considered a failure if it progressed to 38 degrees at maturity. On the other hand, this patient could be considered to have had a successful treatment because he or she is unlikely to require a spine fusion. Possibly, we should reanalyze the natural history in untreated patients and determine the incidence of progression to a surgical range for patients grouped according to presenting curve magnitude and maturity. Subsequently, braced patients should be similarly evaluated for the incidence of surgical indications according to their magnitude and maturity at treatment onset. Only when this information is readily available will we be able to determine whether bracing decreases surgical indications and to what degree. Perhaps only a minority of patients will practically benefit from bracing, and therefore the cost effectiveness of this treatment would need to be critically evaluated. With further genetic and biochemical research, we may be able to identify which patients are likely to progress to a surgical range and thus be more selective in the nonoperative treatment of patients with AIS.

REFERENCES

1. Aaro S, Berg U (1982): The immediate effect of Boston brace on renal function in patients with idiopathic scoliosis. *Clin Orthop* 170: 243–247.
2. Aaro S, Burstrom R, Dahlborn M (1981): The derotating effect of the Boston brace: a comparison between computer tomography and a conventional method. *Spine* 6(5):477–482.
3. Allington NJ, Bowen JR (1996): Adolescent idiopathic scoliosis: treatment with the Wilmington brace. *J Bone Joint Surg Am* 78: 1056–1059.
4. Andrews G, MacEwen GD (1989): Idiopathic scoliosis: an 11-year follow-up study of the role of the Milwaukee brace in curve control and trunco-pelvic alignment. *Orthopedics* 12(6):809–816.
5. Andriacchi TP, Schultz AB, Belytschko TB, et al. (1976): Milwaukee brace correction of idiopathic scoliosis. *J Bone Joint Surg Am* 58: 806–815.
6. Anciaux M, Lenaert A, Van Beneden ML, et al. (1991): Transcutaneous electrical stimulation (TCES) for the treatment of adolescent idiopathic scoliosis: preliminary results. *Acta Orthop Belg* 57:399–405.
7. Apter A, Morein G, Munitz H, et al. (1978): The psychosocial sequela of the Milwaukee brace in adolescent girls. *Clin Orthop* 131:156–159.
8. Axelgaard J, Brown JC (1983): Lateral electrical surface stimulation for the treatment of progressive idiopathic scoliosis. *Spine* 8(3): 242–260.
9. Axelgaard J, Nordwall A, Brown JC (1983): Correction of spinal curvatures by transcutaneous electrical muscle stimulation. *Spine* 8(5): 463–481.
10. Bassett GS, Bunnell WP, MacEwen GD (1986): Treatment of idiopathic scoliosis with the Wilmington brace. *J Bone Joint Surg Am* 68: 602–605.
11. Bassett GS, Bunnell WP (1986): Effect of a thoracolumbosacral orthosis on lateral trunk shift in idiopathic scoliosis. *J Pediatr Orthop* 6: 182–185.
12. Bassett GS, Bunnell WP (1987): Influence of the Wilmington brace on spinal decompensation in adolescent idiopathic scoliosis. *Clin Orthop* 223:164–169.
13. Berg U, Aaro S (1983): Long-term effect of Boston brace treatment on renal function in patients with idiopathic scoliosis. *Clin Orthop* 180:169–172.
14. Blount WP, Schmidt AC, Keever ED, et al. (1958): The Milwaukee brace in the operative treatment of scoliosis. *J Bone Joint Surg Am* 40:511–525.
15. Bobechko WP, Herbert MA, Friedman HG (1979): Electrospinal instrumentation for scoliosis: current status. *Orthop Clin North Am* 10(4):927–941.
16. Bradford DS, Tanguy A, Vanselow J (1983): Surface electrical stimulation in the treatment of idiopathic scoliosis: preliminary results in 30 patients. *Spine* 8(7):757–764.
17. Brown JC, Axelgaard J, Howson DC (1984): Multicenter trial of a noninvasive stimulation method for idiopathic scoliosis: a summary of early treatment results. *Spine* 9(4):382–387.
18. Bunch WH (1997): Comment on "Use of the Milwaukee brace for progressive idiopathic scoliosis." *J Bone Joint Surg Am* 79(6):954.
19. Bunnell WP (1986): The natural history of idiopathic scoliosis before skeletal maturity. *Spine* 11(8):773–776.
20. Bunnell WP, MacEwen D, Jayakumar S (1980): The use of plastic jackets in the non-operative treatment of idiopathic scoliosis. *J Bone Joint Surg Am* 62:31–38.
21. Bylund P, Aaro S, Gottfries B, et al. (1987): Is lateral electric surface stimulation an effective treatment for scoliosis? *J Pediatr Orthop* 7: 298–300.
22. Carman D, Roach JW, Speck G, et al. (1985): Role of exercises in the Milwaukee brace treatment of scoliosis. *J Pediatr Orthop* 5:65–68.
23. Carr WA, Moe JH, Winter RB, et al. (1980): Treatment of idiopathic scoliosis in the Milwaukee brace. *J Bone Joint Surg Am* 62:599–612.
24. Chase AP, Bader DL, Houghton GR (1989): The biomechanical effectiveness of the Boston brace in the management of adolescent idiopathic scoliosis. *Spine* 14(6):636–642.
25. Clayson D, Luz-Alterman S, Cataletto MM, et al. (1987): Long-term psychological sequela of surgically versus non-surgically treated scoliosis. *Spine* 12(10):983–986.
26. Cochran T, Nachemson A (1985): Long-term anatomic and functional changes in patients with adolescent idiopathic scoliosis treated with the Milwaukee brace. *Spine* 10(2):127–133.
27. DiRaimondo CV, Green NE (1988): Brace-wear compliance in patients with adolescent idiopathic scoliosis. *J Pediatr Orthop* 8: 143–146.
28. Durham JW, Moskowitz A, Whitney J (1990): Surface electrical stimulation versus brace in treatment of idiopathic scoliosis. *Spine* 15(9): 888–892.
29. Duval-Beaupere G, Lamireau T (1985): Scoliosis at less than 30 degrees: properties of the evolutivity (risk of progression). *Spine* 19(5): 421–424.
30. Eckerson LF, Axelgaard J (1984): Lateral electrical surface stimulation as an alternative to bracing in the treatment of idiopathic scoliosis: treatment protocol and patient acceptance. *Phys Ther* 64(4):483–490.

31. Edmonson AS, Morris JT (1977): Follow-up study of Milwaukee brace treatment in patients with idiopathic scoliosis. *Clin Orthop* 126:58–61.

32. Eliason ME, Richman LL (1984): Psychological effects of idiopathic adolescent scoliosis. *Dev Behav Pediatr* 5(4):169–172.

33. Emans JB, Kaelin A, Bancel P, et al. (1986): The Boston bracing system for idiopathic scoliosis: follow-up results in 295 patients. *Spine* 8(11):792–801.

34. Fallstrom K, Cochran T, Nachemson A (1986): Long-term effects on personality development in patients with adolescent idiopathic scoliosis: influence on type of treatment. *Spine* 11(7):756–758.

35. Federico DJ, Renshaw TS (1990): Results of treatment of idiopathic scoliosis with the Charleston bending brace. *Spine* 15:886–887.

36. Fernandez-Feliberti R, Flynn J, Ramirez N, et al. (1995): Effectiveness of TLSO bracing in the conservative treatment of idiopathic scoliosis. *J Pediatr Orthop* 15:176–181.

37. Fisher DA, Rapp GF, Emkes M (1987): Idiopathic scoliosis: transcutaneous muscle stimulation versus the Milwaukee brace. *Spine* 12(10):987–991.

38. Focarile FA, Bonaldi A, Giarolo MA, et al. (1991): Effectiveness of non-surgical treatment for idiopathic scoliosis: overview of available evidence. *Spine* 16(4):395–401.

39. Fustier T (1980): *Evolution radiologique spontanee des scolioses idiopathiques de moins de 45 degrees in periode de croissance.* Thesis, Universite Claude-Bernard, Lyon, France, 129:1–64.

40. Galante J, Schultz A, Dewald RL, et al. (1970): Forces acting in the Milwaukee brace on patients undergoing treatment for idiopathic scoliosis. *J Bone Joint Surg Am* 52:498–506.

41. Gardner ADH, Burwell RG, Wozniak AP, (1986): Some beneficial effects of bracing and a search for prognostic indicators in idiopathic scoliosis. *Spine* 11:779.

42. Goldberg CJ, Dowling FE, Fogarty EE, et al. (1988): Electro-spinal stimulation in children with adolescent and juvenile scoliosis. *Spine* 13(5):482–484.

43. Goldberg CJ, Dowling FE, Hall JE, et al. (1993): A statistical comparison between natural history of idiopathic scoliosis and brace treatment in skeletally immature adolescent girls. *Spine* 18(7):902–908.

44. Gratz RR, Papaliu-Finlay D (1984): Psychosocial adaptation to wearing the Milwaukee brace for scoliosis: a pilot study of adolescent females and their mothers. *J Adolesc Health Care* 5:237–242.

45. Green NE (1986): Part-time bracing of adolescent idiopathic scoliosis. *J Bone Joint Surg Am* 68:738–742.

46. Gurnham RB (1983): Adolescent compliance with spinal brace wear. *Orthop Nurs* 2:13–17.

47. Hall J, Miller ME, Schumann W, et al. (1975): A refined concept in the orthotic management of scoliosis: a preliminary report. *Orthot Prosthet* 29(4):7–13.

48. Hanks GA, Zimmer B, Nogi J (1988): TLSO treatment of idiopathic scoliosis: an analysis of the Wilmington jacket. *Spine* 13(6):626–629.

49. Hassan I, Bjerkreim I (1983): Progression in idiopathic scoliosis after conservative treatment. *Acta Orthop Scand* 54:88–90.

50. Heckman-Schatzinger LA, Nash CL, Drotar DD, et al. (1977): Emotional adjustment in scoliosis. *Clin Orthop* 125:145–150.

51. Herbert MA, Bobechko WP (1987): Paraspinal muscle stimulation for the treatment of idiopathic scoliosis in children. *Orthopedics* 10(8):1125–1132.

52. Howard A, Wright JG, Hedden D (1998): A comparative study of TLSO, Charleston, and Milwaukee braces for idiopathic scoliosis. *Spine* 23(22):2404–2411.

53. Jonasson-Rajala E, Josefsson E, Lundberg B, et al. (1984): Boston thoracic brace in the treatment of idiopathic scoliosis: initial correction. *Clin Orthop* 183:37–41.

54. Kahanovitz N, Weiser S (1986): Lateral electrical surface stimulation (LESS) compliance in adolescent female scoliosis patients. *Spine* 11(7):753–755.

55. Karol LA, Johnston III CE, Browne RH, et al. (1993): Progression of the curve in boys who have idiopathic scoliosis. *J Bone Joint Surg Am* 75(12):1804–1810.

56. Katz DE, Richards BS, Browne RH, et al. (1997): A comparison between the Boston brace and the Charleston bending brace in adolescent idiopathic scoliosis. *Spine* 22(12):1302–1312.

57. Keiser RP, Shufflebarger HL (1976): The Milwaukee brace in idiopathic scoliosis: evaluation of 123 completed cases. *Clin Orthop* 118:19–24.

58. Kennedy JD, Robertson CF, Olinsky A, et al. (1987): Pulmonary restrictive effect of bracing in mild idiopathic scoliosis. *Thorax* 42:959–961.

59. Korovessis P, Filos KS, Georgopoulos D (1996): Long-term alterations of respiratory function in adolescents wearing a brace for idiopathic scoliosis. *Spine* 21(17):1979–1984.

60. Labelle H, Dansereau J, Bellefleur C, et al. (1996): Three-dimensional effect of the Boston brace on the thoracic spine and rib cage. *Spine* 21(1):59–64.

61. Laurnen EL, Tupper JW, Mullen MP (1983): The Boston brace in thoracic scoliosis. A preliminary report. *Spine* 8(4):388–395.

62. Lindh M (1980): The effect of sagittal curve changes on brace correction of idiopathic scoliosis. *Spine* 5(1):26–36.

63. Lonstein JE, Carlson JM (1984): The prediction of curve progression in untreated idiopathic scoliosis during growth. *J Bone Joint Surg Am* 66:1061–1071.

64. Lonstein JE, Winter RB (1988): Adolescent idiopathic scoliosis. *Orthop Clin North Am* 19(2):239–246.

65. Lonstein JE, Winter RB (1994): The Milwaukee brace for the treatment of adolescent idiopathic scoliosis: a review of one thousand and twenty patients. *J Bone Joint Surg Am* 76:1207–1221.

66. McCollough NC III (1986): Nonoperative treatment of idiopathic scoliosis using surface electrical stimulation. *Spine* 11(8):802–804.

67. McCollough NC III, Schultz M, Javech N, et al. (1981): Miami TLSO in the management of scoliosis: preliminary results in 100 cases. *J Pediatr Orthop* 1(2):141–152.

68. MacLean WE Jr, Green NE, Pierre CB, et al. (1989): Stress and coping with scoliosis: psychological effects on adolescents and their families. *J Pediatr Orthop* 9(3):257–261.

69. Mellencamp DD, Blount WP, Anderson AJ (1977): Milwaukee brace treatment of idiopathic scoliosis. Late results. *Clin Orthop* 126:47–57.

70. Miller JAA, Nachemson AL, Schultz AB (1984): Effectiveness of braces in mild idiopathic scoliosis. *Spine* 9(6):632–635.

71. Moe JH, Kettleson DN (1970): Idiopathic scoliosis: analysis of curve patterns and the preliminary results of Milwaukee-brace treatment in one hundred sixty-nine patients. *J Bone Joint Surg Am* 52:1509–1533.

72. Montgomery F, Willner S. Prognosis of brace-treated scoliosis. Comparison of the Boston and Milwaukee methods in 244 girls. *Acta Orthop Scand* 1989;60(4):383–385.

73. Montgomery F, Willner S, Appelgren G. Long-term follow-up of patients with adolescent idiopathic scoliosis treated conservatively: an analysis of the clinical value of progression. *J Pediatr Orthop* 1990; 10:48–52.

74. Mulcahy AT, Galante J, DeWald R, et al. A follow-up study of forces acting on the Milwaukee brace on patients undergoing treatment for idiopathic scoliosis. *Clin Orthop Rel Res* 1973;93:53–68.

75. Myers BA, Friedman SB, Weiner IB. Coping with a chronic disability: psychosocial observations of girls with scoliosis treated with the Milwaukee brace. *Am J Dis Child* 1970;120(3):175–181.

76. Nachemson AL, Peterson LE. Effectiveness of treatment with a brace in girls who have adolescent idiopathic scoliosis. *J Bone Joint Surg* 1995;77(A):815–822.

77. Noonan KJ, Dolan LA, Jacobson WC, et al. Long-term psychosocial characteristics of patients treated for idiopathic scoliosis. *J Pediatr Orthop* 1997;17:712–717.

78. Noonan KJ, Weinstein SL, Jacobson WC, et al. (1996): Use of the Milwaukee brace for progressive idiopathic scoliosis. *J Bone Joint Surg Am* 78:557–567.

79. Nordwall A (1973): Studies in idiopathic scoliosis, relevant to etiology, conservative and operative treatment. *Acta Orthop Scand* 150[Suppl]:99–124.

80. O'Donnell CS, Bunnell WP, Betz RR, et al. (1988): Electrical stimulation in the treatment of idiopathic scoliosis. *Clin Orthop* 229:107–113.

81. Olafsson Y, Saraste H, Soderlund V, (1995): Boston brace in the treatment of idiopathic scoliosis. *J Pediatr Orthop* 15:524–527.

82. Peltonen J, Poussa M, Ylikoski M (1988): Three-year results of bracing in scoliosis. *Acta Orthop Scand* 59(5):487–490.

83. Peterson LA, Nachemson AL (1995): Prediction of progression of the curve in girls who have adolescent idiopathic scoliosis of moderate severity. *J Bone Joint Surg Am* 77(6):823–827.

84. Piazza MR, Bassett GS (1990): Curve progression after treatment with the Wilmington brace for idiopathic scoliosis. *J Pediatr Orthop* 10(1):39–43.

85. Picault C, deMauroy JC, Mouilleseaux B, et al. (1986): Natural history of idiopathic scoliosis in girls and boys. *Spine* 11(8):777–778.

86. Price CT, Scott DS, Reed FE Jr, et al. (1990): Nighttime bracing for adolescent idiopathic scoliosis with the Charleston bending brace: preliminary report. *Spine* 15(12):1294–1299.

87. Price CT, Scott DS, Reed FE Jr, et al. (1997): Nighttime bracing for adolescent idiopathic scoliosis with the Charleston bending brace: long-term follow-up. *J Pediatr Orthop* 17(6):703–707.

88. Refsum HE, Naess-Andresen CF, Lange JE (1990): Pulmonary function and gas exchange at rest and exercise in adolescent girls with mild idiopathic scoliosis during treatment with Boston thoracic brace. *Spine* 15(5):421–423.

89. Rogala EJ, Drummond DS, Gurr J (1978): Scoliosis: incidence and natural history. *J Bone Joint Surg Am* 60(2):173–176.

90. Rudicel S, Renshaw TS (1983): The effect of the Milwaukee brace on spinal decompensation in idiopathic scoliosis. *Spine* 8(4):385–387.

91. Sevastikoglou JA, Linderholm H, Lindgren U (1976): Effect of the Milwaukee brace on vital and ventilatory capacity of scoliotic patients. *Acta Orthop Scand* 47:540–545.

92. Stone B, Beekman C, Hall V, et al. (1979): The effect of an exercise program on change in curve in adolescents with minimal idiopathic scoliosis. *Phys Ther* 59(6):759–763.

93. Styblo K (1991): *Conservative treatment of juvenile and adolescent idiopathic scoliosis: a clinical, roentgenological and comparative retrospective study on the effects of conservative treatment by brace in 290 juvenile and adolescent consecutive patients.* Thesis, Aun De Rijksuniversiteit Te Leiden, Leiden, The Netherlands.

94. Sullivan JA, Davidson R, Renshaw TS, et al. (1986): Further evaluation of the scolitron treatment of idiopathic adolescent scoliosis. *Spine* 11(9):903–906.

95. Uden A, Willner S (1983): The effect of lumbar flexion and Boston thoracic brace on the curves in idiopathic scoliosis. *Spine* 8(8): 846–850.

96. Uden A, Willner S, Pettersson H (1982): Initial correction with the Boston thoracic brace. *Acta Orthop Scand* 53:907–911.

97. Upadhyay SS, Nelson IW, Ho EKW, et al. (1995): New prognostic factors to predict the final outcome of brace treatment in adolescent idiopathic scoliosis. *Spine* 20(5):537–545.

98. Watts HG, Hall JE, Stanish W (1977): The Boston Brace system for the treatment of low thoracic and lumbar scoliosis by the use of a girdle without superstructure. *Clin Orthop* 126:87–92.

99. Wickers FC, Bunch WH, Barnett PM (1977): Psychological factors in failure to wear the Milwaukee brace for treatment of idiopathic scoliosis. *Clin Orthop* 126:62–66.

100. Willers U, Normelli H, Aaro S, et al. (1993): Long-term results of Boston Brace treatment on vertebral rotation in idiopathic scoliosis. *Spine* 18(4):432–435.

101. Willner S (1984): Effect of the Boston thoracic brace on the frontal and sagittal curves of the spine. *Acta Orthop Scand* 55:457–460.

102. Winter RB, Lonstein JE, Drogt J, et al. (1986): The effectiveness of bracing in the nonoperative treatment of idiopathic scoliosis. *Spine* 11:790–791.

21

ADOLESCENT IDIOPATHIC SCOLIOSIS: SURGERY

KEITH H. BRIDWELL

Surgical treatment of idiopathic adolescent scoliosis continues to evolve. In the 1960s, Harrington instrumentation was introduced (29,49,50,82). In the late 1970s, sublaminar wires were introduced principally for paralytic deformities (85) but were also applied to idiopathic scoliosis, as were intraspinous Wisconsin wires (31,42,56,57). In the mid-1980s, instrumentation was further segmentalized into the use of two-rod multiple-hook configurations (1,2,26,58,75,78,113,117,119), which have now been expanded to the use of pedicle screws (4,20,47). Most commonly pedicle screws are applied at the thoracolumbar junction and the lumbar spine (4,47), although some authors also favor its use in the thoracic spine (124).

The goal of surgery in idiopathic scoliosis remains the same. It is desirable to obtain a solid fusion and to have the top and the bottom of the fusion balanced within the stable zone (63,67) (Fig. 1). It is desirable in most instances for the top and the bottom of the fusion to be neutral (Fig. 2) and level to the sacrum and pelvis (14,63,67). Autogenous bone works as a source of bone graft (13,51). Some authors have suggested that allograft may work (10,30). Others have suggested that bone graft may not be necessary if a complete facet excision is performed and the spine is immobilized with segmental fixation (37).

Investigators are exploring the role of anterior instrumentation for thoracic curves (9,53,62) as well as lumbar and thoracolumbar curves. Thoracoscopic and other endoscopic techniques for thoracic curves are also being considered (107).

CONSIDERATION FOR SURGICAL TREATMENT

Indications for surgical treatment of idiopathic adolescent scoliosis are relative. In terms of a specific Cobb number, the usual "tide mark" that is considered by most surgeons is 50 degrees (67). At 50 degrees, deformities are usually cosmetically noticeable, and natural history studies such as those by Edgar (34) and Weinstein (133,134) suggest that progression into adulthood is more likely in curves that exceed 50 degrees. We have to remember that idiopathic scoliosis is a three-dimensional deformity;

hence, considerations regarding the axial and sagittal planes play a role in decision making. If conservative or active daytime brace treatment fails and the curve progresses beyond 40 degrees with a substantial amount of growth remaining, recommendation for surgical treatment may be appropriate (13).

The curve pattern is a factor. The tide mark for considering surgery for balanced double major curves is somewhat higher than for a single curve (13). "True" double major curves require long fusions, and most surgeons think twice about fusing both the thoracic and the lumbar curve unless the deformity is more substantial (15,67). Remember that just because the designated tide mark may be 50 degrees, this does not mean that all curves of more than 50 degrees have to be fused and instrumented. It simply means that at 50 degrees, one should consider the pros and cons of surgical treatment.

PREOPERATIVE WORKUP

Idiopathic scoliosis is still a diagnosis of exclusion. We do not have a clear understanding of its etiology. Before defining a curve pattern as idiopathic, one must consider other etiologies, such as neoplasm, inflammation, neurologic disease, muscle disease, central nervous system disorders, and neural axis anomalies, such as syrinx, Chiari malformations, or tethered cords.

If the patient has a left thoracic curve or spinal cord or nerve root signs, appropriate magnetic resonance imaging (MRI) studies should be completed before definitive surgical plans are made (41). If the patient has a substantial thoracic curve, pulmonary function tests may enter into the decision-making process regarding whether it is being treated anteriorly or posteriorly or whether thoracoplasty should be considered (5,8,39,118,123).

Radiographic analysis should include long-cassette standing coronal and lateral radiographs of the spine. These radiographs should be long-cassette 3-foot films and not a series of 14- × 17-inch radiographs because these will not provide an adequate representation of the patient's coronal and sagittal balance. A set of flexibility films should also be performed. Potential flexibility films include right side-bending, left side-bending, push-prone (13,15), and fulcrum-bending radiographs (22). These represent assessments of the flexibility of curves. The purpose of the push-prone radiograph is to apply a maximal force on

K. H. Bridwell, M.D.: Washington University School of Medicine, St. Louis, MO.

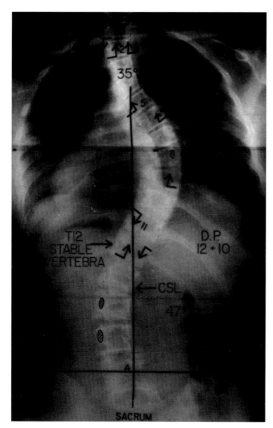

FIGURE 1. Identification of the stable zone, center sacral line, and stable vertebra: The determination is made on a standing coronal long cassette radiograph with the pelvis level. The center sacral line (CSL) is drawn through the midpoint of the sacrum perpendicular to the pelvis. The vertebra bisected by this line is the stable vertebra. Two vertical lines constructed perpendicular to the pelvis intersecting the S1 pedicles represent the stable zone. The center sacral line represents the center of the stable zone.

TABLE 1. PREOPERATIVE WORKUP

Long-cassette standing coronal and lateral radiograph
Side-bending coronal radiographs supine, showing all curves
Long-cassette supine coronal radiograph
Long-cassette coronal "traction" radiograph (for bigger curves)
Long-cassette coronal "push-prone" radiograph (to assess curve correction plus effect on adjacent curves)
Fulcrum-bending coronal radiographs
Supine hyperextension lateral radiograph (to assess flexibility of hyperkyphotic segments)
Magnetic resonance image (skull to sacrum) ⎫
Pulmonary function tests   ⎬ Select patients
Bone scan   ⎭

one curve to see how the other curves above and below respond (13,15). This helps the surgeon decide whether one curve or several curves should be fused and instrumented. Some authors suggest that fulcrum-bending films demonstrate more correction than side-bending radiographs (22). Opinion varies regarding whether a traction film or a supine or standing side-bending radiograph demonstrates more correction (108,127). There are no right or wrong answers regarding which flexibility radiographs should be obtained (Table 1).

The additional value of side-bending radiographs relates to whether certain transitional discs bend two ways or one way, which may be a determinant of where a fusion stops if the fusion and instrumentation is being performed posteriorly. Within a curve, it is advisable to fix all levels within that curve down to the transitional and neutral vertebrae on the top and the bottom. There is some suggestion that with pedicle fixation, it may be possible to limit the fusion to those segments stopping at the neutral and transitional vertebrae both proximally and distally (4,47). With hook constructs, it has been recommended that the distal level be the "stable" vertebra, the one that is intersected or bisected by the center sacral line, which is a line drawn

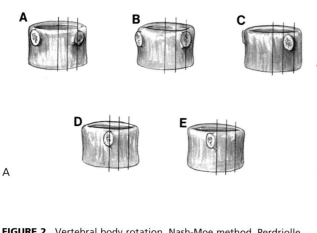

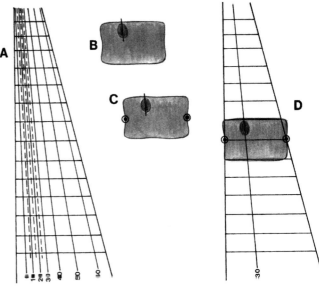

FIGURE 2. Vertebral body rotation, Nash-Moe method, Perdriolle method. **A:** Grade of rotation is determined by the location of the convex pedicle. As more rotation occurs, the concave pedicle disappears, and the convex pedicle moves in to the apparent midpoint of the vertebral body. **B:** Perdriolle method of measurement of vertebral rotation.

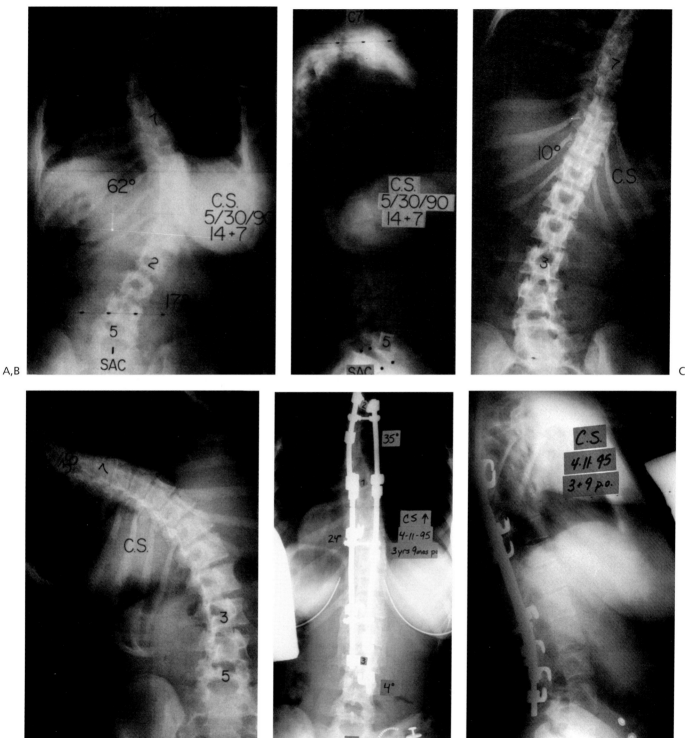

A,B

C

D,E

F

FIGURE 3. This patient presented with characteristics of both a type V and a type IV curve. Because the type IV curve was very flexible and the L3–L4 disc was out of the lower curve and bent both ways on the benders, it was possible to stop at L3. If Harrington instrumentation were used, the construct and fusion would have gone to L4. **A:** Standing coronal radiograph preoperatively. **B:** Standing sagittal radiograph preoperatively. **C:** Right side-bending radiograph preoperatively. **D:** Left side-bending radiograph preoperatively. **E:** Standing coronal radiograph postoperatively. **F:** Standing sagittal radiograph postoperatively.

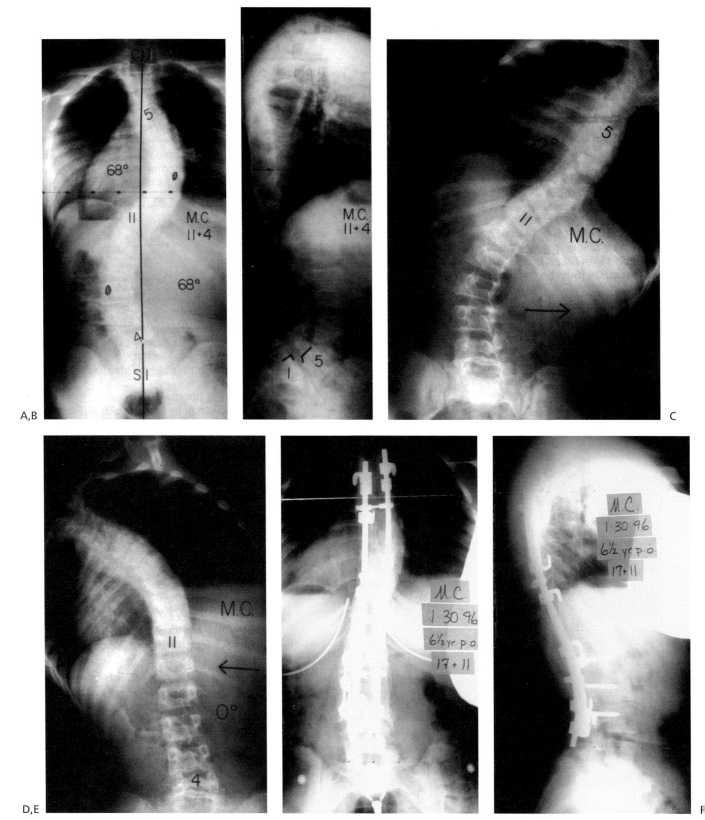

FIGURE 4. This was a double major curve pattern. The thoracic and lumbar curves had equal structural characteristics radiographically, although the lumbar curve was more flexible. Clinically, the thoracic and lumbar curves produced equal amounts of deformity. The L3–L4 segment was quite flexible. L3 was close to being neutral in rotation. It was, therefore, possible to stop at L3. With Harrington or Luque instrumentation, fusion would have been done to L4. **A:** Standing coronal radiograph preoperatively. **B:** Standing sagittal radiograph preoperatively. **C:** Right side-bending radiograph preoperatively. **D:** Left side-bending radiograph preoperatively. **E:** Standing coronal radiograph postoperatively. **F:** Standing sagittal radiograph postoperatively.

TABLE 2. WHEN CAN AN ADDITIONAL LUMBAR LEVEL BE SAVED WITH POSTERIOR DEROTATION SYSTEMS?[a]

1. L3 within 10° of neutral on standing coronal radiograph
2. The L3–L4 disc symmetrical or beginning to open up in the other direction on the standing coronal radiograph
3. The apex of the lumbar or thoracolumbar curve at the L1–L2 disc or higher
4. On the right side bending radiograph (assuming a left lumbar curve) the spine derotates, straightens out, and centralizes from L3 to the sacrum.
5. L4 must be bisected by the center sacral line and have less than 15° of tilt on the standing coronal radiograph.
6. Lumbar curve corrects to less than 30° on the flexibility films.
7. Control of distal lumbar segments is facilitated by either pedicle fixation on the convex side or the four-hook,[b] two-segment Shuf-flebarger technique at the last segment being fused.

[a] Stopping at L3 instead of L4.
[b] See accompanying diagram.

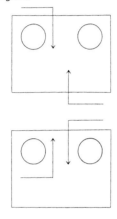

through the center of the sacrum and perpendicular either to the top of the pelvis or the floor (63). To some extent, the appropriate level to fix proximally is determined by the sagittal plane as well. In the sagittal plane, the top and the bottom of the fusion should be transitional, in an area of relative lordosis, and within the weight-bearing line. Established teaching was that posterior fusion should stop two levels above and one level below the transitional segments (49,50), which was appropriate for Harrington instrumentation and systems employing only sublaminar wires or Wisconsin wires. Those levels can at times be shortened if fixation is achieved at every level with hooks or pedicle screws and if the "saving of levels" is compatible with the sagittal plane. Potentially, a disc space that points the opposite way on a standing film and points both ways on side-bending films can be excluded from the fusion (76) (Figs. 3 and 4; Table 2).

DETERMINATION OF FUSION LEVELS: ANTERIOR APPROACH

Anterior-only fusion and instrumentation is considered for thoracic and thoracolumbar-lumbar curves. It is not an option for double thoracic curves or for true double major curves. In considering selective anterior fusion of a right thoracic curve, the surgeon must exclude the structural upper thoracic curve (79). Likewise, if the surgeon is considering a selective anterior fusion of the lumbar or thoracolumbar curve, it is important to assess

the structural characteristics of the thoracic curve above. If a patient has a right thoracic and left lumbar curve pattern and is particularly bothered by a high right shoulder, selective anterior instrumentation and fusion of the thoracolumbar-lumbar curve is unlikely to level the shoulders (13).

Otherwise, picking fusion levels anteriorly is straightforward. One should include all segments within the curve, fusing and instrumenting from the transitional and neutral vertebra above to transitional and neutral vertebra below (9,33,48). All discs that are concave into the curve should be included. Any discs that point the other direction or are symmetric do not need to be included. Anterior-only fixation traditionally has implied screw fixation of every segment (9,33,48).

SURGICAL TREATMENT OF TYPE I, III, AND IV THORACIC CURVES

Recent articles (27,71) have suggested that there is an element of intrarater and interrater variability in assessment of the King classification (63), which is true of all classification systems. Nonetheless, the King classification system has been the most valuable one for classifying thoracic curves in the recent past and, therefore, is used in this chapter (Table 3).

Type I, III, and IV curves are single thoracic curves. A thoracic curve is one with an apex of T10 or higher. A type III curve is the most common pattern in which the stable vertebra is usually L2 (Fig. 5). A type IV curve is a longer thoracic curve in which the stable vertebra is L4 (Fig. 6). The stable vertebra is the one bisected by the center sacral line on the standing long-cassette coronal radiograph. With posterior fixation of these curves, a type III curve is usually stopped at L1 or L2, and a type IV curve is usually stopped at L3. With traditional Harrington instrumentation, a type IV curve would be stopped at L4. We know now that it is often possible to stop at L3 with more modern instrumentation in a type IV curve (1,76) (Fig. 3). Placement of hooks can be defined as either a compression mode or a distraction mode. Compression and distraction modes should be aligned according to the tilt of the disc at that particular segment. In other words, if the disc is convex to the left at a particular level, it makes the most sense to place the hooks in a compression mode on the left side and a distraction mode on the right side. For the most part, hooks are placed in a distraction mode on the concavity and a compression mode on the convexity, but with some reversal of hooks on both the top and the

TABLE 3. CURVE PATTERNS

Thoracic	
Type I	Principal lumbar curve, secondary thoracic curve
Type II	Principal thoracic curve, secondary lumbar curve
Type III	Thoracic curve without structural lumbar curve
Type IV	Long thoracic curve with an apex at T10 but extending to L4
Type V	Double thoracic curve (rotation in the opposite direction from T2–T5 with incomplete correction on the side-bending film)
Double major	Equally structural thoracic and lumbar curves
Lumbar	Curve with apex in the lumbar spine
Thoracolumbar	Curve with apex at the thoracolumbar junction

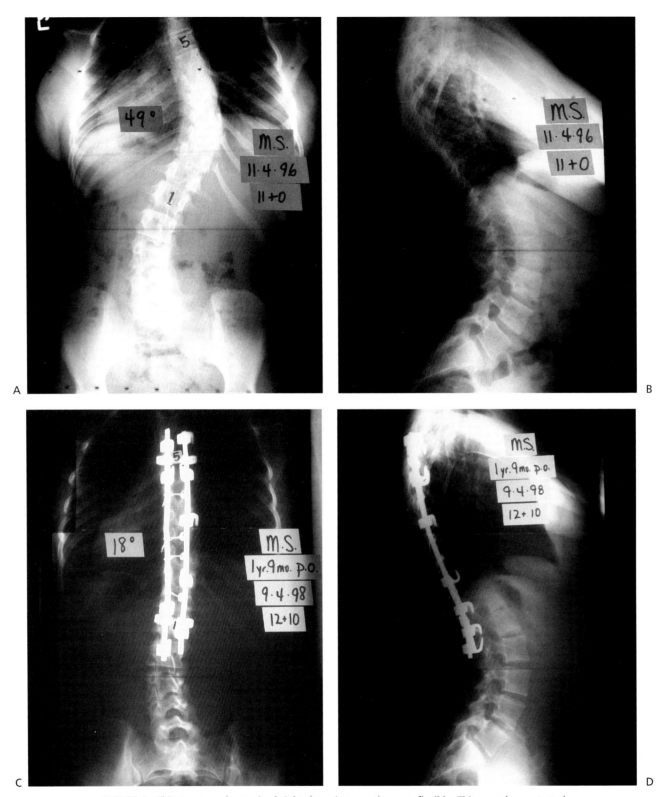

FIGURE 5. This was a moderate-sized right thoracic curve that was flexible. This case demonstrated treatment with posterior instrumentation. Correction was achieved by tightening Wisconsin wires and by in situ contouring of the rod on the left side. Correction was therefore achieved entirely through translation. No distraction was used, and no rod rotation maneuver was used. Initially, the hooks were engaged into the distal two-segment claw, which was then fixed in mild compression. The rod was engaged into the two-segment claw above but was not fixed at those levels. The Wisconsin wires were then sequentially tightened. This was followed by some in situ contouring of the rod, followed by more wire tightening and then a second set of in situ rod recontouring. When final correction was achieved, the proximal two-segment claw was fixed. Using this kind of correction, the incidence of junctional kyphosis and coronal decompensation problems appears to be substantially reduced. **A:** Standing coronal radiograph preoperatively. **B:** Standing sagittal radiograph preoperatively. **C:** Standing coronal radiograph postoperatively. **D:** Standing sagittal radiograph postoperatively.

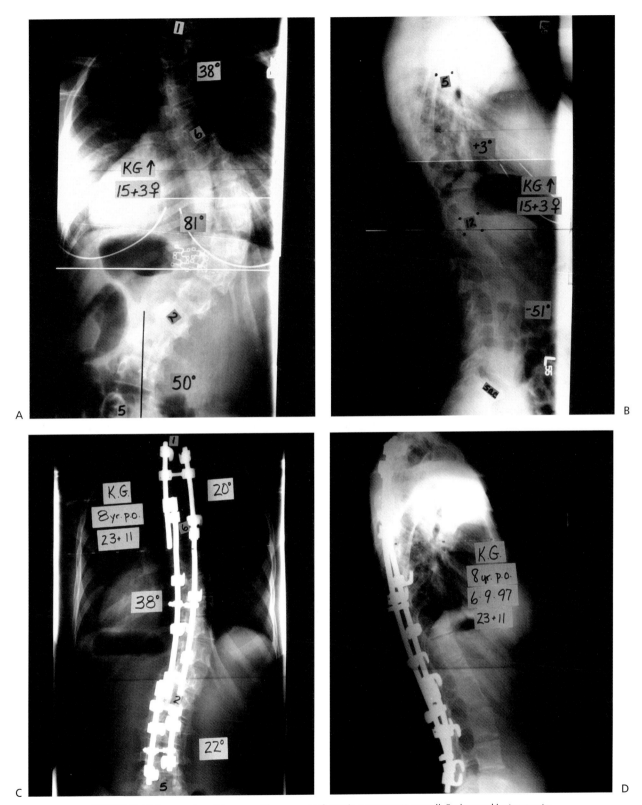

FIGURE 6. This was a type IV curve with an upper thoracic component as well. Fusion and instrumentation were performed down to L4. It is conceivable that the fusion and instrumentation really could have been stopped at L3. Note the hook patterns. Reversal of hooks was accomplished to correlate with reversal of the disc spaces and also with the desired sagittal correction. Note that there was an element of preoperative thoracolumbar kyphosis. With fusions and instrumentations to L3 and L4, it was particularly important to preserve and, in some cases, enhance segmental lordosis. **A:** Standing coronal radiograph preoperatively. **B:** Standing sagittal radiograph preoperatively. **C:** Standing coronal radiograph postoperatively. **D:** Standing sagittal radiograph postoperatively.

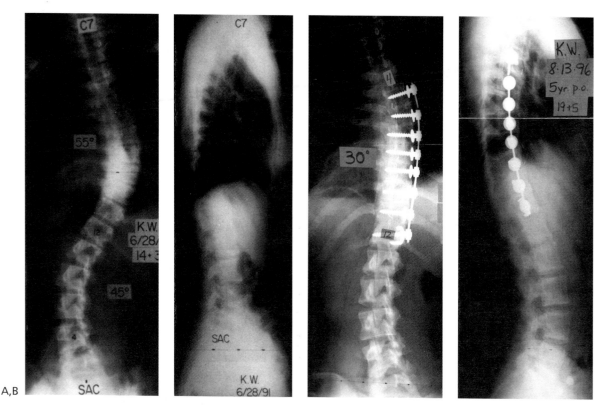

FIGURE 7. This patient presented with a curve pattern that was borderline between being a type II and a type III curve. She was treated with anterior instrumentation using a small flexible threaded rod (Zielke instrumentation). Note that the implant broke at one level. Despite that, she has had an excellent clinical and radiographic result. For idiopathic adolescent scoliosis, a more substantial rod is advisable than what was used in this case. **A:** Standing coronal radiograph preoperatively. **B:** Standing sagittal radiograph preoperatively. **C:** Standing coronal radiograph postoperatively. **D:** Standing sagittal radiograph postoperatively.

bottom (13). For a type III curve, it is going to be advisable to preserve some lordosis from T12 to L1 or L2. For the type IV curve that is fused to L3 or L4, it is extremely important to preserve segmental lordosis, that is, the lordosis from T12 to the last instrumented vertebra.

Type III and type IV curves are amenable to anterior-only instrumentation and fusion. Data for this approach are evolving (9,48,62). It has been suggested that the anterior approach can save one or two distal levels (9). The pseudarthrosis rate using threaded rods anteriorly is unacceptably high (9) (Fig. 7). However, data are evolving on the use of smooth solid rods anteriorly. In smaller patients, a single-screw, single-rod system may suffice. In larger patients, a double-screw, double-rod system may be more advisable (53,62) (Fig. 8). Fixation of a long thoracic curve may require a double thoracotomy. If a double thoracotomy is being strongly considered for a patient, pulmonary function assessment is crucial because some loss of pulmonary function occurs in the postoperative period (132). Fusions to T12 or L1 can be done above the diaphragm. Fusions to L2, as might be attempted in a type IV curve, may require severance of all or part of the peripheral portion of the diaphragm. Anterior convex instrumentation of thoracic curves tends to be kyphosing (9). Therefore, a kyphotic right thoracic curve is a relative contraindication to anterior instrumentation, as opposed to the more com-

mon hypokyphotic thoracic deformity. Instrumentation that crosses the thoracolumbar junction is best managed with structural grafting to the concavity of those disc spaces to preserve lordosis. Options of structural grafting include titanium mesh cages, fresh-frozen tricortical iliac grafts, and fibular allograft wedges supplemented with autogenous rib bone graft (15,125). Many articles discuss the result of fusion and instrumentation of thoracic curves on pulmonary function (64,74,122,130–132, 138,139). There is not universal agreement, but most authors report a positive effect if there is not significant rib cage disruption associated with treatment.

A type I curve implies that the lumbar or thoracolumbar deformity is greater than the thoracic curve. In this circumstance, the structural component of the thoracic curve determine whether both curves are being fixed or fused or just the lumbar-thoracolumbar curve. Assessment factors include which shoulder is higher, the degree of shoulder asymmetry, and the size of the thoracic rib hump. When both curves are to be fused, a posterior approach is preferred. When only the thoracolumbar-lumbar curve is being addressed, either a posterior-only or an anterior-only approach may be considered. The more popular approach for fixing only the thoracolumbar-lumbar curve is the anterior approach, with a thoracoabdominal approach through the ninth or tenth rib (33,40,45,55,59,61,83,101,102,129). In this cir-

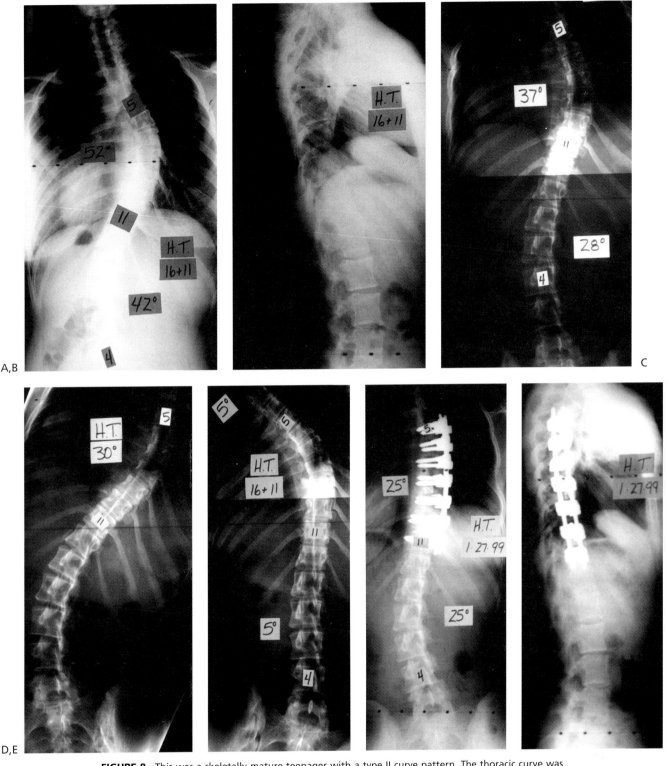

FIGURE 8. This was a skeletally mature teenager with a type II curve pattern. The thoracic curve was somewhat bigger than the lumbar curve. Clinically, the thoracic curve was much more noticeable than the lumbar curve. The patient and the patient's family were unhappy with the appearance of the thoracic deformity. This patient weighed about 175 pounds and was about 5 feet, 10 inches tall. She was treated with a double-screw, double-rod system (the Kaneda/KASS instrumentation). A selective fusion was done of just the thoracic curve. This produced acceptable coronal and sagittal correction as well as a clinical deformity correction that pleased the patient and her family. **A:** Standing coronal radiograph preoperatively. **B:** Standing sagittal radiograph preoperatively. **C:** Supine radiograph preoperatively. **D:** Right side-bending radiograph preoperatively. **E:** Left side-bending radiograph preoperatively. **F:** Standing coronal radiograph postoperatively. **G:** Standing sagittal radiograph postoperatively.

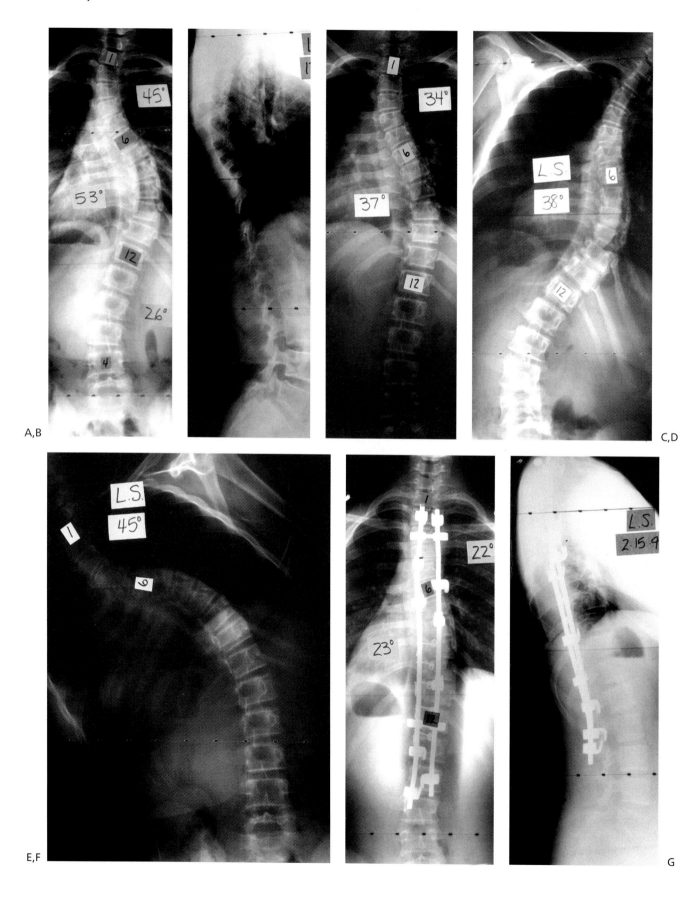

A,B

C,D

E,F

G

cumstance, it is particularly important to preserve lordosis from T12 to the last instrumented vertebra. This is covered in more detail under the section entitled Thoracolumbar and Lumbar Curves.

DOUBLE THORACIC CURVES

A double thoracic curve pattern implies a higher and lower thoracic curve, most commonly a high left thoracic, low right thoracic curve pattern (63,68,79). In this circumstance, the low right thoracic curve is more noticeable because it creates more apical deviation and a larger rib hump. However, the height of the shoulders is determined by the upper curve. In a single right thoracic curve pattern, the right shoulder is higher. In a double thoracic curve pattern, either the shoulders are level, or more commonly, the left shoulder is higher. If the left shoulder is higher, correction of only the lower right thoracic curve further unbalances the shoulders and creates an even higher left shoulder (68,79). With double thoracic curve patterns, the transitional vertebra is usually somewhat lower, that is, T6 rather than T4 to T5. Often, there is somewhat of a junctional kyphosis between the upper and lower curves as well. If the upper thoracic curve exceeds 35 degrees and does not bend out to less than 20 degrees on the opposite side-bending film, these coronal considerations, as well as the sagittal factors, may suggest inclusion of the upper thoracic curve (79). If the left shoulder is higher, the upper thoracic curve should always be included. As in any double curve pattern that is being treated posteriorly, the orientation of the hooks should be reversed as one goes from one curve to the next. If the upper thoracic curve is kyphotic, it is best to apply lordosing compression forces to the convexity first. If the upper thoracic curve is lordotic, it is better to apply forces along the concavity first. In most cases, the upper thoracic curve is kyphotic and the lower thoracic curve is hypokyphotic (13). Double thoracic curves are best treated posteriorly (Fig. 9). If one chooses to treat a double thoracic pattern anteriorly, it is important to limit the correction of the upper portion of the lower thoracic curve and to block correction of the transitional segments so that shoulder asymmetry is not worsened (Table 4).

THORACOLUMBAR AND LUMBAR CURVES

Thoracolumbar and lumbar curves are defined as having an apex at T11 or below. When they are associated with a significantly structural thoracic component (a type I King curve), it may be advisable to fix both thoracic and lumbar curves posteriorly. In

TABLE 4. CHARACTERISTICS OF THE HIGH LEFT THORACIC CURVE IN A DOUBLE THORACIC CURVE

High left shoulder
High left first rib
Rotation T2–T6
T6 transitional
Curve T2–T5/T6 > 35 degrees on standing radiograph
Curve T2–T5/T6 > 20 degrees on side-bending radiograph

most cases, however, the lumbar curve can be treated selectively. This can be accomplished through either a posterior or an anterior approach. Although correction can be accomplished with a posterior approach, for lumbar and thoracolumbar curves, most surgeons today prefer the anterior approach (13,15,61) (Fig. 10).

At times, thoracolumbar curves in particular can be treated by a very short anterior approach if they are extremely flexible (45), the Hall-Millis concept. If the apex is a vertebral body, one segment above and below is included. If the apex is a disc, four vertebral bodies and three discs are included. In this situation, maximal correction or, in some instances, some overcorrection is desirable (Fig. 11).

In most cases, a thoracolumbar or lumbar curve is best treated by fixing and fusing from transitional-neutral to transitional-neutral. This usually entails a T10 or T11 to L3 anterior instrumentation and fusion. The principal advantages of the anterior approach are the abilities to obtain more correction and to stop at L2 or L3 rather than L3 or L4. The type of anterior instrumentation has evolved from Dwyer (33) to Zielke instrumentation (40) and now to solid-rod systems, either a single-screw, single-rod system or a double-screw, double-rod system (61,129). Problems with the Dwyer and Zielke approach include a significant incidence of pseudarthrosis and the kyphogenic nature of the systems (83). Kyphogenic instrumentation may be satisfactory for a hypokyphotic thoracic curve. For lumbar curves, however, one wants to preserve and, in some cases, enhance segmental lordosis. There are those who advocate a rod rotation maneuver anteriorly without application of any compression force to achieve correction but maintain segmental lordosis (129). Others advocate applying some compression, but against anterior structural grafts such as titanium mesh cages, fresh-frozen tricortical iliac grafts, or fresh-frozen or freeze-dried fibular grafts packed with autogenous rib bone (13,15). It has been shown that this approach of using anterior structural grafting or limiting the amount of compression force applied can preserve and, in some instances, even enhance segmental lumbar lordosis (125). With anterior instrumentation of curves, whether they are thoracic or thoracolumbar-lumbar curves, it is crucial that the screw purchase be bicortical at each level (60,61,125). The type of

FIGURE 9. This was a double thoracic curve pattern. Note that there was some rotation and apical deviation from T2 to T5. Note that there was a slight junctional kyphosis between the two curves as well. The left first rib was slightly higher. Therefore, the hooks were reversed between the upper left thoracic and lower right thoracic curve. Correction of the lower thoracic curve was accomplished through translational forces applied through the Wisconsin wires as well as in situ contouring of the rod on the left side. Correction of the upper thoracic curve was accomplished through compression forces being applied. Most correction was achieved with the left-sided rod. Application of compression forces to the left side of the curve addressed the junctional kyphosis. **A:** Standing coronal radiograph preoperatively. **B:** Standing sagittal radiograph preoperatively. **C:** Supine radiograph preoperatively. **D:** Right side-bending radiograph preoperatively. **E:** Left side-bending radiograph preoperatively. **F:** Standing coronal radiograph postoperatively. **G:** Standing sagittal radiograph postoperatively.

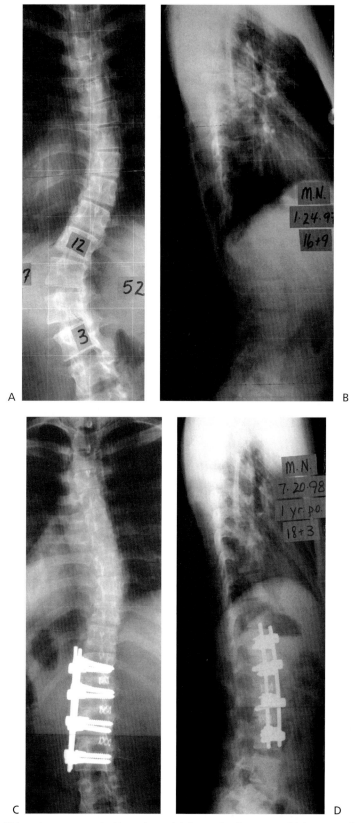

FIGURE 10. This patient presented with a substantial thoracolumbar curve. This boy was 6 feet, 2 inches tall and weighed 185 pounds. He was, therefore, treated with a double-screw, double-rod system (the Kaneda/KASS system) with an acceptable radiographic and clinical result. Note the use of structural cages to preserve segmental lordosis. Also note the residual deformity at the L3–L4 disc 1 year postoperatively. Will this predispose to early disc degeneration at this level? No answer exists in today's literature. **A:** Standing coronal radiograph preoperatively. **B:** Standing sagittal radiograph preoperatively. **C:** Standing coronal radiograph postoperatively. **D:** Standing sagittal radiograph postoperatively.

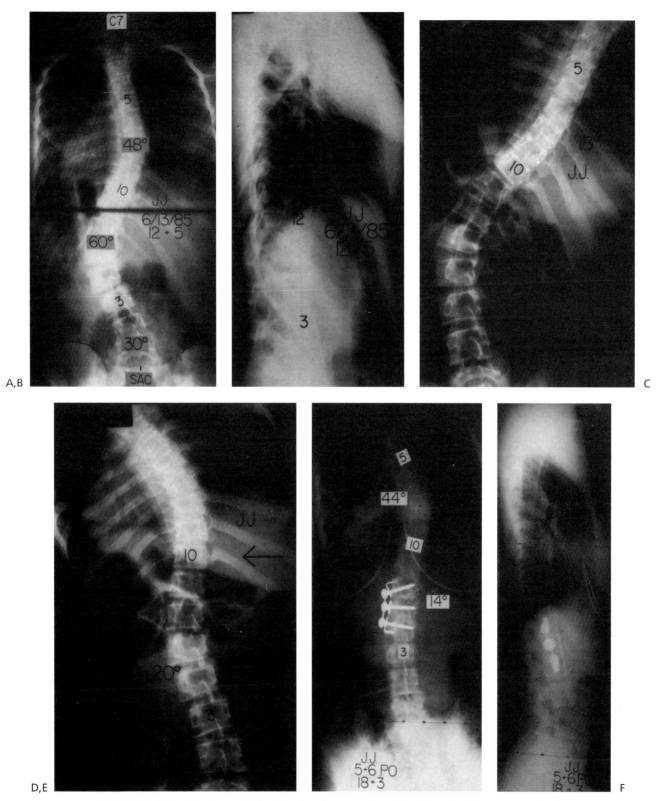

FIGURE 11. This patient presented with a type I curve pattern. The thoracolumbar curve produced substantially more clinical deformity than did the thoracic curve. This thoracolumbar curve was extremely flexible. This case was amenable to very short fixation with overcorrection of the thoracolumbar curve as described by Hall and Millis (45). See the excellent result achieved at 5-year follow-up. **A:** Standing coronal radiograph preoperatively. **B:** Standing sagittal radiograph preoperatively. **C:** Right side-bending radiograph preoperatively. **D:** Left side-bending radiograph preoperatively. **E:** Standing coronal radiograph postoperatively. **F:** Standing sagittal radiograph postoperatively.

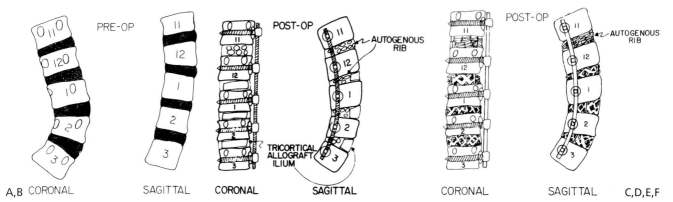

A,B CORONAL   SAGITTAL   **CORONAL**   **SAGITTAL**   CORONAL   SAGITTAL C,D,E,F

FIGURE 12. **A and B:** Preservation of lumbar lordosis with anterior VDS (Zielke instrumentation) and use of anterior allograft struts: a lumbar curve with rotation and some loss of lumbar lordosis. **C and D:** The disc spaces are opened with a laminar spreader, and the largest possible fresh-frozen tricortical allograft iliac graft is placed into each anterior disc space. The Zielke screws are placed in the posterior third of the vertebral body. After an element of derotation has been achieved with the Zielke derotator, the posterior disc space is compressed at each level. This serves to open the anterior disc space and close the posterior disc space, thereby allowing enhancement of lumbar lordosis. An autogenous rib graft is placed in the posterior disc space so that there is autogenous bone graft at each level. Large tricortical grafts must be placed in the anterior disc spaces to keep this column open; simply using rib graft does not provide enough structural support. After the instrumentation is complete, further osteogenesis can be promoted by raising osteal-periosteal flaps anteriorly with a curved osteotome. Additional autogenous rib graft is then placed inside these flaps. **E and F:** The same correction accomplished with a solid-rod system and cages packed with autogenous rib bone rather than structural allograft. (From Bridwell KH [1998]: Surgical treatment of pediatric idiopathic scoliosis. In: An HS, ed. *Principles and techniques of spine surgery.* Baltimore: Williams & Wilkins, pp. 187–212, with permission.)

staple or washer has not proved to be a critical component (Fig. 12).

HOW TO DISTINGUISH A TYPE II FROM A DOUBLE MAJOR CURVE

The most important concept to evolve from the King paper (63) was that of the type II or false double major curve pattern (63), in which it is possible to fuse the thoracic curve selectively and to leave the lumbar curve alone. A typical type II curve has a stable vertebra at T12 or L1. The lumbar curve below has rotation to it, has some structural component, and crosses the midline. However, the thoracic curve is "bigger" than the lumbar curve, and the lumbar curve is more flexible. This definition of a false double major curve has lead to many interpretations (89). The critical point of interpretation is how to define "thoracic curve bigger than lumbar" (Fig. 13, Table 5). Some believe that rod rotation maneuvers are not advisable for false double major curves in which only the thoracic curve is being fused and the fusion is being stopped at T12 or L1, whereas others believe that too much correction of the thoracic curve in this situation is not desirable (18,73,110,112,128,140). Still others believe that anterior surgery for the thoracic curve is the ideal approach (72). Still others advocate fixing both curves and stopping the fusion at L3 if there is a substantial structural component to the lumbar curve (1).

My preference is to fix only the thoracic curve and to stay completely out of the lumbar curve. This is difficult to accomplish if there is a thoracolumbar kyphosis and not at least a 3:2 ratio of thoracic to lumbar apical vertebral rotation, apical translation, and Cobb measurement (15,73) (Figs. 8 and 14).

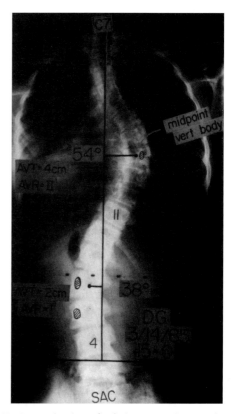

FIGURE 13. Determination of relative curve size: To determine the relative curve sizes (thoracic versus lumbar), one should consider not only the Cobb curve measurement but also the relative apical vertebral rotation (AVR) and the relative apical vertebral translation (AVT) or deviation from the midline.

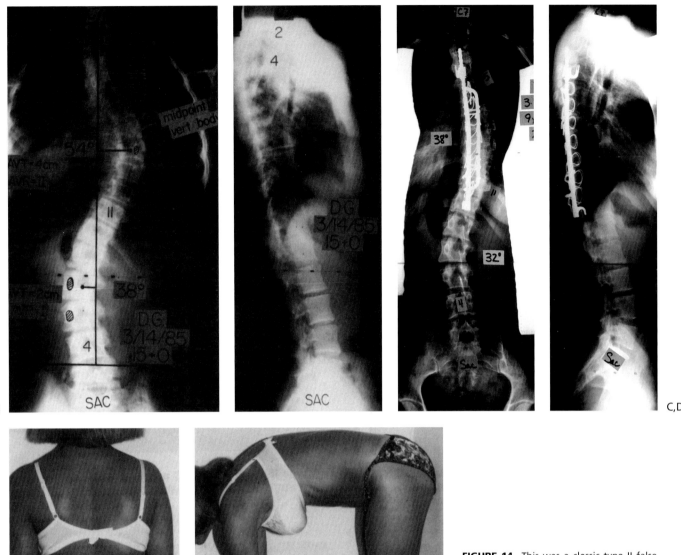

FIGURE 14. This was a classic type II false double major curve pattern. The thoracic curve was roughly 50% bigger than the lumbar curve in Cobb measurement, apical vertebral translation, and apical vertebral rotation. The lumbar curve had structural characteristics. It crossed the midline and had rotation to it and, therefore, a type II curve pattern and not a type III pattern. Note the excellent result 9 years after surgery. Also note how flexible the patient is. **A:** Standing coronal radiograph preoperatively. **B:** Standing sagittal radiograph preoperatively. **C:** Standing coronal radiograph postoperatively. **D:** Standing sagittal radiograph postoperatively. **E and F:** Clinical photographs postoperatively.

If a true double major curve pattern exists, the fixation of the lumbar curve may be accomplished with hooks or pedicle screws. There is a growing body of literature that documents the safety of pedicle screws for the adolescent lumbar spine and suggests that pedicle screws may be used to position the last instrumented vertebra more horizontally and to enhance seg-mental lumbar lordosis (4,20,47). With modern systems, if L3 is relatively neutral (Nash-Moe I or less) on the standing coronal film, if the apex of the lumbar curve is L2 or higher, if the L3 to L4 disc is symmetric or swings the opposite way of the discs within the lumbar curve on the standing coronal film, and if the L3–L4 disc swings both ways on the bending film, the fusion

TABLE 5. DISTINGUISHING BETWEEN A TYPE II (FALSE DOUBLE MAJOR) AND TRUE DOUBLE MAJOR CURVE PATTERN

Radiographic Criteria
Standing film (long-cassette coronal)
Relative curve size by Cobb measurement
Relative apical deviation or translation from:
Plumb line
Center sacral line
Line connecting transitional vertebrae
Relative apical rotation of the thoracic curve versus the lumbar curve
Thoracolumbar junction sagittal plane based on standing sagittal radiograph
Flexibility of the curves (lumbar curve must be more flexible than thoracic curve to consider selective thoracic fusion)

Clinical Criteria
Standing examination: relative thoracic deformity to waistline asymmetry
Forward-bending examination: relative thoracic-to-lumbar hump

and instrumentation may be stopped at L3 rather than L4 (47,76) (Fig. 4). Many articles discuss the aging of segments below a spinal fusion, with a wide spectrum of conclusions (24,25,36,84,93,96,105,126). Nonetheless, it is desirable in most cases to preserve mobile segments and to normalize segmental sagittal curves (7,16,28,52,120,136), especially in the lumbar segments. As distal segments age and lose anterior column height, flatback syndrome is disabling (11,38,65,66)

DECOMPENSATION ASSOCIATED WITH SELECTIVE CURVE FUSION

Treatment of type II curves with selective thoracic fusion is a potential cause for postoperative decompensation (18). There appears to be a higher incidence of decompensation if a rod rotation maneuver is performed (18). Also, if the thoracic and lumbar curves are close in Cobb measurement, apical vertebral rotation, and apical translation on the standing coronal radiograph, there is a significant incidence of decompensation even if the lumbar curve is more flexible than the thoracic (18). Fre-

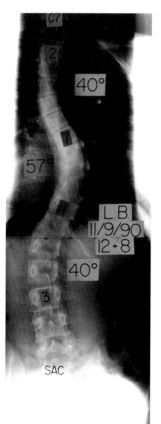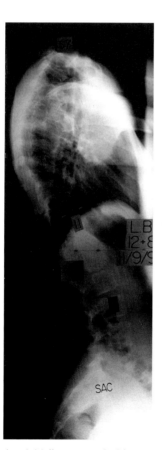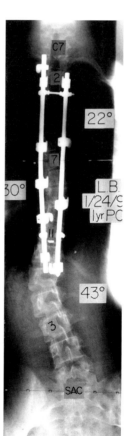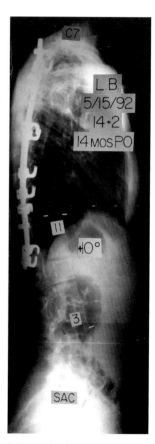

A,B

C,D

FIGURE 15. This patient initially presented with an upper thoracic, lower thoracic, and thoracolumbar curve pattern. She was initially fused and instrumented with a construct addressing the thoracic curves. This produced coronal decompensation and a junctional kyphosis. She then presented to our institution for revision surgery. She was revised by extending her fusion and instrumentation down to include the thoracolumbar curve. Fortunately, it was possible to stop at L3. Note the use of fresh-frozen tricortical iliac grafts in the anterior disc spaces to preserve segmental lordosis. The causes of the patient's initial decompensation were multifactorial. **A:** Standing coronal radiograph preoperatively. **B:** Standing sagittal radiograph preoperatively. **C:** Standing coronal radiograph 1 year postoperatively. **D:** Standing sagittal radiograph 14 months postoperatively. *(Figure continues.)*

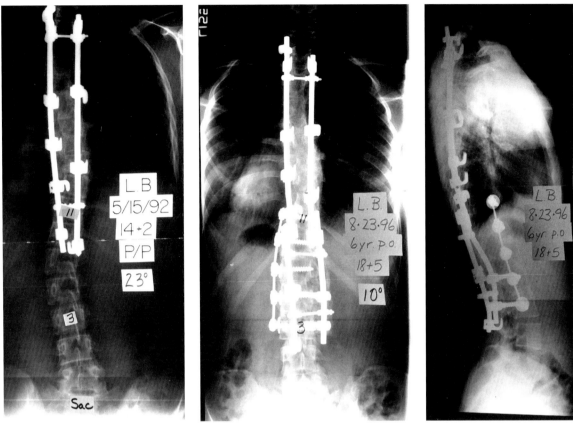

FIGURE 15. *Continued.* **E:** Push prone radiograph 14 months postoperatively. **F:** Standing coronal radiograph 6 years postoperatively. **G:** Standing sagittal radiograph 6 years postoperatively.

quently with true double major curve patterns, the lumbar curve is more flexible than the thoracic curve, even if it is clearly the more structural of the two curves (14,15).

The other curve pattern with an associated incidence of decompensation is the double thoracic pattern. If the upper thoracic curve is not recognized, fusion and instrumentation of only the lower thoracic curve may lead to worsening of shoulder balance (79).

Junctional kyphosis is also an occasional complication of posterior segmental spinal instrumentation (13,15,18,70). The most common causes are (1) not fusing to the end vertebra of a curve, (2) applying an excessive amount of compression to the last instrumented segment, (3) inadvertently disrupting the ligaments at the adjacent segment, (4) applying an excessive cantilever force, and (5) stopping a fusion or instrumentation in an area of kyphosis that is posterior to the weight-bearing line of the spine. Often, junctional kyphosis is a radiographic finding of no apparent clinical significance in the short term. Other times, the junctional kyphosis is progressive and does become clinically significant. Junctional kyphosis of clinical significance usually requires extension of the fusion to a lordotic segment and frequently requires combined surgery.

If it is detected early, coronal plane decompensation, especially in association with type II and type V curves, may be treated by a revision of the instrumentation and applied forces. If it is not revised until the fusion is solid, the fusion should be extended to include the upper thoracic curve if it is a type V or to include the lumbar curve if it is a borderline type II or double major curve pattern (Fig. 15). Occasionally, if the coronal decompensation is mild, a short period of bracing or simply time resolves the problem.

ROLE OF HALO TRACTION

Halo traction is not commonly used for idiopathic adolescent scoliosis. There are not clear guidelines for its use in the literature. If used, the most beneficial traction appears to be halo wheelchair traction. Halo bed, halo femoral, and halo walker traction are options (13). The potential role for traction is when a thoracic curve exceeds 90 degrees or in a patient who has several large curves and is not balanced in the coronal plane.

Halo traction in conjunction with anterior release can help to provide dramatic correction of thoracic curves. It is probably not advisable to start the traction the night after the anterior release procedure. There are significant dangers to halo traction that applies a distractive force to the spine. It is best to begin the halo traction roughly 48 hours after the anterior release when the patient is fully awake and capable of providing feedback about neurologic function and is hemodynamically stable. Although this is anecdotal information, I have been consulted about several cases throughout North America in which halo traction had been employed the night after an anterior release and a neurologic deficit developed. The halo traction should be applied slowly and gradually with small increments and frequent neurologic assessments. The addition of weights should always be performed during daytime waking hours when the patient can provide feedback regarding neurologic status.

The ideal ultimate weight and the time of halo traction have not been clearly established. One would expect that the longer the period of halo traction, the greater the potential for creep and relaxation of the spine.

CONCERNS ABOUT CRANKSHAFT

The concept of the crankshaft phenomenon has been clearly described (32,97). *Crankshaft* refers to the continued growth of the anterior spine after the posterior spine is fused. With continued anterior growth, the spinal deformity progresses despite a solid posterior fusion. It has also been shown that if the triradiate cartilage is closed, the likelihood of a crankshaft phenomenon is extremely remote (46,69).

If the triradiate cartilage is open, there is some chance for crankshaft to occur after posterior fusion. A progression of 10 degrees or more has been described in roughly 35% of patients older than 10 years of age with idiopathic scoliosis and an open triradiate cartilage (46). Sanders and colleagues (115,116) have observed that the patient's proximity to the peak growth velocity is a factor. When patients are at or beyond their peak growth velocity, crankshaft appears not to occur. When they have not yet reached peak growth velocity, the risk is more significant.

A general consensus among most spine surgeons is that the risk for crankshaft in patients 10 to 12 years of age with adolescent idiopathic scoliosis is small. This certainly is a problem in patients younger than 10 years of age with a variety of juvenile deformities and for certain patients with congenital deformities, specifically failures of formation (46).

INDICATIONS FOR CIRCUMFERENTIAL TREATMENT

In most cases, idiopathic adolescent scoliosis curves can be treated with a one-stage approach. If a single curve exists, either an anterior or a posterior approach can be postulated. If structural double curves exist, a posterior approach is advisable. The only reasons for circumferential treatment are either very large curves or significant sagittal plane alterations.

There are no clear-cut tide marks in the literature. In general, thoracic curves between 75 and 100 degrees can benefit from thoracoscopic release anteriorly in order to accomplish more correction with posterior fusion and instrumentation (92,99) (Fig. 16). Thoracic and lumbar curves of more than 100 degrees benefit from formal anterior release and fusion along with poste-

rior treatment (13) (Fig. 17). Patients with significant thoracic lordosis (not hypokyphosis but frank lordosis) benefit from the two-staged approach described by Bradford and colleagues (12) and Winter (137). In this situation, V-shaped kyphosing wedges are created through the disc spaces anteriorly. Posteriorly, the spine is translated to the prebent rods with sublaminar wires. Using two-segment "claws" at the top and bottom of the construct is preferred over Harrington instrumentation or sublaminar wires at the ends of the constructs.

In some patients with idiopathic scoliosis, a substantial thoracolumbar or upper lumbar kyphosis may warrant circumferential treatment. If a patient presents with this coexistent sagittal deformity, it is helpful to perform a supine long-cassette hyperextension lateral radiograph to see whether the sagittal deformity is flexible. If it is flexible, an anterior procedure is not needed. If it is inflexible, it often is advisable to "release" and graft anteriorly. The purpose in this circumstance is to recreate physiologic segmental lordosis.

INDICATIONS FOR ENDOSCOPIC AND THORACOSCOPIC TECHNIQUES

It has been demonstrated that discs can be resected in the thoracic spine through a thoracoscopic approach (92,99) (Fig. 16). This may assist to "loosen up" curves that exceed 75 degrees (Cobb angle) or curves that are very hyperkyphotic. It has not been demonstrated whether there is an endoscopic role for the frankly lordotic thoracic spine.

Investigators are now performing endoscopic anterior instrumentation of the thoracic spine (107). The ultimate fusion and complication rates with this approach will not be fully determined for several years. Although desirable in terms of the short-term morbidity for the patient, the long-term results will only be acceptable if the technique provides as high a fusion rate and comparable correction with as few complications as open anterior or posterior techniques.

SURGICAL TECHNIQUES EXCLUDING INSTRUMENTATION
Posterior Fusion

The technique of posterior fusion has not changed. Decortication from the spinous process to the tip of the transverse process is beneficial. Facet excision and decortication are part of the standard procedure. If segmental instrumentation is being used posteriorly, the fixation points have to be preserved. To some extent, this limits the surface area available for fusion. There are differing philosophies regarding the use of bone graft. The standard has been to use either an autogenous iliac or rib graft that is generated with a concomitant thoracoplasty. However, investigators have reported acceptable results using allograft (10,30) and also using no added bone graft (37). These studies had a minimal 2-year follow-up. A 3- to 5-year follow-up is needed with present-day implants to increase the confidence that spinal fusion is occurring.

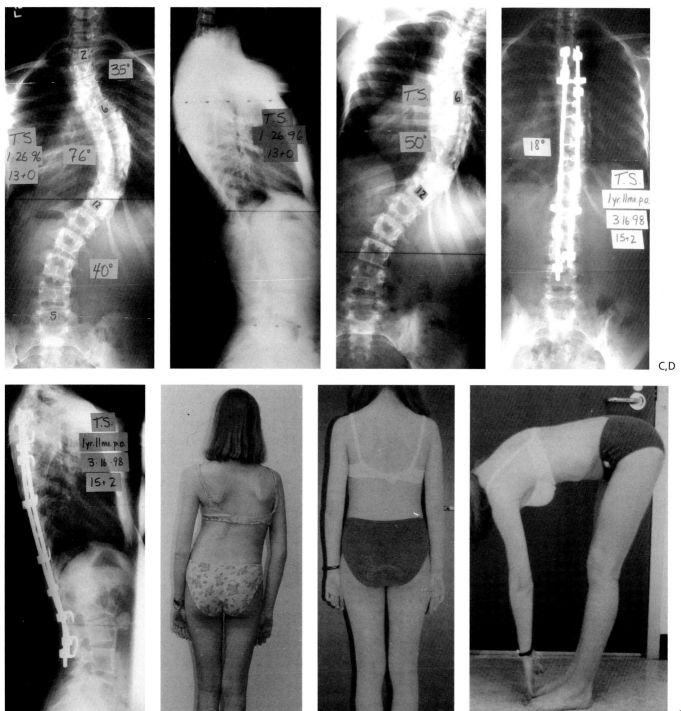

FIGURE 16. This patient presented with a fairly substantial thoracic curve that corrected only from 76 to 50 degrees on side bending. She was, therefore, initially treated with multiple thoracic releases done endoscopically through five portals. This mobilized the apical segments sufficiently that substantially more correction was achieved than what would have been possible without the anterior procedure. **A:** Standing coronal radiograph preoperatively. **B:** Standing sagittal radiograph preoperatively. **C:** Right side-bending radiograph preoperatively. **D:** Standing coronal radiograph postoperatively. **E:** Standing sagittal radiograph postoperatively. **F:** Clinical coronal appearance preoperatively. **G:** Clinical coronal appearance postoperatively. **H:** Patient is still able to touch her toes despite fusion to L3.

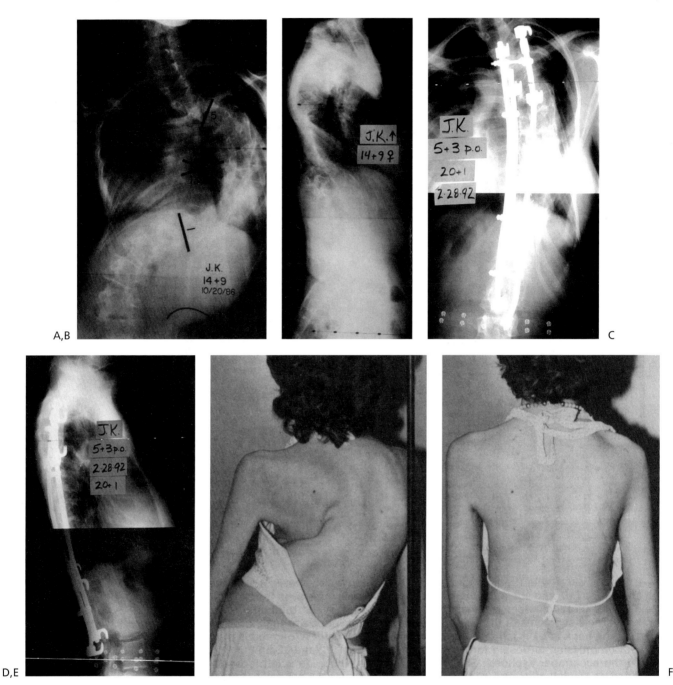

FIGURE 17. This patient presented with a 140-degree right thoracic scoliosis. She was treated with a thoracotomy and open anterior releases at multiple segments, followed by halo traction for 2 weeks, and then by the definitive posterior instrumentation. The patient gained 5 inches in height, and her forced vital capacity improved by nearly 2 liters. **A:** Standing coronal radiograph preoperatively. **B:** Standing sagittal radiograph preoperatively. **C:** Standing coronal radiograph postoperatively. **D:** Standing sagittal radiograph postoperatively. **E and F:** Preoperative and postoperative clinical appearance.

Anterior Fusion

The technique of discectomy and anterior fusion is a standard. It is helpful to excise the disc thoroughly with all of its cartilaginous components back to bony end plate. The most common bone graft placed in the disc space to facilitate fusion is autogenous rib bone, usually harvested during the anterior approach. If the anterior fusion is being performed at the thoracolumbar junction or the upper lumbar spine, there is added benefit to structural grafting anteriorly to maintain lordosis (15). Rib is not the ideal structural graft. Allograft tricortical iliac bone, allograft fibular chunks, and titanium cages filled with autogenous bone are better alternatives to serve that function (125).

Thoracoplasty

If the patient has a substantial rib hump, an anterior or posterior instrumented correction may not significantly improve the axial or tangential deformity. Resection of the prominent ribs can therein improve the cosmetic results (Fig. 18). There are several ways to accomplish this goal. Thoracoplasty can be performed from a posterior (8) or an anterior approach (open or endoscopic) (92,118). From the posterior approach, it is best to expose the rib cage from the midline rather than to make a separate incision over the rib hump. Large sections of the ribs can be resected from the apex of the rib deformity all the way to the transverse processes medially. It is important to resect the medial portions of the ribs as well. Failure to do so results in a noncos-

metic ridge. The other posterior option is to resect the ribs medially close to their vertebral attachments and to suture the cut edge to the transverse process or convex rod. This provides some immediate stability to the rib cage (see Chap. 71).

Thoracoplasty does improve the deformity and therein may improve patient satisfaction (39). However, any chest cage disruption at least temporarily reduces pulmonary function and hence should only be considered in patients with excellent pulmonary function and low pulmonary demands (77,131,132).

Adjuncts

Blood loss during surgery for idiopathic adolescent scoliosis is rarely excessive but may amount to 1 to 3 units of blood if intraoperative losses are combined with losses the first 2 postoperative days. Hypotensive anesthesia, preoperative autologous donations, intraoperative cell-saver, and preoperative use of

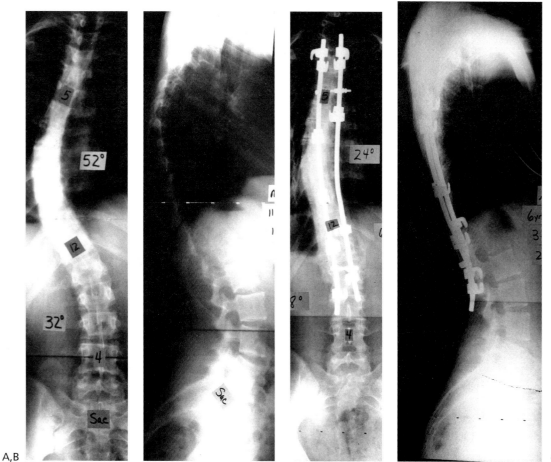

A,B

C,D

FIGURE 18. This was a left thoracic curve that was somewhat hyperkyphotic. Most right thoracic curves are hypokyphotic. The patient's magnetic resonance imaging study was normal. Instrumented forces were applied to the convexity first to correct the sagittal deformity. The correction of the deformity in the coronal plane and sagittal plane was achieved with the instrumentation. The correction in the axial plane was achieved by the thoracoplasty. **A:** Standing coronal radiograph preoperatively. **B:** Standing sagittal radiograph preoperatively. **C:** Standing coronal radiograph postoperatively. **D:** Standing sagittal radiograph postoperatively. *(Figure continues.)*

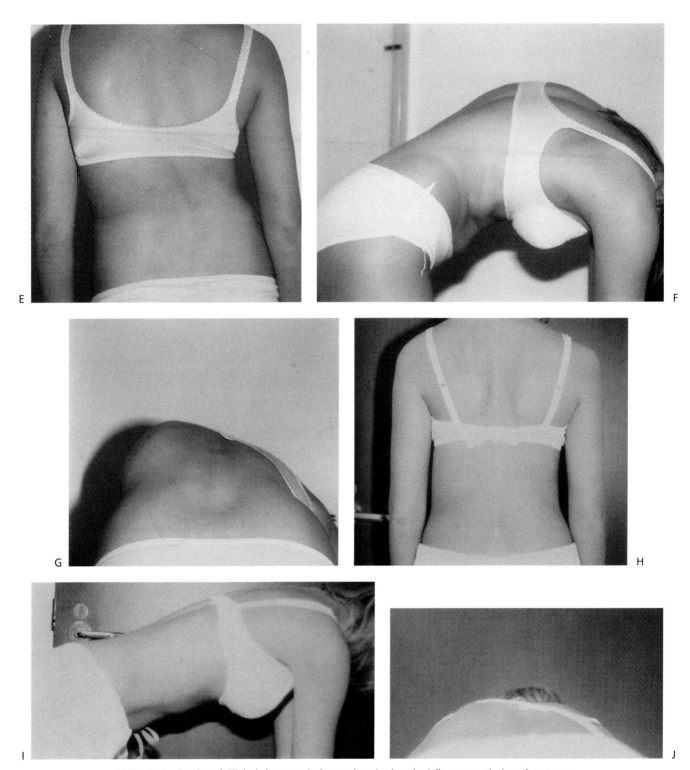

FIGURE 18. *Continued.* Clinical photographs (coronal, sagittal, and axial) preoperatively and postoperatively.

erythropoietin are all potential means of reducing the need for allogenic blood transfusion in patients with idiopathic adolescent scoliosis (3,87,91,95,98,106,114,121).

POSTOPERATIVE MANAGEMENT AND COMPLICATIONS

The average hospital stay for an idiopathic scoliosis patient at our institution in 1999 is 4 to 6 days. We usually stand the patient at the bedside the day after surgery. In most cases, no external protection is used. A brace may be advisable if the patient is very small or judged to be unreliable. This is the exception and not the rule. Recovery from the surgery can be represented as a bell-shaped curve. At the middle of the bell-shaped curve is to be off of all pain medications by 4 to 6 weeks after surgery. During the hospital stay, intravenous narcotics are used during the first 3 days and then the patient is transitioned to oral pain medications.

All patients develop inappropriate antidiuretic hormone syndrome postoperatively (6,88). This usually resolves on the second or third postoperative day without any specific treatment. The tendency is for the patient to retain fluid and have somewhat limited urine output for the first 48 hours and then to have a significant diuresis between 48 and 72 hours after surgery. Most patients develop an ileus, in part from the surgery itself, in part from the anesthesia, and in part from the postoperative pain medication. Uncommonly, a very thin patient, especially with a component of hyperkyphosis, may develop a frank supermesenteric cautery syndrome, which requires several days of a nasogastric tube and intravenous fluids (13).

Postoperative regimens within the first year after the surgery are arbitrary and have not been tested scientifically. I generally tell patients to avoid bending, stooping, twisting, and heavy lifting for the first 4 months after surgery. At 4 postoperative months, some bicycling and swimming is allowed. After 7 months, patients can hit a tennis ball over the net. Running and jumping are restricted until 12 months after surgery. At that time, I generally allow patients to return to noncontact competitive sports, such as soccer and baseball and usually advise against contact sports either indefinitely or until 2 years after surgery. These are all arbitrary guidelines and are not necessarily substantiated by a specific peer-review publication.

The most commonly feared complications with surgical treatment of idiopathic scoliosis include pseudarthrosis, implant failure, decompensation, and neurologic deficit. The exact incidence of pseudarthrosis is not clear and probably can only be determined with present-day instrumentation after a minimal 5-year follow-up. The pseudarthrosis rate with anterior-only constructs may be higher than what it is for posterior-only constructs (9,14).

Wound infections, although uncommon, occur occasionally. If a deep wound infection occurs, it is advisable to return the patient to the operating room, thoroughly irrigate and débride the wound, and close over tubes with an additional period of intravenous antibiotics. The number of days that drainage tubes are used and the length of time that intravenous antibiotics are given has to be individualized to the particular case and offend-

ing organism. In virtually all cases, it is advisable to retain the bone graft and instrumentation until the fusion is solid. Anterior infections, especially in idiopathic scoliosis, are uncommon (90,135). At my institution, we have never had a deep anterior infection in a teenage idiopathic scoliosis patient.

There is an incidence of late infection. Some investigators have referred to this as "fretting corrosion," but most believe this is a low-grade infection (23,111). In some instances, this represents a low-grade infection that was present since the time of the surgery. In other instances, it may represent a late hematogenous seeding of the implants. In both instances, the organism is usually of low virulence, and removal of the implants when the fusion is solid appears to eradicate the infection without the need for long-term antibiotics.

Minor neurologic deficits may occur with surgical treatment of idiopathic scoliosis. There is an incidence of brachial plexus irritation associated with positioning for anterior or posterior approaches (100). These plexopathies usually resolve with time. At my institution, spinal cord monitoring usually includes monitoring of the upper extremities to avoid postoperative deficit of the upper extremities from brachial plexus compression (100). If pedicle screws are being used, there is some potential for irritation of a nerve root. If pedicle screws are used frequently in the lumbar spine, one has to anticipate an occasional, although small, incidence of nerve root irritation (80).

The most dreaded complication with idiopathic scoliosis is a major paraparesis or paraplegia. This is extremely uncommon with idiopathic adolescent scoliosis (17,67,86). Patients at greatest risk are those with either large or hyperkyphotic curves and curves that are treated in a circumferential manner (17). The consequences of a major neurologic deficit in an otherwise healthy idiopathic scoliosis patient are devastating from the social, ethical, medico-legal, and financial perspectives. Therefore, some form of spinal cord monitoring is mandatory during idiopathic scoliosis surgery. Options for monitoring include the Stagnara wake-up test (44), the Hoppenfeld clonus test (54), somatosensory potential monitoring of upper and lower extremities, and motor potential monitoring of lower extremities (21,35,94,103,109). Which combination is most cost-effective is open for debate.

After an instrumented correction of an idiopathic scoliosis deformity, however, it is wise to establish some form of feedback regarding the patient's neurologic function before the wound is closed and the patient is awakened. Our institutional preference is to perform somatosensory and motor evoked potential monitoring. If these tracings are reliable and reproducible throughout the case, we rely on them exclusively (104). If there are any inconsistencies or limitation to the data, we perform a Stagnara wake-up test. In all instances, we rehearse the Stagnara wake-up test with the patient preoperatively to facilitate its performance if it is needed. If a major neurologic deficit does occur after spinal instrumentation for idiopathic scoliosis, advisable considerations include raising the patient's mean blood pressure, removing or revising the instrumentation, and in some cases, transfusing the patient to normalize the oxygen-carrying capacity of the blood (Table 6).

TABLE 6. COMPLICATIONS OF SURGERY

Imbalance (coronal or sagittal)
Junctional kyphosis (proximal or distal)
Pseudarthrosis
Pain at spine and graft sites
Paralysis (spinal cord or nerve root etiology: major or minor)
Lateral femoral cutaneous nerve palsy (from prone positioning on the frame)
Wound infection (superficial or deep)
Superior mesenteric artery syndrome
Scapulothoracic pain
Loss of segmental lumbar lordosis

EVOLUTION OF SPINAL INSTRUMENTATION

From the 1960s to the 1990s, techniques of spinal fusion remained constant; however, instrumentation evolved into greater segmentalization. This provides improved correction in the coronal and sagittal planes, although in most instances, not dramatic correction in the axial plane. On balance, there is no evidence to suggest that greater segmentalization of the instrumentation reduces the fusion rate. When using new technologies, there is always a learning curve. The most commonly used posterior implants are somewhat lower profile today than they were several years ago. There are relative merits to anterior versus posterior instrumentation.

As stated earlier, thoracoscopic fusions and instrumentations are being performed by some investigators. Various methods of spinal deformity correction of lumbar segments, without fusion, are also being investigated (81).

SUMMARY AND THE FUTURE

The goals of surgery for idiopathic scoliosis are to achieve acceptable correction, maintain coronal and sagittal balance, fuse as few segments as possible, and return the patient to function as quickly as possible. Are patients and their families happier if they get 70% versus 50% correction? The answer is probably yes (43), but only if additional correction can be achieved without added complications or morbidity (19). Also, whenever a surgeon recommends a surgical procedure for an adolescent patient, it behooves the surgeon to consider the effect of the surgery on the patient 5, 10, 20, 30, and 50 years after the procedure is completed. Obviously, we do not have all of the answers regarding the effects of scoliosis surgery on aging of the spine.

REFERENCES

1. Asher MA (1997): Isola spinal instrumentation system for scoliosis. In: Bridwell KH, DeWald RL, eds. *The textbook of spinal surgery,* 2nd ed., chap. 39. Philadelphia: Lippincott-Raven, pp. 569–609.
2. Ashman RB, Herring JA, Johnston CE (1991): Texas Scottish Rite Hospital (TSRH) instrumentation system. In: Bridwell KH, DeWald RL, eds. *The textbook of spinal surgery,* 1st ed., chap. 10. Philadelphia: JB Lippincott, pp. 219–248.
3. Bailey TE Jr, Mahoney OM (1987): The use of banked autologous blood in patients undergoing surgery for spinal deformity. *J Bone Joint Surg Am* 69:329–332.
4. Barr SJ, Schuette AM, Emans JB (1997): Lumbar pedicle screws versus hooks: results in double major curves in adolescent idiopathic scoliosis. *Spine* 22:1369–1379.
5. Barrett DS, MacLean JG, Bettany J, et al. (1993): Costoplasty in adolescent idiopathic scoliosis: objective results in 55 patients. *J Bone Joint Surg Br* 75:881–885.
6. Bell GR, Gurd AR, Orlowski JP, et al. (1986): The syndrome of inappropriate antidiuretic hormone secretion following spinal fusion. *J Bone Joint Surg Am* 68:720–724.
7. Bernhardt M, Bridwell KH (1989): Segmental analysis of the sagittal plane alignment of the normal thoracic and lumbar spines and thoracolumbar junction. *Spine* 14:717–721.
8. Betz RR (1997): Thoracoplasty: posterior technique. In: Bridwell KH, DeWald RL, eds. *The textbook of spinal surgery,* 2nd ed., chap. 34. Philadelphia: Lippincott-Raven, pp. 451–461.
9. Betz RR, Harms J, Clements DH III, et al. (1999): Comparison of anterior versus posterior instrumentation for correction of adolescent thoracic idiopathic scoliosis. *Spine* 24:225–239.
10. Blanco JS, Sears CJ (1997): Allograft bone use during instrumentation and fusion in the treatment of adolescent idiopathic scoliosis. *Spine* 22:1338–1342.
11. Booth KC, Bridwell KH, Lenke LG, et al. (1999): Complications and predictive factors for the successful treatment of flatback deformity (fixed sagittal imbalance). *Spine* 24:1712–1720.
12. Bradford DS, Blatt JM, Rasp FL (1983): Surgical management of severe thoracic lordosis: a new technique to restore normal kyphosis. *Spine* 8:420–428.
13. Bridwell KH (1991): Idiopathic scoliosis. In: Bridwell KH, DeWald RL, eds. *The textbook of spinal surgery,* 1st ed., chap. 7. Philadelphia: JB Lippincott, pp. 97–162.
14. Bridwell KH (1994): Surgical treatment of adolescent idiopathic scoliosis: the basics and the controversies. *Spine* 19:1095–1100.
15. Bridwell KH (1997): Spinal instrumentation in the management of adolescent scoliosis. *Clin Orthop* 335:64–72.
16. Bridwell KH, Betz RR, Capelli AM, et al. (1990): Sagittal plane analysis in idiopathic scoliosis patients treated with Cotrel-Dubousset instrumentation. *Spine* 15:644–649.
17. Bridwell KH, Lenke LG, Baldus C, et al. (1998): Major intraoperative neurologic deficits in pediatric and adult spinal deformity patients: incidence and etiology at one institution. *Spine* 23:324–331.
18. Bridwell KH, McAllister JW, Betz RR, et al. (1991): Coronal decompensation produced by Cotrel-Dubousset "derotation" maneuver for idiopathic right thoracic scoliosis. *Spine* 16:769–777.
19. Bridwell KH, Shufflebarger HL, Lenke LG, et al. (9/15/00) Parent/patient preference and concerns in idiopathic adolescent scoliosis: a prospective preoperative analysis. *Spine* (in press).
20. Brown CA, Lenke LG, Bridwell KH, et al. (1998): Complications of pediatric thoracolumbar and lumbar pedicle screws. *Spine* 23:1566–1571.
21. Brown RH, Nash CL, Berilla JA, et al. (1984): Cortical evoked potential monitoring: a system for intraoperative monitoring of spinal cord function. *Spine* 9:256–261.
22. Cheung KM, Luk KD (1997): Prediction of correction of scoliosis with use of the fulcrum bending radiograph. *J Bone Joint Surg Am* 79:1144–1150.
23. Clark C, Shufflebarger H. Late developing infection in instrumented idiopathic scoliosis. *Spine* 24:1909–1912.
24. Cochran T, Irstam L, Nachemson A (1983). Long-term anatomic and functional changes in patients with adolescent idiopathic scoliosis treated by Harrington rod fusion. *Spine* 8:576–584.
25. Connolly PJ, Von Schroeder HP, Johnson GE, et al. (1995): Adolescent idiopathic scoliosis: long-term effect of instrumentation extending to the lumbar spine. *J Bone Joint Surg Am* 77:1210–1216.
26. Cotrel Y, Dubousset J, Guillaumat M (1988): New universal instrumentation in spinal surgery. *Clin Orthop* 227:10–23.
27. Cummings RJ, Loveless EA, Campbell J, et al. (1998): Interobserver reliability and intraobserver reproducibility of the system of King et

al for the classification of adolescent idiopathic scoliosis. *J Bone Joint Surg Am* 80:1107–1111.

28. Davies AG, McMaster MJ (1992): The effect of Luque-rod instrumentation on the sagittal contour of the lumbosacral spine in adolescent idiopathic scoliosis and the preservation of a physiologic lumbar lordosis. *Spine* 17:112–115.

29. Dickson JH, Wendell ED, Rossi D (1990): Harrington instrumentation and arthrodesis for idiopathic scoliosis: a 21 year follow-up. *J Bone Joint Surg Am* 72:678–683.

30. Dodd CAF, Fergusson CM, Freedman L, et al. (1988): Allograft versus autograft bone in scoliosis surgery. *J Bone Joint Surg Br* 70: 431–434.

31. Drummond DS (1988): Harrington instrumentation with spinous process wiring for idiopathic scoliosis. *Orthop Clin North Am* 19: 281–289.

32. Dubousset J, Shufflebarger HL, Herring JA (1989): The crankshaft phenomenon. *J Pediatr Orthop* 9:541–550.

33. Dwyer AF, Schafer MF (1974): Anterior approach to scoliosis: results of treatment in fifty-one cases. *J Bone Joint Surg Br* 56:218–224.

34. Edgar MA, Mehta MH (1988): Long-term follow-up of fused and unfused idiopathic scoliosis. *J Bone Joint Surg Br* 70:712–716.

35. Engler GL, Spielholz NI, Bernhard WN, et al. (1978): Somatosensory evoked potentials during Harrington instrumentation for scoliosis. *J Bone Joint Surg Am* 60:528–532.

36. Fabry G, Van Melkebeek J, Bockx E (1989): Back pain after Harrington rod instrumentation for idiopathic scoliosis. *Spine* 14:620–624.

37. Falatyn SP, Betz RR, Clements DH, et al. (1997): Allograft versus no graft with posterior multisegmented hook systems for the treatment of idiopathic scoliosis. *Orthop Trans* 21:460.

38. Farcy JPC, Schwab FJ (1997): Management of flatback and related kyphotic decompensation syndromes. *Spine* 22:2452—2457.

39. Geissele AE, Ogilvie JW, Cohen M, et al. (1994): Thoracoplasty for the treatment of rib prominence in thoracic scoliosis. *Spine* 19: 1636–1642.

40. Giehl JP, Zielke K (1991): Zielke procedures in scoliosis correction. In: Bridwell KH, DeWald RL, eds. *The textbook of spinal surgery*, 1st ed. Philadelphia: JB Lippincott, pp. 163–182.

41. Goldberg CJ, Dowling FE, Fogarty EE (1994): Left thoracic scoliosis configurations: why so different? *Spine* 19:1385–1389.

42. Guadagni J, Drummond D, Breed A (1984): Improved postoperative course following modified segmental instrumentation and posterior spinal fusion for idiopathic scoliosis. *J Pediatr Orthop* 4:405–408.

43. Haher TR, Merola A, Zipnick RI, et al. (1995): Meta-analysis of surgical outcome in adolescent idiopathic scoliosis: a 35-year English literature review of 11,000 patients. *Spine* 20:1575–1584.

44. Hall JE, Levine CR, Sudhir KG (1978): Intraoperative awakening to monitor spinal cord function during Harrington instrumentation and fusion: description of procedure and report of three cases. *J Bone Joint Surg Am* 60:533–536.

45. Hall JE, Millis MB, Snyder BD (1997): Short segment anterior instrumentation for thoracolumbar scoliosis. In: Bridwell KH, DeWald RL, eds. *The textbook of spinal surgery*, 2nd ed., chap. 43. Philadelphia: Lippincott-Raven, pp. 665–674.

46. Hamill CL, Bridwell KH, Lenke LG, et al. (1997): Posterior arthrodesis in the skeletally immature patient: assessing the risk for crankshaft. Is an open triradiate cartilage the answer? *Spine* 22:1343–1351.

47. Hamill CL, Lenke LG, Bridwell KH, et al. (1996): The use of pedicle screw fixation to improve correction in the lumbar spine of patients with idiopathic scoliosis: is it warranted? *Spine* 21:1241–1249.

48. Harms J, Jeszenszky D, Beele B (1997): Ventral correction of thoracic scoliosis. In: Bridwell KH, DeWald RL, eds. *The textbook of spinal surgery*, 2nd ed., chap. 40. Philadelphia: Lippincott-Raven, pp. 611–626.

49. Harrington PR (1960): Surgical instrumentation for management of scoliosis. *J Bone Joint Surg Am* 42:1448.

50. Harrington PR (1962): Treatment of scoliosis: correction and internal fixation by spine instrumentation. *J Bone Joint Surg Am* 44:591–610.

51. Hibbs RA (1924): A report of 59 cases of scoliosis treated by the fusion operation. *J Bone Joint Surg* 6:3–37.

52. Hilibrand AS, Tannenbaum DA, Graziano GP, et al. (1995): The sagittal alignment of the cervical spine in adolescent idiopathic scoliosis. *J Pediatr Orthop* 15:627–632.

53. Hopf CG, Eysel P, Dubousset J (1997): Operative treatment of scoliosis with Cotrel-Dubousset-Hopf instrumentation: new anterior spinal device. *Spine* 22:618–627.

54. Hoppenfeld S, Gross A, Andrews C, et al. (1997): The ankle clonus test for assessment of the integrity of the spinal cord during operations for scoliosis. *J Bone Joint Surg Am* 79:208–212.

55. Horton WC, Holt RT, Johnson JR, et al. (1988): Zielke instrumentation in idiopathic scoliosis: late effects and minimizing complications. *Spine* 13:1145–1149.

56. Jarvis JG, Greene RN (1996): Adolescent idiopathic scoliosis: correction of vertebral rotation with use of Wisconsin segmental spinal instrumentation. *J Bone Joint Surg Am* 78:1707–1712.

57. Jeng CL, Sponseller PD, Tolo VT (1993): Outcome of Wisconsin instrumentation in idiopathic scoliosis: minimum 5-year follow-up. *Spine* 18:1584–1590.

58. Johnston CE II, Ashman RB, Richards BS, et al. (1997): TSRH universal spine instrumentation. In: Bridwell KH, DeWald RL, eds. *The textbook of spinal surgery*, 2nd ed., chap. 38. Philadelphia: Lippincott-Raven, pp. 535–567.

59. Kaneda K, Fujiya N, Satoh S (1986): Results with Zielke instrumentation for idiopathic thoracolumbar and lumbar scoliosis. *Clin Orthop* 205:195–203.

60. Kaneda K, Shono Y (1997): Kaneda anterior multisegmental instrumentation: two-rod system for the treatment of thoracolumbar and lumbar scoliotic curvatures. In: Bridwell KH, DeWald RL, eds. *The textbook of spinal surgery*, 2nd ed., chap. 42. Philadelphia: Lippincott-Raven, pp. 641–663.

61. Kaneda K, Shono Y, Satoh S, et al. (1996): New anterior instrumentation for the management of thoracolumbar and lumbar scoliosis: application of the Kaneda two-rod system. *Spine* 21:1250–1261.

62. Kaneda K, Shono Y, Satoh S, et al. (1997): Anterior correction of thoracic scoliosis with Kaneda anterior spinal system: a preliminary report. *Spine* 22:1358–1368.

63. King HA, Moe JH, Bradford DS, et al. (1983): The selection of fusion levels in thoracic idiopathic scoliosis. *J Bone Joint Surg Am* 65: 1302–1313.

64. Kinnear WJ, Johnston ID (1993): Does Harrington instrumentation improve pulmonary function in adolescents with idiopathic scoliosis? A meta-analysis. *Spine* 18:1556–1559.

65. Kostuik JP, Maurais GR, Richardson WJ, et al. (1988): Combined single stage anterior and posterior osteotomy for correction of iatrogenic lumbar kyphosis. *Spine* 13:257–266.

66. LaGrone MO, Bradford DS, Moe JH, et al. (1988): Treatment of symptomatic flatback after spinal fusion. *J Bone Joint Surg Am* 70: 569–580.

67. LaGrone MO, King HA (1997): Idiopathic adolescent scoliosis: indications and expectations. In: Bridwell KH, DeWald RL, eds. *The textbook of spinal surgery*, 2nd ed., chap. 33. Philadelphia: Lippincott-Raven, pp. 425–450.

68. Lee CK, Denis F, Winter RB, et al. (1993): Analysis of the upper thoracic curve in surgically treated idiopathic scoliosis: a new concept of the double thoracic curve pattern. *Spine* 18:1599–1608.

69. Lee CS, Nachemson AL (1997): The crankshaft phenomenon after posterior Harrington fusion in skeletally immature patients with thoracic or thoracolumbar idiopathic scoliosis followed to maturity. *Spine* 22:58–67.

70. Lee GA, Betz RR, Clements DH III, et al. (1999): Proximal kyphosis after posterior spinal fusion in patients with idiopathic scoliosis. *Spine* 24:795–799.

71. Lenke LG, Betz RR, Bridwell KH, et al. (1998): Intraobserver and interobserver reliability in the classification of thoracic adolescent idiopathic scoliosis. *J Bone Joint Surg Am* 80:1097–1106.

72. Lenke LG, Betz RR, Bridwell KH, et al. (1999): Spontaneous lumbar curve coronal correction after selective anterior or posterior thoracic fusion in adolescent idiopathic scoliosis. *Spine* 24:1663–1671.

73. Lenke LG, Bridwell KH, Baldus C, et al. (1992): Preventing decompensation in King type II curves treated with Cotrel-Dubousset instru-

mentation: strict guidelines for selective thoracic fusion. *Spine* 17S: 274–281.

74. Lenke LG, Bridwell KH, Baldus C, et al. (1992): Analysis of pulmonary function and axis rotation in adolescent and young adult idiopathic scoliosis patients treated with Cotrel-Dubousset instrumentation. *J Spinal Disord* 5:16–25.

75. Lenke LG, Bridwell KH, Baldus C, et al. (1992): Cotrel-Dubousset instrumentation for adolescent idiopathic scoliosis. *J Bone Joint Surg Am* 74:1056–1067.

76. Lenke LG, Bridwell KH, Baldus C, et al. (1993): Ability of Cotrel-Dubousset instrumentation to preserve distal lumbar motion segments in idiopathic scoliosis. *J Spinal Disord* 6:339–350.

77. Lenke LG, Bridwell KH, Blanke K, et al. (1995): Analysis of pulmonary function and chest cage dimension changes after thoracoplasty in idiopathic scoliosis. *Spine* 20:1343–1350.

78. Lenke LG, Bridwell KH, Blanke K, et al. (1998): Radiographic results of arthrodesis with Cotrel-Dubousset instrumentation for the treatment of adolescent idiopathic scoliosis: a 5 to 10 year follow-up study. *J Bone Joint Surg Am* 80A:807–814.

79. Lenke LG, Bridwell KH, O'Brien MF, et al. (1994): Recognition and treatment of the proximal thoracic curve in adolescent idiopathic scoliosis treated with Cotrel-Dubousset instrumentation. *Spine* 19:1589–1597.

80. Lenke LG, Padberg AM, Russo MH, et al. (1995): Triggered electromyographic stimulation threshold for accuracy of pedicle screw placement: an animal model and clinical correlation. *Spine* 20:1585–1591.

81. Lindseth RE, Kling TF (1999): *Wedge vertebral body osteotomy for correction of lumbar scoliosis.* Paper presented at the 6th International Meeting on Advanced Spine Techniques, Vancouver, BC, Canada, July 8–10.

82. Lovallo JL, Banta JV, Renshaw TS (1986): Adolescent idiopathic scoliosis treated by Harrington rod distraction and fusion. *J Bone Joint Surg Am* 68:1326–1330.

83. Lowe TG, Peters JD (1993): Anterior spinal fusion with Zielke instrumentation for idiopathic scoliosis: a frontal and sagittal curve analysis in 36 patients. *Spine* 18:423–426.

84. Luk KDK, Lee FB, Leong JCY, et al. (1987): The effect on the lumbosacral spine of long spinal fusion for idiopathic scoliosis: a minimum of 10-year follow-up. *Spine* 12:996–1000.

85. Luque ER (1982): Segmental spinal instrumentation for correction of scoliosis. *Clin Orthop* 163:192–198.

86. MacEwen GD, Bunnel WP, Sriram K (1975): Acute neurological complications in the treatment of scoliosis. *J Bone Joint Surg Am* 57:404–408.

87. Macolm-Smith NA, McMaster MJ (1983): The use of induced hypotension to control bleeding during posterior fusion for scoliosis. *J Bone Joint Surg Br* 65:255–258.

88. Mason RJ, Betz RR, Orlowski JP, et al. (1989): The syndrome of inappropriate antidiuretic hormone secretion and its effect on blood indices following spinal fusion. *Spine* 14:722–726.

89. McCance SE, Denis F, Lonstein JE, et al. (1998): Coronal and sagittal balance in surgically treated adolescent idiopathic scoliosis with the King II curve pattern: a review of 67 consecutive cases having selective thoracic arthrodesis. *Spine* 23:2063–2073.

90. McDonnell MF, Glassman SD, Dimar JR II, et al. (1996): Perioperative complications of anterior procedures on the spine. *J Bone Joint Surg* 78:839–847.

91. McNeill TW, DeWald RL, Kuo KN (1974): Controlled hypotensive anesthesia in scoliosis surgery. *J Bone Joint Surg Am* 56:1167–1172.

92. Mehlman CT, Crawford AH, Wolf RK (1997): Video-assisted thoracoscopic surgery (VATS): endoscopic thoracoplasty technique. *Spine* 22:2178–2182.

93. Michel CR, Lalain JJ (1985): Late results of Harrington's operation: long-term evolution of the lumbar spine below the fused segments. *Spine* 10:414–420.

94. Mineiro J, Weinstein SL (1997): Delayed postoperative paraparesis in scoliosis surgery: a case report. *Spine* 22:1668–1672.

95. Moran MM, Kroon D, Tredwell SJ, et al. (1995): The role of autologous blood transfusion in adolescents undergoing spinal surgery. *Spine* 20:532–536.

96. Moskowitz A, Moe JH, Winter RB, et al. (1980): Long-term follow-up of scoliosis fusion. *J Bone Joint Surg Am* 62:364–376.

97. Mullaji AB, Upadhyay SS, Luk KD, et al. (1994): Vertebral growth after posterior spinal fusion for idiopathic scoliosis in skeletally immature adolescents: the effect of growth on spinal deformity. *J Bone Joint Surg Br* 76:870–876.

98. Murray DJ, Forbes RB, Titone MB, et al. (1997): Transfusion management in pediatric and adolescent scoliosis surgery: efficacy of autologous blood. *Spine* 22:2735–2740.

99. Newton PO, Wenger DR, Mubarak SJ, et al. (1997): Anterior release and fusion in pediatric spinal deformity: a comparison of early outcome and cost of thoracoscopic and open thoracotomy approaches. *Spine* 22:1398–1406.

100. O'Brien MF, Lenke LG, Bridwell KH, et al. (1994): Evoked potential monitoring of the upper extremities during thoracic and lumbar spinal deformity surgery: A prospective study. *J Spinal Disord* 7:277–284.

101. Ogiela DM, Chan DPK (1986): Ventral derotation spondylodesis: a review of 22 cases. *Spine* 11:18–22.

102. Ogilvie JW (1988): Anterior spine fusion with Zielke instrumentation for idiopathic scoliosis in adolescents. *Orthop Clin North Am* 19:313–317.

103. Owen JH, Laschinger J, Bridwell KH (1988): Sensitivity and specificity of somatosensory and neurogenic-motor evoked potential in animals and humans. *Spine* 13:1111–1118.

104. Padberg AM, Wilson-Holden TJ, Lenke LG, et al. (1998): Somatosensory- and motor-evoked potential monitoring without a wake-up test during idiopathic scoliosis surgery: an accepted standard of care. *Spine* 23:1392–1400.

105. Paonessa KS, Engler GL (1992): Back pain and disability after Harrington rod fusion to the lumbar spine for scoliosis. *Spine* 17[Suppl]:249–253.

106. Patel NJ, Patel BS, Paskin S, et al. (1985): Induced moderate hypotensive anesthesia for spinal fusion and Harrington-rod instrumentation. *J Bone Joint Surg Am* 67:1384–1387.

107. Picetti GD III, Ertl JP, Bueff UH, et al. (1999): *Correction and fusion of thoracic scoliosis using an endoscopic approach.* Paper No. 151 presented at the annual meeting of the American Academy of Orthopaedic Surgeons, Anaheim, CA, February 4–8.

108. Polly DW Jr, Sturm PF (1998): Traction versus supine side bending. Which technique best determines curve flexibility? *Spine* 23:804–808.

109. Potenza V, Weinstein SL, Neyt JG (1998): Dysfunction of the spinal cord during spinal arthrodesis for scoliosis: recommendations for early detection and treatment. A case report. *J Bone Joint Surg Am* 80:1679–1683.

110. Richards BS (1992): Lumbar curve response in type II idiopathic scoliosis after posterior instrumentation of the thoracic curve. *Spine* 17[Suppl]:282–286.

111. Richards BS (1995): Delayed infections following posterior spinal instrumentation for the treatment of idiopathic scoliosis. *J Bone Joint Surg Am* 77:524–529.

112. Richards BS, Birch JG, Herring JA, et al. (1989): Frontal plane and sagittal plane balance following Cotrel-Dubousset instrumentation for idiopathic scoliosis. *Spine* 14:733–737.

113. Richards BS, Herring JA, Johnston CE, et al. Treatment of adolescent idiopathic scoliosis using Texas Scottish Rite Hospital instrumentation. *Spine* 19:1598–1605.

114. Roye DP Jr, Rothstein P, Rickert JB, et al. (1992): The use of preoperative erythropoietin in scoliosis surgery. *Spine* 17[Suppl]:204–205.

115. Sanders JO, Herring JA, Browne RH (1995): Posterior arthrodesis and instrumentation in the immature (Risser-grade-0) spine in idiopathic scoliosis. *J Bone Joint Surg Am* 77:39–45.

116. Sanders JO, Little DG, Richards BS (1997): Prediction of the crankshaft phenomenon by peak height velocity. *Spine* 22:1352–1356.

117. Sawatzky BJ, Tredwell SJ, Jang SB, et al. (1998): Effects of three-dimensional assessment on surgical correction and on hook strategies in multi-hook instrumentation for adolescent idiopathic scoliosis. *Spine* 23:201–205.

118. Shufflebarger HL (1997): Thoracoplasty: anterior technique. In: Bridwell KH, DeWald RL, eds. *The textbook of spinal surgery,* 2nd ed., chap. 35. Philadelphia: Lippincott-Raven, pp. 463–468.

119. Shufflebarger HL (1997): Moss Miami instrumentation. In: Bridwell KH, DeWald RL, eds. *The textbook of spinal surgery.* 2nd ed., chap. 44. Philadelphia: Lippincott-Raven, pp. 675–693.

120. Shufflebarger HL, King WF (1987): Composite measurement of scoliosis: a new method of analysis of the deformity. *Spine* 12:228–232.

121. Siller TA, Dickson JH, Erwin WD (1996): Efficacy and cost considerations of intraoperative autologous transfusion in spinal fusion for idiopathic scoliosis with predeposited blood. *Spine* 21:848–852.

122. Smith RM, Dickson RA (1994): Changes in residual volume relative to vital capacity and total lung capacity after arthrodesis of the spine in patients who have adolescent idiopathic scoliosis. (Comment). *J Bone Joint Surg Am* 76:153.

123. Steel HH (1983): Rib resection and spine fusion in correction of convex deformity in scoliosis. *J Bone Joint Surg Am* 65:920–925.

124. Suk SI, Lee CK, Jeong ST (1995): Segmental pedicle screw fixation in the treatment of thoracic idiopathic scoliosis. *Spine* 20:1399–1405.

125. Sweet FA, Lenke LG, Bridwell KH, et al. (1999): Maintaining lumbar lordosis with anterior single solid rod instrumentation in thoracolumbar and lumbar adolescent idiopathic scoliosis. *Spine* 24:1655–1662.

126. Takahashi S, Delecrin J, Passuti N (1997): Changes in the unfused lumbar spine in patients with idiopathic scoliosis: a 5- to 9-year assessment after Cotrel-Dubousset instrumentation. *Spine* 22:517–523.

127. Takahashi S, Passuti N, Delecrin J (1997): Interpretation and utility of traction radiography in scoliosis surgery: analysis of patients treated with Cotrel-Dubousset instrumentation. *Spine* 22:2542–2546.

128. Thompson JP, Transfeldt EE, Bradford DS, et al. (1990): Decompensation after Cotrel-Dubousset instrumentation of idiopathic scoliosis. *Spine* 15:927–931.

129. Turi M, Johnston II CE, Richards BS (1993): Anterior correction of idiopathic scoliosis using TSRH instrumentation. *Spine* 18:417–422.

130. Upadhyay SS, Ho EK, Gunawardene WM, et al. (1993): Changes in residual volume relative to vital capacity and total lung capacity after arthrodesis of the spine in patients who have adolescent idiopathic scoliosis. *J Bone Joint Surg Am* 75:46–52.

131. Vedantam R, Crawford AH (1998): The role of preoperative pulmonary function tests in patients with adolescent idiopathic scoliosis undergoing posterior spinal fusion. *Spine* 22:2731–2734.

132. Vedantam R, Lenke LG, Bridwell KH, et al. (2000): A prospective evaluation of pulmonary function in patients with adolescent idiopathic scoliosis relative to surgical approach used for spinal arthrodesis. *Spine* 25:82–90.

133. Weinstein SL (1986): Idiopathic scoliosis: natural history. *Spine* 11:780–783.

134. Weinstein SL, Ponseti IV (1983): Curve progression in idiopathic scoliosis. *J Bone Joint Surg Am* 65:447–455.

135. Weis JC, Betz RR, Clements DH III, et al. (1997): Prevalence of perioperative complications after anterior spinal fusion for patients with idiopathic scoliosis. *J Spinal Disord* 10:371–375.

136. Winter RB (1986): Briefly noted: Harrington instrumentation into the lumbar spine: technique for preservation of normal lumbar lordosis. *Spine* 11:633–635.

137. Winter RB (1992): Surgical correction of rigid thoracic lordoscoliosis. *J Spinal Disord* 5:108–111.

138. Winter RB, Lovell WW, Moe JH (1975): Excessive thoracic lordosis and loss of pulmonary function in patients with idiopathic scoliosis. *J Bone Joint Surg Am* 57:972–977.

139. Wood KB, Schendel MJ, Dekutoski MB, et al. (1996): Thoracic volume changes in scoliosis surgery. *Spine* 21:718–723.

140. Wood KB, Transfeldt EE, Ogilvie JW, et al. (1991): Rotational changes of the vertebral-pelvic axis following Cotrel-Dubousset instrumentation. *Spine* 16[Suppl]:404–408.

SCHEUERMANN KYPHOSIS

ELIO ASCANI
GUIDO LA ROSA
CLAUDIO ASCANI

In 1921, Holger Scheuermann described a typically juvenile kyphotic vertebral disorder that could be distinguished from asthenic (postural) kyphosis on the basis of a peculiar rigidity (94). This condition, known as Scheuermann kyphosis, is radiographically characterized by vertebral wedging and causes a growth disturbance of the vertebral end plates (8,55). Scheuermann kyphosis affects 0.5% to 8% of healthy subjects (4,5,78), with a prevalence in the male population.

ETIOLOGIC FACTORS

The cause of Scheuermann disease has been a matter of controversy and is essentially still unknown. Scheuermann himself described it as a form of aseptic necrosis of the ring apophyses. The observations of Schmorl and Junghans (95) regarding the presence of intraspongy hernias as being typical of the disease led to the hypothesis of a weakening in the consistency of the cartilaginous end plate, with a consequent penetration of disc material and subsequent alteration of the endochondral ossification process, leading to kyphosis. The presence of Schmorl hernias (nodules) in vertebrae located outside the kyphotic areas as well as in patients not affected by Scheuermann kyphosis has challenged the credibility of this theory. Nevertheless, this mechanical theory has been endorsed by some authors who have observed greater tension in the anterior longitudinal ligament and a partial reduction of wedging through the use of corrective braces at a prepubertal age (27,103). Sorensen (98) observed a high familial incidence of the disease. Halal et al. (50) studied the genetic transmission pattern in five families having a high incidence of Scheuermann kyphosis and suggested an autosomal dominant hereditary mode of transmission with a high degree of penetrance and variable expressivity (43). Bradford (24) considers Scheuermann kyphosis to be a form of osteochondrosis. The association of juvenile dorsal kyphosis with dural cysts (1), Legg-Calvé-Perthes disease, hypertonia, hypotonia, polio, infectious processes, hypovitaminosis, and endocrine disorders has been suggested as the cause of Scheuermann kyphosis, but with a lower correlation index.

Hormone Studies

Investigations conducted in our department revealed a growth hormone hyperincretion (elevated levels of growth hormone) in Scheuermann kyphosis–affected patients (6,9). Although the kyphotic deformity was not corrected in these subjects, they were found to be taller than the percentile mean for their ages (97), and their bone age was more advanced than normal for their chronological age. The role of the growth hormone hyperincretion in the etiologic process of Scheuermann disease is still unclear. The increase in height recorded in these patients may be related to growth hormone hyperincretion (at least during the active stage of the disease). Earlier bone aging may be correlated with a qualitative rather than a quantitative alteration (early pubertal spurt) of sexual steroid secretion (6).

It remains to be shown whether the growth hormone hyperincretion is the primary cause of the disease or an attempt at compensation. In a study of 61 adult patients, Murray et al. (78) reported a mean height of 179 cm in men and 162 cm in women. These values are not considered significant in terms of subject height. However, it should be noted that these are real height values; the correction factor due to the severe kyphotic curve (mean Cobb angle for this series is 71 degrees) has not been taken into account.

According to Buckler's height diagrams for the Anglo-Saxon population, the mean values reported by Murray et al. were above the fiftieth percentile for both sexes (28).

It is possible to postulate that the growth hormone hyperincretion is limited to the pubertal period and then returns to normal. Unfortunately, no study has been conducted to assess growth hormone hyperincretion increase over the years. It is widely known that growth cartilage hypertrophy is the physiologic response of bone to growth hormone secretion. Hypertrophic areas have been reported in vertebral growth cartilage in histologic studies of vertebrae in persons with Scheuermann kyphosis.

Other hypotheses have been suggested by Bradford et al. (22), who have considered Scheuermann kyphosis as forms of juvenile osteoporosis and secondary to malabsorption (20,22,29,30). Lopez et al. (71) have confirmed this hypothesis by using dual-photon absorptiometry. Recently, however, Gillsanz et al. (46) studied vertebral bone density in Scheuermann kyphosis–affected patients by using quantitative computed tomography and observed normal ossification in all patients.

E. Ascani and G. La Rosa: Ospedale Bambino Gesu, Cemntro Cura Delle Deformita, Della Colonna, Roma 1 00050, Italy.
C. Ascani: Clinica San Giuseppe, Roma, Italy.

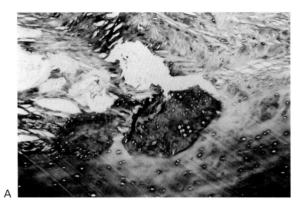

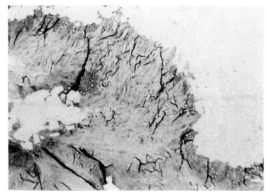

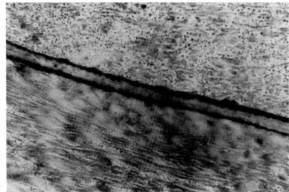

FIGURE 1. A: Vertebral cartilaginous end plate. Two strongly Alcian blue–positive pathologic areas, with many cells assembled in groups. These areas are clearly demarcated from the adjacent mainly period acid–Schiff–positive vertebral plate. **B:** Pathologic growth cartilage with a mosaic-like pattern—on the left, areas of hypertrophy; on the right, interruptions and areas where no cartilage is present. **C:** Matrix of pathologic areas: net reduction in the collagen fibers and an increase in the proteoglycans *(top)* close to the normal area.

Histologic Findings

Histologic studies of affected vertebrae demonstrate vertebral end plate and growth cartilage abnormalities, suggesting that the cause of the juvenile kyphosis may be an alteration of endochondral ossification. Aufdermaur (10,11) and Ippolito and Ponseti (56) have shown the presence of alterations in growth cartilage and in vertebral end plates in the absence of osteoporosis and without evidence of ring apophysis necrosis. The authors (8,9) carried out histologic, histochemical, and ultrastructural studies of vertebrae affected by Scheuermann kyphosis. The findings of these studies may be summarized as follows:

1. In Scheuermann kyphosis, the primary pathologic process is localized to altered areas of the growth cartilage and vertebral end plates according to a mosaic-like pattern (Fig. 1).
2. The alterations probably occur not only in the matrix but in the cells as well.
3. The matrix exhibits a lower number of collagen fibers and a greater proteoglycan content. The collagen fibers are also thinner.
4. The endochondral ossification process is altered: It is slowed down in the altered cartilage growth areas. In some areas it is absent, and direct bone formation on cartilage is seen without the deposition of bone on a necrotic and calcified cartilage model.
5. The longitudinal growth of the vertebra varies according to the variations in different regions.
6. The radiographic appearance of Scheuermann kyphosis

should be interpreted as an "absence of growth" rather than a destructive process (7).

On the basis of recent investigations, the authors believe that Scheuermann kyphosis is caused by disruption of endochondral ossification, which causes a severe alteration in the longitudinal growth of the vertebral end plate. The areas that appear as erosions on radiographs are actually areas of altered ossification, where bone is directly formed from cartilage. The areas that appear "normal" have accelerated growth rates (Fig. 2), as shown

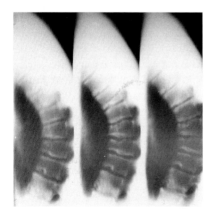

FIGURE 2. Typical radiographic alterations of Scheuermann kyphosis with vertebral end plate erosions, vertebral wedging, Schmorl hernias (nodules), and dorsal hyperkyphosis.

by the hyperplasia of conjugation cartilage. The influence of mechanical factors on this growth disturbance produces increasingly unfavorable effects that lead to a progressive increase in the wedging of vertebral bodies and kyphosis. Genetic factors surely play a role in the etiology of the disorder but are yet to be defined.

According to the studies obtained thus far, growth hormone hyperincretion has not yet been proved to be a primary etiologic factor; rather, it may occur in response to an unidentified metabolic condition. It is difficult to provide unequivocal data on the cause of this condition because the evaluation criteria used in case studies of Scheuermann kyphosis have not always been uniform.

INCIDENCE

Sorensen (98) reported a 0.4% to 8% incidence of Scheuermann kyphosis. Ascani et al. (5) reported a 1% incidence in 19,650 school-aged children (between age 10 and 14 years). Bradford et al. (18) reported an incidence of up to 10% in different levels of severity. Scheuermann reported a predominance in males, with 88% of his cases involving males (male/female ratio of 7.3:1). Murray et al. (78) also reported a male predominance, although the ratio was lower (2.2:1). Montgomery and Erwin (77), Sorensen (98), and Travaglini and Conte (104) reported an equal male/female ratio, and Bradford et al. (18) reported a greater female incidence (2:1). The male/female incidence ratio varies in the literature because of variable inclusion criteria for the studied populations.

CLINICAL PICTURE

The disease onset occurs in the prepubertal phase, at around age 10 years (23). No radiographic evidence of Scheuermann kyphosis has been reported in the literature in any patient younger than 10. In particular, vertebral body wedging has not been identified before age 10 because of the absence of ring apophysis ossification (13), making the vertebral plate profile curvilinear rather than rectilinear. Many forms of Scheuermann kyphosis are probably neglected in the early stages, as they are often labeled asthenic (postural) kyphoses (78). The main clinical difference between asthenic kyphosis and Scheuermann kyphosis is in the rigidity of the kyphotic curve, which in Scheuermann kyphosis makes the voluntary or forced correction of the deformity impossible (Fig. 3). There is also an increase in dorsal kyphosis in the forward flexion of the trunk in Scheuermann kyphosis, compared with a normalization of the lateral spine profile in asthenic kyphosis. Furthermore, patients with Scheuermann kyphosis often have a more athletic body habitus than asthenic patients affected by nonstructural kyphoses. Scheuermann kyphosis patients also frequently present with a contracture of pectoral muscles and hamstrings.

Curve Location

There are two major forms of Scheuermann kyphosis: the more common thoracic type, with the apex localized between T7 and

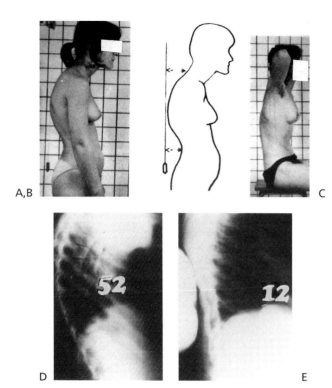

FIGURE 3. Asthenic (postural) kyphosis **(A)**. The clinical attitude may be corrected actively due to the flexibility of the spine **(C)**. The measurement parameters for kyphosis suggested by Stagnara **(B)** (see details in the text). The corresponding radiographs show the absence of lesions typical of Scheuermann kyphosis and the complete reducibility of the hyperkyphosis when the hyperextension test is performed **(D, E)**.

T9, and the so-called thoracolumbar form, with the apex between T10 and T12.

Thoracic Form

Clinical examination reveals an increased dorsal kyphosis. Affected patients develop a compensatory lumbar and cervical lordosis. Stagnara stresses the importance of conducting the clinical examination with the patient flexed forward, with the chest resting on the examination table and the knees slightly flexed. This position makes it possible to better appreciate structural deformities and the sites of pain. Murray et al. (78) conducted an accurate clinical examination in Scheuermann kyphosis patients in which about 30% of patients had significantly greater bilateral hamstring tension in the thoracic form as opposed to the thoracolumbar form.

Murray et al. (78) also observed a slight reduction in the strength of the trunk muscles in extension, with normal trunk strength during flexion. They reported a 90-degree mean trunk flexion (range 45 to 130 degrees) and a 20-degree mean extension (range 0 to 35 degrees). Comparative analysis of the flexibility range compared at the various stages of disease severity demonstrated that increasing curve magnitude is not accompanied by a greater limitation in articular elasticity during flexion and extension (78).

Scheuermann kyphosis is often associated with a moderate

scoliosis (2). The scoliosis usually presents as an angular severity ranging between 10 and 20 degrees in 20% to 30% of affected subjects. Agostini et al. (2) found that the apices of the kyphosis and the scoliosis are the same. There is modest rotation of the vertebra and the gibbus in terms of the lateral deviation. These curves are structural but have a relatively benign natural history (2).

Thoracolumbar Form

The lower curve apex of this form of Scheuermann kyphosis may paradoxically reduce the upper dorsal kyphosis and may actually initiate a thoracic lordosis. This form is characterized by a greater degree of palpable tenderness of the spine. However, Murray et al. (78) have not reported this correlation between the level of kyphosis and increased vertebral tenderness. They found that there was a greater reduction in physical exercise and working activity over time in patients with the thoracolumbar form.

Lumbar Form

Over the past decade, there have been increasing reports of lumbar alterations simulating those typically reported in Scheuermann kyphosis. The peculiarities of this third form are an ever present backache, which causes the patient to present for medical treatment, and the absence of lumbar vertebrae deformations similar to those occurring at a dorsal level (74).

This form seems to occur mostly in male patients who do hard labor or are athletically active. Radiographically, this form is characterized by irregular vertebral end plates, Schmorl nodules, and a reduction in disc space height that is not associated with wedging (15). At times the lesion appears to be preferentially localized to the anterior rim of the vertebral body and resembles the so-called anterior marginal detachment (Fig. 4).

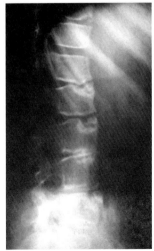
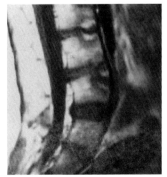

A,B

FIGURE 4. **A:** Tomography of a lumbar Scheuermann kyphosis. **B:** Magnetic resonance imaging demonstrates the anterior marginal detachment.

Pain

In addition to the cosmetic aspects of Scheuermann kyphosis, pain is the predominant clinical symptom of the disease (31). Its distribution and intensity vary according to age, stage of disease, site of kyphosis, and severity of the lesions.

Age

During the growth spurt, pain is uncommon (22% patients), but it reaches maximum incidence (60% of patients) as bone maturity progresses. Some authors believe that pain recedes completely when growth is completed (48,52). At this point, the pain is generally circumscribed and present only in the periapical region of the deformity, with upward or, more often, downward paravertebral radiation (Fig. 5).

By accurately and thoroughly palpating the skin and paravertebral muscle masses in patients presenting without pain symptoms, the physician can trace a latent tenderness map around the apex of the kyphosis and at the upper levels (65). According to our experience, this can be done in about 70% of patients presenting without any subjective painful symptoms. Pain is most frequently localized at the cervicothoracic border and in the interscapular region (9).

In adults, the pain takes the form of a backache, and the previously described periapical pain is not always reported. The pain seems to be localized to the iliac crest region, as evidenced by manually mobilizing T11 and T12. The sensory innervation of the dorsolumbar region presents a typical distribution; the dermatome pattern in the iliac crest region originates from T11 and T12 (Fig. 5B). The loss of mobility of the facet joints and the onset of arthritic degeneration may explain the prevalence of such symptoms in adults (9).

Stage of the Disease

The period of rapid growth, which generally coincides with the time of diagnosis, is when the greatest incidence of symptoms is reported (the so-called florid stage of the disease). Symptoms tend to decrease as vertebral ossification progresses.

Apex Level

Murray et al. (78) did not report any significant correlations between pain incidence and apex level. However, they did note that in patients with high-apex curves, the pain interfered more with day-to-day living than in those with the thoracolumbar form.

Degree of Kyphosis

It would seem logical to expect an increase in painful symptoms proportional to an increase in the angle of the kyphosis. However, Murray et al. (78) found a greater interference with everyday life (attributed to backache or sciatica) in patients affected by kyphosis with average angles (65 to 85 degrees) than those with lesser or greater angles (less than 65 and greater than 85 degrees, respectively). If the degree of the curve is correlated

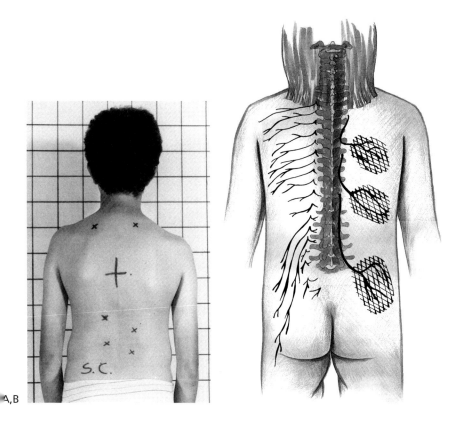

FIGURE 5. A: Typical pain distribution of a Scheuermann patient at a young age. The marker (+) identifies the apex of the kyphosis; the markers (X) show the pattern of pain distribution above and below the apex. **B:** Sensory area supplied by posterior primary division *(left)*. The nerve branches, after having supplied sensitive endings to the facet joints and the dorsal and sacrolumbar muscles, cross the fascia and split into an internal branch and an external branch that leads laterally downward and reaches the cutaneous area at a more caudal level (from three to five levels down) *(right)*. This accounts for the pain manifestation patterns at the level of the iliac crest that are typical in the adult patient.

with the apex level, no significant differences in symptoms are observed. Patients with thoracolumbar Scheuermann kyphosis were found to decrease their activity as the curve magnitude increased (78).

Neurologic Symptoms

Neurologic symptoms are generally absent during the adolescent growth period but may become manifest sporadically in adulthood in the form of backaches and ischialgias (27). Paraparesis has been rarely reported in adolescence due to disc compression, generally at the apex of the kyphosis (107). Thoracic disc herniations in adults are seldom found to be the cause of paraparesis. Bouchez et al. (16) observed that hernia-induced neurologic symptoms in Scheuermann kyphosis patients occur in only 1% of the paralyzing disc hernia cases studied. A vascular pathogenesis, resulting from compression exerted on the spinal artery of Adamkiewicz, seems to be responsible for the onset of acute paraparesis.

Selective spinal arteriography is useful in all cases of a sudden onset of acute paraparesis (66,67). The magnetic resonance scan provides a clear illustration of the cause being investigated. In addition to disc herniation, a compression fracture in a relatively osteoporotic spine (at an adult or senile age) may cause paraparesis. This may lead to an acute paraparesis in patients affected by mildly severe Scheuermann kyphosis (17). Both conditions (dorsal disc hernia and compression fracture) act on spines that have experienced progressive angulation increases over time but in which the spinal cord has previously adapted. However, in

these instances, the spinal cord cannot compensate for these changes and is sensitive to even 1- or 2-degree angle variations (63). One other possible cause of paraparesis has been reported by Lonstein et al. (70). It is typical of wide-angle kyphoses, in which the somatic and vascular compression mechanisms have a role identical to that of congenital curves.

In conclusion, it should be kept in mind that there is a slight possibility that by various pathogenic mechanisms Scheuermann kyphosis may lead to paraparesis in patients who were previously neurologically normal. Paraparesis should not be thought of as occurring exclusively in patients with a severe form of Scheuermann kyphosis (as might seem obvious) or only in adults.

RADIOGRAPHIC STUDIES

The Scoliosis Research Society has established that the normal thoracic kyphosis ranges from 20 to 40 degrees, based on the Cobb method (72). According to many authors, these figures are controversial. For example, Stagnara et al. claim that there is no such thing as a physiologic thoracic kyphosis; rather, each subject has his or her own "spinal profile." Fon et al. (44) studied 316 normal subjects aged 27 years, finding a maximum limit of 45 degrees for a physiologic kyphosis.

Scheuermann kyphosis is diagnosed on the basis of radiographs performed in a left lateral projection. Bradford (23) suggests the following as some of the most accurate criteria for the diagnosis of Scheuermann kyphosis (Fig. 2):

1. Irregular upper and lower vertebral end plates
2. The apparent loss of disc space height
3. Wedging of more than 5 degrees in one or more vertebrae
4. The presence of a hyperkyphosis greater than 40 degrees

It is important to emphasize that the diagnosis of Scheuermann kyphosis does not require the presence of all of the typical radiographic findings associated with the disease. For example, a rigid hyperkyphosis, though it may not have any wedging, may be consistent with the diagnosis of Scheuermann kyphosis. Also, the isolated presence of vertebral end plate irregularities, not accompanied by wedging or hyperkyphosis, could also be indicative of Scheuermann kyphosis. There may be many variants or formes fruste of the disease. According to De Mauroy and Stagnara (36), these forms converge in a separate pathologic picture, which they refer to as idiopathic kyphosis.

The irregular nature of the vertebral end plates is the direct radiographic expression of the previously reported histologic features. Therefore, those areas affected by a longitudinal growth defect look like irregularities and grooves along the rectilinear profile of the vertebral end plate. The thickening and sclerosing of the spongy areas underneath the vertebral end plates are common and typical observations (76). Vertebral wedging is measured by drawing one line along the upper rim of the end vertebrae and another line along the lower rim and measuring the angle at which the lines intersect (105).

Sorensen (98) suggested a widely accepted criterion for the diagnosis of Scheuermann kyphosis that calls for the presence of at least three adjacent vertebrae with a wedging exceeding 5 degrees. Measuring vertebral wedging may be especially complex in patients who have not manifested ring apophyses. In this case, the lateral profile of the vertebra has a curvilinear rather than a rectilinear shape.

Stagnara (102) classifies the ossification stages of the vertebral end plate into six phases, ranging from puberty to bone maturity. In the most advanced stages of growth, the affected vertebra acquires a wedgelike shape, with a greater posterior height and a tendency toward platyspondylisis in both the anteroposterior and the lateral planes (49). The presence of Schmorl nodules, characterized by a depression of the vertebral end plate, is a result of the penetration of nuclear material into the spongy region. This finding is common but is not typical of the disease; it has also been observed in normal subjects (89). The marginal anterior bony detachment that is typical of lumbar localizations may be attributed to the same pathogenetic mechanism (15). The narrowing of the intervertebral space is a typical aspect of the advanced stages of the process. Bradford et al. (26) compare this picture to that of a marshmallow that is compressed between two smooth plates. The metaphor explains the apparently excessive thickness of the intervertebral disc, which seems to exceed that of adjacent vertebrae in the anterior rim.

Reduction of intervertebral disc space seems to be the only persisting radiographic evidence of the lumbar variant of Scheuermann kyphosis. In this form there is no vertebral wedging and kyphosis is constant because the lumbar segment is in lordosis, which maintains the posterior transference of the load-bearing axis (15,33).

A thorough and accurate radiographic investigation should be performed on patients affected by Scheuermann kyphosis and should include the following:

1. *Left-standing lateral radiographic projection of the entire spine.* According to some authors, it is advisable to position the patient so that his or her arms are resting on a support placed in an anterior position with respect to the body at a height not exceeding that of the heart so as to prevent the muscle contraction required to keep the arms suspended from altering the examination. This projection helps evaluate the degree of dorsal kyphosis and lumbar lordosis.

2. *Standing anteroposterior radiographic projection of the entire spine.* This projection helps determine the presence of associated scoliosis (in the various forms previously described) and the bone maturation of the iliac crest according to Risser's sign.

3. *Passive hyperextension test,* which is performed by positioning a wedge of plastic material just below the apex of the kyphosis. The patient is asked to lie in a supine position and release the weight of the head and shoulders in a reclining position. To avoid correction of kyphosis by increasing the compensatory lumbar lordosis, Stagnara (102) suggests that the radiograph be performed with the patient lying down with legs, pelvis, and lumbar spine in maximum flexion. Radiographic investigations performed in this fashion give an estimate of the degree of flexibility of the kyphosis and the percentage correction that may be obtained with standard corrective measures. Special emphasis should be given to positioning of the wedge. The wedge profile should be controlled with respect to the apical vertebra of the kyphotic curve. Incorrect positioning above the apex of the kyphosis will be misleading, giving the appearance of curve rigidity or even a paradoxical curve increase (Fig. 6).

4. *Lateral tomography.* The performance of three to four tomographic cuts at 4-mm intervals at the apical area of the kyphosis reveals in greater detail the irregular nature of the vertebral end plates (Fig. 6C). With this investigation, it is easier to measure the wedging and assess the state of development of the ring apophysis.

5. *Magnetic resonance imaging* (MRI).

Differential Diagnosis

The radiographic differentiation of a postural kyphotic curve is made by the total absence of wedging and vertebral end plate irregularities and the complete reduction of hyperkyphosis with the passive hyperextension test, using wedges as described above. In the clinical entity termed idiopathic kyphosis (35,36), which is probably completely different from Scheuermann kyphosis, the normal vertebral profile is accompanied by rigidity of the hyperkyphotic curve.

Specific or nonspecific spondylitis disorders initially become manifest by an irregular vertebral margin adjacent to the affected disc, and unlike the lesions typical of Scheuermann kyphosis, they do not present sclerotic rims surrounding the eroded areas (Fig. 6). The differentiation from spondyloepiphyseal dysplasias or other forms of osteochondral dystrophies is generally made by the general epiphyseal-metaphyseal involvement of other joints and the fact that the platyspondylisis typical of these conditions is not accompanied by vertebral irregularity or wedging. It may be more difficult to differentiate some forms of type II (failure of segmentation) congenital kyphosis from Scheuermann kyphosis. Kharrat and Dubousset (57) reported some forms of

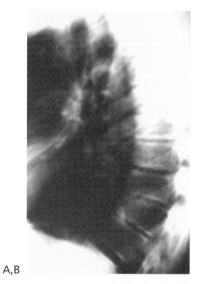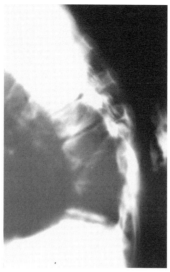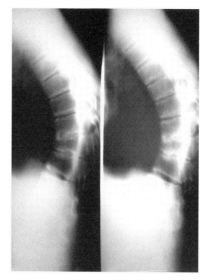

A,B   C

FIGURE 6. **A:** Vertebral kyphosis localized to few disc spaces. **B:** The supine hyperextension test shows that incorrect positioning of the wedge above the apex leads to worsening of the kyphosis. **C:** Tomography shows an apparent intersegment fusion, possibly as a result of spondylitis. No wedging or erosion is observed at other levels.

congenital kyphosis that achieve interbody fusion during the same time that patients typically present with Scheuermann kyphosis. Scheuermann kyphosis rarely exhibits a tendency to interbody fusion, but if fusion does occur it takes place through osteophyte bone bridges that always spare the intervertebral disc.

NATURAL HISTORY

The natural evolution of Scheuermann kyphosis during the growth spurt is quite variable (59). Bradford et al. (21) noted that 96 of 168 patients treated with a Milwaukee brace experienced progression of their deformity prior to the initiation of treatment. Lowe (74) maintains that if the residual kyphotic deformity at skeletal maturity remains under 60 degrees, the patient has an excellent possibility of experiencing little if any discomfort in adult life (74).

Travaglini and Conte (104) studied 50 patients affected by Scheuermann kyphosis with a minimum follow-up of 25 years and noted significant morphologic and structural evolution but insignificant clinical and functional problems. The incidence of pain was moderate in adult life, regardless of the severity of the curve and of the patient's type of work.

Murray et al. (78) observed 61 patients affected by Scheuermann kyphosis with a 31.7-year follow-up and compared them with 34 normal controls. This thorough investigation considered factors such as pain, work, social history, restriction of activities, cardiopulmonary function, vertebral function, and cosmetic aspects. Twenty-eight percent of the affected patients (62% of controls) reported that they had never suffered from vertebral pain. Sixty-four percent of the affected patients (15% of controls) reported that they had suffered from variable forms of backache, which could not be statistically correlated with the

apex of the curve or its magnitude. In the group of Scheuermann kyphosis patients, 6.6% had had spinal surgery, compared with 2.9% of controls. No statistical difference was found between the two groups in terms of the interference of pain with everyday life, lower limb hypoesthesia, fatigue, self-esteem, psychological disorders, type of job chosen, or amount of sick leave required for backache or sciatica. Statistically significant differences were recorded only in the case of pain localization and intensity. A greater incidence of back pain and tenderness was reported in the group of patients affected by Scheuermann kyphosis. The levels of tenderness, however, were not great. No correlation was found with cardiopulmonary insufficiency, except for the most severe cases (curves greater than 110 degrees).

These findings suggest that the clinical and functional natural history of the disease tends to be benign. This is in spite of the morphologic and structural exacerbations that, beyond a certain angle (65 degrees), have to be taken into account even in adult life because of biomechanical imbalances that can lead to curve progression, such as occurs with scoliosis.

One aspect that needs to be addressed is cosmetic appearance and self-esteem, which cannot be easily or adequately quantified on the basis of questionnaires (75a,99).

TREATMENT

According to Stagnara (102), there are four pathologic evolutions or scenarios requiring either nonoperative or surgical treatment:

1. Rapid increase in the curvature of the kyphosis
2. Exacerbation of vertebral lesions and increase of wedging, leading to a progressive kyphosis

3. Pain related to a severe dorsal kyphosis that does not respond to any type of nonoperative treatment
4. Alteration of respiratory function related to the vertebral deformation

Infrequently, these four treatment indications may be accompanied by rapid- or slow-onset spinal cord compromise as a result of dorsal disc hernias and/or compression fractures (90). Generally, adolescents with a slightly increased thoracic kyphosis—between 40 and 50 degrees—with no evidence of progression require only exercise and periodic follow-up. As adults, these patients have an excellent chance of being problem-free.

Nonsurgical Therapy

Physical Therapy

Physical therapy may be helpful, but it should be used only in the early stages of the disease as a complement to more aggressive treatments (Milwaukee brace, casts, and surgery). Physical therapy alone cannot obtain more than improved muscle tone and correction of bad posture. Extension sports, such as swimming, basketball, and volleyball, are advised. Aerobic exercise is an essential adjunct throughout the entire treatment period.

The goals of exercise are to maintain flexibility, correct lumbar hyperlordosis, and strengthen the extensor muscles of the spine. Exercises for stretching the hamstrings should be reserved for patients with clinical evidence of tension in these muscles.

Braces

Scheuermann kyphosis responds positively to treatment with braces, provided the therapy is begun before skeletal maturity is achieved, ideally in the first stages of the disease (at the early diagnosis stage). In general, this approach is indicated for patients with satisfactory back flexibility, with no less than 40% passive correctability in a curvature between 50 and 75 degrees. Flexibility is the crucial factor in making the choice between an active correction system (Milwaukee brace) and a passive correction system (antigravity cast). The reconstitution of the vertebral end plate is possible only if the vertebra maintains its active growth potential for a sufficient time (12).

In spite of good immediate results, if the anterior vertebral height has not been thoroughly reconstituted, considerable loss of correction will be observed in the follow-up period. The most widely used type of brace is the Milwaukee brace (14), which acts as a three-point dynamic orthosis and promotes extension of the thoracic spine. The pelvic girdle stabilizes the lumbar spine, thus reducing the lordosis, while the posterior pads apply corrective pressure at the apex of the kyphosis. Use of this type of brace is indicated predominantly in kyphoses with an apex between T6 and T9. The brace is initially worn on a full-time basis (22 out of 24 hours) for an average of 12 to 18 months. After that, it is usually possible (based on both the correction achieved and the progression of bone maturity) to wear the brace for maintenance purposes on a part-time basis (usually at night) until complete skeletal maturity has been achieved (38).

Generally, brace wear is gradually reduced by progressive 2- to 4-hour daily increments as skeletal maturity approaches. It is difficult to establish in general terms when weaning from the brace should begin. Sachs et al. (91,92) observed that there is no statistical difference between the results of patients who wore the brace on a full-time basis for 11 months and those who wore it for 8 to 10 months. Therefore, they prefer this shorter duration, at least in statistical terms.

The Milwaukee brace's occipital chin ring has often been the cause of psychological problems, which may decrease compliance. For this reason, some authors suggest the use of low-profile braces for thoracic kyphoses with a curve apex below T9 and for thoracolumbar kyphoses. Several types of braces have been suggested. Zielke suggested an orthosis with four valves that act as a double-torque force at the lumbar and thoracic levels (83). At the lumbar level, it provides a pair of opposite thrusts on the sacral promontory and on the anterior part of the iliac crests; at the thoracic level, it provides a couple of thrusts exerted just below the apex of the kyphosis and in the opposite direction on the manubrium sterni.

The lumbar form of Scheuermann disease, characterized by more irregular vertebral end plates, responds well to the application of a lumbar orthosis in which correction of the lordosis is not necessarily complete, as occurs with the Boston brace.

Montgomery and Erwin (77) reported long-term results in 21 patients treated with a Milwaukee brace (full time for 18 months and part time for 6 months). After an initial mean 21-degree improvement at the end of treatment, they observed a mean correction loss of 15 degrees over time. The mean wedging correction amounted to 1.1 degrees. Sachs et al. (91) reported data on 132 patients treated according to this approach with a 5-year minimum follow-up period. The mean full-time wearing period was 14 months, and the part-time mean was 18 months. There was an initial mean correction of about 50% in all curve classes, followed by a constant loss of correction at follow-up of 20 degrees for each group of curves. Sixty-nine percent of the patients who wore the brace faithfully reported improvement of 3 degrees with respect to the initial curvature—an improvement over the natural history of the disease.

There was a trend toward wedging improvement (ranging between 8 and 10 degrees among the various classes), with a reduction in the number of wedged vertebrae from 432 at the beginning of treatment to 266 at the end of treatment. The apical wedging was 8.4 degrees prior to treatment, 7.6 degrees at the end of treatment, and 8.1 degrees at 5-year follow-up. Thirty-two of the patients underwent surgery. The mean apical wedging in these patients amounted to 9.4 degrees, and the mean curvature was greater than 60 degrees.

According to Bradford et al. (21), the indications for brace treatment are initial curves of less than 70 degrees with a Risser sign lower than grade 3 and minimal vertebral wedging in fewer than three vertebrae.

It may thus be concluded, at least from a statistical point of view, that if the goal of brace treatment is to achieve a curvature as close as possible to 50 degrees at maturity in affected patients, there is a good chance of obtaining this goal in immature flexible patients with an initial curvature not exceeding 60 degrees (50% correction = 30 degrees + 20-degree loss at follow-up = 50 degrees).

Casts

When vertebral rigidity is considerable, it is advisable to resort to the preliminary use of corrective casts. De Mauroy and Stagnara (37) developed a therapeutic regime (Lyon method) organized as follows:

1. Physiotherapy in preparation for the cast
2. Application of three antigravity casts
3. Plexidur maintenance braces until skeletal maturity

The plaster casts, changed twice at 45-day intervals, are applied in two stages.

A multicenter trial conducted in France among the members of the Groupe d'Etude de la Scoliose on a total of 255 patients treated with this method showed a 19-degree mean angular correction at the end of the treatment (from an initial 50 degrees to 31 degrees—a 40% correction—with a mean loss of 7 degrees of correction at 2-year follow-up) (83). These findings seem to indicate that although it achieves a lower initial mean correction, the Lyon method guarantees a lower loss of angular correction over time than the Milwaukee brace treatment method.

These studies lead to two conclusions: First, as happens following the treatment of other disorders (e.g., scoliosis), the long-term return to angular values similar to those recorded initially is considered to be a therapeutic success. Second, the goal of treatment is to end up with a curvature in the physiologic range (40 to 50 degrees) at the completion of growth. It is crucial to preserve the correction achieved initially with casts by continuing treatment with the Lyon method or a Milwaukee brace.

Ponte et al. (84,86) treated 3,064 patients affected by kyphosis of various causes, 2,604 of whom presented with wedging greater than 5 degrees in at least one vertebral body, and 1,043 of whom presented with irregular vertebral bodies that were consistent with a diagnosis of Scheuermann kyphosis. Treatment involved the application of antigravity or localizer-type casts for a mean period of 8 months (83% of cases), 12 months (16%), or 16 months (1%). The mean initial curvature was 57 degrees. Forty percent angular improvement was obtained with the antigravity cast and 42% with the localizer cast. This was followed by the application of a Milwaukee brace at night and intense physiotherapy up to maturity. With this therapeutic regime, the authors reported a mean loss of 4 degrees correction at a 3-year mean follow-up. On average, a 62% mean wedging improvement was obtained (from 9 degrees at the beginning of treatment to 3.5 degrees at the end).

This treatment experience with casts confirms that although the initial angular improvement was less, deterioration over time was lessened by use of the brace. There was no correlation between the beginning of treatment, stage of puberty, and degree of wedging. The later the treatment is begun, however, the smaller the chances of reconstituting the vertebral end plates. As a result, even considerable initial angular corrections will not last indefinitely.

Conclusions on Nonsurgical Treatment Methods

The Milwaukee brace is effective in the treatment of Scheuermann kyphosis, provided that treatment is begun in the initial stages of the disorder, with an angle between 45 and 60 degrees, in a skeletally immature patient with at least 40% flexibility.

More rigid kyphoses should be treated with a corrective cast followed by a plexidur or Milwaukee brace to maintain correction. It is not advisable to undertake this treatment at a postpubertal stage, when high loss-of-correction rates are reported. Therefore, in these cases, it may be preferable to resort to surgery, especially in the case of sudden curve increases.

Surgery

Preoperative Techniques

In order to make a decision about the surgical technique to adopt and especially the approach sequence, it is advisable to perform preoperative correction, which will give some idea of the flexibility of the curve and the extent to which it may be improved by surgery.

Lowe (74) suggests analyzing the supine hyperextension lateral radiograph with a wedge. If the kyphosis is not corrected to values under 50 degrees, the procedure should be performed in two stages (anterior-posterior). In patients in which the hyperextension test leads to a decrease in angular values under 50 degrees, a single-stage posterior arthrodesis with instrumentation is advised. Stagnara and Perdriolle (101) recommend a preoperative correction with cast or halo traction to avoid rapid intraoperative correction, which may pose some risk to the spinal cord or a gastrointestinal complication, such as ileus (see Fig. 15). They also suggest the preoperative relaxation of the contracted ligamentous structures in the concavity of the kyphosis. This correction may be achieved according to the flexibility and severity of the kyphosis with either corrective casts or halo traction. These methods are rarely needed in most cases, but will be described for completeness.

Elongation Cast

A pelvic belt resting on the iliac crests is connected to a cervicothoracic belt by means of two Donaldson and Engh elongation screws. The progressive elongation of the screws (1 mm per day) reduces the deformity over an average of 20 to 30 days.

The elongation cast allows for much greater correction than that obtained with the hyperextension test. It is also possible to perform posterior arthrodesis—when this is the only approach planned—without removing the cast for surgery.

Great care should be taken to avoid pressure sores on the iliac crests or chin rests, which must be appropriately padded with soft material.

Halo Traction

The halo system allows for adequate preoperative correction (82). Stagnara (102) suggested a variation of the halo bed or halo wheelchair treatment, which has been found to be effective. This system is rarely used in the curves treated only with a posterior approach. It greatly increases the possibility for correction in combined procedures, in the interval between anterior release and posterior arthrodesis.

Posterior Operative Techniques

According to Stagnara, the general aims of any type of surgical intervention are to shorten the convexity and elongate the concavity (102). The reduction of the convexity may be facilitated by a complete resection of the facet joints in the kyphotic area and may be obtained with the application of surgical instruments.

On the operating table, the patient may have cephalic traction applied, with possible pelvic countertraction. Traction is rarely used in North American centers. Resection of the facet joints must be complete to obtain maximum mobility of the curve. The instrumentation is then positioned, and autologous bone from the iliac crest is added to the joints and lateral transverse process gutter.

The advent of Cotrel and Dubousset's systems and deriving instruments (e.g., Isola), completely supplanted the instruments used up to the early 1980s (Harrington, Cotrel, Luque).

Therefore, we shall illustrate only the advantages and disadvantages of this last type of instrument, which is still in use today.

Cotrel-Dubousset System

The Cotrel-Dubousset system was introduced in 1983 for the treatment of scoliosis. It is currently the most frequently employed system to treat Scheuermann kyphosis (all posterior derotation systems can be used to treat Scheuermann kyphosis). Generally, in Scheuermann kyphosis it is suggested that three or four double pedicular transverse or laminar hook configurations be used on the spine above the apex of the kyphosis; this gives an excellent hold on the posterior arch and minimizes the risk of neurologic impairment. Through an initial levering maneuver (similar to that used with the Luque rod), it is possible to obtain correction of the kyphosis. This allows for the introduction of the rods into the inferior hooks, which are positioned under the lamina of the vertebrae below the apex of the kyphosis and mounted in compression.

Correction is further improved by segmental compression of the hooks. The use of open hooks toward the cranial surface allows for easy positioning of the rod, much more so than with Harrington compression instrumentation. The diameter of the rods (7 mm) is such that lasting correction over time can ensue and postoperative immobilization is unnecessary (Fig. 7). The stability of this system is further enhanced by the application of two transverse interlocks (Cotrel's Device Transverse Traction [DTT]), which convert the instrumentation to a square configuration that cannot be deformed, similar to that proposed by Dove.

All systems similar to the Cotrel-Dubousset system (Isola, Colorado, USS, TSRH) may be used effectively.

The use of a transpeduncular screw in the first two lumbar levels increases the stability of the assembly, provided that the general criteria for the selection of the fusion area are respected. Otherwise, a screw may pull out. The use of sublaminar site at all levels, combined with limited laminectomy of the adjacent vertebral borders, seems to be the most stable assembly scheme.

Biomechanics of Posterior Instrumentation Systems

As for the Cotrel-Dubousset system, biomechanical studies are lacking. However, it appears that the mechanical resistance of the rod increases according to its diameter and that the double

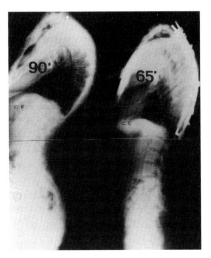

FIGURE 7. Severe 90-degree kyphosis treated with a posterior arthrodesis and Cotrel-Dubousset instrumentation. The curve was corrected to 65 degrees. The rigidity of the system obviates the need for anterior arthrodesis.

hook-claw anchorage system is better biomechanically with regard to the arthrodesis area. The entire curve must be fused (60,61). Shorter fusion areas are subjected to a greater lever arm, created by the weight of the neck and trunk, and are not subjected to arthrodesis (Fig. 8).

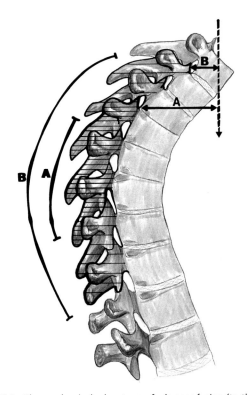

FIGURE 8. The mechanical advantage of a longer fusion (to the upper vertebra) over a shorter one. With the short fusion, there is an effectively longer lever arm *(A)* as opposed to the relatively shorter moment arm *(B)* when the entire kyphotic area is included in the fusion. Reprinted with permission from White AA III, Panjobi MM (1978): *Clinical biomechanics of the spine.* Philadelphia: J.B. Lippincott.

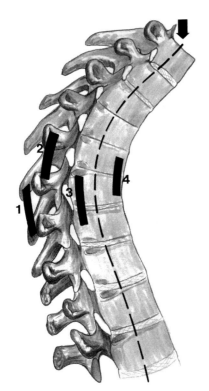

FIGURE 9. In the spine, the graft in position *(1)* is well away from the neutral axis *(dotted line)*. When biologically healed, it can offer tensile resistance against progressive kyphosis. The graft at position *(2)* can do the same but is less effective because it is closer to the neutral axis. The graft at position *(3)* is not likely to be as effective as *(1)* or *(2)* in preventing progression of deformity because it is even closer to the neutral axis. Graft *(4)* is effective because it can immediately begin to resist compression forces. The graft is also some distance away from the neutral axis. (Reprinted with permission from White AA III, Panjobi MM (1978): *Clinical biomechanics of the spine.* Philadelphia: J.B. Lippincott.)

In the most severe cases of kyphosis, which involve angles greater than 45 degrees after correction, the spine is exposed to greater stress in the arthrodesed area, which is under tension. This explains the occurrence of pseudarthrosis when the posterior fusion is not accompanied by an anterior arthrodesis.

With regard to the positioning of bone grafts, their resistance to stress increases with their distance from the neutral axis (Fig. 9). Increase in the kyphotic curvature is accompanied by an increase in the lever arm. Therefore, if reduction of kyphosis is insufficient, the residual tension will bring about such stress that posterior instrumentation may fail and the bone grafts may suffer fatigue fracture.

Bradford et al. observed that patients with vertebral wedging greater than 10 degrees tend to lose the operative correction obtained with posterior approaches more than patients with a wedging less than 10 degrees. The wedging seems to increase angulation and flexion, which in turn increases the eccentric load on the vertebral end plate.

Anterior Operative Techniques

When an anterior arthrodesis is indicated, it is performed by means of an intrathoracic approach for curves with a middorsal apex and by a thoracoabdominal retroperitoneal approach in

thoracolumbar curves (54). The technique makes it possible to resect the anterior longitudinal ligament and to perform multiple discectomies at apical vertebral levels (Fig. 10).

Stagnara (102) suggests that the area arthrodesed be extended to at least two levels above and below the apex of the kyphosis (five to six disc spaces in total). He suggests creating an osteoligamentous flap starting from the anterior and lateral surface of the vertebral bodies within which a fibular strut graft is placed, along with fragments of the rib removed for surgical access (Fig. 11). Other bone fragments, taken from the iliac crest, are positioned in the disc spaces to allow for an interbody fusion. The angular correction obtained is maintained by the fibular strut graft, which is fixed in the apical vertebrae, acting as a mechanical support against flexion forces, until the arthrodesis is achieved. In this case too, the greater the distance from the neutral load axis, the greater the reduction of the lever arm and the better the structural support (60) (Fig. 12A).

Winter (106) described another technique using the rib as an inlay graft, positioning it in a groove excavated on the lateral surface of the vertebral bodies, encasing it in the apical vertebral bodies (26) (Fig. 10).

In cases of extreme vertebral rigidity, there are several distraction devices that may be used intraoperatively that allow for angular reduction when the procedure is performed by an anterior approach. This instrument may be used temporarily and

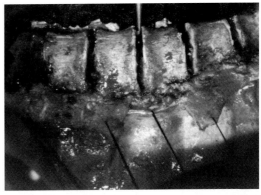

A

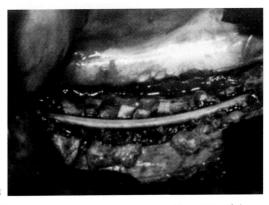

B

FIGURE 10. A: Complete discectomy and obliteration of the vertebral end plates is the best guarantee for successful interbody arthrodesis. **B:** Positioning of the graft in a trench excavated on the lateral aspect of the vertebral bodies; the graft is fitted into the vertebrae at the limits of the arthrodesis area. Other grafts are inserted into the interbody spaces.

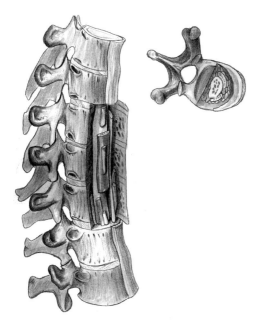

FIGURE 11. The osteoligamentous flap technique of Stagnara (102).

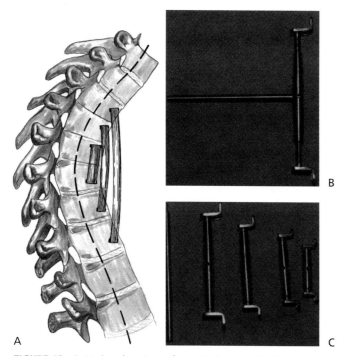

FIGURE 12. A: Various locations of anterior bone grafts for kyphotic deformity. The further one moves away from the neutral axis *(dotted line)*, the more the moments are reduced and the more effective the bony support. (Reprinted with permission from White AA III, Panjobi MM (1978): *Clinical biomechanics of the spine.* Philadelphia: J.B. Lippincott.) **B:** Pinto distractor used in kyphosis. (Courtesy of S. I. Weinstein, M.D., Department of Orthopaedic Surgery, University of Iowa, Ames, Iowa.)

removed following application of the supporting strut grafts (fibula or rib) (Fig. 12B). The use of distraction devices (temporary or permanent) may improve intraoperative correction, which is otherwise reduced because of the integrity of the posterior spine, which promotes maintenance of rigidity.

Various other types of systems have been devised and, according to Dunn (41), may be broken down into two major groups. The first type of system acts by means of two transvertebral body screws connected to a metal bar; the no. 1 Dunn, the Kostuick-Harrington, and the Gardner systems are examples of this type (Fig. 13). This type of system provides no resistance to twisting forces and little resistance to lateral flexion forces. The second type of system acts with the addition of load forces transverse to the apex of the curve and improves the correction capacity that may be obtained with the first type of instrument, which acts according to isolated stretching (Fig. 13).

Planning Surgery

If, in assessing the flexibility of the kyphosis by means of hypercorrection tests or preoperative radiographic techniques, it is possible to correct the curve to values around 50 degrees, it is advisable to plan a single posterior procedure (3,47). If, however, the preoperative assessment of correction reveals a curvature of more than 50 degrees, it is suggested that an anterior procedure be performed first, followed by a posterior arthrodesis and instrumentation (25,53).

Some authors suggest performing the combined procedures (anterior-posterior) at a single operative session; others prefer a 7- to 10-day interval between the two procedures. Concomitant performance of the procedures affords a better control of the angular correction and a shorter hospital stay for the patient. However, it may increase the complexity of surgical interventions and related risks.

Treatment of Paraparesis with a Subacute Onset

The onset of paraparesis has seldom been reported in patients with Scheuermann kyphosis. When it occurs, it may be due to a disc herniation at the apex of the kyphosis or, less frequently, a compression fracture (42,58). In such cases, and especially when a centrally located hernia is present (89), it is advisable to perform a transpedicular decompression to obtain tangential access to the disc space, and to then perform an accurate discectomy, thus avoiding neurologic damage (80).

It is advisable to perform an associated partial osteotomy of the vertebral rims above and below the involved disc in order to broaden the diameter of the vertebral channel. To avoid iatrogenic instability, it is wise to complement this procedure by stabilization of the adjacent levels by means of plates and transpedicular screws. Lesoin et al. (67) suggest that stabilization be achieved by means of a Harrington rod. Bradford (17,25) again advises anterior decompression with circumferential arthrodesis by means of a Harrington compression system (81,88,96). Logroscino et al. (69) prefer to do a costotransversectomy two levels above the lesion and remove the head and neck of the rib and

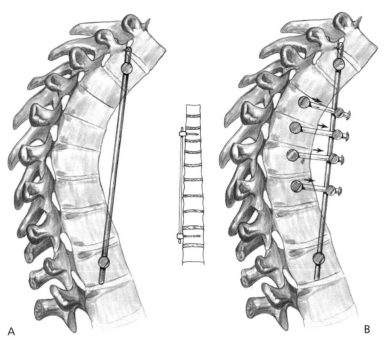

A   B

FIGURE 13. In the area of kyphosis there are two generic types of anterior implants. **A:** This implant gives no resistance to torsion and little or no resistance to lateral bending. **B:** This device applies transverse loading to the apex of the curve. The loading mode is more effective than distraction, as the kyphotic deformity is brought within the normal range. (Reprinted with permission from White AA III, Panjobi MM (1978): *Clinical biomechanics of the spine.* Philadelphia: J.B. Lippincott.)

the transverse process at the lesion level. This makes it possible to effectively visualize the area and perform the discectomy. This anterior costotransversectomy causes less instability and is sufficient to perform a limited arthrodesis in the affected area by means of rib grafts removed to gain surgical access.

It is advisable to perform selective arteriography to localize the emergence of the anterior spinal artery (branch of Adamkiewicz's artery) (39). According to Lazorthes et al. (64), in 75% of cases it is localized between T9 and T12, in 15% it is localized between T7 and T8, and in 10% it is localized between L1 and L2. In 80% of cases, it is localized on the left side (64). Knowing the exact origin of this artery is crucial to avoid cord damage because the anterior spinal artery supplies blood to two thirds of the dorsal medulla.

Results of Surgical Instrumentation

Anterior Arthrodesis and Combined Arthrodeses

Kostuick (62) analyzed the results of 12 patients treated with Kostuick-Harrington anterior instruments. One year after surgery, he reported no cases of pseudarthrosis, one intraoperative vertebral fracture, and one rupture of a transvertebral screw. Using circumferential arthrodesis in 12 cases, Savini et al. (93) obtained a mean correction of 34 degrees, with a 3-degree loss of correction at follow-up.

In 23 cases treated with combined anterior-posterior arthrodeses, Bradford et al. (25) reported excellent results in 80% of the subjects (correction loss less than 6 degrees), and a 15-degree mean loss in the remaining 20%. They observed the total relief of painful symptoms. Herndon et al. (53) evaluated 13 cases treated with anterior and posterior arthrodeses and reported excellent results in 69% (correction loss less than 6 degrees); 11

of these cases had a follow-up period of 3 to 5 years, with a loss of correction of less than 6 degrees in 80%.

Cotrel-Dubousset System

Lowe (73) and Clark and Shufflebarger (32) report results with this system, stressing the low incidence of negative side effects, especially with regard to neurologic problems. Donald et al. (40) compared the ability of the Harrington and Cotrel-Dubousset systems to correct the superior, middle, and inferior segments in the kyphosis. Both systems were found to effectively correct the middorsal section of the kyphosis but were relatively ineffective in correcting the superior section. The Cotrel-Dubousset system achieves a much greater correction on the inferior segment.

Lowe and Kasten (75) analyzed the behavior of sagittal curves subjected to correction with the Cotrel and Dubousset's system in 32 patients affected by Scheuermann disease of more than 75 degrees (range 75 to 105 degrees). The mean correction was 43 degrees (range 26 to 65 degrees). The mean magnitude of the lordosis was 75 degrees (range 58 to 100 degrees), and the mean correction was 20 degrees (range 16 to 35 degrees). Maintenance of the correction was excellent, with a mean loss lower than 5 degrees and a spontaneous reduction of the lordosis following correction of the kyphosis.

The authors observed the appearance of a junctional proximal kyphosis associated with an overcorrection (more than 50%) or a short instrumentation compared with the proximal apical vertebra. When the same situation was observed distally, the authors recommended that overcorrection be avoided (no more than 50% and no less than 40%) to prevent the onset of a proximal junctional kyphosis.

For this purpose, the proximal apical vertebra must always be included in the fusion; distally, the arthrodesis area must include all of the vertebrae included in the kyphotic area plus the transitional area (one or two lordotic vertebrae).

Sagittal balance was measured radiographically by dropping a plumb line from the center of the C7 vertebral body and measuring the distance from this line to the sacral promontory, with a positive value indicating when the plumb line lies anterior to the promontory of the sacrum.

The data indicate that the patients with Scheuermann disease were normally in negative balance and became somewhat more negatively balanced after surgery.

These studies show that the Cotrel-Dubousset system has improved the ease of assembly, in contrast to Harrington's instrument, which has now been abandoned. The larger size of the bars should not lead one to believe that the arthrodesis area may be reduced. The tensions that develop in an excessively short arthrodesis area are not great enough to break the instrument (as used to happen with the Harrington device), but they may cause a loosening of the lamina, as a result of which the hook may become unfastened from the site of the implant. The basic rules must thus be met.

The Cotrel-Dubousset instrument allows for an easier resumption of treatment with an easier extension of fusion area (domino). Therefore, the Cotrel-Dubousset system and its derivatives (Isola, TSRH, and so forth) prove over time to be easier to apply and easier to manage in case of failure, but the basic golden rules (i.e., selection of the fusion area, arthrodesis technique) must not be neglected, as serious problems may ensue if they are not applied (see Figs. 14–16).

This system is the best because of its corrective efficacy, its ability to maintain correction, the absence of neurologic complications associated with its use, and the fact that it does not require postoperative immobilization. Another positive aspect of the Cotrel-Dubousset system is the relatively easy handling of possible complications (such as inferior hook pullout) (Fig. 14).

Complications of Surgery

The complications related to this type of surgery are similar to those observed in major spinal surgery. For posterior procedures, the most frequently occurring complication is pseudarthrosis, followed by hardware failure and secondary loss of the correction. These complications seem to be related to technical defects. It is, however, crucial to perform the arthrodesis of articular processes with great precision (79).

Other complications reported in this type of surgery include pneumothorax, gastrointestinal obstruction, and the onset of postoperative backache or sciatica due to canal encroachment by synthesis devices (e.g., screws, hooks, sublaminar wires). Dural lacerations, infected dural fistulae, and postoperative meningitis and encephalitis may occur sporadically. In their series of 51 patients subjected to various types of corrective procedures, Speck and Chopin (100) reported one Brown-Séquard syndrome, seven vertebral fractures, four deep infections, and one instrument breakage.

In their series of 13 patients treated with combined anterior-posterior arthrodesis, Herndon et al. (53) reported one death,

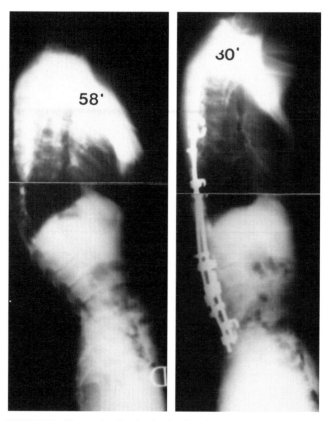

FIGURE 14. Thoracolumbar kyphosis of 58 degrees corrected with the Cotrel-Dubousset system. Perioperative dislodgement of the inferior hook was managed by means of a domino and extension of the fusion distally.

one intraoperative vertebral fracture, one deep venous thrombosis, one transient motor muscle weakness, and one postoperative onset of backache.

As an intraoperative complication, Stagnara (102) reported massive hemorrhage from vertebral venous sinuses and suggested the abundant use of surgical bone wax to avoid such a problem. He also reported frequent pulmonary complications resulting from the ablation of pleural drainage (late postoperative pleuritis and atelectasis). An excessively rapid correction of the kyphotic curve (only posterior) or over-correction may determine the onset of paralytic ileum due the closing of the so-called aortomesenteric compass (cast syndrome) (Fig. 15).

Whatever the instrumentation system used, it is crucial to perform the arthrodesis technique correctly, especially in cases in which the instruments used are cumbersome and hamper implementation of this important part of the procedure.

To avoid progression of kyphosis below the fusion region, it is advisable to extend the procedure one additional level into the area of the inferior neutral vertebra and always include L1 in the arthrodesis. To avoid the onset of a kyphosis above the arthrodesis, fusion and instrumentation should not be discontinued at the lower thoracic region, especially in a thoracolumbar kyphosis; it should be extended well proximal to additional segments.

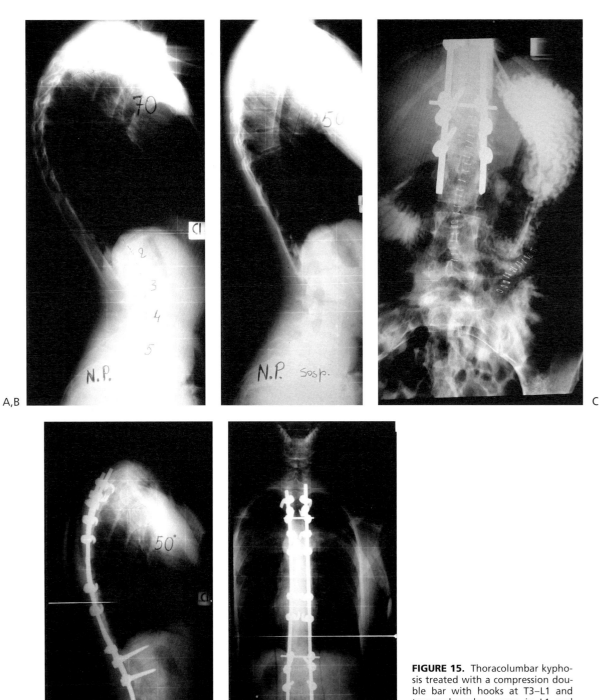

A,B

C

D,E

FIGURE 15. Thoracolumbar kyphosis treated with a compression double bar with hooks at T3–L1 and transpeduncular screws in L1 and D2. The use of the posterior approach alone determined a satisfactory correction with a good reshaping of the thoracolumbar junction. In the postoperative period, there was onset of paralytic ileum (cast syndrome–like), which was resolved by maintenance of the nasogastric tube over the following 2 weeks.

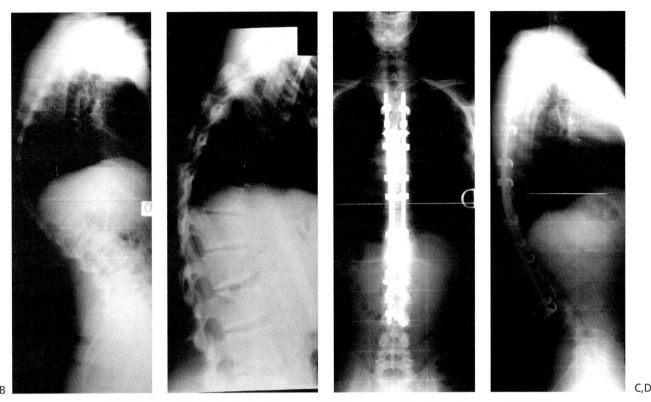

A,B

C,D

FIGURE 16. Thoracolumbar kyphosis with severe sagittal decompensation. Figure shows marked apical rigidity at the wedge hypertension test; anterior release and posterior T3–L2 instruments; sublaminar hooks and L1–2 sublaminar loops. At the end of correction, a sagittal decompensation condition remains.

CONCLUSIONS

About 5% of the Scheuermann kyphosis patients observed and subjected to treatment require a surgical correction and stabilization procedure. According to conventional concepts, surgery should be reserved for adolescents with curvatures exceeding 75 degrees, children with rapidly progressive kyphoses despite treatment with braces or casts (45), and adults with curves greater than 65 degrees.

Our experimental work has shown that it is possible to reconstitute the morphology of a vertebral body affected by Scheuermann kyphosis, depending on the age of the subject, the extent of the lesions, their distribution on the surface of the vertebral end plate, and the extent of wedging. Therefore, it is important to evaluate all of these factors, in addition to the angular level of the kyphosis, to determine the most suitable type of treatment. Surgical treatment for adults with Scheuermann kyphosis must be considered with great caution due to the disorder's benign natural history. The influence of surgical treatment on painful symptoms must also be considered. The rare case of paraparesis with an acute onset in adults requires surgical treatment.

In order to establish the correct approach to treatment, several questions should be addressed:

1. Does the natural history of Scheuermann kyphosis warrant the adoption of some form of preventive treatment? Travaglini and Conte (104) followed 50 cases for more than 25 years, observing that 80% of curves greater than 50 degrees increased in severity in adult life. Murray et al. (78) concluded a long-term clinical study on 62 patients and found that the disease does not bring about a progressive disability at a functional level in relation to pain or pulmonary dysfunction or in cosmetic terms.

2. Will the incidence of pain and its severity be significantly reduced by the treatment? Due to the variability with which pain is manifested (according to age and not in relation to severity of the curvature or the vertebral lesions), there are no proven correlations between a given radiographic or clinical picture and forecasts in terms of therapeutic outcome. Pratelli et al. (87) found that patients suffering from painful symptoms prior to treatment with casts had an 82% chance of suffering from low back pain as adults. In contrast, Murray et al. (78) stated that pain, though present, is never a debilitating symptom in the natural evolution of the disease.

It seems that the presence of pain should not be considered an absolute indication for treatment in view of the disease's benign natural evolution. Thus, the only true indication for treatment is the severity of the angle of the curvature, which has been shown to progress over time.

3. Is it possible to obtain a significant correction of the deformities and maintain that correction over time? It is possible to obtain satisfactory and lasting results both with conservative treatment consisting of a Milwaukee brace associated with casts

and with surgical treatment performed with Cotrel-Dubousset instrumentation (associated with anterior arthrodesis in rigid forms with little preoperative correction).

The authors of this chapter agree with Stagnara (102) in terms of the danger of falling prey to the Procrustes complex (Procrustes was a bandit from Ancient Greece who forced his victims to fit into his own bed by stretching the excessively short and cutting off the legs of the excessively tall). Subjects who enjoy relatively good health and have a relatively benign prospect for adult life must not be "normalized" from a morphologic point of view.

ACKNOWLEDGMENTS

I thank Dr. Sabrina Inciocchi, who contributed substantially to the preparation of this chapter by revising and sharing case photos and case materials.

REFERENCES

1. Adelstein L (1941): Spinal extradural cyst associated with kyphosis dorsalis juvenilis. *J Bone Joint Surg* 23:9.
2. Agostini S, Ferraro C, Mammano S, et al. (1982): La scoliosi nella malattia di Scheuermann. Morfogenesi delle curve di compenso. In: *Progressi in patologia vertebrale. Le cifosi,* vol. 5A. Bologna: Gaggi Editore, p. 265.
3. Allal M, Scheiner JP, Sedat P, et al. (1978): Le traitement chirurgical des formes graves de la maladie de Scheuermann de l'adulte jeune. Presented at Réunion du Groupe d'Etude de la Scoliose, Aix en Provence 1978.
4. Ascani E, Salsano V, Giglio GC (1977): The incidence and early detection of spinal deformities. *J Ital Ort* 3:3.
5. Ascani E, Giglio GC, Salsano V (1979): Scoliosis screening in Rome. In: Zorab PA, Siegler D, eds. *Scoliosis.* New York: Academic Press, p. 39.
6. Ascani E, Borelli P, La Rosa G, et al. (1982): Malattia di Scheuermann. I. Studio ormonale. In: *Progressi in patologia vertebrale. Le cifosi,* vol. 5A. Bologna: Gaggi Editore, p. 97.
7. Ascani E, Montanaro A, La Rosa G, et al. (1982): Malattia di Scheuermann. II. Studio istologico, istochimico e ultrastrutturale. In: *Progressi in patologia vertebrale. Le cifosi,* vol. 5A. Bologna: Gaggi Editore, p. 105.
8. Ascani E, Ippolito E, Montanaro A (1982): Scheuermann's kyphosis: histological, histochemical and ultrastructural studies. Presented at 17th Annual Meeting of the Scoliosis Research Society, Denver.
9. Ascani E, Montanaro A (1985): Scheuermann's disease. In: Bradford D, Hensinger RM, eds. *The pediatric spine.* Berlin: Thieme Verlag, p. 307.
10. Aufdermaur M (1981): Juvenile kyphosis (Scheuermann's disease): radiography, histology and pathogenesis. *Clin Orthop Rel Res* 154:166.
11. Aufdermaur M, Spycher M (1986): Pathogenesis of osteochondrosis juvenilis Scheuermann. *J Pediatr Orthop* 4:452.
12. Bick EM, Copel JW, Spector S (1950): Longitudinal growth of the human vertebra. A contribution to human osteogeny. *J Bone Joint Surg Am* 32:803.
13. Bick EM, Copel JW (1951): The ring apophysis of the human vertebra. Contribution to human osteogeny II. *J Bone Joint Surg Am* 33:783.
14. Blount WP (1972): Use of the Milwaukee brace. *Orthop Clin North Am* 3:3.
15. Blumental S, Roach J, Harring J (1987): Lumbar Scheuermann's. *Spine* 12:929.
16. Bouchez B, Arnott G, Combelles G, et al. (1986): Compression medullaire par hernie discale dorsale. *Rev Neurol (Paris)* 142:154.

17. Bradford DS, Garcia A (1969): Neurological complication in Scheuermann's disease. *J Bone Joint Surg Am* 51:657.
18. Bradford DS, Moe JH, Winter RB (1973): Kyphosis and postural roundback deformity in children and adolescents. *Minn Med* 56:114.
19. Bradford D, Moe J, Montalvo F (1974): Scheuermann's kyphosis and roundback deformity. *J Bone Joint Surg Am* 56:740.
20. Bradford DS, Moe JH (1975): Scheuermann's juvenile kyphosis: a histologic study. *Clin Orthop* 110:45.
21. Bradford DS, Moe JH, Montalvo FJ, et al. (1975): Scheuermann's kyphosis. Result of surgical treatment by posterior spine arthrodesis in twenty-two patients. *J Bone Joint Surg Am* 57:439.
22. Bradford DS, Brown DM, Moe JH, et al. (1976): Scheuermann's kyphosis, a form of juvenile osteoporosis? *Clin Orthop* 118:10.
23. Bradford D (1977): Juvenile kyphosis. *Clin Orthop Rel Res* 128:45.
24. Bradford D (1981): Vertebral osteochondrosis (Scheuermann's kyphosis). *Clin Orthop* 158:83–90.
25. Bradford DS, Khalid BA, Moe JH, et al. (1980): The surgical management of patients with Scheuermann's disease. A review of twenty-four cases managed by combined anterior and posterior spine fusion. *J Bone Joint Surg Am* 62:705.
26. Bradford D, Ganjavian S, Antonious D, et al. (1982): Anterior strut-grafting for the treatment of kyphosis. *J Bone Joint Surg Am* 64:680.
27. Breig A (1964): Biomechanics of the spinal cord in kyphosis and kyphoscoliosis. *Acta Neurol Scand* 40.
28. Buckler JMH (1979): *A reference manual of growth and development.* St. Louis: Blackwell Mosby, pp. 12–16.
29. Burner WL, Badger VM III, Scherman FC (1982): Osteoporosis and acquired back deformities. *J Pediatr Orthop* 2:383.
30. Cann CE, Genant HK, Kolb FO, et al. (1985): Quantitative computed tomography for prediction of vertebral fracture risk. *Bone* 6:1.
31. Carlioz H (1989): Dorsalgie de l'enfant, dos rouds, maladie de Scheuermann. *Ann Pediatr (Paris)* 36:642.
32. Clark CE, Shufflebarger HL (1990): Cotrel-Dubousset instrumentation for Scheuermann's kyphosis. Presented at Annual Meeting of the American Academy of Orthopaedic Surgeons, New Orleans 1990.
33. Cohn S, Akbarnia B, Luisiri A, et al. (1988): Disk space infection versus lumbar Scheuermann's disease. *Orthopaedics* 11: 332.
34. Deacon P, Berkin C, Dickson R (1985): Combined idiopathic kyphosis and scoliosis. An analysis of the lateral spinal curvatures associated with Scheuermann's disease. *J Bone Joint Surg Br* 67:189.
35. De Mauroy JC, Gonon G, Stagnara P (1988): Courbures saggitales, types, morphologiques. Essai de classification. Critères cliniques et radiologiques dans le cyphoses régulières. Réunion du Groupe d'Etude de la Scoliose, Aix en Provence. 1:11.
36. De Mauroy JC, Stagnara P (1978): Cyphose idiopatique: entité pathologique. Réunion du Groupe d'Etude de la Scoliose. Aix en Provence. 1:24.
37. De Mauroy JC, Stagnara P (1978): Résultats à long terme du traitment orthopédique. Réunion du Groupe d'Etude de la Scoliose. Aix en Provence. 1:60.
38. De Smedt A, Fabry G, Mulier JC (1975): Milwaukee brace treatment of Scheuermann's kyphosis. *Acta Orthop Belg* 41:597.
39. Dommisse GF (1974): The blood supply of the spinal cord: a critical vascular zone in spinal surgery. *J Bone Joint Surg Br* 56:225.
40. Donald GD, Nash CL, Wilham MR, et al. (1991): Segmental curve changes following posterior spinal fusion for hyperkyphosis. Presented at 25th Anniversary Meeting of the Scoliosis Research Society, Minneapolis 1991.
41. Dunn HK (1984): Anterior implants for kyphosis and trauma. Presented at 19th Annual Meeting of the Scoliosis Research Society, Orlando 1984.
42. Fau R, Djindjian R, Crouzet G, et al. (1973): Paraplégie régressive et maladie de Scheuermann. Etude radioclinique d'une observation. *Rev Neurol* 129:83.
43. Findlay A, Conner A, Connor J (1989): Dominant inheritance of Scheuermann's juvenile kyphosis. *J Med Genet* 26:400.
44. Fon GT, Pitt MJ, Thies AC Jr (1980): Thoracic kyphosis: range in normal subjects. *AJR Am J Roentgenol* 134:979.
45. Frymoyer J (1989): Are we performing too much spinal surgery? *Iowa Orthop J* 9:32.

46. Gilsanz V, Gibbens D, Carlson M (1989): Vertebral bone density in Scheuermann's disease. *J Bone Joint Surg Am* 71:894.

47. Gonon G, Demauroy JC, Stagnara P (1978): Resultats à long terme du traitement chirurgical des cyphoses régulières. Réunion du Groupe d'Etude de la Scoliose, Aix en Provence. 1:91.

48. Greene T, Hensinger R, Hunter L (1985): Back pain and vertebral changes simulating Scheuermann's disease. *J Pediatr Orthop* 5:1.

49. Hafner RH (1952): Localized osteochondritis, Scheuermann disease. *J Bone Joint Surg Br* 34:38.

50. Halal F, Gledhill R, Fraser C (1978): Dominant inheritance of Scheuermann's juvenile kyphosis. *Am J Dis Child* 132:1105.

51. Heine J, Stauch R, Matthia HH (1984): Ergebnisse der operativen behandlung des morbus Scheuermann. *Z Orthop* 122: 743.

52. Hefti F (1987): Morbus Scheuermann. *Ther Umsch* 44:764.

53. Herndon W, Emans J, Micheli L, et al. (1981): Combined anterior and posterior fusion for Scheuermann's kyphosis. *Spine* 6:125.

54. Hodgson AR, Stock FE (1956): Anterior spinal fusion. *Br J Surg* 44: 226.

55. Ippolito E, Bellocci M, Montanaro A, et al. (1985): Juvenile kyphosis: an ultrastructural study. *J Pediatr Orthop* 5:315.

56. Ippolito E, Ponseti IV (1981): Juvenile kyphosis, histological and histochemical studies. *J Bone Joint Surg Am* 63:175.

57. Kharrat K, Dubousset J (1980): Bloc vertäbra antärieur progressif chez l'enfant. Discussion des blocs vertäbraux acquis au cours de la maladie de Scheuermann. *Rev Chir Orthop* 66:485.

58. Klein D, Weiss R, Allen J (1986): Scheuermann's dorsal kyphosis and spinal cord compression: case report. *Neurosurgery* 18:628.

59. Kling TF Jr, Hensinger RN (1984): Scheuermann's disease: Natural history, current concepts and management. In: Dickson RA, Bradford DS, eds. *Management of spinal deformities.* London: Butterworths.

60. Kostuick JP (1984): Biomechanics of kyphosis using biological grafts. Presented at 19th Annual Meeting of the Scoliosis Research Society, Orlando 1984.

61. Kostuick JP, Gleason TF, Errico TJ (1984): Surgical management in adult Scheuermann's kyphosis. Presented at 19th Annual Meeting of the Scoliosis Research Society, Orlando 1984.

62. Kostuick J, Lorenz M (1982): Longterm follow up of surgical management in adult Scheuermann's kyphosis. Presented at 17th Annual Meeting of the Scoliosis Research Society, Denver 1982.

63. Landingham V (1954): Herniation of thoracic intervertebral disc with spinal cord compression in kyphosis dorsalis juvenilis. *J Neurosurg* 11:327.

64. Lazorthes G, Govaze Q, Zadeh JO, et al. (1971): Arterial vascularization of spinal cord: recent studies of the anastomotic substitution pathway. *J Neurosurg* 35:253.

65. Lehmann TR, Brand RA, Gorman TWO (1983): A low-back rating scale. *Spine* 8:308.

66. Lesoin F, Rousseaux M, Dubois F, et al. (1987): Souffrance radiculomedullaire et maladie de Scheuermann. *Rev Med Interne* 8:39.

67. Lesoin F, Meys D, Rosseaux F, et al. (1987): Thoracic disk herniation and Scheuermann's disease. *Eur Neurol* 26:145.

68. Lesoin F, Rosseaux M, Viaud C, et al. (1985): Syndrome radiculomedullaire au cours de la maladie de Scheuermann. *Rev Rhum Mal Osteoartic* 52:57.

69. Logroscino CA, Bucca C, Paliotta VF (1987): Ernia del disco dorsale: aspetti clinici e orientamenti terapeutici. *Progr Pato Vert* 10:347.

70. Lonstein J, Winter R, Moe J, Bradford DS, Chou S, Pinto W (1980): Neurologic deficits secondary to spinal deformity. *Spine* 5:331.

71. Lopez R, Burke S, Levine D, Schneider R (1988): Osteoporosis in Scheuermann's disease. *Spine* 13:1099.

72. Lowe TG (1987): Mortality-morbidity committee report. Presented at Annual Meeting of the Scoliosis Research Society, Vancouver, British Columbia, Canada 1987.

73. Lowe TG (1990): Combined anterior-posterior fusion with Cotrel-Dubousset instrumentation for severe Scheuermann's kyphosis. Presented at Annual Meeting of the American Academy of Orthopaedic Surgeons, New Orleans 1990.

74. Lowe TG (1990): Current concept review: Scheuermann's disease. *J Bone Joint Surg Am* 72:940.

75. Lowe TG, Kasten MD. An analysis of saggital curves and balance after Cotrel-Dubousset instrumentation for kyphosis secondary to Scheurmann's disease. A review of 32 patients. *Spine* 1994;19; 1680–1685.

75a. McCallum MJ (1984): Scheuermann's disease. The result of emotional stress? (letter). *Med J Aust* 140:184.

76. Moe JH, Winter RB, Bradford DS, et al. (1978): *Scoliosis and other spinal deformities.* Philadelphia: WB Saunders.

77. Montgomery S, Erwin W (1981): Scheuermann's kyphosis long-term results of Milwaukee brace treatment. *Spine* 6:5.

78. Murray PM, Weinstein SL, Spratt KF (1993): The natural history and long-term follow-up of Scheuermann's kyphosis. *J Bone Joint Surg* 75A:236–248.

79. Ostsuka N, Hall J, Mah J (1990): Posterior fusion for Scheuermann's kyphosis. *Clin Orthop Rel Res* 251:134.

80. Patterson RH, Arbi E (1978): A surgical approach through the pedicles to protruded thoracic disks. *J Neurosurg* 148:768.

81. Perot PL, Munro DD (1969): Transthoracic removal of midline thoracic disc protrusions causing spinal cord compression. *J Neurosurg* 31:452.

82. Picault C, Mouilleseaux B, Chavin G (1978): Résultats du traitment orthopédique "Lyonnais" dans les cyphosis dorsales régulières à propos de 105 dossiers 1965–1976. Réunion du Groupe d'Etude de la Scoliose, Aix en Provence. 1:37.

83. Peveraro A, Bertini G, Baccino E, et al. (1988): Il corsetto tipo Zielke nel trattamento del dorso curvo giovanile. *Prog Pat Vert* 11:73.

84. Ponte A, Gebbia F, Eliseo F (1984): Nonoperative treatment of adolescent hyperkyphosis. Presented at 19th Annual Meeting of the Scoliosis Research Society, Orlando 1984.

85. Ponte A, Siccardi GL (1984): Surgical treatment of Scheuermann's hyperkyphosis. Presented at 19th Annual Meeting of the Scoliosis Research Society, Orlando 1984.

86. Ponte A, Vero B, Siccardi GL, et al. (1988): Ipercifosi dell'adolescenza: il trattamento incruento. *Prog Pat Vert* 12:85.

87. Pratelli R, Bartolozzi P, Allegra M, et al. (1982): Valutazione dei risultati a distanza del trattamento del dorso curvo osteocondritico mediante apparecchi gessati in reclinazione tipo Risser. *Prog Pat Vert* 5:157.

88. Ransohoff J, Spencer F, Siew F, et al. (1969): Case reports and technical notes: Transthoracic removal of thoracic disk: report of three cases. *J Neurosurg* 31:459.

89. Reeves DL, Brown HS (1968): Thoracic intervertebral disc protrusion with spinal cord compression. *J Neurosurg* 28:24.

90. Ryan MD, Taylor TKF (1982): Acute spinal cord compression in Scheuermann's disease. *J Bone Joint Surg Br* 64:409.

91. Sachs B, Bradford D, Winter R, Lonstein J, Moe J, Willson S, Orma G (1984): Scheuermann's kyphosis: longterm results of Milwaukee brace treatment of 132 patients. Presented at 19th Annual Meeting of the Scoliosis Research Society, Orlando 1984.

92. Sachs B, Bradford D, Winter R, et al. (1987): Scheuermann kyphosis. *J Bone Joint Surg Am* 69:50.

93. Savini R, Cervellati S, Cioni A, et al. (1988): Il trattamento chirurgico delle cifosi da morbo di Scheuermann. *Progr Pat Vert* 11:95.

94. Scheuermann HW (1921): Kyphosis dorsalis juvenilis. *Orthop Chir* 41:305.

95. Schmorl G, Junghans H (1932): *Die gesunde und kranke wirbelsaeule in roentgenbild.* Leipzig: Thieme Verlag.

96. Sekhar LN, Janetta PJ (1983): Thoracic disc herniation: operative approaches and results. *Neurosurgery* 12:303.

97. Skogland L, Steen H, Trygstad O (1985): Spinal deformities in tall girls. *Acta Orthop Scand* 56:155.

98. Sorensen KH (1964): *Scheuermann's juvenile kyphosis.* Copenhagen: Mundsgaard.

99. Southwick S, White A (1983): The use of psychological tests in the evaluation of low back pain. *J Bone Joint Surg Am* 65:560.

100. Speck G, Chopin D (1986): The surgical treatment of Scheuermann's kyphosis. *J Bone Joint Surg Br* 68:189.

101. Stagnara P, Perdriolle R (1958): Elongation vertebrale continue par platres à tendeurs. Possibilitiés thérapeutiques. *Rev Chir Orthop* 44: 57.

102. Stagnara P (1982): Cyphoses thoraciques regulieres pathologiques. In: *Modern trends in orthopaedics*, Bologna: Gaggi ed. p. 268.

103. Stagnara P, Du Peloux J, Fauchet R (1966): Traitement orthopédique ambulatoire de la maladie de Scheuermann en periode d'evolution. *Rev Chir Orthop* 52:586.

104. Travaglini F, Conte M (1982): Cifosi 25 anni dopo. *Progr Pat Vert* vol. 5A. Gaggi ed. Bologna 163.

105. White AA, Panjabi MM, Thomas CL (1977): The clinical biomechanics of kyphotic deformities. *Clin Orthop Rel Res* 128:8.

106. Winter RB (1978): The spine. In: Lovel WW, Winter RB, eds. *Pediatric orthopaedics,* vol. 2. Philadelphia: JB Lippincott, p. 648.

107. Yablon J, Kasdon D, Levine H (1988): Thoracic cord compression in Scheuermann's disease. *Spine* 13:896.

23

SPONDYLOLYSIS AND SPONDYLOLISTHESIS

SERENA S. HU
DAVID S. BRADFORD

Spondylolisthesis is the slipping forward of one vertebra upon another. It is derived from the Greek words *spondylos,* or "vertebra," and *olisthesis,* meaning "to slip." Spondylolysis is the condition of a bony defect at the pars interarticularis, which may be unilateral or bilateral. Spondylolysis can result in forward slippage, or spondylolisthesis. In the child or adolescent, pars defects are most common at L5, with resultant slippage of L5 on S1.

Spondylolisthesis was first described by the Belgian obstetrician Herbinaux (82) in 1782. He noted on occasion a bony prominence in front of the sacrum that could cause problems during delivery. The presence of a defect at the pars interarticularis was recognized by Robert (156) and then Lambl (101).

There are two types of spondylolisthesis commonly found in children and adolescents. According to the classification system originated by Wiltse in 1969, these are type I (dysplastic) and type II (isthmic) (Fig. 1). Type I, or dysplastic, spondylolisthesis is a congenital deficiency of the superior sacral facets, the inferior fifth lumbar facets, or both, which permits forward slippage of L5 on the sacrum. Isthmic spondylolisthesis is caused by a defect in the pars interarticularis. Type II is further classified as IIA if there is a fatigue fracture of the pars, IIB if there is an elongated but intact pars, and IIC if an acute fracture exists.

More recently, Marchetti and Bartolozzi suggested a new classification system for spondylolisthesis. Their major groups being developmental and acquired types, they divided the developmental type, which encompasses types I and II of Wiltse's classification as well as traumatic, into high dysplastic and low dysplastic, and each of these types could be subdivided to include lysis or elongation of the pars. They felt that their classification was useful with regard to prognosis and treatment (116).

ETIOLOGIC FACTORS

There have been several theories on the cause of spondylolisthesis. Early reports suggested a separate ossification center in the neural arch, with failure to unite, resulting in a defect at the pars interarticularis (128,136). Morphologic studies (29,62,

83,160,163) failed to support this; in fact, there is only one report of this condition in a newborn (15). (This should not be confused with congenital lumbosacral kyphosis.)

The role of upright posture and ambulation in the etiologic process has been suggested, as there are no known cases of spondylolysis or spondylolisthesis in nonambulatory patients (160). Also, although spondylolysis in newborns is virtually nonexistent, the incidence reaches 5% by age 6 years (6), nearing the 6% incidence found in the general population (57).

Repetitive microtrauma has been cited as a likely cause or a contributing factor. This theory is consistent with the belief that upright posture and ambulation are necessary in the development of the spondylolytic defect. Several authors (34,71,86, 88,108,121,132,161,192) have noted an association between loads placed on the lumbar spine in hyperlordosis and the subsequent appearance of a lysis. This occurs specifically in such sports as diving, weight lifting, wrestling, and gymnastics. In 1963, Newman (137) noted the association of spondylolysis with the onset of ambulation in toddlers. The increased incidence (50%) of asymptomatic spondylolysis reported in patients with Scheuermann disease suggests that the compensatory increase in lumbar lordosis is a factor in the development of spondylolysis (144). Biomechanical (45,108,169) and structural studies (99,163) suggest that the pars interarticularis is under the greatest stress in extension. Shear stresses at the pars are greatest in lordosis; this mechanism also may lead to pars fractures (54).

Wiltse (209,211,212,215) and others (3,62,104,178,194, 218) noted the familial incidence of spondylolysis and spondylolisthesis as well as the development of the condition after trauma. These authors believed that there was a congenital defect or dysplasia that when exposed to the stresses of upright posture and lumbar lordosis resulted in development of a pars defect, sometimes with elongation or slippage. The association of spondylolysis and spina bifida occulta also suggests the presence of congenital factors (8,26,57,143). The progressive development of a pars defect has been noted by other authors as well (35,98,127,207).

There is a significantly higher incidence of these conditions in certain populations. Alaskans are reported to have an increased incidence of neural arch defects, ranging from 5% in 6-year-olds to 34% in 40-year-olds (191). Examination of Eskimo skeletons reveals an incidence of spondylolysis in 13% of younger subjects and 54% of adults (183).

S. S. Hu and D. S. Bradford: Department of Orthopaedic Surgery, University of California School of Medicine, San Francisco, California 94143.

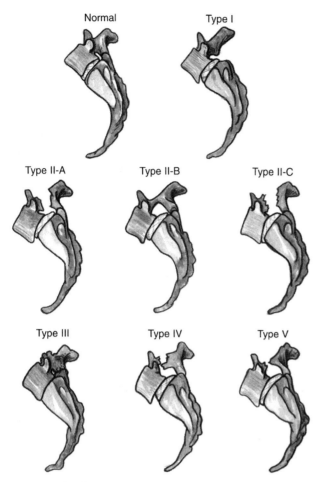

Normal   Type I

Type II-A   Type II-B   Type II-C

Type III   Type IV   Type V

FIGURE 1. Classification of spondylolisthesis according to Wiltse (191). *Type I:* Dysplastic—congenital deficiency of the superior sacral and/or inferior fifth lumbar facets with gradual slipping of the fifth lumbar vertebra. *Type II:* Isthmic—*A:* lytic (fatigue fracture of pars); *B:* elongated but intact pars; *C:* acute fracture. *Type III:* Degenerative—degeneration of joints allowing forward displacement, usually L4 on L5. *Type IV:* Traumatic—acute fracture in areas other than the pars interarticularis. *Type V:* Pathologic—attenuation of the pedicle secondary to structural weakness of the bone. Children and adolescents most commonly demonstrate type I or type II spondylolisthesis.

CLINICAL FINDINGS

Spondylolysis and spondylolisthesis may be completely asymptomatic or present with varying degrees of low back pain (73,115,130,146,180). The patient may note a recent injury or an association with a specific activity. Although the condition probably develops over the first two decades of life, symptoms most commonly present during the preadolescent growth spurt, between the ages of 10 and 15 years (7,37,62,75,80,151,198). The degree of slippage may not correlate with the severity of pain (180). However, some have noted, when comparing supine and standing radiographs, an association between a greater change in the percent of slippage and an increased likelihood of pain (63,114,145).

As noted, the incidence in the population is approximately 6% (57,62). Most reports note a higher incidence of spondylo-

lysis in males, by a ratio of up to 2:1, but females have a higher risk of progression (4,130,174,180). Rowe and Roche (162) noted an overall incidence of 4.2%: 6.4% in white males, 2.8% in black males, 2.3% in white females, and 1.1% in black females.

Athletes participating in certain sports such as gymnastics, wrestling, or football (especially interior linemen) may note low back pain with the activity. The pain may last for varying amounts of time after the activity ceases and may be relieved by avoidance of the particular sport (31,176). Many patients present with acute symptoms related to a specific trauma. These patients may show pathology ranging from normal radiographs with positive bone scans, to a stress fracture, to a pars defect with sclerosis of the fracture edges suggestive of a longstanding process.

Radicular symptoms, bowel or bladder impairment, or both are rare but can occur, particularly with higher degrees of slippage (77). Regardless of the degree of slippage, tight hamstrings and the classic knees-bent, hips-flexed gait—the Phalen-Dickson sign (150)—may be observed. The exact mechanism that causes tight hamstrings is not entirely clear. It is believed by some to be secondary to the vertical position assumed by the sacrum in higher grades of slippage, with resultant flexing of the pelvis, so that the hips cannot extend sufficiently. This results in knees flexed to permit the patient to stand upright (Fig. 2). Such a patient cannot stand upright with his or her knees straight, has limited forward flexion of the spine, and exhibits a characteristic waddling or short-stepped gait (138,187). Tight hamstrings may be caused by nerve root irritation from instability and nerve entrapment (7,42,150).

In patients with spondylolisthesis, careful palpation of the spine may reveal a step-off with a prominent spinous process of L5. With higher degrees of slippage, as the pelvis becomes more flexed and the lumbosacral junction more kyphotic, the trunk appears shortened. The rib cage approaches the iliac crests. Straight leg raising is often limited as well (7).

There are reports that associate scoliosis with spondylolisthesis. It may be secondary to the associated conditions (109) of a rotatory slippage (28,118) or hamstring spasm (155), or it may be a separate condition. The association is reported to exist in 13% to 60% of patients (18,105,109,110,121), with the greater incidences in symptomatic populations.

RADIOLOGIC EVALUATION

Identification of a pars defect is easily done on oblique radiographs of the lumbar spine, with observation of the "collar" on the "Scotty dog" (Fig. 3). Spot lateral views of the lumbosacral junction usually show the defect, particularly with bilateral defects. Isthmic and dysplastic spondylolisthesis are most common at the lumbosacral junction (4), although there are reports of their occurrence in the upper lumbar spine (112,154). Unilateral defects may show sclerosis of the pars or lamina on the contralateral side.

In patients who have a recent onset of pain and in whom no defects are seen on routine radiographs, bone scans may be useful in detecting early stress fractures at the pars interarticularis

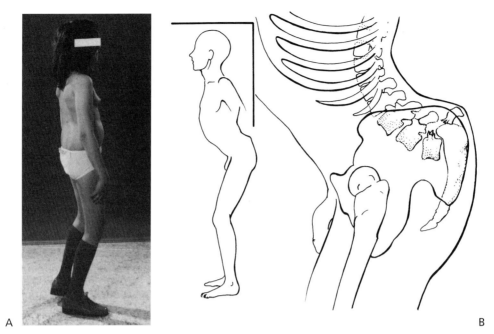

FIGURE 2. **A:** Clinical photograph of a patient with spondylolisthesis exhibiting a short trunk, flattening of lumbosacral lordosis, and flexed hips and knees. **B:** Schematic diagram demonstrating lumbosacral kyphosis. The pelvic tilt results in the inability of the hips to extend sufficiently to permit the patient to stand upright.

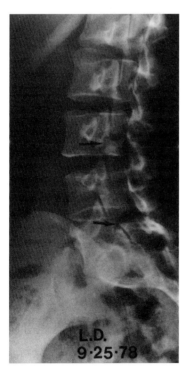

FIGURE 3. Oblique radiograph demonstrating pars defects at L5 and L3, which correspond to the "collar" on the "Scotty dog."

(Fig. 4) or in determining the acuity of the fracture (66,113, 199). Single photon emission computed tomography (SPECT) provides more detail and may be more sensitive (10,33).

A pars defect can be seen on computed tomography (CT) as an incomplete ring; it is occasionally unilateral but more frequently bilateral (103,195) (Fig. 5). If the CT gantry is not tilted to the plane of the L5–S1 disc space, the scan may be difficult to interpret. The pars defect can also be mistaken for a facet joint by the inexperienced observer. Unilateral cases may show sclerosis of the opposite pars, facet degeneration, or contralateral posterior element or pedicle fractures secondary to the increased stresses (2,141).

The actual slippage, or listhesis, can be measured by various parameters. Most commonly, Meyerding's (129) grading system is used: No slippage is grade 0, 1% to 25% slippage is grade I, 26% to 50% is grade II, 51% to 75% is grade III, and 76% to 100% is grade IV; grade V denotes spondyloptosis, or complete slippage past the anterior border of the sacrum (Fig. 6). Slippage is measured as a percentage of the anteroposterior diameter of the sacrum (Fig. 7). Some authors measure percent slippage relative to the inferior aspect of L5 (105). The sacrum may show secondary rounding of its anterosuperior aspect. For accurate and comparable measurements of percent slippage or lumbosacral kyphosis (i.e., slip angle), it is preferable to take radiographs in the standing or loaded position. There can be differences in slippage depending on the loading situation (94,97,114,148). Progression of less than 10% is difficult to detect (38).

In a skeletally immature patient, *slip angle* has been found to be the most useful measure in determining the likelihood of progression to higher grades of slippage (18). Slip angle provides

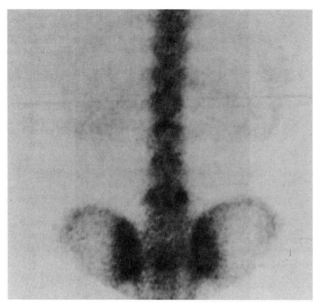

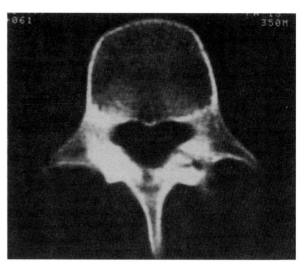

FIGURE 5. CT scan through left pars defect. Note sclerosis on the contralateral pars. (Courtesy of William Carr, M.D.)

FIGURE 4. Bone scan demonstrating increased uptake—more prevalent on the right than on the left side of L4—corresponding to the patient seen in Fig. 5 with a pars defect on the left and a stress reaction on the right.

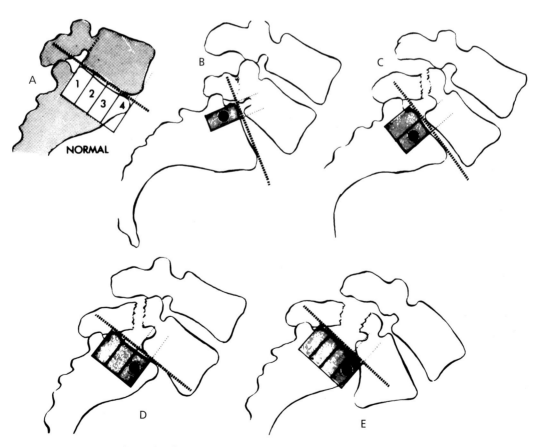

FIGURE 6. Meyerding's classification of spondylolisthesis. **A:** Normal or grade 0. **B:** 1% to 25% slippage is grade I. **C:** Up to 50% is grade II. **D:** Up to 75% is grade III. **E:** 76% to 100% slippage is grade IV.

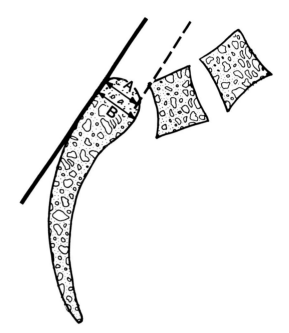

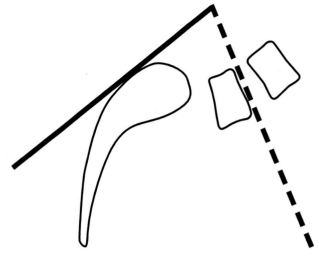

FIGURE 9. The lumbosacral angle is the angle between the posterior wall of the sacrum and the superior end plate of L5.

FIGURE 7. Percent slippage is measured relative to the anteroposterior diameter of the sacrum. As shown, *A/B* × 100 = 72%.

a measure of several radiographic risk factors and the associated compensatory mechanisms. It is determined by drawing a line along the posterior cortex of the sacrum and measuring the angle between its perpendicular and a line drawn along the inferior border of L5 (Fig. 8). Normal angles should be from 0 to −10

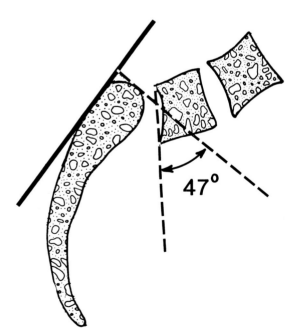

FIGURE 8. The slip angle (47 degrees as shown) is determined by drawing a line along the posterior cortex of the sacrum and measuring the angle between its perpendicular and a line drawn along the inferior border of L5.

degrees. Values greater than 55 degrees correlate with a higher likelihood of progression. Remodeling at the inferior border of L5 may make this measurement difficult; however, most studies that have used slip angle have used the inferior aspect of L5.

The *lumbosacral angle* is the angle measured between the superior end plate of L5 and the posterior border of the sacrum (Fig. 9) (46). Dubousset felt that a lumbosacral angle of less than 100 degrees (vertical sacrum) signified a spondylolisthesis that would always progress.

The *angle of kyphosis* can be measured between the cranial surface of L5 and the caudal surface of S1 (186). Normally, with physiologic lordosis, the value is positive. With spondylolisthesis and lumbosacral kyphosis, this value becomes increasingly negative.

The *lumbar index* is described as the height of the anterior aspect of the L5 vertebra, expressed as a percentage of the height of the posterior aspect of L5. Greater slippages tend to demonstrate lower lumbar indices, and progression of slippage appears to correlate with decreasing index (57,165).

Sagittal rotation is the angle between the posterior surface of the sacrum and the anterior cortex of L5 (Fig. 10). It is also known as *sagittal roll*.

Sacral inclination is determined by drawing a line along the posterior surface of the sacrum and measuring the angle between it and a vertical line from the floor. Normal sacral inclination is greater than 30 degrees, but with higher degrees of slippage the sacrum becomes more vertical and sacral inclination decreases (Fig. 11).

Recently, Schwab et al. (170) described the sagittal pelvic tilt index (SPTI) as a means of quantification of the relationship between S2, the center of the hip, and L5. This measurement is determined from a standing lateral radiograph of the lumbar spine that includes the hip joint. A horizontal line is drawn through the center of S2. A vertical line is drawn from the center of the L5 vertebral body. A second vertical line is drawn through the center of the femoral heads. The distance from the center

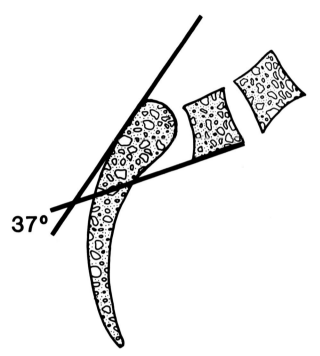

FIGURE 10. Sagittal rotation is the angle measured between the posterior cortex of the sacrum and the anterior cortex of the L5 vertebral body.

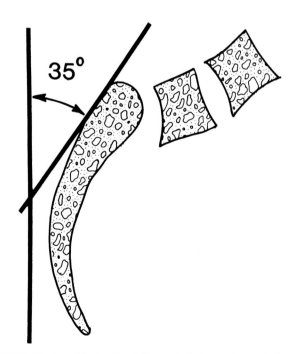

FIGURE 11. Sacral inclination is the angle between the posterior surface of the sacrum and a vertical line drawn from the floor. Normal sacral inclination is greater than 30 degrees.

of S2 to the projection of L5 on the horizontal line is *a* and the distance from the center of S2 to the projection of the femoral head is *b*. Their SPTI is defined as *a/b*. They found that a decreasing SPTI correlated with slip progression and also that those presenting with a lower SPTI (less than 0.7) were more likely to require surgical intervention for their symptoms or progression.

CT scans and magnetic resonance imaging (MRI) studies are used with increasing frequency, particularly in patients whose symptoms suggest cauda equina or nerve root compression. It should be noted that other abnormalities, such as tethered cord, should be sought in such patients (120). It has also been noted that spondylolysis may retard the growth of the facet joints and affect the characteristics of the joint surfaces (131).

Both CT/myelography and operative findings suggest that nerve root compression may occur by one mechanism or by a combination of mechanisms. The L5 arch has been found by some surgeons to pinch the dura. This, as well as compression from the posterior aspect of the upper sacrum, may be seen on CT/myelography or found at the time of surgical exploration (26,68,150).

With significant slippage of the L5 forward on the sacrum, the intervening disc may remain with the sacrum but may appear split or bulging on CT or MRI images, suggesting canal narrowing (11,195).

RISK FACTORS

There is general agreement that low-grade spondylolisthesis can usually be successfully managed with conservative measures (60,171). Progression of spondylolisthesis is more likely in younger or skeletally immature patients because it usually occurs during the preadolescent years or in higher grades of slippage (79,105,125,173,174). Reports indicate that dysplastic spondylo-listhesis is more likely to progress than isthmic spondylolisthesis. Although spondylolysis and spondylolisthesis are more common in young males, progression and advanced slippage are more common in young females (172,174).

Most surgeons agree that spondylolisthesis with slippage greater than 30% to 50% in an adolescent or child is likely to progress and should be fused (105,106,115,125,202). Patients presenting at a younger age appear to be at increased risk for progression.

Patients with greater than 100 degrees of lumbosacral kyphosis (46), decreasing sagittal pelvic tilt indices (170), or higher slip angles also appear to be at risk for progression.

CONSERVATIVE TREATMENT

In patients who have inciting repetitive trauma, such as gymnasts or divers, restriction of the aggravating activity or bed rest often relieves the symptoms of spondylolysis or spondylolisthesis (31). Bracing in neutral lordosis renders good to excellent results in up to 80% of patients with grade 0 or I spondylolisthesis (9,152,190). Brace wear is recommended for 3 to 6 months full time, with gradual weaning as symptoms permit. Occasionally, this treatment regimen permits healing of the stress fracture, particularly with more acute clinical presentations (31,190) (Fig. 12). Physical therapy should emphasize stretching of the lumbodorsal fascia and abdominal strengthening (70,187). Patients

with grade I or II spondylolisthesis are more likely to respond to conservative measures, with only 1 of 12 patients with higher grade slips responding to nonoperative measures (60,152).

Many surgeons allow patients who improve after conservative treatment to resume all activities once they are asymptomatic.

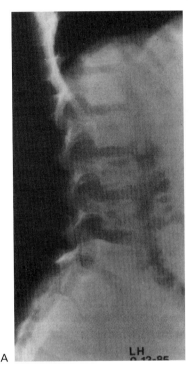

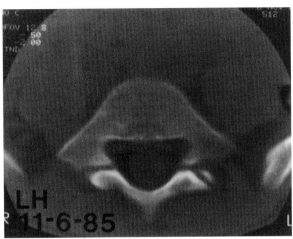

FIGURE 12. A: Lateral radiograph of an 8-year-old patient with symptomatic spondylolysis. **B:** Computed tomography (CT) scan showing bilateral pars defects. **C:** This patient was treated with a cast for 3 months, resulting in healing of the pars defects, as evident on this lateral radiograph. **D:** CT scan showing healed bilateral pars defects after casting.

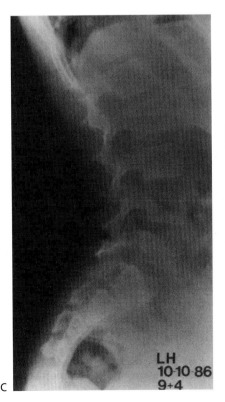

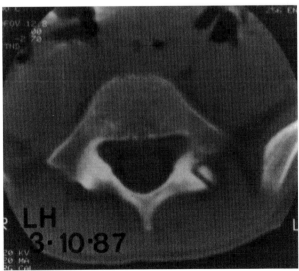

Others do so only if the patient has less than 25% slippage and restrict activities to those who do not load or hyperextend the spine if there is greater than 25% but less than 50% slippage (31,134,210). As will be discussed, fusion is indicated for skeletally immature patients with greater than 50% spondylolisthesis.

Reports tracing the natural history of patients who have spondylolysis or mild to moderate spondylolisthesis note a generally benign course. In one study from Germany (134), competitive athletes from a special school were followed for several years. Although small degrees of progression occurred in some patients, no patient developed any symptoms during the period of study. Most patients who have been managed conservatively as youngsters are satisfied as adults. Progression is rare after adolescence. In fact, progression is rare for those with less than 20% to 30% slippage (57,60,171,173,174).

Pars defects are seen less frequently at L4 and are even more rare in the upper lumbar spine. Male predominance, inciting trauma, and prevalence in young adults compared with adolescents have been noted. Significant slippage at L4 is more uncommon than at the lumbosacral junction. However, neurologic symptoms and spinal stenosis appear to be more common (87,164).

POSTERIOR FUSION

Patients whose symptoms do not resolve with conservative measures, who show progression of their spondylolisthesis, who have greater than 50% slippage, or who have gait or postural abnormalities are candidates for surgical intervention (76,80). For low-grade (less than 50%) slippage, in situ fusion is the treatment of choice. Early reports of interlaminar fusion noted fusion rates of 83% to 84% and improvement of symptoms in 79% to 95% of patients (18,76,78,198). The advent of intertransverse or bilateral lateral fusion has improved fusion rates to 83% to 95% and the clinical outcome to 75% to 100% excellent or good results (37,61,66,73,202).

The need for decompression should be evaluated in patients who have neurologic findings (1,91,102,159,203). Gill (67,69) described good results with his technique of removing the loose lamina as well as the fibrocartilaginous scar at the site of the pars defect. Most surgeons currently recommend removing the residual pars to the base of the pedicle to complete the decompression. It should be noted that for young patients isolated decompression without fusion is contraindicated because it will increase the likelihood of progression (5,100). Several authors (18,39,172) reported an increased probability of slip progression in patients who had L5 laminectomy combined with fusion compared with those who underwent a fusion alone. Nevertheless, patients who undergo fusion without removal of the posterior elements of L5 may also demonstrate progression, particularly prior to consolidation of the fusion mass (16,76,80,104,173,193).

Some surgeons have found that signs of nerve root irritation often resolve with fusion of the spondylolisthetic level, making a formal decompression unnecessary. The time frame for resolution of these signs, including hamstring tightness and sciatic pain, averages 6 to 18 months; however, occasionally these signs do not resolve (80,91,215).

With higher grades of spondylolisthesis, fusion from L5 to the sacrum does not have as high a success rate. This is because the fusion mass is placed on tension and is more likely to fail. Therefore, inclusion of L4 in the intended fusion bed is recommended (153).

Because of the increased cosmetic deformity and gait disturbances that can occur with higher grades of slippage, reduction is recommended by some (this is discussed below). However, Hensinger et al. (80) and others (18,59,76,90) reported satisfactory treatment outcomes in such patients without reduction. Only an occasional patient had residual hamstring tightness or nerve root irritation—three of 16 in the Hensinger et al. (80) series—or complaints related to appearance—two of 14 patients in Freeman and Donati's (59) series, two of 17 in Johnson and Kirwan's study (90), and eight (all females) of 52 in Seitsalo's series (171). Progression may occur after fusion; this phenomenon is more common in higher grades of slippage (17,18, 19,20,22,104,153,172,188). Related to these factors, Newton and Johnston (139) specifically found that poor outcome after in situ fusion was correlated with poor fusion mass and that patients with the greater slip angles had a greater chance of a poor result.

The technique of intertransverse process fusion has been extensively described (122,206,213–214) (Fig. 13). Originally, one transverse incision or two parallel paraspinal skin incisions were described. We prefer a midline skin incision with paraspinal fascial incisions, approximately two fingerbreadths off the midline. Blunt dissection with the index finger can direct one to the transverse processes, and the fibers of the sacrospinalis can be

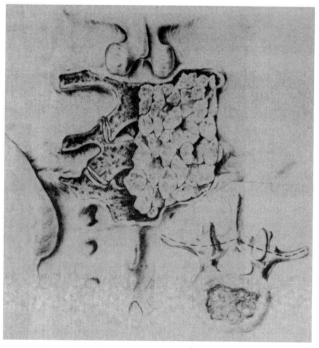

FIGURE 13. Technique of intertransverse process fusion. In this illustration, both midline and lateral bone grafts have been placed.

split, or divided, where needed. Curved self-retaining retractors, such as Gelpis, are often useful to facilitate exposure. The transverse processes, pars interarticularis, and facets of the levels to be fused are exposed using elevators and cautery. If desired, the facet joints may be exposed as well. One should not violate the facet joint at the highest transverse process exposed because its damage may accelerate degenerative changes at this higher level. Iliac crest bone graft is harvested, prepared in corticocancellous strips, and placed over the decorticated bony surface for fusion. Some surgeons advocate the creation of a window or trough in the sacral ala for placement of a larger piece of graft from the sacrum to the upper transverse process to be fused (80).

If decompression is desired, a midline fascial incision should be used to permit removal of the loose posterior elements and exploration and decompression, as described by Gill et al. (69). Not only the loose lamina but also the fibrocartilaginous scar at the site of the defect should be removed.

Postoperative care varies depending on the surgeon's preference. It can range from bed rest for 1 to 2 weeks with application of a pantaloon spica cast (76,80,186) to the use of lumbar corsets (16,66,73), thoracolumbar orthoses (73), or thoracolumbosacral orthoses with leg extensions. After achievement of a solid posterolateral fusion, patients are permitted to return to activities as desired.

DIRECT REPAIR

Direct repair of the pars defect was originally described by Buck (25) in 1970. Screw fixation was used to fix internally the two fragments of the involved vertebra. Since his report, several authors have described their results with this technique (147,157,200,216). Bradford and Iza (23) described their results with transverse process to spinous process wiring, a technique suggested by James Scott (Figs. 14 and 15). Eighty percent of their patients had good to excellent results, with 90% achieving healing of the defect. Kakiuchi (94) described his results in 16 patients with grade I or II spondylolisthesis using a variable-angle Danek screw in the pedicle and a laminar hook, bridging and compressing across the pars defect. He removed all implants

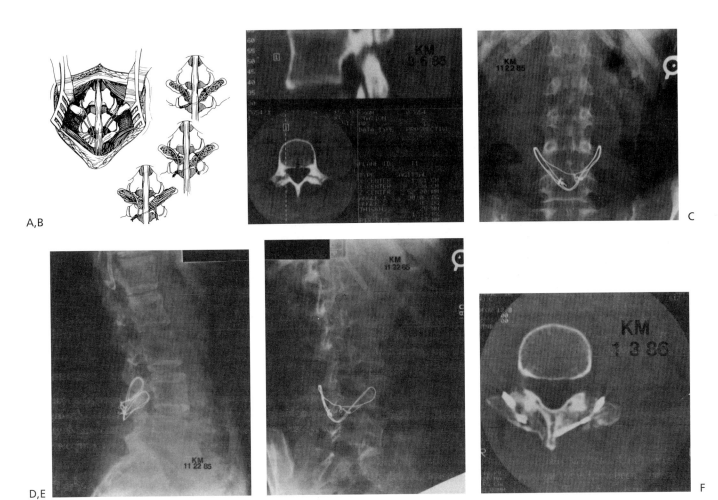

FIGURE 14. A: Diagram showing transverse process to spinous process wiring, for direct repair of the pars defect. **B:** Computed tomography (CT) scan and sagittal reconstruction showing bilateral pars defects at L4. **C:** Anteroposterior radiograph after repair and wiring. **D:** Lateral radiograph after repair and wiring. **E:** Oblique view of direct repair with wiring. **F:** CT scan demonstrating healing of pars defect after direct repair and bone grafting of pars defect.

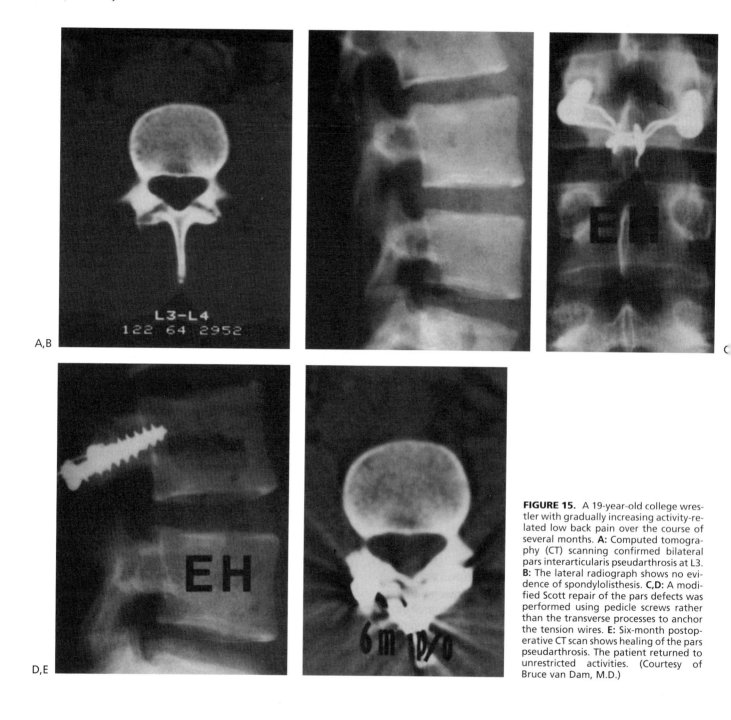

A,B

C

D,E

FIGURE 15. A 19-year-old college wrestler with gradually increasing activity-related low back pain over the course of several months. **A:** Computed tomography (CT) scanning confirmed bilateral pars interarticularis pseudarthrosis at L3. **B:** The lateral radiograph shows no evidence of spondylolisthesis. **C,D:** A modified Scott repair of the pars defects was performed using pedicle screws rather than the transverse processes to anchor the tension wires. **E:** Six-month postoperative CT scan shows healing of the pars pseudarthrosis. The patient returned to unrestricted activities. (Courtesy of Bruce van Dam, M.D.)

and gave radiographic evidence of osseous union in all patients, with all patients noting either complete relief or major improvement of symptoms; 90% obtained healing of their defects. Others have had comparable results with wiring (50,65,72,140) and rigid fixation (111,133), noting 67% to 92% good to excellent results. Pars repair is best considered for L1 to L4 defects in patients younger than 25, with no evidence of disc or facet pathology and no more than 1 to 2 mm of slippage (23). The technique may also be useful for patients with multiple-level pars defects (50).

Biomechanical studies comparing the bending stiffness of the intact spine, the spine with pars defects, and the spine after

transverse process–spinous process wiring indicate that this technique restores the spine to normal stiffness values (72,218).

ANTERIOR FUSION

The anterior approach for spinal fusion as treatment of spondylolisthesis was first proposed by Capener (28) in 1932. Shortly thereafter, Burns (27) reported on his cases with an anterior fusion technique that included placement of a tibial or fibular graft through a drill hole from the L5 vertebral body to the sacrum (Fig. 16A). This technique and that of disc space grafting

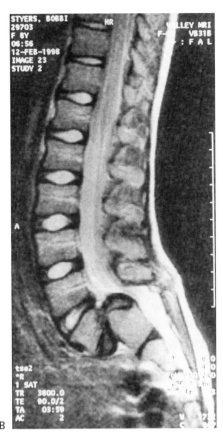

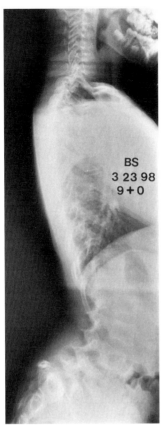

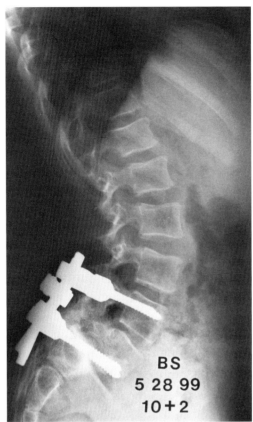

A,B

C

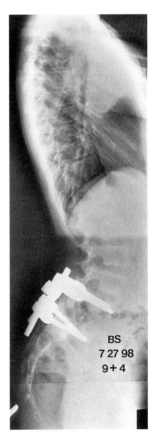

D,E

FIGURE 16. A: Preoperative standing lateral radiograph of 8-year-old female with grade V spondylolysis. **B:** Lateral MRI view. **C,D:** Postoperative anteroposterior and lateral radiographs after partial reduction, placement of transsacral fibular graft, pedicle screw instrumentation, and posterolateral fusion. Note placement of S1 pedicle screws into the body of L5. **E:** Standing lateral radiograph demonstrating improved sagittal balance.

with tricortical iliac crest have been applied successfully (30,40,51,58,84). Adolescents, however, constitute only a small minority of each series. Studies of adolescents who underwent anterior spinal fusion with iliac crest bone grafting reported solid fusion in all patients and complete symptomatic relief in virtually all patients (110,177,201). One of these studies noted gait improvement in all patients; another study did not mention this clinical outcome.

The procedure can be done via either a retroperitoneal or a transperitoneal approach, depending on the surgeon's preference. It has been suggested that for higher grade slips, an anterior fusion places the graft in compression, which is a more biomechanically sound construct (43). The risk of the anterior approach in males has been described, although the actual incidence of postoperative sterility secondary to retrograde ejaculation appears to be low (47,56,92).

Anterior spinal fusion with fibular or other structural graft may also be useful in cases of failed posterolateral arthrodesis (22,93,208).

COMBINED APPROACHES

With variable results from fusion in situ or anterior fusion alone for high-grade spondylolisthesis, some surgeons have advocated combined anterior and posterior approaches for these more challenging cases.

Muschik et al. (135) compared their results of anterior fusion versus anterior fusion combined with posterior instrumented reduction for high-grade spondylolisthesis. They found the pseudarthrosis rate, residual degree of slippage, and residual lumbosacral kyphosis to be lower in patients who had combined approaches rather than anterior fusion alone. However, the clinical outcomes were equivalent and the non-pseudarthrosis-related complications were higher for the patients with combined surgery. A similar study that also compared anterior interbody fusion with combined surgery for high-grade slippages found equivalent results with respect to subjective clinical, functional, and radiographic outcomes, except with respect to progression of sagittal rotation, which occurred in the anterior fusion group (196). The investigators noted that the long-term effect of this improved radiographic result was not known.

POSTERIOR DOWEL GRAFT/POSTERIOR INTERBODY FUSION

Bohlman and associates (13,186) have described a technique, also utilized by others (52,158), for single-stage posterior decompression and interbody fusion in the management of spondyloptosis. After wide decompression and foraminotomy (as needed) and removal of the posterior-superior aspect of the first sacral vertebral body, a drill hole is prepared between the L5 and S1 nerve roots on each side. This hole traverses S1 to the displaced L5 vertebral body, not penetrating the anterior cortex of L5, and is checked with fluoroscopic control. Autograft fibula is then inserted and countersunk longitudinally to avoid dural impingement.

We have successfully used the interbody dowel technique

combined with posterior interpedicular instrumentation in patients who have had partial reduction of a high-grade slippage (Fig. 16) (185).

Posterior lumbar interbody fusion has been successfully applied to young patients with spondylolisthesis (32). However, because of problems with graft resorption and collapse (181), as well as the dangers of perineural scarring, other surgical options are usually preferable.

Harms et al. have promoted the concept of performing an interbody fusion (either via a combined approach or via a transforaminal interbody fusion) in all cases of spondylolisthesis to reduce the shear forces seen at the intervertebral disc and reduce the lumbosacral kyphosis (74). Although we and others (184) have been encouraged by early results of instrumented posterior fusions combined with transforaminal interbody fusion, the selection of young patients for whom this approach is preferable to other techniques available has not been determined.

REDUCTION

Reduction of high-grade spondylolisthesis has received increasing attention in recent years. Reduction of the slip angle is particularly important in the maintenance of correction because those with higher slip angles are more likely to exhibit progression after fusion (18). Residual gait abnormalities in patients fused in situ for high-grade spondylolisthesis, though minor in the young patient (179), may have consequences with maturity, perhaps analogous to flat-back syndrome (205). Spondylolisthesis reduction also appears to improve sagittal alignment, resulting in a more normal gait and trunk appearance.

The technique of closed reduction and fusion was first reported by Jenkins (89) in 1936 and later refined by others (19,21,55,123,193). Preoperative halofemoral or halopelvic traction is applied. Distraction is applied along the axis of the spine; rotation of the pelvis brings the sacrum back to a more normal inclination. Direct pressure is applied to the posterior portion of the sacrum (166) (Fig. 17). This permits gradual reduction with less risk to the neural elements. Careful neurologic assessment is recommended every 4 to 6 hours. A posterior decompression may improve the correction attained, particularly if an elongated pars is present (166). Posterolateral fusion is performed after a period of traction or at the time of decompression. After the additional period of reduction is completed, anterior spinal fusion may be performed if desired. Dubousset recommended anterior interbody fusion if the lumbosacral angle, measured from the superior end plate of L5 and the posterior border of the sacrum, could not be improved to 100 degrees after reduction (46). Casting is performed after acceptable reduction has been attained.

The technique of anterior spinal fusion after reduction is similar to that described previously (43). In addition, the placement of a curved retractor, such as a Homan, within the L5–S1 disc space and the application of a distraction and posterior translation force may permit additional reduction to be achieved. If desired, a structural graft, such as fibula, can be placed through a drill hole from the L5 vertebral body into the sacrum to stabilize the reduction (89).

A period of bed rest after anterior fusion is recommended,

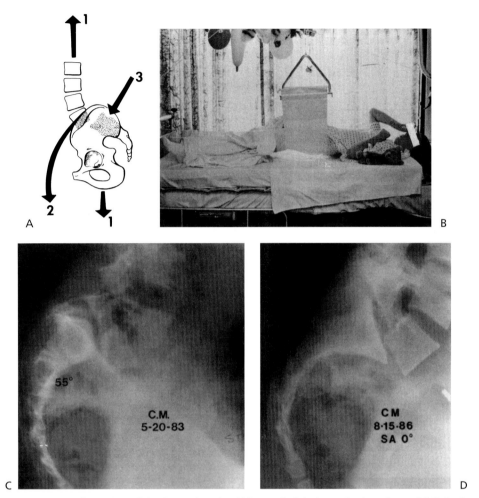

FIGURE 17. A: Illustration of the forces that should be applied during reduction of spondylolisthesis with traction. Axial traction is applied, the pelvis is rotated, and direct pressure is applied to the posterior portion of the scarum. **B:** Photograph of a young girl in traction to reduce her high-grade spondylolisthesis. **C:** Preoperative lateral radiograph demonstrating grade IV spondylolisthesis. **D:** Radiograph after preoperative traction, posterolateral fusion of L4 to the sacrum, and postoperative cast reduction and immobilization.

followed by corrective casting in a pantaloon cast for at least 3 months (43).

Previously, posterior distraction instrumentation from L2 to the sacrum has been used to provide the forces needed for reduction (41,43,75,96,182,204). Because distraction is now understood to flatten the patient's lumbar lordosis and to be a less biomechanically stable construct compared with pedicular screws (181), distraction instrumentation is no longer recommended in the treatment of spondylolisthesis. However, a temporary distraction rod may be used to facilitate reduction.

Interpedicular screws have been applied by several authors (14,44,53,117,126,142,168,182,189). Edwards (48,49) reported on the reduction of high-grade spondylolisthesis via a pedicle screw system that permits gradual distraction, flexion of the sacrum, and posterior translation of the upper lumbar spine. He reported satisfactory results in his patient series, averaging age 25 years, with an average preoperative slip angle of 33 degrees corrected to 4 degrees postoperatively, with only one neurologic deficit and one pseudarthrosis. However, his experience with

spondyloptosis demonstrated a 25% rate of neurologic complications despite the fact that overall improvement of back and leg pain was quite high (36). We have also applied a similar technique to young patients who have failed previous treatment and in skeletally mature but young patients with advanced slippage and a significant cosmetic deformity, tight hamstrings, and the inability to stand erect with the knees straight (85). In this study, preoperative slippage averaged 89%; postoperatively this was improved to 29%. Slip angle averaged 50 degrees preoperatively and was improved to 24 degrees postoperatively. Hardware failure occurred in 25% of patients, all early in the series, and was successfully revised. Later, patients in the series and subsequently have had fibular interbody fusion performed if their slip angle was not adequately reduced. Neurologic complications, occurring in four of the 16 patients, resolved in all but one patient.

A variation of the reduction technique is an L5 vertebrectomy with reduction of L4 onto S1 (64). Surgeons applying this technique believed that it had decreased neurologic risk because the spine is, in effect, shortened. However, their follow-up, larger series (107) demonstrated that despite spinal shortening, the neurologic risk is considerable, with 75% of their 16 patients having early neurologic deficits (seven had preoperative deficits). All of the patients with permanent deficits had had preoperative deficits. Overall, five patients with preoperative deficits improved, six had a worsened neurologic deficit postoperatively, but only one had a permanent worsening of the neurologic deficit. The investigators also noted that the technique restores spinal alignment without the necessity of traction and postoperative casting. Detractors of this method note that the trunk remains shortened and neurologic risks are not avoided.

Results after reduction of high-grade slips have generally been satisfactory, although there have been complications. DeWald et al. (43) performed staged posterior fusion (L4-sacrum) and reduction with Harrington rod instrumentation (L1-sacrum), followed by anterior spinal fusion (L5-sacrum) on 14 young patients with greater than 50% slips. Instrumentation was removed after 6 to 12 months. Only one patient, who had a preoperative 100% slip, developed neurologic problems. This resolved after removal of rods, permitting the patient's spine to fuse in situ. All others went on to solid fusion with normal spinal alignment and gait. The patient who had fusion in situ continued to demonstrate abnormal posture and gait. Muschik's series (135) comparing anterior spinal fusion in situ with combined anterior fusion and posterior instrumented reduction, the fusion rate was greater and better reduction was achieved in patients with combined surgery; however, one neurologic injury (bilateral foot drop) and one vascular injury occurred in the group who underwent reduction.

In Harrington and Tullos's (75) series of nine adolescent patients with grade IV and V slippage treated with Harrington rod reduction, one patient developed cauda equina symptoms, which partially resolved. This patient had preoperative slippage of 90%, which was corrected to 5% at surgery. Some correction was lost in the first year, and the slippage increased to 30% at 3-year follow-up. This was the only patient who lost more than 5 degrees of correction. In Bradford's (21) series of 22 patients who underwent posterolateral fusion and cast reduction, two of six treated in skeletal traction developed unilateral transient L5 weakness. One patient had significant loss of correction secondary to infection and loosening of pelvic fixator pins. Correction of slip angle was well maintained, and only two patients noted mild low back symptoms at follow-up.

Up to a 20% incidence of postoperative sensory deficits and up to a 30% incidence of motor deficits have been noted in some series, although the majority of these have been transient (14,19,44,85,117,142,168). Transient bladder dysfunction was also noted in up to 28% of these patients (55,126). One case report noted paresis of the L2, L3, and L4 nerve roots after reduction of a grade IV spondylolisthesis. This was believed to have occurred because the reduction required posterior and proximal displacement of the proximal spine, with resultant traction on these proximal nerve roots (197). This improved but did not return to normal after reoperation and allowance for a partial loss of reduction.

The extent of L5 nerve stretch in spondylolisthesis reduction has been nicely demonstrated anatomically by Petraco and colleagues (149). They found that the mean nerve strain was 4%

for the first 50% of reduction but increased to 10% for the second half of the reduction. With high grades of slippage, rotation of the L5 vertebral body (i.e., decreasing the lumbosacral kyphosis) resulted in nerve slackening.

COMPLICATIONS

Although fusion in situ is considered a safe and reliable operation for the treatment of spondylolisthesis, cauda equina syndrome has been reported to occur after fusion for grade III or IV spondylolisthesis (61,119,167). This may be related to mechanical factors secondary to impingement at the dome of the sacrum or lamina of L5, as direct iatrogenic injury to the cauda equina was not demonstrated. Early decompression, including removal of the dome of the sacrum and adjacent disc, appears to improve the likelihood of neurologic recovery. The neurologic risk with reduction maneuvers has been delineated above.

It has been suggested that because the lumbar segments above a spinal fusion may be required to bear additional stresses, they are susceptible to disc damage or even spondylolysis (12,24, 73,81). However, when comparing patients who had had L5–S1 fusions for spondylolisthesis with those who had been treated conservatively, Seitsalo and co-workers did not find the rate of disc degeneration at L4–5 to be significantly increased by fusion (175).

Management of patients with significant complaints after surgery for spondylolisthesis is difficult. Jones et al. (93) reported on four patients with grade III or IV slippage who had severe low back pain, gait abnormalities, and neurologic deficit after previous surgery. These patients were then treated by anterior spinal fusion and stabilization using a fibular strut graft, supplemented in two cases by posterolateral fusion. All of the patients in this small series went on to fusion, with improvement of symptoms and gait.

Bradford and Gotfried (22) reviewed 16 patients with grade IV or V spondylolisthesis, all of whom had progressed after previous surgery. These patients presented with severe pain, often with symptoms of neurogenic claudication, and crouched gait. They underwent two- or three-stage surgery, including posterior osteotomy and posterolateral fusion, followed by anterior fusion, partial correction, and grafting. Several patients were treated in traction between stages. When it was deemed indicated, a third stage for application of Harrington compression rods was performed. Three patients in the series had resection of L5 with reduction of L4 onto the sacrum, with the anterior procedure performed first. There were six delayed unions; these were explored and the fusion was augmented, instrumentation was added, or both. There were five neuropathies, three of which resolved, and only one patient with transient difficulty voiding. All patients had excellent or good results and improvement of their deformities. There was marked improvement of percent slippage and slip angle in all patients, which was maintained at follow-up. Although this is a difficult procedure requiring prolonged treatment and with significant associated risks, it is believed to be feasible for patients with significant disability. Note that high rates of pseudarthrosis occurred in series prior to use of transpedicular instrumentation, which would now be considered the instrumentation of choice for these patients.

CONCLUSION

Spondylolysis and spondylolisthesis are common problems. The majority of patients presenting with symptoms can be managed nonoperatively. Continuing back pain, with or without radiculopathy, that is unresponsive to conservative management can usually be managed by posterolateral spinal fusion.

Reduction should be considered only if loss of sagittal alignment is significantly compromising function or if a decompression for a high-grade slippage is believed likely to result in progressive deformity even with arthrodesis in situ. Anatomical reduction is not necessary, and reduction of slip angle rather than complete reduction of the slippage appears less neurologically risky and yields satisfactory results in children, adolescents, and young adults for whom this procedure is indicated.

REFERENCES

1. Adkins EWO (1955): Spondylolisthesis. *J Bone Joint Surg Br* 37: 48–62.
2. Aland C, Rineberg BS, Malberg M, et al. (1986): Fracture of the pedicle of the fourth lumbar vertebra associated with contralateral spondylolysis. *J Bone Joint Surg Am* 68:1454–1455.
3. Albanese M, Pizzutillo PD (1982): Family study of spondylolysis and spondylolisthesis. *J Pediatr Orthop* 2:496–499.
4. Amato M, Totty WG, Gilula LA (1984): Spondylolysis of the lumbar spine: demonstration of defects and laminal fragmentation. *Radiology* 153:627–629.
5. Amuso SJ, Neff RS, Coulson DB, et al. (1970): The surgical treatment of spondylolisthesis by posterior element resection. *J Bone Joint Surg Am* 52:529–536.
6. Baker DR, McHollick W (1956): Spondyloschisis spondylolisthesis in children. *J Bone Joint Surg Am* 38:933–934.
7. Barash HL, Galante JO, Lambert CL, et al. (1970): Spondylolisthesis and tight hamstrings. *J Bone Joint Surg Am* 52:1319–1328.
8. Batts M (1939): The etiology of spondylolisthesis. *J Bone Joint Surg* 21:879–884.
9. Bell DF, Ehrlich MG, Zaleske DJ (1988): Brace treatment for symptomatic spondylolisthesis. *Clin Orthop* 236:192–198.
10. Bellah RD, Summerville DA, Treves ST, et al. (1991): Low back pain in adolescent athletes: Detection of stress injury to the pars interarticularis with SPECT. *Radiology* 180: 509–512.
11. Birch JG, Herring JA, Maravilla KR (1986): Splitting of the intervertebral disc in spondylolisthesis: a magnetic resonance imaging finding in two cases. *J Pediatr Orthop* 6:609–611.
12. Blasier RD, Monson RC (1987): Acquired spondylolysis after posterolateral fusion. *J Pediatr Orthop* 7:215–217.
13. Bohlman HH, Cook SS (1982): One-stage decompression and posterolateral and interbody fusion for lumbosacral spondyloptosis through a posterior approach. *J Bone Joint Surg Am* 64:415–418.
14. Boos N, Marchesi D, Zuber K, et al. (1993): Treatment of severe spondylolisthesis by reduction and pedicular fixation. *Spine* 18: 1655–1661.
15. Borkow SE, Kleiger B (1971): Spondylolisthesis in the newborn. *Clin Orthop* 81:73–76.
16. Bosworth DM, Fielding JW, Demarest L, Bonaquist M (1955): Spondylolisthesis: a critical review of a consecutive series of cases treated by arthrodesis. *J Bone Joint Surg Am* 37:767–785.
17. Boxall D, Bradford DS, Winter RB, et al. (1979): Management of severe spondylolisthesis in children and adolescents. *J Bone Joint Surg Am* 61:479–495.
18. Bradford DS (1979): Spondylolysis and spondylolisthesis. *Curr Pract Orthop* 8:12–37.
19. Bradford DS (1979): Treatment of severe spondylolisthesis: a combined approach for reduction and stabilization. *Spine* 4:423–429.
20. Bradford DS (1983): Spondylolysis and spondylolisthesis in children and adolescents: current concepts in management. In: Bradford DS, Hensinger R, eds. *The pediatric spine.* New York: Thieme Verlag, pp. 403–423.
21. Bradford DS (1988): Closed reduction of spondylolisthesis: an experience in 22 patients. *Spine* 13:580–587.
22. Bradford DS, Gotfried Y (1987): Staged salvage reconstruction of grade IV and V spondylolisthesis. *J Bone Joint Surg Am* 69:191–202.
23. Bradford DS, Iza J (1985): Repair of the defect in spondylolysis or minimal degrees of spondylolisthesis by segmental wire fixation and bone grafting. *Spine* 10:673–679.
24. Brunet JA, Wiley JJ (1984): Acquired spondylolysis after spinal fusion. *J Bone Joint Surg Br* 66:720–724.
25. Buck JE (1970): Direct repair of the defect in spondylolisthesis. *J Bone Joint Surg Br* 52:432–437.
26. Buirski G, McCall IW, O'Brien JP (1984): Myelography in severe lumbosacral spondylolisthesis. *Br J Radiol* 57:1067–1072.
27. Burns RH (1933): An operation for spondylolisthesis. *Lancet* 1:1233.
28. Capener N (1932): Spondylolisthesis. *Br J Surg* 19:374–386.
29. Chandraraj S, Briggs CA (1991): Multiple growth cartilages in the neural arch. *Anat Rec* 230:114–120.
30. Cheng CL, Fang D, Lee PC, et al. (1989): Anterior spinal fusion for spondylolysis and isthmic spondylolisthesis. *J Bone Joint Surg Br* 71: 264–267.
31. Ciullo JV, Jackson DW (1985): Pars interarticularis stress reaction, spondylolysis and spondylolisthesis in gymnasts. *Clin Sports Med* 4: 95–110.
32. Cloward RB (1981): Spondylolisthesis: treatment by laminectomy and posterior interbody fusion. *Clin Orthop* 154:74–81.
33. Collier BD, Johnson RP, Carrera GF, et al. (1985): Painful spondylolysis or spondylolisthesis studied by radiography and single-photon emission computed tomography. *Radiology* 154:207–211.
34. Commandre FA, Raillan B, Gagnerie F, et al. (1988): Spondylolysis and spondylolisthesis in young athletes: 28 cases. *J Sports Med* 28: 104–107.
35. Cope R (1988): Acute traumatic spondylolysis. *Clin Orthop* 230: 162–165.
36. Curcin A, Edwards C: Reduction and fusion of spondylptosis: long term follow up. Presented at the 29th Annual Meeting of the Scoliosis Research Society. *Orthop Trans* 18(2):562.
37. Dandy DJ, Shannon MJ (1971): Lumbosacral subluxation. *J Bone Joint Surg Am* 53:578–595.
38. Danielson B, Frennered K, Selvik G, et al. (1989): Roentgenologic assessment of spondylolisthesis: an evaluation of progression. *Acta Radiol* 30:65–68.
39. Davis IS, Bailey RW (1972): Spondylolisthesis: long-term follow-up study of treatment with total laminectomy. *Clin Orthop* 88:46–49.
40. Debeyre J, Dorat J (1969): Arthrodeses intersomatiques lombosacrees. *Rev Chir Orthop* 55:499–514.
41. Del Torio U (1971): Surgical reduction and stabilization of spondylolisthesis. *Clin Orthop* 75:281–284.
42. Deyerle WM (1961): Lumbar nerve-root irritation in children. *Clin Orthop* 21:125–136.
43. DeWald RL, Faut MM, Taddonio RF, et al. (1981): Severe lumbosacral spondylolisthesis in adolescents and children. *J Bone Joint Surg Am* 63:619–626.
44. Dick WT, Schnebel B (1988): Severe spondylolisthesis: Reduction and internal fixation. *Clin Orthop* 232:70–79.
45. Dietrich M, Kurowski P (1985): The importance of mechanical factors in the etiology of spondylolysis. *Spine* 10:532–542.
46. Dubousset J (1997): Treatment of spondylolysis and spondylolisthesis in children and adolescents. *Clin Orthop Rel Res* 337:77–85.
47. Duncan HJM, Jonck LM (1965): The presacral plexus in anterior fusion of the lumbar spine. *Suid-Afr Tydrkrif Chir* 3:93–96.
48. Edwards CC (1986): Reduction of spondylolisthesis: Biomechanics and fixation. *Orthop Trans* 10:543.

49. Edwards CC (1997): Reduction of spondylolisthesis. In: Bridwell KT, de Wald RL, eds. *The Textbook of Spinal Surgery,* 2nd ed., Philadelphia: JB Lippincott, pp. 1317–1335.

50. Eingorn D, Pizzutillo PD (1985): Pars interarticularis fusion of multiple levels of lumbar spondylolysis. *Spine* 10:250–252.

51. Edvardsen P (1983): Traumatic lumbar spondylolisthesis: anterior fusion by means of a fibular graft. *Injury* 14:366–369.

52. Esses S, Natout N, Kip P (1995): Posterior interbody arrhrodesis with a fibular strut graft in spondylolisthesis. *J Bone Joint Surg Am* 77A: 72–76.

53. Fabris D, Costantini S, Nena U (1996): Surgical treatment of severe L5–S1 spondylolisthesis in children and adolescents. *Spine* 6: 728–733.

54. Farfan HF, Osteria V, Lamy C (1976): The mechanical etiology of spondylolysis and spondylolisthesis. *Clin Orthop* 117:40–55.

55. Ferris LR, Ho E, Leong JCY (1990): Lumbar spondyloptosis: a long term follow up of three cases. *Int Orthop* 14:139–143.

56. Flynn J, Price C (1984). Sexual complications of anterior fusion of the lumbar spine. *Spine* 9:489–92.

57. Fredrickson BE, Baker D, McHolick WJ, et al. (1984): The natural history of spondylolysis and spondy-lolisthesis. *J Bone Joint Surg Am* 66:699–707.

58. Freebody D, Bendall R, Taylor RD (1971): Anterior transperitoneal lumbar fusion. *J Bone Joint Surg Br* 53:617–627.

59. Freeman BL, Donati NL (1989): Spinal arthrodesis for severe spondylolysis in children and adolescents. *J Bone Joint Surg Am* 71:594–598.

60. Frennered AK, Danielson BI, Nachemson AL (1991): Natural history of symptomatic isthmic low-grade spondylolisthesis in children and adolescents: a seven-year follow-up study. *J Pediatr Orthop* 11: 209–213.

61. Frennered AK, Danielson BI, Nachemson AL, et al. (1991): Midterm follow-up of young patients fused in situ for spondylolisthesis. *Spine* 16:409–416.

62. Friberg S (1939): Studies on spondylolisthesis. *Acta Chir Scand* 82: 139.

63. Friberg O (1991): Instability in spondylolisthesis. *Orthopedics* 14: 463–466.

64. Gaines RW, Nichols WK (1985): Treatment of spondyloptosis by two stage L5 vertebrectomy and reduction of L4 onto S1. *Spine* 10: 680–686.

65. Garber JE, Wright AM (1986): Unilateral spondylolysis and contralateral pedicle fracture. *Spine* 11:63–66.

66. Gelfand MJ, Strife JL, Kereiakes JG (1981): Radionuclide bone imaging in spondylolysis of the lumbar spine in children. *Radiology* 140: 191–195.

67. Gill GG (1984): Long term follow-up evaluation of a few patients with spondylolisthesis treated by excision of the loose lamina with decompression of the nerve roots without spinal fusion. *Clin Orthop* 182:215–219.

68. Gill GG, Binder WF (1980): Autoamputation of the first sacral nerve roots in spondyloptosis. *Spine* 5:295–297.

69. Gill GG, Manning JG, White HL (1955): Surgical treatment of spondylolisthesis without spine fusion. *J Bone Joint Surg Am* 37:493–520.

70. Gramse RR, Sinaki M, Ilstrup D (1980): Lumbar spondylolisthesis: a rational approach to conservative treatment. *Mayo Clin Proc* 55: 681–686.

71. Goldberg MJ (1980): Gymnastic injuries. *Orthop Clin North Am* 11: 717–726.

72. Hambly M, Lee CK, Gutteling E, et al. (1989): Tension band wiring-bone grafting for spondylolysis and spondylolisthesis. *Spine* 14: 455–459.

73. Haraldsson S, Willner S (1983): A comparative study of spondylolisthesis in operations on adolescents and adults. *Arch Orthop Trauma Surg* 101:101–105.

74. Harms J, Jeszenszky D, Stoltze D, et al. (1997) True spondylolisthesis reduction and monosegmental fusion in spondylolisthesis. In: Bridwell KW, deWald RL, eds. *The textbook of spinal surgery,* 2nd ed. Philadelphia: Lippincott-Raven Publishers, pp. 1337–1347.

75. Harrington PR, Tullos HS (1971): Spondylolisthesis in children. *Clin Orthop* 79:75–84.

76. Harris IE, Weinstein SL (1987): Long-term follow-up of patients with grade III and IV spondylolisthesis. *J Bone Joint Surg Am* 69: 960–969.

77. Harris RI (1951): Spondylolisthesis. *Ann R Coll Surg Engl* 8:259–297.

78. Henderson ED (1966): Results of surgical treatment of spondylolisthesis. *J Bone Joint Surg Am* 48:619–641.

79. Hensinger RN (1989): Spondylolysis and spondylolisthesis in children and adolescents. *J Bone Joint Surg Am* 71:1098–1107.

80. Hensinger RN, Lang JR, MacEwen GD (1976): Surgical management of spondylolisthesis in children and adolescents. *Spine* 1: 207–215.

81. Henson J, McCall IW, O'Brien JP (1987): Disc damage above a spondylolisthesis. *Br J Radiol* 60:69–72.

82. Herbinaux G (1782): *Traite sur divers accouchemens laborieux, et sur polypes de la matrice.* Brussels: JL De Boubers.

83. Hitchcock HH (1940): Spondylolisthesis. *J Bone Joint Surg* 22:1–16.

84. Hodgson AR, Wong SK (1968): A description of a technic and evaluation of results in anterior spinal fusion for deranged intervertebral disk and spondylolisthesis. *Clin Orthop* 56:133–162.

85. Hu S, Bradford D, Transfeldt E, et al. (1996) Reduction of high-grade spondylolisthesis using Edwards instrumentation. *Spine* 21:367–371.

86. Ichikawa N, Ohara Y, Morishita T, et al. (1982): An aetiological study on spondylolysis from a biomechanical aspect. *Br J Sports Med* 16:135–141.

87. Jackson AM, Kirwan EO, Sullivan MF (1978): Lytic spondylolisthesis above the lumbosacral level. *Spine* 3:260–266.

88. Jackson DW, Wiltse LL, Cirincione RJ (1976): Spondylolysis in the female gymnast. *Clin Orthop* 117:68–73.

89. Jenkins JA (1936): Spondylolisthesis. *Br J Surg* 24:80–85.

90. Johnson JR, Kirwan EO (1983): The long-term results of fusion in situ for severe spondylolisthesis. *J Bone Joint Surg Br* 65:43–46.

91. Johnson LP, Nasca RJ, Dunham WK (1988): Surgical management of isthmic spondylolisthesis. *Spine* 13:93–97.

92. Johnson RM, McGuire EJ (1981): Urogenital complications of anterior approaches to the lumbar spine. *Clin Orthop* 154:114–118.

93. Jones AAM, McAfee PC, Robinson RA, et al. (1988): Failed arthrodesis of the spine for severe spondylolisthesis. *J Bone Joint Surg Am* 70: 25–30.

94. Kakiuchi M (1997) Repair of the defect in spondylolysis. *J Bone Joint Surg Am* 79:818–825.

95. Kalebo P, Kadziolka R, Sward L, et al. (1989): Stress views in the comparative assessment of spondylolytic spondylolisthesis. *Skeletal Radiol* 317:570–575.

96. Kaneda K, Satoh S, Nohara Y, et al. (1985): Distraction rod instrumentation with posterolateral fusion in isthmic spondylolisthesis. *Spine* 10:383–389.

97. Keessen W, During J, Beeker TW, et al. (1984): Recordings of the movement of the intervertebral segment L5–S1: a technique for the determination of the movement in the L5–S1 spinal segment by using three specified postural positions. *Spine* 9:83–90.

98. Klinghoffer L (1982): Spondylolysis following trauma. *Clin Orthop* 166:72–74.

99. Krenz J, Troup JDG (1973): The structure of the pars inter-articularis of the lower lumbar vertebrae and its relation to the etiology of spondylolysis. *J Bone Joint Surg Br* 55:735–741.

100. Lafond G (1962): Surgical treatment of spondylolisthesis. *Clin Orthop* 22:175–179.

101. Lambl W (1858): Das wesen und die entstehung de spondylolisthesis. *Beitrage zur Geburtkunde un Gynakologie,* pp. 1–79.

102. Lance EM (1966): Treatment of severe spondylolisthesis with neural involvement. *J Bone Joint Surg Am* 48:884–891.

103. Langston JW, Gavant ML (1985): "Incomplete ring" sign: a simple method for CT detection of spondylolysis. *J Comp Assist Tomogr* 9: 728–729.

104. Laurent LE (1958): Spondylolisthesis. *Acta Orthop Scand* 35(Suppl): 1–45.

105. Laurent LE, Einola S (1961): Spondylolisthesis in children and adolescents. *Acta Orthop Scand* 31:45–64.

106. Laurent LS, Osterman K (1969): Spondylolisthesis in children and adolescents. *Acta Orthop Belg* 35:717–727.

107. Lehmer S, Steffee A, Gaines R (1994): Spondyloptosis by staged L5

resection with reduction and fusion of L4 onto S1. *Spine* 19: 1916–1925.

108. Letts M, Smallman T, Afanasiev R, et al. (1986): Fracture of the pars interarticularis in adolescent athletes: a clinical-biomechanical analysis. *J Pediatr Orthop* 6:40–46.

109. Libson E, Bloom RA, Shapiro Y (1984): Scoliosis in young men with spondylolysis or spondylolisthesis. *Spine* 9:445–447.

110. Lindholm TS, Ragni P, Ylikoski M, et al. (1990): Lumbar isthmic spondylolisthesis in children and adolescents. *Spine* 15:1350–1355.

111. Louis R (1984): Reconstruction of the pars interarticularis in spondylolysis with little or no alteration of the subjacent intervertebral disc. Presented at the International Society of the Study of the Lumbar Spine, Montreal.

112. Lowe J, Libson E, Ziv I, et al. (1987): Spondylolysis in the upper lumbar spine. *J Bone Joint Surg Br* 69:582–586.

113. Lowe J, Schachner E, Hirschberg E, et al. (1984): Significance of bone scintigraphy in symptomatic spondylolysis. *Spine* 9:653–655.

114. Lowe RW, Hayes TD, Kaye J, et al. (1976): Standing roentgenograms in spondylolisthesis. *Clin Orthop* 117:80–84.

115. Lusskin R (1965): Pain patterns in spondylolisthesis: a correlation of symptoms, local pathology and therapy. Reduction of spondylolisthesis. 40:123–136.

116. Marchetti P, Bartolozzi P (1997): Classification of spondylolisthesis as a guideline for treatment. In: Bridwell KW, deWald RL, eds. *The textbook of spinal surgery,* 2nd ed. Philadelphia: Lippincott-Raven Publishers, pp. 1211–1254.

117. Matthiass HH, Heine J (1986): The surgical reduction of spondylolisthesis. *Clin Orthop* 203:34–44.

118. Mau H (1981): Scoliosis and spondylolysis-spondylolisthesis. *Arch Orthop Trauma Surg* 99:29–34.

119. Maurice HD, Morley TR (1989): Cauda equina lesions following fusion in situ and decompressive laminectomy for severe spondylolisthesis: four case reports. *Spine* 14:214–216.

120. McAfee PC, Yuan HA (1982): Computed tomography in spondylolisthesis. *Clin Orthop* 166:62–70.

121. McCarroll JR, Miller JM, Ritter MA (1986): Lumbar spondylosis and spondylolisthesis in college football players. *Am J Sports Med* 14:404–406.

122. McNab I, Dall D (1971): The blood supply of the lumbar spine and its application to the technique of intertransverse fusion. *J Bone Joint Surg Br* 53:628–637.

123. McPhee IB, O'Brien JP (1979): Reduction of severe spondylolisthesis: a preliminary report. *Spine* 4:430–434.

124. McPhee IB, O'Brien JP (1980): Scoliosis in symptomatic spondylolisthesis. *J Bone Joint Surg Br* 62:155–157.

125. McPhee IB, O'Brien JP, McCall IW, et al. (1981): Progression of lumbosacral spondylolisthesis. *Aust Radiol* 25:91–95.

126. McQueen MM, Court-Brown C, Scott JHS (1986): Stabilization of spondylolisthesis using Dwyer instrumentation. *J Bone Joint Surg Br* 68:185–188.

127. Merbs C (1995): Incomplete spondylolysis and healing: a study of ancient Canadian eskimo skeletons. *Spine* 20:2328–2334.

128. Mercer W (1936): Spondylolisthesis. *Edin Med J* 43:545–572.

129. Meyerding HW (1932): Spondylolisthesis. *Surg Gynecol Obstet* 54:371–377.

130. Meyerding HW (1941): Low backache and sciatic pain associated with spondylolisthesis and protruded intervertebral disc: Incidence, significance and treatment. *J Bone Joint Surg* 23:461–470.

131. Miyake R, Ikata T, Katoh S, et al. (1996) Morphologic analysis of the facet joint in the immature lumbosacral spine with special reference to spondylolysis. *Spine* 21: 783–789.

132. Monticelli G, Ascani E (1975): Spondylolysis and spondylolisthesis. *Acta Orthop Scand* 46:498–506.

133. Morscher E, Gerber B, Fasel J (1984): Surgical treatment of spondylolisthesis by bone grafting and direct stabilization of spondylolysis by means of a hook screw. *Arch Orthop Trauma Surg* 103:175–178.

134. Muschik M, Hahnel H, Robinson P, et al. (1996): Competitive sports and the progression of spondylolisthesis. *J Pediatr Orthop* 16: 364–369.

135. Muschik M, Zippel H, Perka C (1997): Surgical management of severe spondylolisthesis in children and adolescents. *Spine* 22: 2036–2043.

136. Neugebauer FL (1976): The classic: a new contribution to the history and etiology of spondylolisthesis. *Clin Orthop* 117: 4–22.

137. Newman PH (1963): The etiology of spondylolisthesis. *J Bone Joint Surg Br* 45:39–59.

138. Newman PH (1965): A clinical syndrome associated with severe lumbosacral subluxation. *J Bone Joint Surg Br* 47:472–481.

139. Newton P, Johnston C (1997): Analysis and treatment of poor outcomes following in situ arthrodesis in adolescent spondylolisthesis. *J Pediatr Orthop* 17:754–761.

140. Nicol RO, Scott JHS (1986): Lytic spondylolysis: repair by wiring. *Spine* 11:1027–1030.

141. O'Beirne JG, Horgan JG (1988): Stress fracture of the lamina associated with unilateral spondylolysis. *Spine* 13:220–222.

142. O'Brien J, Mehdian H, Jaffray D (1994): Reduction of severe lumbosacral spondylolisthesis: a report of 22 cases with a ten year follow-up period. *Clin Orthop* 300:64–69.

143. Oakley RH, Carty H (1984): Review of spondylolisthesis and spondylolysis in paediatric practice. *Br J Radiol* 57:877–885.

144. Ogilvie JW, Sherman J (1987): Spondylolysis in Scheuermann's disease. *Spine* 12:251–253.

145. Osterman K, Schlenzka D, Poussa M, et al. (1993): Isthmic spondylolisthesis in symptomatic and asymptomatic subjects, epidemiology, and natural history with special reference to disk abnormality and mode of treatment. *Clin Orthop* 297:65–70.

146. Pearcy M, Shepherd J (1985): Is there instability in spondylolisthesis? *Spine* 10:175–177.

147. Pease CN, Najat H (1967): Spondylolisthesis in children. *Clin Orthop* 82:187–198.

148. Pedersen AK, Hagen R (1988): Spondylolysis and spondylolisthesis: treatment by internal fixation and bone grafting of the defect. *J Bone Joint Surg Am* 70:15–24.

149. Petraco D, Spivak J, Cappadona J, et al. (1996): An anatomic evaluation of L5 nerve stretch in spondylolisthesis reduction. *Spine* 21: 1133–1139.

150. Phalen GS, Dickson JA (1961): Spondylolisthesis and tight hamstrings. *J Bone Joint Surg Am* 43:505–512.

151. Pizzutillo PD (1985): Spondylolisthesis: etiology and natural history. In: Bradford DS, Hensinger R, eds. *The pediatric spine.* New York: Thieme Verlag, pp. 395–401.

152. Pizzutillo PD, Hummer CD (1989): Nonoperative treatment for painful adolescent spondylolysis or spondylolisthesis. *J Pediatr Orthop* 9:538–540.

153. Pizzutillo PD, Mirenda W, MacEwen GW (1986): Posterolateral fusion of spondylolisthesis in adolescence. *J Pediatr Orthop* 6:311–316.

154. Ravichandran G (1980): Multiple lumbar spondylolysis. *Spine* 5: 552–557.

155. Risser JC, Norquist DM (1961): Sciatic scoliosis in growing children. *Clin Orthop* 21:137–155.

156. Robert C (1853): Eine cigenthumliche angeborene lordose, wahrscheinlich bedingt durch eine verschiebung des korpers des letzten lendenwirbels avf die vordere fiache des ersten kreuz-beinwirbels (spondololisthesis kiliian) nebst bemerkungen uber die mechanik diser beckenformation. *Monatsschrift Geburt-skunde Frauenkrank* 2: 429–432.

157. Roca J, Moretta D, Fuster S, et al. (1989): Direct repair of spondylolysis. *Clin Orthop* 246:86–91.

158. Roca J, Ubierna M, Caceres E, et al. (1999): One-stage decompression and posterolateral and interbody fusion for severe spondylolisthesis. *Spine* 24:709–714.

159. Rombold C (1966): Treatment of spondylolisthesis by posterolateral fusion, resection of the pars interarticularis, and prompt mobilization of the patient. *J Bone Joint Surg Am* 48:1282–1300.

160. Rosenberg NJ, Bargar WL, Friedman B (1981): The incidence of spondylolysis and spondylolisthesis in nonambulatory patients. *Spine* 6:35–37.

161. Rossi F, Dragoni S (1990): Lumbar spondylolysis: occurrence in competitive athletes. *J Sports Med Phys Fitness* 30:450–452.
162. Rowe GG, Roche MB (1953): The etiology of separate neural arch. *J Bone Joint Surg Am* 35:102–109.
163. Sagi H, Jarvis J, Uhthoff H (1998): Histomorphoic analysis of the development of the pars interarticularis and its association with isthmic spondylolysis. *Spine* 23:13635–1640.
164. Saraste H (1985): The etiology of spondylolysis. *Acta Orthop Scand* 56:253–255.
165. Saraste H (1987): Long-term clinical and radiological follow-up of spondylolysis and spondylolisthesis. *J Pediatr Orthop* 7:631–638.
166. Scaglietti O, Frontino G, Bartolozzi P (1976): Technique of anatomical reduction of lumbar spondylolisthesis and its surgical stabilization. *Clin Orthop* 117:164–175.
167. Schoenecker PL, Cole HO, Herring JA, et al. (1990): Cauda equina syndrome after in situ arthrodesis for severe spondylolisthesis at the lumbosacral junction. *J Bone Joint Surg Am* 72:369–377.
168. Schollner D (1990): One stage reduction and fusion for spondylolisthesis. *Int Orthop* 14:145–150.
169. Schulitz KP, Niethard FU (1980): Strain on the interarticular stress distribution. *Arch Orthop Trauma Surg* 96:197–202.
170. Schwab F, Farcy JP, Roye D (1997): The sagittal pelvic tilt index as a criterion in the evaluation of spondylolisthesis. *Spine* 22:1661–1667.
171. Seitsalo S (1990): Operative and conservative treatment of moderate spondylolisthesis in young patients. *J Bone Joint Surg Br* 72:908–913.
172. Seitsalo S, Osterman K, Hyvarinen H, et al. (1990): Severe spondylolisthesis in children and adolescents. *J Bone Joint Surg Br* 72:259–265.
173. Seitsalo S, Osterman K, Hyvarinen H, et al. (1991): Progression of spondylolisthesis in children and adolescents: a long-term follow-up of 272 patients. *Spine* 16:417–421.
174. Seitsalo S, Osterman K, Poussa M, et al. (1988): Spondylolisthesis in children under 12 years of age: long-term results of 56 patients treated conservatively or operatively. *J Pediatr Orthop* 8:516–521.
175. Seitsalo S, Osterman K, Poussa M (1997): Disc degeneration in young patients with isthmic spondylolisthesis treated operatively or conservatively: a long-term follow-up. *Eur Spine J* 6:393–397.
176. Semon RL, Spengler D (1981): Significance of lumbar spondylolysis in college football players. *Spine* 6:172–174.
177. Sevastikoglou JA, Spangfort E, Aaro S (1980): Operative treatment of spondylolisthesis in children and adolescents with tight hamstrings syndrome. *Clin Orthop* 147:192–199.
178. Shahriaree H, Sajadi K, Rooholamini SA (1979): A family with spondylolisthesis. *J Bone Joint Surg Am* 61:1256–1258.
179. Shelokov A, Haideri N, Roach J (1993): Residual gait abnormalities in surgically treated spondylolisthesis. *Spine* 18:2201–2205.
180. Sherman FC, Rosenthal RK, Hall JE (1979): Spine fusion for spondylolysis and spondylolisthesis in children. *Spine* 4:59–67.
181. Shirado O, Zdeblick TA, McAfee PC, et al. (1991): Biomechanical evaluation of methods of posterior stabilization of the spine and posterior lumbar interbody arthrodesis for lumbosacral isthmic spondylolisthesis. *J Bone Joint Surg Am* 73:518–526.
182. Sijbrandij S (1983): Reduction and stabilization of severe spondylolisthesis. *J Bone Joint Surg Br* 65:40–42.
183. Simper LB (1986): Spondylolysis in Eskimo skeletons. *Acta Orthop Scand* 57:78–90.
184. Shufflebarger, HL: Complex revision spinal surgery: posterior-anterior-posterior sequence. Presented at the 32nd Annual Scoliosis Research Society Meeting. *Orthop Trans* 22(2):612.
185. Smith J, Deviren V, Emani A, et al. Clinical outcome of trans-sacral interbody fusion following partial reduction for high-grade C5-S1 spondylolisthesis. Presented at the annual meeting of the Scoliosis Research Society, October 18–20, 2000, Cairns, Australia.
186. Smith MD, Bohlman HH (1990): Spondylolisthesis treated by single-stage operation combining decompression with in situ posterolateral and anterior fusion. *J Bone Joint Surg Am* 72:415–420.
187. Soren A, Waugh TR (1985): Spondylolisthesis and related disorders. *Clin Orthop* 193:171–177.
188. Stanton RP, Meehan P, Lovell WW (1985): Surgical fusion in childhood spondylolisthesis. *J Pediatr Orthop* 5:411–415.
189. Steffee AD, Sitkowski DJ (1988): Reduction and stabilization of grade IV spondylolisthesis. *Clin Orthop* 227:82–89.
190. Steiner ME, Micheli LJ (1985): Treatment of symptomatic spondylolysis and spondylolisthesis with the modified Boston brace. *Spine* 10:937–943.
191. Stewart TD (1953): The age incidence of neural arch defects in Alaskan natives, considered from the standpoint of etiology. *J Bone Joint Surg Am* 35:937–959.
192. Sward L, Hellstrom M, Jacobsson B, et al. (1989): Spondylolysis and the sacrohorizontal angle in athletes. *Acta Radiol* 30:359–364.
193. Taillard W (1955): Le spondylolisthesis chez l'enfant et l'adolescent. *Acta Orthop* 24:115–144.
194. Taillard W (1969): Traumatisme et spondylolisthesis. *Acta Orthop Belg* 35:703–716.
195. Teplick JG, Laffey PA, Berman A, et al. (1986): Diagnosis and evaluation of spondylolisthesis and/or spondylolysis on axial CT. *Am J Neuroradiol* 7:476–491.
196. Tiusanen H, Schlenzka D, Seitsalo S, et al. (1996): Results of a trial of anterior or circumferential lumbar fusion in the treatment of severe isthmic spondylolisthesis in young patients. *J Pediatr Orthop* 5:190–194.
197. Transfeldt EE, Dendrinos GK, Bradford DS (1989): Paresis of proximal lumbar roots after reduction of L5–S1 spondylolisthesis. *Spine* 14:884–887.
198. Turner H, Bianco AJ (1971): Spondylolisthesis and spondylolysis in children and teenagers. *J Bone Joint Surg Am* 53:1298–1306.
199. van den Oever M, Merrick MV, Scott JH (1987): Bone scintigraphy in symptomatic spondylolysis. *J Bone Joint Surg Br* 69:453–456.
200. van der Werf GJIM, Tonino AJ, Zeegers WS (1985): Direct repair of lumbar spondylolysis. *Acta Orthop Scand* 56:378–379.
201. van Rens TJG, van Horn JR (1982): Long-term results in lumbosacral interbody fusion for spondylolisthesis. *Acta Orthop Scand* 53:383–393.
202. Velikas EP, Blackburne JS (1981): Surgical treatment of spondylolisthesis in children and adolescents. *J Bone Joint Surg Br* 63:67–70.
203. Verbiest H (1979): The treatment of lumbar spondyloptosis or impending spondyloptosis accompanied by neurologic deficit and/or neurogenic intermittent claudication. *Spine* 4:68–77.
204. Vidal J, Fassio B, Buscayret C, et al. (1981): Surgical reduction of spondylolisthesis using a posterior approach. *Clin Orthop* 154:156–165.
205. Wasylenko M, Skinner SR, Perry J, et al. (1983): Analysis of posture and gait following spinal fusion with Harrington instrumentation. *Spine* 6(6):840–845.
206. Watkins MB (1959): Posterolateral bone-grafting for fusion of the lumbar and lumbosacral spine. *J Bone Joint Surg Am* 41:388–395.
207. Weir MR, Smith DS (1989): Stress reaction of the pars interarticularis leading to spondylolysis. *J Adolesc Health Care* 10:573–577.
208. Whitecloud TS, Butler JC (1988): Anterior lumbar fusion utilizing transvertebral fibular graft. *Spine* 13:370–374.
209. Wiltse LL (1957): Etiology of spondylolisthesis. *Clin Orthop* 10:48–60.
210. Wiltse LL (1961): Spondylolisthesis in children. *Clin Orthop* 21:156–163.
211. Wiltse LL (1962): The etiology of spondylolisthesis. *J Bone Joint Surg Am* 44:539–559.
212. Wiltse LL (1969): Spondylolisthesis: classification and etiology. *Symposium on the spine*. Chicago: American Academy of Orthopaedic Surgeons, pp. 143–166.
213. Wiltse LL (1973): The paraspinal sacrospinalis-splitting approach to the lumbar spine. *Clin Orthop* 91:48–57.
214. Wiltse LL, Hutchinson RH (1964): Surgical treatment of spondylolisthesis. *Clin Orthop* 35:116–135.

215. Wiltse LL, Widell EH, Jackson DW (1975): Fatigue fracture: The basic lesion in isthmic spondylolisthesis. *J Bone Joint Surg Am* 57: 17–22.
216. Winter M, Jani L (1989): Results of screw osteosynthesis in spondylolysis and low-grade spondylolisthesis. *Arch Orthop Trauma Surg* 108: 96–99.
217. Wynne-Davies R, Scott JHS (1979): Inheritance and spondylolisthesis. *J Bone Joint Surg Br* 61:301–305.
218. Zimmerman MC, Gutteling E, Langrana NA, et al. (1989): The biomechanical evaluation of a new fixation technique for spondylolysis using single and double tension band wiring. *Bull Hosp Joint Dis* 49:131–139.

HERNIATED NUCLEUS PULPOSUS AND SLIPPED VERTEBRAL APOPHYSIS

VINCENT ARLET
FRANÇOIS FASSIER

The symptoms and clinical signs of herniation of the nucleus pulposus (HNP) and slipped vertebral apophysis (SVA) are very similar in pediatric patients. Hashimoto et al. (41) showed no statistically significant differences in the average age, history of trauma, or symptoms and signs between SVA and HNP. Such differences are the result of a mechanical and or chemical conflict (as recently reported by Olmarker and Myers [66] and Kawakami et al. [47]) between the migration of material inside the spinal canal and the neural structures. For this reason, they should be considered as a consequence of a pathologic entity occurring during the growing years, this being the result of a genetic predisposition, traumatic event, or other causative factors.

A few authors (5,28,32,65,91) have stated that there is little or no difference between adult and pediatric herniations of the nucleus pulposus; this does not correspond to our clinical experience. We therefore reviewed the literature illustrated in Table 1 and summarized the differences between adult and pediatric HNP and SVA. In the sections that follow, the subject will be limited to the aforementioned pathologies. Therefore, problems related to Sheuermann disease, osteochondrodysplasia, and calcification of the intervertebral disc will not be discussed. By "pediatric" we mean patients who are younger than 18 years at the onset of first symptoms.

EPIDEMIOLOGIC FACTORS

Wahren in 1945 (90) was the first to report on the surgical treatment of a herniated nucleus pulposus in a 12-year-old child. In 1954, Begg (4) first reported ring apophyseal fracture associated with a central disc herniation. In 1973, Lowrey (54) first reported a cartilaginous and bony ridge protruding in the spinal canal.

If lumbar disc herniation is common in adults, with a 1.6% of

sciatica prevalent in the adult population as reported by Deoyo et al. (23), its incidence in children is exceptional. The incidence of low back pain leading to hospitalization rises sharply from the age 19, according to Zitting et al. (95). Large series of surgically treated patients with disc herniation report an incidence of only 0.2% to 3.2% occurring in the young patient (27,33,37,73,75,91). In the study by Ramirez et al. (74), only two of 2,442 patients with back pain and scoliosis had disc herniation. However, the incidence of HNP in the Japanese seems higher, with an incidence of 15.4% in one series (49). However, if one considers patients younger than 15 years, the true incidence drops to 4.6%. This was confirmed by Ishihara (44), who reported an incidence of 3% for children younger than 16 years. The age of onset is observed in the second decade, at a mean age of 14.5 years. However, we observed a case in a patient as young as 5 years (Fig. 1), and one can find case reports on patients younger than 12 years (12,13,16,18,91). For most studies, the incidence in males is greater than in females (13,18, 22,37,41,49) by a ratio of 2:1 or 3:1. However, two studies (28,46) found no differences. The sex ratio between girls and boys may vary depending on the age range considered. Girls mature faster than boys and are therefore more likely to have more disc herniations at an earlier age. In the adults likewise, one finds a male preponderance (92).

ETIOLOGIC FACTORS

Several factors can lead to migration of intervertebral contents into the spinal canal.

Trauma

Trauma is reported by patients in most instances (5,14, 21,25,37,38). The reported incidence ranges between 30% and 70% of cases. Trauma may be responsible for an acute disc or ring apophysis migration. On the other hand, repetitive trauma or microtrauma encountered in sports (gymnastics, football, weight lifting) definitely has a role in the etiology of intervertebral materiel migration (Fig. 2).

V. Arlet and F. Fassier: Division of Orthopaedic Surgery, McGill University Health Center, Montreal, Quebec, H3H 1P3 Canada.

TABLE 1. PEDIATRIC VERSUS ADULT HNP & SVA

	Pediatric	Adult
Etiology and Epidemiology		
Overall incidence	Exceptional	Between 1.5 and 5% (23)
% of operated cases	0.8–3.8% (25,27,37,65,67,75)	92–99%
	Japan: 3–15.4% (44,49)	
Male/female ratio	Variable (12,22,27,46,49,67)	2 for 1 (15,48,95)
Trauma history	Acute or repeated microtrauma: 50% (14,21,25,37)	Precipitating factor event on DDD
	No trauma history (75)	
DDD	Classically no. Yes recently (55,72,78)	Yes + + +
Genetics	Identical twins (39,57,64)	
	Family predisposition (50,88,89,94)	Family predisposition for DDD (70,71,82)
Associated Conditions		
Spinal stenosis	Congenital: 12.5% (67)	Acquired and degenerative
Sheuermann	Juvenile discogenic disease (43)	Yes (43)
Transitionnal anomaly	Yes 30% (12–13,28,49,65)	No; only observed in less than 10%
Spondylo	Rare	Yes (degenerative or isthmic)
Clinical Findings		
Time for diagnosis	Delayed (mean delay is 11 months (37,49,50))	Rapid (less than few weeks)
Symptoms	Functional signs less than physical signs (56,75)	Functional signs more than physical signs
Back pain	Less than adult, and less than leg pain	More intense & frequent
Leg pain	Always present (often isolated leg pain) (37), Leg pain often outweights back pain	Intense but rarely isolated leg pain
Physical signs	Spine syndrome takes first place	Less impressive than symptoms
Lumbar lordosis	Decreased + + +	Decrease less obvious
Back stiffness	(+ + + +) (37)	Less pronounced
Gait anomaly	Frequent (21)	Rare
Sciatic scoliosis	Antalgic scoliosis: 55–72% (20,38)	Less frequent
Valsava	(+ + +) in 30%–76% (22)	Less pronounced
SLR	Very limited and present in 85–95% (33,37,21)	Not as limited. Very frequent but not constant despite HNP
	Bilateral SLR more often observed in SVA (41)	
Positive neuro signs	Rare: (34,35,37,50,65)	More frequent
Motor weakness	Classically rare. More frequent in ring #	More frequent (32%) (48)
Sensory deficit	Minor sensory changes	More frequent
Reflexes changes	Rare (possible mild ankle assymmetry)	More frequent
Cauda equina	Exceptional (possible in SVA) (2,50)	Frequence 1.2–2.4%
Imaging		
Plain x-rays	Often normal (in 50% of cases (21))	Often normal or disc space narrowing
	Antalgic scol., ring #, malformations (13,21,22,49)	Signs of spondylolysis
CAT scan	Better for ring #. Tanaka classification. Spinal stenosis	Inferior to MRI
Myelo CT	Rarely indicated	Prior surgery or stenosis or cauda equina syndrome
Discogram	Rarely indicated	Far lateral disc herniation (with CT) or discogenic back pain
MRI	Best for HNP (45), but inferior to CT for ring #	Yes (best for HNP). Often multiple level DDD
	Assess state of disc (degenerated) in ring #, & HNP	MRI + gadolinium: for postoperative radiculopathy.
	Disc can be normal in ring apohysis # (2,52).	
	MRI can show intact Sharpey's fibers in SVA (3)	
	Multilevel disease in 3/4 patients with HNP (36)	
Location HNP	L4–L5 & L5–S1 equally affected; 2 levels HNP: 3.2% (79)	L4–L5 and L5–S1 equally affected; 2 levels HNP: 5.1% (79)
Location ring #	L4–L5: 55% L3–L4: 24% and L5–S1: 21%	L4–L5 and L5–S1 (sup. aspect of S1) (30,31)
Differential Diagnosis	Clinical, x-rays, CT and MRI & bone scan	Clinical, x-rays, bone scan, CT, MRI
Neoplasms	Primary tumors: age<11, bilat. leg pain, neuro. findings (56)	Secondary tumors and nonback syndromes
Spondylolysis	Yes	Yes

(continued)

TABLE 1. *Continued.*

	Pediatric	Adult
Discitis	Yes	Rare
Spinal stenosis	Yes (congenital)	Yes (acquired)
Tethered cord	Yes (MRI)	No
Spinal tumors	Yes	Yes
Natural History		
Short-term	Conservative treatment fails in 75% of cases (21,46,49)	Resolution in 50–75% of cases within a month (15)
Recurrence	Frequent if conservative treatment successful	Recurrence in 8–15% (63)
Long term	May lead to restriction of activity (sports)	70% still report sciatica (63)
MRI changes	Spectrum of MRI changes same as adult (55)	Decrease size of HNP, migration of HNP, DDD at other levels (59,86)
Operative Findings		
Disc degeneration	35% of normal disc on microscopic exam (49)	Degeneration
Herniated disc	Often disc protrusion, extruded free fragment rare (25,46)	Disc more often extruded or even sequestred
	Fragment is larger than in adult.	
	Disc more hydrated	Disc with decreased water content
	Herniated disc often attached to PLL or Sharpey fibers	Bony compression often associated
# Ring	19–32% of fractured vertebral rim (3,55)	Rare, can be observed to the 40s (30,31)
	Sharpey's fibers intact	
	Pathogenesis is the fragility of the end plate (84)	
	Mostly Takata 1 and 2	Mostly Takata 3 (84)
	Mostly associated with central disc herniation (54,83,85)	
	May require extended uni. or bilat. laminotomy (2,29,30,31)	Same as pediatric
	Remove avulsed fragment only or further discectomy? (52)	Same as pediatric
Treatment (Mainstay)	Open discectomy (after trial of conserv. treatment)	Mostly conservative
	Epidural, nerve root block?	Epidural steroids not superior to placebo injections (17)
	Fusion not recommended (13,27,46,49,67)	Fusion rarely recommended.
	Only few authors advocate chemonucleolysis (11,53)	Open discectomy sup. to chemonucl. or percut. discectomy (61)
	Microdiscectomy or conventional open discectomy	Microdiscectomy or conventional open discectomy
Outcome of Surgery		
Initial	Excellent or good: 73–95% (9,21,22,25,33,37,78,81)	Guarded: (24,63)
Long-term	Poor result in 9–26% (21,22,25,32)	70% still complaining of LBP (24)
Recurrence	4–10% (9,22,32)	45% still have residual sciatica (24)
Reoperation	21–28% with a 28 or 34 years f.up (25,67)	12–17% (4–17 years f.up) (24,63,87)

DDD, Degenerative disc disease; HNP, Herniated nucleus pulposus; LBP, Low back pain; NP, Nucleus pulposus; SVA, Slipped vertebral apophysis; SLR, Straight leg raising; PLL, Posterior longitudinal ligament.

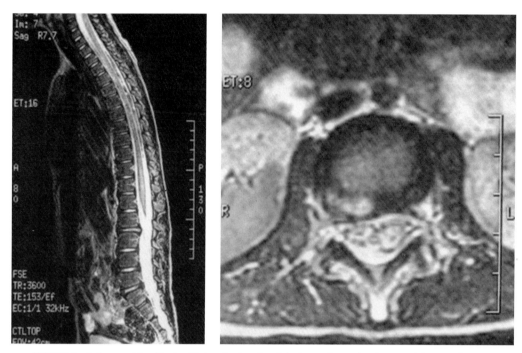

FIGURE 1. A 5-year-old patient with low back pain, right leg pain, and a decreased knee reflex. Her symptoms persisted despite one year of conservative treatment. The radiographs were read as normal. The magnetic resonance image showed a right posterolateral herniated L2–3 disc but with only partial dehydration (disc still white). At surgery, a large disc bulge contained by the posterior longitudinal ligament was identified. After incision of the disc, outer annulus disc material emerged under pressure "like toothpaste." The pathology report referred to "fragments of degenerated disc." (Courtesy of J. P. Farmer, M.D.)

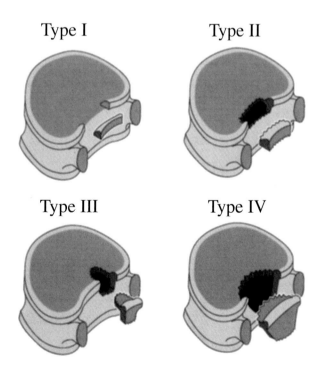

FIGURE 2. Classification of the ring apophysis fracture. Limbus vertebral fractures have been classified by Takata in type I, II, and III. Epstein later added the type IV. In children most of the ring apophysis fractures are type 1. (Redrawn from Takata et al. [84] and Epstein et al. [29]).

Disc Degeneration

Disc degeneration has always been thought to be one of the characteristics of the adult disc and its well-described degenerative disc disease (DDD). The advent of magnetic resonance imaging (MRI) has shown that early disc degeneration is observed at many other levels in teenagers complaining of sciatica or low back pain (36,55,72,76,78). At this age, as opposed to in adulthood, it is rare for asymptomatic individuals to show signs of disc degeneration on MRI (36). Poussa et al. (72) showed that after a 10-year follow-up patients operated before age 15 for an HNP had multiple level lumbar DDD on the MR image. This was further confirmed by Luukkonen et al. (55), who showed that 6 years after lumbar discectomy the MR images of 67% of patients indicated DDD at other lumbar levels. In this series, of nine patients with disc herniation, the intradiscal contents were normal in five and degenerated in four. Savini et al. (78) reported that early-onset disc degeneration was one of the most significant etiologic factors, along with trauma and lumbosacral malformation (Fig. 1). Gibson et al. (36) compared a control group of healthy asymptomatic teenagers with a matched group of patients with a disc herniation and found that there were multiple-level disc abnormalities in 75% of patients in the latter group. Heithoff (43) found a high incidence of lumbar DDD in patients with Sheuermann's disease. This suggests an underlying degenerative diathesis in patients with disc herniation. Salminen et al. (76), in a prospective 3-year follow-up study of low back pain in the young, found a causal relationship between degenerative process and frequent low back pain.

Congenital Malformation

Congenital anomaly or malformation of the lumbar spine has been recognized as a predisposing factor. This is observed in as many as 30% of young patients with lumbar disc herniation (13,22,27,28,49,65) and may consist of a transitional anomaly, such as 6 lumbar vertebrae, or complete or incomplete sacralization of the L5 vertebra. Spina bifida occulta has been reported in 15% of cases, an incidence higher than that of the general population. Congenital spinal stenosis has been recognized as a very important contributing factor in the clinical manifestations of HNP or SVA (69,8,10,26,28,42,67). The incidence of a congenital narrow canal was reported to be 12.5% (67). Small disc protrusions in a normal size canal may be little or mildly symptomatic, whereas their occurrence in a narrow canal may be a different situation entirely.

Genetic Predisposition

Gunzburg et al. (39), Matsui et al. (57), and Obukhov et al. (64) have separately reported on monozygote teenaged twins who developed at the same age a disc herniation. Varlotta et al. (88) in studying 63 patients younger than 21 years with sciatica found an incidence of 32% of first-degree relatives with sciatica. A control group had an incidence of only 7% of sciatica in first-degree relatives. This strong family predisposition has also been stressed by other authors (58,60) and in the adult population

(70,71,82). The possibility of a congenital narrow canal as a predisposing factor and its genetic incidence must be kept in mind. Varughese and Quartey (89) reported on four brothers with such a condition.

Environmental Factors

Nutritional status, weight, and postural habits also have been suggested as causative factors.

PATHOANATOMY

Intervertebral Disc and End Plate

The intervertebral disc space is occupied by the nucleus pulposus, the annulus fibrosis, and the cartilaginous end plates. The end plate of the immature spine consists of hyaline cartilage adjacent to the nucleus pulposus and a physeal cartilage adjacent to the bony vertebral body (Fig. 3). The physeal cartilage is further subdivided into a physeal plate (responsible for vertical growth) and a traction apophysis or ring apophysis. We refer the reader to the work of Bick and Copel (6,7) and to Fig. 3 for development of the end plate. The disc is constituted of the nucleus pulposus and the annulus fibrosis. The disc is attached to the ring apophysis (Fig. 4) by the curved Sharpey fibers. As the ring ossifies the Sharpey fibers insert into the vertebral bony

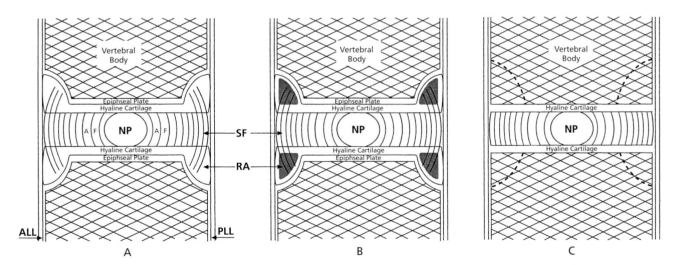

FIGURE 3. Drawing of the disc–vertebral end plate development, based on the original work of Bick and Copel (7,8). **A:** Age 6 years—The vertebral body grows longitudinally by enchondral ossification due to the growth plate. First foci of calcification determine the histology of the ring apophysis, which is separated from the vertebral body by the epiphyseal plate. The Sharpey fibers (which are the outer expansions of the annulus fibrosus) insert into the ring apophysis. The ring apophysis is a traction apophysis. **B:** Between ages 10 and 14 years—At age 10 there is a condensation of cartilage determining the triangular shape of the ring apophysis. At age 14 the ring apophysis starts to ossify. The Sharpey fibers become embedded in the bone of the ring apophysis. The ring, which is still separated from the vertebral body by the epiphyseal plate, appears on radiographs as a small triangular piece of bone separated from the vertebral body. **C:** At age 18 years—The ring apophysis fuses to the vertebral body when the epiphyseal plate disappears. *NP*, nucleus pulposus; *AF*, annulus fibrosus; *SF*, Sharpey's fibers; *ALL*, Anterior longitudinal ligament; *PLL*, Posterior longitudinal ligament; *RA*, ring apophysis.

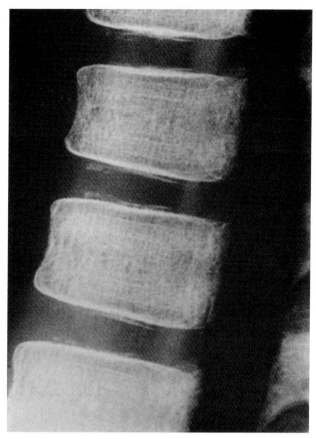

FIGURE 4. Ring apophysis at age 7 years (upper thoracic spine). (Reprinted from Ogden JA (1990): *Spine.* In: *Skeletal injury in the child.* Philadelphia: WB Saunders, with permission.)

end plate as the vertebra matures. The Sharpey fiber attachments to the ring are stronger than the junction between the ring and the vertebral body. Therefore, the osteocartilaginous junction is a weak point until it ossifies. As a result, in children one can observe migration into the spinal canal of disc material, cartilage, fibrous tissue, or bone, as opposed to the adult, in whom the pathology is almost exclusively migration of disc contents.

Ring Apophysis Fracture

The advent of computed tomography (CT) has confirmed the higher incidence of ring apophysis migration into the spinal canal of what was thought to be a simple HNP. Likewise, careful review of the MR image and histologic examination of the excised disc will often reveal the presence of pieces of cartilage and/or bone. The pathology of slipped vertebral apophysis includes common histologic features: Part of the ring has displaced into the spinal canal with or without cancellous bone from the vertebral body. The classification of such lesions was described by Takata et al. (84). Epstein and colleagues (29,30,31) added a further subgroup (Fig. 2). Type 1 lesions occur more in the younger group. Most of these lesions seem to be located at the inferior aspect of L4 (40). Adjacent to it there is most often a

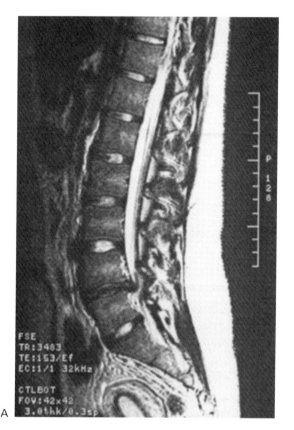

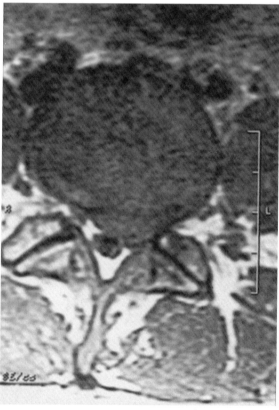

FIGURE 5. A 15-year-old girl with predominantly left leg pain for the last 9 months attributed to a hamstring pull. The magnetic resonance image shows the typical subligamentous L4–5 disc **(A and B)** herniation, which is posterolateral. At surgery, the herniated disc was subligamentous.

central disc herniation (41). The fragment remains attached to the posterior longitudinal ligament by the outer expansions of the Sharpey fibers.

Herniation of the Nucleus Pulposus

According to Garrido (34), herniation of the nucleus pulposus rarely is completely extruded into the epidural space (free fragments) but rather is a disc protrusion in continuity with the rest of the nucleus pulposus and is covered by a thin membrane formed by the annulus and posterior longitudinal ligament. The herniation is mostly posterolateral (Fig. 5) (41). However, there is a clinical form wherein the disc protrusion is central and usually subligamentous too (79). These forms give more low back pain symptoms than true sciatica. The juvenile disc is quite moist, elastic, and gelatinous, and usually only a few pieces can be removed with the pituitary rongeur (34). The histologic evaluation of all excised specimens shows serious degeneration of the disc tissue (50) (Fig. 1). However, the degree of disc degeneration is not as great as that in the adult. Conversely, in the adult the hernia is more often extruded or even sequestered than in the juvenile. We think that this may be due to the stronger resistance of the outer fibers of the annulus fibrosus. The nucleus in the child is more gelatinous than the myxomatous nucleus observed in the older patient.

Chemical Factors Responsible for the Painful Radiculopathy

Recently, Olmarker and Myers (66), Kawakami et al. (47), and Yabuki et al. (93) have reported strong evidence of the role of chemical factors in the possible mechanism of painful radiculopathy. Mechanical factors were thought for a long time to be the only explanation for the pathogenesis of the radiculopathy. It seems that nucleus pulposus–related chemical substances sensitize the nerve root, producing pain even in the absence of compression. However, in children, because most of the hernia is subligamentous, chemical factors may not be as relevant to the pain pathogenesis as in the adult.

CLINICAL PRESENTATION

Table 1 compares the pediatric disease to the adult version. We emphasize only the most striking features between pediatric and adult HNP and SVA: In children, the diagnosis is often delayed (33,37,49,50) because it is rare and the pain does not preclude functioning. Clinically, the radiculopathy (with Lasegue sign) is almost constant, the stiffness of the back is often impressive, and the patient may have sciatic scoliosis (Figs. 6 and 7). There is generally a lack of neurologic deficit. In contrast to the adult, the physical signs in children are usually more impressive than the clinical symptoms. However, in central disc protrusion the symptomatology may be limited to back pain, but without any

sciatica (79). Neurologic complications in children seem to be more related to ring apophysis fractures (77).

IMAGING TECHNIQUES

Imaging studies have recently emphasized the presence of slipped vertebral apophysis that was not recognized previously. It is now recognized that between 19% (55) and 32% (3) in the 13- to 14-year subgroup of what was thought to be a simple HNP are in fact an SVA. The presence of associated anomalies, such as spondylolysis (Fig. 8) and spinal stenosis (Fig. 9), is also a common feature. MRI will typically show a posterolateral subligamentous hernia for the HNP (Fig. 5) and a central disc herniation in SVA (16,41,83,85) (see Fig. 6). CT scanning is bested for SVA (1,3) and MRI best for HNP (45). MRI alone can fail to detect an SVA (68). It is the authors' opinion that when treating children one should request assessment of both the state of the discs and the possibility of a ring fracture (Figs. 10 and 11).

DIFFERENTIAL DIAGNOSIS

In children, sciatica is rare and one must rule out other causes of back and leg problems. In children before their teens the diagnosis of HNP or SVA remains unusual but possible (Fig. 1). One must rule out other conditions, such neoplasms, tethering of the cord, infections, discitis, and spondylolisthesis (74). In the teenager, spondylolysis typically does not produce a true radiculopathy. The diagnosis of these conditions may require a bone scan, MRI, and CT, but MRI is the examination of choice.

NATURAL HISTORY

Most authors recognize that conservative treatment is not very effective in children (94). According to DeLuca et al. (21), failure of conservative treatment was observed in 75% of cases. Kurihara and Kotaoka (49) reported that nonsurgical treatment was ineffective in 60% of cases. In a number of cases, conservative treatment that was at first successful is no longer effective once the child has resumed all sports activities. Some studies have focused on the state of the disc and the herniation by following the patients with sequential MRI (48,59). These studies have been done mostly in adults and have showed that the cases corresponding to protrusion showed little or no change on follow-up MRI. By contrast, migration of HNP frequently was associated with an obvious decrease in size and even disappearance. As to DDD, it seems to involve all age groups. Tullberg et al. (86) reported a 90% incidence of DDD at another level in the adult 1 year after lumbar discectomy. Luukkonen et al. (55) in his pediatric group found that with a mean follow-up of 6 years, 65% had disc degeneration at another lumbar level. The natural history as observed on MRI does not seem different from that of the adult. The natural history of SVA is more like a fracture type of pattern with callus forming at the fracture site, end plate irregularities, and possible late spinal stenosis as reported (41).

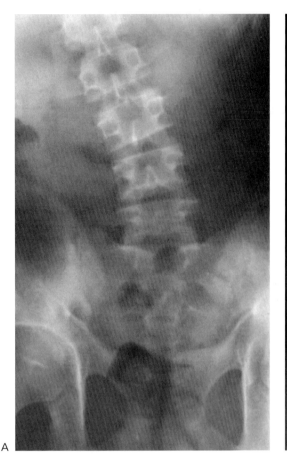
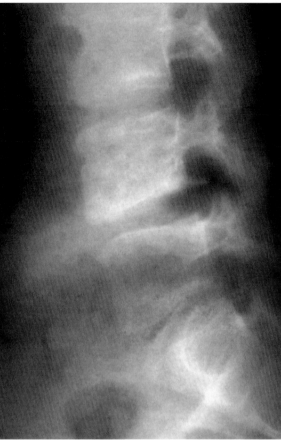
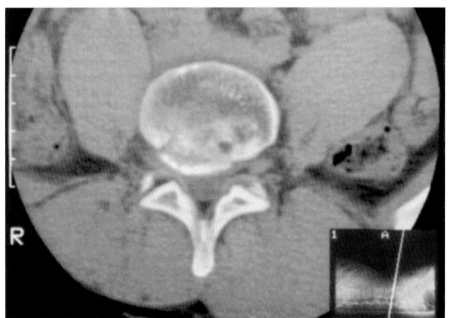

FIGURE 6. A 15-year-old patient complaining for several months of a severe right sciatica after having lifted a heavy weight. Radiographs show an impressive sciatic scoliosis without any rotation **(A)**. The spot lateral lumbar spine shows a localized kyphosis at L4–5 and an avulsed piece from the inferior border of L4 **(B)**. The CT scan demonstrates an arcuate avulsed fragment of the ring apophysis here classified as a type 1 in the Takata classification **(C)**. (At operation, removal of the fragment required an extended exposure, including a unilateral partial medial facetectomy.)

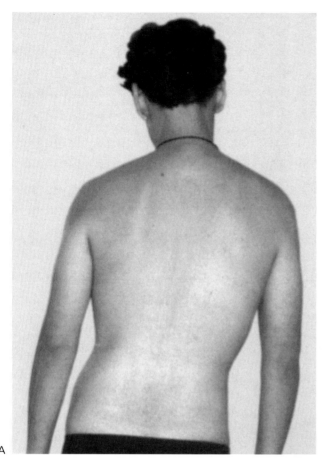

A

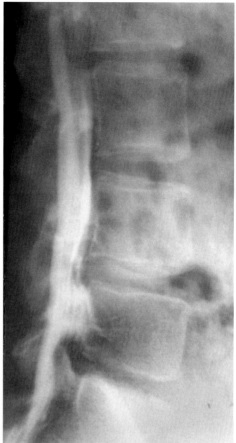

B

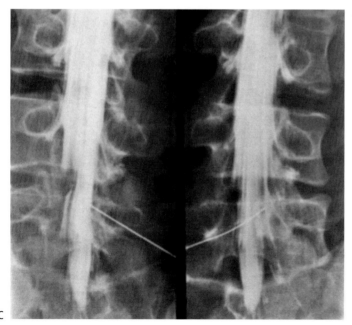

C

FIGURE 7. A 17-year-old boy with marked postural scoliosis and a left sciatica of 2 years duration **(A)**. Note that the patient is listing away from the sciatica. A myelogram was done at the time (old case). Lack of filling of the left L5 and S1 nerve root is evident with an extrinsic compression **(B and C)**. A two-level discectomy relieved the boy's symptoms.

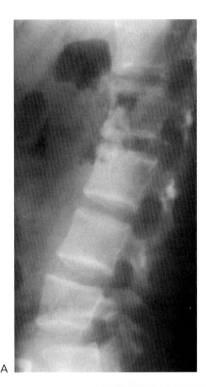

A

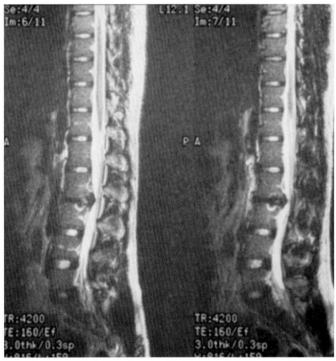

B

FIGURE 8. A 16-year-old patient with a longstanding history of low back pain after weight training. The lateral radiograph shows a sagittal malalignment of the lumbar spine with a spondylolysis L5–S1 and a triangular chip calcification in the canal at the L2–3 level **(A)**. The magnetic resonance image shows posterior Schmorl nodes and a black triangular shape corresponding to the avulsed ring apophysis still attached to the Sharpey fibers at the L2–3 level **(B)**. This case illustrates the possibility of a combined pathology and the question of the pain generator.

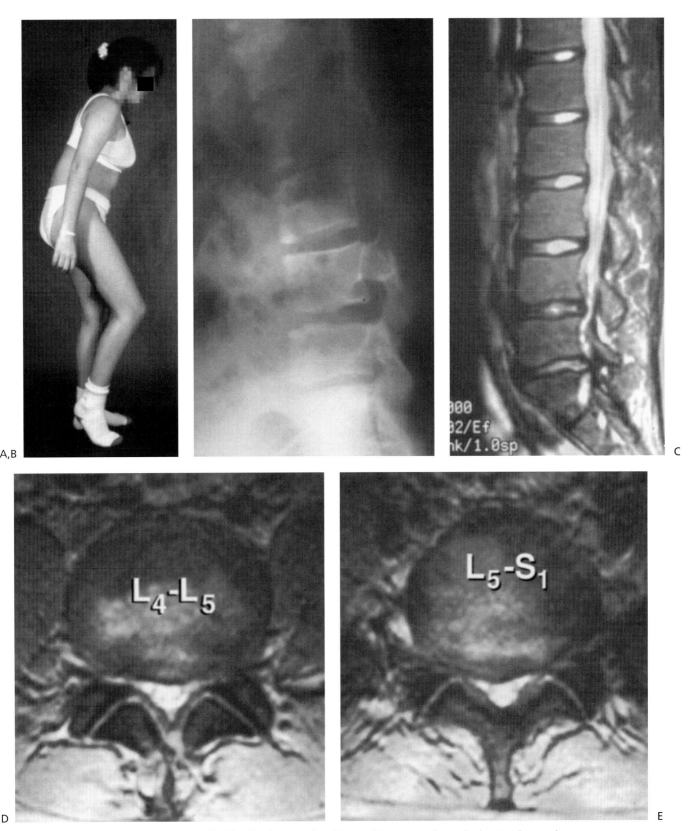

FIGURE 9. A 15-year-old girl with a longstanding history of leg pain and a marked postural anomaly without back pain **(A)**. The radiographs demonstrate a local kyphosis L4–5 and very short pedicles **(B)**. The magnetic resonance image shows L4–5 and L5–S1 disc herniation with severe spinal stenosis **(C–E)**. Her symptoms were relieved after L4–5 and L5–S1 discectomy.

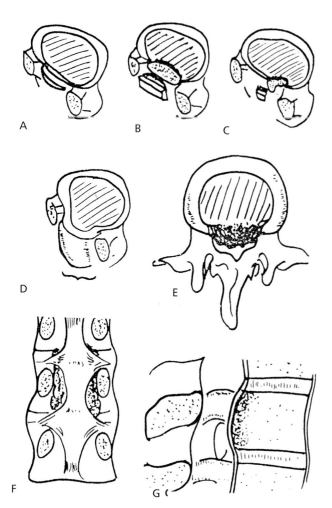

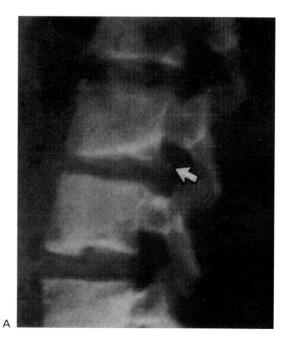

FIGURE 10. Schematic diagram of fractures of the vertebral limbus. **A:** Type I—simple separation of the entire posterior vertebral margin. **B:** Type II—avulsion fracture of some of the substance of the vertebral body, including the margin. **C:** Type III—more localized lateral fracture of the posterior margin of the vertebral body. **D–G:** Type IV—fracture that extends both beyond the margins of the disc and for the full length of the vertebral body between the end plates. The type IV fracture effectively displaces bone in the posterior direction, filling the floor of the spinal canal with a combination of reconstituted cortical and cancellous bone accompanied in part by scar formation. (Reprinted from Epstein NE, Epstein JA (1991): Limbus lumbar vertebral fractures in 27 adolescents and adults. *Spine* 16:962–966, with permission.)

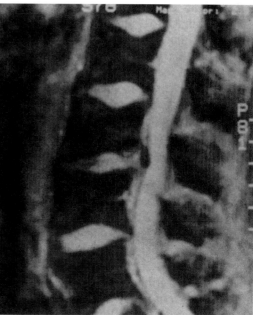

FIGURE 11. A 13-year-old boy scaled a high fence and jumped. He subsequently complained of back pain and presented with radicular symptoms with an L4–5 distribution. Removal of the large osteocartilaginous apophysis of the inferior aspect of L3 gave him immediate relief. **A:** A true lateral radiograph of the lumbar spine showing an ossific density in the spinal canal *(arrow)* posterior of the inferior margin L3. **B:** Magnetic resonance imaging illustrates the rim fracture of the posteroinferior end plate of the L3 vertebra with posterior displacement of the fragment into the spinal canal. The child underwent excision of the vertebral end plate apophysis and experienced complete relief. (Reprinted with permission from Crawford AH. (1990): Operative treatment of spine fractures in children. *Orthop Clin North Am* 21: 325–339, with permission.)

TREATMENT

As disk problems are common in adults, conservative treatment is often advocated immediately without a proven diagnosis. In children and adolescents, disc problems are so rare that it is mandatory to make a diagnosis (and rule out other causes of back pain) before deciding which treatment is indicated.

Nonoperative Treatment

Conservative treatment is similar to that in the adult with a disc herniation. It includes the following:

- *Rest.* Complete bed rest in the acute phase or relative rest, with little or no physical activity in the rehabilitation period.
- *Medications.* Analgesics and muscle relaxants are indicated to help relieve the muscle spasms in the acute phase. Administration of local steroids by epidural injection has mostly been reported in adults (15). It remains an option in the acute phase if rest does not alleviate the symptoms and the patient has a contraindication for surgery. However, in a large prospective randomized study, Carette et al. (17) demonstrated that epidural steroids have not shown their superiority to a placebo-saline epidural injection.
- *Physiotherapy.* In the acute phase, massage, local heat, and transcutaneous electrical nerve stimulation can help reduce the muscle contracture. But it is in the rehabilitation period that these modalities are more helpful; the program may include strengthening muscles (including abdominal muscles), regaining motion (around the hips), and preventing bad postures and habits.
- *Bracing.* The use of thoracolumbosacral orthosis in HNP or SVA is not well documented and not advocated by the authors.
- *Chemonucleolysis.* Bradbury et al. (11) in a series of 60 pediatric patients reported 81% good or excellent results in his surgical group compared with 64% in his chymopapain group. However, they concluded that the patients were more likely to be employed after chemonucleolysis than after primary surgery. They favored chemonucleolysis as a first-line treatment, with surgery reserved for the failures. Lorenz and McCulloch (53) in a series of 55 pediatric cases had a failure of chemonucleolysis in 20% of the cases. However, most centers do not use chymopapain for adolescent disc protrusion. This may be due to the possible complications of treatment (mostly anaphylactic reaction) (62,63), the higher failure rate of chymopapain (19), and a lower success rate than open discectomy (63). In the authors' opinion, this is more true in the pediatric population, where surgery gives usually excellent result with little or no morbidity.

Conservative treatment must always be used first in the absence of neurologic deficit. However, results are controversial in the pediatric age group. Some authors report a satisfactory or good success rate in their conservatively treated group of patients (35,50,94), but a large majority agree that it is most often unsuccessful (21,37,46,49,56).

OPERATIVE TREATMENT

Before surgery is performed, the following questions have to be answered:

1. Does the compression involve one or two levels? (See Figs. 7 and 9.)
2. Is the compression central? (This applies most often to an SVA.) In this case, the requirement of the decompression requires a bilateral approach and an extended laminotomy (Fig. 6). Is the compression posterolateral with a subligamentous HNP?
3. Is there a sequestered fragment? (This is rare in children.)
4. What is the size and shape of the canal when spinal stenosis is present?
5. Is there a fracture of the ring apophysis and is it old or new? (It will be easier to remove if new.)
6. What is the state of the disc (degenerated or not) and of the discs above and below it?
7. Is there an associated anomaly (spondylolysis, transitional anomaly, spina bifida occulta)?
8. Have other conditions, such as a tethered cord, been ruled out?

When all of these questions have been answered, the goal in treatment is to decompress the nerve root. In the absence of very clear scientific data regarding whether the discectomy should be complete or incomplete, the rationale for treatment is to perform a microdiscectomy that decompresses the nerve root. We believe that if MRI shows the disc to be not degenerated or only mildly degenerated, then removal of the hernia is sufficient. If, on the other hand, the disc is degenerated, a more complete removal of the disc on the side of the hernia should be done. In fracture of the ring apophysis this information is even more crucial because the disc may not be degenerated as mentioned (2,52). Therefore, removal of only the ring fracture is necessary if the disc is healthy on the preoperative MR image and adequate nerve decompression has been achieved.

Disc Excision

Whether the technique is a standard or a microsurgical approach, radiography is necessary to localize the proper level. The surgery then consists of opening of the ligamentum flavum, associated with a limited laminotomy if necessary to excise all compressing material. The herniation should be removed, but complete removal of the intervertebral disc is more difficult (and not necessary) than in the adult because the disc is not dehydrated and is more resistant (20). Cartilaginous fragments and bone fragments must be cut away, and if the diagnosis is delayed (as is often the case) local fibrous and remodeling make this part of the surgery harder and dangerous in terms of the dural sac and nerve roots. In the case of SVA, there is often a need to do a bilateral approach and an extended laminotomy (2,78) (Fig. 6). We have no experience with percutaneous nucleotomy or arthroscopic discectomy, both of which, in our opinion, are rarely indicated for treatment of HNP in children and are contraindicated in SVA or spinal stenosis.

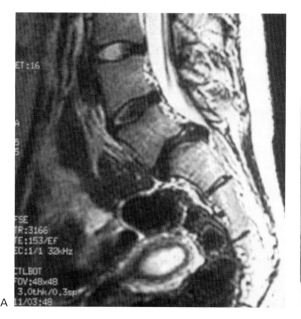

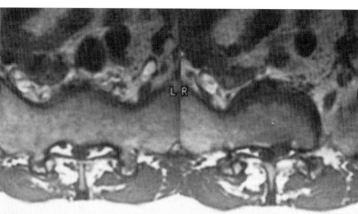

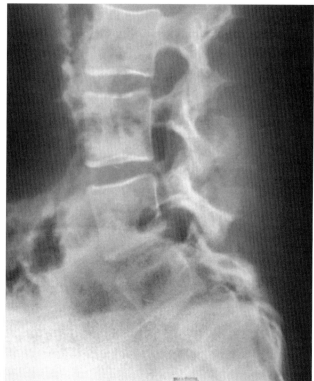

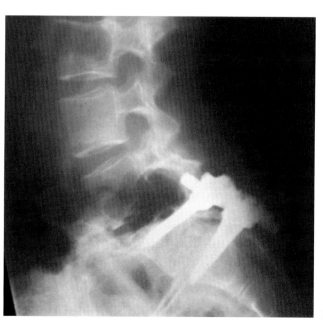

FIGURE 12. **(A)** Magnetic resonance image (MRI) from a 15-year-old girl who presented with left side sciatica of several months duration. MRI had confirmed the diagnosis of subligamentous disc herniation at L5–S1 **(B)**. A review of the magnetic resonance image and the radiograph **(C)** shows clearly a spondylol-isthesis with a positive slip angle. At surgery, the hernia was subligamentous and compressing the left S1 nerve root. Because of the spondylolisthesis, an L5–S1 fusion was added **(D)**. This case illustrates the rare occurrence of a true herniation of the nucleus pulposus (HNP) and a spondylolisthesis. In our minds this is the only indication for a spine fusion in HNP in the pediatric spine.

Spinal Fusion

Most authors (12,13,27,28,46,49,81) (except Leong et al. [51] and Ishihara et al. [44] in selected cases) recommend that spinal fusion not be performed at the time of the discectomy. As the results of spinal fusion are not superior to those of simple discectomy, we do not advocate fusion. However, in the case of true sciatica due to HNP in a spondylolisthesis case, we strongly recommend that spinal fusion be performed at the time of the decompression (Fig. 12).

Results of Surgical Treatment

In contrast to adults, in whom the initial outcome is guarded (24,63), most authors agree that in the pediatric population surgical treatment gives good or excellent initial results in more than 85% of cases. The radicular pain and back pain disappear rapidly in the postoperative period (9,21,22,25,33,37,78,81).

Long-term results tend to endure but a certain number of reoperations are needed (78,81,72,22): In Ebersold and colleagues' (25) series of 74 patients, 16 patients (21%) had to undergo a second spine operation over a 34-year follow-up. For DeLuca et al. (21), there were poor results (9%) at 6.3 years follow-up. Fisher and Saunders (32) reported that 10% of patients required reoperation within 3 years. DeOrio and Bianco (22) reported 26.5% poor results at a mean of 19 years follow-up. Luukkonen et al. (55) had poor results in 10% of their cases.

RECOMMENDATIONS

In a child with symptomatic HNP or SVA one should rule out other causes of sciatica and obtain a CT scan and an MRI. A trial of conservative treatment consisting of rest, muscle relaxants, and anti-inflammatories should be started. Unfortunately, in the pediatric age group this treatment often is insufficient, and symptoms may persist. In more than 90% of such cases, surgical treatment can achieve a very satisfactory outcome. However, very long-term results may follow the spectrum of DDD.

REFERENCES

1. Albeck MJ, Madsen FF, Wagner A, et al. (1991): Fracture of the lumbar vertebral ring apophysis imitating disc herniation. *Acta neurochir* 113(1–2):52–56.
2. Baba H, Uchida K, Furusawa N, et al. (1996): Posterior limbus vertebral lesions causing lumbosacral radiculopathy and the cauda equina syndrome. *Spinal Cord* 34(7):427–432.
3. Banerian KG, Wang A, Samberg LC, Kerr HH, Wesolowski DP (1990): Association of vertebral end plate fracture with pediatric lumbar intervertebral disk herniation: value of CT and MRI imaging. *Radiology* 177:763–765.
4. Begg AC (1954): Nuclear herniations of the intervertebral disc: The radiologic manifestations and significance. *J Bone Joint Surg Br* 36: 180–193.
5. Beks JW, ter Weeme CA (1975): Herniated lumbar discs in teenagers. *Acta Neurochir* 31:195–199.
6. Bick EM, Copel JW (1950): Longitudinal growth of the human vertebra. *J Bone Joint Surg Am* 32:803–814.
7. Bick EM, Copel JW (1951): The ring apophysis of the human vertebra. Contribution to human osteogeny II. *J Bone Joint Surg Am* 33: 783–787.
8. Birkenfeld R, Kasdon DL. Congenital lumbar ridge causing spinal claudication in adolescents. Report of two cases. *J Neurosurg* 1978 49(3): 441–444.
9. Borgesen SE, Vang PS (1974): Herniation of the lumbar intervertebral disc in children and adolescents. *Acta Orthop Scand* 45:540–549.
10. Bowen V, Shannon R, Kirkaldy-Willis WH. (1978): Lumbar spinal stenosis: a review article. *Child's Brain* 4(5):257–277.
11. Bradbury N, Wilson LF, Mulholland RC (1996): Adolescent disc protrusions. A long-term follow-up of surgery compared to chymopapain. *Spine* 21(3):372–377.
12. Bradford DS, Garcia A (1971): Lumbar intervertebral disc herniations in children and adolescents. *Orthop Clin North Am* 2:583–592.
13. Bradford DS, Garcia A (1969): Herniations of the lumbar intervertebral disc in children and adolescents. *JAMA* 210:2045–2051.
14. Bulos S (1973): Herniated intervertebral lumbar disc in the teenager. *J Bone Joint Surg Br* 55:273–278.
15. Bush K, Cowan N, Katz DE, et al. (1992). The natural history of sciatica associated with disc pathology. *Spine* 17(10):1205–1212.
16. Callahan DJ, Pack LL, Bream RC, et al. (1986): Intervertebral disc impingement syndrome in a child. Report of a case and suggested pathology. *Spine* 11(4):402–404.
17. Carette S, Leclaire R, Marcoux S, et al. (1997): Epidural corticosteroid injections for sciatica due to herniated nucleus pulposus. *N Engl J Med* 336(23):1634–1640.
18. Clarke NMP, Cleak DK (1983): Intervertebral lumbar disc prolapse in children and adolescents. *J Pediatr Orthop* 3:202–206.
19. Crawshaw C, Frazer A, Merriam WF, et al. (1984): A comparison of surgery and chemonucleolysis in the treatment of sciatica: a prospective randomized trial. *Spine* 9:195.
20. Czorny A, Forlodou P, Kilic K, et al. [Lumbar disk hernia in children. A propos of 12 cases]. *Neurochirurgie* 1988;34(6):389–393.
21. DeLuca PF, Mason DE, Weiand R, et al. (1994): Excision of herniated nucleus pulposus in children and adolescents. *J Pediatr Orthop* 14(3): 318–322.
22. DeOrio JK, Bianco AJ Jr (1982): Lumbar disc excision in children and adolescents. *J Bone Joint Surg Am* 64:991–996.
23. Deoyo RA, Loeser J, Bigos S. (1986): Herniated lumbar intervertebral disc. *Ann Intern Med* 315:1064.
24. Dvorak J, Gauchat MH, Valach L. (1988): The outcome of surgery for lumbar disc herniation. I.A 4–17 years' follow-up with emphasis on somatic aspects. *Spine* 13(12):1418–1422.
25. Ebersold MJ, Quast LM, Bianco AJ Jr (1987): Results of lumbar discectomy in the pediatric patient. *J Neurosurg* 67(5):643–647.
26. Eisenstein S (1976): Measurements of the lumbar spinal canal in 2 racial groups. *Clin Orthop* 115:42–46.
27. Epstein JA, Lavine LS (1964): Herniated lumbar intervertebral discs in teenage children. *J Neurosurg* 21:1070–1075.
28. Epstein JA, Epstein NE, Marc J, et al. (1984): Lumbar intervertebral disc herniation in teenage children: recognition and management of associated anomalies. *Spine* 9:427–432.
29. Epstein NE, Epstein JA, Mauri T. Treatment of fractures of the vertebral limbus and spinal stenosis in five adolescents and five adults. *Neurosurgery* 1989 24(4):595–604.
30. Epstein NE, Epstein JA (1991): Limbus lumbar vertebral fractures in 27 adolescents and adults. *Spine* 16:962–966.
31. Epstein NE (1992): Lumbar surgery for 56 limbus fractures emphasizing noncalcified type III lesions. *Spine* 17(12):1489–1496.
32. Fisher RG, Saunders RL (1981): Lumbar disc protrusion in children. *J Neurosurg* 54(4):480–483.
33. Furnes O, Boe A, Sudmann E (1996): [Lumbar intervertebral disk

prolapse in adolescents]. *Tidsskr Nor Laegeforen* 20;116(25): 2993–2995.

34. Garrido Eddy (1983): Lumbar disc herniation in the pediatric patient. *Neurosurg Clin North Am* 4(1).

35. Ghabrial YA, Tarrant MJ (1989): Adolescent disc prolapse. *Acta Orthop Scand* 60(2):174–176.

36. Gibson MJ, Szypryt EP, Buckley JH, et al. (1987): Magnetic resonance imaging of adolescent disc herniation. *J Bone Joint Surg Br* 69(5): 699–703.

37. Giroux JC, Leclercq TA (1982): Lumbar disc excision in the second decade. *Spine* 7:168–170.

38. Grobler LJ, Simmons EH, Barrington TW (1979): Intervertebral disc herniation in the adolescent. *Spine* 4:267–278.

39. Gunzburg R, Fraser RD, Fraser GA (1990): Lumbar intervertebral disc prolapse in teenage twins. *J Bone Joint Surg Br* 72:914–916.

40. Handel SF, Twiford TW, Reigel DH, et al. (1979): Posterior lumbar apophyseal fracture. *Radiology* 130:629–633.

41. Hashimoto K, Fujita K, Kojimoto H, et al. (1990): Lumbar disc herniation in children. *J Pediatr Orthop* 10:394–396.

42. Hasso AN, McKinney JM, Killeen J, et al. (1987): Computed tomography of children and adolescents with suspected spinal stenosis. *J Comput Assist Tomogr* 11(4):609–611.

43. Heithoff KB, Gundry CR, Burton CV, et al. (1994): Juvenile discogenic disease. *Spine* 19(3):335–340.

44. Ishihara H, Matsui H, Hirano N, et al. (1997): Lumbar intervertebral disc herniation in children less than 16 years of age. Long-term follow-up study of surgically managed cases. *Spine* 22(17):2044–2049.

45. Jackson RP, Cain JE Jr, Jacobs RR, et al. (1989): The neuroradiographic diagnosis of lumbar herniated nucleus pulposus: II. A comparison of computed tomography (CT), myelography, CT-myelography, and magnetic resonance imaging. *Spine* 14(12):1362–1367.

46. Kamel M, Rosman M. (1984): Disc protrusion in the growing child. *Clin Orthop* 185:46–52.

47. Kawakami M, Tamaki T, Hayashi N, et al. (1998): Possible mechanism of painful radiculopathy in lumbar disc herniation. *Clin Orthop* (351): 241–251.

48. Komori H, Shinomiya K, Nakai O, et al. (1996): The natural history of herniated nucleus pulposus with radiculopathy. *Spine* 15(2):225–229.

49. Kurihara A, Kotaoka O (1980): Lumbar disc herniation in children and adolescents. A review of 70 operated cases and their minimum 5-year follow-up studies. *Spine* 5:443–451.

50. Kurth AA, Rau S, Wang C, et al. (1996): Treatment of lumbar disc herniation in the second decade of life. *Eur Spine J* 5(4):220–224.

51. Leong JCY, Hooper G, Fang D, et al. (1982): Disc excision and anterior spinal fusion for lumbar disc protrusion in the adolescent *Spine* 7: 626–628.

52. Liquois F, Demay P, Filipe G (1987): Sciatica caused by avulsion of the vertebral limbus in children. *Rev Chir Orthop Reparatrice Appar Mot* 83(3):210–216.

53. Lorenz M, McCulloch J (1985): Chemonucleolysis for herniated nucleus pulposus in adolescents. *J Bone Joint Surg Am* 67(9):1402–1404.

54. Lowrey JJ (1973): Dislocated lumbar vertebral epiphysis in adolescent children. Report of three cases. *J Neurosurg* 38:232–234.

55. Luukkonen M, Partanen K, Vapalahti M (1997): Lumbar disc herniations in children: a long-term clinical and magnetic resonance imaging follow-up study. *Br J Neurosurg* 11(4):280–285.

56. Martinez-Lage JF, Martinez Robledo A, Lopez F, Poza M (1997): Disc protrusion in the child. Particular features and comparison with neoplasms. *Child's Nerv Syst* 13(4):201–207.

57. Matsui H, Tsuji H, Terahata N. (1990): Juvenile lumbar herniated nucleus pulposus in monozygotic twins. *Spine* 15(11):1228–1230.

58. Matsui H, Terahata N, Tsuji H, et al. (1992): Familial predisposition and clustering for juvenile lumbar disc herniation. *Spine* 17(11): 1323–1328.

59. Modic MT, Ross JS, Obuchowski NA, et al. (1995): Contrast-enhanced MR imaging in acute lumbar radiculopathy: a pilot study of the natural history. *Radiology* 195(2):429–435.

60. Nelson CL, Janecki CJ, Gildenberg PL, et al. (1972): Disc protrusions in the young. *CORR Clin Orthop* 88:142–150.

61. Nordby EJ, Wright PH (1994): Efficacy of chymopapain in chemonucleolysis. A review. *Spine* 19(22):2578–2583.

62. Nordby EJ, Fraser RD, Javid MJ (1996): Chemonucleolysis. *Spine* 21(9):1102–1105.

63. Nykvist F, Hurme M, Alaranta H, et al. (1995): Severe sciatica: a 13 years follow-up of 342 patients. *Eur Spine J* 4(6):335–338.

64. Obukhov SK, Hankenson L, Manka M, et al. (1996): Multilevel lumbar disc herniation in 12-year-old twins. *Child's Nerv Sys* 12(3): 169–171.

65. O'Connell JEA (1960): Intervertebral disc protrusions in children and adolescents. *Br J Surg* 47:611–616.

66. Olmarker K, Myers RR (1998): Pathogenesis of sciatic pain: role of herniated nucleus pulposus and deformation of spinal nerve root and dorsal root ganglion. *Pain* 78(2):99–105.

67. Panayiotis J, Papagelopoulos PJ, Shaughnessy WJ, et al. (1998): Long-term outcome of lumbar discectomy in children and adolescents sixteen years of age or younger. *J Bone Joint Surg Am* 80(5):689–698.

68. Peh WC, Griffith JF, Yip DK, et al. (1998): Magnetic resonance imaging of lumbar vertebral apophyseal ring fractures. *Australas Radiol* 42(1):34–37.

69. Perron O, Fassier F, Joncas J (1996): Herniated disk and congenital spinal stenosis in the adolescent. *Rev Chir Orthop Rep Appar Mot* 82(1): 29–33.

70. Porter RW, Thorp L (1986): Familial aspects of disc protrusion. *Orthop Trans* 10:524.

71. Postaccini F, Lami R, Pugliese O (1988): Familial predisposition to discogenic low back pain. An epidemiologic and immunogenetic study. *Spine* 13:1403–1406.

72. Poussa M, Schlenzka D, Maenpaa S, et al. (1997): Disc herniation in the lumbar spine during growth: long-term results of operative treatment in 18 patients. *Eur Spine J* 6(6):390–392.

73. Raaf J (1959): Some observations regarding 905 patients operated upon for protruded lumbar intervertebral disc. *Am J Surg* 97:388–399.

74. Ramirez N, Johnston CE, Browne RH (1997): The prevalence of back pain in children who have idiopathic scoliosis. *J Bone Joint Surg Am* 79(3):364–368.

75. Rugtveit A (1966): Juvenile lumbar disc herniations. *Acta Orthop Scand* 37:348–356.

76. Salminen JJ, Erkintalo M, Laine M, et al. (1995): Low back pain in the young. A prospective three-year follow-up study of subjects with and without low back pain. *Spine* 20(19):2101–2107.

77. Savini R, Di Silvestre M, Gargiulo G, et al. (1991): Posterior lumbar apophyseal fracture. *Spine* 16:1118–1123.

78. Savini R, Martucci E, Nardi S, et al. (1991): The herniated lumbar intervertebral disc in children and adolescent. Long term follow-up of 101 cases treated by surgery. *Ital J Orthop Traumatol* 17(4):505–511.

79. Schindler OS, Fairbank JC (1996): Two-level intervertebral disc herniation in an adolescent. *Br J Clin Pract* 50(3):171–173.

80. Schillito J (1996): Pediatric lumbar disc surgery: 20 patients under 15 years of age. *Surg Neurol* 46(1):14–18.

81. Silvers HR, Lewis PJ, Clabeaux DE, et al. (1994): Lumbar disc excisions in patients under the age of 21 years. *Spine* 19(21):2387–2391.

82. Simmons ED Jr, Guntupalli M, Kowalski JM, et al. (1996): Familial predisposition for degenerative disc disease. A case control study. *Spine* 21(13):1527–1529.

83. Sovio OM, Bell HM, Beauchamp RD, et al. (1985): Fracture of the lumbar vertebral apophysis. *J Pediatr Orthop* 5:550–552.

84. Takata K, Inoue S, Takahashi K, et al. (1988): Fracture of the posterior margin of a lumbar vertebral body. *J Bone Joint Surg Am* 70:589–594.

85. Techakapuch S (1981): Rupture of the lumbar cartilage plate into the spinal canal in an adolescent. *J Bone Joint Surg Am* 63:481–482.

86. Tullberg T, Grane P, Isacson J (1994): Gadolinium-enhanced magnetic

resonance imaging of 36 patients one year after lumbar disc resection. *Spine* 19:176–182.

87. Valen B, Rolfsen LC (1998): Quality assurance of back surgery. A follow up of 350 patients treated for sciatica by means of survival analysis. *Tidsskr Nor Laegeforen* 118(14):2136–2139.

88. Varlotta GP, Brown MD, Kelsey JL, et al. (1991): Familial predisposition for herniation of a lumbar disc in patients who are less than twenty-one years old. *J Bone Joint Surg Am* 73:124–128.

89. Varughese G, Quartey GR (1979): Familial lumbar spinal stenosis with acute disc herniations. Case reports of four brothers. *J Neurosurg Aug* 51(2):234–236.

90. Wahren H (1945): Herniated nucleus pulposus in a child of twelve years. *Acta Orthop Scand* 16:40–42.

91. Webb JH, Svien HJ, Kennedy RLJ (1954): Protruded lumbar intervertebral discs in children. *JAMA* 154:1153–1154.

92. Wisneski RJ, Garfin SR (1992): Lumbar disc disease. In: Rothman RH, Simeone S, eds. *The spine,* 3rd ed. Philadelphia: WB Saunders, pp. 671–746.

93. Yabuki S, Kikuchi S, Olmarker K, et al. (1998): Acute effects of nucleus pulposus on blood flow and endoneurial fluid pressure in rat dorsal ganglia. *Spine* 23(23):2517–2523.

94. Zamani MH, MacEwen GD (1982): Herniation of the lumbar disc in children and adolescents. *J Pediatr Orthop* 2:528–533.

95. Zitting P, Rantakallio P, Vanharanta H (1998): Cumulative incidence of lumbar disc diseases leading to hospitalization up to the age of 28 years. *Spine* 23(21):2337–2343; discussion 2343–2344.

25

NEUROFIBROMATOSIS

ALVIN H. CRAWFORD

HISTORICAL REVIEW

Neurofibromatosis is a spectrum of multifaceted diseases involving not only neuroectoderm and mesoderm but also endoderm. It presents with a wide range of clinical manifestations that have in common the presence of schwannomas, neurofibromas, and/or café-au-lait spots (8). Clinically, this multisystemic, hereditary disease may manifest as abnormalities of the skin, nervous tissue, bones, and soft tissues. The primary pathologic process is believed to be a hamartomatous disorder of neural crest derivation. Common findings in pediatric neurofibromatosis type 1 (NF-1) are noted in Table 1. Reports in the orthopaedics literature have dealt primarily with specific entities such as spinal deformity, pseudarthrosis of the tibia, paraplegia, hemihypertrophy, and neoplasia. Scoliosis is the most common musculoskeletal complication of NF-1 (2,31). This chapter deals with the primary and secondary effects of NF-1 on the pediatric spine.

DIAGNOSTIC PROBLEMS

Most investigators now accept four clinical forms of neurofibromatosis: peripheral (NF-1), central (NF-2), segmental, and mixed. A variety of eponyms have been used to describe all forms, although subsequent information has made these names technically inaccurate or incomplete. The most common type, NF-1, was previously known as von Recklinghausen disease and is an autosomal dominant disorder affecting about one in 4,000 persons; multiple hyperpigmented areas (café-au-lait macules) and neurofibromas are characteristic.

The 1987 Consensus Development Conference of the National Institutes of Health on NF-1 concluded that the diagnosis of NF-1 was established when two or more of the following diagnostic criteria were found: (a) six or more café-au-lait macules greater than 5 mm in widest diameter in prepubertal children and more than 15 mm in widest diameter in postpubertal individuals; (b) two or more neurofibromas of any type or one plexiform neurofibroma; (c) freckling in the axillary or inguinal regions; (d) optic glioma; (e) two or more Lisch nodules (iris hamartomas); (f) a distinctive osseous lesion, such as sphenoid dysplasia or thinning of a long bone cortex with or without pseudarthrosis; and (g) a first-degree relative (parent, sibling, or offspring) with NF-1 identified by the above criteria. Other disorders of pigmentation, such as McCune-Albright or Watson's syndrome, can be confused with NF-1 (49).

GENETICS

NF-1 is the most common human single-gene disorder. It affects at least one million people throughout the world. It is seen in all racial and ethnic groups. It would be conservative to estimate that half of all people with NF-1 will suffer serious medical and social complications. The gene is fairly large (about 300,000 base pairs). (Most genes are several tens of thousands of base pairs, and the largest known, the gene for Duchenne muscular dystrophy, extends over 2.5 million base pairs.)

In 1990, the gene locus of NF-1 in humans was cloned and its protein product, neurofibromin, was identified (25). The gene is very large and has been linked to the long arm of chromosome 17. The NF-2 locus is probably linked to the long arm of chromosome 22; this genetic linkage is useful for the accurate diagnosis in families that have a high risk for NF-1. Given the fact that several hundred families with NF-1 have shown linkage to DNA markers on 17q (11,20), prenatal diagnosis for NF-1 is possible. For the time being, NF-1 prenatal diagnosis requires the genetic linkage approach, which means that only families in which two or more generations are already involved can use this exciting new aspect of health care (52). Continued rapid scientific progress is expected in molecular genetics for both NF-1 and NF-2. Such studies should lead to the development of a direct diagnostic test for NF-1, which would be especially helpful in establishing the diagnosis in uncertain cases, such as young children with only café-au-lait spots. This will directly influence classification, patient care, counseling of families, and research.

CLINICAL FINDINGS
Café-au-lait Spots

Café-au-lait spots are present in well over 90% of all patients with NF-1. The pigmentation is tan, macular, and melanotic in origin and is located in and around the basal layer of the epidermis; the lesions may vary in shape, size, number, and loca-

A. H. Crawford: Department of Pediatric Orthopaedic Surgery, Children's Hospital Medical Center, Cincinnati, Ohio 45229

TABLE 1. COMMON FINDINGS IN PEDIATRIC NEUROFIBROMATOSIS TYPE 1

Finding	Percent
Café-au-lait (CAL) and cutaneous tumors by adolescent years	72–90
Positive family history	45–48
Central nervous system lesions	16–26
Scoliosis (as high as 60% in orthopaedic literature)	20–26
Skull and facial deformities	20
Significant CAL alone (not a true diagnosis of NF-1)	17
Failure to thrive in infancy	16
Aqueductal stenosis	16
Breast enlargement	13
Seizures	13
Hemihypertrophy	13
Tibial pseudarthrosis	12
Benign tumors alone	11
Extracranial malignancy (dramatic increase with age)	11–20
Vascular disease (dramatic increase with age)	10
Mediastinal tumors	8

Modified from Fienman NL (1981): Pediatric neurofibromatosis: review. *Compr Ther* 7:66–72.

tion. In NF-1, these spots are frequently found in areas of the skin not exposed to the sun (Fig. 1).

Lisch Nodules

Lisch nodules, or iris-pigmented hamartomas, are present in 94% of patients with NF-1 who are 6 years of age or older; 28% of younger patients have them (42). They increase in number with age (39) but do not become symptomatic. The lesions appear to be specific for NF-1; they are not seen in non-NF-1 individuals.

Neurofibromas

Neurofibromas mostly involve the skin, but they may be seen in deeper peripheral nerves. They may be nodular and discrete, or diffuse with interdigitation with surrounding tissues. Highly vascular plexiform neurofibromas may cause segmental or localized hypertrophy. Puberty or pregnancy may cause an increase in the size and number of the lesions (12).

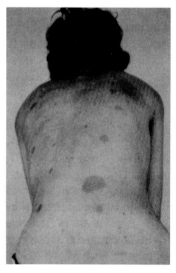
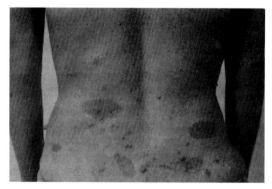

A,B

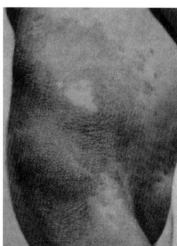
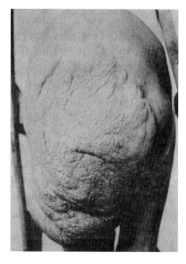

C,D

FIGURE 1. Cutaneous lesions of neurofibromatosis seen in children include café-au-lait spots, fibroma molluscum, pigmented nevi, and verrucous hyperplasia. **A:** Multiple café-au-lait spots in a young patient with scoliosis. Note the variation in size and shape of lesions. These lesions tend to increase in size and number as the child matures. **B:** Multiple café-au-lait spots in an older patient who also has subcutaneous nodules (fibroma molluscum), that is, pedunculated lesions that occur in the postpubescent adolescent. This patient also has several subcutaneous neurofibromas of the intercostal nerves, which are sessile. **C:** This large nevus, occurring on only one side of the trunk, is the nevus lateralis. It can be quite sensitive, and several patients who had spinal curvatures could not tolerate external corrective devices (e.g., Milwaukee brace or orthoplast jacket) because of this extreme sensitivity, which is believed to be related to an underlying plexiform neurofibroma. **D:** Verrucous hyperplasia of the skin over the left buttocks. This is the most grotesque of all cutaneous lesions. (Reprinted with permission from Crawford AH [1990]: NF-1. In: Morrissy RT, ed. *Lovell and Winters pediatric orthopaedics,* 3rd ed. Philadelphia: JB Lippincott.)

Cutaneous Neurofibroma

Cutaneous neurofibromas, formerly called fibroma molluscum, are found in subcutaneous tissues after puberty. They are usually manifestations of longstanding or adult disease and do not occur with any frequency (12%) in childhood (53). Recent electron microscopy studies have demonstrated that axons and Schwann cells are present in these tumors; therefore, it is appropriate that they be called dermal neurofibroma (30).

Elephantiasis

Frequently, large soft-tissue masses are seen in NF-1. These masses have been termed *pachydermatocele* or *elephantiasis neuromatosa* and are characterized by a rough, raised, villous type of skin hypertrophy presenting an unmistakable appearance.

Pigmented Nevi

Eight percent of all patients presenting with NF-1 have pigmented nevi, some presenting with geographic descriptions (e.g., "nevus lateralus"). "Bathing trunk" nevi or hyperpigmentation may be present in up to 6% of children with NF-1 (53). Some nevi are quite sensitive, often the result of an underlying subcutaneous plexiform neurofibroma.

Plexiform Neurofibroma

Plexiform neurofibromas are subcutaneous neurofibromas that have a ropy, "bag of worms" feeling. Their cutaneous involvement may cause decreased sensation, causing sores to develop under a brace or cast without the patient's knowledge, or they may be hypersensitive. The plexiform neurofibroma has the potential for malignant degeneration (53).

Optic Gliomas

Although optic gliomas account for only 2% to 5% of all brain tumors in childhood, as many as 70% of cases are found in persons with NF-1. In many NF-1 patients these tumors change little in size over many years, but a small percentage of such tumors may enlarge rapidly, leading to exophthalmos and visual impairment.

Verrucous Hyperplasia

Verrucous hyperplasia is an uncommon, unsightly, extensive overgrowth of the skin, with thickening of a velvety-soft papillary quality. Many crevices form and tend to break down easily, with some weeping occurring in the skin folds.

Axillary and Inguinal Freckling

Freckles—diffuse, small, hyperpigmented spots up to 2 to 3 mm in diameter found in the armpits and inguinal region (areas not usually exposed to sunlight)—are helpful diagnostic criteria for NF-1.

Spinal Deformities

Spinal deformities have been noted to occur only in NF-1. The deformities include nondystrophic and dystrophic changes. The dystrophic changes may be intrinsic or associated with spinal canal anomalies secondary to abnormalities of the spinal cord dura mater.

The relative incidence of spinal deformities in NF-1 is unknown. Patients having some disorder of the spine will vary from 2% to 36% (3,60). Of the approximately 10,000 scoliosis patients seen by Winter et al. (73), only 102 were found to fit the traditional criteria for diagnosis of NF-1. Functional scoliosis resulting from limb hypertrophy or long-bone dysplasia must be ruled out in patients with NF-1. All preadolescent children with NF-1 should be evaluated by the scoliosis screening or Adam's "bend test" to rule out the presence of a spinal deformity, which usually occurs earlier in children with NF-1 (15). The characteristic deformity tends to a short segmented, sharply angulated curvature; it usually includes four to six vertebrae. It may be noticed in early childhood.

Recent investigators have suggested that there is no standard pattern of spinal deformity in NF-1; the types of curvature found are variable.

RADIOLOGY

Routine posteroanterior and lateral cervical, thoracolumbar, and sacral radiographs are necessary when studying the deformed spine because of the potential for occult deformity in each location. Careful attention is directed on plain radiographs to the sagittal plane for evidence of abnormal lordosis, kyphosis, or dystrophic changes.

Computed tomography (CT) has been used extensively to identify the occasional abnormal structure of the spine in NF-1; it allows one to assess the spinal canal, its contents, and the associated anatomy. Three-dimensional reconstruction enhances the explicitness of the bony detail. The addition of contrast myelography to CT has allowed the surgeon to identify lesions found in and about the spinal canal. Magnetic resonance imaging (MRI) has recently been utilized to determine the internal contents of the spinal canal and will show the presence of lesions within and about the spinal cord itself. There are occasional problems interpreting magnetic resonance image of severe deformities because of distortion brought on by the complex three-plane deformity of kyphoscoliosis (5).

MANAGEMENT OF DEFORMITIES
Cervical Deformities

The cervical spine deformity is usually kyphosis. Until recently, only casual references to the cervical spine have been evident in studies of other manifestations of NF-1. Many patients with cervical spine deformities are asymptomatic and clinically not apparent. Even so, curves in this area are more frequently associated with dysplastic lesions than in other areas of the spine (37).

Yong-Hing et al. (76) reviewed 56 patients with NF-1 specifi-

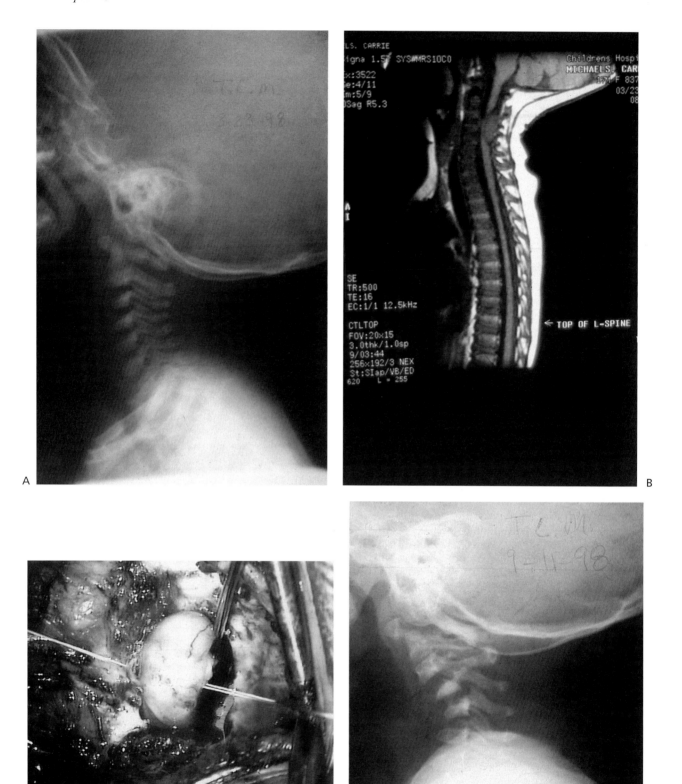

FIGURE 2. Spinal instability following laminectomy in a very young child who complained of neck pain and decreased range of motion. **A:** Presenting lateral cervical spine radiograph with slightly decreased lordosis. **B:** Magnetic resonance image illustrating extradural neurofibromatosis at C3–4 with spinal cord indentation. **C:** Operative view of neurofibroma excision. **D:** Lateral cervical spine radiograph 6 months following laminectomy and neurofibroma excision illustrating significant kyphosis of entire cervical spine.

cally for abnormalities of the cervical spine and found 17 to have lesions. Of 37 patients who had thoracic scoliosis or kyphosis, 15 (44%) had cervical spine lesions; many of these patients were asymptomatic. Adkins and Ratvich (1) reviewed 85 patients with NF-1 and found that head and neck masses were responsible for 22% of the patients' complaints. Five cases of atlantoaxial dislocation have been reported in patients with NF-1, two of whom were noted to have neurofibromas between the odontoid and anterior arch of C1 (57,68,76).

The clinical consequences of cervical NF-1 tend to be less marked than in other regions because the cord versus canal diameter is commonly reported to be less critical. Because of its gener-

ally asymptomatic nature, the problem is probably underreported. However, these lesions should not be disregarded because the tendency of the disease to progress has led to severe neurologic deficits in several cases (24,28).

Most patients with cervical spine anomalies seen by the orthopaedist have already had excision of a neck mass by other surgical services (Fig. 2) The preceding workup has most likely included radiographs of the cervical spine showing considerable bony anomalies, but orthopaedic or neurosurgical consultations have not been obtained. Any evidence of bony deformity noted on cervical spine radiographs requires orthopaedic consultation (Fig. 3). Other reasons for consulting an orthopaedist and ob-

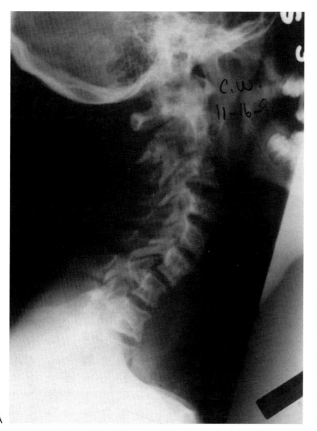

A

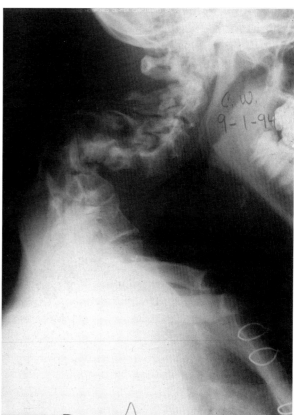

B

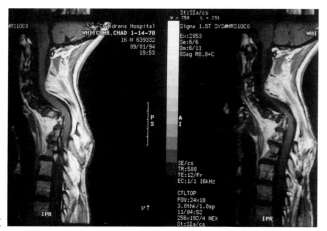

C

FIGURE 3. Spinal instability in 17-year-old following laminectomy for cervical neurofibrosarcoma. **A:** Lateral cervical spine x-ray taken prior to laminectomy. **B:** Lateral cervical spine radiograph taken 3 years following laminectomy illustrating significant (>90 degrees) kyphosis at time of referral to orthopaedic surgery. The child was neurologically intact. **C:** Preoperative magnetic resonance image illustrating dural sac expansion in area of kyphosis and absence of the posterior elements.

taining cervical spine radiographs in an NF-1 patient include torticollis and dysphagia. Both conditions may be related to intraspinal as well as extraspinal neurofibromas.

Anteroposterior and lateral radiographs of the cervical spine are recommended at the time of original evaluation of all spinal deformities in NF-1 patients. If dystrophic changes are noted, oblique radiographs to rule out dumbbell lesions (enlargement of neuroforamina due to intraspinal meningoceles, solitary tumors, or interstitial hypertrophic neuritis) and lateral flexion and extension radiographs to rule out instability should be obtained. One should be suspicious of scalloping of the vertebral bodies or an increase in the size of the neural foramina. If found, MRI should be performed to evaluate the intraspinal contents. All cases seen by the author following decompression laminectomies without fusion demonstrated instability with progressive kyphotic deformities.

Posterior spinal fusion is recommended for cervical spine deformity with instability. Autologous bone graft and halo immobilization are usually adequate, and a solid fusion can be expected. If there has been previous surgery, such as laminectomy, it may be necessary to perform anterior surgery as well. With the use of laser technology, neurofibromas in this region can be removed without compromise to the spinal cord. Because of the extent of bone removal required to completely excise the tumor and the resulting instability, posterior and anterior spinal fusion should always be carried out. The level of instability often requires an occipitocervical fusion. A halo-assisted orthosis may be utilized to stabilize the occipitocervicothoracic area until fusion takes place. Multiple view radiographs of the cervical spine are mandatory before general anesthesia or halo traction to rule out dystrophic deformity and possible instability.

Thoracic Scoliosis

Thoracic scoliosis is the most common osseous defect associated with NF-1. Gould (26) and Weiss (70) were the first to point out the associated spinal deformities in this disease; many authors have subsequently done so (5,13,32,64). The cause of spinal deformity is unknown, but it has been suggested to be secondary to osteomalacia, localized neurofibromatous tumor–related erosion and infiltration of bone, endocrine disturbances, or mesodermal dysplasia (7,26,29,64).

There have been relatively few clinical studies discussing the treatment of spinal deformities in patients with NF-1. Winter et al. (72) reviewed the natural history, associated anomalies, and responses to operative and nonoperative treatment in 102 patients with NF-1 and spinal deformity. Eighty patients were found to have curvature associated with dystrophic changes in vertebrae or ribs. The presence of dystrophic changes, such as rib rotation in the anteroposterior direction resulting in an abnormally thin appearance, spindling of the transverse processes, vertebral scalloping, severe apical vertebral rotation, foraminal enlargement, and adjacent soft-tissue neurofibromas, were found to be highly significant in terms of prognosis and management. Brace treatment has not been effective in the management of progressive dystrophic curves and should not be used, even in young children. Early fusion causes minimum stunting of truncal height because the curves are usually short, with poor growth

potential in the involved vertebrae; therefore, one need not wait for the child to attain a certain physiologic or chronologic age (73).

Chaglassian et al. (10) reported a 6.5% incidence of pseudarthrosis following 23 operations in 15 patients; there was no separation of dystrophic and nondystrophic curves. Crawford (14) reported a 15% incidence of pseudarthrosis in 46 patients. Savini et al. (58) performed 56 operations on 26 patients. They recommended anterior fusion and complete disc excision in addition to repeat bone grafting for relapse after posterior fusion. Betz et al. (5) reported the results of surgery performed on 23 patients; 20 obtained solid fusion, but 13 required one or more posterior augmentations because of progressive deformity. Three patients with dystrophic kyphoscoliosis obtained solid fusion with no further progression following primary anterior-posterior fusion.

Shufflebarger (65) used Cotrel-Dubousset instrumentation on 12 patients with NF-1: ten with nondystrophic NF-1, one with dystrophic NF-1, and another following multiple laminectomies. Follow-up averaged 33 months. The fusion on the dystrophic deformity failed and required repeat anterior-posterior fusion. He advocated immobilization following Cotrel-Dubousset instrumentation in patients with poor bone stock. More importantly, he stressed the necessity of performing the anterior procedure from the concave side utilizing multiple strut grafts. Convex discectomies tend to further destabilize the spine, and it is technically difficult, if not impossible, to properly place struts from the convex approach.

Holt and Johnson (33) treated five patients with dystrophic scoliosis with Cotrel-Dubousset instrumentation; surgery included posterior, anterior-posterior, and multistaged fusion.

Hsu et al. (34) reported on 13 patients with dystrophic spinal deformities treated by anterior-posterior fusion. Anterior-posterior fusion achieved satisfactory results in patients with smooth kyphoscoliosis or scoliosis without excessive kyphosis, but it was unsatisfactory in patients with an angular kyphoscoliosis. Five patients had angular kyphoscoliosis; one had persistent pseudarthrosis after operation, and all had progression of the kyphosis despite the treatment.

Sirois and Drennan (66) reviewed 32 patients with NF-1 and spinal deformity, 23 (72%) of whom had dystrophic curve patterns. The incidence of pseudarthrosis was 38% for the dystrophic group undergoing isolated posterior fusion. Retrospective curve extension following surgery was noted in three patients; one required extension of the fusion mass. The average curve progression was 12.7 degrees and required an average of 1.7 procedures to achieve solid posterior fusion. They recommend treatment of kyphoscoliotic curves with anterior-posterior fusion.

The author agrees with others that spinal deformities in NF-1 should be divided into two groups: those with dystrophic changes and those with no apparent dystrophy. The most serious spinal deformity complicating NF-1 is dystrophy of the vertebral bodies, posterior arches, and spinal canal. The clinical problems associated with these deformities are most common in the thoracic area, possibly because the canal-to-cord-diameter ratio is more critical in the thoracic region.

Nondystrophic Scoliosis

The nondystrophic curvature is the most common spinal deformity in NF-1, and findings are believed to be similar to those of idiopathic scoliosis. The nonprogressive curvatures can usually be managed in the same manner as other idiopathic curvatures. When following patients with what appear to be nondystrophic spinal deformities over an extended period, there is a higher incidence of progressive deformity, including possible pseudarthrosis following instrumentation and fusion, than that found in idiopathic scoliosis. *There is the distinct possibility of modulation across a spectrum of nondystrophic to dystrophic curvatures, but this tendency shows no consistent pattern (25).* These patients are also subject to spinal canal neurofibromas that may grow and give rise to pressure-induced expansion of the canal, as well as dystrophy of the vertebral bodies.

The author's recommendations for managing nondystrophic scoliosis accompanying NF-1 are to treat the curvature as an idiopathic curvature (i.e., the patient should be observed for curvatures of less than 20 degrees). If there are no dystrophic changes, a brace is applied following progression of the deformity up to 35 degrees. For those deformities exceeding 35 to 45 degrees, a posterior spinal fusion of all articular facets and segmental spinal instrumentation is strongly recommended. Patients whose deformities exceed 60 degrees should routinely have anterior disc excision with bone grafting of the area of curvature followed by posterior spinal fusion of all articular facets, segmental spinal instrumentation, and autogenous iliac crest bone graft.

There is a definite tendency of nondystrophic curves to become dystrophic in some patients, with a coexistent higher incidence of pseudarthrosis and loss of correction following attempts at surgical stabilization.

Dystrophic Scoliosis

The short segmented, sharply angulated curvature is the most common identifiable spinal deformity associated with NF-1. Specific vertebral body changes, such as scalloping of the vertebral bodies, wedging of the vertebral margins (Fig. 4), severe rotation (Fig. 5), widening of the interpediculate distance, widening of the intervertebral foramina, "penciling" of the ribs, a spindled appearance of the transverse processes, and the presence of a paravertebral mass are characteristic.

Canal widening is believed to be the result of either an intraspinal tumor or dural ectasia, that is, an increase in the width of the thecal sac subsequent to an increase in hydrostatic pressure, causing expansive and erosive deformity to the surrounding spinal canal and vertebral bodies. Because of spinal canal widening and expansion, there may be tremendous angular deformity and distortion without spinal cord compromise or neurologic deficit.

There are no universally acceptable criteria for spinal dystrophy. We feel that there is a definite potential for what appears to be idiopathic deformities to become dystrophic (i.e., to modulate or transform to dystrophic). We studied the relationship of dystrophy to progression (18). Ninety-one patients were studied—48 male and 43 female—who presented at 2 months to 26 years of age, with an average follow-up of 6.5 years. There

were 43 thoracic, 20 thoracolumbar, 14 cervicothoracic, and 14 double curves. There were 37 left convex and 32 right convex. We analyzed for dystrophic features (Table 2) and found 62% rib penciling, 51% vertebral rotation, 31% posterior vertebral scalloping, 36% vertebral wedging, 31% spindling of the transverse processes, 31% anterior wedging, 29% widened interpedicular distances, 25% enlarged intervertebral foraminae, and 13% lateral vertebral scalloping. We reviewed the natural history and described three types.

Type I: No dystrophy at presentation or follow-up (N = 13).

Type II: Dystrophy at presentation with (A) no progression (N = 18), (B) progression (N = 21), (C) progression and extension (N = 9).

Type III: Acquired dystrophy not present when first seen (A), with no progression (N = 6), (B) progression (N = 14), (C) progression and extension (N = 10). A total of 31 patients showed no tendency to modulate.

We reviewed such risk factors as the patient's age, patient's sex, extent of curve (number of vertebral segments), location of curve, and side of curve for evidence of progression and dystrophy. Multiple regression analysis of radiographic dystrophy to progression was carried out. Our results revealed that 81% of patients diagnosed with deformity prior to 7 years showed modulation, whereas only 25% diagnosed after 7 years modulated. Age was the most significant finding of our series. The extent, number of vertebral segments greater or less than six, was not a predictor; neither was sex, location, or side. No other single dystrophic feature was significant; however, when three or more dystrophic features were present progression was significant in 85%. We concluded that spinal deformities in NF-1 are dynamic in terms of both modulation and progression. Deformities presenting before age 7 should be observed for modulation if no dystrophy is present initially because 81% did eventually modulate. Gender, location, side, and extent of deformity did not influence the propensity to modulate. Rib penciling was the only singular dystrophic feature statistically linked to progression. The presence of three or more dystrophic features statistically increases the risk of progression (18).

It is most important to recognize the dystrophic curve and to distinguish it from the nondystrophic one. It is equally important to determine the degree of kyphosis and/or lordosis. Brace treatment is not effective in the management of dystrophic curves, and an aggressive approach to management is recommended. There is no justification for passively observing the progression of the dystrophic spinal deformity of NF-1 (73). The dystrophic deformity has a strong tendency to progress even following fusion.

Those patients with a curvature of less than 20 degrees should be observed for progression at 6-month intervals. For patients with greater than 20 to 40 degrees of angulation, a posterior spinal fusion of all articular facets using autogenous iliac crest graft and segmental spinal instrumentation should be performed. The pernicious course of the dystrophic curve justifies early stabilization. Early aggressive surgical intervention, even in young children, is strongly recommended. Early fusion does not lead to significant trunkal height loss because the curves are usually

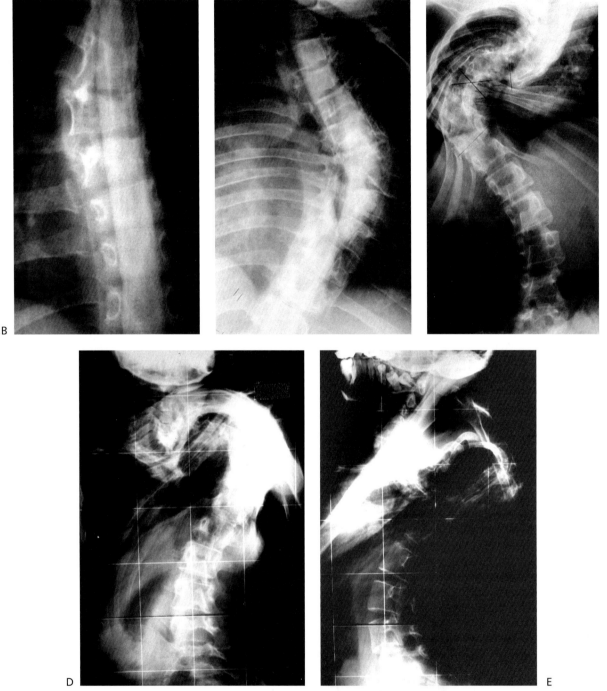

A,B

C

D

E

FIGURE 4. Examples of dystrophic scoliosis at ages 6, 9, 16, and 21 years. None of these patients had neurologic deficits when they presented to the orthopaedic surgeon. **A:** A left dorsal curvature in a 6-year-old with scalloping of the vertebral bodies and irregular sclerotic margins demonstrating dystrophic changes of neurofibromatosis scoliosis. Note the widening of the spinal canal that is not in conformity with scoliosis angulation. **B:** Right dorsal curve in a 9-year-old. Myelogram shows widening of the spinal canal and vertebral bodies rotating into the convexity. **C:** Left dorsal curve in a 16-year-old. The curvature is short segmented, sharply angulated, and kinky. Anteroposterior radiograph of the spine reveals scalloping of the vertebral margins, gross rotation of the apical vertebra, and penciling of the ribs in the concavity. Note proximity of the apical vertebrae to the ribs. The widening of the spinal canal is believed to be secondary to dural ectasia. (Courtesy of Dr. Michael Schaefer, Chicago, IL. Reprinted with permission of Crawford AH [1981]: Neurofibromatosis in childhood. *Instr Course Lect* 30:56–74.) **D:** Anteroposterior radiograph of a 21-year-old with severe rotation and angulation. **E:** Lateral radiograph of the person shown in D. The kyphosis is striking in its severity, as is the scoliosis. (Courtesy of Dr. Klaus Zielke Badwildengen, West Germany.)

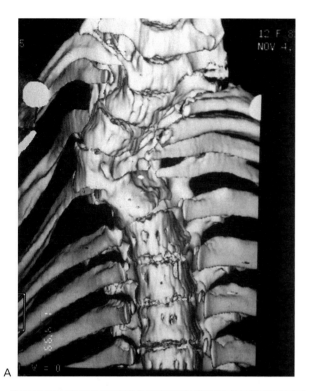

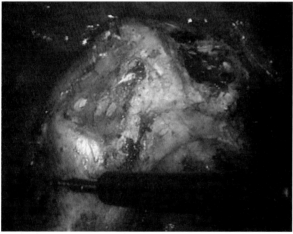

FIGURE 5. A 9-year-old child with dysplastic thoracic scoliosis who underwent anterior release and fusion by video-assisted thoracoscopic surgery. **A:** Three-dimensional reconstructed computed tomogram of a child with dysplastic scoliosis illustrating significant rotation of thoracic vertebra. **B:** Thoracoscopic view of anterior apical vertebrae. The anterior longitudinal ligament has rotated completely posterior and is attached to the concave rib heads. The vertebrae appear to have spun around toward the convex side.

TABLE 2. DYSTROPHIC FEATURES NOTED IN 91 PATIENTS

Feature	Percent
Rib penciling	62
Vertebral rotation	51
Posterior vertebral scalloping	31
Vertebral wedging	36
Spindling of transverse processes	31
Anterior wedging	31
Widened interpedicular distances	29
Enlarged intervetebral forminae	25
Lateral vertebral scalloping	13

Modified from Durrani AA, Morley TR, Choudhary SN, et al. (2000): Modulation of spinal deformitive in NF. *Spine* 25(1):69–75.

neutral vertebra above to the neutral vertebra below. Postoperative orthotic immobilization is recommended, and the patient should be radiographed at 6 months post surgery; oblique views should be taken to assess the fusion of the facet joints and to rule out pseudarthrosis. Patients with dystrophic curvatures that exceed 40 degrees should undergo anterior discectomy, intervertebral fusion, and posterior fusion and stabilization with segmental instrumentation as a primary procedure. A postoperative Risser cast or thoracolumbosacral orthosis is recommended for all patients with dystrophic deformity following fusion.

Kyphoscoliosis

Kyphoscoliosis in NF-1 is distinguished by the predominance of kyphosis (more than 50 degrees on the lateral radiograph) associated with scoliosis; acute posterior angulation is a typical sign. The vertebral bodies are frequently so deformed and attenuated at the apex that it may be impossible to identify them on routine radiographs. Hsu et al. (34) described a progressive dystrophy of the apical vertebral body that led to an angular kyphosis and a sideways slip or subluxation of the spine such that the upper and lower limbs of the kyphosis were in bayonet apposition. Tredwell has theorized this deformity to be related to instability of the pedicle. Curtis et al. (17) believe that kyphosis contributed more to the production of paraplegia in their patients than did scoliosis. This view is supported by the biomechanical studies of Breig (6), which showed that flexion of the spine causes elongation of the spinal canal and deformation of the spinal cord. Pathologically increased spinal flexion, as by kyphotic deformity, leads to excessive axial tension of the spinal cord parenchyma and may result in neurologic impairment. Miller (47) found that among 20 patients with paraplegia associated with NF-1, severe angulation of the spine was responsible for the paraplegia in more than half of cases. Lonstein et al. (40) reviewed 45 patients with cord compression due to spinal curvature and found NF-1 to be second only to congenital kyphosis as the cause of spinal cord compression.

Winter et al. (72) reviewed 33 patients with NF-1 and kyphosis averaging 132 degrees. Six patients had paraparesis and six had respiratory distress; 27 patients had operative treatment. Laminectomy was useless for the treatment of paraparesis resulting from angulated spine deformity. Combined anterior and

short, with poor growth potential in the involved vertebra; therefore, one need not wait for the child to reach a certain physiologic or chronologic age. Thoracic lordosis is less often associated with intracanal lesions but should be treated as aggressively as kyphosis. Care should be taken during the exposure because some of the laminae may be extremely thin or eroded as a result of subjacent neurofibroma or dural ectasia, and the spinal cord could be injured directly. The fusion should be carried out from the posterior spinal fusion, using abundant amounts of autogenous bone for both, coupled with a prolonged rigid immobilization gave the best results. Halo traction and halo casts were invaluable for the most severe deformities. Instrumentation was often impossible due to the severity of the deformity. All of the reported patients eventually achieved solid union.

Patients with dystrophic angular kyphosis respond poorly to posterior fusion alone. This is a potentially malignant deformity and should be aggressively pursued. Good results are consistently obtained only in those patients who have both anterior and posterior fusion; however, not every patient obtains solid fusion follow-

ing these procedures (Fig. 6). Some patients require repeat operative procedures. Technically inadequate implementation of anterior procedures has been considered the usual reason for failure; however, pressure erosion from enlarging neurofibromas, dural ectasia, and meningoceles may play a role. Most important (Treatment A), the entire structural area of the deformity should be fused anteriorly with complete disc excision and strong strut grafting, preferably from the fibula, as well as rib and iliac crest graft. No soft tissue should be allowed to interpose between the grafts (Fig. 7), and all grafts should have contact with each other and with the spine. Those grafts surrounded by soft tissue tend to resorb in the

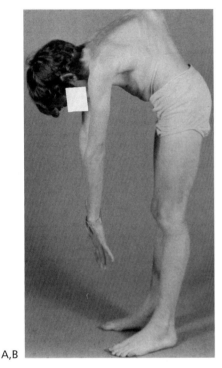
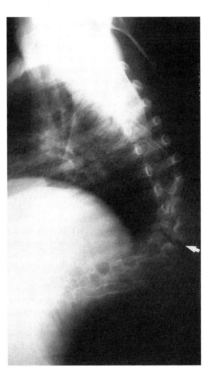
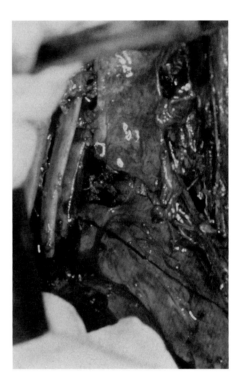

A,B   C

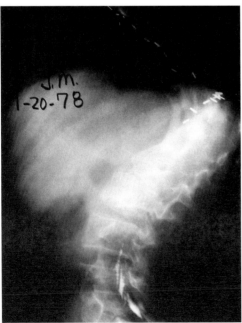

D

FIGURE 6. This boy presented with a severe kyphoscoliosis after having undergone three attempts at posterior spinal fusion. The kyphosis was in excess of 100 degrees. He underwent an anterior spinal fusion with fibular and rib strut grafts. The fusion subsequently failed, probably due to resorption of the grafts by neurofibromatous tissue. **A:** Clinical photographs of side view while the child is bending show severe gibbus or kyphotic deformity. The trunk is significantly foreshortened. **B:** Lateral radiographic view of thoracic spine showing one of the areas of pseudarthrosis *(arrow).* **C:** An operative photograph at the time of thoracotomy demonstrating the nesting of the fibular and rib grafts across the apex of the kyphos. **D:** One-year postoperative radiograph showing incorporation of grafts with loss of correction and bending.

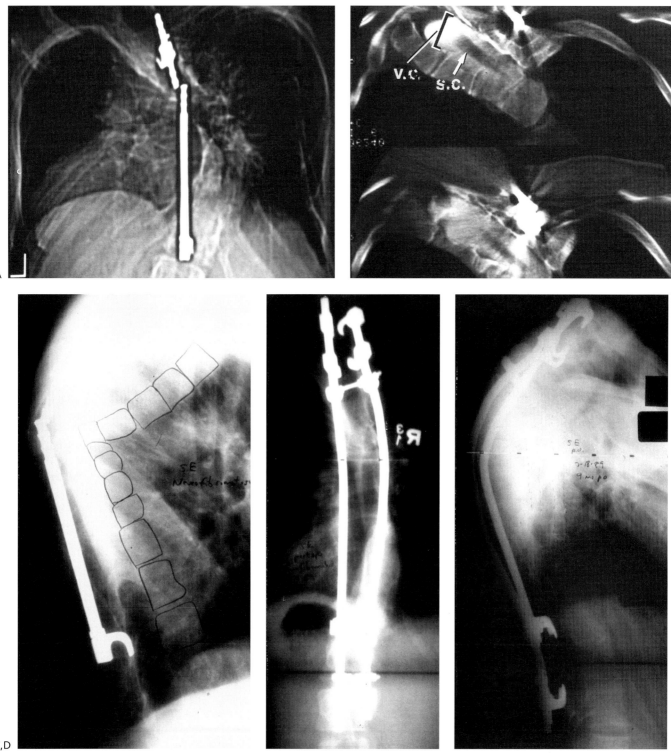

FIGURE 7. A 16-year-old patient with a dystrophic kyphoscoliotic curvature who encountered a pseud-arthrosis following initial attempt at spinal fusion. He subsequently underwent anterior fusion with rib and fibular strut grafting followed by posterior spinal fusion with Cotrel-Dubousset instrumentation. **A:** Anteroposterior digital radiograph of the spine illustrating right dystrophic scoliosis with broken Harrington rod. **B:** Frontal computed tomogram illustrating the angular distortion of the spinal column. There is widening of the vertebral canal (V.C.). The myelographic dye outlines the scalloping of the posterior vertebral bodies as well as the shadow of the spinal cord (S.C.). Because of the widening of the canal, the cord is rarely injured even though there may be a severe angular deformity. **C:** Lateral thoracic spine radiograph revealing significant angular kyphosis at the site of the broken Harrington rod. Note the widening of the spinal canal at the level of the inferior hook purchase site. **D:** Anteroposterior thoracolumbar spine radiograph following anterior and posterior spinal fusion with Cotrel-Dubousset instrumentation. **E:** Lateral thoracic spine radiograph illustrating fibular and rib strut grafts used for anterior fusion. (Courtesy of Jame Lehner, M.D., Dayton, Ohio.)

midportion (73). Two of the author's patients with kyphoscoliosis have had a total of seven procedures each, both anterior and posterior, and have not obtained a stable spine as of this writing. Eight of 74 patients with kyphoscoliosis have had a total of 24 procedures to date. Only two of these eight patients have what appears to be a bona fide fusion and are asymptomatic, and only one patient has reached skeletal maturity; therefore, more problems can be expected.

Because of the association of paraplegia with kyphoscoliosis, there has been a tendency to perform laminectomies. Laminectomy alone for kyphoscoliosis cord compression is *absolutely contraindicated*; the inciting lesion is usually anterior, and the compression cannot be made visible from behind. Also, the removal of the posterior element predisposes the patient to unstable postlaminectomy kyphosis and removes valuable bone stock required for posterior spinal fusion. Because the majority of these patients with neurologic problems are seen first by neurosurgeons, orthopaedists should endeavor to inform them that spinal stability is critical following posterior decompression procedures; *all should undergo arthrodesis*. One of the benefits of the author's NF-1 clinic is the establishment of a multidisciplinary team approach to these problems in an attempt to eliminate subsequent problems (60).

Some authors have stratified dystrophic curves with kyphosis into two categories: type I kyphosis of less than 50 degrees; type II kyphosis of more than 50 degrees and recommended treatment (A). They recommended posterior fusion only for kyphosis less than 50 degrees and anterior posterior fusion for kyphosis greater than 50 degrees. This author strongly recommends anterior and posterior fusion for all dystrophic curvatures greater than 40 degrees coronal Cobb angle. If the kyphosis is greater than 50 degrees, a strong anterior strut graft (preferably fibula) should also be performed.

A complete spine MRI or a complete high-volume CT myelogram in the prone, lateral, and supine positions should be performed prior to surgical treatment. If there is spinal cord impingement, the problem should be approached directly—anteriorly with partial corpectomy for anterior lesions and a hemilaminectomy for posterior ones, both to be followed by anterior and posterior fusions. Finally, an anterior disc excision with tibial or fibular strut bone graft followed by posterior arthrodesis and instrumentation should be performed if the kyphotic angle is greater than 50 degrees; the anterior fusion should be extended one to two levels past both end vertebrae. The patient should be reexplored posteriorly at 6 months postsurgery, with augmentation of the fusion mass if polytomography or bone scan shows any evidence of weakness of the fusion mass. The curvature may be such that conventional or even hybrid instrumentation cannot be utilized, and prolonged halo casting may be necessary. Prolonged immobilization is required until the fusion is absolutely solid (possibly up to a year).

Lordoscoliosis

Lordoscoliosis has been reported in a small percentage of patients with NF-1. However, the lack of reporting should not be taken as proof that the problem is rare. Kyphoscoliosis has been closely observed and documented for some time in scoliosis evaluation, whereas lordosis has been well documented only over the last decade. It is well known that thoracic lordosis (hypokyphosis) predisposes to a significant decrease in pulmonary function and mitral valve prolapse (32,74).

The dystrophic thinning of the posterior elements and the possible presence of intracanal dural ectasia make planning instrumentation to correct the deformity a challenge. The author has used anterior intervertebral fusion and posterior spinous process wiring to a contoured Harrington rod to achieve correction of dystrophic scoliosis, a paravertebral mass, and thoracic lordosis.

Spondylolisthesis

Few cases of spondylolisthesis due to NF-1 have been reported (13,35,44,45,73,75). The deformity is usually the result of increased diameter of the spinal canal, with pathologic elongation and thinning of the pedicles giving rise to a pathologic forward progression of the anterior elements of the spinal column. Dural ectasia with meningoceles, or interstitial hypertrophic neurofibromas with involvement of the lumbosacral roots exiting the spinal canal through the neuroforaminae, is the cause of the problem (Fig. 8). MRI or large-volume CT myelography is necessary to identify the character of the soft tissue affecting and surrounding the vertebral elements before considering surgery. The vertebral bodies are secondarily affected and appear to be thin and dystrophic; the smaller vertebral bodies and narrower pedicles preclude reduction with pedicle screws. A posterior fusion may be inadequate because of the forward traction effect of the vertebral bodies, causing a tension field unsuitable for fusion. The author recommends a posterior fusion using autogenous bone and postoperative hyperextension pantaloon cast correction rather than instrumentation. The fusion mass should be evaluated for stability at 6 months and reinforced if necessary.

Paraplegia

Most articles on NF-1 and spinal deformities have included cases of paraplegia (17,40,47). It is possible that neurologic compromise may be related to tumor, structural instability of the vertebral column complex, dural ectasia, vertebral destruction, neurofibromas, neurosarcomas, fibrofatty tissue reaction, severe kyphosis, vertebral subluxation, dislocation, protrusion of ribs into the spinal canal, or progressive dystrophy of the bony elements of the spine. A neoplasm is usually responsible for paraplegia in older patients, whereas spinal malalignment or rib displacement into the spinal canal is the most common cause in younger individuals. Kyphosis contributes more than scoliosis to neurologic impairment. Rockower et al. (55) reported two patients who, because of vertebral body instability and displacement secondary to neurofibromatous tissue encroachment, developed paraplegia. The problem was solved by carefully monitored traction and spinal fusion. Traction should be used very rarely when the deformity is mostly kyphotic. Traction should be used only with *flexible* kyphosis—never if the kyphosis is rigid. If the kyphosis is rigid, an anterior release, disc excision, and fusion followed by posterior spinal fusion are recommended.

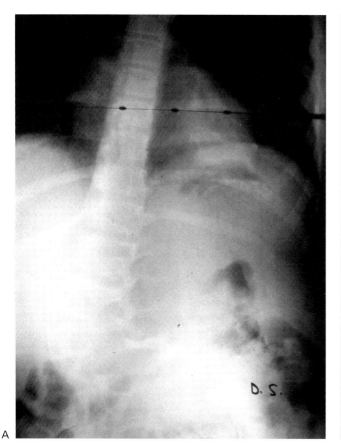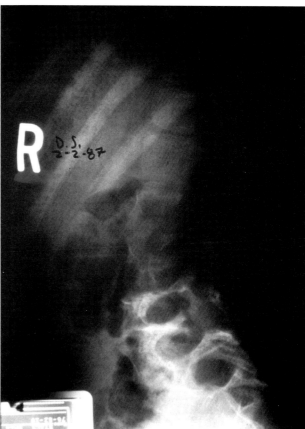

FIGURE 8.   This child was noted to have hypertrophy of the left lower extremity, spondylolisthesis, and a right lumbar scoliosis. **A:** Anteroposterior thoracolumbar spine radiograph illustrating short segmented, sharply angulated, and rotated lumbosacral scoliosis. **B:** Lateral thoracolumbar spine radiograph showing dystrophic spondylolisthesis with elongation and thinning of the lumbar pedicles and widening of neuro-foramina.

Using CT, Major and Huizenga (43) and Tredwell (69) were able to demonstrate that the rib heads had penetrated the enlarged neuroforamina, entered the spinal canal, and compressed the thoracic spinal cord directly (Fig. 9). Neither patient encountered permanent neurologic sequelae. It could be speculated that occult rib penetration into the spinal canal with spinal cord compromise could be a source of paraplegia that, prior to current imaging technology (CT, MRI), was thought to be the natural course of NF-1 with kyphoscoliosis.

With the advent of hardware systems that can apply considerable force to the spine, there is a clear risk of neurologic injury in the presence of instability of the rib end and potential spinal canal protrusion. Preoperative high-volume CT or MRI should prevent this consequence.

For patients with paraplegia one must first rule out an intraspinal lesion (tumor, meningocele) as opposed to kyphotic angular cord compression (54). Those with severe spinal curvatures without significant kyphosis and with evidence of paraplegia should be assumed to have intraspinal lesions until proven otherwise. MRI or high-volume CT myelography is done in the prone, lateral, and supine positions. The author has not been able to perform adequate MRI studies in patients with severe

deformities because of distortion. If the kyphosis is mobile and no intraspinal tumor is present, the patient should be placed in halo-assisted traction. This must be done with extreme caution and neurologic monitoring; it should definitely not be performed if the kyphosis is rigid. Even if the kyphosis is mobile and there is paraplegia, the author recommends somatosensory evoked potential monitoring during traction. If a tumor is anterior, immediate anterior excision, spinal cord decompression, and fusion should be carried out; if the lesion is posterior, a hemilaminectomy with tumor excision and posterior spinal fusion should be performed. If total laminectomy is required, posterior spinal fusion is mandatory. The posterior fusion should be performed with the addition of universal instrumentation if possible; if not, a halo cast should be applied. Deep hemovac drainage is necessary in all patients having spinal canal exploration because of the significant bleeding that may occur once the patient is normotensive. The patient should be observed for development of pseudarthrosis, and augmentation of the fusion mass should be carried out directly if such evidence is present.

Spinal instrumentation and fusion in the face of unrecognized intracanal neurofibroma or structural instability of the laminae due to dural ectasia can cause serious neurologic compromise.

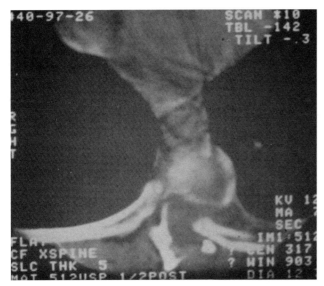

FIGURE 9. Thoracic cross-sectional computed tomogram of a patient with acute paraparesis. Computed tomography revealed that the head of a rib had entered the spinal canal through the neural foramina, with subsequent compression of the spinal cord. The paraparesis was transient and had resolved spontaneously prior to removal of the rib. (Courtesy of Drs. Huizenga and Major, Milwaukee, Wisconsin. Reprinted with permission from Crawford AH [1990]: NF-1. In: Morrissy RT, ed. *Lovell and Winters pediatric orthopaedics*, 3rd ed. Philadelphia: JB Lippincott.)

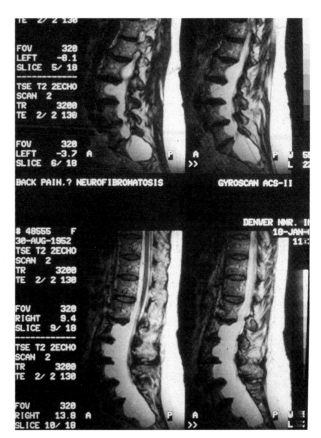

FIGURE 10. Four-level magnetic resonance image of a 47-year-old patient who complained of back pain. Image illustrates significant erosion of the lower lumbosacral spine from dural ectasia (Courtesy of Dr. Courtney Brown, Denver, Colorado.)

Therefore, preoperative neuroradiographic evaluation of the spinal canal is warranted.

PROBLEMS RELATED TO SOFT-TISSUE INVOLVEMENT

Dural Ectasia

A finding unique to NF-1 is an expansion of the dural sac, which often causes deformity of the adjacent spinal canal and vertebral bodies. It expands the spinal canal at the expense of the bony and ligamentous elements (Fig. 10). This wide expanse of the spinal canal may explain why, in spite of the severe progressive deformities of the spine seen in NF-1, the spinal cord is rarely injured (Fig. 11). The same does not hold true if a neurofibroma develops in the spinal canal, where it can provoke medullary compression, as can any space-occupying lesion. This expansion is responsible for the destabilization of the vertebra, giving rise to spontaneous dislocation (55) of the vertebra as well as penetration of the canal by ribs that have separated from the costotransverse ligaments (22,43). The continuation of this expanding dural sleeve more than likely gives rise to meningocele.

Intrathoracic Meningocele

Intrathoracic meningocele is relatively rare (19,38,46,50). A meningocele in this instance is a protrusion of the spinal meninges through an intervertebral foramen or bony defect of the vertebra; it contains an extension of the subarachnoid space filled with cerebrospinal fluid. Meningocele in association with NF-1 can occur at any level of the spine. A posterior mediastinal mass in a patient with NF-1, particularly if associated with kyphoscoliosis, is most likely a lateral meningocele. With contrast myelography, ultrasonography, or MRI, a well-demarcated soft-tissue cystic mass is seen protruding from the spinal canal into the posterior mediastinum (Fig. 12). Structural defects in the pedicles, enlargement of the intervertebral foramina, rib deformities including costotransverse dislocation, and scalloping of the vertebral bodies may accompany the mass. Several etiologies for the condition have been implicated, including nerve root sleeve elongation (63) (similar to a hernia of the meninges through the neuroforamina), cystic degeneration in a neurofibroma (48), trauma (16), dural dysplasia, bone dysplasia, regional dystrophy, and congenital derangement. The more likely explanation is that regional dysplasia affecting both bone and meninges is responsible for the formation of the meningocele (9,56).

The posterior scalloping of the vertebral bodies, with deformities of the pedicle and widening of the intervertebral foramina, could be caused either by the presence of a dumbbell tumor (intraspinal neurofibroma) or by saccular dilatations of the dura (dural ectasia). There is a distinct potential spinal instability due to the loss of supporting bone structure when associated with kyphoscoliosis. It is possible that neurofibromatous meningo-

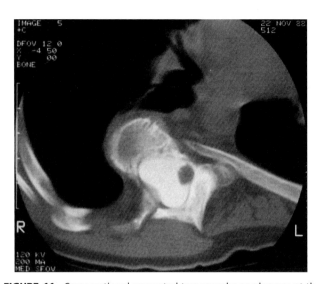

FIGURE 11. Cross-sectional computed tomography myelogram at the apex of a thoracic curve showing the deformity of the vertebral body with elongation of the pedicle on the concavity. There is a significant widening of the spinal canal from intrinsic pressure on the lamina, pedicles, and posterior vertebral body. The spinal cord is notched into the concavity of the spinal canal to the left. Neurofibromatous tissue has caused a widening of the spinal canal and is itself a tremendous space-occupying lesion. There is a paravertebral soft-tissue mass on the concavity. At surgery, the tissue from the neuroforamina proved to be fibrofatty, encapsulated material surrounding the spinal nerves. (Reprinted with permission from Crawford AH [1989]: Pitfalls of spinal deformities associated with NF-1 in children. *Clin Orthop Rel Res* 245:29–42.)

celes and dural ectasia are variations of the same phenomenon, with the meningocele being more localized and possibly related to its exit through the neuroforamina and the dural ectasia being more diffuse. Thoracic and sacral meningoceles in patients with NF-1 may develop secondary to the growth of ectatic dural outpouchings through preexisting bony deformities, such as enlarged neuroforamina, when exposed to changing cerebrospinal fluid pressures (4).

Most meningoceles (60%) are discovered incidentally on routine radiologic examination of the chest. Pain, though not a characteristic feature, was noted by Miles et al. (46) in 23% of cases; in all but one case, kyphoscoliosis was noted.

Pulmonary symptoms (cough 10%, dyspnea 11%) have been associated only with massive intrathoracic lesions. Only two cases of pulmonary problems as a direct result of the lesion have been reported; one meningocele ruptured during a bout of coughing when it was penetrated by a previously fractured rib. The patient died from medullary coning due to leakage of cerebrospinal fluid into the pleural cavity. Another patient presented with spontaneous hemothorax originating from the very vascular wall of the meningocele; the patient survived.

Because intrathoracic meningoceles are often symptomless, the question of treatment is difficult. If it is a chance radiologic finding and causes no symptoms, the right course would be observation. If there is definite progressive enlargement, an initial attempt should be made to ligate the sac. It may be feasible to occlude the neck of the sac by plicating sutures via videoassisted thoracoscopy. Excision of the lesion is indicated for pro-

A

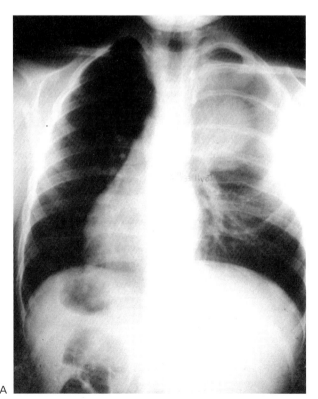

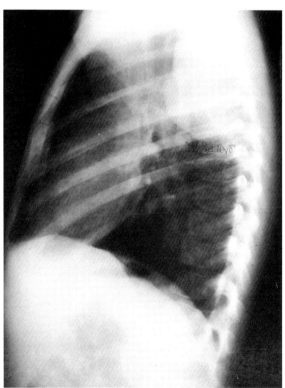

B

FIGURE 12. Intrathoracic meningocele associated with neurofibromatosis. **A:** Anteroposterior view showing increased shadow density in upper right chest cage. **B:** Lateral view illustrating superior posterior mediastinal mass. The lesion was removed by thoracotomy. (Courtesy of Anthony Herring, M.D., Dallas, Texas.)

gressive excavation of the vertebra, neurologic injury, respiratory distress, or if there is evidence of rapid progression in size.

Dumbbell Lesions

The classic dumbbell lesion is one in which the neurofibroma is constricted as it exits the neuroforamina, giving it the appearance of a weight lifter's dumbbell (Fig. 13A). Love and Dodge (41) defined dumbbell neurofibroma of the spine as a benign neoplasm that arises from a nerve root and grows in such a way that two or more portions of the tumor are connected by a narrow stalk through an intervertebral foramen, through the interlaminar space of the vertebra, or through the dura mater. They may be intradural and extradural, intradural, extradural, or extradural and extraspinal. The tumors may occur at any level of the cord, but the cervical and thoracic levels are most often involved. The tumors may present as nodules arising from the sheath along the nerve, or they may actually invade the nerve. If the tumor invades the nerve with consequent interstitial hypertrophy, then "the nerve becomes the tumor and the tumor becomes the nerve" (Fig. 13B, C). In this case, resecting the tumor results in a neurologic deficit. The incidence of malignant degeneration of peripheral neurofibromas is unknown.

We recently reviewed 260 pediatric patients with NF-1 and noted that nine patients (3.5%) had extrapleural thoracic tumors. Ninety-five of these patients were primarily screened by chest radiographs, and many patients might have asymptomatic thoracic tumors that have yet to be diagnosed. All patients were 6 years of age or older, six were asymptomatic, and three presented with respiratory symptoms. A clue to thoracic involvement in two patients was the presence of a visible plexiform neurofibroma in the neck, which later was found to have extended into the chest. Focal scoliosis was a significant clue to an underlying tumor in four patients, and bony changes such as narrowing of ribs were often seen in the area of tumor involvement. Malignant transformation of a benign plexiform neurofibroma occurred in one patient. Signs on physical examination that should raise suspicion of an underlying thoracic tumor include a plexiform neurofibroma of the neck or a focal area of scoliosis. When reviewed retrospectively, eight of the nine patients had either a symptom or a sign on physical examination that was a clue to the underlying tumor. Surgical management of these tumors can be difficult because of frequent involvement of nerves and blood vessels (61).

Vertebral Column Dislocation

Complete dislocation of the spine in NF-1 is rare. In one review of 55 patients who had NF-1 and spinal deformity, only two had a lateral subluxation or dislocation of the spine (59); one of the dislocations involved a thoracic vertebra and posterior arch with destruction of the latter, and the other patient had destruction of the articular part of the apophysis. In another study of eight patients who had NF-1 and paraplegia, five patients had a vertebral subluxation or dislocation (17). Involvement of the cervical spine by NF-1 was noted in one study in which five patients had subluxation of a cervical vertebral body (31). In a second study of 56 patients, 17 had abnormal cervical

spines; one patient had a fixed subluxation of the second cervical vertebra on the third, and another had an atlantoaxial rotatory instability (76). Isu et al. (36) reported on three patients (two with hemiparesis) who had atlantoaxial dislocation due to NF-1. They pointed out that laxity of capsular and ligamentous structures in patients with NF-1 may contribute to a predisposition to instability of the cervical spine. Scott's (62) study of scoliosis associated with NF-1 showed a cervical thoracic dislocation, but no details were provided of the history and physical findings. Rockower et al. (55) reported two cases of spinal dislocation after minor trauma in children who had NF-1. One patient had a dislocation of the fourth thoracic vertebra on the fifth and no neurologic deficit. At surgery, neurofibromatous tissue was found to envelop the vertebral bodies anteriorly but not posteriorly. The second patient had a dislocation of the sixth cervical vertebra on the seventh and was quadriparetic. Stone et al. (67) reported a 9-year-old child with NF-1 who had complete dislocation of the first thoracic vertebra on the second anteriorly, with the body of the seventh cervical vertebra situated completely anterior to that of the second thoracic vertebra following a 2-day history of pain in the lower neck. Complete reduction following traction and manipulation was not successful. Surgery resulted in the child having a solid union with no neurologic deficits. They believed that dural ectasia produced erosion of the middle column of the spine, with dissociation of the posterior elements from the body of the first thoracic vertebra and complete dislocation of the first thoracic vertebra on the second. They speculated that the child was spared neurologic damage by virtue of the pathologically enlarged spinal canal (67).

Significant subluxation or dislocation of the spine in patients who have NF-1 can occur with little radiographic or clinical warning because the osseous erosion is so extensive (Fig. 14). This diagnosis should be considered in any patient who has NF-1 and unexplained pain in the neck or back. The mechanism of dural expansion and osseous erosion is unknown. When seen at operation, the dura in the area of ectasia is extremely thin and fragile. Therefore, every effort should be made to avoid entry into the region of the dural ectasia. Aggressive surgical stabilization should be carried out when radiographic examination reveals instability of the spine, which may precede dislocation (71).

Plexiform Venous Channels

McCarroll (45) pointed out that a plexiform type of venous anomaly may be encountered in the soft tissues; these may surround the spine, impeding the operative approach to the vertebral bodies. In one of Hsu's patients with angular kyphosis, the venous anomalies were so dense that the anterior approach to the internal kyphos had to be abandoned due to excessive bleeding (34). Greene et al. (27) described vascular NF-1 in two categories according to the diameter of the vessel: the larger (greater than 1 mm, such as the aorta, carotid, and proximal renal arteries), which are surrounded by or involved with neurofibromatous tissue, reveal intimal hypertrophy, fragmentation of the medial and elastic laminae, and a fibrous adventitial reaction leading to stenosis or aneurysm formation. The author has not experienced excessive venous bleeding while performing anterior

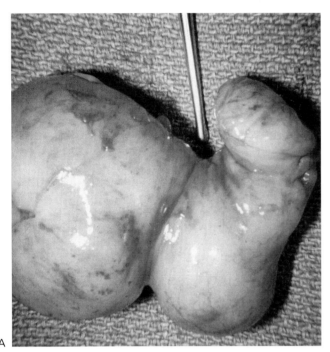

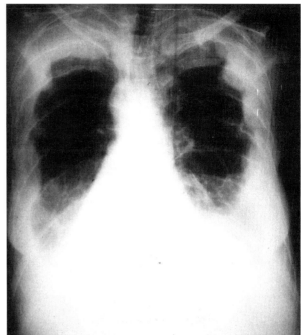

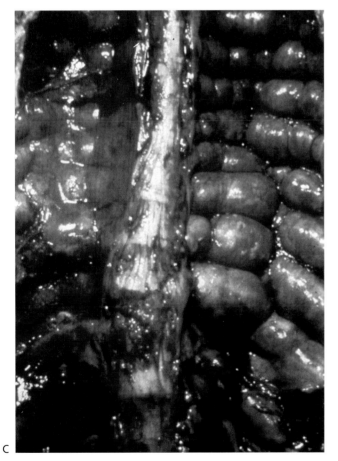

FIGURE 13. A: Example of a dumbbell-shaped tumor removed from the neuroforamina of a 17-year-old patient at time of exposure for posterior spinal fusion. The dumbbell appearance results from the constriction of the neurofibroma that occurs when the tumor exits the spinal canal. **B:** This 44-year-old woman was hospitalized for pneumonia and subsequently expired. The chest radiograph showed bony hypertrophy of the ribs in addition to increased soft-tissue densities in the intercostal spaces and surrounding the lung fields. **C:** At necropsy the intercostal spaces were found to be filled with neurofibromas that had infiltrated and replaced all of the intercostal nerves. (Courtesy of B. Van Damm, M.D., San Diego, California.)

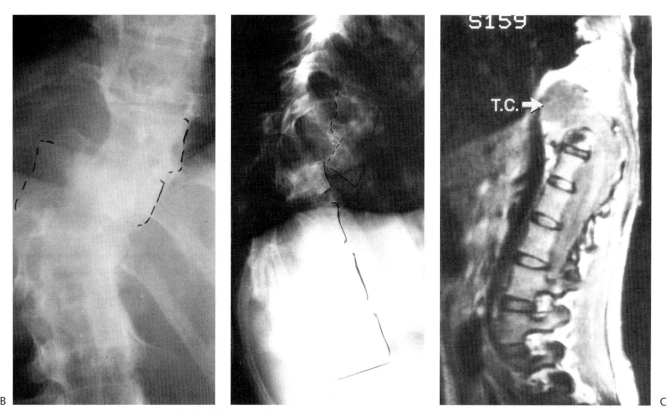

A,B   C

FIGURE 14. Example of a dislocation of the spine noted in a patient with neurofibromatosis. **A:** Note the sharply angulated deformity on anteroposterior radiograph, with some translation of the vertebral bodies. **B:** The lateral radiograph shows a short-segment kyphosis with anterior dislocation of the thoracic spine. **C:** The sagittal plane magnetic resonance image through the spine shows complete separation of the thoracic segment of the spine from the lumbar segment. The area of increased signal intensity just above and posterior to the lumbar segment *(arrow)* is a thoracic meningocele. The patient experienced a minor neurologic deficit. (Courtesy of Robert Winter, M.D., Minneapolis, Minnesota. Reprinted with permission from Crawford AH [1990]: NF-1. In: Morrissy RT, ed. *Lovell and Winters pediatric orthopaedics,* 3rd ed. Philadelphia: JB Lippincott.)

removal of neurofibromatous tissue and strut grafting, but warns the reader of the possibility. Wound hematomas following surgery have not been a problem; however, meticulous hemostasis and wound drainage should be carried out when performing surgery on patients with NF-1.

Pseudarthrosis

Pseudarthrosis occurs more commonly following attempted spinal fusion for both dystrophic and nondystrophic curvatures than for idiopathic ones. The incidence is higher in those associated with kyphosis of greater than 50 degrees. Prior to the use of universal spinal instrumentation and anterior-posterior combined surgeries, reexploration was routine for patients with neurofibromatous spinal deformities. The best results are obtained by planning a double (anterior and posterior) arthrodesis from the start. Even the increased strength of the instrumentation is insufficient to obtain stability at the time of surgery when dealing with deformed dystrophic posterior elements.

DISCUSSION

Careful attention should be paid to the vertebral body shapes on the posteroanterior and lateral spine radiographs. When one sees scalloping and indentation of vertebral bodies, a careful investigation should be carried out for intraspinal pathology, such as dural ectasia, meningocele, or dumbbell lesion. The scalloping has been associated with intraspinal NF-1 as well as with the expansion of the dural sac, suggesting dural ectasia or meningocele. Scalloping can exist only with one of the aforementioned eroding factors. The implication that the deformity is primarily a vertebral or developmental defect associated with NF-1 and not dependent on pressure erosion is incorrect. Because some intraspinal myelography studies have shown that the contrast material does not conform to the posterior scalloped surfaces of the vertebrae, there is a suggestion of an intervening intradural mass. These masses have been clearly elucidated by modern diagnostic technologies, such as CT, myelography, and especially MRI. The vertebral scalloping and dysplasia represent an indirect manifestation of a proximal tumor. Because of the possibility of an intraspinal tumor or dural ectasia being present, it is strongly recommended that contrast CT or MRI be performed on those patients with dystrophic vertebral bodies and curvatures requiring instrumentation and fusion (13). Angtuaco et al. (4) recommend CT myelography for patients with NF-1. Myelography alone can help differentiate between a mass lesion and the pseudomeningocele-like pattern of dural ectasia. With CT, additional details, such as displacement of the spinal cord and the extent of involvement of the subarachnoid compartment by tumor, can be assessed. Klatte et al. (38) attempted to elucidate the cause of posterior scalloping of the vertebrae in NF-1 with CT. They believe that eccentric unilateral scalloping favors a neurofibroma whereas central scalloping occurs more frequently in dural ectasia. The author recommends MRI assessment of any areas demonstrated by CT myelogram to be suspicious, as well as any areas that are poorly demonstrated.

Careful evaluation of the cervical spine is indicated prior to instrumentation of the thoracic or lumbar spine. The most dangerous situation for the neurologically intact NF-1 patient and the surgeon is the instrumentation and manipulation of the spine in the presence of unrecognized intraspinal lesions. More often than not, the patient presents to the spinal surgeon with a significant deformity with or without an intraspinal tumor or expansive dura, with no evidence of a neurologic disorder or paraplegia. This author currently utilizes four methods of spinal cord monitoring: SSEVP, NMEP, electromyography, and the gold standard, the "wake-up" test.

While correction is the goal of the spine surgeon in idiopathic scoliosis, halting the progression of the deformity, even with a small correction, can be considered a good result in the case of NF-1 spinal deformities. The surgeon's responsibility is to stabilize the spine in the most expedient, permanent, and safest way without causing permanent neurologic injury.

ACKNOWLEDGMENT

The author thanks Tiffany Whatley for assisting in the preparation of this manuscript.

REFERENCES

1. Adkins JC, Ratvich MD (1977): Children's Hospital of Pittsburgh. The operative management of von Recklinghausen's NF-1 in children, with special reference to regions of the head and neck. *Surgery* 82:343.
2. Allibone DC, Illingworth RS, Wright T (1960): NF-1 (von Recklinghausen disease) of the vertebral column. *Arch Dis Child* 35:153–158.
3. Akbarnia BA, Gabriel KR, Beckman E, et al. (1992): Prevalence of scoliosis in NF-1. *Spine* 17:5244.
4. Angtuaco EJ, Binet EF, Flanigan S (1983): Value of computer tomographic myelography in NF-1. *Neurosurgery* 13:666–671.
5. Betz R, Iorio R, Lombardi AV, et al. (1989): Scoliosis surgery in NF-1. *Clin Orthop Rel Res* 245:53.
6. Breig A (1960): *Biomechanics of the central nervous system: some basic and normal pathological phenomena concerning spine, disc and cord.* Stockholm: Almquist and Wiskel. p. 1960.
7. Brooks B, Lehman EP (1924): The bone changes in Recklinghausen's NF-1. *Surg Gynecol Obstet* 28:587–595.
8. Calzavara PG, Caralion A, Anzola GP, Pasolini MP (1988): Segmental neurofibromatosis: case report and review of the literature. *NF-1 J* 1: 318–322.
9. Casselman ES, Mandell GA (1979): Vertebral scalloping in NF-1. *Radiology* 131:89–94.
10. Chaglassian JH, Risborough EJ, Hall JE (1976): NF-1 scoliosis: natural history and results of treatment of 37 cases. *J Bone Joint Surg Am* 58: 695.
11. Collins FS, Ponder BAJ, Seizinger BR, et al. (1989): The von Recklinghausen NF-1 region on chromosome 17: genital and physical maps come into focus. *Am J Hum Genet* 44:1–5.
12. Crawford AH (1990): NF-1. In: Morrissy RT, ed. *Lovell and Winters pediatric orthopaedics,* 3rd ed. Philadelphia: JB Lippincott. pp 175–201.
13. Crawford AH (1989): Pitfalls of spinal deformities associated with NF-1 in children. *Clin Orthop Rel Res* 245:29–42.
14. Crawford AH (1986): NF-1 in children. *Acta Orthop Scand (Suppl)* 218:57.
15. Crawford AH, Schorry EK: Neurofibromatosis in children for the orthopaedist (review article). *J Am Acad Orthop Surg* 1999, 7:217–230.
16. Cross JO, Reavis JR, Saunders WB (1949): Lateral interthoracic meningocele. *J Neurosurg* 6:423–432.
17. Curtis BH, Fisher RL, Butterfield WL, Saunders FP (1969): NF-1 with paraplegia: report of 8 cases. *J Bone Joint Surg Am* 51:843.
18. Durrani AA, Morley TR, Choudhury SN, et al.: Modulation of spinal deformities in NF. *Spine* 25(1):69–75.
19. Erkulurawatra S, Gammal TE, Hawkins J, et al. (1979): Interthoracic meningoceles in NF-1. *Arch Neurol* 36:557–559.
20. Fialkow PJ, Sagebiel RW, Gartler SM, et al. (1971): Multiple cell origin of hereditary NF-1. *N Engl J Med* 284:298–300.
21. Fienman NL (1981): Pediatric neurofibromatosis: review. *Compr Ther* 7:66–72.
22. Flood BM, Butt WP, Dickson RA (1986): Rib penetration of the intervertebral foraminae in NF-1. *Spine* 11:172–174.
23. Funasaki H, Winter RB, Lonstein JB, Denis F (1994): Pathophysiology of spinal deformities in neurofibromatosis: an analysis of seventy-one patients who had curves associated with dystrophic changes. *J Bone Joint Surg* 76-A:692.
24. Goffin J, Grob D (1999): Spondyloptosis of the cervical spine in neurofibromatosis: a case report. *Spine* 24;6:587–590.
25. Goldberg NS, Collins FS (1991): The hunt for the neurofibromatosis gene. *Arch Dermatol* 127:1705–1707.
26. Gould EP (1918): The bone changes occurring in von Recklinghausen's disease. *Q J Med* 11:221.
27. Greene JF, Fitzwater JE, Burgess J (1974): Arterial lesions associated with NF-1. *Am J Clin Pathol* 62:481.
28. Haddad FS, Williams RL, Bentley G (1995): The cervical spine in neurofibromatosis. *Br J Hosp Med* 1995:53:318–319.
29. Hagelstrom L (1946): Deformities of the spine and multiple neurofibromatoses (von Recklinghausen). *Acta Chir Scand* 93:169.
30. Harkin JC, Reed RJ (1969): *Tumors of the peripheral nervous system.* Washington, DC: Armed Forces Institute of Pathology, 2nd series, fascicle 3.
31. Heard GE, Holt JE, Naylor B (1962): Cervical vertebral deformities in von Recklinghausen disease of the nervous system. A review of necropsy findings. *J Bone Joint Surg Br* 44:880–885.
32. Hirschfeld SS, et al. (1982): Incidence of mitral valve prolapse in adolescent scoliosis and thoracic hypokyphosis. *Pediatrics* 70:451–454.
33. Holt RT, Johnson JR (1989): Cotrel-Dubousset instrumentation in NF-1 in spine curves: a preliminary report. *Clin Orthop Rel Res* 245: 19.
34. Hsu LCS, Lee PC, Leong JCY (1980): Dystrophic spinal deformities in NF-1, treated by anterior and posterior fusion. *J Bone Joint Surg Br* 66:495.
35. Hunt JC, Pugh DC (1961): Skeletal legions in NF-1. *Radiology* 76: 12.
36. Isu T, Miyasaka K, Abe H, et al. (1953): Atlantoaxial dislocation with NF-1. *J Neurosurg* 58:451–453.
37. Kim HW, Weinstein SL (1997): Spine update: the management of Scoliosis in neurofibromatosis. *Spine* 22:2770–2776.

38. Klatte EC, Franken EA, Smith JA (1976): The radiographic spectrum in NF-1. *Semin Roentgenol* 11:17–33.
39. Lewis RA, Riccardi VM (1981): von Recklinghausen's NF-1. Incidents of iris hamartomata. *Ophthalmology* 88:348.
40. Lonstein JE, Winter RB, et al. (1980): Neurologic deficit secondary to spinal deformity. *Spine* 5:331.
41. Love JG, Dodge HW (1952): Lumbar (hourglass) neurofibroma affecting the spinal cord. *Surg Gynecol Obstet* 94:161–172.
42. Lubs MLE, et al. (1991): Lisch nodules in NF-1 type I. Brief report. *N Engl J Med* 328:1264–1285.
43. Major MR, Huizenga BA (1988): Spinal cord compression by displaced ribs in NF-1. A report of three cases. *J Bone Joint Surg Am* 70:1101–1102.
44. Mandell GA (1978): The pedicle in NF-1. *Am J Radiol* 130:575.
45. McCarroll HR (1950): Clinical manifestations of congenital NF-1. *J Bone Joint Surg Am* 32:601–617.
46. Miles J, Pennybacker J, Sheldon P (1969): Interthoracic meningocele: its development and association with NF-1. *J Neurol Neurosurg Psychiatry* 32:99–110.
47. Miller A (1936): NF-1 with reference to skeletal changes, compression myolytis and malignant degeneration. *Arch Surg* 32:109.
48. Nanson EM (1957): Thoracic meningocele associated with NF-1. *Thorac Surg* 33:650–652.
49. National Institutes of Health Consensus Development Conference (1988): NF-1. *NF-1* 1:172–178.
50. O'Neil P, Whatmore WJ, Booth AE (1983): Spinal myelomeningocele in association with NF-1. *J Neurosurg* 13:82–84.
51. Parisini P, DiSilvestre M, Greggi T, et al. (1999): Surgical correction of dystrophic spinal curves in neurofibromatosis: a review of 56 patients. *Spine* 24(21):2247–2253.
52. Riccardi VM (1989): NF-1 update. *NF-1* 2:284–291.
53. Riccardi VM (1981): von Recklinghausen's NF-1. *N Engl J Med* 305:1617.
54. Robin GC (1983): Scoliosis in neurological disease. *J Med Sci* 9:578.
55. Rockower S, McKay D, Nason S (1982): Dislocation of the spine in NF-1. A report of two cases. *J Bone Joint Surg Am* 64:1240–1242.
56. Salerno NR, Edeiken J (1970): Vertebral scalloping in NF-1. *Radiology* 97:509–510.
57. Samoto T, Wantanabe Y, Suda A (1981): Atlantoaxial dislocation with NF-1: a case report. *Orthop Traumatol Surg (Jpn)* 24:289.
58. Savini ED, Parisini P, et al. (1983): Surgical treatment of vertebral deformities in NF-1. *Ital J Orthop Traumatol* 9:13.
59. Savini R, Vicenzi G. Le deformita del rachide nella neurofibromatosi. Studio clinico e radiografico, d: 46 casi. *J Orthop Trauma* 2:37–50.
60. Schorry EK, Stowens DW, Crawford AH, et al. (1989): Summary of patient data from a multidisciplinary NF-1 clinic. *NF-1* 2:129–134.
61. Schorry EK, Crawford AH, Egelhoff JC, et al. (1997): Thoracic tumors in children with neurofibromatosis-1. *Am J Med Genet* 74:533–537.
62. Scott JC (1965): Scoliosis in NF-1. *J Bone Joint Surg Br* 47:240.
63. Sengpiel JW, Ruzicka FF, Lodmell EA (1948): Lateral interthoracic meningocele. *Radiology* 50:515–520.
64. Seville PD, et al. (1955): Osteomalacia in von Recklinghausen's NF-1: metabolic study of a case. *Br Med J* 1:1311.
65. Shufflebarger HL (1989): Cotrel-Dubousset instrumentation in NF-1 spinal problems. *Clin Orthop Rel Res* 245:24–29.
66. Sirois JL, Drennan JC (1990): Distrophic spinal deformities in NF-1. *J Pediatr Orthop* 10:525–526.
67. Stone JW, et al. (1987): Dural ectasia associated with spontaneous dislocation of the upper part of the thoracic spine in NF-1. A case report and a review of the literature. *J Bone Joint Surg Am* 69:1083–1097.
68. Toyohido I, Miyasaka K, Hiroshi A (1983): Atlantoaxial dislocation associated with NF-1. *J Neurosurg* 68:451.
69. Tredwell S (1994): Complications of spinal surgery. In: Weinstein, ed. *The pediatric spine.* Philadelphia: Lippincott-Raven Publishers, p. 1766.
70. Weiss RA (1921): Curvature of the spine in von Recklinghausen's disease. *Arch Dermatol Syphilol* 3:144.
71. Winter RB (1991): Spontaneous dislocation of a vertebra in a patient who had NF-1 (report of a case with dural ectasia). *J Bone Joint Surg Am* 9:1402–1404.
72. Winter RB, Lonstein JE, Anderson M (1988): NF-1 hyperkyphosis: a review of 33 cases with hyperkyphosis with 80 degrees or greater. *J Spinal Disord* 1:39.
73. Winter RB, Moe JH, Bradford DS, et al. (1979): Spine deformities in NF-1. *J Bone Joint Surg Am* 61:677.
74. Winter RB, Lovell WW, Moe JH (1975): Excessive thoracic lordosis and loss of pulmonary function in patients with idiopathic scoliosis. *J Bone Joint Surg Am* 57:972–977.
75. Wong-Chung J, Gillespie R (1991): Lumbosacral spondyloptosis with NF-1. *Spine* 16:986.
76. Yong-Hing K, Kalamchi A, MacEwen GD (1979): Cervical spine abnormalities in NF-1. *J Bone Joint Surg Am* 61:695.

IATROGENIC SPINAL DEFORMITIES

JOSEPH H. PERRA

Study principles rather than methods. The mind that understands principles will develop its own methods.—A. Bruce Gill

DEFINITIONS

Iatrogenic

From the Greek, -genic is "to produce," iatro- denotes a relation to a physician or to medicine. Iatrogenic may be anything resulting from the activity of physicians or medicine. More commonly it denotes any adverse condition caused by treatment given by a physician or surgeon. These adverse results do not imply improper management or technique but only that a certain percentage of cases can have an untoward outcome.

Spinal Deformity

Spinal deformity is abnormal coronal or sagittal curvature or imbalance of the spine in the coronal or sagittal plane. This includes scoliosis, kyphosis, and decompensation of the normal balance position of the head over the pelvis in the upright, standing position.

INTRODUCTION

Iatrogenic Spinal Deformities

An iatrogenic deformity can consist of scoliosis, kyphosis, or an imbalance in the sagittal or coronal plane that develops as the result of therapy for another condition that does not include the "new" deformity. By definition, this excludes residual deformity or progressing deformity believed to exist before treatment. Numerous causes of these iatrogenic deformities exist. Understanding the principles of production of deformity will assist physicians in understanding when a deformity may develop. With this knowledge, physicians may be able to reduce the incidence of deformity or minimize the severity of deformity to optimize patient outcomes. When a condition is encountered that may produce a deformity, it is incumbent on the physician to make certain that the child is observed for the development

of the deformity. If a deformity develops, appropriate treatment should be instituted to minimize the consequences.

Information regarding iatrogenic spinal deformities usually deals with specific causes related to the diagnosis, such as post-laminectomy kyphosis. Information about specific causes of iatrogenic spinal deformities should help clinicians understand the risk of deformity and responses to previous treatments. This specific information, on top of the foundation of a good understanding of the principles of development of deformity, should help clinicians treating patients who are prone to iatrogenic spinal deformity.

Treatment

Treatment of patient with spinal deformities can be operative or nonoperative. Nonoperative treatment usually consists of observation or bracing. With the recognition that some conditions cause iatrogenic deformities, another treatment option exists—prevention. Operative treatment usually consists of spinal fusion and can include instrumentation for correction and stability. Some deformities may necessitate osteotomy to obtain satisfactory balance and a good long-term outcome.

ETIOLOGIC PRINCIPLES

Spinal deformity can be caused by an imbalance of vertebral growth or spinal instability that cannot withstand normal physiologic forces. Deformities also can be caused directly by manipulation of the spine or its supporting structures, the pelvis and lower extremities. By understanding these principles, we can determine whether iatrogenic deformity is likely to occur, observe the patient for development of deformity, and recommend appropriate treatment if deformity does occur.

Classification of Iatrogenic Spinal Deformities on the Basis of Etiologic Principle

I. Growth imbalance
  A. Growth arrest
    1. Direct
    2. Indirect
  B. Growth acceleration

J.H. Perra: Twin Cities Spine Center, Minneapolis, Minnesota 55404.

II. Instability
    A. Posterior column
        1. Bilateral
        2. Unilateral
    B. Anterior column
    C. Loss of muscular support—spinal cord injury
III. Direct manipulation of the spine
    A. Manipulation away from physiologic contour
    B. Manipulation toward physiologic contour
IV. Manipulation of the foundation for the spine
    A. Pelvis
    B. Lower extremities
        1. Length differences
        2. Range of motion

Type I: Growth Imbalance

Growth imbalance implies either interruption of normal growth or acceleration of growth. Deformity occurs only when alteration of growth potential is asymmetric. Asymmetric growth is caused by surgical manipulation of growth centers, formation of tethering anterior or posterior vertebral bony bars or rib tethers, or partial removal of a growth center in one portion of a vertebra and leaving the other portion intact. Irradiation of a growing spine can interfere with normal growth and cause deformity. For example, stimulation of growth by extrinsic growth hormone can cause deformity, but it is likely that a smaller deformity had existed and was made worse or more noticeable after acceleration of growth. Unlike findings about the long bones, there is no clear evidence of stimulation of growth centers of vertebrae by trauma or hyperemia that causes deformity or marked asymmetry, although it is conceivable that this could occur and produce deformity. Typical deformities from growth imbalance are scoliosis, kyphosis, lordosis, and crankshaft phenomenon (rotation). Treatment is based on restoration of balance of growth, usually by means of fusion and when necessary by means of release, osteotomy, external immobilization, or internal fixation.

Type II: Instability

Instability implies loss of structural integrity of the spinal column or cylinder. Mechanically, the articulated spine can be thought of as a curved column. Each segment has components that provide axial support and tensile resistance. In the anterior aspect, the vertebral body and disc resist the compressive load, and the anterior and posterior longitudinal ligament and disc anulus resist distractive forces. In the posterior aspect, the facet joint complex resists axial load, lateral bending, and depending on the level, shear forces. The ligament complex (supraspinal, interspinal, capsular facet ligaments, and ligamentum flavum) act as tension wires to stabilize the spine. Normal muscle tone in the paraspinal muscles complements the posterior ligament complex. Gravity normally exerts a flexion force on the cervical and thoracic portions of the spine, which is counteracted by the posterior ligament complex and spinal extensor muscles.

Removal of or injury to any of the supporting structures of the spine alters the stability of the spine. Depending on the degree of change, permanent alterations can occur. The most obvious alteration occurs when the spine is rendered unstable and subluxation occurs. Growth disturbances can occur when an increase in the load on the cartilaginous ossification center causes wedged vertebrae.

Spinal deformity can occur after removal of a portion of the anterior supporting column or the posterior stabilizing complex or by means of alteration of the facet joints. In a high percentage of cases, loss of muscular control of the trunk following spinal cord or neurologic injury causes deformity in the growing child. Kyphosis, lordosis, scoliosis, and combinations thereof are possible, but kyphosis is most common after laminectomy. When scoliosis occurs, it usually is associated with kyphosis. If the anterior column is not reconstructed after partial or complete vertebrectomy, collapse into kyphosis should be expected. If the resection is not symmetric, lateral angulation and scoliosis will occur in addition to the kyphosis.

The best treatment remains avoiding the deformity by restoring stability, which is done by replacing or augmenting weakened structures. Stability can be restored by means of internal fixation or external stabilization with braces. Late treatment necessitates fusion of the deformity and possibly correction of the deformity, possibly with osteotomy or internal fixation.

Type III: Direct Manipulation of the Spine

Manipulation of the spine implies application of distractional, compressional, rotational, or translational forces to one or more motion segments. Application of these forces can be external or internal. Examples of external forces are casts, braces, or even positioning at the time of surgery. Internal forces usually are applied with fixation devices during surgery, frequently for the correction of a deformity or instability. Application of these forces has direct consequences to the area treated and indirect consequences to the compensatory areas of the spine. Depending on the nature and magnitude of the force vectors, not all direct changes are desirable. Some of the changes are likely to be in a physiologic plane, and others may direct the spine out of a physiologic plane. For example, correction of scoliosis by means of distraction within the concavity of a curve on the dorsal side of the spine also induces kyphosis. This can be desirable in the thoracic spine but is deleterious in the lumbar spine. Anterior compression of a scoliotic curve likewise reduces scoliosis and produces kyphosis, which would be in the physiologic plane of the thoracic spine but away from the physiologic contour in the thoracolumbar and lumbar spine. Even translation, whether by cantilever forces, in situ bending, or rod rotation, imparts stress on the next adjacent segment and is likely to cause junctional kyphosis or scoliosis if the force applied is too powerful. Indirect changes occur either when correction of a curve is greater than the ability of the compensatory curve to compensate or when the curve is corrected to an inappropriate end fusion level. These changes usually result in truncal decompensations that were not present earlier, and they represent a new deformity.

Type IV: Manipulation of the Foundation for the Spine

The spine terminates in the sacrum, and the sacrum is wedged as a keystone in the pelvis. The pelvis and legs therefore are the foundation of the spine. Alteration of the foundation by means of manipulation of the pelvis or leg length may produce spinal deformity. In the treatment of patients with fractures and leg length discrepancies, failure to maintain balance by keeping the foundation level can cause deformity. Contractures of the knee and hip alter the orientation of the pelvis and can imbalance and deformity. Tumors of the sacrum or pelvis may require extensive resection. If reconstruction is not possible, collapse of the spine into the void produced by resection can cause a new deformity.

DESCRIBED ETIOLOGIC FACTORS

Spinal Fusion

The most common and direct cause of tethering is spinal fusion. Partial fusion for preexisting deformities or instabilities caused by tumor excision stops growth in the area fused. Although this fused area of the spine has had the growth potential removed, other growth centers of the vertebrae in the fusion can cause the spine to bend in conjunction with their growth. If the fused area is unilateral, this in essence is a unilateral bar. If the fusion is posterior and the growth potential of the anterior column is great, lordosis or crankshaft deformity can occur, as described by Dubousset (22). The direction of the deformity and its effect on the patient vary depending on many factors. The deformity can be kyphotic, lordotic, or rotational and scoliotic depending on the area tethered and the area that can grow. The resulting change can be in appearance alone or can have an effect on function and spinal balance.

Whenever arthrodesis is performed on a growing child, the child should be observed to maturity. If the chance of progressive deformity is identified, an attempt should be made to determine whether this deformity has clinical significance. If there is evidence that progression of this deformity will cause undesirable consequences, further surgery to stop growth is necessary. This surgery usually takes the form of an anterior fusion, but if the resulting deformity has been allowed to proceed too far, osteotomy of the fusion may be necessary.

Spinal Deformity following Radiation Therapy

Vertebral bodies grow axially by means of endochondral ossification, as do the epiphyseal plates of long bones. Epiphyseal cartilage is radiosensitive tissue, and growth zone cartilage cells in immature bones become disorganized after irradiation. Radiation in sufficient concentration prevents normal endochondral maturation (3,4,82). The degree of growth inhibition with higher doses is related to the age of the child and the dose. The younger the bone and the greater the radiation dosage, the greater is the ultimate deformity (24,40,41,66,73,85,88, 105,106).

Therapy for numerous malignant tumors of childhood includes the use of radiation therapy. Neuroblastoma and Wilms tumor occur close to the vertebral column, and thus the spinal column can be included in the treatment beam. Low linear energy transfer radiation, such as gamma and roentgen rays, can be associated with serious disturbances of skeletal growth. Alterations of vertebral growth patterns can be found as early as 6 months after therapeutic irradiation. Any patient with an immature skeleton who receives more than 1,000 cGy radiation to the vertebral column is at risk of spinal deformity. Less than 1,000 cGy usually produces no detectable changes in the vertebral body (60). Mild curves occur frequently among patients who 2,000 cGy, and the most severe spinal deformities have been associated with 3,000-cGy exposure. Irradiation to asymmetric fields has been associated with increased number and severity of spinal deformities, whereas use of symmetric portals for spinal irradiation more commonly causes kyphosis (61,70,82).

The most severe changes occur among patients 2 years or younger at the time of irradiation. Permanent growth plate inhibition manifests as irregularity or scalloping of vertebral end plates with diminished axial height or as gross abnormalities with flat-beaked vertebral bodies. These changes are produced by 2,000 to 3,000 cGy radiation or more (41,73,84,85,88,93,103). There is little correlation between the individual changes in the vertebral body and the severity of the curvature, but a direct relation exists between absorbed radiation and subsequent spinal deformity.

It is well established that the younger the patient at exposure, the greater is the probability of spinal deformity. Patients who undergo irradiation when they are younger than 2 years have the most serious disturbances. Patients older than 4 years undergoing radiation treatment rarely have appreciable spinal deformity unless the spine has been surgically destabilized, either with laminectomy or through bony erosion of the primary tumor. Any child undergoing therapeutic irradiation to the spine should undergo follow-up examinations until skeletal maturity.

The incidence and importance of spinal deformity after radiation therapy was studied by Riseborough et al. (85), who found that among 81 patients who had undergone irradiation for Wilms tumor, 59 with scoliosis, 19 had kyphoscoliosis, and 2 had kyphosis alone. Fourteen of those patients had curves greater than 25 degrees. Riseborough et al. also found that no child younger than 10 years had a curvature more than 20 degrees. Donaldson and Wissinger (20) conducted a study with 37 children who had undergone radiation therapy for Wilms tumor or neuroblastoma. They found that scoliosis had developed among 70% of the patients and that 2 of these patients needed surgery. Other authors have reported that as many as 40% of patients have scoliosis and 65% have kyphotic deformities (Fig. 1).

Spinal deformity among patients who have received radiation is not always caused by vertebral body distortion from growth abnormalities. The cause of the deformity can be soft-tissue fibrosis and contractures, rib and iliac hypoplasia, or a primary result of the tumor or the surgical intervention. Deformities clearly can develop among patients with Wilms tumor who do not receive radiation. In one study, such patients treated with radiation had scoliosis seven times more often (35 of 57) than did those who did not undergo radiation (5 of 53) (68).

Spinal deformity can occur later in life among patients with spinal tumors who received radiation therapy many years previously. In this situation, the deformity can be caused by the tumor itself or even the surgery, rather than the radiation therapy (87). It is difficult to determine the precise cause.

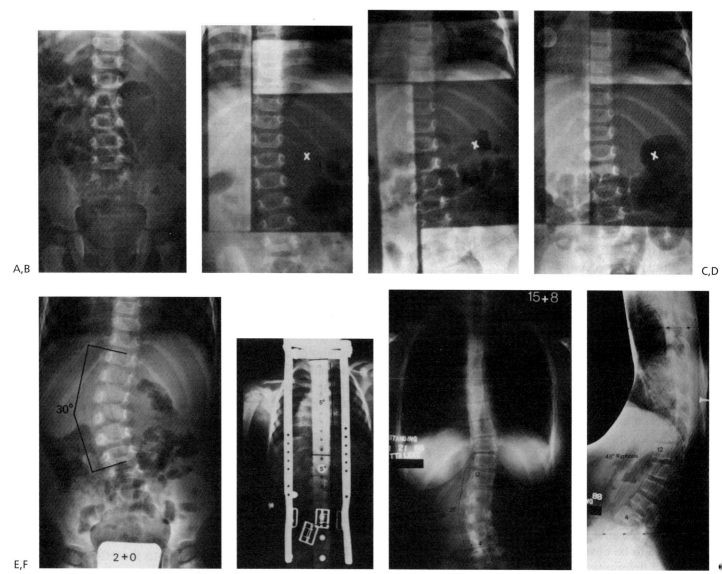

A,B

C,D

E,F

FIGURE 1. A girl with Wilms' tumor treated by nephrectomy and irradiation developed scoliosis controlled by a brace. **A:** Age 1 year 2 months; preoperative anteroposterior radiograph of lumbar spine and pelvis. Bone structures are normal; note straight spine and symmetry of vertebrae, particularly pedicles. At time of right nephrectomy, tumor was found to extend outside kidney. **B, C, and D:** Posteroanterior scout radiographs taken on the fourteenth, fifteenth, and nineteenth postoperative days to aid in determining portals for radiation therapy. Primary treatment field (x) lay lateral to the spine, but a portion of the spine was included within the area to be irradiated, as determined by these scout films. Presumably, the portals were altered to exclude or include the entire spine after these scout films were made. However, a second scout film was not made before radiation therapy, and a portion of spine may still have been included in radiation field. Mild lumbar scoliosis in **B** could be positional or related to the opertive wound. Dosage was 1,975 rads in 12 doses over 20 days. **E:** Age 2 years 0 months; posteroanterior radiograph made 8 months after irradiation. Note lumbar scoliosis, minimal vertebral rotation, pedicle size discrepancy, and asymmetry of each vertebra (vertebral body shape is irregular, and the height of each vertebral body is less on the right side than on the left). A Milwaukee brace was applied. **F:** Age 3 years 6 months; posteroanterior radiographs after wearing of Milwaukee brace with only a left lumbar pad for 16 months. Note satisfactory alignment of spine. Milwaukee brace was changed to a body jacket at age 6 years 3 months. The body jacket was discontinued at age 14 years 9 months. **G:** Age 15 years 8 months. Mild (21-degree) residual left lumbar scoliosis. **H:** The patient is normally active but has occasional low back pain, possibly related to residual upper lumbar kyphosis (48 degrees). Note sagittal wedging of lumbar vertebral bodies 1, 2, and 3. (Figures A–F reproduced with permission from Peterson HA (1985): Spinal deformity secondary to tumor, irradiation, and laminectomy. In: Bradford DS, Hensinger RN, eds. *The pediatric spine.* New York: Thieme-Stratton, pp. 273–285.)

Treatment

Marked scoliosis rarely is present before the age of 10 years. As a patient enters adolescent growth acceleration, curves that have been relatively static in previous years can have a dramatic increase. As with idiopathic scoliosis, when a curve exceeds 25 degrees as measured by the Cobb method, orthotic treatment is used. Whether this prevents progression of certain curves or merely delays progression is unclear. Prolonged observation of a progressive radiation-induced spinal deformity is not indicated. Careful assessment of the soft tissue is necessary for each patient, and extensive scarring or contracture may obviate use of an orthosis. Bracing continues until skeletal maturity. The age at which skeletal maturity occurs does not differ from that among patients with spines that have not been exposed to radiation. If the coronal plane deformity exceeds 45 degrees, surgical intervention should be considered; however, the risk of pseudarthrosis and infection increases when surgery is performed on a previously irradiated spine (41). The choice of fusion limits does not differ from that for idiopathic scoliosis. This generally includes the caudalmost vertebra that rests within the stable zone and one level cephalic to the upper neutral vertebra. Careful attention to the sagittal plane deformity must be used in determining fusion and instrumentation levels.

Healing normally takes a great deal of time. If there is poor evidence of posterior fusion, repetition of bone grafting 6 months after the initial operation has been recommended. The use of third-generation spinal fixation provides sufficient strength and fixation, so pseudarthrosis may be difficult to detect. Therefore a high index of suspicion must be maintained. Use of an autogenous cancellous bone graft from a donor site that has not been irradiated is desirable.

Circumferential anteroposterior fusion is required when the kyphotic component of the deformity is greater than 35 degrees in the lumbar area. A vascularized rib graft transferred from an area that has not been irradiated is ideal as an autogenous, rapidly healing anterior bone strut. Supplemental grafting seldom is needed in circumferential fusion.

A total contact, low-profile orthosis has been routinely used for the 6 months after the operation. The use of newer segmental spinal instrumentation provides good fixation and may allow brace-free convalescence. It is suspected that this type of management improves the fusion rate, but the improvement cannot be confirmed. If fixation is questionable or if fusion healing has not advanced satisfactorily, bracing can be continued or supplementary bone grafting can be performed.

Spinal Deformity following Thoracotomy or Rib Resection

The rib cage provides stability to the spine because of its composite structure and because it is a cylinder with a large radius rather than because of its many articulations and ligamentous connections. The cause of spinal deformity following thoracotomy or rib resections seems to be either instability or tethering.

Several ribs or articulations have to be removed to reduce the stability of the spine. Although mild lateral deviation of the thoracic spine can occur in cases of rib resection, it is rare for the deviation to produce a deformity of clinical importance (10,23,94). It has been difficult to predict who will have a substantial curve, but it has been observed that a direct correlation exists between the number of ribs resected and the curve produced (the more resected, the greater the deformity). Resection of upper ribs produces smaller curves than resection of lower ribs (18,94). In addition, the major curve is limited to the segments of the thoracic spine adjacent to the resected ribs, and the apex of the curve is centrally placed in the region of the resected ribs (94). Patients who undergo transversectomy have greater curvature.

The age of the patient is also a factor (18,23). In adult patients, most of the angular deformity develops 1 week after surgery, and there is almost no progression after 1 year (94). Scoliosis among children who undergo chest wall resection is progressive during growth. The degree of curvature is related to the number of ribs resected (15). Anterior resection of ribs does not produce marked scoliosis, but posterior resection of the ribs promptly produces scoliosis that is convex toward the side of the ribs resected (instability) (18,51). The scoliosis is concave toward the side operated on if there is chest wall resection with scarring, tethering or marked pleural thickening caused by recurrent tumor, radiation scarring, or underlying pulmonary metastasis (18). Scoliosis associated with empyema and chest wall osteomyelitis is likewise concave toward the side operated on and may respond to removal of this tether in a growing child.

That scoliosis follows open heart surgery among patients with congenital heart disease is well known. Some authors have assumed that thoracotomy is responsible for the development of the curve. In one large study, however, no correlation was found between the appearance or side of the scoliosis and either the number and type of thoracotomy incisions or the number and side of ribs removed (81). No more than two ribs were removed from any patient in this study.

Prevention of scoliosis after major en bloc chest wall excision is difficult. Autogenous tissue such as fascia lata, contralateral rib graft, transposed omentum, or a latissimus dorsi muscle flap can be used, as can prosthetic materials such as metallic plates, acrylics, and synthetic mesh fabrics, such as Marlex, Prolene, Silastic, Teflon, or Gortex. Gortex allows incorporation of tissue, is soft and easy to use, and does not fragment (31).

Once deformity is substantial, spinal fusion with instrumentation is the usual treatment. This may improve pulmonary function (34). The correction may be maximized by rib osteotomy or resection on the contralateral concave side (34,59,95,100) (Fig. 2).

Spinal Deformity following Multilevel Laminectomy

With aggressive management of malignant tumors by means of laminectomy and excision, radiation therapy, and chemotherapy, a large number of children survive and come to orthopedic surgeons with severe postlaminectomy spinal deformity. Overall, the younger the patient and the more cephalic the laminectomy (excluding the occiput, C1, and C2), the more likely is deformity (78,96).

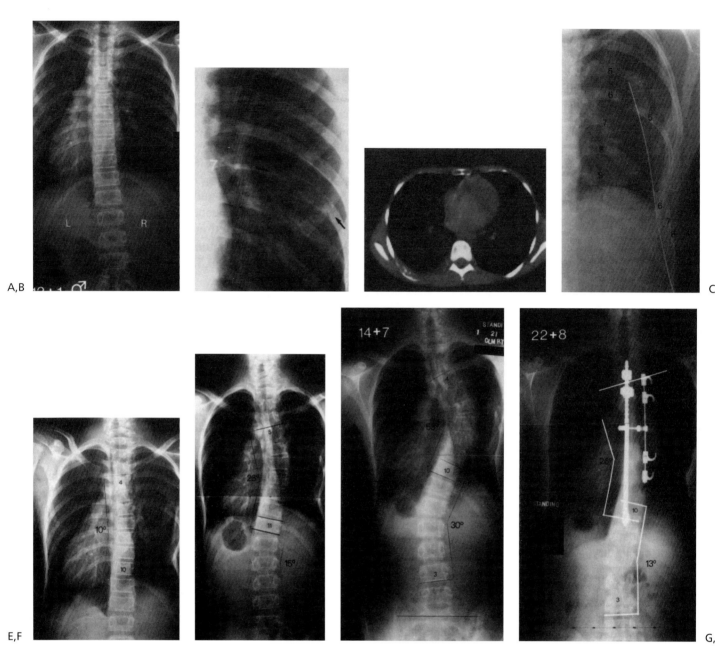

A,B

C,

E,F

G,H

FIGURE 2. Scoliosis following rib resection. **A:** Boy aged 13 years 1 month with lytic lesion in posterior aspect of right seventh rib. Note straight spine. **B:** Close-up radiograph. Note lytic destruction of seventh rib (between *arrows*). This was regarded as malignant. **C:** Computed tomographic appearance also suggested malignancy. **D:** Operative radiograph at time of en bloc excision of posterior portions of ribs 6 through 9, and osteotomy of fifth rib. Thoracic wall reconstruction utilized silastic sheeting. Note straight spine. **E:** Eight weeks postop. Beginning of scoliosis. **F:** Eight months postop. Note little, if any, vertebral body rotation. **G:** Eighteen months postop. Posterior fusion with Harrington distraction and compression rods was performed three days later. **H:** Age 22 years 8 months; 9 years 7 months after rib resection, 8 years 1 month after spinal fusion.

Incidence

Spinal deformity following multilevel laminectomy is rare among adults but occurs among approximately 50% of children treated for spinal cord tumors. Bette and Englehardt (8) first reported this problem in 1955 with three cases of postlaminectomy deformity. In 1959, Haft et al. (32) reported the cases of

30 children who had undergone laminectomy for spinal cord tumors. Among 17 children who underwent complete follow-up evaluation, 10 (33% of the total) experienced spinal deformity. In Tachdjian and Matson's (98) series of 115 children with spinal cord tumors, 46 (40%) acquired spinal deformity. Boersma (12) reported that 50% of the 51 children in his series had spinal deformity after laminectomy for spinal cord tumor.

In 1970, Dubousset et al. (21) reported on 55 children, 78% of whom had late postlaminectomy spinal deformity. Fraser et al. (26) reported in 1977 that 35% of 29 children acquired postlaminectomy spinal deformity. Yasuoka et al. (111) reported that 46% of patients younger than 25 years who underwent laminectomy acquired postlaminectomy deformity. Taking all these series together, the incidence of deformity is 50%.

The most common deformity following multiple-level laminectomy among children is kyphosis, although scoliosis and rotatory deformities can occur (99). The incidence of spinal deformity caused by multiple-level laminectomy alone is difficult to determine, because many laminectomies are performed for conditions that in themselves can cause progressive spinal deformity (78). In one large study, all cases in which the underlying condition was one that could cause spinal deformity were excluded (112). It was found that the occurrence of spinal deformity after multiple-level laminectomy correlated with two factors—the age of the patient (spinal deformity following laminectomy is in part dependent on growth) and the anatomic level of the laminectomy. In the study, 46% of the patients younger than 15 years had deformity, but only 6% of those between 15 and 24 years of age did so, and all those who did were 18 years or younger. Spinal deformity occurred in all patients who underwent cervical laminectomy, 36% of those who underwent thoracic laminectomy, and none of the patients who underwent lumbar laminectomy. No correlation was found between occurrence of the deformity and sex of the patient, number of laminae removed, neurologic condition after laminectomy, or length of time after surgery. Deformity was found as late as 6 years after surgical intervention (32,112). Long-term follow-up evaluation is necessary to identify all cases.

Among children, three types of kyphosis can develop after laminectomy: instability after facetectomy, wedging of vertebral bodies caused by abnormal compressive forces on immature, growing structures, and hypermobility between vertebral bodies associated with gradual rounding of the spine. The importance of facets for stability of the spine is well recognized and has been demonstrated in animal and cadaver experiments (69,74). Facet injury can cause spinal instability with vertebral body subluxation in both children and adults, even without laminectomy or facetectomy. During laminectomy, the facet joints and their capsule should be preserved in their entirety whenever possible. Use of the technique of Dubousset et al. shows a correlation between facet integrity and the deformity (21). If the facets are completely removed at one level, sharp, angular kyphosis develops with the apex at this level. If the facet is partially removed on one side, sharp, angular scoliosis develops in addition to the kyphosis. If the facets are preserved, either completely or in part, gradual rounding kyphosis develops (see later). With careful evaluation of postlaminectomy x-ray films and examination of the facet joints, an accurate prediction of the potential deformity can be made.

Removal of the posterior supporting structures causes transmission of more of the weight load to the anterior column. The immature vertebral body is composed of a relatively small ossification center and a large proportion of cartilage. The compressive force is greatest anteriorly, inhibits cartilage growth and ossification, and produces gradual vertebral body wedging as the more posterior aspects of the body and of the vertebra continue

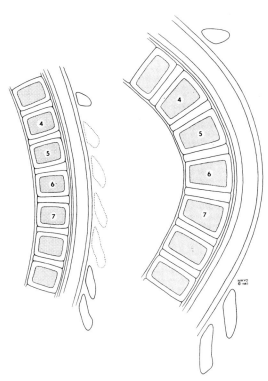

FIGURE 3. Thoracic vertebrae, theoretical drawing. Left: Before laminectomy. Note rectangular configuration of ossified portion of vertebral body, entire vertebral body (ossification center and surrounding growth cartilage), and intervertebral discs. Right: After laminectomy of T4–T7 and subsequent growth. Note kyphosis and wedging of ossified portions of involved vertebrae. Growth plates have been under increased compression anteriorly because of loss of posterior supporting (tension) structures. This compression allows less growth on anterior portion of body than on posterior portion. With time, vertebral end plates and intervertebral discs also become wedge shaped. (Reproduced with permission from Peterson HA (1985): Spinal deformity secondary to tumor, irradiation, and laminectomy. In: Bradford DS, Hensinger RN, eds. *The pediatric spine.* New York: Thieme-Stratton, pp. 273–285.)

to grow. The deformity is short, angular, and limited to the level of the laminectomy. This mechanism of deformity depends on growth and therefore occurs more often among more immature patients (Figs. 3–6).

Hypermobility associated with gradual rounding of the spine can occur without deformation or actual subluxation of vertebral bodies. This is called *pseudosubluxation.* The plane of facet joints is more horizontal in children and becomes more vertical with maturity. The ligamentous and capsular tissues also are more viscoelastic in children than in adults. After removal of the posterior supporting complex by means of laminectomy, the load shifts anteriorly. The viscoelastic capsular tissue around the facet joints and remaining ligaments gradually stretches to allow gradual rounding of the spine that may extend cephalad and caudad to exceed the actual levels of the multilevel laminectomy. If the vertebral bodies are very immature, wedging can occur.

These same mechanisms do not seem to occur in the lumbar spine when it has a normal lordotic curve. Removal of the posterior tension band does not place an abnormally high compressive load on the anterior supporting column. Thus kyphosis is much less likely to occur (112).

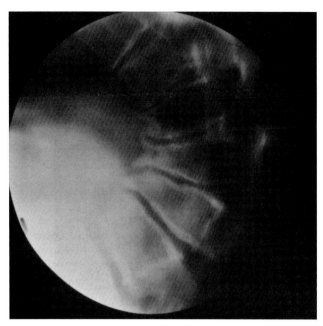

FIGURE 4. Girl aged 16 years 9 months. Thoracic spine was normal when the patient underwent laminectomy at T9–L1 at age 5 years for an astrocytoma. Rdiograph, taken 11 years after multilevel laminectomy, shows wedged vertebrae with only mildly irregular disc spaces. There has been compensatory increased circumferential growth of vertebral bodies (noted anteriorly on this lateral radiograph), much like the increased circumferential growth of the femoral head and neck after early closure of proximal femoral physis with Perthes' disease. (Reproduced with permission from Yasuoka S, Peterson HA, Laws ER Jr, et al. (1981): Pathogenesis and prophylaxis of postlaminectomy deformity of the spine after multiple level laminectomy: difference between children and adults. *Neurosurg* 9:145–152.)

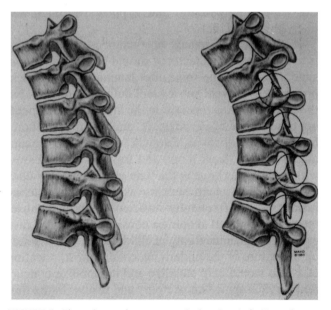

FIGURE 5. Thoracic vertebrae, anatomic drawing. Left: Normal vertebrae before laminectomy. Note congruent apposition of opposing facet joints. Right: After four-level laminectomy, loss of posterior (tension) supporting structures has allowed each involved facet joint surface to slide and subluxate on its opposing surface (circles) and produce increased compressive force on the anterior portion of each vertebral body. There is no deformation or subluxation of vertebral bodies. (Reproduced with permission from Peterson HA (1985): Spinal deformity secondary to tumor, irradiation, and laminectomy. In: Bradford DS, Hensinger RN, eds. *The pediatric spine.* New York: Thieme-Stratton, pp. 273–285.)

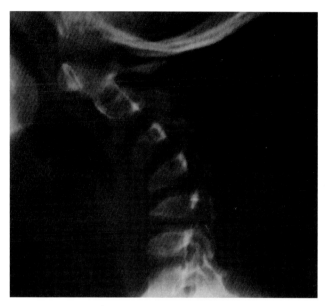

FIGURE 6. Boy aged 12 years 9 months, who had a normal cervical spine before laminectomy of C2–C6 at age 10 years. Two years after laminectomy, there is gradual rounding of the spine, with shearing distraction of the facet joints but not the vertebral bodies. With growth, compressive force on the anterior portion of vertebral bodies will cause them to become wedged also. (Reproduced with permission from Yasuoka S, Peterson HA, Laws ER Jr, et al. (1981): Pathogenesis and prophylaxis of postlaminectomy deformity of the spine after multiple level laminectomy: difference between children and adults. *Neurosurg* 9: 145–152.)

Treatment

Prevention is the best way to manage postlaminectomy deformity. Facetectomy should be avoided if possible. Although bracing of the spine after laminectomy has been proposed to prevent subsequent deformity (92,96), no series reported in the literature documents this method of prophylaxis, and its efficacy remains unproven. Surgical fusion of the remaining structures (facet joints and transverse processes) with autogenous bone at the time of laminectomy usually is sufficient to prevent subsequent deformity and should be considered in every case of multilevel laminectomy on a child. Whether this procedures is used depends on the nature of the underlying condition. Application of external immobilization helps stabilize and immobilize concurrent laminectomy and fusion. Instrumentation is sometimes appropriate in the thoracic and lumbar spine and, when the anatomic configuration allows, in the cervical spine (36,71). Winter (108) even recommends prophylactic anterior spinal fusion after posterior laminectomy in certain circumstances.

Laminoplasty is another procedure that can prevent deformity after operations on the spinal canal (63,69,79,91,96). In this procedure, both laminae are divided as close to the pedicle as possible at each level. The two laminae and the connecting spinous process of each vertebra are removed as one piece and preserved. At the conclusion of the procedure, they are reinserted and sutured in place. The procedure is followed by immobilization with a brace or cast to prevent deformity and instability. The effectiveness of the procedure for prevention of deformity among children has not been established, and additional experience and follow-up study are necessary. The aforementioned hypothesis about the mechanism of development of kyphosis among children supports the rationale for this procedure.

If fusion in situ at the time of laminectomy is not feasible, the patient should be observed closely with repeated radiographic examinations of the spine in the standing position. Early intervention with surgical fusion is recommended as soon as deformity is recognized, especially among young children.

Once spinal deformity has appeared after laminectomy, bracing does not correct it. Correction and stabilization of the deformity necessitate surgical fusion. The surgical approaches are the posterior, the anterior, and the combined approach. Only a small amount of bone surface is available posteriorly after wide laminectomy. This makes fusion difficult. A review of the treatment of 48 patients at my center showed the pseudarthrosis rate was 50% with posterior fusion alone, 25% with anterior fusion alone, and 9.5% with combined anterior and posterior fusions (60). The combined approaches are thus the treatment of choice.

For anterior fusion in an immature patient, the entire disc must be excised back to the posterior longitudinal ligament to eliminate posterior vertebral growth because posterior fusion tends to be thin. This growth causes pseudarthrosis or increasing deformity, the anterior fusion acting as the bar in type 2 congenital kyphosis. The disc and cartilage are thus completely removed, and the fusion is performed with the rib as an inlay strut graft. The vertebral bone and any additional chips of rib bone are placed in the disc spaces. Posterior fusion is performed either during the same operation or 1 week later. This fusion extends into the compensatory lordotic curve. Posteriorly instrumentation frequently is impossible because the bony anatomic features have been altered, the bone is too soft in a young child, or the angle of kyphosis is too great.

A halo cast often is used postoperatively because the deformity is frequently in the high thoracic area, and internal fixation is extremely difficult. When instrumentation cannot be performed or if kyphosis is unstable, the patient may need to stay nonambulatory for 3 to 4 months. After this time, the cast is removed and the patient can walk in a Milwaukee brace. In the cervical spine, anterior fusion with bone grafts between the vertebral bodies usually produces a satisfactory outcome. In the thoracic spine, mild early deformity can be stabilized by means of posterior fusion alone (Fig. 7).

Spinal Cord and Central Nervous System Injury

Whether spinal cord injury causes spinal deformity in a growing child depends on the level of the injury and the growth remaining. Iatrogenic causes of spinal cord injury among children are far less common than traumatic or neoplastic causes. Possible iatrogenic causes include spinal cord ischemia and stretch or trauma from surgical manipulation. The loss of muscular control of the trunk is the presumed primary mechanism for the develop-

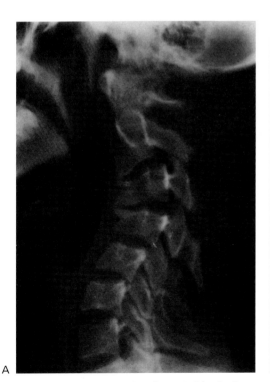 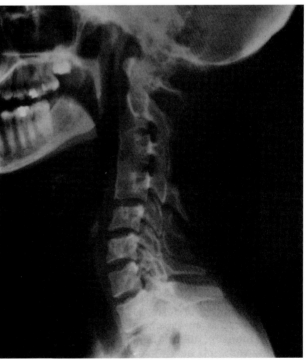

A   B

FIGURE 7. Girl with cervical kyphosis successfully treated with anterior interbody fusion. **A:** Age 15 years 8 months, two year after suboccipital craniectomy and laminectomy at C1–C3 for syringomyelia with Arnold Chiari malformation. Note normal anterior portions of C1 and C2 but wedging of the bodies of C3 and C4 due to asymmetric growth of vertebral bodies. **B:** Age 18 years 8 months, three years after anterior interbody fusion at C2–C4. Cervical spine motion is 75% of normal. (Reproduced with permission from Yasuoka S, Peterson HA, MacCarty CS. (1982): Incidence of spinal column deformity after multilevel laminectomy in children and adults. *J Neurosurg* 57:441–445.)

ment of spinal deformity. Central nervous system injuries can change the muscle tone of a child. The changes are well known to be associated with and probably cause spinal deformities, such as those associated with cerebral palsy.

Spinal Cord Ischemia

Spinal cord ischemia with resultant paraplegia usually is accompanied by substantial progressive spinal deformity. The deformity usually is scoliosis, and lumbar lordosis or lumbar kyphosis can be associated with it. Iatrogenic causes of spinal cord ischemia include clamping or compression of the aorta during a surgical procedure, hypotension during or after a surgical procedure, altered vascular supply to the spinal cord due to surgical ligation of segmental vessels and hypotension, and transumbilical catheter injection of the aorta (6,33,47).

The primary treatment of spinal cord ischemia is avoidance. A common cause of spinal cord injury during operation on the spine is believed to be ischemia due to hypotension and the altered blood flow dynamics of surgery. Avoidance of induced hypotension and appropriate monitoring and fluid resuscitation can minimize the likelihood of spinal cord ischemia.

Umbilical artery catheterization frequently is used for both maintenance of fluid balance and administration of medications in neonatal intensive care units. If the catheter is advanced cephalad to T12, it is believed that a large bolus of fluid can cause ischemia owing to spasm, thrombosis, embolization of the anterior spinal vasculature or so-called artery of Adamkiewicz, or injection of hypertonic fluids or drugs into the spinal cord circulation (5,27,33,90). If the insult is of sufficient degree, spinal cord ischemia or infarction can occur (50). To avoid this complication, a catheter with a radiopaque tip is used, and a radiograph is obtained to ascertain the superior location of the tip of the catheter. If it is caudad to T12, spinal cord ischemia is unlikely.

Spinal Manipulation

Manipulation of the spine has direct consequences to the area treated and indirect consequences to the compensatory areas of the spine. Depending on the nature and magnitude of the force vectors, the changes may not all be desirable. For example, correction of scoliosis by means of distraction on the dorsal side of the spine induces kyphosis. This may be desirable in the thoracic spine but is deleterious in the lumbar spine. Correction of a scoliotic curve that is greater than the ability of the compensatory curve to compensate or that is corrected to an inappropriate end fusion level can cause truncal decompensation not present earlier and represents a new deformity. Spinal fusion for spinal deformity once was performed without instrumentation. Von Lackum (104), of the New York Orthopaedic Hospital, was among the pioneers and was highly aware of the risk of decompensation following spinal fusion. He started to apply surgical casts with the patient in the prone position to maintain lumbar lordosis and avoid a flat back.

Flat-back Syndrome

Doherty (19) first described the problem of flat-back syndrome in 1973. In 1976, Moe and Denis (64) described a series of 16

patients with iatrogenic loss of lumbar lordosis; they coined the term *flat-back syndrome*. Moe and Denis commented on the little attention given to the flattening of the normal lumbar lordosis that occurs when a straight Harrington distraction rod is used to correct lumbar or thoracolumbar lateral curvature of the spine. When the entire lumbosacral spine is flattened, the patient cannot assume a normal erect stance and stoops forward, finding it necessary to bend both knees to bring the trunk into alignment with the pelvis. Moe and Denis found that this problem became particularly troublesome in the presence of pseudarthrosis or whenever the thoracic or thoracolumbar spine showed an increased amount of kyphosis. Denis (17a) later discussed the importance of hip flexion contracture in the pathogenesis of symptomatic flat-back syndrome.

Few children or adolescents are bothered by the typical syndrome as described, probably because they are flexible and have good compensatory mechanisms. Patients often compensate until they reach the middle of the fourth decade of life and then tend to stoop forward more, possibly because of decreasing muscle tone. This posture often is associated with evidence of early disc narrowing at the levels below the fusion; the result is an increasingly flat back. The lower the lumbar fusion, the more marked is the flattening (75,97). An increase in lordosis below the fusion does not compensate for the overall loss of lordosis (97). As patients age, the symptoms develop with a deformity characterized by decreased or absent lumbar lordosis, fixed forward inclination of the trunk, compensatory hyperextension of the cervical spine, inability to stand erect without flexion of the knees, and increasing fatigue and pain as the day progresses. The pain is muscular and is located in the upper back, lower cervical area, and knees. The most common problem, however, is inability to stand erect (48,49).

The primary cause of iatrogenic loss of lumbar lordosis is posterior distraction instrumentation of the lumbar spine that produces flexion forces. Several authors have examined the specific effects of posterior distraction on lumbar lordosis. Aaro and Ohlen (1) analyzed a series of 96 patients specifically in regard to the effect of Harrington distraction instrumentation on lumbar lordosis. The authors found that the loss of lumbar lordosis was proportional to the chosen distal level of fusion—the best case scenario being fusion that stopped at T12 and the worse case scenario being fusion that stopped at the sacrum. Other authors described the importance of positioning during instrumented fusions into the lumbar spine. Jackson and Denis (36a) both advocate placing the legs in extension to maintain lumbar lordosis. Third-generation, segmental instrumentation used to its potential should decrease the likelihood of loss of lordosis.

Loss of lordosis is not limited to posterior instrumentation. It has been found to occur after anterior Dwyer and Zielke instrumentation. The use of rigid rod anterior systems should decrease the kyphogenic nature of the older anterior instrumentation and thus maintain more physiologic lordosis.

Treatment

Maintenance of physiologic lordosis and, when possible, avoiding fusion into the lumbar spine can decrease the likelihood of development of flat-back syndrome later in life. Precautions taken during the operation, such as careful attention to detail, preservation of lumbar lordosis, hyperextension of the spine and hips, avoidance of distraction for correction, and appropriate contouring of the rods, pays dividends in the long run. Segmental fixation with hooks, wires, or screws secures and maintains lordosis. When anterior surgical intervention and fixation are indicated, solid rod designs and good interbody grafting techniques should minimize the kyphosing tendency of anterior correction of scoliosis.

Conservative therapy for symptomatic flat-back syndrome has proved over time to be less than satisfactory and usually is insufficient in relieving symptoms. Extensor strengthening exercises, hip capsule stretching, and analgesics can be prescribed in an attempt to decrease the symptoms in the hope that this might decrease the tendency to stoop. Bracing rarely is indicated unless the brace is expected to stabilize pseudarthrosis and decrease the related symptoms. Whenever bracing temporarily alleviates the symptoms, it tends to further weaken the extensor musculature and thus contribute to the problem.

Treatment of flat-back syndrome has been directed at restoring an upright position. Bilateral innominate osteotomy has been used, but no long-term results have been documented (19). Primary surgical treatment consists of realigning the spine in the sagittal plane by means of posterior closing wedge osteotomy or combined anterior spinal fusion (frequently to the sacrum because of degeneration in the lumbosacral discs) and multiple closing wedge osteotomies. Failure to restore balance in the sagittal plane predisposes to pseudarthrosis, which is associated with recurrent deformity.

Posterior closing wedge osteotomy is indicated in cases of mild to moderate iatrogenic loss of lumbar lordosis in the absence of marked thoracic hyperkyphosis. Return to true lordotic alignment of the lumbar spine after osteotomy is more likely to lead to solid fusion. Incomplete correction with persisting lumbar kyphosis is known for its greater likelihood of being complicated by pseudarthrosis, particularly among patients with osteoporosis.

Anterior spinal fusion combined with one or more closing wedge osteotomies is used when the lumbosacral discs have degenerated and iatrogenic loss of lumbar lordosis exists, particularly when there is a large amount of lumbar kyphosis. Anterior fusion combined with posterior osteotomy is more likely to maintain correction of lordosis (49). Anterior fusion is performed to decrease the rate of pseudarthrosis and to allow multiple levels for correction. Vertebrectomy or pedicle subtraction osteotomy can be used to obtain greater correction at one level. Some surgeons have recommended a simultaneous anterior and posterior approach, making it possible to use anterior struts after correction through a posterior osteotomy. Other surgeons recommend a three-stage procedure to allow for anterior structural grafts with less chance of displacement. Still other surgeons have not found this to be necessary and prefer cancellous grafts for the anterior fusion to avoid the risk of secondary displacement of anterior struts at the stage of posterior extension immediately after osteotomy.

Junctional Problems

Junctional problems are the presence of an angular change between two vertebrae. They usually occur at the end of an instru-

mented fusion between two curves. Junctional problems are most commonly occur and are described as a kyphotic problem, but a lateral change can be caused by the same mechanism. When a junctional problem is sharp forward angulation, it typically occurs at the cephalic or caudal end of a fused spine or between two scoliotic curves, usually at the thoracolumbar junction. Junctional kyphosis usually is associated with instrumented fusion and typically is associated with distraction against the end vertebra of the fusion. It can occur, however, with any type of instrumentation. In the transition between curves of different directions, forces are concentrated on opposing sides of the neutral axis and usually are in balance. Distraction or compression forces applied by instrumentation can upset the balance of forces on a motion segment and causes the sharp angular change. It appears plausible that these problems may be related to changes that affect the ability of the spine to maintain equilibrium of the forces on a spinal motion segment. Patients with underlying neurologic disorders or collagen diseases in which the tensile strength of tissue is reduced may be more prone to this deformity than are others (1a) (Fig. 8). The changes can be made worse if surgical exposure destabilizes the area. Imbalance also occurs if the correction of one curve exceeds the ability of a compensatory curve to correct, thus focusing stress on the transition vertebra. The change can occur immediately after the operation or many years thereafter, because the fusion can allow a concentration of stress at the ends of the fusion, which can cause early degenerative changes or instability.

Junctional kyphosis is most likely to occur at the site of preexisting kyphosis. It is therefore more likely to occur at the mid- or upper thoracic spine, where kyphosis normally is present. Use of distraction hooks that apply an excessive distraction force to the most cephalic vertebra can increase kyphosis. Excessive

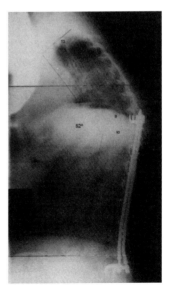

FIGURE 8. Junctional kyphosis in a 17-year-2-month-old nonambulatory female with myelodysplasia fused six years previously for a 58-degree right thoracolumbar scoliosis. Even though mild lumbar lordosis was maintained, junctional kyphosis occurred at the site of normal thoracic kyphosis apex.

intraoperative distraction can tear the supraspinous, intraspinous, and posterior longitudinal ligaments of the upper- or lowermost vertebra. This was much more common in the era of the Harrington rod and is less so with use of third-generation spinal instrumentation, which does not depend on distraction as the primary method of correction. If ligamentous injury is suspected, wiring of the two adjacent end spinous processes has been advocated as a way to prevent this complication.

Treatment

Prevention remains the best treatment to avoid the potential need for additional reconstructive surgery. To prevent these junctional problems from developing, the surgeon must attempt to identify situations that cause risk and take steps to avoid the complication. These steps should include avoidance of overdistraction, overcorrection beyond the compensatory curve, and an attempt to not terminate instrumentation at the mid- or low thoracic level (1a,54,83). If junctional kyphosis exists between two curves, the fusion should cross this kyphosis and represent an attempt to correct it when possible. Neutral coronal and sagittal alignment should be obtained to minimize decompensation and excessive stress on the fusion or instrumentation; the stress can cause instrumentation failure and pseudarthrosis. Late reconstruction of junctional curves necessitates extension of the fusion and possibly osteotomy for correction of the curve and restoration of balance to the spine (13).

Wrong Levels and Overcorrection

Judgment errors in the choice of level of fusion in correction of spinal deformities can cause new deformities. The choice of which curves to fuse, which levels to include, and which mechanism to use for correction and stabilization is not without controversy (54). The controversy arises from the problems some patients have had with decompensation and new deformity after correction of scoliosis. The two curve patterns that have the most controversy surrounding them are the King II and King V curves. King and Moe (41a) described the King V curve, also known as the *double thoracic curve pattern* to bring attention to the high thoracic curve and the problems that occur if this curve is not identified and addressed. When the structurally high thoracic curve is not corrected and is fused along with the larger lower thoracic curve, the left shoulder typically becomes noticeably elevated (52). Although this elevation may not be evident to the family and others before the operation, it usually is evident afterward. Inclusion of this curve with fusion to T2 avoids this problem.

The King II curve has been the subject of controversy related to decompensation with third-generation spinal instrumentation (54). The controversy is not yet resolved but seems to relate to the correction power and mechanism of the newer instrumentation systems and the size and flexibility of the lumbar curve. Several reports regarding decompensation after third-generation instrumentation at the fusion levels recommended by King have caused some authors to advocate new "rules" for the management of these curves (see Chapter 21). If decompensation occurs after surgery for the King II curve, the options for treatment include bracing to see whether the spine becomes balanced over time and extension of the fusion further caudad to obtain balance (13).

Alteration of the Base of the Spine (Pisa Principle)

The spine arises from its base, the sacrum, as a tower. The sacrum is suspended in the pelvis as the foundation for the spine. Changes in the orientation of this foundation cause deformity of the spine. The spine attempts to hold the head erect above the pelvis. If the sacrum starts to incline to the right, the spine either decompensates to the right or develops a curve to bring the head back in line. Lordosis and kyphosis likewise usually keep the head above the sacrum. Flexing or extending the sacral inclination changes the lordosis or kyphosis and can take the head out of balance.

A stable foundation for the spine necessitates symmetry in leg length and pelvis and symmetric and normal motion of the hips and knees. Changes to the foundation can cause iatrogenic deformities. Contractures of the hips and knees and leg length discrepancy are the most likely causes of this deformity. Changes in the size of the pelvis, possibly after surgical treatment, also can cause deformity. Treatment is aimed at restoring a stable and balanced spine and pelvis. This can be done with lifts or with adjustment of leg length by means of growth arrest or other lengthening or shortening procedures. Joint contractures should be addressed with stretching and, when necessary, surgical release.

REFERENCES

1a. Aaro S, Ohlen G (1983): The effect of Harrington instrumentation on the sagittal configuration and mobility of the spine in scoliosis. *Spine: State of Art Reviews* 8:570–575.

1. Amis J, Herring JA (1984): Iatrogenic kyphosis: a complication of Harrington instrumentation in Marfan's syndrome. *J Bone Joint Surg Am* 66:460–464.

2. Arkin AM, Pack GT, Ransohoff NS, et al. (1950): Radiation induced scoliosis: a case report. *J Bone Joint Surg Am* 32:401–404.

3. Arkin AM, Simon N (1950): Radiation scoliosis: an experimental study. *J Bone Joint Surg Am* 32:396–401.

4. Arkin A, Simon N, Siffert R (1948): Asymmetrical suppression of vertebral epiphyseal growth with ionizing radiation. *Proc Soc Exp Biol Med* 69:171–173.

5. Atkinson JP (1969): Transverse myelopathy secondary to injection of penicillin. *J Pediatr* 75:867–869.

6. Aziz EJ, Robertson AF (1973): Paraplegia: a complication of umbilical artery catheterization. *J Pediatr* 82:1051–1052.

7. Barrera M, Roy LP, Stevens M (1989): Long-term follow-up after unilateral nephrectomy and radiotherapy for Wilms' tumor. *Pediatr Nephrol* 3:430–432.

8. Bette H, Englehardt H: Folgezustande von Laminektomie an der Halswirbelsaule. *Z Orthop* 85:564–573, 1955.

9. Bisgard JD (1934): Thoracogenic scoliosis: influence of thoracic disease and thoracic operations on the spine. *Arch Surg* 29:417–445.

10. Bisgard JD (1935): Experimental thoracogenic scoliosis. *J Thorac Surg* 4:435–442.

11. Boersma G (1969): *Verkrommingen van de Wervelkolom na Laminectomie bij Kinderen: Een Klinisch Onderzoek en een Literatuurstudie Over Normale en Mechanisch Verstoorde Wervelgroei.* Amsterdam: Born.

12. Boersma G (1969): *Curvatures of the spine following laminectomies in children.* Amsterdam: Born.

13. Bridwell KH (2000): Reconstruction for failed fusion. *Spine: State Art Rev* 14:141–161.

14. Butler MS, Robertson WW Jr, Rate W, et al. (1990): Skeletal sequelae of radiation therapy for malignant childhood tumors. *Clin Orthop* 251:235–240.

15. Callahan RA, Johnson RM, Margolis RN, et al. (1977): Cervical facet fusion for control of instability following laminectomy. *J Bone Joint Surg Am* 59:991–1002.

16. Cattell HS, Clark GL Jr (1967): Cervical kyphosis and instability following multiple laminectomies in children. *J Bone Joint Surg Am* 49:713–720.

17. Cerisoli M, Vernizzi E, Giulioni M (1980): Cervical spine changes following laminectomy. *J Neurosurg Sci* 24:63–70.

17a. Denis FD (1994): The iatrogenic loss of lumbar lordosis. *Spine: State of Art Reviews* 8:659–672.

18. DeRosa GP (1985): Progressive scoliosis following chest wall resection in children. *Spine* 10:618–622.

19. Doherty JH (1973): Complications of fusion in lumbar scoliosis. *J Bone Joint Surg Am* 55:438 (abst).

20. Donaldson WF, Wissinger HA (1967): Axial skeletal changes following tumor dose radiation therapy. *J Bone Joint Surg Am* 49:1469–1470.

21. Dubousset J, Guillaurnat J, Mechin JF (1973): In: Rougerie J, ed. *Les compressions medullaires non traumatiques de VenJunt.* Paris: Masson.

22. Dubousset J, Herring JA, Shufflebarger H (1989): The crankshaft phenomenon. *J Pediatr Orthop* 9:541–550.

23. Durning RP, Scoles PV, Fox OD (1980): Scoliosis after thoracotomy in tracheoesophageal fistula patients. *J Bone Joint Surg Am* 62:1156–1159.

24. Engel D (1986): Can juvenile scoliosis be corrected by circumscribed radium-irradiation of the spine? *Med Hypotheses* 19:161–168.

25. Evans AE, Norkool P, Evans L, et al. (1991): Late effects of treatment for Wilms' tumor. *Cancer* 67:331–336.

26. Fraser RD, Paterson DC, Simpson DA (1977): Orthopaedic aspects of spinal tumours in children. *J Bone Joint Surg Br* 59:143–151.

27. Gammel JA (1927): Arterial embolism: an unusual complication following the intramuscular administration of bismuth. *JAMA* 88:998–999.

28. Goetzman BW, Stadalnik RC, Bogren HG, et al. (1972): Thrombotic complications of umbilical artery catheters: a clinical and radiographic study. *Pediatrics* 56:1–2.

29. Graham JJ (1989): Complications of cervical spine surgery: a five-year report on a survey of the membership of the Cervical Spine Research Society by the Morbidity and Mortality Committee. *Spine* 14:1046–1050.

30. Grobler LJ, Moe JH, Winter RB (1978): Loss of lumbar lordosis following surgical correction of thoracolumbar deformities. *Orthop Trans* 2:38.

31. Grosfeld JL, Rescorla FJ, West KW, et al. (1988): Chest wall resection and reconstruction for malignant conditions in childhood. *J Pediatr Surg* 23:667–673.

32. Haft H, Ransohoff J, Carter S (1959): Spinal cord tumors in children. *Pediatrics* 23:1152–1159.

33. Haldeman S, Fowler GW, Ashwal S, et al. (1983): Acute flaccid neonatal paraplegia: a case report. *Neurology* 33:93–95.

34. Halsall AP, James DF, Kostuik JP, et al. (1983): An experimental evaluation of spinal flexibility with respect to scoliosis surgery. *Spine* 8:482–488.

35. Haritonova KI, Tzivian JL, Ekshtadt NK (1974): Orthopaedic sequelae of laminectomy. *Ortop Travmatol Protez* 11:32–36.

36. Hopf C, Heine J (1990): Operative therapy in metastases and primary tumors of the spine. *Neurosurg Rev* 13:205–210.

36a. Jackson RP (1994): Jackson intrasacral fixation and segmental corrections with adjustable contoured translating axes, *Spine: State of Art Reviews* 8:307–341.

37. Jaffe N, McNeese M, Mayfield JK, et al. (1980): Childhood urologic cancer therapy: related sequelae and their impact on management. *Cancer* 45[Suppl 7]:1815–1822.

38. Jenkins DH (1973): Extensive cervical laminectomy: long-term results. *Br J Surg* 60:852–854.

39. Katsumi Y, Honma T, Nakamura T (1989): Analysis of cervical instability resulting from laminectomies for removal of spinal cord tumor. *Spine* 14:1171–1176.

40. Katz LD, Lawson JP (1990): Radiation-induced growth abnormalities. *Skeletal Radiol* 19:50–53.

41. Katzman H, Waugh T, Berdon W (1969): Skeletal changes following irradiation of childhood tumors. *J Bone Joint Surg Am* 51:825–842.

41a. King HA, Moe JH, Bradford DS, et al. (1983): The selection of fusion levels in thoracic idiopathic scoliosis. *J Bone Joint Surg* 65A:1302–1313.

42. King J, Stowe S (1982): Results of spinal fusion for radiation scoliosis. *Spine* 7:574–585.

43. Kostuik JP (1990): Anterior Kostuik-Harrington distraction systems for the treatment of kyphotic deformities. *Spine* 15:169–180.

44. Kostuik JP (1988): Treatment of scoliosis in the adult thoracolumbar spine with special reference to fusion to the sacrum. *Orthop Clin North Am* 19:371–381.

45. Kostuik JP, Errico TJ, Gleason TF (1986): Techniques of internal fixation for degenerative conditions of the lumbar spine. *Clin Orthop* 203:219–231.

46. Kostuik JP, Maurais GR, Richardson WJ, et al. (1986): Combined single stage anterior and posterior osteotomy for correction of iatrogenic lumbar kyphosis. *Spine* 13:257–266.

47. Krishnamoorthy KS, Fernandez RJ, Todres ID, et al. (1976): Paraplegia associated with umbilical artery catheterization in the newborn. *Pediatrics* 58:443–445.

48. LaGrone MO (1988): Loss of lumbar lordosis: a complication of spinal fusion for scoliosis. *Orthop Clin North Am* 19:383–393.

49. LaGrone MO, Bradford SD, Moe JH, et al. (1988): The treatment of symptomatic flatback after spine fusion. *J Bone Joint Surg Am* 70:569–580.

50. Laguna J, Carioto H (1973): Spinal cord infarction secondary to occlusion of the anterior spinal artery. *Arch Neurol* 28:134–136.

51. Langenskibld A, Michelsson JE (1961): Experimental progressive scoliosis in the rabbit. *J Bone Joint Surg Br* 43:116–120.

52. Lee CK, Denis F, Winter RB, et al. (1993): Analysis of the upper thoracic curve in surgically treated idiopathic scoliosis: a new concept of the double thoracic curve pattern. *Spine* 18:1599–1608.

53. Lemerle J (1982): Complications and sequelae of the treatment of Wilms' tumor. *Prog Clin Biol Res* 100:119–121.

54. Lenke LG, Bridwell KH, Baldus C, et al. (1992): Preventing decompensation in King II curves treated with Cotrel-Dubousset instrumentation: strict guidelines for selective thoracic fusion. *Spine* [Suppl 8]:S274–S281,

55. Lettice J, Ogilvie J, Transfeldt E, et al. (1991): Proximal junctional kyphos following Cotrel-Dubousset instrumentation in adult scoliosis. Presented at the Meeting of the Scoliosis Research Society, Minneapolis.

56. Lonstein JE (1977): Post-laminectomy kyphosis. *Clin Orthop* 128:93–100.

57. Lonstein JE (1978): Postlaminectomy kyphosis. In: Chou SN, Seljeskog EL, eds. *Spinal deformities and neurological dysfunction.* New York: Raven Press, pp 53–63.

58. Lonstein JE, Winter RB, Moe JH, et al. (1976): Post-laminectomy spine deformity. *J Bone Joint Surg Am* 58:727.(abst).

59. Mann DC, Nash CL Jr, William MR, et al. (1989): Evaluation of the role of concave rib osteotomies in the correction of thoracic scoliosis. *Spine* 14:491–495.

60. Matsumoto M, Cho JL, Lonstein JE, et al. (1993): Postlaminectomy spine deformity. *Orthop Trans* 17:125.

61. Mayfield JK, Riseborough EJ, Jaffe N, et al. (1981): Spinal deformity in children treated for neuroblastoma. *J Bone Joint Surg Am* 63:183–193.

62. Mikawa Y, Shikata J, Yamamuro T (1987): Spinal deformity and instability after multilevel cervical laminectomy. *Spine* 12:6–11.

63. Milhorat TH (1978): *Pediatric neurosurgery: contemporary neurology.* Philadelphia: FA Davis.

64. Moe JH, Denis F (1977): The iatrogenic loss of lumbar lordosis. *Orthop Trans* 1:131.

65. Moe JH, Winter RB, Bradford DS, et al. (1978): Postlaminectomy spine deformity. In: *Scoliosis and other spinal deformities.* Philadelphia: WB Saunders, pp. 595–600.

66. Moe JH, Winter RB, Bradford DS, et al. (1978): Spine deformity following irradiation. In: *Scoliosis and other spine deformities.* Philadelphia: WB Saunders, pp. 303–314.

67. Mohrohisky ST, Levine RL, Blumhagen JD, et al. (1978): Low positioning of umbilical-artery catheters increases associated complications in newborn infants. *N Engl J Med* 299:561–564.

68. Moss WT, Brand WN, Battifora H (1979): The bone: response of normal bone to irradiation. In: *Radiation oncology: rationale, techniques, results,* 5th ed. St. Louis: CV Mosby.

69. Munechica Y (1973): Influence of laminectomy on the stability of the spine: an experimental study with special reference to the extent of laminectomy and the resection of the intervertebral joint. *J Jpn Orthop Assoc* 47:111–126.

70. Murphy FD, Blount VVT (1962): Cartilaginous exostoses following irradiation. *J Bone Joint Surg Am* 44:662.

71. Natelson SE (1966): The injudicious laminectomy. *Spine* 11:966–969.

72. Neal WA, Reynolds JW, Jarvis CW, et al. (1972): Umbilical artery catheterization: demonstration of arterial thrombosis by aortography. *Pediatrics* 50:6–13.

73. Neuhauser EBD, Wittenborg MH, Berman CZ, et al. (1952): Irradiation effects of roentgen therapy on the growing spine. *Radiology* 59:637–650.

74. Panjabi MM, White AA III, Johnson RM (1975): Cervical spine mechanics as a function of transection of components. *J Biomech* 8:327–336.

75. Paonessa K, Engler G (1991): Back pain and disability following Harrington rod fusion to the lumbar spine for scoliosis: how flat is the flat back? Presented at the Meeting of the Scoliosis Research Society, Minneapolis.

76. Pastore G, Antonelli R, Fine W, et al. (1982): Late effects of treatment of cancer in infancy. *Med Pediatr Oncol* 10:369–375.

77. Peter JC, Hoffman EB, Arens LJ, et al. (1990): Incidence of spinal deformity in children after multiple level laminectomy for selective posterior rhizotomy. *Childs Nerv Syst* 6:30–32.

78. Peterson HA (1985): Spinal deformity secondary to tumor, irradiation, and laminectomy. In: Bradford DS, Hensinger RN, eds. *The pediatric spine.* New York: Thieme-Stratton, pp. 273–285.

79. Raimondi AJ, Gutierrez FA, Di Rocco C (1976): Laminotomy and total reconstruction of the posterior spinal arch for spinal canal surgery in childhood. *J Neurosurg* 45:555–560.

80. Rand C, Smith MA (1989): Anterior spinal tuberculosis: paraplegia following laminectomy. *Ann R Coll Surg Engl* 71:105–109.

81. Reckles LN, Peterson HA, Bianco AJ, et al. (1975): The association of scoliosis and congenital heart disease. *J Bone Joint Surg Am* 57:449–455.

82. Reidy JA, Lingley JR, Gall EA, et al. (1947): The effect of roentgen irradiation on epiphyseal growth, II: experimental studies upon the dog. *J Bone Joint Surg Am* 29:853–873.

83. Richards BS, Birch JG, Herring JA, et al. (1989): Frontal plane and sagittal plane balance following Cotrel-Dubousset instrumentation for idiopathic scoliosis. *Spine* 14:733–737.

84. Riseborough EJ (1977): Irradiation induced kyphosis. *Clin Orthop* 128:101–106.

85. Riseborough EJ, Grabias SL, Burton RL, et al. (1976): Skeletal alterations following irradiation for Wilms' tumor: with particular reference to scoliosis and kyphosis. *J Bone Joint Surg Am* 58:526–536.

86. Riseborough EJ, Herndon JH (1975): Irradiation scoliosis. In: *Scoliosis and other deformities of the axial skeleton.* Boston: Little, Brown, pp. 257–258.

87. Rubin P, Duthie RB, Young LW (1962): The significance of scoliosis in postirradiated Wilms' tumor and neuroblastoma. *Radiology* 79:539–558.

88. Rutherford H, Dodd GD (1974): Complications of radiation therapy: growing bone. *Semin Roentgenol* 9:15–27.

89. Shah M, Eng K, Engler GL (1980): Radiation enteritis and radiation scoliosis. *NY State J Med* 80:1611–1613.

90. Shaw EB (1966): Transverse myelitis from injection of penicillin. *Am J Dis Child* 111: 548–551.

91. Shikata J, Yamamuro T, Shimizu K, et al. (1990): Combined laminoplasty and posterolateral fusion for spinal canal surgery in children and adolescents. *Clin Orthop* 259:92–99.

92. Sim FH, Svien HJ, Bickel WH, et al. (1974): Swan-neck deformity following extensive cervical laminectomy: a review of twenty-one cases. *J Bone Joint Surg Am* 56:564–580.

93. Smith R, Davidson JK, Flatman GE (1982): Skeletal effects of orthovoltage and megavoltage therapy following treatment of nephroblastoma. *Clin Radiol* 33:601–613.

94. Stauffer ES, Mankin HJ (1966): Scoliosis after thoracoplasty: a study of thirty patients. *J Bone Joint Surg Am* 48:339–348.

95. Steel HH (1983): Rib resection and spine fusion in correction of convex deformity in scoliosis. *J Bone Joint Surg Am* 65:920–925.

96. Steinbok P, Boyd M, Cochrane D (1989): Cervical spinal deformity following craniotomy and upper cervical laminectomy for posterior fossa tumors in children. *Childs Nerv Syst* 5:25–28.

97. Swank SM, Mauri TM, Brown JC (1990): The lumbar lordosis below Harrington instrumentation for scoliosis. *Spine* 15: 181–186.

98. Tachdjian MO, Matson DD (1965): Orthopaedic aspects of intraspinal tumors in infants and children. *J Bone Joint Surg Am* 47:223–248.

99. Taddonio RF Jr, King AG (1982): Atlantoaxial rotatory fixation after decompressive laminectomy: a case report. *Spine* 7:540–544.

100. Taylor JF, Roaf R, Owen R, et al. (1983): Costodesis and contralateral rib release in the management of progressive scoliosis. *Acta Orthop Scand* 54:603–612.

101. Thomas PRM, Griffith KD, Fineberg BB, et al. (1983): Late effects of treatment for Wilms' tumor. *Int J Radiat Oncol Biol Phys* 9:651–657.

102. Tooley WH (1972): What is the risk of an umbilical catheter? *Pediatrics* 50:1–2.

103. Vaeth JM, Levitt SH, Jones MD, et al. (1962): Effects of radiation therapy in survivors of Wilms' tumor. *Radiology* 79:560–567.

104. Von Lackurn WH, Miller JP, (1949): Critical observations on the result in the operative treatment of scoliosis. *J Bone Joint Surg Am.* 31A:102–106.

105. Wallace WHB, Shalet SM, Morris-Jones PH, et al. (1980): Effect of abdominal irradiation on growth in boys treated for a Wilms' tumor. *Med Pediatr Oncol* 18: 441–446.

106. Whitehouse WM, Lampe L (1953): Osseous damage in irradiation of renal tumors in infancy and childhood. *Am J Roentgenol* 70:721–729.

107. Winter RB (1978): Postirradiation spinal deformity. In: Lovell WW, Winter RB, eds. *Pediatric orthopaedics,* vol 2. Philadelphia: JB Lippincott, pp. 646–647.

108. Winter RB (1978): Postlaminectomy kyphosis. In: Lovell WW, Winter RB, eds. *Pediatric orthopaedics,* vol 2. Philadelphia: JB Lippincott, pp. 645–646.

109. Winter RB (1986): Harrington instrumentation into the lumbar spine: technique for preservation of normal lumbar lordosis. *Spine* 11:633–635.

110. Winter RB, McBride GG (1984): Severe postlaminectomy kyphosis: treatment by total vertebrectomy (plus late recurrence of childhood spinal cord astrocytoma). *Spine* 9:690–694.

111. Yasuoka S, Peterson HA, Laws ER Jr, et al. (1981): Pathogenesis and prophylaxis of postlaminectomy deformity of the spine after multiple level laminectomy: difference between children and adults. *Neurosurgery* 9:145–152.

112. Yasuoka S, Peterson HA, MacCarty CS (1982): Incidence of spinal column deformity after multilevel laminectomy in children and adults. *J Neurosurg* 57:441–445.

113. Zajtchuk R, Bowen TE, Seyfer AE, et al. (1980): Intrathoracic ganglioneuroblastoma. *J Thorac Cardiovasc Surg* 80: 605–612.

114. Zdeblick TA, Bohlman HH (1989): Cervical kyphosis and myelopathy. *J Bone Joint Surg Am* 71:170–182.

MARFAN SYNDROME

S. JAY KUMAR
JAMES T. GUILLE

Marfan syndrome is a generalized disorder of connective tissue that affects the supporting structures of the body, especially those in the musculoskeletal system. In 1896, Marfan published his report of a girl who had the features of what is now eponymically known as *Marfan syndrome* (29,32). The syndrome is defined by the clinical features that have become the hallmark of the condition, especially the phenotypic body habitus. Because of the wide pleiotropic expression of this autosomal dominant disorder, patients usually are considered to belong to one of two groups—those having Marfan syndrome and those having the Marfan habitus (marfanoid). The variability in this expression can make prognostication and genetic counseling difficult and indecisive (8,40,42). Marfan syndrome often is misdiagnosed as homocystinuria, Ehlers-Danlos syndrome, congenital contractural arachnodactyly, and many other conditions because of the wide expression of the gene (3,6,7,19,26,56). Ligamentous laxity and joint hypermobility with muscular underdevelopment can appear as primary myopathy among children (15). Patients with Marfan syndrome are of normal intelligence. Any variations in this factor should lead one to suspect another cause of the condition, such as homocystinuria, in which mental retardation is common. Careful examination and history taking, with special attention to specific diagnostic details, should avoid any errors in diagnosis. A collaborative multidisciplinary approach should be used in the care of these patients.

EPIDEMIOLOGY

The prevalence of Marfan syndrome has been estimated to be one case among in 10,000 persons in the United States (14). Because there is considerable variability in this syndrome, one must question the true incidence, considering the possible inclusion of those with the Marfan habitus or misdiagnoses in older studies. There is no ethnic or racial predilection for Marfan syndrome, and men and women are affected equally. Marfan syndrome is inherited as an autosomal dominant gene, and spontaneous new mutations account for approximately 25% of cases

among persons who do not have a family history of the disorder (37). The average life expectancy among persons with Marfan syndrome once was 40 years for men and 45 years for women. These figures may be inaccurate today. They were calculated before improvements were made in treatment modalities, especially in cardiovascular surgery, that can extend the life span of these individuals (36).

ETIOLOGY

The genetic defect that causes Marfan syndrome has been identified (10,23,30,31). A mutation of the fibrillin gene seems to be the key factor, and the specific locale of the gene FBN1 has been mapped to the q arm of chromosome 15 (15q21.1). Fibrillin is a large glycoprotein component of the microfibrillar system associated with elastin and is thus present in connective tissues.

CLINICAL FEATURES

Even though there is extensive phenotypic variation, Marfan syndrome has one of the most recognizable of all phenotypes. Recognition of the characteristics of this phenotype is of the utmost importance, because the syndrome is defined predominantly by its clinical features. A diagnostic tree has been published by the American Academy of Pediatrics that lists major and minor criteria of the following areas: skeletal system, ocular system, cardiovascular system, pulmonary system, skin and integument, dura, and family and genetic history (8). The requirements for the diagnosis of Marfan syndrome are as follows. If there is no family history, there needs to be a major criterion in two different organ systems and involvement of a third organ system. If there is a family history, there need be only one major criterion in an organ system and involvement of a second organ system. Patients who have the phenotypic features but who do not meet the aforementioned criteria are considered to have the Marfan habitus. Patients who are evaluated in the orthopaedic clinic with typical findings should be referred for pediatric, genetic, cardiac, and ophthalmologic evaluations as well.

SPINAL DEFORMITIES
Scoliosis

The spine is involved in most patients with Marfan syndrome. Scoliosis is the most common spinal deformity among these

S.J. Kumar: Departments of Orthopaedics, Thomas Jefferson University Hospital, Philadelphia, Pennsylvania 19107.

J.T. Guille: Medical College of Pennsylvania–Hahnemann University Program in Orthopaedic Surgery, Philadelphia, PA 19120.

patients, and it is also the most insidious (1,5,22,43,44). It is difficult to assess the exact prevalence of scoliosis in Marfan syndrome, because many of the reports are from tertiary referral centers for scoliosis, and different studies use different terms and diagnostic criteria. Scoliosis is common among the infantile and juvenile age groups, and 50% of patients who have scoliosis have it by 6 years of age; almost all have it by 9 years of age (15). Many curves progress early and rapidly. The curve types have been said to resemble those of patients with idiopathic scoliosis. They include single curves, double structural curves, triple curves, or long, sweeping C-shaped thoracolumbar curves. Unlike idiopathic scoliosis, however, these curves continue to progress throughout adolescence (Fig. 1). Many of these curves are quite rigid, although one would expect flexible curves because of ligamentous laxity. Ligamentous laxity is considered one of the causes of scoliosis (15,44). Lateral subluxation and dysplasia of vertebrae are frequent (Fig. 2).

The following sections on scoliosis have been divided as they relate to patients with Marfan syndrome and those with the Marfan habitus (so-called marfanoid), because the two should be considered as separate entities. Treatment, however, is standard for patients in either category.

Marfan Syndrome

Course of Condition

The course of spinal deformity in Marfan syndrome is not well delineated. Many studies are flawed by the inclusion of patients with Marfan habitus. Despite this shortcoming, several tenets are generally accepted. It appears that men and women are affected almost equally. The curve patterns are similar to those of idiopathic scoliosis, although double major curves seem to be more common in Marfan syndrome. Scoliosis manifests itself during the infantile and juvenile periods, and some children may come to medical attention early adolescence with curves of large magnitude. Most authors on the subject have found that scoliosis in Marfan syndrome is severe, painful, progressive, and can cause respiratory problems (5,28,43,44). Scoliosis among patients with Marfan syndrome should not be considered idiopathic scoliosis; it behaves more as neuromuscular scoliosis.

The prevalence of scoliosis among patients with Marfan syndrome ranges from 52% to 100% (5,20,28,39,43,47). The curves are progressive. If the patients are left untreated, it is not uncommon to see curves of 180 degrees (43,44,52). The average age at diagnosis of the scoliosis has ranged from birth to 15 years, most cases being diagnosed in the late juvenile period (28,43,44,46–48,52).

Presentation

Pain was a presenting symptom for 20 of the 27 patients (74%) in the series of Makin et al. (28). The combined data for both patients with Marfan syndrome and patients with Marfan habitus in the series of Robins et al. (43) revealed that 74% of patients had pain. The patients in the series of Sponseller et al. (48) reported their back pain to be localized to the area of the curve, not in the low back. The subject of back pain among these patients appears inconsistently in the literature, and its nature is vague and unknown. The importance of the pain is unclear

other than that Marfan syndrome may be one cause of painful scoliosis.

Curve Types

There is debate in the literature whether single or double curves are more common, although it is generally accepted that double major curves often are severe and rigid. Double major curves predominate in most series, and when single curves exist, the apex is usually in the right thoracic area. There is also an increased prevalence of triple curves and thoracolumbar curves among these patients (5,20,22,28,43,44,47,52,57). Fixed pelvic obliquity has not been reported among Marfan patients (43,52,59).

Curve Magnitude and Progression

Curve progression in patients with Marfan syndrome is rapid, often to the point of severe deformity. In LeDelliou's (22) series of 59 patients, 11 patients had curves greater than 100 degrees, 19 had curves less than 50 degrees, and only eight had curves less than 30 degrees. The average curve magnitude at the time of presentation (average age, 9.3 years) was 53.5 degrees for the patients with Marfan syndrome in the series of Taneja and Manning (52), who calculated an average rate of progression of 10.2 degrees per year. Robins et al. (43) did not differentiate the values for patient with Marfan syndrome and those with Marfan habitus, but for both groups the mean preoperative curve was 72 degrees and rigid, as demonstrated by a side-bending correction of only 50%. They also found curve progression to be most rapid during the early adolescent period. In Daudon's series (9), the greatest curve progression was observed during the adolescent period. Male patients had an average curve progression of 7.2 degrees per year and female patients 5.8 degrees per year. Sponseller et al. (47) calculated the mean yearly progression of scoliosis for different age groups. There was a mean progression of 19 ± 17 degrees in the 0 to 3 years age group, 3 ± 4 degrees in the 4 to 10 years age group, 6 ± 9 degrees in the 11 to 16 years age group, 1 ± 2 degrees in the 17 to 30 years age group, 1 ± 7 degrees in the 31 to 40 years age group, 1 ± 1 degree in the 41 to 50 years age group, and 3 ± 5 degrees in patients older than 50 years. These authors showed that all curves greater than 30 degrees progressed at least 10 degrees, and all curves were at least 40 degrees by skeletal maturity.

Infantile Scoliosis

Sponseller et al. (48) reported on 14 patients with scoliosis diagnosed before the patient was 3 years old. Unlike idiopathic infantile scoliosis, no curve resolved spontaneously, there was no left thoracic curve, and there was an almost equal distribution of boys and girls. Thirteen of the 14 patients did not have a family history of Marfan syndrome, and all 14 had exaggeration of the syndromic features. The mean curve magnitude was 38 degrees, and 11 of the curves were double major. Bracing had no effect, and instrumentation without fusion was recommended only for patients without marked kyphosis. These authors suggested that surgery not be performed on children younger than 4 years, because many with large curves die of cardiac problems early in life.

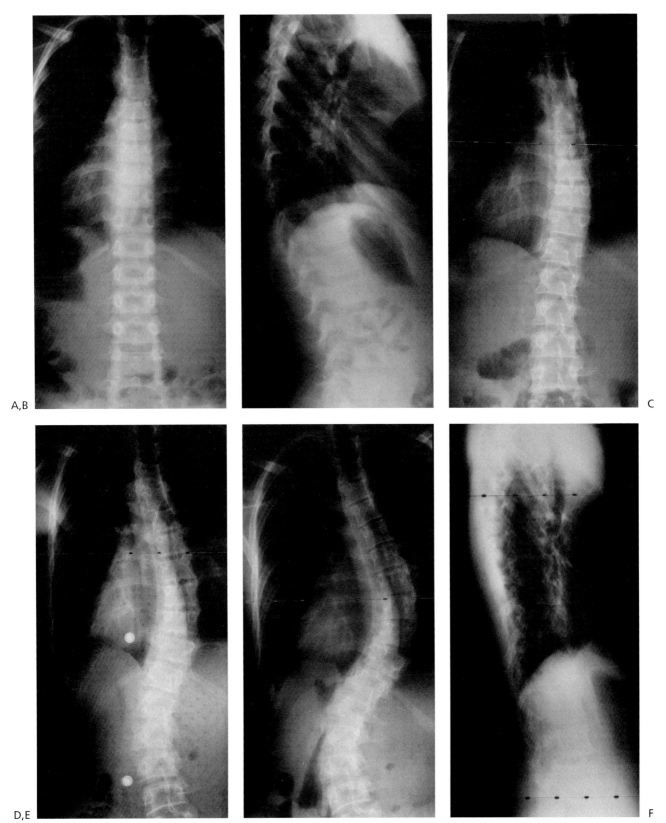

A,B

C

D,E

F

FIGURE 1. Anteroposterior **(A)** and lateral **(B)** radiographs of a 4-year-old girl with Marfan syndrome show no scoliosis and normal sagittal alignment. **C:** At age 12 years, there is a right thoracic curve of 17 degrees, and the patient was placed in a Wilmington jacket. **D:** At age 13 years, the right thoracic curve has progressed to 29 degrees despite compliant use of the brace. There is now a left lumbar curve of 30 degrees. Anteroposterior **(E)** and lateral **(F)** radiographs at the age of 14 years show a right thoracic curve of 62 degrees, a left lumbar curve of 52 degrees, and loss of thoracic kyphosis and lumbar lordosis.

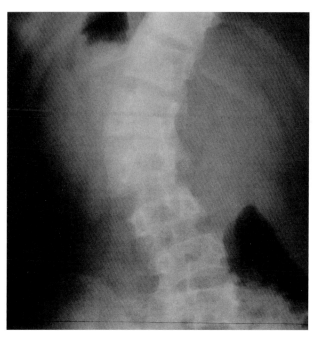

FIGURE 2. Anteroposterior radiograph shows dysplasia, subluxation, and marked rotation of the lumbar vertebrae. This situation can be exacerbated if the distal extent of the fusion ends amid these vertebrae or if a derotation maneuver is performed.

Patients with Marfan Habitus

Natural History

The prevalence of scoliosis among persons with Marfan habitus ranges from 34% to 88% (12,20,28,43,52).

Age at Onset

The age at onset of scoliosis among patients with Marfan habitus is similar to that among patients with the true syndrome. In this group, the average age at presentation ranges from 8.7 years to 10.5 years (43,52). In one series the scoliosis of seven of eight patients became apparent in the adolescent age period (43).

Presentation

No patient with the Marfan habitus in the series of Makin et al. (28) had back pain. In the series of Robins et al. (43), eight of 19 patients (42%) had scoliosis, and five of these had back pain. Fixed pelvic obliquity has not been reported among these patients.

Curve Types

Whereas double curves appear to predominate among patients with Marfan syndrome, patients with Marfan habitus appear to have a predominance of single curve patterns, especially right thoracic and thoracolumbar curves.

Curve Magnitude and Progression

The average curve at presentation (average age, 11.3 years) was 53.6 degrees in the series of Taneja and Manning (52), who also found curve progression (average, 10.5 degrees per year) to be slightly more rapid among patients with Marfan habitus than among those with Marfan syndrome. On the contrary, the patients with Marfan habitus in the report of Joseph et al. (20) appeared to have less rapid progression.

Treatment Recommendations

Nonoperative

Although it is generally accepted that the scoliosis associated with Marfan syndrome is probably recalcitrant to treatment with orthotic devices, an initial attempt should be made to manage the curves with an appropriate brace. We believe that once the curve reaches 20 degrees, consideration should be given to fitting a brace. Many patients experience difficulty in brace wear because of their asthenic body type or the presence of anterior chest wall deformities (52). Many authors believe that bracing is effective in holding in place a curve in a younger child until spinal fusion can be performed at an older age (35,43,44,52). Most researchers, however, have come to the conclusion that brace treatment is generally ineffective in preventing the need for spinal fusion.

Operative

Posterior spinal fusion should be considered once a curve reaches a magnitude greater than 40 degrees or if there is a rapid or documented progression of curve magnitude. Savini et al. (44) suggested fusion for curves greater than 50 degrees. There appears to be a higher than normal occurrence of mechanical problems with instrumentation and of pseudarthrosis (1,4,5,43,44), although this issue is debatable (52,60). For concomitant kyphosis, most authors recommend the addition of an anterior procedure (1,4,5,44). Most of these patients can safely undergo the rigors of spinal surgery if a thorough preoperative evaluation is performed.

Preoperative Considerations. Preoperative cardiac and pulmonary examinations should be meticulously performed and the results carefully weighed. Hemodynamic changes usually are poorly tolerated by patients with mitral and aortic regurgitation or aortic aneurysm. Goldberg (15) mentioned the theoretical possibility that overdistraction of the spine may transmit forces to the mediastinum and an intrinsically weak aortic root. Curve correction should not exceed the correction observed on preoperative side-bending radiographs. Patients with concomitant thoracic lordosis and pectus excavatum may encounter respiratory insufficiency at the time of the operation because of the compromise in chest space. Most surgeons agree, however, that the presence of cardiovascular abnormalities is not an absolute contraindication to spinal surgery. Mesrobian and Epps (33) believe that the preoperative evaluation should include elicitation for a history of dyspnea in various positions, a review of the tracheal air column on preoperative radiographs, and pulmonary function tests with flow volume loops in standing, prone, and supine positions.

The blood needs of these patients can be met safely with the use of predeposited autologous blood and meticulous hemostasis. MacEwen et al. (27) showed that the blood needs of patients weighing even less than 45 kg can be met by an autologous blood program without a concomitant increase in morbidity. Loder et al. (25) published an article concerning the use of somatosensory evoked potentials in operations on patients with nonidiopathic scoliosis. In their series, three patients had scoliosis associated with Marfan syndrome. In every instance, a somatosensory evoked potential was elicited. Thus this intraoperative monitoring modality should be used in operations on patients with Marfan syndrome in a manner comparable with its use in operations on patients with idiopathic scoliosis along with the monitoring of motor-evoked potentials. A wake-up test should be performed in the absence of motor-evoked potentials.

Surgical Options. Posterior spinal fusion with autogenous iliac crest bone graft and instrumentation is the mainstay in the treatment of scoliosis. Many studies report the use of no instrumentation or of Harrington distraction rods with good results (43,44,52,57). Isolated reports have appeared concerning the use of segmental fixation and multihook systems. Sublaminar wires, whether used in conjunction with Harrington rods or standard Luque or Unit rod instrumentation, have the advantage of restoring kyphosis to the hyperlordotic thoracic spine in selected patients. Wisconsin wiring can be used in conjunction with Harrington rods for added stability. Because these curves often are quite rigid, the effectiveness of the derotation maneuver with the Cotrel-Dubousset technique is not certain. Fusion to the sacrum has not been reported and is probably rarely indicated. Rigid curves may require anterior release and fusion before the posterior procedure, however, no patient in our series needed an anterior procedure. Preoperative traction is rarely effective and is not used. Side-bending radiographs should be used to determine curve flexibility and fusion levels. We disagree with Donaldson and Brown (11), who recommend using the same guidelines for choosing fusion levels as for patients with idiopathic scoliosis. It is mandatory that all curves, including compensatory curves, be fused. Use of the criteria set forth by King et al. (21) for the selection of fusion levels is not applicable to the patient population with Marfan syndrome (Fig. 3).

The role of subcutaneous Harrington instrumentation in the care of very young children with much growth potential is debatable. Joseph et al. (20) described a 4-year-old girl with a 90-degree curve that had progressed despite bracing. The girl was treated with limited posterior fusion and a subcutaneous Harrington rod. Fifty percent correction was achieved, but the patient still had complications. Sponseller et al. (47) treated three patients with a Harrington rod without fusion at a mean age of 3 years. The curves ranged from 60 to 80 degrees before surgery, and the treatment lasted an average of 30 months. Two cases of inferior rod dislodgment occurred.

Postoperative Management. Important considerations should be given to the postoperative management of these patients. Although the guidelines are essentially the same as those for any operation of this magnitude, careful attention should be given to the type of immobilization used. Hook displacement and dislodgment and pseudarthrosis have been reported among patients who received inadequate or no postoperative immobilization (1,62). Even patients who have supplemental sublaminar wires or multihook systems should have some form of postoperative immobilization.

Complications. There is debate whether patients with Marfan syndrome have a higher incidence of complications after spinal surgery than do other patients (5,60). It is important to analyze whether the complications are caused by extraneous factors, such as the type of instrumentation, or whether intrinsic factors of the syndrome are responsible for the complications.

Mechanical problems with instrumentation have been reported, although these may be related to the type of instrumentation and lack of postoperative immobilization rather than the patient's condition.

Amis and Herring (1) reported a case of iatrogenic kyphosis following operative correction of 50-degree right lumbar scoliosis managed with Harrington compression and distraction rods from T10 to L5. Forceful distraction caused dislocation of the facet joint and disruption of the disc space, which caused severe progressive kyphosis. The curve had corrected completely, which was 25 degrees more than that achieved on the side-bending radiographs. The patient was immobilized postoperatively with a Jewett brace. A postoperative lateral radiograph showed iatrogenic kyphosis with posterior wedging of the disc space between T11 and T12, facet joint distraction, and an avulsed fragment from the body of T11. Eighteen months later the kyphosis measured 70 degrees. The instrumentation was removed, and anterior discectomy with rib strut grafting was performed. Two weeks later posterior spinal fusion was performed with with Harrington instrumentation and autogenous iliac crest bone grafting. Two pseudarthroses were found at the operation. The authors speculated that if a body cast had been used, the pseudarthroses might not have developed. They concluded that in the care of patients with ligamentous laxity, compression instrumentation should extend through the uppermost instrumented vertebra, excessive distraction forces should not be used, and the degree of correction should not exceed that obtained on the preoperative side-bending radiographs.

Winter and Anderson (62) reported that one patient with Marfan syndrome underwent posterior spinal fusion with a Harrington distraction rod and sublaminar wires. The curve had been corrected to 2 degrees. No postoperative immobilization was used, and the patient subsequently dislodged the inferior hook, lost the curve correction, and had pseudarthrosis. These authors suggested wiring the two most distal spinous processes together to prevent this complication.

Taneja and Manning (52) had a patient in whom the upper Harrington hook cut through the facet joint. Savini et al. (44) treated four patients who had rotation of the upper Harrington hook and three who had dislodgment of the lower hook, two of which dislodged after rupture of the laminae due to pseudarthrosis. Savini et al. concluded that Harrington instrumentation is useful but that vertebral dysplasia causes a higher frequency of mechanical problems.

Hutchinson and Bassett (18) reported a case of superior mesenteric artery syndrome in a girl with Marfan syndrome who underwent posterior spinal fusion in situ. The girl was in the eightieth percentile for height and the seventh percentile for weight. One week after the operation, the patient was placed in

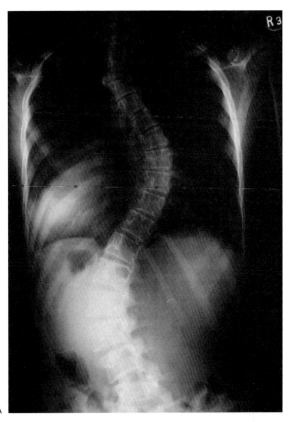

A

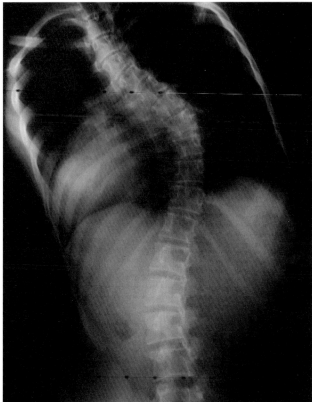

B

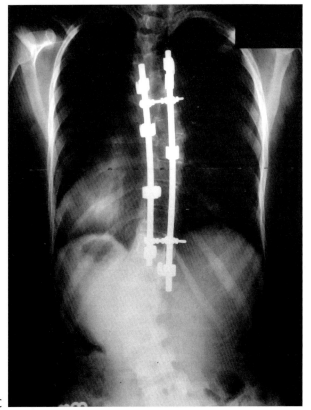

C

FIGURE 3. A: Anteroposterior radiograph of a 14-year-old girl with a 40-degree left cervicothoracic curve, 62-degree right thoracic curve, and 56-degree left lumbar curve. **B:** Preoperative side-bending radiographs show correction of the lumbar curve to 22 degrees. **C:** Two years postoperatively the lumbar curve has progressed to 44 degrees. Fusion should have been performed at the beginning.

a body cast, which corrected the curve to 35 degrees. The patient was treated with intravenous fluids and nasogastric suctioning, and the cast was removed, thus resolving the symptoms.

It is a commonly held belief that patients with Marfan syndrome tend to have a higher incidence of pseudarthrosis than do other patients. Although pseudarthrosis has been reported in many series, the true incidence remains unknown. Birch and Herring (5) were able to achieve only three solid fusions in nine patients who underwent posterior spinal fusion. The rest of the patients had pseudarthrosis and complications. Five patients with pseudarthrosis occurred in the series of Robins et al. (43), even though the surgeons had used meticulous technique and autogenous bone graft. Makin et al. (28) and Taneja and Manning (52) each described one patient with this complication. Winter (57) had treated three patients who had pseudarthrosis; all patients had double curves. In the series of Savini et al. (44), two patients treated with bank bone had pseudarthrosis. Amis and Herring (1) attributed the two cases of pseudarthrosis that occurred in their patient to the lack of adequate postoperative immobilization. Winter and Anderson (62) also treated a patient who had no postoperative immobilization and who had multiple pseudarthroses. Sponseller et al. (48) had only one young patient who had pseudarthrosis. There was no case of pseudarthrosis or

hardware failure in our series. We attributed this to meticulous exposure and decortication with facet fusion and the use of autogenous iliac crest bone and postoperative immobilization in an underarm orthosis (Fig. 4).

Respiratory failure caused by kyphoscoliosis led to cor pulmonale in a patient with scoliosis greater than 100 degrees, kyphosis greater than 20 degrees, and a vital capacity less than 1 L (54). This was therefore not a complication of the operation but of the patient's condition. Mesrobian and Epps (33) reported a midthoracic tracheal obstruction caused by Harrington rod displacement in a boy who underwent posterior spinal fusion with Harrington compression and distraction rods for severe scoliosis. Preoperative radiographs revealed that the patient had thoracic lordosis with close approximation of the sternum and thoracic vertebrae at the level of the thoracic outlet. A postoperative radiograph showed complete loss of the tracheal air column at the same level. The authors speculated that the combination of structural weakness of the cartilaginous sternochondral junction and trachea, dilatation of the aortic root, and abnormal vertebral curvature contributed to this problem.

Results Obtained or to Be Expected. In the report of Taneja and Manning (52), the average correction obtained was 38.2%,

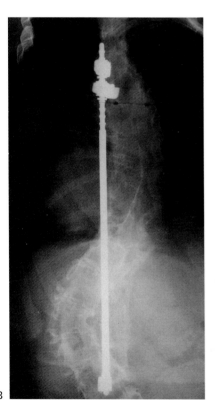 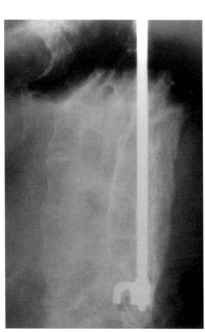 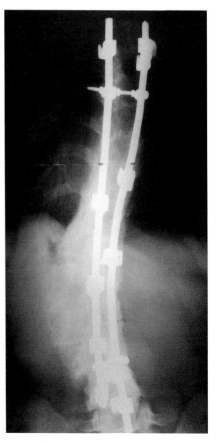

A,B
C

FIGURE 4. Anteroposterior **(A)** and lateral **(B)** radiographs of Harrington instrumentation. **C:** Anteroposterior radiograph of Cotrel-Dubousset instrumentation. Solid fusion mass is present in both cases, regardless of the type of instrumentation, with no hardware failure or pseudarthrosis at long-term follow-up evaluation.

the final curve showing an average loss of 9.9 degrees of correction. Robins et al. (43) reported an overall average correction of 41%, which they believed to be comparable with that seen in idiopathic scoliosis. The patient of Makin et al. (28) had an average 44% correction, whereas correction ranged from 10% to 81% in the series of Joseph et al. (20). Winter (57) reported almost no loss of postoperative correction at follow-up evaluations in his series. Winter and Anderson (62) reported the results of posterior spinal fusion with sublaminar wiring for 100 patients, five of whom had Marfan syndrome. The average preoperative curve among these patients was 52 degrees, and the average curve at follow-up evaluations was 29 degrees, representing an average curve correction of 33 degrees. Sponseller et al. (48) reported the results for nine children who underwent surgery at a mean age of 6.6 years. The mean immediate postoperative correction was 51%; however, after a mean follow-up period of 4 years, this correction was only 20%. The five patients treated with segmental fixation and Luque rods had a mean correction of 29%, whereas those treated with Harrington rod instrumentation had a mean correction of only 3%.

Miscellaneous Deformities

Sinclair et al. (45) reported the skeletal manifestations in 40 Marfan patients according to those thought to be caused by tissue and ligamentous laxity and those that were incidental findings. These included loss of normal lordosis in the cervical spine; thoracic kyphosis, scoliosis, rotation, "slipping" of vertebrae, compression fractures, and osteochondral dystrophy; and lumbar spondylolisthesis and vertebral dysplasia. Incidental findings included cervical spina bifida and congenital fusion, thoracic epiphysitis, and lumbar spina bifida. Seven patients had back pain. Additional problems listed included sacroiliac sclerosis, lumbar scoliosis, congenital fusion of sacroiliac joints, flattening of the thoracic vertebrae, and osteochondritis of the thoracic and lumbar vertebrae. There was no mention of treatment or subsequent outcome. Tallroth et al. (51) reported an 18% prevalence of lumbosacral transitional vertebra in their series (4% to 6% in the normal population) as well as the appearance of biconcave vertebral bodies, also known as *codfish vertebra.*

Thoracic Lordosis

Patients with Marfan syndrome may have a reversal of the normal sagittal alignment of the spine (Fig. 5). Thoracic lordosis or lumbar kyphosis occurs in some of these patients. Thoracic lordosis, especially in combination with pectus excavatum, can cause respiratory difficulty because of the narrowed anteroposterior (sternovertebral) diameter of the chest. The thoracic lordosis usually is associated with concomitant loss of normal lumbar lordosis (Fig. 6). Approximately two thirds of patients with Marfan syndrome have thoracic lordosis, regardless of the presence of scoliosis (15). Sponseller et al. (47) reported five variations in the sagittal alignment of the spine among these patients. Winter (61) reported the results of treatment of two patients for thoracic lordoscoliosis. The operative technique entailed the use of paired, square-ended Harrington distraction rods, square-

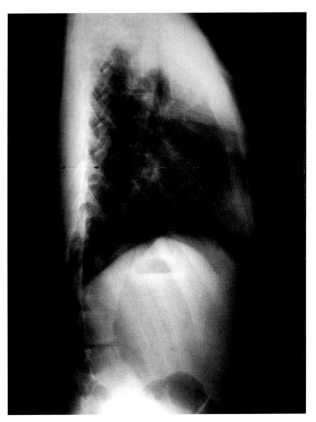

FIGURE 5. Lateral radiograph shows reversal of normal sagittal alignment, thoracic lordosis, and lumbar kyphosis.

ended hooks, and sublaminar wires. In no instance did wire cut through the laminae or did postoperative wire breakage occur.

Thoracic and Thoracolumbar Kyphosis

Approximately 10% of patients with Marfan syndrome have thoracic and thoracolumbar kyphosis, which usually manifests late in infancy or early in childhood and is most obvious when the child is sitting. Exercises to improve muscle tone often result in improvement, but many cases persist and progress during adolescence (15). Radiographically this deformity can mimic Scheuermann disease in that end plate irregularities often are noticed; Scheuermann disease, however, rarely occurs in the thoracolumbar spine.

Kyphosis of the thoracic spine has been reported among patients with Marfan syndrome, although Winter stated that it is rare (57). Sponseller et al. (47) reported that 41% of their patients had kyphosis greater than 50 degrees. It is usually part of the scoliotic deformity, causing kyphoscoliosis. Taneja and Manning (52) found a 45% incidence of "marked" kyphosis among their patients with Marfan syndrome and 11% among the patients with Marfan habitus. Savini et al. (44) had three patients with kyphosis that ranged from 50 to 100 degrees. Makin et al. (28) and Joseph et al. (20) each had three patients with kyphosis. Concomitant kyphosis can cause difficulties in treatment, as evidenced by the cases of Amis and Herring (1)

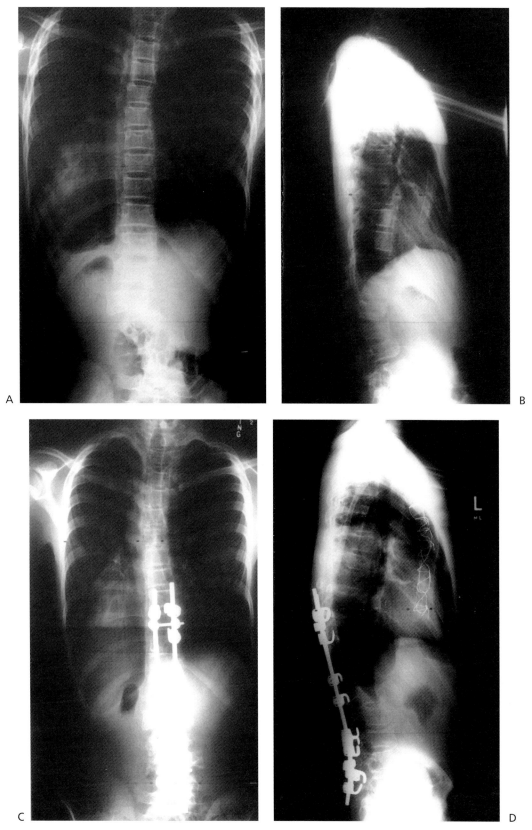

FIGURE 6. A 14-year-old boy with Marfan syndrome and progressive lumbar kyphosis and scoliosis. **A:** Anteroposterior view shows marked rotation in the lumbar curve with translatory shifts of L2 on L3 and L3 on L4. **B:** Marked lumbar kyphosis is visible with posture subluxation of L3 on L4 and secondary adaptive changes in vertebral shape. **C, D:** The patient was successfully treated by posterior spinal fusion and instrumentation. (Courtesy of Stuart Weinstein, M.D.)

and Birch and Herring (5). In the report of Birch and Herring, Luque instrumentation failed in one patient with thoracolumbar kyphosis, leading to pseudarthrosis. They suggested anterior and posterior fusion for kyphosis. However, this method of treatment was not without problems; four patients with pseudarthrosis and kyphosis who had anterior and posterior operations had a total of 19 procedures, leading the surgeons to recommend segmental fixation with massive amounts of bone graft.

Cervical Spine Deformities

Levander et al. (24) reported the case of a woman with Marfan syndrome who had exaggerated deep tendon reflexes and paresthesia and weakness in all extremities when her head was flexed. Functional stenosis with flexion was found to be the cause of the neurologic symptoms, and occipitocervical stabilization relieved the symptoms. Nelson (38) reported the case of a patient with vertebral dysplasia in the cervical spine. The bodies of C3, C4, and C5 were tall and narrow with posterior scalloping, the importance of which was not discussed. Sinclair et al. (45) also described anomalies in the cervical spine. Yajnik et al. (63) reported the case of a patient with basilar impression. Hobbs et al. (17) reported a prevalence of focal kyphosis of 16%, and 35% of the patients had a loss of normal cervical lordosis. Hobbs et al. also found increased atlantoaxial translation in 54% of the patients and basilar impression in 36%. There was no increased frequency of developmental spinal stenosis or neck pain.

Congenital Spine Deformities

There is no report in the literature that deals solely with the topic of congenital spinal deformity in association with Marfan syndrome. It would seem that the appearance of scoliosis with congenital dysplasia of the vertebrae is incidental.

Spondylolisthesis

Spondylolisthesis has been reported infrequently among patients with Marfan syndrome (Fig. 7). Taylor (53) speculated that it is a result of the ligamentous laxity and poor musculature that occurs among these patients. In most reported cases, the deformity is described as severe (44,53,58). Makin et al. (28) described four patients who had either spondylolisthesis or spondylolysis; however, these authors did not differentiate between patients with true Marfan syndrome and those with Marfan habitus, nor did they comment on treatment or outcome. In the report by Sinclair et al. (45), spondylolisthesis is mentioned; one patient was found to have posterior slipping of L2 on L3. Sponseller et al. (47) reported a prevalence of spondylolisthesis of 6% among patients with Marfan syndrome, compared with 3% among the general population. The average slip was 30%, compared with 15% among otherwise healthy patients. Patients with the typical findings of lumbosacral step-off, flat buttocks, tight hamstrings (limited straight leg raising), and radicular pain in the backs of the legs should have undergo additional studies to delineate the cause. We believe that among children, posterolateral fusion in situ with autogenous iliac crest bone graft yields

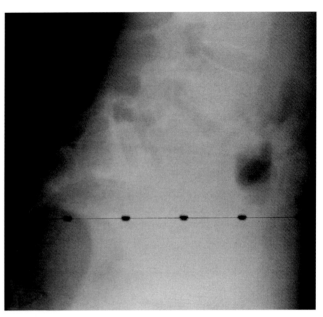

FIGURE 7. Lateral radiograph of a 15-year-old boy with a grade II spondylolisthesis.

satisfactory results without the associated risk of neurologic injury from reduction maneuvers or instrumentation. Patients should be immobilized postoperatively for at least 4 months in a pantaloon spica cast.

Scheuermann Disease

Makin et al. (28) and Sinclair et al. (45) described patients with Scheuermann disease, but no details were given concerning its importance, characteristics, or treatment.

Scoliosis and Chest Wall Deformity

Waters et al. (55) conducted a study to define the incidence and characteristics of scoliosis among patients with pectus carinatum and pectus excavatum. They found that there is an association between Marfan syndrome, scoliosis, and anterior chest wall deformity. Of the patients with pectus excavatum, three had Marfan syndrome. Of the patients with pectus carinatum, two had Marfan syndrome. Waters et al. concluded that the presence of pectus deformities and scoliosis is a risk factor for Marfan syndrome.

Dural Ectasia and Meningocele

Dural ectasia, or widening of the spinal canal, appears to be a relatively common finding among patients with Marfan syndrome (49). Pyeritz et al. (41) found that 33 of 51 patients who underwent computed tomography had dural ectasia in the lower lumbar and sacral areas. The cause is thought to be an abnormality in the dura, which stretches with cerebrospinal fluid pressure. Intrasacral meningocele has been reported to occur in a few patients (2,13,16,34,50). Although most reports in the literature concern adult patients, it is worth mentioning this condition should a patient have low back pain or radicular pain. We prefer magnetic resonance imaging over myelography in the diagnosis of sacral meningocele because of its better resolution and noninvasive nature.

SUMMARY

The disorder of connective tissue first described by the French pediatrician Marfan in 1896 is still an enigma. There is no way to reverse its effects on various systems, and treatment is mainly symptomatic. Until strict diagnostic criteria are used by researchers writing on the subject, exact details concerning the syndrome and its variants will remain elusive. Although the lifelong prognosis differs for patients with true Marfan syndrome and for those with Marfan habitus, management of spinal deformities for either group is relatively consistent. Scoliosis among patients with Marfan syndrome should be detected early and controlled by means of bracing. Although bracing may not be totally effective in preventing an operation, it can help postpone surgery until the child's condition is medically stable or the child is closer to skeletal maturity. All patients need a thorough preoperative cardiovascular evaluation. All curves should be fused, because the criteria of King et al., set forth for patients with idiopathic scoliosis, are not applicable to the patient population with Marfan syndrome or habitus. Standard posterior spinal fusion with rigid internal fixation should be performed. The value of derotational maneuvers is questionable and may even exacerbate the deformity. Copious amounts of autogenous iliac crest bone graft should be harvested. Postoperative immobilization in an underarm orthosis should be used until the fusion mass is solid. In spite of the pessimism in the literature regarding results of the operative management of scoliosis, with proper attention to details in the technique, selection of proper fusion levels, and appropriate instrumentation, good results can be obtained.

REFERENCES

1. Amis J, Herring JA (1984): Iatrogenic kyphosis: a complication of Harrington instrumentation in Marfan syndrome. *J Bone Joint Surg Am* 66:460–463.
2. Arroyo JF, Garcia JF (1989): Case report 582. *Skeletal Radiol* 18: 614–618.
3. Beals RK, Hecht F (1971): Congenital contractual arachnodactyly: a heritable disorder of connective tissue. *J Bone Joint Surg Am* 53: 987–993.
4. Beneux J, Rigault P, Poliquen JC (1978): Les deviations rachidiennes de la maladie de Marfan chez l'enfant. Etude de 20 cas. *Rev Chir Orthop* 64:471–485.
5. Birch JG, Herring JA (1987): Spinal deformity in Marfan syndrome. *J Pediatr Orthop* 7:546–552.
6. Birkenstock WE, Louw JH, Maze A, et al. (1973): Combined Ehlers-Danlos and Marfan syndromes. *S Afr Med J* 10:2097–2102.
7. Brenton DP, Dow CJ, James JIP, et al. (1972): Homocystinuria and Marfan syndrome: a comparison. *J Bone Joint Surg Br* 54:277–298.
8. Committee on Genetics (1996): Health supervision for children with Marfan syndrome. *Pediatrics* 98:978–982.
9. Daudon DP (1972): *Contribution a l'etude du syndrome de Marfan: les deviations vertebrales de ce syndrome propos de 21 observations du centre de Massues* [doctoral thesis]. Lyon, France.
10. Dietz HC, Cutting GR, Pyeritz RE, et al. (1991): Marfan syndrome caused by a recurrent de novo missense mutation in the fibrillin gene. *Nature* 352:337–339.
11. Donaldson DH, Brown CW (1996): Marfan's spinal pathology. In: Bridwell KH and DeWald RL, eds. *Textbook of spinal surgery,* 2nd ed. Philadelphia: Lippincott-Raven, pp. 299–306.
12. Fahey JJ (1939): Muscular and skeletal changes in arachnodactyly. *Arch Surg* 39:741–760.
13. Fishman EK, Zinreich SJ, Kumar AJ, et al. (1983): Sacral abnormalities in Marfan syndrome. *J Comput Assist Tomogr* 7:851–856.
14. Francke U, Furthmayr H (1994): Marfan's syndrome and other disorders of fibrillin. *N Engl J Med* 330:1384–1385.
15. Goldberg MJ, ed. (1987): Marfan and the marfanoid habitus. In: *The dysmorphic child: an orthopaedic perspective.* New York: Raven Press, pp. 83–108.
16. Harkens KL, El-Khoury GY (1989): Intrasacral meningocele in a patient with Marfan syndrome. *Spine* 15:610–612.
17. Hobbs WR, Sponseller PD, Weiss AP, et al. (1997): The cervical spine in Marfan syndrome. *Spine* 22:983–989.
18. Hutchinson DT, Bassett GS (1990): Superior mesenteric artery syndrome in pediatric orthopedic patients. *Clin Orthop* 250:250–257.
19. Jaffer J, Beighton P (1983): Syndrome identification case report 98: arachnodactyly, joint laxity, and spondylolisthesis. *J Clin Dysmorph* 1: 14–15.
20. Joseph KN, Kane HA, Milner RS, et al. (1992): Orthopedic aspects of the Marfan phenotype. *Clin Orthop* 277:251–261.
21. King HA, Moe JH, Bradford DS, et al. (1983): The selection of fusion levels in thoracic idiopathic scoliosis. *J Bone Joint Surg Am* 65: 1302–1313.
22. LeDelliou M (1983): *Contribution a l'etude du syndrome de Marfan* [thesis]. Universite Claude Bernard, Lyon, France.
23. Lee B, Godfrey M, Vitale E, et al. (1991): Linkage of Marfan syndrome and a phenotypically related disorder to two different fibrillin genes. *Nature* 352:330–334.
24. Levander B, Mellstrom A, Grepe A (1981): Atlantoaxial instability in Marfan syndrome: diagnosis and treatment. *Neuroradiology* 21:43–46.
25. Loder RT, Thomson GJ, LaMont RL (1991): Spinal cord monitoring in patients with nonidiopathic spinal deformities using somatosensory evoked potentials. *Spine* 16:1359–1364.
26. Lowry RB, Guichon VC (1972): Congenital contractural arachnodactyly: a syndrome simulating Marfan syndrome. *Can Med Assoc J* 107: 531–532.
27. MacEwen GD, Bennett E, Guille JT (1990): Autologous blood transfusion in patients with low body weight undergoing spinal surgery. *J Pediatr Orthop* 10:750–753.
28. Makin M, MacEwen GD, Steel HH (1984): Marfan syndrome and its marfanoid SAJ variant. *Journal of the Western Pacific Orthopaedic Association* 21:29–36.
29. Marfan AG (1896): Un cas de deformation congenitale des 4 membres plus pronouncee aux extremities, caracterisee par l'allongement des os avec un certain degre d'amincissement. *Bull Soc Med Hop Paris* 13: 220–226.
30. Maslen CL, Corson GM, Maddox BK, et al. (1991): Partial sequence of a candidate gene for the Marfan syndrome. *Nature* 352:334–337.
31. McKusick VA (1991): The defect in Marfan syndrome. *Nature* 352: 279–281.
32. Mery H, Babonneix L (1902): Un cas de deformation congenitale des quatre membres: hyperchondroplasie. *Bull Soc Med Hop Paris* 19: 671–676.
33. Mesrobian RB, Epps JL (1986): Clinical reports: midtracheal obstruction after Harrington rod placement in a patient with Marfan syndrome. *Anesth Analg* 65:411–413.
34. Mitchell GE, Lourie H, Berne AS (1967): The various causes of scalloped vertebrae with notes on their pathogenesis. *Radiology* 89:67–74.
35. Moe JH (1977): Marfan disorder in scoliosis. In: Zorab PA, ed. *Scoliosis.* London: Academic Press, pp. 257–260.
36. Murdoch JL, Walker BA, Halpern BL, et al. (1972): Life expectancy and causes of death in the Marfan syndrome. *N Engl J Med* 286: 804–808.
37. Murdoch JL, Walker BA, McKusick VA (1972): Parental age effects

on the occurrence of new mutations for the Marfan syndrome. *Ann Hum Genet* 35:331–336.

38. Nelson JD (1958): The Marfan syndrome, with special reference to congenital enlargement of the spinal canal. *Br J Radiol* 31:561–564.
39. Orcutt FV, DeWald RL (1974): The special problems which the Marfan syndrome introduces to scoliosis. *J Bone Joint Surg Am* 56:1763.
40. Pyeritz RE (1982): The Marfan phenotype: pleiotropy and variability as clues to genetic heterogeneity. In: Akeson WH, Bornstein P, Glimcher MJ, eds. *Symposium on heritable disorders of connective tissue.* St. Louis: CV Mosby, pp. 114–121.
41. Pyeritz RE, Fishman EK, Bernhardt BA, et al. (1988): Dural ectasia is a common feature of the Marfan syndrome. *Am J Hum Genet* 43: 726–732.
42. Pyeritz RE, Murphy EA, McKusick VA (1979): Clinical variability in the Marfan syndrome. *Birth Defects* 15:155–178.
43. Robins PR, Moe JH, Winter RB (1975): Scoliosis in Marfan syndrome: its characteristics and results of treatment in thirty-five patients. *J Bone Joint Surg Am* 57:358–368.
44. Savini R, Cervellati S, Beroaldo E (1980): Spinal deformities in Marfan syndrome. *Ital J Orthop Traumatol* 6:19–40.
45. Sinclair RJG, Kitchin AH, Turner RWD (1960): The Marfan syndrome. *Q J Med* 113:19–53.
46. Sliman N (1971): A propos de 16 cas de scoliosis-Marfan. *Tunis Med* 2:93.
47. Sponseller PD, Hobbs W, Riley LH, et al. (1995): The thoracolumbar spine in Marfan syndrome. *J Bone Joint Surg Am* 77:867–876.
48. Sponseller PD, Sethi N, Cameron DE, et al. (1997): Infantile scoliosis in Marfan syndrome. *Spine* 22:509–516.
49. Stern WE (1988): Dural ectasia and the Marfan syndrome. *J Neurosurg* 69:221–227.
50. Strand RD, Eisenberg HM (1971): Anterior sacral meningocele in association with Marfan syndrome. *Radiology* 99:653–654.
51. Tallroth K, Malmivaara A, Laitinen ML, et al. (1995): Lumbar spine in Marfan syndrome. *Skeletal Radiol* 24:337–340.
52. Taneja DK, Manning CW (1977): Scoliosis in Marfan syndrome and arachnodactyly. In: Zorab PA, ed. *Scoliosis.* London: Academic Press, pp. 261–281.
53. Taylor LJ (1987): Severe spondylolisthesis and scoliosis in association with Marfan syndrome: case report and review of the literature. *Clin Orthop* 221:207–211.
54. Wanderman KL, Goldstein MS, Faver J (1975): Cor pulmonale secondary to severe kyphoscoliosis in Marfan syndrome. *Chest* 67: 250–251.
55. Waters P, Welch K, Micheli LJ, et al. (1989): Scoliosis in children with pectus excavatum and pectus carinatum. *J Pediatr Orthop* 9:551–556.
56. Wilner HI, Finby N (1964): Skeletal manifestations in the Marfan syndrome. *JAMA* 187:490–495.
57. Winter RB (1977): The surgical treatment of scoliosis in Marfan syndrome. In: Zorab PA, ed. *Scoliosis.* London: Academic Press, pp. 283–299.
58. Winter RB (1982): Severe spondylolisthesis in Marfan syndrome: report of two cases. *J Pediatr Orthop* 2:51–55.
59. Winter RB (1987): Marfan syndrome. In: Bradford DS, ed. *Moe's textbook of scoliosis.* Philadelphia: WB Saunders, pp. 554–560.
60. Winter RB (1988): Letters to the editors. *J Pediatr Orthop* 8:507.
61. Winter RB (1990): Thoracic lordoscoliosis in Marfan syndrome: report of two patients with surgical correction using rods and sublaminar wires. *Spine* 15:233–235.
62. Winter RB, Anderson MB (1985): Spinal arthrodesis for spinal deformity using posterior instrumentation and sublaminar wiring. *Int Orthop* 9:239–245.
63. Yajnik VH, Kshatriya PK, Vaidya MH, et al. (1975): Marfan syndrome, ventricular septal defect and basilar impression in one patient. *J Indian Med Assoc* 64:242–244.

28

CHIARI MALFORMATIONS, SYRINGOMYELIA, AND THE TETHERED CORD SYNDROME

PAUL A. GRABB
VIRINDER NOHRIA
W. JERRY OAKES

The emphasis of this chapter is on the clinical aspects and management of Chiari malformations, syringomyelia, and tethered spinal cord. Although traditionally considered products of dysembryogenesis, all three of these entities can be acquired as well, through inflammatory, infectious, neoplastic, or iatrogenic mechanisms. At times two or three of these entities occur simultaneously as part of a constellation of malformations or as interrelated pathophysiologic processes (17). This interrelationship makes dividing a chapter neatly into three components each addressing a single entity somewhat artificial. For the sake of discussion however, we address each entity separately and highlight any associations between or among Chiari malformations, syringomyelia, and tethered spinal cord.

CHIARI MALFORMATIONS

Although four types of Chiari malformations have been described, types I and II account for 99% of the clinical cases. Chiari I malformation involves descent of the cerebellar tonsils below the plane of the foramen magnum (Fig. 1). The cerebellar tonsils can be situated below the foramen magnum as a normal finding called *cerebellar ectopia.* This tends to occur more commonly between 5 and 15 years of age. The presence of up to 5 mm of cerebellar ectopia in this age group is considered by many investigators to fall within the normal range (10). The distinction between innocent cerebellar ectopia and true symptomatic Chiari malformation can be difficult in evaluations of a children. Chiari I malformations are not associated with myelomeningocele but infrequently may be associated with occult spinal dysraphism, such as spinal lipoma. Chiari II malformations are hindbrain hernias associated with myelomeningocele. In Chiari II malformation, the descent cerebellar vermis may be

associated with caudal displacement of the medulla and the lower pons (Fig. 2). Often there is caudal displacement of the fourth ventricle and of the inferior cerebellar vermis into the upper cervical spinal canal and sometimes as low as the level of T4. Chiari III malformations are herniation of the posterior fossa contents through a bifid upper cervical canal. Chiari IV malformations involve agenesis of the cerebellum and no herniation of structures. Chiari IV malformation is not a surgical entity.

Etiology

Chiari I

The pathologic changes and the disordered anatomic features that occur among patients with Chiari malformation encompass an imaging and clinical spectrum from asymptomatic mild tonsillar ectopia to profound crowding of the foramen magnum and upper cervical canal with life-threatening symptoms and signs. During a surgical procedure the tonsils can be recognized readily because of the vertical orientation of their folia. The tonsillar loop of the posterior inferior cerebellar artery usually accompanies the cerebellum in its caudal descent. With long-standing compression, the tips of the tonsils may lose their fine pial vascularity and foliar pattern and appear pale. The tips of the tonsils can be tough and histologically gliotic. In Chiari I malformation, the denticulate ligaments, cervical nerve roots, fourth ventricle, and brain stem are in their normal positions. There are multiple mechanisms by which tonsillar descent can cause Chiari I malformation. Increased intracranial pressure from a supratentorial tumor or hydrocephalus gradually can lead to tonsillar herniation and the clinical signs and symptoms of Chiari malformation (Fig. 3). The presence of a lumboperitoneal shunt inserted to manage hydrocephalus can cause symptomatic tonsillar herniation (Fig. 4), especially among children (14,15,60).

These first two mechanisms clearly show that abnormal pressure gradients over time can cause Chiari I malformation. Multiple studies have addressed the possibility that the posterior fossa cranial volume can be relatively small for its contents, hence

P.A. Grabb and W.J. Oakes: Department of Surgery, Division of Neurosurgery, University of Alabama at Birmingham, Children's Hospital of Alabama, Birmingham, Alabama 35233.

V. Nohria: DevCo Pharmaceuticals Incorporated, Durham, North Carolina 27703.

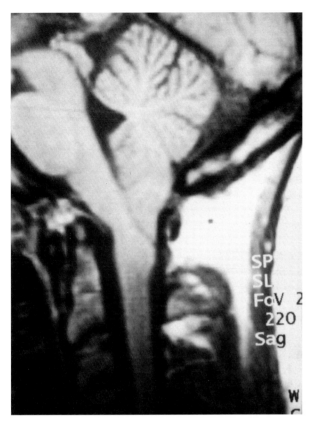

FIGURE 1. Sagittal, T1-weighted magnetic resonance image shows a typical Chiari I malformation. Crowded foramen magnum and cerebellar tonsil tips at the lower border of C1 are evident.

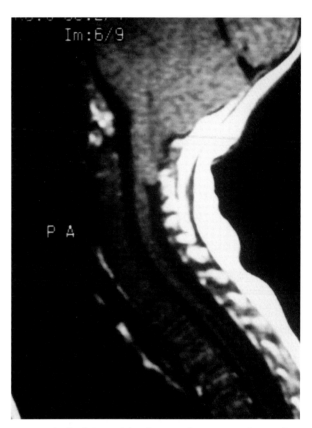

FIGURE 2. Sagittal, T1-weighted magnetic resonance image shows a typical Chiari II malformation. The entire posterior fossa is crowded, and the fourth ventricle is compressed and caudally situated. The caudal end of the pons is at the level of the basion, and the medulla is in the upper cervical canal.

growth of the neural tissue follows the path of least resistance out the foramen magnum. In multisuture craniosynostosis when both lambdoid sutures have premature synostosis there is a high likelihood of tonsillar herniation. It is presumed that synostosis of the lambdoids does not allow adequate bony expansion of the posterior fossa to accommodate the neural contents (16). Acquired malformations of the skull base that reduce posterior fossa volume from progressive basilar invagination, such as osteogenesis imperfecta, can be associated with Chiari I malformation. The infrequent but real association of Chiari I malformation with occult spinal dysraphism suggests an embryologic event or condition that leads to tonsillar herniation. There are clearly multiple causes of Chiari I malformation. Determining which one is operative for an individual patient however, may not be obvious.

Chiari II

Whereas Chiari I malformation can have multiple causes, Chiari II malformation is almost exclusively associated with myelomeningocele. The mechanism of formation, however, remains disputed. The degree of neural malformation usually is much greater with Chiari II malformation because much of the posterior fossa contents, such as the brain stem, fourth ventricle, and vermis, are situated caudally. The caudal shift of the medulla

may distort and compress the fourth ventricle and obstruct the flow of cerebrospinal fluid (CSF) through the foramina of Magendie and Luschka into the subarachnoid space. The choroid plexus may be outside the fourth ventricle. The descended vermis may appear yellow and gliotic with or without loss of the normal horizontal foliar pattern over its caudal portion. The dorsal surface of the displaced vermis may be hypovascular or hypervascular. The course of the upper cervical nerve roots can be upward or horizontal, and the denticulate ligaments can be taut and angled upward. The entire upper cervical spine usually appears crowded. A posterior extradural band may greatly constrict the neural structures under the arch of C1. This band usually corresponds to the periosteum of C1. The foramen magnum is often enlarged. Within the posterior fossa, the transverse sinuses and the torcular herophili (confluence of the sinuses) may be displaced downward. They may be displaced to such a degree as to lie at the foramen magnum, making operative exposure of the posterior fossa potentially hazardous. The upper portion of the cerebellar vermis may rise through the enlarged tentorial notch. Fusion of the superior and the inferior colliculi on both sides into a single beaked structure is common (1). The petrous ridges and the clivus are concave, again emphasizing the reduced volume of the bony posterior fossa in relation to its crowded neural contents.

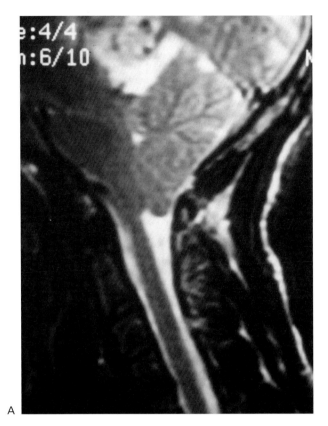

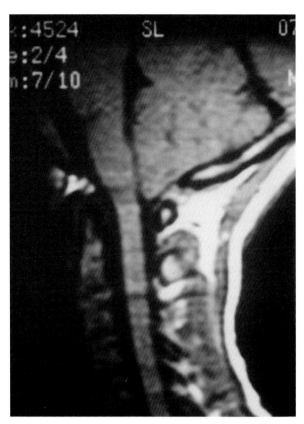

FIGURE 4. Sagittal, T1-weighted magnetic resonance image shows pointed tonsils below the foramen magnum in an 11-year-old child with neck pain and diplopia who had a lumboperitoneal shunt placed at 3 years of age.

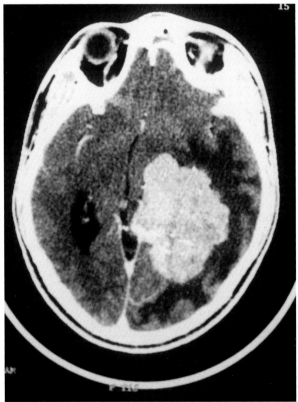

FIGURE 3. Sagittal, T2-weighted magnetic resonance image shows tonsillar herniation in a child with severe neck pain **(A)**. A contrasted computed tomographic scan of the head shows a huge intracranial tumor as the cause of elevated intrcranial pressure and tonsillar herniation **(B)**.

Hydrodynamic Theory

Chiari proposed that the herniation of the posterior fossa contents was the result of supratentorial hydrocephalus (13). Gardner has been the major proponent of the hydrodynamic theory (26). He suggested that the foramina of Magendie and Luschka are either delayed in embryonic opening or remain functionally closed. Thus the pulsatile flow of CSF from the fourth ventricle is obstructed, and a water hammer pulse effect is generated. The pulsatility of the anterior choroid plexus in the lateral ventricles may push the tentorium too far inferiorly, diminish the size of the posterior fossa, extrude the cerebellum and the hindbrain, kink the cervicomedullary junction, and further aggravate the embryonic hydrocephalus. Progression of the hydrocephalus may then cause other supratentorial and infratentorial abnormalities.

Patients with Chiari I malformation have a high incidence of traumatic delivery and presumed subarachnoid hemorrhage and cerebral compression (52,72). This is thought to result in the development of subarachnoid adhesions that restrict equilibration of intracranial and intraspinal CSF pressures associated with Valsalva maneuvers. This results in impaction of cerebellar tonsils and further aggravates the difficulty of achieving pressure equilibration. Evidence against this theory comes from animal studies in which arachnoiditis and subarachnoid adhesions were

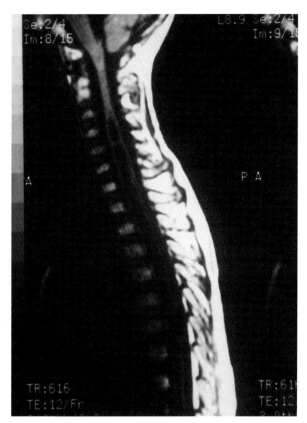

FIGURE 5. Sagittal, T1-weighted magnetic resonance image shows syringomyelia and an enlarged fourth ventricle in a child with a functioning ventriculoperitoneal shunt and a history of meningitis.

and posterior fossa content volume (neural elements) in adults with Chiari I malformation. They did not find any significant differences in these measurements compared with measurements of controls. When a ratio of neural content volume to osseous-dural defined volume was calculated, however, a difference was detected. This finding suggested that the patients with Chiari I malformation had relative overcrowding of the posterior fossa. Milhorat et al. (49) did find evidence of small posterior fossa volumes, reduced CSF volumes, and normal brain volumes in the posterior fossae of 364 patients with symptomatic Chiari I malformation.

McLone et al. (44,46) put forward a unified theory of Chiari II malformation based on their observations of genetic mutant mice with a sacral neural tube defect. The authors suggested that abnormal neurulation is an a priori feature of Chiari II malformation. Failure of correct timing of apposition and transient occlusion of spinal neuroceles lead to failure to maintain distention of the primitive ventricular system with CSF. Lack of distention of the rhombencephalic vesicles alters the inductive effect of pressure on the surrounding mesenchyma and endochondral bone formation and results in a small posterior fossa. Consequently, development of the cerebellum and the brain stem within the small posterior fossa leads to upward herniation, which produces an enlarged incisural opening and a dysplastic tentorium; downward herniation, which produces a large foramen magnum; and cerebellar vermis and brain stem displacement into the cervical spine. Hydrocephalus is caused by maldevelopment of the CSF pathways in the posterior fossa. This theory, supported with an animal model, seems the most compelling for explaining the pathogenesis of Chiari II malformation.

Clinical Features

The clinical signs and symptoms of Chiari malformation are truly protean and correlate with age at presentation (20,49,54,59). The symptoms can best be understood by remembering the anatomic structures that pass through the foramen magnum and upper cervical spine. There also may be symptoms referable to the accompanying syringomyelia and, in the case of the Chiari II malformation, the accompanying supratentorial anomalies, hydrocephalus, or myelomeningocele.

In a review of 39 patients with symptomatic Chiari I malformation, 30 of whom were younger than 19 years (54), there was a diversity of symptoms and signs (Tables 1, 2). The most common symptom was pain, and the most common site of pain was the occiput or neck. In a number of patients, the pain was exacerbated by laughing, coughing, running, or, in one case, by heading the ball while playing soccer. These episodic exacerbations are often electric shock–like in nature. The other sites of pain include the shoulder, back, and upper or lower extremities. Such pain is typically not dermatomal in distribution but is deep and usually burning. Movement of the neck also may elicit pain, and because the pain is not dermatomal, the initial symptoms are easily cast aside. Other common symptoms are attributable to lower cranial nerve dysfunction. The most common signs were those of motor and sensory deficit. Two patients had been labeled as having cerebral palsy at birth. One of the two had

caused by intracisternal injection of contrast agents and kaolin (77). In this model, cord cavities, which were in communication with the central canal or the fourth ventricle, were observed, but no hindbrain herniation was seen. Patients with basilar meningitis (Fig. 5) likewise may go on to have syringomyelia without Chiari malformation (5). Further support for the differential pressure theory has come from observations of progressive herniation of the well-developed cerebellar tonsils through the foramen magnum, which occurs years after insertion of a lumboperitoneal shunt (14,15,60).

Developmental Theories

Marin-Padilla and Marin-Padilla (42) proposed a small posterior fossa theory based on the concept of primary paraxial mesodermal insufficiency as a cause of Chiari II malformation. They observed that among in hamsters treated with vitamin A, underdevelopment of the occipital bone resulted in a small, short posterior fossa. The overall consequence is that the cerebellum must grow toward the foramen magnum, the pontine flexure is reduced, and the angle of the cervical flexure is increased. No experimental embryo, however, had displacement of the posterior fossa elements below the foramen magnum, and there were no other manifestations of Chiari malformation. Nishikawa et al. (53) measured posterior fossa volume (osseous-dural confines)

TABLE 1. SYMPTOMS AMONG 39 PATIENTS WITH CHIARI I MALFORMATION

Symptom	Number (%)
Pain	27 (69)
Weakness	29 (74)
Upper extremity	12 (31)
Lower extremity	7 (18)
Hemiparesis	7 (18)
Quadriparesis	3 (8)
Sensory changes	20 (50)
Numbness	17 (44)
Painless ulcers and fractures	5 (13)
Paresthesia	6 (15)
Clumsiness	6 (15)
Respiratory dysrhythmia	4 (10)
Dysphagia	4 (10)
Dysarthria	2 (5)
Hoarseness	3 (8)
Facial numbness	3 (8)
Hiccups	3 (8)
Severe snoring	2 (5)
Drop attacks	2 (5)
Urinary incontinence	2 (5)

fisting of both hands, and the other had varus deformity of both feet. The nystagmus that is characteristic among these patients is downbeat on down gaze and rotatory on lateral gaze. Esotropia without abducens paresis is a reversible deficit among this patient population (41).

Chiari II malformation is associated almost invariably with myelomeningocele, so most of these patients come to medical attention at birth for closure of their back lesions. However,

TABLE 2. CLINICAL SIGNS AMONG 39 PATIENTS WITH CHIARI I MALFORMATION

Sign	Number (%)
Weakness	36 (92)
Upper extremity	20 (51)
Lower extremity	6 (15)
Hemiparesis	7 (18)
Quadriparesis	3 (8)
Atrophy	5 (13)
Sensory loss	29 (74)
Fewer than three dermatomes	7 (18)
More than three dermatomes	22 (56)
Posterior columns	9 (23)
Charcot joints	2 (5)
Hyporeflexia	15 (38)
Upper extremity	13 (33)
Lower extremity	2 (5)
Hyperreflexia	17 (44)
Lower-extremity clonus	7 (18)
Babinski response	11 (28)
Ataxia	9 (23)
Nystagmus	9 (23)
Absence of gag reflex	8 (20)
Facial sensory loss	5 (13)
Tongue atrophy	3 (8)
Vocal cord palsy	3 (8)

only 20% of children with myelomeningocele have symptoms of Chiari II malformation (59). The symptoms and signs are more likely to be attributable to brain stem dysfunction with Chiari II malformation than they are with type I malformation.

A typical sequence of events in an infant with myelomeningocele and Chiari II malformation may be as follows. The spinal lesion is repaired in the neonatal period, and a ventriculoperitoneal shunt is inserted to manage progressive hydrocephalus. On the return visit, at 4 to 6 weeks of age, the mother reports that the infant is feeding poorly and is episodically arching the head backward. Nasal regurgitation of milk or formula may occur as evidence of palatal dysfunction. Neurogenic dysphagia should be considered an urgent problem and addressed promptly (63,64). When angered or agitated, the infant may develop an inspiratory wheeze or stridor, sometimes described as *crowing*, which may develop into actual periods of apnea and anoxic seizure (34). On examination, the infant may have coarse downbeat or lateral gaze nystagmus, a diminished gag reflex, or fixed retrocollis. Examination of the vocal cords may show abductor paralysis with intact adduction (34). Long tract signs may develop.

No stereotypical development of symptoms and signs has been recognized to allow the determination of the importance of any single symptom. What is important to remember is that patients with myelodysplasia have a stable neurologic lesion and, on the whole, do not have new symptoms that are not attributable to either raised intracranial pressure or local complications from their spinal lesions. New symptoms attributable to either brain stem or long tract dysfunction among children with myelodysplasia of any age should alert the clinician to the possibility that Chiari II malformation can become symptomatic. It is of great importance to ensure the shunt is functioning because control of hydrocephalus reverses the symptoms of a Chiari II malformation for many of these children.

In addition to the signs and symptoms attributable to the Chiari malformation, patients may have symptoms of the associated syringomyelia (see later). Relapse and remission and diffuse involvement of the motor and sensory systems may lead to the diagnosis, particularly in adolescents and young adults, of demyelinating disease. If the motor symptoms and signs predominate and there is a paucity of sensory dysfunction, the patient may be thought to have motoneuron disease. Thus the protean manifestations of Chiari malformation and syringomyelia can confuse even an astute clinician.

Management

Diagnostic Evaluation

With the advent of magnetic resonance imaging (MRI), previous methods of diagnosing Chiari malformation, such as angiography, air myelography, and computed tomography (CT) with water-soluble contrast medium, rarely are necessary. MRI should be the initial investigation in the care of patients with suspected Chiari malformation (Figs. 2, 3) (27,54). Both the brain and the spinal cord can be easily imaged in multiple planes. In addition to its high sensitivity and specificity, MRI is noninvasive in nature. This imaging modality also is useful for follow-up evaluations. Because MRI accurately delineates the size of the syrinx cavity, it can easily be used to monitor treatment failure as evidenced by increasing or lack of reduction in syrinx size. Other associated features such as syringomyelia, tethered cord, lipomyelomeningocele, and craniocervical junction abnormalities are easily seen at MRI. Infants and small children however, must be sedated so that they will lie still while the information is acquired to construct the images.

It occasionally is necessary to perform cisternography on patients who have syringomyelia with questionable hindbrain anomalies (6). In these cases, the cause of syringomyelia can be a CSF block caused by arachnoid adhesions at the foramen of Magendie. Conventional metrizamide myelography combined with delayed CT has been useful in defining anatomic details and in appreciating the dynamics of CSF flow in the region. There is no role for CT without subarachnoid contrast enhancement to exclude the presence of Chiari malformation. CSF flow studies performed with MRI are a noninvasive way of obtaining similar information (35). The reliability of this new technology, however, is yet to be proved.

As experience accumulates, gradations in the caudal descent of the cerebellar tonsils are becoming increasingly clear. Caudal descent of the tonsils more than 5 mm below the plane of the foramen magnum is considered by almost all authors to be pathologic. Caudal descent between 0 and 5 mm must be put in the perspective of the individual patient. Marginal caudal descent in conjunction with syringomyelia without another cause may well prove to be clinically significant. Minor degrees of cerebellar ectopia among patients without symptoms, however, usually warrant simple observation.

Treatment

Once the initial suspicion of a Chiari malformation has been confirmed, the question is what therapeutic alternatives are available and would be best suited to the patient's needs. Because these are structural abnormalities, no medical treatment is available for correction. All the therapeutic options consist of surgical intervention. If the patient has symptoms, clinical observation may be an option. It must be kept in mind, however, that the course of syringomyelia is progressive loss of neurologic function over years or decades (4). Some patients with asymptomatic Chiari I or Chiari II malformation experience sudden brain stem dysfunction and die without warning (70,83).

Patients with no symptoms referable to the craniocervical junction and 2 to 3 mm of caudal displacement of the cerebellar tonsils are being recognized with increasing frequency (Fig. 4). In general, this special group of patients without syringomyelia should simply be observed. At the other end of the spectrum are elderly patients with severe disabilities who have little chance of improvement after surgical intervention. Supportive measures may be provided to this group. In most instances, however, therapeutic intervention is indicated (Fig. 5). Patients with symptomatic Chiari I malformation and especially those with Chiari II malformation must have evidence of normal intracranial pressure before surgical decompression of the posterior fossa can be considered. Shunt revision or insertion is a much more appropriate therapeutic option for patients with increased intracranial pressure.

A number of studies have analyzed the effect of surgical treatment of patients with Chiari I malformation and syringomyelia (19,20,40,54). A direct comparison of studies is difficult because of the different clinical features emphasized and the varied operative procedures performed. Most patients, however, have improvement or stabilization of symptoms after decompressive surgery (54). The improvement is more marked in symptoms such as head and neck pain, cranial nerve dysfunction, and long tract signs. There usually is a stabilization of sensory and motor symptoms, but there is rarely a return of lost tendon reflexes, muscle wasting, or sensory loss. A retrospective study showed that there was either stabilization or improvement for 70% of patients with Chiari I malformation after decompression of the posterior fossa, but there was rarely complete resolution (54). Among patients who also had syringomyelia, there was a positive correlation between clinical improvement and improvement in the extent of the syrinx cavity (Fig. 6). Several authors showed improvement or stabilization of progressive scoliosis after surgical treatment of patients with Chiari I malformation and syringomyelia (50).

In contrast are neonates or infants with myelomeningocele, an adequately functioning shunt, and difficulty with respiration or swallowing. Despite operative intervention, this group continues to have a grave prognosis for survival (63,64). Chiari II malformation continues to be the leading cause of death among treated patients with myelodysplasia.

Operative Technique

Once the decision has been made to surgically treat a patient with a Chiari I malformation, a range of posterior decompressive procedures are used by various surgeons. Simple bony decompression of the occipital bone and upper cervical canal can be done. Intraoperative ultrasonography is used to document normal tonsillar motion. If there is not normal tonsillar motion, dural decompression is performed. Some surgeons open the dura without opening the arachnoid so as to avoid contamination of the CSF with blood. At the more aggressive end of the spectrum is opening of the arachnoid followed by microsurgical dissection of the tonsils and fourth ventricular outlet. To further lower any resistance to fourth ventricular outflow of CSF, the surgeon can coagulate and shrink the medial aspect of one cerebellar tonsil with bipolar cautery. In 95% of Chiari I decompressions, removal of the foramen magnum–occipital bone and C1 is adequate bony removal. In only 5% of our patients has removal of C2 been necessary for an adequate decompression. Restricting the bony removal to the foramen magnum and posterior arch of C1 decreases postoperative pain and increases the patient's long-term spinal stability. We have found that restricting the opening to this area has not led to any substantial spinal deformity. When the decompression needs to be caudal to the upper margin of C2, the surgeon can undercut the lamina and spinous process with rongeurs while leaving the C2 elements intact. Plugging of the obex and fourth ventricular stents are not only passe but also carry an unjustified high morbidity in the care of this patient population.

A small number of patients with Chiari I malformation have ventral brain stem compression from extradural osseous and soft-

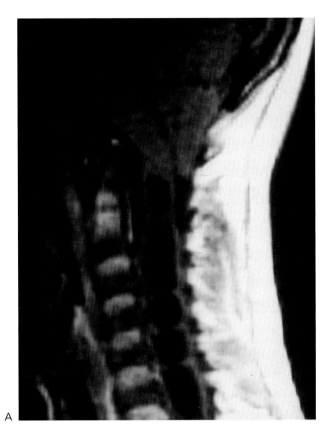

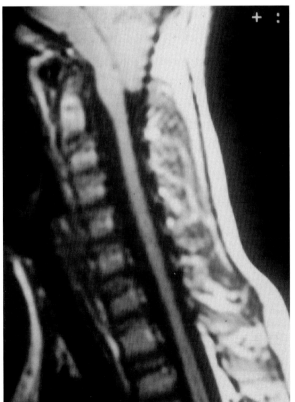

FIGURE 6. Preoperative sagittal, T1-weighted magnetic resonance image shows Chiari I malformation and cervical syringomyelia **(A)**. After posterior fossa decompression, the syringomyelia resolved **(B)**.

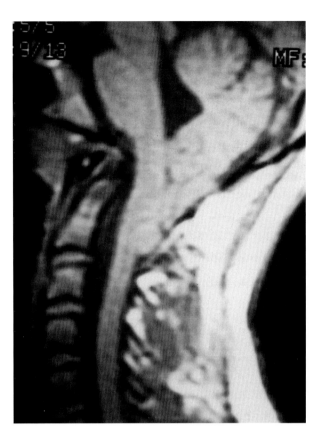

FIGURE 7. Sagittal, T1-weighted magnetic resonance image shows a Chiari I malformation with ventral brain stem compression even though there is no basilar invagination.

tissue anomalies that should be addressed before any posterior decompression is performed (Fig. 7) (27). The excepted approach to substantial ventral compression is to attempt reduction with halo traction. If the traction is successful, posterior decompression and fusion with internal fixation are performed. If the traction is not successful, then the ventral vector must be removed before any dorsal procedure is performed. This ventral decompression often is performed through the transoral route.

We routinely observe patients in a monitored setting the night of the operation and then transfer them to a regular floor the following day. Complications are infrequent but are severe when they occur. Intraoperative bleeding from an uncontrolled venous sinus is the most feared intraoperative complication. A small child can quickly exsanguinate from an uncontrolled venous sinus. Suturing of the dural leaves or approximating them with titanium hemostatic clips is at times invaluable when it is necessary to open a vascular dura. Lower cranial nerve dysfunction following posterior decompression in the face of ventral compression can occur when ventral compression has not been adequately addressed (27). Vertebral artery injury from craniocervical instability can cause thromboembolic complications among these patients. Leakage of CSF and meningitis can occur when increased intracranial pressure from hydrocephalus has not been controlled. Cerebellar slump can occur when a large posterior decompression is performed and the cerebellum sags into the decompression to produce traction on the brain stem or cranial nerves or recurrent crowding of the cervicomedullary junction. These mechanisms cause cranial neuropathy, brain stem dysfunction, or syringomyelia. One of our patients had postoperative bilateral posterior fossa subdural fluid collections that produced a mass effect and caused obstructive hydrocephalus (Fig. 8). "Expected" morbidity is neck pain and some nausea, which usually clears quickly.

For Chiari II decompression the most important preoperative information is the relation between the torcular herophili and the foramen magnum. Because the torcular can be situated at the foramen magnum, removal of the foramen magnum in these cases (a) usually does nothing to relieve the compression and (b) can cause catastrophic bleeding (Fig. 9). Usually the maximal compression is at the level of the cervicomedullary kink, which often is situated anywhere from the rostral cervical to rostral thoracic spinal canal. Therefore, unlike Chiari I malformation, for which a very stereotypical procedure often is performed, Chiari II malformation necessitates customization that depends on the MRI and intraoperative findings. Most Chiari II malformation are most effectively managed with multilevel laminectomy centered over the medullary kink and little if any foramen magnum decompression. This decompression should include the laminae over the caudally descended brain stem and fourth ventricle. There are little advantage and much risk in being too aggressive in the extent of this laminectomy. The medullary kink

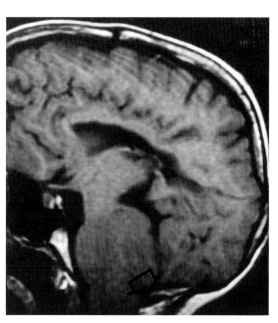

FIGURE 9. Sagittal T1-weighted magnetic resonance image of a child with a Chiari II malformation shows the torcular herophili (confluence of sinuses) situated at the foramen magnum.

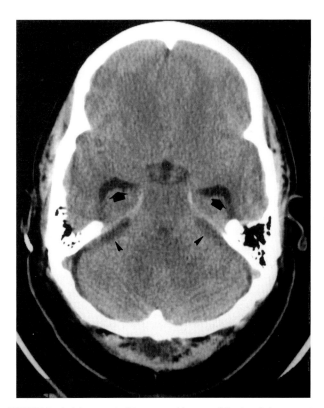

FIGURE 8. Axial computed tomographic scan of the head shows posterior fossa subdural hygromas (*arrowheads*) causing obstructive hydrocephalus (*arrows* show dilated temporal horns) 10 days after uneventful posterior decompression for Chiari I malformation.

usually can be differentiated from the distal fourth ventricle and vermis. The laminectomy need not extend below the caudal fourth ventricle. In the presence of a large syrinx and an extensive laminectomy, there exists a real risk of development of severe kyphosis (swan-neck deformity). Restricting the bony opening to the smallest area necessary to allow a dural opening and to reestablish the foramen of Magendie lessens this risk.

SYRINGOMYELIA

Accumulation of CSF within the spinal cord has multiple causes. The most common is Chiari malformation followed by posttraumatic syringes and intramedullary spinal cord tumors. Syringes also occur in association with basilar meningitis and tethered spinal cord without Chiari malformation. There have been many theories as to how CSF accumulates within the spinal cord to cause syringomyelia. The underlying unifying pathogenesis seems to relate to a disturbance of CSF circulation in the subarachnoid space at either the foramen magnum or within the spinal canal.

Spinal cord cavitations traditionally have been considered hydromyelia if they are ependyma-lined dilatations of the central canal and considered syringomyelia if the cavitation is not ependyma-lined. The clinical practicality of this differentiation may be moot given the necessity of histopathologic examination to make the differentiation. We simply refer to all cavities as *syringomyelia*. Autopsy studies have shown that communication of the syrinx with the rostral central canal occurs almost exclusively among young children with myelodysplasia or other congenital anomalies. In the setting of Chiari I malformation and syringomyelia, there is more often a segment of cord without a patent central canal between the fourth ventricle and syrinx. This noncommunicating form of syringomyelia usually is associated with Chiari I malformation, trauma, intramedullary spinal cord tumor, or arachnoiditis. Among humans without syringomyelia, autopsy studies have shown a patent central canal in 97% of infants, 12% of adolescents and young adults, 4% of middle-aged adults, and 0% of adults older than 65 years (49).

The hydrodynamic theory proposed by Gardner (26) is that because the physiologic outlets of the fourth ventricle are obstructed, the CSF pulsations transmit down the central canal through a persistent communication between the fourth ventricle and the central canal and cause the canal to dilate. This theory may be operative among infants or fetuses with a Chiari II malformation. This situation is further exacerbated by the cranial spinal pressure dissociation theory proposed by Williams (75,76). Williams suggested that with a Valsalva maneuver, the intraspinal pressure increases owing to engorgement of the epidural veins. This causes displacement of CSF into the intracranial subarachnoid space. When spinal venous pressure returns to normal, the reverse occurs, and there is flow out of the intracranial cavity. If this equilibrium is delayed by adhesions or tissue in the foramen magnum, a pressure differential is produced between the intracranial and the intraspinal compartments, and alternative pathways of decompression are encouraged. One such pathway that allows reduction of pressure is through a patent rostral central canal; the result is dilatation of the central canal of the spinal cord. The other pathway is progressive caudal displacement of the posterior fossa tissue; the result is worsening of the Chiari malformation. Williams refers to this as the *suck hypothesis.* He provided support for this hypothesis by measuring CSF pressures simultaneously within the cranial cavity and the spinal canal of subjects with and those without Chiari malformation (75,76).

We have successfully treated patients with syringomyelia and no Chiari malformation with posterior fossa decompression. Our theory is that a disturbance of CSF flow at the foramen magnum despite no history of meningitis or trauma was the cause of the syringomyelia (35). This suggests that an anatomic abnormality need not be obviously present at MRI to cause the pathophysiologic features of Chiari malformation.

A cause of noncommunicating syringomyelia is intrinsic spinal cord tumor. Proteinaceous fluid may be secreted by the tumor cells. As the fluid accumulates, it dissects the spinal cord tissue at the pole of the neoplasm. With increasing accumulation the cavity enlarges, and the clinical worsening can be explained by expansion under pressure. But expansion of the syringomyelic cavity may be caused by other mechanisms. One such explanation is that CSF can dissect along the arteries and the Virchow-Robin spaces (7); macroscopic and microscopic openings provide the connections to fill the cyst with fluid. Evidence of such a mechanism came from studies in which water-soluble contrast medium injected into the subarachnoid space commonly opacified the syringomyelic cavity on delayed scanning (6). This suggests that obstruction of normal bulk flow of CSF by either a hydrodynamic mechanism or extramedullary compression can lead to syringomyelia. Bulk flow of CSF in the spinal canal goes from the spinal subarachnoid space into the central canal and then flows rostrally.

Another explanation for expansion of noncommunicating syringomyelia is provided by Williams and is once again based on the theory of differential pressures (75,76). In this instance, the differential pressure is within the spinal subarachnoid space. As before, a Valsalva maneuver causes engorgement of epidural veins and compression of a focal area of subarachnoid space. The change in pressure is dissipated throughout the subarachnoid space and causes a sudden upward surge within the cyst cavity. The cavity returns to the pre-Valsalva position because of the elastic properties of the cord tissue. Such a "sloshing" of the fluid within the spinal cord cavity may dissect additional portions of the spinal cord during this surge. This concept is clinically supported by the fact that patients with known syringomyelia can have sudden neurologic worsening during attacks of coughing or sneezing. Such a dynamic process may explain why more than one cyst may run in parallel within the spinal cord or why there may be several transverse septations within one syringomyelic cavity (75,76).

The incidence of syringomyelia among patients with posttraumatic paraplegia is between 2% and 8% (78). Posttraumatic syringomyelia can develop after severe or moderate spinal cord injury. The clinical symptoms can develop years or even decades after the injury. An intramedullary hematoma or hematomyelia can develop at the site of trauma. The spinal cord can become fixed by arachnoid adhesions, which reduce the mobility of the CSF around the cord. Such adhesions and reduced mobility can contribute to delayed ischemia of the cord. Both posttraumatic and delayed ischemia can cause myelomalacia and cyst formation (65). These cysts may move during a Valsalva maneuver. Pathologic examination shows that the area around the syringomyelic cavity can be affected by mild reactive gliosis, but typically there is no evidence of acute inflammation or vascular compromise.

Clinical Features

There is extreme variation in the clinical presentation and objective signs of syringomyelia, and the progression is relentless but protracted (22,32,75,80). In the past, it was because of this long interval of progression that syringomyelia was categorized as a chronic neurodegenerative disease (47). Syringomyelia associated with hindbrain herniation is the form of spinal cord cavitation most frequently seen by clinicians. It can be difficult to differentiate the symptoms caused by the cyst from those caused by the Chiari malformation, particularly among patients who may have cephalic dissection of the syrinx into the brain stem, which causes syringobulbia.

Well-recognized clinical features of syringomyelia include suspended and dissociated sensory loss, cervical and occipital pain, lower motoneuron weakness of the upper extremities, and neurogenic arthropathy (Charcot joints). Although prominently discussed, painless joint destruction occurs among only 5% to 7% of patients with syringomyelia. Numbness frequently is the initial symptom; the sensory disturbance usually is in the upper extremities and may be asymmetric. Typically there is loss of pain and temperature sensation with preservation of touch and proprioception. Dysesthesia and disturbance of proprioception may occur with advanced disease. The pain may be radicular in distribution or be more diffuse. Headache and posterior cervical pain are thought to be caused by distortion of the descending fibers of the trigeminal nerve or upper cervical nerve roots or by distortion of the C2 sensory roots by the caudal tonsils. The pain may be exacerbated or caused by coughing or sneezing. A Valsalva maneuver can alter neurologic findings among patients with syringomyelia of any cause. The disturbance in motor function is manifested by difficulty in performing motor tasks with the upper extremities. This may be followed by atrophy in both distal and proximal muscle groups. There may be fasciculations in the affected muscles, and deep tendon reflexes may be diminished or absent in the arms. The lower extremities can become spastic with ankle clonus and extensor plantar responses. A lower motoneuron syndrome in the lower extremities occasionally occurs. Bowel and bladder function usually is normal, and complete or partial Horner syndrome may be present. If there has been cephalic dissection of the syrinx into the brain stem, there may be cranial nerve and brain stem dysfunction.

The causal relation between syringomyelia and scoliosis is well recognized (61). Twenty percent to 25% of patients with syringomyelia have scoliosis. Scoliosis among this patient population is atypical in that it is midthoracic and convex to the left, unlike idiopathic scoliosis, which is more often convex to the right and involves the lower thoracic or lumbar region. In a series of 43 patients with Chiari I malformation, 50% of patients without scoliosis had syringomyelia, but syringomyelia was present in 95% of patients with scoliosis (54). Williams (75,76) and Foster (22) analyzed the clinical features of large numbers of patients with syringomyelia (Table 3).

The prognosis of syringomyelia is determined by the cause of the fluid accumulation. Patients with syringomyelia from a spinal cord neoplasm or arteriovenous malformation are best served with therapy for the underlying cause of the fluid accumulation and not the cyst itself. In general, for patients with spinal arachnoiditis or trauma, it is most effective to drain the cyst into the pleural or peritoneal cavity and not the subarachnoid space—this opinion is not universal.

Improvement after shunting for posttraumatic syringomyelia is seldom dramatic. Major neurologic deficits usually are permanent; however, there often is lasting improvement in pain. When considering surgery in the care of patients with posttraumatic syringomyelia, it is worth remembering that the course of the disease is progressive deterioration among about 50% to 70% of the patients. Barbaro (9) analyzed the results of various published reports and concluded that at least 50% of patients who underwent surgical treatment had signs of improvement and that an additional 30% had stabilization. In view of the course of this entity and the encouraging results, surgical intervention for posttraumatic syringomyelia is indicated when patients have symptoms or when there is MRI evidence of progressive enlargement of the syrinx.

Management

Diagnostic Evaluation

MRI is the ideal means of detecting and evaluating syringomyelia. Not only is it a noninvasive means of defining a syrinx, but also it adequately delineates most associated entities, such as Chiari malformation, intraspinal tumor, and occult spinal dysraphism. It occasionally is necessary to perform cisternography for patients who have syringomyelia with questionable hindbrain anomalies (6). In these cases, the cause of syringomyelia may be CSF block caused by arachnoid adhesions at the foramen magnum. Conventional metrizamide myelography combined with delayed CT has been useful in defining anatomy details and in appreciating the dynamics of CSF flow in the region. MRI can be used to generate CSF flow studies. Standardization of these noninvasive techniques is in evolution. Whether the specificity and sensitivity are as good as those of CT cisternography remains a question.

Treatment

When syringomyelia is detected, the clinician must determine the cause of the syrinx. It usually is most appropriate to direct treatment at the cause of the syrinx rather than to conduct a direct attack on the syrinx. If the patient has symptoms, clinical observation may be an option. It must be kept in mind, however, that the course of syringomyelia is progressive loss of neurologic function over years or decades (4).

More than 90% of syringes associated with Chiari I malformation shrink after posterior fossa decompression alone. Establishment of normal CSF circulation at the foramen magnum resolves the syringomyelia. Among patients with myelomeningocele, inadequate function of a CSF shunt can cause syringomyelia. It is of great importance, therefore, to ensure adequate shunt function. If syringomyelia continues to be a problem for a patient with Chiari II malformation a functioning shunt, posterior fossa decompression alone is unlikely to resolve the syringomyelia. For these patients, arachnoidal scarring in association with tethered spinal cord or Chiari II malformation may be important factors (Fig. 10). We perform Chiari II decompression in concert with some form of syrinx shunt (usually syringopleural) with good success. Syringes associated with tumors or vascular malformations are addressed by treating the tumor or vascular malformation. Syringes associated with trauma probably are caused by a cavitating cord injury and arachnoidal scarring from hemorrhage. Therefore aggressive release of arachnoidal scarring along with a shunt from the syrinx to an extraarachnoidal site is the preferred treatment.

TABLE 3. CLINICAL SYMPTOMS AND SIGNS AMONG 100 PATIENTS WITH SYRINGOMYELIA

Symptom	No. of Cases	Sign	No. of Cases
Stiffness of the legs	42	Scoliosis	22
Hand numbness	28	Hydrosyringomyelia	78
Neck pain	24	Spastic paraparesis	58
Arm pain	16	Hydrocephalus	11
Headache	14	Brain stem signs	29
Oscillopsia	6	Proprioceptive loss	20
Diplopia	4	Neurogenic arthropathy	7
Vertigo	3	Horner syndrome	5
Drop attacks	2		

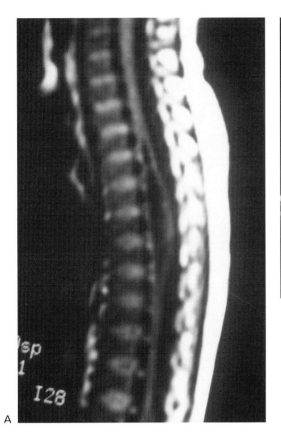

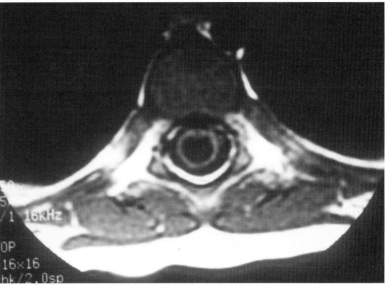

FIGURE 10. Sagittal **(A)** and axial **(B)** T1-weighted magnetic resonance images show syringomyelia of the thoracic cord in association with spina bifida.

TETHERED CORD SYNDROME

The term *tethered cord syndrome* has been used to describe a constellation of symptoms and signs thought to be caused by traction on the conus medullaris. This tension or traction usually causes caudal displacement of the conus. One can still have a functionally tethered spinal cord with the conus at a normal position. The cause of the tethering may be a variety of intradural congenital anomalies or previous surgical procedures. The tethering can be caused by a thickened or tight filum terminale; intradural lipoma, which usually extends into the subcutaneous tissues; intradural fibrous adhesions; split cord malformation; dermal sinus tract; occult meningocele; or previous myelomeningocele closure. Until recently, tethered cord syndrome usually referred to the lumbosacral cord exclusively, but a number of cases of tethered cervical cord have now been described (18,21,56,57,81).

Embryology and Pathophysiology

Congenital tethered cord syndrome is considered to be a form of occult spinal dysraphism. To understand the pathophysiology, it is important to review the development of the normal spinal cord. There are multiple reviews on this subject and we only briefly highlight the stages of spinal development (43,56). The vertebral column and spinal cord match segment for segment, and the spinal nerve roots exit through the intervertebral foramina directly opposite the point of origin until 9 weeks of gesta-

tion. Thereafter, the neural tube "ascends" within the vertebral column. Two processes are involved in this ascension of the spinal cord and the associated development of the cauda equina and filum terminale (38). The first process is regression or dedifferentiation of already formed structures. This causes the distal portions of the neural tube, formed by canalization, to undergo cellular necrosis between 40 to 48 days of gestation and form the future filum terminale.

The central canal immediately cephalic to the area of necrosis dilates to form the ventriculus terminalis. This lies at the entry zone of the fifth sacral nerve root and marks the junction of the future conus medullaris and the filum terminale. The distal end of the future filum terminale is attached to the posterior aspect of the fifth coccygeal vertebral segment. The second process involved in the ascension of the spinal cord is differential growth of the vertebral column and neural tube. Because the cephalic portion of the neural tube is fixed in position, relative cephalic migration of the caudal cord occurs. The lumbosacral nerves are attached to the spinal cord and lengthen to form the cauda equina. The filum terminale lengthens because of the growth of its fibrous components and mechanical stretching. Between 9 and 17 weeks of gestation, the conus ascends from the midcoccygeal level to the fourth lumbar level. After this the ascent is slow. The conus reaches the third lumbar vertebral body by term and the adult level of the L1–2 intervertebral disc space by 2 months of postnatal development.

Thus it is possible that during this complicated process, several errors can occur that lead to tethering of the lower part of the spinal cord (23). Tethering by a lipoma may be the result of inclusion of adipose tissue within the dural sac during early development, similar to the formation of more complex lumbosacral lipoma. An abnormality of canalization or regression may cause abnormalities in the filum terminale. The errors in closure of other midline structures, such as dura, vertebral body, or skin, may cause adhesion or fibrous bands and interfere with ascension of the cord. The result is tethering.

Breig (11) studied the biomechanics of the central nervous system in human cadavers. He established the dynamics of the spinal cord and described elongation of the cervical cord in flexion and slackening in extension. He showed that in the neutral position the cord folds as does an accordion and is under slight tension. During flexion the spinal cord first unfolds then undergoes elastic deformation near full flexion. Conversely, during extension, it simply folds and undergoes elastic compression. The change in length measured on the dorsal aspect in flexion and extension was 1.8 to 2.8 cm for the cervical cord, 0.9 to 1.3 cm for the thoracic cord, and 1 to 2 cm for the lumbar cord. Thus any interference with the mobility of the spinal cord can cause imbalance of traction forces and changes in blood supply.

Reigel (66) demonstrated attenuation of the spinal cord exacerbated by pelvic flexion. This observation suggested that intermittent stretch may occur with sitting, standing, and other daily activities. It also was found that the spinal cord vasculature often was attenuated and linear. This suggested that any process leading to lengthening or stretching of the spinal cord may cause intermittent or progressive ischemia and spinal cord dysfunction. The slow rate of progression of symptoms may further support vascular insufficiency as an etiologic factor in tethered cord syndrome. Experimental traction on the spinal cords of cats decreases local blood flow and impairs oxidative metabolism (82). It also increases the vulnerability of the spinal cord to compressive injuries (24). Among patients with tethered cord syndrome, oxidative metabolism improved after untethering (82). Vulnerability of spinal cord gray matter to ischemia during experimental tethering in animals was further confirmed in horseradish peroxidase studies (25).

Clinical Syndrome

Swift and Carmel (69) analyzed data from a number of studies and drew up a table of common causes of spinal cord tethering (Table 4). Pang and Wilberger (58) compared tethering lesions

TABLE 4. CAUSES OF SPINAL CORD TETHERING

Cause	No. of Cases
Thickened filum terminale	8
Lumbosacral lipoma	34
Adhesions	7
Diastematomyelia, diplomyelia	13
Prior myelomeningocele closure	22
Occult meningomyelocale	1
Neurenteric cyst	1
Dermoid, epidermoid	8
Dermal sinus tract	1
Multiple causes	7

From Swift DM, Carmel PW (69).

found at operation in the adult population with those found by Anderson (3) in children. There also are an increasing number of reports of tethering of the cervical cord, which may be associated with cervical cutaneous lesions (81), cervical split cord malformation (56,57), or cervical dermal sinus (21).

Cutaneous manifestations (Fig. 6) are present among 54% of patients with tethered cord syndrome of congenital origin: 22% have hypertrichosis; 15% have subcutaneous lipoma; and 17% have hemangiomatous discoloration, congenital dermal sinus, or multiple manifestations (23). The converse has not been analyzed; thus the incidence of spinal cord tethering among the population with minor midline cutaneous lesions, such as hemangiomatous discoloration, is not known. Because of the availability of noninvasive imaging of the spinal cord (MRI), there is increasing awareness of the association between tethered cord and midline cutaneous lesions (2).

The incidence of tethered cord in the overall incidence of occult spinal dysraphism is unknown. There is a 2:1 female preponderance. The symptoms of tethered cord syndrome vary considerably in time and mode of presentation and generally suggest progressive myelopathy. French (23) analyzed a number of published reports of tethered cord syndrome and suggested that most patients are younger than 20 years at the time of initial presentation. He found that 31% came to medical attention between birth and 5 years of age, 21% between 6 and 10 years, 42% between 11 and 20 years, and 6% after 21 years of age.

Hoffman et al. (30,31) commented on the "protean manifestations" of tethered spinal cord among children. The most common presentation in their population was progressive motor dysfunction with hyperreflexia and a positive Babinski sign. Other features included orthopaedic deformities of the feet and legs and bladder and bowel dysfunction and scoliosis. Pain at presentation is uncommon among children with tethered cord syndrome. In contrast, back pain was the most common presenting symptom among the adult population (58). Analysis of data from many studies showed that 93% of patients had gait difficulty, 63% having possible muscle atrophy, a short limb, or ankle deformity. Sensory deficit was present among 70%, and bladder dysfunction in 40% of patients. Only 4% of patients had bladder dysfunction in the absence of motor, sensory, or skeletal abnormalities. Most of these patients with bladder dysfunction alone were children (37). Pain in the back or leg or in the arches of the feet occurred among 37% of patients.

Pang and Wilberger (58) compared the presentation of tethered cord syndrome among children with that among adults. The study also suggested a clear-cut precipitating factor for presentation among 6% of the adult population. Among the pediatric population, tethered cord syndrome may become apparent during periods of growth spurt (39), but repetitive trauma associated with spinal flexion is a more reasonable explanation for progressive symptoms.

Among adults the pain of tethered cord syndrome is dramatic and often is localized to the anal, perineal, or medial gluteal region (58). It occasionally is diffuse over one or both lower extremities. Shocklike sensations (Lhermitte sign) are characteristic of dorsal column demyelination. Urinary symptoms include urgency, frequency, dribbling, or stress incontinence (58). Urodynamic abnormalities include detrusor hyperactivity, low-compliance bladder, and sphincter detrusor dyssynergia (37,84). Orthopaedic deformities include kyphoscoliosis, leg length discrepancies, and foot deformities (31,66). The common sensory deficit is saddle anesthesia (58) or hyperesthesia with variable involvement of the feet.

Patients with tethering of the cervical spinal cord may have progressive cervical myelopathy (21). There may be progressive loss of fine motor skills in the hands, increasing clumsiness, and intermittent sensory symptoms in the upper and lower extremities. These patients usually do not have bladder dysfunction, and pain may be absent. On occasion, arm symptoms may be caused by lumbar spinal cord tethering. Although somewhat controversial, this phenomenon has clearly appeared in our practice both from myelomeningocele tethering and from a thickening of the filum terminale. These arm symptoms may be modestly reversible after untethering.

Management

Diagnostic Evaluation

In view of the protean manifestations of tethered cord syndrome, the patient be brought to a pediatrician, dermatologist, orthopedist, neurologist, or in rare instances directly to a neurosurgeon. Such patients need a multidisciplinary evaluation to ascertain the anatomic cause of tethering and the extent of the functional deficits. A detailed neurologic examination is the cornerstone of such an evaluation.

Radiologic assessment should begin with plain radiographs of the spine. In a series of 30 patients with surgically confirmed tethered cord (48), 28 were found to have open lumbar or sacral vertebral arches (Fig. 7), seven had fused arches, three block vertebra, one butterfly vertebra, five bony spurs, 11 sacral hypoplasia, nine scalloping of the vertebra, and eight scoliosis. MRI has revolutionized imaging of the spinal cord. The imaging features that suggest tethered cord include low position of the conus (68,79), thickened filum terminale (68), fatty infiltration of the filum terminale (Fig. 11) (55), split cord malformation (Fig. 12) (48,56), asymmetric location of the cord (48), intraspinal lipoma (Fig. 13), dorsal location of the cord (68), and abnormal movement of the cord from prone to supine position (68). Scatliff et al. (68), using metrizamide myelography with CT, showed that among 14 patients with tethered cord, 12 had an abnormally low conus medullaris, nine had thickened filum terminale (ranging from 1.5 to 4 mm in transverse diameter at L5), and all (including the two with normal position of the conus) had a decrease in movement of the cord as the myelographic position changed from prone to supine (normal movement is thought to be 5 mm or greater).

The normal position of the conus medullaris continues to be debated. In a study using MRI, Wilson and Prince (79) concluded that a conus level of L2–3 or above is normal at any age. A conus level at L3 is indeterminate, because it is possible for a normal or tethered conus to be located at this level. Merx et al. (48) analyzed several features seen at metrizamide myelography with CT of 30 patients who had surgically proven tethered cords. The authors estimated the sensitivity, specificity, and predictive value of these features. On the basis of the data, they

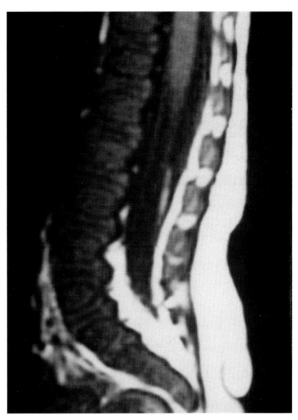

FIGURE 11. Sagittal T1-weighted magnetic resonance image of an infant with cutaneous dermal sinus shows lipomatous elements in a thickened filum terminale.

suggested that contrast myelography with CT be used as a standard of reference for preoperative evaluation for tethered cord syndrome. The main limitations of myelography, however, are its invasive nature and the amount of ionizing radiation needed to complete the study. Because of the noninvasive nature of MRI and its availability, it should be the first line of investigation for patients who may have tethered cord syndrome. A number of studies have emphasized the specificity and sensitivity of spinal MRI (29). Ultrasonography has been proposed as a useful tool to screen infants for low conus, but use of this modality is limited to patients with incomplete posterior elements of the spine and to infants (51). The availability of an acoustic window in the developing lumbar spine usually is limited to the first 6 months of life. When available, ultrasonography can give clear visualization of the important anatomic features and add dynamic information concerning spinal cord mobility.

Children with tethered cord syndrome may come to medical attention with bladder dysfunction (37,84). Zoller et al. (84) performed urodynamic studies for 14 children with tethered cord syndrome. Seven of these 14 children did not have any clinical signs of bladder dysfunction. Urodynamic studies, however, showed neurogenic bladder in three of the seven children. The studies showed overactive detrusor function in two children and reflexic detrusor function in the third. Other authors have emphasized the high incidence of bladder dysfunction among

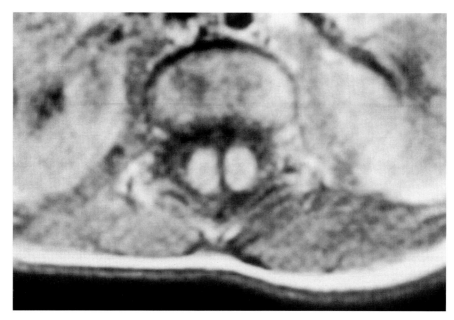

FIGURE 12. Axial, T2-weighted magnetic resonance image of an infant with a pronounced hairy patch in the lumbar region shows split cord malformation.

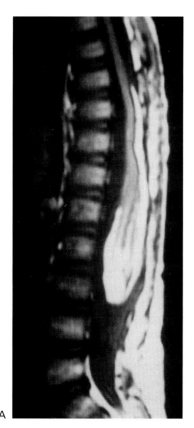

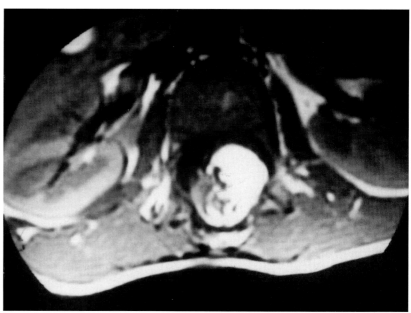

FIGURE 13. Sagittal **(A)** and axial **(B)** T1-weighted magnetic resonance images show large lipomyelomeningocele. Axial image shows how the conus and nerve roots are completely engulfed by lipoma, making simple debulking a treacherous undertaking.

children with tethered cord syndrome (31,66). It is therefore generally recommended that all children with tethered cord syndrome undergo preoperative urodynamic evaluation.

The usefulness of electrophysiologic studies (somatosensory evoked potentials) in evaluating patients with tethered cord syndrome is not fully established. Kang et al. (36) studied sensory evoked potentials and regional spinal cord blood flow in an experimental model of the tethered spinal cord in growing cats. They showed that tethering caused reduction in blood flow and suppression of early components of sensory evoked potentials. They suggested that early untethering can normalize sensory evoked potentials and improve blood flow. Similarly, Roy et al. (67) were able to show that somatosensory evoked potentials from the lower extremity were altered among patients with tethered cord syndrome. Roy et al. (67) also showed a significant correlation ($r = 0.81$) between the severity of neurologic impairment and the extent of the abnormality of posterior tibial somatosensory evoked potential. Electrophysiologic studies alone should not be used to evaluate for the presence of tethered cord syndrome.

Treatment

Operative intervention should be considered for patients with spinal cord fixation from split cord malformation or from thickened filum terminale and symptoms attributable to that level of the spinal cord. The purpose of operation is to release the cord from its point of fixation. This would include resection of bony or cartilaginous septum with its dural sleeve or section of the filum terminale. In operations on patients without clear evidence of progressive dysfunction, the risks of operative intervention must be contrasted with the risks of the course of the condition. Guthkelch (28) provided a classic natural historical study in which 37 cases were diagnosed with myelography and followed. The conditions of 83% of the patients worsened in the 15 years of follow-up study. Continued observation of patients who have undergone surgical treatment shows them to have a high likelihood of remaining in neurologically stable condition after adequate surgical intervention. With this simple analysis, there appears little justification for a conservative approach to infants and children with these conditions.

A more difficult problem exists in the care of patients with symptoms referable to the conus medullaris and fat in the filum

terminale but a distal conus only over the lower border of L2. We conducted an analysis with a group of 14 patients who had evidence of appropriate symptoms and associated findings of congenital malformation in which the conus could be considered in the lower limits of the normal position (71). Our view is that in a risk-benefit analysis, this select group of patients should be considered for operation if the clinical and radiographic evidence is strong.

Early operative intervention also should be considered for patients with lipomyelomeningocele. For decades, neurosurgeons shunned this group of children, thinking that if the condition remained clinically stable or if the lesion did progress, an operation would have little chance of altering the process. Within the past 15 years, inevitable progressive neurologic decline has been accepted as the natural course of these lesions, and operative intervention to release the cord and remove most of the infiltrating adipose tissue has become markedly safer (12,62). A large number (approximately 10%) of patients with this lesion, however, have recurrence of the cord fixation symptoms over several years. Operative intervention improves on the course of the lesions but can be associated with adhesions at the operative site, which secondarily cause cord fixation.

Tethered cord syndrome caused by closure of myelomeningocele is much more controversial. It is recognized that patients in this group are at risk of deterioration with respect to progressive weakness, scoliosis, pain, and bladder dysfunction. Even upper-extremity dysfunction has been attributed to caudal tension. The problem is not recognition of symptoms but the risk of the operative procedure to release the cord and the ability of any untethering procedure to keep the patient's condition neurologically stable for a long time. The results of untethering procedures among this population are still under study, and no general recommendation can be made at this time. For a large number of these patients, the intradural soft tissues are densely adherent. Surgically releasing these tissues without undue damage appears problematic, much less maintaining these tissues in a free state within a restricted and scarred dura. It seems logical at this point to reserve surgical treatment for the group of patients with documented progressive loss of neurologic function (8).

With regard to outcome (Table 5), numerous authors have documented their results. It appears that fixed deficits in children older than 4 years are unlikely to improve (33). Back pain is

TABLE 5. RESULTS OF UNTETHERING OF THE SPINAL CORD

Author	Year	No. of Patients Operated On	No. Improved	No. Unchanged	No. Worse
Anderson	1975	69	50	17	2
Hoffman et al.	1976	31	26	3	2
Pang and Wilberger	1982	23	15	7	1
Reigel	1983	102	60	29	13
Hendrick et al.	1983	86	64	22	0
Pierre-Kahn et al.	1986	64	14	48	2
McLone and Neidich	1986	50	20	27	3
Khoury et al.	1990	31	21	10	0
Zoller et al.	1991	14	3	10	1
Total		470	273 (58%)	173 (37%)	24 (5%)

very likely to improve. Motor recovery improves among 40% and urinary continence among only 12% of patients (45). With this limited improvement in urinary dysfunction, early intervention appears justified if the operative risks are sufficiently low and the likelihood of long-term neurologic stability after the operation is high

REFERENCES

1. Adeloye A (1976): Mesencephalic spur (beaking deformity of the tectum) in Arnold Chiari malformation. *J Neurosurg* 45:315–320.
2. Albright AL, Gartner JC, Weiner ES (1989): Lumbar cutaneous hemangiomas as indicators of tethered spinal cord. *Pediatrics* 83:977–980.
3. Anderson FM (1975): Occult spinal dysraphism: a series of 73 cases. *Pediatrics* 55:826–835.
4. Anderson NE, Willoughby EW, Wrighson P (1975): The natural history and the influence of surgical treatment in syringomyelia. *Acta Neurol Scand* 71:472–479.
5. Appleby A, Bradley WG, Foster JB, et al. (1969): Syringomyelia due to chronic arachnoiditis at the foramen magnum. *J Neurol Sci* 8:451–464.
6. Aubin ML, Vignaud J, Jardin C, et al. (1981): Computed tomography in 75 cases of syringomyelia. *AJNR Am J Neuroradiol* 2:199–204.
7. Ball MJ, Dayan AD (1972): Pathogenesis of syringomyelia. *Lancet* 2: 799–801.
8. Banta JV (1991): The tethered cord in myelomeningocele: should it be untethered? *Dev Med Child Neurol* 33:173–178.
9. Barbaro NM (1991): Surgery for primary spinal syringomyelia. In: Batzdorf U, ed. *Syringomyelia: current concepts in diagnosis and treatment.* Baltimore: Williams & Wilkins, pp. 183–199.
10. Barkovitch AJ (1995). In: Barkovitch AJ, ed. *Pediatric neuroimaging,* 2nd ed. New York: Raven Press, pp 238–239.
11. Breig A (1960): *Biomechanics of the central nervous system: some basics, normal and pathological phenomena.* Stockholm: Almquist and Wiksell.
12. Bruce D, Schut L (1979): Spinal lipomas in infancy and childhood. *Childs Brain* 5:19–203.
13. Chiari H (1896): Uber Veranderungen des Kleinhirns, des Pons und der Medulla Oblongata infolge von congenitaler Hydrocephalie des Grosshirns. *Denkschrift Kais Adad Wiss Math Naturn* 63:71–116.
14. Chumas PD, Armstrong DC, Drake JM, et al. (1993): Tonsillar herniation: the rule rather than the exception after lumboperitoneal shunting in the pediatric population. *J Neurosurg* 78:568–573
15. Chumas PD, Drake JM, Del Bigio MR (1992): Death from chronic tonsillar herniation in a patient with lumboperitoneal shunt and Crouzon's disease. *Br J Neurosurg* 6:595–599.
16. Cinalli G, Renier D, Sebag G, et al. (1995): Chronic tonsillar herniation in Crouzon's and Apert's syndromes: the role of premature synostosis of the lambdoid suture. *J Neurosurg* 83:575–582.
17. Cleland J (1883): Contribution to the study of spina bifida, encephalocele, and anencephalus. *J Anat Physiol* 17:257–292.
18. Dias MS, Pang D (1995): Split cord malformations. *Neurosurg Clin N Am* 6:339–358.
19. Dyste GN, Menezes AH (1988): Presentation and management of pediatric Chiari malformations without myelodysplasia. *Neurosurgery* 23:589–597.
20. Dyste GN, Menezes AH, Van Gilder JC (1989): Symptomatic Chiari malformations. *J Neurosurg* 71:159–168.
21. Eller TW, Berstein LP, Rosenberg RS, et al. (1987): Tethered cervical spinal cord. *J Neurosurg* 67:600–602.
22. Foster JB (1991): Neurology of syringomyelia. In: Batzdorf U, ed. *Syringomyelia: current concepts in diagnosis and treatment.* Baltimore: Williams & Wilkins, pp. 91–115.
23. French BN (1990): Midline fusion defects and defects of formation. In: Youmans JR, ed. *Neurological surgery.* Philadelphia: WB Saunders, pp. 1081–1235.
24. Fujita Y, Yamamota H (1989): An experimental study on spinal cord traction effect. *Spine* 14:698–705.
25. Fuse T, Patrickson JW, Yamada S (1989): Axonal transport of horserad-ish peroxidase in the experimental tethered spinal cord. *Pediatr Neurosci* 15:296–301.
26. Gardner WJ (1965): Hydrodynamic mechanism of syringomyelia: its relationship to myelocele. *J Neurol Neurosurg Psychiatry* 28:247–259.
27. Grabb PA, Mapstone TB, Oakes WJ (1999): Ventral brainstem compression in children and young adults with Chiari I malformations. *Neurosurgery* 44: 520–528.
28. Guthkelch AN (1974): Diastematomyelia with median septum. *Brain* 97:729–742.
29. Hall WA, Albright AL, Brumberg JA (1988): Diagnosis of tethered cord by magnetic resonance imaging. *Surg Neurol* 30:60–64.
30. Hendrick EB, Hoffman HJ, Humphreys RP (1983): The tethered spinal cord. *Clin Neurosurg* 30:457–463.
31. Hoffman HJ, Hendrick EB, Humphreys RP (1976): The tethered spinal cord: its protean manifestations, diagnosis and surgical correction. *Childs Brain* 2:145–155.
32. Hoffman HJ, Neill J, Crone KR, et al. (1987): Hydrosyringomyelia and its management in childhood. *Neurosurgery* 21:347–351.
33. Hoffman HJ, Talcholarn C, Hendrick EB, et al. (1985): Management of lipomyelomeningoceles. *J Neurosurg* 62:1–8.
34. Holinger PC, Holinger LD, Reichert TJ, et al. (1978): Respiratory obstruction and apnea in infants with bilateral abductor vocal cord paralysis, meningocele, hydrocephalus, and Arnold Chiari malformation. *J Pediatr* 92:368–373.
35. Iskandar BJ, Hedlund GL, Grabb PA, et al. (1998): The resolution of syringomyelia without hindbrain herniation by posterior fossa decompression. *J Neurosurg* 89:212–216.
36. Kang JK, Kim MC, Kim DS, et al. (1987): Effects of tethering on regional spinal cord blood flow and sensory evoked potential in growing cats. *Childs Nerv Syst* 3:35–39.
37. Khoury AE, Hendrick EB, McLorie GA, et al. (1990): Occult spinal dysraphism: Clinical and urodynamic outcome after division of the filum terminale. *J Urol* 144:426–429.
38. Kunitomo K (1918): The development and reduction of the tail and of the caudal end of the spinal cord. *Contrib Embryol* 8:161–198.
39. Lassman LP, James CCM (1967): Lumbosacral lipomas: critical survey of 26 cases submitted to laminectomy. *J Neurol Neurosurg Psychiatry* 30:174–181.
40. Levy WJ, Mason L, Hahn JF (1983): Chiari malformation presenting in adults: a surgical experience in 127 cases. *Neurosurgery* 12:377–390.
41. Lewis AR, Kline LB, Sharpe JA (1996): Acquired esotropia due to Arnold-Chiari malformation. *J Neuroophthalmol* 16:49–54.
42. Marin-Padilla M, Marin-Padilla TM (1981): Morphogenesis of experimentally induced Arnold-Chiari malformation. *J Neurol Sci* 50:29–55.
43. McLone DG, Dias MS (1994): Normal and abnormal development of the spine. In: Cheek WR, ed. *Pediatric neurosurgery.* Philadelphia: WB Saunders, pp.40–50.
44. McLone DG, Knepper PA (1989): The cause of Chiari II malformations: a unified theory. *Pediatr Neurosci* 15:1–12.
45. McLone DG, Naidich TP (1986): Laser resection of fifty spinal lipomas. *Neurosurgery* 18:611–615.
46. McLone DG, Nakahara S, Knepper PA (1991): Chiari II malformation: pathogenesis and dynamics. *Concepts Pediatr Neurosurg* 11:1–17.
47. Merritt HH (1973): *A textbook of neurology,* 5th ed. Philadelphia: Lea & Febiger.
48. Merx JL, Bakke-Niezen SH, Thijssen HOM, et al. (1989): The tethered spinal cord syndrome: a correlation of radiological features and preoperative findings in 30 patients. *Neuroradiology* 31:63–70.
49. Milhorat TH, Chou MW, Trinidad EM, et al. (1999): Chiari I malformation redefined: clinical and radiographic findings for 364 symptomatic patients. *Neurosurgery* 44:1005–1017.
50. Muhonen MG, Menezes AH, Sawin PD, et al. (1992). Scoliosis in pediatric Chiari malformations without myelodysplasia. *J Neurosurg* 77:69–77.
51. Naidich T, Fernbach S, McLone DG, et al. (1984): Sonography of the caudal spine and back: congenital anomalies in children. *AJR Am J Roentgenol* 142:1229–1242.
52. Newman PL, Terenty TR, Foster JB (1981): Some observations on the pathogenesis of syringomyelia. *J Neurol Neurosurg Psychiatry* 44: 964–969.

53. Nishikawa M, Sakamoto H, Hakuba A, et al. (1997): Pathogenesis of Chiari malformation: a morphometric study of the posterior cranial fossa. *J Neurosurg* 86:40–47.

54. Nohria V, Oakes WJ (1992): Chiari I malformation: a review of 43 patients. *Pediatr Neurosurg* 16:222–227.

55. Okumura R, Minami S, Asato R, et al. (1990): Fatty filum terminale: assessment with MR imaging. *J Comput Assist Tomogr* 14:571–573.

56. Pang D, Dias MS (1992). Split cord malformation, I: a unified theory of embryogenesis for double spinal cord malformations [review]. *Neurosurgery* 31:451–480.

57. Pang D, Dias MS (1993). Cervical myelomeningoceles. *Neurosurgery* 33:363–372.

58. Pang D, Wilberger JE (1982): Tethered cord syndrome in adults. *J Neurosurg* 57:32–47.

59. Park TS, Hoffman HJ, Hendrick EB, et al. (1983): Experience with surgical decompression of the Arnold-Chiari malformation with myelomeningocele. *Neurosurgery* 13:147–152.

60. Payner TD, Prenger E, Berger TS, et al. (1994). Acquired Chiari malformations: incidence, diagnosis, and management [review]. *Neurosurgery* 34:429–434.

61. Phillips WA, Hensinger RN, Kling TF (1990): Management of scoliosis due to syringomyelia in childhood and adolescence. *J Pediatr Orthop* 10:351–354.

62. Pierre-Kahn A, Lacombe J, Pichon J, et al. (1986): Intraspinal lipomas with spina bifida: prognosis and treatment in 73 cases. *J Neurosurg* 65:756–761.

63. Pollack IF, Pang D, Albright AL, et al. (1992): Outcome following hindbrain decompression of symptomatic Chiari malformations in children previously treated with myelomeningocele closure and shunts. *J Neurosurg* 77:881–888.

64. Pollack IF, Pang D, Kocoshis S, et al. (1992): Neurogenic dysphagia resulting from Chiari malformations. *Neurosurgery* 30:709–719.

65. Reddy KKV, Del Bigio MR, Sutherland GR (1989): Ultrastructure of the human post traumatic syrinx. *J Neurosurg* 71:239–243.

66. Reigel DH (1983): Tethered spinal cord. *Concepts Pediatr Neurosurg* 4:142–164.

67. Roy MW, Gilmore R, Walsh JW (1986): Evaluation of children and young adults with tethered spinal cord syndrome: utility of spinal and scalp somatosensory evoked potentials. *Surg Neurol* 26:241–248.

68. Scatliff JH, Kendall BE, Kingsley DPE, et al. (1989): Closed spinal dysraphism: analysis of clinical, radiological, and surgical findings in 104 consecutive patients. *AJR Am J Roentgenol* 152:1049–1057.

69. Swift DM, Carmel PW (1990): Congenital intradural pathology. *Neurosurg Clin N Am* 1:551–567.

70. Tomaszek DE, Tyson GW, Bouldin T, et al. (1984): Sudden death in a child with an occult hindbrain malformation. *Ann Emerg Med* 13:136–138.

71. Warder D, Oakes WJ (1993): Tethered cord syndrome and the conus of normal position. *Neurosurgery* 33:374–378.

72. Williams B (1977): Difficult labour as a cause of communicating syringomyelia. *Lancet* 2:51–53.

73. Williams B (1981): Simultaneous cerebral and spinal fluid pressure recordings, I: technique, physiology and normal results. *Acta Neurochir (Wien)* 58:167–185.

74. Williams B (1981): Simultaneous cerebral and spinal fluid pressure recordings, II: cerebrospinal dissociation with lesions at the foramen magnum. *Acta Neurochir (Wien)* 59:123–142.

75. Williams B (1990): Syringomyelia. *Neurosurg Clin N Am* 1:653–685.

76. Williams B (1991): Pathogenesis of syringomyelia. In: Batzdorf U, ed. *Syringomyelia: current concepts in diagnosis and treatment.* Baltimore: Williams & Wilkins, pp. 59–90.

77. Williams B, Bentley J (1980): Experimental communicating syringomyelia in dogs after cisternal kaolin injection, I: morphology. *J Neurol Sci* 48:93–107.

78. Williams B, Terry AF, Jones F, et al. (1981): Syringomyelia as a sequela to traumatic paraplegia. *Paraplegia* 19:67–80.

79. Wilson DA, Prince JR (1989): MR imaging determination of the location of the normal conus medullaris throughout childhood. *AJR Am J Roentgenol* 152:1029–1039.

80. Wisoff JH (1988): Hydromyelia: a critical review. *Childs Nerv Syst* 4:1–8.

81. Wu JK, Scott RM (1990): Myelopathy presenting decades after surgery for congenital cervical cutaneous lesions. *Neurosurgery* 27:635–638.

82. Yamada S, Zinke DE, Sanders D (1981): Pathophysiology of the "tethered cord syndrome." *J Neurosurg* 54:494–503.

83. Zager EL, Ojemann RE, Poletti CE (1990): Acute presentations of syringomyelia: report of three cases. *J Neurosurg* 72:133–138.

84. Zoller G, Schoner W, Ringert RH (1991): Pre and postoperative urodynamic findings in children with tethered spinal cord syndrome. *Eur Urol* 19:139–141.

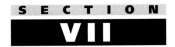

TRAUMATIC CONDITIONS

29

CELL BIOLOGY
OF SPINAL CORD INJURY

VINCENT J. CAIOZZO

One of the key concepts underlying cell physiology is the concept of cellular homeostasis. In essence, this principle states that the survival of a cell depends on its ability to maintain a constant internal environment. From a mechanistic perspective, the cell is isolated from its external environment by the cell membrane, which is composed of a lipid bilayer that contains many different kinds or classes of proteins. The physical-chemical properties of the lipid bilayer and associated membrane proteins are essential in maintaining a homeostatic environment. If the function of these different systems becomes impaired, then the very ability of the cell to regulate its internal environment becomes compromised. The result is consequential cell injury or death. As shown in Fig. 1, the major components of the cell membrane responsible for maintaining the precarious balance between intracellular and extracellular compartments include (a) the phospholipids that provide the backbone of the cell membrane; (b) receptor-gated ion channels; (c) voltage-gated ion channels; (d) Na^+-Ca^{2+} exchangers; and (e) pumps such as the Na^+-K^+-ATPase pump and Ca^{2+}-ATPase pump.

When the functions of these different components become disrupted, there seem to be two major pathways by which cellular injury or death may occur. The first of these pathways is elevation in intracellular calcium concentration. As shown in Fig. 1, elevated concentrations of calcium ion are known to overactivate a number of key enzymes that produce hydrolysis of the cell membrane, degradation of key cytoskeletal proteins, digestion of deoxyribonucleic acid (DNA), and evolution of free radicals. The second pathway involves lysis of the cell by unregulated influx of sodium and chloride ions.

Over the past 5 years, a great amount of attention has been devoted to studying programmed cell death, that is *apoptosis*. The concept of programmed cell death is thought to be in stark contrast to that of necrosis. It is entirely possible, however, that there may be hybrid forms of cell death that share features of apoptosis and necrosis. Hence, the first part of this chapter contrasts the morphologic, biochemical, and molecular features associated with apoptosis and necrosis. This is especially appropriate given the tremendous amount of scientific interest in

apoptosis that has occurred during the past 5 years. This is followed by a discussion on the role of calcium, sodium, and chloride ions and free radicals in the cell death of neurons of the spinal cord. Efficacious management of spinal cord injury requires a molecular model of the cellular components involved in promoting spinal cord injury and paralysis. This review is intended to provide an overview of current knowledge regarding the cellular and molecular events involved in spinal cord injury and to introduce various animal models developed to address these issues.

PROGRAMMED CELL DEATH (APOPTOSIS) AND NECROSIS

Cell death is a fundamental biologic process that occurs under a variety of conditions, such as development, the adult steady-state condition, and disease. Programmed cell death occurs continuously during the adult state. It is well known to occur, for instance, where there is slow or rapid proliferation of cells, as in the intestine.

Many years ago it was suggested that physiologic cell death was much different from that which occurs after trauma or disease. At least two different terms—*apoptosis* and *necrosis*—were developed to differentiate these types of cell death from one another. Apoptosis has received much attention over the past 5 to 10 years and is thought to have a signature distinct from that of necrosis that varies in morphologic, biochemical, and molecular features. Physiologic cell death often is referred to as *apoptosis* and is mediated by active intrinsic factors. In contrast, pathologic cell death resulting from trauma or disease results in extrinsic insults to cells. For example, the insult can be osmotic, traumatic, toxic, or thermal in nature. Features of cell necrosis include disruption of cell membrane integrity, uncontrolled influx of calcium ion and water, and lysis and dissolution of the cell.

The foregoing scheme suggests that there are only two forms of cell death. However, there are forms of cell death that clearly share properties of both apoptosis and cellular necrosis. Hence, differentiating one form of cell death from another may not always be a simple task. It has been suggested that there can be an apoptosis-necrosis continuum based on the findings that

V.J. Caiozzo: Neuromuscular Research Laboratory, Department of Orthopaedics, College of Medicine, University of California, Irvine, California 92717.

537

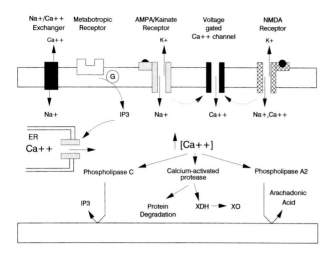

FIGURE 1. Mechanisms proposed as responsible for elevated intracellular Ca^{2+} concentration after injury and the possible pathways by which elevated intracellular Ca^{2+} concentration may produce cell injury or death. *G*, G protein; *XDH*, xanthine dehydrogenase; *XO*, xanthine oxidase.

excitotoxic neuronal cell death has features common to both apoptosis and necrosis. Other schemes of classifying the various types of cell death differentiate on the basis of nuclear or cytoplasmic degeneration.

Morphologic Features of Apoptosis and Cellular Necrosis

From a morphologic perspective, the phenotype of apoptosis is distinctive. The earliest phenotypic alteration typically occurs in the nucleus (43,44). Nuclear alterations include condensation of chromatin that abuts the nuclear envelope. Nucleolar dissolution occurs concomitantly with condensation of the chromatin. A number of alterations occur within the cytoplasm. The cytoplasm is known to condense with a consequential shrinkage in cell size. The mitochondria appear normal during this period, and it is thought that they are essential for apoptosis to continue. Subsequently, the nuclear and cellular membranes become convoluted in such a manner that it often is described as *budding.* So-called apoptotic bodies are then formed. Apoptotic bodies are membrane bound and can contain rough endoplasmic reticulum and mitochondria (42,115). The cellular debris then undergoes phagocytosis by neighboring cells without an inflammatory response. Hence, one of the key features of apoptosis is that infiltration of neutrophils does not occur (115). This is in contrast to cellular necrosis.

Unlike apoptosis, cellular necrosis usually occurs when there is a rapid departure from steady-state conditions, as can occur during anoxic-ischemic or traumatic events. The causal events that initiate cellular necrosis typically occur before the morphologic features of cell injury and death are detected. Perturbations that alter cell-volume homeostasis and mitochondrial function typically culminate in cellular necrosis (15,48,49,61). Such perturbations typically affect the integrity of the cell membrane and alter the ability to regulate the movement of ions. Perturbations

that produce cellular necrosis affect oxidative phosphorylation and deplete high-energy phosphates. During apoptosis, there appears to be well-organized dismantling of the cell. In contrast, during cellular necrosis, cellular dysfunction appears to occur at many different nuclear and cytoplasmic levels. With respect to ultrastructural changes, clumping of chromatin, swelling and degeneration of organelles, and destruction of membrane integrity are key events. The progression of cellular necrosis contracts the mitochondria and condenses the inner membrane. Ribosomes are known to disengage from the rough endoplasmic reticulum and become dispersed throughout the cytoplasm. Unlike apoptosis, cellular necrosis culminates in the release of antigenic cellular debris that produces an inflammatory response characterized by leukocytic infiltration, edema, and a gross change in the histologic appearance of the tissue.

DNA Fragmentation during Apoptosis and Cellular Necrosis

One of the key approaches developed for classifying cellular death has been the so-called DNA ladder. During the process of cellular death, Ca^{2+}-Mg^{2+} endonucleases are known to be activated, and this phenomenon leads to digestion of DNA. The process of DNA digestion signifies an irreversible stage of cell death (3,109,115). It is generally believed that activation of endonucleases produces digestion of DNA that yields fragments that are uniform in length (180 bp). One of the proteins involved in the digestion of DNA during apoptosis is DNA fragmentation factor 45. This protein functions downstream of caspase-3 and causes internucleosomal DNA digestion during apoptosis (55). This type of digestion produces the DNA ladder, which can be identified with gel electrophoresis. In contrast, the digestion of DNA that occurs during cellular necrosis is much less uniform and produces a smear pattern (115). There are exceptions to these general rules. For example, internucleosomal DNA fragmentation occurs in ischemic liver necrosis and *N*-methyl D-aspartate (NMDA)–induced excitotoxicity.

DNA fragmentation can be detected in situ with several different techniques involving the end-labeling of either single-strand or double-strand DNA breaks (28,112). In the in situ nick translation technique DNA polymerase is used to catalyze the transfer of deoxyuridine triphosphate, which is conjugated with a reporter molecule. The TUNEL technique derives its name from the fact that it involves terminal transferase-mediated D-uridine triphosphate nick end labeling. Both techniques are highly sensitive to identifying nicked DNA. However, DNA repair might also lead to end labeling. Neither of these techniques can be used to differentiate apoptotic from necrotic cell death.

Molecular Aspects of Apoptosis

Two major gene families are believed to play critical roles in mediating apoptosis. The caspases are one of these families and belong to a group of so-called cysteine proteases. To date, at least ten different caspases have been identified. The caspases are proenzymes that undergo proteolytic cleavage and rearrangement of subunits to produce active enzymes that interact with substrates at the nuclear level, the cytoskeletal level, and the inflammatory level. A second group of apoptotic regulatory genes is the *bcl*-2 protooncogene family. Within this family *bcl*-2, *bcl*-xl, and *mcl*-1 are antiapoptotic. Other members of this family are proapoptotic and include *bax, bcl*-xs, *bad, bak,* and *bik.*

A number of lines of evidence indicate that the mitochondria play a key role in the apoptotic process. For example, it has been shown that during apoptosis the mitochondria remain intact and that *bcl*–2 localizes on the outer membrane of the mitochondria (52). Additionally, it has been shown that the mitochondria of *Xenopus* eggs contain a dense organelle essential for apoptosis. Cytochrome *c* also has been shown (51,54) to be an essential component of the apoptotic program. The suggestion is that the mitochondria release cytochrome *c* during apoptosis. One model (51) is used to propose that cytochrome *c*, also called apoptotic protease activating factor 2, is a potent activator of caspases. Subsequent involvement of caspases leads to cleavage of a protein with deoxyribonuclease activity, which causes internucleosomal fragmentation of genomic DNA. The antiapoptotic proteins *bcl*–2 and *bcl*-xl are thought to prevent release of cytochrome *c* from the mitochondria. This prevents activation of caspase-3. The role of *bcl*–2 and *bcl*-xl in preventing the release of cytochrome *c* from the mitochondria may involve inhibition of *bax*-related channels, proapoptotic activity of the outer membrane of the mitochondria, or the regulation of mitochondrial membrane potential.

CALCIUM PARADOX

Large differences in ion concentration exist across the cell membrane. For example, the extracellular concentration of sodium ion is approximately tenfold greater than the intracellular concentration. In contrast, the extracellular concentration of potassium is approximately 30-fold less than the intracellular concentration. Of all the main ions, however, the 10,000-fold concentration difference for calcium is the most prominent. Although the cytoplasmic concentration of calcium ion is regulated at very low concentrations, calcium is an extremely important ion that is essential for normal cellular function.

The role of intracellular calcium was first elucidated in 1883 by Sidney Ringer, who showed that calcium is essential for the contraction of cardiac muscle. The role of calcium in modulating neurotransmitter release was elucidated by Bernard Katz during the 1950s and 1960s. We now know that calcium ions play a key role in regulating a vast array of cellular processes under normal physiologic conditions. It plays a key role in regulating actin-myosin interaction, which is essential for locomotion, breathing, and cardiac function. It serves a pivotal role in regulating the release of neurotransmitters from synaptic vesicles. It plays an important role in the allosteric regulation of calmodulin, and calcium serves a key function in exocytosis.

As shown in Fig. 1, the intracellular concentration of calcium is normally regulated by a variety of systems, which include plasma membrane proteins such as the Ca^{2+}-ATPase pump, Na^+-Ca^{2+} ion exchanger, voltage-gated calcium ion channels, receptor-gated ion channels, and second-messenger systems.

Within the cell, organelles such as the endoplasmic reticulum and mitochondria play a key role in maintaining calcium ion concentration at micromolar levels (68).

Under conditions of anoxia or toxicity, each of these systems potentially represents a failure point that can disturb the homeostasis of intracellular calcium ion (68). Evidence of the involvement of calcium ion in promoting cell injury and death has come from the study a number of different cell types. For example, Dayton et al. (14) showed that calcium ion plays a central role in the dissolution of Z lines in skeletal muscle. Schanne et al. (84) examined the effects of ten different toxins on hepatocyte viability. In each instance, the investigators concluded that calcium ion is essential for promoting cell death induced by the toxins. In the presence of these ten different toxins but in the absence of calcium ion, almost all hepatocytes survived. These investigators concluded that cell injury or death occurs in a two-step process. The first phase is disruption of the integrity of the cell membrane; the second is influx of extracellular calcium ion into the cytoplasm of the cell. The latter phase was described as the final common pathway for cell death.

With respect to neurons, Schlaepfer et al. (85–92) as early as 1973 reported that degeneration of axons depends on a calcium-mediated process. Schlaepfer et al. (85–92) later identified this degenerative process as degradation of microtubules and the neurofilament triplet. The neurofilament triplet is composed of three subunits with molecular weights of 200 kd (heavy subunit), 150 kd (medium subunit), and 68 kd (light subunit). Using the calcium ionophore A23187, Schlaepfer (85) showed that peripheral nerves exposed to the ionophore in the absence of calcium exhibited little degradation of the neurofilaments. When calcium was added to the bathing medium, degradation of the neurofilament triplet was substantial.

With respect to spinal cord injury, Young (117) reported that impact trauma causes the extracellular concentration of calcium ion to decrease from a normal value greater than 1 mmol to less than 0.001 mmol. The marked decrease in extracellular calcium ion concentration is the result of cellular injury, which allows calcium ion to flow into the cytoplasm in an unregulated manner. Consistent with these findings was the finding by Happel et al. (31) that spinal cord intracellular calcium levels are elevated as early as approximately 30 minutes after injury induced by the weight-drop technique. Regan and Choi (77) explored the importance of calcium ion in promoting cellular injury. These investigators used spinal cord cultures and found that the cellular damage induced by high concentrations of glutamate (see later) depends on the presence of calcium. When calcium was not included in the bathing medium, the rate of cellular injury decreased by approximately 80%. Banik et al. (4) reported that at the protein level neurofilament degradation in the spinal cord was evident as early as 15 minutes after injury. Degradation of neurofilaments is a calcium-dependent process. The observation that neurofilament degradation occurs very early during injury demonstrates that unregulated calcium influx occurs early in the evolution of spinal cord injury. My colleagues and I (25) found that 4 hours of anoxia was sufficient to decrease the neurofilament triplet content of the spinal cord approximately 60%.

As shown in Fig. 1, uncontrolled influx of calcium ion can mediate cellular injury through a number of pathways. These include overactivation of (a) calcium-activated neutral proteases, (b) phospholipase C, (c) phospholipase A_2, and (d) endonucleases. This represents the *calcium paradox*. Under normal conditions, calcium ions play key roles in regulating a number of important biochemical pathways. However, if the intracellular homeostasis of calcium ion becomes disrupted, cell death is a likely consequence.

The pivotal role of calcium ion in mediating cellular injury has stimulated investigators to examine a number of potential pathways by which extracellular calcium ion enters neurons during episodes of anoxia or ischemia.

ROLE OF EXCITATORY AMINO ACID RECEPTORS IN PROMOTING SPINAL CORD INJURY

Excitatory Amino Acids as Neurotransmitters

Excitatory amino acids such as glutamate and aspartate are major neurotransmitters within the central nervous system. These excitatory amino acids are normally released from the axon terminal of a neuron and bind to excitatory amino acid receptors on the postsynaptic membrane, producing depolarization of the postsynaptic neuron. Under normal conditions, excitatory amino acids play important roles in processes such as synaptogenesis, neuronal plasticity, learning, memory, and central pattern generators (9,21,101,102).

Paradoxically, under conditions of anoxia, extracellular calcium ion may leak into the axon terminals of presynaptic neurons and cause glutamate to be released in large, uncontrolled quantities. Under these conditions, the glutamate concentration in the synaptic cleft may reach concentrations approaching 10 mmol, a concentration two orders of magnitude greater than that needed to cause extensive neuronal damage (12). The ensuing neuronal damage is thought to be caused by the unregulated release of these excitatory amino acids, which overactivates the respective receptors on the postsynaptic cell. This process of overactivation has been called *excitotoxicity*. Olney and Rothman (67,81) initially developed the concept of excitotoxicity, which is that exposure of neurons to excitatory amino acids such as glutamate produces excess depolarization. This excessive depolarization was hypothesized to produce altered ionic flux across the cell membrane. This hypothesis was supported further when it was shown that excitatory amino acids induce swelling of the cell bodies and dendrites, regions of the neurons that have high concentrations of excitatory amino acid receptors (60). The swelling that accompanied exposure to excitatory amino acids was later shown to be related to the uncontrolled influx of sodium and chloride ions. When these ions were replaced with impermeable ions, the swelling that accompanied exposure to excitatory amino acids was abolished.

A cornerstone to the concept that spinal cord injury may be mediated by the unregulated release of excitatory amino acids is the observation that spinal cord injury does produce elevations in extracellular concentrations of glutamate and aspartate, two of the major excitatory amino acids in the spinal cord (19,53,74). Panter et al. (74) reported that the concentrations of glutamate

and aspartate were markedly (approximately 300%) elevated above baseline values immediately after impact trauma. Liu et al. (53) found large increases in the extracellular concentrations of glutamate and aspartate after impact trauma. In both studies, the increases in extracellular concentrations of excitatory amino acids were rapid (within several minutes after trauma) and remained at toxic levels for several hours after impact trauma. These two key studies showed that trauma to the spinal cord can produce toxic concentrations of excitatory amino acids.

Major Classes of Excitatory Amino Acid Receptors

Four major classes of excitatory amino acid receptors have been identified. Each of these receptors can play a role in promulgating spinal cord injury. The four excitatory amino acid receptors are the NMDA receptor, the α-amino-3-hydroxy-5-methyl-4-isoxazole propionate receptor (AMPA), the kainate receptor, and the metabotropic receptor. The NMDA, AMPA, and kainate receptors have been classified as ionotropic receptors because they are associated with an ion channel. The ion channels associated with each of these three kinds of excitatory amino acid receptors are typified by different permeabilities to sodium, potassium, and calcium ions (21,60,64).

NMDA Receptor and Its Possible Role in Spinal Cord Injury

The NMDA receptor is a macromolecular complex that contains a transmitter-binding site, a modulatory site that binds the allosteric activator glycine, and an ion channel permeable to sodium, potassium, and calcium ions (21,59,60,64). It has been hypothesized that during ischemic or anoxic episodes, the NMDA receptor may become overactivated by means of unregulated release of the neurotransmitter glutamate from presynaptic vesicles or by means of impaired uptake of glutamate by glial cells. Both of these mechanisms are attractive because they can account for the pathways by which calcium and sodium ions may gain access to the cytoplasm after events that induce spinal cord injury.

Overactivation of the NMDA receptor provides a secondary pathway by which calcium ion homeostasis can be disturbed. Overaction of the NMDA receptor is known to depolarize the cell. As a consequence, the voltage-gated calcium ion channels become activated and allow calcium ion to enter through this additional pathway.

The spinal cord is known to contain NMDA receptors. Studies by Jansen et al. (39), Mitchell and Anderson (62), Monaghan et al. (64), and Shaw et al. (95) have shown the existence of NMDA receptors in the spinal cords of cats, rats, and humans. Shaw et al. (95) found that the greatest density of NMDA receptors occurs in the lumbar and sacral segments of the spinal cord. With respect to the distribution of NMDA receptors in the gray matter, Mitchell and Anderson (62) and Shaw et al. (95) found that the greatest density of NMDA receptors occurs in the dorsal horns. Shaw et al. (95) found that the density of NMDA receptors in the substantia gelatinosa was approximately twofold greater than throughout the rest of the gray matter. The remaining regions of gray matter appear to have a uniform density of

NMDA receptors. Shaw et al. (95) also found focal areas of high concentration of NMDA receptors in the ventral horn. These focal areas had NMDA receptor concentrations twofold greater than the substantia gelatinosa. Shaw et al. (95) suggested that the distribution and size of these foci were similar to those of the cell bodies of motor neurons.

The potential role of NMDA receptors in promoting cellular injury in the central nervous system was highlighted by the finding that NMDA antagonists protect the hippocampal region of the brain from ischemic insult (100). Simon et al. (100) induced ischemic brain damage by occluding the carotid arteries for 30 minutes. They found that the NMDA antagonist 2-amino-phosphonoheptanoic acid (APH) markedly attenuated ischemia-induced injury. The NMDA antagonist was found to be so effective that some of the APH-protected hippocampal regions appeared normal. The findings of Simon et al. (100) provided a strong stimulus for examining the potential role of the NMDA receptor in promoting spinal cord injury.

Faden and Simon (19) were one of the first groups of investigators to examine the role of excitotoxicity in spinal cord injury. Using a weight drop model of inducing spinal cord injury, these investigators examined the extent of spinal cord injury in animals that were treated with an NMDA antagonist, MK-801, or a control solution of saline. Faden and Simon (19) found that the NMDA antagonist was effective in minimizing the extent of spinal cord injury. Four weeks after the initial injury, 45% of animals treated with MK-801 had regained the ability to walk; 20% of the animals used as controls had the same result. Gomez-Pinilla et al. (29) found that MK-801 provided a moderate neuroprotective effect after injury induced with a weight-drop technique.

Yum and Faden (118) examined the efficacy of using MK-801 after spinal cord ischemia induced with a catheter balloon. As did earlier investigators, these investigators found that administration of MK-801 was followed by motor scores and a greater survival rate of neurons within the ventral horn of the spinal cord.

Regan and Choi (77) showed that the NMDA receptor can play a powerful role in promoting cellular injury and death. Using cultured neurons obtained from the spinal cords of mice, these investigators found that high concentrations of glutamate markedly elevated the lactate dehydrogenase (LDH) concentration of the bathing medium. When the noncompetitive NMDA receptor antagonist dextrorphan was added to the bathing medium containing high concentrations of glutamate, the LDH concentration in the bathing medium was markedly reduced. These investigators also found that high levels of glutamate in the absence of calcium ion in the bathing medium produced little cellular injury. This finding in combination with those observed with dextrorphan suggests that high concentrations of glutamate induce death of spinal cord neurons by means of excessive calcium influx.

Gardner et al. (25) showed that at the protein level, neurofilament degradation in anoxic spinal cords can be amplified when the spinal cord is bathed in a medium containing high concentrations of glutamate or NMDA. When ketamine, an NMDA receptor antagonist, is included in the bathing medium, the extent of neurofilament degradation decreases.

The NMDA Paradox: Its Role in the Neurogenesis of Locomotion

It is ironic that although the NMDA receptor can play such powerful role in promoting cell injury within the spinal cord under abnormal conditions, it is essential for the neurogenesis of locomotion under normal conditions—hence the NMDA paradox. In studies of the spinal cords of lampreys, Brodin and Grillner (9) showed that when the spinal cord was exposed to NMDA receptor agonists a rhythmic swimming motion was initiated. Smith et al. (101,102), using a neonatal rat model, found that all forms of locomotion depended on activation of the NMDA receptor. Locomotion initiated by activating the command center in the brain stem can be blocked with application of a competitive inhibitor of the NMDA receptor, AP5, to the solution bathing the spinal cord. Smith et al. also showed that the application of AP5 to the bathing solution abolished locomotion initiated by sensorimotor circuits. They (102) concluded that all locomotor activity ultimately depends on activation of the NMDA receptors in the spinal cord.

Potential Role of the AMPA Excitatory Amino Acid Receptor in Spinal Cord Injury

As shown in Fig. 1, the AMPA receptor is permeable to sodium and potassium ions (21,64). As with the NMDA receptor, during episodes of spinal cord trauma, elevated toxic levels of glutamate may occur. Overactivation of this receptor consequently depolarizes spinal cord neurons. This depolarization causes the voltage-gated calcium ion channels to open and allows unregulated influx of calcium ions. In this scenario, the AMPA receptor is thought to be capable of inducing cell death through overactivation of calcium-mediated pathways as well as through cellular swelling and lysis.

The investigations of Jansen et al. (39) and Mitchell and Anderson (62) indicated that the greatest density of AMPA receptors is within lamina II region of the dorsal horn. Using a quantitative radiographic technique, Mitchell and Anderson (62) found that the lamina III-V region of the dorsal horn has a receptor density approximately 70% of that in the lamina II region. In the ventral horn, AMPA receptor density was approximately 50% of that in lamina II.

The presence of AMPA receptors and their potential for mediating neuronal injury by means of unregulated influx of sodium ions and activation of voltage-gated calcium ion channels raises the possibility that these receptors might be involved in promoting spinal cord injury. We do not know of any studies examining the role of the AMPA receptor in promoting spinal cord damage after anoxic insult or trauma after weight drop. However, the AMPA receptor has been implicated in promoting motor neuron death associated with human neurolathyrism. Neurolathyrism is characterized by irreversible spastic paralysis of the lower limbs (8,80,103). Neurolathyrism occurs as a result of excessive consumption of seeds (*Lathyrus sativus*, the chickling pea) that contain the neurotoxin β-N-oxalylamino-L-alanine (L-BOAA). L-BOAA is a very potent excitotoxic glutamate analogue. Spencer et al. (103) found that subconvulsive doses of L-BOAA produced motor deficits among other primates similar to those among humans. Ross et al. (80) later showed that the excitotoxic effect of L-BOAA can be attenuated by antagonists of the AMPA receptor.

Neurolathyrism provides an important model to establish the potential role of the AMPA receptor in spinal cord injury. However, no studies have directly examined the role of this excitatory amino acid receptor in the promulgation of spinal cord injury. This issue needs to be specifically addressed as does the mechanism by which overactivation of this receptor induces cellular injury (cellular swelling through influx of sodium ions, unregulated influx of calcium ion).

Recent studies have showed that the extent of cellular injury in the brain after an ischemic insult can be minimized with AMPA antagonists. For example, Buchan et al. (10) used a four-vessel occlusion rat model to produce severe forebrain ischemia. The AMPA antagonist reduced the amount of cellular injury from a control value of approximately 75% down to approximately 25% of the CA1 cells examined. A similar effect was found by Sheardown et al. (96). In both studies, investigators used the AMPA antagonist 2,3-dihydroxy-6-nitro-7-sulfamoyl-benzo-(f)-quinoxaline (NBQX). These studies provide encouraging possibilities with respect to the potential involvement of AMPA receptors in promoting spinal cord injury.

Although the AMPA receptor may play a role in the pathogenesis of spinal cord injury, the findings of Regan and Choi (77) suggest that the NMDA receptor plays the central role among excitatory amino acid receptors in promoting this process. Regan and Choi (77) found that spinal cord neurons in culture are extensively damaged when incubated with a high concentration of glutamate and physiologic concentration of calcium ion. When the NMDA receptor antagonist dextrorphan was included in the bathing medium, the extent of cellular damage was reduced by approximately 80%, as indicated by LDH levels. Because of this finding, it would appear as if most of the cellular injury induced by elevated levels of glutamate occurs through the NMDA receptor and that at most the combined effect of the AMPA and kainate receptors can account for only approximately 20% of cell damage.

Possible Involvement of Kainate Receptors in Promoting Spinal Cord Injury

Like the AMPA receptor, the kainate receptor is believed to be permeable to both sodium and potassium ions (21,64). Overactivation of this receptor consequently can produce excitotoxicity by allowing excessive influx of sodium ion and producing cellular swelling and lysis. Elevation of the resting membrane potential caused by influx of sodium ions through the kainate receptor may act through a secondary pathway, that is, voltage-gated calcium ion channels. As with the NMDA and AMPA receptors, the kainate receptor is capable of promoting cellular injury and death by two different pathways.

The spinal cord has been shown to contain a large number of kainate receptors. Monaghan et al. (64), Jansen et al. (39), and Mitchell and Anderson (62) have consistently found that the greatest density of kainate receptors occurs in the dorsal horn of the spinal cord. In a quantitative study, Mitchell and Anderson (62) found that the greatest density occurred in lamina

I-II with the lowest density occurring in the ventral horn. The general pattern of receptor density is similar to that of the NMDA and AMPA receptors.

Regan and Choi (77) have provided strong evidence that in the presence of elevated concentrations of glutamate, the NMDA receptor plays a key role in modulating the extent of neuronal injury in the spinal cord. However, Urca and Urca (111) showed that intrathecal injection of high concentrations of kainate (the preferred agonist of the kainate receptor) were capable of producing nonselective destruction of neurons in the lumbar region of the spinal cord. However, when low doses of kainate were intrathecally injected there was limited damage to motor neurons and little motor deficit.

Most studies examining the importance of excitatory amino acid receptors in the pathogenesis of spinal cord injury have been focused on the NMDA receptor. More work is needed to better define the role of AMPA and kainate receptors in this process.

Potential of the Metabotropic Receptor for Promoting Spinal Cord Injury

As shown in Fig. 1, the endoplasmic reticulum is known to sequester calcium. Therefore the concentration of calcium ion within the endoplasmic reticulum is much higher than the cytosol concentration. The endoplasmic reticulum is known to regulate the content of calcium through the interaction of two endoplasmic reticulum membrane proteins, the Ca^{2+}-ATPase pump and a calcium ion release channel. The Ca^{2+}-ATPase pump moves calcium ions against a large concentration gradient into the endoplasmic reticulum. In contrast, the open calcium ion release channel allows calcium ion to diffuse from the endoplasmic reticulum compartment into the cytoplasm. The endoplasmic reticulum calcium ion release channel is known to be activated by a second messenger, inositol triphosphate. Elevation of inositol triphosphate level during ischemic or anoxic events can cause the endoplasmic reticulum to release a large amount of calcium ion into the cytoplasm of the affected neuron.

As shown in Fig. 1, overaction of the metabotropic receptor because of the presence of elevated concentrations of glutamate may play a role in promoting spinal cord injury by producing abnormal levels of inositol triphosphate. We know of no studies, however, in which investigators have attempted to examine the role of the metabotropic receptor in spinal cord injury. The findings of Madden et al. (57) and Regan and Choi (77) seem to indicate that the disruption of calcium ion homeostasis that occurs during anoxia or elevated glutamate exposure occurs as a result of overaction of the NMDA receptor. Although the metabotropic receptor does have the potential for disrupting calcium ion homeostasis, it would seem to play a minor role at best.

Na^+-Ca^{2+} Exchanger

Overactivation of excitatory amino acid receptor potential may alter calcium ion homeostasis by acting on the Na^+-Ca^{2+} exchanger. Under normal conditions, the high concentration gradient for sodium ion that exists causes sodium ions to move inward through this membrane protein. In exchange, calcium ions move from the intracellular to the extracellular compartment, thereby maintaining intracellular concentration of calcium ion at a low level. The high concentrations of intracellular sodium ion that accompany exposure to elevated levels of glutamate, however, can reduce the concentration gradient for sodium ion and may actually cause the Na^+-Ca^{2+} exchanger to work in a reverse direction, moving extracellular calcium ions into the intracellular compartment.

Potential Role of Voltage-gated Calcium Ion Channels in Promoting Spinal Cord Injury

As shown in Fig. 1, voltage-gated calcium channels have been postulated to play a role in the pathogenesis of spinal cord injury. Any mechanism capable of elevating the resting membrane potential of a spinal cord neuron is thought to be capable of activating the voltage-gated calcium channels and producing an unregulated influx of calcium ions. It has been proposed that overactivation of the NMDA, AMPA, and kainate receptors may play a role in this process.

Voltage-gated calcium ion channels normally play a vital part in intracellular calcium homeostasis. These calcium ion channels, which open in response to membrane depolarization, have been found to be ubiquitous among vertebrates. With the aid of pharmacologic tools such as dihydropyridines and natural toxins, it has been possible to identify a number of subtypes of voltage-gated calcium ion channels. At least three different kinds of voltage-gated calcium ion channels are present in neurons. These have been classified as the L (long lasting), T (transient), and N (neither L or T) types (97). The N type is thought to be specific to neurons, whereas the L type has been found in a number of other excitable tissues, such as skeletal and cardiac muscle (97). These channels differ from one another with respect to conduction properties and activation-inactivation properties. The L-type channel is located on the cell bodies and dendrites of neurons in the spinal cord (97). The N type of voltage-gated calcium ion channel is believed to be predominately located in the axon terminal that corresponds to sites where neurotransmitter release is known to occur. The different locations of the L (postsynaptic) and N (presynaptic) types of channels suggest different roles for these subtypes of voltage-gated calcium ion channels. It has been proposed that the location of the N-type channel on the presynaptic membrane indicates that this type of channel plays a key role in regulating neurotransmitter release (97). In contrast, the postsynaptic localization of the L type has been suggested to reflect its role in a number of activities specific to the cell body, such as cytoskeletal organization and gene expression.

A small peptide has been isolated from the venom of a marine snail (*Conus geographus*) and has been shown to be a potent and highly specific inhibitor of the N-type voltage-gated calcium ion channel. Madden et al. (57) used this peptide to explore the role of the N-type channel in pathogenesis of spinal cord injury. They found that when the N-type channel was blocked with this peptide, there was a small effect on the calcium accumulation that occurred under hypoxic conditions. They also found that blockade of the N-type channel had little effect on calcium

accumulation when neurons were exposed to high concentrations of glutamate. When ketamine was added to the bathing medium, however, it was found that all of the glutamate-induced calcium accumulation could be prevented. The findings of this study are important in two respects. First, they suggest that the N-type voltage-gated calcium ion channel does not have an important role under injurious conditions such as hypoxia or high levels of glutamate. Second, the investigators found that all of the calcium accumulation during exposures to high glutamate concentrations could be prevented when cells were bathed with the NMDA receptor antagonist ketamine. This is powerful evidence that the AMPA and kainate receptors have a much less important role in the pathogenesis of spinal cord injury than does the NMDA receptor. However, the N-type channel is thought to be located in the region of the axon terminal that might preclude the N-type channel from playing an important role in neuronal death. It might be possible that the L-type channels more proximal to the cell body play a greater role in the pathogenesis of spinal cord injury.

Some studies of the L-type channel (98) have shown that antagonists of this channel can be effective in minimizing the extent of cerebral damage after ischemia. However, results of these studies seem to indicate that antagonists such as nimodipine exert influence by acting on the blood vessels and producing vasodilatation rather than preventing an unregulated influx of calcium ion through L-type channels. These findings are consistent with those of Regan and Choi (77) and Madden et al. (57). The combination of the latter two studies strongly suggest that the large influx of calcium ion associated with hypoxia or elevated levels of glutamate occurs through the NMDA receptor (11). At most, it appears as if 20% of the calcium ion influx can be explained by the involvement of voltage-gated calcium ion channels.

CALCIUM-MEDIATED CELL DEATH: THE FINAL COMMON PATHWAY

Calcium may act in a variety of ways to produce cell death. The different pathways include activation of calcium-activated proteases I and II (calpains I and II), phospholipase A_2, phospholipase C, or endonucleases.

Calcium-activated Neutral Proteases (Calpains)

As early as 1964, Guroff (30) described a calcium-activated neutral protease responsible for degrading a number of proteins in the cytoplasm of neurons. Dayton et al. (14) later were able to develop a purified preparation of calcium-activated neutral proteases. They showed that these proteases were capable of degrading cytoskeletal proteins such as α-actinin, which makes up the Z line in skeletal muscle. These calcium-activated neutral proteases are now called *calpains*.

Calpains are calcium ion–activated cysteine proteases. At least two isoforms exist. These have been classified as calpain I and calpain II. Calpain I is known to be activated at micromolar concentrations of calcium ion. Calpain II requires millimolar concentrations of calcium ion to become activated. Both calpain I and II are heterodimers composed of a heavy catalytic subunit (approximately 80 kd) and a light regulatory subunit (approximately 30 kd). The heavy subunits of calpains I and II each contain four domains. The first domain represents the N terminus and is composed of 79 residues. The second domain (240 residues) has a high degree of homology with papain. The third domain is also approximately 240 residues long. The fourth domain has a calmodulin-like sequence (145 residues long) and binds calcium ions.

In contrast to the heavy chain, the light chain contains two subunits. The first subunit comprises the N terminus, whereas the second subunit contains a calmodulin-like sequence at the C terminus. Site-directed mutagenesis has shown that the first domain is not essential for the catalytic activity of the 80-kd subunit. However, the second subunit of the light chain seems to play an essential role in the activation of the 80 kd catalytic subunit.

The common properties of calpains are that (a) activation requires calcium ion and a sulfhydryl reducing agent, (b) these substances are principally located in the cytosol, (c) molecular weight is approximately 110,000 composed of two subunits with molecular weights of 72 to 82 kd and 25 to 30 kd, respectively, (d) these substances are specifically inactivated by endogenase inhibitor calpastatin and microbial inhibitor leupeptin, and (e) the optimum pH is 7.0 to 8.5. The active site is known to be located within the heavy subunit. Calpains and their endogenous inhibitor are present in a wide variety of cell types, including neurons, cardiac and skeletal muscle, hepatocytes, and erythrocytes.

As shown in Fig. 1, calpains are known to play an important role in promoting cell death. Overactivation of calpain has been shown to degrade a number of proteins essential for normal cellular function and possibly to promote production of superoxide free radicals by means of activation of xanthine dehydrogenase.

Membrane-associated Protein Substrates of Calpain

Calpains have been shown to act on a number of membrane-associated proteins. These include spectrin, fodrin, ankyrin, Ca^{2+}-ATPase, α-adrenergic receptors, and the phospholipid-binding protein lipocortin (33,35). Spectrin is known to be a major calpain substrate. Spectrin is of particular interest because it seems to play an important role in the cytoskeletal architecture of neurons, providing a link between proteins such as actin and neurofilaments (22,23). Spectrin is known to be composed of two large subunits classified as alpha and beta (22,23). Specifically, the β subunit has been shown to contain binding sites for both actin and neurofilaments (22). Both the α and β subunits are known to be degraded by calpain (33,94). Overactivation of calpain by an unregulated influx of calcium ions has the potential for disrupting the cytoskeletal architecture of neurons. Seubert et al. (94) found that the spectrin meshwork is essential for maintaining membrane lipid bilayer asymmetry and that loss of this asymmetry has been shown to result in engulfment of

erythrocytes by macrophages. Seubert et al. (94) suggested that a similar scenario may occur in neurons.

Cytoskeletal Substrates of Calpain

Overaction of the calpain system is capable of disrupting the normal cytoskeletal architecture not only by acting on spectrin but also by degrading important cytoskeletal proteins, such as neurofilaments, microtubule-associated proteins, tubulin, and vimentin. Neurofilaments are known to be located in axons and are thought to play a role in axonal transport of key molecules. The neurofilament is known to be composed of three subunits. These have been identified as the heavy (200 kd), medium (160 kd), and light (68 kd) subunits. Schlaepfer et al. (85–92) initially described the susceptibility of the three neurofilament subunits to calcium-mediated protein degradation. The initial studies were performed on peripheral nerve. These investigators later were able to confirm similar findings in the spinal cord. The neurofilaments were shown to be selectively degraded by calcium-activated neutral proteases (38,71–73).

Tsujinaka et al. (110) synthesized an inhibitor of calcium-activated proteases that they called *calpeptin*. The strategy of these investigators was twofold: (a) to develop an inhibitor directed at the active site of calpain and thus very specific and (b) to chemically modify such an inhibitor to enhance its permeability. Following this scheme, Gardner et al. (26) synthesized calpeptin in a similar manner. Using this inhibitor, Gardner et al. (26) examined the role of calpain in producing the neurofilament degradation that accompanies anoxic events in the spinal cord. These investigators used three different indexes to assess the effectiveness of calpeptin. These were total neurofilament pellet weight, total protein, and quantitative assessment of each of the individual neurofilament triplets. By every account, calpeptin proved to be extremely effective in preventing loss of the neurofilament triplet. For example, the heavy, medium, and light subunits were reduced by only 24%, 23%, and 16%, respectively, which compares with losses of 92%, 92%, and 86% under conditions in which the spinal cords was exposed to an anoxic calcium ion solution.

In addition to the neurofilament, calpain also has been shown to degrade microtubule-associated protein 2 (MAP2). The α and β tubulins form the structural backbone of mircrotubules. Microtubules are long, unbranched macromolecules. The presence of microtubules and neurofilaments in the axon suggests that these macromolecules play a role in axonal transport. MAPs are thought to play a role in determining the polymerization of tubulins, their association with other cytoskeletal proteins, and the treadmill-like activity associated with microtubules. MAP2 is thought to be restricted to the dendritic and cell body regions of neurons, where it plays an important role in morphogenesis. Inuzuka et al. (35) used a calpain inhibitor, E-64c, to examine the degradation of MAP2 after cerebral ischemia. These investigators found that ischemia reduced the MAP2 content approximately 70%. When E-64c was injected into the animals before the ischemic episode, loss of MAP2 decreased, demonstrating the potential role of calpain in mediating disassembly of microtubules after ischemic insult.

Role of Phospholipases in Producing Membrane Dysfunction

Although elevated levels of intracellular calcium ion are capable of producing cell injury by acting on calcium-activated neutral proteases, the elevation of intracellular calcium ion concentrations can produce extensive membrane damage by acting on two key enzymes, phospholipase A_2 and phospholipase C. Phospholipases are known to catalyze hydrolysis of the phospholipids that make up the cell membrane (62). The membrane plays a key role in maintaining intracellular homeostasis. Activation of these two enzymes has the potential for disrupting normal membrane function.

Phospholipase A_2 and the Arachidonic Acid Cascade

As shown in Fig. 2, activation of phospholipase A_2 catalyzes a reaction that splits arachidonic acid off from the phospholipids of the cell membrane. Once formed, arachidonic acid is converted by one of two enzymes, cyclooxygenase or lipoxygenase, into a class of chemical messengers known as *eicosanoids*. As shown in Fig. 2, cyclooxygenase converts arachidonic acid into one of three classes of cyclic endoperoxides. These are prostaglandins, thromboxanes, and prostacyclin. In contrast, lipoxygenase converts arachidonic acid into leukotrienes. Arachidonic acid and its metabolic by-products have been shown to play key roles in such neuronal processes as modulating ion channel activity, modulating ligand binding, modulating neurotransmitter release, and interacting with other cellular messenger systems (79). Under normal conditions, the concentration of arachidonic acid is relatively low (99). However, under conditions that produce cellular injury, it has been observed that the intracellular concentration of arachidonic acid increases rapidly. Prostaglandins, thromboxanes, and leukotrienes are known mediators of inflammatory reactions. More important, it is known that the

synthesis of prostaglandins from the precursor arachidonic acid produces oxygen free radicals (46).

Phospholipase A_2 and the Arachidonic Acid Cascade

The role of phospholipase A_2 in promoting neuronal damage was first described by Bazan (5) who found that arachidonic acid levels were markedly elevated after ischemia of the brain. At that time, however, it was not clear which phospholipases played key roles. Over the past several years, it has been shown that the activity of phospholipase A_2 increases dramatically with cerebral contusion or ischemia. Shohami et al. (99) found that phospholipase A_2 activity was elevated 175% 15 minutes after cerebral contusion. These investigators also found an increase of approximately 100% in prostaglandin E levels. Rordorf et al. (79) induced 10 minutes of cerebral ischemia by occluding the common carotid arteries; they found 10 minutes later that the activity of phospholipase A_2 was elevated approximately 60%. Rordorf et al. (79) identified three different phospholipase A_2 isoforms, which they classified as cytosolic, mitochondrial, and microsomal. The activity of each of these forms of phospholipase A_2 was elevated after the induction of ischemia. These investigators found that the mitochondrial membranes are rich with unsaturated fatty acids, which are good substrates for phospholipase A_2. They also found that mitochondrial phospholipase A_2 acts on cardiolipin, which plays an important role in the electron transport chain.

Phospholipase C and Disruption of Normal Membrane Function

The role of phospholipase C in promoting spinal cord injury has not been studied. However, results of studies of the role of phospholipase C in myocardial ischemia suggest that this enzyme may be involved in the pathogenesis of spinal cord injury. Prasad et al. (75) showed that phospholipase C is capable of converting phosphatidylinositol, a membrane phospholipid, into inositol triphosphate and diacylglycerol. The overactivation of phospholipase C can further elevate intracellular levels of calcium ion by acting on the calcium ion release channel of the endoplasmic reticulum through the action of inositol triphosphate. This causes the calcium ion sequestered within the endoplasmic reticulum to be emptied into the cytoplasm.

Free Radicals

Formation of highly reactive molecules containing oxygen is a normal consequence of a number of biochemical pathways. If such a molecule contains one or more unpaired electrons, the molecule is called a *free radical*. The intracellular production of free radicals evolves from the activity of cyclooxygenases, lipoxygenases, dehydrogenases, oxidases, and peroxidases (37). Sources of free radicals include the lipid bilayer of the cell, mitochondria, endoplasmic reticulum, peroxisomes, and the nucleus. It has been proposed that during ischemic events, the catabolism of adenosine triphosphate (ATP) increases the level of hypoxanthine. Xanthine oxidase then acts on hypoxanthine in the pres-

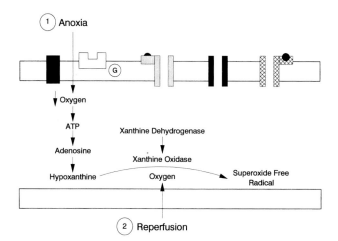

FIGURE 2. Pathway by which superoxide free radical may be formed after anoxia (*1*) and subsequent reperfusion (*2*). (Modified from McCord JM [1987]: Oxygen-derived radicals: a link between reperfusion injury and inflammation. *Fed Proc* 46:2402–2406 with permission.)

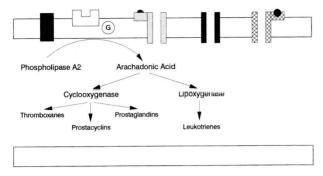

FIGURE 3. Arachidonic acid cascade.

ence of molecular oxygen to produce the superoxide free radical (Fig. 3).

The prime targets of free radicals include the unsaturated bonds in membrane lipids (64). Free radicals thereby disturb the fluid mosaic motif of membranes by altering the fluidity of membranes and altering the alignment of proteins within these membranes. Free radicals also can cause tissue damage by means of cross-linking and denaturation of proteins.

McCord (58) proposed that elevated intracellular concentrations of calcium ion can increase superoxide formation by activating calcium-activated proteases. These proteases were hypothesized to convert xanthine dehydrogenase to xanthine oxidase. Xanthine oxidase then would generate the superoxide radical by means of univalent reduction of molecular oxygen. Given the potential role of free radicals in exacerbating the extent of spinal cord injury, free radical scavengers may play an important role in inhibiting the production of free radicals.

Xu et al. (116) found that the activity of xanthine oxidase was elevated by approximately 100% 4 hours after spinal cord injury induced with the weight-drop model. These investigators showed that the increase in xanthine oxidase activity could be prevented with allopurinol, a strong xanthine oxidase inhibitor. The scavenging enzyme superoxide dismutase also is known to inhibit xanthine oxidase and as a consequence has been shown to be effective in preventing injury that would usually occur as a result of this cascade. Agee et al. (1) attempted to induce paraplegia by occluding the abdominal aorta. Paralysis developed in 30% of animals given superoxide dismutase. In contrast, 90% of the control animals had paralysis.

ANIMAL MODELS

A tremendous amount of research has accumulated on the subject of the experimental management of spinal cord injury. The basic premise for this research has been mounting evidence of a reversible component of neuronal injury caused by a derangement in the metabolic cascade (4). Because of lack of standardization of animal models, results of most of these pharmacologic studies claiming success of treatment cannot be verified or compared. This flaw in basic clinical research is becoming more obstructive as a host of new and mechanism-specific agents are being evaluated for use in the treatment of patients with spinal

cord injuries. From neurotransmitter antagonism to proteolytic enzyme inhibition, the mechanism of these compounds have been developed through painstaking neuroscientific research with molecular biologic techniques. The ability of the agent to reduce neuronal injury in vitro usually is well established. However, the ability to diminish spinal cord damage after traumatic injury may be difficult to evaluate given the present status of animal models as screening studies for these compounds. The ideal model should mimic the human condition of spinal cord trauma, be reproducible, and allow precise biochemical and physiologic quantification of the degree of residual spinal cord damage. Recognizing the limitations of each model in achieving this ideal goal may provide useful information to clinicians struggling with the decision to treat pharmacologically a patient with spinal cord injury. This section describes the various techniques for studying experimental spinal cord injury and points out the shortcomings and advantages of each model.

General Considerations

Until the last decade, most spinal cord research was performed with large animals, such as dogs, cats, or monkeys (56). Because of protests from increasingly powerful animal rights groups, experimental spinal cord injury research is currently performed with rabbits, mice, or especially laboratory rats as the animal model. Strict attention to the guidelines of the animal studies committee at each institution is imperative in this work. General nursing care for paraplegic animals can be time consuming and frustrating; all the complications that occur among humans with spinal cord injury can occur with experimental spinal cord injury. Surgical technique should be meticulous and blood loss compulsively controlled. Blood pressure is an extremely important variable and should be kept normal during the procedure. Hypotension has been shown to produce detrimental effects on the porcine cauda equina during compression studies (27). In addition to physiologic monitoring, in vivo studies can be affected by the type of anesthetic. Halothane is recommended over pentobarbital or nitrous oxide (82). Ketamine may have protective effects owing to its NMDA antagonist properties (see earlier).

Surviving animals usually are evaluated at regular intervals with a series of standard motor tasks described first by Tarlov et al. (106,107). A limitation of the Tarlov scoring system is the difficulty in reproducing consistent data between laboratories. The inclined-plane test of Rivlin and Tator (78) is less subjective, but only one complex motor function can be analyzed. Gale et al. (24) developed a complex system that combines evaluation of both sensory and motor function with multiple behavioral tests. This combined behavioral score is more consistent and predictive of functional deficits.

In addition to behavioral analysis, histologic examination of the spinal cord is performed. Central necrosis is the hallmark of impact studies and of most other forms of experimental spinal cord injury. Quantification of necrosis with analysis of cross-sectional area makes it difficult to depend on intraobserver variability for comparison of data.

Electrodiagnostic studies have been used to assess the severity of trauma after graded spinal cord impact. Somatosensory evoked potential area and amplitude reduction 4 weeks after injury have been found to correlate with the combined behavioral score (76). No correlation between latency and injury was found. In another study evoked potentials returned among animals sustaining only petechial hemorrhages but not those with central cavitation (13).

Impact Studies

Initially described by Allen (2) with various modification since (7,16,17,41,47,56,63,66,70,113), impact or contusive spinal cord injury classically is produced with a weight of a specific mass in grams dropped down a cylinder or over a metal shaft from a specific height in centimeters onto an exposed posterior spinal cord (usually thoracic). This standardized load is calculated as the product of the mass and height or gram-centimeter force.

This technique appears sound at first glance. It is believed that the main advantage of the impact model of Allen is its similarity to human spinal cord injury. However, the posterior spinal cord is injured in the model, and human spinal cords are most often injured anteriorly. Using high-speed scintigraphy, Koozekanani et al. (47) found that a single weight drop produces several collisions between spinal cord and impounder and that the impounder weight varies between studies. Dohrmann et al. (16,17) and Molt et al. (63) showed that the actual trauma dose can vary widely even when the products of various gram-centimeter combinations are equal. Dohrman et al. (16,17) concluded that calculated injury values consisting of impulse, energy, and velocity of deformation correlate more closely with the response to injury than the gram-centimeter product. A wide variability of the effects of various gram-centimeter forces between different animal species also is evident. Hashemi et al. (32) showed that the amount of cord compression varies inversely with the square root of cord stiffness; therefore, a smaller cord will suffer a greater degree of compression than a larger cord for a given drop-mass energy with all other factors being equal. This may explain the relative resistance to spinal cord injury among large animals (400 g-cm required energy for dogs verses 25 to 100 g-cm for rats). That is out of proportion to the difference in size of the animals. Other difficulties involved with this test are the importance of controlling vertebral motion during impact (73) and difficulty controlling rate and amount of compression (17).

Difficulty with the weight-drop test has led investigation into other forms of spinal cord impaction. Models of anterior injury have been developed but used sporadically. Kearney et al. (40) developed a model that allows independent control of rate depth and duration variables. The velocity of impact and duration are controlled with a pneumatic impactor, thus allowing for a situation of constant velocity and compression.

Compression Studies

Ability to control the rate of cord displacement has intrigued investigators since Tarlov's first report of a compression model with dogs (6,34,36,93,108). An implantable inflatable balloon was attached to a movable guide, and the dog was allowed to walk in the cage during spinal cord compression. The dog was examined while awake for acute effects of compression. This ingenious device would be difficult to reproduce because of the present state of animal rights activities on most university campuses.

A compression models of a circumferential balloon in monkeys was described by Tator (108). This technique involved passing a polymeric silicone cuff around the spinal cord and then rapidly filling the cuff. The pressure in the cuff was recorded with a Taylor aneroid sphygmomanometer. This technique was thought to represent a more clinically applicable model because spinal cord injury usually produces impingement of both posterior and anterior structures. However, the degree of dissection and the possibility of surgical injury to the cord have discouraged wide use of this model.

A number of investigators have used slow, graded compression. Each technique is a modification of a template that slowly compresses the posterior thoracic spine. Hukuda and Wilson (34), however, used a screw to transmit force to the anterior cervical spine. These techniques provide more precise control over the force applied to the cord but lack clinical correlation to acute spinal cord injury. Use of these techniques for the neuropathologic study of neoplastic or other slower compressive states and the investigation of cord recovery with varying rates is a promising area for this model.

Various orthopaedic laboratories have used cauda equina compression with a plastic band. In these studies, rapid circumferential restriction was used to simulate acute cauda equina syndrome. Elaborate modifications of these studies with cystometrographic analysis have shown a potential for nerve root recovery even with late decompression. Other models of spinal cord injury using "pinch" technique are rarely used and are not described herein.

Distraction Studies

Of most importance to pediatric spinal surgeons are distraction studies that presumably mimic scoliosis surgery. Dolan et al. (18) described use of a distraction device in a cat model. Circumferential clamps were used around adjacent vertebral bodies, and a central screw moved a clamp along a threaded rod. This technique produced considerable displacement of the vertebrae, and thus spinal cord distraction. Spinal cord blood flow and evoked potentials were recorded. The authors believed their data supported the view of spinal cord ischemia as the mechanism of cord injury. The results of spinal cord blood flow and histologic studies were not conclusive, however.

Perhaps the ideal model for studying the effects of spinal distraction on a scoliotic spine and cord was described by Salzman et al. (82). They initially produced scoliotic deformities in Sprague-Dawley rats by suturing the scapula to the pelvis. After 8 weeks of tethering, permanent kyphoscoliosis had developed. The mean scoliotic curves of 51 rats was 31.7 degrees. The rats were then subjected to incremental (5.0 mm over 2.5 minutes) distraction with a modified Harrington distraction device until the upper laminae separated. Twenty-nine rats with kyphoscoliosis were used in this experiment. Twenty-four sustained complete hindlimb paralysis, and five severe paraparesis. A strain gauge was used to measure the force on the upper hook, and force to failure was similar for all rats. The authors performed this experiment to assay for concentrations of serotonin and its metabolite 5HIAA at various sites in the spinal cord. Their results showed an increase in serotonin concentration at the level of distraction and long-term depletion of serotonin below the site of injury. An elaborate hypothesis for serotonin-induced spinal cord injury involving platelet-derived serotonin and the raphe-spinal tract was hypothesized. The hypothesis of serotonin-induced cellular injury requires more validation. However, the model for distraction and the attempt at quantifying the degree of neuronal injury with a molecular marker represent an important step in the study of iatrogenic spinal cord injury. This model may prove useful in examining the integrity of the cytoskeleton (neurofilament composition) and the role of excitotoxicity.

Occlusion Studies

Because the incidence of paraplegia after operations on the thoracic or thoracoabdominal aorta ranges from 2.2% to 24% (45), much of the work using arterial occlusion spinal cord injury models has been performed in vascular surgery laboratories (50). Various animal species have been studied. Apparently, because of the variability of the spinal cord blood supply in rats, dogs, and nonhuman primates, models with these species have produced only inconsistent spinal cord ischemia. Rabbits are the most widely used species and their unique vascular anatomic features allow infrarenal aortic cross-clamping to produce paraplegia (119). However, the behavioral repertoire of rabbits is extremely limited. Large animals are more easily examined behaviorally, but long-term maintenance of paretic dogs or primates is extremely difficult. Rats have been subjected to cord ischemia by means of a median sternotomy incision for cross clamping of the descending aorta.

In Vitro Spinal Cord Model

Although each of these models has yielded interesting and valuable results, our ability to understand and intercede in the events that lead to paralysis after spinal cord injury would be facilitated by a model that allows the cellular and molecular mechanisms responsible for both normal locomotion and pathologic damage to be studied in the same preparation. In this respect, an isolated in vitro spinal cord preparation may offer several advantages because (a) cord function can be directly assessed before, during, and after a variety of insults; (b) the environment surrounding the cord can be carefully regulated and easily modified; and (c) the cord is readily available for rapid biochemical analysis. Considerable progress has been made in the development of in vitro spinal cord preparations and in the elucidation of the transmitter systems that participate in the generation of locomotion (9). Several studies have identified the excitatory amino acid systems, the NMDA receptor in particular, as the primary transmitter system involved in locomotion. It has been established that in addition to participating in normal function, under pathologic conditions the NMDA receptor can contribute to neuronal damage and loss through the process of excitotoxin-mediated cell death (11,12).

The presence of NMDA receptors in the spinal cord and their role in locomotion and excitotoxicity raise several questions regarding the potential involvement of the NMDA receptor in pathologic conditions of the spinal cord. We (105) are attempting to answer these questions with a modification of the model developed by Smith et al. (101,102). Twenty-two neonatal rats ages 0 to 4 days were used in four series of experiments. The experiments were performed by means of dissecting the brain stem–spinal cord and hindlimbs of each animal and perfusing the preparations with physiologic solution and bubbled oxygen. These preparations were viable for up to 8 hours with the ability to generate locomotion (coordinated hindlimb movement that can be observed, videotaped, and neurodiagnostically monitored with electromyography and lumbar spine peripheral nerve condition). Experimental conditions such as hypoxia also can be produced, and the ability of the preparation to withstand these conditions with various pharmacologic agents can be tested. Mechanical conditions can be produced that provide compression or distraction.

Our preliminary results with this model have shown that excitatory amino acids can cause excitotoxic damage in neonatal spinal cords. We view the advantages of this model as follows: (a) the neural circuitry in the brain stem motor command center, in the spinal cord central pattern generators, and in the sensorimotor circuits can be selectively activated; (b) the conditions of the medium bathing the spinal cord can be selectively controlled; (c) hindlimb movement represents a powerful functional bioassay that provides important information about the integrity of the neural circuits responsible for generating locomotion; (d) the preparation can be partitioned so that injury can be induced at any level of the brain stem–spinal cord; (e) diffusional limitations are minor, and consequently the preparation is robust; (f) the model is ideally suited for studying issues related to injury and the developmental state; (g) anoxic injury can be carefully controlled; (h) the preparation can be easily adapted for distraction or compression studies, yet the conditions of the bathing medium can be controlled; (i) the model can be easily adapted for impact studies; and (j) this preparation is one of the few spinal cord models ideally suited for examining issues related to excitotoxicity.

Limitations of this model are that (a) the brain stem–spinal cord–hindlimb preparation cannot be used to examine issues related to long-term recovery; and (b) the applicability of this preparation to the adult condition is yet to be determined. It may be that there are substantial ontogenic differences between neonates and adults that limit the applicability of this preparation to the adult condition.

SUMMARY

Injury to and death of neurons in the spinal cord occur when these cells lose the ability to regulate their internal environment. Although calcium ion plays a critical role in regulating the molecular events of neurons within the spinal cord under normal conditions, it also has become apparent over the past 10 to 15 years that calcium ion paradoxically plays a central role in promoting cellular injury to and death of these neurons. Because of the involvement of calcium ion in this process, investigators have focused on the cell membrane and various receptors, ion channels, and second-messenger systems. It appears as if excitatory amino acid receptors may play a major role in regulating the influx of calcium ion during periods of hypoxia and anoxia. Of the four kinds of excitatory amino acid receptors (NMDA, AMPA, kainate, metabotropic), studies indicate that the NMDA receptor can play a prominent role in facilitating the influx of calcium ion under injurious conditions such as hypoxia and anoxia. Therefore, damage to the spinal cord and ensuing paralysis appears to involve not only the calcium paradox but also the NMDA paradox. Under normal conditions, the NMDA receptor seems to play a key role in the neurogenesis of locomotion. More complete understanding of the events involved in spinal cord injury will evolve as understanding of molecular events continues to progress. Good experimental models are needed to facilitate this understanding. We believe that in vitro spinal cord models capable of generating locomotion will play a key role in this process.

ACKNOWLEDGMENTS

This work was funded in part by a grant from the Orthopaedic Research and Education Foundation.

REFERENCES

1. Agee JM, Flanagan T, Blackbourne LH, et al. (1991): Reducing post-ischemic paraplegia using conjugated superoxide dismutase. *Ann Thorac Surg* 51:911–915.
2. Allen AR (1911): Surgery of experimental lesion of spinal cord equivalent to crush injury of fracture dislocation of spinal column: a preliminary report. *JAMA* 57:878–880.
3. Arends MJ, Morris RG, Wyllie AH (1990): Apoptosis: the role of endonuclease. *Am J Pathol* 136:593–608.
4. Banik NL, Hogan EL, Hsu CY (1987): The multimolecular cascade of spinal cord injury. *Neurochem Pathol* 7:57–76.
5. Bazan NG (1970): Effects of ischemia and electroconvulsive shock on fatty acid pool in the brain. *Biochim Biophys Acta* 218:1–10.
6. Bennett MH (1983): Effects of compression and ischemia on spinal cord evoked potentials. *Exp Neurol* 80:508–519.
7. Black P, Markowitz RS, Cooper V, et al. (1986): Models of spinal cord injury, 1: static load technique. *Neurosurgery* 19:752–766.
8. Bridges RJ, Stevens DR, Kahle JS, et al. (1989): Structure-function studies on *N*-oxalyl-diamino-dicarboxylic acids and excitatory amino acid receptors: evidence that B-L-ODAP is a selective non-NMDA agonist. *J Neurosci* 9:2073–2079.
9. Brodin L, Grillner S (1985): The role of putative excitatory amino acid neurotransmitters in the initiation of locomotion in the lamprey spinal cord, I: the effects of excitatory amino acid antagonists. *Brain Res* 360:139–148.
10. Buchan A (1992): Advances in cerebral ischemia: experimental approaches. *Neurol Clin* 10:49–61.
11. Choi DW (1987): Ionic dependence of glutamate neurotoxicity. *J Neurosci* 7:369–379.
12. Choi DW (1988): Calcium-mediated neurotoxicity: relationship to specific channel types and role in ischemic damage. *Trends Neurosci* 11:465–469.
13. D'Angelo CM, VanGilder JC, Taub A (1973): Evoked cortical potentials in experimental spinal cord trauma. *J Neurosurgery* 38:332–336.
14. Dayton WR, Reville WJ, Goll DE, et al. (1976): A Ca^{2+}-activated protease possibly involved in myofibrillar protein turnover: partial characterization of the purified enzyme. *Biochemistry* 15:2159–2167.
15. Dean RT (1987): Some critical membrane events during mammalian cell death. In: Potten CS, ed. *Perspectives on mammalian cell death.* New York: Oxford University Press, pp. 18–38.
16. Dohrmann GJ, Panjabi MM, Tech D, et al. (1977): Biomechanics of the thoracic spinal cord and thorax in experimentally produced trauma. *Surgical Neurology* 28:448–450.
17. Dohrmann GJ, Panjabi MM, Tech D, et al. (1978): Biomechanics of experimental spinal cord trauma. *J Neurosurgery* 48:993–1001.
18. Dolan EJ, Transfeldt EE, Tator CH, et al. (1980): The effect of spinal distraction on regional spinal cord blood flow in cats. *J Neurosurgery* 53:756–764.
19. Faden AI, Salzman S (1992): Pharmacological strategies in CNS trauma. *Trends Pharmacol Sci* 13:29–35.
20. Faden AI, Simon RP (1988): A potential role for excitotoxins in the pathophysiology of spinal cord injury. *Ann Neurol* 23:623–626.
21. Farooqui AA, Horrocks LA (1991): Excitatory amino acid receptors neural membrane phospholipid metabolism and neurological disorders. *Brain Res Brain Res Rev* 16:171–191.
22. Frappier T, Derancourt J, Pradel L. (1992): Actin and neurofilament binding domain of brain spectrin B subunit. *Eur J Biochem* 205:85–91.
23. Frappier T, Stetzkowski-Marden F, Pradel L (1991): Interaction domains of neurofilament light chain and brain spectrin. *Biochem J* 275:521–527.
24. Gale K, Kerasidis H, Wrathall JR (1985): Spinal cord contusion in the rat:behavioral analysis of functional neurologic impairment. *Exp Neurol* 88:123–134.
25. Gardner VO, Caiozzo VJ, Munden SK, et al. (1990): Excitotoxins can produce protein degradation in the spinal cord. *Spine* 15:858–863.
26. Gardner VO, Caiozzo VJ, Munden SK, et al. (1992): Inhibition of neurofilament degradation in the spinal cord using a new calpain inhibitor: calpeptin. *Spine.*
27. Garfin SR, Cohen MS, Massie JB, et al. (1990): Nerve-roots of the cauda equina. *J Bone Joint Surg Am* 72:1185–1192.
28. Gold RM, Schmied G, Giegerich H, et al. (1994). Differentiation between cellular apoptosis and necrosis by combined use of in situ tailing and nick translation techniques. *Lab Invest* 71:219–225.
29. Gomez-Pinilla F, Tram H, Cotman CW, et al. (1989): Neuroprotective effect of MK-801 and U-50488H after contusive spinal cord injury. *Exp Neurol* 104:118–124.
30. Guroff G (1964): A neutral calcium-activated proteinase from the soluble fraction of rat brain. *J Biol Chem* 239:149–155.
31. Happel RD, Smith KP, Banik NL, et al. (1981): Ca^{2+}-accumulation in experimental spinal cord trauma. *Brain Res* 211:476–479.
32. Hashemi RM, Koozekanani SH, McGhee RB (1975): A lumped parameter computer model for the mechanics of experimental spinal cord injury by the method of Allen. Technical Note no. 17 Comm. Con. Sys. Lab. Columbus OH: Ohio State University.
33. Hu R, Bennett V. (1991): In vitro proteolysis of brain spectrin by calpain I inhibits association of spectrin with ankyrin-independent membrane binding site(s). *J Biol Chem* 266:18200–18205.
34. Hukuda S, Wilson CB (1972): Experimental cervical myelopathy: effects of compression and ischemia on the canine cervical cord. *J Neurosurgery* 37:631–652.
35. Inuzuka T, Tamur A, Sato S, et al. (1990): Suppressive effect of E-64c on ischemic degradation of cerebral proteins following occlusion of the middle cerebral artery in rats. *Brain Res* 526:177–179.
36. Iizuka H, Yamamoto H, Iwasaki Y, et al. (1987): Evolution of tissue damage in compressive spinal cord injury in rats. *J Neurosurgery* 66:595–603.
37. Iwasa K, Ikata T, Fukuzawa K (1989): Protective effect of vitaminute E on spinal cord injury by compression and concurrent lipid peroxidation. *Free Radic Biol Med* 6:599–606.
38. Iwasaki Y, Yamamoto H, Iizuka Yamamoto T, et al. (1987): Suppression of neurofilament degradation by protease inhibitors in experimental spinal cord injury. *Brain Res* 406:99–104.
39. Jansen KLR, Faull RLM, Dragunow M, et al. (1990): Autoradiographic localisation of NMDA quisqualate and kainic acid receptors in human spinal cord. *Neurosci Lett* 108:53–57.
40. Kearney PA, Ridella SA, Viano DC, et al. (1988): Interaction of

contact velocity and cord compression in determining the severity of spinal cord injury. *J Neurotrauma* 5:187–208.

41. Kerasidis H, Wrathall JR, Gale K (1987): Behavioral assessment of functional deficit in rats with contusive spinal cord injury. *J Neurosci Methods* 20:167–189.

42. Kerr JF, Gobe G, Winterford CM, et al. (1995): Anatomical methods in cell death. In: Schwartz LM, Osborne BA, eds. *Cell death.* New York: Academic Press, 1–27.

43. Kerr JF, Harmon BV (1991). Definition and incidence of apoptosis: an historical perspective. In: Tomei LD, Cope FO, eds. *Apoptosis: the molecular basis of cell death.* Cold Spring Harbor, NY: Cold Spring Harbor Laboratory Press, 5–29.

44. Kerr JF, Wyllie AH, Currie AR (1972). Apoptosis: a basic biological phenomenon with wide-ranging implications in tissue kinetics. *Br J Cancer* 26:239–257.

45. Kirshner DL, Kirshner RL, Heggeness LM, et al. (1989): Spinal cord ischemia: an evaluation of pharmacologic agents in minimizing paraplegia after aortic occlusion. *J Vasc Surg* 9:305–308.

46. Kontos HA, Wei EP, Povlishock JT, et al. (1980): Cerebral arteriolar damage by arachidonic acid and prostaglandin G2. *Science* 209:1242–1245.

47. Koozekanani SH, Vise WM, Hashemi RM, et al. (1976): Possible mechanisms for observed pathophysiological variability in experimental spinal cord injury by the method of Allen. *J Neurosurgery* 44:429–434.

48. Laiho KU, Shelburne JD, Trump RJ (1971): Observations on cell volume ultrastructure mitochondrial conformation and vital-dye uptake in Ehrlich ascites tumor cells. *Am J Pathol* 65:203–230.

49. Laiho KU, Trump BJ (1975): Studies on the pathogenesis of cell injury: effects of inhibitors of metabolism and membrane function on the mitochondria of Ehrlich ascites tumor cells. *Lab Invest* 32:163–182.

50. LeMay DR, Neal S, Zelenock GB, et al. (1987): Paraplegia in the rat induced by aortic cross-clamping: model characterization and glucose exacerbation of neurologic deficit. *J Vasc Surg* 6:383–390.

51. Li PD, Nijhawan L, Budihardjo SM, et al. (1997): Cytochrome c and dATP-dependent formation of Apaf-1/caspase-9 complex initiates an apoptotic protease cascade. *Cell* 91:479–489.

52. Linden R (1994): The survival of developing neurons: a review of afferent control. *Neuroscience* 58:671–682.

53. Liu D, Thangnipon W, McAdoo DJ (1991): Excitatory amino acids rise to toxic levels upon impact injury to the rat spinal cord. *Brain Res* 547:344–348.

54. Liu X, Kim CN, Jemmerson R, et al. (1996): Induction of apoptotic program in cell-free extracts: requirement for dATP and cytochrome c. *Cell* 86:147–157.

55. Liu X, Zou H, Slaughter C, et al. (1997): Dff: a heterodimeric protein that functions down-stream of caspase-3 to trigger DNA fragmentation during apoptosis. *Cell* 8:175–184.

56. Lucas JH, Wolf A (1991): In vitro studies of multiple impact injury to mammalian CNS neurons: prevention of perikaryal damage and death by ketamine. *Brain Res* 543:181–193.

57. Madden KP, Clark WM, Marcoux FW, et al. (1990): Treatment with conotoxin and "N-type" calcium channel blocker in neuronal hypoxic-ischemic injury. *Brain Res* 537:256–262.

58. McCord JM (1987): Oxygen-derived radicals: a link between reperfusion injury and inflammation. *Fed Proc* 46:2402–2406.

59. McDonald JW, Johnston MV (1990): Physiological and pathophysiological roles of excitatory amino acids during central nervous system development. *Brain Res Brain Res Rev* 15:41–70.

60. Meldrum B, Garthwaite J (1990): Excitatory amino acid neurotoxicity and neurodegenerative disease. *Trends Pharmacol Sci* 11:379–387.

61. Mergner WJ, Jones RT, Trump BJ (1990): *Cell death: mechanisms of acute and lethal cell injury.* New York: Field and Wood.

62. Mitchell JJ, and Anderson KJ, (1991): Quantitative autoradiographic analysis of excitatory amino acid receptors in the cat spinal cord. *Neurosci Lett* 124:269–272.

63. Molt JT, Nelson LR, Poulos DA, et al. (1979): Analysis and measurement of some sources of variability in experimental spinal cord trauma. *J Neurosurgery* 50:784–791.

64. Monaghan DT, Bridges RJ, Cotman CW (1989): The excitatory amino acid receptors: their classes pharmacology and distinct properties in the function of the central nervous system. *Annu Rev Pharmacol Toxicol* 29:365–402.

65. Naftchi NE (1991): Treatment of mammalian spinal cord injury with antioxidants. *Int J Dev Neurosci* 9:113–126.

66. Noble LJ, Wrathall JR (1987): An inexpensive apparatus for producing graded spinal cord contusive injury in the rat. *Exp Neurol* 95:530–533.

67. Olney JW (1969): Brain lesions obesity and other disturbances in mice treated with monosodium glutamate. *Science* 164:719–721.

68. Orrenius S, McConkey DJ, Bellomo G, et al. (1989): Role of Ca^{++} in toxic cell killing. *Trends Pharmacol Sci* 10:281–285.

69. Osterholm JL (1974): The pathophysiological response to spinal cord injury. *J Neurosurgery* 40:5–33.

70. Panjabi MM, Dicker DB, Dohrmann GJ (1977): Biomechanical quantification of experimental spinal cord trauma. *J Biomech* 10:681–687.

71. Pant HC (1988): Dephosphorylation of neurofilament proteins enhances their susceptibility to degradation by calpain. *Biochem J* 256:665–668.

72. Pant HC, Gainer H (1980): Properties of calcium-activated protease in squid axoplasm which selectively degrades neurofilament proteins. *J Neurobiol* 11:1–12.

73. Pant HC, Gallant PE, Gould R, et al. (1982): Distribution of calcium-activated protease activity and endogenous substrates in the squid nervous system. *J Neurosci* 2:1578–1587.

74. Panter SS, Yum SW, Faden AI (1990): Alteration in extracellular amino acids after traumatic spinal cord injury. *Ann Neurol* 27:96–99.

75. Prasad MR, Popescu LM, Moraru II, et al. (1991): Role of phospholipase A_2 and C in myocardial ischemic reperfusion injury. *Am J Physiol* 260:H877–H883.

76. Raines A, Dretchen KL, Marx K, et al. (1988): Spinal cord contusion in the rat: somatosensory evoked potentials as a function of graded injury. *J Neurotrauma* 5:151–160.

77. Regan RF, Choi DW (1991): Glutamate neurotoxicity in spinal cord cell culture. *Neuroscience* 43:585–591.

78. Rivlin AS, Tator CH (1977): Objective clinical assessment of motor function after experimental spinal cord injury in the rat. *J Neurosurgery* 47:577–581.

79. Rordorf G, Uemura Y, Bonventre JV (1991): Characterization of phospholipase A_2 (PLA_2) activity in gerbil brain: enhanced activities of cytosolic mitochondrial and microsomal forms after ischemia and reperfusion. *J Neurosci* 11:1829–1836.

80. Ross SM, Roy DN, Spencer PS (1989): β-N-oxalylamino-L-alanine action on glutamate receptors. *J Neurochem* 53:710–71.

81. Rothman SM, Olney JW (1986): Glutamate and the pathophysiology of hypoxic-ischemic brain damage. *Ann Neurol* 19:105–111.

82. Salzman SK, Mendez AA, Dabney KW, et al. (1991): Serotonergic response to spinal distraction trauma in experimental scoliosis. *J Neurotrauma* 8:45–54.

83. Salzman SK, Mendez AA, Sabato S, et al. (1990): Anesthesia influences the outcome from experimental spinal cord injury. *Brain Res* 521:33–39.

84. Schanne FAX, Kane AB, Yound EE, et al. (1979): Calcium dependence of toxic cell death: a final common pathway. *Science* 206:700–702.

85. Schlaepfer WW (1977): Structural alterations of peripheral nerve induced by the calcium ionophore A23187. *Brain Res* 136:1–9.

86. Schlaepfer WW (1979): Nature of mammalian neurofilaments and their breakdown by calcium. *Prog Neuropathol* 4:101–123.

87. Schlaepfer WW, Bunge RP (1973): Effects of calcium ion concentration on the degeneration of amputated axons in tissue culture. *J Cell Biol* 59:456–470.

88. Schlaepfer WW, Freeman LA (1978): Neurofilament proteins of rat peripheral nerve and spinal cord. *J Cell Biol* 78:653–662.

89. Schlaepfer WW, Freeman LA (1980): Calcium-dependent degradation of mammalian neurofilaments by soluble tissue factor(s) from rat spinal cord. *Neuroscience* 5:2305–2314.

90. Schlaepfer WW, Lee C, Lee MY, et al. (1985): An immunoblot study

of neurofilament degradation in situ and during calcium-activated proteolysis. *J Neurochem* 44:502–509.

91. Schlaepfer WW, Micko S (1978): Chemical and structural changes of neurofilaments in transected rat sciatic nerve. *J Cell Biol* 369–378.

92. Schlaepfer WW, Micko S (1979): Calcium-dependent alterations of neurofilament proteins of rat peripheral nerve. *J Neurochem* 32:211–219.

93. Schramm J, Hashizume K, Fukushima T, et al. (1979): Experimental spinal cord injury produced by slow graded compression. *J Neurosurgery* 50:48–57.

94. Seubert P, Nakagawa Y, Ivy G, et al. (1989): Intrahippocampal colchicine injection results in spectrin proteolysis. *Neuroscience* 31:195–202.

95. Shaw PJ, Ince PG, Johnson M, et al. (1991): The quantitative autoradiographic distribution of [3H]MK-801 binding sites in the normal human spinal cord. *Brain Res* 539:164–168.

96. Sheardown MJ, Nielsen EO, Hansen AJ (1990): 2,3-Dihydroxy-6-nitro-7-sulfamoyl-benzo(F)quinoxaline: a neuroprotectant for cerebral ischemia. *Science* 247:571–574.

97. Sher E, Biancardi E, Passafaro M, et al. (1991): Physiopathology of neuronal voltage-operated calcium channels. *FASEB J* 5:2677–2683.

98. Shi R, Lucas JH, Wolf A, et al. (1989): Calcium antagonists fail to protect mammalian spinal neurons after physical injury. *J Neurotrauma* 6:261–276.

99. Shohami E, Shapira Y, Yadid G, et al. (1989): Brain phospholipase A$_2$ is activated after experimental closed head injury in the rat. *J Neurochem* 53:1541–1546.

100. Simon RP, Swan JH, Griffiths T, et al. (1988): Blockade of *N*-methyl-D-aspartate receptors may protect against ischemic damage in the brain. *Science* 226:850–852.

101. Smith JC, Feldman JL (1987): In vitro brainstem-spinal cord preparations for study of motor systems for mammalian respiration and locomotion. *J Neurosci* Methods 21:321–333.

102. Smith JC, Feldman JL, Schmidt BJ (1988): Neural mechanisms generating locomotion studied in mammalian brain stem-spinal cord in vitro. *FASEB J* 2:2283–2288.

103. Spencer PS, Roy DN, Ludolph A, et al. (1986): Lathyrism: evidence for role of the neuroexcitatory amino acid BOAA. *Lancet* 2:1066–1067.

104. Stark K, Seubert P, Lynch G, et al. (1989): Proteolytic conversion of xanthine dehydrogenase to xanthine oxidase: evidence against a role for calcium-activated protease (calpain). *Biochem Biophys Res Commun* 165:858–864.

105. Takeda H, Caiozzo VJ, Gardner VO (1993): A functional in vitro model for studying the cellular and molecular basis of spinal cord injury. *Spine* 18:1125–1133.

106. Tarlov IM (1954): Spinal cord compression studies. *AMA Arch Neurol Psychiatry* 71:588–597.

107. Tarlov IM, Klinger H, Vitale S (1953): Spinal cord compression studies. *AMA Arch Neurol Psychiatry* 70:813–819.

108. Tator CH (1973): Acute spinal cord injury in primates produced by an inflatable extradural cuff. *Can J Surg* 16:222–231.

109. Tominaga T, Dure S, Narisawa K, et al. (1993). Endonuclease activation following focal ischemic injury in rat brain. *Brain Res* 608:21–26.

110. Tsujinaka T, Kajiwara Y, Kambayashi J (1988): Synthesis of a new cell penetrating calpain inhibitor (calpeptin). *Biochem Biophys Res Commun* 153:1201–1208

111. Urca G, Urca R (1990): Neurotoxic effects of excitatory amino acids in the mouse spinal cord: quisqualate and kainate but not *N*-ethyl-D-aspartate induce permanent neural damage. *Brain Res* 529:7–15.

112. Wood KA, Dipasquale B, Youle RJ (1993): In situ labeling of granule cells for apoptosis-associated DNA fragmentation reveals different mechanisms of cell loss in developing cerebellum. *Neuron* 11:621–632.

113. Wrathall JR, Pettegrew RK, Harvey F (1985): Spinal cord contusion in the rat: production of graded reproducible injury groups. *Exp Neurol* 88:108–122.

114. Wyllie AH (1980): Glucocorticoid-induced thymocyte apoptosis is associated with endogenous endonuclease activation. *Nature* 284:555–556.

115. Wyllie AH, Kerr JF, Currie AR (1990): Cell death: the significance of apoptosis. *Int Rev Cytol* 68:251–306.

116. Xu J, Beckman JS, Hogan EL, et al. (1991): Xanthine oxidase in experimental spinal cord injury. *J Neurotrauma* 8:11–18.

117. Young W (1986): Ca paradox in neural injury: a hypothesis. *Cent Nerv Syst Trauma* 3:235–251.

118. Yum SW, Faden AI (1990): Comparison of the neuroprotective effects of *N*-methyl-D-aspartate antagonist MK-801 and the opiate-receptor antagonist nalmefene in experimental spinal cord ischemia. *Arch Neurol* 47:277–281.

119. Zivin JA, DeGirolami U (1980): Spinal cord infarction: a highly reproducible stroke model. *Stroke* 11:200–202.

30

CERVICAL SPINE INJURIES IN CHILDREN

NATHAN H. LEBWOHL
FRANK J. EISMONT

Injuries to the cervical spines of children are relatively uncommon. There are few large series reported in the literature, and most major medical centers treat only one or two patients each year. Despite this, the need to evaluate children for possible injury to the cervical spine is common. In the care of very young children, this task is complicated by the inability to obtain a complete history and by the radiographic appearance of the vertebral column, which changes during development. The delay in diagnosis commonly cited in reports of treatment of series of patients attests to these difficulties. Familiarity with the developmental anatomy of the spine and with the usual patterns of injury should help the physicians confidently arrive at an accurate diagnosis.

EPIDEMIOLOGY

In 1969, Melzak (65) reported that only 2% of patients admitted to a spinal cord injury center in Great Britain were children. Burke (19) found only 29 children with spinal cord injury admitted to Rancho Los Amigos Hospital over an 18-year period; 13 of those had a injury to the cervical spine. Kewalramani and Tori (50) reviewed admissions to the Institute for Rehabilitation Research in Houston. They found that 13.2% of all patients with spinal cord injury were younger than 16 years. Two thirds of the injuries were to the cervical spinal cord. In a study spanning 41 years at the Mayo Clinic, McGrory et al. (63) estimated the incidence of injury to the cervical spine among patients living in Olmsted County, Minnesota, to be 1.19 per 100,000 for children younger than 11 years. For children between 11 and 15 years of age the incidence was 13.24 per 100,000. In this series, 62 of 143 patients (43%) had neurologic injury, and there was no difference in frequency between the younger and older groups.

Motor vehicle accidents are responsible for most injuries to cervical spine among children (58). These are followed by falls,

athletic injuries, and gunshot wounds in most series (Fig. 1). Among the youngest patients, falls are the most common cause of injury (44,83). Diving is the sport most commonly associated with injury to the cervical spine. Gymnastics, football, wrestling, rugby, and trampoline also are common causes (38).

The incidence of birth injury to the spinal cord is not known. In the past, most such injuries were associated with breech delivery. From 5% to 25% of breech deliveries are associated with spinal cord injury (1,3,14). Injury also can occur with cephalic presentations (89). The use of forceps has been associated with an increased incidence of spinal cord injury. Evidence of spinal cord injury has been identified in as many as 50% of neonatal deaths (1,4).

Child abuse is another important cause of pediatric injury to the cervical spine. Once again, the true incidence is not known. An infant's large head, combined with poor control of cervical musculature predisposes the cervical spine to injury from violent shaking. Vigilance for associated musculoskeletal injuries should help identify abuse among these children (23,51,100).

EARLY MANAGEMENT

Whenever a spinal injury is suspected, the patient must be immediately immobilized and transported carefully to avoid neurologic injury. Injury to the cervical spine should be considered whenever a patient is unconscious after trauma or reports numbness, weakness, or neck pain. Even transient neurologic symptoms after trauma warrant immobilization until instability is ruled out.

Because young children have a large head in comparison with the rest of the body, positioning on a standard backboard forces the cervical spine into relative kyphosis. Herzenberg et al. (46) described ten patients with unstable cervical spine injuries in whom the kyphotic deformity increased with positioning on a standard backboard. They recommended use of a double mattress pad to raise the chest or use of a recess for the occiput (Fig. 2). This discrepancy between the circumference of the head and the circumference of the chest exists until 8 years of age, when the chest attains 50% of its adult size (91). Ogden (69) advocates placing a small support under the lumbar spine to maintain normal lordosis and to prevent malalignment.

N.H. Lebwohl and **F.J. Eismont:** Department of Orthopaedics and Rehabilitation, University of Miami School of Medicine, Miami, Florida 33101.

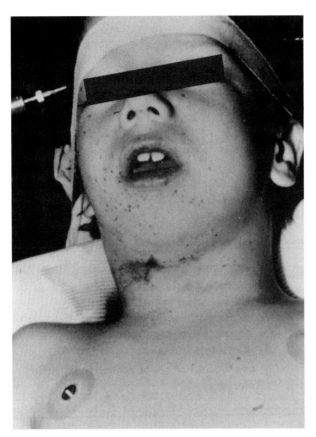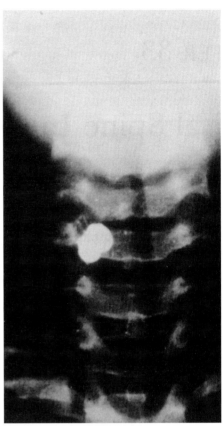

FIGURE 1. Gunshot wounds are an increasingly common cause of pediatric spinal cord injury in inner cities in the United States.

Athletic injuries are a common cause of injuries to the cervical spine among older pediatric patients. Spine boards always should be present at playing fields and gymnasiums where high-risk sports such as football and gymnastics take place. The combination of tape and sandbags provides much more effective immobi-

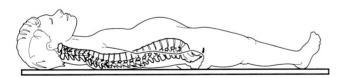

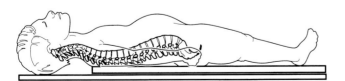

FIGURE 2. Because a child's head is large in proportion to its chest, immobilization on a standard backboard pushes the cervical spine into kyphosis. This may increase fracture deformity among patients with unstable spines. The use of a double mattress pad allows the head to fall backward and allows the spine to assume a more normal lordosis.

lization of the head and neck than does use of a hard collar. In helmeted sports, the face mask should be cut away to provide access to the airway. The patient should be transported with the helmet in place, because it is difficult to remove the helmet without causing neck flexion. Removal of the helmet usually is best accomplished when the patient arrives in the emergency department. The helmet is spread open and pulled off while the head is manually stabilized (105).

As in all emergency care, initial attention must be given to the airway, breathing, and circulation. Children with injury to the cervical cord commonly have compromised respiratory function and need endotracheal intubation. There is controversy about the safety of various techniques to establish an airway. Aprahamian et al. (5), in a radiographic study of cadavers, found that cervical collars did not immobilize the spine during orotracheal intubation. Nasotracheal intubation, however, caused minimal motion of the spine. Majernick et al. (57) likewise found that cervical collars did not adequately immobilize the spine during orotracheal intubation. In-line traction, however, minimized spinal motion during intubation. In contrast, Bivins et al. (12), Turner (103), and Joyce (49) argued against the use of in-line traction during intubation because of the danger of overdistraction of a highly unstable injury. In combined clinical series of 136 patients with fractures of the cervical spine who underwent oral intubation and 143 patients who underwent nasal intubation, Holley and Jorden (47) and Suderman et al. (97) found no patients with neurologic deterioration attributable to intubation technique. In the series described by Suderman et al., 83 of the patients underwent intubation after induction of general anesthesia.

Other techniques that have been advocated for airway management in the care of patients with injuries to the cervical spine include fiberoptics-guided intubation and intubation over a wire placed percutaneously through the cricothyroid membrane and guided retrograde into the mouth (8). None of these studies has specifically addressed airway management in the care of injured pediatric patients.

PHYSICAL ASSESSMENT

An unresponsive child with a head injury always should be considered to have a spinal injury until proved otherwise. The presence of clonus in a child with a brain injury without the finding of decerebrate rigidity strongly suggests spinal cord injury (90). Facial abrasions and scalp wounds also should direct attention to the cervical spine and suggest the direction of forces that could have caused injury (10,55). Palpation of a gap between the spinous processes implies severe ligamentous disruption and a highly unstable injury. A history of cardiopulmonary arrest after trauma should alert the physician to the possibility of an injury to the upper part of the cervical spine (13).

Evaluation of an awake child who is unable or unwilling to cooperate with an examination can be difficult. Determining the extent of paralysis, or even determining its presence for an infant, is challenging. A child with paralysis may have reflex mass flexion withdrawal movements in response to stimulation. These movements may be indistinguishable from the normal movements of an infant. In examinations of older, cooperative patients, absence of voluntary movement in the extremities, or sensory deficit, makes the diagnosis of spinal cord injury obvious. It is important, however, to elicit a history of transient neurologic deficit for children who appear to have normal findings. These patients may have occult instability, identification of which can make the difference between no injury and neurologic catastrophe.

Tenderness to palpation of the neck, muscle guarding, cervical rigidity, and torticollis all suggest injury to the cervical spine. Injured children may support their heads with their hands. Seimon (86) described two children with fractures of the odontoid process whose only symptom was neck pain when changing from a lying to a sitting position. Missed and delayed diagnosis is commonly reported in series of pediatric spinal fractures, and a conservative approach to management with immobilization and reexamination is prudent.

PATTERN OF INJURY

Although injuries to adolescents are similar to those to adults, injuries to young children are distinctly different. Allen and Ferguson (2) classified pediatric injuries into three groups: infantile, young juvenile, and old juvenile.

Infantile injuries are those that occur before the development of good head control. These children lack adequate voluntary muscle strength and cannot protect their spines from external forces. They are susceptible to traction and torsion injuries during birth and to flexion and extension injuries inflicted by parental shaking (20). Radiographs are commonly unrevealing, perhaps because of the large proportion of the infantile spine that is cartilaginous and therefore difficult to evaluate radiographically (35) or because of the elasticity of the infant's spinal column, which can be deformed or stretched. The stretching allows injury to the less elastic spinal cord, which is tethered by exiting nerve roots and the dentate ligaments. In the laboratory, the infantile spinal column can be stretched more than 2 inches (5 cm) without injury, although the adult spinal cord ruptures when stretched more than $\frac{1}{4}$ inch (6.25 mm) (29,54). Stretching and disruption of the vertebral arteries also may be important in fatal neurologic injuries owing to distraction of the cervical spine and craniospinal junction (24,110).

Young juvenile injuries are classified as those occurring after the development of good head control until about 8 years of age. Unlike injuries in older age groups, most injuries to these children occur in the upper cervical spine, above C4 (11). The fulcrum of normal cervical spinal motion among children younger than 8 years is at the C2–3 interspace rather than at C5–6 (67). This is attributed in part to the disproportionate largeness of the heads of young children but also to the relatively horizontal orientation of the upper cervical facet joints of children, which allows hypermobility of the upper cervical spine (98). Ligamentous laxity also contributes to the hypermobility of the juvenile spine. Some authors have identified the anteriorly wedged appearance of the normal child's cervical vertebral bodies as a contributing factor in cervical instability (95); however, this is merely a radiographic finding caused by the pattern of vertebral ossification. The vertebral body itself is not wedged.

In the lower cervical spines of young children, the joints of Luschka are incompletely developed. The absence of a well-developed uncinate process may predispose children in this age group to separation of the vertebral end plate, an injury that may play an important role in the syndrome of spinal cord injury without radiographic abnormality.

After the age of 8 years, a child's spine begins to take on a more adult appearance, and the pattern of injuries is similar to that of adults. Injuries in the midcervical spine become more frequent. The proportion of head size to torso size decreases. The cervical facet joints become more vertical and reach the adult shape by the age of 10 years. These changes combine to reduce the hypermobility of the upper cervical spine and move the fulcrum of spinal motion down toward the midcervical spine. By the age of 8 years, all of the ossification centers have appeared and fused, with the exception of the apical odontoid epiphysis and the ring apophysis and other secondary ossification centers at the tips of the spinous, transverse, and mammillary processes, which appear in puberty. Thus Salter-Harris type I physeal separations (84) of the synchondroses or the basilar odontoid growth cartilage can no longer occur. In this age group, sports injuries become a more frequent cause of spinal injury than they are younger children.

SPECIFIC INJURIES

Occipitoatlantal Dislocation

Traumatic dislocation of the occiput from the atlas occurs commonly in fatal craniospinal injuries (Fig. 3). Bucholz and Burkhead et al. (17,18) reported an incidence of 8% among victims of fatal traffic accidents, making it the single most common injury encountered. The injury was more than twice as frequent among infants and children (15%) as it was among adults (6%). This finding is consistent with the higher incidence of injuries to the upper cervical spine among children than among adults.

Occipitoatlantal dislocation with survival is rare. This is because of the neurologic deficits caused by injury to the upper cervical cord, brain stem, and cranial nerves. Dislocation usually is the result of high-energy trauma, commonly involving a motor vehicle. Severe associated injury is common. Survival is being reported with increasing frequency, in part because better emergency care results in early cardiopulmonary resuscitation and ventilatory support of these patients, who previously would not have lived.

The degree of neurologic injury to patients who survive occipitoatlantal dislocation varies. In rare instances, patients have normal neurologic findings or minimal deficit. In a series described by Montane et al. (66), two patients had minor weakness and

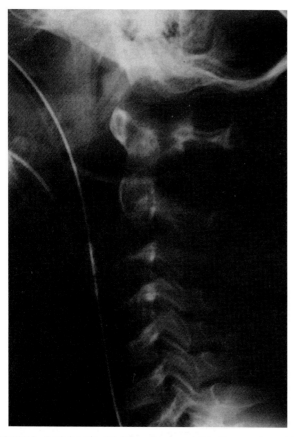

FIGURE 3. Occipitoatlantal dislocation in a child after a motor vehicle accident. This usually is a fatal injury because of the associated trauma to the high cervical spinal cord.

hyperreflexia, and one patient had a more severe neurologic injury, retaining only unilateral antigravity strength in her extremities. The latter patient also had several episodes of heart block and respiratory arrest, suggesting injury to the cardiorespiratory centers in the brain stem. A fourth patient, who did not live, had complete cord transection at C1 and severe head injury. The patient described by Zigler et al. (112) lived with complete paralysis at the C1 level and palsy of the spinal accessory nerve. This resulted in a flail neck, which necessitated fusion from the occiput to the thoracic spine to avoid the need for external support. The patient also needed tracheostomy because he was ventilator dependent. Ogden (69) described a 6-year-old girl with irregular pulse and respiration, which resolved with extension of the neck. Page et al. (72) described a patient with C5 quadriplegia and palsy of the tenth and twelfth cranial nerves at initial presentation with ascent to a C2 level. Przybylski et al. (80) summarized the findings in the published reports of 79 patients who survived atlantooccipital dislocation: 18% had normal neurologic findings, 10% had isolated cranial nerve deficits, 34% had unilateral limb deficits, and 38% had quadriparesis or quadriplegia.

The radiographic diagnosis of occipitoatlantal dislocation may not be apparent until traction is applied to the skull. It is important to examine a lateral radiograph of the cervical spine immediately after applying traction to avoid overdistraction of this or other ligamentous injuries. Wholey et al. (108) studied the relation between the basion and the dens on 600 lateral radiographs of the cervical spine. They found that that the distance between the basion and the dens should not exceed 5 mm in adults and 10 mm in children. The greater distance in children was attributed to incomplete ossification of the dens. Powers et al. (78), however, found that in a randomly selected population of 100 adults and 50 children, the dens-basion distance exceeded those values in 85% of patients. Powers et al. devised a ratio based on two simple measurements: the distance between the basion (B, the anterior margin of the foramen magnum) and the posterior arch (C) of the atlas divided by the distance between the opisthion (O, the posterior margin of the foramen magnum) and the anterior arch (A) of the atlas. Values greater than 1.0 are definitely abnormal, values less than 0.9 are definitely normal (Fig. 4). The advantage of this ratio is that it is dimensionless and thus unaffected by magnification of the radiograph. If the landmarks are not easily identified on a lateral radiograph of the cervical spine, they can be measured on a midline sagittal reconstruction of a computed tomographic (CT) scan. The ratio is sensitive to anterior occipitoatlantal dislocation because one line, BC, parallels the direction of dislocation, and the second, OA, is almost perpendicular to it. The Powers ratio may be insensitive to posterior occipitoatlantal dislocation, as described by Eismont and Bohlman (31) and is not valid if there is a fracture of the atlas or congenital anomaly of the foramen magnum (22,79).

Another measurement that can be used to evaluate the stability of the occipitoatlantal joint is horizontal translation on flexion and extension. The basion should not translate more than 1 mm relative to the odontoid process. This value has only been established for adults, however, and has not been validated for children (106). This measurement should not be made if there

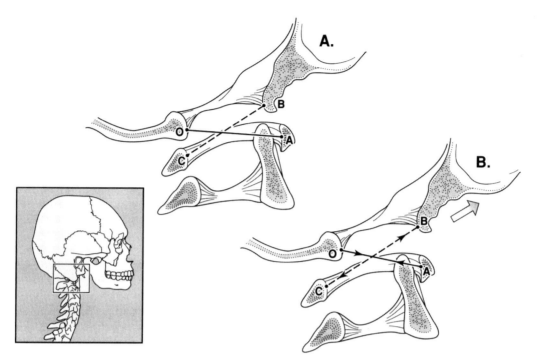

FIGURE 4. The Powers ratio is determined by means of drawing a line from the basion (*B*) to the posterior arch of the atlas (*C*) and a second line from the opisthion (*O*) to the anterior arch of the atlas (*A*). The length of the line *BC* is divided by the length of line *OA*. **A:** Values less than 0.9 are definitely normal. **B:** A ratio greater than 1.0 confirms the diagnosis of anterior occipitoatlantal dislocation.

is evidence of spinal instability on the plain radiographs or if the patient is not able to cooperate. Flexion-extension radiographs never should be obtained when the patient is comatose or otherwise unresponsive.

There is controversy regarding management of occipitoatlantal dislocation. Some authors have advocated immobilization in a halo or Minerva cast. Most recent authors advocate operative treatment with posterior occipitocervical fusion. Because traction can distract the occipitocervical junction, halo immobilization is recommended as soon as this injury is identified. This device provides the most secure stabilization and should be placed preoperatively.

Atlas Fractures

Burst fractures of the C1 ring can occur among children (70,102), although they are infrequently described. The mechanism of injury is believed to be similar to that for adults. A blow to the head transmits an axial compressive force. The occipital condyles push down onto the lateral masses of the atlas, which are displaced centripetally (69). If the force is severe enough, the transverse ligament ruptures or is avulsed at its point of attachment. Among young children, the fracture can occur through neurocentral synchondroses (42), which may remain unfused until 7 years of age (7). CT scanning usually is the most helpful diagnostic study. It is important not to confuse normal synchondroses with fractures. In addition, anomalous ossification centers of the anterior arch are common and should not be confused. Ogden (69) recommends treatment in a Minerva

cast for 6 months followed by a brace. Sponseller and Herzenberg advocate treatment in a less restrictive cervical orthosis (92). Allen and Ferguson (2) advocate an initial 4- to 6-week period in traction if more than 4 mm lateral displacement of the lateral masses is present. After treatment, stability of the atlantoaxial articulation should be confirmed on flexion-extension radiographs.

Atlantoaxial Instability

Traumatic atlantoaxial subluxation due to rupture of the transverse ligament of the atlas among children may be more common than previously believed. McGrory et al. (63) reported an incidence of 10% in their large series of injuries to the cervical spine. DeBeer et al. (26) reported that rupture of the transverse ligament was the second most common type of injury to the cervical spine. Among young children, one would expect the synchondrosis at the base of the dens to fail, rather than the transverse ligament. An atlantodens interval measuring more than 5 mm on a lateral radiograph after trauma suggests the diagnosis of rupture of the transverse ligament (Fig. 5). An atlantodens interval up to 4 mm is normal for children (56). Fielding (35) recommends 8 to 12 weeks of immobilization for management of acute traumatic rupture of the transverse ligament. DeBeer reported excellent results for all 3 patients treated in this way in his series. In contrast, Floman et al. (39) reported that immobilization did not adequately reduce subluxation and argued that atlantoaxial arthrodesis is the treatment of choice.

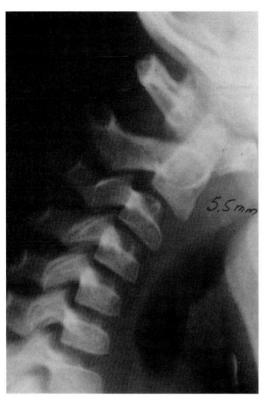

FIGURE 5. An atlantodens interval greater than 5.0 mm suggests rupture of the transverse ligament in a child injured in a motor vehicle accident.

Atlantoaxial Rotatory Subluxation

Rotatory instability of the atlantoaxial joint is probably the most fascinating abnormality of the pediatric cervical spine. Although it can occur as the result of minor or major trauma, its cause is commonly atraumatic. Most cases not involving trauma follow upper respiratory infections (28). Other predisposing conditions include rheumatoid arthritis and a history of head or neck surgery. A small number of patients have no obvious predisposing factor. Sir Charles Bell is credited with first describing this condition, in 1830 (33). Grisel in 1930 described two cases of torticollis following pharyngeal inflammation (43). In the same year an additional case was reported by Desfosses with the description *maladie de Grisel.* Since that time, the eponym *Grisel syndrome* has been used.

Parke et al. (74) described a venous plexus, the pharyngovertebral veins, which drain the posterosuperior nasopharynx and anastomose with the epidural plexus and periodontoidal plexus. Lymphatic vessels from the nasopharynx enter directly into the pharyngovertebral veins. It is believed that inflammatory exudates can be transported via these veins to the ligaments that support the atlantoaxial complex, resulting in inflammation and secondary ligamentous laxity. Once ligamentous laxity exists, rotation of the neck can result in subluxation of the atlantoaxial joints. A combination of muscle spasm and infolding with interposition of swollen capsular and synovial tissue are believed to be responsible for blocking reduction of the subluxation.

Patients have painful torticollis, and neurologic deficit is uncommon. Conventional radiographs can be used to confirm the diagnosis, but interpretation is difficult. Dynamic CT scanning with the head turned to the right and the left is the best examination; evidence of loss of normal rotation between C1 and C2 confirms the diagnosis (Figs. 6, 7).

When the injury is diagnosed early, most patients respond well to a simple treatment program. Once other injuries have been ruled out, treatment protocols are the same whether or not the onset was traumatic or atraumatic. Immobilization in a collar and bed rest may be adequate to allow resolution of muscle spasm and torticollis. If symptoms persist for more than 1 week, cervical traction with a head halter or tongs should be used until the spasm resolves and the subluxation is reduced. Fielding (35) recommended an arbitrary maximum weight of 6.8 kg for children. Once reduction is achieved, immobilization for 4 to 6 weeks is recommended. If subluxation reoccurs, the prognosis for successful nonoperative treatment is poor (96). If symptoms have been present for more than 1 month, reduction with traction is less likely (75), and operative treatment is appropriate. Manipulative reduction under general anesthesia is controversial because of the risk of spinal cord injury. El-Khoury et al. (32) described three children with more severe rotational abnormalities at C1–2 after trauma. They called this condition *atlantoaxial dislocation* and recommended immediate reduction with traction and manipulation. They found reduction easy to accomplish. Reduction was followed by immobilization for 10 to 16 weeks in a cervical orthosis with good results for all three patients treated.

Fielding and Hawkins (37) described a subgroup of patients with long-standing torticollis and irreducible atlantoaxial rotatory subluxation. They called this condition *rotatory fixation.* Among their patients, there was an average delay in diagnosis of more than 11 months, underscoring the importance of early recognition of this entity. Fielding and Hawkins recommended an initial period of traction followed by posterior cervical fusion. If reduction is not achieved, fusion in situ should be performed rather than reduction under general anesthesia, which can cause neurologic deficit.

Odontoid Fracture

Fractures of the odontoid process in young children always occur as epiphyseal separation of the growth plate at the base of the dens. Most cases are caused by severe falls or motor vehicle accidents, but separation of the growth plate can occur with minor trauma as well. Most authors report that neurologic deficit is uncommon. In the series reported by Sherk et al. (88), the only patients with neural deficit were those who had sustained concomitant head injury. In contrast, Odent et al. (68) reported neurologic involvement in eight of 15 patients; four of the eight had high thoracic paraplegia and three had quadriplegia. None of these patients had associated head injury. Fracture displacement of at least 50% was universal among the patients described by Sherk et al. If displacement is not present, identification of the fracture on radiographs can be difficult. Tomograms may show widening of the growth plate. Anterior angulation of the odontoid fragment is an almost constant finding and may help

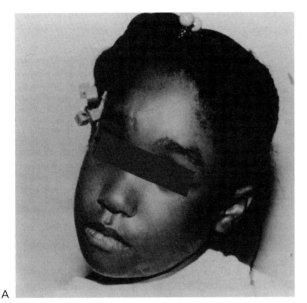
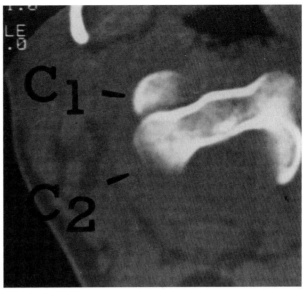

A   B

FIGURE 6. A: Cock robin appearance of a child with atlantoaxial rotatory subluxation. **B:** Computed tomographic scan through the C1–2 facet joint demonstrates subluxation. Diagnosis is confirmed if subluxation persists when scan is repeated with the head turned in the direction opposite the subluxation. (CT scan courtesy of Dr. Stephen Stricker. From Grobman LR, Stricker S [1990]: Grisel's syndrome. *Ear Nose Throat J* 69:799–801, with permission.)

identify the nondisplaced fracture. As in other injuries to the upper cervical spine, occipital pain, muscle spasm, and resistance to movement are common symptoms and physical findings (Fig. 8).

Postural reduction with cast or halo immobilization is the appropriate management of this injury, and 6 to 8 weeks of immobilization is required. When the patient is appropriately immobilized, nonunion is rare, as is avascular necrosis or growth disturbance of the odontoid fragment. Fractures of the odontoid process among older children after closure of the growth plate at the base of the dens are extremely uncommon. When they

occur, such fractures follow the patterns seen among adults. It is important not to confuse the epiphyseal scar at the base of the odontoid process with a fracture.

Failure to recognize and immobilize an odontoid fracture in a child may be responsible for the clinical syndrome of os odontoideum. It once was believed that os odontoideum was a congenital anomaly caused by failed fusion of the odontoid process to the vertebral centrum (30,109). Several case reports in the literature, however, document os odontoideum or disappearance of the odontoid process after trauma to the cervical spine (36,41,45,48,85). In nine cases, radiographic documentation ex-

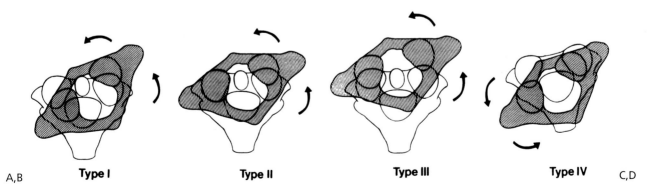

A,B   **Type I**   **Type II**   **Type III**   **Type IV**   C,D

FIGURE 7. Fielding and Hawkins classification of C1–2 rotatory subluxation. **A:** Type 1 rotation without anterior displacement (transverse ligament intact). **B:** Type 2 rotation with 3 to 5 mm anterior displacement (transverse ligament deficient). **C:** Type 3 rotation with greater than 5 mm anterior displacement (transverse and secondary ligaments insufficient). **D:** Type 4 rotation with posterior displacement (odontoid deficiency). (From Grobman LR, Stricker S [1990]: Grisel's syndrome. *Ear Nose Throat J* 69:799–801, with permission.)

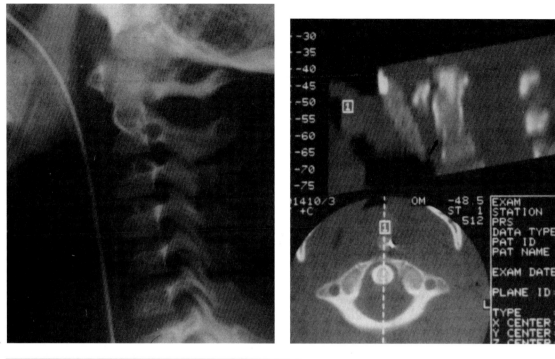

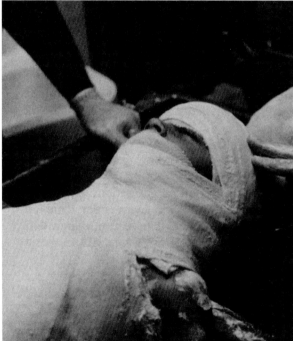

FIGURE 8. **A:** Fracture through basal growth plate of the odontoid process is appreciated only on computed tomographic sagittal reconstruction. **B:** Anterior displacement at the fracture site is evident. **C:** Application of Minerva cast to immobilize the patient.

ists of a normal odontoid with the development of an os odontoideum after trauma. Fielding et al. (36,37) wrote that injury to the blood supply combined with retraction of the dens by the alar ligaments contributed to nonunion of the odontoid. Os odontoideum causes atlantoaxial instability because the odontoid can no longer function as a post with which the anterior atlas and the transverse ligament can articulate. When a patient has symptoms or a patient without symptoms has documented instability, treatment is by means of posterior cervical fusion.

C2 Pedicle Fracture

Fracture of the C2 pedicle, better known as *hangman's fracture,* has been reported in an infant as young as 7 weeks old (99).

No data exist regarding the mechanism of injury among children, but it is believed to be similar to that for adult hangman's fractures (40). In most reported cases, there is no associated neurologic deficit. Weiss and Kaufman (107) reported the case of a 12-month-old child with central cord syndrome, which had almost completely resolved after 1 year of follow-up evaluation. In the series of Pizzutillo et al. (76), only one of five patients had a neurologic deficit, which had resolved completely after 1-year of follow-up evaluation.

Radiographic evaluation of C2 pedicle fracture is complicated by two factors. The neurocentral synchondroses can mimic a fracture on oblique radiographic views (82) and may persist beyond the age of 7 years, by which time it usually is closed (59). The more difficult problem in radiographic evaluation is differentiating physiologic subluxation at C2–3 from pathologic subluxation caused by disruption of the pedicles of C2. Hypermobility at C2–3 is common among children up to about the age of 8 years (21). This is the result of ligamentous laxity and horizontal alignment of the facet joints. The posterior cervical line of Swischuk (101) is useful in evaluating hypermobility at this level. The posterior laminar line is identified at the base of the spinous process at C1, C2, and C3. A line is drawn connecting this landmark at C1 and C3. The posterior laminar line of C2 should lie within 1 mm of this line. If it lies more than 1.5 mm posterior to the Swischuk line, a fracture may separate the anterior body and posterior lamina. If the distance is more than 2 mm, a fracture is almost certainly present. Anterior displacement greater than 2 mm implies pathologic subluxation without pedicle fracture. If the static view is normal, the same criteria should be applied to the flexion radiograph. A true lateral radiographic view is essential for this technique to be used reliably (Fig. 9).

Treatment of infants with hangman's fracture is similar to treatment of adult. If the body of C2 is not significantly displaced on C3, immobilization in a collar or custom-fabricated splint should be adequate. If there is more than 3-mm anterior displacement of C2 on C3, more rigid immobilization is indicated (2). A Minerva cast or a halo would be appropriate for 8 to 12 weeks.

Subaxial Injuries

Among children older than 8 years, most injuries occur below C2. Injury patterns are similar to those among adults. Flexion injuries predominate. Complete facet dislocations appear to be uncommon until late adolescence. Simple compression fracture is the most common injury. Residual kyphosis after flexion injury may be less well tolerated by growing children than by adults. Some authors advocate posterior fusion to prevent late disability (34,61). In contrast, Ogden (69) stated that surgical treatment rarely is necessary in the care of young children, even with ligamentous instability. He advocated reduction in traction followed by rigid immobilization for these injuries.

With the exception of burst fractures and other injuries in which anterior surgery is needed to remove bone fragments that compress the spinal cord (87), there is a relative contraindication to anterior fusion in a growing child. Anterior fusion destroys the anterior growth potential. Posterior growth continues, and a

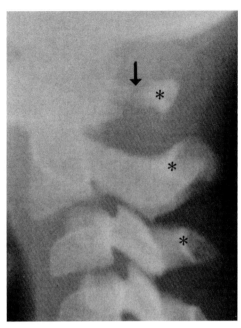

FIGURE 9. Pseudosubluxation of C2–3 is common among children younger than 8 years. *Asterisks* denote posterior laminar lines at C1, C2, and C3. The posterior laminar line of C2 should lie within 1 mm of a line drawn from C1–3, the posterior cervical line described by Swischuk. Greater than 2 mm posterior displacement of the C2 posterior laminar line implies C2 pedicle fracture. If anterior displacement is more than 2 mm, pathologic subluxation is implied. This patient also has incomplete ossification of the posterior arch of C1 (*arrow*), a common anomaly.

kyphotic deformity may result (94). If posterior fusion is needed, autogenous bone graft should be used. The use of allograft bone is associated with a high rate of pseudarthrosis (93). For posterior fusions, we routinely use iliac crest bone graft. We take care to minimize injury to the cartilaginous iliac apophysis. The use of rib graft has also been described, and the results have been good (64). The use of allograft bone in anterior fusion with instrumentation was reported to be successful in a small series (15). In posterior fusion, care must be taken to avoid exposure of levels not to be included in the arthrodesis to avoid spontaneous extension of the fusion. This occurred among 38% of patients described by McGrory and Klassen (62). (Figs. 10, 11).

Physeal Injuries

One important type of subaxial injury does occur among young children. Separation of the vertebral end plate from the vertebral body can occur through the epiphysis; it is similar to a physeal injury to a long bone. Salter-Harris type I injuries occur among infants and young children; type III injuries occur among older adolescents as the physis begins to close (53). The true incidence of this injury is not known because it is difficult to identify on radiographs. The fracture may recoil after injury and return to normal alignment, making radiographic identification impossible. The most likely radiographic finding is widening of the intervertebral disc space. Physeal separation can play an important role in injuries in which neurologic deficit has occurred,

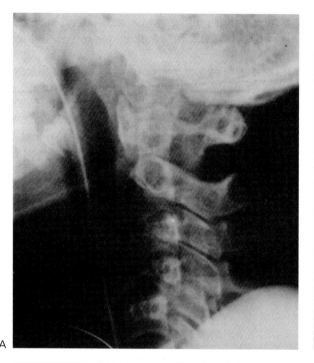

A

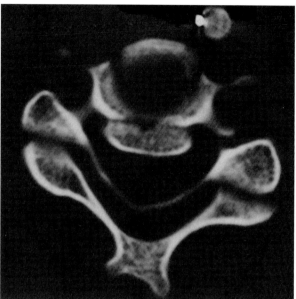

B

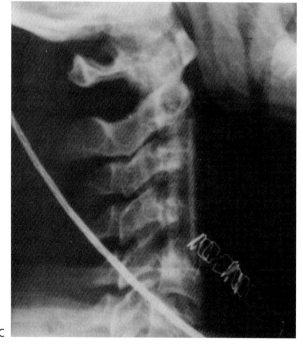

C

FIGURE 10. Subaxial injuries are more common among older than among young children. **A:** Image of a 16-year-old girl shows severe burst fracture of C4 with neurologic injury. **B:** Computed tomographic scan shows retopulsed bone in canal and posterior subluxation of the facet joint. **C:** Lateral radiograph obtained after anterior decompression and reconstruction with fibular allograft. (Courtesy of Barth Green, M.D.)

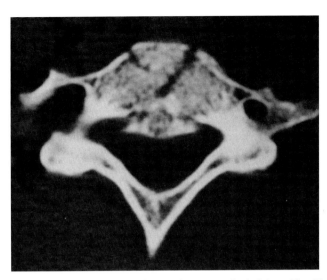

FIGURE 11. Burst fracture of C7 without neurologic injury. The 15-year-old boy was treated with initial traction followed by halo immobilization.

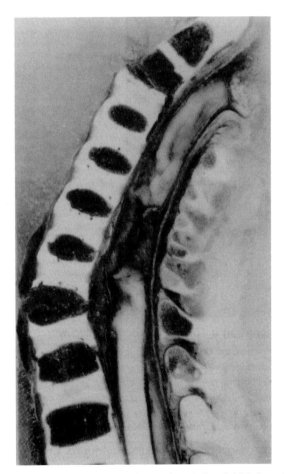

FIGURE 12. Cryosection of spine from infant victim of child abuse demonstrates end plate separation at C3–4, disruption of cord, and separation through vertebral body at T1. (Courtesy of Richard Bunge, M.D., and Bill Puckett, Miami Project to Cure Paralysis.)

but no radiographic abnormality is seen. Aufdermaur (6) found this injury in 12% of juvenile autopsy specimens and then reproduced the injury by applying an extension force to the spines of cadavers. In the cervical spine, the injury usually involves the inferior end plate. This has been attributed to a protective effect of the uncinate process, which may stabilize the end plate (Fig. 12).

Subaxial type I injuries are extremely unstable. If identified in a surviving child, Ogden (69) advocated operative stabilization. In contrast, type III injuries do not completely separate the physis from the vertebra. Therefore stability is maintained, and these injuries heal quickly if immobilized.

SCIWORA

The syndrome of spinal cord injury without radiographic abnormality (SCIWORA) after trauma is the single most common severe injury to the pediatric spine among patients who survive. The incidence in various reports ranges from 4% to 66% of all children with spinal cord injury (27). The incidence among younger children is higher (71). In most series, injury at the cervical level is slightly more common than injury at the thoracic level. Incomplete neurologic injuries have a good prognosis for recovery of function. Complete neurologic injuries have a dismal prognosis. There is a trend to more severe injury among younger children. When myelography or magnetic resonance imaging has been performed, there has been no consistent finding to explain the neurologic injury. In some cases, no abnormality can be identified. Cord swelling, cord disruption, leak of myelographic contrast medium, and epidural hematoma all have been described (111). Normal findings are common, but magnetic resonance imaging was used infrequently in the reported series.

The mechanism of injury is not known. More than one mechanism is likely. Theories proposed include traction injury to the spinal column and cord, end plate separation, transient disc herniation, and vascular compromise with infarction of the cord (104). Because the mechanism is not known, all patients should be treated initially as if their spines are unstable. Routine immobilization is appropriate. Careful radiographic evaluation is essential with special attention to spinal stability and compressive lesions that can be removed. There is no place for routine laminectomy to decompress the cord unless a compressive lesion is identified.

One of the most important observations was that of Pang and Wilberger (73). These authors found that 52% of children with SCIWORA had delayed onset of paraplegia, up to 4 days after the injury. Most of these children recalled transient symptoms at the time of injury. If instability is the mechanism of injury, it is possible that progressive deficit can be prevented by means of immobilization. The physician must be vigilant to identify these patients, in the hope of preventing more severe injury. Pollack et al. (77) advocate rigid cervical immobilization for 3 months for all of these patients, even if there is no radiographic evidence of instability. This recommendation is made on the basis of their finding that recurrent cord injury occurred among eight of 42 patients within 2 months after the initial injury. A clearly defined traumatic episode, usually trivial, was identified in seven of these eight cases. The incidence of SCIW-ORA after spinal cord concussion, as occurs among athletes, is not known (81). The role of steroids in preventing progressive deficit has not been studied.

LONG-TERM EFFECTS OF SPINAL CORD INJURY

Children who sustain spinal cord injuries share all the problems of their adult counterparts. Sphincter dysfunction, pulmonary insufficiency, autonomic dysreflexia, joint contractures, pressure sores, and spasticity are just a few of the chronic complications of spinal cord injury. In addition, children with spinal cord injury commonly have spinal deformity at or below the level of the injury. Age at injury is the single most important factor in the development of scoliosis (52). Among patients injured before the onset of the adolescent growth spurt, the development of severe deformity is almost universal. Deformity may progress more rapidly among patients with high cord lesions, but a low thoracic lesion does not exempt the patient from the development of deformity (60). Bracing delays the progression of deformity, but the use of bracing must be weighed against limitation of mobility (16,25).

Paraplegic and quadriplegic patients with scoliosis are predisposed to ischial pressure sores because of uneven weight bearing while sitting. Correction of the deformity is required once it exceeds 40 degrees. If a curve progresses rapidly, the cord should be screened for the development of a posttraumatic syrinx. If surgery is needed, limited fusion is not successful. Fusion must extend into the upper thoracic spine to prevent the development of late kyphosis above the instrumentation. The lower end of fusion is subject to much controversy. Most authors advocate extending the fusion to the sacrum and anchoring the instrumentation in the pelvis. This is to prevent the progression of pelvic obliquity. Some authors describe stopping at L5 to maintain lumbosacral mobility and avoid pseudarthrosis. At present there have been no results of a prospective series large enough to guide this decision.

REFERENCES

1. Abroms IF, Bresnan MJ, Zuckerman JE, et al. (1973): Cervical cord injuries secondary to hyperextension of the head in breech presentation. *Obstet Gynecol* 41:369–378.
2. Allen BL, Ferguson RL (1985): Cervical spine trauma in children. In Bradford DS, Hensinger RN, eds. *The pediatric spine.* New York: Thieme Medical Publishers.
3. Allen JP (1970): Birth injury to the spinal cord. *Northwest Med* 69:323–336.
4. Allen JP, Myers GG, Condon VR (1969): Laceration of the spinal cord related to breech delivery. *JAMA* 208:1019–1022.
5. Aprahamian C, Thompson BM, Finger WA, et al. (1984): Experimental cervical spine injury model: evaluation of airway management and splinting techniques. *Ann Emerg Med* 13:584–587.
6. Aufdermaur M (1974): Spinal injuries in juveniles. *J Bone Joint Surg Br* 56:513–519.
7. Bailey DK (1952): The normal cervical spine in infants and children. *Radiology* 59:712–719.
8. Barriot P, Riou B (1988): Retrograde technique for tracheal intubation in trauma patients. *Crit Care Med* 16:712–713.
9. Beighton P, Craig J (1973): Atlanto-axial subluxation in Morquio syndrome. *J Bone Joint Surg Br* 55:478–581.
10. Bertolami CN, Kaban LB (1982): Chin trauma: a clue to associated mandibular and cervical spine injury. *Oral Surg* 53:122–126.
11. Birney TJ, Hanley EN (1989): Traumatic cervical spine injuries in childhood and adolescence. *Spine* 14.1277–1282.
12. Bivins HG, Ford S, Bezmalinovic Z, et al. (1988): The effect of axial traction during orotracheal intubation of the trauma victim with an unstable cervical spine. *Ann Emerg Med* 17:25–29.
13. Bohn D, Armstrong D, Becker L, et al. (1990): Cervical spine injuries in children. *J Trauma* 30:463–469.
14. Bresnan MJ, Abroms IF (1974): Neonatal spinal cord transection secondary to intrauterine hyperextension of the neck in breech presentation. *J Pediatr* 5:734–737.
15. Brockmeyer D, Apfelbaum R, Tippets R, et al. (1995): Pediatric cervical spine instrumentation using screw fixation. *Pediatr Neurosurg* 22:147–157.
16. Brown JC, Swank SM, Matta J, et al. (1984): Late spinal deformity in quadriplegic children and adolescents. *J Pediatr Orthop* 4:456–461.
17. Bucholz RW, Burkhead WZ (1979): The pathological anatomy of fatal atlantooccipital dislocations. *J Bone Joint Surg Am* 61:248–250.
18. Bucholz RW, Burkhead WZ, Graham W, et al. (1979): Occult cervical spine injuries in fatal traffic accidents. *J Trauma* 19:768–771.
19. Burke DC (1974): Traumatic spinal paralysis in children. *Paraplegia* 11:268–276.
20. Caffey J (1974): The whiplash shaken infant syndrome. *Pediatrics* 54:396.
21. Cattell HS, Filtzer DL (1965): Pseudosubluxation and other normal variations in the cervical spine in children. *J Bone Joint Surg Am* 47:1295–1309.
22. Collalto PM, Demuth WW, Schwentker EP, et al. (1986): Traumatic atlanto-occipital dislocation. *J Bone Joint Surg Am* 68:1106–1109.
23. Cullen JC (1975): Spinal lesions in battered babies. *J Bone Joint Surg Br* 57:364–366.
24. Davis D, Bohlman H, Walker AE, et al. (1971): The pathologic findings in fatal craniospinal injuries. *J Neurosurg* 34:603–613.
25. Dearolf WW, Betz RR, Vogel LC, et al. (1990): Scoliosis in pediatric spinal cord injured patients. *J Pediatr Orthop* 10:214–218.
26. DeBeer JDV, Hoffman EB, Kieck CF (1990): Traumatic atlantoaxial subluxation in children. *J Pediatr Orthop* 10:397–400.
27. Dickman CA, Zambranski JM, Hadley MN, et al. (1991): Pediatric spinal cord injury without radiographic abnormalities: report of 26 cases and review of the literature. *J Spinal Disord* 4:296–305.
28. Donaldson JS (1956): Acquired torticollis in children and young adults. *JAMA* 160:458–461.
29. Duncan JM (1874): Laboratory note: on the tensile strength of the fresh adult foetus. *Br Med J* 2:763.
30. Dyck P (1978): Os odontoideum in children: neurological manifestations and surgical management. *Neurosurgery* 2:93–99.
31. Eismont FJ, Bohlman HH (1978): Posterior atlanto-occipital dislocation with fractures of the atlas and odontoid process. *J Bone Joint Surg Am* 60:397–399.
32. El-Khoury GY, Clark CR, Gravett AW (1984): Acute traumatic rotatory atlanto-axial dislocation in children: a report of three cases. *J Bone Joint Surg Am* 66:774–777.
33. Englander O (1942): Non-traumatic occipito-atlanto-axial dislocation: a contribution to the radiology of the atlas. *Br J Radiol* 15:341–345.
34. Evans DL, Bethem D (1989): Cervical spine injuries in children. *J Pediatr Orthop* 9:563–568.
35. Fielding JW (1989): Cervical spine injuries in children. In: Sherk HH, et al., eds. *The cervical spine: the Cervical Spine Research Society Editorial Committee.* Philadelphia: JB Lippincott.
36. Fielding JW, Griffin PP (1974): Os odontoideum: an acquired lesion. *J Bone Joint Surg Am* 56:187–190.
37. Fielding JW, Hawkins RJ (1977): Atlanto-axial rotatory fixation. *J Bone Joint Surg Am* 59:37–44.
38. Finch GD, Barnes MJ (1998): Major cervical spine injuries in children and adolescents. *J Pediatr Orthop* 18:811–814.
39. Floman Y, Kaplan L, Elidan J, et al. (1991): Transverse ligament

rupture and atlanto-axial subluxation in children. *J Bone Joint Surg Br* 73:640–643.

40. Francis WR, Fielding JW, Hawkins RJ, et al. (1981): Traumatic spondylolisthesis of the axis. *J Bone Joint Surg Br* 63:313–318.
41. Frieberger RH, Wilson PD, Nicholas JA (1965): Acquired absence of the odontoid process: a case report. *J Bone Joint Surg Am* 47:1231–1236.
42. Galindo MJ, Francis WR (1983): Atlantal fracture in a child through congenital anterior and posterior arch defects: a case report. *Clin Orthop* 178:220–222.
43. Grobman LR, Stricker S (1990): Grisel's syndrome. *Ear Nose Throat J* 69:799–801.
44. Hadley MN, Zabramski JM, Browner CM, et al. (1988): Pediatric spinal trauma. *J Neurosurg* 68:18–24.
45. Hawkins RJ, Fielding JW, Thompson WJ (1976): Os odontoideum, congenital or acquired: a case report. *J Bone Joint Surg Am* 58:413–414.
46. Herzenberg JE, et al. (1989): Emergency transport and positioning of young children who have an injury of the cervical spine. *J Bone Joint Surg Am* 71:15–22.
47. Holley J, Jorden R (1989): Airway management in patients with unstable cervical spine fractures. *Ann Emerg Med* 18:1237–1239.
48. Hukuda S, Ota H, Okabe N, et al. (1980): Traumatic atlantoaxial dislocation causing os odontoideum in infants. *Spine* 5:207–210.
49. Joyce SM (1988): Cervical immobilization during orotracheal intubation in trauma victims. *Ann Emerg Med* 17:88.
50. Kewalramani LS, Tori JG (1980): Spinal cord trauma in children, neurologic patterns, radiologic features, and pathomechanics of injury. *Spine* 5:11–18.
51. Kleinman PK, Zito JL (1984): Avulsion of the spinous process caused by infant abuse. *Radiology* 115:389–391.
52. Lancourt JE, Dickson JH, Carter RE (1981): Paralytic spinal deformity following traumatic spinal-cord injury in children and adolescents. *J Bone Joint Surg Am* 63:47–53.
53. Lawson JP, Ogden JA, Bucholz RW, et al. (1987): Physeal injuries of the cervical spine. *J Pediatr Orthop* 7:428–435.
54. Leventhal HR (1960): Birth injuries of the spinal cord. *J Pediatr* 56:447–453.
55. Lewis VL, Manson PN, Morgan RF, et al. (1985): Facial injuries associated with cervical fractures: recognition, patterns, and management. *J Trauma* 25:90–93.
56. Locke GR, Gardner JI, Van Epps EF (1966): Atlas-dens interval (ADI) in children: a study based on 200 normal cervical spines. *AJR Am J Roentgenol* 97:135–140.
57. Majernick TG, Bieniek R, Houston JB, et al. (1986): Cervical spine movement during oro-tracheal intubation. *Ann Emerg Med* 15:417–420.
58. Mann DC, Dodds JA (1993): Spinal injuries in 57 patients 17 years or younger. *Orthopedics* 16:159–164.
59. Mathews LS, Vetter WL, Tolo VT (1982): Cervical anomaly simulating hangman's fracture in a child. *J Bone Joint Surg Am* 64:299–300.
60. Mayfield J, Erkkila JC, Winter RW (1981): Spine deformity subsequent to acquired childhood spinal injury. *J Bone Joint Surg Am* 63:1401–1411.
61. Mazur JM, Stauffer ES (1983): Unrecognized spinal instability associated with seemingly "simple" cervical compression fractures. *Spine* 8:687–692.
62. McGrory BJ, Klassen, RA (1994): Arthrodesis of the cervical spine for fractures and dislocations in children and adolescents: a long term follow-up study. *J Bone Joint Surg Am* 76:1606–1616.
63. McGrory BJ, Klassen RA, Chao EYS (1993): Acute fractures and dislocations of the cervical spine in children and adolescents. *J Bone Joint Surg Am* 75:988–995.
64. McWhorter JM, Alexander E, Davis CH, et al. (1976): Posterior cervical fusion in children. *J Neurosurg* 45:211–215.
65. Melzak J (1969): Paraplegia among children. *Lancet* 2:45–48.
66. Montane I, Eismont FJ, Green BA (1991): Traumatic occipitoatlantal dislocation. *Spine* 16:112–116.
67. Murphy MJ, Ogden JA, Bucholz RW (1981): Cervical spine injury in the child. *Contemp Orthop* 3:615–623.

68. Odent MD, Langlais J, Glorion C, et al. (1999): Fractures of the odontoid process: a report of 15 cases in children younger than 6 years. *J Pediatr Orthop* 19:51–54.
69. Ogden JA (1990): *Skeletal injury in the child.* Philadelphia: WB Saunders.
70. Oller DW, Boone S (1991): Blunt cervical spine Brown-Séquard injury: a report of three cases. *Am Surg* 57:361–365.
71. Osenbach RK, Menezes AH (1989): Spinal cord injury without radiographic abnormality in children. *Pediatr Neurosci* 15:168–175.
72. Page CP, Story JL, Wissinger JP, et al. (1973): Traumatic atlantooccipital dislocation: case report. *J Neurosurg* 39:394–397.
73. Pang D, Wilberger JE (1982): Spinal cord injury without radiographic abnormalities in children. *J Neurosurg* 57:114–129.
74. Parke WW, Rothman RH, Brown MD (1984): The pharyngovertebral veins: an anatomical rational for Grisel's syndrome. *J Bone Joint Surg Am* 66:568–574.
75. Phillips WA, Hensinger RN (1989): The management of rotatory atlanto-axial subluxation in children. *J Bone Joint Surg Am* 71:664–668.
76. Pizzutillo PD, Rocha EF, D'Astous J, et al. (1986): Bilateral fracture of the pedicle of the second cervical vertebra in the young child. *J Bone Joint Surg Am* 68:892–896.
77. Pollack IF, Pang D, Sclabassi R (1988): Recurrent spinal cord injury without radiographic abnormalities in children. *J Neurosurg* 69:177–182.
78. Powers B, Miller MD, Kramer RS, et al. (1979): Traumatic anterior atlanto-occipital dislocation. *Neurosurgery* 4:12–17.
79. Price AE (1991): Unique aspects of pediatric spine injuries. In: Errico TJ, Bauer RD, Waugh T, eds. *Spinal trauma.* Philadelphia: JB Lippincott.
80. Przybylski GJ, Clyde BL, Fitz CR (1996): Craniocervical junction subarachnoid hemorrhage associated with atlantooccipital dislocation. *Spine* 21:1761–1768.
81. Rathbone D, Johnson G, Letts M (1992): Spinal cord concussion in pediatric athletes. *J Pediatr Orthop* 12:616–620.
82. Ruff SJ, Taylor TKF (1986): Hangman's fracture in an infant. *J Bone Joint Surg Br* 68:702–703.
83. Ruge JR, Sinson GP, McLone DG, et al. (1988): Pediatric spinal injury: the very young. *J Neurosurg* 68:25–30.
84. Salter RB, Harris WR (1963): Injuries involving the epiphyseal plate. *J Bone Joint Surg Am* 45:587–622.
85. Schuler TC, Kurz L, Thompson E, et al. (1991): Natural history of os odontoideum. *J Pediatr Orthop* 11:221–225.
86. Seimon LP (1977): Fracture of the odontoid process in young children. *J Bone Joint Surg Am* 59:943–948.
87. Shacked I, Ram Z, Hadani M (1993): The anterior cervical approach for traumatic injuries to the cervical spine in children. *Clin Orthop* 292:144–150.
88. Sherk HH, Nicholson JT, Chung SMK (1978): Fractures of the odontoid process in young children. *J Bone Joint Surg Am* 60:921–924.
89. Shulman SI, Madden JD, Easterly JR, et al. (1971): Transection of spinal cord: a rare obstetrical complication of cephalic delivery. *Arch Dis Child* 46:291.
90. Sneed RC, Stover SL (1988): Undiagnosed spinal cord injuries in brain injured children. *Am J Dis Child* 142:965–967.
91. Snyder RG, Schneider LW, Owings CL, et al. (1977): Athropometry of infants, children, and youths to age 18 for product safety design SP-450. Warrandale, PA: Society of Automative Engineers.
92. Sponseller PD, Herzenberg JE (1998): Cervical spine injuries in children. In: *The cervical spine: the Cervical Spine Research Society Editorial Committee.* Philadelphia: JB Lippincott.
93. Stabler CL, Eismont FJ, Brown MD, et al. (1985): Failure of posterior cervical fusions using cadaveric bone graft in children. *J Bone Joint Surg Am* 67:370–375.
94. Stauffer ES, Kelly EG (1977): Fracture dislocation of the cervical spine. *J Bone Joint Surg Am* 59:45–48.
95. Stauffer ES, Mazur JM (1982): Cervical spine injuries in children. *Pediatr Ann* 11:502–511.
96. Subach BR, McLaughlin MR, Albright AL, et al. (1998): Current

management of atlantoaxial rotatory subluxation. *Spine* 20: 2174–2179.

97. Suderman VS, Crosby ET, Lui A (1991): Elective oral tracheal intubation in spine-injured adults. *Can J Anaesth* 38:785–789.

98. Sullivan CR, Bruwer AJ, Harris LE (1958): Hypermobility of the cervical spine in children: a pitfall in the diagnosis of cervical dislocation. *Am J Surg* 95:636–640.

99. Sumchai AP, Sternbach GL (1991): Hangman's fracture in a 7-week-old infant. *Ann Emerg Med* 20:119–122.

100. Swischuk LE (1969): Spine and spinal cord trauma in the battered child syndrome. *Radiology* 92:733–738.

101. Swischuk LE (1977): Anterior displacement of C2 in children: physiologic or pathologic? a helpful differentiating line. *Pediatr Radiol* 122: 759–763.

102. Tolo VT, Weiland AJ (1979): Unsuspected atlas fracture and instability associated with oropharyngeal injury: case report. *J Trauma* 19: 278–280.

103. Turner LM (1989): Cervical spine immobilization with axial traction: a practice to be discouraged. *J Emerg Med* 7:385–386.

104. Walsh JW, Stevens DB, Young AB (1983): Traumatic paraplegia in children without contiguous spinal fracture or dislocation. *Neurosurgery* 12:439–445.

105. Watkins RG (1986): Neck injuries in football players. *Clin Sports Med* 5:215–246.

106. Weisel SW, Rothman RH (1979): Occipitoatlantal hypermobility. *Spine* 4:187–191.

107. Weiss MH, Kaufman B (1973): Hangman's fracture in an infant. *Am J Dis Child* 126:268–269.

108. Wholey MH, Bruwer AJ, Baker HL (1958): The lateral roentgenogram of the neck. *Radiology* 71:350–356.

109. Wollin DG (1963): The os odontoideum: separate odontoid process. *J Bone Joint Surg Am* 45:1459–1471.

110. Yates PO (1959): Birth trauma to the vertebral arteries. *Arch Dis Child* 34:436–441.

111. Yngve DA, Harris WP, Herndon WA, et al. (1988): Spinal cord injury without osseous spine fracture. *J Pediatr Orthop* 8:153–159.

112. Zigler JE, Waters RL, Nelson RW, et al. (1986): Occipito-cervico-thoracic spine fusion in a patient with occipito-cervical dislocation with survival. *Spine* 11:645–646.

THORACIC, LUMBAR, AND SACRAL SPINE FRACTURES AND DISLOCATIONS

HENRY G. CHAMBERS
BEHROOZ A. AKBARNIA

Fractures of the thoracic, lumbar, and sacral spine are rare in children. Fractures that are significant in adults may be less so in children, who have more elastic soft tissue, the potential for remodeling, and normal mineralization of their bones. Certain injuries are unique to children, including posterior limbus injuries, most cases of spinal cord injury without radiographic abnormalities (SCIWORA), and, unfortunately, child abuse. This chapter discusses the anatomy, pathomechanics, clinical presentation, and treatment of injuries of the thoracic, lumbar, and sacral spine in children.

INCIDENCE

The true incidence of thoracic and lumbar fractures in children is difficult to ascertain. Because of biases inherent in reporting methods, data collection systems, and classifications, the number of fractures is underreported and underestimated (21). Most of the literature on this subject is related to traumatic quadriplegia or paraplegia in childhood, and many articles include cases of cervical spine injuries (8,15,21,30,46). Twenty-six to 75% of all spine fractures in children are in the thoracic or lumbar spine (15,36). Our experience is that about 50% of pediatric spine fractures are in this region. These are relatively infrequent fractures, constituting only 2% to 3% of all injuries in children. The incidence of pediatric spine injuries peaks in two age groups: children 5 years old or younger, and children older than 10 years of age (15,41,42).

The most common cause of spinal injury in children is motor vehicle accidents in which they are either passengers or pedestrians (8). Other common causes of spine fractures are falls from heights (46), sports-related activities, and child abuse (2,5,54). Spinal cord injuries are common in accidents involving motorcycles and all-terrain vehicles (53). Boys and girls have an equal incidence of nonosseous injury, but boys have a greater incidence of bony involvement (59). There are other associated injuries in about half of patients, and 20% of those who have a spinal fracture have an associated neurologic injury (7).

ANATOMY

The differences in the anatomy between adult's and children's bone determine the different manifestations of trauma to the thoracic and lumbar spine. Children have a greater capacity for growth and remodeling and are much more resilient to trauma. The osseous, ligamentous, cartilaginous, and neurologic anatomy must be completely understood before interpreting clinical, radiographic, and other imaging studies (see Chapter 1.)

CLINICAL PRESENTATION

The force necessary to create a spinal fracture is considerable and is often dissipated throughout the body, involving not only adjacent neural elements and ligamentous structures but also chest and abdominal organs. Half of patients with spinal fractures have associated injuries, and 20% to 30% have neurologic injuries (7,59).

The history should determine the mechanism of injury. Automobile accidents, crush injuries, and sports injuries involve much higher energy than a fall from a chair. Child abuse must be contemplated when the history given does not correlate with the clinical picture. Flexion-distraction spinal injuries and abdominal injuries are common in patients wearing seat belts in automobile accidents.

Examination of the spine often demonstrates posterior tenderness of both the spinous processes and the paravertebral musculature. There may or may not be a palpable step-off. Crepitus may be elicited in spinous process fractures. The neurologic examination is extremely important. A complete examination must be performed initially and at frequent intervals, even in neurologically normal children, because delayed neurologic deterioration may occur (47). The neurologic examination is difficult in small children, but every attempt to perform a complete exami-

H. G. Chambers and B. A. Akbarnia: Department of Orthopaedic Surgery, University of California, San Diego, California.

nation should be made. A rectal examination should be performed in all patients. In those who have neurologic involvement, the bulbocavernosus test must be performed to determine the presence of spinal shock. All patients with a significant spinal injury should have evaluation of their bladder function, usually by a postvoid straight catheterization.

Associated injuries, such as cardiac contusion, pneumothorax, hemothorax, aortic injury, abdominal visceral ruptures, and renal and bladder injuries, are all life-threatening insults that may present with spinal injuries. These associated injuries may not manifest on the initial trauma evaluation but may present later. Awareness and prompt treatment of such associated injuries may save the child's life.

IMAGING OF SPINAL FRACTURES

Crawford (15) believes that there are three "must know" categories in the management of spinal injuries: alignment, displacement, and extent of canal compromise. There are six major imaging studies to ascertain this information: plain radiography, computed tomography (CT) with or without contrast and with or without three-dimensional reconstruction, tomography, magnetic resonance imaging (MRI), myelography, and technetium bone scan.

Plain radiography permits a good evaluation of fractures, overall alignment, and displacement (33). Because of the complex anatomy of the vertebra, this two-dimensional image may not completely demonstrate the extent of the injury. In many severe injuries, especially SCIWORA (by definition), the plain radiographs are normal.

The CT scan should be used when bony injuries are suspected or known to exist to help determine the extent of canal impingement. Vertebral end plate fractures are imaged better by this modality than by any other (16). The addition of contrast, either intravenously or myelographically, can often enhance the lesion (bone or end plate) impinging on the canal or neuroforamina. Cystic lesions may be seen in the cord. The addition of computer software enables CT images to be converted to a three-dimensional reconstruction, which is extremely helpful in the planning of both surgical and nonsurgical treatment.

Plain tomography, although not as readily available as previously, can be helpful in determining the extent of canal compromise. The widespread availability of CT scans with sagittal reconstruction makes this modality less useful. However, it may still be the best imaging modality in flexion-distraction (seatbelt) injuries.

MRI is best used when soft tissue injuries are suspected; these include herniated disc, neuroforaminal encroachment, hematoma, spinal cord edema, or posttraumatic spinal cord cyst (25). The MRI may help find a lesion when the clinical presentation does not match the radiographic examination. A soft tissue or cord injury at a level different from that of the bony lesion may be present. Therefore, every child who has a neurologic deficit should have an MRI in addition to other imaging modalities. Myelography has a limited role in children's thoracic and lumbar fractures and should not be used if MRI is available.

Radionuclide imaging using technetium-99m phosphate can be helpful in diagnosing stress fractures of the spine, especially in spondylolysis of the pars intraarticularis. It may also be helpful, when combined with laboratory studies and the clinical presentation, in differentiating trauma from other entities that might present as back pain, such as infection or tumor. It has been used successfully to evaluate children who have been abused. The single-photon emission computed tomography (SPECT) scan is an important adjunct to the diagnosis of stress fractures, especially of the pars intraarticularis, because it may have positive results even in the presence of "normal" bone scans.

The clinical examination and knowledge of the pathophysiology of thoracic and lumbar trauma determine which imaging modality is used. Because of the inherent elasticity of the soft tissue in children's spines, trauma can cause damage that will not be evident on plain radiography. Other factors, such as the need for anesthesia for MRIs in young children, exposure to radiation, and the judicious use of financial resources must also be considered when imaging thoracic and lumbar spine injuries. The determination of alignment, displacement, and extent of canal compromise must occur with the fewest possible tests.

DIFFERENTIAL DIAGNOSIS

Children can sometimes sustain spinal fractures—usually anterior compression fractures—with seemingly minor trauma, such as falling out of bed. The radiographic appearance may suggest a fracture, but several other diagnoses must be entertained before beginning treatment.

Congenital Hemivertebra

Although congenital hemivertebra is typically not painful, generalized back pain with an anterior wedge hemivertebra (congenital kyphosis) could be confused with acute trauma. Other vertebrae are often involved to a lesser or greater degree. There are often abnormalities of the end plate and disc. There would not be localized tenderness over the paravertebral musculature. The bone scan would be normal to confirm the diagnosis of a congenital problem.

Infection

Occasionally, a pathologic fracture can occur through an osteoporotic infected vertebral body. Wedging can also occur in adjacent vertebrae as a result of discitis (56). The plain radiographs often demonstrate narrowing. Patients with vertebral osteomyelitis are usually very ill, but this is not always the case. The cause of this pathologic fracture may be trauma, but other pertinent information from the history, such as fever, antecedent back pain, and a concurrent infection, should raise suspicion. There is often fever, leukocytosis, and an increased erythrocyte sedimentation rate. A blood culture is often positive. Bone scan may not differentiate among fracture, tumor, or infection. MRI may show replacement or edema of the marrow elements. Occasionally, biopsy may be necessary to obtain a correct diagnosis.

Neoplasm

Primary tumors, both benign and malignant, involve the thoracic and lumbar spine. As the marrow and cancellous bone become replaced by tumor, pathologic fractures can occur. Metastatic tumor may occur in the vertebral body, leading to weakened bone and subsequent fracture. Biopsy is often necessary to confirm these diagnoses. Treatment is dependent on the tumor: some can be treated by support and observation (e.g., eosinophilic granuloma); others may require radiation therapy or even excision. Often, the spine needs to be supported while treatment is underway (e.g., for leukemia) (31).

Metabolic Disease

Any of the metabolic diseases that lead to osteopenia significantly weaken the vertebrae, so that minor trauma can lead to a pathologic fracture. Osteogenesis imperfecta patients often have spine fractures at different levels. The mucopolysaccharidoses often involve the spine; Morquio syndrome is characterized by involvement of all the vertebrae. The radiographic appearance is similar to that of spondyloepiphyseal dysplasia with platyspondia (44). A careful history and physical examination, as well as laboratory investigations, usually help make the diagnosis of metabolic bone disease.

Scheuermann Disease

Scheuermann disease is characterized by wedging of multiple thoracic vertebrae. These patients have a characteristic round back deformity with chronic thoracic spine pain and a rigid kyphoses. The radiographic picture is one of narrowed disc space, increased anteroposterior diameter of the apical thoracic vertebra, loss of normal height of the involved vertebrae, and end plate irregularity (14). Schmorl nodules may be present, but their presence is not necessary to make the diagnosis. Classically, the wedging is described as three consecutive vertebrae with wedging of at least 5 degrees (58). The clinical and radiographic presentation of Scheuermann disease usually eliminates trauma as a cause of the wedging of the vertebrae.

When evaluating a child with vertebral wedging, all the diagnoses described previously must be considered. The reader is referred to other chapters in this text discussing these entities in greater detail. Trauma, albeit minor, may be involved in the occurrence of pathologic fractures.

EVALUATION AND TREATMENT OF MAJOR SPINAL FRACTURES

Evaluation

In an effort to describe the biomechanics of the spine and the pathomechanics of spine fractures, Holdsworth (34) developed the two-column theory of the spine. This theory allows for the understanding of many spine injuries but does not describe canal impingement, which is the most devastating aspect of spinal fractures. Denis (17,18) described the three-column spine, which has proved more useful in understanding spinal fractures.

Although developed for the adult spine, this system can be extrapolated to children and adolescents with adjustments for anatomic and biomechanical differences. The pediatric spine has most of the adult radiographic features by 8 years of age, although juvenile features occasionally persist until 11 or 12 years of age (51). The physis may continue to grow even after damage, and restoration of the height of the vertebral body may occur in young children whose physes are not damaged (36).

The posterior column consists of the posterior laminar arch, supraspinous ligament, interspinous ligament, posterior lateral capsule, and ligamentum flavum. The middle column includes the posterior longitudinal ligament, posterior annulus fibrosis, and posterior wall of the vertebral body. The anterior column consists of the anterior vertebral body, anterior annulus fibrosis, and anterior longitudinal ligament (17) (Fig. 1).

The three-column system permits injuries to be divided into four major types: *a compression fracture*, which is a failure of the anterior column with an intact middle column; *a burst fracture*, which is a failure under compression (usually axial) of both the anterior and middle columns; *a seat-belt fracture*, which is a compression injury of the anterior column, with distraction of the middle and posterior columns through either bony or ligamentous elements; and *a fracture-dislocation*, in which all three columns fail in compression, with rotation and shear of the anterior column, distraction with shear of the middle column, and distraction with rotation and shear of the posterior column (15,17,18). Spinal stability has many definitions, but Denis (18) groups instability into three main types: *first-degree instability,* which is a mechanical instability with risk for kyphosis; *second-degree instability,* which is a neurologic instability, such as a collapsing "stable" burst fracture; and *third-degree instability,* which is both mechanical and neurologic instability, such as an unstable burst fracture or a fracture-dislocation.

Another way to group fractures in terms of stability is acute versus chronic. Those fractures in which there is either bony

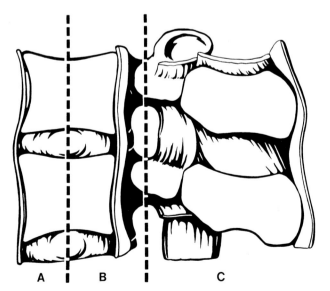

FIGURE 1. The three-column concept. *A,* Anterior column. *B,* Middle column. *C,* Posterior column.

instability or progression of neurologic deficit are labeled *acute instabilities*. Fractures in which there will be a predictable increase in angulation (kyphosis or scoliosis) and a potential for late neurologic compromise are *chronic instabilities*.

General Principles of Treatment

The goal of operative treatment of spine fractures is threefold: to provide an environment for maximal neurologic recovery, to preserve maximal spinal mobility, and to provide long-term stability in a balanced spine.

Management of thoracic and lumbar spine fractures in children is not significantly different from that in adults. However, there are some aspects of childhood fractures of the spine that differ. There is immature muscle development, and the support of the posterior ligamentous complex is often lost. If a kyphotic deformity is allowed to remain after treatment of spine fractures, it may spontaneously progress. This is more likely when there has been crushing of the vertebral body and epiphyseal plate, similar to postlaminectomy kyphosis. On the positive side, the growth potential may help remodeling and reconstitution of the deformity (48). This is often seen in compression fractures. Spinal canal compromise seen in burst fractures has more potential for remodeling in a child than in an adult. If the fragments have not caused neurologic deficit, they may often be left alone; further remodeling can be expected if the spine is otherwise stable.

The alternatives in surgical management of spine fractures in children are reduction, fusion, decompression, and instrumentation. The assessment of a child's spine fracture should include evaluation of spinal alignment, spinal stability, and degree of canal compromise (15). If initial imaging studies show that the alignment of the spine is satisfactory, there is no displacement at the fracture site, and the spinal canal has not been violated by bony or disc fragments, no reduction is necessary. The need for surgical stabilization depends on the degree of stability after reduction. In cases of neurologic deficit, the spinal canal should be evaluated by imaging studies such as MRI or CT contrast. Patients with complete neurologic deficits who have no apparent spinal fractures (e.g., those with SCIWORA) or whose spines are aligned and stable do not require surgical intervention. Patients with incomplete neurologic deficits and spinal canal compromise and patients who are worsening neurologically are candidates for spinal canal decompression.

In the thoracic spine, the arthrodesis and instrumentation can be extended a few levels above and below the fracture. Longer posterior instrumentation may be necessary to correct and maintain kyphosis in this region. In addition, mobility of the thoracic spine is not significantly affected by longer instrumentation and fusion.

In the lumbar spine, shorter instrumentation is desirable to preserve maximum mobility. Fixation must be secure. A pedicle screw system may be of benefit for the lumbar spine (3). Thoracolumbar fractures (T12 to L2), especially when associated with increased kyphosis and neurologic deficit, may be approached with anterior decompression, grafting, and instrumentation, or posteriorly by posterolateral decompression, posterior interbody grafting, and posterior instrumentation. If the loss of anterior vertebral height is significant, anterior strut grafting is preferable to posterolateral interbody fusion. In the case of burst fractures, decompression can be done anteriorly or posterolaterally (13,39).

The surgical approach and the choice of instrumentation depend on the type of fracture, location, neurologic deficit, and surgeon's experience.

Flexion (Compression) Fractures

Compression fractures of the thoracic spine are relatively common. Fractures in the thoracolumbar region occur more frequently than those in the thoracic or lumbar spine. The compression is usually 20% or less and may occur over several levels. This results from the strong normal disc and end plates. There is an additional support from the rib cage, which prevents excessive translational movements during trauma.

The elasticity of the entire segment permits compression of only the anterior column. The end plates may be involved in fractures, with a superior end plate sustaining injury twice as often as an inferior end plate (24). Even in those fractures with 50% compression, the posterior elements are often not involved. Although there may be pain and tenderness in the posterior spine, there is usually no palpable defect of the interspinous ligament.

The wedge, if in the sagittal plane, usually reconstitutes the vertebral height, especially if the child is younger than 10 years of age (Fig. 2). Frontal plane wedges do not correct as well. If the end plates are fractured, there is usually no correction. Slight axial deviations are corrected by growth of adjacent vertebral bodies.

Compression fractures that do not have posterior involvement or apophyseal ring fractures are usually stable, both mechanically and neurologically. If there is any middle or posterior column involvement, there is some potential for instability.

Most compression fractures—except for some severe compressions and multiple fractures in the thoracic spine—can be treated conservatively. Compression fractures heal quickly and do not tend to progress. If the compression is mild, the patient can be treated symptomatically by bed rest and immobilization with or without external support. Children are usually symptom free within 1 or 2 weeks. Posterior tenderness at the level of fracture may continue for several weeks but often responds to symptomatic treatment. If there is an end plate fracture or disc herniation, symptoms may persist a little longer. The outcome of conservative treatment with casting and bed rest has been satisfactory (35). Compression fractures with less than 50% loss of anterior body height are good candidates for nonoperative treatment. Increase in kyphosis is rare after 3 months (32). Patients with multiple compression fractures should be watched closely because further deformity—in both the coronal and the sagittal planes—can develop.

When there is more than 50% loss of anterior height or there are multiple compression fractures leading to an increased kyphosis, posterior instrumentation may be necessary. Contoured (to the sagittal alignment) Harrington rods or any of the newer rod-hook systems may be used (6). Instrumentation

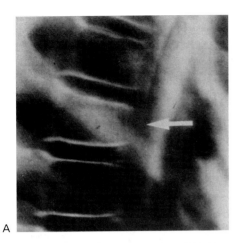

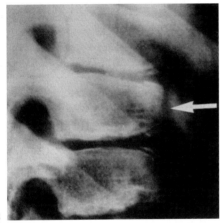

FIGURE 2. **A:** Mild compression fracture *(arrow)* of a thoracic vertebra. **B:** Appearance one year later; reconstitution of the anterior height is beginning.

should be long enough in the thoracic spine to encompass the kyphosis and apply compression force by multiple anchors.

Axial (Burst) Fractures

Holdsworth (34) introduced the concept of "burst" fractures in 1970. When a vertical (axial) compression force is applied, the vertebral end plate fractures and the nucleus of the disc are forced into the vertebral body, which explodes and shatters. Burst fractures usually occur in the lower thoracic region, thoracolumbar junction, and lumbar region, where axial loading is possible. Holdsworth stated that these are stable but painful injuries.

Some of these burst fractures are both mechanically unstable—with collapse and painful kyphosis—and neurologically unstable—both acutely and chronically, with a retropulsed middle column into the spinal canal and neural foramina (45). Those fractures in which the end plate is damaged are prone to physeal damage and may progress to kyphosis with further growth. The extent of bursting cannot always be appreciated on plain radiography. CT scanning has proved invaluable in the evaluation of burst fractures, both as an aid to diagnosis and as a guide to further treatment (20,45,57).

"Stable" burst fractures may be treated conservatively if the kyphosis is less than 20 degrees (23). If the fracture is deemed "unstable," surgical treatment is necessary. For a burst fracture in the thoracic spine, the length of the instrumentation may be similar to that used for compression fractures, without compression force. Contouring the rods and using three-point fixation help the reduction and restore spinal alignment. In the lumbar region, instrumentation can be short, using pedicle fixation (pedicle screw fixation in children has not been approved by the U.S. Food and Drug Administration) or hooks. After reduction, if there is a significant loss of anterior body height (more than 60%), anterior grafting—from either a posterior or an anterior approach—may be required.

It is often possible to use one screw at the fracture level in one pedicle. This adds to the strength of the construct. If required, decompression, especially in the lower lumbar spine, can be accomplished through one pedicle, including anterior interbody grafting (4) (Fig. 3). Pedicle screw devices are usually extended one level above and one level below the fracture. Harrington instrumentation can be used for longer instrumentation levels to reduce the fractures, with contoured rods and application of three-point fixation, distraction, and short (two-disc and even one-disc) fusion to preserve mobility. Rods are usually removed 6 months after surgery (6,18,22).

At the thoracolumbar junction, in fractures with severe anterior angulation of the vertebral body, anterior instrumentation with the Kaneda device or other similar instrumentation allows reconstitution of vertebral height and a short fusion (one vertebra above and one vertebra below) (39). In cases of neurologic deficit, anterior decompression is possible at the same time (13,38) (Fig. 4).

Flexion-Distraction (Seat-belt) Injuries

Chance (12) described three fractures of the lumbar spine in which the fracture went through the vertebral bodies, exiting through the neural arches and the pedicle. He thought that the fracture was secondary to a flexion injury, but Smith and Kaufer (52), and later Rennie and Mitchell (50), described what is now the accepted pathomechanics of flexion and distraction as the cause of the fraction (Figs. 5, 6, and 7).

Gumley and colleagues (29) suggested a classification based on the location of the fracture in the posterior elements of the vertebra. Type I extends through the spinous process and travels symmetrically forward through all the posterior bony elements to emerge in a variable position in the vertebral body. Type II is identical, except that the fracture line traverses the posterior elements between the spinous processes. Type III is asymmetric, involving the posterior elements more on one side than the other, which is possibly associated with a rotational force occurring around a seat-belt strap (27,29).

Gertzbein and Court-Brown (27) extended this classification to describe the trauma to the anterior vertebral column, the posterior elements, and the resulting axially loaded spine (Fig. 8). The anterior lesion may be a fracture or a combination of soft tissue injury and bony injury. Type A injuries, involving the disc, may not heal sufficiently to restabilize the spinal segment. Similarly, type C injuries involve only a small area of bone as

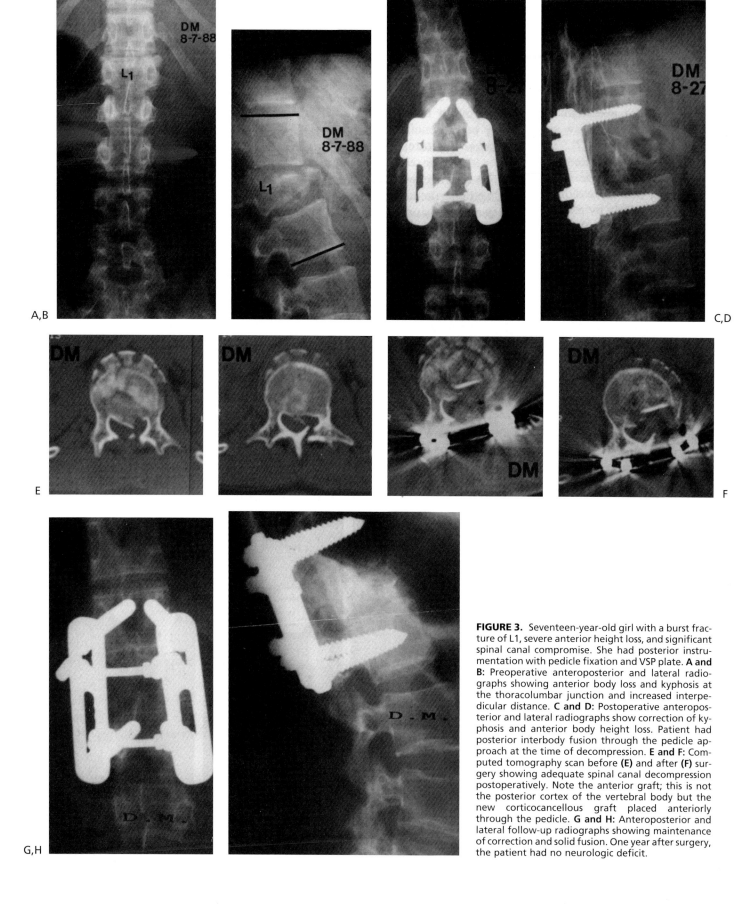

A,B

C,D

E

F

G,H

FIGURE 3. Seventeen-year-old girl with a burst fracture of L1, severe anterior height loss, and significant spinal canal compromise. She had posterior instrumentation with pedicle fixation and VSP plate. **A and B:** Preoperative anteroposterior and lateral radiographs showing anterior body loss and kyphosis at the thoracolumbar junction and increased interpedicular distance. **C and D:** Postoperative anteroposterior and lateral radiographs show correction of kyphosis and anterior body height loss. Patient had posterior interbody fusion through the pedicle approach at the time of decompression. **E and F:** Computed tomography scan before **(E)** and after **(F)** surgery showing adequate spinal canal decompression postoperatively. Note the anterior graft; this is not the posterior cortex of the vertebral body but the new corticocancellous graft placed anteriorly through the pedicle. **G and H:** Anteroposterior and lateral follow-up radiographs showing maintenance of correction and solid fusion. One year after surgery, the patient had no neurologic deficit.

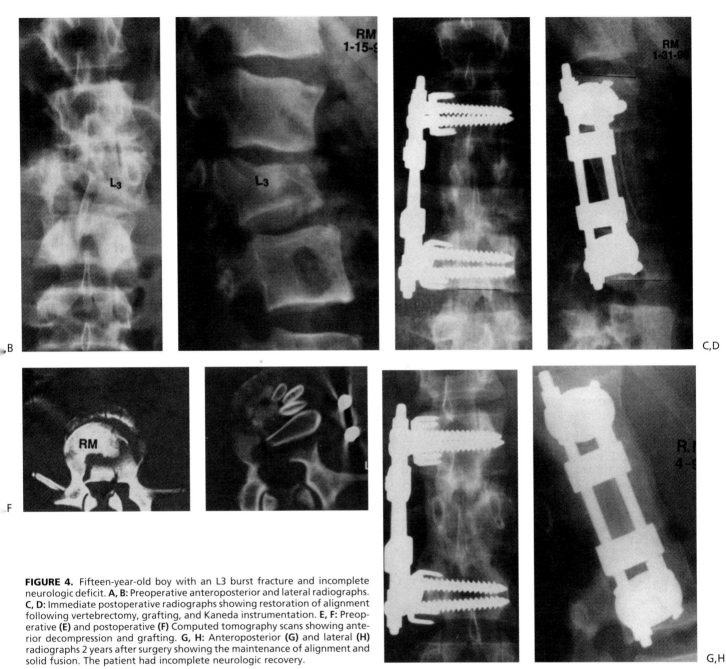

FIGURE 4. Fifteen-year-old boy with an L3 burst fracture and incomplete neurologic deficit. **A, B:** Preoperative anteroposterior and lateral radiographs. **C, D:** Immediate postoperative radiographs showing restoration of alignment following vertebrectomy, grafting, and Kaneda instrumentation. **E, F:** Preoperative **(E)** and postoperative **(F)** Computed tomography scans showing anterior decompression and grafting. **G, H:** Anteroposterior **(G)** and lateral **(H)** radiographs 2 years after surgery showing the maintenance of alignment and solid fusion. The patient had incomplete neurologic recovery.

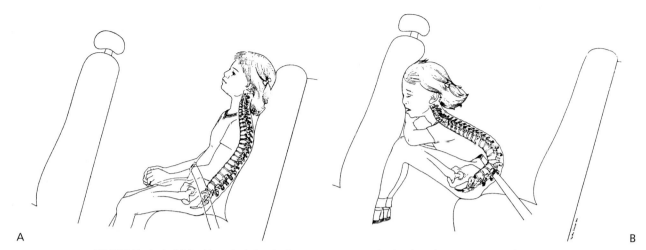

FIGURE 5. **A:** A child with typical slouched posture; note poorly developed anterosuperior iliac spine. **B:** Frontal collision; lap belt slips over iliac crests to focus bending force in the midlumbar region.

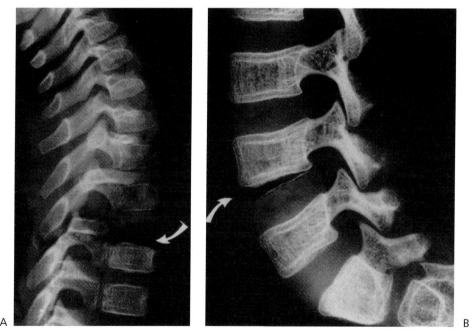

FIGURE 6. Experimental flexion-distraction injuries of immature spines. **A:** Thoracic. **B:** Lumbar.

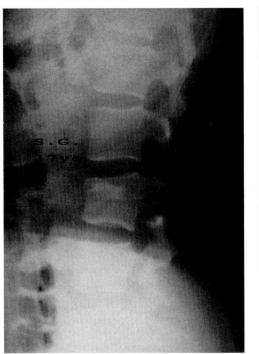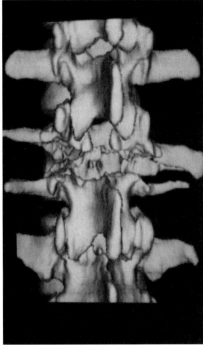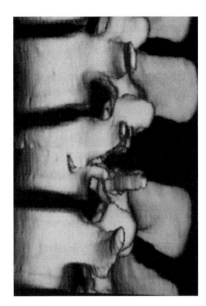

A,B   C

FIGURE 7. Seventeen-year-old girl who sustained an L3 flexion-distraction injury. **A:** Lateral radiograph. **B:** Anteroposterior three-dimensional reconstruction. **C:** Lateral three-dimensional reconstruction.

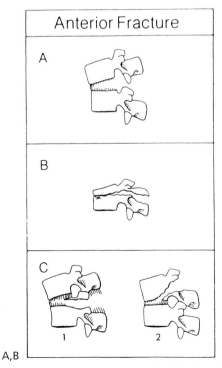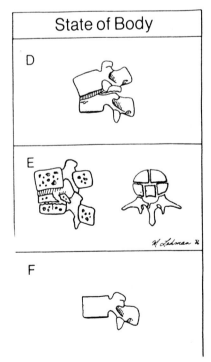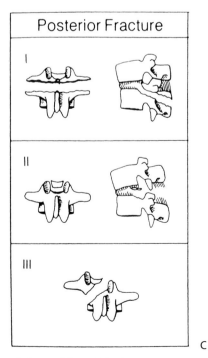

A,B   C

FIGURE 8. Classification of flexion-distraction injuries. **A:** Anterior disruption. **B:** State of the vertebral body. **C:** Injuries of the posterior elements. (From Gertzbein S, Court-Brown C (1988): Flexion-distraction injuries of the lumbar spine: mechanisms of injury and classification. *Clin Orthop* 227:52–60.).

the injury proceeds through the end plate. Type B injuries through the vertebral body, compression fractures (type D), and burst injuries (type E) are all associated with major bony trauma and usually heal with little surgical intervention. Classification of these injuries allows one to identify the degree of soft tissue involvement and thereby plan for management, either surgical or nonoperative (27).

Many state laws require that children use seat-belt restraints while traveling in automobiles. None of these laws requires the use of shoulder belts, which would decrease the incidence of lap belt injuries but might increase neck injuries in severe crashes. Children are particularly susceptible to the seat-belt injury because they have a large head relative to their body length, a high center of gravity compared with that of adults, poor protection of thoracic and abdominal organs by the chest and abdominal

wall, and underdevelopment of the anterior iliac crests, which serve to anchor the body to the seat belt (11). The National Transportation Safety Board suggested that the use of seat belts may be more harmful than no seat belt because "in many cases the lap belts induce severe to fatal injuries that would not have occurred if the lap belt had not been worn" (28). Therefore, the seat belt must be worn correctly.

Agran and associates (1) reported on 191 patients who were wearing seat belts when they were involved in motor vehicle accidents in the Los Angeles area. This study represented only 12% of the 1,642 patients who were involved in motor vehicle accidents. The children were divided into the following groups:

Infants and toddlers (0 to 3 years). These children have proportionally larger heads and a higher center of gravity than older

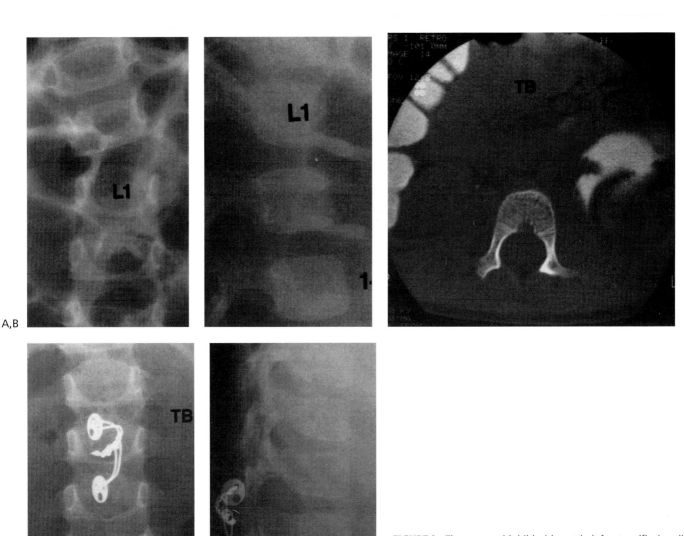

A,B

C

D,E

FIGURE 9. Three-year-old child with seat-belt fracture (flexion-distraction) that is mostly posterolateral, with obvious separation at L1 to L2. **A, B:** Injury radiograph showing the separation between L1 and L2. **C:** Computed tomography scan showing the "naked facet sign" (absence of articulating facet), indicating facet dislocation. **D, E:** Radiograph showing internal fixation with Wisconsin wires in compression correcting the deformity. At surgery, the facets were found to be dislocated. No fracture was found. There was leakage of cerebrospinal fluid.

children. Internal chest and abdominal organs are less protected by overlying bony structures and muscles. In motor vehicle crashes, these children tend to undergo rotational movement, become airborne more easily, and move head-first toward the side of impact. Child safety seats are designed for children in this age group.

School-aged children (4 to 9 years). During these growth years, the center of gravity moves toward the umbilicus, thus reducing the top-heaviness evident in the younger group. Nonetheless, the iliac crests are not adequately developed at this age to serve as a lap-belt anchor point. Also, proper upright seated posture is difficult to maintain because of lordosis in this age group. The seat belt tends to slide up and lie over the abdomen. Although these children have outgrown child safety seats, a booster seat is available to be used in conjunction with the seat belt to assure proper positioning of the belt on the child's body.

Adolescents (10 to 14 years). The physical characteristics of this age group are more like those of an adult. By 10 years of age, the anterior iliac crests are adequately developed to serve as anchor points for the lap portion of the belt. In addition, an upright seated position can be maintained.

Johnson and Falci (37) described nine patients who had lumbar spine injuries caused by rear lap seat belts. Four of the nine had associated severe abdominal injuries. One had a skull fracture caused by the forward thrust of the unrestrained upper body against the poorly padded interior of the car. There is also a possibility of a bony injury at one level and a disc injury at another level. This must be thoroughly evaluated with MRI.

Seat-belt fractures can be treated nonoperatively if satisfactory reduction can be obtained and maintained in a cast or a rigid orthosis. Conservative treatment appears to be more efficient when the fracture crosses through the bone. In burst fractures, if the lesion involves the end plates, progressive deformity may result; children should be observed carefully for this complication. Spontaneous interbody fusion seldom occurs and should not be depended on to provide long-term stability (36). Satisfactory results in burst fractures with or without neurologic deficit have been reported after nonoperative treatment, with excellent long-term functional results (49,55). Children who are treated nonoperatively for their spine fractures should be followed longer to make sure no subsequent deformity develops.

If reduction is not achieved by nonoperative methods of casting or postural reduction, surgery may be indicated. A posterior compression force is required to reduce the fracture. This can be achieved by wiring in small children or by pedicle screws in older patients. Instrumentation is usually extended one level above and one level below the level of injury using hooks (18,27) (Fig. 9).

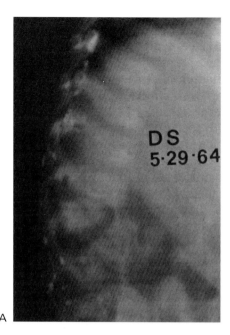

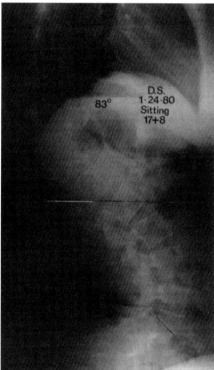

FIGURE 10. Fracture-dislocation of the spine in a 2-year-old abused child who became paraplegic. **A:** Injury. **B:** Sixteen-year follow-up. (Courtesy of Robert Winter M.D., Twin Cities Scoliosis Spine Center, Minneapolis, Minnesota.)

Fracture-Dislocation Injuries

These rare fractures usually occur at the thoracolumbar junction. There are often associated neurologic injuries of either the conus medullaris or nerve roots. This injury is always unstable, requiring operative stabilization (and decompression) as dictated by the individual patient's clinical presentation (10) (Fig. 10).

Fracture-dislocation injuries are unstable and require rigid fixation with long instrumentation levels and multiple anchors, starting close to the fracture level. Long instrumentation ensures increased stability. In addition, if the patient has complete neurologic deficit, longer fusion and instrumentation may help prevent subsequent paralytic deformity (Fig. 11). If short segmental

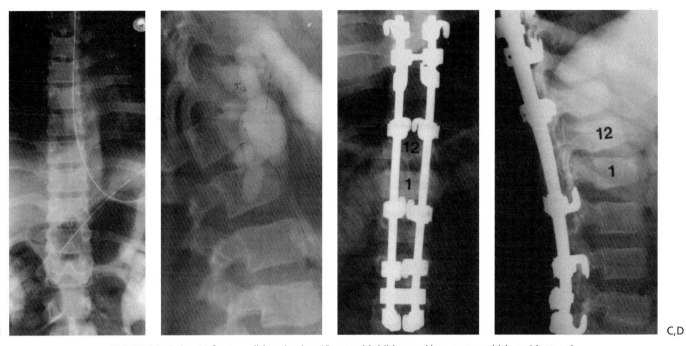

A,B
C,D

FIGURE 11. T12 to L1 fracture-dislocation in a 15-year-old child caused by a motor vehicle accident and resulting in complete paraplegia. **A, B:** Anteroposterior and lateral injury radiographs. **C, D:** Radiographs showing reduction of dislocation with Cotrel-Dubousset instrumentation. (Courtesy of Steven Marjetko, M.D., Illinois Bone and Joint Institute, Des Plaines, Illinois.)

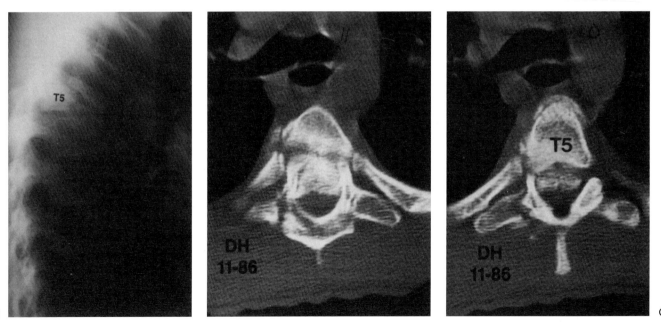

A,B
C

FIGURE 12. Fifteen-year-old boy with a burst fracture of T5. **A:** Lateral injury radiograph. **B, C:** Preoperative computed tomography scans showing significant canal compromise. *(Figure continues.)*

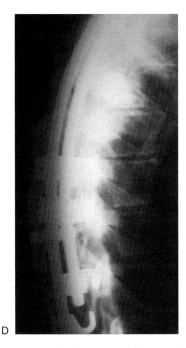

D

FIGURE 12. *Continued.* **D**: Radiograph after posterior spinal fusion and Cotrel-Dubousset instrumentation throughout the kyphosis. No decompression was performed. **E and F**: Computed tomography scans 1 year after injury showing excellent remodeling and restoration of the spinal canal.

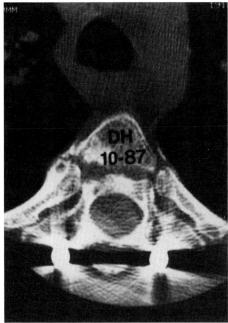

E

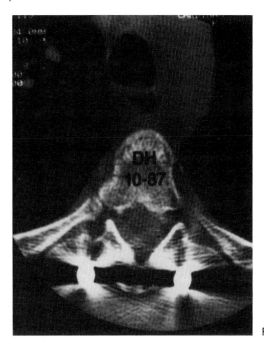

F

instrumentation is used, it should be extended at least two levels above and two levels below, with postoperative bracing.

The Role of Spinal Decompression

The indications for decompression in patients with spine fractures who are neurologically intact are controversial. There is a significant potential for remodeling of the spinal canal in children (40). Therefore, decompression in neurologically intact patients who have spinal canal compromise may not always be necessary. If patients require anterior grafting for correction of kyphosis, decompression can be done at the same time (Fig. 12).

Patients who have incomplete return of neurologic function and have no change in this status or are getting worse are candidates for decompression. There is evidence that early anterior decompression may lead to an improved neurologic recovery (13).

Posterolateral decompression includes removal of the entire pedicle at the fracture level and the disc superior to the level of the fracture; it also includes an "eggshell" procedure of the vertebral body to allow room for fragments to reduce. Special instruments are necessary to accomplish this goal (Fig. 13).

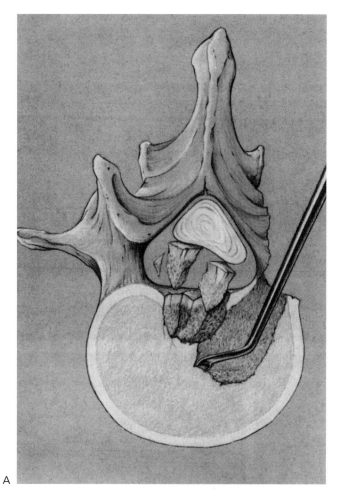

A

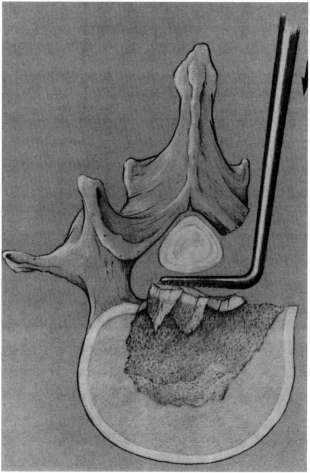

B

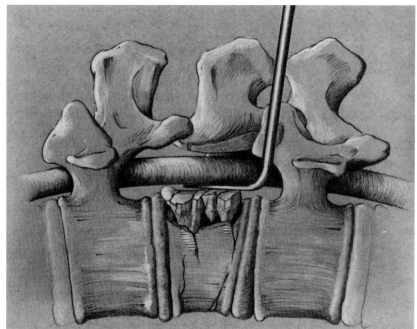

C

FIGURE 13. The technique of posterolateral decompression. **A:** Removal of the pedicle and lateral cortex, leaving the medial cortex intact to protect the dura while special currettes are used to "eggshell" the vertebral body. **B:** Removal of medial cortex of the pedicle and beginning of impaction. **C:** Impaction of the protruded fragments into the vertebral body. Interbody grafting can be done after disc removal if necessary.

MINOR SPINAL FRACTURES

Fractures of the spinous and transverse processes are often encountered with blunt trauma to the back. Although the fractures themselves may be minor, the associated injuries may be severe. Transverse process fractures of the thoracic region may be associated with significant pleural cavity trauma; those in the thoracolumbar region may be associated with renal damage; and those in the lower lumbar region may have an accompanying unstable pelvic fracture. Associated injuries must be thoroughly investigated before these "minor" injuries are treated symptomatically.

FRACTURES RESULTING FROM CHILD ABUSE

The true incidence of spinal injuries as a result of child abuse is not known, but it ranges from 0% to 3% in large series (2,5,7,26). One of the reasons for this discrepancy may be the lack of consistency in obtaining a skeletal survey among different institutions. Most radiology departments include an anteroposterior radiograph of the entire spine in a skeletal series, but the lateral radiograph is often not included. Furthermore, abused children with spinal injuries occasionally show mild kyphosis, but most patients do not have significant clinical findings referable to their spine. It is not unusual that many of these injuries go unrecognized, and they may be more common than is reported in the literature. Because these injuries are likely to be silent but associated with extremely violent assaults, routine evaluation of the spine is mandatory.

The average age reported by Kleinman (43) of 45 children with 85 spinal fractures was 22 months. Most spine fractures caused by abuse involve vertebral bodies. Posterior elements are involved only occasionally. Varying degrees of anterior compression are seen. There may be anterior notching of the vertebral body near the superior end plate (54). There may be decreased disc space caused by disc herniation.

Severe injuries, such as fracture-dislocations with or without neurologic deficit, have also been reported. Spinal cord injury or hematoma may be seen without bony involvement. Significant fracture-dislocations, especially those not associated with neurologic deficit, may go unrecognized and result in significant spinal deformity later in life (Fig. 10).

The mechanism of injury in most cases is hyperflexion, extension, or a combination of the two. Multiple compression fractures are not unusual findings. Fractures of the upper extremities may be seen in association with spine fractures. For example, children are held above a table or counter and their buttocks are slammed down, they use their outstretched arms to break the impact, causing fractures of the upper extremities. Most fractures are in the region of the thoracolumbar and lumbar spine. However, fractures and fracture-dislocations of the cervical region are also seen.

In evaluating the changes in vertebral bodies and the disc space in child abuse, one should consider developmental changes or infection. Disc space narrowing caused by infection is usually more severe than that caused by trauma and disc herniation. The value of the bone scan in detecting spinal injuries in child abuse is not clear, and it is generally believed that the standard

radiographic studies are the primary method of detecting spinal trauma in child abuse.

According to Kleinman (43), vertebral body fractures and subluxations are fractures with moderate specificity for child abuse, but if the history of trauma is absent or inconsistent with the injuries, they become high-specificity lesions. After child abuse is detected, the principles of diagnosis and treatment of victims should be followed (2,5).

SACRAL FRACTURES

Sacral fractures are usually associated with pelvic injuries and are not common in children. They may also occur in association with more obvious thoracolumbar spinal fractures and as such they are frequently underdiagnosed.

Fractures of the sacrum may involve the sacral nerve roots and cause neurologic deficit. Higher-level sacral injuries (S1 to S2 or S2 to S3) are more likely to cause bladder paralysis than lower injuries, such as S4 to S5. The foraminal entrapment of S3 and S4 is less likely than that of S1 and S2 because of the size of the nerve root relative to the foramen at these levels (19). If sacral fractures are undiagnosed and untreated, they may result in neurologic symptoms and deficits in the lower extremities and in urinary, rectal, and sexual dysfunction. These neurologic problems often remain the major chronic sequelae after the more obvious pelvic trauma has healed (19).

Denis and colleagues (19) studied 236 patients with sacral fractures in a series of 776 patients with pelvic injuries (30.4%) and introduced a new classification system. Previous classifications did not provide a simple anatomic-clinical correlation, particularly for bladder involvement (9). Denis divided the sacral fractures into three zones (Fig. 14). A zone I (alar zone) fracture,

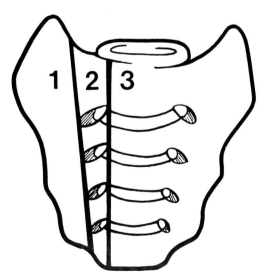

FIGURE 14. Classification of sacral fractures: the region of the ala (zone I); the region of the foramina (zone II); the central sacral canal region (zone III) (From Denis F, Davis S, Comfort T [1988]: Sacral fractures: an important problem. Retrospective analysis of 236 cases. *Clin Orthop* 227:67–81, with permission.)

by definition, involves a fracture through the ala without any damage to either the foramina or the central sacral canal. A zone II (foraminal zone) fracture involves one or several foramina. It may also go through the ala without impinging on the central sacral canal. A zone III (central zone) fracture involves primarily the central sacral canal. The fracture line may involve two zones or, in the case of a transverse fracture, all three zones. Any fracture involving multiple zones and the central canal is considered a zone III fracture because the central canal is the most significant component of the injury. Most sacral fractures are not associated with neurologic deficit.

Zone I fractures are rarely associated with neurologic deficit resulting from sacral nerve root entrapment, although they may occasionally involve the L5 nerve root or the sciatic nerve. Vertical shear-type fractures may compress the L5 nerve root between the ala and the transverse process of L5. Initial traction may be helpful in reducing the compression, but if displacement and neurologic deficit continue, open reduction may be necessary. When the sacral fracture has been displaced vertically by 2 cm or more for more than 72 hours, it is difficult to reduce because the paravertebral musculature has contracted.

Zone II fractures may involve one or several foramina. Neurologic injuries are found in 28% of these fractures; they may include bowel and bladder dysfunction and L5, S1, S2, and nerve injuries. If the CT scan shows reduction of the sacral foraminal size by at least 50%, early surgical decompression may be indicated. In the case of unstable fractures, open reduction posteriorly in conjunction with anterior pelvic external fixation may be required.

Zone III fractures involve primarily the central sacral canal. Neurologic damage occurs in more than half of these cases and involves the bowel and bladder in most cases. It may also involve L5 and S1 nerve roots independently or in combination. Transverse sacral fractures may be associated with thoracolumbar burst fractures. Treatment of zone III fractures without neurologic deficit is aimed at pelvic stabilization. Neurologically involved patients require careful evaluation, including CT scans with thin cuts and tilted gantry and reconstruction. Three-dimensional CT programs are invaluable for this purpose. Cystometrograms are also helpful in determining bladder function before and after surgery.

Decompression of sacral roots in the acute phase may be necessary to improve neurologic function. Delayed decompressions are often difficult and may not lead to significant recovery.

REFERENCES

1. Agran PF, Dunkle DE, Winn DG (1987): Injuries to a sample of seatbelted children evaluated and treated in a hospital emergency room. *J Trauma* 27:58–64.
2. Akbarnia B (1990): The role of the orthopedic surgeon in child abuse. In: Morrisey RT, eds. *Pediatric orthopedics.* Philadelphia, JB Lippincott.
3. Akbarnia B, Gains R, Marenda J, et al. (1990): Surgical treatment of spine fractures and fracture dislocations using pedicular screws and plate fixation. *Orthop Trans* 14:3.
4. Akbarnia B, Mardjetko S, Kostial P (1992): *Results of anterior spinal fusion and Kaneda instrumentation using tricorticate iliac allograft.* Presented at the Scoliosis Research Society, Kansas City, Missouri, 1992.
5. Akbarnia B, Torg JS, Kirkpatrick RT (1974): Manifestations of the battered-child syndrome. *J Bone Joint Surg Am* 56:1159.
6. Akbarnia BA, Fogerty JP, Tayob AA (1984): Contoured Harrington instrumentation in the treatment of unstable spinal fractures: the effect of sublaminar wires. *Clin Orthop* 189:186–191.
7. Anderson M, Schutt A (1980): Spinal injury in children: a review of 156 cases seen from 1950–1978. *Mayo Clin Proc* 55:499–504.
8. Babcock J (1975): Spinal injuries in children. *Pediatr Clin North Am* 22:487–500.
9. Bonnin J (1945): Sacral fractures and injuries of the cauda equina. *J Bone Joint Surg* 27:113–122.
10. Brenner B, Moiel R, Dickson J, et al. (1977): Instrumentation of the spine from fracture-dislocations in children. *Child's Brain* 3:249–255.
11. Burdi AR, Huelke DF (1969): Infant and children in the adult world of automobile safety design: pediatric and anatomic considerations for design of child restraints. *Biomechanics* 2:267–280.
12. Chance G (1948): Note on a type of flexion fracture of the spine. *Br J Radiol* 21:452–453.
13. Clohisy J, Akbarnia B, Bucholz R. Neurologic recovery associated with anterior decompression of spine fractures at the thoracolumbar junction (T12–L1). *Spine* 17:S325–S330.
14. Cohn S, Akbarnia B, Luisiri A, et al. (1988): Disc space infection versus Scheuermann's disease. *Orthopedics* 2:330–335.
15. Crawford AH (1990): Operative treatment of spine fractures in children. *Orthop Clin North Am* 21(2):325–339.
16. Dake M, Jacobs R, Margolin F (1985): Computed tomography of posterior lumbar apophyseal ring fractures. *J Comput Assist Tomogr* 9:730–732.
17. Denis F (1983): The three column spine and its significance in the classification of acute thoracolumbar spinal injuries. *Spine* 8:817–831.
18. Denis F (1984): Spinal instability as defined by the three column concept in acute spinal trauma. *Clin Orthop* 189:65–76.
19. Denis F, Davis S, Comfort T (1988): Sacral fractures: an important problem: retrospective analysis of 236 cases. *Clin Orthop* 227:67–81.
20. DeWald R (1984): Burst fractures of the thoracic and lumbar spine. *Clin Orthop* 189:150–161.
21. Dickman C, Rekate H, Sonntag V (1989): Pediatric spinal trauma: vertebral column and spinal cord injuries in children. *Pediatr Neurosci* 15:237–256.
22. Dickson J, Harrington P, Erwin W (1973): Harrington instrumentation in the fractured, unstable thoracic and lumbar spine. *Tex Med* 69:91–97.
23. Domenicucci M, Preite R, Ramieri A, et al. (1996): Thoracolumbar fractures without neurosurgical involvement: surgical or conservative treatment. *J Neurosurg Sci* 40:1–10.
24. Ferguson R (1992): Thoracic and lumbar spinal trauma of the immature spine. In: Rothman RH, ed. *The spine.* Philadelphia: WB Saunders, pp. 501–512.
25. Gabriel K, Crawford A (1988): Identification of an acute spinal cord cyst by MRI: a case report and review of the literature. *J Pediatr Orthop* 8:710–714.
26. Galleno H, Oppenheim W (1982): The battered child syndrome. *Clin Orthop* 162:11.
27. Gertzbein S, Court-Brown C (1988): Flexion-distraction injuries of the lumbar spine: mechanisms of injury and classification. *Clin Orthop* 227:52–60.
28. Goldman P (1984): A summary of the National Transportation Safety Board child passengers' safety. No. 840520. *Advances in belt restraint systems: design performance and usage.* Warrendale, PA, Society of Automotive Engineers, pp. 341–351.
29. Gumley G, Taylor T, Ryan M (1982): Distraction fractures of the lumbar spine. *J Bone Joint Surg Br* 64:520–525.
30. Hadley MN, Zabramski J, Browner C, et al. (1988): Pediatric spinal trauma: review of 122 cases of spinal cord and vertebral column injuries. *J Neurosurg* 68:18–24.
31. Hann I, Gupta S, Palmer M, et al. (1979): The prognostic significance of radiological and symptomatic bone involvement in childhood acute lymphocytic leukemia. *Med Pediatr Oncol* 6:51–55.
32. Hazel W, Jones R, Morrey B, et al. (1988): Vertebral fractures without neurological deficit. a long-term follow-up study. *J Bone Joint Surg Am* 70:1319–1321.
33. Hegenbarth R, Ebel K-D (1976): Roentgen findings in fractures of

the vertebral column in childhood: examination of 35 patients and its results. *Pediatr Radiol* 5:34–39.

34. Holdsworth F (1970): Fractures, dislocations and fracture-dislocations of the spine. *J Bone Joint Surg* 52:1534–1551.

35. Horal J, Nachemson A, Scheller S (1972): Clinical and radiological long term follow-up of vertebral fractures in children. *Acta Orthop Scand* 42:471–503.

36. Hubbard D (1974): Injuries of the spine in children and adults. *Clin Orthop* 100:56–65.

37. Johnson D, Falci S (1990): The diagnosis and treatment of pediatric lumbar spine injuries caused caused by rear seat lap belts. *Neurosurgery* 26:434–441.

38. Kaneda K, Abumi K, Fujiya M (1984): Burst fractures with neurologic deficits of the thoracolumbar spine: results of anterior decompression and stabilization with anterior instrumentation. *Spine* 9:788–795.

39. Kaneda K, Taneichi H, Abumi K, et al. (1997): Anterior decompression and stabilization with the Kaneda device for thoracolumbar burst fractures associated with neurological deficits. *J Bone Joint Surg Am* 79(1): 69–83.

40. Karlsson MK, Hasserius R, Sundgren P, et al. (1997): Remodeling of the spinal canal deformed by trauma. *J Spinal Disord* 10(2):157–61.

41. Kewalramani L, Kraus J, Sterling H (1980): Acute spinal cord lesions in a pediatric population: epidemiological and clinical features. *Paraplegia* 18:206–219.

42. Kewalramani L, Tori J (1980): Spinal cord trauma in children: neurologic patterns, radiologic features and pathomechanics of injury. *Spine* 5:11–18.

43. Kleinman P (1987): *Diagnostic imaging of child abuse.* Baltimore, Williams & Wilkins.

44. Kopits S (1976): Orthopedic complications of dwarfism. *Clin Orthop* 114:153–159.

45. McAfee P, Yuan H, Lasda N (1982): The unstable burst fracture. *Spine* 7:365–373.

46. McPhee I (1981): Spinal fractures and dislocations in children and adolescents. *Spine* 6(533–537).

46A. Ogden JA (1990): Spine. In: *Skeletal injury in the child.* Philadelphia: WB Saunders, pp. 571–626.

47. Pang D, Wilberger J (1982): Spinal cord injury without radiographic abnormalities in children. *J Neurosurg* 57:114–129.

48. Pouliquen JC, Kassis B, Glorion C, et al. (1997): Vertebral growth after thoracic or lumbar fracture of the spine in children. *J Pediatr Orthop* 17(1):115–120.

49. Reid D, Ju R, Davis LA, et al. (1988): The nonoperative treatment of burst fractures of the thoracolumbar junction. *J Trauma* 28: 1188–1194.

50. Rennie WMN, Mitchell N (1973): Flexion distraction fractures of the thoracolumbar spine. *J Bone Joint Surg Am* 55-A 386–390.

51. Ruge J, Sinson G, McLone DG, et al. (1988): Pediatric spinal injury: the very young. *J Neurosurg* 68:25–30.

52. Smith W, Kaufer H (1969): Patterns in mechanisms of lumbar injury associated with lap seatbelts. *J Bone Joint Surg Am* 51:239–254.

53. Sneed R, Tover S, Fine P (1986): Spinal cord injury associated with all-terrain vehicle accidents. *Pediatrics* 77:271–274.

54. Swischuk L (1969): Spine and spinal cord trauma in the battered child syndrome. *Radiology* 92:733–738.

55. Weinstein J, Collalto P, Lehmann T (1988): Thoracolumbar burst fractures treated conservatively: a long-term followup. *Spine* 13:33–38.

56. Wenger D, Bobechko W, Gilday D (1978): The spectrum of intervertebral disc space infection in children. *J Bone Joint Surg Am* 60:100–108.

57. White R, Newberg A, Seligson D (1980): Computed tomographic assessment of the traumatized dorsolumbar spine before and after Harrington instrumentation. *Clin Orthop* 146:150–156.

58. Winter R (1990): Spinal problems in pediatric orthopedics. In: Morrisey R, ed. *Lovell and Winter's pediatric orthopedics.* Philadelphia: JB Lippincott, pp. 676–680.

59. Yngve D, Harris W, Herndon, WA, et al. (1988): Spinal cord injury without osseous spine fracture. *J Pediatr Orthop* 8:153–159.

SPINAL CORD INJURY AND POSTTRAUMATIC DEFORMITIES

THOMAS S. RENSHAW

Up to 10,000 spinal cord injuries (SCIs) occur in the United States each year, or almost 40 cases per 1 million people (22,47,81,87). Perhaps half again those many do not survive the trauma and are not included in occurrence figures (88). An estimated 200,000 Americans are alive with their SCI. The mean age at the time of injury is about 30 years, with only 3% to 5% of SCIs occurring in children younger than 15 years of age (59,69,88).

Spinal cord injured children who initially survive the trauma and are hospitalized have an overall mortality risk of 5% to 10% during the first year, with most early deaths occurring in the first 2 weeks after the injury as the result of cardiac or pulmonary complications (33). Fatalities from cervical spine injuries in children correlate directly with the level of the lesion: the more cephalad the injury, the worse the prognosis. Most atlantoaxial injuries result in death, and injury levels of C1, C2, C3, and C4 had fatality rates of 17%, 9%, 4.3%, and 3.7%, respectively, in a study of 227 treated children (62). This study also showed that the younger the child, the more cephalad the cervical injury.

The causes of SCI in children vary with the age of the child and where he or she lives. Among the most common causes are falls and automobile-related injuries (46,72,85). Falls are a particularly frequent cause in younger children (less than age 6 years); even falls from low heights (less than 5 feet) can result in C1 to C2 subluxation, odontoid fracture, and C2 fracture (75). Motor vehicle accidents most commonly involve occupants of automobiles or pedestrians and bicyclists struck by automobiles. Airbags and seat belts, although major advances in saving lives, may nevertheless produce SCI when used improperly (31,34). Gunshot wounds account for a disproportionate share of SCIs in some cities (3), and other acts of violence and sports-related injuries, particularly diving accidents, each account for a double digit percentage in most series. Much less common are sports injuries related to football, wrestling, and horseback riding (6,24,59,60). Other uncommon causes are shaken baby syndrome (76), birth trauma, industrial and agricultural accidents, infections, and vascular episodes.

Older boys are more likely to be injured than older girls (60,72,85), but under 3 years of age, the sex incidence is nearly equal (88). SCIs occur more commonly in the summer months and near the end of the week or on weekends (88). Resultant incomplete neurologic lesions are more common in most reports (72,85), but in some, complete and incomplete lesions are about equal in frequency (33,60). High-velocity injuries have a worse prognosis than low-velocity injuries; open fractures do worse than closed fractures; higher levels of paralysis have more complications than lower levels; and older patients have a poorer outcome than younger patients.

Considering all injuries to children's spines, the cervical region is the most commonly injured and most dangerous site. Fractures here carry a risk of neurologic injury of up to 53%, compared with a 15% to 20% risk in the thoracolumbar region (9,24,60). Children 10 years of age and younger have a predominance of ligamentous injuries in the cephalic portion of the cervical spine. Those 11 years of age and older are likely to have a more caudal cervical injury, with a pattern similar to that seen in adult trauma (3,59).

Whenever the spine is fractured, it is essential to look for more than one lesion. A report on more than 800 patients includes a 6.4% incidence of noncontiguous spine fractures (45); another report lists noncontiguous abnormalities and spinal cord injury without radiographic abnormality (SCIWORA) as the most common injuries in very young patients (53). Contiguous and noncontiguous injuries can occur in 15% to 24% of spine trauma patients (20,33,37,49).

ANATOMY AND PATHOPHYSIOLOGY

The spinal cord occupies about half of the space in the bony spinal canal, except at the level of C1, where it fills one third of the cross-sectional area. The cord expands in the cervical and lumbar regions because of the concentration of nerve roots to the extremities, but this expansion is accompanied by widening of the canal. Cervical nerve roots arise from the cord opposite their corresponding vertebrae and exit through foramina above those vertebral bodies. Because there are seven cervical vertebrae and eight cervical nerve roots, the C8 nerves exit between C7 and T1. The thoracic roots originate from segments of spinal cord about one level cephalad to the corresponding numbered

T. S. Renshaw: Department of Orthopaedics, Yale University School of Medicine, New Haven, Connecticut 06510.

vertebral body and exit through the foramina just caudal to the corresponding vertebra (9). The lumbar and sacral nerve roots originate from the cord between the levels of T10 and L1, the conus medullaris. The spinal cord normally ends at the level of the L1 to L2 intervertebral disc. Caudal to the conus is the cauda equina. This group of free nerve roots has ample space in the spinal canal and, therefore, is less susceptible to injury than is the spinal cord.

Most SCIs in children are the result of crushing, contusion, or stretching of the cord, often with hemorrhage, rather than complete disruption. The injury sets off a cascade of events, including ischemia, hypoxia, edema, and necrosis (38). Experimental evidence has shown that spinal cord distraction can generate cord tissue pressures that could cause a spinal cord compartment syndrome and thus impair spinal cord blood flow (42).

In the initial minutes after SCI, neurogenic shock may be present. It has been reported to occur in 69% of cervical spine injured patients (77) and is characterized by hypotension and bradycardia. The magnitude of neurogenic shock is directly proportional to the magnitude of the SCI (67). It is believed to be the result of unopposed vagal parasympathetic activity that is manifest because sympathetic function from the thoracic and lumbar spinal cord has been interrupted (36).

Spinal shock is different from neurogenic shock but also occurs directly after SCI. It is a physiologic phenomenon that almost always lasts less than 24 hours (78). Rarely, it can persist for as long as a few weeks (92). It is characterized by flaccid paralysis and areflexia and is thought to result from interruption of descending inhibitory fibers of the caudatospinal, reticulospinal, cerebelloreticular, and corticobulboreticular pathways (81). After spinal shock resolves, the upper motor neuron lesion findings of hypertonia, hyperreflexia, and clonus can be elicited through stimulation of monosynaptic reflex pathways in the intact spinal cord caudal to the lesion. Other reflexes, such as the bulbocavernosus, cremasteric, and anal wink, also return.

CARE OF THE SPINAL CORD INJURED PATIENT

Prehospital Management

The mortality and morbidity of SCI in children can depend on the patient's management at the scene of the accident. At the accident site, the ABCs (airway, breathing, circulation) of trauma management begin. Assessment of the airway must include careful handling of the cervical spine, the assumption being that there is an unstable injury. Respiratory and cardiovascular evaluation and resuscitation, if necessary, are done simultaneously with immobilization of the spine in the neutral supine position on a spine board or rigid stretcher. It must be remembered that before 6 years of age, a child's head size is relatively greater than his or her chest size, so that immobilization on a flat board can produce flexion or anterior translation of an unstable cervical injury and cause further spinal cord damage. This is avoided by using a child-specific spine board with a cutout for the occipital area or by placing a folded sheet or blanket under the chest so that the top-center area of the shoulders is horizontally level with the external auditory meatus (39).

Sterile dressings are placed on open wounds, fractures are splinted in a position of function, and a screening motor and sensory examination is done and recorded. If a cervical injury is suspected, the head should be taped to sandbags or towels and then to the backboard, or an appropriate pediatric cervical orthosis should be applied and then the head taped to the backboard. To avoid distracting an unstable spine and further injuring the spinal cord, cervical traction should never be applied during transportation.

Venous access should be established with two large lines. Next, a Foley catheter is placed in the bladder and a nasogastric tube is carefully inserted, taking great care not to move the neck from the neutral position. Hypovolemic shock is a frequent occurrence and is treated with volume replacement. Neurogenic shock is initially treated with volume replacement; if bradycardia and hypotension persist, vasopressors should be given. It is important to remember that in patients with neurogenic shock, further vagal stimulation, caused by endotracheal intubation or suctioning, may produce cardiac arrest. Overhydration in patients with neurogenic shock can precipitate pulmonary edema. Continued monitoring and resuscitation occur during transport to the emergency department.

Patients with SCI may be equally safely transported by ground or air. The distance and the extent of associated injuries should dictate the means of transport. Using standard methods of stabilization, it is exceptionally rare for an ascending level of injury to result from the transfer (13).

Emergency Department Treatment

While pulmonary and cardiovascular management and spinal immobilization continue, more sophisticated monitoring equipment is applied. A rapid but detailed history is obtained from the patient (if possible), the emergency medical technicians, and any eyewitnesses to the accident who may provide information about the type or direction of forces involved. Thorough general physical, neurologic, and musculoskeletal examinations are performed and recorded. Venus blood and arterial oxygen samples are obtained, and a urinalysis is collected. At this time, prevention of hypoxia and hypotension may be critical in preserving spinal cord function. When an SCI is confirmed, the steroid protocol discussed later in this chapter should be immediately initiated (11). Although acute life-threatening injuries have priority over spinal cord trauma, it is ideal to manage all problems simultaneously.

Meaningful data on specific associated injuries in other systems in children are few, but such injuries have been reported in up to 31% of spine trauma cases and are more common in older children (24,58,77). A study of associated injuries in 508 consecutive spinal injury admissions, mostly adults, showed that 47% of patients had such injuries, the most common being head, chest, and long bone trauma. Single associated injuries occurred in 22%; 15% had two associated injuries; and 10% had three or more. These injuries were more common with thoracic and lumbar fractures, and patients with associated injuries were surprisingly less likely to have a neural deficit (73).

Neuromusculoskeletal examination begins with observation of voluntary or spontaneous extremity motion, particularly in unconscious or intoxicated patients. With the spine immobi-

TABLE 1. GRADING SYSTEM FOR VOLUNTARY MUSCLE STRENGTH

Grade	Description
0	Complete paralysis
1	The least detectable voluntary contraction; only a flicker
2	More than a flicker but less than antigravity strength
3	Able to maintain position against gravity
4	Stronger than antigravity, but less than full strength[a]
5	Full strength

[a] Grade 4 is a wide range and may be separated into 4$^-$ and 4$^+$.

lized, the patient should be rolled to one side and the entire spine inspected for deformity and obvious traumatic lesions. The spinous processes are palpated to detect any tenderness, widening, or step-off between them.

A conscious patient can relate the location of any pain and voluntarily cooperate with motor and sensory examinations. Motor evaluation should assess all major extremity muscle groups using the universal grading system of grades 0 to 5 (Table 1). Keep in mind that children are not as strong as adults.

Sensory evaluation should include both dorsal and lateral column assessments. The lateral columns, which carry pain and temperature perception, are of greater prognostic value regarding the return of motor function than are the dorsal columns, which carry touch, vibration, and position sense (32) (Fig. 1). The sensory examination should test dermatomal patterns (Fig. 2), and the findings should be recorded on a time-oriented flow sheet.

Rectal examination is part of the neurologic evaluation of all SCI patients. Voluntary motor sparing, as indicated by sphincter contraction and perianal sensation to pinprick, indicates an incomplete lesion with implications for treatment and prognosis.

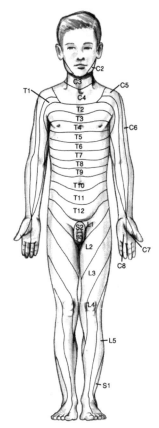

FIGURE 2. A chart of the sensory dermatome segments is invaluable for recording sensory function. This should be done during the initial evaluation and then periodically, as indicated, throughout the treatment process.

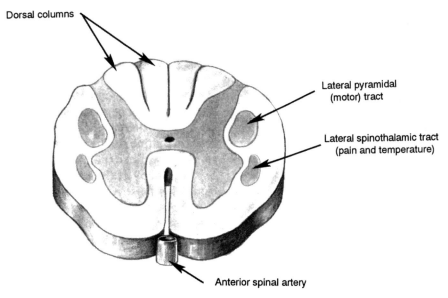

FIGURE 1. This cross-section of the spinal cord shows the major descending and ascending motor and sensory tracts.

It is important to differentiate voluntary motor function from reflex withdrawal. Evaluation of stretch reflexes is important but is less reliable than motor and sensory examinations. Spinal shock may obliterate all reflexes for up to 24 hours or more. The absence of stretch reflexes in an unconscious patient suggests either spinal shock or a lower motor neuron injury; exaggerated stretch reflexes imply an intracranial or other upper motor neuron lesion.

Other reflexes are important as indicators of the status of spinal shock. Continued paralysis in the presence of intact caudal reflex arcs implies a poor prognosis. The bulbocavernosus reflex produces contraction of the anal sphincter and reflects the integrity of the third and fourth sacral roots. It is dependent on a horizontal sensory-motor reflex arc and is, therefore, independent of a cord lesion at a higher level. A similar contraction of the anal sphincter, the anal wink, is elicited by stroking the skin of the perianal area. This reflex tests roots S2 through S4. The cremasteric reflex is elicited by stroking the proximal medial thigh with an instrument and eliciting elevation of the scrotal sac by cremasteric muscle contraction. This tests roots T12 and L1.

Radiographic Evaluation

Plain radiographs most often provide the definitive diagnostic information regarding injuries to the vertebral column. It is essential to obtain anteroposterior and lateral images of the entire spine. This helps detect spinal injuries at multiple levels. If the lower cervical vertebrae are not seen on standard views, a swimmer's view or plain tomogram or a computed tomography (CT) scan may be obtained.

To interpret cervical radiographs correctly in children, knowledge of the normal cervical anatomy, ossification process, and normal variants is essential. The following are some important considerations:

Anterior soft tissue spaces: Increase in the prevertebral space between the anterior vertebral body of C3 and the laryngeal air column may not be a useful marker in children. Although the distance is increased with bleeding, infection, or edema, the normal space varies with neck flexion, extension, and respiration, and baseline values are lacking (49). On the other hand, the normal amount of retropharyngeal soft tissue space between the air column and the anterior body of C2 has been reported as great as 7 mm in children. The retrotracheal space anterior to the body of C6 is normally as wide as 14 mm (9).

Atlas-odontoid interval: An interval of more than 5 mm on a lateral flexion radiograph indicates instability. In extension, 20% of normal children have riding up of the anterior arch of the atlas to the top of the odontoid (15).

Space available for the cord: The space from the posterior odontoid cortex to the anterior cortex of posterior arch of C1 should be greater than 13 mm in older children. In young children, it should be equal to or greater than the width of the odontoid.

Facet joints: The planes of the facet surfaces change with growth, becoming more vertical. Upper facets (C2 to C4) change from 30 to 70 degrees and lower facets from 55 to 70 degrees (63).

C2 to C3 and C3 to C4 displacement: Until middle childhood, substantial anterior displacement of C2 on C3 and C3 on C4 can normally occur in flexion. The Swischuk line is helpful in delineating pathologic displacement (82). The C3 and C4 vertebral bodies are commonly wedged anteriorly in childhood, and their facets are more horizontal, contributing to the hypermobility.

Sagittal cervical contours: Angulation at a single interspace, absence of normal cervical lordosis, and absence of cervical kyphosis from C2 to C7 on maximal flexion can be normal in 14% to 16% of children (15). Widening of more than 10 mm between the spinous processes of C1 to C2 on a neutral lateral radiograph should alert the physician to the potential for cervical SCI (2).

Ossification variants: Spina bifida occulta can occur throughout the cervical spine, especially in the lower levels. It is also seen at C1, where multiple ossification centers may be present and are differentiated from fractures by their smooth cortical margins (49). The dens has its major ossification centers joined by the dentocentral synchondrosis and has another small center at the apical epiphysis of the odontoid. Fusion of these centers can occur at any time over a span from at least 3 to 11 years. The spinous processes of a vertebra may have secondary ossification centers that can be confused with fractures and are differentiated by lack of focal tenderness (49).

When assessing the spine by radiograph, it is important to remember that substantial soft tissue injury with resultant instability can be masked by spontaneous reduction, protective myospasm, or immobilization devices. Subtle signs, such as reversal of normal cervical, thoracic, or lumbar sagittal curves and evidence of soft tissue swelling, may indicate significant ligamentous disruption. If cervical spine instability is strongly suspected but is not seen on routine still radiographic views, careful, gentle, slow active flexion and extension lateral radiographs or fluoroscopy of the neck may reveal an unstable lesion. This must only be done with the patient awake, alert, and cooperative and must be stopped immediately if any symptoms of spinal cord impingement occur. Anteroposterior and lateral radiographs are usually adequate for the thoracic and lumbar spine.

Cervical immobilization must be carefully monitored at all times when the patient is in the radiology department. A soft collar does not provide adequate immobilization; the cervical spine should be immobilized using a rigid collar or a four-poster or other cervicothoracic orthosis or by taping the forehead to bilateral sandbags and a spine board. Most physicians believe that the spine board provides adequate immobilization for the thoracic, thoracolumbar, and lumbar spine.

Other imaging techniques can be invaluable when plain radiographs do not clearly define a spinal injury. Plain tomography allows visualization of the cervicothoracic junction, the occiput, C1, and C2, including the odontoid, unilateral cervical facet dislocations, and subtle fractures elsewhere in the spine. A CT scan is valuable for identifying these injuries as well as lesions of the facets and posterior elements, defining burst fractures of vertebral bodies, and assessing the spinal canal. Reconstructed CT scans in the coronal, sagittal, or oblique planes can also be helpful.

Magnetic resonance imaging (MRI) is the technique of choice for imaging soft tissues, particularly the spinal cord. Accurate assessment of spinal cord parenchymal lesions improves the accuracy of prognostication. An MRI study can also demonstrate extrinsic cord compression from bony fragments, vertebral canal malalignment, and disc extrusion. Studies have shown that early MRI findings correlate well with outcome in SCI (49). Spinal cord transection is presently irreversible, and cord hemorrhage is nearly so; however, patients with edema have potential for recovery of neurologic function. Contusion is often associated with an incomplete lesion, whereas compression patterns are likely to be associated with either complete paralysis or an incomplete lesion with little likelihood of improvement (68). When MRI is not available or cannot be done, myelography with water-soluble contrast material may be helpful in assessing extrinsic cord compression, particularly in patients with incomplete lesions.

Evoked Potentials

Another prognostic technique that is sometimes useful in SCI is the early assessment of evoked motor and sensory potentials. Good correlations have been noted between the severity of the cord injury and sensory evoked potential grading. For motor potentials, the assessment of intercostal responses to cervical and cortical stimulation is a good prognostic indicator. In incomplete lesions, both types of potentials can be found in areas that are clinically deficient. Patients with complete lesions and absent sensory and motor responses have a poor outcome (17).

Mitigating Spinal Cord Damage

Directly after an acute mechanical SCI, secondary chemical changes take place in the cord. Oxidative enzymes produce further necrosis, and neurotoxicity results from excitatory amino acids and free radicals (8). There is much research emphasis on attempts to reverse or prevent this chemical neurologic damage, and some positive beneficial interventions have been established.

A multicenter study showed that for patients with acute SCI, treatment with methylprednisolone in the early hours after injury improves neurologic recovery. The dose given is 30 mg/kg in a 15-minute bolus infusion, followed by a 45-minute pause, and then a maintenance infusion of 5.4 mg/kg per hour for either 24 or 48 hours (11). Patients who receive methylprednisolone within 3 hours of injury should be maintained on the treatment regimen for 24 hours. When methylprednisolone is initiated 3 to 8 hours after injury, patients should be maintained on the regimen for 48 hours (11). The steroid regimen is based on studies of patients aged 14 years and older, but until a pediatric age group can be studied, it seems prudent to extrapolate the beneficial results to children (54).

Another study showed an increase in neurologic return by giving the ganglioside GM-1 within 72 hours of injury (30). The use of methylprednisolone, however, may negate the effects of ganglioside (18). Hyperbaric oxygen has been shown to accelerate peroxide formation and the generation of free radicals. This should increase the secondary injury and, therefore, is not indicated in SCI (8). Ongoing research is evaluating hypother-

mia for reducing the production of excitatory amino acids and the activity of degradative enzymes (55).

Treatment Plan

If the initial radiographs suggest a cervical spine injury, a halo or tongs may be elected for stabilization. In children, these are applied under general anesthesia. A child's skull is smaller, thinner, and more elastic than an adult skull, and halo application is different. Skull thickness can vary substantially, even up to 10 years of age; therefore, a CT scan of the skull is wise before halo application (91). In young children, six or eight pins may be necessary, each tightened to 2 to 4 inches per pound of torque. In infants, 10 pins tightened to 2 inches per pound are appropriate (61). Later retightening of pins is not recommended in children, although this point is controversial (6). Proper cervical spine alignment in children is with the external auditory meatus centered over the midsagittal shoulder. This position should be confirmed radiographically. The child with a halo should be followed frequently, with special attention to pin loosening, infection, or increased pin penetration as well as to skin breakdown beneath the vest or cast. If the halo is not tolerated, use of a Minerva cast or Minerva cervicothoracolumbosacral orthosis (CTLSO) is the best alternative.

After emergency department evaluation is complete, the patient is transferred either to the operating room, the intensive care unit, or the ward. The absolute indications for emergency surgery in spinal injuries are documented deterioration of an incomplete neurologic lesion, open fractures or penetrating wounds of the spine, and life-threatening injuries to other systems. As a rule, those injuries with spinal column instability of a pure ligamentous nature that cannot be reduced or in which the reduction cannot be maintained, those with an overtly unstable fracture pattern, those with unreducible kyphosis, and those with associated neurologic or intraabdominal injury should undergo operative reduction and internal fixation with fusion (34). In patients with complete or incomplete but stable cord lesions, the spine must be initially immobilized and may be electively stabilized by surgical means within 7 to 10 days or, if appropriate, treated with orthoses or by other closed means. Regardless of the type of initial treatment, patients with SCI should have repeated neurologic evaluations performed and recorded on a flow sheet at appropriate intervals dependent on their neurologic status.

Long-term follow-up studies of acutely performed surgical fusion in children with SCI are few, but at least one has indicated that for cervical fractures and dislocations, lasting stability is established, the fusion mass remains intact, and deformity does not recur (57). Overall neck mobility does decrease, however, and significant osteoarthritic changes occur in the adjacent unfused segments as follow-up time increases. Spontaneous extension of the fusion mass was seen in 38% of cases (46).

Problems and Complications

After the acute phase of treatment, patients who have complete or severe incomplete spinal cord lesions may develop multiple problems related to the paralysis. Spinal deformity (discussed

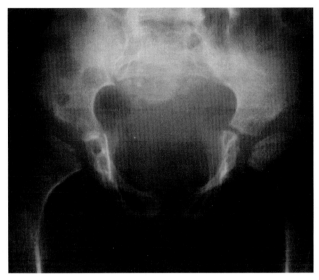

FIGURE 3. Anteroposterior radiograph of the pelvis of a child with long-standing thoracic paraplegia. There is severe bilateral acetabular dysplasia and hip subluxation.

later in this chapter) and hip subluxation or dislocation are the most common orthopaedic problems in younger patients (23,70,94). Children with prolonged spasticity are at particular risk for progressive acetabular dysplasia, hip subluxation, or dislocation, either unilateral or bilateral (Fig. 3). The cause of the hip instability may be pelvic obliquity, asymmetric spasticity, flexion-adduction contracture, or flaccidity with a paralytic pattern. Despite this, it is rare for patients to have functional problems related to the hip abnormality. Soft tissue releases may be needed for spastic contractures with hip dysplasia to improve sitting or hygiene. Bony surgery or operative reductions are rarely necessary, even with subluxation or dislocation (70). Lower extremity osteopenia (44,71), low-energy fractures (27,86), hypercalcemia, joint contractures, and heterotopic bone formation, usually at the hip (29), can also occur.

Spasticity and pain have been reported by more than 25% of SCI survivors (43). In adolescents and adults, the continuous intrathecal infusion of baclofen has been effective in reducing spasticity and mitigating pain caused by cramps. Accommodation to the drug often occurs, so that increasingly larger doses may be necessary to maintain the clinical effect (7). The use of baclofen in children younger than 12 years of age has not been thoroughly studied. As an alternative, a shorter-term treatment of spasticity and pain by intramuscular injections of botulinum toxin, type A may be beneficial (1). Spasticity can be treated by surgical means, such as tendon lengthening, tenotomy, or rhizotomy. The use of implanted spinal cord stimulators has not been shown to be effective (8).

Chronic pain is a common, potentially devastating problem; it may be classified as central or neurogenic, musculoskeletal, or syringomyelic pain. Its quality and location suggest confirmatory studies that may reveal correctable causes (28).

Another important consideration is the development of a latex allergy, the likelihood of which increases with the time from injury. Latex allergy has been reported in 18% of children with SCI (90). Because of this, all children with SCI should be provided with a latex-free environment (8).

Common nonorthopaedic problems are discussed in Chapter 33 and have been well-reviewed (25,69,89). It is wise to reevaluate SCI patients periodically, looking for multisystem problems as well as the development of spinal deformity and hip problems.

SPINAL CORD INJURY SYNDROMES

SCI may produce complete neurologic loss or any of a wide variety of incomplete or transient patterns of neurologic deficit. Although "classic" patterns of incomplete injury are described here, it is unusual to see pure patterns. The most widely used classification of functional neurologic deficit is that of Frankel and colleagues (26) (Table 2).

Complete Lesions

Complete lesions show immediate and total loss of motor and sensory function caudal to the injury and, during spinal shock, absence of segmental reflex responses caudal to the lesion. With initially complete lesions, some functional motor recovery is seen in only 3% of patients during the first 24 hours and, thereafter, drops to virtually zero (3). Complete cervical injuries produce predictable motor involvement patterns in the upper extremities (Table 3).

After the resolution of spinal shock, which occurs within 24 hours in 99% of patients (35), caudal spinal cord reflexes return. Lack of neurologic function below the level of the injury after the return of such reflexes identifies a complete lesion. Nerve roots immediately proximal to the level of the SCI may be contused and initially appear nonfunctional. Recovery over a period of several months may occur, a phenomenon known as *root escape.*

If spinal cord and root impingement is demonstrated, late surgical decompression, even up to 24 months after injury, has been shown to afford some benefit in terms of root recovery in selected cases (10,84). Because the spinal cord ends at L1 to L2, lesions caudal to this level damage the cauda equina instead of the cord. Delayed recovery of these lower motor neuron lesions is more likely than when the conus medullaris or the spinal cord is injured.

TABLE 2. FRANKEL CLASSIFICATION OF FUNCTIONAL NEUROLOGIC DEFICIT

Grade	Description
A	Absent motor and sensory function
B	Sensation present, motor absent
C	Sensation present, motor active but not useful
D	Sensation present, motor active and useful
E	Normal motor and sensory function

From Frankel HL, Hancock DO, Hyslop G, et al. (1969): The value of postural reduction in the initial management of closed injuries of the spine with paraplegia and tetraplegia. *Paraplegia* 77:179–192, with permission.

TABLE 3. MOTOR FUNCTION IN CERVICAL SPINAL CORD LESIONS

Lowest Functioning Motor Level	Weak	Paralyzed
C1–C2	—	Diaphragm
C3–C4	Diaphragm	Elbow flexors
C5	Elbow flexors	Wrist extensors
C6	Wrist extensors	Elbow extensors
C7	Elbow extensors	Hand intrinsics
C8	Hand intrinsics	—

Incomplete Lesions

Incomplete lesions have a better prognosis than complete lesions, and greater functional motor return is often seen. These lesions are defined by patterns of partial neurologic loss. As a general rule, the more distal the lesion and the greater the function distal to the lesion, the more rapid the recovery and the better the prognosis (51). The following are the most common incomplete spinal cord lesions.

Brown-Séquard Syndrome

A Brown-Séquard syndrome results from a unilateral SCI and is characterized by unilateral weakness or paralysis and bilateral, but dissociated, sensory loss. The clinical picture, therefore, is ipsilateral motor loss, ipsilateral loss of posterior column position and vibratory sensation, often vasomotor changes, and contralateral loss of pain and temperature sensation (Fig. 4). Because light touch and pressure are conducted bilaterally, they are spared. The syndrome is most commonly seen in the cervical spinal cord and is usually not a pure lesion. Most patients demonstrate partial to complete recovery and maintain ambulatory

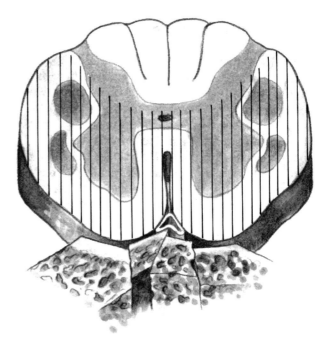

FIGURE 5. Anterior cord syndrome. This lesion is characterized by motor loss and interference with pain and temperature perception. Posterior column function is preserved.

ability and normal or near-normal bowel and bladder function (16,74,78).

Anterior Cord Syndrome

Anterior spinal cord damage is usually caused by cervical flexion injuries. It may also occur from vertebral body fracture or the acute posterior herniation of a disc (Fig. 5). The anterior part of the spinal cord (supplied by the anterior spinal artery) is involved, including motor neurons and the corticospinal and spinothalamic tracts. The patient shows caudal motor loss, usually with flaccid paralysis or weakness; atrophy; areflexia; and interference with pain and temperature sensation. Other sensations usually remain intact. Unless recovery begins within 24 hours of injury, this syndrome has a poor prognosis (74) (Fig. 6). Only about 10% of patients show functional motor recovery (79,81).

Central Cord Syndrome

Central cord syndrome is the most common incomplete neurologic injury (78). It almost always occurs in the cervical region and is seen after hyperextension injuries, although it may occur with any injury pattern (Fig. 7). Chiari I malformations, syringomyelia, and central spinal cord parenchymal tumors may be associated with this syndrome (80). The clinical presentation is substantial weakness of the arms with lesser paresis in the lower extremities, although almost complete quadriplegia can occur (78). Sacral sparing is the rule. This occurs because in the motor tracts, the sacral and lower-extremity fibers are most peripheral and cervical fibers most central. Because of edema and irregular

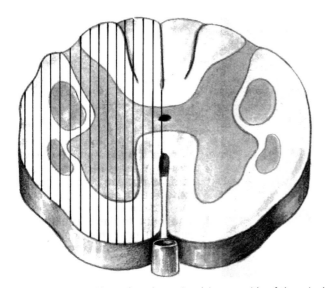

FIGURE 4. Brown-Séquard syndrome involving one side of the spinal cord. With this lesion, ipsilateral motor and position senses are compromised, as are contralateral pain and temperature perceptions.

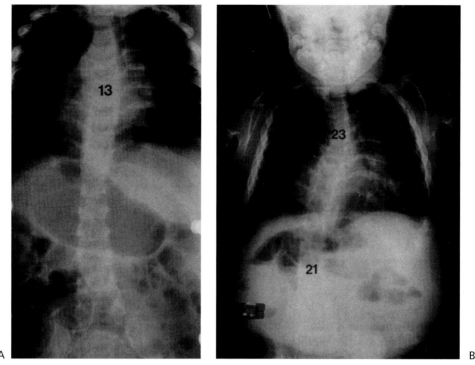

FIGURE 6. A: Posteroanterior radiograph of the spine of a 6-year-old boy who sustained an anterior cord syndrome from cervical spine trauma 1 year previously. The radiograph shows a 13-degree right thoracic scoliosis. **B:** One year later, his scoliosis has progressed to 23 degrees.

parenchymal vascular damage, pure symmetric central lesions are unusual. Incomplete lesions with variable sensory loss have a reasonably good prognosis, with about 50% to 75% of patients showing functional motor recovery. Recovery begins with improvement of function in the lumbar-innervated structures. The

likelihood of return of upper extremity function is remote, however (74,81).

Posterior Cord Syndrome

Posterior cord syndrome is a rare lesion, usually the result of a hyperextension cervical injury. Posterior column function is compromised, which results in loss of proprioception, deep pain, and deep pressure sensation (Fig. 8). Recovery is likely in most cases (33).

Cervical Cord Neurapraxia

Cervical cord neurapraxia is a transient phenomenon, characterized by paresthesias such as numbness, tingling, or burning in any distribution pattern, including quadrimelic. It is seen mostly during athletic activities such as football and wrestling and can last from seconds to several minutes. Congenital or degenerative narrowing of the sagittal diameter of the cervical spinal canal is the major contributing causative factor. Neurapraxia is then produced by excessive flexion, extension, compression or other combined motions. In a study of 110 cases, there were no instances of permanent neurologic injury, even with a recurrence rate of 56% in those who returned to contact sports. The smaller the canal, however, the greater the likelihood of recurrence (83).

Root Syndromes

Spinal nerve root injuries may occur as isolated phenomena but are more commonly associated with SCIs in the region. Unless

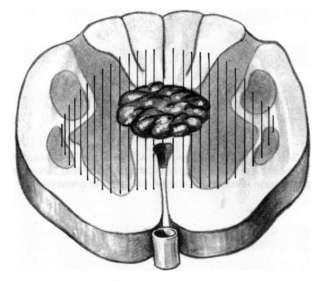

FIGURE 7. Central cord syndrome. This lesion produces bilateral involvement, with greater weakness of the upper extremities than the lower extremities.

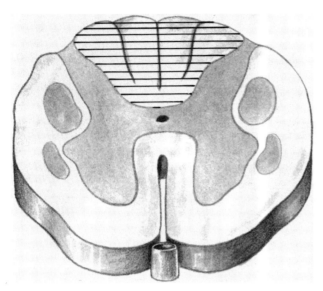

FIGURE 8. Posterior cord syndrome. Pain and temperature sensation and motor function are preserved in this lesion.

the root is transected, partial or complete recovery is possible. Most lower cervical SCIs show recovery of at least one root level, and midcervical lesions have about a 60% chance of some root recovery. The prognosis is not as good with high cervical lesions (80).

Conus Medullaris Injuries

The conus medullaris is the caudal end of the spinal cord, and an injury to this area usually is a sacral cord injury. This may produce an areflexic bladder and bowel. Lumbar roots may be injured at the same time, resulting in lower motor deficits in the lower extremities.

Cauda Equina Lesions

Cauda equina lesions interfere with function in lumbar and sacral innervated regions and may be overlooked if anal sphincter tone, perineal sensation, and distal lower-extremity motor function are not clinically assessed. The cauda equina is composed of peripheral nerves; thus, an injury produces a lower motor neuron type of flaccid paralysis. The lesion is usually patchy and may produce areflexia in the bowel and bladder and limb weakness or paralysis. Some roots can escape injury, resulting in asymmetric neurologic deficit in the lower extremities. Because the cauda equina consists of peripheral nerves, recovery is possible unless complete disruption has occurred.

Sacral Sparing

In patients with severe SCIs, sacral sparing with retention of perineal sensation, voluntary anal sphincter tone, and often flexor hallucis longus muscle activity is an indication of an incomplete lesion. This indicates that the peripheral white matter

of the spinal cord remains intact and that further functional recovery may occur. Sacral sparing may be the only early indication of an incomplete lesion (6).

SPINAL CORD INJURY WITHOUT RADIOGRAPHIC ABNORMALITY

In children younger than 10 years of age, the spine is considered biomechanically immature (4,40). The elasticity of the spinal column exceeds that of the spinal cord, and severe injury can overstretch the cord or impinge it on bony elements and produce substantial cord injury. Instantaneous reduction then occurs, preventing a radiographically recognizable lesion, referred to as SCIWORA (65,66). Flexion and extension are the most common causative mechanisms, not only in cases of single major trauma, but also with repetitive microtrauma, as seen in the shaken baby syndrome.

SCIWORA most often involves the cervical spinal cord, with the peak age at injury ranging from 3 to 6 years (64,66,73,93). Such injuries reportedly constitute 21% to 35% of SCIs in children. The likelihood of a complete neurologic lesion is about 40%, and children younger than 8 years of age are at greatest risk for severe neurologic injury (64,65,72). The younger the child, the more cephalad the level of injury. Thoracic, thoracolumbar, and lumbar SCIWORA can occur, usually in older children subjected to high-energy trauma. In these cases, there is a high incidence of associated trunk injuries.

It is important to realize that the onset of neurologic deficit or the increased deterioration of neurologic status can be delayed for up to several days (65,66). A history of transient neurologic symptoms or the presence of neck or other spine pain should raise one's awareness of this possibility.

The diagnosis is confirmed either by carefully supervised dynamic flexion and extension radiographs in a fully awake, alert, cooperative child or by MRI studies. The MRI findings, both neural and extraneural, are well reviewed by Pang (65). In some cases, evoked sensory and motor potentials can detect a lesion in an unconscious patient.

Treatment of the injury consists of immediate institution of the high-dose steroid protocol (11) and immobilization of the involved spinal region. Cervical immobilization is by means of an appropriate orthosis or a halo vest until adequate healing has occurred, as documented by stability on flexion and extension lateral radiographs. This requires a minimum of 3 months of immobilization. Recurrent SCIWORA has been reported in cases in which adequate healing did not occur (65). The indications for surgery to stabilize an unstable vertebral lesion in SCIWORA are the inability of an orthosis to maintain a stable reduction, and late instability after an adequate period of immobilization.

POSTTRAUMATIC SPINAL DEFORMITY

Spinal deformity in a paralyzed child may result from the following:

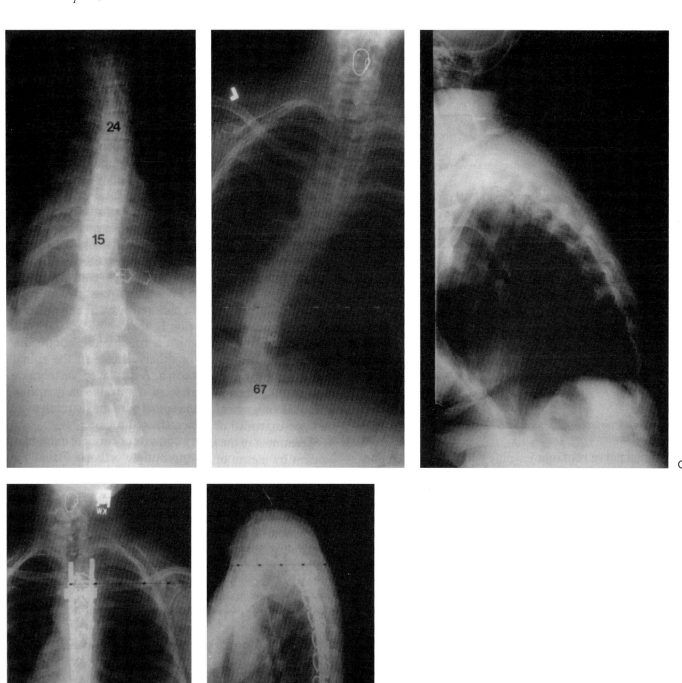

A,B

C

D,E

FIGURE 9. Exacerbation of preexisting idiopathic scoliosis in a skeletally mature adolescent after a complete traumatic cervical spinal cord lesion. **A:** Preinjury posteroanterior radiograph obtained at the time of discharge from the idiopathic scoliosis follow-up clinic. The patient is a 15-year-old girl with double thoracic scoliosis measuring 24 degrees and 15 degrees. **B:** Two years after injury, the left curve has progressed to 67 degrees. **C:** Lateral radiograph showing paralytic kyphosis. **D:** Postoperative radiograph showing stabilization of the scoliosis with a segmental fixation system from T4 to the pelvis. **E:** Lateral view showing restoration of the normal sagittal spinal contours.

- Chronic instability with progressive deformity at the site of the vertebral trauma
- Muscle weakness with paralytic collapse of the column into scoliosis, kyphosis, or lordosis involving much larger segments of the spine
- Injury to the vertebral growth plates producing asymmetric growth arrest (41)
- Postlaminectomy deformity, especially after multilevel laminectomies at or above the thoracolumbar junction (5,92) (Fig. 9)
- Exacerbation of a preexisting idiopathic spinal deformity (Fig. 10)

The most significant factor influencing the development of scoliosis is the age of the patient when the paralysis occurs (69). The incidence of scoliosis has been reported to be up to 100% in children injured before 10 years of age, 19% in children injured between 10 and 16 years of age, and 12% in patients older than 17 years (48). Another study reports scoliosis developing in 97% of children with SCIs incurred before the adolescent growth spurt and in 52% of those injured after the growth spurt (19). The presence of spasticity is another factor increasing the

TABLE 4. ETIOLOGIC FACTORS IN PARALYTIC SPINAL DEFORMITY

Acquired neurologic lesions
Trunk muscle paralysis
Asymmetric fractures
Gravity
Osteopenia
Pelvic obliquity
↓
Loss of trunk muscle support
Loss of spinal column end support
Increased spinal flexibility
Increased spinal length with growth
Asymmetric growth
↓
Paralytic spinal deformity

risk for deformity, but the level of injury does not appear to be a factor (19,48). In younger patients, scoliosis is more common than kyphosis, but in postadolescent patients, the most common lesion is kyphosis at the fracture site. When laminectomy has been performed at or above the thoracolumbar junction, the risk for kyphosis is substantially increased (5,56) (Fig. 11).. Older children with preexisting but static idiopathic scoliosis or kyphosis may experience significant curve progression when paralysis is superimposed (69).

The pathogenesis of paralytic spinal deformity in children is probably multifactorial (Table 4). Spasticity, particularly asymmetric spasticity, is likely a major factor. Deformity may relate to lack of spinal support because of muscle weakness or paralysis, the effect of gravity, asymmetric trunk muscle imbalance, fascial contractures, osteoporosis with loss of vertebral strength, and asymmetric growth based on the Heuter-Volkmann principle. Pelvic obliquity, pelvic rotation contractures, and hip flexion and adduction contractures may also predispose to the development of scoliosis. Conversely, progressive scoliosis may lead to suprapelvic obliquity and continue a vicious circle. Other etiologic factors include progressive neurologic lesions, such as syringomyelia and cord necrosis (35), and asymmetric fractures of vertebrae with imperfect reduction or malunion (52). Investigation of the cause of scoliosis in SCI continues, with emphasis on basic neurophysiology and neuropharmacology. A recent study suggested that in spinal cord injured experimental animals, clenbuterol, a β_2-adrenoceptor agonist, can retard loss of muscle contractility and bone mineralization caused by denervation and reduce the magnitude of resultant scoliosis (95).

Early Treatment

Children with paralysis caused by SCI should be assumed to be developing spinal deformities until proved otherwise. Periodic clinical and, if indicated, radiographic assessment is therefore advisable throughout childhood (Fig. 11). Prevention of deformity may not be possible; in fact, half or more of spinal cord injured preadolescent children require later spinal fusion surgery

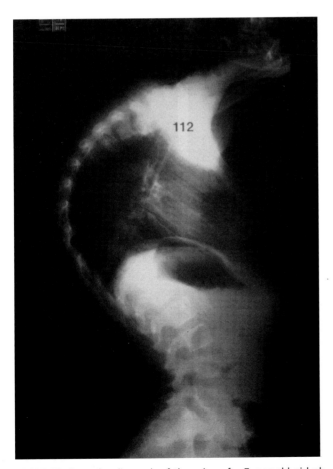

FIGURE 10. Lateral radiograph of the spine of a 7-year-old girl obtained 3 months after complete bilateral laminectomy from T3 to T9. Before surgery, her sagittal plane contour was normal.

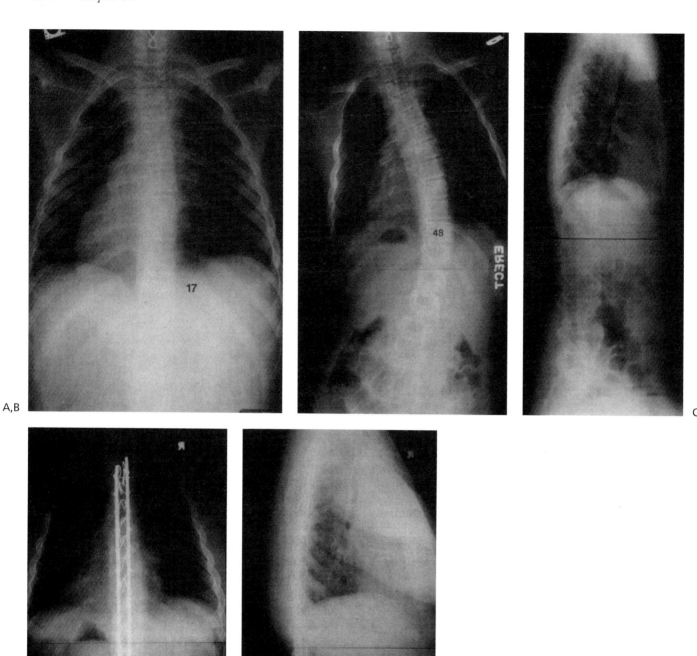

A,B

C

D,E

FIGURE 11. Progression of paralytic spinal deformity in a boy who sustained a traumatic cervical cord lesion at 12 years of age. **A:** Two years later, he had developed a 17-degree right thoracic scoliosis. **B:** Four years after injury, the curve had progressed to 48 degrees, and surgery was performed. **C:** Lateral radiograph of the spine showing a mild low thoracic kyphosis. **D:** Postoperative radiograph after posterior spinal fusion from the upper thoracic spine to the pelvis. **E:** Lateral radiograph after spinal fusion.

(23,56). Nevertheless, perfect reduction of the initial vertebral injury is wise. Prevention of major lower extremity joint contractures and measures to reduce spasticity may also be helpful.

Although orthotic treatment of early spinal deformity is rarely successful in halting curve progression (19), it may help in slowing curve progression to "buy time" while further useful growth of the spine occurs. In this situation, treatment is usually initiated when the curve reaches 20 to 30 degrees, but there are no objective data to support this intervention. Most surgeons agree that by 10 years of age, the spinal growth is sufficient to proceed with the definitive spinal fusion surgery (50). A thoracolumbosacral orthosis (TLSO) can improve sitting balance and allow freer use of the arms and hands (14). If orthotic treatment is undertaken, attention to detail is necessary to prevent skin breakdown and thermoregulation problems. The orthosis should be easily removable, well padded, and perfectly fitted. Although Milwaukee brace treatment may be successful, most physicians prefer a total-contract TLSO. Children who are obese or who have rigid curves usually do not benefit from an orthosis but rather are uncomfortable and risk pressure ulcers of their skin.

Surgical Treatment

When paralytic scoliosis exceeds 45 to 50 degrees in a child older than about 10 years of age, surgical treatment is indicated. The treatment of choice is a long posterior spinal fusion with a segmental fixation system incorporating rigid rods that are cross-linked together and attached to the spine by sublaminar wires, multiple hooks, or vertebral body or sacral screws. Instrumentation from T2 to the pelvis is often appropriate (Fig. 12), but taking away the flexibility of the paralytic spine may hamper function in activities of daily living and transfers. Preserving motion by not fusing the entire lumbar spine is theoretically desirable but may only lead to increased pelvic obliquity with its attendant problems and is probably best reserved for those few patients with incomplete lesions who are able to walk. A particular challenge is the child, younger than 9 or 10 years of age, with a large and progressing curve not controllable by a TLSO. In this case, a short segment fusion may be preferred, with the knowledge that adding on will occur and extension of the fusion will be necessary years later when further beneficial spine growth has occurred.

Anterior surgery is indicated for correctability in rigid curves that are larger than about 60 degrees on a correction film, such as with bending or traction; in spines with deficient posterior elements, for example, after extensive laminectomy; and to prevent the crankshaft phenomenon in children younger than 10 years of age. Whether it also has a role in preserving lumbar segments is yet to be determined. Anterior fusion may also be required in treating pseudoarthroses and in cases in which previous spine surgery, often at the time of the injury, has been performed and subsequent deformity has developed.

Surgery may be indicated for a rigid paralytic kyphosis of greater than 70 or 80 degrees or for shorter angular kyphoses

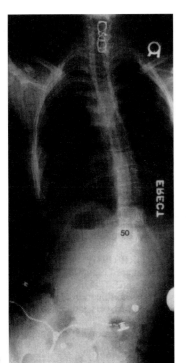
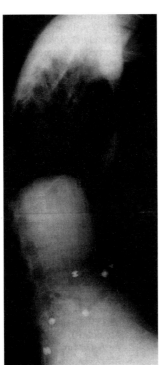
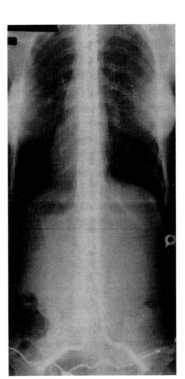
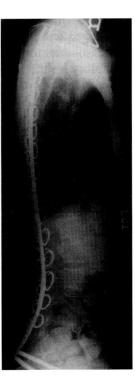

A,B

C,D

FIGURE 12. Surgical treatment of paralytic scoliosis after a cervical fracture-dislocation. **A:** Fifty-degree right thoracolumbar curve 2 years after a complete traumatic spinal cord lesion in the lower cervical region. **B:** Lateral radiograph showing paralytic kyphosis. **C:** Postoperative radiograph showing stabilization of the scoliosis. **D:** Lateral radiograph showing normal sagittal spinal contour.

TABLE 5. PREOPERATIVE CONSIDERATIONS IN PARALYTIC SPINAL DEFORMITY

General condition
Ambulatory status
Pulmonary status
Cardiac status
Renal function
Liver function
Nutritional status
Serum electrolytes
Coagulation studies
Pelvic obliquity
Spinal flexibility
Posterior versus circumferential fusion
Extent of fusion
Implants
Postoperative management

of lesser magnitudes, but this is a case-by-case consideration. In kyphosis, an anterior fusion is usually necessary in addition to a posterior procedure.

The objectives of surgery are to halt progression of deformity, obtain correction, and balance the spine over a level pelvis in order to distribute the sitting skin pressure equally and to prevent or at least minimize the occurrence of pressure ulcers (21). Grafting allograft bone or bone-extender substances to augment the local autogenous bone is necessary to maximize the development of an adequate fusion mass. Preoperative considerations are numerous before such surgery (69) (Table 5).

Patients with SCI and spinal deformity are often nutritionally and metabolically disadvantaged and have poor muscle tone, osteopenia, poor vasomotor tone (so that bleeding is often profuse), respiratory insufficiency, and chronic urinary tract infections. Postoperative complications are more common in this population than in patients with most other neuromuscular disorders or in idiopathic scoliosis patients and include an increased risk for infection, pseudarthrosis formation, and delayed wound healing (12,56,69). Postoperatively, unless profound osteopenia has been encountered and the integrity of the internal fixation is questionable, external orthotic support is usually not necessary. Postoperative mobilization and rehabilitation should be rapid and vigorous.

REFERENCES

1. Al-Khodairy AT, Gobelet C, Rossier AB (1998): Has botulinum toxin type A a place in the treatment of spasticity in spinal cord injury patients? *Spinal Cord* 36:854–58.
2. Allington NJ, Zembo M, Nadell J, et al. (1990): C1–C2 posterior soft-tissue injuries with neurologic impairment in children. *J Pediatr Orthop* 10:596–601.
3. Apple DF Jr, Anson CA, Hunter JD, et al. (1995): Spinal cord injury in youth. *Clin Pediatr* 34:90–95.
4. Apple JS, Kirks DR, Merten DF, et al. (1987): Cervical spine fractures and dislocations in children. *Pediatr Radiol* 17:45–49.
5. Bell DF, Walker JL, O'Connor G, et al. (1994): Spinal deformity after multiple-level cervical laminectomy in children. *Spine* 19:406–411.
6. Benson DR, Keenan TL (1990): Evaluation and treatment of trauma to the vertebral column. *Am Acad Orthop Surg* 39:577–589.
7. Berg-Johnsen J, Roste GK, Solgaard T, et al. (1998): Continuous intrathecal infusion of baclofen: a new therapeutic method for spasticity. *Tidsskr Nor Laegeforen* 118:3256–3260.
8. Betz RR, Mulcahey MJ (1996): *The child with a spinal cord injury.* Rosemont, IL: American Academy of Orthopaedic Surgeons, pp. 803–878.
9. Bohlman HH (1979): Acute fractures and dislocations of the cervical spine: an analysis of three hundred hospitalized patients and review of the literature. *J Bone Joint Surg Am* 61:1119–1142.
10. Bohlman HH, Kirkpatrick JS, Delamarter RB, et al. (1994): Anterior decompression for late pain and paralysis after fractures of the thoracolumbar spine. *Clin Orthop* 300:24–29.
11. Bracken MB, Shepard MJ, Holford TR, et al. (1998): Methylprednisolone or tirilazad mesylate administration after acute spinal cord injury: 1-year follow up. Results of the 3rd National Acute Spinal Cord Injury randomized controlled trial. *J Neurosurg* 89:699–706.
12. Brown JC, Swank SM, Matta J, et al. (1984): Late spinal deformity in quadriplegic children and adolescents. *J Pediatr Orthop* 4:456–461.
13. Burney RD, Waggoner R, Maynard FM (1989): Stabilization of spinal injury for early transfer. *J Trauma* 29:1497–1499.
14. Campbell J, Bonnett C (1975): Spinal cord injury in children. *Clin Orthop* 112:114–123.
15. Cattell HS, Filtzer DL (1965): Pseudosubluxation and other normal variations in the cervical spine in children: a study of one hundred and sixty children. *J Bone Joint Surg Am* 83:1295–1309.
16. Cawley MF (1996): Incomplete spinal cord Injury. In: Betz RR, Mulcahey MJ, eds. *The child with a spinal cord injury.* Rosemont, IL: American Academy of Orthopaedic Surgeons, pp. 791–802.
17. Cheliout-Heraut F, Loubert G, Masri-Zada T, et al. (1998): Evaluation of early motor and sensory evoked potentials in cervical spinal cord injury. *Neurophysiol Clin* 28:39–55.
18. Constantini S, Young W (1994): The effects of methylprednisolone and ganglioside GM-1 on acute spinal cord injury in rats. *J Neurosurg* 80:97–111.
19. Dearolf WW III, Betz RR, Vogel LC, et al. (1990): Scoliosis in pediatric spinal cord-injured patients. *J Pediatr Orthop* 10:214–218.
20. Dekutoski MB, Green B (1996): Overview, evaluation, modulation and principles of treatment of spinal stability. In: Betz RR, Mulcahey MJ, eds. *The child with a spinal cord injury.* Rosemont, IL: American Academy of Orthopaedic Surgeons, pp. 35–46.
21. Drummond DS, Narechama RG, Rosenthal AN, et al. (1982): A study of pressure distributions measured during balance and unbalanced sitting. *J Bone Joint Surg Am* 64:1034–1039.
22. Ergas Z (1985): Spinal cord injury in the United States: a statistical update. *Cent Nerv Syst Trauma* 2:19–32.
23. Farley FA, Hensinger RN, Herzenberg JE (1992): Cervical spinal cord injury in children. *J Spinal Disord* 5:410–416.
24. Finch GD, Barnes MJ (1998): Major cervical spine injuries in children and adolescents. *J Pediatr Orthop* 18:811–814.
25. Fletcher DJ, Taddonio RF, Byrne DW, et al. (1995): Incidence of acute care complications in vertebral column fracture patients with and without spinal cord injury. *Spine* 15:1136–1146.
26. Frankel HL, Hancock DO, Hyslop G, et al. (1969): The value of postural reduction in the initial management of closed injuries of the spine with paraplegia and tetraplegia. *Paraplegia* 77:179–192.
27. Freehafer AA (1995): Limb fractures in patients with spinal cord injury. *Arch Phys Med Rehabil* 76:823–827.
28. Frisbie JH, Aguilera EJ (1990): Chronic pain after spinal cord injury: an expedient diagnostic approach. *Paraplegia* 28:460–465.
29. Garland DE, Shimoyama ST, Lugo C, et al. (1989): Spinal cord insults and heterotopic ossification in the pediatric population. *Clin Orthop* 245:303–310.
30. Geisler FH, Dorsey FC, Coleman WP (1993): Past and current clinical studies with GM-1 ganglioside in acute spinal cord injury. *Ann Emerg Med* 22:1041–1047.
31. Giguere JF, St-Vil D, Turmel A, et al. (1998): Airbags and children: a spectrum of C-spine injuries. *J Pediatr Surg* 33:811–816.
32. Green BA, Callahan RA, Klose KJ, et al. (1981): Acute spinal cord injury: current concepts. *Clin Orthop* 154:125–135.
33. Green BA, Klose KJ, Eismont FJ, et al. (1991): Immediate management of the spinal cord injured patient. In: Lee BY, Ostrander LE, Cochran

G, et al., eds. *The spinal cord injured patient: comprehensive management.* Philadelphia: WB Saunders, pp. 24–33.

34. Greenwald TA, Mann DC (1994): Pediatric seatbelt injuries: diagnosis and treatment of lumbar flexion-distraction injuries. *Paraplegia* 32: 743–751.

35. Griffiths EF, McCormick CC (1981): Post-traumatic syringomyelia (cystic myelopathy). *Paraplegia* 19:81–88.

36. Grundy D, Swain A, Russell J (1986): ABC of spinal cord injury: early management and complications, part I. *Br Med J* 292:44–47.

37. Hadden WA, Gillesie WJ (1985): Multiple level injuries of the cervical spine. *Injury* 16:628–633.

38. Hall ED, Braughler JM (1987): Non-surgical management of spinal cord injuries: A review of studies with the glucocorticoid steroid methylprednisolone. *Acta Anesthesiol Belg* 38:405–409.

39. Herzenberg JE, Hensinger RN, Dedrick DK, et al. (1989): Emergency transport and positioning of young children who have an injury of the cervical spins. *J Bone Joint Surg Am* 71:15–22.

40. Hill SA, Miller CA, Kosnik EJ, et al. (1984): Pediatric neck injuries: a clinical study. *J Neurosurg* 60:700–706.

41. Jani L (1987): Spinal fractures in children and adolescents. *Z Kinderchir* 42(6):333–338.

42. Jarzem PF, Kostuik JP, Filiaggi M, et al. (1991): Spinal cord distraction: an in vitro study of length, tension and tissue pressure. *J Spinal Disord* 4:177–182.

43. Johnson RL, Gerhart KA, McCray J, et al. (1998): Secondary conditions following spinal cord injury in a population-based sample. *Spinal Cord* 36:45–50.

44. Kannisto M, Alaranta H, Merikanto J, et al.(1998): Bone mineral status after pediatric spinal cord injury. *Spinal Cord* 36:641–646.

45. Keenan TL, Antony J, Benson DR (1990): Non-contiguous spinal fractures. *J Trauma* 30:489–491.

46. Klassen RH, McGrory BJ (1996): Management of C3–C7 Injuries. In: Betz RR, Mulcahey MJ, eds. *The child with a spinal cord injury.* Rosemont, IL: American Academy of Orthopaedic Surgeons, pp. 97–108.

47. Kraus JF, Franti CE, Riggins RS, et al (1975): Incidence of traumatic spinal cord lesions. *J Chronic Dis* 28:471–492.

48. Lancourt JE, Dickson JH, Carter RE (1981): Paralytic spinal deformity following traumatic spinal cord injury in children and adolescents. *J Bone Joint Surg Am* 63:47–53.

49. Loder RT (1996): Imaging of the pediatric spine. In: Betz RR, Mulcahey MJ, eds. *The child with a spinal cord injury.* Rosemont, IL: American Academy of Orthopaedic Surgeons, pp. 47–60.

50. Lubicky JP, Betz RR (1996): Spinal deformity in children and adolescents after spinal cord injury. In: Betz RR, Mulcahey MJ, eds. *The child with a spinal cord injury.* Rosemont, IL: American Academy of Orthopaedic Surgeons, pp. 363–370.

51. Lucas JT, Ducker TB (1979): Motor classification of spinal cord injuries with mobility, morbidity and recovery indices. *Am Surg* 45: 151–158.

52. Malcolm BW (1979): Spinal deformity secondary to spinal injury. *Orthop Clin North Am* 10:943–952.

53. Mann DC, Dodds JA (1993): Spinal injuries in 57 patients 17 years or younger. *Orthopedics* 16:159–164.

54. Marks RM, Cotler JM (1996): Early closed reduction for pediatric fracture-dislocations. In: Betz RR, Mulcahey MJ, eds. *The child with a spinal cord injury.* Rosemont, IL: American Academy of Orthopaedic Surgeons, pp. 109–112.

55. Martinez-Arizala A, Green BA (1992): Hypothermia in spinal cord injury. *J Neurotrauma* 2[Suppl]:S497–S505.

56. Mayfield JK, Erkkila JC, Winter RB (1981): Spine deformity subsequent to acquired childhood spinal cord injury. *J Bone Joint Surg Am* 63:1401–1411.

57. McGrory BJ, Klassen RA (1994): Arthrodesis of the cervical spine for fractures and dislocations in children and adolescents: a long-term follow-up study. *J Bone Joint Surg Am* 76(11):1606–1616.

58. McGrory BJ, Klassen RH (1996): Outcome of pediatric cervical spine trauma. In: Betz RR, Mulcahey MJ, eds. *The child with a spinal cord injury.* Rosemont, IL: American Academy of Orthopaedic Surgeons, pp. 113–121.

59. McGrory BJ, Klassen RA, Chao EY, et al. (1993): Acute fractures and dislocations of the cervical spine in children and adolescents. *J Bone Joint Surg Am* 75:988–995.

60. McPhee IB (1981): Spinal fractures and dislocations in children and adolescents. *Spine* 6:533–537.

61. Mubarak SJ, Camp JF, Vuletich W, et al. (1989): Halo application in the infant. *J Pediatr Orthop* 9:612–614.

62. Nitecki S, Moir CR (1994): Predictive factors of the outcome of traumatic cervical spine fracture in children. *J Pediatr Surg* 29:1409–1411.

63. Ogden JA (1990): *Skeletal injury in the child,* 2nd ed. Philadelphia: WB Saunders, pp. 571–625.

64. Osenbach RK, Menezes AH (1989): Spinal cord injury without radiographic abnormality in children. *Pediatr Neurosci* 15:168–175.

65. Pang D (1996): Spinal cord injury without radiographic abnormality (SCIWORA) in children. In: Betz RR, Mulcahey MJ, eds. *The child with a spinal cord injury.* Rosemont, IL: American Academy of Orthopaedic Surgeons, pp. 139–160.

66. Pang D, Pollack IF (1989): Spinal cord injury without radiographic abnormality in children: the SCIWORA syndrome. *J Trauma* 29: 654–664.

67. Piepmeier JM, Lehmann KB, Lane JG (1985): Cardiovascular instability following acute cervical spinal cord trauma. *Cent Nerv Syst Trauma* 2:153–160.

68. Ramon S, Dominguez R, Ramirez L, et al. (1997): Clinical and magnetic resonance imaging correlation in acute spinal cord injury. *Spinal Cord* 35:664–673.

69. Renshaw TS (1985): Paralysis in the child: orthopaedic management. In: Bradford DS, Hensinger RM, eds. *The pediatric spine.* New York: Thieme, pp. 118–128.

70. Rink P, Miller F (1990): Hip instability in spinal cord injury patients. *J Pediatr Orthop* 10:583–587.

71. Roberts D, Lee W, Cuneo RC, et al. (1998): Longitudinal study of bone turnover after acute spinal cord injury. *J Clin Endocrinol Metab* 83:415–422.

72. Ruge JR, Sinson GP, McLone DG, et al. (1998): Pediatric spinal injury: the very young. *J Neurosurg* 68:25–30.

73. Saboe LA, Reid DC, Davis LA, et al. (1991): Spine trauma and associated injuries. *J Trauma* 31:43–48.

74. Schneider RC, Crosby EC, Russo RH, et al. (1973): Traumatic spinal cord syndromes and their management. *Clin Neurosurg* 20:424–492.

75. Schwartz GR, Wright SW, Fein JA, et al. (1997): Pediatric cervical spine injury sustained in falls from low heights. *Ann Emerg Med* 30: 249–252.

76. Shannon P, Smith CR, Deck J, et al. (1998): Axonal injury and the neuropathology of shaken baby syndrome. *Acta Neuropathol* 95: 625–631.

77. Soderstrom CA, McArdle DQ, Ducker TB, et al. (1983): The diagnosis of intra-abdominal injury in patients with cervical cord trauma. *J Trauma* 23:1061–1065.

78. Stauffer ES (1975): Diagnosis and prognosis of acute cervical spinal cord injury. *Clin Orthop* 112:9–15.

79. Stauffer ES (1984): Neurologic recovery following injuries to the cervical spinal cord and nerve roots. *Spine* 9:532–534.

80. Stern J (1991): Neurologic evaluation and neurologic sequelae of the spinal cord injured patient. In: Lee BY, Ostrander LE, Cochran G, et al., eds. *The spinal cord injured patient: comprehensive management.* Philadelphia: WB Saunders, pp. 115–123.

81. Stover SL, Fine PR (1986): *Spinal cord injury: the facts and figures.* Birmingham, AL: University of Alabama.

82. Swischuk LE (1977): Anterior displacement of C2 in children: physiologic of pathologic? *Radiology* 122:759–763.

83. Torg JS, Corcoran TA, Thibault LE, et al. (1997): Cervical cord neurapraxia: classification, pathomechanics, morbidity, and management guidelines. *J Neurosurg* 87(6):843–850.

84. Transfeldt EE, White D, Bradford DS, et al. (1990): Delayed anterior decompression in patients with spinal cord and cauda equina injuries of the thoracolumbar spine. *Spine* 15:952–959.

85. Turgut M, Akpinar G, Akalan N, et al. (1996): Spinal injuries in the pediatric age group: a review of 82 cases of spinal cord and vertebral column injuries. *Eur Spine J* 5:148–152.

86. Vestergaard P, Krogh K, Rejnmark L, et al. (1998): Fracture rates and risk factors for fractures in patients with spinal cord injury. *Spinal Cord* 36:790–796.

87. Vogel LC, Betz RR (1996): Introduction. In: Betz RR, Mulcahey MJ, eds. *The child with a spinal cord injury.* Rosemont, IL: American Academy of Orthopaedic Surgeons, pp. xxi–xxiv.

88. Vogel LC, DeVivo MJ (1996): Etiology and demographics. In: Betz RR, Mulcahey MJ, eds. *The child with a spinal cord injury.* Rosemont, IL: American Academy of Orthopaedic Surgeons, pp. 3–12.

89. Vogel LC, Klaas SJ, Lubicky JP, et al. (1998): Long-term outcomes and life satisfaction of adults who had pediatric spinal cord injuries. *Arch Phys Med Rehabil* 79:1496–1503.

90. Vogel LC, Schrader T, Lubicky JP (1995): Latex allergy in children and adolescents with spinal cord injuries. *J Pediatr Orthop* 15:517–520.

91. Wong WB, Haynes RJ (1994): Osteology of the pediatric skull: considerations of halo pin placement. *Spine* 19:1451–1454.

92. Yasuoka S, Peterson HA, Laws ER Jr, et al. (1991): Pathogenesis and prophylaxis of postlaminectomy deformity of the spine after multiple level laminectomy: difference between children and adults. *Neurosurgery* 9:145–152.

93. Yngve DA, Harris WP, Herndon WA, et al. (1988): Spinal cord injury without osseous spine fracture. *J Pediatr Orthop* 8:153–159.

94. Yoshimura O, Takayanagi K, Kawaguchi K, et al. (1996): Spinal cord injuries in children observed over many years. *Hiroshima J Med Sci* 45:37–41.

95. Zeman RJ, Zhang Y, Etlinger JD (1997): Clenbuterol, a beta2-adrenoceptor agonist, reduces scoliosis due to partial transection of rat spinal cord. *Am J Physiol* 272:E712–715.

33

SPINAL CORD INJURY REHABILITATION

RANDAL R. BETZ
M. J. MULCAHEY

From an orthopaedic standpoint, the comprehensive care of a child with a spinal cord injury (SCI) is an ongoing process beginning at the time of injury and lasting not only through the rehabilitation and discharge phases but for the remainder of the patient's life. A common misconception held by many orthopaedists and neurosurgeons is that their role is an active one during only the acute phase, and then the child's care is turned over to rehabilitation specialists. But treatment and prevention of soft tissue contractures, pressure ulcers, spine deformity, hip dislocation, upper extremity pain, spinal cord tethering, syrinx formation, and so forth, as well as upper extremity reconstruction, must start immediately after injury and continue indefinitely, and the orthopaedist must continue to be a key member of the patient care team long after the acute phase has passed.

The concept of early rehabilitation has led to the development of hospitals and hospital units that specialize in treating patients with SCI. As a result of a patient's early transfer to one of these specialty units (preferably the day of the injury), the number of complications and days spent in the hospital are greatly reduced (46).

Discharge planning should begin immediately on a patient's admission to a hospital and must consist of more than a tentative plan for rehabilitation. Discharge planning must address both the human environment (people in the discharge setting) and the nonhuman environment (architectural and geographic barriers). Evaluation of the nonhuman environment should begin immediately so that arrangements can be made for proper equipment and modifications to the home, school, or workplace. Architectural evaluations and home visits should be scheduled throughout the rehabilitation period. Education for people in the child's discharge environment (family members, school personnel, and fellow students) should also begin immediately so that the stigmas and preconceptions that are often associated with disabilities are minimized as the child reenters the community.

If at all possible, a child or adolescent with an SCI should undergo rehabilitation in a pediatric rehabilitation facility, where health care providers are specifically trained to address their ever-changing needs. Adult rehabilitation centers provide for a population with a wide range of disabilities and ages, and it is difficult for a child to feel comfortable in a place where his or her needs and normal development are so different from those of most of the other patients. Also, peer interaction with other children with SCI allows a newly injured child or adolescent to talk to and model himself or herself after someone who has adjusted to a similar injury.

Family-centered care (24,146), which actively involves the family members in the care and rehabilitation of the child, should be employed.

DEMOGRAPHICS
Prevalence

There are roughly 200,000 people living in the United States with some degree of spinal cord impairment resulting from trauma (47,74). It is estimated that there are 7,800 to 11,000 new cases of SCI each year (129) and that 4% to 14% of such injuries occur in patients younger than 15 years of age (30,64,83). Forty percent have tetraplegia, and 60% have paraplegia. Thirty to 40% have incomplete lesions.

Causes of pediatric SCI include motor vehicle accidents in about 40% of patients, diving in 13%, other sports in 24%, gunshot wounds in 8%, falls in 8%, transverse myelitis in 4% (49), and spinal cord tumors in 3% (147). Causes unique to the pediatric population include birth injury (1,68), child abuse, high cervical injuries secondary to skeletal dysplasias, Down syndrome, and juvenile rheumatoid arthritis. With improvements in medical technology, a child with paraplegia or tetraplegia may now survive through normal adulthood (22,45,48).

Brain injury concomitant with SCI occurs in 25% to 50% of patients (41,142). Careful history of the injury should be obtained because unrecognized brain injury can significantly affect the rehabilitation process. Patients with both brain injury and SCIs may have perceptual deficits, speech deficits, and other associated disabilities that may affect the rehabilitation course.

Unique to pediatrics is SCI without radiographic abnormalities (SCIWORA), which occurs in about 16% to 20% of children's injuries (133,169). Diagnosis is delayed for up to 4 days in about half of these patients (4). The neurologic level in most children with complete lesions and SCIWORA does not im-

R.R. Betz and M.J. Mulcahey: Shriners Hospitals for Children, Philadelphia, Pennsylvania 19140.

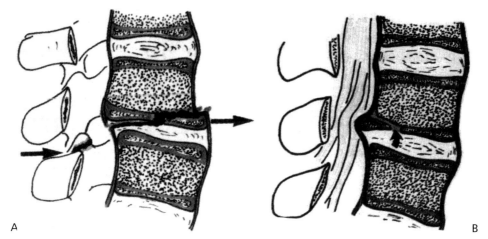

FIGURE 1. Schematic drawings of injury pattern of ring apophysis. **A:** Displaced anteriorly. **B:** Displaced posteriorly.

prove (4). Isolated examples of physeal injury have been reported (80,91,131). Magnetic resonance imaging (MRI) of the spine should still be done in children with SCIWORA to exclude a displaced ring apophysis (Fig. 1).

Classification of Injury

Most spinal cord lesions are initially described as complete or incomplete at a given bony level (the level of injury) of the spinal column. A system promoted by the American Spinal Injury Association (ASIA) to describe a patient's functional level of injury defines the level of function as that at which there is minimal muscle power of 3 and intact sensation to pinprick (2). The next proximal muscle must be grade 5. The muscles affected that are tested at each level of the spinal cord are listed in Table 1. The use of this motor classification system allows for a total motor index, which then allows for accurate comparison of neurologic recovery from either natural history or surgical intervention (Table 2). In addition, patients are classified by the ASIA Impairment Scale A through E. This is similar to the old Frankel grading system but now to be classified as incomplete there

TABLE 1. KEY MUSCLES FOR MOTOR LEVEL CLASSIFICATION

Motor Level	Muscles
C5	Elbow flexors (biceps, brachialis, brachioradialis)
C6	Wrist extensors (extensor carpi radialis longus and brevis)
C7	Elbow extensors (triceps)
C8	Finger flexors (flexor digitorum profundus to the middle finger)
T1	Small finger abductors (abductor digiti minimi)
L2	Hip flexors (iliopsoas)
L3	Knee extensors (quadriceps)
L4	Ankle dorsiflexors (tibialis anterior)
L5	Long toe extensors (extensor hallucis longus)
S1	Ankle plantar flexors (gastrocnemius, soleus)

TABLE 2. MOTOR EXAMINATION: REQUIRED ELEMENTS

Grade	Description
0	Total paralysis
1	Palpable or visible contraction
2	Active movement, full range of motion (ROM) with gravity eliminated
3	Active movement, full ROM against gravity
4	Active movement, full ROM against moderate resistance
5	(Normal) active movement, full ROM against full resistance
NT	Not testable

must be evidence of sacral sparing either by perianal sensation or voluntary anal contraction. With the ASIA Impairment Scale, A is complete, B is sacral sparing plus preserved sensation only, C is sacral sparing plus motor preservation distal to the level of injury but nonfunctional, D is sacral sparing plus motor preservation and functional, and E is normal.

MEDICAL PROBLEMS

Deep-Vein Thrombosis

Kewalramani (82) noted a 50% risk for thrombosis in children but only a rare occurrence of pulmonary embolus. Most cases of DVT occur during the first 3 months after injury, but it should be considered a risk whenever a patient is kept on bed rest after plastic surgery for decubitus or for any subsequent spinal column surgery. Preventive measures include antiembolism stockings, compression boots, subcutaneous heparin (enoxaparin sodium [Lovenox]) or low-dose warfarin sodium (Coumadin).

Immobilization Hypercalcemia

Hypercalcemia is a risk for any patient who is immobilized but especially for children on bed rest after SCI (35,90). Nand and

Goldschmidt (124) reported a 19.8% incidence of hypercalcemia as defined by a serum calcium level of greater than 10.6 mg%. Symptoms include nausea, vomiting, abdominal cramps (if the patient has sensation), and distinct personality changes. Diagnosis is confirmed with a high serum calcium level but must be differentiated from primary and secondary hyperparathyroidism by a parathyroid hormone assay. Treatment consists of intravenous hydration and early mobilization of the patient. Temporarily, a diet including less than 400 mg of calcium per day may also help. Additional treatment aimed at retarding any osteoclastic-mediated bone resorption includes biphosphates and calcitonin (135).

Autonomic Dysreflexia

Patients with injuries above T6 are at risk for autonomic dysreflexia as a result of the traumatic sympathectomy. Autonomic dysreflexia is triggered by noxious afferent stimuli to the skin and viscera below the level of the SCI. The sympathetic reaction cannot be modulated by higher levels of the central nervous system because the response is blocked at the level of the spinal cord lesion. The autonomic reflex through the lateral horn cells in the spinal cord below the level of injury remains intact and unchecked, causing reflex arteriolar spasm and blood pressure elevation. The hypertension is recognized by baroreceptors in the carotid sinus, aortic arch, and cerebral vessels. These receptors send impulses to the vasomotor center in the brain stem through the ninth and tenth cranial nerves. The vasomotor center sends efferent vagal stimulus to slow the heart rate and cause dilation of the skin vasculature, which can occur only above the level of injury (144) (Fig. 2).

Signs and symptoms include hypertension, bradycardia, pounding headaches, vasodilation, flushing, blotching of the skin, and cold sweating above the level of the spinal cord lesion. The major differential diagnosis is anxiety. If the pulse is elevated instead of decreased, the episode is more likely an anxiety attack. If there is evidence of bradycardia, it is most likely autonomic dysreflexia.

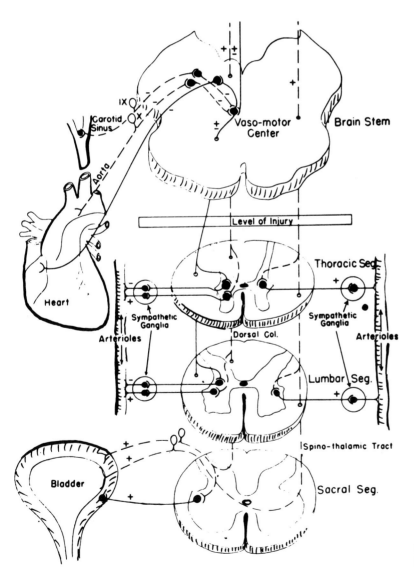

FIGURE 2. Diagram demonstrating the neuroanatomic pathways relevant to autonomic dysreflexia.

Dysreflexia is a medical emergency. The initial step is to detect and eliminate the cause of the noxious stimuli. In general, the most common cause is an overfull bladder, and the second most common cause is fecal impaction (83). If the cause cannot be found and alleviated, medical treatment with an antihypertensive agent should be initiated. The treatment of choice is 10 to 20 mg of nifedipine in a bite-and-chew capsule or sublingually. If this fails and arterial blood pressure monitoring is available, a nitroprusside drip works well. If not, Arfonad (ganglionic blocker), hydralazine hydrochloride, or intrathecal tetracaine hydrochloride is an acceptable treatment option (52).

Respiratory Insufficiency

Depending on the level of injury, respiratory inefficiency of tetraplegia and high-level paraplegia can occur. Decreased inspiratory ventilation is the result of lost intercostal muscles. Decreased expiratory pressure occurs because the diaphragm cannot be passively pushed upward by the contracting abdominal muscles. These patients are at risk for aspiration pneumonia and bronchopneumonia. Prevention of respiratory infections, including pneumococcus and yearly influenza vaccines, is crucial. Postural maneuvers and breathing exercises are essential to train accessory muscles to assist in breathing and to help clear secretions.

Cardiovascular Problems

Bradycardia is the primary cardiac problem in patients with tetraplegia. It results from the loss of sympathetic control of the vagovagal reflex (33). In the acute setting, this can account for 66% of the mortality rate in adult patients with cervical SCI. The cardiovascular system readjusts itself within 3 to 5 weeks, and the patient does not require a pacemaker. If needed, vagolytic therapy with either atropine or propantheline is effective (165). Hypotension in patients with tetraplegia can occur when they attempt to sit. The use of an abdominal binder can decrease venous pooling and help control this.

Vertebral Artery Injury

Although rare, vertebral artery injury can occur with cervical spine trauma. Phenomena not ordinarily associated with cervical trauma, such as altered consciousness, nystagmus, swallowing difficulties, ataxia, and dysarthria, should arouse suspicion (98).

Urologic Problems

The major goals of urologic management of children with SCI are continence and the prevention of urogenital complications, primarily urinary tract infections, urolithiasis, and renal damage. A bladder management program must accommodate the physical and psychosocial development of children and should be convenient and economical, foster independence, and provide for adequate privacy.

During the acute phase of an SCI, an indwelling urinary catheter is usually used to monitor the patient closely. As soon as possible after the injury, an intermittent catheterization program should be implemented, which is initially performed by the hospital staff with sterile equipment and technique. If the neurologic level and developmental age permit, the patient is taught a clean intermittent self-catheterization program (89), otherwise, caregivers are instructed in the procedure. Some children can start to learn to catheterize themselves at about 5 years of age. A clean intermittent catheterization program results in complete emptying of the bladder, which is integral in preventing infections and consequent renal damage. The frequency of catheterization ranges from four to six times a day and is adjusted to maintain continence, maximize convenience, and prevent overdistention. Catheterized volumes approximate 100 to 150 mL in preschool-aged children, 200 to 250 mL in school-aged children, and 400 to 500 mL in adolescents (Vogel LC, personal communication).

To remain continent between catheterizations, some patients require pharmacologic intervention. Commonly used medications include parasympatholytics such as oxybutynin, which relax the bladder detrusor, and α-adrenergic agents such as ephedrine or pseudoephedrine, which increase bladder outlet resistance. Pharmacologic intervention is most effective after a urodynamic evaluation of the detrusor-sphincter dysfunction using a functional classification of the neuropathic bladder (99).

Management of bacteriuria with the use of prophylactic antibiotics is not recommended. Routine culturing of urine from symptom-free patients and treatment of asymptomatic bacteriuria in patients without any significant urologic abnormalities should probably be avoided (154).

Patients should have a baseline renal ultrasound, urodynamics, and follow-up renal ultrasound every 12 months.

Kidney and bladder stones are common in children because of the increased incidence of hypercalcemia and subsequent hypercalciuria, especially if there is a urinary tract infection. Stones are less common in patients who practice intermittent catheterization (157).

Adjunct surgical procedures are available for children with bladder management problems. Patients with incontinence associated with high bladder pressure or refractory to oral medication are candidates for augmentation cystoplasty. In this procedure, a piece of bowel is sewn into the bivalved bladder, which increases the bladder volume and lowers intravascular pressure (63,79,85,95,148). Problems reported with augmentation have included cases of acidosis secondary to absorption of urine across the bowel wall (which can be treated by oral alkalyzing agents) and a few isolated cases of colonic cancer in the bladder.

For some patients with cervical level injuries, clean intermittent catheterization still requires dependence on a caregiver. In these cases, a continent diversion can be an excellent option to facilitate independence. In the Mitrofanoff procedure (111), the appendix is implanted into the bladder and the other end brought out to the skin (most commonly near the umbilicus) to function as a continent, catheterizable stoma.

For patients with upper level tetraplegia who cannot independently cath because they cannot remove their clothing, reconstruction of the hands for grasp and pinch along with a continent diversion such as the Mitrofanoff can make them independent in bladder care.

Another option is a device recently approved by the U.S.

TABLE 3. DIFFERENTIAL DIAGNOSIS OF FEVER OF UNKNOWN ORIGIN

Most common possibilities
- Urinary tract infection
- Upper respiratory infection
- Atelectasis
- Pneumonia
- Deep-vein thrombosis
- Extremity fracture
- Early heterotopic ossification
- Viral gastroenteritis
- Grade III pressure ulcers
- Otitis media
- Wound infection
- Thermoregulator insufficiency

Less common possibilities
- Drug fever
- Hepatitis
- Pancreatitis
- Cholecystitis
- Appendicitis
- Perforated ulcer
- Autonomic dysreflexia
- Abscess

Food and Drug Administration called the Vocare system (NeuroControl, Inc., Cleveland, Ohio), which is a sacral root electrical stimulator. A dorsal root rhizotomy desensitizes the bladder, increasing bladder capacity and improving continence, thus allowing for electrically stimulated control of bladder contractions. The electrical leads from the sacral roots are channeled from the spine at the S1 to S3 laminectomy, subcutaneously around the trunk, to the implant on the abdominal wall. Through a radio frequency antenna, power and stimulus controls are transmitted to the implanted receiver, giving the patient control over bladder contractions. In a series by Egon and colleagues (50), continence was obtained in more than 90% of patients secondary to the rhizotomy, and bladder emptying occurred in 90% of the patients using the stimulator. Bowel programs are a secondary adjunct to this procedure, and bowel times are reduced by 50%.

Fever of Unknown Origin

Fever is a common problem in children with SCI. Evaluation includes history (checking for recent urine culture and sensitivity or recent surgery), physical examination (routine thigh and calf measurements for swelling, crepitus in the extremity, skin lesions), laboratory studies (urinalysis, urine culture and sensitivity, complete blood count with differential, sedimentation rate, chest radiograph, bilirubin, liver enzymes, and sometimes amylase), and other studies (radiographs of extremities and abdomen, bone scan, and venous imaging study of the lower extremities). A sample differential diagnosis is listed in Table 3.

ORTHOPAEDIC PROBLEMS

Halo Fixators

As with adults, proper halo ring application in children is crucial in preventing problems with pin loosening and infection. Ante-

rior pins should be placed superior to the middle or lateral one third of the orbit (to avoid the supraorbital and supratrochlear nerves) and below the greatest circumference of the cranium (59). For the patient older than 12 years, pins should be torqued to 8 lb/in^2, which has been shown to reduce pin loosening and infection as compared with 5 to 6 lb/in^2 (21). If a pin starts to drain fluid, a culture should be obtained, antibiotics started, and the torque on the pin checked. The pin should tighten within three turns; if not, it should be removed and a new one inserted (59).

Children younger than 12 years of age present a unique problem with halo fixation. Multiple pins (10, as compared with 4 in adults) with low torque (2 lb/in^2) have been shown to be safe in infants (115) (Fig. 3). For children 2 to 12 years of age, the torque used may range from 4 to 6 lb/in^2. For children younger than 6 years of age, computed tomography (CT) scanning of the skull is recommended for pin placement because of the great variability in skull thickness (60,93). When halo fixation fails because of loosening or infection, a Minerva-type cervicothoracolumbosacral orthosis (CTLSO) is effective.

Use of Crutchfield tongs in patients younger than 12 years of age is associated with skull penetration and dural fluid leaks. Use of the halo ring for traction, using the principles outlined previously, can be an effective alternative.

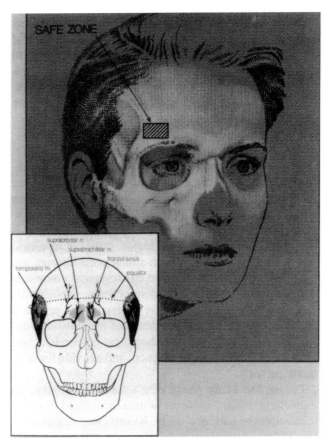

FIGURE 3. Schematic drawing of the ideal position for the anterior pins in the halo, avoiding the superorbital and supertrunclear nerves and the temporalis muscle.

TABLE 4. RIGID CONVENTIONAL BRACES THAT PROVIDE THE BEST CONTROL OF FLEXION AND EXTENSION AT DIFFERENT LEVELS OF THE CERVICAL SPINE

Segmental Levels	Brace	Mean Motion Allowed (degrees)
C1 C2	Halo	3.4
C2–C3	Halo	2.4
	Four poster	3.7
	Cervicothoracic	3.8
Middle (C3–C5)	Cervicothoracic	4.6
Lower (C5–T1)	Cervicothoracic	4.0

From Johnson RM, Hart DL, Simmons EF, et al. (1977): Cervical orthoses: a study in comparing their effectiveness in restricting cervical motion in normal subjects. *J Bone Joint Surg Am* 59: 332–339.

Halo vests can cause severe pressure ulcers in a paralyzed patient. Frequent skin inspection beneath the entire halo vest by the nursing staff initially and then by the care provider at home is essential.

Bracing for Spinal Instability

Data on bracing the cervical spine are available for adults and extrapolated to children, but no actual pediatric data are available (78). Recommended bracing by level of injury reported by Johnson and colleagues (78) is reported in Table 4. For thoracic and lumbar injuries, a custom thoracolumbosacral orthosis (TLSO) is the preferred choice for bracing.

Spasticity

Whenever an upper motor neuron SCI exists, spasticity is present. Spasticity is a condition of excessive reflex activity associated with involuntary movements and clonus accompanied by increased muscle tone. It becomes apparent about 6 weeks after injury and appears to plateau after 6 months. Unique to pediatrics is a higher incidence of patients with flaccid rather than spastic paralysis. In a review of 169 pediatric patients (147), only 74% had spasticity, with 26% being flaccid. Of adults with SCI, most (more than 90%) have spasticity. This may be due to a more severe SCI secondary to the flexible condition of a child's spinal column. Although spasticity may be annoying to the patient, it is thought to preserve muscle mass, which may aid in preventing pressure ulcers. Spasticity may increase with nociceptive complications such as a urinary tract infection, kidney stones, pressure ulcers, bowel impaction, tight clothes, or underinflated wheelchair cushions.

Treatment involves prevention of noxious stimuli and putting the paralyzed joints through a full range of motion. Drug treatment is the mainstay of therapy and includes diazepam (Valium), baclofen (Lioresal), tizanidine (Xanoflex), and dantrolene sodium (Dantrium). Dantrolene sodium is potentially toxic to the liver; therefore, liver function tests are necessary at regular intervals (109). It also causes muscle weakness. Patients for whom drug treatment is not effective may be candidates for a baclofen pump.

Heterotopic Ossification

Heterotopic ossification occurs in 16% to 53% of patients with SCI of all ages and is most commonly seen at the hips, knees, elbows, and shoulders (161). It usually develops during the first 14 months after injury in children, as compared with 6 months in adults (62), and is most common in patients with tetraplegia. Heterotopic ossification may present subtly as an inflammatory reaction of increased redness, warmth, swelling, and gradual loss of joint motion. In pediatrics, the only finding commonly seen is decreased range of motion (62). Several patients have presented with knee and hip joint effusions. Three-phase bone scans are often positive 4 to 6 weeks before there is evidence of ossification on plain radiographs (31). Treatment involves maintaining range of motion and indomethacin. Didronel (etidronate disodium) can be effective, but the dose must be 20 mg/kg per day (initially intravenously). Didronel should be used with caution in children because it may cause growth abnormalities (153). Radiation therapy has been effective in adults, but it is not used in children except for the second occurrence because of the risk for sarcomatous changes.

Heterotopic ossification can be a significant problem, especially at the hips, in that it can prevent a patient from sitting (Fig. 4). It appears to become mature after about 18 months, but maturity can be assessed by bone scan and alkaline phosphatase level. The timing of surgery is crucial. In the past, it was believed that an abnormal serum alkaline phosphatase level and an abnormal three-phase bone scan were predictors of recurrence (156). As a result, it used to be recommended that the bone

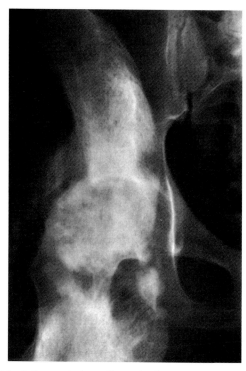

FIGURE 4. Anteroposterior radiograph of an 18-year-old patient with quadriplegia and severe heterotopic ossification of the right hip. The patient's hip was fixed in 20 degrees of flexion.

scan and alkaline phosphatase level be repeated and surgery delayed until they returned to normal. Garland (61) strongly recommends resecting the heterotopic ossification 1.5 years after SCI. Waiting any longer for the bones scan and alkaline phosphatase to return to normal increases the risk for severe intraarticular fibrosis and femoral neck osteoporosis, which prevent return of hip motion or increase the risk for hip fracture during surgery.

Spine Deformity

There is a high prevalence of spine deformity in children and adolescents with SCI. If a child is injured more than a year before reaching maturity, the child has a 98% chance of developing scoliosis and a 67% chance of requiring surgery (43,88,102). In contrast, if an adolescent is injured less than a year before reaching maturity, there is only a 20% chance that he or she will develop scoliosis, with a 5% risk of progressing to surgery (43).

Prophylactic bracing in the form of a lightweight TLSO may be effective in delaying surgery. In a comparison series reported by Lieberman and Betz (94), 24 patients who underwent prophylactic bracing showed an 80% success rate in maintaining their curvature versus a 20% failure rate, progressing over 50 degrees. In comparison, in a group of 5 patients who were never braced, scoliosis in 4 of the 5 (80%) progressed past 50 degrees and required surgery. In that study, further analysis of the data showed that starting a brace before the curve progressed to more than 20 degrees or before 1 year after injury had an excellent success rate in maintaining a curvature as compared with with later bracing, which had a much higher rate of progression.

For patients with tetraplegia, a brace can sometimes provide trunk support, which may help increase upper extremity work space but may cause problems in other areas, such as dressing and transfers. The child's and family's goals for rehabilitation may need to be redefined because of the TLSO, and expectations for independence in some activities may not be met. For example, it is self-defeating to train a child in dressing if the child is to be discharged in a TLSO because a primary requirement of independent dressing is trunk movement. In this case, rehabilitation may need to emphasize parent training in dressing as the patient verbally instructs the activity. When the TLSO is discontinued at skeletal maturity, the patient can then participate in a self-dressing and self-transfer rehabilitation program. For the long term, sacrificing a few years of independence while wearing a TLSO for the benefit of a flexible spine, versus a rigid, instrumented spine (T2 to sacrum) for a lifetime seems more appropriate.

Before reaching skeletal maturity, a child should be seen every 3 months for observation of paralytic spine deformities. For children older than 10 years of age, surgery is recommended when curves progress past 40 degrees. For those younger than 10 years of age, curves of up to 80 degrees are tolerated if they are somewhat flexible and temporarily decrease while in a brace; otherwise, surgery is recommended regardless of age.

Dislocated or Subluxated Hips

In an unpublished review of pediatric patients with SCI (136), there was a 43% prevalence of nonseptic subluxated or dislocated hips in growing children followed a minimum of 3 years. Age at injury correlated with hip deformities, with a 100% incidence of instability in those injured before 5 years of age and 83% of those injured before 10 years of age. It appears to be equally prevalent in patients with tetraplegia and paraplegia and in boys and girls (9). The onset of hip instability after SCI varies widely, from 7 months to 15 years after injury. Hip instability has been seen in patients with spastic and flaccid SCI. Several skeletally mature patients have been seen at our center with rapid onset of noninfected hip subluxation. Untreated, these hips can develop into a Charcot joint. As the hip dislocates and relocates with spasticity, a vicious circle is created; increased fragmentation of the joint results in further spasticity, until the hip socket is totally destroyed (Fig. 5).

In the past, the hips of children with SCI have not routinely been treated. One report of a small series notes no functional deficits in children with SCI with subluxated or dislocated hips (137), but diminution in sitting tolerance has been reported (6). With the development of functional neuromuscular stimulation for computerized standing and walking and the future potential for spinal cord regeneration, more aggressive treatment of hip deformities must be considered. Prophylactic abduction bracing starting at the onset of injury should be instituted in all patients younger than 5 years of age to help prevent subluxation or dislocation. No reports are yet available on this treatment.

Treatment of a patient with a subluxated or dislocated hip is complex. Spasticity needs to be addressed with medication, nerve blocks, a baclofen pump, or rhizotomies (either thermal or open). Soft-tissue contractures must be released. After the spasticity and contractures are addressed, bony stability should be achieved. The hip instability is usually posterior; therefore, a posterior capsulorrhaphy and an acetabular augmentation posteriorly (12) or a Chiari osteotomy should be considered.

Pain

Chronic pain after SCI can be disabling and can have negative effects on successful school, work, and social interactions (26). Pain can originate from the area of trauma, either in a radicular pattern (specifically from compression of the nerve root at the level of injury) or from mechanical instability of an unhealed fracture, or it can consist of central pain (also known as *spinal cord pain* or *dysesthesia*) (55).

Spinal cord dysesthesias constitute a perplexing problem involving numbness, tingling, burning, and pain felt below the level of injury, similar to phantom pain after amputation. The dysesthesias are diffuse and do not conform to a dermal distribution. The incidence of dysesthesias in patients with SCI ranges from 82% to 94% (42), and they are influenced by many factors, including depression, anxiety, weather, smoking, alcohol, exercise, and fatigue. Drugs are occasionally effective, including nonsteroidal antiinflammatory agents, amitriptyline (Elavil), carbamazepine (Tegretol), phenytoin (Dilantin), and gabapentin (Neurontin). A transcutaneous electrical nerve stimulation (TENS) unit can be helpful on occasion (55).

Upper extremity pain is common (31% to 55%) among patients with tetraplegia, especially at the C5 level (7,149). This can occur because of muscle deconditioning and shortening,

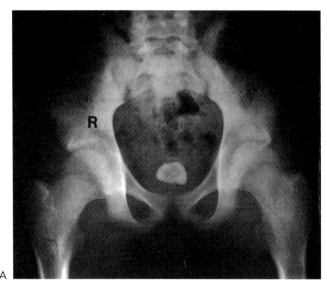 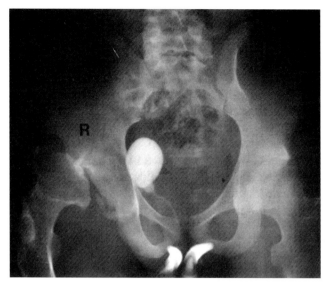

FIGURE 5. A: This 17-year-old boy with T8 complete paraplegia had severe flexor and adductor spasms. He was instructed to perform range-of-motion exercises, sleep prone with a pillow between the legs, and take antispasmodic medication. The patient refused to utilize the recommendations and did not follow-up. **B:** The patient was seen 9 months later with the right hip dislocated posteriorly and no evidence of sepsis. Fragmentation of the joint confirmed the diagnosis of a Charcot joint.

overuse, or cervical radiculopathy. Treatment most often requires muscle strengthening and stretching (145) and alternative ways of performing functional tasks (149).

Reflex Sympathetic Dystrophy

Reflex sympathetic dystrophy has been seen in patients with tetraplegia who complain of diffuse pain, swelling, and stiffness in their upper extremity. A prospective series by Gellman and associates (67) showed a prevalence of 12% in adults. Three-phase bone scan is considered the most sensitive and specific diagnostic study (105), and the diagnosis is confirmed by a response to a stellate ganglion block.

Carpal Tunnel Syndrome

Gellman and colleagues (66) reported that 38 of 77 patients (49%) with paraplegia whose level of injury was at or caudad to the second thoracic vertebra were found to have signs and symptoms of carpal tunnel syndrome.

Osteopenia

Osteopenia occurs in all patients with SCI. It starts immediately and appears to plateau between 6 months and 1 year after injury. Children and adolescents with SCI appear to have bone density that is about 60% of that in normal age- and gender-matched controls (14).

Fractures Secondary to Osteopenia

The prevalence of pathologic fractures occurring secondary to osteopenia in patients with SCI ranges from 10% to 20%

(37,107,130,158). In a review of 176 children and adolescents with SCI (147), 25 patients had 54 pathologic fractures. The etiology in 40% included gait training, range-of-motion exercises, and minor trauma. Sixty percent presented with no etiology, and presentation included fever of unknown origin or redness and swelling around the lower extremities. The most frequent locations of fracture were the supracondylar region of the femur and the proximal tibia. Fractures also occurred at the hip and the ankle.

Treatment of pathologic fractures is usually best managed by soft dressings and splints because of the high prevalence of decubitus ulcers beneath casts (51,106). If casts are essential, they should be foam padded over all bony prominences, and spasticity must be controlled. Because the bone is osteoporotic, long bones typically do not hold internal or external fixation very well. Surgical fixation may be necessary to obtain or maintain bony alignment, but supplemental immobilization may also be needed. For fractures around the hip, internal fixation is necessary and has been reported to be successful (103). If internal fixation of long bone fractures is needed, intramedullary fixation should be used. Fortunately, exuberant callus is generated within 3 to 4 weeks, at which time the splinting and soft tissue dressing can be minimized and general range of motion resumed. Generally, ambulation in braces must be delayed for 6 to 8 weeks after any fracture.

Posttraumatic Syrinx

Posttraumatic syrinx after SCI has been reported (5,138). In the past, the prevalence was thought to be very low (2% to 3%), and diagnosis by CT myelography was required (138). However, recent studies with MRI report an incidence averaging 50% (5). Therefore, because the cysts are extremely common, it is essential that a patient's symptoms be established and related to a progressive cyst before decompression is considered. Symptoms that may necessitate decompression of a cyst include ascending neurologic level, increasing pain, increased spasticity, and change in bladder management and hyperhidrosis. Surgical treatment may include aspirations or shunting through a catheter into either the intrapleural or the intraperitoneal cavity (138). Detethering the scarred area with dural patching has been helpful (54).

Brachial Plexus Palsy

A brachial plexus injury may be seen concomitant with SCI (71). The clinical features suggesting an associated brachial plexus palsy include lower motor neuron paralysis, absent reflexes, variable sensory changes, and occasionally Horner syndrome.

ANESTHESIA ISSUES

Surgical procedures are relatively common in patients with SCI, including children. Genitourinary tract procedures, such as removal of calculi, repair of urinary fistulae, or procedures for bladder emptying, are most common. Plastic and orthopaedic procedures for decubitus and spine and extremity deformities are also common.

It should not be assumed that because a patient with SCI has no sensation distal to the level of the injury there is no need for anesthesia when performing surgical procedures (27). Autonomic dysreflexia is a life-threatening situation that can occur intraoperatively as a result of a noxious stimulus, especially in patients with injury levels above T6. Severe hypertension may result in fatal cerebrovascular hemorrhage (44). It is probably best to assume that the patient is at risk for autonomic dysreflexia and that an invasive procedure should be performed under controlled general or spinal anesthesia.

Schonwald and colleagues (141) documented the reliability of halothane and enflurane in preventing autonomic dysreflexia. Succinylcholine has been associated with acute cardiac arrest secondary to massive release of potassium from the muscle after induction of muscle relaxation in patients with SCI (125).

THE REHABILITATION PROCESS

Establishment of Realistic Goals

Traditionally, goals for rehabilitation of children with SCI have been based on charts of adult function with complete SCI (97,164). These functional level charts should be considered indicators of minimal levels of function as opposed to the traditional perspective of maximal levels of function for the following reasons: About half of SCIs are incomplete lesions (170), suggesting increased potential for independence. Also, there is a great deal of anatomic variation regarding what muscles are innervated and denervated at specific injury levels, and children, because of their size, weight, flexibility, and apparent resiliency, may excel beyond established levels of adult outcome. In addi-

tion, with improved acute management, increased technical developments, advances in orthoses, functional electrical stimulation (FES), biofeedback, environmental modifications, and public laws, previously unobtainable functional levels are now possible for some patients (166–168). In the past, most discussions of rehabilitation focused on adults, but there is an emerging body of literature on children (3,8,11,118,120,132,141, 151,155,162). Although discussions of most of these issues are beyond the scope of this chapter, we review several pertinent topics related to pediatric SCI rehabilitation.

Prevention of Deformity

The primary goal is to obtain pain-free functional range and mobility in all affected joints, including those of the rib cage and spinal column. All children and adolescents with paraplegia should be able to range both lower extremities independently. Problems such as the hip flexors can be addressed not only by daily ranging but also by prone positioning when sleeping or lying prone for part of the day. Patients who cannot perform range-of-motion exercises themselves should be taught to instruct others in this task. The shoulders also need to be ranged, especially while the patient is in a halo.

Traditional approaches of SCI rehabilitation have encouraged specific patterns of joint limitation because they actually enhance function. The most prevalent example concerns the intentional tightening of the finger flexors in patients with C5 or C6 tetraplegia. With tightening of the long finger flexors, when the wrist is flexed by means of gravity, the fingers passively extend for hand opening. With voluntary wrist extension, the fingers pull into the palm, creating a passive pinch. This tenodesis action (Fig. 6) enables the patient to grasp and release small, light objects and, with the assistance of a wrist-driven flexor hinge orthosis, control the thumb and strengthen the pinch (Fig. 7). Although encouragement of tight finger flexors has been the traditional standard of care for the hands of patients with a C5- or C6-level injury, the contractures prove to be a difficult obstacle to overcome in the event that FES or tendon transfers are desirable. Splinting the hand in an intrinsic-plus posture at night prevents flexion contractures and preserves the hand for future FES or tendon transfers.

Return to Vertical Positioning

Tolerance of vertical sitting and, when appropriate, standing, should be considered soon after an injury but may not always be achieved during the early stages, especially when patients have undergone spine surgery. One barrier to obtaining a vertical position soon after injury is postural hypotension, which is manifested by decreased blood pressure, increased pulse, pallor, and dizziness. Initially, this can be managed by a reclining wheelchair, and most patients respond to progressive attempts to sit or stand. On occasion, pressure-gradient stockings or abdominal binders are necessary.

Prevention of Pressure Ulcers

Patients with paralysis resulting in insensate areas must understand the importance of skin care, safety, hygiene, skin checks,

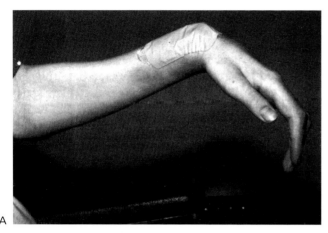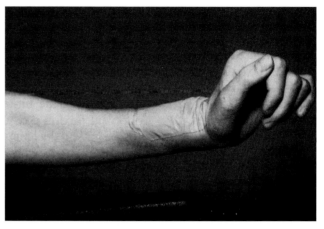

A B

FIGURE 6. Tenodesis action of the fingers with wrist flexion and extension. **A:** With passive flexion of the wrist, the fingers extend. **B:** With active extension of the wrist, because of the contractures of the flexor digitorum superficialis and profundus, the fingers are pulled into the palm, enabling the patient to grasp and release small, light objects. Usually, the thumb pinch is weak, requiring either a tenodesis orthosis or a flexor pollicis longus (FPL) tenodesis to the distal radius.

and pressure reliefs. With advances in technology, sophisticated pressure mapping and monitoring can aid in decisions concerning appropriate seating systems and prevention of shearing forces. In the event of a pressure ulcer, a program consisting of progressive sitting or weight bearing should be implemented.

Prevention of pressure ulcers is of utmost importance and involves pressure relief skills, frequent skin inspections, and avoidance of trauma while transferring. The patient also needs to be taught to protect the skin from extreme heat or cold. Burns can easily occur during bathing or from cigarettes, heating pads, or car heaters.

Respiratory and Cardiovascular Function

Rehabilitation goals include training in more efficient coordinated breathing patterns, maintaining chest mobility, and bron-

chial hygiene. Use of an incentive spirometer and group games, including sipping through straws and blowing bubbles, are helpful. Specific training of the diaphragm and the secondary accessory muscles, such as the sternocleidomastoid, trapezius, levator scapula, and scalene muscles, can also improve function. An elastic abdominal binder may also assist with respiratory function. Maintenance or improvement of chest mobility should be attempted with counterrotation trunk exercises. Patients should be taught assisted coughing, postural drainage, and deep-breathing exercises.

Tendon Transfers for Volitional Arm and Hand Function

Static and dynamic splints and a variety of orthoses are available to improve hand function of patients with tetraplegia (87), even

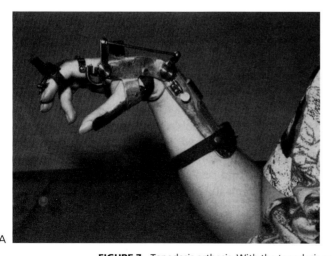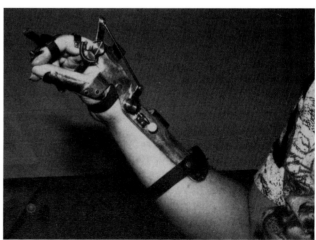

A B

FIGURE 7. Tenodesis orthosis. With the tenodesis action, the orthosis controls the thumb, index finger, middle finger. **A:** With passive flexion of the wrist, the thumb is abducted out of the palm. **B:** With active extension of the wrist, the fingers and thumb are drawn together, producing a pinch.

TABLE 5. INTERNATIONAL CLASSIFICATION OF HAND SURGERY IN TETRAPLEGIA

Group	Characteristics[a]	Function
0	No muscle below elbow suitable for transfer	—
1	Brachioradialis	Flexion and supination of the elbow
2	Extensor carpi radialis longus	Extension of the wrist (weak or strong)
3[b]	Extensor carpi radialis brevis	Extension of the wrist
4	Pronator teres	Extension and pronation of the wrist
5	Flexor carpi radialis	Flexion of the wrist
6	Finger extensors	Extrinsic extension of fingers (partial or complete)
7	Thumb extensor	Extrinsic extension of the thumb
8	Partial digital flexors	Extrinsic flexion of the fingers (weak)
9	Lacks only intrinsics	Extrinsic flexion of the fingers
X	Exceptions	Extrinsic flexion of the fingers

[a] Key muscles must be tested as grade 4. Note that this is different from the ASIA functional level, in which muscles are tested as grade 3. A sensory prefix is also needed: O, ocular intact; Cu, sensation <10 mm on two-point discrimination in thumb and index finger.
[b] It is not possible to determine strength of the extensor carpi radialis brevis without surgical exposure.

for children (117). Typically, however, splints and orthoses are abandoned after discharge because of the cosmesis, the added stigma, and the burden of carrying equipment to and from different settings. Many children and adolescents with tetraplegia could benefit from surgical restoration of hand function by means of tendon transfers. Although the literature is extensive with regard to results and procedures for adults (75,104,112), literature describing the results of tendon transfers in children and adolescents with SCI is just recently emerging (116,121).

Candidates for upper extremity reconstruction are evaluated based on the International Classification System for Surgery of the Hand in Tetraplegia (104). As shown in Table 5, surgical reconstruction of the upper extremity in tetraplegia has been performed to restore elbow extension (29,34,75), wrist extension (57,108), finger flexion (53,58,75,81), and thumb pinch (75,76). Restoration of these functions is made possible by transferring the tendons of muscles under voluntary control to the tendons of muscles that are paralyzed. Often, other procedures, such as an arthrodesis, tenodesis, or the New Zealand flexor pollicis longus split tendon transfer (113), are performed in conjunction to enhance hand function.

Functional Electrical Stimulation of the Upper Extremities

Functional electrical stimulation (FES) applications have concentrated on restoration of grasp and release in adults and adolescents with C5 and weak C6 function who do not meet the criteria for reconstructive surgery according to the international classification (122,134).

The success with the research-grade percutaneous systems (13,118,134,150) has led to development and market approval of the Freehand System, an eight-channel hand stimulation system with totally implantable electrodes. The Freehand system involves implantation of electrodes onto select muscles of the arm and hand. The electrode leads are tunneled subcutaneously to the stimulator that is sutured onto the subcutaneous fascia in the chest. Control of stimulated grasp and release is achieved with a sensor that is typically mounted onto the contralateral shoulder. Outcomes data on the Freehand system with both adults (84) and adolescents (116) show increased independence in activities and improved satisfaction level of activity performance.

Applications of FES in patients with high-level tetraplegia (C4) are also under investigation (13,73,123,126–128). Restoration of elbow flexion and grasp and release by means of FES has enabled one adolescent with a C4-level injury to feed himself and drink with minimal assistance and little external bracing (13). Although patients with high-level tetraplegia will always require some level of attendant care, FES may provide a higher degree of independence and autonomy.

Standing and Ambulation

Most children and adolescents with SCI desire to stand and walk. The importance of standing as a component of the rehabilitation process, especially with children, cannot be overemphasized. The following physiologic benefits of standing have been described (28,40,56,92,160):

- Maintenance of range of motion in both lower extremities
- Reduction of hypercalciuria and osteoporosis of the long bones
- Improvement of organ position and bowel and bladder function
- Improvement in skin condition as a result of pressure relief of pelvic bony prominences
- Improvement in regulation of orthostatic circulation
- Reduction in spasticity

In very young children with a SCI, standing also has developmental significance for perceptual, cognitive, and emotional growth (114,160). In the past, patients with injury levels of T10 or below were routinely fitted with some form of standing brace (139). In children and adolescents, there are few guidelines for upright mobility (11).

Methods for providing standing and walking ability fall into five categories: orthoses, standing frames, specialized wheelchairs, FES, and hybrid systems. The general advantages and disadvantages of each method are considered elsewhere (39,77). The most frequently prescribed method of standing is the knee-ankle-foot orthosis (KAFO). Several studies of adults with SCI addressed the long-term use of KAFOs after discharge from rehabilitation (38,110). In all these studies, most adults had abandoned their orthoses for a variety of reasons, including time spent donning and doffing, pressure problems related to extended wear, impracticality, energy expenditure, inability to rise independently, and poor cosmesis.

A survey of young patients with SCIs assessed their attitudes about standing (36). One hundred five individuals responded, with 48 responses coming from patients with T4- to T12-level paraplegia. In this subgroup, 85% reported that they used a lightweight sport wheelchair—50% without armrests and 35% with. Sixty percent of the subgroup reported that they had KAFOs, but only half reported using their KAFOs more than 3 days a week for exercise, standing, or ambulation. When asked to rank the most important reasons for standing, 39% chose getting an object stored out of reach; 35% chose being eye to eye with another person; and 27% chose transferring more easily.

The fact that more than one third of the respondents chose being eye to eye with another person as the most important reason to stand is testimony to the powerful psychological benefit associated with standing. An assistive device is necessary to achieve standing with all portable standing methods, and the preference for lightweight sport wheelchairs dictates careful consideration of an appropriate device. In adolescents, choosing to convert from upright mobility to wheeled mobility should be viewed as a transition rather than a failure.

For young children, one alternative to KAFOs is the parapodium, which allows sitting and standing. For a child with tetraplegia, a swivel walker may allow standing and ambulation for a short distance in the home, but the time necessary to don and doff the orthosis typically makes it impractical for daily and spontaneous use. Other common orthoses include the hip-knee-ankle-foot orthosis (HKAFO) and the reciprocating gait orthosis (RGO), which are described in detail elsewhere (39).

Functional electrical stimulation for standing and walking has been under investigation for several decades (40,100,101, 119,152). The Parastep I (Sigmedics, Inc., Northfield, IL) (86), a surface stimulation system, is available on the market and provides short-distance walking ability to persons with mid-thoracic injuries. In our study of an investigational device (114), adolescents used FES to stand at home between two and four times a week. Common activities while standing included reaching high places, accessing environments, and exercise.

In another study (19), we showed that FES was comparable or better than braces in facilitating independence and that FES was preferred over braces for most activities. Research is underway on totally implantable FES devices for upright mobility (10).

Denervation of lower extremity muscles excludes 23% of patients from FES (159) because only upper motor neuron innervated muscles can be stimulated. This problem could be overcome by transferring spastic muscles, which can then be stimulated, as has been done in the upper extremity (163). Orthopaedic problems, such as hip dislocation, severe scoliosis, and muscle flaps for pressure ulcers, will continue to affect future FES candidates and should be addressed prophylactically.

RESEARCH

It is important that the care provider organizing a patient's rehabilitation be up to date on research being conducted on SCIs. Patients and parents are likely to ask about the status of research regarding a cure. Current research strategies are focused on protection, enhancement, and regeneration.

A large portion of research is working toward minimizing the trauma at the time of the acute injury. Trauma alone causes the anatomic transection of the spinal cord in less than 15% of cases (18). The neurologic deficits caused by microscopic physical disruption of the axons transversing the injury site are compounded by local infarction, microhemorrhages, or edema. Laboratory studies of chronically injured spinal cords indicate that even a few remaining intact axons (5% to 18%) can support functional recovery (15,16). Although axons remain, they may be dysfunctional, and demyelination is probably responsible for most of this dysfunction (17).

To minimize this secondary damage after trauma, high-dose methylprednisolone (30 mg/kg of body weight followed by an infusion of 5.4 mg/kg per hour for 23 hours started within 8 hours of injury) is used (23). No patients under 13 years of age have been studied. Gangliosides (Sygen) present in central nervous system cell membranes augment neurite outgrowth in vitro and induce regeneration and sprouting of neurons (69,70). Melsher and associates (65) reported results of a randomized, prospective study of Sygen in about 1,000 patients. They showed no change in patients classified as ASIA A, but there was improvement in patients classified as ASIA B and earlier recovery in those classified as ASIA C and D.

Research in regeneration of injured spinal cords has focused on ways to stimulate axonal growth. Brain-derived neurotrophic factor and Schwann cells from peripheral nerves in tissue culture have been found to stimulate neurite outgrowth in a rat model (72). The axonal proteins that appear to inhibit regeneration of the spinal cord, in contrast to peripheral nerve regeneration, have been identified (32,143). Attempts in laboratories to modulate these protein productions have been through immunologic manipulation (140) and enzymatic alteration, both of which appear to be promising. In animal studies, electrical stimulation of regenerating axons has been performed (20), as has embryonic transfer of fetal tissue (25,96).

Even when regeneration of the spinal cord becomes possible, there will be patients with SCI whose injury is either so severe or of such a nature that regeneration will never be possible. Such injuries include gunshot wounds that completely destroy the spinal cord, massive infections that leave the spinal cord completely necrotic, and severe trauma with documented total transection of the spinal cord. These patients will need other means to restore them to more functional lives. Functional neuromuscular stimulation of both the upper and lower extremities will probably be the most promising treatment for these patients.

REFERENCES

1. Abroms IF, Bresnan MJ, Zuckerman JE, et al. (1973): Cervical cord injuries secondary to hyperextension of the head in breech presentations. *Obstet Gynecol* 41:369–378.
2. American Spinal Injury Association (1991): *Standards for neurologic classification of spinal injury patients.* Atlanta: Author.
3. Anderson CJ (1997): Unique management needs of pediatric spinal cord injury patients: psychosocial issues. *J Spinal Cord Med* 20:21–24.
4. Anderson JM, Schutt AH (1980): Spinal injury in children: a review of 156 cases seen from 1950 through 1978. *Mayo Clin Proc* 55:499–504.
5. Backe HA, Betz RR, Mesgarzadeh M, et al. (1991): Post-traumatic spinal cord cysts evaluated by magnetic resonance imaging. *Paraplegia* 29:607–612.

6. Baird RA, DeBenedetti MJ, Eltorai I (1986): Non-septic hip instability in the chronic spinal cord injury patient. *Paraplegia* 24:293–300.

7. Bayley JC, Cochran TP, Sledge CB (1987): The weight-bearing shoulder: the impingement syndrome in paraplegics. *J Bone Joint Surg Am* 69:676–678.

8. Betz RR (1997): Orthopaedic problems in the child with spinal cord injury. *Top Spinal Cord Inj Rehabil* 3(2):9–19.

9. Betz RR, Beck T, Huss GK, et al. (1994): *Hip instability in children with spinal cord injury.* Presented at the American Spinal Injury Association annual meeting, Philadelphia, April 1994.

10. Betz RR, Johnston TE, Mulcahey MJ, et al (1999): *Implantable functional electrical stimulation for upright mobility in children: preliminary experience.* Presented at the American Spinal Injury Association annual meeting, Atlanta, April 1999.

11. Betz RR, Mulcahey MJ, eds. (1996): *The child with a spinal cord injury.* Rosemont, IL: American Academy of Orthopaedic Surgeons.

12. Betz RR, Mulcahey MJ, Smith BT, et al. Implications of hip subluxation for FES-assisted mobility in patients with spinal cord injury. *Orthopedics* (in press).

13. Betz RR, Mulcahey MJ, Smith B, et al. (1992): Bipolar latissimus dorsi transposition and functional neuromuscular stimulation to restore elbow flexion in an individual with C4 tetraplegia and C5 denervation. *J Am Paraplegia Soc* 15(4):220–228.

14. Betz RR, Triolo RJ, Hermida VM, et al. (1991): *The effects of functional neuromuscular stimulation on the bone mineral content in the lower limbs of spinal cord injured children.* Presented at the American Spinal Injury Association annual meeting, Seattle, April 1991.

15. Blight AR (1983): Cellular morphology of chronic spinal cord injury in the cat: analysis of myelinated axons by line sampling. *Neuroscience* 10:521–543.

16. Blight AR, DeCrescito V (1986): Morphometric analysis of experimental spinal cord injury in the cat: the relation of injury intensity to survival of myelinated axons. *Neuroscience* 19:321–341.

17. Blight AR, Young W (1989): Central axons in injured cat spinal cord recover electrophysiological function following remyelination by Schwann cells. *J Neurol Sci* 91:15–34.

18. Bohlman HH (1979): Acute fractures and dislocations of the cervical spine. *J Bone Joint Surg Am* 61:1119–1142.

19. Bonaroti D, Akers J, Smith BT, et al. (1999): Comparison of functional electrical stimulation to long leg braces for upright mobility in children with complete thoracic level spinal injuries. *Arch Phys Med Rehabil* 80:1047–1053.

20. Borgens RB, Blight AR, McGinnis ME (1987): Behavioral recovery induced by applied electric fields after spinal cord hemisection in guinea pig. *Science* 238:366–369.

21. Botte MJ, Byrne T, Garfin SR (1987): Application of the halo device for immobilization of the cervical spine using an increased torque pressure. *J Bone Joint Surg Am* 69:750–753.

22. Bracken MB, Collins WF, Freeman DF, et al. (1984): Efficacy of methylprednisolone in acute spinal cord injury. *JAMA* 251:45–52.

23. Bracken MB Shepard MJ, Collins WF, et al. (1990): A randomized controlled trial of methylprednisolone or naloxone in the treatment of acute spinal-cord injury: results of the Second National Acute Spinal Cord Injury Study. *N Engl J Med* 322:1405–1411.

24. Bray GP (1978): Rehabilitation of the spinal cord injured: a family approach. *J Appl Rehabil Counseling* 9:70–78.

25. Bregman BS, Kunkel-Bagden E (1990): Fetal tissue transplants promote functional recovery in rats. *Prog Res* 23:11.

26. Brittell CW, Mariano AJ (1991): Chronic pain in spinal cord injury. *Phys Med Rehabil: State of the Art Rev* 5:71–82.

27. Brodsky RC, Stehling LC (1984): Anesthesia update 17. Autonomic hyperreflexia. *Orthop Rev* 13:101–104.

28. Bromley I (1981): *Tetraplegia and paraplegia: a guide for physiotherapists,* 2nd ed. Edinburgh: Churchill Livingstone, pp. 160–161.

29. Bryan RS (1977): The Moberg deltoid-triceps replacement and key-pinch operations in quadriplegia: preliminary experience. *Hand* 9: 207–220.

30. Burke DC (1976): Injuries of the spinal cord in children. In: Vinken PJ, Bruyn GW, eds. *Handbook of clinical neurology,* vol. 25. New York: American Elsevier Publishers.

31. Campbell J, Bonnett C (1975): Spinal cord injury in children. *Clin Orthop* 92:114–123.

32. Caroni P, Schwab ME (1989): Codistribution of neurite growth inhibitors and oligodendrocytes in rat CNS: appearance follows nerve fiber growth and precedes myelination. *Dev Biol* 136:287–295.

33. Carter RE (1979): Medical management of pulmonary complications of spinal cord injury. *Adv Neurol* 22:261.

34. Castro-Sierra A, Lopez-Pita A (1983): A new surgical technique to correct triceps paralysis. *Hand* 15:42–46.

35. Christofaro RL, Brink JD (1979): Hypercalcemia of immobilization in neurologically injured children: a prospective study. *Orthopedics* 2: 486–491.

36. Cohn JC, Moynahan M, Triolo RJ, et al. (1992): *A survey of the pediatric spinal cord injured population on attitudes towards standing.* Presented at the American Spinal Injury Association annual meeting, Toronto, May 1992.

37. Comarr AE, Hutchinson RH, Bors E (1962): Extremity fractures of patients with spinal cord injuries. *Am J Surg* 103:732–739.

38. Coughlan JK, Robinson CE, Newmarch B, et al. (1980): Lower extremity bracing in paraplegia: a follow-up study. *Paraplegia* 18:25–32.

39. Creitz L, Nelson VS, Haubenstricker L, et al. (1996): Orthotic prescriptions, ch. 46. In: Betz RR, Mulcahey MJ, eds. *The child with a spinal cord injury.* Rosemont, IL: American Academy of Orthopaedic Surgeons, pp. 537–554.

40. Cybulski GR, Penn RD, Jaeger RJ (1984): Lower extremity functional neuromuscular stimulation in cases of spinal cord injury. *Neurosurgery* 15:132–146.

41. Davidoff G, Morris J, Roth E, et al. (1985): Cognitive dysfunction and mild closed head injury in traumatic spinal cord injury. *Arch Phys Med Rehabil* 66:489–491.

42. Davis R (1975): Pain and suffering following spinal cord injury. *Clin Orthop* 112:76.

43. Dearolf WW III, Betz RR, Vogel LC, et al. (1990): Scoliosis in pediatric spinal cord-injured patients. *J Pediatr Orthop* 10:214–218.

44. Desmond J (1970): Paraplegia: problems confronting the anesthesiologist. *Can Anaesth Soc J* 17:435–451.

45. DeVivo MJ (1990): Life expectancy and causes of death for persons with spinal cord injuries. Research Update. Birmingham: University of Alabama.

46. DeVivo MJ, Kartus PL, Stover SL, et al. (1990): Benefits of early admission to an organised spinal cord injury care system. *Paraplegia* 28:545–555.

47. DeVivo MJ, Fine PR, Maetz HM, et al. (1980): Prevalence of spinal cord injury: a reestimation employing life table techniques. *Arch Neurol* 37:707–708.

48. DeVivo MJ, Stover SL, Black KJ (1992): Prognostic factors for 12-year survival after spinal cord injury. *Arch Phys Med Rehabil* 73: 156–162.

49. Dunne K, Hopkins IJ, Shield LK (1986): Acute transverse myelopathy in childhood. *Dev Med Child Neurol* 28:198–204.

50. Egon G, Barat M, Colombel P, et al. (1998): Implantation of anterior sacral root stimulators combined with posterior sacral rhizotomy in spinal injury patients. *World J Urol* 16:342–349.

51. Eichenholtz S (1963): Management of long-bone fractures in paraplegic patients. *J Bone Joint Surg Am* 45:299–310.

52. Erickson RP (1980): Autonomic hyperreflexia: pathophysiology and medical management. *Arch Phys Med Rehabil* 61:431–440.

53. Failla JC, Peimer CA, Sherwin FS (1990): Brachioradialis transfer for digital palsy. *J Hand Surg Br* 15:312–316.

54. Falci S, Lammertse D, Seiger A, et al. *Surgical treatment of post-traumatic syringomyelia and tethered spinal cords.* Presented at the American Spinal Injury Association annual meeting, Atlanta, April 1999.

55. Farkash AE, Portenoy RK (1986): The pharmacological management of chronic pain in the paraplegic patient. *J Am Paraplegia Soc* 9:41–50.

56. Fitzsimmons AS (1996): The physiologic benefits of standing, ch. 45. In: Betz RR, Mulcahey MJ, eds. *The child with a spinal cord injury.* Rosemont, IL: American Academy of Orthopaedic Surgeons, pp. 533–535.

57. Freehafer AA, Peckham PH, Keith MW (1988): New concepts on treatment of the upper limb in the tetraplegic. *Hand Clin* 4:563–574.

58. Gansel J, Waters R, Gellman H (1990): Transfer of the pronator tendon to the tendons of the flexor digitorum profundus in tetraplegia. *J Bone Joint Surg Am* 72:427–432.

59. Garfin SR, Botte MJ, Waters RL, et al. (1986): Complications in the use of the halo fixation device. *J Bone Joint Surg Am* 68:320–325.

60. Garfin SR, Roux R, Botte MJ, et al. (1986): Skull osteology as it affects halo pin placement in children. *J Pediatr Orthop* 6:434–436.

61. Garland DE (1991): A clinical perspective on common forms of acquired heterotopic ossification. *Clin Orthop* 263:13–29.

62. Garland DE, Shimoya ST, Lugo C, et al. (1989): Spinal cord insults and heterotopic ossification in the pediatric population. *Clin Orthop* 245:303–310.

63. Gearhart JP, Albertsen PC, Marshall FF, et al. (1986): Pediatric applications of augmentation cystoplasty: The Johns Hopkins experience. *J Urol* 136:430–432.

64. Gehrig R, Michaelis LS (1976): Statistics of acute paraplegia and tetraplegia on a national scale. *Paraplegia* 10:232.

65. Geisler FH, Grieco G, Dorsey FC, et al. (1999): *GM1 Ganglioside Acute Spinal Cord Injury Study II: efficacy and safety.* North American Spine Society annual meeting, October 1999.

66. Gellman H, Chandler DR, Petrasek J, et al. (1988): Carpal tunnel syndrome in paraplegic patients. *J Bone Joint Surg Am* 70:517–519.

67. Gellman H, Eckert RR, Botte MJ, et al. (1988): Reflex sympathetic dystrophy in cervical spinal cord injury patients. *Clin Orthop* 233:126–131.

68. Gordon N, Marsden B (1970): Spinal cord injury at birth. *Neuropadiatrie* 2:112–118.

69. Gorio A, DiGuillo AM, Young W, et al. (1986): GM1 effects on chemical, traumatic and peripheral nerve induce lesions to the spinal cord. In: Goldberger ME, Gorio A, Murray M, eds. *Development and plasticity of the mammalian spinal cord,* vol 3. Padua, Italy: Liviana Press, pp. 227–242.

70. Gorio A, Ferrari G, Fusco M, et al. (1984): Gangliosides and their effects on rearranging peripheral and central neural pathways. *Cent Nerv Syst Trauma* 1:29–37.

71. Grundy DJ, Silver JR (1983): Combined brachial plexus and spinal cord trauma. *Injury* 15:57–61.

72. Guest JD, Roa A, Olson L, et al. (1997): The ability of human Schwann cell grafts to promote regeneration in the transected nude rat spinal cord. *Exp Neurol* 148:502–522.

73. Handa Y, Naito A, Ichie M, et al. (1987): *EMG-based stimulation patterns of FNS for the paralyzed upper extremities.* Presented at the 9th International Symposium on Advances in External Control of Human Extremities, Dubrovnik, Yugoslavia, pp. 329–337.

74. Harvey C, Rothschild BB, Asmann AJ, et al. (1990): New estimates of traumatic SCI prevalence: a survey-based approach. *Paraplegia* 28:537–544.

75. Hentz VR, House J, McDowell C, et al. (1992): Rehabilitation and surgical reconstruction of the upper limb in tetraplegia: an update. *J Hand Surg* 17A:964–967.

76. House J (1985): Reconstruction of the thumb in tetraplegia following spinal cord injury. *Clin Orthop* 195:117–128.

77. Jaeger RW, Yarkony GM, Roth EJ (1989): Rehabilitation technology for standing and walking after spinal cord injury. *Am J Phys Med Rehabil* 68:128–133.

78. Johnson RM, Hart DL, Simmons EF, et al. (1977): Cervical orthoses: a study in comparing their effectiveness in restricting cervical motion in normal subjects. *J Bone Joint Surg Am* 59:332–339.

79. Kass EJ, Koff SA (1983): Bladder augmentation in the pediatric neuropathic bladder. *J Urol* 129:552–555.

80. Keller RH (1974): Traumatic displacement of the cartilaginous vertebral rim: a sign of intervertebral disc prolapse. *Radiology* 110:21–24.

81. Kelly CM, Freehafer AA, Peckham PH, et al. (1985): Post-operative results of opponensplasty and flexor tendon transfer with spinal cord injured patients. *J Hand Surg Am* 10:890–894.

82. Kewalramani LS (1979): Neurogenic gastroduodenal ulceration and bleeding associated with spinal cord injuries. *Trauma* 19:259–265.

83. Kewalramani LS (1980): Autonomic dysreflexia in traumatic myelopathy. *Am J Phys Med* 59:1–21.

84. Kilgore KL, Peckham PH, Keith MW, et al. (1997): An implanted upper-extremity neuroprosthesis: follow-up of five patients. *J Bone Joint Surg Am* 79:533–541.

85. King LR, Webster GD, Bertram RA (1987): Experiences with bladder reconstruction in children. *J Urol* 138:1002–1006.

86. Klose KJ, Jacobs PL, Broton JG, et al. (1997): Evaluation of a training program for persons with SCI paraplegia using the Parastep 1 ambulation system: part 1. Ambulation performance and anthropometric measures. *Arch Phys Med Rehabil* 78:789–793.

87. Krajnik S, Bridle M (1992): Hand splinting in tetraplegia: current practice. *Am J Occup Ther* 46:149–156.

88. Lancourt JE, Dickson JH, Carter RE (1981): Paralytic spinal deformity following traumatic spinal-cord injury in children and adolescents. *J Bone Joint Surg Am* 63:47–53.

89. Lapides J, Diokno AC, Lowe BS, et al. (1974): Follow up on unsterile, intermittent self-catheterization. *J Urol* 111:184–187.

90. Lawrence GD, Loeffler RG, Martin LG, et al. (1973): Immobilization hypercalcemia: some new aspects of diagnosis and treatment. *J Bone Joint Surg Am* 55:87–94.

91. Lawson JP, Ogden JA, Bucholz RW, et al. (1987): Physeal injuries of the cervical spine. *J Pediatr Orthop* 7:428–435.

92. Leo K (1985): The effects of passive standing. *Paraplegia News* November: 45–47.

93. Letts M, Kaylor D, Gouw G (1988): A biomechanical analysis of halo fixation in children. *J Bone Joint Surg Br* 70:277–279.

94. Lieberman GS, Betz RR (1998): *Bracing for delaying the progression of scoliosis in the immature patient with spinal cord injury.* Presented at the American Spinal Injury Association annual meeting, Cleveland, OH, April 1998.

95. Linder A, Leach GE, Raz S (1983): Augmentation cystoplasty in the treatment of neurogenic bladder dysfunction. *J Urol* 129:491–493.

96. Lindvall O, Bjørkland A (1990): Fetal tissue implant in Sweden leads to significant recovery in Parkinson's disease. *Prog Res* 23:5.

97. Long C, Lawton E (1955): Functional significance of spinal cord lesion level. *Arch Phys Med Rehabil* 36:299–302.

98. Lyness SS, Simeone FA (1978): Vascular complications of upper cervical spine injuries. *Orthop Clin North Am* 9:1029–1038.

99. Madersbacher H (1990): The various types of neurogenic bladder dysfunction: an update of current therapeutic concepts. *Paraplegia* 28:217–229.

100. Marsolais EB, Kobetic R (1986): Implantation techniques and experience with percutaneous intramuscular electrodes in the lower extremities. *J Rehabil Res Dev* 23:1–8.

101. Marsolais EB, Kobetic R (1987): Functional electrical stimulation for walking in paraplegia. *J Bone Joint Surg Am* 69:728–733.

102. Mayfield JK, Erkkila JC, Winter RB (1981): Spine deformity subsequent to acquired childhood spinal cord injury. *J Bone Joint Surg Am* 63:1401–1411.

103. McCarthy JJ, Betz RR (1999): *The treatment of hip fractures in children with existing spinal cord injuries.* Presented at the Howard H. Steel Conference on Pediatric Spinal Cord Injury: Contemporary Principles and New Directions. Palm Springs, CA, December 1999.

104. McDowell C, Moberg E, House J (1986): The second international conference on the surgical rehabilitation of the upper limb in tetraplegia. *J Hand Surg* 11:604–608.

105. McKinnon SE, Holder LE (1984): The use of three-phase radionuclide bone scanning in the diagnosis of reflex sympathetic dystrophy. *J Hand Surg Am* 9:556.

106. McMaster W, Stauffer ES (1975): The management of long bone fracture in the spinal cord injured patient. *Clin Orthop* 112:44–52.

107. Meinecke FW, Rehn J, Leitz G (1967): Conservative and operative treatment of fractures of the limbs in paraplegia. *Proc Annual Clinical Spinal Cord Injury Conference* 17:77–91.

108. Mendelson LS, Peckham PH, Freehafer AA, et al. (1988): Assessment of tendon transfer surgery in the tetraplegic extremity. *Innov Tech Biol Med* 9:281–292.

109. Merritt JL (1981): Management of spasticity in spinal cord injury. *Mayo Clin Proc* 56:614–622.

110. Mickelberg R, Reid S (1981): Spinal cord lesions and lower extremity bracing: an overview and follow-up study. *Paraplegia* 19:379–385.

111. Mitrofanoff P (1980): Trans-appendicular continent cystotomy in the management of the neurogenic bladder. *Chir Pediatr* 21:297–305.

112. Moberg E (1990): Surgical rehabilitation of the upper limb in tetraplegia. *Paraplegia* 28:330–334.

113. Mohammad KD (1992): Upper limb surgery for tetraplegia. *J Bone Joint Surg Br* 74:873–879.

114. Moynahan MA, Mullin C, Cohn J, et al. (1996): Home use of a FES system for standing and mobility in adolescents with spinal cord injury. *Arch Phys Med Rehabil* 77:1005–1013.

115. Mubarak SJ, Camp JF, Vuletich W, et al. (1989): Halo application in the infant. *J Pediatr Orthop* 9:612–614.

116. Mulcahey MJ (1996): Rehabilitation and outcomes of upper extremity tendon transfer surgery, ch. 37. In: Betz RR, Mulcahey MJ, eds. *The child with a spinal cord injury.* Rosemont, IL: American Academy of Orthopaedic Surgeons, pp. 419–448.

117. Mulcahey MJ (1996): Upper extremity orthoses and splints, ch. 34. In: Betz RR, Mulcahey MJ, eds. *The child with a spinal cord injury.* Rosemont, IL: American Academy of Orthopaedic Surgeons, pp. 375–392.

118. Mulcahey MJ (1992): Returning to school following spinal cord injury: perspectives from four adolescents. *Am J Occup Ther* 46:305–313.

119. Mulcahey MJ, Betz RR (1997): Upper and lower extremity applications of functional electrical stimulation: a decade of research with children and adolescents with spinal injuries. *Pediatr Phys Ther* 9:113–122.

120. Mulcahey MJ, Betz RR (1997): Considerations in the rehabilitation of children with spinal cord injury. *Top SCI Rehabil* 3:31–36.

121. Mulcahey MJ, Betz RR, Smith BT, et al. (1999): A prospective evaluation of upper extremity tendon transfers in children with cervical spinal cord injury. *J Pediatr Orthop* 19:319–328.

122. Mulcahey MJ, Betz RR, Smith BT, et al. (1997): Implanted FES hand system in adolescents with SCI: an evaluation. *Arch Phys Med Rehabil* 78:597–607.

123. Mulcahey MJ, Smith BT, Betz RR (1999): Evaluation of the lower motor neuron integrity of upper extremity muscles in high level spinal cord injury. *Spinal Cord* 37:585–591.

124. Nand S, Goldschmidt JW (1976): Hypercalcemia and hyperuricemia in young patients with spinal cord injury (Abstract). *Arch Phys Med Rehabil* 57:553.

125. Nash CL Jr, Haller R, Brown RH (1981): Succinylcholine, paraplegia, and intraoperative cardiac arrest: a case report. *J Bone Joint Surg Am* 63:1010–1011.

126. Nathan RH (1986): Electrostimulation of the upper limb: programmed hand function. *Proceedings of the IEEE 8th Annual Conference Eng Med Biol Soc* 8:653–655.

127. Nathan RH (1989): An FNS-based system for generating upper limb function in the C4 quadriplegic. *Med Biol Eng Comput* 27:549–556.

128. Nathan RH, Ohry A (1990): Upper limb functions regained in quadriplegia: a hybrid computerized neuromuscular stimulation system. *Arch Phys Med Rehabil* 71:415–421.

129. National Spinal Cord Injury Association (1988): Fact sheet #2: spinal cord injury statistical information. Summarized and excerpted from: *Spinal cord injury: the facts and figures* [1986]. Birmingham: Spinal Cord Injury Statistical Center, University of Alabama.

130. Nottage W (1981): A review of long-bone fractures in patients with spinal cord injuries. *Clin Orthop* 155:65–70.

131. Ogden JA (1982): Skeletal injury in the child. Philadelphia: Lea & Febiger, pp. 385–395.

132. Pact V, Sirotkin-Roses M, Beatos J (1984): The muscle testing handbook. Boston: Little, Brown, pp. 123–143.

133. Pang D, Wilberger JE Jr (1982): Spinal cord injury without radiographic abnormalities in children. *J Neurosurg* 57:114–129.

134. Peckham PH, Marsolais EB, Mortimer JT (1980): Restoration of key grip and release in the C6 tetraplegia patient through functional neuromuscular stimulation. *J Hand Surg* 5:462–469.

135. Pezeshki C, Brooker AF Jr (1977): Immobilization hypercalcemia: report of two cases treated with calcitonin. *J Bone Joint Surg Am* 59:971–973.

136. Pierre-Jacques H, Betz RR, Berman AT, et al. (1995): *Hip instability in children with spinal cord injuries.* Presented at the American Academy of Orthopaedic Surgeons annual meeting, Orlando, February 1995.

137. Rink P, Miller F (1990): Hip instability in spinal cord injury patients. *J Pediatr Orthop* 10:583–587.

138. Rossier AB, Foo D, Shillito J, et al. (1985): Post traumatic cervical syringomyelia: incidence, clinical presentation, electrophysiological studies, syrinx protein, and results of conservative and operative treatment. *Brain* 108:439–461.

139. Rusk H (1977): *Rehabilitation medicine,* 4th ed. St. Louis: CV Mosby.

140. Schnell L, Schwab ME (1990): Axonal regeneration in the rat spinal cord produced by an antibody against myelin-associated neurite growth inhibitors. *Nature* 343:269–272.

141. Schonwald G, Fish KJ, Perkash I (1981): Cardiovascular complications during anesthesia in chronic spinal cord injured patients. *Anesthesiology* 55:550–558.

142. Schueneman AL, Morris J (1982): Neuropsychological deficits associated with spinal cord injury. *SCI Dig* 35–36.

143. Schwab ME, Caroni P (1988): Oligodendrocytes and CND myelin are nonpermissive substrates for neurite growth and fibroblast spreading in vitro. *J Neurosci* 8:2381–2393.

144. Shea JD, Gioffre R, Carrion H, et al. (1973): Autonomic hyperreflexia in spinal cord injury. *South Med J* 66:869–872.

145. Sheldon GM (1988): Treatment options for shoulder pain in quadriplegia. *Am Occup Ther Assoc* 11:1–3.

146. Shelton T, Jeppson E, Johnson B (1989): Facilitation of parent/professional collaboration at all levels of health care. In: *Family centered care: an early intervention resource manual.* Rockville, MD: American Occupational Therapy Association. pp. 2:3–2:8.

147. Shriners Hospitals (1998): *Shriners Hospital's annual pediatric SCI statistical report for the Shrine units.* Birmingham: University of Alabama.

148. Sidi AA, Aliabadi H, Gonzalez R (1987): Enterocystoplasty in the management and reconstruction of the pediatric neurogenic bladder. *J Pediatr Surg* 22:153–157.

149. Sie IH, Waters RL, Adkins RH, et al. (1992): Upper extremity pain in the postrehabilitation spinal cord injured patient. *Arch Phys Med Rehabil* 73:44–48.

150. Smith BT, Mulcahey MJ, Triolo RJ, et al. (1992): The application of a modified neuroprosthetic hand system in a child with a C7 spinal cord injury. *Int J Paraplegia* 30(8):598–606.

151. Smith C (1985): Adolescent spinal cord injury and paralysis: understanding the psychosocial aspects. *Division of Physically Handicapped Journal* 8:16–23.

152. Solomonow M, Baratta R, Hirokawa S, et al. (1989): The RGO generation II: muscle stimulation powered orthosis as a practical walking system for thoracic paraplegics. *Orthopedics* 12:1309–1315.

153. Stover SL, Hahn HR, Miller JM III (1976): Disodium etidronate in the prevention of heterotopic ossification following spinal cord injury. *Paraplegia* 14:146–156.

154. Stover SL, Lloyd LK, Waites KB, et al. (1989): Urinary tract infection in spinal cord injury. *Arch Phys Med Rehabil* 70:47–54.

155. Strax T (1988): Psychological problems of disabled children and young adults. *Pediatr Ann* 17:756–761.

156. Tibone J, Sakimura I, Nickel VL, et al. (1978): Heterotopic ossification around the hip in spinal cord injured patients: a long-term follow-up study. *J Bone Joint Surg Am* 60:769–775.

157. Tori JA, Kewalramani LS (1979): Urolithiasis in children with spinal cord injury. *Paraplegia* 16:357–365.

158. Tricot A, Hallot R (1968): Traumatic paraplegia and associated fractures. *Paraplegia* 5:211–215.

159. Triolo R, Reilley B, Freedman W, et al. (1993): Development and standardization of a clinical evaluation of standing function: the functional standing test. *IEEE Trans Rehabil Eng* 1:18–25.

160. Umphred DA (1990): *Neurological rehabilitation,* 2nd ed. St Louis: CV Mosby, 413.

161. Venier LJ, Ditunno JF Jr (1971): Heterotopic ossification in the paraplegic patient. *Arch Phys Med Rehabil* 52:475–479.

162. Vogel L, Mulcahey MJ, Betz RR (1997): The child with a spinal cord injury. *Dev Med Child Neurol* 39:202–207.

163. Weiss AA, Betz RR (1991): *Transfer of paralyzed but not denervated*

muscles for functional nerve stimulation: restoration of prehensile activity in spinal cord injury patients. Presented at the American Academy of Pediatrics Orthopaedics Section, New Orleans, October 1991.

164. Welch R, Lobley SJ, O'Sullivan SB, Freed M (1986): Functional independence in quadriplegia: critical levels. *Arch Phys Med Rehabil* 67:235–240.

165. Winslow EBJ, Lesch M, Talano JV, et al. (1986): Spinal cord injuries associated with cardiopulmonary complications. *Spine* 11:809–812.

166. Yarkony GM, Roth EJ, Heinemann AW, et al. (1988): Rehabilitation outcomes in C6 tetraplegia. *Paraplegia* 26:177–185.

167. Yarkony GM, Roth EJ, Heinemann AW, et al. (1987): Benefits of rehabilitation for traumatic spinal cord injury: multivariate analysis in 711 patients. *Arch Neurol* 44:93–96.

168. Yarkony GM, et al. (1987): Rehabilitation outcomes in 120 patients with C5 quadriplegia (abstract). *Arch Phys Med Rehabil* 68:672.

169. Yngve DA, Harris WP, Herndon WA, et al. (1988): Spinal cord injury without osseous spine fracture. *J Pediatr Orthop* 8:153–159.

170. Young JS, Northrup NE (1979): *Statistical information pertaining to some of the most commonly asked questions about SCI* (Monograph). Phoenix: National Spinal Cord Injury Data Research Center.

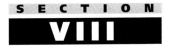

SECTION
VIII

INFLAMMATORY AND INFECTIOUS CONDITIONS

34

PYOGENIC INFECTIOUS SPONDYLITIS IN CHILDREN

DENNIS R. WENGER
DAVID RING
GREGORY V. HAHN

Infections involving the spinal column in children produce confusing symptoms and findings, which historically have led to delay in diagnosis. The evolution to current understanding of this condition is outlined in Table 1. Modern imaging techniques have blurred the distinction between infection of the disc space and vertebral osteomyelitis. Pyogenic infections in patients of all ages characteristically involve a single disc and both adjacent vertebral bodies. The persistent belief in alternative etiologies for what has been termed "discitis" in children is puzzling when one considers that the insidious onset, disc space narrowing, magnetic resonance imaging appearance, and difficulty isolating the causative organism observed in pediatric infectious spondylitis are almost identical to the clinical situation encountered in adults. The unusual feature of pediatric spinal infections is that, in many cases, the infection resolves without specific antibiotic therapy and with few long-term sequelae. Nonetheless, treatment with antibiotics rapidly diminishes symptoms, decreases the risk for recurrence, and may limit the potential for development of psoas or epidural abscesses.

ETIOLOGY AND PATHOPHYSIOLOGY

Anatomy

The distinction between disc space infection in children and vertebral osteomyelitis in adults has long been reinforced by observations of a vascular supply to the intervertebral disc that is present in children but disappears after adolescence; however, the vascular anatomy of the intervertebral disc is disputed. The published experiments claiming to demonstrate either the presence or the absence of a vascular supply to the intervertebral disc in children are consistent in that they demonstrate vascular channels in the hyaline cartilage of the vertebral end plate in children, but not in adults (10,22,33,42,46,59,60) (Fig. 1).

They differ simply on the anatomic definition of the intervertebral disc, with those authors who include the hyaline cartilage of the end plate as an anatomic portion of the disc claiming that the disc is vascular in children (10,22,33,46) and those who restrict the definition of the intervertebral disc to the annulus fibrosus and the nucleus pulposus claiming that the disc is avascular throughout development (42,59). They also differ on the estimated age at which the vascular supply to the hyaline cartilage of the vertebral end plate is lost.

Modern imaging modalities have demonstrated early involvement of the intervertebral disc in pyogenic infections at all ages, making considerations of vascular anatomy less important (3,13,16,17,23,34,43,44,45,52,57) (Fig. 2). Current pathophysiologic theories propose that, in both children and adults, hematogenous bacterial emboli lodge in either the subchondral bone or the hyaline cartilage of the vertebral end plate and spread rapidly to the intervertebral disc and the opposite vertebral end plate (42,54,59) (Fig. 3). The mechanism of such progression is speculative but most likely involves direct spread through the disc, facilitated by bacterial or inflammatory enzymes or perforations in the vertebral end plate (25,37).

The differences between the usual course of such infections in children and adults remains incompletely explained. It has been suggested that differences in the vascularity of the vertebrae (which may influence the spread of septic thromboses) are important (54,59). Other important factors may include differences in the source of bacteremia (believed to be small, transient, and incidental in the context of cuts, abrasions, or pharyngitis in otherwise healthy children as opposed to more substantial, repeated episodes in intravenous drug–abusing adults and the debilitated elderly) and the overall health of the patient. A third unexplained subgroup occurs in bacteremic neonates, in whom pyogenic infectious spondylitis can be quite destructive (15).

Bacteriology

Because many cases of spondylitis have been treated successfully without antibiotics, some authors have proposed that the disc narrowing and adjacent reactive bony changes are a result of some other developmental or reactive process (11,27,50,55). A careful consideration of alternative causes of symptomatic disc narrowing in children, however, finds little support for any other

D. R. Wenger: Department of Pediatric Orthopedics, Children's Hospital San Diego, San Diego, California 92123.

D. R. Ring: Department of Orthopaedic Surgery, Massachusetts General Hospital and Harvard Combined Orthopaedic Program, Boston, Massachusetts 02114.

G. V. Hahn: Department of Orthopaedic Surgery, All Children's Hospital, St. Petersburg, Florida 33701.

619

TABLE 1. THE EVOLUTION OF UNDERSTANDING PYOGENIC INFECTIOUS SPONDYLITIS

Date	Event	Results
c. 1880	Koch's experiments with the anthrax bacillus establish the germ theory of disease. Koch also discovers tubercle bacillus.	Vertebral caries are understood to represent tuberculous osteomyelitis
	Pasteur isolates *Staphylococcus* species from a superficially draining spinal abscess in the setting of an acute febrile illness.	Pyogenic vertebral osteomyelitis distinguished from tuberculous osteomyelitis
c. 1896	Roentgen and advent of radiography	Increased recognition of infectious spondylitis before death and autopsy
c. 1900–1960	Improved clinical recognition of infectious spondylitis	Description of "benign" forms of vertebral osteomyelitis
		In 1940, Ghormley and colleagues (19) proposed the concept of intervertebral disc infection
		The concept of discitis in children gains in popularity.
c. 1940	Development of antibiotics	Minimal influence on vertebral osteomyelitis noted initially, mainstay of treatment remains prolonged brace immobilization and surgery when necessary.
c. 1950–1980	High percentage of sterile cultures of direct biopsy specimens noted in many musculoskeletal infections	As an explanation of this observation in discitis, alternative, nonbacterial causes are proposed.
c. 1970	Improved treatment of musculoskeletal infections with parenteral antibiotics	Vertebral osteomyelitis in adults becomes a medically treated disease for which prolonged immobilization and operative intervention are rarely required. Traditional treatments (immobilization) are still advocated for discitis in children.
c. 1980	Computed tomography	Substantial bone and soft issue involvement are noted in so-called "discitis."
c. 1985	Magnetic resonance imaging	The appearance of pyogenic infections of the spine in adults and children is noted to be essentially identical.

Adapted from Ring D, Wenger DR (1996): Pyogenic infectious spondylitis in children: the evolution to current thought. *Am J Orthop* 25: 342–348, with permission.

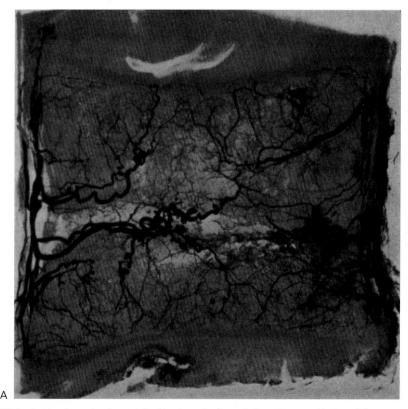

FIGURE 1. A: Blood supply of a vertebral body and adjacent discs above and below. *(Figure continues.)*

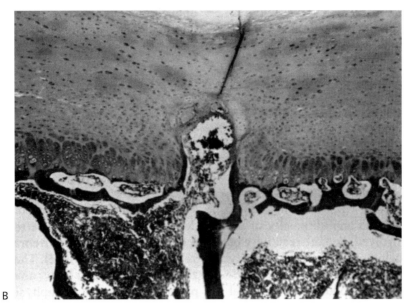

B

FIGURE 1. *Continued.* **B:** Vertebral end plate (cartilage), adjacent disc, and cancellous bone of the vertebral body in an autopsy histologic specimen from a child. Note the vascular channel traversing the end plate. Such channels allow bacterial infection to involve the disc. (**A** from Menelaus MB [1964]: Discitis: an inflammation affecting the intervertebral discs in children. *J Bone Joint Surg Br* 46:16–23, with permission.)

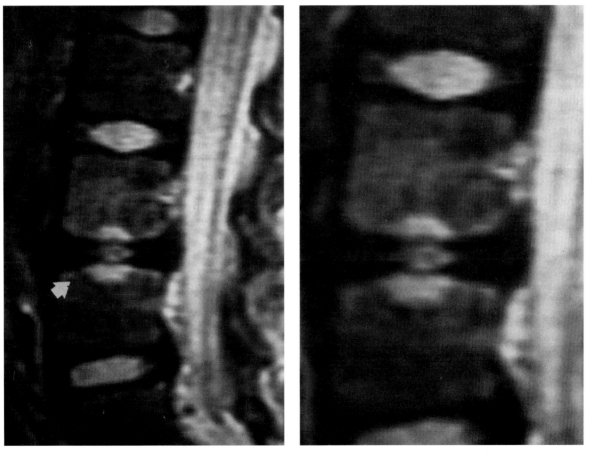

A

B

FIGURE 2. **A:** Magnetic resonance imaging study in a 4-year-old with *Staphylococcus aureus* spondylitis (later proved by biopsy). Note asymmetric involvement of the end plates of the affected disc *(arrow)*. **B:** Close-up view. The end plate below the disc appears to be more involved.

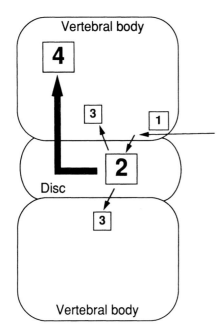

FIGURE 3. Proposed sequence of intervertebral disc infection and evolution to osteomyelitis: (*1*) microabscess in "metaphysis" (adjacent to end plate), (*2*) disc colonized and infected, (*3*) reactive process (or low-grade infection of opposite end plate), (*4*) diagnosis and treatment delayed—development of vertebral osteomyelitis.

process as a cause of the radiographic changes seen in infectious spondylitis. A number of authors have cited the large percentage of negative cultures as further support for a nonbacterial etiology in many cases of disc space narrowing in children. Among the numerous small case series that comprise the existing literature documenting pyogenic infections of the spine in children, the reported rate of successful isolation of a causative organism has ranged from 27% to 88% (average, 60%) (8,11–13,26,32,35, 48,50,55,58).

The bacteriologic data from the Toronto study (58) is one of the most comprehensive available. Biopsy was performed in nine patients in an attempt to establish an accurate diagnosis. There were four needle and five open biopsies. Six of the nine biopsy specimens were positive for *Staphylococcus aureus,* and one of the six also grew α-hemolytic *Streptococcus* species. The other three biopsy specimens showed no growth. Histologic examination showed acute inflammation in a few cases, with subacute and chronic inflammation in the remainder. Blood specimens were cultured for 22 patients. Positive cultures for *S. aureus* were obtained in nine patients and for diphtheroids in one. The diphtheroid culture was considered a probable contaminant. One patient had both a positive blood culture and a positive culture from biopsy material. Few patients had cultures of both blood and biopsy tissue. Most of the biopsies performed were in patients in the early years of the study, when only occasional blood specimens were drawn for culture; in more recent years, when blood was cultured in most patients, few patients underwent biopsy. Organisms were identified in 14 of the 28 patients (50%) who had cultures of blood or biopsy material.

In considering all of the bacteriologic data, one must keep in mind that direct biopsy material for culture and organism isolation has rarely been sought in cases of inflammatory disc narrowing in children. The organism has most often been identified from blood cultures. Such difficulty with organism isolation is typical of other pyogenic musculoskeletal infections (48,56). Therefore, alternative, nonbacterial, etiologies such as viral infection, trauma, or a nonspecific inflammatory disorder are unlikely (1,4,5,11,14,26,31,35,47,53,55).

Imaging

In children, the appearance of pyogenic infectious spondylitis on standard radiographs rarely progresses beyond disc space narrowing with erosion or sclerosis of the adjacent vertebral end plates (Fig. 4).

The radiology literature on pyogenic infectious spondylitis affirms the usefulness of computed tomography (CT) and magnetic resonance imaging (MRI) in both managing and understanding this disease. Studies have confirmed the findings of Crawford and colleagues (11) and Szalay and associates (57) that MRI and CT are more sensitive than bone scan for diagnosing infectious spondylitis (13,49,54). The extent of the inflammatory process is also better depicted, with frequent demonstration of paravertebral inflammatory masses, intraspinal soft tissue extension, psoas involvement with abscess formation, and advanced bony destruction. In a review of the CT scans of seven patients with spondylitis, paravertebral masses were present in all seven, intraspinal extension was noted in six of seven, and a psoas abscess was appreciated in one, demonstrating that the inflammatory process may be more extensive than demonstrated by conventional radiographic studies and thus more consistent with an infectious etiology (49).

The MRI findings recognized as characteristic of vertebral osteomyelitis in adult patients (diffusely decreased signal in adjacent vertebral bodies, with loss of distinction of the intervertebral disc, on T1-weighted images; increased signal in the disc and loss of the intranuclear cleft on T2-weighted images; and increased signal in the adjacent vertebral body end plates on T2-weighted images) have also been found to be characteristic of infectious spondylitis in children (13,54,57). In fact, it is difficult to distinguish between the imaging appearance of pyogenic infectious spondylitis in children and adults (29) (Fig. 5). As a result, the concept of a noninfectious inflammatory disc space narrowing in children has become less appealing.

Clinical Observations

Despite the fact that a large percentage of cases of inflammatory disc space narrowing in children have been proved to be of bacterial etiology, the process resolves spontaneously in many children (9,14,19,21,26,30,32,40). This is an interesting observation of the ability of the immune response in young patients to resolve a pyogenic skeletal infection, but not a reason to suggest alternative, nonbacterial etiologies. Denying a bacterial etiology may be risky because some children with pyogenic infectious

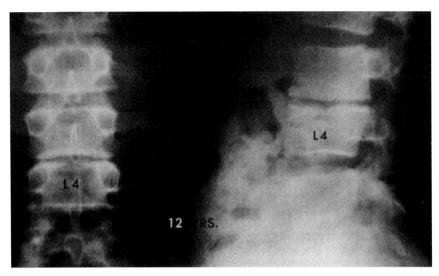

FIGURE 4. Classic pyogenic infectious spondylitis changes. The child had onset at 4 years of age and is now 12 years of age. Note the disc narrowing and vertebra magna but absence of vertebral wedging.

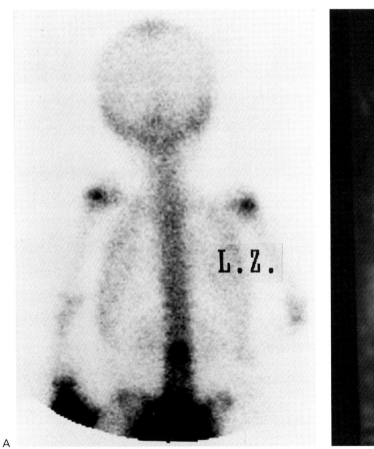

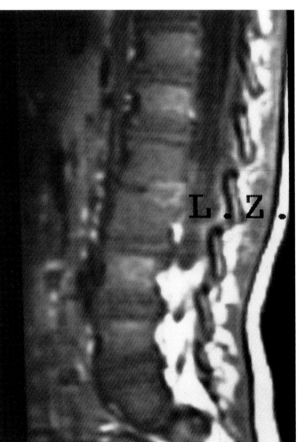

FIGURE 5. A 17-month-old girl presented with a 3-day history of refusal to ambulate and was found to have an increased erthyrocyte sedimentation rate. A lateral radiograph demonstrated narrowing of the disc space between the second and third lumbar vertebral bodies (not shown). **A:** Technetium-99m methylene diphosphonate bone scan demonstrates increased uptake in the second and third vertebral bodies. **B:** T1-weighted image demonstrates decreased signal throughout the second and third lumbar vertebra-disc-vertebra unit. *(Figure continues.)*

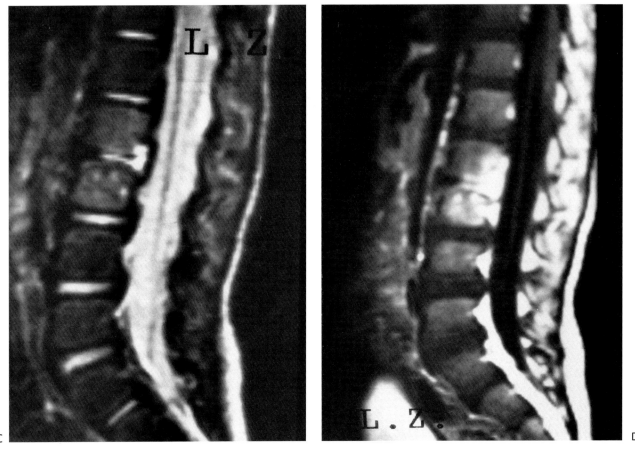

C
D

FIGURE 5. *Continued.* **C:** T2-weighted image demonstrates narrowing of the intervertebral disc be-tween the second and third lumbar vertebral bodies with increased signal in the adjacent end plates and posterior soft tissues. **D:** Gadolinium-enhanced T1-weighted image demonstrates high-intensity signal in areas corresponding to those enhancing on T2-weighted images. The patient was ambulating normally within 48 hours of the initiation of treatment with parenteral cefazolin.

spondylitis occasionally develop an abscess requiring operative drainage (24,31,49,51).

DIAGNOSIS

History

Young children cannot communicate their symptoms, and often the presentation is nonspecific. The clinical subgroups described by Puig Guri continue to be useful (41,58).

Failure to Walk Syndrome

Children younger than 3 years of age who cannot accurately verbalize their complaints often present with apparent dysfunc-tion of the lower extremities or failure to walk. The alarming chronology of a previously normal child suddenly being unable to walk often led to an extensive, misguided workup in the era before bone scans. Occasionally, the child was admitted to the neurology service because of a fear of impending paraplegia, and studies such as myelograms were performed. The series of

clinical, radiographic, and even exploratory abdominal proce-dures used to evaluate these patients is, in retrospect, quite re-markable.

Abdominal Pain Syndrome

Somewhat older children (3 to 8 years of age) often have pain referred to the abdomen, particularly with low thoracic lesions. In the past, these children underwent a variety of complex studies including upper and lower gastrointestinal studies, intravenous pyelograms, even inferior venacavograms (Fig. 6). Occasionally, these patients had exploratory laparotomies for a suspected in-flamed retrocecal appendix or psoas abscess (58). The prevalence of psoas inflammation noted on MRI may explain, in part, the presentation with abdominal symptoms.

Back Pain Syndrome

Teenagers with spondylitis are more likely to have specific back pain, but those with lumbar involvement often present with a "disc pattern," with discomfort radiating into the legs.

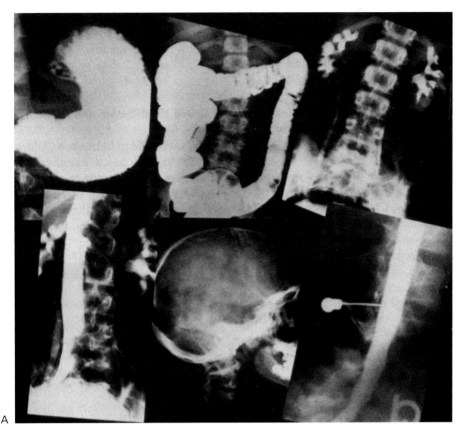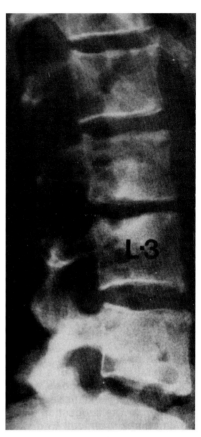

A

B

FIGURE 6. A: Multiple studies (including an inferior venacavogram) ordered in a 10-year-old with abdominal pain in the era before bone scanning. **B:** The patient was later found to have L2 to L3 pyogenic infectious spondylitis.

Physical Examination

A child with possible pyogenic infectious spondylitis should have a clinical examination, which often demonstrates tight hamstrings or positive straight-leg raising test (Fig. 7). The child often has a characteristic loss of normal "spinal rhythm." When the child is asked to pick up a toy from the floor, the back is held in an abnormally stiff posture rather than the usually smooth flexion and extension.

Diagnostic Tests

Although younger children often present with a nonspecific presentation, the possibility of a skeletal infection is usually considered, particularly if the erythrocyte sedimentation rate or C-reactive protein level is elevated. If symptoms or signs can be localized to the spine, radiographs should be ordered; however, during the early stages of the illness, the process may not be apparent (Fig. 8).

This nonspecific presentation makes a bone scan the best choice for diagnostic imaging (Fig. 9). MRI is more specific, may be more sensitive, and can define the extent of the process, but it should not be obtained before the bone scan unless the process can be clearly localized to the spine by history or examination.

It is important to draw blood cultures because they may isolate the causative organism in many patients. A direct biopsy is probably not necessary on a routine basis because most of the organisms known to cause pyogenic infectious spondylitis in children are sensitive to first-generation cephalosporins. In areas with a large percentage of cases of methacillin-resistant *S. aureus,* needle biopsy may need to be considered to confirm the antibiotic sensitivity of the organism.

DIFFERENTIAL DIAGNOSIS

Although classic pyogenic infectious spondylitis has a relatively distinct clinical and radiographic pattern, other disorders to consider include Scheuermann kyphosis, tuberculosis, atypical bacterial or fungal infection, spinal epidural abscess, vertebra plana (Fig. 10), kyphosis (failure to segment anteriorly), osteoid osteoma, and rarely a malignant disease (primary vertebral body malignancy, metastatic disease, or leukemia with vertebral involvement).

Tuberculosis

Not all infectious spondylitis is bacterial. In the border regions of the Southwest United States, tuberculosis is still relatively

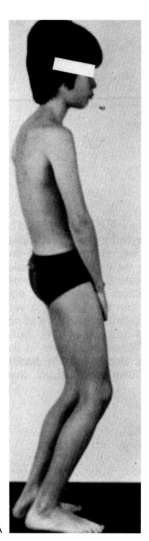

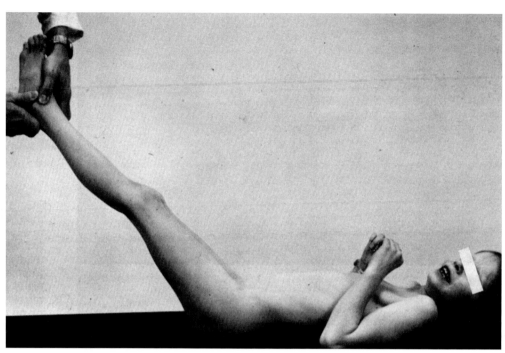

FIGURE 7. A: Child with pyogenic infectious spondylitis and abnormal posture due to tight hamstrings. **B:** Another child with pyogenic infectious spondylitis and a markedly positive straight-leg raising test.

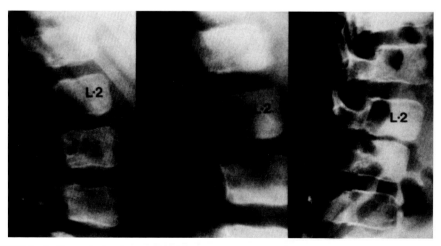

FIGURE 8. Radiographs in a 5-year-old with L2 to L3 pyogenic infectious spondylitis. The original films *(left)* and tomogram *(center)* were interpreted as normal. Two months later, marked disc narrowing was noted *(right)*.

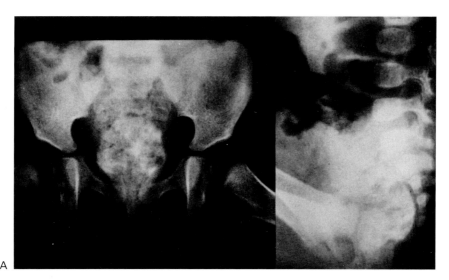

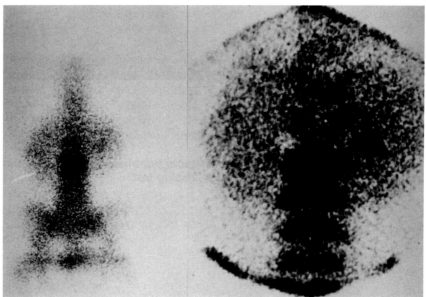

FIGURE 9. Pyogenic infectious spondylitis in a 2-year-old child. **A:** The initial films, ordered by an experienced pediatric orthopaedist who was worried about the child's hip, included a pelvis radiograph and lateral view of the lumbosacral junction. In retrospect, disc narrowing can be seen at the very top on the lateral view. This was not recognized until after the bone scan. **B:** Classic bone scan in the same case. Bone scans in pyogenic infectious spondylitis are sometimes less distinct than this.

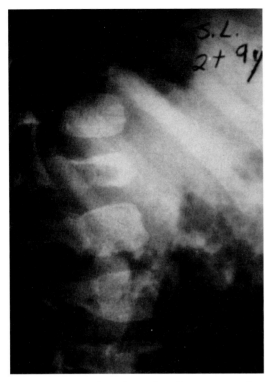

FIGURE 10. Three-year-old with vertebra plana. Because of an uncertain clinical picture (elevated sedimentation rate), the diagnosis of eosinophilic granuloma was confirmed by a computed tomography–guided needle biopsy.

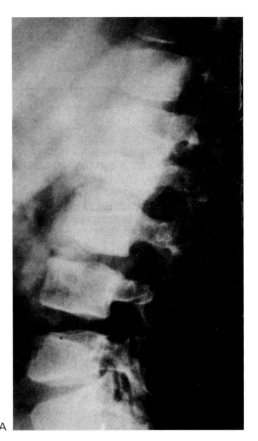

A

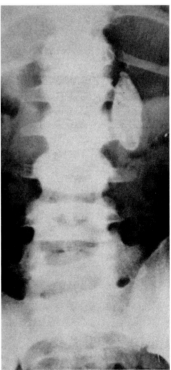

B

FIGURE 11. Ten-year-old with backache. **A:** The lateral radiograph shows loss of the disc space in the upper lumbar spine plus early vertebral wedging. **B:** The anteroposterior view shows a calcified psoas abscess, characteristic of established tuberculosis.

common (Fig. 11). Before 1985, tuberculosis was considered to be under control in the United States, with most tuberculosis sanatoriums having been closed or reduced in size years earlier. However, a substantial increase in the incidence of new cases was reported in the late 1980s and early 1990s, with 26,283 new active cases reported in the United States in 1991, a 2.3% increase over 1990. In California, 3,500 active cases were reported in 1990, rising to 5,273 active cases in 1991 (38). Many social factors have caused the recent rapid increase in the incidence of tuberculosis, including immigration of infected foreign nationals, increased intravenous drug use, greater homelessness, the AIDS epidemic, and increased poverty (especially among children). These factors have led us to have a much higher suspicion of tuberculosis in children with back disorders. The most recent data suggest that increased awareness of these factors led to a stabilization of the incidence of tuberculosis in the late 1990s. The clinical history, a tuberculin skin test, and a chest radiograph help make the diagnosis. Other chronic granulomatous infections, such as brucellosis, must also be considered. In the era of empiric antibiotic treatment for spondylitis, physicians must remember that patients who fail to respond may require further diagnostic workup, including aspiration, open biopsy, or both, to establish the bacteriologic agent.

Other Disorders

Other disorders may present as back pain and require clarification by a bone scan. Disorders of the genitourinary tract are commonly identified, and the patient is referred to a urologist. Sacroiliac joint infections also cause obscure back pain and are best diagnosed by a bone scan. These patients have back, hip, and buttock pain; a positive Faber test; and pain with pelvic compression. The bone scan is often classic and diagnostic; sometimes, however, the scan is only minimally asymmetric, and a gallium scan or MRI may be required to confirm the diagnosis. We have seen several children whose early bone scans were normal but whose subsequent MRI studies demonstrated classic sacroiliac joint infection. Neoplasms may also present as nonspecific back pain. The history, physical examination, laboratory, and—in particular—imaging studies (notably MRI) are usually characteristic for these disorders and distinct from pyogenic infectious spondylitis. Any case that features substantial collapse, involvement of a single vertebra, or other uncharacteristic findings may merit a diagnostic biopsy.

Treatment

After the diagnosis of spondylitis has been established by a bone scan or MRI, blood cultures should be drawn and tuberculosis excluded by a skin test and chest radiograph if indicated. Because blood cultures are often negative and needle aspiration or biopsy is usually not indicated, an empiric course of intravenous antibiotics that covers *S. aureus* (usually a first-generation cephalosporin) is begun. Parenteral antibiotics are continued until the symptoms are largely relieved and the laboratory values approach normal. In most cases, after 3 or 4 days, a child who was unable to walk before treatment will be moving freely around the bed and, if allowed, walking around the room. Parental antibiotic therapy is followed by a 4- to 6-week course of oral antibiotics.

Large oral doses of cephalosporins have been recommended for the outpatient treatment of skeletal infections. It is unclear whether or not this is important in the treatment of pediatric pyogenic infectious spondylitis (6,7). The data from our series suggest that standard doses may suffice after appropriate treatment with parenteral antibiotics (45). Treatment with oral antibiotics alone may increase the risk for prolonged or recurrent symptoms or for development of an abscess requiring operative drainage. Compliance is always an issue with oral antibiotic regimens in children, particularly when large doses are prescribed.

A few cases will not respond to antibiotics and require acute surgical drainage. Figure 12 demonstrates a child with a classic bone scan for spondylitis who was placed on intravenous cephalosporin but continued to have a high fever and refused to walk. An MRI study showed a probable paraspinal abscess. Anterior exploration through a retroperitoneal approach revealed chronic edema and granulation tissue both near and within the disc, which was curetted and drained. The patient rapidly became afebrile and resumed walking. In a few cases, the disc narrowing is marked and the patient continues to have low-grade classic symptoms (Figs. 13 and 14). In two of 38 patients in our Toronto series, late anterior disc curettement and fusion were required to relieve symptoms. One case was in the cervical spine and the other in the midlumbar spine. In both cases, *S. aureus* was cultured from the anterior approach.

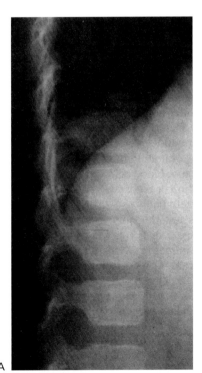 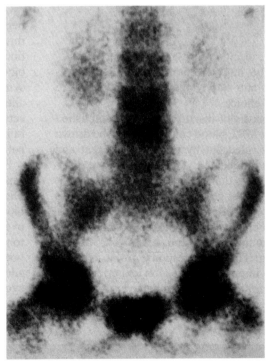

FIGURE 12. Several studies in a 4-year-old child with pyogenic infectious spondylitis who failed to respond to intravenous antibiotics. **A:** Plain lateral lumbar spine films were read as normal. **B:** The bone scan shows classic changes of L3 to L4 pyogenic infectious spondylitis, with a question of increased uptake in L2 as well. *(Figure continues.)*

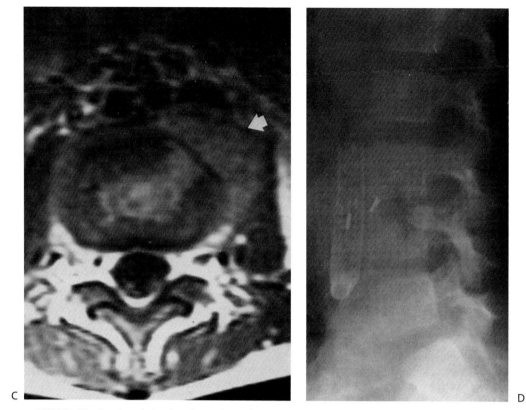

C   D

FIGURE 12. *Continued.* **C:** After the patient's failure to respond to antibiotic treatment, a magnetic resonance image was ordered, which demonstrates a paravertebral abscess *(arrow).* **D:** Lateral radiograph after surgical drainage through an anterolateral retroperitoneal approach. The Jackson-Pratt drain is noted. The L3 to L4 disc is now narrowed. The culture grew *Staphylococcus aureus.*

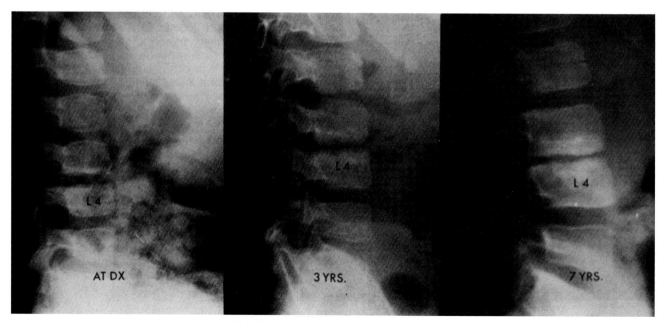

FIGURE 13. Early and late radiographs in a 6-year-old boy who continued to have back pain 9 months after onset. He eventually required anterior spinal fusion, and *Staphylococcus aureus* grew on the culture of the débrided L3 to L4 disc material.

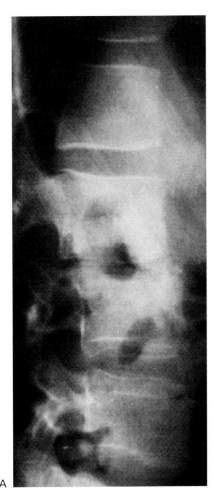

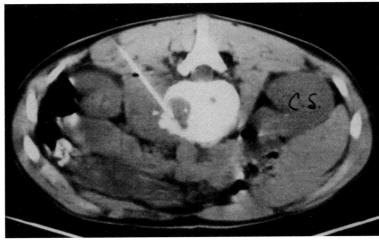

FIGURE 14. Fifteen-year-old boy with pyogenic infectious spondylitis. **A:** Plain radiographs show marked loss of disc space and suggested vertebral body involvement. **B:** Computed tomography–guided needle biopsy of lytic process in vertebral body near the end plate. *Staphylococcus aureus* grew on culture.

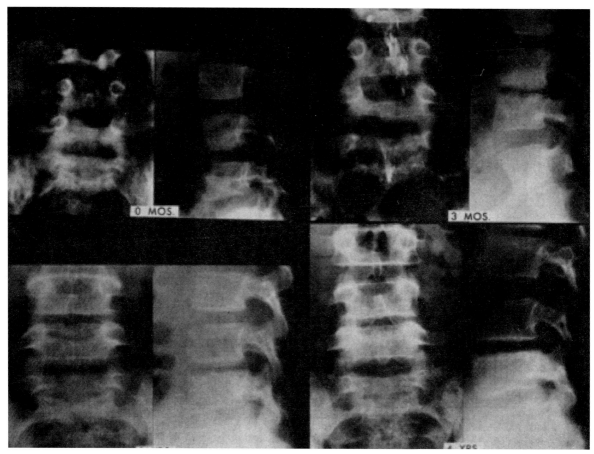

FIGURE 15. Radiographic chronology of L4 to L5 pyogenic infectious spondylitis in a child diagnosed at 4 years of age treated with antibiotics. The radiographic changes at baseline, 3 months, 2 years, and 4 years after onset are shown. The partial but not complete restoration of disc space height is typical of pyogenic infectious spondylitis in children.

Because deformity is uncommon and symptoms resolve rapidly with intravenous antibiotics, there appears to be little role for immobilization of the spine with a cast or brace (2,18,20,28,36,39). We prescribe temporary bracing for symptomatic relief on occasion. In juveniles and adolescents, back pain may be more prolonged and a corset or back brace may be required for several weeks. All patients should be followed for at least 1 year, with serial radiographs usually showing a continued but not complete narrowing of the disc (Fig. 15). In rare cases, the disc narrowing is marked; in others, there is partial reconstitution.

ophysiology of the disorder with both vertebral body and disc involvement. The MRI is now the most specific noninvasive diagnostic tool for evaluating childhood spinal infection; however, the bone scan remains the best screening study when the presentation and symptoms are not specific.

The rapid response of severely symptomatic spondylitis patients to intravenous antibiotics that cover *S. aureus* provides convincing evidence that the condition is bacterial in most cases. Although a few centers continue to treat this condition with immobilization alone, we believe that such treatment is not specific and should not be the first choice.

SUMMARY

The evaluation and treatment of pyogenic infectious spondylitis in children has greatly improved. The ability to make an early diagnosis has been aided by an increased awareness of the disorder and an understanding of its presenting patterns. The use of the radionuclide bone scan was a landmark event that has made early diagnosis more likely. The MRI has further advanced the ability to make an early correct diagnosis to understand the path-

REFERENCES

1. Alexander CV (1970): The aetiology of juvenile spondyloarthritis (discitis). *Clin Radiol* 21:178.
2. Ambrose GB, Meyer A, Neer CS (1966): Vertebral osteomyelitis: a diagnostic problem. *JAMA* 197:619–622.
3. An HS, Vaccaro AR, Dolinskas C, et al. (1991): Differentiation between spinal tumors and infections with magnetic resonance imaging. *Spine* 16:S334–338.
4. Atar D, Gdalia A, Galil A, et al. (1992): Discitis in children. *Contemp Orthop* 25:493–497.

5. Atar D, Lehman WB, Grant AD (1992): Discitis in children. *Orthop Rev* 21:931–933.

6. Bolivar R, Kohl S, Pickering LK (1978): Vertebral osteomyelitis in children: report of four cases. *Pediatrics* 62(4):549–553.

7. Bonfiglio M, Lange TA, Kim YM (1988): Pyogenic vertebral osteomyelitis: disk space infections. *Clin Orthop* 96:234–247.

8. Boston HC, Bianco AJ, Rhodes KH (1975): Disk space infections in children. *Orthop Clin North Am* 6:953–964.

9. Bremner AE, Neligan GA (1953): Benign form of acute osteitis of the spine in young children. *Br Med J* 1:856–860.

10. Coventry MB, Ghormley RK, Kernohan JW (1945): The intervertebral disc: its microscopic anatomy and pathology. Part I. Anatomy, development and physiology. *J Bone Joint Surg Am* 27:105–112.

11. Crawford AH, Kucharzyk DW, Ruida R, et al. (1991): Diskitis in children. *Clin Orthop* 266:70–79.

12. Doyle JR (1960): Narrowing of the intervertebral-disc space in children: presumably an infectious lesion of the disc. *J Bone Joint Surg Am* 42:1191–1200.

13. Du Lac P, Panuel M, Devred P, et al. (1990): MRI of disc space infection in infants and children. *Pediatr Radiol* 20:175–178.

14. Dupont A, Andersen H (1956): Non-specific spondylitis in childhood. *Acta Paediatr* 45:361–366.

15. Eismont FJ, Bohlman HH, Soni PL, et al. (1982): Vertebral osteomyelitis in infants. *J Bone Joint Surg Br* 64:32–35.

16. Forster A, Pothmann R, Winter K, et al. (1987): Magnetic resonance imaging in non-specific discitis. *Pediatr Radiol* 17:162–163.

17. Gabriel KR, Crawford AH (1988): Magnetic resonance imaging in a child who had clinical signs of discitis. *J Bone Joint Surg Am* 70:938–941.

18. Garcia A, Grantham SA (1960): Hematogeneous pyogenic vertebral osteomyelitis. *J Bone Joint Surg Am* 42:429–436.

19. Ghormley RK, Bickel WH, Dickson DD (1940): A study of acute infectious lesions of the intervertebral discs. *South Med J* 33:347–352.

20. Griffiths HED, Jones DM (1971): Pyogenic infection of the spine: a review of twenty-eight cases. *J Bone Joint Surg Br* 53:383–391.

21. Grimes HA, Keiser RP (1963): Nonspecific Infections of the disk space in children. *South Med J* 56:511–517.

22. Hassler O (1970): The human intervertebral disc: a microangiographical study on its vascular supply at various ages. *Acta Orthop Scand* 40:765–772.

23. Heller RM, Szalay EA, Green NE, et al. (1988): Disc space infection in children: magnetic resonance imaging. *Radiol Clin North Am* 26(2):207–209.

24. Holliday PO, Davis CH, Shaffner LD (1980): Intervertebral disc space infection in a child presenting as a psoas abscess: case report. *Neurosurgery* 7:395–397.

25. Inoue H (1981): Three-dimensional architecture of lumbar intervertebral discs. *Spine* 6:139–146.

26. Jamison RC, Heimlich EM, Miethke JC, et al. (1961): Nonspecific spondylitis of infants and children. *Radiology* 77:355–367.

27. Jansen BRH, Wimpeter H, Schreuder O (1993): Discitis in childhood: 12–35-year follow-up of 35 patients. *Acta Orthop Scand* 64(1):33–36.

28. Jordan MC, Kirby WMM (1971): Pyogenic vertebral osteomyelitis: treatment with antimicrobial agents and bed rest. *Arch Intern Med* 128:405–410.

29. Kemp HBS, Jackson JW, Jeremiah JD, et al. (1973): Pyogenic infections occurring primarily in intervertebral discs. *J Bone Joint Surg Br* 55:698–714.

30. Matthews SS, Wiltse LL, Karbelnig MJ (1957): A destructive lesion involving the intervertebral disk in children. *Clin Orthop* 9:162.

31. Menelaus MB (1964): Discitis: an inflammation affecting the intervertebral discs in children. *J Bone Joint Surg Br* 46:16–23.

32. Milone FP, Bianco AJ, Ivins JC (1962): Infections of the intervertebral disk in children. *JAMA* 181:1029–1033.

33. Mineiro JD (1965): *Coluna vertebral humana: alguns aspectos da sua estrutura e vascularizacao.* Lisboa, Dissertaco de Doutoramento.

34. Modic MT, Feiglin DH, Piraino DW, et al. (1985): Vertebral osteomyelitis: Assessment using MR. *Radiology* 157:157–166.

35. Moes CAF (1964): Spondylarthritis in childhood. *Am J Roentgenol* 91:578–587.

36. Musher DM, Thorsteinsson SB, Minuth JN (1976): Vertebral osteomyelitis: still a diagnostic pitfall. *Arch Intern Med* 136:105–110.

37. Nachemson A, Lewis T, Maroudas A, et al. (1970): In vitro diffusion of dye through the endplates and the annulus fibrosus of human intervertebral discs. *Acta Orthop Scand* 41:589–607.

38. Nelson H (1992): Officials scramble to deal with resurgence of tuberculosis. *Los Angeles Times* July 9, 1992, San Diego County ed., sec. A: 5.

39. Osenbach RK, Hitchon PW, Menezes AH (1990): Diagnosis and management of pyogenic vertebral osteomyelitis in adults. *Surg Neurol* 33:266–275.

40. Pritchard AE, Thompson WAL (1960): Acute pyogenic infections of the spine in children. *J Bone Joint Surg Br* 42:86–89.

41. Puig Guri J (1946): Pyogenic osteomyelitis of the spine: differential diagnosis through clinical and roentgenographic observations. *J Bone Joint Surg Am* 28:29–39.

42. Ratcliffe JF (1985): Anatomic basis for the pathogenesis and radiologic features of vertebral osteomyelitis and its differentiation from childhood discitis: a microarteriographic investigation. *Acta Radiol* 26:137–143.

43. Ring D, Wenger DR (1996): Pyogenic infectious spondylitis in children: the evolution to current thought. *Am J Orthop* 25:342–348.

44. Ring D, Wenger DR (1994): Magnetic resonance imaging scans in discitis: sequential studies in a child requiring operative drainage. *J Bone Joint Surg Am* 76:596–601.

45. Ring D, Wenger DR, Johnston CE (1995): Infectious spondylitis: the convergence of discitis and osteomyelitis. *J Pediatr Orthop* 15:652–660.

46. Rudert M, Tillmann B (1993): Lymph and blood supply of the human intervertebral disc: cadaver study of correlations to discitis. *Acta Orthop Scand* 64(1):37–40.

47. Saenger EL (1950): Spondylarthritis in children. *Am J Roentgenol* 64(1):20–31.

48. Sapico FL, Montgonmerie JZ (1990): Vertebral osteomyelitis. *Infect Dis Clin North Am* 4(3):539—550.

49. Sartoris DJ, Moskowitz PS, Kaufman RA, et al. (1983): Childhood diskitis: computed tomographic findings. *Radiology* 149:701–707.

50. Scoles PV, Quinn TP (1982): Intervertebral discitis in children and adolescents. *Clin Orthop* 162:31–36.

51. Short DJ, Webley M, Hadfield J (1983): Septic discitis presenting as a psoas abscess. *J R Soc Med* 76:1066–1068.

52. Smith AS, Weinstein MA, Mizushima A, et al. (1989): MR imaging characteristics of tuberculous spondylitis vs. vertebral osteomyelitis. *AJR Am J Roentgenol* 153:399–405.

53. Smith RF, Taylor TKF (1967): Inflammatory lesions of intervertebral discs in children. *J Bone Joint Surg Am* 49:1508–1520.

54. Song KS, Ogden JA, Ganey T, et al. (1997): Contiguous discitis and osteomyelitis in children. *J Pediatr Orthop* 17:470–477.

55. Speigel PG, Kengla KW, Isaacson AS, et al. (1972): Intervertebral disc-space inflammation in children. *J Bone Joint Surg Am* 54:284–296.

56. Syriopoulou VP, Smith AL (1992): Osteomyelitis and septic arthritis. In: Feigin RD, Cherry JD, eds. *Textbook of pediatric infectious disease,* 3rd ed. Philadelphia: WB Saunders, pp. 727–745.

57. Szalay EA, Green NE, Heller RM, et al. (1987): Magnetic resonance imaging in the diagnosis of childhood discitis. *J Pediatr Orthop* 7:164–167.

58. Wenger DR, Bobechko WP, Gilday DL (1978): The spectrum of intervertebral disc-space infection in children. *J Bone Joint Surg Am* 60:100–108.

59. Whalen JL, Parke WW, Mazur JM, et al. (1985): The intrinsic vasculature of developing vertebral end plates and its nutritive significance to the intervertebral discs. *J Pediatr Orthop* 5:403–410.

60. Wiley AM, Trueta J (1959): The vascular anatomy of the spine and its relationship to pyogenic vertebral osteomyelitis. *J Bone Joint Surg Br* 41:796–809.

TUBERCULOSIS OF THE SPINE

KEITH D. K. LUK
JOHN C. Y. LEONG
ERIC K. W. HO

The history of treatment of tuberculosis of the spine has gone through several stages. The classic scientific description of the disease by Percival Pott in 1779 (35) was an important step in its recognition as a distinct entity. Advances in treatment of tuberculosis of the spine were marked by two events. First was the description of the anterior surgical approach to the spine, a direct approach to the disease focus, first described by Ito and colleagues (20) in 1934. The second major event was the introduction of antituberculous chemotherapy in 1954.

Today, spinal tuberculosis poses the following problems:

- Diagnostic difficulty in industrialized countries because of its rarity, although the disease is appearing again in immunocompromised patients with chronic alcoholism and AIDS. In third-world countries, the disease is common, often involving complications and gross deformity. In children, when a significant number of vertebrae are involved, spinal deformity ultimately appears; with time, paraplegia of healed disease may also occur.
- Drug resistance in endemic areas
- Controversy over the best modality of treatment, that is surgical versus conservative management, especially in children in relation to spinal deformity progression

EPIDEMIOLOGY

The prevalence of this disease is inversely proportional to the socioeconomic background of the patient and the standard of public health in the area.

Despite advances in medical technology, the diagnosis of spinal tuberculosis is sometimes missed. Because the initial presentation is varied, its inclusion in the differential diagnosis of any spinal pathology is essential in industrialized countries. In third-world countries, the cases usually present late, with little diagnostic problem. In these late-presenting cases, however, the surgeon faces the problems of a patient with significant disease involvement, possible neurologic complications, and gross spinal deformity. These patients require expert management, which is usually available only in specialized centers with access to chemotherapy and experienced spinal surgeons.

Spinal tuberculosis is common in children, particularly in countries in which the disease is prevalent. The "childhood" type of disease is more malignant in extent and degree of abscess formation but has less associated paraplegia; the reverse is usually the case in the adult type (19). This may be related to differences in the immunologic response of children and adults.

BACTERIOLOGY AND PATHOLOGY

Spinal tuberculosis is the result of infection by *Mycobacterium tuberculosis.* It is usually a secondary infection, with the primary extraspinal lesion usually occurring in the chest or genitourinary system. These primary sites may be quiescent (9). Spread of the organism through the lymphatics at the corresponding anatomic levels—for example, tuberculosis of the kidney spreading to the dorsolumbar junction—is possible. It may also spread by direct adjacent visceral extension.

In a vertebral segment, three patterns of involvement are recognized: paradiscal, anterior, and central lesions. The understanding of these patterns is important in appreciating the presentation of this disease. A *paradiscal* lesion is a lesion on either side of the intervertebral disc, usually with some narrowing of the intervertebral disc space. It is the most common pattern and is more common in adults than children. Bone infarction, necrosis, and impaction lead to decrease in vertebral size, which, if significant, may cause a kyphotic deformity. Paravertebral abscesses may develop (Fig. 4A). When the disease is healed, osseous interbody fusion occurs, especially in the presence of sinus discharge and superinfection by pyogenic bacteria.

An *anterior* lesion occurs with bony destruction under the anterior longitudinal ligament. With increasing accumulation in the abscess, tension rises and strips off the anterior longitudinal ligament and periosteum from the anterior surface of the vertebral body. Anterior scalloping occurs most commonly in the thoracic spine in children (Fig. 1B). There is minimal bone destruction, and kyphotic deformity is rare.

The *central* lesion, which is more common in children than

K.D.K. Luk, J.C.Y. Leong, and E.K.W. Ho: Department of Orthopaedic Surgery, University of Hong Kong, Queen Mary Hospital, Hong Kong.

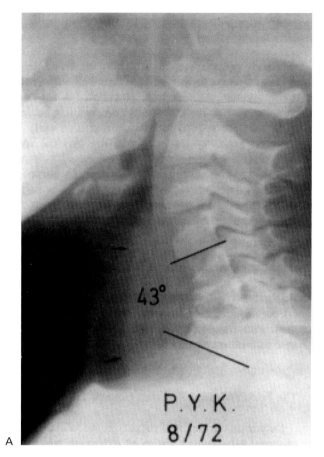

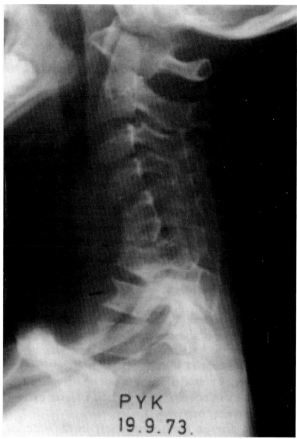

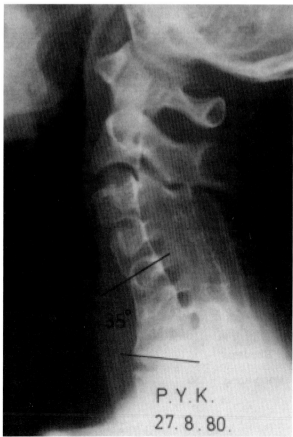

FIGURE 1. A: Preoperative radiograph of a 3-year-old boy with tuberculous involvement of C5 to C7. He presented with fever and refusal to eat. There is extensive prevertebral soft tissue swelling, indicating abscess formation *(arrow)*. There is significant corporeal destruction of C5, C6, and the upper part of C7, which resulted in a kyphosis. Speckles of calcification are present just in front of the C6–7 disc space. **B:** Radiograph taken 1 year after staged anterior and posterior spinal fusion from C4 to C7. There is spontaneous posterior fusion of C3 to C4 *(arrow)*. Some correction of kyphos has been obtained by insertion of oversized graft. Scalloping of T1 is present *(arrow)*. **C:** Postoperative radiograph at 7 years showing solid fusion circumferentially over C4 to C7 and posterior fusion over C3 to C4. The initial preoperative kyphos has been reduced. The aneurysmal effect of the abscess on T1 has resolved.

in adults, generally involves the whole body. Vertebral collapse occurs (vertebra plana). This pattern of involvement is most likely to produce a kyphosis. The more vertebral bodies affected, the greater the severity of the kyphosis (37) (Fig. 6A).

Tuberculous infection of the posterior elements of the spine is rare. The use of computed tomography (CT) scanning or magnetic resonance imaging (MRI) is helpful in making the diagnosis of posterior involvement (2).

The most frequent site of spinal tuberculosis is the thoracolumbar junction and the adjacent segments. Involvement of more than one segment is common (Fig. 4A). Sometimes, there is concomitant infection of the lumbar spine and the hip, especially in fulminating cases. Classically, a localized kyphosis at the thoracic or thoracolumbar junction appears. In the lumbar spine, there is loss of lumbar lordosis. Scoliosis may appear if bony destruction is asymmetric. A bayonet deformity and subluxation or dislocation may occur. With gross vertebral destruction, a reverse spondylolisthesis type of malalignment may also occur.

Unlike pyogenic infections, which destroy tissues by proteolytic enzymes, tuberculous infections causes destruction through a delayed hypersensitivity reaction of the body. This explains the typical low bacterial count within an active lesion. The actual sequence of infection in a spinal segment progresses from the "pre-pus" phase to paraspinal abscess formation. As the abscess expands, propagation of the abscess along the plane of least resistance (causing superficial abscess formation) or rupture into adjacent organs can occur. Healing produces fibrosis and bony reactions. If these consequences of healing take place in front of the vertebral body, bony bridging occurs. When the posterior part of the vertebral body is involved, paraplegia may result.

The pre-pus phase is the initial stage, characterized by granulation tissue proliferation. Histologically, epithelioid, round, and giant cells are evident. With proliferation of these cells and their disintegration, pus forms, leading to a paraspinal abscess.

The presence of a paraspinal abscess indicates an active disease. An abscess should be easy to diagnose. Hodgson (11) pointed out that about 10% of abscesses were missed clinically and were subsequently diagnosed at surgery. In the early stage, the pus is usually yellowish fluid; it eventually turns solid white and caseous. A large abscess, because of its mechanical effect, strips off the periosteum circumferentially. The blood supply of the peripheral portion of the vertebral body suffers, and a scalloping effect is produced in the form of an aneurysmal effect (aneurysmal syndrome) (Fig. 1B). The abscess may rupture into adjacent organs, which then produce symptoms of their own. A thoracic abscess may discharge into any organ in the mediastinum. The lung is most commonly involved (10%). Before actual rupture into adjacent organs, the space-occupying effect of the abscess may cause compression of adjacent structures (Fig. 1A); for example, a cervical spinal abscess may compress the trachea, causing inspiratory stridor in a child.

With advanced disease, intervertebral disc space narrowing occurs, partly because of the lack of nutrition from the subchondral bone. The detached disc may cause compression of the spinal cord or cauda equina. Multiple-level weakening of the vertebral body results in a "concertina" type of collapse. Profound destruction of multiple vertebral segments anteriorly re-

sults in a sharp kyphosis, which is especially marked at the thoracic or thoracolumbar junction (Fig. 6A). Under favorable conditions, the granulation tissue becomes fibrotic and subsequently calcifies and then ossifies. During this process of revascularization, bone reossifies and becomes dense. All these maturing fibrotic and bony elements may cause paraplegia of healed disease (see later). Spontaneous calcification of the intervertebral disc and paravertebral ligament may also occur. The corresponding posterior elements at the level of the disease may fuse spontaneously, especially in children.

CLINICAL PRESENTATION IN CHILDREN

Probably because of their low immunity, tuberculosis in young children is relatively malignant in its clinical course. However, in children there is a lower incidence of paraplegia. Aside from the usual systemic manifestations of chronic infection, there are interesting and important local manifestations unique to spinal tuberculosis in children. High thoracic spinal involvement with paraspinal abscess formation in children may cause significant bronchial compression and irritation. These symptoms may simulate asthmatic bronchitis (Millar asthma), especially when the patient lies down at night. With extensive destruction of the anterior elements of the spine, a significant angular kyphos appears. With differential growth of the intact posterior elements, progressive increase in the kyphos occurs, causing more deformity and restriction of visceral function. In severe cases, this may lead to restrictive lung disease or even secondary congestive heart failure.

The actual clinical presentation depends on the stage of the disease, the location of spinal involvement, the formation of a paraspinal abscess and its associated features, any associated obvious primary tuberculous manifestation (e.g., tuberculosis of the genitourinary tract), the immunologic status of the child, and prior antituberculous therapy. Neurologic involvement further complicates presentation by producing signs of meningitis, gait disturbance (psoas irritation), or frank paraparesis or tetraparesis and paraplegia or tetraplegia. Extreme spasticity in the limbs is associated with meningomyelitis caused by direct invasion of the meninges and neural tissue by the infected material. In patients with excessive systemic reactions, spinal involvement is part of disseminated tuberculosis.

Pott's paraplegia is a serious complication whose incidence averages about 10% (12). It is actually becoming rare in affluent countries, where presentation and diagnosis are made early and treatment is begun promptly. Classification into early and late types has been used by other authors (10,39), but we propose a more clinicopathologically oriented classification (15) (Table 1).

Healed disease often still harbors active infection. In a review of 22 cases of paraplegia of late onset (18), two thirds of patients still had active disease. This active disease group with late-onset paraplegia has a slightly better prognosis than the inactive healed disease group, in which neural compression is strictly mechanical in origin (because of fibrosis or anterior bony bridge).

TABLE 1. CLINICAL-PATHOLOGIC CLASSIFICATION OF POTT'S PARAPLEGIA

Pathology	Cause of Paraplegia	Presentation	Prognosis
Active disease	Pus, sequestra, sequestrated disc, granulation tissue; increased contents, subluxation, dislocation, vertebral collapse	Paraparesis or paraplegia	Good with early treatment especially surgical decompression.
Active disease	Dural penetration, direct neural involvement; pachymeningitis, meningomyelitis	Signs of meningitis, extreme spasticity	Poor
Active disease	Compression from diseased posterior elements; data lacking	Same as for anterior element destruction	Rare
Healed disease	New bone healing replaces diseased bone, especially in spontaneous healing; anterior bony bridge is retropulsed and matures	Paraplegia (late onset)	Poor
Healed disease	Maturation of fibrous component of granulation tissue; slow mechanical strangulation of cord	Distal sensory and motor symptoms	Poor

DIAGNOSIS

Diagnosis may be difficult in children, especially in the early stages of the disease. Systemic symptoms are similar to those of pyogenic infections, including malaise, easy fatigability, weight and appetite loss, and sometimes fever. Frank septicemia is uncommon. The most common local manifestation is pain over the involved spinal segment and a kyphosis. Advanced disease in a child may also produce a limping gait as a result of psoas irritation or weakness caused by Pott's paraplegia. A child presenting with additional respiratory embarrassment may have one of three complications: concomitant pulmonary tuberculosis, rupture of thoracic paraspinal abscess into the lung, or Millar asthma.

Radiologic manifestations can be bizarre and mimic many spinal lesions. The classic radiologic description depends on the site of infection. In central disease, which is common in children, a concertina type of collapse may appear, and clinically, there is paraplegia. Occasionally, a ballooning effect is seen instead. Because most parts of the vertebral body are affected, the products of inflammation expand the weakened vertebral wall, depicting an expansile lesion on the radiograph. Paradiscal disease is less common in children. Narrowing of intervertebral disc mimics discitis. Anterior disease signifies a spreading abscess. This phenomenon is common in children, especially in the thoracic spine, but it may be present anywhere in the spinal column. In healed disease, vertebral bodies sometimes have spontaneous fusion, simulating a hemivertebra (Fig. 2C, D). The vertebra-within-a-vertebra phenomenon (manifestation of arrested bone growth) may also be seen on radiographs. These radiologic features of tuberculosis of the spine have been well described by Hodgson and colleagues (16). Buchelt and associates (4), however, reported that many of these findings in plain radiographs are not pathognomonic of tuberculous infection and thus that differentiation from pyogenic spondylitis can sometimes be difficult.

There are other interesting changes in the segments of the spine adjacent to the acute kyphosis, especially in growing children. The vertebral bodies just above the kyphos lie more horizontally than usual. Because of a weight-relieving effect, the vertebral body increases in height. The anterior length of the vertebral body is also longer than its posterior length. This phenomenon is observed both radiologically and morphologically in postmortem studies. In addition to early narrowing of the intervertebral disc, calcification of the nucleus pulposus may occur but is rare. In children with gross thoracic kyphotic deformity, there may be lengthening of ribs and narrowing of their posterior portions.

In addition to plain radiographs, other useful investigations include myelographic studies, which are essential in patients with neurologic compression when compression at the internal kyphos needs to be demonstrated (Fig. 5A). Tomograms are useful to visualize the kyphos and ascertain the presence of a spontaneous posterior fusion. They are also useful at the upper dorsal and sacral areas to delineate the overlapping effect of the overlying bone. CT scans are helpful in demonstrating the extent of bony involvement, and sagittal reconstructions are useful in delineating the internal kyphos (Fig. 5B). Involvement of the posterior elements is also demonstrated by CT scan. An MRI investigation is useful to delineate the soft tissue involvement, concomitant abscess formation, and neural compression. A rim enhancement with contrast on a T2-weighted image helps in differentiating infections from a malignant condition (17) (Fig. 3A–D). A chest radiograph is necessary in cases of suspected pulmonary tuberculosis or rupture of abscess into the lungs.

Scintigraphic studies have low specificity and sensitivity, and the pattern of uptake can be similar to that seen in metastatic disease (43).

The erythrocyte sedimentation rate is a simple test that is useful for monitoring the progress of the disease. The Tine skin test is not specific in diagnosis, especially in endemic areas, where the chance of previous subclinical exposure to tuberculous infection is high.

The definitive diagnosis for inclusion into the MRC trial requires a positive culture and histology report on specimens obtained during surgery. With the advent of CT guidance and thoracoscopic or endoscopic assistance, biopsies can now be obtained easily in doubtful cases. Ziehl-Neelsen staining is helpful but was positive in only 47% of histologically proven specimens. Of these 47%, only 85% yielded a positive culture for the mycobacterium. Of the remaining 53% negative but histologically proven specimens, 87% yielded a positive culture for the myco-

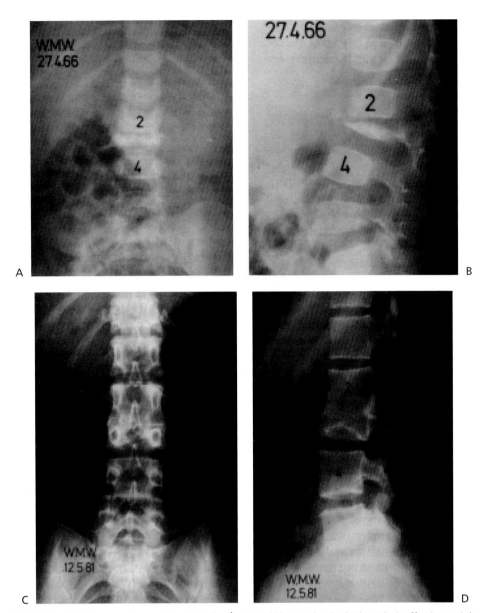

FIGURE 2. A, B: Preoperative radiographs of a 5½-year-old boy with spinal tuberculosis affecting mainly L3. Only the lower portion of L3 remains. The abscess detected at surgery was hardly visible on preoperative radiographs. **C, D:** Postoperative radiographs at 15 years follow-up after the Hong Kong operation at L2 to L3, showing total solid fusion simulating a congenital block vertebra. The inferior portion of L3 appears to have regenerated to some extent despite gross initial destruction. There is minimal kyphosis.

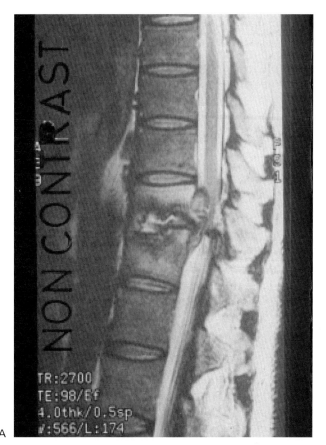

A

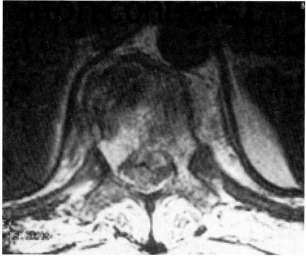

B

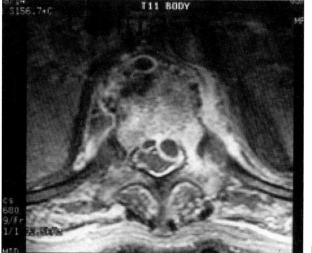

D

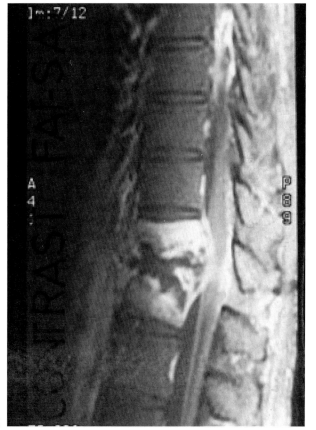

C

FIGURE 3. Magnetic resonance imaging study of a 25-year-old man with tuberculosis of the thoracic spine presenting with paraparesis of both lower limbs. Sagittal **(A)** and cross-section **(B)** T2-weighted images showing an abscess opposite T11 compressing the spinal cord. Note the hypointense signal of the abscess. Sagittal **(C)** and cross-section **(D)** images at the same levels after intravenous gadolinium infusion with fat-saturation sequence. The enhancement at the rim of the abscess is diagnostic of an infection.

bacterium. A positive bacterial culture is thus indicative but not absolutely essential for a firm diagnosis of spinal tuberculosis. The confirmation of spinal tuberculosis is especially difficult for healing of chronic lesions. This is partly explained by the presence of fewer bacilli in osseous tuberculosis than in tuberculosis of organs such as the lung. In these cases with a low bacterial load, the polymerase chain reaction test (3,34,40), which involves amplification of the mycobacterium DNA in biopsy specimens, has been considered the most important breakthrough in the field of diagnostic mycobacteriology. The technique, however, still has limitations, especially in detecting extrapulmonary lesions (5).

TREATMENT

The basic treatment of all forms of active spinal tuberculosis is a complete course of chemotherapy. This consists of an initial first-line drug regimen: streptomycin, isoniazid, and rifampicin. The second-line regimen (ethambutol, pyrazinamide) may be necessary in cases of poor clinical-hematologic response, side effects, or demonstrable resistance of bacillus to the first-line drugs. (Readers are advised to consult pharmaceutical texts for dosage, side effects, and duration of the drugs mentioned.) The first-line drug regimen should be started 1 week before surgery, if feasible. Close collaboration between orthopedic surgeons and physicians improves the efficiency of drug delivery and patients' compliance with this prolonged chemotherapy. A short-course chemotherapy regimen has also been accepted (1). In a prospective controlled trial conducted in Korea by the Medical Research Council (MRC) on the duration of chemotherapy, 265 patients were randomly allocated to four chemotherapy regimens. The conclusion was that isoniazid plus rifampicin for 6 or 9 months was effective and as successful as the 18-month regimen of isoniazid plus paraaminosalicylic acid or ethambutol (31). This recommendation of a shorter regimen may improve the drug compliance of the patients.

Indications for chemotherapy alone (without surgery) are few. The medically unfit, high-risk patient should be treated conservatively initially. Those with early proven disease, little bony destruction, and minimal abscess formation may fare well with chemotherapy alone. Classically, chemotherapy and surgery to immobilize the spine were the standard treatment. A regimen of chemotherapy without immobilization was advocated by some authors in the early 1960s, partly because of lack of hospital beds and, to a lesser extent, lack of surgical expertise.

With advances in surgery and anesthetic technique, various surgical procedures to treat spinal tuberculosis have been developed over the years. Except in cases of demonstrated posterior element involvement (which is rare), almost all posterior surgery has been abandoned, and posterior decompression alone is mentioned to be condemned. Modified costotransversectomy still has a place when decompression of the internal kyphos is necessary in an extremely kyphotic spine. In these cases, the internal kyphos is deeply seated and therefore difficult to approach anteriorly. A costotransversectomy also avoids a formal thoracotomy in patients with already compromised lung function.

Because the disease focus lies mainly in the anterior bony column, it is rational to use an anterior approach. Hodgson and Stock (13) popularized such an approach in spinal tuberculosis in nearly all segments of the spine. The concept of having a direct approach to the disease focus satisfies the following aims: complete extirpation of the disease focus and the ability to place a strut graft into the débrided cavity.

Extirpation of the disease focus obtains diseased material for diagnosis. After evacuation of the abscess and thorough débridement, pain relief is almost immediate, and the general condition of the patient often improves markedly. Early complete débridement also prevents spread of the abscess to adjacent spinal segments. Débridement quickly decompresses any neural or visceral compression. During an anterior spinal approach, exposure and confirmation of organ penetration can be made and sometimes dealt with simultaneously.

The placement of a strut graft into the débrided cavity under compression allows for hypertrophy of the graft according to Wolff's law. Early fusion generally results (Fig. 4B, C). After solid anterior fusion has been achieved, late recurrence is rare; increasing spinal deformity and paraplegia of healed disease are avoided. Moreover, a slightly oversized graft produces some correction of kyphosis (Fig. 1A–C). Using this regimen, Hodgson and Stock (14) achieved complete recovery from spinal disease in almost all cases. The fusion rate was 93%.

An absolute indication for surgery is paraplegia of active disease. The operation achieves rapid relief of cord compression and thus early and complete recovery (especially in the cervical spine) (19). In fact, this surgery for active disease is relatively simple, and the results are rewarding. In paraplegia of healed disease, surgical decompression is usually difficult partly because of the gross deformity and partly because the compression is caused by hard bony ridges or diffuse fibrosis. In special cases of technical difficulty, stabilization procedures without decompression to prevent further deterioration of the paraparesis may be the solution of last resort. In children with extensive disease who are critically ill, radical excision may not be practical. In these cases, débridement with drainage of the abscess should be the initial goal as a life-saving measure.

The British Medical Research Council Trial

Debate on the merits of surgery in the total treatment of spinal tuberculosis led to an extensive multicenter study in 1965, initiated by the Medical Research Council of the United Kingdom (23–32). This study was based on well-controlled clinical trials comparing various modes of treatment (Table 2). The results of subsequent 10-year and 15-year follow-ups have clearly defined the role of surgery in spinal tuberculosis.

Groups of patients from Korea, Rhodesia, and Hong Kong were studied. All patients had at least 18 months of either a two-drug (INAH and PAS) or a three-drug (streptomycin, INAH, and PAS) regimen. These three groups were fairly homogeneous in their pretreatment factors, except that the Korean patients were all children; 82% of Rhodesian and 54% of Hong Kong patients were adults. The criterion for inclusion in the study was the presence of clinical and radiologic evidence of active spinal tuberculosis at any level except the cervical spine. Four categories of patients were excluded:

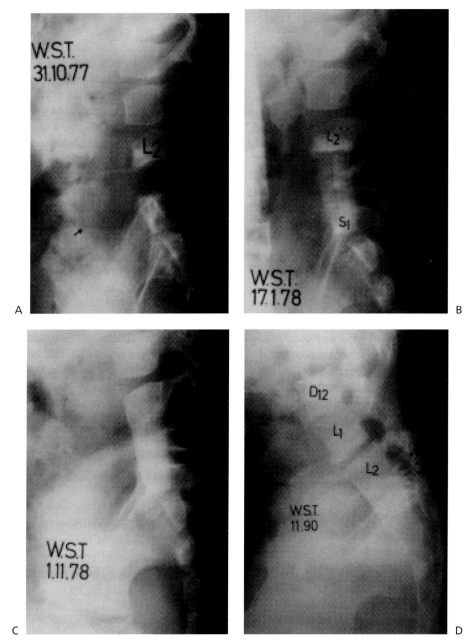

FIGURE 4. A: Preoperative radiograph of a 7-year-old boy with tuberculous involvement of the lower border of L2 to probably S2. The parents noticed a swelling over the child's back at 4 years of age, when a complete course of antituberculous chemotherapy was given. He developed a discharging groin sinus at about the time this radiograph was taken. This preoperative radiograph shows gross bony destruction of L3, L4, L5, and S1, with sparing of the posterior elements. A soft tissue swelling *(arrow)* is present. There is no significant kyphosis. **B:** Postoperative radiograph taken 4 months after anterior spinal débridement and circumferential fusion. The anterior grafts used were ribs obtained during thoracotomy. **C:** Radiograph taken 1 year postoperatively, showing no collapse of the graft. It also shows very good graft incorporation. There is no kyphosis. **D:** Radiograph at 13 years follow-up showing solid circumferential fusion from L2 to the sacrum. The remnant of the posterior element of the missing segments is still visible *(arrow)*. The patient is totally asymptomatic except for a shortened trunk.

TABLE 2. BRITISH MEDICAL RESEARCH COUNCIL PROTOCOL

Location	Number of Patients	Treatment Modality
Masan, South Korea	350 (total)	Inpatient bed rest for 6 months, then outpatient treatment; or, ambulatory outpatient treatment from the start
Pusan, South Korea	—	Outpatient treatment with a plaster jacket for 9 months, or ambulatory treatment without any support
Bulawayo, Rhodesia	130	Randomly, by débridement of spinal focus or by ambulatory treatment
Hong Kong	150	Randomly, by radical resection of lesion and insertion of autogenous bone grafts, or by débridement

1. Those with significant paralysis, such that the patient could not walk across a room
2. Patients having 1 year or more of antituberculous chemotherapy
3. Those in whom the presence of concomitant serious extraspinal disease was likely to affect the total management of a patient
4. In Hong Kong, those with extensive destruction of three or more vertebral bodies because fusion by itself was justified in those patients

The results presented at the 5-year report (28) already showed the advantage of the Hong Kong operation over other modalities of treatment, and this continued to hold true at the 10-year (29) and 15-year (32) follow-ups. Although at the final MRC report, all three groups of patients treated ([1] conservatively in Korea, [2] with débridement alone, and [3] with radical débridement plus fusion in Hong Kong) achieved the same 87% of favorable clinical results, 85% of the radical surgery group in Hong Kong had complete radiologic union at 18 months. This figure increased to 92% at 5 years, 97% at 10 years, and 94% at 15 years. The corresponding figures in Korea showed that, with conservative treatment, 54% of patients still had no signs of fusion at 5 years. The bony fusion rate remained at 73% and 72% at 10 and 15 years, respectively (Table 3).

TABLE 3. BONY FUSION RATE (%) AT 5, 10, AND 13 TO 15 YEARS

	0–18 mo	0–5 y	0–10 y	13–15 y
Korea				
Chemotherapy alone	15	46	73	72
Hong Kong				
Débridement alone	52	84	90	94
Débridement plus fusion	85	92	97	94

Modified from the Medical Research Council Working Party on Tuberculosis of the Spine (1998): A 15-year assessment of controlled trials of the management of tuberculosis of the spine in Korea and Hong Kong. *J Bone Joint Surg Br* 80:456–462, with permission.

Vertebral reconstitution was actually positive (0.2 of a vertebra) at 5 years in the Hong Kong group, contrasting with increased vertebral loss of 0.18 of a vertebra in the débridement group and 0.44 of a vertebra in the ambulatory chemotherapy group. These results were maintained at the 15-year follow-up.

The angle of kyphosis of the conservatively treated group showed an increase to 21 degrees at 5 years and further increased to 25 degrees at 15 years (32). About 5% of this group suffered an alarming increase in their final angles, which ranged from 51 to 70 degrees. The corresponding figures for the débridement group were 8 and 11 degrees, respectively. In contrast, the radical surgery group showed an improvement of 3 degrees at 5 years, and this was maintained at the final follow-up of 15 years. This preservation of the sagittal curvature is particularly important for the lumbar spine, where there is normally a lordosis.

Healing of sinuses and abscesses occurred in all the Hong Kong patients by 18 months. In Korea, 3% of the patients still had sinus tracts or abscesses after 5 years. There was no neurologic involvement during treatment in the Hong Kong group. In the ambulatory chemotherapy group, 5% of patients developed neurologic deficits during treatment.

The long-term follow-up report of the MRC trial confirms that the radical Hong Kong surgical approach can fulfill the aims of treatment in spinal tuberculosis. It produces rapid decompression and fusion, prevents late recurrence once healing has occurred, and, most important, prevents the development of progressive and severe deformity, which may be further complicated by paraplegia of healed disease (Fig. 2A–D).

Spinal Growth and Deformity After Fusion in Children

The MRC trial has a number of limitations. First, the results from children and adults were analyzed together; second, the long-term effect of fusion during early childhood on spinal growth was not studied; and third, diseases involving three or more bodies were excluded.

The only prospective longitudinal study on the long-term outcome of deformity in children who received radical or débridement surgery was by Upadhyay and colleagues in 1993 (41). They followed 80 children in the MRC trial in Hong Kong who underwent surgery before 10 years of age to maturity. Forty-seven had radical surgery and bone grafting at a mean age of 7.6 years, and the remaining 33 patients had débridement alone at a mean age of 5.1 years. Six months after surgery, 56% of the radical surgery group showed an improvement in the deformity angle of 5 degrees or more compared with the preoperative evaluation, whereas 69% showed deterioration after débridement surgery. At the final follow-up at a mean of 17 years after surgery, the status of the deformity was virtually unchanged. They also found that the problem of kyphosis was particularly important in patients who had lumbar tuberculosis in that 60% of patients in the débridement group had a 10-degree or more kyphus angle, whereas only one patient in the radical group had a kyphotic lumbar spine as a result of graft failure. The findings from this study further strengthen the merits of radical surgery in children.

The same group of researchers studied longitudinally the

growth of the fused spinal segment in 33 patients who underwent radical surgery before 10 years of age. They found no difference in the growth pattern when compared with that in 71 patients who had surgery when 18 years or older. The authors concluded that there was no disproportionate posterior spinal growth after anterior spinal fusion and that routine posterior spinal fusion after anterior surgery in children was not necessary (42).

In contrast to the findings of Upadhyay and colleagues (42), Schulitz and associates in 1997 (38) reported in a series of 117 children that anterior fusion alone resulted in worsening of the kyphotic angle by an average of 12 degrees after 10 years, compared with an unchanged kyphotic angle in the posterior spinal fusion group. In the combined anteroposterior fusion and simple anterior débridement group, there were decreases in the kyphotic angle of −7 and −4 degrees, respectively. These investigators believed that destruction of the anterior growth potential and continued growth in the posterior neural arch reduced the remodeling power of the spine. This is especially true when the lesion is located in the thoracic spine and when several segments are involved. Although the difference in findings in these two series could be explained by the fact that the patients in Schulitz's series were on average 2.5 years younger than those in Upadhyay's series, one can see that there are still ongoing controversies regarding this issue.

Infections in Special Regions

Three regions of the spine deserve special consideration in treatment.

Tuberculosis of the upper cervical spine has special features of local pain and stiffness, paralysis, swelling of the retropharyngeal soft tissue, and atlantoaxial subluxation. This region is much less commonly affected than the subaxial region. Six patients with tuberculosis of the upper cervical spine were studied (8), with the above-mentioned features present in varying combinations. Cervical lymphadenopathy was present in all cases. Treatment necessitates transoral anterior débridement and often concomitant atlantoaxial fusion for stability. Halo immobilization is recommended at all stages of management and is also useful in some cases to achieve reduction. The transoral route also decompresses the large retropharyngeal abscess, thus avoiding acute dysphagia and asphyxia.

Tuberculosis of the subaxial cervical spine has been studied in detail in 40 patients (19). There is a distinct difference in the disease before and after 10 years of age. At a younger age, disease involvement is extensive and large abscesses form; the contrary occurs after 10 years of age. The incidence of paraplegia is much less in the childhood type (before 10 years of age) than in the adult type (after 10 years of age). Besides chemotherapy, anterior débridement and grafting are highly recommended; such a regimen gives rapid pain relief, decompresses abscesses that cause respiratory symptoms, and relieves paraplegia quickly. This operation also corrects kyphotic deformity significantly, ranging from 5.4 to 25.5 degrees (Fig. 1A–C).

Tuberculosis of the lumbosacral junction is a unique condition. Twenty-six cases have been studied, with an average follow-up of 20 years (36). Patients younger than 10 years of age presented with a discharging sinus or a pointing abscess and a visible kyphosis. Older patients presented with low back pain. Neurologic involvement was uncommon. Anterior débridement and strut fusion, although technically difficult, reduced the incidence and size of kyphosis (Fig. 4A–D). Conservative treatment resulted in a higher incidence of back pain, truncal shortening, and complications in pregnancy. Irrespective of their mode of treatment, all cases had radiologic fusion. The authors stressed the biomechanical importance of preserving the normal lumbosacral angle in management of this condition.

Surgical Management of Active Tuberculosis of the Spine

Management is divided into preoperative, operative, and postoperative management, including early and late surgical complications. Relevant details of the surgical approach to the spine are contained in a description by Leong (22).

Preoperative Management

Chemotherapy should be started a few days before surgery. Sometimes, in a dire emergency, when there is a neurologic or visceral complication, surgery can be performed before commencement of chemotherapy without added morbidity. Other preoperative assessments include checking vestibular nerve function because streptomycin may have an adverse effect on the eighth cranial nerve. Thrombocytopenia caused by rifampicin treatment should be watched for in patients receiving surgery. Preoperative halo immobilization may be necessary in infection of the cervical (especially the upper cervical) region. A prefabricated plaster shell is often required for an uncooperative child; it facilitates postoperative nursing and immobilization. The erythrocyte sedimentation rate should be evaluated before surgery. Radiologic investigation to delineate the site and extent of the lesion and to detect any complications (e.g., MRI scan for Pott's paraplegia, chest radiograph for rupture of thoracic abscess in lung) is necessary. CT is especially useful to study the anatomy of the kyphos before surgical decompression.

Operative Management

The operation is usually done using an anterior approach (22). Identification of the paraspinal abscess is easy unless the anatomy has been disturbed by a previous operation. The abscess is opened in a T-shaped fashion. Segmental vessels nearby have to be ligated if they are not already thrombosed. The abscess is evacuated and the diseased vertebra exposed. Radical excision is performed until fresh bleeding bone is obtained. The contralateral side abscess should be evacuated by suction and curettage as much as possible. This is done when the far side of the diseased vertebral bodies is reached. The excision sometimes leaves end plates exposed, in which case the normal disc and cartilage end plate of the adjoining healthy vertebra have to be removed to create a healthy bed for graft placement. The subchondral plate remnant is totally removed toward the back of the vertebral body until the posterior longitudinal ligament is visible. This ensures

TABLE 4. EARLY COMPLICATIONS

Complication	Cause	Treatment
Worsening of neurologic deficit	Surgical neurapraxia of spinal cord	Observation; steroids for edema
Slippage of graft (especially long ones) impinging onto spinal cord	Graft replacement and better external immobilization	
Horner syndrome	Injury to cervical sympathetics	Observe; most will recover
Warm leg	Injury to lumbar sympathetic	Usually transient
Hemothorax, pneumothorax, atelectasis	Thoracotomy complication; poor drainage or intrinsic lung disease	General resuscitation, chest physiotherapy, and improved drainage of chest cavity; antibiotics if necessary
Paralytic ileus	Reflex reaction with surgery around dorsolumbar or lumbar spine	Usually transient; observation, fasting, and nasogastric suction
Residual abscess	Incomplete evacuation of contralateral abscess	Continue effective chemotherapy; exclude drug-resistant bacteria

complete decompression and removal of remnants of subchon-dral plate in the posterior part of the vertebra. Slightly oversized graft is used and inserted after springing open the kyphos by gentle manual pressure over the kyphos apex posteriorly. The available graft sources commonly come from the excised rib or iliac crest blocks. Neck wounds are routinely drained, and chest tubes are used after thoracotomy. Occasionally, an extrapleural approach is used in thoracic disease, especially in patients with marked restriction of lung function. In this case, chest drainage is not necessary.

Postoperative Management

Management at this stage includes fluid replacement and pain relief. Proper care of any drains to prevent fluid accumulation at the operative site is important. Prefabricated body jackets are useful for immobilization and for nursing children postopera-tively. Halo immobilization should be incorporated into a body vest or plaster cast so that patients can be mobilized early. Staged supplementary posterior spinal fusion may be necessary when two or more vertebrae were diseased or removed anteriorly (21).

Postoperative complications may be early or late in onset. Complications are related to the spinal segment involved and may be neurologic or visceral in origin and related to the graft insertion or the residual disease (Tables 4 and 5).

TABLE 5. LATE COMPLICATIONS

Complication	Cause	Treatment
Nonunion at graft site	Persistent infection—disease reactivation or resistant organism	Spinal restabilization if kyphosis increases; alter chemotherapy regime if necessary
Graft fracture (long graft at midportion) 12–18 mo after surgery	Stress fracture	Spinal immobilization
Graft reabsorption 6–12 wk after operation	Persistent infection (resistant organism)	Alter chemotherapy regimen if necessary reexplore if conservative treatment fails

Management of Paraplegia of Healed Disease

Paraplegia of healed disease is caused by impingement of the spinal canal by a sharp internal bony kyphos or from a constric-tion effect caused by fibrosis resulting from maturing granulation tissue around neural elements. Paraplegia can occur many years after the initial active infection, when the clinical deformity is apparently already nonprogressive. The documentation of compression requires early myelographic studies (Fig. 5A, B) or MRI.

Approach to the kyphos for surgical decompression requires detailed knowledge and surgical skill in anterior spinal surgery. An alternative is modified costotransversectomy with pediculec-tomy, which is particularly useful in a very severe angular kyphos. Anterior access to the apex of the internal kyphos is best obtained by tracing a nerve root proximally to the intervertebral foramen. The bony and fibrous material in front of the spinal cord must be removed carefully. The dura at the apex should be adequately exposed and protected. After thorough decompression, the dura should displace forward without tension and pulsate. Approach-ing the apex of the kyphos is fraught with dangers of injury to the spinal cord or dura. These complications occurred in 36% of patients with paraplegia of late onset treated surgically (18). Using better operating instruments, including high-speed burr, and intraoperative spinal cord monitoring, the operative mor-bidity has decreased significantly in our recent experience. Most of the cases of surgical complications occurred in paraplegia of late onset without concomitant active disease. Thus, the presence of active disease in this particular condition is of prognostic significance.

The overall prognosis of paraplegia of healed disease is poor, even with adequate decompression; recovery is usually prolonged and incomplete. The presence of active disease calls for addi-tional chemotherapy. After adequate decompression, anterior strut graft fusion is performed using either the removed rib or an iliac crest graft.

Management of Severe Kyphotic Deformity

Significant angular kyphosis is a difficult problem that is com-mon after spinal tuberculosis, especially in children with exten-sive anterior disease. The kyphosis is unsightly and, more impor-

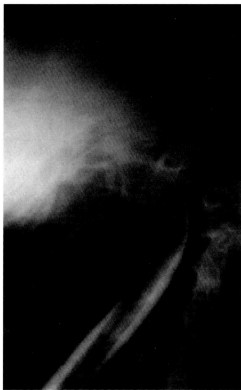

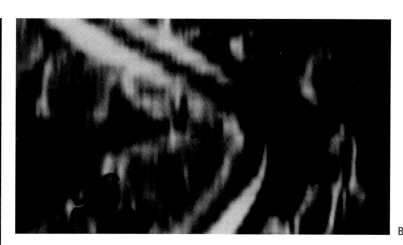

A

B

FIGURE 5. A: Myelogram of an 11-year-old girl with paraplegia of healed disease. Progressive paraplegia occurred 6 months before this investigation. There was multisegmental high thoracic disease that had been quiescent for many years. This myelogram showed a near right-angle kink of the contrast column, with significant anterior indentation *(arrow)*. The blockade is only partial, and the contrast column is visible above the kyphos. **B:** Computed tomography reconstruction demonstrated the internal kyphos remarkably well. This patient had an uneventful anterior decompression and fusion, with near total recovery of her neurologic function.

A,B

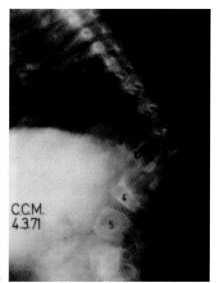

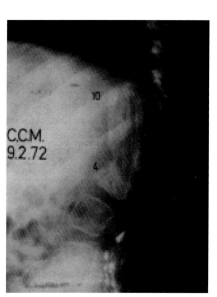

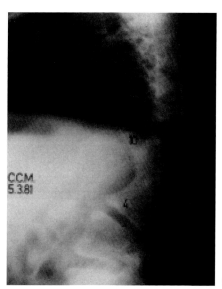

C

FIGURE 6. A: Preoperative radiograph of a 6-year-old boy with gross kyphotic deformity due to active spinal tuberculosis destroying the T11 to L4 vertebral bodies. He underwent anterior drainage and débridement followed by gradual halo-pelvic distraction. This was followed by a circumferential fusion after maximal gradual correction. **B:** Significant correction is noticed in the radiograph taken 9 months after fusion. The rib graft is still visible. **C:** At 10 years follow-up, the radiograph shows solid anterior fusion with some loss of correction. However, the final deformity is much less than the original.

tant, may compromise visceral function. It may be associated with paraplegia of healed disease with or without residual active disease. Besides the deformity itself, the adjacent spinal segments develop compensatory hyperlordosis, which may pose additional problems in the future. There may also be secondary rib changes, sternal deformity, and spontaneous posterior fusion.

Surgical correction is technically difficult because of the aforementioned problems in the anterior approach to the kyphos apex. The cephalad and caudad limbs of the kyphos may be in different planes, constituting a bayonet type of deformity. In multisegmental disease, the vertebral bodies intended to receive the graft may differ significantly in size after thorough débridement, making proper and adequate placement of strut grafts difficult.

The development of halo-pelvic distraction (33) enabled the circumferentially osteotomized spine to be distracted in a slow, controlled fashion. Strain gauges can be incorporated into the bars of the apparatus to register total tension in the spine, which should be at most one fourth to one third of the patient's body weight. During gradual distraction, frequent neurologic assessment is necessary. Avascular necrosis of the dens and spontaneous fusion of cervical segments are late consequences of prolonged traction in the cervical spine (6,7). The cervical spine should be radiographed before starting halo-pelvis distraction.

After achieving the required distraction, circumferential fusion is performed (Fig. 6A–C). This form of staged procedure needs a prolonged hospital stay and constant monitoring of the patient. There is significant mortality and morbidity associated with this treatment. Yau and colleagues (44) reported on a series of 30 patients who underwent such correction. There were three deaths, and complications in the cervical spine were common. The mortality and morbidity occurred mainly in the very early surgical experience. Cosmetic and pulmonary improvement were observed, however. This operation should be done only in specialized spine centers with the relevant expertise.

REFERENCES

1. Antituberculosis regimens of chemotherapy (1988): *Bull Int Union Tuberc Lung Dis* 63:60–64.
2. Arthornthurasrok A, Chongpieboonpatana A (1990): Spinal tuberculosis with posterior element involvement. *Spine* 15:191–194.
3. Brisson-Noel A, Aznar C, Churea C, et al. (1991): Diagnosis of tuberculosis by DNA amplification: clinical practice evaluation. *Lancet* 338: 364–366.
4. Buchelt M, Lack W, Kutschera HP, et al. (1993): Comparison of tuberculous and pyogenic spondylitis: an analysis of 122 cases. *Clin Orthop* 296:192–199.
5. Chan CM, Yuen KY, Chan KS, et al. (1996): Single-tube nested PCR in the diagnosis of tuberculosis. *J Clin Pathol* 49:290–294.
6. Dove J, Hsu LCS, Yau ACMA (1980): The cervical spine after halo-pelvic traction: an analysis of the complications in 83 patients. *J Bone Joint Surg Br* 62:158–161.
7. Dove J, Hsu LCS, Yau ACMC (1982): Avascular necrosis of the dens: a follow-up study. *Spine* 7:408–411.
8. Fang D, Leong JCY, Fang HSY (1983): Tuberculosis of the upper cervical spine. *J Bone Joint Surg Br* 65:47.
9. Friedman B (1966): Chemotherapy of tuberculosis of the spine. *J Bone Joint Surg Am* 48:451.
10. Griffiths DL, Seddon HJ, Roaf R (1956): *Pott's paraplegia.* London: Oxford University Press.
11. Hodgson AR (1975): Infectious disease of the spine. In: Rothman RH, Simeone, eds. *Spine,* 1st ed. Philadelphia: WB Saunders, pp. 567–598.
12. Hodgson AR, Skinsnes OK, Leong JCY (1967): The pathogenesis of Pott's paraplegia. *J Bone Joint Surg Am* 49:1147.
13. Hodgson AR, Stock FE (1956): Anterior spinal fusion. *Br J Surg* 44: 266.
14. Hodgson AR, Stock FE (1960): Anterior spinal fusion for the treatment of tuberculosis of the spine: the operative findings and results of treatment in the first one hundred cases. *J Bone Joint Surg Am* 42:295.
15. Hodgson AR, Yau AC (1967): Pott's paraplegia: a classification based upon the living pathology. *Paraplegia* 5:1–16.
16. Hodgson AR, Wong W, Yau A (1969): X-ray appearances of tuberculosis of the spine. Springfield: Charles C Thomas.
17. Hoffman EB, Crosier JH, Cremin BJ (1993): Imaging in children with spinal tuberculosis: a comparison of radiography, computed tomography and magnetic resonance imaging. *J Bone Joint Surg Br* 75:233–239.
18. Hsu LCS, Cheng CL, Leong JCY (1988): Pott's paraplegia of late onset. *J Bone Joint Surg Br* 70:534–538.
19. Hsu LCS, Leong JCY (1984): Tuberculosis of the lower cervical spine (C2–7): a report on forty cases. *J Bone Joint Surg Br* 66:1.
20. Ito H, Tsuchiya J, Asami G (1934): A new radical operation for Pott's disease. *J Bone Joint Surg* 16:499.
21. Jenkins DHR, Hodgson AR, Yau ACMC, et al. (1975): Stabilization of the spine in the surgical treatment of severe spinal tuberculosis in children. *Clin Orthop* 110:69.
22. Leong JCY (1991): Operations for infections of the spine. In: *Rob & Smith's operative surgery. Part I. Orthopaedics.* London, U.K.: Butterworth-Heinemann, pp. 559–570.
23. Medical Research Council Working Party on Tuberculosis of the Spine (1973): A controlled trial of ambulant outpatient treatment and inpatient rest in bed in the management of tuberculosis of the spine in young Korean patients on standard chemotherapy: a study in Masan, Korea. *J Bone Joint Surg Br* 55:678–697.
24. Medical Research Council Working Party on Tuberculosis of the Spine (1973): A controlled trial of plaster-of-Paris jackets in the management of ambulant outpatient treatment of tuberculosis of the spine in children on standard chemotherapy: a study in Pusan, Korea. *Tubercle* 54: 261–282.
25. Medical Research Council Working Party on Tuberculosis of the Spine (1974): A controlled trial of debridement and ambulatory treatment in the management of tuberculosis of the spine in patients on standard chemotherapy. *J Trop Med Hyg* 77:72–79.
26. Medical Research Council Working Party on Tuberculosis of the Spine (1974): A controlled trial of anterior spinal fusion and debridement in the surgical management of tuberculosis of the spine in patients on standard chemotherapy: a study in Hong Kong. *Br J Surg* 61:853–866.
27. Medical Research Council Working Party on Tuberculosis of the Spine (1976): A five-year assessment of controlled trials of inpatient and outpatient treatment and of plaster-of-Paris jackets for tuberculosis of the spine in children on standard chemotherapy: studies in Masan and Pusan, Korea. *J Bone Joint Surg Br* 58:399–411.
28. Medical Research Council Working Party on Tuberculosis of the Spine (1978): Five-year assessments of controlled trials of ambulatory treatment, debridement and anterior spinal fusion in the management of tuberculosis of the spine: studies in Bulawayo (Rhodesia) and in Hong Kong. *J Bone Joint Surg Br* 60:163–177.
29. Medical Research Council Working Party on Tuberculosis of the Spine (1982): A ten-year assessment of a controlled trial comparing debridement and anterior spinal fusion in the management of tuberculosis of the spine in patients on standard chemotherapy in Hong Kong. *J Bone Joint Surg Br* 64:393–398.
30. Medical Research Council Working Party on Tuberculosis of the Spine (1985): A ten-year assessment of controlled trials of inpatient and outpatient treatment and of plaster-of-Paris jacket for tuberculosis of the spine in children on standard chemotherapy: studies in Masan and Pusan, Korea. *J Bone Joint Surg Br* 67:103–110.
31. Medical Research Council Working Party on Tuberculosis of the Spine (1993): Controlled trial of short-course regiments of chemotherapy in the ambulatory treatment of spinal tuberculosis: results at three years of a study in Korea. *J Bone Joint Surg Br* 75:240–248.

32. Medical Research Council Working Party on Tuberculosis of the Spine (1998): A 15-year assessment of controlled trials of the management of tuberculosis of the spine in Korea and Hong Kong. *J Bone Joint Surg Br* 80:456–462.

33. O'Brien JP, Yau ACMC, Smith TK, et al. (1971): Halo pelvic traction. *J Bone Joint Surg Br* 53:217–229.

34. Pierre C, Lecossier D, Boussougant Y, et al. (1991): Use of a reamplification protocol improves sensitivity of detection of mycobacterium tuberculosis in clinical samples by amplification of DNA. *J Clin Microbiol* 29:712–717.

35. Pott P: *Remarks on that kind of palsy of the lower limbs which is frequently found to accompany a curvature of the spine.* London: J. Johnson, 1779.

36. Pun WK, Chow SP, Luk KDK, et al. (1990): Tuberculosis of lumbosacral junction: longterm follow-up of 26 cases. *J Bone Joint Surg Br* 72:675–678.

37. Rajasekaran S, Shanmugasundaram TK (1987): Prediction of the angle of gibbus deformity in tuberculosis of the spine. *J Bone Joint Surg Am* 69:503–509.

38. Schulitz KP, Kothe R, Leong JCY, et al. (1997): Growth changes of solidly fused kyphotic bloc after surgery for tuberculosis: comparison of four procedures. *Spine* 22:1150–1155.

39. Seddon HJ (1935): Pott's paraplegia: prognosis and treatment. *Br J Surg* 22:769.

40. Shawer RM, El-Zaatari AK, Nataraj A, et al. (1993): Detection of mycobacterium tuberculosis in clinical samples by two-step polymerase chain reaction and nonisotopic hybridization methods. *J Clin Microbiol* 31:61–65.

41. Upadhyay SS, Sell P, Saji MJ, et al. (1993): 17-Year prospective study of surgical management of spinal tuberculosis in children: Hong Kong operation compared with debridement surgery for short- and long-term outcome of deformity. *Spine* 18:1704–1711.

42. Upadhyay SS, Saji MJ, Sell P, et al. (1994): The effect of age on the change in deformity after radical resection and anterior arthrodesis for tuberculosis of the spine. *J Bone Joint Surg Am* 76:701–708.

43. Weaver P, Lifeso RM (1984): The radiological diagnosis of tuberculosis of the adult spine. *Skel Radiol* 12:178–186.

44. Yau ACMC, Hsu LCS, O'Brien JP, et al. (1974): Tuberculous kyphosis: correction with spinal osteotomy, halo-pelvic distraction and anterior and posterior fusion. *J Bone Joint Surg Am* 56:1419–1434.

FUNGAL INFECTIONS OF THE SPINE

TEDDY S. GOVENDER

DEFINITION

Fungi are plantlike organisms that are obligatory or facultative aerobes. Morphologically they appear either as single cells (yeasts), such as *Cryptococcus neoformans* and *Candida albicans*, or as multicellular filamentous colonies (molds), such as *Aspergillus* (6,10). The cells are larger and genomically more complex than bacteria, with a highly organized nucleus bounded by a nuclear membrane. Actinomycetes superficially resemble fungi but are a heterogeneous gram-positive filamentous bacteria.

Isolated fungal infection of the spine is uncommon in children, although spinal involvement may occur in systemic disease in the immunocompromised host (18,19,27,43,52). Spinal infections due to aspergillosis, candidiasis, cryptococcosis, blastomycosis, and coccoidioidomycosis have been reported in both immunocompetent and immunocompromised patients (1,3,5,7, 8,11,14,16,22,23,26,28,36,45).

EPIDEMIOLOGIC FACTORS

Yeasts and mycelial fungi are ubiquitous organisms found in almost all types of organic substrates. They behave as pathogens by invading the tissues of patients whose normal immunologic defenses are impaired as a effect of the prolonged use of antibacterial or immunosuppressive drugs (6,8,10). Invasion may occur in patients with lowered resistance due to cancer, uncontrolled diabetes, organ transplantation, AIDS, chronic granulomatous disease (CGD), and long-term steroid therapy (8,21,25,36, 38,51).

Candida albicans, the most common yeast pathogen, is a normal colonizer of the gastrointestinal and urogenital tracts (6). Candidiasis is undoubtedly one of the most widespread and prevalent mycotic diseases in humans, and this is especially true of the infections caused by the endogenous species (e.g., *C. albicans*) (1,28). The common predisposing factors in candidiasis are burns, infected central venous catheters, and intravenous drug abuse (1,28,39). Pigeon roosts are a common source of *Cryptococcus neoformans*, and the only known source of *C. neoformans* var. *gattii* is *Eucalyptus camaldulensis*. *C. neoformans* var.

gattii has a propensity for causing disease in immunocompetent hosts (37,49). Aspergilli, which are opportunistic mycelial organisms, live as saprophytes by deriving nutrients from dead plants and animal matter (10). Because threshing areas and mills have high concentrations of aspergilli, which are readily disseminated into the air by wind currents, farm laborers are at increased risk of developing the infection (50).

Coccidioides and *Blastomyces* are true pathogenic infections, and inhalation of their spores results in a primary acute self-limiting respiratory infection (27,43). In the immunocompromised patients a fatal systemic mycosis may develop. *Coccidioides* is endemic to the arid southwestern United States, and in parts of South America. The infection is seen more frequently outside the traditional geographic areas due to the increasing number of immunocompromised patients (27). Blastomycosis is a systemic illness caused by the dimorphic fungus *Blastomyces dermatitides*, which is endemic in the midwestern, south central, and parts of the southeastern United States (2–4). Exposure to the infection begins insidiously and may be contracted during travel through an endemic area. The prevalence of osseous involvement due to blastomycosis ranged from 6% to 48% (32,43). Basset and Tindall (3) reported on 31 cases of blastomycosis of bone, and 26% (eight patients) included vertebral involvement.

PATHOANATOMY

Cryptococcosis is a subacute or chronic infection usually involving the lungs, brain, meninges, and skeleton (8,11,25). The infectious organism enters the respiratory tract by inhalation, producing a primary pulmonary infection that is usually transitory, mild, and unrecognized (6,11). The tissue reaction of the host to *C. neoformans* is very broad and may vary from little or no inflammation to a purely granulomatous reaction with varying degrees of necrosis (22,29). In the immunocompetent patient the infection that is subclinical resolves rapidly, with minimal symptoms. In the immunocompromised patient the infection spreads to involve multiple organs, with a predilection for the central nervous system (CNS), which is affected in about 8% of AIDS patients in the United States (8). The lesion may have a glistening appearance and a slimy consistency on gross examination and can mimic both sarcoidosis and tuberculosis (11,34).

Aspergillus fumigatus is the most common isolated species associated with invasive and noninvasive aspergillosis. It may pro-

T.S. Govender: Department of Orthopaedic Surgery, University of Natal, Durban, South Africa.

duce an allergic response, such as asthma, or bronchopulmonary aspergillosis (49). Invasive pulmonary aspergillosis is due to the *A. niger*. In chronic lesions, the center of the granuloma may become necrotic and/or liquefy, forming a cavity (50). Secondary, noninvasive pulmonary aspergillosis is characterized by the presence of a "fungal ball" or aspergilloma. This mycelial mass is usually located within a preformed pulmonary cavity (e.g., tuberculosis or bronchietatsis) (24).

Sixty percent of patients with coccidioidomycosis are asymptomatic and manifest only a positive skin test. However, 33% will develop a primary pneumonia and subsequently be at risk for extrapulmonary dissemination. Cutaneous, osseous, prostatic, and CNS involvement are the next most common in descending order (27).

Candidiasis is a relatively common mycosis of worldwide distribution and in the immunocompromised may manifest as endocarditis, meningitis, fungemia, or infections caused by other organisms (8). In recent years, the increasing incidence of infection due to *Candida* species in humans may be attributed to the use of broad-spectrum antibiotics, corticosteroids, immunosuppressive therapy, as well as the wider use of parenteral hyperalimentation and indwelling catheters (28,39).

CLINICAL FEATURES

Fungal infections of the spine are uncommon in children and the clinical presentation is often subtle. The relatively nonspecific nature of the physical findings and the difficulty children have in communicating their symptoms frequently results in a delayed diagnosis. A detailed history from the child and the parents is essential in the evaluation of a child with back pain. The patient and the family should be questioned about alterations in neurologic functions, including changes in bladder and bowel habits and gait pattern. The young child may present with back pain, abdominal pain, and difficulty in walking or standing. Primary involvement of the psoas muscle may present as a swelling over the flank, with a pronounced limp (8, 20,23,43). In children, a mass in the right flank may mimic an inflamed appendix, and an inadequate clinical evaluation may result in unnecessary surgery and a delay in the diagnosis (18). The psoas abscess can present as a presacral mass or extend inferiorly beneath the inguinal ligament into the thigh. In the older child, the presenting features include back rigidity, muscle spasm, excessive lordosis, or scoliosis. The back rigidity results in loss of the normal spinal rhythm. The spine may be tender to palpation, and progression of symptoms from local back pain to root pain, weakness, and paralysis is typical of an epidural abscess (8). The neurologic examination should be thorough, although the sensory examination may not be reliable in young children. In addition, these children may have spasm, tightness of the hamstrings, or a positive straight-leg raising test. These infections are more common in patients who are immunocompromised due to CGD, malignancy, immunosuppressive therapy, rheumatoid arthritis, organ transplantation, steroid therapy, and AIDS. The relatively low virulence of fungal organisms and the debilitated state of the compromised host can mask the physical findings of fungal infections (8,35). In patients for whom

an antecedent *Candida* septicemia was documented, a striking delay was found between the septicemia and the onset of symptoms as well as the time of diagnosis. An average of 4.7 months elapsed between the septicemia and the time of definitive diagnosis by culture of the organism. Patients sought treatment for their back pain at an average of 5.3 months following the septicemia (1). *Aspergillus* osteomyelitis is a well-recognized, life-threatening infection in children who have CGD (21,23). In CGD of childhood, pulmonary aspergillosis involving the superior mediastinum may present with paraplegia due to contiguous involvement of the thoracic spine (45). Paraplegia may be due to mycotic spinal arachnoiditis or meningitis causing signs and symptoms of spinal cord neoplasm and is frequently associated with recent pregnancy, and the abuse of alcohol and narcotics (46). Mycotic thrombosis of the anterior spinal artery resulting in paraplegia due to *Aspergillus* has been reported in a formerly healthy patient (41).

Cryptococcosis presenting as a painful neck mass with weakness of the upper extremities due to contiguous involvement of the cervical spine may mimic tuberculosis (44). In areas where tuberculosis is endemic the fungal infection is normally due to secondary infection of a tuberculous cavitation and subsequent hematogenous spread to the spine (10,24). Depending on the extent of spinal involvement, these patients may have pain, deformity, and neurologic deficit and may present with concurrent tuberculosis and fungal infection (14). Very rarely isolated osseous involvement may occur in patients who are immunocompetent (11,15,20,52). CNS involvement often has an insidious onset characterized by headache and alteration in mental status (36). In addition, cough and hemoptysis following pulmonary invasion are common symptoms in patients with systemic involvement. Constitutional symptoms are nonspecific and include fever, weight loss, malaise, and fatigue (48).

RADIOGRAPHIC FEATURES

Young children may require sedation or general anesthesia to obtain an optimum evaluation of computed tomography (CT) and magnetic resonance imaging (MRI) studies. Adequate communication between the clinician and the radiologist is essential in establishing a diagnosis (15,27,43). The thoracic and lumbar spine are the most common regions involved (Fig. 1A, B). Children commonly develop discitis, and in the early stages of the infection the anteroposterior and lateral spinal radiographs may be normal (20). Radioisotope bone scanning is sensitive in detecting lesions not seen on conventional radiographs and is important in the diagnosis of occult lesions or multiple sites of involvement (8,27,43). In established infections, disc space narrowing may be accompanied by erosive changes in the end plates (Fig. 2A, B). The radiologic features are nonspecific and include single-body involvement with a permeative lesion resulting in a platyspondyly (Fig. 3A). In established infection the radiographs may reveal lytic lesions often mimicking malignancies or bacterial osteomyelitis. Fungal infection can also mimic spinal tuberculosis, with two adjacent bodies (Fig. 4A, B) being involved with narrowing of the disc space and a paraspinal abscess. The paraspinal soft-tissue swelling may be present with cystic lesions

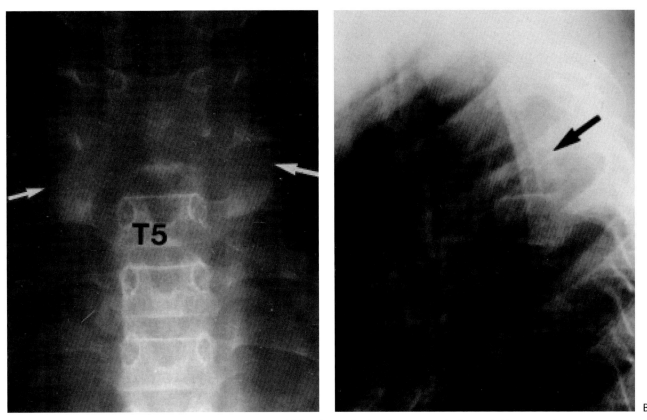

FIGURE 1. Anteroposterior **(A)** and lateral **(B)** radiographs showing a paraspinal mass *(white arrows)* and destruction of T4 *(black arrow)* in a 9-year-old child with paraplegia due to *Cryptococcus neoformans.*

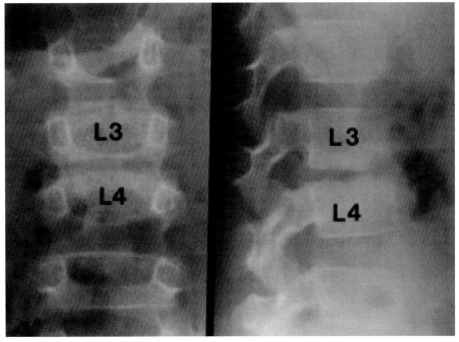

FIGURE 2. **A:** Disc space narrowing with irregular end plates (L3–4) in a 5-year-old child who presented with back pain. Three months prior to presentation the child sustained second-degree burns to the lower back. Closed-needle biopsy cultured *Candida albicans. (Figure continues.)*

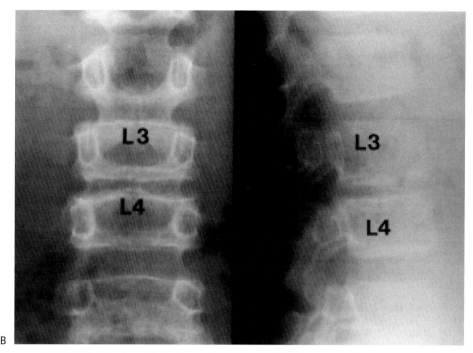

FIGURE 2. *Continued.* **B:** Radiographs at 15 months following antifungal treatment.

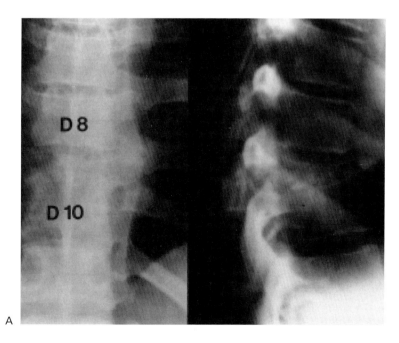

FIGURE 3. **A:** An 18-year-old girl developed paraplegia following collapse of D9 due to *Aspergillus fumigatus*. The patient had been treated for pulmonary tuberculosis 7 years previously. *(Figure continues.)*

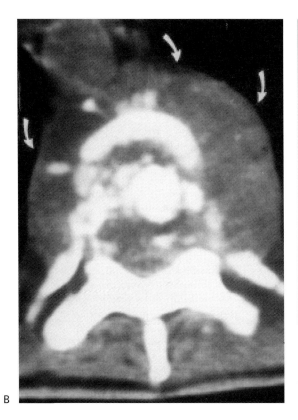

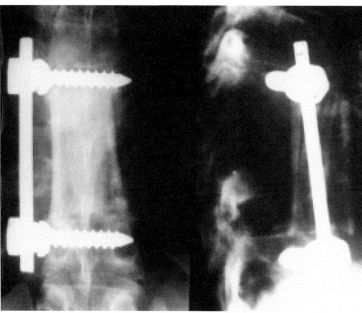

FIGURE 3. *Continued.* **B:** Computed tomography scan demonstrating paraspinal swelling *(white arrows)* with cord compression. **C:** Anterior spinal instrumentation with allograft at 27 months. There was complete neurologic recovery following surgical and antifungal treatment.

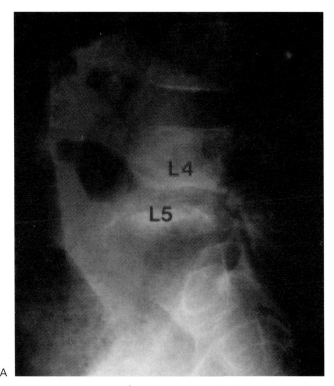

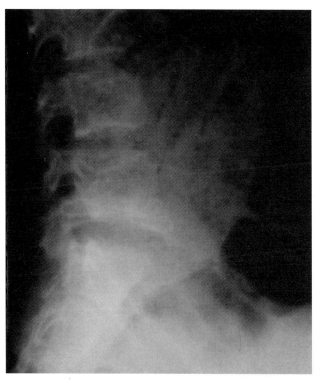

FIGURE 4. **A:** A 7-year-old child presented with low backache (L4–5), mass over left flank, and fixed-flexion deformity of the left hip. *Blastomyces dermatitides* was isolated following drainage of left psoas abscess and débridement of L4–5 disc space. **B:** Follow-up at 14 months following antifungal treatment.

surrounded by sclerosis. The lumbar spine could be involved secondarily, with infection tracking along the psoas muscle, resulting in scalloping of the vertebral bodies. Dissection under the anterior longitudinal ligament may cause seeding to other vertebral bodies and skip lesions without involvement of the disc space (20). Spinal involvement in the immunocompromised patients may be extensive, involving multiple bodies and resulting in kyphosis (25,34). Cryptococcal infection involving the posterior elements of the lumbar spine and mimicking sciatica have been reported (30). The plain roentgenograms of the spine may be normal in patients with arachnoiditis or meningitis and in patients with an extradural abscess (46).

Although the CT findings are nonspecific, they will define the extent of the lesions, provide information on the site of biopsy and aspiration, show evidence of extradural cord compression, and delineate the paraspinal soft-tissue mass (Fig. 3B). Gadolinium-enhanced MRI is useful in delineating the extent of the epidural abscess, facilitating the differentiation between solid inflammatory tissue and abscesses, and highlighting cases of paraplegia due to arachnoiditis and meningitis in which the conventional radiographs may be normal. In addition, gadolinium-enhanced MRI increases observer confidence in the diagnosis of disc space infection and osteomyelitis in patients with equivocal noncontrast MRI (40,42,43). The enhanced scans may differentiate active infections from those that responded adequately to medical treatment. The CT and MRI features of fungal infections are nonspecific and may mimic those of other granulomatous diseases, such as tuberculosis and brucellosis. Biopsy and culture are essential to establishing the diagnosis (42). The chest radiograph may show active pulmonary involvement or a healed focus of tuberculosis.

DIAGNOSTIC TESTS

To avoid contamination all biopsy material should be placed in sterile containers for laboratory examination. The fungus should be demonstrated microscopically in clinical material, cultured repeatedly from clinical specimens, and if possible confirmed by serologic tests (6).

Cryptococcus is readily seen in India ink mounts of the material as round to oval, thin-walled, budding cells ranging from 5 to 20 μm in diameter (6,10). The organisms are usually surrounded by wide, refractile, polysaccharide, gelatinous capsules. The yeast can be cultured on Sabouraud glucose agar at room temperature, and in tissue sections the organism can be demonstrated with hematoxylin-eosin (H&E) stain. Serologic tests for cryptococcal antibodies include indirect fluorescent antibody (IFA) techniques, enzyme immunoassay (EIA), and tube agglutination (TA). Procedures for detecting cryptococcal antigens are the latex agglutination (LA) test and enzyme immunoassay (EIA) tests. The antibody tests are useful in the detection of either early or localized cryptococcosis and to determine prognosis (6). However, the LA test is very specific and of diagnostic and prognostic value, and is useful in detecting cryptococcal antigens in the sera and cerebrospinal fluid. A titer of 1:4 or lower is suggestive of cryptococcal infection, but titers of 8 or more are indicative of acute cryptococcosis (35). Cryptococcal antigens were not detected in the cerebrospinal fluid and sera in an immunocompetent child with cryptococcal osteomyelitis (19). A commercially developed DNA probe is useful for easy, rapid, and accurate identification of this encapsulated yeast from a primary culture (6).

Microscopically, aspergilli appear as fragments of dichotomously branched septate hyphae 4 to 6 μm in diameter. Colonies can be isolated readily on Sabouraud glucose agar at 30°C to 37°C (6,10). The immunodiffusion (ID) test is an effective and specific method for the diagnosis of aspergillosis in patients with an intact immune system. In patients suspected of having invasive aspergillosis with serum negative for antibody, counter-immunoelectrophoresis (CIE) and radioimmunoassay (RIA) should be performed (6).

Wet mounts of *Candida* in 10% KOH show small, oval, thin-walled, budding cells, and the pseudohyphae are 2 to 6 μm in diameter (6,10). Colonies of *C. albicans* on Sabouraud glucose agar are cream-colored, smooth, and glistening and have a yeasty odor. The addition of penicillin and streptomycin or chloramphenicol to the medium reduces contamination in the cultures (6). LA, ID, and CIE are useful in detecting antibodies to *Candida* species in the sera of immunocompromised patients. A titer of 1:8 or greater by LA is diagnostic of systemic candidiasis (6).

Coccidioides can be cultured in Sabouraud glucose agar or blood agar. It appears as round, refractile, thick-walled spherules 20 to 80 μm in diameter, and with many small endospores (10,49). The culture develops into moist, membranous, gray colonies that later produce abundant white mycelia (6). The coccidioidin skin test is of limited diagnostic value but is of considerable importance in epidemiologic studies (27). The immunodiffusion complement test detects IgG antibodies, and a titer of 1:16 is significantly associated with the presence of extrapulmonary lesions (6,27). The test could be used to follow the progress of the disease. The sensitivity and specificity for *Coccidioides immitis* is 99% and 100%, respectively with commercially available gene probes (6).

Blastomycosis can be identified as a dimorphic fungus by its typical "shoe print" morphology with the periodic acid–Schiff (PAS) stain (9). In uncertain culture results, more sensitive serologic techniques and DNA probes have significantly improved the sensitivity of laboratory diagnosis (2,3,6).

Sputum examination is essential in patients with a cough and in those with radiologic evidence of pulmonary involvement. Anemia and a decreased lymphocyte and neutrophil count are frequently observed in immunocompromised patients. The erythrocyte sedimentation rate (ESR), though nonspecific, is frequently raised. The liver function is usually deranged, and the albumin levels are often less than 30 g % in most immunocompromised patients. Blood cultures are essential in patients presenting with fever.

NATURAL HISTORY

Isolated osteomyelitis due to fungal infections may occur without evidence of systemic disease and in the absence of a detectable underlying disorder (5,7,9,11,18). The prognosis is good in patients who have localized infections without gross pulmonary involvement (19,27). Patients with clinical features of AIDS and other immunosuppressive disorders develop a fulminating fungal infection and die (8,21,35). Meningitis is the most common cause of death in patients with disseminated cryptococcal infection (35). Tack et al. (47) concluded that isolated fungal infections are due to silent dissemination from a pulmonary source that had not been established. They found that the difference in survival rates between compromised and immunologically competent patients was statistically significant ($p < 0.00025$, ψ^2). The presence of an underlying immunosuppressed state correlates highly with the ultimate survival rate. In children with CGD, spinal involvement due to aspergillosis is usually a result of contiguous spread from an adjacent pulmonary focus, and the prognosis in these patients is poor (23,38,51).

TREATMENT RECOMMENDATIONS

Fungal infections should be included in the differential diagnosis of spondylitis, especially in immunocompromised patients, those with CGD of childhood, and those who spent time in places where tuberculosis is endemic (8,35). The rising prevalence of human immunodeficiency virus (HIV) and intravenous drug abuse has increased the awareness and concern for the diagnosis and treatment of spinal infections in the immunocompromised host. The delay in diagnosis and treatment, especially in children, is commonly due to the insidious presentation of physical signs and symptoms of the disease. This diagnostic delay may create a more complex problem and a difficult solution because the disease may be well advanced at the time of initial diagnosis (18,20). Malnutrition, which is frequently associated with immunodeficiencies, is due to a decrease in the number of circulating T cells with impaired lymphokine production (8). In patients with no obvious underlying predisposing factors an immunologic survey is essential to exclude immunodeficiency (26). Children with CGD should have supportive immunotherapy to control and prevent fungal infections (23). Patients undergoing major decompressive and reconstructive surgery of the spine require adequate nutritional support prior to surgery because postoperative morbidity is significantly increased in malnourished patients (8).

SURGICAL TREATMENT

In patients who are neurologically intact, tissue diagnosis can be obtained by a needle biopsy using the CT-guided technique or with fluoroscopy. Percutaneous CT-guided technique is recommended for drainage of a psoas abscess for both diagnostic and therapeutic reasons (27,40). Open biopsy is indicated in all patients who have neurologic deficit or painful deformity, those whose histologic examination following the needle biopsy is inconclusive, those who are not improving on antifungal medication, and those who relapse after initial improvement (47). Adequate tissue samples for diagnostic purposes in children with lesions involving the cervical and upper thoracic spine are best obtained from an open biopsy. Because the vertebral bodies are commonly involved, an anterior approach is advocated to allow

for thorough debridement and provide adequate tissue samples for histologic diagnosis. In patients who are compromised neurologically it is essential to perform a meticulous decompression of the spinal cord that is compressed by exuberant granulation tissue, sequestra, and disc (15). Tissue diagnosis is essential because the granulomatous tissue may resemble that of tuberculosis, although granulation tissue in cryptococcosis and aspergillosis has a slimy consistency. Antituberculosis medication has been administered to patients on the basis of clinical evaluation alone and following an inadequate survey of biopsy samples (18). In children, rib grafts, iliac crest grafts, and allografts have been successfully used in attempts to reconstitute the anterior column (Fig. 3C) (15,17). In children with CGD, surgical débridement of *Aspergillus* vertebral osteomyelitis is difficult due to the contiguous pulmonary lesion. Multiple surgical procedures have been performed in these patients using bone grafts and instrumentation for stabilization of the spine (12,38,45). Peripheral and posterior abscesses of the lung should be treated aggressively both medically and with operative debridement to prevent extension to the spine. Surgical treatment (debridement, radical excision) without antifungal agents has been successful with isolated lesions in immunocompetent patients, avoiding the potential side effects associated with antifungal medication (11,16). In young children with multiple vertebral involvement due to blastomycosis, a satisfactory outcome followed aspiration and drug therapy (20). In skeletal coccidioidomycosis it is now well accepted that surgical débridement is mandatory, as the results following surgical débridement and medical therapy are significantly better than the results of medical therapy alone (27). A delay in the diagnosis of more than 1 month increased the recurrence, which required further surgical intervention. Posterior spinal decompression is recommended when draining an epidural abscess and in lesions involving the posterior elements (29). In the immunocompromised patient, additional spinal stabilization with instrumentation may be necessary to promote fusion and facilitate rehabilitation (45). Following transthoracic procedures in children, it is essential that adequate postoperative analgesia and chest physiotherapy be implemented to prevent potential pulmonary complications (15).

MEDICAL TREATMENT

Once the diagnosis is confirmed by microscopy, culture, and serologic testing, the immunocompetent patient's status should be reassessed to confirm or exclude the presence of an underlying disorder (19,20). The infective process should be monitored clinically, radiologically, and by serial serology during treatment.

The antifungal agents amphotericin B and flucytosine, which work synergistically, have been recommended for treatment of aspergillosis candidiasis, cryptococcosis, blastomycosis, and coccidioidomycosis (35). The recommended daily dosage of amphotericin B, which is given intravenously, ranges from 0.25 mg/kg to 0.7 mg/kg and flucytosine (200 to 400 mg/kg) is administered orally. Amphotericin B combines with sterols in the plasma membrane, resulting in an increase in permeability and cell death. The intravenous route is recommended, as absorption is negligible following oral administration. Fungal cells are susceptible if they convert flucytosine to fluorouracil, which inhibits DNA synthesis (11,16,22,50). It is important to monitor the full blood count and liver and renal functions, as amphotericin B depresses bone marrow function and is toxic to the liver and kidneys. Other potential side effects include alopecia, vomiting, and diarrhea. The duration of medical treatment is unknown and must be individualized with respect to side effects and therapeutic response (47), and the drug is temporarily discontinued when side effects occur. Amphotericin B remains the initial drug of choice for patients who are severely ill, have life-threatening disease, or have CNS involvement (8).

Due to the poor oral absorption and toxic side effects of amphotericin B, antifungal imidazoles and triazoles have been introduced. The synthetic antifungal imidazoles and triazoles (ketoconazole, fluconazole, and itraconazole) inhibit fungal growth by blocking the biosynthesis of fungal lipids, especially ergosterol, in cell membranes (13,22,35,50). Fluconazole is well absorbed from the gastrointestinal tract and diffuses readily into body fluids, including cerebrospinal fluid and saliva. Concentrations in cerebrospinal fluid are 50% to 90% of simultaneous values in plasma following a daily oral dose of 100 to 400 mg. Apart from being administered orally, these drugs have been shown to have a good blood-brain barrier and are effective in AIDS patients with meningitis (8).

Amphotericin B has been shown to be the most effective agent in the treatment of musculoskeletal coccidioidomycosis and blastomycosis. Generally up to a cumulative dose of 1 g is given, and further therapy may be completed with an oral azole agent (27). Satisfactory results were obtained with intravenous intraconazole for 7 days (200 mg twice daily for 2 days and then once daily followed by oral administration for 6 months). Combination therapy of an antifungal agent and surgical debridement of involved bone and joint has been significantly more effective than medical treatment alone (7). The treatment is monitored by serial evaluation of complement fixation titers. The treatment is continued until the titers fall below a ratio of 1:8. The titers are more accurate than sedimentation rates and white cell counts in following the disease progress and treatment response (27). Vertebral osteomyelitis in children with CGD is usually due to aspergillosis. Unfortunately, despite aggressive medical and surgical therapy, reported cases have been associated with treatment failure, recurrence, severe neurologic complications, and death (21,38,51). Reports have suggested the beneficial effects of granulocyte transfusions in patients with aspergillosis that did not respond to antifungal therapy (23). However, Cohen et al. (12) were unable to demonstrate a significant reduction in the rate of infection in CGD patients treated with granulocyte infusions as an adjunct to antifungal chemotherapy for disseminated infection. In a controlled clinical trial recombinant interferon-γ was found to reduce the frequency of serious infections in patients with CGD. Recombinant interferon-γ can augment the ability of CGD neutrophils to destroy *Aspergillus* hyphae in vitro (23).

Ambisome, a liposomal formulation of amphotericin B, has been used to treat aspergillosis, candidiasis, and cryptococcal infections refractory to amphotericin B (35). Early initiation of high-dose Ambisone therapy should be considered in patients with CGD and *Aspergillus* osteomyelitis of the spine (23). Treat-

ment should be administered for 6 months or longer. Because of the risk of recurrence, a long-term treatment regimen with an oral antifungal agent should be prescribed. In the neutropenic patient with fungal infection, the administration of cytokines such as granulocyte-monocyte colony-stimulating factor (GM-CSF) and granulocyte colony-stimulating factor (G-CSF) has reduced the degree and duration of neutropenia (23).

Prevention of fungal infections should be a high priority in the management of all at-risk patients in a hospital environment (33). In candidiasis it is important not to disturb the resident flora by limiting the use of broad-spectrum antibiotics (28). People visiting endemic areas where blastomycosis and coccidioidomycosis is common should be counseled for possible pulmonary infection.

SUMMARY

The history must be thorough with respect to the endemic area of exposure and the state of immunocompromise. Immunocompromised patients with HIV, history of intravenous drug abuse, organ transplantation, long-term steroid treatment, diabetes, and CGDs are prone to develop fungal infections. Decreased host immune response and the paucity of signs and symptoms in younger children may lead to a delayed diagnosis of spinal infections. With a timely diagnosis and appropriate treatment, the outcome of extrapulmonary fungal infection in the immunocompetent host is usually excellent, though some fatalities do occur. The physical examination should emphasize identification of pulmonary and additional foci. The overriding symptoms of back pain, radiculopathy, myelopathy, and sensory loss may accompany local pain and tenderness. Radiologic evaluation, including radioisotope bone scanning, CT, and MRI, is invaluable in planning treatment. The mainstays of treatment are identification of the responsible pathogen and implementation of appropriate medical and surgical treatment.

REFERENCES

1. Almekinders LC, Greene WB (1991): Vertebral *Candida* infections. A case report and review of the literature. *Clin Orthop* 267:174–178.
2. Areno JP, Campbell GD Jr, George RB (1997): Diagnosis of blastomycosis. *Semin Respir Infect* 12:252–262.
3. Basset FH, Tindall JP (1972): Blastomycosis of bone. *S Med J* 65:547–555.
4. Baumgardner DJ, Buggy BP, Mattson BJ, et al. (1992): Epidemiology of blastomycosis in a region of high endemicity in North Central Wisconsin. *Clin Infect Dis* 15:629–635.
5. Behrman RE, Masci JR, Nicholas P (1990): Cryptococcal skeletal infections: case report and review. *Rev Infect Dis* 12:181–190.
6. Beneke ES, Rogers AL, eds (1996): *Medical mycology and human mycoses.* California: Star Publishing Company.
7. Bried JM, Galgiani JN (1986): *Coccidioides immitis* infections in bones and joints. *Clin Orthop* 211:235–243.
8. Broner FA, Garland DE, Zigler JE (1996): Spinal infections in the immunocompromised host. *Orthop Clin N Am* 27:37–46.
9. Chao D, Steier KJ, Gomila R (1997): Update and review of Blastomycosis. *J Am Osteopath Assoc* 97:525–532.
10. Chandler RW, Kaplan W, Ajello L, eds (1980): *A colour atlas and textbook of the histopathology of mycotic diseases.* Ilsted, Netherlands: Wolfe Medical Publications.

11. Chleboun J, Nade S (1977): Skeletal cryptococcosis. *J Bone Joint Surg Am* 59:509–514.

12. Cohen MS, Isturiz RE, Malech HL, et al. (1981): Fungal infection in chronic granulomatous disease. *Am J Med* 71:59–66.

13. Dismukes WE, Bradsher RW, Cloud GA, et al. (1992): Itraconazole therapy for blastomycosis and histoplasmosis. *Am J Med* 93:489–497.

14. Govender S, Charles RW (1987): Cryptococcal infection of the spine. A case report. *S Afr Med J* 71:782–783.

15. Govender S, Rajoo R, Goga IE, et al. (1991): *Aspergillus* osteomyelitis of the spine. *Spine* 16:746–749.

16. Govender S, Ganpath V, Charles RW, et al. (1988): Localized osseous cryptococcal infection: report of 2 cases. *Acta Orthop Scand* 59: 720–722.

17. Govender S, Parbhoo AH (1999): Support of the anterior column with allografts in tuberculosis of the spine. *J Bone Joint Surg Br* 81:106–109.

18. Guler N, Palanduz A, Ones U, et al. (1995): Progressive vertebral blastomycosis mimicking tuberculosis. *Pediatr Infect Dis* 14:816–818.

19. Hammerschlag MR, Domingo J, Haller JO, et al. (1981): Cryptococcal osteomyelitis: report of a case and a review of the literature. *Clin Pediatr* 21:109–112.

20. Hardjasudarma M, Willis B, Black-Payne C, et al. (1995) Pediatric spinal blastomycosis: case report. *Neurosurgery* 37:534–536.

21. Heinrich SD, Finney T, Craver R, et al. (1991): *Aspergillus* osteomyelitis in patients who have chronic granulomatous disease. Case report. *J Bone Joint Surg Am* 73:456–460.

22. Hoeprich PD (1994): Cryptococcosis. In: Hoeprich PD, Jordan C, Ronald AR, eds. *Infectious diseases.* Philadelphia: Lippincott-Raven Publishers, pp. 1132–1140.

23. Kline MW, Bocobo FC, Paul ME, Rosenblatt, et al. (1993): Successful medical therapy of *Aspergillus* osteomyelitis of the spine in an 11-year-old boy with chronic granulomatous disease. *Pediatrics* 5:830–835.

24. Korovessis P, Repanti M, Katsandis T, et al. (1994): Anterior decompression and fusion for *Aspergillus* osteomyelitis of the lumbar spine associated with paraparesis. *Spine* 19:2715–2718.

25. Kromminga R, Staib F, Thalmann U, et al. (1999): Osteomyelitis due to *Cryptococcus neoformans* in advanced age. Case report and review of literature. *Mycoses* 33:157–166.

26. Kumlin U, Elmqvist LG, Granlund M, et al. (1997): CD4 lymphopenia in a patient with cryptococcal osteomyelitis. *Scand J Infect Dis* 29: 205–206.

27. Kushwaha VP, Shaw BA, Gerardi JA, et al. (1996): Musculoskeletal coccidioidomycosis: a review of 25 cases. *Clin Orthop* 332:190–199.

28. Lafont A, Olive M, Gelman M, et al. (1994): *Candida albicans* spondylodiscitis and vertebral osteomyelitis with intravenous heroin drug addiction. Report of 3 new cases. *J Rheumatol* 15:953–956.

29. Lie KW, Yu YL, Cheng IK, et al. (1989): Cryptococcal infection of the lumbar spine. *J R Soc Med* 82:172–173.

30. Litvinoff J, Nelson M (1978): Extradural lumbar cryptococcosis. Case report. *J Neurosurg* 49:921–923.

31. Liu PY (1998): Cryptococcal osteomyelitis: case report and review. *Diag Microbiol Infect Dis* 30:33–35.

32. MacDonald PB, Black GB, MacKenzie R (1990): Orthopaedic manifestations of blastomycosis. *J Bone Joint Surg Am* 72:860–864.

33. Manuel JR, Kibbler CC (1998): The epidemiology and prevention of invasive aspergillosis. *J Hosp Infect* 39:95–109.

34. Matsushita T, Suzuki K (1985): Spastic paraparesis due to cryptococcal osteomyelitis: a case report. *Clin Orthop* 196:279–284.

35. Minamoto GY, Rosenberg AS (1997): Fungal infections in patients with acquired immunodeficiency syndrome. *Med Clin N Am* 81: 381–409.

36. Mitchell DH, Sorrell TC, Allworth AM, et al. (1995): Cryptococcal disease of the CNS in immunocompetent hosts: influence of cryptococcal variety on clinical manifestations and outcome. *Clin Infect Dis* 20: 611–616.

37. Moore RM, Green NE (1982): Blastomycosis of bone: a report of six cases. *J Bone Joint Surg Am* 64:1097–1101.

38. Mouy R, Fischer A, Vilmer E, et al. (1989): Incidence, severity and prevention of infections in chronic granulomatous disease. *Pediatrics* 114:555–560.

39. Mullins RF, Still JM, Savage J, et al. (1993): Osteomyelitis of the spine in a burn patient due to *Candida albicans.* *Burns* 19:174–176.

40. Olson EM, Duberg AC, Herron LD, et al. (1998): Coccidioidal spondylitis: MR findings in 15 patients. *Am J Roentgenol* 171:785–789.

41. Pfausler B, Kampfl A, Berek K, et al. (1995): Syndrome of the anterior spinal artery as the primary manifestation of aspergillosis. *Infection* 23: 240–244.

42. Post MJ, Sze G, Quencer RM, et al. (1990): Gadolinium-enhanced MR in spinal infection. *J Comp Assist Tomogr* 14:721–729.

43. Saccente M, Abernathy RS, Paas PG, et al. (1998): Vertebral blastomycosis with paravertebral abscess: report of eight cases and review of the literature. *Clin Infect Dis* 26:413–418.

44. Schmidt DM, Kevorkian KF, Sercarz JA, et al. (1995): Cryptococcosis presenting as a neck mass. *Ann Otol Rhinol Laryngol* 104:711–714.

45. Sponseller PD, Malech HL, McCarthy EF Jr, et al. (1991): Skeletal involvement in children who have chronic granulomatous disease. *J Bone Joint Surg Am* 73:37–51.

46. Stein SC, Corrado ML, Friedlander M (1982): Chronic mycotic meningitis with spinal involvement: a report of five cases. *Ann Neurol* 11: 519–524.

47. Tack KJ, Rhame FS, Brown B, et al. (1982): *Aspergillus* osteomyelitis: report of four cases and review of the literature. *Am J Med* 73:295–300.

48. Thomas GM (1992): Blastomycosis. In: Feigin RD, Cherry JD, eds. *Textbook of pediatric infectious diseases.* Philadelphia: WB Saunders, pp. 1898–1906.

49. Von Lichtenberg F, ed. (1991): *Pathology of infectious diseases.* New York: Raven Press.

50. Walsh TJ, Pizzo PA (1994): Aspergillosis. In: Hoeprich PD, Jordan C, Ronald AR, eds. *Infectious diseases.* Philadelphia: Lippincott-Raven Publishers, pp. 541–547.

51. White CJ, Kwon-Chung KJ, Gallin JI (1988): Chronic granulomatous disease of childhood: an unusual case of infection with *Aspergillus nidulans* var. *echinulatus*. *Am J Clin Pediatr* 90:312–316.

52. Zach T, Penn RG (1986): Localized cryptococcal osteomyelitis in an immunocompetent host. *Pediatr Infect Dis* 5:601–603.

RHEUMATIC DISEASES

MARY D. MOORE

The term *rheumatic diseases* refers to a diverse group of inflammatory conditions primarily involving the peripheral joints and axial skeleton. With the exception of cervical spine disease in juvenile rheumatoid arthritis (JRA), spinal involvement is much less common in the childhood rheumatic diseases than in the adult rheumatic diseases. Spinal disease may be present at onset but more commonly develops during the course of the illness, often years later. The two most common childhood rheumatic conditions with spinal involvement are JRA and the spondyloarthropathies. Both of these conditions will be described in greater detail in this chapter. JRA usually involves only the cervical spine, whereas the spinal involvement in the spondyloarthropathies usually starts in the lumbar sacral spine and sacroiliac joints, and involvement of the cervical and thoracic spine occurs decades after onset.

Primary involvement of the spine is not typical in the other rheumatic diseases of childhood. However, spinal involvement may occur as a complication of the disease process or its treatment. Many of the rheumatic diseases are characterized by decreased bone mineral content with the problem of osteoporosis and the secondary complication of vertebral stress fractures. Back pain can be a presenting symptom of nonrheumatic conditions (e.g., malignancy), chronic pain syndromes, as well as referred pain from abdominal or renal diseases. The child who presents with nonorganic back pain can be a diagnostic challenge. It is important to identify those children early to avoid putting the child through an extensive and unnecessary evaluation and to focus on symptom control and return to school and normal functioning.

In evaluating all children with rheumatic complaints, the importance of a detailed history and physical examination, including a comprehensive family history, cannot be overemphasized. The working impression from the history and examination will greatly assist in the development of a well-considered, logical, and appropriate diagnostic and treatment plan. General goals of management include determination of the patient's diagnosis, control of pain, prevention of disability, adequate rest, and appropriate exercise. The family and child need to be educated in terms of the disease process, its treatment, and a realistic assessment of disease outcome.

JUVENILE RHEUMATOID ARTHRITIS

JRA encompasses a heterogeneous group of idiopathic disorders, the hallmark of which is chronic synovitis, predominantly of peripheral joints. JRA refers to children under 16 years old; this age distinction is somewhat arbitrary, as adult rheumatoid arthritis (RA) can present in children, particularly in older female adolescents. The American College of Rheumatology has established classification criteria for a diagnosis of JRA. JRA is further subdivided into three main subtypes: systemic onset, polyarticular (more than five affected joints), and pauciarticular (four or fewer joints). JRA subtypes are based on the clinical course 6 months after onset (9,25). The different subtypes and the major distinctions between the JRA subtypes and spondyloarthropathy are summarized in Table 1. Some U.S. pediatric rheumatology centers further divide the subtypes based on the results of serologic studies and the presence or absence of the histocompatibility locus antigen B27 (HLA-B27). The American College of Rheumatology classification is used extensively in North and South America. European investigators use the criteria of the European League Against Rheumatism, which reserve the term "rheumatoid" for children with a positive serum rheumatoid factor (37).

Epidemiologic and Etiologic Factors

In the United States and Europe, JRA occurs in approximately 1 to 22 per 100,000 children, with an estimated prevalence of 86.1 per 100,000, of which half would represent inactive cases (14,27). Epidemiologic studies of JRA have been mainly descriptive and are further complicated by the differences in diagnostic criteria, the marked heterogeneity in disease expression, as well as the inability to identify specific etiologic agents (14). Despite major advances in understanding of the inflammatory response, the cause of most rheumatic diseases remains unknown. Stress, infection, and trauma can all play a role in triggering the onset of arthritis, as well as causing exacerbations of existing disease. However, the actual contribution of each factor is not known. Genetic factors also contribute to development of JRA, but the association is much less consistent than the strong association of HLA-B27 in the spondyloarthropathies (17).

JRA probably encompasses several diseases of differing causes. In addition, other types of inflammatory arthritis, such as reactive arthritis and Lyme arthritis, can be difficult to distinguish from pauciarticular JRA. Another difficulty is that inflammatory

M. D. Moore: Department of Pediatrics, University of Iowa, Iowa City, Iowa 52246.

TABLE 1. OVERVIEW OF JUVENILE RHEUMATOID ARTHRITIS AND SPONDYLOARTHROPATHY

Factor	Systemic	Pauciarticular	Polyarticular	Spondyloarthropathy
Gender	M=F	F>>M	F>M	M>>F
Age of onset (yr)	1–6	1–4	1–8	8–18
Laboratory studies				
Rheumatoid factor	−	−	+	−
Antinuclear antibody	−	+++	++	−
HLA B27	−		−	+++
Sites of joint disease				
Peripheral arthritis	+++	++	+++	+
Cervical spine	+	−	+	−
Lumbosocral spine/sacroiliac disease	−	−	−	++
Extraarticular manifestations				
Chronic iritis	−	+++	+	−
Acute iritis	−	−	−	+
Fever, weight loss, leukocytosis	++	−	+	−
Rashes	+++	−	−	++

−, not found; +, occasional; ++, frequent; +++, often.

conditions evolve over time, and it might be decades later that another rheumatic disease becomes evident. The typical example of this process would be a young boy diagnosed as having pauciarticular JRA who develops typical spinal involvement, intestinal disease, or psoriasis in adult life and is then correctly diagnosed as having a spondyloarthropathy.

Clinical Features of Cervical Spine Disease

The typical child with JRA will be a preschool-age girl who presents with an asymmetrical pauciarthritis. Pain will be mild; most children are identified by persistent swelling, limp, and/or contracture of peripheral joints. Morning stiffness may be prominent, and joint symptoms typically improve later in the day. Arthritis is often in the large joints of the lower extremities. Occasionally, children present with abrupt onset of inflammatory arthritis and fever, but the initial presentation is usually more indolent. Physical examination shows inflammatory arthritis. Joints are not usually red; pain and tenderness are mild to moderate. Acute phase reactants, such as the erythrocyte sedimentation rate (ESR) and C-reactive protein, will be mildly elevated. The peripheral white blood cell count may be elevated, and the child may have a mild anemia. However, these blood tests often are completely normal. Synovial fluid will show inflammatory fluid, with cell counts ranging from 1,000 to 50,000 cells per mm³. On serologic testing, many JRA patients, especially those with pauciarticular JRA, have a low titer of antinuclear antibody (ANA). However, in contrast to adult RA, rheumatoid factor is present in only 10% of JRA cases overall. Children with systemic JRA (also called Still disease) present with systemic signs and symptoms, such as rash, fever, lymphadenopathy, serositis, leukocytosis, and marked increases in acute-phase reactants, and may be quite ill at presentation (9,20,46,55).

Cervical spine disease is common in JRA and occurs in 50% to 60% of children with polyarticular and systemic disease. Cervical spine disease is virtually absent in children who have a pauciarticular course (9,22). Rarely, cervical spine disease can be the sole initial presentation of JRA; and the child will subsequently develop signs of peripheral arthritis. Usually, however, peripheral arthritis presents first and the cervical spine disease appears later in the clinical course (52). Although cervical spine involvement is more common in JRA than in RA, complaints of neck pain and serious complications are less common in JRA than in RA (47). Isolated cervical spine arthritis is extremely rare in JRA, and careful evaluation will reveal involvement of other joints. The child with cervical spine involvement may present initially with torticollis, although the usual presenting complaint is stiff neck (especially in the morning) and decreased neck motion on examination (52). Thoracic or lumbosacral spinal involvement is extremely uncommon in JRA and would represent another disease, a complication from therapy of concurrent osteoporosis, or an overuse syndrome triggered by arthritis at other sites. Cervical spine complications can include fractures, erosions, subaxial subluxation, and atlantoaxial subluxation (which can lead to basilar invagination), resulting in neurologic impingement (Fig. 1). Rare spinal complications of JRA include spinal lipomatosis, developing as a complication of increased weight gain from glucocorticoid use (2) and rotary subluxation of the cervical spine (44).

Severe complications are rare in JRA cervical spine disease but should be watched for, especially in systemic or polyarticular JRA patients with severe and/or advanced disease in peripheral joints. Any history of neck pain, neurologic symptoms, or trauma to the neck (even relatively trivial injury) should be taken seriously in these patients, as they are at higher risk of fracture or dislocation resulting from concurrent osteopenia or ligamentous damage resulting from chronic inflammation. Pain and neurologic symptoms may be subtle and overlooked, particularly if the child has significant underlying inflammatory arthritis and concomitant pain. In the evaluation of suspected neurologic compromise, the child and parent should be specifically questioned about trauma, subjective weakness, gait changes, or urinary retention or incontinence. The child should be examined carefully for signs of myelopathy. Red flags would include persistent torticollis, progressive or acute paresis, weakness, spasticity,

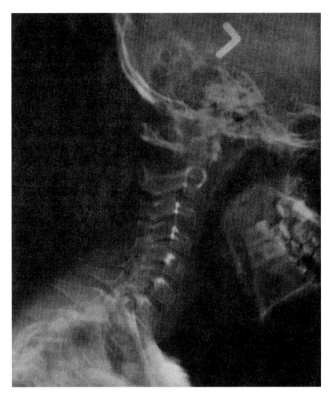

FIGURE 1. Anterior subluxation of C2 on C3 in an 11-year-old girl with seronegative polyarticular juvenile rheumatoid arthritis.

sensory loss, bladder symptoms, change in deep-tendon reflexes, or incoordination, and would call for immediate assessment (39). Plain radiographs should be obtained, followed by computed tomography (CT) or magnetic resonance imaging (MRI) as indicated (21).

Radiographic Features

Standard radiographs are normal at onset of JRA joint disease. Typical destructive changes may take years to develop or not develop at all. Radiographs are obtained at onset for baseline studies for comparison and, more importantly, to rule out other causes of the articular symptoms. The first evident radiographic changes are soft-tissue swelling and juxtaarticular osteoporosis, followed by bone erosion and, later, loss of articular cartilage, decreased joint space, and bone destruction. A distinct feature in the developing child is regional overgrowth or undergrowth in joints with persistent disease. The most common example of this feature is a leg length discrepancy in a child with pauciarticular JRA of one knee. The chronic inflammatory process and increased blood flow in synovial tissue leads to advanced bone maturation, with the result that the involved leg is longer than the uninvolved extremity (9,25,30).

The most common radiographic findings of cervical spine disease in JRA are calcification of the anterior aspect of the first cervical vertebra, anterior erosion of the odontoid, and ankylosis of the apophyseal joint. Other radiographic features include growth disturbances of the vertebral bodies, spondylitis of the

cervical spine, and micrognathia (22). To evaluate children for cervical spine disease or for preoperative assessment of the neck, the child should have routine anteroposterior, open-mouth, lateral, and extension-flexion radiographs of the cervical spine. Radiographic findings in advanced disease may include osteoporosis, abnormalities of the cervical curves, and erosion of vertebral end plates. This may be followed by spondylitis, vertebral subluxation, and destructive arthritis of the apophyseal joints with ankylosis (Fig. 2) (22,47,52). To evaluate for neurologic impingement or cervical spine fractures, radionuclide scanning or MRI can be particularly useful (21).

Natural History

The hallmark of the rheumatic diseases is inflammation of synovial tissue. There is a marked increase in macrophages and T lymphocytes, local production of inflammatory mediators, recruitment of neutrophils into the joint space leading to synovial hypertrophy, increased vascularity, and joint fluid secretion. Over time, the inflammatory process extends from the synovium, with local invasion of cartilage followed by erosion of bone. If inflammation does not remit or cannot be controlled by treatment, the final result may be end-stage joint damage and ankylosis (9,20,22,25,46,55).

The inflammatory process in the cervical spine is similar to that in the peripheral joints. The normal cervical spine has 32 synovial articulations. There is a synovial-lined bursa between the odontoid process and the transverse ligament. The three most common lesions that result in cervical instability are atlantoaxial subluxation, basilar invagination, and subaxial subluxa-

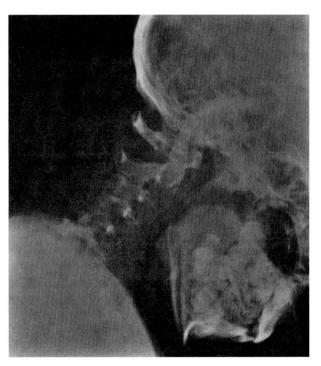

FIGURE 2. Fusion of C2–C3 in the cervical spine of an 8-year-old boy with systemic-onset juvenile rheumatoid arthritis.

tion, or a combination. Expansion from synovitis may lead to distention and finally to rupture of the transverse ligament or to odontoid fracture, resulting in cervical instability; the atlas then slides anteriorly, and atlanto-axial subluxation is considered when the distance between the odontoid process and the anterior arch of the atlas in adults exceeds 4 mm. However, in children, the atlantoaxial distance is longer (up to 4 to 4.5 mm) (39,47,52). Although cervical spine involvement is more common in JRA than in adult RA, the children have less pain and a much lower incidence of neurologic involvement and complications (22). Overall, in adult RA, subaxial subluxation occurs in 20% to 25% of patients, with neurologic progression in up to one third of untreated patients (39).

The natural course of JRA is extremely variable. However, most children do well with early recognition and management. Remission rates vary from 26% to 65%, and severe disability occurs in 20% to 45%. This marked variation in outcome is due to differences in clinical criteria, length of follow-up, and types of treatment. Children with pauciarticular JRA do best, although this subtype is at high risk of inflammatory eye disease, with the additional risk of severe vision loss or even blindness if untreated. Those with the most severe outcome are systemic JRA patients with persistent polyarthritis and patients who have positive rheumatoid factor. Chronic inflammatory arthritis of more than 5 years duration is also predictive of more severe disability (9,13,20,46). An important consideration is that children initially diagnosed with JRA may be rediagnosed years later with a different rheumatic disease; this was seen in one series in 22% of JRA patients followed for decades, and most of those children were ultimately diagnosed with spondyloarthropathy (18).

Treatment Recommendations

All children with JRA need an individualized treatment plan and should be managed by a practitioner skilled in the treatment of these disorders. Pain should be controlled with appropriate nonnarcotic analgesics, with narcotics reserved for severe pain (26). Conservative therapies should not be overlooked and include moist heat, splinting or casting for comfort, use of crutches or canes, sufficient rest, and an appropriate exercise program (19). Younger children generally do not like topical medications and find the burning sensation or texture of many of these agents unacceptable. However, such agents can be useful in adolescents. Virtually all patients will be started on a nonsteroidal antiinflammatory drug (NSAID) for control of symptoms. NSAIDs reduce joint swelling, relieve pain, and have a modest effect on the overall inflammatory process. There are several NSAIDs from which to choose. In general, a NSAID that needs to be taken only once or twice daily is preferred, especially for the school-age child (5,9,25). Several selective inhibitors of cyclooxygenase-2 have been recently marketed in the United States and abroad, and can be useful in the child who cannot tolerate the usual NSAIDs. These agents (celecoxib, rofecoxib, among others) are similar to the other NSAIDs with a good safety profile, but they are more expensive and do not have the cardiovascular protective effect of the earlier NSAIDs (32). Salicylates, the first group of NSAIDs developed, are less commonly used in children due to

increased risk of gastrointestinal toxicity, the small risk of Reyes syndrome, and the need for more frequent laboratory studies, including salicylate levels. Serum levels of the other NSAIDs are not useful clinically. In general, patients on chronic NSAIDs should have laboratory studies every 3 to 4 months, including a complete blood count, measurement of liver enzymes, and a urinalysis to monitor for drug toxicity (5). Short courses and/or low doses of glucocorticoid can be useful for rapid and sustained control of inflammation. However, glucocorticoids have the potential for significant long-term side effects; long-term use and high doses are reserved for children with severe systemic disease or incapacitating polyarthritis. Intraarticular injection of glucocorticoids is safe and a very useful tool for management of arthritis, especially in the child with involvement of only a few joints (36).

The past decade has seen major advances in the understanding and treatment of chronic inflammatory arthritis. There is increasing emphasis on early identification of patients at risk of severe disease and aggressive control of inflammation, often involving simultaneous use of several pharmacologic agents. Medications include methotrexate, leufludomide, hydroxychloroquine, sulfasalazine, and novel biologic agents that specifically inhibit inflammatory mediators, specifically interleukin-1 and tumor necrosis factor. Detailed discussion of these agents is beyond the scope of this chapter, and the reader is referred to the end-of-chapter references for more detailed information (24,35,43,49).

For children with cervical spine involvement, symptomatic treatment is similar to management of peripheral arthritis and would include analgesics, immobilization (in this case with a cervical collar or, rarely, by traction), and various physical therapy modalities. A short course of oral glucocorticoids may be useful for immediate relief of symptoms in the child with new onset of neck disease. Indications for surgery are neurologic abnormality, intractable pain, and impending neurologic deficit. Procedures include laminectomy, decompression of nerve roots or spinal canal, and spinal fusion. These procedures are described in other chapters in this textbook. The choice of procedure, anatomical location, and timing of the specific surgical procedure will be individualized and based on the child's clinical signs, symptoms, and radiologic evaluation. In general, outcome is favorable, and early identification of neurologic impingement and prompt surgical treatment provide the best outcome (9,22,39).

SPONDYLOARTHROPATHIES

The spondyloarthropathies encompass a group of diseases, with considerable overlap in clinical features. The majority of these conditions have in common the presence of HLA-B27 (overall about 75% to 90% of individuals with a spondyloarthropathy) and enthesitis (inflammation at sites of attachment to bone). The current American College of Rheumatology classification is spondyloarthropathy with the following diagnostic subcategories: ankylosing spondylitis, reactive arthritis (also called Reiter syndrome), psoriatic arthropathy, and enteropathic arthropathy (arthritis associated with inflammatory bowel disease) (7,9,25).

TABLE 2. SPONDYLOARTHROPATHIES

Ankylosing spondylitis
Reactive arthritis/Reiters syndrome
Psoriatic arthropathy
Enteropathic arthropathy
Undifferentiated spondyloarthropathy

There is also a subset called "unclassified" or "undifferentiated" spondyloarthropathy for patients who do not yet meet diagnostic criteria for definite diagnosis (Table 2). Classic ankylosing spondylitis does not occur in young children. The child may present with an asymmetrical pauciarthritis and only later in adult life be correctly diagnosed; children presenting with isolated hip arthritis are particularly likely to develop a spondyloarthropathy (3). Some investigators define juvenile spondyloarthropathy as disease occurring in youngsters less than 16 years of age (6,13). Difficulties in the diagnosis include the considerable overlap in clinical features and the fact that decades may elapse before a specific spondyloarthropathy can be diagnosed.

Epidemiologic and Etiologic Factors

The spondyloarthropathies are ancient disorders; ankylosing spondylitis in skeletal remains dating to the thirtieth century BC has been described. In contrast, adult RA appeared during the Renaissance (8,25). The incidence of ankylosing spondylitis is 2.1 in 1,000, with a male/female ratio of 3–9:1, depending on the series (8,27). Anklylosing spondylitis represents about half of all cases of spondyloarthropathy. In children, the spondyloarthropathies account for one third of cases of chronic arthritis, and most of these children fulfill JRA criteria as well (13,37).

The cause of the spondyloarthropathy is still unknown. There have been tremendous advances in the last two decades in the understanding of the immune response, in identification of microbial triggers of inflammation, and in delineation of the contributions of HLA antigens and enteric infections in these diseases. The actual role of HLA-B27 is still not entirely clear. Patients can have a spondyloarthropathy without the presence of this antigen. Theories of the role of HLA-B27 include molecular mimicry (where a bacterial antigen is similar in structure to B27) and posttranslational modification of the B27 molecule (resulting in an altered structure and subsequent autoimmune response); or the B27 molecule might be associated with a deficient or altered host response to various infectious agents, resulting in the triggering of a chronic immune response. A transgenic HLA-B27 rat model has also contributed to our understanding of these disorders.

Clinical Features

The hallmark of the spondyloarthropathies is enthesitis, which refers to inflammation at the sites of attachment of connective tissue (tendons, fascia, ligaments) to bone. Typical sites of involvement include the lower extremities (e.g., heel, plantar fascia) and the sacroiliac joints. Pathologically, sites of enthesitis show non-specific inflammatory changes, with lymphocytic in-

flammation and destructive changes in adjacent bone (34). In addition to enthesitis, these conditions may also be associated with synovitis, tendonitis, spinal disease (especially at the sacroiliac joint), as well as mucocutaneous features. The importance of a careful history and physical examination cannot be overstated. The patient should be specifically asked about symptoms of inflammatory pain, such as morning stiffness, nighttime and early-morning pain, and improvement of pain with exercise. The patient or parents should be specifically asked about a family history of any of the spondyloarthropathies, psoriasis, and inflammatory bowel diseases. For the busy practitioner, a checklist can be useful if completed before the physician examines the patient; this list can also be useful for clinical studies and has been tested in a variety of settings (46). Enthesitis, especially of the lower extremities, is often misdiagnosed as an overuse syndrome, and it may be decades before the youngster has a definable spondyloarthropathy (34). In one large series, the diagnosis of a spondyloarthropathy was made at a mean of 7.3 years (6).

For many young children, the initial presentation may be hip involvement. Indeed, isolated hip involvement is distinctly uncommon in JRA (3). In general, youngsters with spondyloarthropathy are older males. Other clinical features that are useful in distinguishing spondyloarthropathy from JRA are the presence of enthesitis and tarsal disease. In children later diagnosed with a spondyloarthropathy, the discriminative value of either enthesitis or tarsal disease approached that of the gold standard of diagnosis: axial disease (6). Back involvement in children with spondyloarthropathy usually originates from inflammation of the sacroiliac joints. Symptoms may be bilateral. Pain is inflammatory in nature: worse in the morning, associated with morning stiffness, and often relieved by exercise and improved by the end of the day. Pain is usually mild to moderate and persists for months. A careful and thorough physical examination should be done. The mouth should be inspected for lesions and the skin examined for psoriasis (especially the nape of the neck, elbows, knees, and umbilicus). Shoes should be removed and the feet examined carefully for nail pits, sausage toes (dactylitis), and signs of enthesitis. In addition to the standard examination of the back, a useful procedure is the Schober test (Fig. 3), which can indicate spinal limitation and suggest the presence of a spondyloarthropathy (25,50).

Determination of the presence or absence of HLA-B27 can be helpful, particularly when combined with the patient's medical history and examination, family history, and radiographic evaluation. However, this antigen can be negative and can only be used to support a clinical diagnosis. It is not a useful screening tool in asymptomatic individuals. In many patients, especially those with involvement of few joints, laboratory studies may be completely normal. Tests for rheumatoid factors and ANAs will almost always be negative. Patients with significant inflammation may have a low-grade anemia and elevation of acute-phase reactants, such as C-reactive protein and the ESR.

Ankylosing Spondylitis

Ankylosing spondylitis is uncommon in children younger than 16 years. Onset is usually in young adulthood, again primarily

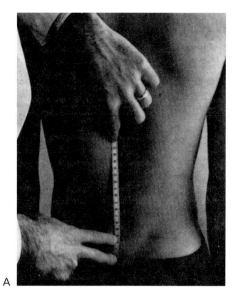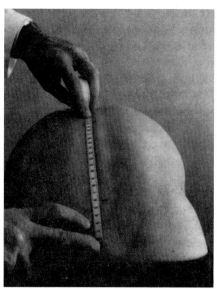

A   B

FIGURE 3. Measurement of spinal mobility in children using the Schober test. **A:** With the child upright, a line is drawn across the lumbosacral junction. A mark is placed 5 cm below and 10 cm above this point. **B:** With the child bending forward, the total excursion between the lower and upper points is measured. The normal measurement is 6 cm or greater.

in males. Most patients will present with insidious, persistent, chronic low back pain. Other features include enthesitis, peripheral arthritis, and, less commonly, extraarticular manifestations. Typical radiographic spinal changes will not be present for years (53).

Reactive Arthritis (Reiter Syndrome)

Reactive arthritis, also called Reiter syndrome, refers to an acute reactive arthritis occurring after an enteric infection or, less commonly, after a genitourinary infection, predominantly occurring in young white males. Onset will be quite abrupt, within a few days of the infection, and a large weight-bearing joint of the lower extremity is most often involved. The original description of Reiter syndrome is a triad of peripheral arthritis, conjunctivitis, and urethritis, but most patients present at first with peripheral arthritis alone. The arthritis will be self-limited, lasting for weeks to months, and patients can experience recurrences. Enthesitis is quite common. Similarly, most patients will develop conjunctivitis, low back pain, and mucocutaneous manifestations (mouth ulcers, rashes, nail changes). Back pain is most often attributable to sacroiliac involvement and is often unilateral; progression to clinically evident ankylosing spondylitis occurs in about 10% of cases (9,25).

Psoriatic Arthropathy

The arthropathy associated with psoriasis can be manifested in extremely varied ways, from peripheral asymmetrical arthritis, to a polyarthritis resembling RA, to spinal and sacroiliac disease, or even to a combination of these manifestations. Most patients will have typical psoriasis skin lesions before developing arthritis, but the psoriasis may appear at onset of the arthritis or, in a small

percentage, years later. Psoriatic arthropathy is more common in adults, again with a male predominance, but does occur in children as well (14,16,25).

Enteropathic Arthropathy

Arthropathy occurs in about one third of patients with inflammatory disease and may be the initial manifestation. Acute arthritis in peripheral joints usually coincides with active bowel inflammation and will subside once the gastrointestinal disease is controlled. Ten percent of patients eventually develop spinal disease, usually sacroiliitis or, occasionally, ankylosing spondylitis. Other features include mouth ulcers, skin lesions (erythema nodosum, pyoderma gangrenosa), and uveitis. Interestingly, a substantial proportion of patients with other arthropathies have occult gastrointestinal inflammation (25,29,33).

Undifferentiated Arthropathy

Accurate classification of a spondyloarthropathy may not be possible for several years following onset of characteristic symptoms, as it will be years before the classic radiographic findings of sacroiliitis or spondylitis are present. This is particularly true in younger patients. This group of patients will again be predominantly male. Most will have HLA-B27 and will not have rheumatoid factor or other autoantibodies. An earlier term for the spondyloarthropathies was "seronegative arthritis." However, RA and JRA patients can also be seronegative, and this designation is now used infrequently. A subgroup of undifferentiated spondyloarthropathy was previously called seronegative enthesopathy, or SEA syndrome, and these patients were primarily young males with chronic enthesitis. Most of these individuals followed over time will develop one of the spondyloarthropathies discussed above (7,25,53).

Radiographic Features

Routine radiographs will be normal early on, except for soft-tissue changes. The most common radiographic changes in the spondyloarthropathies are caused by enthesitis and by disease in the sacroiliac joints. At first enthesitis is characterized radiographically by bony erosion, then by sclerosis, and with long-standing disease by ankylosis of the adjacent bone. In sacroiliac disease, which can be unilateral, changes are similar and appear first on the iliac side of the joint (Fig. 4). Before significant radiographic changes can be seen on plain films, MRI will show profound alterations in the sacroiliac joint or, in the case of enthesitis, alterations in involved bone and attached connective tissues. Spondylitis occurs from a combination of arthritis and enthesitis; it begins in the lower spine and slowly progresses to involve the entire spine. Erosions develop at the vertebral corners, followed by formation of syndesmophytes and ultimately leading to the "bamboo spine" appearance. A late feature is ankylosis (12). For diagnosis of early disease, the more useful imaging procedure is MRI. Other useful procedures include ultrasonography and radionuclide scanning, particularly for evaluation of enthesitis. CT scanning is not useful for enthesitis but can be quite useful for evaluation of sacroiliac disease (34).

Natural History

Most youngsters presenting with a spondyloarthropathy do quite well, and permanent disability is not common. Long-term studies showing marked variation in progression to classic ankylosing spondylitis of 9% to 92%, mainly due to differences in classifica-

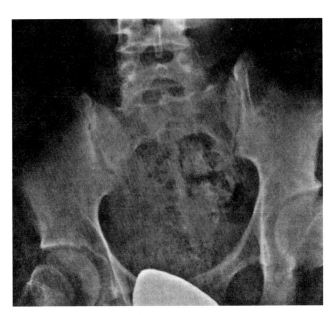

FIGURE 4. Bilateral sacroiliitis, as seen by hazy iliac margins in a 16-year-old boy with juvenile ankylosing spondylitis.

tion criteria and length of follow-up. In a recent series of patients with childhood-onset spondyloarthropathy of at least 10 years duration, those with enteropathic or psoriatic arthropathy had remission rates of 50% to 70%, whereas no patient with ankylosing spondylitis was in remission (13); however this was a very small series. In a study of 100 adults with typical ankylosing spondylitis, more than 80% had daily pain, even after 20 years of disease, suggesting that ankylosing spondylitis does not "burn out," as previously suggested (18). Similar findings were reported in a study of 328 patients with either ankylosing spondylitis or another spondyloarthropathy. In that series, factors associated with a more severe outcome included presence of oligoarthritis, sausage digits, hip or lumbar spine disease, young age of symptom onset (younger than 15 years), poor response to NSAIDs, and persistently elevated ESR. Severe outcome was much more likely with hip involvement and/or three of the above factors (1).

Treatment

Similar to treatment for the child with JRA, the initial focus is on pain control, appropriate balance of rest and exercise, use of analgesics, and a trial of NSAIDs. Exercises to preserve back flexibility, an appropriate exercise program, and inserts to protect heels or plantar fascia can all be useful. For reactive arthritis, this is usually sufficient to control disease. Many rheumatologists also treat an acute exacerbation of reactive arthritis with a course of doxycycline, as this has been shown to reduce the duration of the exacerbation (25). For more recalcitrant and persistent peripheral arthritis, other agents can be added, and the dose and types of agents are similar to those used to treat RA and JRA. Medications include sulfasalazine, methotrexate, doxycycline, chronic NSAIDs, low-dose prednisone, and potentially some of the newer biologic agents may control spondyloarthropathy as well (24,25,35). Injection of glucocorticoids into involved joints and bursae may provide considerable and longstanding relief of symptoms. Vertebral compression fractures (discussed below) are a common but often undiagnosed complication in adults with ankylosing spondylitis, as many such patients have significant osteoporosis of the spine as a complication of the disease process (38).

SYSTEMIC LUPUS ERYTHEMATOSUS

Systemic lupus erythematosus (SLE) is an inflammatory disorder of unknown cause, occurring predominantly in young women, with an increased incidence in certain ethnic groups (Asian, Hispanic, and African American women in particular). In the United States, the overall incidence is about 1 in 2,000 individuals (27). The hallmark of SLE is the production of multiple autoantibodies, vasculitis, and inflammation of multiple organ systems. Disease expression and long-term prognosis are quite unpredictable and variable. Diagnosis is based on exclusion of other rheumatic diseases and the presence of 4 of 11 specific classification criteria, including rashes, presence of certain serologic markers, arthritis, nephritis, serositis, and neurologic or hematologic abnormalities. As in many other rheumatic diseases (including JRA), most patients have positive ANA. Antibodies to double-stranded DNA and various cytoplasmic antigens are much more sensitive and specific for a diagnosis of lupus. A detailed discussion of autoantibodies is beyond the scope of this chapter.

A lupus patient presenting with back or neck pain should be carefully evaluated, as these patients are at high risk of unusual infections, fractures, and central nervous system (CNS) complications from active lupus. The differential diagnosis of neck or back pain is quite extensive in these patients. Cervical spine pain could result from lupus or from a concomitant infection. Meningeal inflammation with stiff neck and headache can occur in lupus vasculitis as the result of an opportunistic CNS infection (e.g., cryptococcal disease) or as an adverse effect of therapy (e.g., ibuprofen can cause aseptic meningitis in lupus patients). Back pain may be caused by an unusual infection, an inflammatory neuropathic process, or referred pain stemming from pleuritis, pericarditis, or an intraabdominal process. Patients with herpes zoster infections can present with burning radicular back pain several days before developing the typical vesicular eruption. Neurologic manifestations of lupus include transverse myelitis, polymyositis, aseptic meningitis, and peripheral neuropathies. A lupus patient may have back pain from osteoporotic stress fractures or mechanical back pain from muscle weakness or immobility. Consultation with a specialist who has expertise in lupus can be helpful in directing the evaluation of the patient's symptoms, as well as in determining therapy (9,25,27,41).

NONINFLAMMATORY CONDITIONS

Fibromyalgia

Fibromyalgia is common, particularly in older female adolescents. These patients have diffuse, longstanding, chronic pain and often cannot identify a single site of pain. Review of systems reveals multiple diffuse somatic symptoms, including sleep disturbance, fatigue, mood disorders, generalized joint and muscle aches, backache, abdominal pain and chronic headaches. These children often have a lifelong history of vague chronic symptoms and positive family history of fibromyalgia or irritable bowel syndrome. Physical examination is completely normal, except for tender points across the back and anterior chest wall. The patient may occasionally have pain on joint motion but should have no clinical signs of inflammation. Laboratory studies should be completely normal, including serologic studies, acute-phase reactants, radiographs, and routine blood tests. There is significant overlap of this condition with chronic fatigue syndrome, as well as with the mood and somatization disorders (54). School problems and other stresses are often present. Treatment of these adolescents can be extremely challenging and, at times, frustrating. The diagnosis of fibromyalgia is based on the typical history of chronic, stable, diffuse pain; normal laboratory investigations; and the presence of tender points on physical examination. The focus is on pain control, use of nonnarcotic analgesics, physical therapy, stress reduction, and normalization of sleep schedules. Referral to support groups and treatment of any concomitant mood disturbance can be quite helpful. In the evaluation of these patients, an appropriate and limited workup is indicated,

followed by a trial of conservative therapies and an agreement as to what types of symptoms would warrant further evaluation. Careful and consistent follow-up with a supportive health care provider can prevent a prolonged and unnecessary evaluation. In general, adolescents have a better prognosis than adults with fibromyalgia (9,25,45).

Osteoporotic Vertebral Compression Fractures

The past two decades has seen an explosion of research and new information on osteoporosis, in both the prevention and treatment of established bone loss. Approximately half of adult bone mass is acquired during adolescence, with bone mass increasing 8% each year during the adolescent growth spurt. Achievement of normal peak bone mass during childhood is important, as it may not be possible to correct this deficiency later in life (10). All children should be counseled about adequate calcium and vitamin D intake, as well as the importance of sufficient regular physical exercise. Children at high risk for decreased bone mass include amenorrheic female athletes, children with eating disorders (anorexia nervosa, in particular), metabolic diseases, and children with any disorder limiting physical mobility or requiring prolonged glucocorticoid administration. JRA patients have diminished bone mass, even in the absence of glucocorticoid use (4). Glucocorticoids are frequently used in the treatment of the rheumatic diseases. The risk and severity of glucocorticoid-induced osteoporosis is related to both the cumulative dose and the duration of treatment. A careful balance between disease control and use of the lowest dose of glucocorticoids is necessary. If the steroid dose cannot be reduced, other antiinflammatory agents should be added for disease control and to allow for a reduction in the daily steroid dose (steroid-sparing effect). Children identified with significant osteopenia from any cause should be referred for treatment, which may include estrogen (in estrogen-deficient girls), vitamin D, and treatment with one of the bisphosphonates, such as alendronate or etidronate. Although the bisphosphonates have been studied and are effective in postmenopausal osteoporosis and in steroid-induced osteoporosis in adults (42), there are few studies on the use of these agents in children or young adults. The treatment recommendations for osteoporosis are in considerable flux, and several large-scale trials are under way to determine optimal doses and duration of therapy, as well as to determine the indications in younger patients.

Children with glucocorticoid-induced compression fractures usually present with vague chronic back pain (Fig. 5). Occasionally, pain is more severe and abrupt. Physical examination is often normal, whereas the radiographs show dramatic changes. Progressive fractures can lead to significant kyphosis and poor posture. Management consists of administration of analgesics, bracing for comfort, physical therapy, as well as a focus on reducing the glucocorticoid dose if possible and referring the patient for treatment of the osteoporosis.

The Child with Nonorganic Back Pain

Back pain is discussed in more extensively in an earlier chapter, but will be briefly reviewed here. Back pain is an extremely

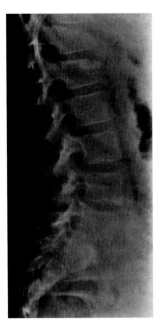

FIGURE 5. Multiple compression fractures in an 8-year-old boy with systemic-onset juvenile rheumatoid arthritis managed with oral glucocorticoids for 4 years.

common symptom and increases markedly with age. The incidence and prevalence in older adolescents is similar to adults. In adults, at any one time, 20% to 40% will have experienced back pain (defined as any back pain lasting longer than 24 hours) in the past month (51), and adults have a lifetime 70% to 90% probability of experiencing back pain (18). Over half of children have experienced episodes of back pain, and 8% to 30% have reported the presence of chronic back pain. Most of these children do not seek medical evaluation (28,48). Of those seeking evaluation, a specific cause will be found in only about half. A specific cause is more often found in younger children, particularly those younger than 10 years. In a large series of children presenting to a pediatric orthopedic clinic with back pain, no organic cause was found in 57%. Interestingly, the group of patients in this series with nonorganic pain had a higher incidence of psychosocial problems, disability claims, and pending litigation (11); similar findings have been seen in studies in adults with chronic back pain. The inability to find an organic cause is even higher in patients presenting to the general practitioner, and the cause is assumed to be myofascial in origin in most cases. In general, functional back pain is more common in patients with lower socioeconomic status, high stress, and in those patients with a higher incidence of self-reported physical or sexual abuse (11,51). Nonorganic back pain can be one of the more challenging conditions to evaluate, as patients can have severe pain, prolonged symptoms, and seek evaluation from multiple health care providers. Parents may become upset when no organic cause of their child's pain can be found.

All children with back pain should have a careful history and physical examination, including a family and social history. Red flags for an organic cause include young age (under 10 years), the presence of systemic symptoms (e.g., fever and weight loss),

pain that interferes with sleep, inflammatory pain (worse in the morning with relief at the end of the day), neurologic signs or symptoms, and constant pain (23,48). Malingering and/or factitious causes are not common in children and can usually be ascertained by careful investigation. Nonorganic back pain is an important differential diagnosis to consider as it may spare the child an unnecessary and costly evaluation. Nonorganic pain should be considered in the older child presenting with extreme school absence; psychosocial stresses; bizarre, diffuse, and/or vague symptoms; and a normal physical examination. Often the child's reported disability and dysfunction is out of proportion to the physical examination. For these children, a limited diagnostic evaluation and careful observation and symptom control may be indicated as the first line of management. A trial of physical therapy, analgesics, and/or NSAIDs is recommended, and the child should be scheduled for a reexamination in 4 to 8 weeks. The child can keep a diary of symptoms and should be reassured in a sympathetic tone. The child should be strongly encouraged to return to school and to normal physical activity.

PREOPERATIVE CONSIDERATIONS IN RHEUMATIC DISEASES

The rheumatic diseases are complex, chronic conditions, and a careful preoperative evaluation is important for all children recommended for surgery (Table 3). Medications and other health problems should be reviewed, and consultations with anesthesiologists, nurses, surgeons, and other health care providers recommended as indicated. Steps should be take to reduce the child's fear and anxiety. Anesthesia can be particularly challenging for the child with severe JRA and polyarthritis. These children often have limited mouth opening, small mandibles, limited cervical spine extension, and osteoporotic bone, all of which lead to increased risks from anesthesia and endotracheal intubation. A careful preoperative examination of the neck should be performed on all children with JRA. Any child with neck pain or limited cervical spine movement should have cervical spine films (extension and flexion) obtained to expose possible subluxation or another abnormality. Consideration should be given to

TABLE 3. PREOPERATIVE ASSESSMENT OF CHILDREN WITH RHEUMATIC DISEASES

All Cases
History and physical examination
    Anesthetic history, prior anesthetic difficulties
    Careful attention to cervical spine and jaw examination
Medication history
Complete blood count
If indicated
Cervical spine x-rays—any child with neck symptoms or limitation of
    motion (especially patients with polyarthritis)
Corticosteroid stress coverage—children on corticosteroids for more
    than 1 mo the past 6 mo
Hold aspirin, consider holding other nonsteroidal antiinflammatory
    drugs for 5–7 d
Hold methotrexate and other immune suppressants for 1 wk

fiberoptic intubation and consultation with the anesthesiologist to determine the most appropriate choices of anesthesia (31,55).

A child on chronic glucocorticoid therapy (more then 10 mg daily for more than 30 days) should receive intravenous stress coverage during the surgery and until he or she can resume the usual oral steroid dose. Antibiotic prophylaxis for endocarditis is not necessary unless the child also has a heart defect. Any NSAID medications may be stopped a few days before the surgery and then restarted a few days later due to the small risk of an effect on platelet function. Some rheumatologists recommend withholding methotrexate or other immune suppressants during the week of surgery because of the small potential for a delay in wound healing or an increased the risk of infection, though there are no firm data to confirm these risks. Omitting most rheumatic medications for a few days will have no long-term consequences on the underlying disease (31,47).

REFERENCES

1. Amor B, Santos RS, Nahal R, et al. (1994): Predictive factors for the long-term outcome of spondyloarthropathies. *J Rheumatol* 21:1883–7.
2. Arroyo IL, Barron KS, Brewer EJ (1988): Spinal cord compression by epidural lipomatosis in juvenile rheumatoid arthritis. *Arthritis Rheum* 38:447–451.
3. Bowyer S (1995): Hip contracture as the presenting sign in children with HLA B27 arthritis. *J Rheumatol* 22:165–167.
4. Brik R, Keidar Z, Schapira D, et al. (1998): Bone mineral density and turnover in children with systemic juvenile chronic arthritis. *J Rheumatol* 25:990–992.
5. Brooks P (1998): Use and benefits of nonsteroidal anti-inflammatory drugs. *Am J Med* 104:9S–13S.
6. Burgos-Vargas R, Vazquez-Mellado J (1995): The early clinical recognition of juvenile-onset ankylosing spondylitis and its differentiation from juvenile rheumatoid arthritis. *Arthritis Rheum* 38:835–844.
7. Cabral DA, Malleson PN, Petty RE (1995): Spondyloarthropathies of childhood. *Pediatr Clin N Am* 42:1051–1070.
8. Carbone LD, Cooper C, Michet CJ, et al. (1992): Ankylosing Spondylitis in Rochester, Minnesota, 1935–1989. *Arthritis Rheum* 35:1476–1482.
9. Cassidy JT, Petty RE (1995): *Textbook of pediatric rheumatology,* 3rd ed. Philadelphia: WB Saunders.
10. Cassidy JT, Langman CB, Allen SH, et al. (1995): Bone mineral metabolism in children with juvenile rheumatoid arthritis. *Pediatr Clin N Am* 42:1017–1033.
11. Combs JA, Caskey PM (1997): Back pain in children and adolescents: a retrospective review of 648 patients. *S Med J* 90:789–92.
12. El-Khoury GY, Kathol MH, Brandser EA (1996): Seronegative spondyloarthropathies. *Radiol Clin N Am* 34:343–357.
13. Flato B, Aasland A, Vinje O, Forre O (1998): Outcome and predictive factors in juvenile rheumatoid arthritis and juvenile spondyloarthropathy. *J Rheumatol* 25:366–375.
14. Gare BA (1998): Epidemiology. *Bailliere's Clin Rheumatol* 12:191–208.
15. Gillette RD (1996): A practical approach to the patient with back pain. *Am Fam Phys* 53:670–78.
16. Gladman DD (1998): Psoriatic arthritis. Rheum Dis Clin N Am 24:829–844.
17. Graham TB, Glass DN (1997): Juvenile rheumatoid arthritis: ethnic differences in diagnostic types. *J Rheumatol* 24:1677–1679.
18. Gran JT, Skomsvoll JF (1997): The outcome of ankylosing spondylitis: a study of 100 patients. *Br J Rheumatol* 36:766–71.
19. Guccione AA (1996): Physical therapy for musculoskeletal syndromes. *Rheum Dis Clin N Am* 2:551–562.
20. Hafner R, Truckenbrodt H, Spamer M (1998): Rehabilitation in children with juvenile chronic arthritis. *Bailliere's Clin Rheumatol* 12:329–361.
21. Haldeman S (1996): Diagnostic tests for the evaluation of back and neck pain. *Neurol Clin N Am* 14:103–117.
22. Hensinger RN, DeVito PD, Ragsdale CG (1986): Changes in the cervical spine in juvenile rheumatoid arthritis. *J Bone Joint Surg* 68A:189–198.
23. Hollinsworth P (1996): Back pain in children. *Br J Rheumatol* 35:1022–1028.
24. Jones RE, Moreland LW (1999): Tumor necrosis factor inhibitors for rheumatoid arthritis. *Bull Rheum Dis* 48(3):1–5.
25. Klippel JH, ed. (1997): *Primer on the rheumatic diseases.* Atlanta: Arthritis Foundation.
26. Kuis W, Heijnen CJ, Sinnema G, et al. (1998): Pain in childhood rheumatic arthritis. *Bailliere's Clin Rheumatol* 12:229–244.
27. Lawrence RC, Helmick CG, Arnett FC, et al. (1998): Estimates of the prevalence of arthritis and selected musculoskeletal disorders in the United States. *Arthritis Rheum* 41:778–799.
28. Leboeuf-Yde C, Kyvik KO (1998): At what age does low back pain become a common problem? *Spine* 23:228–234.
29. Leirisalo-Repo M, Turunen U, Stenman S, et al. (1994): High frequency of silent inflammatory bowel disease in spondyloarthropathy. *Arthritis Rheum* 37:23–31.
30. Lovell D (1997): JRA and juvenile spondyloarthropathies. In: Klippel JH, ed. *Primer on the rheumatic diseases.* Atlanta: Arthritis Foundation, pp. 393–398.
31. MacKenzie CR, Sharrock NE (1998): Perioperative medical considerations in patients with rheumatoid arthritis. *Rheum Dis Clin N Am* 24:1–17.
32. Mandell BF (1999): Cox 2-selective NSAIDs: biology, promises, and concerns. *Cleveland Clin J Med* 66:285–292.
33. Munch H, Purrmann J, Reis HE, et al. (1986): Clinical features of inflammatory joint and spine manifestations in Crohn's disease. *Hepatogastroenterolgy* 33:123–127.
34. Olivieri I, Barozzi L, Padula A (1998): Enthesiopathy: clinical manifestations, imaging and treatment. *Bailliere's Clin Rheumatol* 12:665–678.
35. Olsen NJ, Strand V, Kremer JM (1999): Leflunomide for the treatment of rheumatoid arthritis. *Bull Rheum Dis* 48(8):1–4.
36. Padeh S, Passwell JH (1998): Intraarticular corticosteroid injection in the management of children with chronic arthritis. *Arthritis Rheum* 14:1210–1214.
37. Petty RE (1998): Classification of childhood arthritis: a work in progress. *Bailliere's Clin Rheumatol* 12:181–190.
38. Ralston SH, Urquhart GDK, Brzeski M, et al. (1990): Prevalence of vertebral compression fractures due to osteoporosis in ankylosing spondylitis. *Br Med J* 300:563–565.
39. Rawlins BA, Girardi FP, Boachie-Adjei O (1998): Rheumatoid arthritis of the cervical spine. *Rheum Dis Clin N Am* 24:55–65.
40. Reveille JD (1998): HLA-B27 and the seronegative spondyloarthropathies. *Am J Med Sci* 316:239–249.
41. Roberts NW (1997): Keys to managing systemic lupus erythematosus. *Hosp Practice* February 15:113–126.
42. Saag KG, Emkey R, Schnitzer TJ, et al. (1998): Alendronate for the prevention and treatment of glucocorticoid-induced osteoporosis. *N Engl J Med* 339:292–299.
43. Schaller JG (1997): Juvenile rheumatoid arthritis. *Pediatr Rev* 18:337–349.
44. Sherk H, Pasquariallo P, Watters W (1992): Multiple dislocations of the cervical spine in a patient with JRA and Down's syndrome. *Clin Orthop Rel Res* 162:37–39.
45. Siegel DM, Janeway D, Baum (1998): Fibromyalgia syndrome in children and adolescents: clinical features at presentation and status at follow-up. *Pediatrics* 101:377–382.
46. Singh G, Athreya BH, Fries JF, et al. (1994): Measurement of health status in children with juvenile rheumatoid arthritis. *Arthritis Rheum* 37:1761–1769.
47. Skues MA, Welchew EA (1993): Anaesthesia and rheumatoid arthritis. *Anesthesia* 48:989–997.
48. Sponseller PD (1996): Evaluating the child with back pain. *Am Fam Physician* 54:1933–1941.
49. Szer IS (1997): Chronic arthritis in children. *Compreh Ther* 23:124–129.

50. Tucker LB, Miller LC, Schaller JG (1994): Rheumatic diseases. In: Weinstein SL, ed. *The pediatric spine: principles and practice.* New York: Raven Press, pp. 851–69.

51. Urwin M, Symmons D, Allison T, et al. (1998): Estimating the burden of musculoskeletal disorders in the community: the comparative prevalence of symptoms at different anatomical sites, and the relation to social deprivations. *Ann Rheum Dis* 57:649–655.

52. Uziel Y, Rathaus V, Pomeranz A, et al. (1998): Torticollis as the sole initial presenting sign of systemic onset juvenile rheumatoid arthritis. *J Rheumatol* 25:166–168.

53. Van der Linden S, Van der Heijde D (1998): Ankylosing spondylitis: clinical features. *Rheum Dis Clin N Am* 24:663–676.

54. Wallace DJ (1999): Lupus for the non-rheumatologist. *Bull Rheum Dis* 48(9):1–4.

55. Woo P, White PH, Ansell BM (1990): *Paediatric rheumatology update.* Oxford: Oxford University Press.

INFLAMMATORY DISEASES OF THE SPINAL CORD, LEPTOMENINGES, AND DURA

RUSSELL D. SNYDER

This chapter considers inflammatory and infectious conditions of the spinal cord, the leptomeninges (the surrounding pia and arachnoid membranes), and the dura mater. Meningitis and epidural abscess are caused by bacteria. Arachnoiditis is an inflammatory response established by an agent, infectious or otherwise, that irritates the leptomeninges. Transverse myelitis has diverse etiologic factors, and frequently no specific cause can be determined. All of these conditions are rare but have major unfavorable consequences when left untreated—and sometimes even when they are appropriately treated. The chronic orthopaedic management of an individual who recovers from one of these conditions with significant deficit is not considered here. Also, other inflammatory and infectious conditions of structures surrounding the spinal cord, such as disc space infection and vertebral osteomyelitis, are considered elsewhere in this volume.

BACTERIAL MENINGITIS

Bacterial meningitis is a bacterial infection involving the pia, the arachnoid, and the subarachnoid space. The infection is usually acute.

Epidemiologic Factors

The peak attack rate was between 6 and 12 months of age until the introduction of *Haemophilus influenzae* immunization at an early age, when the median age shifted to 25 years (74). Bacterial meningitis is more common in winter except that *H. influenzae* type b peaks in spring and fall. Risk factors for *H. influenzae* type b include male sex, black race, Native American heritage, household crowding, and attendance at day-care centers (12,18).

Etiologic Factors

In the neonate, *Escherichia coli*, *Listeria monocytogenes*, and various gram-negative organisms are found. Between 1 and 3

R. D. Snyder: Department of Neurology and Pediatrics, University of New Mexico School of Medicine, Albuquerque, New Mexico 87131–5281.

months of age, similar organisms are cultured along with *H. influenzae*, *Streptococcus pneumoniae*, and *Neisseria meningitidis*. Between 3 months and 10 years of age, *H. influenzae*, *S. pneumoniae*, and *N. meningitidis* are the common organisms. In adolescence, *N. meningitidis* is an important organism. *Staphylococcus aureus* and *Staphylococcus epidermidis* are important etiologic agents in surgically acquired infections, as are *Klebsiella* and *Pseudomonas* species. With immunization against *H. influenzae* reducing the incidence of this organism, *S. pneumoniae* is gaining in importance. Infection with unusual organisms, such as *Mycobacterium tuberculosis*, must be considered in every case (97).

Clinical Features

Fever with neurologic signs or symptoms, especially if accompanied by a seizure, should raise a suspicion of meningitis (Table 1). The classic finding of fever and stiff neck is useful. Stiff neck is tested by flexion of the neck and not by rotation. In the very young and in the debilitated, neck stiffness may not be present. Other findings of meningeal irritation include Kernig sign (inability to fully straighten the leg that is flexed at the hip) and Brudzinski sign (flexion at the hips with passive flexion of the neck) (92). Headache is less common in children than in adults.

A history of a preceding upper respiratory or gastrointestinal infection is common. Instead of recovery from the initial illness, as is the usual occurrence in common childhood infections, the child becomes progressively more ill, developing septicemia and then meningitis. There is never a precise moment when a respiratory or gastrointestinal infection evolves into meningitis. The symptoms of bacterial meningitis usually run a rapid course, with progressive deterioration of neurologic function over several hours and seldom over more than a day or two

Seizures may be focal or generalized. Depressed consciousness is present, which may rapidly evolve into coma. A bulging fontanel and fever in a small child or infant is a strong indication of meningitis, especially if trauma is excluded. Focal neurologic signs, such as hemiparesis or cranial nerve deficits, occur later and are unusual as part of the presentation. The lack of specific neurologic symptoms or of meningeal signs in a febrile child who is lethargic or irritable does not exclude the possibility of meningitis.

TABLE 1. SIGNS AND SYMPTOMS OF BACTERIAL MENINGITIS

Acute progression
Depressed consciousness
Fever
Stiff neck
Bulging fontanelle
Headache
Seizure
Focal neurologic signs

Purpuric skin lesions may be found in *N. meningococcus* meningitis and, less often, in other forms of meningitis. Purpuric skin lesions may be a manifestation of meningitis complicated by disseminated intravascular coagulation.

The infectious process surrounds the spinal cord, and the diagnosis of meningitis is made by recovery of organisms from the region of the cauda equina. However, clinical signs relating to the spinal cord are surprisingly rare. Paresis of one or more limbs and sphincter involvement secondary to spinal cord lesions can be found (34,86). A cauda equina syndrome with paraplegia, saddle anesthesia, and bladder and bowel dysfunction has been reported in *S. pneumoniae* meningitis (45). Children with meningitis may have such significant involvement of the brain that spinal findings may be hidden or overlooked.

Meningitis is an important consideration in any infant or child with a fever and neurologic symptoms or signs.

Differential Diagnosis

A common concern in differential diagnosis is the benign febrile seizure of childhood. Febrile seizures occur between 6 months and 4 years of age. They are usually single seizures, are generalized, and last for less than 5 minutes. Cerebrospinal fluid (CSF) and the electroencephalogram are normal.

Occasionally, head trauma is mistaken for bacterial meningitis. A child with head trauma may be depressed, have neurologic signs, have a full fontanel and fever. The presence of retinal hemorrhage is strongly suggestive of trauma and would be most unusual in meningitis. Associated evidence of trauma may be present in the skin or long bones.

Other concerns in differential diagnosis include sepsis, brain or epidural abscess, viral central nervous system (CNS) infection, intoxication, Reye syndrome, and tonsillar herniation.

Radiographic and Imaging Studies

Head imaging should be performed in any meningitis patient with an unfavorable clinical course to exclude extraaxial fluid collection, ventricular enlargement, vascular involvement (such as infarction or necrosis), empyema, and venous thrombosis (28). Vascular changes can be arterial or venous.

Magnetic resonance imaging (MRI) offers little advantage over computed tomography (CT) in the evaluation of acute bacterial meningitis, although experience is limited. The child with complicated meningitis may be acutely ill and on a ventilator, rendering MRI difficult.

Other Diagnostic Studies

Lumbar puncture with examination of CSF is the definitive test for meningitis. However, it should not be performed without consideration of possible adverse effects (59). In certain situations, the pressure changes produced by removal of CSF at lumbar puncture can result in shifts of intracranial contents and even brain herniation. Although the presence of increased intracranial pressure is a relative contraindication to lumbar puncture, the diffuse increased pressure of meningitis in infants or children seldom leads to difficulties. Papilledema or focal findings on examination suggest a mass lesion, a situation that may result in complications from lumbar puncture.

Brain imaging before lumbar puncture provides some assurance that lumbar puncture can be performed safely. In selected situations, sedation of the child prior to lumbar puncture may be indicated.

Initial antibiotic treatment can be started prior to lumbar puncture so that there is no delay in starting therapy directed against a suspected meningitis. A short regimen of antibiotics prior to CSF examination will not significantly interfere with the results.

Lumbar puncture should not be performed through an area of abscess or cellulitis. If the patient has a bleeding diathesis, correction of the diathesis should be undertaken before performance of the lumbar puncture. Inadvertent needle entry into the disc space can lead to subsequent pain and collapse of the disc space. The amount of CSF necessary for performance of testing will vary from one facility to another and according to the specific testing requested.

Headache 1 to 4 hours after the lumbar puncture is a troublesome but usually benign complication. This complication occurs in 10% to 25% of adults and appears less common in preadolescent children (59). The headache is frontal and is exaggerated by movement from a lying to a sitting or standing position. Post-lumbar puncture headache appears to be caused by continued leak of CSF from the site of lumbar puncture, with resulting low CSF pressure and pulling of the brain on pain-sensitive structures. The problem can be minimized by use of a small-bore needle and removal of a minimal amount of fluid. Pain in the lower back or legs occurs occasionally after lumbar puncture. This pain is of uncertain cause and usually resolves spontaneously in several days (80).

Opening pressure at lumbar puncture, a frequently overlooked procedure in infants and children, can easily be obtained if the patient is not struggling. It provides useful information as the opening pressure is usually elevated in bacterial meningitis.

The CSF may have a cloudy appearance. The cell count is increased, with the predominant cell being polymorphonuclear. On the initial lumbar puncture at the onset of illness, a predominance of polymorphonuclear cells may be found in bacterial or viral meningitis. In aseptic meningitis of viral origin, a predominance of polymorphonuclear cells on the second or third day is distinctly unusual (1). Protein is increased with depression of sugar content. Gram staining should be carried out. Cultures of CSF and blood should be obtained for bacteria and, in certain circumstances, for other organisms. Immunoassays for bacterial antigen can provide a rapid diagnosis. These antigen tests can be performed on CSF, blood, and urine. Both Gram staining and antigen testing are rapid, providing results in about 15 minutes, and become useful in guiding initial therapy. Culture of the CSF is the gold standard for etiology and can provide information concerning antibiotic sensitivities. When CSF is normal and a suspicion of meningitis persists, the lumbar puncture should be repeated. Blood culture can recover the organism of bacterial meningitis in about 70% of cases.

Pathoanatomy

The sequence of events in the pathogenesis of bacterial meningitis begins with bacterial colonization of the nasopharynx. From there the organism enters the bloodstream or, rarely, enters directly into the cranial vault. The bloodstream can carry the organism to the CNS. Direct spread is possible from a focus in the skin or sinuses, from a brain abscess, or from osteomyelitis of adjacent bone (57). Trauma from a surgical or diagnostic procedure involving the CNS may lead to entry of the organism. The purulent exudate in bacterial meningitis is within the subarachnoid space between the pia and arachnoid, which contains the CSF (Fig. 1). The basal cisterns, sylvian fissure, rolandic sulci, and perivascular spaces are prime locations for the infection (8). Vascular changes may be marked because of an associated vasculitis from the infection surrounding major vessels entering and leaving the brain (29,61).

Although bacterial meningitis is a disease of the brain and surrounding structures, the spinal cord and its surrounding structures are involved with the subarachnoid exudate. Historically, a bacterial infection of the subarachnoid space was called "spinal meningitis," although this term has fallen into disuse. In severe cases, the spinal cord can be encased in purulent exudate (8). The recovery of organisms and inflammatory cells on lumbar puncture shows the widespread nature of the infection.

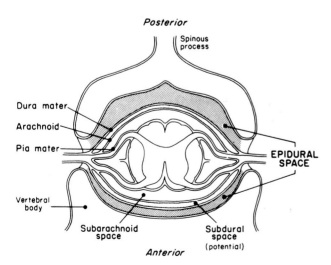

FIGURE 1. Transverse section of spinal cord showing relation of the spinal cord to the leptomeninges, the bone, and the various spaces mentioned in the text. (From Beland B, Prien T, Vanaken H [1997]: Spinal and epidural anaesthesia in bacteremic patients. *Anaesthesist* 46: 536–547, with permission.)

The low incidence of clinical signs and symptoms referable to the spinal cord is surprising. Spinal cord findings appear related to cord infarction or necrosis (34,86).

Replication of the organism within the CNS occurs easily. Pus accumulates, edema develops, and the CSF circulation becomes compromised. All blood vessels entering or leaving the brain must pass through the subarachnoid space. When this space is inflamed, vasculitis develops with ischemia and infarction.

Natural mechanisms and bactericidal antibiotics used in the treatment of meningitis result in the release of lipopolysaccharide endotoxin. Endotoxin in the CSF induces the production of cytokines that can initiate an inflammatory response even in the absence of bacteria. These cytokines are found in increased amounts in the CSF in experimental and human meningitis, especially after treatment with bactericidal antibiotics. They damage the CNS by direct cellular toxicity and by changes in the vascular milieu (72,84). Improvement in outcome depends on the development of techniques to counteract these mechanisms.

Complications

Complications occur in the management of bacterial meningitis, even when the diagnosis is prompt and appropriate therapy is rapidly instituted. Seizures are found in approximately 30% of children, usually early in the illness (68). Seizures may be caused by toxic products of bacteria or leukocytes, inflammation, vasculitis, fever, electrolyte imbalance, or an unrecognized process.

Focal signs, such as hemiparesis, may be found. Cranial nerve palsies occur. The eighth cranial nerve is involved in 5% to 20% of cases and may result in hearing loss, which usually has an early onset and is permanent (70).

Collections of extraaxial fluid, the so-called subdural effusions, are found over the brain convexities in some younger children. These collections seldom cause symptoms and can be followed on brain imaging until they regress or until intervention becomes necessary because of pressure or displacement of brain parenchyma. Hydrocephalus may occur. However, ventricular widening may also be the result of parenchymal loss. Surgical intervention should not be undertaken until the surgeon is assured that elevated intraventricular pressure is present. Temporary external drainage with serial brain imaging can determine if a shunt will be effective.

Disseminated intravascular coagulation is a complication in those who are severely ill with meningitis. Septic shock, cerebral edema, and the syndrome of inappropriate secretion of antidiuretic hormone also occur.

Natural History

Without treatment, bacterial meningitis is fatal in almost all cases. Following treatment most children recover without sequelae (87). In a series of children, 37% had neurologic abnormalities 1 month after meningitis. Within a year only 14% had persistent deficits (68). Subtle cognitive and learning problems may be found (88). Recovery from spinal cord involvement is poor (76).

Treatment

Nonsurgical

Antibiotics remain the mainstay of specific treatment. Recommendations change frequently, and expert advice may be needed. Initial empirical treatment is determined by the suspected organism. Once an organism is identified by immunologic means, Gram stain, or culture, the antibiotics can be adjusted to achieve ideal therapy.

In newborns the therapy is directed to organisms acquired during delivery. Empirical therapy includes ampicillin plus an aminoglycoside or a third-generation cephalosporin. Between 1 month and 3 months of age, ampicillin and cefotaxime or ceftriaxone are recommended. Between 3 months and 10 years of age, cefotaxime or ceftriaxone alone is used. In older children, ampicillin alone or penicillin G is appropriate. If *Staphylococcus* is a likely offender, methicillin can be utilized. Strains of *S. pneumoniae* are found that are resistant to penicillin and ceftriaxone (3). Research has suggested that steroids may reduce the suspected harmful effects of rapid bacterial lysis within the subarachnoid space and the associated release of biologically active products, at least in *H. influenzae* meningitis (43). Also, moderate and severe hearing loss may be decreased by dexamethasone after initial antibiotics (50). Dexamethasone decreases the duration of fever and CSF pleocytosis. Cytokines in the CSF are reduced when glucocorticoids are administered prior to the initial antibiotic (2). In a trial of dexamethasone administered 15 to 20 minutes prior to institution of antibiotic therapy, the CSF opening pressure was lower; 12 hours later, the evidence of inflammation in the spinal fluid had begun to disappear, the CSF contained lower concentrations of cytokines, and neurologic sequelae were less marked (66). Dexamethasone has not demonstrated similar effectiveness in *S. pneumoniae* meningitis (3) and probably should not be used routinely except in *H. influenzae* meningitis (67).

When seizures are severe or prolonged, lorazepam is effective. The intravenous (IV) dose is 0.05 to 0.1 mg/kg up to a maximum of 4 mg administered no more rapidly than 2 mg/min. Fosphenytoin may be effective in this situation in an initial dose of 10 to 20 mg/kg IV, administered no more rapidly than 100 mg/min; cardiac function must be monitored for signs of bradycardia or dysrhythmia. Phenobarbital can be administered in the dose of 10 to 20 mg/kg IV or intramuscularly. Once initial control is achieved, continuous anticonvulsant administration with phenobarbital or phenytoin can be undertaken for more prolonged coverage. The self-limited seizures that are found early in bacterial meningitis may not be an indication for prolonged anticonvulsant treatment.

Cerebral edema requires traditional management, with elevation of the head, osmotic agents, diuretics, and possibly hyperventilation. Supportive care is indicated, with attention to the skin and joints.

Recommendations change frequently. The physicians undertaking treatment of bacterial meningitis should check for current recommendations regarding antibiotics, fluid management, steroid use, brain imaging, and management of cerebral edema.

Surgical

Extraaxial collections must be drained if significant compression or shift of brain parenchyma is occurring, if the child remains symptomatic in spite of a good response to antibiotics, or if the extraaxial fluid becomes infected. Repeated tapping through the fontanel or continuous external drainage is appropriate if the collection is liquid. Shunting of the extraaxial space should be reserved for those cases refractory to more conservative measures (83). Rapid removal of large volumes of extraaxial fluid may have a deleterious effect secondary to shifts in intracranial contents. Continuous ventricular drainage or shunting is indicated in selected cases with persistent increased intraventricular pressure.

Neurosurgical intervention may also be necessary if the infection progresses to brain abscess or cerebral epidural abscess (17).

SPINAL ARACHNOIDITIS

Spinal arachnoiditis is a noninfectious or postinfectious chronic aseptic inflammatory process of the leptomeninges (94). The condition is not usually seen in isolation but occurs as part of another disease of the spinal cord, spinal subarachnoid space, or surrounding structures, or as sequelae of a procedure around the leptomeninges.

Epidemiologic Factors

Spinal arachnoiditis is unusual before adolescence. Males are affected more commonly than females.

Etiologic Factors

Many agents produce arachnoiditis. The common theme is violation of the arachnoid. Aseptic arachnoiditis is initiated by a variety of chemical and physical agents in the subarachnoid space and is seen as a sequela of a spinal or paraspinal infectious process including tuberculosis (47). Myelographic contrast material has been a particular offender, although newer contrast materials present less of a problem (22). Intrathecal steroids are implicated (40). Spinal arachnoiditis has been reported after epidural and spinal anesthesia (33,81), and after back surgery (25) and other forms of trauma.

Extrinsic or intrinsic spinal cord disease, including neoplasms and syringomyelia, can produce arachnoiditis. Arachnoiditis occurs following subarachnoid hemorrhage. Intervertebral disc disease can produce the condition. Aseptic and purulent infections of the meninges or adjacent areas of the spine can lead to spinal arachnoiditis; chronic infections, such as tuberculosis, cryptococcosis, and syphilis, have been offenders. Spinal arachnoiditis is found in adolescents with tuberculous meningitis (51).

A familial form of spinal arachnoiditis has been described (21). Arachnoiditis may appear in developmental disorders of the spine or spinal cord, such as meningomyelocele, neurofibromatosis type 1, and syringomyelia (15). Many cases remain idiopathic.

TABLE 2. SIGNS AND SYMPTOMS OF ARACHNOIDITIS

Chronic progression
Spotty and localized pain
Migratory paresthesias
Weakness
Spastic paraparesis
Sphincter disturbance
Symptoms out of proportion to signs

Clinical Features

The symptoms of spinal arachnoiditis are produced by cord compression, adhesions about nerve roots, constriction of blood vessels supplying cord and roots, and the formation of cysts (Table 2). The cord may become fixed from adhesions and then damaged by constant spine movement (15).

Onset may be rapid or gradual. Fever and other systemic manifestations are usually absent. Remissions occur. Symptoms may not appear for months or years after the initiating event. The first symptoms are pain and paresthesia (69). The pain is aching or burning and is poorly localized; it may follow a broad radicular pattern or be spotty. Movement and straining, as with coughing or sneezing, may increase the pain. Bed rest may also increase the pain. In some patients, the pain is worse upon rising. The paresthesias are described as tingling, numbness, the sensation of heat or cold, or a constricting sensation. The paresthesias may be in a neurologically inconsistent distribution and migratory. Sensory examination may be normal or may reveal areas of hyperesthesia or hypesthesia. Trophic changes are rare.

Weakness eventually appears, and the course then becomes one of slowly progressive spastic paraparesis. Painful muscle spasms and muscle atrophy develop with the passage of time. Sphincter problems evolve in one third of cases. Muscle stretch reflexes are increased or decreased depending on the location, duration, and nature of the lesions.

The straight-leg raising test is often positive. The back is tender and stiff, with limitation of motion. Symptoms are frequently out of proportion to signs. Arachnoiditis is responsible for the symptoms in some "failed back surgery" patients (79).

Differential Diagnosis

The differential diagnosis includes extramedullary cord tumor and syringomyelia.

Radiographic and Imaging Studies

The diagnosis of arachnoiditis should be made by clinical findings, with imaging providing supportive evidence. Arachnoiditis can be present on imaging without clinical symptomatology (40). Gadolinium-enhanced MRI is now the appropriate imaging examination in spinal arachnoiditis, as it is for all infectious and inflammatory diseases of the spinal cord (33,91). Partial or complete obstruction is present with irregularity of the thecal sac plus thickening and clumping of the nerve roots. The area of abnormality may have a considerable longitudinal extent.

Arachnoid cysts can develop, compressing and distorting the cord (41).

Other Diagnostic Studies

Imaging should usually precede lumbar puncture, which is contraindicated if spinal block is present. The lumbar CSF is usually under normal pressure or, when a block is present, under reduced pressure. Fluid constituents are normal, or there may be a slight pleocytosis and slight elevation of protein. The pleocytosis can be either mononuclear or polymorphonuclear. The CSF protein will be markedly elevated below the level of a complete block (Froin syndrome).

Pathoanatomy

The arachnoid is a thin membrane throughout the CNS between the pia and dura. A potential space separates the arachnoid from the dura. CSF is located between the arachnoid and pia (Fig. 1). The pia is adherent to the CNS.

The arachnoid is relatively avascular and thus has difficulty participating in an inflammatory reaction. In response to chronic irritation, fibrosis with proliferation and thickening of the arachnoid is found, and adhesions develop between the arachnoid, pia, and dura, which may produce an associated compromise of circulation. The fibrotic bands may form cystic structures communicating with the subarachnoid space or containing loculated CSF. Constriction of the cord can develop as can compromise of nerve roots. The area of pathology is localized or diffuse. Arachnoiditis is one cause of arachnoid cyst (11). The midthoracic spine is most commonly involved, followed by the midcervical spine.

With time, a constrictive phase develops with obliteration of the subarachnoid space and a block of CSF pathways. Blood vessel walls become thickened. The constrictive and vascular effects result in intramedullary changes in the cord. The associated vasculitis can produce infarction of the cord. Compression of the spinal cord from arachnoid cysts also produces these changes. In tuberculous arachnoiditis, the spinal cord can be encased in a fibrous or gelatinous exudate (16).

Natural History

Progression of symptomatology commonly develops. Although cessation of progression may occur spontaneously, improvement is usually minimal (30).

Treatment

Neither medical nor surgical treatment is satisfactory (11).

Nonsurgical

Antiinflammatory agents, including steroids, are the mainstays of treatment. However, significant improvement is seldom realized. Of particular interest is the fact that intrathecal steroids may also incite the process of arachnoiditis (40). Antibiotics probably have no place in the management of this condition. Supportive care should be undertaken with physical therapy and other appropriate measures.

Surgical

The results of surgery have not been encouraging and remain controversial (23). A tangle of fibrous meninges and neural structures is found at surgery, and any attempt at dissection has the risk of producing further neurologic impairment and further compromise of vascular function. Surgery should only be considered when the process involves a small circumscribed area or when an arachnoid cyst is producing symptoms.

SPINAL EPIDURAL ABSCESS

An epidural abscess is a collection of pus between the dura and overlying bone. The terms *epidural* and *extradural* are interchangeable.

Epidemiologic Factors

The incidence of epidural abscess is 2 in 10,000 hospital admissions (36). Epidural abscess is more common in males except during childhood when females predominate 2:1 (71). All age groups are affected from infancy on (19). A review of 45 cases from the English language literature was reported in 1974 (6).

Etiologic Factors

Spinal epidural abscess is usually a complication of bacteremia. Urinary tract infections and furuncles are common sources of the infection, although decubitus ulcers, pulmonary infection, and dental infection are implicated. Altered immune status predisposes to epidural abscess (36). It has been reported secondary to intravenous substance abuse (82). Considering the frequency with which lumbar puncture is performed, epidural abscess is extremely rare after that procedure (7). Trauma to the back, back surgery, vertebral osteomyelitis, and spinal or epidural anesthesia (14,96) are sometimes associated findings. The abscess may develop by spread from a contiguous osteomyelitis (78). A focus cannot always be identified.

Staphylococcus aureus is the most common organism recovered, responsible for at least 50% of cases in both children and adults (71). Gram-negative organisms, such as *E. coli* and *Proteus,* are other etiologic factors. Tuberculosis is always a consideration.

Clinical Features

Spinal epidural abscess is a "painful, febrile, spinal syndrome" (31) (Table 3). A preexisting remote infection is usually present. Pain is the most consistent symptom, and discomfort evolves rapidly from localized back pain to radicular pain and is frequently severe. The radicular pain is appropriate for the dermatomes involved in the infection. There may be swelling and

TABLE 3. SIGNS AND SYMPTOMS OF SPINAL EPIDURAL ABSCESS

Rapid progression
Fever
Tenderness and swelling about spine
Localized and radicular pain
Paresis
Sphincter involvement
Headache
Stiff neck

tenderness in the area of back pain. Headache and nuchal rigidity may be present.

Progression can be extremely rapid. Clinical symptoms progress through four phases—(a) spinal ache, (b) root pain, (c) partial neurologic dysfunction, and (d) paralysis (35)—often within 24 hours of onset. The weakness is the result of spinal cord compression and ischemia. Bladder dysfunction, especially urinary retention, is an ominous sign. A sensory level is a late finding. When the cause is tuberculosis, symptoms evolve more slowly.

In children, back pain and fever may be the only symptoms preceding precipitous development of neurologic signs (71). In infants, the condition may present as fever and diminished limb movements. Prior antibiotic therapy masks symptoms. A high index of suspicion is necessary to make the diagnosis of spinal epidural abscess. Early diagnosis and treatment are of paramount importance (54).

To make the diagnosis the clinician must recognize that an acute spinal syndrome is present. Cardinal clinical features include fever, back pain, numbness, tingling, weakness, and bladder dysfunction. Imaging establishes that the condition is an epidural abscess.

Differential Diagnosis

Acute transverse myelitis can be confused with spinal epidural abscess. Fever and back pain are usually less prominent in acute transverse myelitis, and a sensory level is an early finding (27). Meningitis, spinal tumors, spondylitis, and herniated discs need to be considered. Spinal trauma, acute back strain, and Pott disease can all mimic spinal epidural abscess, but none of these conditions has a significant febrile response or other sign of infection. In the infant or young child, an acute discitis can present with diminished movements of the lower extremities and pain.

Radiographic and Imaging Studies

Immediate gadolinium-enhanced spinal MRI is indicated and should precede lumbar puncture (93). MRI shows a fluid collection between neural structures and bone. The entire spine should be imaged, even if symptoms are localized. MRI is noninvasive, readily available in the United States, and has the advantage of being able to detect other conditions, such as disc herniation, joint space infection, vertebral osteomyelitis, syrinx, intramedul-

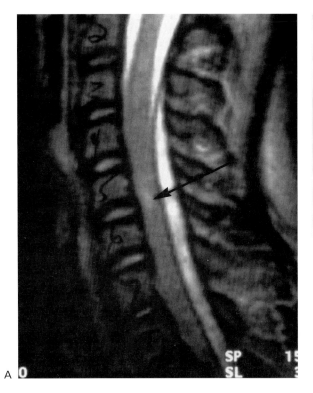
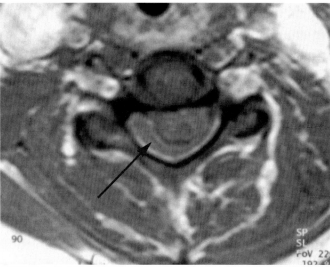

FIGURE 2. A 12-year-old girl with acute back pain, fever, incontinence, and numbness and weakness of arms and legs. **A:** Magnetic resonance image of cervical spinal cord in sagittal planes (TR: 4,000; TE: 90). There is increased signal in the central cord on longitudinal image that does not enhance with contrast and does not have mass effect, probably ischemia secondary to vasculitis *(arrow)*. Also, there is increased signal surrounding the cord secondary to *S. aureus* epidural abscess. **B:** On axial image, epidural mass *(arrow)* is compressing the spinal cord and displacing it anteriorly, secondary to *S. aureus* epidural abscess (TR: 700; TE: 17).

lary spinal tumor, spinal hematoma, and transverse myelitis (36). MRI is superior to CT-myelography in delimiting the extent of the lesion (Fig. 2).

Other Diagnostic Studies

The sedimentation rate is consistently elevated. The peripheral white count may be slightly elevated with a left shift or the white count may be normal (96).

Lumbar puncture is contraindicated because of the possibility of increased symptomatology when either a partial or a complete spinal block is present (37). Also, lumbar puncture can inadvertently carry infectious material into the subarachnoid space, thus causing meningitis. If lumbar puncture is performed and purulent material is found before entry into the subarachnoid space, the needle should not be advanced further.

CSF may be turbid or xanthochromic, with elevation of protein, polymorphonuclear pleocytosis, and normal sugar (44). Normal CSF does not rule out the diagnosis of epidural abscess. As spinal epidural abscess is associated with bacteremia, the etiologic organism can sometimes be recovered by blood culture.

Pathoanatomy

Bacteremia underlies most cases of spinal epidural abscess, especially when the presentation is acute. Infection usually occurs by hematogenous spread and produces rapid neurologic dysfunction and purulence in the epidural space (Fig. 1). Batson's plexus is a low-pressure epidural network of veins. Bacteria from the pelvis may seed into the area of Batson's plexus during straining, such as in a Valsalva maneuver, and thus initiate the process of formation of an epidural abscess. Debilitation is a predisposing factor. The abscess produces neurologic symptomatology by nerve root and cord compression, by vascular changes induced by the inflammation with spinal cord infarction, and by obstruction of CSF flow (13). An infection of the epidural space may be produced by spread from contiguous structures such as bone or soft tissues. Purulent meningitis is surprisingly rare in spinal epidural abscess.

The epidural space consists mostly of fat and, similar to other fatty tissues, has a lowered resistance to infection (63). Epidural abscesses usually occur in the mid-thoracic and upper lumbar area, dorsal to the spinal cord where the epidural space is more capacious. Epidural abscess is less common in the cervical area, perhaps because the dura is more closely applied to the vertebral bodies in that area.

Natural History

Epidural abscess is a condition with a poor prognosis and a high mortality. Progression is frequently rapid, requiring early diagnosis with urgent appropriate intervention to achieve a favorable outcome (54). The outcome is related, at least in part, to the condition of the patient at the time of diagnosis. Appropriate management may prevent progression but does not always reverse the clinical deficits present at the time of surgery. Permanent neurologic sequelae result when treatment is delayed (60), and recovery may be incomplete (85). Preoperative paralysis is an especially ominous sign (36). Children and adolescents probably recover more completely than older individuals (75). If not promptly treated, an epidural abscess may spread beneath the dura and expand to produce spinal cord compression and CSF block.

Treatment

Spinal epidural abscess is a medical and surgical emergency (58).

Nonsurgical

Appropriate antibiotics should be started immediately after recognition of the condition, with initial empirical therapy directed against *S. aureus.* The physician is advised to consult appropriate sources for current antibiotic recommendations (53).

The role of glucocorticoids in the medical management of this condition is uncertain, although glucocorticoids are frequently used. Glucocorticoid treatment is associated with a poor outcome, although the most seriously ill patients are more likely to be placed on steroids (20). The use of very high-dose glucocorticoids in this condition has not been reported.

Claims have been made that spinal epidural abscess can be successfully treated by intravenous antibiotics without surgical intervention (55,62,82). Nonoperative treatment with antibiotics should only be considered when the pathogenic organism is known, antibiotic sensitivities are available, the neurologic condition is stable, and MRI is readily available for reevaluation (32). Nonsurgical treatment avoids the spinal deformities that develop in children after extensive laminectomies and is probably appropriate for patients who are poor surgical risks. No data are available concerning the epidural penetration of antibiotics.

Supportive care is appropriate with attention to skin, joints, and bladder.

Surgical

Epidural abscess with cord compression remains a surgical emergency. Aggressive surgical treatment is the mainstay of successful therapy (26,39). Immediate drainage and decompression are indicated, with culture of the purulent material. Antibiotic coverage is essential.

ACUTE TRANSVERSE MYELOPATHY

Acute transverse myelopathy is an acute monophasic intramedullary dysfunction of the spinal cord not related to trauma or extrinsic pressure in an individual without preexisting neurologic disease.

Epidemiologic Factors

Persons of any age between 18 months and 80 years may be affected. The peak incidence occurs between 10 and 19 years of age. In children, the condition is more common during spring, summer, and fall (24).

Etiologic Factors

Acute transverse myelopathy has multiple causes, such as postinfectious processes (64,90), response to immunization, vascular factors (4), direct infection by a virus (e.g., herpes, mumps [65], varicella-zoster, Epstein-Barr) or by bacteria, including Lyme borreliosis (52) and perhaps some instances of *Mycoplasma pneumoniae* infection. However, when transverse myelitis is found in association with *M. pneumoniae,* the neurologic lesions are frequently an immune response. Retrovirus infection is associated with a myelopathy that does not have an acute onset. Some cases of acute transverse myelopathy are clearly autoimmune (49), and acute transverse myelopathy is often a feature of acute disseminated encephalomyelitis. Acute transverse myelopathy has been found in a child with lupus erythematosus (5). Fibrocartilaginous emboli must be considered (95). Many cases remain idiopathic.

Multiple sclerosis is usually considered as a separate category and not as a cause of acute transverse myelopathy. Acute transverse myelopathy is rarely the first sign of multiple sclerosis (10,89). Acute transverse myelopathy with acute or subacute optic neuropathy, so-called Devic disease, may also not be a form of multiple sclerosis (56).

Clinical Features

Acute pain, usually interscapular, is the most common initial complaint (46) (Table 4). Paresthesias and leg weakness follow. The arms may be involved if the lesion is cervical. Urinary retention and overflow incontinence are almost universal findings. Progression is usually rapid, with maximum deficit present within 2 hours. However, progression has been reported for as long as 10 days (48).

To make the diagnosis of transverse myelopathy the clinician must recognize that an acute spinal syndrome is present. Cardinal clinical features include localized back pain, numbness, tingling, a sensory level, weakness, and bladder dysfunction. Imaging establishes that the condition is transverse myelitis.

Differential Diagnosis

Diagnostic difficulty occurs in differentiating acute transverse myelopathy and Guillain-Barré syndrome, disc disease, spinal epidural abscess, trauma, neoplasm, multiple sclerosis, poliomyelitis, and malingering. Urinary retention, common in transverse myelitis, is not a prominent feature of Guillain-Barré syndrome.

TABLE 4. SIGNS AND SYMPTOMS OF TRANSVERSE MYELOPATHY

Rapid progression
Back pain, often interscapular
Paresthesias
Leg weakness
Sphincter disturbance
Sensory level

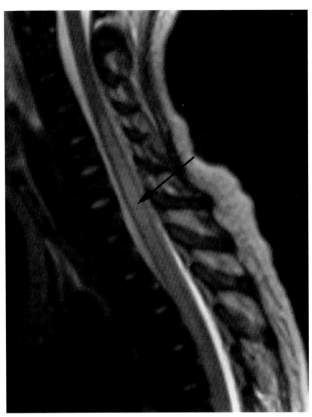

FIGURE 3. A 14-year-old girl with lupus and acute myelopathy. Post-gadolinium-pentetic acid T2-weighted magnetic resonance image of cervical and upper thoracic spinal cord (TR: 4,000; TE: 102). There is a large longitudinal area of increased signal within the substance of the cord from C4 through T2, probably representing edema within the cord *(arrow)*. There is also transverse myelopathy caused by vasculitis or inflammatory changes.

Radiographic and Imaging Studies

Exclusion of an alternative diagnosis, such as a mass lesion, is an important aspect of management. An acute compressive cord lesion is a surgical emergency, whereas surgery is contraindicated in acute transverse myelopathy. MRI offers a noninvasive technique to determine the location and extent of the spinal cord lesion (38). MRI may show high signal in the area of the lesion on T2-weighted imaging and cord swelling, or may be normal. Gadolinium-enhanced MRI provides more precise clarification of the extent of the lesion (Fig. 3).

Other Diagnostic Studies

Examination of CSF should be postponed until imaging is obtained. The fluid will be normal or have an elevated protein with a pleocytosis, predominantly lymphocytic. Somatosensory evoked potentials are useful in diagnosis and follow-up. Visual evoked potentials and brain stem auditory evoked potentials should be normal. Electromyelography is claimed to be of value (42).

Pathoanatomy

The thoracic cord is the site of the lesion in 80% of the cases with the remainder of the lesions in the cervical or lumbar cord (24). The cord involvement is transverse (partial or complete) and may have considerable longitudinal extent. The pathology is necrotizing rather than demyelinating raising further doubt of its relation to multiple sclerosis (56). With the passage of time, cystic changes appear within the cord. Pathology is often not obtained until months after onset, adding additional confusion regarding characteristic pathology (4).

Natural History

Rapid onset of disability is associated with an unfavorable outcome. Recovery continues for many months. A significant return of function occurs in about half of cases (73). Prolonged bladder and sexual dysfunction may persist despite recovery of other neurologic function (9).

Treatment

Nonsurgical

Supportive care is indicated, with attention to skin, joints, and bladder. The place of steroids in the management of acute transverse myelopathy remains uncertain. High-dose methylprednisolone may lead to more rapid and more complete recovery (46,48,77). Appropriate antibiotics must be given when the cause is bacterial or an immune response to a bacteria, as in *M. pneumoniae* infection.

Surgical

No surgical treatment exists for this condition.

REFERENCES

1. Amir J, Harel L, Frydman M, et al. (1991): Shift of cerebrospinal polymorphonuclear cell percentage in the early stage of aseptic meningitis. *J Pediatr* 119:938–941.
2. Arditi M, Ables L, Yogev R (1989): Cerebrospinal fluid endotoxin levels in children with *H. influenzae* meningitis before and after administration of intravenous ceftriaxone. *J Infect Dis* 160:1005–1011.
3. Arditi M, Mason EO, Bradley JS, et al. (1998): Three-year multicenter surveillance of pneumococcal meningitis in children: clinical characteristics and outcome. *Pediatrics* 102:1087–1097.
4. Arlazoroff A, Klein C, Blumen N, et al. (1989): Acute transverse myelitis: a possible vascular etiology. *Med Hypoth* 30:27–30.
5. Baca V, Sanchezvaca G, Martinexmuniz I, et al. (1996): Successful treatment of transverse myelitis in a child with systemic lupus-erythematosus. *Neuropediatrics* 27:42–44.
6. Baker AS, Ojemann RG, Swartz MN, et al. (1975): Spinal epidural abscess. *N Engl J Med* 293:463–468.
7. Beland B, Prien T, Vanaken H (1997): Spinal and epidural-anaesthesia in bacteremic patients. *Anaesthesist* 46:536–547.
8. Bell WE, McCormick WF (1981): *Neurologic infections in children*, 2nd ed. Philadelphia: WB Saunders, pp. 27–40.
9. Berger Y, Blaivas JG, Oliver L (1990): Urinary dysfunction in transverse myelitis. *J Urol* 144:103–105.
10. Berman M, Feldman S, Alter M, et al. (1981): Acute transverse myelitis: Incidence and etiologic considerations. *Neurology* 31:966–971.

11. Bourne IH (1990): Lumbo-sacral adhesive arachnoiditis: a review. *J R Soc Med* 83:262–265.
12. Broome CV (1987): Epidemiology of Haemophilus influenzae type b infections in the United States. *Pediatr Infect Dis J* 6:779–782.
13. Browder J, Meyers R (1941): Pyogenic infections of the spinal epidural space: a consideration of the anatomic and physiologic pathology. *Surgery* 10:296–308.
14. Bulow PM, Biering-Sorensen F (1999). Paraplegia, a severe complication to epidural analgesia. *Acta Anaesthesiol Scand* 43:233–235.
15. Caplan LR, Norohna AB, Amico LL (1990): Syringomyelia and arachnoiditis. *J Neurol Neurosurg Psychiatry* 53:106–113.
16. Chang HS, Han MH, Choi YW, et al. (1989): Tuberculous arachnoiditis of the spine: findings on myelography, CT, and MR imaging. *AJNR Am J Neuroradiol* 10:1255–1262.
17. Chang YC, Huang CC, Wang ST, et al. (1997): Risk factor of complications requiring neurosurgical intervention in infants with bacterial meningitis. *Pediatr Neurol* 17:144–149.
18. Cochi SL, Fleming DW, Hightower AW, et al. (1986): Primary invasive *Haemophilus influenzae* type B disease: a population-based assessment of risk factors. *J Pediatr* 108:887–896.
19. D'Angelo CM, Whisler WW (1978): Bacterial infections of the spinal cord and its coverings. In: Vinken PJ, Bruyn GW, eds. *Handbook of clinical neurology,* Vol. 33. Amsterdam: North-Holland, pp. 187–194.
20. Danner RL, Hartman BJ (1987): Update of spinal epidural abscess: 35 cases and review of the literature. *Rev Infect Dis* 9:265–274.
21. DeJong RN (1981): Arachnoiditis, spinal familial (familial arachnoidal fibrosis with secondary ischemic radiculomyelopathy). In: Vinken PJ, Bruyn GW, eds. *Handbook of clinical neurology,* Vol. 42. Amsterdam: North-Holland, pp. 107–108.
22. Delamarter RB, Ross JS, Masaryk TJ, et al. (1990): Diagnosis of lumbar arachnoiditis by magnetic resonance imaging. *Spine* 15:304–310.
23. Dolan RA (1993): Spinal adhesive arachnoiditis. *Surg Neurol* 39:479–484.
24. Dunne K, Hopkins IJ, Shield LK (1986): Acute transverse myelopathy in childhood. *Dev Med Child Neurol* 28:198–204.
25. Elzayat SG, Elzayat IM (1995): Failed back surgery: a prospective study. *J Neurol Orthop Med Surg* 16:165–166.
26. Enberg RN, Kaplan RJ (1994): Spinal epidural abscess in children: early diagnosis and immediate surgical drainage is essential to forestall paralysis. *Clin Pediatr* 13:247–253.
27. Ericsson M, Algers G, Schliamser SE (1990): Spinal epidural abscesses in adults: review and report of iatrogenic cases. *Scand J Infect Dis* 22:249–257.
28. Gilman S (1998): Imaging the brain. *N Engl J Med* 338:889–896.
29. Grau AJ (1997): Infection, inflammation, and cerebrovascular ischemia. *Neurology* 49(Suppl 4):S47–S51
30. Guyer DW, Wiltse LL, Eskay ML, et al. (1989): The long-range prognosis of arachnoiditis. *Spine* 14:1332–1341.
31. Hancock DO (1973): A study of 49 patients with acute spinal extradural abscess. *Paraplegia* 10:285–288.
32. Hanigan WC, Asner NG, Elwood PW (1990): Magnetic resonance imaging and the nonoperative treatment of spinal epidural abscess. *Surg Neurol* 34:408–413.
33. Hardjasudarma M, Davis DR (1993): Neuroimaging of arachnoiditis induced by spinal anesthesia. *S Med J* 86:1293–1296.
34. Haupt HM, Kurlinski JP, Barnett NK, et al. (1981): Infarction of the spinal cord as a complication of pneumococcus meningitis. *J Neurosurg* 55:121–123.
35. Heusner AP (1948): Nontuberculous spinal epidural infections. *N Engl J Med* 239:845–853.
36. Hlavin ML, Kaminski HJ, Ross JS, et al. (1990): Spinal epidural abscess: a ten-year perspective. *Neurosurgery* 27:177–184.
37. Hollis PH, Malis LI, Zappulla RA (1986): Neurological deterioration after lumbar puncture below complete spinal subarachnoid block. *J Neurosurg* 64:253–256.
38. Holtas S, Basibuyuk N, Fredricksson K (1993): MRI in acute transverse myelopathy. *Neuroradiology* 35:221–226.
39. Jacobsen FS, Sullivan B (1994): Spinal epidural abscesses in children. *Orthopedics* 17:1131–1138.
40. Johnson A, Ryan MD, Roche J (1991): Depo-Medrol and myelographic arachnoiditis. *Med J Aust* 155:18–20.
41. Johnson CE, Sze G (1990): Benign lumbar arachnoiditis: MR imaging with gadopentetate dimeglumine. *AJNR Am J Neuroradiol* 11:763–770.
42. Kalita J, Misra UK, Mandal SK (1998): Prognostic predictors of acute transverse myelitis. *Acta Neurol Scand* 98:60–63.
43. Kaplan SL (1990): Corticosteroids in bacterial meningitis. *Scand J Infect Dis* 73(Suppl):43–54.
44. Kaufmann DM, Kaplan JG, Litman N (1980): Infectious agents in spinal epidural abscess. *Neurology* 30:844–850.
45. Kikuchi M, Nagao KMY, Ohnuma S, et al. (1999): Cauda equina syndrome complicating pneumococcal meningitis. *Pediatr Neurol* 20:152–154.
46. Knebusch M, Strassburg HM, Reiners K (1998): Acute transverse myelitis in childhood: nine cases and review of the literature. *Dev Med Child Neurol* 40:631–639.
47. Kumar A, Montanera W, Willinsky R, et al. (1993): MR features of tuberculous arachnoiditis. *J Comp Assist Tomogr* 17:127–130.
48. Lahat E, Pillar G, Ravid S, et al. Rapid recovery from transverse myelopathy in children treated with methylprednisolone. *Pediatr Neurol* 19:279–282.
49. Lavalle C, Pizarro S, Drenkard C, et al. (1990): Transverse myelitis: a manifestation of systemic lupus erythematosus strongly associated with antiphospholipid antibodies. *J Rheumatol* 17:34–37.
50. Lebel MH, Freij BJ, Syrgiannopolos GA, et al. (1988): Dexamethasone therapy for bacterial meningitis: results of 2 double-blind placebo-controlled trials. *N Engl J Med* 319:964–971.
51. Leonard JM, Des Prez RM (1990): Tuberculous meningitis. *Infect Dis Clin N Am* 4:769–787.
52. Linssen WHJP, Gabreels FJM, Weavers RA (1991): Infective acute transverse myelopathy: report of 2 cases. *Neuropediatrics* 22:107–109.
53. Lowy FD (1998): *Staphylococcus aureus* infections. *N Engl J Med* 339:520–532.
54. Mackenzie AR, Laing RBS, Smith CC, et al. (1998): Spinal epidural abscess: the importance of early diagnosis and treatment. *J Neurol Neurosurg Psychiatry* 65:209–212.
55. Mampalam TJ, Rosegay H, Andrews BT, et al. (1989): Nonoperative treatment of spinal epidural infections. *J Neurosurg* 71:208–210.
56. Mandler RN, Davis LD, Jeffrey DR, et al. (1993): Devic's neuromyelitis optica: a clinicopathological study of 8 patients. *Ann Neurol* 34:162–168.
57. Markus HS, Allison SP (1989): Staphylococcus aureus meningitis from osteomyelitis of the spine. *Postgrad Med J* 65:941–942.
58. Martin RJ, Yuan HA (1996): Neurosurgical care of spinal epidural, subdural, and intramedullary abscesses and arachnoiditis. *Orthoped Clin N Am* 27:125–136.
59. Marton KI, Gean AD (1986): The diagnostic spinal tap. *Ann Intern Med* 104:880–885.
60. McGee-Collette M, Johnson IH (1991): Spinal epidural abscess: presentation and treatment. *Med J Aust* 155:14–17.
61. Merkelbach S, Muller M, Huber G, et al. (1998): Alteration of cerebral blood flow in patients with bacterial and viral meningoencephalitis. *AJNR Am J Neuroradiol* 19:433–438.
62. Nordberg G, Mark H (1998): Epidural abscess after epidural analgesia treated successfully with antibiotics. *Acta Anaesthesiol Scand* 42:727–731.
63. North JB, Brophy BP (1979): Epidural abscess: a hazard of spinal epidural anesthesia. *Aust N Z J Surg* 49:484–485.
64. Nussinovitch M, Brand N, Frydman M, et al. (1992): Transverse myelitis following mumps in children. *Acta Paediatr* 81:183–184.
65. Nussinovitch M, Volovitz B, Varsano I (1995): Complications of mumps requiring hospitalization in children. *Eur J Pediatr* 154:732–734.
66. Odio CM, Faingezicht I, Paris M, et al. (1991): The beneficial effects of early dexamethasone administration in infants and children with bacterial meningitis. *N Engl J Med* 324:1525–1531.
67. Peltola H (1997): Controversies in the management of childhood meningitis. *J Med Microbiol* 46:901–902.
68. Pomeroy SL, Holmes SJ, Dodge PR, et al. (1990): Seizures and other

neurologic sequelae of bacterial meningitis in children. *N Engl J Med* 323:1651–1657.

69. Quiles M, Marchisello PJ, Tsairis P (1978): Lumbar adhesive arachnoiditis. *Spine* 3:45–50.

70. Richardson MP, Reid A, Tarlow MJ, et al. (1997): Hearing loss during bacterial meningitis. *Arch Dis Child* 76:134–138.

71. Rockney R, Ryan R, Knuckey N (1989): Spinal epidural abscess. An infectious emergency. Case report and review. *Clin Pediatr* 28: 332–334.

72. Roos KL (1995): The use of adjunctive therapy to alter the pathophysiology of bacterial meningitis. *Clin Neuropharmacol* 18:138–147.

73. Ropper AH, Poskanzer DC (1978): The prognosis of acute and subacute transverse myelopathy based on early signs and symptoms. *Ann Neurol* 4:51–59.

74. Schuchat A, Robinson K, Wenger JD, et al. (1997): Bacterial meningitis in the United States in 1995. *N Engl J Med* 337:970–976.

75. Schweich PJ, Hurt TL (1992): Spinal epidural abscess in children: two illustrative cases. *Pediatr Emerg Care* 8:84–87.

76. Seay AR (1984): Spinal cord dysfunction complicating bacterial meningitis. *Arch Neurol* 41:545–546.

77. Sebire G, Hollenberg H, Meyer L, et al. (1997): High dose methylprednisolone in severe acute transverse myelopathy. *Arch Dis Child* 76: 167–168.

78. Shen WC, Lee SK (1991): Chronic osteomyelitis with epidural abscess; CT and MR findings. *J Comp Assist Tomogr* 15:839–841.

79. Shipton EA (1989): Low back pain and the post-laminectomy pain syndrome. *S Afr Med J* 76:20–23.

80. Silberstein SD (1998): Post-lumbar puncture headache. *Cephalagia* 18: 72.

81. Sklar EML, Quencer RM, Green BA, et al. (1991): Complications of epidural anesthesia: MR appearance of abnormalities. *Radiology* 181: 549–554.

82. Slade WR, Lonano F (1990): Acute spinal epidural abscess. *J Natl Med Assoc* 82:713–716.

83. Snedeker JD, Kaplan SL, Dodge PR, et al. (1990): Subdural effusion and its relationship with neurologic sequelae of bacterial meningitis in infancy: a prospective study. *Pediatrics* 86:163–170.

84. Spellerberg B, Tuomanen EI (1994): The pathophysiology of pneumococcal meningitis. *Annals of Medicine* 26:411–418.

85. Statham P, Gentleman D (1989): Importance of early diagnosis of acute spinal extradural abscess. *J R Soc Med* 82:584–587.

86. Tal Y, Crichton U, Dunn HG, et al. (1980): Spinal cord damage: a rare complication of purulent meningitis. *Acta Paediatr Scand* 69: 471–474.

87. Taylor HG, Mills EL, Ciampi A, et al. (1990): The sequelae of *Haemophilus influenzae* meningitis in school-aged children. *N Engl J Med* 323: 1657–1663.

88. Taylor HG, Schatschneider C, Watters GV, et al. (1998): Acute-phase neurologic complications of *Haemophilus influenzae* type b meningitis: association with developmental problems at school age. *J Child Neurol* 13:113–119.

89. Tippett DS, Fishman PS, Panitch HS (1991): Relapsing transverse myelitis. *Neurology* 1991;41:703–706.

90. Tsutsumi H, Kamazaki H, Nakata S, et al. (1994): Sequential development of acute meningoencephalitis and transverse myelitis caused by Epstein-Barr virus during infectious mononucleosis. *Pediatr Infect Dis J* 13:665–667.

91. Vantassel P (1994): Magnetic resonance imaging of spinal infections. *Topics Magn Reson Imaging* 6:69–81.

92. Verghese A, Gallemore G (1987): Kernig's and Brudzinski's signs revisited. *Rev Infect Dis* 9:1187–1192.

93. Weingarten K, Zimmerman RD, Becker RD, et al. (1989): Subdural and epidural empyemas: MR imaging. *AJR Am J Roentgenol* 152: 615–621.

94. Whisler WW (1978): Chronic spinal arachnoiditis. In: Vinken PJ, Bruyn GW, eds. *Handbook of clinical neurology,* 33rd ed. Amsterdam: North-Holland, pp. 263–274.

95. Wilmshurst JM, Walker MC, Pohl KRE (1999): Rapid onset transverse myelitis in adolescence: implications for pathogenesis and prognosis. *Arch Dis Child* 80:137–142.

96. Wong D, Raymond NJ (1998): Spinal epidural abscess. *N Z Med J* 111:345–347.

97. Yaramis A, Gurkan M, Elevli E, et al. (1998): Central nervous system tuberculosis in children: a review of 214 cases. *Pediatrics* 102: E491–E495.

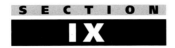

NEOPLASMS AND MALFORMATIONS

39

SPINE NEOPLASMS

JAMES N. WEINSTEIN
STEFANO BORIANI
LAURA CAMPANACCI

Back pain in a child should make the family doctor, pediatrician, or spine surgeon take note. A high index of suspicion is essential. It is easy to pass off back pain as nothing and to tell the patient and parents that it will get better. In the pediatric population, a history of persistent back pain always warrants further investigation and begins with a good history and physical examination (6). One should have a list of differential diagnoses (Table 1). Indeed, as compared with adults, in whom more than 80% of back pain is self-limited, fewer than 30% of children with back pain have a self-limited problem and in most cases there is a skeletal cause.

In children with persistent back pain, preliminary studies at least should be performed, including anteroposterior and lateral radiographs of the thoracolumbar spine and sacrum. Initial laboratory tests should include a complete blood count and determination of erythrocyte sedimentation rate (ESR).

DIAGNOSIS

Early diagnosis of a tumor can be challenging, and misdiagnosis is an unfortunate reality in many cases. Most cases of back pain in children are believed to be due to recreational accidents, and the presence of a tumor is seldom expected as a cause of pain. In a series of 1,971 patients with musculoskeletal neoplasms in a 17-year period, only 29 patients, including eight children, had primary osseous tumors of the thoracic or lumbar spine (19). Spinal tumors are extremely rare and thus often unsuspected. However, common symptoms of spinal tumors do exist and should lead physicians to consider this in the differential diagnosis.

SYMPTOMS

The most common symptom is pain (6). Although pain is a very nonspecific complaint, that associated with a tumor tends to be progressive and unrelenting, and is not closely related to activity. Night pain is a particular cause for worry. Pain occurs due to several causes. Tumor growth may cause expansion of the bony cortex of the vertebral body, which results in pathologic fracture and invasion of paravertebral soft tissues. Pain is also associated with acute or chronic compression of the spinal cord, resulting in focal and radicular symptoms of pain, paraparesis, or paraplegia. Spinal deformity may also be linked with pain and tumors.

Clinical Presentation

Clinical symptoms were nonspecific in 94 cases of bone tumors of the spine observed in pediatric patients at Rizzoli Institute during the period 1928–1994. Pain was the presenting symptom in all of the malignant lesions and in 69 of 74 benign tumors (93%); the average duration of pain was 29 weeks. Severe neurologic deficits (paraparesis) were reported in seven cases (7.5%), always in benign aggressive or malignant tumors. A palpable mass was observed in five cases (5.5%), arising from the posterior elements (e.g., osteoblastomas, aneurysmal bone cysts, or osteochondromas).

Weakness, usually in the lower extremities, may manifest sometime after pain is felt but is rarely the first symptom. Thus, maintaining a high index of suspicion when following patients is a necessity (86). Bowel and bladder dysfunction may also be a sign of a spinal tumor. The most important part of a correct diagnosis is the ability to evaluate the symptoms and to remain suspicious of a spinal neoplasm. In children, pain is not always expressed, but a change in personality, lethargy, instability, fever, limping, or bruising may be signs that must be taken seriously and investigated.

IMAGING

Plain radiographs are the first step in the search for a spinal tumor. Anteroposterior and lateral radiographic views are often useful in determining the nature and behavior of the lesion and can help identify specific tumor types. Bone scans are used to locate the site of the tumor when a standard radiograph is negative; they distinguish between monostotic and polyostotic pro-

J.N. Weinstein: Dartmouth Medical School, Hanover, New Hampshire 03755.

S. Boriani and L. Campanacci: Department of Orthopaedics and Traumatology, Ospedal Maggiore, Bologna, Italy 40133.

TABLE 1. DIFFERENTIAL DIAGNOSIS FOR PEDIATRIC BACK PAIN

Scheuermann disease
Spondylolysis/spondylolisthesis
Herniated nucleus pulposus
Spondylolysis
Disc space infection/osteomyelitis
Spondyloarthropathies (i.e., ankylosing spondylitis, psoriatic arthritis, Reiter syndrome, spondyloepiphyseal dysplasia)
Trauma
Benign bone tumors
Malignant bone tumors
Spinal cord tumors, intra- and extramedullary
Metastatic tumors, neuroblastoma, and Wilms tumor

cesses and are also helpful in identifying the most accessible biopsy site in polyostotic disease. In the spine, computed tomography (CT) and magnetic resonance imaging (MRI) are probably the most helpful procedures for early detection of a tumor. Likewise, in surgical preparation and perioperative planning, CT often remains the most beneficial imaging method (85). MRI has replaced myelography and is a useful tool in the diagnosis and treatment of spinal neoplasms. MRI is often used as the primary diagnostic imaging tool, whereas CT is often an adjunctive modality in planning. MRI has several advantages: there is no radiation, sagittal views of the entire spine are possible, and tumorous and nontumorous conditions can be more easily distinguished. MRI is probably best for describing the spinal cord in relation to its surrounding structures.

In evaluation of spinal tumors, MRI can help classify tumors by location as (a) intramedullary, (b) intradural extramedullary, (c) extradural, and (d) osseous. Tumors can be located in more than one of these sites and in more than one site in the spine, particularly in metastatic disease involving the vertebral bodies and extending into or throughout the extradural space. Intramedullary cord tumors are especially easy to identify by MRI. The microstructure of bone marrow consists of a bone framework surrounding fat cells, hematopoietic cells, reticulum cells, nerves, and vascular channels. The magnetic resonance image of the bone marrow depends on the chemical composition of the marrow. Red marrow is approximately 40% water, 40% fat, and 20% protein. Yellow marrow is 15% water, 80% fat, and 5% protein (28). T1-weighted images optimize the signal from fat and provide excellent anatomical detail of bone. Processes that replace fat in the bone marrow are best visualized on T1-weighted images. T2-weighted images help characterize abnormal tissue. Pathologic processes that increase the free water demonstrate increased activity on T2-weighted images as compared with normal fatty marrow. Disease processes that infiltrate or replace the red or yellow marrow can be delineated accurately on standard T1- and T2-weighted images. Such processes include benign and malignant tumors, leukemia, lymphoma, myeloma, infection, marrow abnormalities with degenerative disease, and avascular necrosis (7,82). MRI is also an excellent technique for delineating vertebral and paravertebral extension of tumor. This helps the surgeon in planning surgical intervention, surgical margins, and/or radiation therapy. Depending on the types of resec-

tions and instrumentation used, MRI may also be useful in detecting tumor recurrences and in distinguishing between benign and malignant processes associated with vertebral compression fractures.

TERMINOLOGY AND STAGING

The lack of a logically organized paradigm contributes to the confusion associated with evaluating the results of treatment for primary spinal tumors. There is no common terminology (26), and there are difficulties in applying the current oncologic staging system (24) that is widely accepted for the study and treatment of bone tumors involving the limbs. The result is that the limb salvage procedures are performed for the treatment of different spinal tumors (51), notwithstanding the techniques of vertebral resection that are well known, at least for the thoracolumbar spine (68,76,78,80). What remains unclear in this evolution is the transfer of information to a common terminology. We purposefully use a common terminology throughout this chapter, and it is hoped that all in our profession will see this as the only way to efficiently and effectively measure outcomes in these difficult cases.

TERMINOLOGY

Excision is piecemeal removal of a tumor ("curettage"). This is an intralesional procedure.

Resection refers to the attempt to remove the tumor en bloc. The pathologist must confirm that the resections around the tumor mass can be defined as intralesional, marginal-wide (10,13,24).

Radical resection refers to the en bloc removal of the tumor together with the complete compartment of origin. It is obvious that this is possible for a tumor arising in the scapula, or even in the femur, but is absolutely impossible for a vertebral tumor unless the spinal cord is sectioned above and below.

All of the surgical procedures that are directed to a functional response (e.g., cord decompression and fracture stabilization), with or without partial (piecemeal) removal of the tumor, are called "palliative." In general, these procedures are only intended to facilitate a diagnosis, decrease pain, and possibly improve function.

The terms *vertebrectomy* and *corpectomy* (removal of all elements of the vertebra), and *somectomy* (removal of the vertebral body) have no significance from an oncologic viewpoint if they are not specified according to the aforementioned terminology.

Oncologic Staging

The oncologic staging system proposed by Enneking et al. (24) defines the biologic behavior of primary tumors and has proven effective in defining a relationship between tumor aggressiveness, surgery (intralesional, marginal-wide, or radical), and results for limb lesions. This system (24) divides benign tumors into three stages (S1, S2, S3) and localizes malignant tumors into four

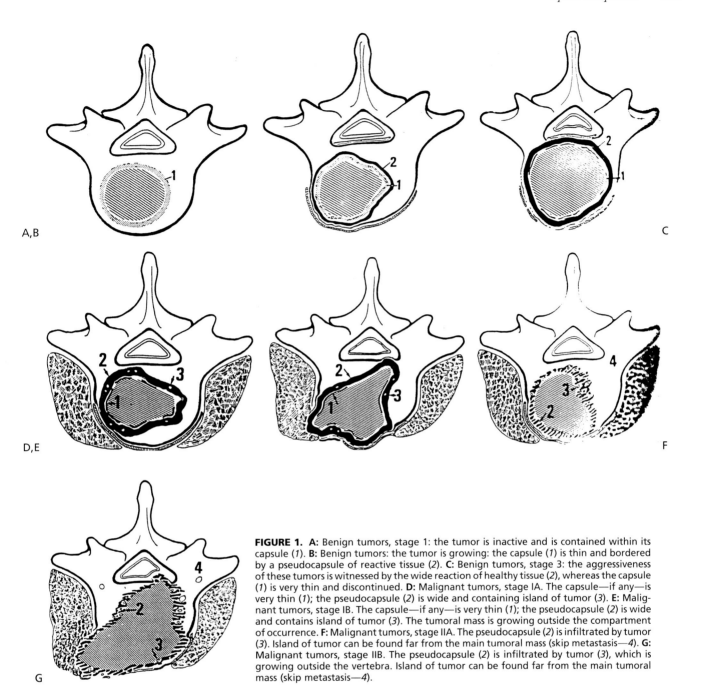

FIGURE 1. **A:** Benign tumors, stage 1: the tumor is inactive and is contained within its capsule (*1*). **B:** Benign tumors: the tumor is growing: the capsule (*1*) is thin and bordered by a pseudocapsule of reactive tissue (*2*). **C:** Benign tumors, stage 3: the aggressiveness of these tumors is witnessed by the wide reaction of healthy tissue (*2*), whereas the capsule (*1*) is very thin and discontinued. **D:** Malignant tumors, stage IA. The capsule—if any—is very thin (*1*); the pseudocapsule (*2*) is wide and containing island of tumor (*3*). **E:** Malignant tumors, stage IB. The capsule—if any—is very thin (*1*); the pseudocapsule (*2*) is wide and contains island of tumor (*3*). The tumoral mass is growing outside the compartment of occurrence. **F:** Malignant tumors, stage IIA. The pseudocapsule (*2*) is infiltrated by tumor (*3*). Island of tumor can be found far from the main tumoral mass (skip metastasis—*4*). **G:** Malignant tumors, stage IIB. The pseudocapsule (*2*) is infiltrated by tumor (*3*), which is growing outside the vertebra. Island of tumor can be found far from the main tumoral mass (skip metastasis—*4*).

stages (IA, IB, IIA, IIB) (Fig. 1). Two additional stages include metastatic high-grade intra- and extracompartmental malignant tumors (IIIA and IIIB, respectively). This classification is based on clinical features, radiographic pattern, CT scan/MRI data, and histologic findings. It was formerly applied to bone tumors and applied to spinal tumors in some reports (8,10,14,34).

Benign Tumors

The first stage of benign tumor (S1, latent, inactive) includes asymptomatic lesions bordered by a true capsule (Fig. 1A), which is usually seen as a sclerotic rim on plain radiographs. These

tumors do not grow, or grow very slowly. No treatment is required unless palliative surgery is needed for decompression or stabilization.

Benign S2 (active) tumors grow slowly, causing mild symptoms. The tumor is bordered by a thin capsule and by a layer of reactive tissue (Fig. 1B), sometimes seen on plain radiographs as an enlargement of the tumor outline. Bone scan is positive. Intralesional excision can be performed with a low rate of recurrence (8). The incidence of recurrences can be lowered further by use of local adjuvants (e.g., cryotherapy, embolization, or radiation therapy).

The third stage of benign tumors (S3, aggressive) includes

rapidly growing benign tumors; the capsule is very thin, discontinued, or absent (Fig. 1C). The tumor invades neighboring compartments, and a wide reactive hypervascularized tissue (pseudocapsule) is often found, sometimes permeated by neoplastic digitations. Bone scan is highly positive, plain films show fuzzy limits, CT scan shows compartmental extension, and magnetic resonance images clearly define a pseudocapsule and its relationship to the neurologic structures. Intralesional curettage, even if augmented by radiation, may be associated with a significant rate of recurrence (14,34). En bloc excision is the treatment of choice.

Malignant Tumors

Low-grade malignant tumors are included in stage I, subdivided into IA (the tumor remains inside the vertebra) and IB (tumor invades paravertebral compartments). No true capsule is associated with these lesions, but a thick pseudocapsule of reactive tissue permeated by small microscopic islands of tumor is seen (Fig. 1D, E). A resection performed along the pseudocapsule often leaves residual foci of active tumor; megavoltage radiation or proton-beam therapy can be added to reduce the risk of recurrence (77). The treatment of choice, if feasible, is wide resection. High-grade malignancies are defined as IIA or IIB. The neoplastic growth is so rapid that the host has no time to form a continuous reactive tissue (Fig. 1F, G). There is continuous seeding with neoplastic nodules (satellites). Moreover, these tumors can have neoplastic nodules at some distance from the main tumor mass (skip metastases). These malignancies are generally seen on plain radiographs as radiolucent and destructive; in many cases, they are associated with a pathologic fracture. Invasion of the epidural space is rapid in stage B, particularly in small-cell tumors characterized by semifluid tissue (e.g., Ewing sarcoma, lymphomas), and able to occupy the epidural space after infiltrating the cortical border of the vertebra.

The margin of the resection must be wide (it is not possible in the spine to achieve a "radical" margin), and courses of radiation and chemotherapy (according to the tumor type) must be considered for local control and for the avoidance of distant spread. Stages IIIA and IIIB describe the same lesions as IIA and IIB, with distant metastasis.

Surgical Staging

For correct application of the above described grading, a complete preoperative workup must be performed. The first attempt to propose such a staging for surgical purposes of primary spinal tumors was introduced by Weinstein (85) and subsequently modified in collaboration with the Rizzoli Institute (10) to identify each lesion in a systematic computerized fashion. This staging system, called the WBB (Weinstein-Boriani-Biagini) system, has been subjected to clinical evaluation (34).

On the transverse plane, the vertebra is divided into 12 radiating zones (numbered 1 to 12 in a clockwise order) and into 5 layers (A to E from the prevertebral to the dural involvement). The longitudinal extent of the tumor is recorded. This system (Fig. 2) should allow for a more rational approach to the surgical planning, provided that all efforts are made to perform surgery along the required margins. The basic concept of a clock-face radiating zone system is that the crucial problem in performing en bloc resections in the spine is due to the presence of the cord in the longitudinal median axis of the vertebra. To save such a structure, the surgeon is compelled to resect circular sectors of the vertebra. For example, it is impossible to perform an en bloc resection of the vertebral body without first removing the posterior arch because the margins are the pedicles. Conversely,

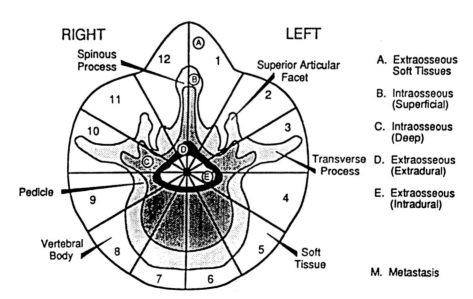

FIGURE 2. The transverse extension of the vertebral tumor is described with reference to 12 radiating zones (numbered 1 to 12 in a clockwise order) and to 5 concentric layers (A to E from the prevertebral to the dural involvement). The longitudinal extent of the tumor is also recorded.

if the tumor occupies an eccentric area, the surgeon is compelled to remove the healthy contralateral parts of the vertebra, dislocate the dural sac, and perform radiating sections by chisel/osteotome.

BENIGN TUMORS

Spinal tumors of any type are uncommon in children. In most cases, they are benign. Nearly 70% of primary bone tumors in children are benign. Osteoid osteoma, osteoblastoma, osteochondroma, and aneurysmal bone cyst account for more than 40% of all primary spinal lesions in younger patients (86). Out of 74 cases collected at the Rizzoli Institute, 53% affected females and the mean age at onset was 9.3 years (ranged 1 to 14 years). The thoracic spine was most frequently affected; nine patients had multiple locations (Fig. 3A–D).

Osteoid Osteoma

In 1953, Dr. H. Jaffee defined osteoid osteoma as a benign bone tumor characterized by a nidus of bone surrounded by fibrovascular tissue and a dense sclerotic bone margin (40). These lesions account for approximately 11% of all primary benign bone tumors, and 10% of them occur in the spine (18).

Osteoid osteoma is most prevalent between the ages of 6 and 17 years (3). In one review of 36 patients with osteoid osteoma, nine tumors were located in the spine, all in the posterior elements (42). Unrelenting pain, most noticeable at night (in about 60% of cases), is the common complaint of patients with osteoid osteoma. The lesions are usually 1.52 cm or smaller, with a small radiolucent nidus surrounded by osteosclerosis (2). The small size causes difficulty in identifying and locating the tumor. Bone scan is the most sensitive method of locating an osteoid osteoma (Fig. 4). Technetium bone scanning provides accurate localization of the lesion, decreasing the average duration of symptoms by providing an early diagnosis and allowing prompt treatment (61). In about 70% to 80% of patients, the diagnosis is made within 2 years of symptom onset. Prostaglandin activity or venous congestion is believed to be responsible for the night symptoms (35). Although aspirin is believed to provide symptomatic relief, it does not always do so. Osteoid osteomas can be associated with severe spinal deformities. Indeed, osteoid osteomas are probably the most common cause of painful scoliosis in adolescence (58). The lumbar spine is the most common location (more than 50%), followed by the cervical, thoracic, and sacral spine. Most osteoid osteomas are located in the posterior elements, lamina, or pedicles; rarely do osteoid osteomas occur in the vertebral body. Seventeen cases were observed at the Rizzoli Institute (11 males, averaging 8.2 years old). Nocturnal pain was the chief complaint in all cases, occurring in the lumbar spine in nine cases, in the cervical spine in five, in the thoracic spine in three. Only four cases arose anteriorly (sectors 4, 5, 8, and 9); all other cases arose in sectors 2, 3, 10, and 11.

Treatment

Long-term administration of nonsteroidal antiinflammatory drugs can often be as effective as excision for treatment of osteoid osteomas, without the morbidity associated with surgery, especially in patients in whom operative treatment would be complex or might lead to disability. Pain treated with antiinflammatory agents resolves in 30 to 40 months (38). Because there have been no reports of malignant transformation or metastases, non-

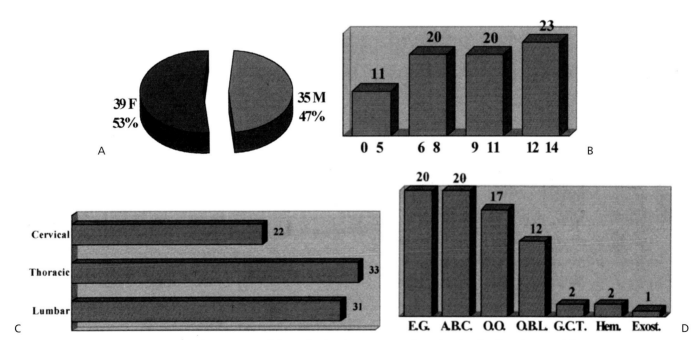

FIGURE 3. Benign bone tumors of the pediatric spine: 74 cases collected at the Rizzoli Institute. Demographics: **A**, sex; **B**, age; **C**, location; **D**, diagnosis.

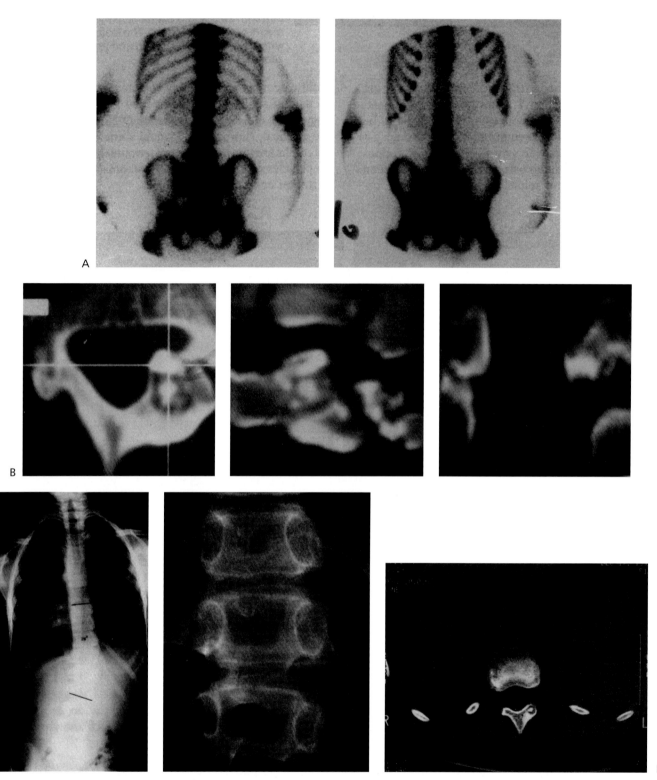

FIGURE 4. Osteoid osteoma. **A:** Posterior *(left)* and anterior *(right)* prone technetium bone scan of an 8-year-old boy who had night pain relieved by aspirin for approximately 6 months; however, the pain was interfering with activities of daily living. He constantly complained of pain during school, but more often at night. Increased uptake is evident at L5 *(left).* **B:** A multiplanar computed tomography (CT) scan of the same patient identifying the nidus of the osteoid osteoma in the posterior elements in the axial *(left),* sagittal *(center),* and coronal *(right)* views. **C:** A 13-year-old boy with back pain caused by osteoid osteoma. Anteroposterior radiograph demonstrates thoracolumbar scoliosis. **D:** A 13-year-old boy with thoracolumbar scoliosis and pain. Coned-down radiograph demonstrates a probable nidus in the posterior elements of T12 on the left. **E:** CT scan of a 13-year-old boy with painful scoliosis demonstrates a nidus consistent with an osteoid osteoma in the posterior elements of T12 on the right. The lesion was excised with complete relief of pain and resolution of the scoliosis.

operative treatment remains a viable option. Radiation therapy is not necessary and may be harmful.

Surgical treatment can produce almost immediate pain relief in more than 95% of cases. On the other hand, incomplete excision is often followed by recurrence of pain. If the lesion does recur (one recurrence after incomplete excision in 17 pediatric patients treated at Rizzoli Institute), additional attempts at complete excision are recommended. Early diagnosis and complete excision frequently leads to relief of symptoms. Painful scoliosis that develops as a result of an osteoid osteoma is often relieved after excision of the benign lesion if it has not been existed for more than 15 months. Lesions that exist for more than 15 months are believed to have more fixed deformities that may not resolve after excision of the benign tumor (15, 58). This is not confirmed by the experience collected at the Rizzoli Institute: 16 patients had osteoid osteoma-associated scoliosis (94% of cases); 12 deformities improved or disappeared, and four remained unchanged, irrespective of symptom duration.

Osteoblastoma

Enneking's stage 2 osteoblastomas are histologically indistinguishable from osteoid osteomas and differ mainly in size. Osteoblastomas are larger than osteoid osteomas. They are usually more than 2 cm in diameter. Stage 3 osteoblastomas are clinically and radiographically similar to other aggressive conditions, such as giant cell tumors (5). Osteoblastomas account for less than 1% of all bone tumors, and 5% of primary bone tumors are osteoblastomas. Osteoblastomas have a distinct predilection for the spine, especially the posterior elements. They occur most frequently in the lamina and pedicle and exhibit progressive growth (2). More than 40% of reported tumors have been located in the spine (49). Although osteoblastomas are less painful than osteoid osteomas, in a series of nine patients, all patients with osteoblastoma had back pain for 6 weeks to 36 months duration at the time of diagnosis (4). Osteoblastomas usually affect patients aged 10 to 15 years (4). Twelve cases were observed at the Rizzoli Institute in patients 4 to 14 years of age (average 11 years). In all cases, the presenting symptom was pain (average 54 weeks); in only two cases was there concomitant abrupt paraparesis, confirming that myelopathy is uncommon, whereas radiculopathy occurs in up to 50% of patients. Aspirin and nonsteroidal antiinflammatory agents do not relieve pain associated with osteoblastomas as effectively as they relieve the pain of osteoid osteoma. Scoliosis with a convex side away from the involved side of the vertebra, generally related to pain-producing lesions in the thoracic spine, is reported in up to two thirds of affected patients. The thoracic and lumbar spine are the most common sites involved, each accounting for about 30% to 40% of cases, followed by the cervical spine and sacrum. In the series collected at the Rizzoli Institute, two cases arose in both the cervical spine and in the lumbar spine, whereas 10 involved the thoracic spine. The posterior arch (sectors 10 to 3) was involved in all cases; the pedicles (sectors 4 and 9) in three; the vertebral body was never involved. The tumor invaded layer D in all five stage 3 tumors. This confirms that epidural expansion, as well as paraspinous soft-tissue involvement, is common.

In about 5% of the cases reported in the literature, adjacent vertebrae are involved.

Radiographically, stage 3 osteoblastomas are destructive expansile lesions. Calcification is evident mostly in stage 3 lesions (approximately one third of all series) and, as in osteoid osteomas, radionuclide bone scanning is a reliable screening technique.

CT may be the best imaging procedure for defining the location and extent of osteoblastomas with regard to their osseous involvement. CT is also the best aid to surgical planning for extirpation and reconstruction. With radiculopathy or myelopathy, one may consider performing CT myelography or MRI (Fig. 5A–C).

Treatment

Osteoblastomas are slowly growing lesions that are locally expansive and destructive, yet it is said that complete surgical extirpation of the lesions appears to be curative (2,9,31,35,36,39, 61,63,85,86). In the vertebrae, intralesional curettage is often used as the only possible technical solution (Figs. 5 and 6). However, the authors recommend selecting the treatment according to the oncologic stage (24). This makes it possible to significantly reduce the rate of recurrence (8), which in the literature is reported to be around 10%. Radiation therapy remains controversial and has been reported by some investigators to be ineffective (39,55). Malignant transformation, spinal cord necrosis, and aggravation of spinal cord compression has been reported (18,69). The author believes that radiation therapy should be used as an adjuvant to intralesional excision in stage 3 tumors not suitable for en bloc excision.

Aneurysmal Bone Cyst

Aneurysmal bone cyst is a pseudotumoral condition that typically arises in the spine during early life. The usual age of patients with aneurysmal bone cyst is 5 to 20 years, and females are affected more commonly than males. In 60% of cases, the cysts are localized to the posterior elements of the vertebra and occasionally expand directly into the vertebral bodies (45) (Fig. 7). Radiographs typically show an expansile osteolytic cavity, with strands of bone forming a bubbly appearance. The cortex is often eggshell thin and blown out (18). The lesion is often extremely vascular, but this feature is not often appreciated angiographically even though it is apparent pathologically.

Twenty patients were observed at the Rizzoli Institute, including those reported by Capanna et al. (8). This series includes 7 males and 13 females; their ages ranged from 5 to 14 years, with an average age of 10 years. The lesions occurred mostly in the lumbar spine (10 cases) and the cervical spine (7 cases). They involved only the posterior sectors (10 to 3) in 9 cases (a palpable mass was present in 3 cases), and both vertebral body and arch in the remaining cases. The epidural space (layer D) was invaded in 10 cases; in only 1 case was cord compression seen following the initial complaint.

Treatment

Excision and curettage are the best treatments for aneurysmal bone cyst. The procedures are frequently risky and sometimes

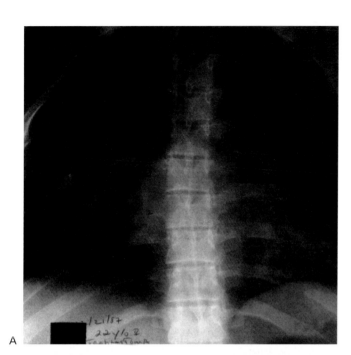

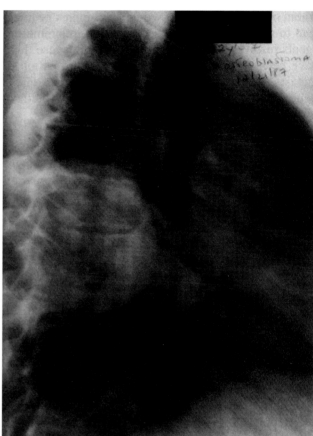

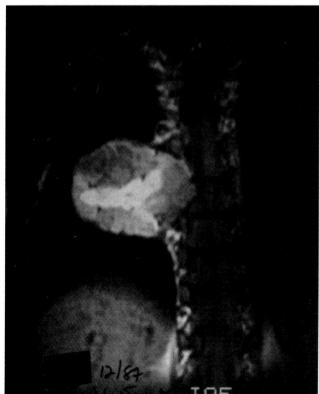

FIGURE 5. A T7 osteoblastoma. **A:** Anterior radiograph shows the expansile lesion from the body of T7 including and up to the body of T6; the ribs of T7 and 8 are clearly involved. Some calcification of the lesion is apparent. **B:** Lateral image shows a large expansile mass in the area of T6, T7, and T8, with some calcification. **C:** Coronal magnetic resonance image shows growth of a large osteoblastoma off the vertebral bodies of T6 and T7 with some central calcification.

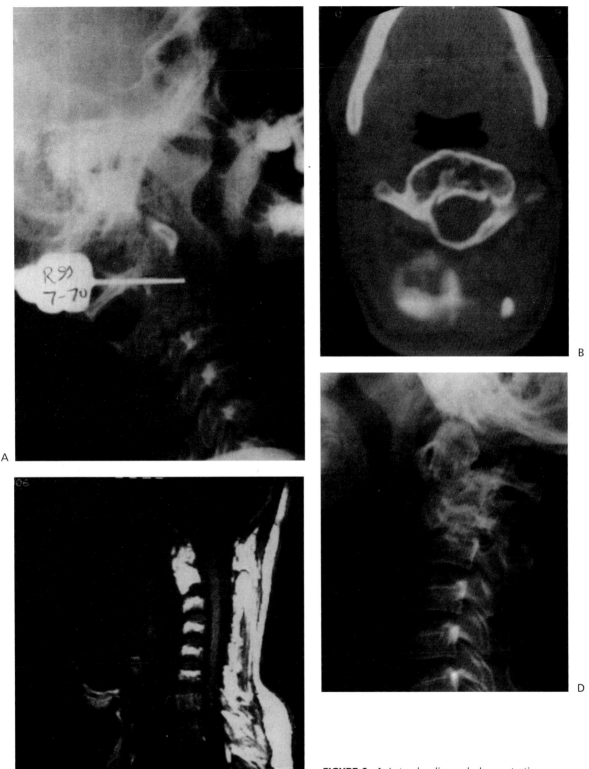

FIGURE 6. A: Lateral radiograph demonstrating a percutaneous biopsy of a C2 osteoblastoma. **B:** Axial computed tomography scan 15 years after curettage and bone grafting of C2. **C:** Magnetic resonance image of the patient 18 years after curettage and bone grafting. **D:** Radiograph 23 years after curettage and bone grafting of C2.

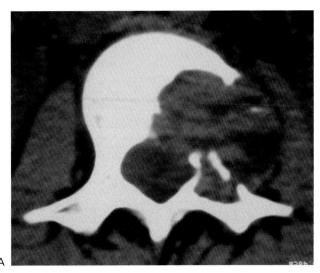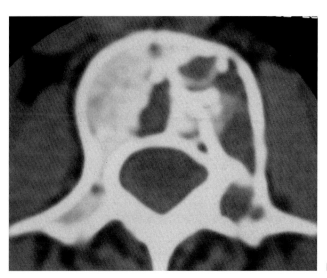

FIGURE 7. A: Aneurysmal bone cyst of L3 in a 12-year-old girl. It is interesting to note the double density levels within the radiolucent area occupying the vertebral body and eroding the cortex. The patient was submitted to selective arterial embolization. Biopsy was achieved by trocar computed tomography-guided biopsy. There was no surgery or radiation therapy. **B:** Five-year follow-up. No other treatment was given. The girl has no pain and has normal function.

prevented by a significant interoperative hemorrhage, which can be controlled by rapid removal of the lining wall of the cyst at the time of surgery. Preoperative selective embolization with polyvinyl alcohol (Ivalon) or absorbable gelatin (Gelfoam) can significantly reduce the bleeding (75) and is itself a treatment option (20) (Fig. 7). Recurrence rates have been reported in the range 10% to 25% (8). Recurrence developed in 13% of cases in the review of Hay et al., but all cases were successfully treated by a second curettage or excision procedure (33).

Irradiation of these lesions has limited effectiveness and is associated with poor results (8) unless done as an adjuvant. One should remember that radiation also has an adverse effect on growth in children, with consequent late deformities and possible later effects on the spinal cord itself (e.g., myelopathy, myelitis, or sarcomas) (59,79).

The excision required is frequently so destructive and the effect of radiation so important that instrumented fusion must be considered in the operative planning.

At the Rizzoli Institute, two patients were treated by selective arterial embolization, one by radiation therapy, nine by intralesional excision, and eight by intralesional excision combined with radiation. Selective arterial embolization as a preoperative adjuvant was performed in eight cases. Only one recurrence was observed, after incomplete excision (performed without adjuvants), and healed following further intracapsular excision and radiation therapy. The patient affected by neurologic deficit (Frankel B) improved to Frankel D3. Five of 12 preoperative deformities (scoliosis and/or kyphosis) worsened, and two were worse after treatment that did not include stabilization. Surgery was performed in both cases.

Giant Cell Tumor

Giant cell tumors are extremely rare before the growth spurt. These tumors generally are histologically benign, but their clinical behavior is sometimes unpredictable, with a high recurrence rate if not correctly staged and treated. Prolonged disease-free survivals have been reported after curettage and radiotherapy, although some patients require two or more additional procedures owing to local recurrence (21); en bloc excision, when feasible, is curative (34). A high-grade sarcoma occurs in 5% to 15% of irradiated patients. On the other hand, benign giant cell tumors can produce pulmonary metastases without clear biologic relation to their radiographic appearance of aggressiveness. These metastases occasionally may regress spontaneously; they have been controlled by marginal excision. They can be lethal in 25% of cases.

In 70 years of survey, only two cases of giant cell tumor of the spine in the pediatric age group were observed at the Rizzoli Institute, both occurring in the thoracic spine. During the same period, 876 giant cell tumors were diagnosed and treated in the same institution, 34 of them occurring in the spine. Both of the pediatric patients had paraparesis as the presenting symptom. The first child died in 1928 after emergency decompression. The second child is disease-free with recovery of the neurologic functions 6 years after a second excision and one course of megavoltage radiation for multiple recurrences (en bloc surgery was not feasible).

Treatment

Based on CT and MRI (Fig. 8), followed by trocar biopsy under CT control, oncologic and surgical staging are helpful for the decision making process. Complete (extracapsular) excision seems to be effective for stage 2 giant cell tumor, whereas en bloc excision (or intralesional excision plus radiation therapy) are required for local control in stage 3 giant cell tumor (18,21,34).

Selective arterial embolization will reduce intraoperative bleeding and is therefore mandatory before intralesional excision

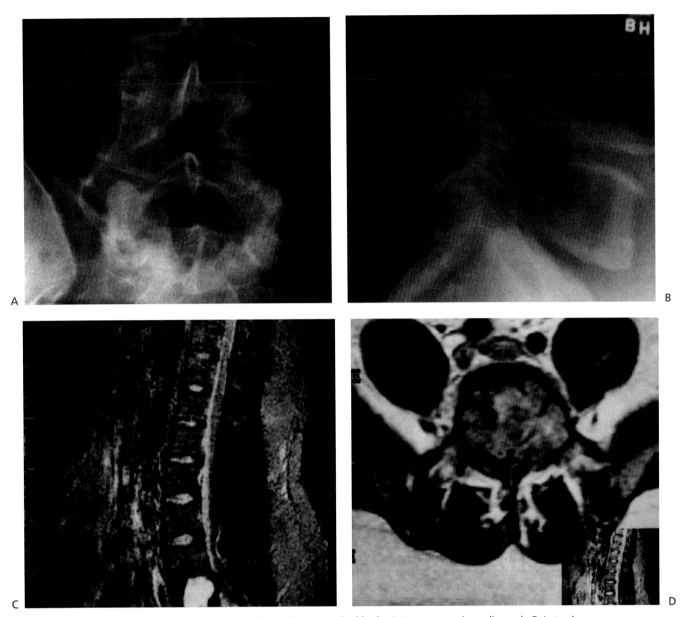

FIGURE 8. Giant cell tumor involving the L5 vertebral body. **A:** Anteroposterior radiograph. **B:** Lateral radiograph. **C, D:** Magnetic resonance image on T2 scale shows same giant cell tumor involving the vertebral body of L5 on both the sagittal and axial views with some encroachment of the vertebral canal evident on the axial images.

can be performed. Radiation therapy must be considered only as an adjuvant after complete excision.

Eosinophilic Granuloma

Eosinophilic granuloma is a benign, self-limiting neoplasm that produces destruction of bone (38). This condition usually occurs in children younger than 10 years, and vertebral involvement occurs in 10% to 15% of cases. This disease has onset as one of a triad of syndromes: (a) isolated eosinophilic granulomas; (b) Hand-Schüller-Christian disease; or (c) Letterer-Siwe disease (27,57). Eosinophilic granuloma is the most benign form of

histiocytosis and thus is not a true neoplasm. The lesion consists of an abnormal proliferation of lipid-containing histiocytes from the reticulo-endothelial system. Spinal eosinophilic granulomas can affect multiple spinal levels. They often present with localized pain but rarely with neurologic deficits. The vertebral body is often involved, particularly the lumbar or thoracic spine, and is usually partially or totally destroyed. The destruction of the bone often leads to significant pain, and neurologic symptoms may be associated. The degree of compression is dependent on the extent of vertebral body involvement. In younger children, there is often rapid vertebral body collapse because most of the body is involved, resulting in complete flattening or "vertebra plana." In older children or adolescents, lesser amounts of vertebral body involvement can cause a wedge-shaped deformity or punched-out lytic lesion of the vertebral body. Adjacent intervertebral disc spaces are often well maintained, and extraosseous paravertebral soft-tissue masses are rare.

Treatment

The "coin-on-end" appearance, or vertebra plana, is a classic description of eosinophilic granuloma of the spine, which actually represents the final evolution of the disease. It is sometimes observed incidentally on a radiograph, as eosinophilic granulomas often are self-limited and may heal spontaneously (57). The initial pattern is a lytic image that requires one to rule out infection, benign tumor, or malignancy such as Ewing sarcoma. Laboratory tests, well-marginated borders, and the presence or absence of a tumoral mass in the surrounding soft tissues are the most important elements to distinguish those conditions. Biopsy is mandatory before any treatment is instituted, unless it presents as a completely asymptomatic vertebra plana without any soft-tissue mass.

Vertebral reconstitution is greater for younger patients and occurs regardless of treatment (71) (Fig. 9). Spontaneous reconstitution of vertebral height has been attributed to the sparing of areas of enchondral ossification (71).

The series collected by the Rizzoli Institute includes 20 patients (10 males, 10 females) with a total of 28 vertebral locations (6 multiple sites in the spine); 9 patients presented or developed extraaxial involvement. The lesion always occurred in the vertebral body, mostly in the thoracic spine (14 of 28). The vertebra plana was the initial pattern in 54% of cases. Five lesions were observed incidentally; all of the other patients complained of pain and 3 of them had neurologic symptoms (root compression). In 6 cases the lesion healed by othesic treatment in 12 to 45 months (average 28 months). In 6 other cases, chemotherapy was added due to systemic spread. Intralesional excision was performed in 8 cases, for diagnostic purpose. Radiation therapy (21 Gy) was added in 1 case, local corticosteroids in 4. Only one recurrence was observed, after incomplete excision followed by chemotherapy; 7 years later, no evidence of disease was found. The other 19 patients have been disease-free for an average of 70 months after treatment (range 24 to 183 months). Ten of

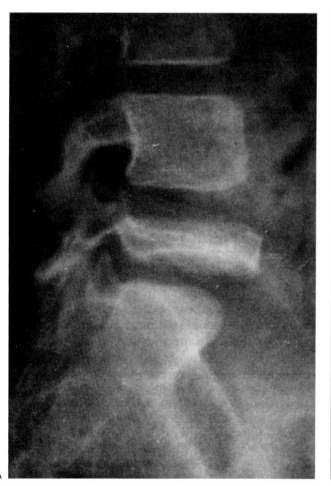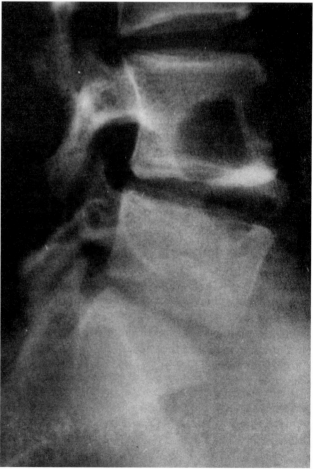

A

B

FIGURE 9. Eosinophilic granuloma. **A:** Lateral radiograph of a 5-year-old boy with an eosinophilic granuloma of L5. **B:** Follow-up radiograph of the same patient 7 years later, without treatment, shows reconstitution of the vertebral body.

12 vertebra plana patients who were followed for a minimum of 37 months showed vertebral height restoration (10% to 90% of original height). One thoracic hyperkyphosis developed after conservative treatment.

The best treatment for this disease is not known. For acute pain, a short period of bed rest followed by use of an orthosis or body jacket often provides symptomatic relief. Local corticosteroid injection has been successfully performed. For patients with neurologic deficits, biopsy followed by low-dose irradiation and immobilization is indicated (30).

Multifocal occurrence is a sign of systemic disease; the patient should be referred to a pediatric oncologist for corticosteroids and chemotherapy.

Osteochondroma

Osteochondromas are very common lesions of bone. Solitary osteochondromas are noninherited malformations and are not true neoplasms. They are cartilage-capped bony growths on either a broad base or a stalk, first appearing in relation to the epiphyseal growth plate. Most are painless and are noted during the first two decades of life. Benign lesions are often elongated and point to the metaphysis of the involved bone. After closure of the growth plates, these lesions usually stop growing in 12 years. Vertebral involvement is very rare, around 7%, occurring mostly in the cervical or upper thoracic spine. A palpable mass is the most prominent symptom. Neurologic compromise is rare; only 16 osteochondromas have been reported to be associated with symptomatic cord compression.

Treatment

Biopsy is indicated when malignant transformation is suspected, and must include the cartilage component. Tumor excision should include the perichondral soft-tissue covering and all cartilage extending to normal cortical bone. It is indicated when the patient complains of pain and dysfunction resulting from pressure on adjacent soft tissues, such as nerves or blood vessels, or when malignant transformation has been confirmed. Adjuvant treatment is not indicated (Fig. 9A, B).

PREMALIGNANT LESIONS IN CHILDREN

Neurofibromatosis

The presence of multiple schwannomas is virtually diagnostic of neurofibromatosis. The involved nerves are often swollen, with margins indistinct from the tumor. Two distinct forms of neurofibromatosis have been identified. Both show autosomal dominance in transmission with high penetrance. If a person possesses this genetic defect, a characteristic condition is usually expressed. The classic picture is one of multiple cutaneous or subcutaneous neurofibromas that are pathopneumonic of the disease (18). Café-au-lait spots occur due to the abnormality of large melanosomes in the skin. This may be associated with kyphoscoliosis in about 2% of cases. Associated pheochromocytomas occur in 1% of cases.

Bilateral acoustic neuroma is the second form of neurofibromatosis. In this form, the gene is located on chromosome 22, whereas patients with type 1 neurofibromatosis, referred to also as von Recklinghausen disease, have a defect on chromosome 17. Both types are autosomal dominant and have high penetrance. Other abnormalities associated with neurofibromatosis are spinal and intracranial meningiomas along with astrocytomas. Whereas sporadic neurofibromas are almost always benign, it is estimated that 3% to 30% of lesions in von Recklinghausen disease undergo malignant transformation. Changes in spinal anatomy are related to neurofibromas of spinal nerves, spinal meningiomas, sympathetic chain neurofibromas, and sometimes neuroblastomas. Enlargement of the neural foramen, thinning of a rib, or deformation of the bone secondary to these soft-tissue tumors is common.

Treatment

Surgical treatment typically consists of fully exposing these tumors both interspinally, foraminally, and extraspinally through laminectomy and facetectomy. If the involved roots are not crucial, they are often sacrificed. However, if they are important, the schwannoma may be dissected free of the nerve fascicles using microsurgical techniques and intraoperative electrophysiologic recordings. Long-term results of dissectable lesions are generally good. More than 90% of patients can be cured of these nerve sheath tumors. If neurofibromas become malignant, they are generally locally destructive and resistant to radiation or adjuvant chemotherapy.

Multiple Hereditary Osteochondromatosis

Multiple hereditary osteochondromatosis (MHO) is inherited through an autosomal dominant gene and is characterized by multiple cartilaginous bony protrusions with cartilaginous caps ("exostoses") that are radiographically and histologically indistinguishable from solitary osteochondromas. Malignant transformation to a chondrosarcoma occurs rarely, but is possible and more common than in solitary osteochondromas due to the greater number of lesions exposed to risk.

Treatment

As for solitary lesions, surgical excision is indicated for symptomatic or enlarging lesions.

Enchondroma

Solitary enchondromas are benign intramedullary tumors composed of hyaline cartilage arising from growth plate rests that rarely occur in the vertebral column (less than 1%). These benign tumors usually do not require treatment. Chondrosarcomatous degeneration is rare but is not uncommon in patients with Maffucci's syndrome (i.e., multiple enchondromas associated with hemangiomas). Those suspected of malignant degeneration should undergo biopsy, followed by appropriate treatment.

MALIGNANT TUMORS

Malignant spinal tumors in children are rare. Fewer than 30% of all primary bone tumors in children are malignant; an even smaller percentage is associated with the vertebral spine (86). Spinal malignancies in children generally have a very poor prognosis, and treatments to date have not been very effective. Of 20 cases collected at the Rizzoli Institute in the last 10 years, 60% involved males and the mean age at onset was 9 years (range 1.5 to 14 years). The thoracic and lumbar spines were equally affected, and five patients had two tumoral locations. The total number of tumor sites was 25 (Fig. 10).

Ewing Sarcoma

Ewing sarcoma is the most common malignant bone tumor in children and is most prevalent in patients aged 5 to 15 years (2). Approximately 3.5% of all Ewing tumors originate in the spinal column, mostly in the sacrum (87), and account for only about 0.5% of all primary malignant tumors of bone (65,67,88). The average time from onset of symptoms to diagnosis is about 8 months. The common symptom is pain; other symptoms are related to the proximity of the tumor to the spinal cord and/or nerve roots. Fever occurs in less than 25% of cases, and a mass may be palpated in 25%. Laboratory studies are generally nonspecific, but increased ESR occurs in slightly less than 50% of cases. The permeative appearance of Ewing tumors on radiographs can make diagnosis difficult, and a collapse of the vertebral body may produce a vertebra plana that is difficult to differentiate from eosinophilic granuloma (62,72) (Fig. 10) if not on the basis of the soft-tissue mass expanding quickly outside the site of occurrence. MRI is the preferable imaging study, as the tumors so quickly that frequently no destruction of the vertebra outline is appreciated even in presence of a large soft-tissue mass.

Treatment

Modern therapies have made local control and disease-free survival obtainable in terms of the spine, but the long-term outlook is still poor (43). There is no known best cure for this disease. Ewing tumors of the spine can be very large, with significant soft-tissue invasion (11). En bloc excision with appropriate margins is seldom feasible, and the risk of leaving an island of tumor behind is very high. Protocols of combined chemotherapy and radiation therapy must be considered as the first option to make en bloc excision feasible and oncologically appropriate (Fig. 11).

Metastases commonly involve the lungs and/or other locations in the spine, as well as ribs, lymph nodes, brain, and abdominal viscera.

Eight pediatric patients with Ewing sarcoma were observed at the Rizzoli Institute; most were referred before the 1980s and were treated only by palliative radiation therapy. More recently, two patients treated by combined radiation and chemotherapy who then submitted to en bloc excision are disease-free 4 and 5 years after the vertebrectomy (Fig. 11).

Osteogenic Sarcoma

Osteogenic sarcoma ("osteosarcoma") is the most common primary malignant tumor of bone, with the exception of myeloma.

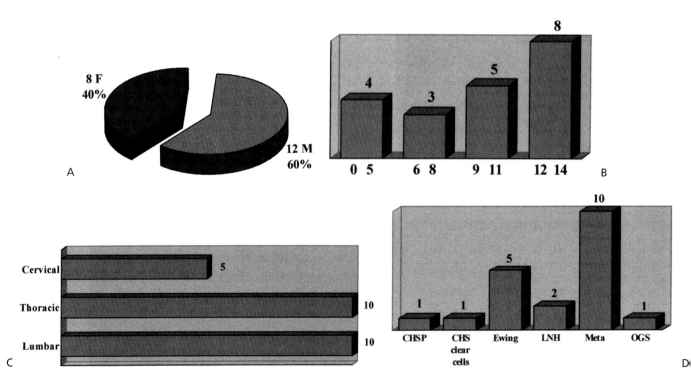

FIGURE 10. Malignant bone tumors of the pediatric spine: 20 cases collected at the Rizzoli Institute in the latest 10 years. Demographics: **A,** sex; **B,** age; **C,** location; **D,** diagnosis.

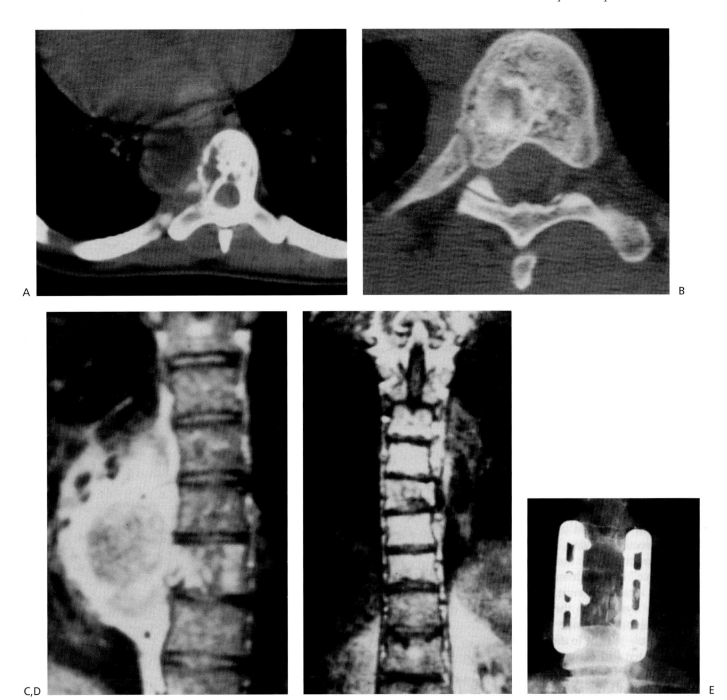

FIGURE 11. Ewing sarcoma arising from T7 and expanding in the mediastinum. **(A)** CT scan before and **(B)** after chemotherapy and radiation therapy. **(C)** Magnetic resonance image before and after chemotherapy and radiation therapy. **D:** Resected specimen after en bloc excision (wide margin) by double-approach vertebrectomy. **E:** Reconstruction achieved by variable spinal plates and carbon fiber prosthesis filled with autogenous cancellous bone graft.

It accounts for approximately 20% to 25% of the bony neoplasms. It is more than twice as common as chondrosarcoma and three times more common than Ewing sarcoma. In the United States, there are approximately two cases per million, or approximately 1,000 to 1,500 new cases diagnosed annually (18,37,47). Approximately 50% of cases occur between the ages of 10 and 20 years, especially during the adolescent growth spurt.

Although the cause of osteosarcoma remains unknown, it occurs not only in rapidly growing adolescents but as a secondary neoplasm in Paget disease, post irradiation, and in some benign bone tumors (22,23,36,56,81,83).

Retinoblastoma, a malignant tumor that occurs in the eyes of newborns and young children, is associated with an increased risk of developing osteosarcoma. This risk in children is approxi-

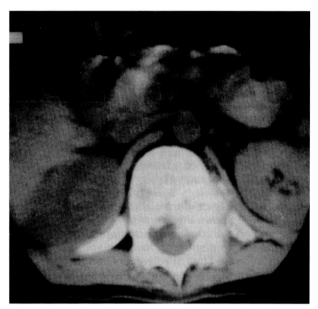

FIGURE 12. Osteosarcoma of T12 involving the vertebral body pedicle and entering the epidural space is evident on axial computed tomography scan of soft-tissue window.

mately 2,000 times greater than that in the rest of the population and is independent of radiation administration (1). Osteosarcoma may be polyostotic and involve multiple skeletal sites at the same time or consecutively (60).

Osteogenic sarcoma of the vertebral column is extremely rare and very deadly. Approximately 10% of osteosarcomas arise in the axial skeleton, including the vertebra as well as skull, ribs, and pelvis. Those specifically in the spine are believed to occur in 0.8% to 3% of cases (12,81). The lesions often originate in the lower portions of the vertebral column, causing pain as well as sensory and motor disturbances (Fig. 12). Two thirds of the patients reported in the literature had neurologic deficits at initial examination. Those with epidural extension of their tumor at time of diagnosis obviously are adversely affected because of some surgical limitations and the nature of the tumor. Radiographically, these tumors can be variable in their presentation. The most common finding in the spine is a mixed osteolytic and sclerotic lesion of the vertebral body. In 90% of cases, the tumor is located in the vertebral body, but the posterior elements also may be affected (Fig. 12). In children, one must distinguish osteosarcomas from osteoblastomas or aneurysmal bone cysts, more rarely from giant cell tumors and metastatic lesions. MRI is the preferred diagnostic imaging modality for the evaluation of soft-tissue masses, although CT/myelography is acceptable. Bone scans are of help in demonstrating skip or satellite lesions. Bone scans may also be used in follow-up treatment for residual or persistent or recurrent tumor.

Treatment

No prospective and/or standardized protocols exist for treatment of malignant lesions of the spine (e.g., osteosarcoma). After bi-

opsy-proven diagnosis, usually by a CT-directed procedure, chest CT scans and bone scans should be obtained to rule out metastatic disease.

Rosen et al. (64) propose that surgery be delayed up to 16 weeks before resection of primary tumors while preoperative chemotherapy is given. The rationale for this treatment comprises several considerations. The first is that systemic micrometastases exist at the time of initial diagnosis; thus, chemotherapy is most effective when the burden of tumor is relatively small. Because the doubling time of osteosarcoma is estimated at 30 to 40 days, this is very important. Second, primary tumor regression and shrinkage potentially allows for more effective and less morbid surgical intervention. In spinal tumors, this may be extremely important because sometimes en bloc excision is possible. Finally, the effects of chemotherapy on tumors have been quantified histologically (66).

Local radiation therapy could be used when surgery is not oncologically appropriate and should be considered only after appropriate wound healing has taken place, generally in 3 to 4 weeks. Treatment also includes many postoperative courses of chemotherapy.

Outcome of Treatment

In the Mayo Clinic series of 27 cases, median survival was 10 months, and only seven patients survived for more than a year. One patient survived for more than 5 years (73). Similar results were reported by Barwick et al. (5). In their series, only one patient, a 3-year-old boy who had a thoracic tumor treated by external-beam radiation and chemotherapy and who survived for 6 years and 2 months, was considered a long-term survivor. Ogihara et al. reported a 15-year-old boy with a T4 osteosarcoma who, after laminectomy and three courses of adjunctive chemotherapy at 6-week intervals, was free of disease at follow-up 6 years later (58). In the Shives study from the Mayo Clinic, no patient had been treated intensively with the modern chemotherapy regimens currently available (73).

Metastatic disease exists at diagnosis in about 10% to 20% of patients. This does not necessarily preclude long-term survival. Current recommendations for treatment of metastatic disease suggest aggressive resection of pulmonary metastases, which may involve multiple thoracotomies. Forty-one percent of patients with pulmonary metastases can be rendered disease-free and achieve long-term survival (29). Recent data obtained with flow cytometry of the tumors has been of considerable help in predicting metastatic potential and the need for more intensive therapy (50). Patients with near-diploid stem lines have considerably better prognosis and decreased potential for metastatic disease than those with marked aneuploidy. With this knowledge and more advanced surgical techniques, better 5-year survivals may be achievable.

Leukemia

Leukemia is the most common cancer in children and can affect all organ systems. In 6% of children with leukemia, back pain and vertebral collapse are the initial findings at the time of presentation (9) (Fig. 13). Correct diagnosis is very difficult because

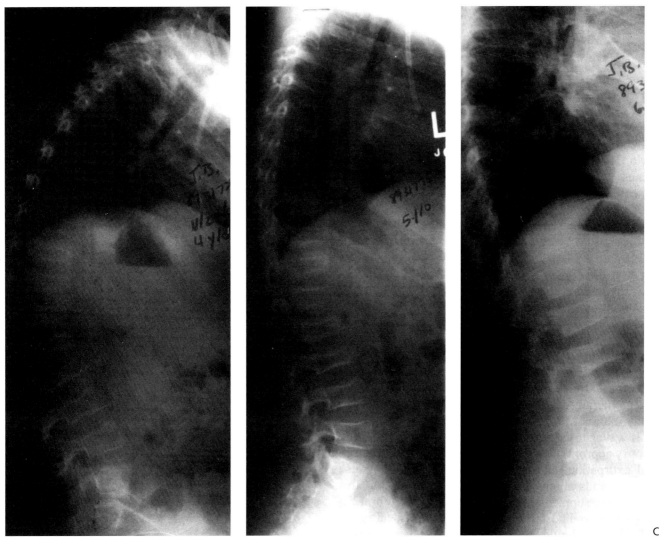

A,B   C

FIGURE 13. Leukemia. **A:** Lateral radiograph of a 4-year-old boy at time of diagnosis. Osteopenia and numerous compression fractures are apparent. **B:** Lateral radiographs during treatment. **C:** Lateral radiographs 2 years after diagnosis and treatment. Some vertebral height has been restored.

patients often have several nonspecific symptoms. Lethargy, anemia, fever, and increased peripheral leukocyte count are all common symptoms (9). A very high index of suspicion is the key to correct diagnosis of this disease. Radiographs may not demonstrate any focal abnormality or may show focal lytic lesions, occasional sclerotic lesions, or isolated periosteal reactions (72). At some time during the disease process, approximately 10% to 15% of children will have at least one pathologic fracture of the spine. A seemingly insignificant injury or fall that has unexpected consequences should make the treating physician highly suspicious. If radiographs of the involved extremity are negative, a complete blood count and ESR should be obtained. The peripheral white blood cell count will be increased, as will the ESR; the platelet count often is decreased. This is enough to warrant further investigation. Radiography and/or other spinal investigations may not be diagnostic. Misdiagnosis of a septic joint or osteomyelitis is not at all uncommon. Bone scan generally is not useful. Again, a high index of suspicion is imperative.

Treatment

Treatment of the specific types of leukemia with appropriate chemotherapy and/or radiation is the key. Spinal care is supportive in most cases.

Metastatic Spinal tumors in Children

Although the metastatic diseases of adulthood do not generally occur in children, metastasis and/or contiguous invasion of certain tumors does occur in children, and one must be cognizant of such tumors. Neuroblastomas, embryonal carcinomas, and various sarcomas are all metastatic in children (Fig. 14). These lesions often have a poor prognosis, and most are treated nonoperatively with adjuvant therapy. Surgical experiences in such cases other than Ewing sarcoma has been limited. In the series of Fraser et al. (28), 30% of pediatric spinal tumors were metastatic neuroblastomas, and in the series of Leeson et al. (48), 41%

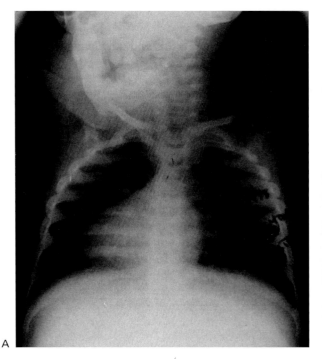

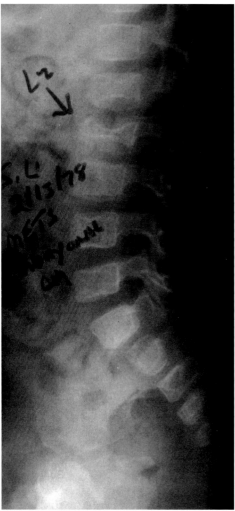

FIGURE 14. **A:** Posteroanterior chest radiograph of a patient with metastatic embryonal carcinoma to T3 shows changes of the vertebral body and pedicle. **B:** Lateral radiograph of same patient with metastatic embryonal carcinoma to L2. There is an obvious compression fracture of L2.

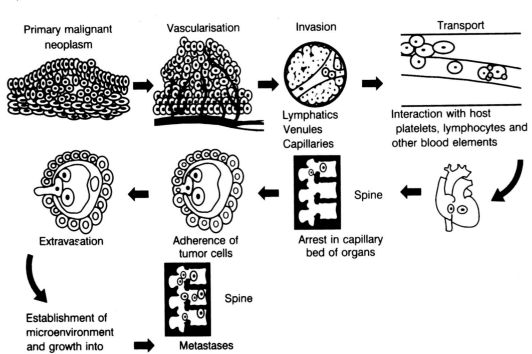

FIGURE 15. The pathogenesis of metastasis (16,25,46).

were neuroblastomas. Unfortunately, treatment in these cases is often delayed because of misdiagnosis (17). The pathogenesis of a metastasis is controlled by several factors, some of which are contact inhibition, cell adhesiveness, and cell membrane mediation. Tumor cell survival is dependent on antigen-stimulated macrophage response, nonspecific immunologic response to fibrin clot, and permeability of endothelial and basement membranes, lymph vessels, and capillaries (16,25) (Fig. 15).

TREATMENT

Appropriate treatment of children with spinal tumors only results from accurate diagnosis. A high index of suspicion, followed by appropriate diagnostic studies and biopsy at specialized institutions, is essential, as is the contribution of surgeons who can treat these children. Inappropriate biopsy and diagnostics can profoundly affect not only the short-term outlook but long-term survival as well. Today there are specialized centers for the diagnosis and treatment of childhood cancers. Experienced spine surgeons must work closely with their oncology colleagues to offer the best possible outcome for these children and their families. A mistake can be life threatening. To this end, an algorithmic approach may be helpful (Table 2). It is important to remark

that spinal tumors in children are more frequently benign than those in adults. Therefore, the priority is to prevent permanent cord damage over the need to perform en bloc surgery in an uncontaminated lesion.

Spinal Fixation in Childhood Tumors

Most benign tumors can be resected and bone grafted with the patient's own iliac crest as graft material. On the other hand, some of the more aggressive tumors require extensive bone and soft-tissue resection, necessitating an adjunctive internal fixation device, or even a prosthesis for the reconstruction of the vertebral body. A sound reconstruction of the anterior column allows for immediate function recovery and long-term stability. To this purpose, the author's (SB) experience suggests the use of carbon fiber implants filled with autogenous bone cancellous chips (Fig. 11E). This system, connected with the posterior plates or rods, is rigid enough to allow for immediate weight bearing, whereas the piezoelectric features of carbon fiber implants enhance bone formation inside the prosthesis. However, more study is needed.

Spinal fixation devices today have evolved to a state wherein nearly any surgical extirpation can be reconstructed. Figure 16 shows the case of an 8-year-old boy who had mesenchymal chon-

TABLE 2. ALGORITHM: PEDIATRIC SPINE TUMORS

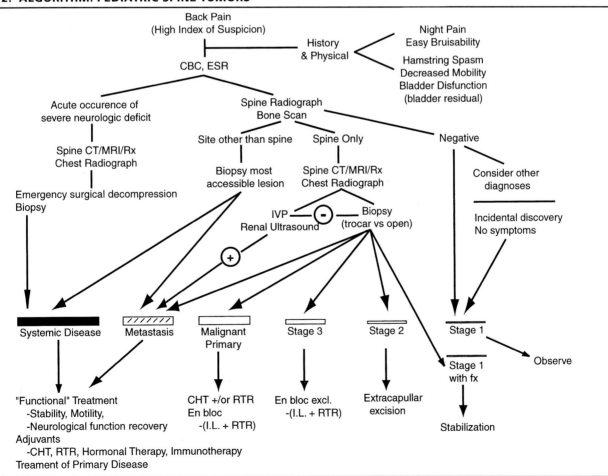

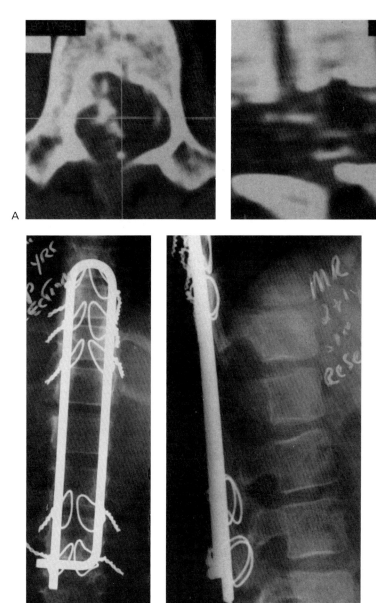

A

B,C

FIGURE 16. Mesenchymal chondrosarcoma of T12 in an 8-year-old boy who had progressive paraplegia. **A:** Computed tomography scan: axial, sagittal, and coronal cuts. **B, C:** Anteroposterior and lateral radiographs show Luque instrumentation from T9 to L3, 2 years after surgical extirpation.

drosarcoma of T12 and progressive paraplegia. Surgical intervention involved a laminectomy of T12 with en bloc excision of the lesion, including the right T12 pedicle. In this case, Luque instrumentation was used along with autogenous iliac bone graft from T9 to L3. The patient had 2 years of chemotherapy; now, 5 years after his resection, he has no signs of tumor recurrence.

Tumor resections, whether anterior, posterior, or both, often necessitate posterior instrumentation. On the other hand, anterior devices are not commonly used in the reconstruction of childhood tumors. Although Luque instrumentation has been used in almost all spinal regions, newer devices allowing distraction and compression and/or a combination using pedicular fixation, hooks, rods, plates, and various cross-linking devices offer experienced spinal tumor surgeons adequate alternatives for reconstructing childhood spinal tumors. Owing to the increased risk of infection and complications associated with cement and/or allograft, these materials are not generally indicated.

Complications

It is important to consider the complications in these most difficult cases, as sometimes management of complications is more difficult than management of the primary tumor. Second chances are often too late. The first chance not only is the most important but it may be the only chance. The ability to interface the best surgical and nonsurgical treatments can affect not only the immediate care of the patient but, more importantly, his or her long-term survival (86).

Several series have implicated acquired instability and deformity as the cause of lack of neurologic improvement and, occasionally, the progression of neurologic dysfunction. Hypermobility or acquired instability may be the result of inadequate reconstruction or stabilization at the time of initial surgery or of late failure of fixation owing to disease progression and/or implant failure. Obviously, attention to the mechanics of reconstruction is important. In Harrington's series of 77 patients treated with posterior stabilization and adjuvant methylmethacrylate, five patients had loss of fixation and required restabilization. In addition, six patients subsequently developed spinal hypermobility due to metastatic disease at adjacent levels of the spine (32). Of the 24 complications reported by McAfee et al. (53), only five occurred after anterior stabilization using methylmethacrylate. Of the 19 patients with posterior stabilization, 15 had loss of fixation and several developed significant kyphosis. Six patients developed deep infections; three had associated significant neurologic deterioration (53). In the series of Kostuik et al. (44), among 100 patients there were 3 cases of instrumentation failure; one occurred in a patient who had anterior reinforced methylmethacrylate with metastatic disease in the cervical spine. Failure occurred because it was not recognized that the disease extended into the proximal vertebral body. A second procedure was successful. Two other major failures occurred; both were in the thoracic spine, and both were associated with use of Harrington instrumentation without use of sublaminar wires. A proximal hook pulled out in one patient, and both lower hooks pulled out in another. Both patients underwent reconstruction without sequelae (44). In children for whom long-term survival may be possible, the author recommends using either autogenous bone graft and/or autogenous bone graft supplemented with various synthetic vertebral replacements, of which several are now available, rather than methylmethacrylate.

The complications of radiation have already been alluded to: sarcomatous degeneration and/or neurologic dysfunction, and stunted growth. Before surgery, radiation has a significant effect. Radiation can increase the risk of infection at the time of surgery by 36%.

In a review of technical considerations and complications in tumor surgery by McLain et al. (54), pedicle fixation was noted to confer significant technical advantages in spinal reconstruction, with complications comparable to those of other methods of posterior segmental fixation, although operative times were slightly longer. With this system, fewer levels had to be fused as compared with systems using sublaminar hooks or wires. Preoperatively irradiated patients experienced 42% of all complications and had 70% of the major complications. Wound infections occurred in 18%, vascular injuries occurred in 18%, and transient neurologic deficits occurred in 36%. Clinical pseudarthrosis developed in two patients, and tumor progression produced late instability in two patients with renal carcinoma. Thecal compression and late collapse led to therapeutic failure in four patients 12 to 18 months after surgery. Fixation failure occurred in four patients, resulting in loosening of the hardware devices. Failure to adequately address the anterior column disease was the primary cause of treatment failure in these patients; had it been addressed, the fixation devices may have remained intact throughout the illness. However, appropriate instrumentation provided rigid fixation and allowed more extensive tumor resection with sparing of vertebral motion segments. However, failure to address key technical and biomechanical principles can lead to serious complications. In the pediatric population, pedicle fixation may not be possible; but when it is, it appears to have the advantage of involving fewer motion segments.

SUMMARY

In the United States, approximately 2,000 malignant tumors of bone are diagnosed each year (74). Of these, between 4% and 20% are primary spinal tumors (80 to 400). Therefore, it would be unusual if not impossible for any one institution to acquire the necessary understanding of the natural history of these tumors and their response to various forms of treatment. Therefore, the authors would prefer that an international registry be organized through which centers with special interest in these cases can work together. To this end, adopting the same terminology and possibly using the same oncologic and surgical staging system is mandatory (Fig. 2). Only through a collaborative effort will enough information be obtained to allow rational surgical and nonsurgical decision making on behalf of our patients.

Treatments for vertebral spinal tumors in children have evolved over the years. More aggressive treatment has helped tremendously, as have improved diagnostic techniques. Diagnosis is the most important factor in treatment of tumors. The earlier the diagnosis, the more beneficial treatment will be. Although no single technique has emerged as superior, combinations of techniques based on individual cases have given the best results. However, many problems in treating cancer, especially in children, remain. Many neoplasms still are not curable, and treatments for these tumors can in and of themselves lead to problems (e.g., excision of tumors in children may result in spinal deformity and instability of the spine). The younger the patient, the more susceptible to severe deformity he or she is. Complete excision is the best cure, although in the spine this can be very difficult. Radiation and/or chemotherapy may not only affect growth but can be responsible for sarcomatous degeneration and/or development of secondary neoplasms.

In the future, the origin of human cancer as explained by molecular and cellular mechanisms in the various stages of carcinogenesis may provide the most effective means for cancer prevention and treatment. The mechanisms by which normal cell growth fails and cells become malignant is believed to be related in part to the absence of tumor suppressor genes or an activated oncogene (70,84). The suppressor genes are involved in cell cycle control, signal transmission, angiogenesis, and development, indicating that they contribute to normal cell and tumor cell functions. These suppressor genes are believed to provide an untapped resource for anticancer treatment (70). It is hoped that this technology will bring us closer to understanding the cellular mechanism of cancer and that our currently crude methods will give way to a more basic and reasonable approach to patients with spinal neoplasms. Clearly, time will tell, but while we wait we must not intervene without cause or delay without reason. Surgical intervention can be a valuable adjunct and at times constitutes the primary treatment for spinal neoplasms. Although there are times when intervention may be worse for the patient than no intervention, at other times strong intervention is the best alternative.

REFERENCES

1. Abramson DH, Ellsworth RM, Zimmerman LE (1976): Nonocular cancer in retinoblastoma survivors. *Trans Acad Ophthalmol Otolaryngol* 81:454–457.
2. Afshani E, Kuhn JP (1991): Common causes of low back pain in children. *Radiographics* 11:277–287.
3. Amacher AL, Eltomey A (1985): Spinal osteoblastoma in children in adolescence. *Child's Nerv Syst* 1:29–32.
4. Azouz EM, Kozlowski K, Martin D, et al. (1986): Osteoid osteoma and osteoblastoma of the spine in children. *Pediatr Radiol* 16:25–31.
5. Barwick KW, Huvos AG, Smith J (1980): Primary osteogenic sarcoma of the vertebral column: a clinical pathologic correlation of 10 patients. *Cancer* 46:595–604.
6. Beer SJ, Menezes AH (1997): Primary tumors of the spine in children. Natural history, management, and long term follow-up. *Spine* 22: 649–659.
7. Boden SD, Lee RR, Herzog RJ (1997): Magnetic resonance imaging of the spine. In: Frymoyer JW, ed. *The adult spine: principles and practice*, 2nd ed. Philadelphia: Lippincott-Raven Publishers, pp. 563–630.
8. Boriani S, Capanna R, Donati D, et al. (1992): Osteoblastoma of the spine. *Clin Orthop* 278:37–45.
9. Boriani S, Weinstein JN (1997): Differential diagnosis and surgical treatment of primary benign and malignant neoplasms. In: Frymoyer JW, ed. *The adult spine: principles and practice*, 2nd ed. Philadelphia: Lippincott-Raven Publishers, pp. 951–987.
10. Boriani S, Weinstein JN, Biagini R (1997): Spine update. A surgical staging system for therapeutic planning of primary bone tumors of the spine. A contribution to a common terminology. *Spine* 22:1036–1044.
11. Brown AP, Fixsen JA, Plowman PN (1987): Local control of Ewing's sarcoma: an analysis of sixty-seven patients. *J Radiol* 60:261–268.
12. Campanacci M, Cervellati G (1975): Osteosarcoma. A review of 345 cases. *Ital J Orthop Traumatol* 1:522.
13. Campanacci M, Boriani S, Savini R (1983): Staging, biopsy, surgical planning of primary spine tumors. *Chir Org Mov* 75:99–103.
14. Campanacci M, Boriani S, Giunti A (1990): Giant cell tumors of the spine. In: Sundaresan SN, Schmidek HH, Schiller AL, eds. *Tumors of the spine: diagnosis and clinical management*. Philadelphia: WB Saunders, pp. 163–172.
15. Capanna R, Albisinni U, Picci P, et al. (1985): Aneurysmal bone cyst of the spine. *J Bone Joint Surg Am* 67:527–531.
16. Coman DR, deLong RP (1951): The role of the vertebral venous system in the metastasis of cancer to the spinal column: experiments with tumor cell suspensions in rats and rabbits. *Cancer* 4:610–618.
17. Conrad E, Olszewski A, Berger M, et al. (1992): Pediatric spine tumors with spinal cord compromise. *J Pediatr Orthop* 4:454–460.
18. Dahlin DC (1967): *Bone tumors: general aspects and data on 6,221 cases*, 3rd ed. Springfield, IL: Charles C Thomas.
19. Delamarter RB, Sachs BL, Thompson GH, et al. (1889): Primary neoplasms of the thoracic and lumbar spine: analysis of 29 consecutive cases. *Clin Orthop* 256:87–100.
20. DeRosa G, Graziano G, Scott J (1990): Arterial embolization of aneurysmal bone cyst of the lumbar spine. *J Bone Joint Surg Am* 72:777–780.
21. DiLorenzo N, Spallone A, Nolletti A, et al. (1980): Giant cell tumors of the spine: a clinical study of six cases, with emphasis on the radiological features, treatment, and follow-up. *Neurosurgery* 6:29–34.
22. Dorfmann HD (1977): Malignant transformation of benign bone lesions. *Proc Natl Cancer Conf* 7:901–913.
23. Dowdle JA Jr, Winter RB, Dehner LP (1977): Postradiation osteosarcoma of the cervical spine in childhood. *J Bone Joint Surg Am* 59: 1968–1971.
24. Enneking WF, Spanier SS, Goodmann M (1980): A system for surgical staging of musculoskeletal sarcoma. *Clin Orthop* 153:106–120.
25. Fidler IJ, Gersten D, Hart I (1978): The biology of cancer invasion and metastasis. *Adv Cancer Res* 28:149–150.
26. Fidler MW (1994): Radical resection of vertebral body tumours. A surgical technique used in ten cases. *J Bone Joint Surg Br* 76:765–772.
27. Fowles JV, Bobechko WP (1970): Solitary eosinophilic granuloma in bone. *J Bone Joint Surg Br* 52:238–243.
28. Fraser RD, Paterson DC, Simpson DA (1977): Orthopedic aspects of spinal tumors in children. *J Bone Joint Surg Br* 59:143–151.
29. Goorin AM, Delorey MJ, Lack EE, et al. (1984): Prognostic significance of complete surgical resection of pulmonary metastases from osteogenic sarcoma: analysis of 32 patients. *J Clin Oncol* 2:425–431.
30. Green NE, Robertson WW Jr, Kilroy AW (1980): Eosinophilic granuloma of the spine with associated neural deficit. Report of three cases. *J Bone Joint Surg Am* 62:1198–1202.
31. Griffin JB (1978): Benign osteoblastoma of the thoracic spine. Case report with fifteen year followup. *J Bone Joint Surg Am* 60:833–835.
32. Harrington KD (1988): Metastatic disease of the spine. In: Harrington KD, ed. *Orthopaedic management of metastatic bone disease*. St. Louis: Mosby, pp. 309–383.
33. Hay MC, Patterson D, Taylor TK (1978): Aneurysmal bone cysts of the spine. *J Bone Joint Surg Br* 60:406–411.
34. Hart RA, Boriani S, Biagini R, et al. (1977): A system for surgical staging and management of spine tumors. A clinical outcome study of giant cell tumors of the spine. *Spine* 22:1773–1782.
35. Healy JH, Ghelman B (1986): Osteoid osteoma and osteoblastoma: Current concepts and recent advances. *Clin Orthop* 204:76–85.
36. Huvos AG (1979): *Bone tumors: diagnosis, treatment and prognosis*. Philadelphia: WB Saunders, pp. 47–93.
37. Huvos AG, Butler A, Bretsky SS (1983): Osteogenic sarcoma associated with Paget's disease of bone: a clinical pathologic study of 65 patients. *Cancer* 52:1489–1495.
38. Ippolito E, Farsetti P, Tadisco C (1984): Vertebra plana. Long term follow-up in five patients. *J Bone Joint Surg Am* 66:1364–1368.
39. Jackson RP (1978): Recurrent osteoblastoma. *Clin Orthop* 131: 229–233.
40. Jaffee HL (1953): Osteoid osteoma. *Proc R Soc Med* 46:1007–1012.
41. Kneisl J, Simon M (1992): Medical management compared with operative treatment for osteoid osteoma. *J Bone Joint Surg Am* 72:179–185.
42. Keim HA, Regina EG (1975): Osteoid osteoma as a cause of scoliosis. *J Bone Joint Surg Am* 57:159–163.
43. Kornberg M (1986): Primary Ewing's sarcoma of the spine. A review and case report. *Spine* 11:54–57.
44. Kostuik JP, Errico TJ, Gleason TF, et al. (1988): Spinal stabilization for vertebral tumors. *Spine* 13:250–256.
45. Kozlowski K, Beluffi G, Masel J, et al. (1984): Primary vertebral tumors in children: report of twenty cases with brief literature review. *Pediatr Radiol* 14:129–139.
46. Lane H, Parada L, Weinberg R (1987): Cellular oncogenes and multistep carcinogenesis. *Science* 237:1340–1343.
47. Larsson SE, Lorentzon R (1974): The incidence of malignant primary bone tumors in relation to age, sex and site. A site of osteogenic sarcoma, condrosarcoma and Ewing sarcoma diagnosed in Sweden from 1958 to 1968. *J Bone Joint Surg Br* 56:534–540.
48. Leeson MC, Makley JT, Carter JR (1985): Metastatic skeletal disease in the pediatric population. *J Pediatr Orthop* 5:261–267.
49. Loftus CM, Michelsen CB, Rapoport F, et al. (1983): Management of plasmacytomas of the spine. *Neurosurgery* 13:30–36.
50. Look AT, Douglass EC, Meyer WH (1988): Clinical importance of near diploid tumor stemlines in patients with osteosarcoma of an extremity. *N Engl J Med* 318:1567–1572.
51. Magerl F, Coscia MF (1988): Total posterior vertebrectomy of the thoracic and lumbar spine. *Clin Orthop* 232:62–69.
52. Marsh BW, Bonfiglio M, Brady LP, et al. (1975): Benign osteoblastoma: range of manifestations. *J Bone Joint Surg Am* 57:19.
53. McAfee P, Bohlman H, Ducker T, et al. (1986): Failure of stabilization of the spine with methylmethacrylate. A retrospective analysis of twenty four cases. *J Bone Joint Surg Am* 68:1145–1157.
54. McLain R, Kabins M, Weinstein J (1991): VSP stabilization of lumbar neoplasms: technical considerations and complications. *J Spinal Disord* 4:359–365.
55. McLeod RA, Dahlin DC, Beabout JW (1976): The spectrum of osteoblastoma. *Am J Radiol* 126:321–335.

56. Merryweather R, Middlemiss JH, Sanerkin NG (1980): Malignant transformation of osteoblastoma. *J Bone Joint Surg Am* 62:381–384.

57. Nesbit ME, Kieffer S, D'Angio GJ (1969): Reconstitution of vertebral height in histiocytosis X: a longterm followup. *J Bone Joint Surg Am* 51:1360–1368.

58. Ogihara Y, Sckiguchi K, Tsureta T (1984): Osteogenic sarcoma of the fourth thoracic vertebra. Long term survival by chemotherapy only. *Cancer* 53:2615–2618.

59. Palmer JJ (1972): Radiation myelopathy. *Brain* 95:109–122.

60. Parham DM, Pratt CB, Parvey LS, et al. (1985): Childhood multifocal osteosarcoma: clinical-pathologic and radiologic correlates. *Cancer* 55:2653–2658.

61. Pettine KA, Klassen RA (1986): Osteoid osteomas and osteoblastomas of the spine. *J Bone Joint Surg Am* 68:354–361.

62. Poulsen JO, Jensen JT, Thommesen P (1975): Ewing's sarcoma simulating vertebral plana. *Acta Orthop Scand* 46:211–215.

63. Raskas DS, Graziano GP, Herzenberg JE, et al. (1992): Osteoid osteoma and osteoblastoma of the spine. *J Spinal Disord* 5:204–211.

64. Rosen G, Caparros B, Huvos AG, et al. (1982): Preoperative chemotherapy for osteogenic sarcoma: selection of postoperative adjuvant therapy based on the response of the primary tumor to preoperative chemotherapy. *Cancer* 49:1221–1230.

65. Rosen G, Caparros B, Nirenberg A, et al. (1982): Ewing's sarcoma: ten year experience with adjuvant chemotherapy. *Cancer* 47:2204–2213.

66. Rosen G, Marcove RC, Huvos AG, et al. (1983): Primary osteogenic sarcoma: eight year experience with adjuvant chemotherapy. *J Cancer Res Clin Oncol* 106:55–67.

67. Rosen G, Wollner N, Tan C, et al. (1974): Disease-free survival in children with Ewing sarcoma treated with radiation therapy and adjuvant four drug sequential chemotherapy. *Cancer* 33:384–393.

68. Roy-Camille R, Monpierre H, Mazel C, et al. (1990): Technique de vertebrectomie totale lombaire. In: Roy-Camille R, ed. *Rachis Dorsal et Lombaire. Septieme Journees d'Orthopedie de la Pitié.* Paris: Masson, pp. 49–52.

69. Sabinas AO, Bickel WH, Moe JH (1970): Natural history of osteoid osteoma of the spine. Review of the literature and report of three cases. *Am J Surg* 1:880–889.

70. Sager R (1989): Tumor suppressor genes: the puzzle and the promise. *Science* 246:1406–1412.

71. Seimon LP (1981): Eosinophilic granuloma of the spine. *J Pediatr Orthop* 1:371–376.

72. Sharafuddin M, Haddad F, Hitchon P, et al. (1992): *Neurosurgery* 30:610–619.

73. Shives TC, McLeod RA, Unni KK, et al. (1996): Chondrosarcoma of the spine. *J Bone Joint Surg Am* 68:660–668.

74. Silverberg B, Lubera J (1987): Cancer statistics. *CA Cancer J Clin* 37:12.

75. Smith TP, Cragg AH (1991): Angiography of the spine. In: Frymoyer JW, ed. *The adult spine: principles and practice.* New York: Raven Press, pp. 511–525.

76. Stener B, Jensen E (1971): Complete removal of three vertebrae for giant cell tumor. *J Bone Joint Surg Br* 53:278–287.

77. Suit HD, Goiten M, Munzenreider J, et al. (1982): Definitive radiation therapy for chordoma and chondrosarcoma of base of skull and cervical spine. *J Neurosurg* 56:377–385.

78. Sundaresan N, DiGiacinto GV, Krol G, et al. (1989): Spondilectomy for malignant tumors of the spine. *J Clin Oncol* 7:1485–1491

79. Tillman BP, Dahlin DC, Lipscomb PR, et al. (1968): Aneurysmal bone cyst: an analysis of ninety-five cases. *Mayo Clin Proc* 93:478–495.

80. Tomita K, Kawahara N, Baba H, et al. (1994): Total en bloc spondylectomy for solitary spinal metastases. *Int Orthop (SICOT)* 18:291–298.

81. UribeBotero G, Russell WD, Sutow WW (1977): Primary osteosarcoma of bone. A clinical pathological investigation of 243 cases, and the necroscopy studies in 54. *Am J Clin Pathol* 67:427–435.

82. Vogler JB III, Murphy WA (1988): Bone marrow imaging. *Radiology* 168:679–693.

83. Weatherby RP, Dahlin DC, Ivins JC (1981): Post radiation sarcoma of bone: review of 78 Mayo Clinic cases. *Mayo Clin Proc* 56:294–306.

84. Weinstein B (1988): The origins of human cancer: molecular mechanisms of carcinogenesis and their implications for cancer prevention and treatment. *Cancer Res* 48:4135–4143.

85. Weinstein JN (1989): Surgical approach to spine tumors. *Orthopedics* 12:897–905.

86. Weinstein JN, McLain RF (1987): Primary tumors of the spine. *Spine* 12:843–851.

87. Whitehouse GH, Griffiths GJ (1976): Roentgenologic aspects of spinal involvement by primary and metastatic Ewing's tumor. *Can Assoc Radiol J* 27:290–297.

88. Wilkens RM, Pritchard DJ, Burgert EO Jr, et al. (1986): Ewing's sarcoma of bone. Experience with 140 patients. *Cancer* 58:2551–2555.

SPINAL CORD TUMORS

J. GORDON MC COMB
MARK A. LIKER
MICHAEL L. LEVY

The incidence of spinal cord tumors in comparison to brain tumors varies from series to series and is influenced by what is included under this heading (40). For instance, many series have included closed neural tube defects (NTDs) with lipomatous malformations under the category of lipomas, which in reality are hamartomatous rather than neoplastic lesions and are not included in this chapter. However, other closed NTDs, such as dermoids and neurenteric cysts, although not neoplastic, steadily expand in size and produce symptoms that are comparable to other benign neoplastic lesions in the spinal canal. Because the clinical presentation of dermoids, neurenteric cysts, vascular lesions and syringes are similar to that of other neoplastic lesions, they will be included in this chapter. Excluded are tumors of bony mesenchymal origin, which are discussed in another chapter. The incidence and types of spinal cord tumors are influenced significantly by referral patterns. For instance, a center that has an active neurofibromatosis program will have a disproportionate number of neurofibromas. If there is a very active oncology service, there will be a much higher incidence of epidural malignant tumors. Thus, although the incidence of spinal cord tumors is much lower compared with that of brain tumors, it varies considerably based on what is included and the nature of the referral patterns to a given center.

The classification of spinal cord tumors can also vary to a degree, although most reports divide tumors into extradural, intradural, extramedullary, and intramedullary categories (Fig. 1) based on location, as noted in Tables 1 and 2. Some tumors can be in more than one location, such as neurofibromas, which are often intradural extramedullary, as well as extradural. On rare occasions, an intradural extramedullary tumor, such as a primitive neuroectodermal tumor (PNET), can spread to become extradural. It is even rarer yet, however, for extradural tumors to penetrate the dural barrier and become intradural. In Table 3, the presenting signs and symptoms are listed in a rough order of decreasing frequency. Although some generalizations can be made, as seen in Table 4, there is enough overlap so that

the clinical presentation does not specify the position of the tumor with respect to the dura mater or spinal cord.

As noted in the generalizations in Table 4, this group of lesions is fairly uniformly distributed throughout the pediatric age group and is fairly equally divided as to sex. Also, as another generalization, the location of tumors along the spinal axis is by and large in proportion to the length of the spinal segment.

Although there still is often a fair delay between the onset of symptoms and the time that the definitive diagnosis is made, the advent of magnetic resonance imaging (MRI) in addition to computerized tomographic (CT) scanning has made remarkable strides in being able to detect and assess the treatment of this group of lesions. Improved surgical techniques have also significantly improved the outcome in patients with these tumors. As noted in Table 4, approximately two thirds of the neoplastic lesions are benign in the pediatric age group, whereas just the reverse is true for adults. This chapter provides an overview of this group of lesions, be they neoplastic or nonneoplastic masses that have the commonality of all being expanding lesions that will produce progressive neurologic deterioration if not addressed. In most, but not in all, instances, the best outcome will be obtained with a high degree of collaboration among a number of pediatric specialties residing at centers where these problems are frequently encountered.

CLINICAL SYMPTOMS AND SIGNS

Spinal cord tumors are notorious, in all but a small percentage of cases, for their indolent course because it is often months, if not years, before the correct diagnosis is made (39). With the advent of noninvasive MRI, however, the time between the onset of symptoms and diagnosis has been shortened considerably. In some cases, the progression of symptoms is relentless, whereas in many, the course is variable. The more malignant the tumor, the more likely that the progression is rapid and the time to diagnose shorter. A sudden change in spinal cord function can occasionally be seen in the face of hemorrhage, bony collapse, or extramedullary spinal cord compression that causes an ischemic stroke to the spinal cord.

Occasionally, the onset of symptoms is presumed to be the result of a minor traumatic injury, such as a fall. It may be

J. G. McComb, M. A. Liker, and M. L. Levy: Division of Neurosurgery, Children's Hospital Los Angeles, Los Angeles, CA 90027.

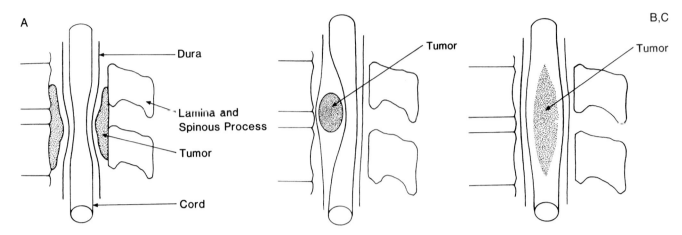

FIGURE 1. Different categories of spinal cord tumors. **A:** Extradural tumor lying outside of the thecal sac but within the bony confines of the spinal canal. **B:** Intradural extramedullary tumor lying within the thecal sac but outside of the spinal cord. **C:** Intramedullary tumor entirely in the substance of the spinal cord, causing cord widening.

TABLE 1. INTRAMEDULLARY TUMORS

Astrocytoma—low grade
Astrocytoma—high grade
Ependymoma
Ganglioglioma
Mixed glioma
Primitive neuroectodermal tumor (PNET) (same as medulloblastoma)
Lipoma
Neurenteric cyst
Syrinx

TABLE 3. SYMPTOMS AND SIGNS

Weakness	Reflex changes
Back pain	Tenderness
Radicular pain	Atrophy
Gait abnormality	Visible/palpable mass
Kyphoscoliosis	Muscle spasm
Torticollis	Hydrocephalus
Urinary incontinence/retention	Meningitis
Loss of or delayed milestones	Subarachnoid hemorrhage
Sensory changes	

TABLE 2. EXTRAMEDULLARY TUMORS

Intradural	Extraneural
Congenital	Lymphoma
Dermoid	Leukemia
Teratoma	Other
Neurenteric cyst	**Extradural**
Other	Neural Crest
Epidermoid	Neuroblastoma
Lipoma	Ganglioneuroma
Ependymoma	Mesenchymal—soft tissue
Nerve Sheath	Ewing Sarcoma
Neurofibroma	Rhabdomyosarcoma
Schwannoma	Unidentified sarcoma
Malignant nerve sheath tumor	Lymphoma
Meningeal	Leukemia
Meningioma	Germ cell
Arachnoid cyst	Wilms tumor
Vascular	Other
Arteriovenous malformation	Mesenchymal-bone (See other
Aneurysm	chapter)
Hemangioblastoma	
Hemangioendothelioma	
Metastatic	
Neural	
PNET	
Glioma	
Melanomatosis	

TABLE 4. GENERALIZATIONS

Tumor versus location
  Overall distribution of tumors in the spine is proportional to spinal segment length
  Fairly well distributed as to location among the intramedullary, intradural extramedullary and extradural spaces
Tumor versus gender
  Overall equal distribution between sexes
Tumor versus age
  < 18 years – 2/3 benign
  > 18 years – 2/3 malignant
  Fairly evenly distributed throughout the first 18 years
  Gliomas are seen fairly consistently across all age groups
  Neuroblastomas, teratomas and PNETs seen more frequently in the very young
  Neurofibromas, schwannomas and hemangioblastomas seen more commonly in older children
Location versus presentation
  Extradural or intradural extramedullary tumors are more likely to present with pain
  Intramedullary tumors have a higher incidence of kyphoscoliosis
Age versus presentation
  Pain more likely to herald a tumor in older age group
  Weakness and bladder dysfunction more frequently noted in the younger age group

that the preexisting myelopathy made the child clumsy and thus resulted in the fall. On the other hand, a minor injury could be enough to exacerbate the underlying pathophysiology, leading to spinal cord edema, microscopic hemorrhage in the spinal cord or surrounding tissues, and so on. It is frequent that the parents will pick up a very subtle abnormality long before any objective findings are noted. Many patients are often seen for orthopaedic evaluation because of gait abnormality or the development of kyphoscoliosis or back pain. Pain can be a significant factor, and many of the children have been prescribed various pain and antiinflammatory nonsteroidal medications for some time before the diagnosis being made.

The signs and symptoms are roughly in frequency to the listing in Table 3. In Table 4, there are some generalizations, such as the extradural or intradural extramedullary tumors are more likely to present with pain, whereas intramedullary tumors have a higher degree of kyphoscoliosis as the initial symptoms. Also, pain is more likely to herald the presence of a tumor in the older age group, whereas weakness and bladder dysfunction are more frequently noted in those who are younger. In the infant, irritability or general fussiness may be all that is indicative of a spinal cord tumor. A tumor located in the cervical region can often present with a head tilt or torticollis. If there is upper extremity neurologic involvement from a cervical tumor, an infant or young child may switch hand dominance.

Pain is more commonly reported to be present at night. This presumes that the horizontal position may alter the pressure on the spinal cord or exiting nerve roots secondary to venous congestion or, perhaps, the absence of cerebrospinal fluid (CSF) hydrostatic pressure to distend the spinal subarachnoid space (SAS), or possibly, that fewer stimuli are present to act as distraction from pain that is present during the day but is less noted.

The striking feature is the subtlety, the variability, the often indolent nature of the process, and the lack of early objective findings that make it so difficult to diagnose spinal cord tumors and leads to the delay between the initial onset of symptoms and the establishment of a definitive diagnosis.

The ready availability of noninvasive high-quality MRI has, once again, markedly shortened the time from onset of symptoms to diagnosis, as well as providing examiners with the ability to exclude other entities that can be confused with spinal cord tumors.

DIAGNOSTIC STUDIES

Imaging Modalities

MRI has revolutionized our ability to detect the presence of various forms of spinal cord tumors and has largely replaced other modalities (1). The signal characteristics of a tumor and its response to contrast enhancement, as well as the superior anatomic detail, give precise information as to the size, location, and to a fair degree, the likelihood of the histology of the lesion. Postoperative studies will document the degree of tumor excision and provide a non-invasive way for subsequent monitoring.

Because MRI does not image bone well, CT scanning is particularly helpful with tumors that primarily involve the bone or

significantly change the configuration of the surrounding normal bony structures. In some cases, three-dimensional reconstruction adds additional information that is beneficial in making clinical decisions. In some cases, it is helpful to obtain both MRI and CT images.

Myelography, with or without CT, is rarely needed for diagnostic purposes. The main indication at this point would be to determine if an area within the SAS is or is not in communication with the rest of the SAS, as with an arachnoid cyst, and cine-MRI is either not available or helpful.

Although abnormalities can be detected on plain spine x-rays (Fig. 2) their role is limited in detecting spinal cord tumors and they are used to assess the overall structural relationships and alignment of the vertebral column. Plain x-rays are of value to monitor the presence or progression of a kyphosis, scoliosis, or kyphoscoliosis of the spine.

Ultrasound does not readily penetrate through bone. This modality plays a minor role in making the diagnosis of an intraspinal lesion. In the first few months of life, the contents of the spinal canal can be imaged and, in some cases, used for screening purposes. If operative intervention is contemplated, MRI would also be indicated. The spinal canal can be imaged at the site of a laminectomy, although few clinical situations arise when this is clinically helpful and would not be better served with MRI. Intraoperatively, ultrasound is particularly useful for intramedullary tumors. The cystic and solid components can be readily detected once the spinal cord is exposed. In addition to helping with localization, intraoperative ultrasound may evaluate the presence of remaining solid tumor following excision in cases in which the echogenicity of the tumor is different from that of the normal spinal cord.

Bone scans, using various radiopharmaceuticals, can be helpful in detecting primary bone tumors before changes can be seen on plain x-ray studies, as well as detecting the presence of metastatic disease that involves the bone. A case in point is that of eosinophilic granuloma of the spine in a young child who is at risk of having multiple lesions. Bone scanning may also be helpful in monitoring the response of diffuse metastatic disease to chemotherapy and radiation therapy.

An angiogram is indicated when a vascular lesion, such as an arteriovenous malformation (AVM) or aneurysm, is suspected. Super selective catheter techniques and better equipment have greatly improved the ability to image vascular lesions.

Other Modalities

Much attention was previously given to the analysis of CSF and the response to manometric maneuvers before the advent of MRI and CT imaging. Modern imaging has rendered the examination of CSF unnecessary in all but a few select situations. In some cases, lumbar puncture may be contraindicated because it could lead to neurologic deterioration caused by the pressure differential created by removing CSF below a complete spinal canal block. Some cancer protocols still call for CSF cytologic determinations. Mounting evidence has shown this to be of limited value, because CSF cytology can be normal in spite of obvious lesions in the SAS on MRI (Fig. 3). However, CSF cytology can be helpful in ascertaining the presence or absence of

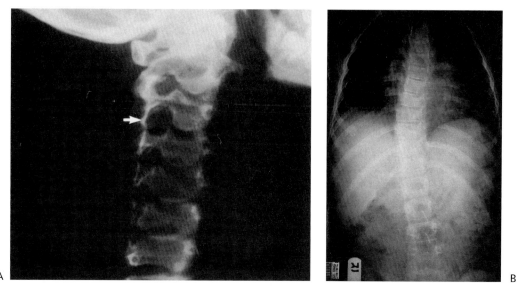

FIGURE 2. **A:** Plain radiograph of the cervical spine demonstrating widening of the C2–3 foramen by a neurofibroma *(arrow).* **B:** Anteroposterior spine x-ray studies showing thinning of the pedicles in the thoracic region and scoliosis secondary to an intramedullary tumor and syrinx.

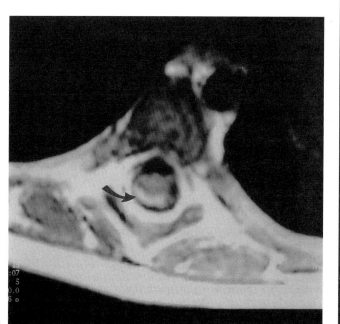
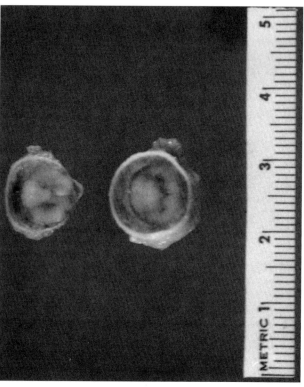

FIGURE 3. **A:** Contrast-enhanced magnetic resonance image of the spine showing the presence of a metastatic primitive neuroectodermal tumor (PNET) in the subarachnoid space *(arrow).* **B:** Autopsy specimen demonstrating diffuse subarachnoid tumor. The subarachnoid space surrounding the spinal cord is completely filled with metastatic tumor, in this case a PNET.

central nervous system (CNS) involvement with leukemia and lymphoma. CSF protein levels may rise or fall in response to advancing or receding disease, but these levels are only a very gross indicator of change and often in a much delayed fashion. Once again, MRI is a much better measure. Alpha-fetoprotein and beta-human chorionic gonadotropin levels in CSF may help with the diagnosis as well as monitoring the response to treatment, in certain malignant teratomas and germ cell tumors, but these lesions are usually intracranial in location. Congenital dermal sinuses and associated dermoid tumors can produce both an infective as well as a sterile inflammatory response that would be reflected by a pleocytosis and positive bacterial cultures.

Examination of the peripheral blood as well as bone marrow aspiration can be helpful in lymphomas, leukemias, and other metastatic disease entities. Measurement of the levels of the catecholamine breakdown products associated with neural crest tumors is often useful as a diagnostic tool, as well as a monitoring adjunct.

DIFFERENTIAL DIAGNOSIS

In addition to mesenchymal bony tumors, which are covered elsewhere, discitis (intravertebral disc infection) and osteomyelitis of the spine can present in similar fashion to that of spinal cord tumors.

Discitis is usually limited to the lumbar region in children younger than 5 years of age who present with progressive lower extremity weakness, refusal to walk, local tenderness, and either no fever or a low-grade fever. Vertebral osteomyelitis can present anywhere on the spine in an older group of children who primarily complain of back pain and are often febrile. In both entities, there is usually elevation of the peripheral white blood cell (WBC) count and erythrocyte sedimentation rate. Plain x-ray studies, CT scanning, and bone scans may all show changes depending on the stage of the disease. Once again, MRI will provide the most definitive information in distinguishing between discitis and osteomyelitis, as well as establishing that the process is not related to the spinal cord itself (11).

Demyelinating disease is uncommon in the pediatric age group and is only rarely a consideration in the differential diagnosis of spinal cord tumors. The onset of symptoms is usually much more rapid than with typical spinal cord tumors. Often, there are motor and sensory findings, with pain usually not being a significant factor. Also, the group most likely to be affected with a demyelination process is teenage girls. Once again, findings on MRI are the most helpful in making such a diagnosis, which is confirmed with CSF analysis.

Herniated discs are another entity that is uncommon in the pediatric age group and are most frequently encountered in the teenage group. The herniated discs are lumbar in location, present with back pain with or without radiculopathy, and occasionally, a neurogenic bladder. Once again, MRI is the diagnostic study of choice.

In the pediatric age group, brachial plexus, lumbar plexus, or peripheral nerve disease processes are rarely confused with spinal cord tumors and thus usually not a problem in the differential diagnosis, as is also true with myopathic entities. However, if there is any question, it is always better to image the spine with MRI.

Occasionally, a situation arises wherein an infant shows regression of milestones (i.e., stops walking or develops ataxia). The spinal cord is imaged, and nothing is found. Under these circumstances, it is necessary to image the head, because occasionally hydrocephalus by itself or associated with an intracranial tumor can present with symptom that could be confused with a spinal cord tumor.

INTRAMEDULLARY TUMORS

Astrocytoma—Low Grade

Low-grade astrocytomas are by far the most frequent intramedullary tumors seen in the pediatric age group (5,9). As the tumor slowly grows, it can reach considerable size before being diagnosed. As noted in Table 4 of generalizations, these tumors are fairly evenly distributed across all age groups and show no significant predilection for gender. They also tend to have a higher incidence of kyphoscoliosis and present less with pain (4, 44). The tumor involvement can be localized to one or two spinal cord segments, or it may extend the entire length of the spinal cord from the medulla to the conus medullaris. A majority of these tumors are associated with syringes that are rostral to the tumor (Fig. 4), caudal to the tumor (Fig. 5), or often even both.

MRI shows diffuse widening of the spinal cord with areas of high and low signal intensity, depending on the presence or absence of cystic formation or hemorrhage in addition to the solid component. The enhancement is inhomogeneous and often is irregular. The MRI characteristics do not differentiate between high-grade and low-grade astrocytomas. These tumors have a low-grade histology, some of which will contain features that are pilocytic in nature.

Laminectomy or laminotomy begins at the midportion of the tumor and extends both rostrally and caudally as needed to gain access to the solid component. The cystic portion of the tumor either above or below the solid component need not be exposed, thereby limiting the amount of bony removal. Once the upper or lower limits of the solid component are reached, one will enter the cystic cavity and drain its contents, which usually consists of highly proteinaceous fluid that often congeals at room temperature. On opening the dura mater, one can see thickened arachnoid, with an increase in the vasculature on the dorsal surface of the spinal cord. The cord may be rotated by the tumor, so the midline may be off to one side. With careful inspection, the area that appears to be most in the midline is chosen for the site of myelotomy. Using the operating microscope, the myelotomy is made and extended over the solid portion of the tumor. The ultrasonic aspirator is used to debulk the tumor. The presence of the cyst at the end of the tumor makes it easy to know that the end of the tumor has been reached. In those cases without a cyst, the tumor tends to taper, making the extent of the myelotomy deeper. In such a case, it is helpful to angle the microscope considerably in order to remove the tumor from within the cord, without extending the

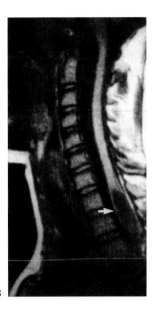
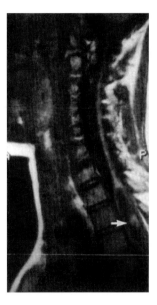

A,B

FIGURE 4. Intramedullary low-grade astrocytoma. **A** and **B:** Magnetic resonance image demonstrating the upper extent of tumor and associated cyst *(arrow)*. No postoperative adjuvant therapy was given after gross total removal of this tumor. This patient required an extensive spine stabilization procedure. Her neurologic condition remains stable, and there has been no evidence of tumor recurrence for almost 10 years.

myelotomy further. We have found it helpful to go over the length of the tumor many times, tilting the table and microscope in many directions so as to gain better exposure and feeling for where the interface between the tumor and spinal cord resides. Intraoperative ultrasound may be helpful in some situations. Localization of the cystic component in some cases can guide one's myelotomy, particularly if the tumor involves a very short segment of the spinal cord. When many segments are involved, it is just as easy to start where one knows solid tumor to be

present and extend the dissection in either direction. If the signal characteristics of the tumor are similar to those of the spinal cord, the ultrasound will not help in determining the degree of tumor removal. Small residual amounts of tumor can also be eliminated with bipolar cauterization. If possible, the goal is to perform a gross total removal of the tumor. Following debulking of the tumor, the dura mater is usually easily closed with a running absorbable suture. The wound is then closed in a standard fashion.

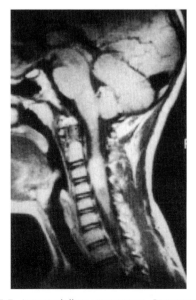
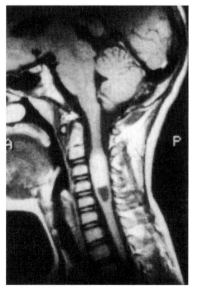

FIGURE 5. Intramedullary astrocytoma. Preoperative magnetic resonance image (MRI) with contrast enhancement. Note enhancing intramedullary mass with associated cyst.

Postoperative imaging studies are obtained to determine the degree of resection. If tumor is left behind, consideration should be given for an additional procedure to remove the remaining tumor (33). Postoperative radiation or chemotherapy are not indicated. Although there are undoubtedly viable tumor cells left behind, it would appear that, if their number is reduced to a certain threshold, the body's defense mechanisms appear to keep them in check from further growth. The long-term outcome can be quite favorable, with many patients being neurologically stable for years to decades following tumor excision (16,18,19,26,37,41). Surveillance imaging is indicated at progressively less frequent intervals if no change is noted on serial studies.

If the neurologic deficit is worse immediately postoperatively, often there will be a progressive improvement, such that the patient is the same as or better than before operative intervention was undertaken (6,8). There is no evidence that there can be any improvement in function for a patient who is paraplegic or quadriplegic before the operative procedure. In those situations in which recurrence does occur, consideration can be given to re-resection. Occasionally, although not common, these tumors can become progressively more malignant in histologic appearance. On occasion, low-grade astrocytomas can be present throughout the SAS, even before operative intervention. If enough of the SAS is filled with tumor, hydrocephalus develops, requiring CSF diversion. Although radiation therapy or chemotherapy is often initiated under these circumstances, the benefit of such is unknown and probably variable (13).

Astrocytoma—High Grade

Roughly 10% of intramedullary astrocytomas are classified as anaplastic astrocytoma or glioblastoma multiforme and thus are classified as high grade. The clinical progression is usually more rapid, although one cannot use this factor to distinguish between high-grade and low-grade astrocytomas. Imaging by MRI cannot discern the difference between high-grade and low-grade astrocytomas with any degree of reliability.

On opening the dura mater, one cannot always ascertain whether a tumor is high grade or low grade. Even while probing within the tumor, it may not be possible. Availability of reliable intraoperative neuropathologic assessment is key to knowing the nature of the tumor and how aggressive one needs to be with tumor resection. Less aggressive debulking of the tumor may be called for with high-grade astrocytomas, because it has not been shown to influence the prognosis positively, which in this group of patients is very poor. Also, the plane of demarcation between the tumor and spinal cord may be even more difficult to define compared with a low-grade astrocytoma (Fig. 6). In this situation, the dura mater is left open for decompression and oxidized cellulose is placed over the exposed spinal cord and dura mater before beginning closure. Radiation therapy, or chemotherapy, or both, are appropriate in these situations, with the outcome being similar to that of intracranial tumors with the same histology (32,38). Often, these tumors will disseminate widely

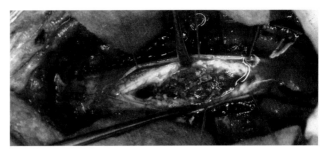

FIGURE 6. Intraoperative photograph of a high-grade astrocytoma. The tumor is diffusely infiltrating the spinal cord. There is no clear cut demarcation between tumor and spinal cord. The tumor was debulked, and the patient was given a course of chemotherapy and radiation. The patient subsequently died of disseminated disease.

through the SAS and result in increased resistance to CSF drainage, requiring CSF diversion.

Ependymomas

Ependymomas are the most common intramedullary tumors in adults (6,7,29) and the second most common in children. Nothing clinically distinguishes an ependymoma from an astrocytoma. The appearance of ependymomas on MRI is comparable to that of an astrocytoma in many respects, with the notable difference that the area of enhancement tends to be fairly uniform and better demarcated than most astrocytomas. Ependymomas grow in the spinal cord, mainly by displacing rather than invading neural structures, producing a well-demarcated plane around the tumor. This makes it easier to achieve a gross total removal with less possibility of causing neurologic damage. Following gross total removal of ependymoma, long-term survival without recurrence is the rule (18). If residual tumor is seen on the postoperative imaging study, consideration need be given to reexplore the spinal cord, with an attempt to remove the residual tumor unless deemed otherwise by the first operative procedure. In some cases, observation with serial imaging studies may be an alternative. There is little role for chemotherapy or radiation therapy in a grossly resected ependymoma. The benefits of these modalities in incompletely resected tumors remains uncertain (14).

Ganglioglioma

These are uncommon tumors that constitute but a small fraction of intramedullary tumors. It is a slow-growing tumor and has an indolent clinical course. On MRI, there is nothing specific that distinguishes this tumor from any other intramedullary tumor. The optimum treatment is gross total excision, which is easier in some cases than others, as the line of demarcation between tumor and surrounding spinal cord may be similar to that of a low-grade astrocytoma. As with an ependymoma, there is no need for adjuvant therapy in a completely resected tumor. For those tumors that are not completely resected, the same guidelines hold as for ependymomas.

Mixed Gliomas

A percentage of intramedullary tumors have mixed glial elements and thus are classified as low-grade astrocytoma and ependymoma, or low-grade astrocytoma and oligodendroglioma. As long as all of the components are low grade, the clinical course is similar to that of a low grade astrocytoma. Ideal treatment consists of gross total resection without adjuvant therapy. With an incomplete resection, the same considerations hold for that discussed under low-grade astrocytomas.

Primitive Neuroectodermal Tumors

On rare occasions, PNETs can present as an isolated intramedullary tumor of the spinal cord. On some occasions, they can be a direct extension into the spinal cord from the posterior fossa or be a discreet tumor mass separated from that in the region of the fourth ventricle (Fig. 7). The surgical goal for these tumors is gross total resection, followed by either chemotherapy or radiation therapy, or both. These tumors can widely disseminate in the SAS, like those whose primary is in the posterior fossa.

Lipomas

These intramedullary tumors are usually found in the thoracic region, although they may extend to the cervical and lumbar regions to involve a large segment of the spinal cord (Fig. 8).

They are most likely congenital in nature and may or may not be truly neoplastic. They are not associated with any cutaneous markers for dysraphism. This type of tumor is different from that of the lipomatous malformation associated with a closed NTD that results in tethering of the spinal cord. The symptoms from this type of lipoma are that of spinal cord compression and may become manifest after weight gain or a growth spurt. The findings on MRI are typical of fat.

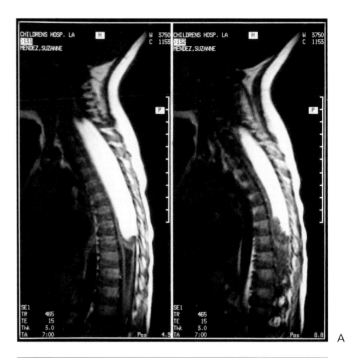

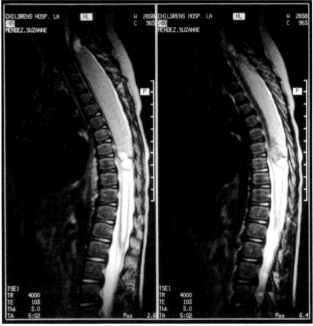

FIGURE 8. Fibrolipoma. **A:** This noncontrast T1-weighted magnetic resonance imaging study shows the presence of an intramedullary tumor, which is hyperintense to the spinal cord. It did not enhance with contrast. At the bottom of the tumor, one can appreciate the presence of a syrinx. **B:** The T2-weighted image shows the mass to have similar characteristics to adipose tissue. The syrinx is even better seen on this image. This 3-year-old child presented with developmental delay, scoliosis, weakness in her right lower extremity, and hyperactive reflexes. This patient underwent a thoracic laminectomy, with resection of over 50% of the mass. A postoperative scan showed a decrease in the syrinx. Her neurologic function remained stable. She did develop progressive kyphosis, which required stabilization.

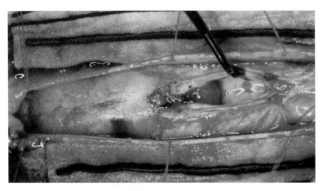

FIGURE 7. Intramedullary primitive neuroectodermal tumor (PNET). This patient had a posterior fossa PNET resected previously followed by chemotherapy and radiation therapy. On follow-up imaging studies, he was found to have an intramedullary mass in the cervical region, remote from the original posterior fossa tumor. This tumor had a clear-cut margin, and it was possible to grossly resect what was a histologically similar PNET. Note the syrinx rostral to the tumor. The patient died secondary to recurrence of the intracranial tumor component.

The goal of surgery is to decompress the spinal cord through a subtotal removal of the lipomatous tissue using the ultrasonic aspirator. No attempt is made to perform a gross total excision, because these tumors appear to have limited growth potential and there is no clear-cut plane of separation between the fat and the adjacent neural tissue. The long-term prognosis is usually excellent.

Neurenteric Cysts

Neurenteric cysts may be intramedullary, extramedullary, or a combination of both. Because it is more common for them to be extramedullary, they are discussed in the section below.

Syrinx

Owing to the availability of noninvasive MRI of the spinal cord, syringes are being diagnosed with increasing frequency and earlier in the course of progression. The vast majority of these syringes result from a Chiari I malformation, a downward herniation of the cerebellar tonsils through the foramen magnum into the spinal canal that interferes with the normal movement of CSF between the cranial and spinal SAS. This alteration in CSF dynamics can result in CSF accumulating within the spinal cord to produce a syrinx. If the fluid accumulation is confined to the dilated central canal, it is referred to as hydromyelia, whereas if the fluid collection extends into the parenchyma of the spinal cord, it is termed syringomyelia. In practice, those syringes that are large enough to produce symptoms are a combination of both hydromyelia and syringomyelia for which the term hydrosyringomyelia is used and often referred to simply as a syrinx. Those syringes that are a few millimeters in diameter are of no clinical significance, whereas those in which the syrinx is larger than the diameter of the normal spinal cord definitely are significant (Fig. 9).

In our experience, the presenting symptom in the majority of these patients is a progressive scoliosis (24,27). Other symptoms in decreasing frequency were headache, upper extremity weakness, sensory abnormality, gait disturbance, and cranial nerve involvement. Hydrocephalus is rarely a factor. The diagnosis is easily made with MRI. Treatment consists of a cervicomedullary decompression to restore the normal CSF dynamics, whereupon in all but a few cases, the diameter of the syrinx slowly diminishes with time. Serial MRI is used to follow these patients, and reoperation is indicated should the syrinx recur.

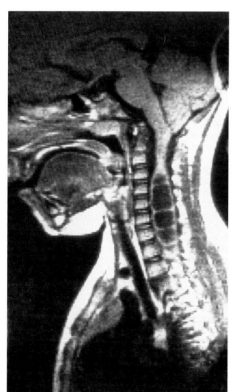
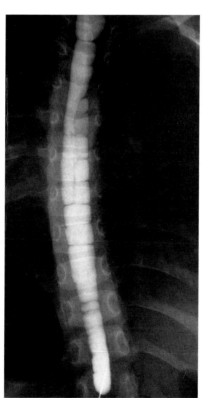
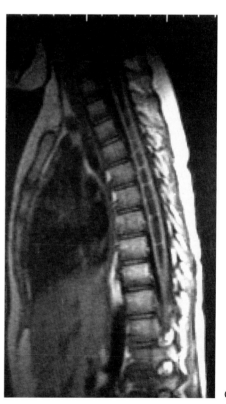

,B

C

FIGURE 9. **A:** Sagittal T1 magnetic resonance image (MRI) showing the presence of a Chiari I malformation and marked dilatation of the spinal cord by a syrinx. **B:** A syringogram was performed during the period when MRI was first being used to evaluate syringes. This large holocord syrinx has multiple septated regions; however, there is complete communication from the rostral to caudal end of the syrinx. **C:** Definitive decrease in the size of the syrinx 2 weeks after a cervicomedullary decompression. Subsequent MRI scans showed nearly complete collapse of the syrinx. This 6-year-old boy presented only with scoliosis. The scoliosis did not progress and, in fact, with bracing, markedly diminished.

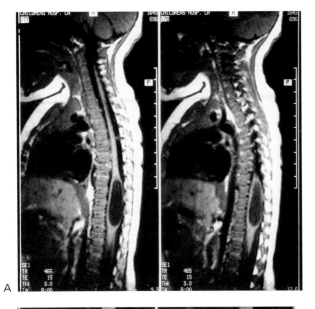

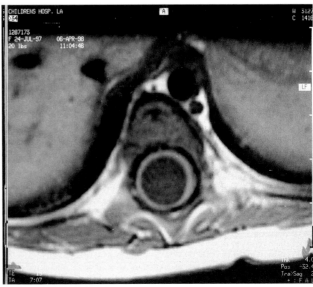

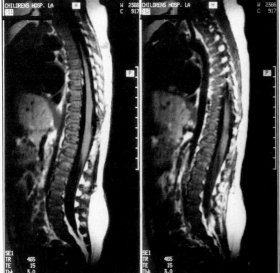

FIGURE 10. Isolated spinal cord syrinx. Sagittal **(A)** and transverse magnetic resonance images **(B)** showing an isolated syrinx in the spinal cord. There was no enhancement. **C:** Following a myelotomy, the syrinx collapsed and has not recurred. This 8-month-old infant presented with a 3-cm region of cutis aplasia and hypertrichosis in the lumbar region, which had remained unchanged since birth. Imaging of the rest of the central nervous system was normal. The patient had a normal neurologic examination preoperatively and postoperatively.

These patients also need close orthopaedic follow-up of their scoliosis.

Occasionally, isolated syringes of the spinal cord not associated with a Chiari I malformation may also be encountered following MRI imaging for suspected spinal cord abnormality (Fig. 10) (35). These lesions are surgically treated by making a myelotomy in the spinal cord, allowing communication between the syrinx and the SAS.

EXTRAMEDULLARY TUMORS—INTRADURAL

Congenital

Dermoid

Dermoids, which contain both dermal and epidermal elements, can present anywhere along the spinal axis but overwhelmingly

are found at the level of the conus medullaris or cauda equina and are associated with a congenital dermal sinus. These lesions are thought to arise from an abnormal adhesion or failure of normal separation between the ectoderm destined to form the neural tube and that which will form skin. Depending on the extent of the incomplete separation, the tract may end in the subcutaneous tissue or extend any distance inward to its ultimate embryologic terminus, which is the conus medullaris for lesions in the lumbosacral region and the central canal of the spinal cord for tracts at the thoracic or cervical levels (Fig. 11).

As noted in Figure 11A, those near the tip of the coccyx end in the fascia and do not extend to the SAS and, therefore, are usually of little consequence. The tract may be readily visible and be associated with other cutaneous markers, such as capillary telangiectasia, pigmentation changes of the surrounding skin, hair or debris exiting the orifice (Fig. 12), or with none of these markers, making it harder to detect. The capsule of dermoid

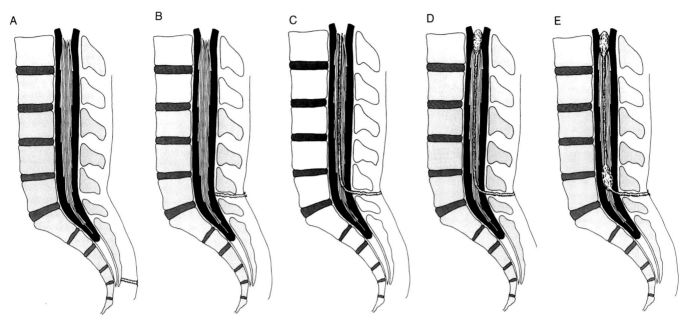

FIGURE 11. The varying anatomy of dermal sinuses and dermoid tumors. **A:** The tract ends at the coccyx and does not involve the neural elements. **B:** Dermal sinus. The sinus passes between spinous processes and ends at the dura mater. No dermoid tumor is present. **C:** Dermal sinus. The sinus enters the thecal sac and ends at the tip of the conus medullaris. No dermoid tumor is present. **D:** Dermal sinus and dermoid tumor. A dermoid tumor is present at the termination of the sinus at the conus medullaris. **E:** Dermal sinus and dermoid tumors. Two dermoid tumors are present along the course of the dermal sinus, one in the cauda equina and one at the conus medullaris.

usually adheres to the surrounding neural structures and becomes even more densely adherent in cases of inflammation from an infection or from the fatty acids of the degenerating material within the capsule should they enter the SAS. All tumors associated with a congenital dermal sinus should be dermoids embryologically; however, confusion exists because some reports, particularly in the older literature, do not correctly differentiate

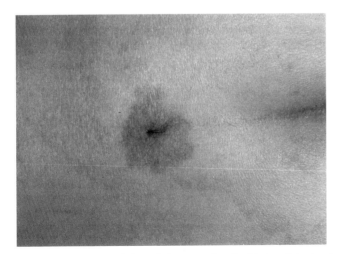

FIGURE 12. Congenital dermal sinus associated with two intradural dermoid tumors. Photograph showing congenital dermal sinus with hair coming from the orifice. There is an area of capillary telangiectasia surrounding the orifice.

between dermoids and epidermoids and, in addition, the tissue sent for histopathologic examination may not reflect the lesion in its entirety or the dermal elements may have been destroyed by inflammation. Malignant change in these lesions is not a factor. The depth to which the congenital dermal sinus penetrates and whether it is associated with one or more dermoids will determine the clinical manifestations. A congenital dermal sinus may go unnoticed until the patient presents with infection, either meningitis or an extradural or intradural abscess. The usual hallmarks of a local infection may be present or, in some cases, completely absent when a deeper lying abscess or meningitis exists. Even without infection, the contents of the dermoid cyst can produce a chemical meningitis or dense arachnoiditis. Hydrocephalus can develop secondary to increased resistance of CSF absorption as a result of one or more bouts of bacterial or chemical meningitis. A progressively enlarging dermoid cyst along the tract will eventually result in compression of the conus medullaris or cauda equina, and the patient's symptoms will depend on the level of compression.

A diagnosis of congenital dermal sinus and associated dermoid is clinical, and the imaging studies, particularly MR, is only augmentive (28). Negative findings on MRI do not exclude the need to explore the tract to its end and excise it along with any accompanied dermoid tumors (Fig. 13). The most important factor influencing the outcome in cases of congenital dermal sinuses and dermoids is total excision of the lesion before the development of infection or irreversible neural neurologic damage.

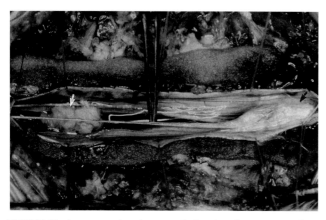

FIGURE 13. Intraoperative photograph showing the presence of two intradural dermoids, the first being in the lower lumbar region *(white arrow)* and the second being embedded in the conus medullaris *(black arrow)*. This patient presented with bacterial meningitis. Both of these tumors were subsequently removed, and the patient had a complete recovery.

As shown in Figure 14, dermoids can also be seen in association with an anterior sacral meningocele.

Teratoma

The vast majority of teratomas present as sacrococcygeal teratomas, are extradural in location, and are characteristic enough in that they are rarely confused with intraspinal tumors. Occasionally, teratomas can be present with anterior sacral meningoceles and other NTDs just like dermoid tumors (15).

The overwhelming number of teratomas present as masses of varying size extending outward from the sacrum and coccyx, often with involvement of one or both buttocks (Fig. 15). The overlying skin is perfectly normal unless the tumor has grown to such an extent that there is necrosis of tumor and the overlying skin. A small percentage can be totally intrapelvic without the presence of an anterior sacral meningocele and can be identified only on rectal examination. In most cases, it is easy to differentiate teratoma from an NTD.

Sacrococcygeal teratomas may consist of either cystic or solid components and may have completely mature tissue that is benign, a mixture of benign elements and tissue having malignant potential, or components that are frankly malignant. The prog-

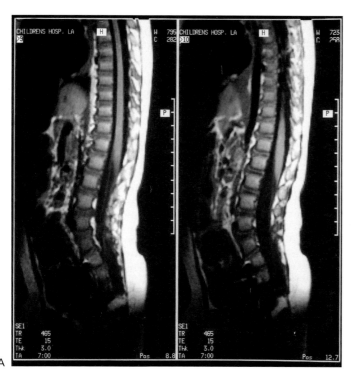

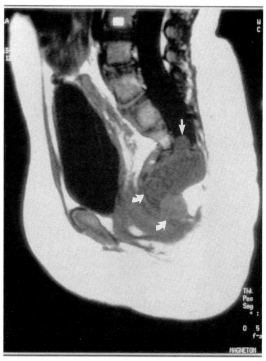

FIGURE 14. Anterior sacral meningocele with a dermoid. This infant was born with an anteriorly displaced rectum. Because of the known association of closed neural tube defects and rectal anomalies, a magnetic resonance image (MRI) study was obtained when she was 6 months of age. **A:** Sagittal T1-weighted MRI study showing the presence of a low-lying and tethered cord. The presence of the anterior meningocele was initially missed on this imaging study. **B:** Subsequent T1-weighted sagittal MRI study of the pelvis showed the presence of the anterior sacral meningocele and associated dermoid tumor. The *straight arrow* is at the interface between the dermoid and the subarachnoid space. The *curved arrows* demarcate the interface between the meningeal sac containing dermoid tumor with the surrounding pelvic structures. At the time of surgery, the dermoid was partially resected, the meningocele was closed, and the spinal cord untethered. Several months later, at the time of the definitive procedure to repair the rectum, the remainder of the dermoid, located anterior to the sacrum, was excised.

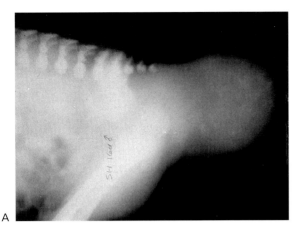
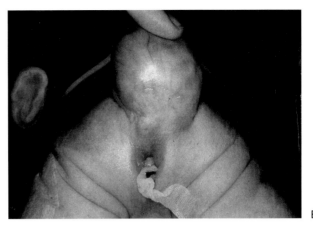

A   B

FIGURE 15. Sacral coccygeal teratoma. **A:** Sagittal plain x-ray study of a 16-day-old boy with a partially calcified mass distal to the tip of the coccyx. **B:** Operative photograph showing the relationship of this tumor to the anus. This was a benign teratoma that was completely resected. Postoperatively, the patient did well and had no neurologic deficit.

nosis depends on the histopathology of the tumor. The longer the tumor remains beyond early infancy, the higher the incidence of malignant transformation. Treatment consists of removal of tumor and the coccyx. Most of these lesions are excised by or in conjunction with a pediatric surgical specialist.

Neurenteric Cysts

The embryologic disorder responsible for neurenteric cysts appears to occur during gastrulation similar to that for a split cord malformation (diastematamyelia). These two types of NTDs can occur together.

Neurenteric cysts occur most frequently in the low cervical or upper thoracic region (Fig. 16) (34) and, occasionally, at the conus medullaris. The neurenteric cyst can be extradural or intradural, and if it is intra-dural, it can be anterior to, within, or posterior to the spinal cord or even between, as in the case of a split cord malformation (Fig. 17). The histopathologic features of the cyst can vary in complexity, but most cysts are lined by a single layer of stratified or pseudostratified or columnar

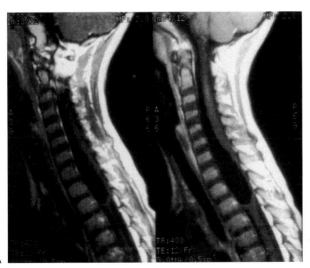
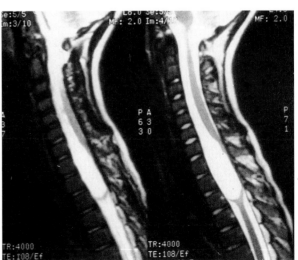

A   B

FIGURE 16. Neurenteric cyst. This 5-year-old girl presented with back pain and early symptoms of a neurogenic bladder. On examination, her back was normal without cutaneous markers for dysraphism. The neurologic examination was normal except for brisk reflexes in the lower extremities. **A:** Sagittal T1-weighted magnetic resonance image showing intraaxial and extraaxial characteristics of a cyst, which did not enhance with contrast. **B:** The T2-weighted image shows that the fluid content has similar density to cerebrospinal fluid. A midline myelotomy was made, and clear viscous fluid was encountered. The cyst wall was found to be neurenteric in origin and completely excised. In addition, there was an anteriorly located extramedullary arachnoid cyst that was fenestrated. Postoperatively, the patient had dyesthesia that subsequently cleared. At present, she is neurologically normal and free of pain.

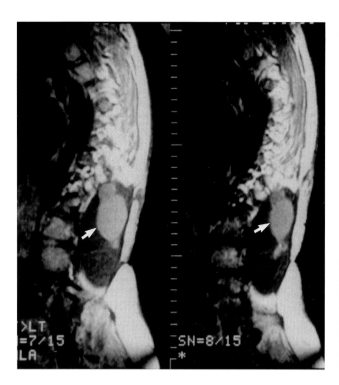

FIGURE 17. Neurenteric cyst. This is a sagittal T1-weighted magnetic resonance imaging (MRI) study, showing the presence of a mass *(arrow)*, which is hypointense to fat. This child had an open neural tube defect (myelomeningocele), closed at birth. He had a CSF diverting shunt placed. Despite the fact that his hydrocephalus was under good control, he had progressive loss of neurologic function. An MRI study was obtained and showed the presence of a neurenteric cyst and a split cord malformation. The bony spur was removed. His cord was untethered and the neurenteric cyst excised. Postoperatively, his neurologic deficit was worse and did not improve to his preoperative level.

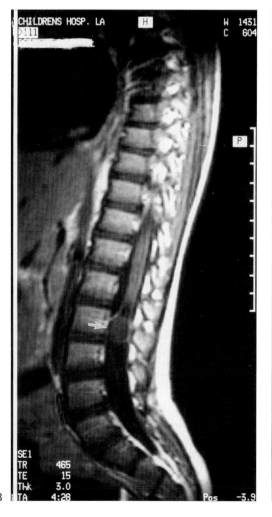
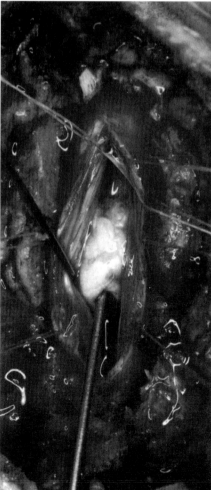

FIGURE 18. Epidermoid tumor. **A:** Magnetic resonance imaging (MRI), noncontrast T1-weighted, sagittal image shows a mass distal to the cauda equina that is hypointense to the spinal cord and did not enhance with contrast *(arrow)*. On a T2-weighted image (not shown) it was difficult to visualize the mass. **B:** Intraoperative photographs of a dermoid tumor among the roots of the cauda equina. *(Figure continues.)*

A,B

epithelium that stains positive for mucin. The vertebral column can be completely normal or may have significant segmentation abnormalities. Neurenteric cysts that are not associated with other NTDs will have no neurocutaneous markers for dysraphism. They are more common in males. Most neurenteric cysts have symptoms of a spinal cord compression, often with pain localized at the level of the cyst. Discharge of the cyst contents into the SAS can result an aseptic meningitis.

As usual, MRI is the modality of choice. The contents of the cyst usually have a higher signal intensity on T1- and T2-weighted images than that of CSF. The capsule may enhance or be too thin to be seen. Spine and chest x-ray studies are indicated to assess for bony abnormalities and the possible presence of a paraspinal or intrathoracic mass.

Depending on the location of the cyst, the approach will vary. The goal is to completely remove the capsule if possible.

Other

Epidermoid

Unlike dermoids, these tumors have no dermal elements but only that of epidermal origin. The overwhelming majority of these tumors are located in the cauda equina and result from a lumbar puncture in the neonatal or early infancy period to rule out meningitis (Fig. 18). Often, a lumbar puncture is performed with a fine-gauge needle without a stylet, which allows the introduction of epidermal elements into the SAS. This technique is to be highly discouraged.

The presence of an epidermoid tumor is usually made known by compression of the adjacent nerve roots with pain at the level of the lesion. The goal of surgery is complete excision without leaving any remnants behind. The outcome, obviously, should be most favorable.

Lipoma

Lipomas can be either intradural intramedullary or intradural extramedullary and, thus, are placed in both these categories. Intramedullary tumors are discussed earlier. The extramedullary lipoma is a true neoplasm with progressive increase in the number of adipose cells rather than being a hamartomatous malformation, as is the case with closed NTDs. These extradural tumors usually have a clear plane of demarcation from the spinal cord and dura mater, and usually are easily excised. They present

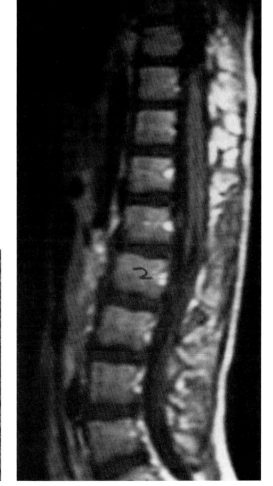
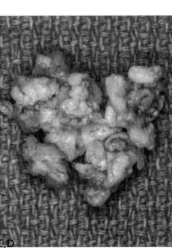

FIGURE 18. *Continued.* **C:** Material from the epidermoid tumor. **D:** Postoperative MRI demonstrating no evidence of residual tumor. This 6-year-old child presented with progressive back pain. No neurologic deficit was present. As a neonate, this patient had a lumbar puncture for suspected meningitis.

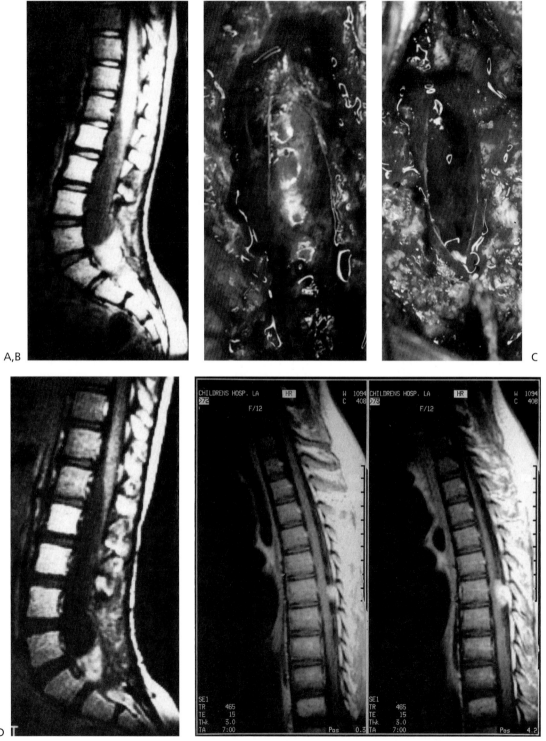

FIGURE 19. Myxopapillary ependymoma. **A:** Preoperative magnetic resonance image (MRI) with contrast demonstrating an enhancing mass filling the distal thecal sac. **B:** Intraoperative photograph demonstrating large intradural mass. **C:** Intraoperative photograph at the end of tumor resection. The unencapsulated ependymoma diffusely filled the subarachnoid space enveloping the entire cauda equina and thus negating the opportunity to excise this neoplasm completely. **D:** Postoperative MRI demonstrating degree of tumor resection. Residual tumor is present. This 10-year-old girl presented with back pain. There was local tenderness and limited mobility to spinal movement but no neurologic deficits. She received a postoperative course of localized radiation therapy. Two years later, she developed midthoracic back pain. **E:** An MRI showed the presence of a uniformly enhancing intradural extramedullary mass rostral to the field of radiation at T6–7, compressing the spinal cord. This mass, a myxopapillary ependymoma, was completely excised, and the thoracic spinal cord was radiated. The patient is now 19 years of age. *(Figure continues.)*

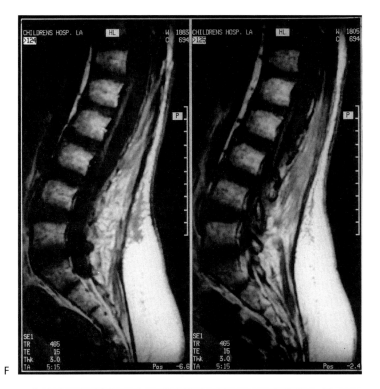

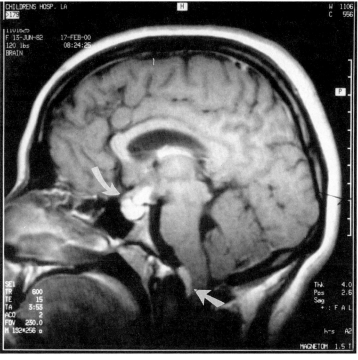

FIGURE 19. *Continued.* **F:** A follow-up MRI study showed no residual tumor at the sacral, lumbar or thoracic levels. **G:** She has an enhancing mass anterior to the medulla and cervical spinal cord at the cervicomedullary junction *(straight arrow)* and a second lesion enveloping the hypothalamic-pituitary area *(curved arrow)*. No attempt was made to resect these tumors, which are presumed to be myxopapillary ependymomas. The patient has just completed a course of radiation therapy to the head and cervical spine.

with spinal cord compression. On MRI, they have the typical features of adipose tissue. Following excision, the outcome should be excellent.

Ependymoma

These tumors can be intramedullary or extramedullary in location and are commonly found in the region of the conus medul-laris and cauda equina in the pediatric age group. The histology of these tumors in this location is usually that of a myxopapillary variety and somewhat less aggressive than those ependymomas with a more malignant histologic appearance. These tumors present with evidence of either conus medullaris or cauda equina compression. The course is, as with most slowly growing tumors, indolent. The MRI characteristics are noted in Figure 19.

In those cases in which the tumor is completely encapsulated, gross total removal can most often be accomplished. In such situations, postoperative radiation is not indicated. In some cases, the tumor is not encapsulated but completely fills the SAS and is intimately adherent to all of the nerve roots of the cauda equina (Fig. 19C). In such situations, it is not possible to remove the tumor completely but an extensive debulking should be un dertaken, followed by a course of radiation. In this situation, long-term follow-up is indicated, as shown by the patient in Figure 19E, who had recurrence of tumor above the field of radiation.

This tumor was subsequently removed, but the patient then developed intracranial extension of tumor 9 years later (Fig. 19G). Thus, even though the histology of myxopapillary ependymomas is relatively benign, they can biologically behave in a more aggressive fashion. At present, chemotherapy has not be proven to be of any benefit in treating this type of ependymoma.

Nerve Sheath Tumors

The terminology for this group of tumors is confusing with the interchangeable terms, such as neurofibromas, schwannomas, neurinomas, neuromas, and neurilemomas being used. It is generally agreed that there are basically two types of tumors, namely neurofibromas and schwannomas. Neurofibromas appear to be derived from mesenchymal cells of fibroblastic origin, whereas schwannomas arise from Schwann cell precursors.

Histopathologically, they present different appearances that allow for separation into the two categories. Because the nerve fascicles are intimately intermingled with tumor tissue, it is almost always necessary to sacrifice the nerve root when removing a neurofibroma, whereas it may be possible to spare some or all of the fascicles when excising a schwannoma. In the pediatric age group, neurofibromas are much more frequent than schwannomas. The incidence of neurofibromas will vary directly with the presence of an active neurofibromatosis (NF) program. Although reports that roughly a quarter of neurofibromas are

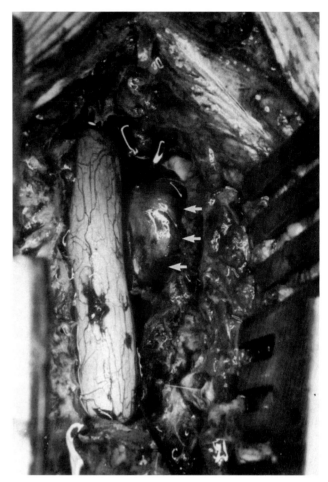

FIGURE 21. Neurofibroma at T12. Intraoperative photograph demonstrating a large extradural mass at T12 *(arrows)*.

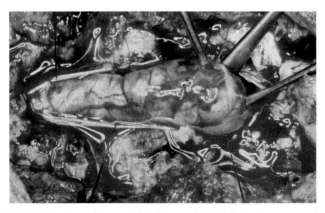

FIGURE 20. Neurofibroma. This 10-year-old child did not have neurofibromatosis but presented with back pain and limitation of forward flexion. There was no neurologic deficit. This operative photo shows the neurofibroma being completely removed from the region of the cauda equina. The patient made an uneventful recovery without any neurologic deficit.

found in association with NF, in our experience, it has been the majority of patients with neurofibromas that have NF.

Nerve sheath tumors can be intradural (Fig. 20), extradural (Fig. 21) or, as often the case, a combination of both (Fig. 22). Symptoms are usually the result of a spinal cord compression or individual nerve root irritation. On MRI, they appear as discreet lesions that fairly uniformly enhance with contrast.

The vast majority of these tumors can be excised from a posterior approach with complete excision of the tumor. Some will extend into the foramen. It is possible to excise all of the tumor if it does not extend beyond the foramen. Occasionally, it will be necessary to remove the dumb-bell portion of the tumor extending beyond the foramen through another approach (Fig. 22).

The spectrum of NF varies widely. NF is often subdivided into NF I when there is primarily peripheral nerve involvement and an alteration in chromosome 17, whereas NF II tends to be more central and is particularly characterized by bilateral acoustic tumors and has an alteration of chromosome 22. There is, however, a considerable degree of variation and overlap, so as to make the difference in categories only relative. In NF, neurofibromas are frequently multiple, with occasionally

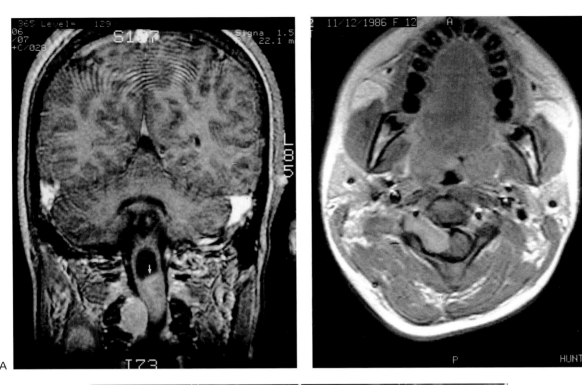

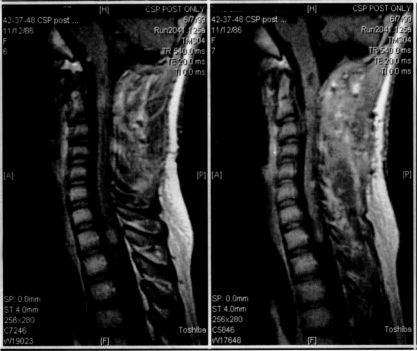

FIGURE 22. Multiple lesions in a patient with neurofibromatosis. Contrast-enhanced T1-weighted magnetic resonance image. Coronal **(A)** and sagittal **(B)** images showing an intramedullary contrast-enhancing tumor that has a rostrally located cyst *(arrow at tumor cyst interface)* and an extramedullary intradural and extradural neurofibroma at C2–3, which is compressing the spinal cord. As seen on the sagittal and axial images, the neurofibroma extended through an enlarged foramen to the cervical region. In addition to these spinal lesions, the patient also had multiple intracranial lesions associated with her neurofibromatosis. She presented with progressive weakness on the right side with long tract signs. At the time of surgery, both tumors were excised. The intramedullary tumor was a mixed astroependymoma. The neurofibroma was removed as far into the foramen as possible. **C:** Postoperative image showing complete removal of the intramedullary tumor, which has not recurred in spite of receiving no postoperative adjuvant therapy. The extension of the neurofibroma into the neck progressively enlarged. *(Figure continued.)*

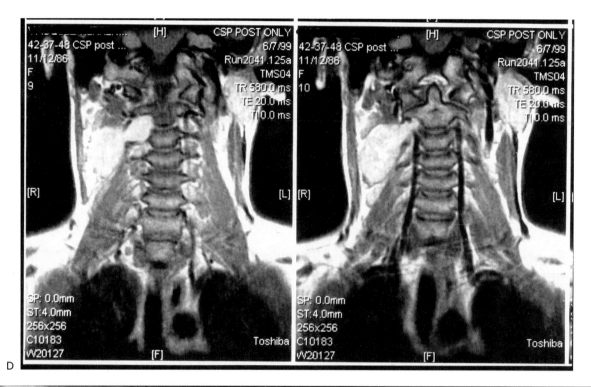

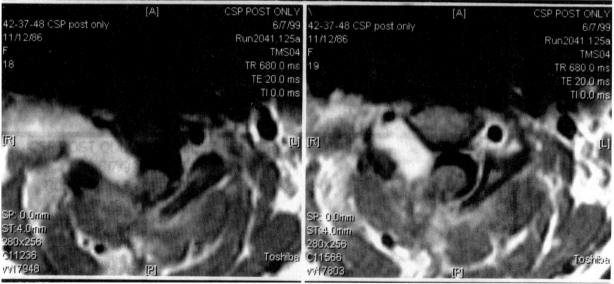

FIGURE 22. *Continued.* T1-weighted contrast-enhanced anteroposterior **(D)** and axial images **(E)** 5 months later showing regrowth of the tumor into the foramen, as well as the large neck mass. *(Figure continued.)*

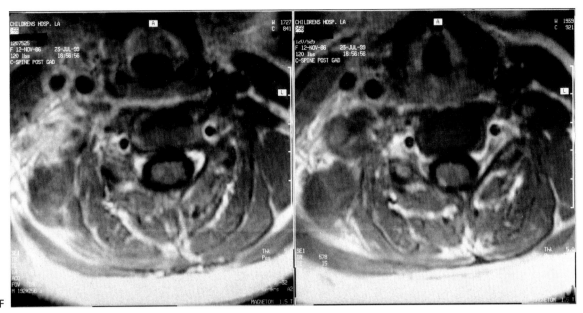

FIGURE 22. *Continued.* From a cervical approach, the remainder of the tumor was excised, as shown on the postoperative image **(F)**. The patient has received no adjuvant therapy. She is now developing brain stem compression from one of her bilateral acoustic tumors for which she will undergo surgery.

hundreds of tumors of varying size present throughout the spinal canal (Fig. 23). Only tumors that are symptomatic need to be excised. The other indication for excision is when there is rapid growth in a given tumor, because this could herald a malignant transformation that occurs in somewhat under 10% of patients with this disease entity. Every time a neurofibroma is excised,

there is loss of a nerve root. At one level, there will usually be only a mild deficit; however, with multiple tumors removed at adjacent levels, the deficit can become profound.

Another type of neurofibroma seen with NF is that of the plexiform neurofibroma (Fig. 24), which is usually seen in the cervical or thoracic region and can cause spinal cord compression either

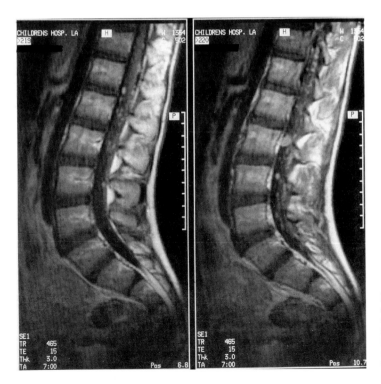

FIGURE 23. Neurofibromatosis. A sagittal T1-weighted contrast-enhanced magnetic resonance image (MRI) showing the presence of multiple neurofibromas in the regions of the cauda equina. This 8-year-old boy with neurofibromatosis previously had a neurofibroma removed from the thoracic region. Surveillance MRI studies have been used to monitor the other neurofibromas present. Only if the tumors show a significant increase in size would they be excised.

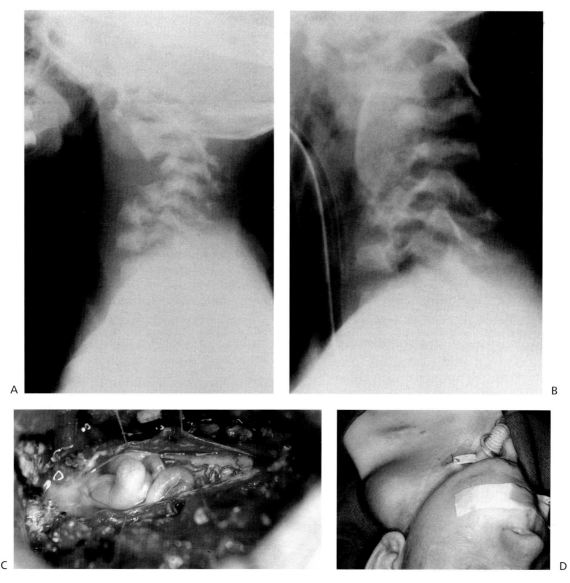

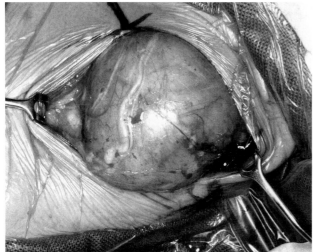

FIGURE 24. Plexiform neurofibroma degenerating into a sarcoma. This 3-year-old boy was rendered nearly quadriplegic by a fall from a swing. Multiple café au lait spots indicated that he had neurofibromatosis. **A:** Admitting lateral C-spine x-ray studies showing a marked gibbus deformity involving C2–3–4. **B:** Halo traction was applied, and the patient had an anterior approach with resection of the bodies of C2–3–4 and a strut graft inserted. This lateral spine x-ray study shows the postoperative result. **C:** The patient then underwent a posterior decompression and stabilization with the removal of the intradural portion of a plexiform neurofibroma. The patient's neurologic condition improved mildly postoperatively, and he was able to have functional use of one upper extremity. **D:** Ten years later, the patient developed rapid enlargement of a mass in the neck. His neurologic condition continued to be stable. **E:** Intraoperative photograph showing a portion of the tumor, which contained a malignant peripheral nerve sheath tumor arising from the plexiform neurofibroma. The sarcoma had diffusely infiltrated surrounding structures, so it was not possible to perform a gross total excision. The patient has received a course of focal radiation; however, he continues to deteriorate.

from tumor within the spinal canal or as a result of involvement of the vertebral columns, leading to a progressive deformity that narrows the spinal canal. The plexiform neurofibroma diffusely involves all of the surrounding structures, thus making it impossible to excise completely. Often, they will envelop structures in the neck and mediastinum and lead to progressive disability and ultimately death over a course of years to decades even without the malignant transformation seen in a small percentage of cases. Radiation and chemotherapy have been used to treat malignant nerve sheath tumors with only very limited success.

With NF, intramedullary spinal tumors have an increased frequency over that of the normal population, such as astrocytomas and ependymomas, as seen in Figure 22.

It is recommended that patients with NF have routine surveillance MRI at regular intervals.

Meningeal Tumors

Meningioma

Meningiomas are exceedingly rare tumors in the pediatric age group. Their presentation, location, and MRI characteristics are similar to those of neurofibromas. They can occur in isolation or be multiple, and if they are multiple, they are much more likely to associated with NF. Treatment is total excision with an excellent outcome. Although meningiomas in the pediatric age group tend to be more aggressive when compared with those in adults, malignant transformation occurs but rarely.

Arachnoid Cysts

Arachnoid cysts can be either intradural (Fig. 25) or extradural (Fig. 26) (10,36) in location but are not a combination of both. The intradural cyst results from an alteration of the arachnoid trabeculi that produces a loculation that traps CSF and results in slow enlargement over time to compress the adjacent neural structures. The extradural cyst arises from a hole in the dura mater that allows the arachnoid membrane to herniate through the dural defect, followed by slow enlargement that, with time, produces local symptoms. Many of these cysts appear to be congenital in nature but they may also be acquired as a result of arachnoid adhesions that develop following surgery. In our experience, there has been an association between intradural arachnoid cysts with previously operated open (myelomeningoceles) and closed NTDs (42).

The presentation varies widely and is dependent on location and the degree of compression of adjacent neural elements. The

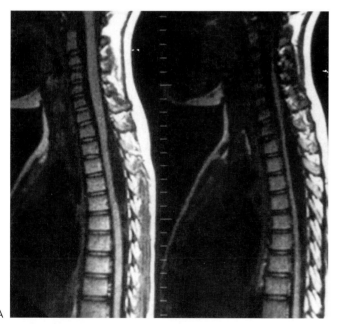

A

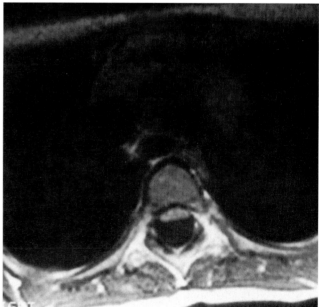

B

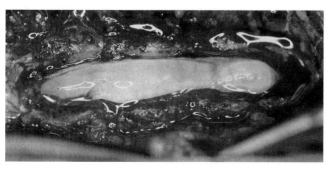

C

FIGURE 25. Intradural arachnoid cyst. Sagittal **(A)** and axial **(B)** T1-weighted magnetic resonance imaging demonstrating anterior displacement of the spinal cord by an intradural mass with the signal characteristics of cerebrospinal fluid. **C:** Intraoperative photograph of the intradural arachnoid cyst. This 8-year-old child presented with recurrent urinary tract infections and progressive constipation. The neurologic examination was normal. Her symptoms resolved postoperatively.

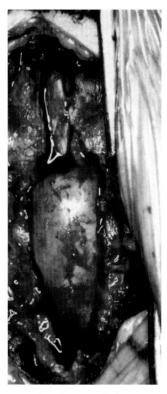

FIGURE 26. Intraoperative photograph demonstrating a large extradural arachnoid cyst. This 18-year-old female presented with S1 radiopathy that resolved postoperatively.

MRI appearance is that of a cyst containing CSF without enhancement of the wall.

Treatment of intradural arachnoid cysts is fenestration. It is important to make certain that there is good communication into the surrounding SAS, both above and below the arachnoid cyst. If the cyst covers multiple levels, placement of an endoscope in the canal can aid in the fenestration while limiting the number of levels that require a laminectomy or laminotomy or both. With extradural cysts, it is necessary to find the defect in the dura mater through which the arachnoid has herniated and eliminate the area of communication. The outcome is generally excellent. Recurrence can be seen in some cases, especially of repaired NTD (21,22). If there is a question, either cine-MRI or CT myelography would be helpful in establishing that the area in question is isolated from the surrounding SAS (12).

Vascular Lesions

Arteriovenous Malformations (AVMs)

AVMs can been seen anywhere along the length of the spinal cord. They may be extramedullary, intramedullary, or a combination of both, as well as being associated with dural fistulae. They also can be seen in conjunction with some neurocutaneous syndromes, as shown in Figure 27. Occasionally, they will pre-

sent with an acute onset secondary to hemorrhage and resulting local compression or from blood within the SAS. More commonly, however, there is an insidious progression of a neurologic deficit.

MRI shows the presence of signal flow voids that are typical for such a lesion. The AVM also enhances. However, once such a lesion is suspected, angiography is the imaging modality of choice. Better equipment and super selective catheterization has allowed not only better visualization of these lesions but also the ability to embolize the feeders to the lesion. If embolization is a consideration, then arrangements should be made for such at the time of the initial angiogram, thereby saving the patient an additional procedure. Following embolization, the remainder of the AVM is surgically removed. The outcome is variable, depending on the extent of spinal cord involvement.

Aneurysms

Most spinal cord aneurysms are associated with AVMs, although isolated aneurysms of the spinal cord do occur. Although these previously have been classified as true aneurysms, a more recent examination suggests that many of these lesions are more correctly classified as intrathecal perimedullary AV fistulas with giant venous dilatation (Fig. 28) (23).

Hemorrhage is a rare occurrence, and these lesions usually make their presence known by a compression of adjacent neural structures.

As with AVMs, angiography is undertaken with the expectation of endovascular treatment of the lesion at the same procedure. These lesions may have a single large feeder, which may be occluded, thereby permanently blocking the inflow and thus eliminating the need for surgical intervention. The prognosis in these cases has generally been quite good.

Hemangioblastomas

These tumors are frequently classified as being intramedullary. They actually form on the pial surface and can extend both into and out of the spinal cord (Fig. 29). Frequently, they are associated with a cystic cavity, which is intramedullary in location. They are uncommon tumors in the pediatric age group and can be seen anywhere along the spinal cord, be single or multiple, and in our experience more likely to be associated with the Von Hippel–Lindau complex.

On imaging, the solid part is well circumscribed and shows a decreased signal intensity on T1, whereas the intensity will be increased on T2, and they will uniformly enhance with contrast. If a cystic cavity is present, the solid component will be as a mural nodule. Angiography is not indicated.

The lesions can be completely excised because there is a plane of demarcation between the lesion and the adjacent spinal cord. The outlook is excellent. Often, in the presence of Von Hippel–Lindau disease, multiple lesions are present. As with neurofibromatosis, some lesions remain small and do not increase in size with time and should not be surgically addressed. Only those

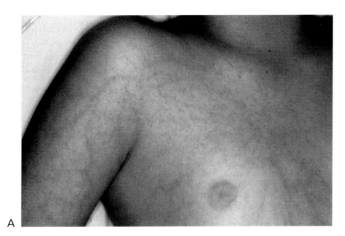

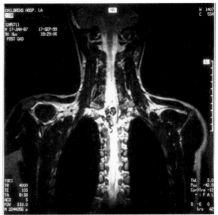

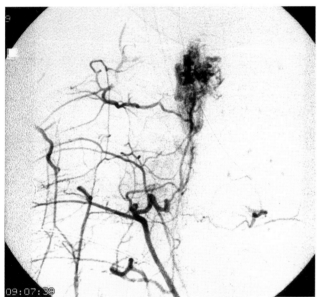

FIGURE 27. Spinal cord arteriovenous malformation (AVM). **A:** Photograph of a 13-year-old boy with Klippel-Trenaury-Webber syndrome. The right upper extremity was hypertrophic, and there was superficial dilatation of the blood vessels. The patient developed a progressive myelopathy. **B:** A T2-weighted magnetic resonance imaging study showed the presence of a large AVM at the cervicothoracic junction. Most of the lesion was intradural, but had some extramedullary components. **C:** An angiogram showed feeders from both vertebral arteries, the thyrocervical trunk, and the intercostal arteries. He underwent embolization with partial obliteration of the malformation. **D:** Intraoperative photograph showing a thickened arachnoid and dilated blood vessels. **E:** Operative photograph at the completion of removal of all of the malformation. Postoperative angiogram showed no evidence of a residual AVM. The patient's neurologic deficit was more pronounced following the operative procedure, but function has gradually returned and the patient has less neurologic deficit than preoperatively.

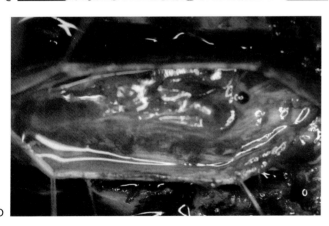

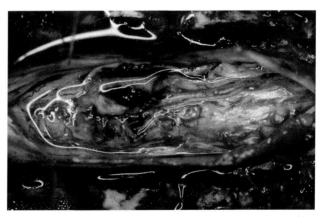

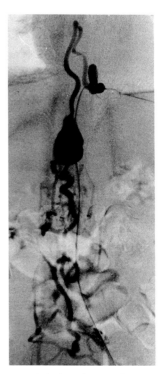

FIGURE 28. Aneurysm. Spinal angiogram showing the presence of an arterial feeder to a giant venus pseudo aneurysm. Using endovascular technique, the arterial feeder was occluded with a balloon, obliterating the flow to the aneurysm. This 3-year-old child presented with back pain and progressive myelopathy that nearly completely resolved over the course of many months.

hemangioblastomas that show progressive increase in either the solid or cystic portion of the tumor with successive imaging studies should be excised. Hemangioblastomas are much more commonly found in the cerebellum. However, if the patient presents with initial spinal cord symptoms, imaging of the head is indicated. In select cases, it is also appropriate to perform an MRI study on close family members.

Hemangioendotheliomas

Hemangioendotheliomas are rare vascular tumors that are histologically intermediate in appearance between a hemangioma and an angiosarcoma (2). These lesions can appear anywhere either inside or outside of the central nervous system (CNS), although CNS involvement is quite uncommon. The MRI signal characteristics are similar to that of a hemangioblastoma. Patients with these lesions may present with hydrocephalus because of elevated CSF protein content. Treatment is gross total excision, if possible. The use of interferon alpha may be of benefit in treating those lesions that are incompletely excised. The prognosis appears to be variable.

Metastatic

Neural

PNET is the most likely tumor to metastasize widely through the SAS. It is best detected with contrast enhancement MRI.

This is more reliable than obtaining CSF for cytologic evaluation. The presence of diffuse spread of PNET into the SAS at initial presentation carries a poor prognosis, as does its presence at the time of intracranial tumor recurrence. Often, the patient will develop hydrocephalus and require CSF diversion.

Although high-grade gliomas are much more likely to metastasize than those that are low grade, occasionally one can see extensive spread of tumor in the SAS of low-grade astrocytomas. Thus, the biologic behavior does not always reflect the histologic characteristics of the tumor. These patients have a very poor prognosis and often develop hydrocephalus that requires CSF diversion.

Melanomatosis

The meninges have cells that contain melanin. On rare occasions, there will be a proliferation of these cells to produce a diffuse involvement of the SAS (Fig. 30). Initially, it can be difficult to make the diagnosis, and understandably, other etiologies are suspected before the correct diagnosis is obtained. On some occasions, the CSF can even be discolored by the presence of melanin. Usually, a biopsy is needed to make the diagnosis. Inspection of the meninges finds that they are thickened and dark or black in color. The histopathology shows the presence of considerable melanin, although the cells themselves may not have all of the characteristics of melanoma. There is an increased incidence of this particular problem that is associated with giant hairy nevus syndrome (Fig. 31).

Extraneural

Lymphoma And Leukemia

In addition to presenting as extradural lesions, lymphomas and leukemias can also be intradural. The CSF cytology is quite useful and very frequently diagnostic. It is rare that either lymphomas or leukemias in the SAS cause mass effect producing spinal cord compression. It is only occasionally that CSF resistance is elevated by the disease process to the extent that CSF diversion is required. Chemotherapy and radiation modalities are achieving ever-greater success in treating this constellation of disease.

Other

Infection with the human immunodeficiency virus (HIV) predisposes patients to many malignancies, particularly Kaposi's sarcoma and CNS lymphoma. In children, HIV infection has been associated with leiomyosarcomas and leiomyomas (3). With an ever-growing number of pediatric patients with HIV, these entities will likely to be encountered with increasing frequency. If such a tumor is encountered and the patient is not known to have HIV, such testing should be undertaken.

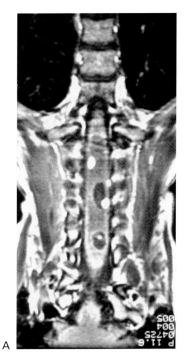

FIGURE 29. Hemangioblastoma. **A:** T1-weighted magnetic resonance imaging (MRI) study with an anteroposterior view of the cervical and upper thoracic spine, showing four uniformly contrast-enhancing intramedullary lesions, two of which are associated with cystic formation. **B:** Transverse MRI section showing one of the cystic lesions with a uniformly enhancing neural nodule located on the anterior aspect of the cervical spinal cord. This 15-year-old patient with Von Hippel–Landau disease presented with a progressive neurologic deficit involving the upper and lower extremities; however, she had no bladder or bowel involvement. All of the lesions were subsequently resected. The patient has generated no new lesions and is stable 6 years after the initial operative procedure.

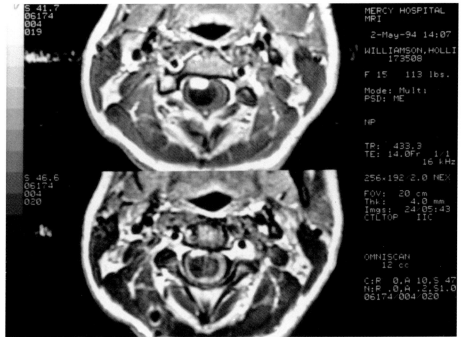

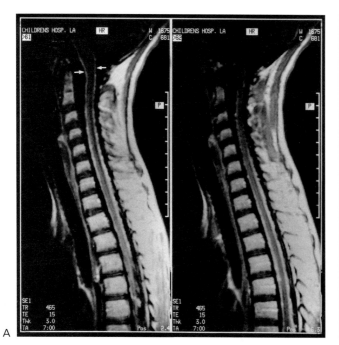
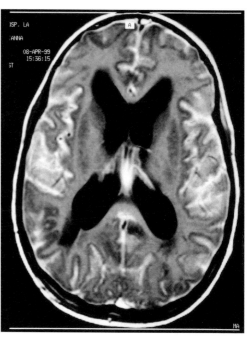

FIGURE 30. Melanomatosis. Contrast-enhanced T1-weighted sagittal spine **(A)** and axial head **(B)** magnetic resonance imaging studies showing diffuse enhancement of the leptomeningies *(arrows)*. The patient also developed hydrocephalus secondary to impairment of cerebrospinal fluid (CSF) absorption. This 10-year-old female had a 6-week history of progressive headaches, nausea, vomiting, and intermittent diplopia. Multiple CSF samples were abnormal but inconclusive. A single level laminectomy was performed for biopsy purposes. The leptomeninges, as anticipated, were quite thickened; however, they were also black and consistent with melanomatosis, which was subsequently confirmed histopathologically. Because of progressive hydrocephalus she required a CSF diverting shunt. Despite a course of intensive chemotherapy, the patient died 2 months later.

EXTRAMEDULLARY TUMORS—EXTRADURAL

The vast majority of extradural tumors of childhood are of the metastatic variety. They can however, be divided into three groups: those derived from neural crest tissue, such as neuroblastomas and ganglioneuromas; those arising from mesenchymal soft tissue, such as sarcomas, germ cell tumors, lymphomas, leukemias, and Wilms tumor; or those derived from mesenchymal bony origins. Of this group, sarcoma and neuroblastoma (Fig. 32) are the most frequent owing to their overall higher incidence in the pediatric population.

Epidural spinal cord compression by malignant tumors occurs infrequently in children. Back pain is the most common symptom, and weakness and bladder dysfunction the most common signs. In our series of children with rapid progressive myelopathy, in which there was extensive encroachment of tumor into the spinal canal (50% or more), surgical decompression obtained better neurologic outcome than radiation or chemotherapy alone (43). Our patients had no morbidity or mortality from surgical decompression, and the pain of laminectomy was significantly less than that caused by the spinal cord compression. In adults, common epidural tumors causing spinal cord compression are lung, breast, and prostate carcinomas and result from tumor extension from a metastatic lesion in the vertebral bodies. The mass compressing the spinal cord is frequently anteriorly located and often associated with spinal instability. Most epidural compression in children with epidural malignant tumors occurs by direct extension of the tumor through the vertebral foramen without significant bony involvement. The tumor mass is primarily lateral in location and is readily accessibly via a posterior approach. Spine stability is usually not a factor. As a group, the children rarely had diffuse metastatic disease, and their overall health was much better than that of a typical group of adults with a similar profile. The consideration for operative intervention is based on the general condition of the child; the degree of spinal canal compromise; the location of the tumor relative to the spinal cord; the tumor type, if known; and the sensitivity of the tumor to radiation or chemotherapy.

Neural Crest

Neuroblastomas originate either from the adrenal medulla or the sympathetic chain; thus, the majority arise in the retroperitoneal region. Those from adrenal sources are most likely to be found in younger children. Approximately two thirds of these cases are identified in children younger than 4 years of age. Interestingly, there is evidence that in some young infants, the tumor may spontaneously regress. The incidence is equal in males and females. Histologic examination of a neuroblastoma specimen reveals sheets of blue cells similar to those of a PNET but with a greater component of fibroblastic stroma. High levels of homovanillic acid and vanillymandelic acid may be identified in the

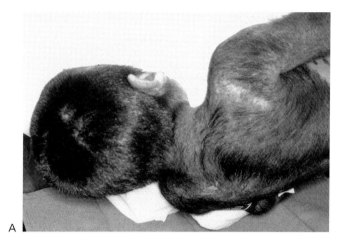

A

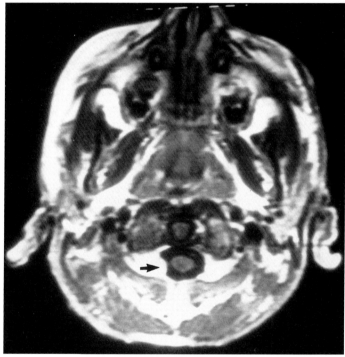

B

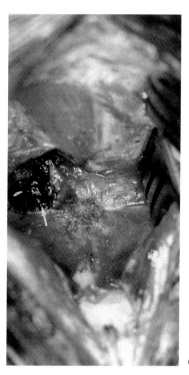

C

FIGURE 31. Melanomatosis. **A:** This 5-year-old had giant hairy nevus syndrome. The patient presented with an initial onset of seizures. There were no other neurologic symptoms and no focal neurologic deficit. **B:** In the workup, there was noted to be an enhancing mass in the high cervical region *(arrow)*. **C:** Intraoperative photograph showing melanoma tissue present *(arrow)*. The patient was treated with chemotherapy but subsequently died of his disease.

serum and 24-hour urine samples in more than 75% of patients (6). Cystathionine has been reported to be found in the urine in these patients in direct relation to the degree of malignancy. In the absence of marked spinal cord compression, these tumors are treated with chemotherapy or radiation therapy.

Ganglioneuromas are less common than neuroblastomas but are believed to represent the benign end of this spectrum of tumors that also includes ganglioneuroblastomas as an intermediary between the two. Gangliogliomas are also located in the retroperitoneum or retropleural spaces and are often asymptomatic until they become quite large. In contrast to neuroblastomas, older children and young adults in the second decade of life and females have a greater incidence. In addition, owing to the degree of differentiation, the survival rate is higher than that of patients with neuroblastomas (17). Involvement of the spinal canal is usually by direct extension. Treatment of gangliogliomas involves surgical resection only if there is spinal cord compression.

Mesenchymal—Soft Tissue

Approximately one quarter of pediatric extradural spinal tumors are metastatic either through distant or contiguous spread (1). Infrequently encountered metastatic tumors include genitourinary tumors such as malignant teratomas, embryonal carcinomas, renal cell carcinoma, and Wilms tumor. The thoracic spine is the most common site of spread for these because of its length.

Although bony changes can be noted on plain films or CT, MRI is the modality of choice for the evaluation of metastatic disease.

Leukemias and lymphomas are also common sources of meta-

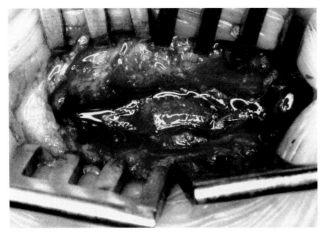

FIGURE 32. Operative photograph of an epidural neuroblastoma. This infant presented with irritability, and refused to stand. An MRI study showed the presence of a perivertebral mass with extension of tumor through the adjacent foramen to occupy more of 50% of the spinal canal. The patient underwent an emergency decompressive laminectomy with improved neurologic function.

static disease to the pediatric spine. Of the leukemias, acute myelogenous leukemnia is the one most frequently associated with spinal metastatic disease and may be present in a third of newly diagnosed cases (30). The acute lymphocytic variety will metastasize to the spine often unless treated appropriately, after which the incidence of spinal involvement falls to under 10%. Spinal metastasis through vascular pathways occurs along dural or arachnoid planes. Lymphomas may histologically fall within the non-Hodgkin's or Hodgkin's varieties and either as a primary or secondary lesion. Non-Hodgkin's lymphomas are the more common of the two to metastasize to the spinal axis and more commonly seen as a primary lesion. Epidural involvement is the rule due to contiguous spread from bony or soft tissue sites.

Most leukemias and lymphomas do not require surgical intervention but respond well to adjuvant therapy, whereas sarcomas are much more likely to require a decompressive laminectomy. If operative intervention is undertaken, no attempt is made to remove as much tumor as possible but just to decompress the spinal cord (Fig. 32), as well as obtaining adequate tissue for the various diagnostic studies.

The other indication for surgery is if the histology of the tumor is unknown and the primary site is not discernible or is less accessible.

Mesenchymal—Bone

Primary bone tumors of the spinal column include osteomas, osteoblastomas, osteochondromas, osteosarcomas, giant cell tumors, eosinophilic granulomas, hemangiomas, and aneurysmal bone cysts. Surgical treatment requires complete *en bloc* resection, often followed by some form of fusion to address the problem of instability. They are discussed in another chapter.

SURGICAL ADJUNCTS AND CONSIDERATIONS

Ultrasonic Aspiration

Ultrasonic aspiration has proved to be particularly useful for intramedullary tumors. At higher settings, it can rapidly debulk large tumors. When approaching the interface between the tumor and spinal cord, the power of the ultrasonic aspirator can be diminished in order to reduce the chance of injuring normal adjacent neural structures. Some units also have a pulse mode, which provides for very gentle aspiration at the interface between tumor and spinal cord. However, it is the neurosurgeon and not the ultrasonic aspirator that distinguishes normal from abnormal tissue and both types of tissue can be readily removed with this device.

The ultrasonic aspirator is a much less useful for non intramedullary tumors with the exception of a dumb-bell neurofibroma in which its use to resect tumor extending into the foramen can be quite helpful.

Laser

Soon after the introduction of laser technology to the operating room, there ensued a tremendous popularity in its use. This wave of enthusiasm has markedly subsided, and now lasers are only infrequently used for removal of spinal cord tumors. The laser's role is limited almost exclusively to that of intramedullary tumors.

Some neurosurgeons prefer making a myelotomy in the spinal cord with the laser because it will reduce or eliminate the bleeding at the myelotomy site, which can interfere with visualization of the underlying tumor. Only a small quantity of tumor tissue can be removed in a given interval of time. Thus, it is much more efficient to use the ultrasonic aspirator to debulk the vast majority of tumor tissue. Some neurosurgeons advocate use of the laser to remove the last residual tumor at its margin with the spinal cord. We have found that the use of bipolar coagulation is just as effective and see little advantage to use of the laser.

Evoked Potentials

In some centers, somatosensory evoked potentials (SSEPs) are customarily used to monitor spinal cord function during tumor removal. In those patients in whom the dorsal columns are preoperatively affected by the tumor, the SSEPs are often abnormal at the beginning of the procedure and thus of less value. Also, during an operative procedure, the SSEPs may change in response to a myelotomy, manipulation with tumor removal, or irrigation with lower than body temperature solutions. On some occasions, the decreased amplitude of the SSEPs during surgical manipulation does not reflect any permanent postoperative changes in the patient's neurologic function. On the other hand, the loss of signal or significant diminution of amplitude can indicate a permanent neurologic deficit. We believe that surgical judgement during intramedullary tumor resection is a better guideline than the responses seen on SSEPs. The use of SSEPs during intramedullary tumor resection is an option and is, by no means, a standard of care.

More recently, techniques have been developed to monitor motor evoked potentials (MEPs). We have no experience in their use. Reports state that they can be greatly influenced by the degree and type of anesthesia, surgical manipulation, and interpretation by the electrophysiologist. MEPs will require further evaluation to determine their usefulness.

Like with SSEPs, the use of MEPs can detect damage to the spinal cord; however, it is not able to distinguish that which is reversible or irreversible, and at this juncture, there is no way for any monitoring technique to alert the neurosurgeon in advance so as to avoid causing a permanent neurologic deficit.

Spinal Deformity

In a number of children, it is the presence of a progressive kyphoscoliosis that heralds the presence of tumor, particularly one that is intramedullary. The efficacy of a laminotomy over that of a laminectomy to prevent the progression of a kyphosis or kyphoscoliosis following tumor resection has been debated (25). As a general rule, the higher on the spinal axis, the more likely that there will be a progressive deformation (20). Laminectomies in the lumbosacral region are rarely associated with any deformity, whereas those in the cervical region are very frequently associated with a progressive kyphosis or swan neck appearance. As a general rule, bony removal is limited to as few segments as necessary, and the width of the bony removal is minimized only to the extent that is necessary to gain adequate exposure for tumor removal. The facets are kept intact. A laminectomy is less time consuming than a laminotomy, which can add additional operative time to what already can be a lengthy procedure. When performing a laminotomy, it is important not to generate too much heat while cutting the bone, because this can cause an injury to the adjacent nerve roots, resulting in a postoperative dysesthesia that can be profound. Also, care must be taken when replacing the posterior elements so as not to compromise the size of the spinal canal and thereby produce a postoperative stenosis. In addition to the loss of posterior elements, a deformity may result because of weakening or imbalance of the paraspinous muscles by the involvement of the nerves that innervate this musculature (31). Radiation to the spine can be a factor in causing a deformity as well. In spite of undergoing a laminaplasty, some children still develop a progressive deformity to the spine. However, the incidence may be less than when compared with a laminectomy. A longer term for follow-up of a larger number of patients is needed to clarify this issue further. As a generalization, however, there appears to be little need to do a laminotomy in the lower end of the vertebral column, whereas it is probably a worthy consideration when operating in the upper thoracic and cervical region.

General Considerations

For obvious reasons, most of the operative procedures are performed with the patient in a prone position. If the cervical or upper thoracic regions are the sites of operation, the patient's head is placed in a horseshoe. Care must be taken to pad the rest well and position it correctly so as not to cause any injuries

to the face or globes. The authors do not advocate the use of the sitting position under any circumstance, because it offers little advantage and is associated with the risk of air embolism and hypotension. The lateral decubitus position is an option in certain situations; however, its main disadvantage is that the anatomic structures are not midline centered.

After initial paralyzation for intubation, the patients are kept in a nonparalyzed state until beginning the closure. This allows for intraoperative monitoring with a nerve stimulator, if needed.

Before coming to the operating room or at the beginning of the procedure, the patients are given a high dose of corticosteroids that are maintained in the initial post-operative period. Also, for whatever neuroprotective effect it may have, phenobarbital is used. With the exception of emergency situations such as from epidural spinal cord compression with rapid loss of neurologic function, dehydrating agents, such as mannitol, do not appear to play any significant role. Antibiotics are routinely administered for a day or two.

We do not advocate the use of any presently available synthetic dural substitutes. If it is necessary to leave the dura mater open, we cover it with a sheet of gelatin. Even under these circumstances, postoperative CSF leaks have rarely been a problem. In those cases in which CSF accumulation at the wound site is a factor, it may signal impaired absorption of CSF from the CNS and may indicate the need for a CSF diverting shunt. Closure techniques vary from center to center. We have rarely found it necessary to use drains or rotational flaps. If postoperative chemotherapy or radiation therapy needs to be given, it is preferable to wait approximately a week for sufficient wound healing before beginning adjuvant therapy if the patient's condition can tolerate this delay.

REFERENCES

1. Brotchi J, Dewitte O, Levivier M, et al. (1991): A survery of 65 tumors within the spinal cord: surgical results and the importance of preoperative magnetic resonance imaging. *Neurosurgery* 29:651–657.
2. Chen TC, Gonzalez-Gomez I, Gilles FH, McComb JG (1997): Pediatric intracranial hemangioendotheliomas. *Neurosurgery* 40:410–414.
3. Choi S, Levy ML, Krieger MD, McComb JG (1997): Spinal extradural leiomyoma in a pediatric patient with acquired immunodeficiency syndrome: case report. *Neurosurgery* 40:1080–1082.
4. Citron N, Edgar MA, Sheehy J, et al. (1984): Intramedullary spinal cord tumours presenting as scoliosis. *J Bone Joint Surg Br* 66:513–517.
5. Constantini S, Houten J, Miller DC, et al. (1996): Intramedullary spinal cord tumors in children under the age of 3 years. *Neurosurgery* 85:1036–1043.
6. Cooper PR (1989): Outcome after operative treatment of intramedullary spinal cord tumors in adults: intermediate and long-term results in 51 patients. *Neurosurgery* 25:855–859.
7. Cooper PR, Epstein F (1985): Radical resection of intramedullary spinal cord tumors in adults. Recent experience in 29 patients. *Neurosurgery* 63:492–499.
8. Cristante L, Herrmann HD (1994): Surgical management of intramedullary spinal cord tumors: functional outcome and sources of morbidity. *Neurosurgery* 35:69–76.
9. Epstein F, Epstein N (1982): Surgical treatment of spinal cord astrocytomas of childhood. A series of 19 patients. *J Neurosurg* 57:685–689.
10. Ersahin Y, Yildizhan A, Seber N (1993): Spinal extradural arachnoid cyst. *Childs Nerv Syst* 9:250–252.
11. Fernandez M, Carrol CL, Baker CJ (2000): Discitis and vertebral osteomyelitis children: an 18-year review. *Pediatrics* 105:1299–1304.

12. Fobe JL, Nishikuni K, Gianni MA (1998): Evolving magnetic resonance spinal cord trauma in child: from hemorrhage to intradural arachnoid cyst. *Spinal Cord* 36:864–866.

13. Garcia DM (1985): Primary spinal cord tumors treated with surgery and postoperative irradiation. *Radiol Oncol Biol Phys* 11:1933–1939.

14. Goh KY, Velasquez L, Epstein FJ (1997): Pediatric intramedullary spinal cord tumors: is surgery alone enough? *Pediatr Neurosurg* 27: 34–39

15. Hader WJ, Steinbok P, Poskitt K, et al. (1999): Intramedullary spinal teratoma and diastematomyelia. Case report and review of the literature. *Pediatr Neurosurg* 30:140–145.

16. Hardison HH, Packer RJ, Rorke LB, et al. (1987): Outcome of children with primary intramedullary spinal cord tumors. *Childs Nerv Syst* 3: 89–92.

17. Hoover M, Bowman LC, Crawford SE, et al. (1999): Long-term outcome of patients with intraspinal neuroblastoma. *Med Pediatr Oncol* 32:353–359.

18. Innocenzi G, Raco A, Cantore G, et al. (1996): Intramedullary astrocytomas and ependymomas in the pediatric age group: a retrospective study. *Childs Nerv Syst* 12:776–780.

19. Innocenzi G, Salvati M, Cervoni L, et al. (1997): Prognostic factors in intramedullary astrocytomas. *Clin Neur Neurosurg* 99:1–5.

20. Inoue A, Ikata T, Katoh S (1996): Spinal deformity following surgery for spinal cord tumors and tumorous lesions: analysis based on an assessment of the spinal functional curve. *Spinal Cord* 34:536–542.

21. Jean WC, Keene CD, Haines SJ (1998): Cervical arachnoid cysts after craniocervical decompression for Chiari II malformations: report of three cases. *Neurosurgery* 43:941–944.

22. Kazan S, Ozdemir O, Akyuz M, et al. (1999): Spinal intradural arachnoid cysts located anterior to the cervical spinal cord. Report of two cases and review of the literature. *J Neurosurg* 91:211–215.

23. Khoo TL, Teitelbaum GP, Stanley P, et al. Familial occurrence of an arteriovenous fistula with a giant perimedullary pseudoaneurysm of the thoracic spinal cord in 2 young siblings. *Pediatr Neurosurg* 28:286–292.

24. Krieger DM, McComb JG, Levy ML (1999): Toward a simpler surgical management of Chiari I malformation in a pediatric population. *Pediatr Neurosurg* 30:113–121.

25. Lonstein JE (1977): Postlaminectomy kyphosis. *Clin Orthop Rel Res* 128:93–100.

26. Lunardi P, Licastro G, Missori P, et al. (1993): Management of intramedullary tumors in children. *Acta Neurochir (Weir)* 120:59–65.

27. Maiocco B, Deeney VF, Coulon R, et al. (1997): Adolescent idiopathic scoliosis and the presence of spinal cord abnormalities. Preoperative magnetic resonance imaging analysis. *Spine* 22:2537–2541.

28. McComb JG (1995): Congenital dermal sinus. In Pang D, ed. *Disorders of the Pediatric Spine* New York: Raven Press, pp. 349–360.

29. McCormick PC, Torres R, Post KD, et al. (1990): Intramedullary ependymoma of the spinal cord. *Neurosurgery* 72:523–532.

30. McElwain TJ, Clink HM, Jameson B, et al. (1979): Central nervous system involvement in acute myelogenous leukemia. In: Whitehouse JMA, Kay HE, eds. *Central nervous system complications of malignant disease.* London: Macmillan, pp. 91–96.

31. Mehlman CT, Crawford AH, McMath JA (1999): Pediatric vertebral and spinal cord tumors: a retrospective study of musculoskeletal aspects of presentation, treatment, and complications. *Orthopedics* 22:49–55.

32. Merchant TE, Nguyen D, Thompson SJ, et al. (1999): High grade pediatric spinal cord tumors. *Pediatr Neurosurg* 30:1–5.

33. Minehan KJ, Shaw EG, Scheithauer BW, et al. (1995): Spinal cord astrocytoma: pathological and treatment considerations. *Neurosurgery* 83:590–595.

34. Mittler MA, McComb JG (1999): Adjacent thoracic neuroenteric and arachnoid cysts. *Pediatr Neurosurg* 30:164–165.

35. Mittler MA, McComb JG (1999): Idiopathic thoracolumbar syrinx with cutaneous marker. *Pediatr Neurosurg* 30:100–101.

36. Myles LM, Gupta N, Armstrong D, et al. (1999): Multiple extradural arachnoid cysts as a cause of spinal cord compression in a child. Case report. *Neurosurgery* 91:116–120.

37. Nadkarni TD, Rekate HL (1999): Pediatric intramedullary spinal cord tumors. Critical review of the literature. *Childs Nerv Syst* 15:17–28.

38. OSullivan C, Jenkin RD, Doherty MA, et al. (1994): Spinal cord tumors in children: long-term results of combined surgical and radiation treatment. *Neurosurgery* 81:507–512.

39. Parker AP, Robinson RO, Bullock P (1996): Difficulties in diagnosing intrinsic spinal cord tumours. *Arch Dis Child* 75:204–207.

40. Pascual-Castroviejo I (1990): Epidemiology of spinal cord tumors in children. In Pascual-Castroviejo I, ed. *Spinal tumors in children and adolescents.* New York: Raven Press, pp. 1–10.

41. Przybylski GJ, Albright AL, Martinez AJ (1997): Spinal cord astrocytomas: long-term results comparing treatments in children. *Childs Nerv Syst* 13:375–382.

42. Rabb CH, McComb JG, Raffel C, et al. (1992): Spinal arachnoid cysts in the pediatric age group: an association with neural tube defects. *Neurosurgery* 77:369–372.

43. Raffel C, Neave VCD, Lavane S, McComb JG (1991): Treatment of spinal cord compression by epidural malignancy in childhood. *Neurosurgery* 28:349–352.

44. Samuelsson L, Lindell D (1995): Scoliosis as the first sign of a cystic spinal cord lesion. *Eur Spine J* 4:284–290.

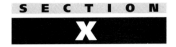

METABOLIC DISEASE

IDIOPATHIC JUVENILE OSTEOPOROSIS

WALTER B. GREENE

DEFINITION

Idiopathic juvenile osteoporosis (IJO) is a rare and poorly understood pediatric disease that was first described by Schippers (54) in 1939. The 1965 report of six cases by Dent and Friedman (12) firmly established the validity of the disorder. Idiopathic juvenile osteoporosis, the term used by Dent and Friedman, is the preferred nomenclature, even though some authors have used terms such as idiopathic osteoporosis, juvenile osteoporosis, and even Dent-Friedman syndrome.

Generalized osteoporosis is the hallmark of IJO. However, the diagnosis can be made only after other causes of osteoporosis in children have been excluded (Table 1). Trabecular bone is more readily and dramatically affected by osteoporosis. Therefore, the spine and the metaphysis of long bones are prime targets in these patients.

Fewer than 100 cases of IJO have been reported in the English literature. For that and other reasons, IJO can be challenging to review. Some patients have been recycled through more than one report (5,25,29,38,45,52,55,56,60). Some cases were probably misdiagnosed. For example, one case report involved an 8-year-old girl who developed pain and osteoporosis limited to her feet after she was hit by a stone thrown by another girl (33). Her exam was characterized by painful passive and active movements of the foot. With encouragement to walk, this girl's problem completely resolved in 9 months. Reflex sympathetic dystrophy is a more plausible diagnosis for this case (13). Another probable misdiagnosis is found in the case of a 11-year-old boy, described by Jowsey and Johnson (29), who had a 9-year history of fractures and progressive osteoporosis. This patient also had a history of blindness and bilateral enucleation at age 6 weeks. Osteoporosis pseudoglioma syndrome is a more likely diagnosis for this patient (42,57).

Clinical symptoms in patients with IJO resolve over a period of several years. Therefore, even the landmark article by Dent and Friedman (12) and a recent review of 21 patients by Smith (56) include patients who were probably misdiagnosed. These atypical patients had multiple fractures and progressive osteoporosis that continued into adult life. They probably have a form of osteogenesis imperfecta.

EPIDEMIOLOGIC FACTORS

Table 2 summarizes the presentation and treatment of patients with IJO reported in the English literature (1,3,10,12,14,18, 21,23,24,27,29,32,33,38,39,52,55,56,59,61). Excluded from Table 2 are patients whose diagnoses were questionable, series that did not provide adequate demographic information (31), and multiple reports about the same patient.

Age at presentation is typically prepubertal (1,3,43,56). The oldest patient included in Table 2 (Case 23) was noted to have delayed bone age, with onset of secondary sexual characteristics at age 17 years (28). Some authors (59) think that very young patients should not be diagnosed as having IJO; however, if other causes of generalized osteoporosis have been excluded and if the disorder resolves, then this author thinks that young children should be included. Patients younger than 5 years at diagnosis may have less pain and quicker remission of their symptoms; however, this is not always true.

Although IJO affects both sexes, the cases tabulated in Table 2 show a slight male predominance, with the male-to-female ratio being 1.5 : 1. The published cases of IJO mostly come from northern European centers, and no cases have been reported from institutions located in the southern part of the United States, South America, or Africa. Furthermore, no African American, native American, or African child has been noted with this disorder.

PATHOANATOMY

Osteoporosis can result from increased bone resorption, decreased bone formation, or a combination of these factors.

Iliac crest biopsies from patients with IJO typically show thin, mature trabeculae with normal osteoid seams and normal marrow elements. Microradiographic evaluations of iliac crest biopsies were interpreted as showing an increase in osteoclastic resorption in two reports from the same institution (27,29); however, two other studies observed no evidence of excessive resorption on quantitative histomorphometry (17,56).

W. B. Greene: Department of Orthopedic Surgery, University of Missouri–Columbia, Columbia, Missouri 65212.

TABLE 1. DISEASES CAUSING OSTEOPOROSIS IN CHILDREN

Blood disorders
  Leukemia
  Lymphoma
  Thalassemia
Chromosome disorders
  Down syndrome
  Turner syndrome
Endocrine disorders
  Cushing syndrome
  Juvenile diabetes
  Growth hormone deficiency
  Hypogonadism
  Hyperparathyroidism
Genetic defects of bone formation/bone resorption
  Hypophosphatasia
  Osteogenesis imperfecta
  Osteolytic disease
    Acroosteolysis
    Cranioskeletal dysplasia with acroosteolysis
    Multicentric osteolysis
    Winchester syndrome (skin lesions, corneal opacities, osteoporosis, and osteolysis)
  Osteoporosis pseudoglioma syndrome
Idiopathic disorders
  Juvenile idiopathic osteoporosis
  Regional transient osteoporosis
  Reflex sympathetic dystrophy

Immune disorders
  Hyperimmunoglobulinemia E syndrome
  Suppressor T-cell hyperactivity
Immobilization
  Cast therapy
  Paralysis secondary to myelomeningocele, spinal cord injury, severe cerebral palsy, etc.
  Painful skeletal disorders ranging from tarsal coalition to juvenile rheumatoid arthritis
Metabolic disorders
  Homocystinuria
  Lysinuric protein intolerance
  Renal osteodystrophy
  Rickets
Medications
  Steroids
  Retinoids
  Antineoplastic agents
Nutritional disorders
  Anorexia nervosa
  Malabsorption
  Cystic fibrosis
  Protein deficiency
  Scurvy
Radiation therapy
  Cranial irradiation for leukemia, etc.

TABLE 2. REPORTS OF JUVENILE OSTEOPOROSIS IN ENGLISH LANGUAGE DOCUMENTS

Case	Ref.	Year	Location	Age at presentation	Sex	Chief complaint	Long-bone fracture	Vertebral collapse fracture	Therapy
1	3	1960	Sweden	12	M	Pain feet	NR	+	Calcium, vitamins, anabolic steroids
2			Sweden	12	M	Back pain	NR	+	Corset
3	12	1965	Great Britain	8	F	Pain hips, back	Multiple	+	Vitamin D, stilbestrol
4			Great Britain	9	F	Pain legs	Multiple	+	Vitamin D, stilbestrol
5			Great Britain	9	M	Pain back	−	+	None
6			Great Britain	11	M	Pain arms, back, legs	−	+	Calcium, vitamin D
7			Great Britain	9	F	Pain feet, back	Multiple	+	None
8	10	1967	Minn., USA	11	F	Stiffness, back pain	NR	+	Hyperextension brace
9	21	1969	Calif., USA	13	F	Pain ankles	−	+	Calcium, pharmacologic doses of vitamin D
10	33	1971	Greece	11	M	Low back pain	−	+	Calcium, vitamin D
11	29	1972	Minn., USA	13	M	Back pain	Two	+	Not stated
12	32	1977	Austria	12	F	Low back pain	−	+, but limited	Corset
13	59	1979	India	12	M	Low back pain	Multiple	+	Calcium
14			India	10	F	Pain feet	Multiple	+	Calcium, 5,000 IU vitamin D/d
15			India	13	M	Pain legs, back	−	+	Calcium, 10,000 IU vitamin D/d
16			India	12	M	Pain feet	−	+	None
17	55	1980	Great Britain	4	F	Intermittent back pain	−	+	Calcium

(continued)

TABLE 2. *Continued.*

Case	Ref.	Year	Location	Age at presentation	Sex	Chief complaint	Long-bone fracture	Vertebral collapse fracture	Therapy
18			Great Britain	7	M	Foot pain, limp	Multiple	+	None
19			Great Britain	7	M	Round back	−	+	Laminectomy, physiotherapy
20			Great Britain	7	M	Back pain	−	+	None
21			Great Britain	9	F	Back pain	−	+	None
22	28	1981	Mich., USA	12	M	Back pain	−	+	Milwaukee brace
23		1981	Mich., USA	17	M	Back pain	−	+	Milwaukee brace
24	1	1982	Conn., USA	6	M	Scoliosis	−	+	Milwaukee brace, total-contact orthosis
25	38	1982	Ohio, USA	11	F	Extremity fractures	Multiple	+	Calcitriol 0.5 µg bid
26	18	1984	Switzerland	3	F	Limited walking	NR	+	None
27	23	1985	Netherlands	12	M	Foot, knee, back pain	Multiple	+	Bisphosphonate
28	27	1988	Ky., USA	8	M	Limp	Multiple	+	Calcitonin, calcitriol
29	52	1991	Italy	12	M	Diffuse back pain	Multiple	+	None
30			Italy	2	M	Knee, foot pain	−	+	0.25 µg calcitriol qd
31			Italy	12	F	Back, leg pain	Multiple	+	0.25 µg calcitriol bid
32			Italy	9	M	Back, leg pain	Multiple	+	0.25 µg calcitriol bid
33	39	1993	Norway	7	M	Back pain	−	+	None
34	14	1995	Ky., USA	13	M	Back pain	−	+	Pulsed oral phosphate, calcitonin, clamshell brace
35	56	1995	Great Britain	13	M	Back pain	−	concave vertebra	N.S.
36			Great Britain	7	F	Fractures	Multiple	+	N.S.
37			Great Britain	11	F	Back pain	Multiple	+	N.S.
38			Great Britain	8	F	Difficulty walking	Metatarsal	+	N.S.
39			Great Britain	8	M	Fractures	Multiple	+	N.S.
40			Great Britain	5	M	Fractures	Fingers and toes	+	N.S.
41			Great Britain	11	M	Difficulty walking	Multiple	Biconcave vertebrae	N.S.
42			Great Britain	9 mo	M	Fractures	Multiple	+	N.S.
43			Great Britain	5	F	Back Pain	−	+	Estrogen, anabolic steroids, clodronate
44			Great Britain	9	F	Foot pain	+	Biconcave vertebrae	Calcitonin
45			Great Britain	11	M	Back pain	−	Biconcave vertebrae	N.S.
46			Great Britain	1.5	M	Fractures	Multiple	+	N.S.
47	24	1995	Taiwan	9	M	Fracture	Humerus	+	Brace
47	61	1998	Spain	8	F	Back, leg pain	Multiple	Biconcave vertebrae	Calcitonin, calcium, vit D
48			Spain	10	M	Leg pain	−	+	Calcitonin, calcifediol

NR, not reported.

ETIOLOGIC FACTORS

By definition, the cause of IJO is unknown. Serum levels of calcium, phosphorus, alkaline phosphatase, thyroid hormone, and parathyroid hormone are consistently normal.

Calcitonin levels were low in one case report (27) but normal in others (52,61). Furthermore, treatment with calcitonin has not been helpful (5,27). Osteocalcin, a bone matrix protein that is typically elevated in diseases characterized by high bone turnover, has been reported to be normal in IJO (52). Collagen ratios from skin fibroblast cultures were normal in six patients with IJO (46). The serum level of certain collagen peptides was reduced (46,47), but the significance of these findings is unclear. Normal osteoblast function as determined by a 1,25-dihydroxyvitamin D_3 stimulation test was observed in six patients with IJO (2).

In an early study of patients who were extensively analyzed, Dent and Friedman (12) observed a negative calcium balance at presentation and a positive calcium balance on remission of the disease. Negative calcium balance at presentation has also been reported by other authors (3,31,59), but positive accretion of calcium by isotope studies has been described as well (32). Brenton and Dent (5) noted that a negative calcium balance was typically seen in those with moderate or severe involvement, and a positive calcium balance was seen in mildly affected patients and in those who were studied after menarche.

In three studies, decreased serum levels of 1,25-dihydroxyvitamin D were observed in seven patients (38,51,52). Furthermore, treatment with calcitriol apparently decreased the incidence of fractures in these patients. Other authors, however, have reported normal serum levels of both 1,25-dihydroxyvitamin D and 25-hydroxyvitamin D (24,27,36,39,56).

One can speculate that a mild deficiency of 1,25-dihyroxyvitamin D, either from a seasonal deficiency (15) or from a partial defect of either renal α-hydroxylase or insulin-like growth factor I (62), could play a pivotal role in the development of IJO. If the increased levels of 1,25-dihydroxyvitamin D needed during periods of rapid growth are unavailable, then calcium absorption would be mildly suboptimal, and bone formation would be affected. Bone resorption, an activity also stimulated by 1,25-dihydroxyvitamin D, could also be decreased. As a result, the bone-remodeling system would become uncoupled or slowed down, causing a further decrease in bone formation. A parallel situation may be observed in early postmenopausal osteoporosis, where reduced levels of 1,25-dihydroxyvitamin D are thought to retard bone resorption and uncouple the bone-remodeling system (11). The increased production of sex hormones during puberty—a significant factor in the increased bone density that occurs during adolescence (20)—would subsequently overcome the effect of this mild 1,25-dihydroxyvitamin D deficiency and allow remission of the osteoporosis. If IJO is truly absent in warmer climates, a possible explanation is that the greater sunlight exposure in these areas provides enhanced conversion of 7-dehydrocholesterol to vitamin D_3 and ergosterol to vitamin D_2.

CLINICAL FEATURES

Symptoms typically begin during the prepubertal years with the insidious onset of back pain, lower extremity pain, or fractures.

Knee and ankle pain are more common than hip discomfort. The child may walk with a limp or stiff-legged gait. Extreme difficulty with walking occurs in severe forms.

Back pain may be limited to the lumbar region, or the spine may be diffusely involved. Vertebral collapse or wedging is typical, but some patients only develop biconcave vertebra. Multiple thoracic and lumbar vertebrae are frequently involved. Kyphosis is common, but the degree of kyphosis has not been documented in the literature. Scoliosis has also been noted, but a severe spinal curvature has been reported in only one patient whose spinal deformity apparently preceded the onset of IJO (1). Spondylolisthesis was noted in two of the 14 patients reviewed by Houang et al. (25), but the degree of vertebral slippage did not require treatment.

Fractures of the long bones may be multiple or may not occur at all. The incidence of fractures is higher in the lower extremities, but the upper extremities may also be affected. Many of the injuries are of the low-impact type, most frequently causing nondisplaced or unicortical metaphyseal fractures; however, displaced fractures of the diaphysis and of the femoral neck may also occur (25). Some fractures, particularly those in the feet or those characterized by metaphyseal buckling, have only been recognized after skeletal radiographic surveys have been obtained.

Brenton and Dent (5) classified their series of 17 patients into mild, moderate, and severe categories. Those in the mild category typically had pain limited to the back and had a limited number of collapsed vertebra. Their activity was only temporarily restricted, and their ultimate loss of height averaged 4 cm.[1] Patients in the moderate category presented with back and extremity pain and had numerous vertebral and metaphyseal fractures. Activity restriction was prolonged, and many of these patients required temporary use of a wheelchair. The ultimate height loss ranged from 4 to 12 cm, but these patients eventually recovered full activity levels. Those in the severe category had numerous vertebral and metaphyseal fractures and frequently demonstrated diaphyseal fractures. Their ultimate loss in height ranged from 12 to 35 cm. Although cessation of spontaneous fractures ultimately occurred, these patients demonstrated only partial recovery to normal activity levels. As previously noted, some of these patients may have actually had a type of osteogenesis imperfecta.

RADIOGRAPHIC FEATURES

Generalized osteoporosis is the hallmark radiographic feature of IJO. Loss of trabecular bone in the vertebrae and metaphyses is particularly striking. On plain radiographs, the skull appears to be spared.

Cortical thinning is noted in the long bones of the appendicular skeleton. Unlike osteogenesis imperfecta, the long tubular bones in IJO do not become thin and gracile. Two of the 14

---

[1] Loss of height in this series was measured as the difference between standing height and arm span. Because the ratio of arm span to height is normally 1.03:1, the ultimate loss was probably overestimated.

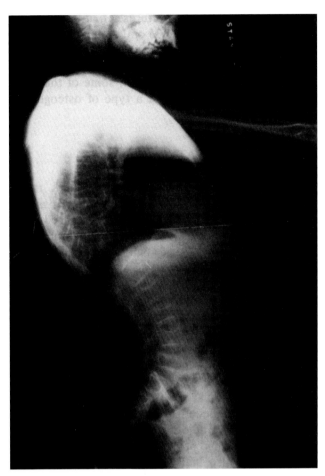

FIGURE 1. Standing lateral radiograph of a 10-year-old girl with idiopathic juvenile osteoporosis. Note diffuse osteopenia, multiple "codfish" vertebrae in the thoracic and lumbar spine, and "coin" vertebrae in the upper thoracic spine secondary to extreme collapse. (Courtesy of Stuart L. Weinstein, M.D., Department of Orthopedic Surgery, University of Iowa.)

patients in the radiographic review by Houang et al. (25) demonstrated protrusio acetabuli. Two patients in this review also had coxa vara associated with a fracture of the femoral neck.

Radiographic features in the vertebrae range from wedging to collapse, with the vertebral body having a "codfish" deformity with biconcave superior and inferior borders. With extreme collapse, the vertebral body has a "coin" appearance (Fig. 1) (25).

OTHER IMAGING STUDIES

Routine radiographs permit limited assessment of osteoporosis. In the spine approximately 50 percent of the bone mass must be lost before osteoporosis can be consistently diagnosed on plain radiographs (48).

Bone densitometry studies have revolutionized our ability to quantify osteoporosis and should be obtained in all patients with IJO. Dual-energy x-ray absorptiometry (DXA) is preferred. In comparison with quantitative CT measurement of bone density, DXA has superior precision, lower cost, and minimal absorbed doses of radiation (16). Furthermore, age-adjusted DXA standards are available to determine bone mineral density Z scores (standard deviation above or below the age-matched normal mean). This is important because gender and race do not affect bone mineral density (g/cm^2) in children, but age is a significant factor that must be taken into account. Of note, the difference in bone mineral content between males and females at the end of growth is mostly related to differences in bone width (19).

For patients with IJO, bone mineral density should be measured in both the lumbar spine and proximal femur. The DXA lumbar study assesses axial skeletal trabecular bone density, whereas the proximal femur reflects appendicular trabecular bone strength. Although measurements in these two areas correlate highly, for the individual patient the difference is often significant, particularly when the bone mineral density is abnormal (22).

Although DXA studies are preferred, limited data are available on these measurements in IJO. Villaverde et al (61) observed a -4.21 DXA lumbar Z score in a 8.5-year-old girl 2 years after onset of symptoms and a -5.30 DXA lumbar Z score in 10-year-old boy at presentation. Similar strikingly low values have been noted in two patients in the series reported by Smith (56).

Single-photon absorptiometry measurements performed in the standard fashion at the midradius have been reported in at least seven patients with IJO (27,38,52). Midradius absorptiometry primarily measures cortical bone density, but these studies provide some insight into the variability and natural history of IJO. In the patient reported by Jackson et al. (31), the bone density was 6 standard deviations (SD) below the mean for age. This patient's recurrent fractures ceased at the onset of puberty, but the bone density measurements had increased to only 4 SD below the mean by that time. In a patient treated with calcitriol, the bone density was markedly depressed at presentation, steadily improved while the patient was receiving the medication, but showed a precipitous increase at menarche (38). Serial measurements were helpful in monitoring medical treatment in the series reported by Saggese et al. (52). Two of their patients were taking calcitriol and achieved normal bone density of the midradius. The third patient was not on medication, never achieved normal bone density, and had continued problems with fractures at the 30-month follow-up visit.

OTHER DIAGNOSTIC STUDIES

The diagnosis of IJO is one of exclusion. Therefore, in the workup of a patient with IJO, it is necessary to perform diagnostic studies for disorders that cause osteoporosis in children. Screening studies should include a complete blood count, as well as measurement of serum calcium, phosphate, alkaline phosphatase, parathyroid hormone, calcitonin, 25-hydroxyvitamin D, and 1,25-dihydroxyvitamin D levels.

It is most important to exclude *leukemia* in a child who presents with generalized osteoporosis (53) (Fig. 2). Patients with leukemia have decreased bone mineral density at diagnosis (34), but fortunately, only a small percentage present with generalized osteoporosis and vertebral compression fractures. This scenario occurred in only one of 250 children in the study by Leheup et al. (35). However, it is this type of patient who is particularly

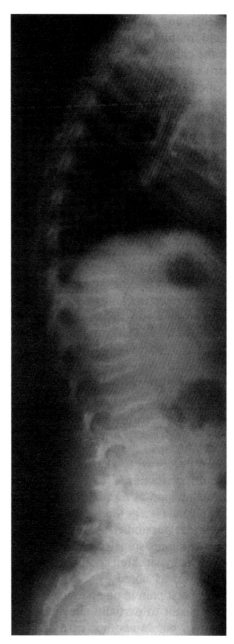

FIGURE 2. This 6-year-old girl presented with severe back pain and inability to walk. Note diffuse osteopenia and multiple compression fractures. Diagnostic evaluation revealed acute leukemia. (Courtesy of Stuart L. Weinstein, M.D., Department of Orthopedic Surgery, University of Iowa.)

Cushing syndrome, or hyperadrenocorticism, may also cause generalized osteoporosis in children. Twenty-four-hour measurement of total free urinary cortisol and an 8 a.m. determination of serum plasma cortisol level are usually adequate screening for Cushing syndrome. If these two laboratory measurements are abnormal, then a more complete workup to localize the source of the hyperadrenocorticism is indicated.

Lysinuric protein intolerance should be considered in a young child who presents with osteopenia and fractures (8,58). This autosomal recessive disease results from defective transport of cationic amino acids. Measurement of urinary amino acids in these children demonstrates hyperlysinuria. Osteoporosis in this disorder is thought to result from defective matrix protein synthesis caused by protein deprivation and deficiency of cationic amino acids. Although these patients are often recognized by their aversion to protein and frequent vomiting, these symptoms may not be present or obvious; therefore, urinary amino acid levels should be obtained in children with unexplained generalized osteoporosis. Diagnosing lysinuric protein intolerance is important because citrulline supplementation therapy not only increases protein intake but improves bone density as well (8).

Type I homocystinuria, a disorder that is phenotypically similar to Marfan syndrome, also causes osteoporosis in children. The screening study for this disease is measurement of urinary levels of homocystine. The diagnosis of type I homocystinuria can then be confirmed by demonstrating increased serum levels of methionine (63).

Hyperimmunoglobulinemia E syndrome can also cause osteoporosis and recurrent fractures in young children (30). Monocytes from patients with hyperimmunoglobulinemia E syndrome probably increase bone resorption by abnormal production of prostaglandins (37). This syndrome is associated with recurrent pyogenic infections, chronic eczematoid dermatitis, and mucocutaneous candidiasis. The diagnosis is confirmed by marked elevation of serum immunoglobulin E levels.

Osteogenesis imperfecta is another disorder that must be differentiated from IJO. The typical patient with osteogenesis imperfecta has the onset of fractures during infancy or early childhood; but some of these children do not have fractures until they are older than 5 years (44). Because the features of IJO and osteogenesis imperfecta overlap, it is reasonable to obtain skin fibroblast cultures for collagen type evaluation in any child who presents with generalized osteoporosis and fractures of unknown cause.

NATURAL HISTORY

The natural history of IJO is eventual remission, typically at the onset of puberty (12). The associated kyphosis typically improves, but measurements of thoracic kyphosis on standing films have not been performed. Recurrent fractures also cease, and apparent reconstitution of bone occurs. However, long-term studies have not documented whether the bone density returns to normal. This is critical because it is now apparent that development of an adequate bone mass at the completion of growth is critical (7,9,40,41,49). The variance of peak vertebral bone density in young adults is high—in the range of 25% (26). By comparison, the subsequent rate of bone loss, ranging from less

prone to be misdiagnosed as having IJO, a situation that has occurred in at least two patients (12,35). Children with leukemia who present with generalized osteoporosis and vertebral compression fractures typically have no organomegaly and a low-normal white blood cell count (4,12,53). Such parameters obviously do not permit differentiation of IJO from leukemia. A bone marrow biopsy should be part of the evaluation of any child with generalized osteoporosis unless a pediatric hematology consultant believes that leukemia can be ruled out by other means.

than 1% to 2% per year, is relatively small (7,50). Therefore, if patients with IJO have low bone mineral density at completion of growth, they are at significant risk for developing recurrent osteoporosis during their later adult years.

The variable severity and the rarity of IJO make evaluation of medical therapies difficult. Recent reports have advocated the use of calcitriol or bisphosphonates (23,38,52), but whether any medication influences the natural history of IJO remains to be proved.

TREATMENT

Nonsurgical

Treatment includes modification of activities, dietary counseling, consideration of calcium and vitamin D supplements, and supportive therapy for spinal deformities and fractures. The orthopaedic surgeon must work with the child and the family to outline activities that will strike a reasonable balance between those that cause repeated fractures and those that restrict physical activities to such an extent that the osteoporosis is exacerbated. This program obviously has to be individualized, depending on the severity of the disease and whether remission of the osteoporosis has commenced.

A nutritional assessment should be done to confirm that the patient is getting adequate dietary calcium (12,29). Because phosphates may affect intestinal absorption of calcium, it is appropriate to ensure that the patient does not have excessive phosphate intake. Judicious restriction of soft drinks not only decreases phosphate intake but also helps control obesity, a problem that may develop in children with IJO (12,59).

A trial with calcitriol may be indicated if 1,25-dihydroxyvitamin D levels are depressed. Marder et al. (38) noted better results when calcitriol was given in two divided doses, as opposed to 1.0 μg given as a single daily dose. Saggese et al. (52) recommended 0.50 μg/d in two divided doses for two older children and 0.25 μg/d in a 2-year-old patient. Of note, single-photon absorptiometry measurement of midradius cortical bone mineral density normalized in two IJO patients in this study (52). Optimal therapy requires ongoing assessment of 1,25-dihydroxyvitamin D levels to maintain normal limits for the child's age. Hypercalcemia is a possible side effect of calcitriol therapy, and that possibility should be monitored.

Bisphosphonates (oral pamidronate) has been used to treat six children with IJO (6,23). Symptomatic improvement as well as normalization of calcium balance and significant improvement in DXA lumbar spine bone mineral density z scores were observed. Radiologic changes during treatment included a striking sclerosis at the metaphysis of the long bones and vertebrae. No change in skeletal maturation was observed, and the bisphosphonates were well tolerated. These studies have impressive early results but can be criticized because all patients underwent treatment during puberty. The authors speculated that IJO resulted from excessive bone resorption and that the bisphosphonates suppressed the hyperactive osteoclasts.

The most common spinal problems are back pain and kyphosis. A hyperextension brace worn only during the daytime was noted by Cloutier et al. (10) to control lower back pain in one

patient. A lumbosacral corset was thought to partially alleviate back pain in one report (32), but in another case it did not seem to help (3). Jones and Hensinger (28) noted gratifying results after using a Milwaukee brace in two children with IJO and kyphosis.

A lumbosacral corset should be tried if the patient's main complaint is low back pain. If increased thoracic kyphosis is present, a Milwaukee brace should minimize progression of the kyphotic deformity. A rigid total-contact spinal orthosis is contraindicated, as this type of brace might accentuate or cause bony deformity. Rapid weaning from the brace is recommended (28); this minimizes the effect of stress shielding on the osteoporotic bone.

As most fractures in IJO are of the unicortical or nondisplaced pattern, short-term immobilization with coaptation splints usually constitutes satisfactory treatment. Displaced fractures require longer immobilization, but prolonged casting should be avoided to minimize the osteoporotic effect of immobilization. For a child who has recurrent fractures or painful ambulation, the use of a light-weight orthosis will protect the extremity while maintaining weight-bearing function. In this situation, bracing will provide a better environment for improving bone strength.

Surgical

Operative treatment of spinal deformity has been reported in only one patient with IJO (1). A posterior spinal fusion was performed at age 13 years for progressive scoliosis, apparently before the osteoporosis was recognized. The operation was fraught with difficulty. The laminae were so soft that Harrington instrumentation could not be utilized. Despite obtaining a solid fusion, this patient's curvature continued to increase from apparent bending of the osteoporotic bone. After bone densitometry studies demonstrated recovery, this patient underwent a two-stage operation at age 17 that included osteotomies of the fusion mass during the first operation followed by halo traction, followed by repeat posterior spinal fusion with multiple Harrington rods.

Operative therapy was apparently successful in stabilizing a metaphyseal fracture of the femoral neck in one patient with IJO (25). Villaverde et al. (61) reported that surgical realignment of genu varum was helpful in one case but provided no other details. The extreme osteoporosis associated with the active phase of the disease narrowly restricts the indications for surgical treatment. Bony deformity that results from either vertebral collapse or recurrent fractures should be operated on after remission of the disease, if possible. By then, the bone strength would be improved, and internal fixation would be more reliable.

REFERENCES

1. Bartal E, Gage J (1982): Idiopathic juvenile osteoporosis and scoliosis. *J Pediatr Orthop* 2:295–298.
2. Bertelloni S, Baroncelli GI, Di Nero G, et al. (1992): Idiopathic juvenile osteoporosis: evidence of normal osteoblast function by 1,25-dihydroxyvitamin D$_3$ stimulation test. *Calc Tissue Int* 51:20–23.
3. Berglund G, Lindquist B (1960): Osteopenia in adolescence. *Clin Orthop* 17:259–264.
4. Blatt J, Martini SL, Penchansky L (1985): Characteristics of acute lymphoblastic leukemia in children with osteopenia and vertebral compression fractures. *J Pediatr* 105:280–282.

5. Brenton DP, Dent CE (1976): Idiopathic juvenile osteoporosis. In: Bickel H, Stern J, eds. *Inborn errors of calcium and bone metabolism.* Baltimore: University Park Press, pp. 222–238.

6. Brumsen C, Hamdy NAT, Papapoulos SE (1997): Long-term effects of bisphosphonates on the growing skeleton. *Medicine* 76:266–283.

7. Burckhardt P, Michel C (1989): The peak bone mass concept. *Clin Rheumatol* 8(Suppl 2):16–21.

8. Carpenter TO, Levy HL, Holtrop ME, et al. (1985): Lysinuric protein intolerance presenting as childhood osteoporosis. *N Engl J Med* 312:290–294.

9. Carrie Fassler AL, Bonjour JP (1995): Osteoporosis as a pediatric problem. *Pediatr Clin N Am* 42:811–824.

10. Cloutier MD, Hayles AB, Riggs BL, et al. (1967): Juvenile osteoporosis: report of a case including a description of some metabolic and microradiographic studies. *Pediatrics* 40:649–655.

11. DeLuca HF (1990): The vitamin D story: a success of basic science in the treatment of disease. In: Castells S, Finberg L, eds. *Metabolic bone disease in children.* New York: Marcel Dekker, pp. 1–41.

12. Dent CE, Friedman M (1965): Idiopathic juvenile osteoporosis. *Q J Med* 134:177–210.

13. Dietz FR, Mathews KD, Montgomery WJ (1990): Reflex sympathetic dystrophy in children. *Clin Orthop* 258:225–231.

14. Dimar JR, Campbell M, Glassman SD, et al. (1995): Idiopathic juvenile osteoporosis: an unusual cause of back pain in an adolescent. *Am J Orthop* 24:865–869.

15. Docio S, Riancho DS, Perez A, et al. (1998): Seasonal deficiency of vitamin D in children: a potential target for osteoporosis-preventing strategies? *J Bone Min Res* 13:544–548.

16. Einhorn TA, Gill SS (1999): Bone metabolism and metabolic bone disease. In: Beatty JH, ed. *Orthopaedic knowledge update,* 6th ed. Rosemont, IL: American Academy of Orthopaedic Surgeons, pp. 149–165.

17. Evans RA, Dunstan CR, Hills E (1983): Bone metabolism in idiopathic juvenile osteoporosis: a case report. *Calcif Tissue Int* 35:5–8.

18. Exner U, Prader A, Elsasser U, et al. (1984): Idiopathic osteoporosis in a three-year-old girl. *Helv Paediatr Acta* 39:517–528.

19. Gilsanz V, Gibbens DT, Roe TF, et al. (1988): Vertebral bone density in children: effect of puberty. *Radiology* 166:847–850.

20. Gilsanz V, Roe TF, Gibbens DT, et al. (1988): Effect of sex steroids on peak bone density of growing rabbits. *Am J Physiol* 255:E416–E420.

21. Gooding CA, Ball JH (1969): Idiopathic juvenile osteoporosis. *Radiology* 93:1349–1350.

22. Henderson RC (1997): The correlation between dual-energy X-ray absorptiometry measures of bone density in the proximal femur and lumbar spine of children. *Skeletal Radiol* 26:544–547.

23. Hoekman K, Papapoulos SE, Peters ACB, et al. (1985): Characteristics and bisphosphonates treatment of a patient with juvenile osteoporosis. *J Clin Endocrinol Metab* 61:952–956.

24. Hou JW, Wang TR (1995): Idiopathic juvenile osteoporosis: five-year case follow-up. *J Formos Med Assoc* 94:277–280.

25. Houang MTW, Brenton DP, Renton P (1978): Idiopathic juvenile osteoporosis. *Skeletal Radiol* 3:17–23.

26. Hui SL, Slemenda CW, Johnston CC, et al. (1987): Effects of age and menopause on vertebral bone density. *Bone Min* 2:141–146.

27. Jackson EC, Strife CF, Tsang RC, et al. (1988): Effect of calcitonin replacement therapy in idiopathic juvenile osteoporosis. *Am J Dis Child* 142:1237–1239.

28. Jones ET, Hensinger RN (1981): Spinal deformity in idiopathic juvenile osteoporosis. *Spine* 6:1–4.

29. Jowsey J, Johnson KA (1972): Juvenile osteoporosis: bone findings in seven patients. *J Pediatr* 81:511–517.

30. Kirchner SG, Sivit CJ, Wright PF (1985): Hyperimmunoglobulinemia E syndrome: association with osteoporosis and recurrent fractures. *Radiology* 156:362.

31. Kooh SW, Cumming WA, Fraser D, et al. (1973): Transient childhood osteoporosis of unknown cause. In: Frame B, Partiff AM, Duncan H, eds. International Congress Series No. 270: *Clinical aspects of metabolic bone disease.* Amsterdam: Excerpta Medica, pp. 329–332.

32. Lachmann D, Willvonseder R, Hofer R, et al. (1977): A case-report of idiopathic juvenile osteoporosis with particular reference to 47-calcium absorption. *Eur J Pediatr* 125:265–273.

33. Lapatsanis P, Kavadias A, Vretos K (1971): Juvenile osteoporosis. *Arch Dis Child* 146:66–71.

34. Leeuw JA, Piers DA, Kamps WA (1990): Osteoporosis in children with leukemia: a potentially debilitating anomaly? *Haem Blood Trans* 33:580–582.

35. Leheup B, Membre H, Gerard H, et al. (1985): Lymphoblastic leukemia with osteopenia and vertebral compression fractures. *J Pediatr* 106:860.

36. Leroy D, Garabedian M, Guillozo H, et al. (1981): Evolution des concentrations seriques en metabolites de la vitamine D [25-OH-D, 24,25(OH)2D, 1,25(OH)2D] dans un case d'osteoporose juvenile idiopathique. *Arch Fr Pediatr* 38:165–170.

37. Leung DYM, Key L, Steinberg J, et al. (1988): Increased in vitro bone resorption by monocytes in the hyper-immunoglobulin E syndrome. *J Immunol* 140:84–88.

38. Marder HK, Tsang RC, Hug G, et al. (1982): Calcitriol deficiency in idiopathic juvenile osteoporosis. *Am J Dis Child* 136:914–917.

39. Marhaug G (1993): Idiopathic juvenile osteoporosis. *Scand J Rheumatol* 22:45–47.

40. Matkovic V (1992): Osteoporosis as a pediatric disease: role of calcium and heredity. *J Rheumatol* 33:54–59.

41. Mazess RB, Cameron JR (1971): Skeletal growth in school children: maturation and bone loss. *Am J Phys Anthropol* 35:399–407.

42. McDowell CL, Moore JD (1992): Multiple fractures in a child: the osteoporosis pseudoglioma syndrome. *J Bone Joint Surg* 74(A):1247–1249.

43. Nizankowska BT, Bijak M (1987): Samoistna modziencza osteoporoza (zespo Dent-Friedman) u 8-letniejdziewczynki. *Pediatr Pol* 62:185–187.

44. Penttinen R, Sipola E, Kouvalainen K, et al. (1980): An arthropathic form of osteogenesis imperfecta. *Acta Paediatr Scand* 69:263–267.

45. Perri G, Calderazzi A, Grassi L, et al. (1987): L'osteoporosi idiopatica giovanile. *Radiol Med (Torino)* 74:399–403.

46. Pocock AE, Francis MJO, Smith R (1995): Type I colagen biosynthesis by skin fibroblasts from patients with idiopathic juvenile osteoporosis. *Clin Sci* 89:69–73.

47. Prósyzńska K, Wieczorek E, Olszaniecka M, et al. (1996): Collagen peptides in osteogenesis imperfecta, idiopathic juvenile osteoporosis and Ehlers-Danlos syndrome. *Acta Paediatr* 85:688–691.

48. Poznanski AK (1990): Radiologic evaluation of bone mineral. In: Favus MJ, ed. *Primer on the metabolic bone diseases and disorders of mineral metabolism.* Kelseyville, CA: American Society for Bone and Mineral Research, pp. 79–87.

49. Rigotti NA, Nussbaum SR, Herzog DB, et al. (1984): Osteoporosis in women with anorexia nervosa. *N Engl J Med* 311:1601–1606.

50. Rodin A, Murby B, Smith MA, et al. (1990): Premenopausal bone loss in the lumbar spine and neck of femur: a study of 225 Caucasian women. *Bone* ll:1–5.

51. Rosskamp R, Sell G, Emons D, et al. (1987): Idiopathische juvenile Osteoporose—Bericht uber zwei Falle. *Klin Padiatr* 199:457–461.

52. Saggese G, Bartelloni S, Baroncelli GI, et al. (1991): Mineral metabolism and calcitrol therapy in idiopathic juvenile osteoporosis. *Am J Dis Child* 145:457–462.

53. Samuda GM, Cheng MY, Yeung CY (1987): Back pain and vertebral compression: an uncommon presentation of childhood acute lymphoblastic leukemia. *J Pediatr Orthop* 7:175–178.

54. Schippers JC (1939): Over een geval van "spontane" algemeene osteoporose bij een klein meisje. *Maandschrift voor Kindergeneeskd* 8:108–117.

55. Smith R (1980): Idiopathic osteoporosis in the young. *J Bone Joint Surg Br* 62:417–427.

56. Smith R (1995): Idiopathic juvenile osteoporosis: experience of twenty-one patients. *Br J Rheumatol* 34:68–77.

57. Spriggs DW (1990): Case report 613: Osteoporosis pseudoglioma syndrome. *Skeletal Radiol* 19:302–304.

58. Svedstrom E, Parto K, Marttinen M, et al. (1993): Skeletal manifestations of lysinuric protein intolerance. A follow-up study of 29 patients. *Skeletal Radiol* 22:11–16.

59. Teotia M, Teotia SPS, Singh RK (1979): Idiopathic juvenile osteoporosis. *Am J Dis Child* 133:894–900.
60. Towbin R, Dunbar JS (1981): Generalized osteoporosis with multiple fractures in an adolescent. *Invest Radiol* 16:171–174.
61. Villaverde V, De Inocencio J, Merino R, et al. (1998): Difficulty walking. A presentation of idiopathic juvenile osteoporosis. *J Rheumatol* 25:173–176.
62. Wright NM, Metzger DL, Key LL (1995): Extrogen and diclofenac sodium therapy in a prepubertal female with idiopathic juvenile osteoporosis. *J Pediatr Endocrinol Metab* 8(2):135–139.
63. Zaleske DJ (1996): Metabolic and endocrine abnormalities. In: Morrissy RT, Weinstein SL, eds. *Lovell and Winter's Pediatric orthopaedics,* 4th ed. Philadelphia: Lippincott-Raven Publishers, pp. 137–201.

THE SPINE IN OSTEOGENESIS IMPERFECTA

JOHN P. LUBICKY

Osteogenesis imperfecta is a heritable disease of connective tissue in which the chief abnormality is in the collagen matrix of bone. It is a genetically heterogeneous condition. For this reason, both the type of inheritance and the severity of involvement can vary from patient to patient. The chief feature of this condition is the brittleness of the bones throughout the body; there are abnormalities in other tissue as well. Patients with osteogenesis imperfecta characteristically are of short stature and have peculiar triangle-shaped faces. They often have blue sclerae, abnormal teeth, deafness, and frequent fractures. They also have ligamentous laxity (11,19,35,36,38,45) (Fig. 1). Because the bones are weak, bowing of the long bones takes place and may be accelerated by fractures in the area of bowing. Deformities of other bones occur, including molding deformities of the skull and distortion of the pelvis. Ligamentous laxity and weak bone both contribute to the development of spinal deformities (Fig. 2).

The currently accepted classification system for osteogenesis imperfecta is that proposed by Sillence (35,36) (Table 1). It incorporates the clinical features with the mode of inheritance. Although this classification is not perfect, it is a good working scheme for this condition. Additional features of the condition may sort out the type in the Sillence classification. Versfeld et al. (41) found that all of 16 patients with type III osteogenesis imperfecta had markedly elongated vertebral pedicles. They did not find this true of other types. They also found posterior rib angulation in type III.

A complete discussion of the genetics and pathophysiologic mechanisms of osteogenesis imperfecta is beyond the scope of this chapter. Osteogenesis imperfecta can be transmitted by both autosomal dominant and autosomal recessive modes (35,36). In the biochemistry of the disease, calcium, phosphorus, magnesium, vitamin D, and parathormone levels all are normal. The abnormality is in the composition and architecture of the collagen matrix. There seem to be abnormally high amounts of types III and V collagen in bone. There is also an abnormality of the cross-linking of the collagen chains (45). With this background of the general features of osteogenesis imperfecta, this chapter examines the various spinal problems associated with it.

INCIDENCE AND PATHOGENESIS OF SPINAL DEFORMITY

Although repeated fractures and bowing of the long bones are the chief orthopaedic problems associated with osteogenesis imperfecta, spinal deformities have been discussed frequently in the literature. A review of various series reveals that the incidence of spinal deformities is 20% to 80% among patients with osteogenesis imperfecta (2–4,7,9,11,17,25,32). A number of factors influence the development and progression of spinal deformities, including severity of the disease, age, history of long bone fractures, and ambulatory status.

Two reports on spinal deformities in osteogenesis imperfecta were the result of a review of more than 100 patients from the Shriners Hospitals for Children, Chicago (3,4). The authors found that patients with severe disease who could not walk, had numerous long-bone fractures, and had chest deformities were at risk of development of scoliosis. They also found that the incidence varied with age. Among patients younger than 5 years, the incidence of scoliosis was 26%, but among those older than 12 years, the incidence was about 80%. Cristofaro et al. (7) also found that the severity of osteogenesis imperfecta seemed related to the incidence of scoliosis. Among their patients with osteogenesis imperfecta congenita and osteogenesis imperfecta tarda type I, 80% had scoliosis with an average curve of 47 degrees. The patients with osteogenesis imperfecta tarda type II had a 50% chance of having scoliosis with an average curvature of 26 degrees. Engelbert et al. (10) found in a group of 47 children that severe spinal problems are more likely in types III and IV rather than in type I. Children in this study who had dentinogenesis imperfecta also seemed more prone to scoliosis than those who did not (10). Similar findings were reported by others (2,11,27).

Hanscom and Bloom (17) devised a classification system (grades A through E) that correlated the patient's degree of osteogenesis imperfecta and the risk of scoliosis. Again, this system indicated that severity of the disease correlates with risk of development and severity of scoliosis. As with other forms of scoliosis, continued progression is possible after skeletal maturity (2). One of the possible mechanisms of the pathogenesis is additional compression fractures due to superimposition of osteoporosis on already weak bone in an already deformed spine.

J.P. Lubicky: Department of Orthopaedic Surgery, Rush Medical College, Shriners Hospitals for Children, Chicago, Illinois 60707.

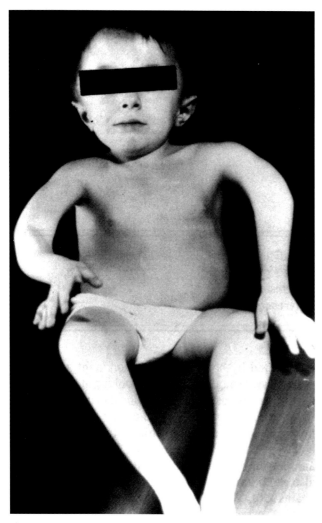

FIGURE 1. Child with osteogenesis imperfecta with typical features of triangular face, distorted trunk, and bowed extremities.

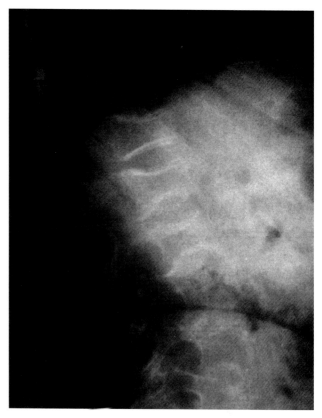

FIGURE 2. Lateral spinal radiograph shows multiple compression fractures with preservation of the discs, giving the typical appearance of codfish vertebrae.

A number of curve patterns occur with or without kyphosis. Cristofaro et al. (7) found that 43% patients had double curves, 28% had thoracic curves, 26% had thoracolumbar curves, and 3% had cervicothoracic curves. Renshaw et al. (32) found that 14 patients with osteogenesis and scoliosis had thoracic curves, nine of 28 had lumbar curves, and 4 of 28 had thoracolumbar curves. Almost one half had kyphosis greater than 45 degrees.

Engelbert et al. (10) also found a rather high incidence of a kyphotic component to the scoliosis, 18 of 22 patients. Benson et al. (3) found little rotation in the scoliotic spines of their patients.

The pathogenesis of spinal deformities in osteogenesis imperfecta seems to be a combination of weak bone and ligamentous laxity. This weak bone is prone to microfractures, which may involve the vertebral growth plates, which then do not grow normally. This abnormal growth may produce abnormally shaped vertebrae. Additional macroscopic compression fractures may further alter vertebral shape, perpetuating the deformity. This explanation is compatible with the finding that in general, the incidence and severity of the spinal deformity correlate with

TABLE 1. CLASSIFICATION OF OSTEOGENESIS IMPERFECTA

Type	Blue Sclerae	Bone Fragility	Hearing Loss	Dentinogesis Imperfecta
IA	Present	Mild	20–30 y of age	Absent
IB	Present	Mild	20–30 y of age	Present
II	Unknown	Severe	Absent	Unknown
III	Less blue with age	Severe	Absent	Absent
IVA	Absent	Moderate to severe	Absent	Absent
IVB	Absent	Moderate to severe	Absent	Present

Modified from Sillence D (1981): Osteogenesis imperfecta: an expanding panorama of variants. *Clin Orthop* 159:11–25, with permission.

the severity of involvement of osteogenesis imperfecta. Results of a number of studies have indicated that the incidence increases with age. This may have something to do with upright posture and the effect of axial loading on the weak spinal column (2,3,17,27). It has been found (2–4,32) that the intervertebral discs are stronger than the bone of the vertebral bodies and that compression fractures give the vertebrae a codfish appearance. Progression eventually stops and may be related to settling of the deformed rib cage onto the pelvis.

Information obtained with various imaging techniques can help identify and quantify abnormal bone in vertebrae affected by osteogenesis imperfecta. Moore et al. (24) found that decreased bone mineral density as identified with dual-energy x-ray absorptiometry (DEXA) may be associated with osteogenesis imperfecta. Patients with osteogenesis imperfecta had a low bone mineral density and bone mineral content for weight and age as determined (8). Fredricks et al. (14) used quantitative computed tomography to assess trabecular bone mineral concentration. All three patients with osteogenesis imperfecta in the multidiagnosis study had abnormally low values. Frater et al. (13) used bone and DEXA to examine a woman with type I osteogenesis imperfecta and back pain. The findings were intense uptake in several vertebral bodies that had no deformity and osteopenia. Glorieux et al. (16) used DEXA to evaluate the effectiveness of medical therapy for osteogenesis imperfecta. They found evidence to suggest that a lower z score was associated with greater likelihood of having more severe scoliosis. The results of all these studies give credence to the fact that the weak bone of the vertebra contributes to the development of spinal deformity.

MANAGEMENT OF SPINAL DEFORMITIES

As with other types of spinal deformities, both nonoperative and operative methods have been used. In general, criteria used for other types of scoliosis, such as curve magnitude, age, patient maturity status, have been applied to curves associated with osteogenesis imperfecta.

Observation is one form of nonoperative treatment. All children with osteogenesis imperfecta, especially those with extensive disease involvement, should undergo regular clinical and radiographic spinal evaluations. Although it is not 100%, the incidence of scoliosis does increase with age.

Because the weak bone of osteogenesis imperfecta has a large part to play in the development of spinal deformities, strengthening the bone to help prevent deformity or to facilitate brace or surgical treatment may be helpful. Nagant de Deuxchaisnes et al. (26) in 1990 described the use of enteric-coated sodium fluoride and calcium in the treatment of a group of 101 patients who had low bone mineral density as determined by dual-photon absorptiometry of the lumbar spine; three of the patients had osteogenesis imperfecta. The investigators found that bone mineral density increased in a linear manner with time, regardless of the diagnosis.

In a more recent report, Glorieux et al. (16) described an uncontrolled observational study with 30 children and adolescents who had severe osteogenesis imperfecta. The patients were treated with cyclic administration of pamidronate. The drug was administered intravenously at 4 to 6 month intervals. The investigators found decreases in serum alkaline phosphate levels and in urinary excretion of calcium and type I collagen *N*-telopeptide. There was a mean annualized increase in bone mineral density of almost 42%, and the z score improved from -5.3 to -3.4. The investigators also found increases in cortical width in the metacarpals and in the size of the vertebral bodies, both suggesting that new bone had been formed. There was a statistically proved decrease in radiographically documented fractures. The children expressed a sense of improved well-being from relief of pain and fatigue. The results of this study suggest that medical treatment may correct some of the metabolic abnormalities of the bone that contribute to the development of spinal deformities. Another implication may be that medical treatment of those who have substantial spinal deformity before surgical intervention may aid in achieving better correction and security of the implants.

Brace treatment has been reviewed in a number of series (2,4,17,32,44). Bathgate and Moseley (2) stated that there may be a place for bracing—perhaps in management of smaller curves—but that exact indications are unclear. In their study, bracing was generally unsuccessful because it either was started too late or had to be stopped because of brace-related complications, especially rib deformities. Benson and Newman (4) found that bracing did not control curve progression and caused chest and rib deformities. Recommendations for bracing and for electrical stimulation—a treatment now not generally used, were put forth by Hanscom and Bloom (17), but no results were given. Renshaw et al. (32) found that some patients had chest deformities with bracing. Except for two patients treated in suspension orthoses, the patients were treated with conventional braces and had progression of the curve. Yong-Hing and Mac-Ewen (44) reviewed the records of 73 patients treated with a variety of braces. Fifty-eight patients had curve progression, and 15 patients had a decrease in or stabilization of the curve. Early bracing for smaller curves did not give better curve control. A number of complications occurred, and most patients were still in braces at the time the report was written.

In summary, it appears that bracing does not change the course of scoliosis in osteogenesis imperfecta and frequently causes complications. Use of this modality must be questioned in light of these findings.

Surgical treatment, usually consisting of at least posterior spinal fusion, has become popular as a means of controlling scoliosis in osteogenesis imperfecta (2,4–6,15,17,40,44). Bathgate and Moseley (2) pointed out that marked correction cannot be expected with surgery, and loss of correction is greater without instrumentation. The best results combined Harrington instrumentation and segmental wires. Benson and Newman (4) recommended spinal fusion with instrumentation and local bone grafting for progressive curves. They found that loss of correction was twice that among those who underwent fusion without instrumentation (Fig. 3).

Eight patients underwent surgery in the series by Cristofaro et al. (7). All underwent posterior spinal fusion, five with instrumentation. One also had an anterior spinal fusion. Gitelis et al. (15) combined the use of halo gravity traction, anterior spinal fusion with Dwyer instrumentation, and posterior spinal fusion

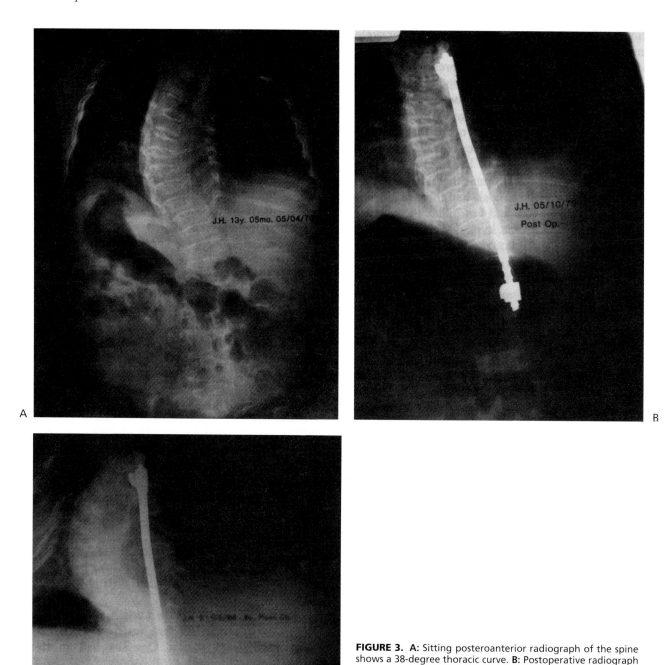

FIGURE 3. A: Sitting posteroanterior radiograph of the spine shows a 38-degree thoracic curve. **B:** Postoperative radiograph shows Harrington instrumentation supplemented with methyl methacrylate. Improvement in the curvature is evident. **C:** Posteroanterior radiograph obtained 9 years postoperatively shows the instrumentation in place and progression of the thoracic curve. Even in the presence of instrumentation—in this case, nonsegmental instrumentation—increasing curvature can occur postoperatively.

with Harrington instrumentation to treat a patient with severe scoliosis (Fig. 4).

Hanscom and Bloom (17) recommend fusion for curves greater than 45 degrees in patients with mild osteogenesis imperfecta and for curves greater than 35 degrees in patients with more severe disease. They also advise the use of segmental instrumentation. Trotter (40) found segmental instrumentation superior to fusions in situ and fusion with nonsegmental instru-

mentation in maintaining spinal alignment and preventing progression (Fig. 5).

Yong-Hing and MacEwen (44) described 60 patients undergoing surgical treatment. Fifty-five patients underwent posterior spinal fusion, 39 with instrumentation. Three of four patients undergoing anterior spinal fusion had Dwyer instrumentation as well. A modest increase in the amount of correction was found among patients who underwent instrumentation. A

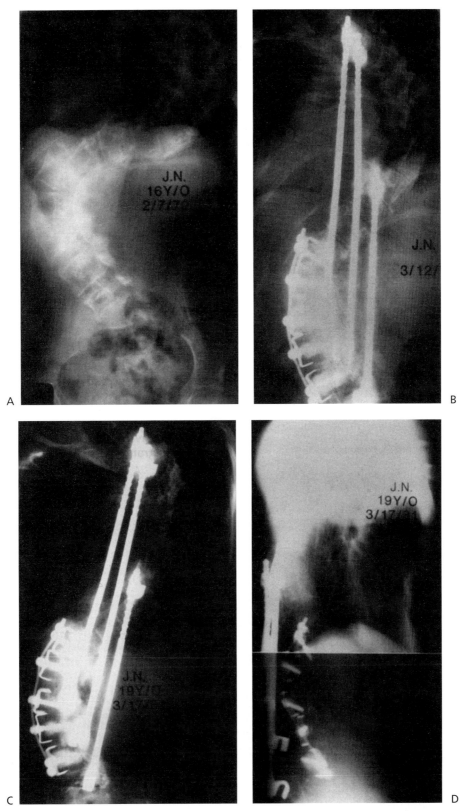

FIGURE 4. A: Posteroanterior upright thoracolumbar spinal radiograph shows severe double curve. **B:** Postoperative posteroanterior radiograph shows several posterior Harrington rods supplemented with methyl methacrylate and the anterior Dwyer instrumentation. Marked correction, particularly of the lower curve, has been achieved, although there is still substantial deformity of the trunk. Posteroanterior **(C)** and lateral **(D)** upright radiographs obtained 2 years after the operation show that there has been some loss of alignment on the frontal image. However, instrumentation has not completely failed. The kyphosing effect of the Dwyer instrumentation is evident in the anterior aspect.

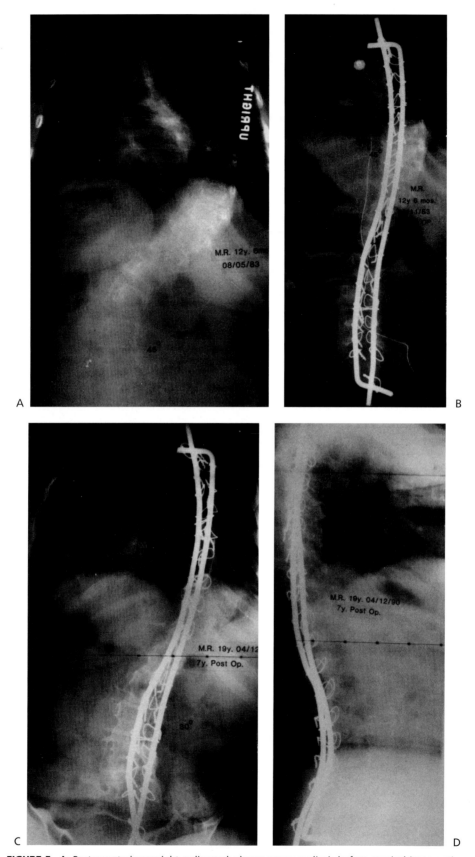

FIGURE 5. **A:** Posteroanterior upright radiograph shows severe scoliosis before surgical intervention. **B:** Postoperative anteroposterior radiograph shows Luque instrumentation in place and considerable correction of both curves. Posteroanterior **(C)** and lateral **(D)** upright radiographs obtained 7 years postoperatively show some loss of correction of both curves and some disruption of the instrumentation.

number of complications occurred, the most frequent of which were excessive blood loss and instrumentation problems. The authors found that in addition to stabilization of the curve, many patients achieved better sitting balance.

Poor bone stock provides poor purchase for instrumentation. Herron and Dawson (19) found that methylmethacrylate used around Harrington hook sites reinforces the construct. Methylmethacrylate has become an accepted adjunct to the use of hook-rod instrumentation in osteogenesis imperfecta (2,4,5,15,17,40) (Figs. 6, 7). However, the use of totally segmental instrumentation may obviate use of methylmethacrylate.

Although the main deformity described in all these series is scoliosis, many patients have associated kyphotic deformities—either true kyphosis or rotational kyphosis. Collapse into this kyphotic position is an additional deformity to be considered. It may play a role in the development of instrumentation problems, such as instrumentation cutout caused by continued kyphotic forces over the posterior instrumented segment (Figs. 8, 9).

It can be seen from this review that bracing is ineffective in controlling scoliosis in osteogenesis imperfecta and has some rather serious side effects. Surgical stabilization is the management of choice of progressive curves. The operation should entail posterior spinal fusion with segmental instrumentation and local and bank bone graft. A great deal of correction cannot be expected, however. Although instrumentation should be planned for all patients, the bone sometimes is so soft that instrumentation cannot be used. In such cases, in situ fusion is the only recourse. Therefore, when a curve has evidence of progression and has reached 35 to 40 degrees, it should be fused regardless of the age of the patient. Progression usually starts at approximately 8 years of age. Waiting for continued spinal growth in the face of unrelenting curve progression does not lengthen the trunk, even after surgical treatment, because significant correction of the curvature and elongation of the trunk cannot be expected. Attention also should be given to the sagittal plane. For patients with marked kyphosis, consideration should be given to anterior spinal fusion to ensure healing of the fusion and curve control.

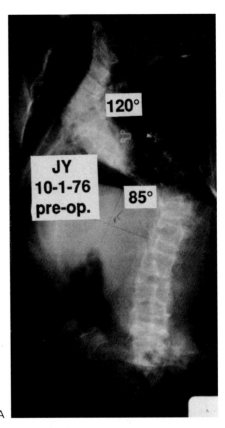

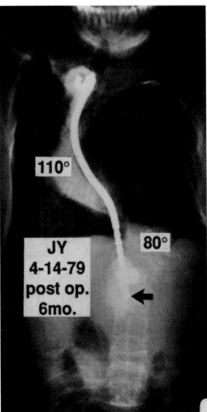

FIGURE 7. A: Preoperative posteroanterior upright radiograph shows severe scoliosis. **B:** Postoperative radiograph shows a contoured Harrington rod in place and hook sites supplemented with methylmethacrylate (*arrows*).

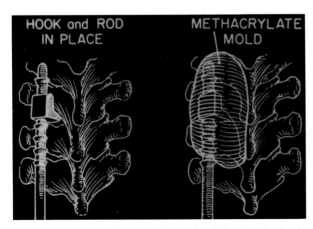

FIGURE 6. Illustration shows Harrington hook in place in the facet joint, which later was supplemented with the use of methylmethacrylate around the hook and onto the lamina.

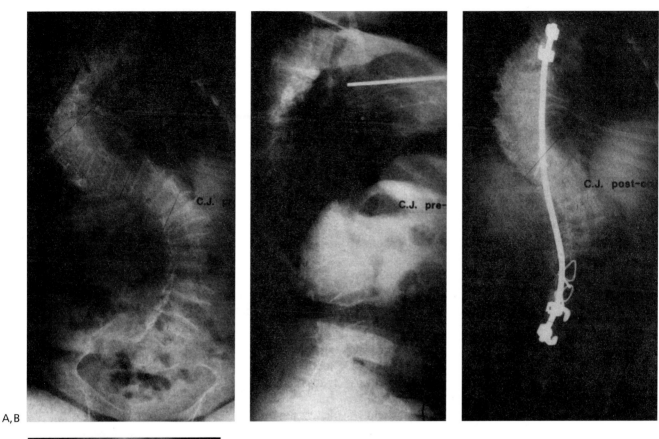

A,B   C

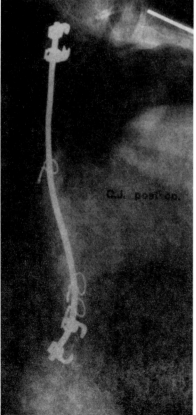

D

FIGURE 8. Preoperative posteroanterior **(A)** and lateral **(B)** upright radiographs of a 13-year-old girl with severe osteogenesis imperfecta. Sitting caused back pain. Postoperative posteroanterior **(C)** and lateral **(D)** upright radiographs show moderate correction and balance with the use of limited Cotrel-Dubousset instrumentation. Bone quality was quite poor. Lateral radiograph shows preservation of normal sagittal contour.

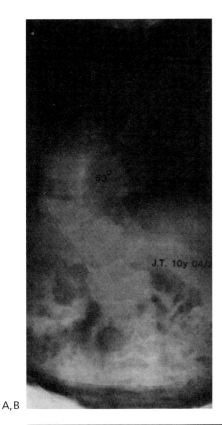
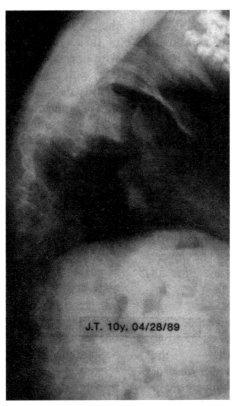

A,B

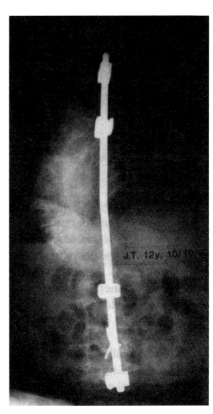

C

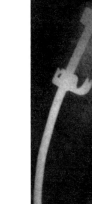
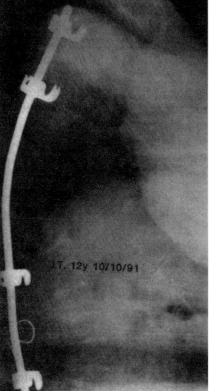

D

FIGURE 9. Posteroanterior **(A)** and lateral **(B)** sitting radiographs of the spine show severe curvature. Posteroanterior **(C)** and lateral **(D)** sitting radiographs obtained 2½ years postoperatively show limited Cotrel-Dubousset instrumentation supplemented with a sublaminar wire in the lumbar spine. Only minimal correction was achieved because of the quality of the bone. Lateral radiograph shows contouring of the rod. Adequate contouring prevents hook cutout from excessive kyphotic forces against a straight rod.

Complications, especially instrumentation problems, should be anticipated (37). (Medical pretreatment to improve bone stock may decrease some of these bone-instrument interface problems.) Because most of the patients are small and have low physical demands, postoperative immobilization may not be necessary, especially with the use of segmental instrumentation. However, a removable plastic brace may provide some support during healing of the fusion.

ANESTHETIC CONSIDERATIONS

Anesthetic management for patients with osteogenesis imperfecta can be challenging, especially for those undergoing major spinal surgery. Libman (22), drawing on extensive experience with patients with osteogenesis imperfecta at Shriners Hospitals for Children, Chicago, defined several areas of particular concern.

First, because of their fragility, these patients can sustain fractures during transfer from the stretcher to the operating table or while being positioned on the surgical frame. Intraoral manipulation can easily fracture abnormal teeth. Even the use of tourniquets for insertion of intravenous catheters and the use of blood pressure cuffs can cause fractures. Second, airway problems can be caused by the relatively large heads and tongues and short necks of these patients. Third, chest deformities interfere with normal respiratory mechanics and often impair pulmonary function. Because of deformities of the spine and extremities, normal measurements for the prediction of lung volumes may be inaccurate, making pulmonary function test results suspect. Last, there is a tendency toward hyperthermia and diaphoresis. This is not true malignant hyperthermia, but it can be nearly as severe and can be managed as such if it becomes serious. Hyperthermia is thought to be caused by hyperthyroidism among some patients. The hyperthermia can be induced by certain anesthetic agents and may be triggered by atropine. These children tend to be high-strung, and their natural nervousness and tendency to sweat seem to be exacerbated by atropine. In addition to avoidance of triggering agents, the usual methods for temperature control should be used. Dantrolene also can be used to prevent hyperthermia, but it is not recommended for routine use.

Standard anesthetic regimens can be used for patients with osteogenesis imperfecta, including controlled hypotension. When used as a paralyzing agent, however, succinylcholine can cause muscle fasciculation, which may cause fractures among patients with severe osteogenesis imperfecta. Therefore, succinylcholine should not be used at all or should be used only with pretreatment with a nondepolarizing agent. Although regional blocks can be used in operations on older patients, the deformities and bone fragility may make such use difficult. Close monitoring and careful handling are essential to avoid iatrogenic problems.

CRANIOCERVICAL AND CERVICAL ABNORMALITIES

Although there is a fair amount of information regarding deformity of the thoracolumbar spine (2–6,11,15,27,32,40,44),

fewer reports address problems of the craniocervical area and the cervical spine in osteogenesis imperfecta (6,11,12,18,21,29, 30,34,39,42,46). Most of the large series already cited either do not mention this area at all or state that no particular problems were seen. It is thus difficult to know the true incidence of such problems.

One of the most serious abnormalities that can occur is basilar impression, although many patients may have no symptoms. Pozo et al. (29) looked at three patients with basilar impression and reviewed their clinical histories. The weak bone of the craniocervical junction and the relatively large head often of patients with osteogenesis imperfecta both probably contribute to the development of basilar impression. When basilar impression occurs, the foramen magnum invaginates into the posterior fossa. This and medial migration of the occipital condyles cause stenosis and interfere with cerebrospinal fluid dynamics; the interference with flow of cerebrospinal fluid causes internal hydrocephalus. Direct compression of the cerebellum, brain stem, and upper cervical cord, various cranial nerve abnormalities, long-tract signs, and respiratory depression also can occur. Pozo et al. (29) found that their patients with basilar impression were not severely affected by osteogenesis imperfecta.

Harkey et al. (18) described the surgical management of basilar impression. They found that although the classic treatment is posterior decompression, this technique does not decompress the area sufficiently and often causes instability. These authors described the technique of anterior transoral decompression of the anterior arch of C1, the odontoid process, and part of the clivus. They suggested that the procedure be accompanied by a posterior occiput to cervical fusion with instrumentation. Unfortunately, they reported on only four patients. As an alternative to the transoral approach to anterior decompression, they also described the possibility of using LeFort midface osteotomy combined with the midline hard and soft palate split. They also suggested using internal fixation as an adjunct to posterior fusion. Recovery of function seems to be related to both the severity and duration of the symptoms.

Ziv et al. (46) reported on a patient who with paraplegia that developed at the thoracic level after a fall. The patient had been an independent ambulator. Because of neck pain and a history of low back pain, he underwent chiropractic manipulation but soon had progressive paralysis with sacral sparing. Evaluation showed C7–T1 spondyloptosis. The authors performed anterior decompression, but after walking in a halo vest, the patient again became paralyzed. Posterior decompression and fusion resulted in progressive improvement.

Ransford et al. (30) described posterior internal fixation from the skull to the cervical spine for patients with severe instability after decompression of basilar impression. They used a specially contoured Luque rod secured to the skull with wires through burr holes and sublaminar wires in the cervical spine. Because of subsequent spinal collapse, rendering the craniocervical junction unstable through decompression may cause recurrence of the neurologic deficit that was initially improved with the original decompression. This "second insult" should be avoided with stabilization of the spine at the index operation.

Frank et al. (12) and Wang et al. (42) described patients with respiratory depression due to basilar impression. Decompression

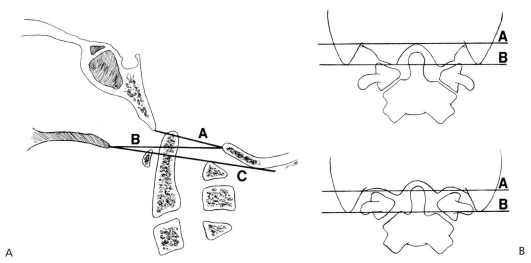

FIGURE 10. **A:** Drawing of lateral view of the craniocervical junction in basilar impression. Image shows position of the tip of the odontoid process with respect to the McRae line (*A*), Chamberlain line (*B*), and McGregor line (*C*). **B:** Drawing of open-mouth anteroposterior view of the craniocervical junction shows a line connecting the digastric grooves (*A*) and the Fishgold line (*B*), which joins the tips of the mastoid processes. The normal situation is depicted in the *top* drawing, and basilar impression in the *bottom.*

of the brain stem and shunting of the hydrocephalus resulted in improvement (12). The association of basilar impression, hydrocephalus, and hydrosyringomyelia has been reported by a number of authors (6,12,34,39)

The diagnosis of basilar impression is a radiographic one. A number of radiographic features are common to basilar impression from osteogenesis imperfecta and other causes. Upward migration of the cervical spine into the base of the skull (or descent of the skull onto the cervical spine) may be obvious, particularly on lateral cervical spinal radiographs. When the deformity is more subtle, however, various measurements on the

radiographs help make the diagnosis. The Chamberlain, McRae, and McGregor lines can be drawn on lateral cervical spinal radiographs (Fig. 10A). Protrusion of the odontoid process above these lines indicates basilar impression. On an anterior open-mouth radiograph or tomogram of the base of the skull, the Fishgold line can be drawn and should pass through the occiput-C1 junction (18) (Fig. 10B).

Somewhat more characteristic of basilar impression with osteogenesis imperfecta is the shape of the skull. Basically, two patterns are seen—the "tam-o'-shanter" and the "Darth Vader" (10,18) (Fig. 11A, B). The tam-o'-shanter skull is reminiscent

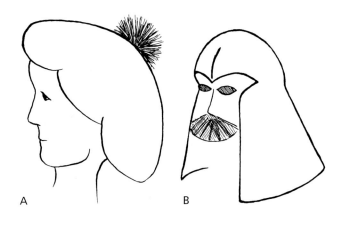

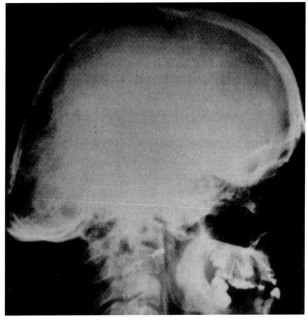

FIGURE 11. Drawing shows "tam-o'-shanter" **(A)** and a "Darth Vader" helmet **(B)**. **C:** Lateral radiograph of the skull and cervical spine of a child with severe osteogenesis imperfecta. Distortion of the craniocervical junction and overhang of the occipital bones of the skull (tam-o'-shanter) are evident.

of the floppy cap worn in Scotland. The anatomic reason for this appearance is overhang of the temporal and occipital bones (Fig. 11C). When the overhang is more acute and angular, flattening of the interparietal area gives the appearance of the helmet worn by Darth Vader of *Star Wars* fame (17).

In summary, even though patients with osteogenesis imperfecta may have severe thoracolumbar spine deformities, evaluation of the craniocervical junction and the cervical spine is especially important if such patients have neurologic signs and symptoms. Patients with mild forms of osteogenesis imperfecta may be the very ones to have such problems. The role of prophylactic decompression in the care of patients with radiographic evidence of basilar impression without appreciable symptoms is unclear. However, for patients with documented basilar impression with neurologic deficits, appropriate imaging studies followed by decompression of the neural elements and spinal stabilization are recommended.

SPONDYLOLYSIS AND SPONDYLOLISTHESIS

Because the bone of patients with osteogenesis imperfecta is weak enough to cause multiple compression fractures of the vertebrae, an increased incidence of spondylolysis and spondylolisthesis (with pars defect or elongation of pars or pedicles) is expected (Fig. 12). It makes sense that an isthmic type—Wiltse type ID (28)—fracture could easily occur with the usual stresses found at the lumbosacral junction. A number of authors have described a few cases of spondylolysis and spondylolisthesis (2,17,20,29,41,43). Many series dealing with spinal deformity in osteogenesis imperfecta do not mention problems of spondy-

lolysis or spondylolisthesis at all. Rask (31) described a single case of a 4-year-old with mild osteogenesis imperfecta, but disorder was probably traumatic. Wiltse (43) stated that "defects in the pars in children with [osteogenesis imperfecta] seem to occur too frequently," but he did not have any statistics to support that statement. Barrack et al (1) described spondylolysis in a patient who had undergone posterior spinal fusion with instrumentation, but the spondylolysis probably was iatrogenic. It is evident from this review that either the incidence of spondylolysis and spondylolisthesis is truly low or these conditions are just not recognized or do not cause symptoms.

The literature contains no reports of specific therapy for these problems in osteogenesis imperfecta. However, Barrack et al. (1) mentioned that among their patients the preexisting fusion was extended to the sacrum. Isolated spondylolysis or spondylolisthesis that is progressive or symptomatic (unresponsive to nonoperative measures) should be managed by means of appropriate posterior lateral spinal fusion after appropriate imaging studies (5). The use of instrumentation is dictated by the size of the vertebrae and the quality of bone. Posterior spinal fusion for scoliosis that extends low into the lumbosacral spine probably should extend across the lumbosacral junction in an effort to eliminate the stress of a long fusion over only one or two mobile segments. The loss of these motion segments, particularly by a patient who does not walk who has severe involvement, would do little to decrease function. However, this approach may decrease the likelihood of development of either spondylolysis or spondylolisthesis or compression injury below the fusion. The incidence of pseudarthrosis across the lumbosacral junction in these situations cannot be determined with the available literature.

SPINAL FRACTURES

The abnormal bone of osteogenesis imperfecta is said to be weak, and that fact is offered as one of the causes of spinal deformity. The typical ligamentous laxity and repeated microfractures without substantial trauma cause progressive collapse of the vertebral bodies. This gives them a typical codfish appearance, which can progress to a wedge shape with further deformity (2–4,23). It is also observed, at least among younger patients, that the intervertebral discs are stronger than the vertebral bodies, and their shape is preserved even in the presence of surrounding vertebral body compression.

None of the references cited at the end of this chapter mention anything about truly traumatic fractures of the thoracolumbar spine. Two reports, however, described fractures of the cervical spine (23,33). The progressive collapse of the spine caused by compression fractures often is mentioned. It is common knowledge that postmenopausal osteoporosis can cause recurrent compression fractures, even among women without other systemic diseases. This process can be extensive. In the presence of preexisting scoliosis or kyphosis, it can cause severe deformity. Paterson et al. (28) reviewed the records of 65 adult patients with osteogenesis imperfecta and found that the incidence of fractures of all types increased after menopause. The fracture rate among postmenopausal women was seven times that of the

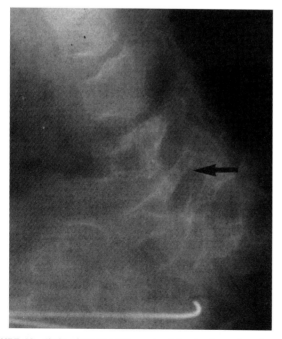

FIGURE 12. Sitting lateral radiograph of the lumbar spine shows severe elongation of the pedicle of the lower lumbar spine (*arrow*).

general population. The incidence of backache, loss of height, and scoliosis was higher among women than among men. The authors concluded that spinal fractures are a major cause of disability among older women with osteogenesis imperfecta. Even those who had apparently mild disease as children can have severe problems after menopause. Girls with osteogenesis imperfecta should therefore be counseled and should seek the help of an endocrinologist to begin early treatment to avoid age- and hormone-related bone loss.

There is no reason to believe that patients with osteogenesis imperfecta cannot sustain traumatic spinal fractures. No series of such patients is mentioned in the literature. Among the many patients treated at the Shriners Hospitals for Children, Chicago, including those with compression fractures, only one had an unstable fracture that necessitated surgical treatment (Fig. 13).

Patients with acute compression fractures that are not believed to be unstable after appropriate imaging should be treated with the usual measures. These measures include an initial period of bed rest with gradual mobilization with external support. When there are preexisting compression and osteoporosis, it is sometimes difficult to determine when healing has occurred. In these situations, an arbitrary period of support can be prescribed and correlated with symptoms of back pain. Patients with unstable fractures or who have neurologic deficits should be treated

as any other patient with a spinal fracture. The technical points mentioned with regard to scoliosis should be applied to those with fractures. Adequate anterior column support must be provided to patients with traumatic kyphosis and vertebral body crush. Segmental posterior instrumentation offers the most secure fixation. Even in situations in which segmental spinal instrumentation of one kind or another is used, postoperative external support may be indicated.

SUMMARY

Spinal problems in osteogenesis imperfecta run the gamut of spinal deformity, craniocervical abnormalities, spondylolysis or spondylolisthesis, and spine fractures. It appears that bracing is not effective in controlling progressive spinal deformity. In such situations, spinal fusion with instrumentation, preferably segmental instrumentation, should be used to control the deformity. This should be done when curves demonstrate that they are progressive and before severe deformity occurs, because significant correction cannot be anticipated (Figs. 14, 15). Craniocervical problems are uncommon but may cause catastrophic neurologic problems. Early recognition of basilar impression and prompt decompression and stabilization of the craniocervical

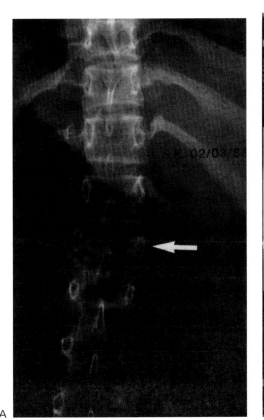

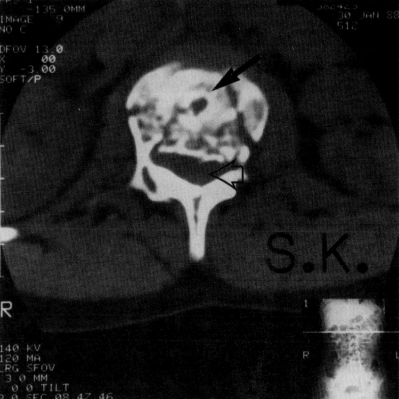

A   B

FIGURE 13. **A:** Supine anteroposterior radiograph of the thoracolumbar spine of an 18-year-old patient with mild to moderate osteogenesis imperfecta. Widening of the pedicles of L1 (*arrow*) and loss of height of L1 are evident. **B:** Axial computed tomographic (CT) image at L1 shows the burst component of the vertebral body (*solid arrow*) and canal compromise (*open arrow*). *(Figure continues.)*

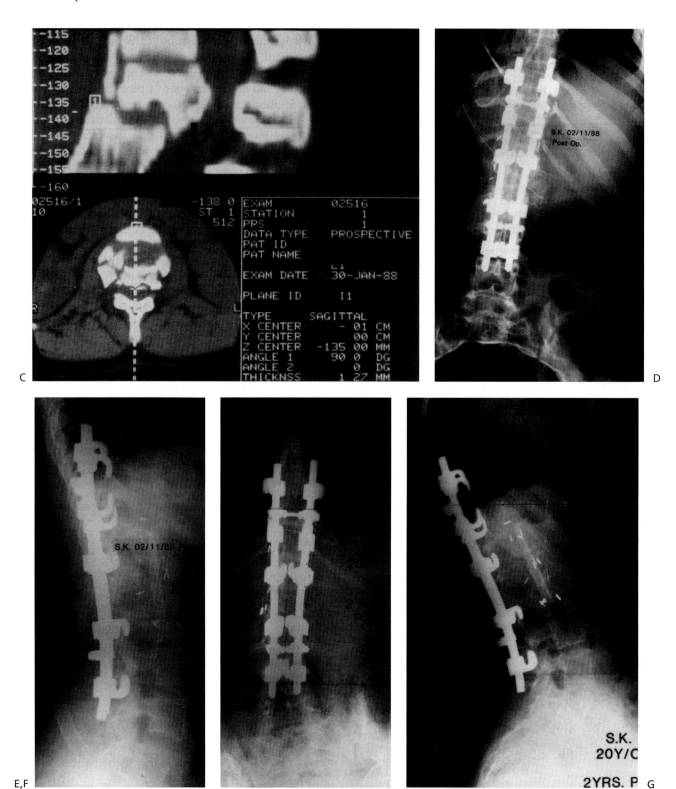

FIGURE 13. *Continued.* **C:** Lateral CT reconstruction shows the canal compromise (*arrow*) and the overall kyphotic alignment at that level. Anteroposterior **(D)** and lateral **(E)** radiographs after posterior instrumentation and realignment of the spine and anterior decompression with strut grafting. Anatomic alignment is evident on the anteroposterior image and preservation of the sagittal contour on the lateral image. Posteroanterior **(F)** and lateral **(G)** standing radiographs 2 years after the operation. In the area of previous instrumentation, the spine remains in the correct anatomic position. Pelvic obliquity due to leg length discrepancy is present on the posteroanterior image (the patient sustained a tibial fracture with shortening about 1 year after the spinal fracture). The lateral image shows preservation of the sagittal contour and incorporation of the fibular graft.

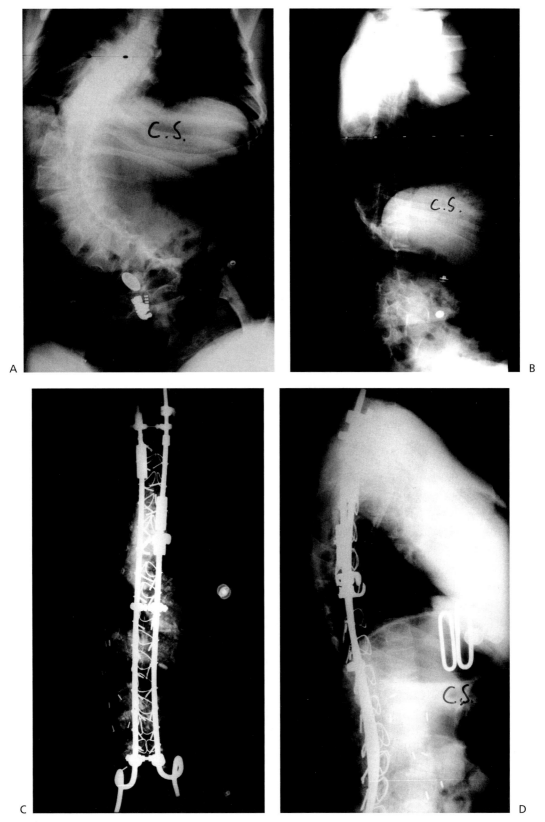

FIGURE 14. Images of a 16 year-old girl with osteogenesis imperfecta who had progressive thoracolumbar scoliosis. Although she had many long-bone fractures and had undergone surgical therapy for them, the patient could walk. Posteroanterior **(A)** and lateral **(B)** radiographs show severe left thoracolumbar scoliosis with pelvic obliquity and an abnormal sagittal contour, respectively. The sacrum is deformed and horizontally oriented, the L5 pedicles are elongated, and the L5–S1 disc is oriented vertically. Posteroanterior **(C)** and lateral **(D)** radiographs after staged anterior release and fusion followed by posterior fusion and Cotrel-Dubousset instrumentation supplemented with sublaminar wires. Coronal correction is excellent, and the sagittal contour has normalized. Dunn-McCarthy pelvic fixation was used in this construct.

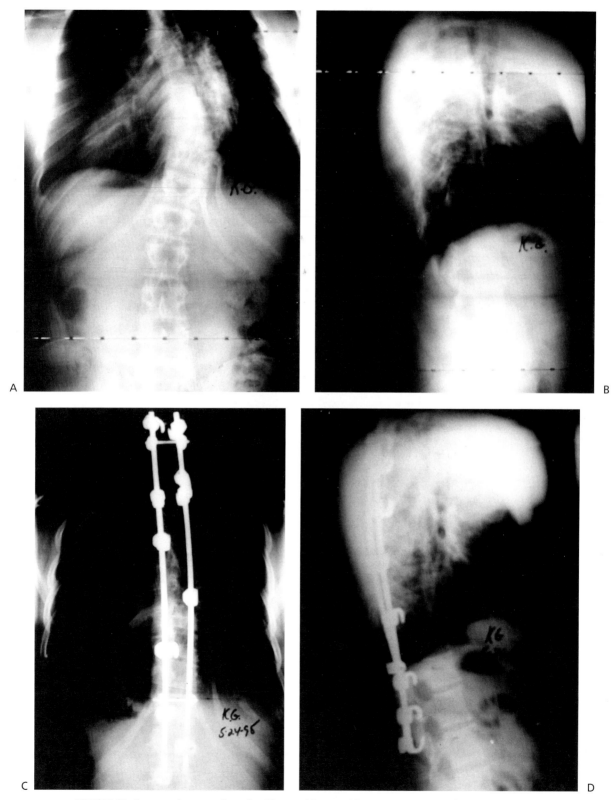

FIGURE 15. Images of a normally active 18-year-old man with osteogenesis imperfecta show normal stature despite multiple long-bone fractures as a child. The scoliotic deformity gradually increased and was associated with a large right rib hump. Posteroanterior **(A)** and lateral **(B)** radiographs show right thoracic curve with a structural left upper thoracic component. The normal thoracic kyphosis is flattened. Posteroanterior **(C)** and lateral **(D)** radiographs show the correction and balance achieved after posterior fusion, right thoracoplasty, and use of Moss-Miami instrumentation. Coronal correction and balance are quite good, and the sagittal contour has been improved.

junction improve symptoms and prevent the instability of the upper cervical spine that occurs with decompression only. Commonsense management of spondylolysis or spondylolisthesis and spinal fractures is indicated in the care of patients with osteogenesis imperfecta. Patients with osteogenesis imperfecta have peculiar physiologic characteristics that necessitate special attention during anesthesia. Careful handling of these fragile patients is essential. A whole new era of medical management of osteogenesis imperfecta appears to be dawning. Improvement in the quality of bone may preclude the development of deformity, lessen its severity, or at least make the bone stronger so that spinal instrumentation can be more secure if surgery is needed. Only time will tell how effective this kind of therapy will be.

REFERENCES

1. Barrack R, Whitecloud TS, Skinner HB (1984): Spondylolysis after spinal instrumentation in osteogenesis imperfecta. *South Med J* 11: 1453–1454.
2. Bathgate B, Moseley CF (1990): Scoliosis in osteogenesis imperfecta. *Spine State Art Rev* 4:121–130.
3. Benson DR, Donaldson DH, Millar EA (1978): The spine in osteogenesis imperfecta. *J Bone Joint Surg Am* 60:925–929.
4. Benson DR, Newman DC (1981): The spine and surgical treatment in osteogenesis imperfecta. *Clin Orthop* 159:147–153.
5. Bradford DS (1987): Osteogenesis imperfecta. In: *Moe's textbook of scoliosis and other spinal deformities,* 2nd ed. Philadelphia: WB Saunders.
6. Charnas LR, Marini JC (1993): Communicating hydrocephalus, basilar invagination and other neurologic features in osteogenesis imperfecta. *Neurology* 43:2603–2608.
7. Cristofaro RL, Hoek KJ, Bonnett CA, et al. (1979): Operative treatment of spine deformities in osteogenesis imperfecta. *Clin Orthop* 139: 40–48.
8. Davie MWJ, Haddaway MJ (1994): Bone mineral content and density in healthy subjects and in osteogenesis imperfecta. *Arch Dis Child* 70: 331–334.
9. Donaldson DH (1991): Spinal deformity associated with osteogenesis imperfecta. In: Bridwell KH, DeWald RL, eds. *Textbook of spinal surgery.* Philadelphia: JB Lippincott, pp. 491–498.
10. Engelbert RH, Gerver WJM, Breslau-Sideris LJ, et al. (1998): Spinal complications in osteogenesis imperfecta. *Acta Orthop Scand* 69: 283–286.
11. Falvo K, Root L, Bullough P (1974): Osteogenesis imperfecta: clinical evaluation and management. *J Bone Joint Surg Am* 56:783–793.
12. Frank E, Berger T, Tew Jr JM (1982): Basilar impression and platybasia in osteogenesis imperfecta. *Surg Neurology* 17:116–119.
13. Frater CJ, Murray IPC, Calligeros D (1995): Multiple flexion-stress vertebral end-plate fractures: an osteogenesis imperfecta presentation. *Clin Nucl Med* 20:1055–1057.
14. Fredericks BJ, de Campo JF, Sephton R, et al. (1990): Computed tomographic assessment of vertebral bone mineral in childhood. *Skeletal Radiol* 19:99–102.
15. Gitelis S, Whiffen J, DeWald RL (1983): The treatment of severe scoliosis in osteogenesis imperfecta: case report. *Clin Orthop* 175: 56–59.
16. Glorieux FH, Bishop NJ, Plotkin H, et al. (1998): Cyclic administration of pamidronate in children with severe osteogenesis imperfecta. *N Engl J Med* 339:947–952.
17. Hanscom DA, Bloom, BA (1988): The spine in osteogenesis imperfecta. *Orthop Clin North Am* 19:449–458.
18. Harkey HL, Crochard HA, Stevens JM, et al. (1990): The operative management of basilar impression in osteogenesis imperfecta. *Neurosurgery* 27:782–785.
19. Herron LD, Dawson EG (1977): Methylmethacrylate as an adjunct in spinal instrumentation. *J Bone Joint Surg Am* 59:866–868.
20. King JD, Bobechko WP (1971): Osteogenesis imperfecta: an orthopaedic description and surgical review. *J Bone Joint Surg Br* 53:72–89.
21. Kurimoto M, Ohara S, Takaku A (1991): Basilar impression in osteogenesis imperfecta tarda: a case report. *J Neurosurg* 74:136–138.
22. Libman RH (1981): Anesthetic considerations for the patient with osteogenesis imperfecta. *Clin Orthop* 159:123–125.
23. Meyer S, Villarreal M, Zio I (1986): A three-level fracture of the axis in a patient with osteogenesis imperfecta. *Spine* 11:505–506.
24. Moore MS, Minch CM, Kruse RW, et al. (1998): The role of dual energy x-ray absorptiometry in aiding the diagnosis of pediatric osteogenesis imperfecta. *Am J Orthop* 27:797–801.
25. Moorefield WG, Miller GR (1980): Aftermath of osteogenesis imperfecta: the disease in adulthood. *J Bone Joint Surg Am* 62:113–119.
26. Nagant de Deuxchaisnes CN, Devogelaer JP, Depresseux G, et al. (1990): Treatment of vertebral crush fracture syndrome with enteric-coated fluoride tablets and calcium supplements. *J Bone Miner Res* [5 Suppl]:S5–26.
27. Norimatsu H, Mayuzumi T, Takahashi H (1982): The development of spinal deformities in osteogenesis imperfecta. *Clin Orthop* 162:20–25.
28. Paterson CR, McAllion S, Stellman JL (1984): Osteogenesis imperfecta after the menopause. *N Engl J Med* 310:1694–1696.
29. Pozo JL, Crockard A, Ransford AO (1984): Basilar impression in osteogenesis imperfecta: a report of three cases in one family. *J Bone Joint Surg* 66:233–238.
30. Ransford AO, Crockard HA, Pozo JL, et al. (1986): Craniocervical instability treated by contoured loop fixation. *J Bone Joint Surg Br* 68: 173–177.
31. Rask MR (1979): Spondylolisthesis resulting from osteogenesis imperfecta. *Clin Orthop* 139:164–166.
32. Renshaw T, Cook R, Albright J (1979): Scoliosis in osteogenesis imperfecta. *Clin Orthop* 145:163–167.
33. Rush GA, Burke SW (1984): Hangman's fracture in a patient with osteogenesis imperfecta. *J Bone Joint Surg Am* 66:778–779.
34. Sawin PD, Menezes AH (1997): Basilar invagination in osteogenesis imperfecta and related osteochondrodysplasias: medical and surgical management. *J Neurosurg* 86:950–960.
35. Sillence D (1981): Osteogenesis imperfecta: an expanding panorama of variants. *Clin Orthop* 159:11–25.
36. Sillence D, Sean A, Denha DM (1979): Genetic heterogenecity in osteogenesis imperfecta. *J Med Genet* 16:101–116.
37. Sperry K (1989): Fatal intraoperative hemorrhage during spinal fusion for osteogenesis imperfecta. *Am J Forensic Med Pathol* 10:54–59.
38. Stoltz MR, Dietrich GL, Marshall JG (1989): Osteogenesis imperfecta: perspectives. *Clin Orthop* 242:120–136.
39. Tanaka T, Yamazaki Y, Mii K, et al. (1996): Syringomyelia with basilar impression in osteogenesis imperfecta. *Acta Neurochir (Wien)* 138: 888–889.
40. Trotter D (1986): Spinal fusion for scoliosis in osteogenesis imperfecta: the Chicago Shriners Hospital experience [abstract]. *Orthop Trans* 10: 28.
41. Versfeld GA, Beighton PH, Katz K, et al. (1985): Costovertebral anomalies in osteogenesis imperfecta. *J Bone Joint Surg Br* 67:602–604.
42. Wang TG, Yang GFW, Alba A (1994): Chronic ventilator use in osteogenesis imperfecta congenita with basilar impression: a case report. *Arch Phys Med Rehabil* 75:699–702.
43. Wiltse LL (1977): Spondylolisthesis and its treatment. In: Ruge D, Wiltse LL, eds. *Spinal disorders, diagnosis and treatment.* Philadelphia: Lea & Febiger, p. 193–217.
44. Yong-Hing K, MacEwen GD (1982): Scoliosis associated with osteogenesis imperfecta. *J Bone Joint Surg Br* 64:36–43.
45. Zaleske DJ, Doppelt SH, Mandin HJ (1990): Metabolic and endocrine abnormalities of the immature skeleton. In: Morrissy RT, ed. *Lovell and Winter's pediatric orthopaedics.* Philadelphia: JB Lippincott, 229–233.
46. Ziv I, Rang M, Hoffman HJ (1983): Paraplegia in osteogenesis imperfecta: a case report. *J Bone Joint Surg Br* 65:184–185.

MUCOPOLYSACCHARIDOSIS, MUCOLIPIDOSIS, AND HOMOCYSTINURIA

JOHN F. SARWARK
CARL DIRAIMONDO

MUCOPOLYSACCHARIDOSIS

Mucopolysaccharidosis (MPS), Hurler syndrome in particular, presents unmistakable signs and symptoms. These include blindness, hoarseness, pasty complexion, large ears, bushy eyebrows, hypertelorism, a snub nose, open mouth, prognathism, hirsutism, clawed fingers, a pot belly, knock knees, flat feet, knobby jointed, dwarfism, and mental retardation. Abnormality of a macromolecular storage substance causes the nonosseous features of this fatal recessive disease (30,38,53,118,121,125).

MPS is a family of recessively inherited diseases that have as a common feature a defect in lysosomal storage (83,84,96,126). Mucopolysaccharides accumulate as a result of deficiencies of specific degradative enzymes. There is a wide spectrum of clinical severity not only from one type to another but also within the various types (16,57) (Fig. 1).

Mucopolysaccharides are linked to specific noncollagenous proteins and in combination with collagen form the matrix of connective tissue. The mucopolysaccharide unit or glycosaminoglycan consists of a core protein to which side chains of polysaccharides are attached. The polysaccharide chains consist of repeating disaccharide units. The polymers of disaccharides are specific to each type of glycosaminoglycan.

The three mucopolysaccharides that accumulate in the MPS syndromes are dermatan sulfate, heparan sulfate, and keratan sulfate (108). The sites of specific enzyme defects on a portion of the polysaccharide chain of dermatan sulfate and heparan sulfate are shown in Table 1. Morquio syndrome (type IV MPS) is a defect of catabolism of keratan sulfate (50,55,101), which is present only in cartilage, nucleus pulposus, and cornea (57). The characteristics of all types of MPS are summarized in Table 2.

Hurler Syndrome and Scheie Syndrome

Hurler syndrome (type IH MPS) is synonymous with gargoylism, dysostosis multiplex, or lipochondrodystrophy. Scheie syndrome (type IS MPS, formerly type V) is a relatively milder variant of Hurler syndrome. There is also an intermediate form—Hurler-Scheie compound (type I H/S MPS). Recessive mutations are responsible for these disorders, and they rarely occur. The incidence of type IH MPS is estimated to be 1: 100,000, type I H/S MPS to be 1:112,000 to 1:500,000, and type IS MPS to be 1:500,000 (35,40,77,133).

Etiology

Hurler and Scheie syndromes are caused by an enzyme deficiency in the same enzyme, α-L-iduronidase, required to degrade both heparin sulfate and dermatan sulfate (9,10,110,129,144). The degree of enzyme deficiency varies, resulting in the three forms of the disorder.

Clinical Features and Pathologic Anatomy

Hurler syndrome is characterized by short stature, severe and progressive mental deterioration, and grotesque facies with protruding eyes, thick jaws, and a large tongue. The joints are stiff and cannot be fully extended. A thoracolumbar kyphotic deformity is common because the vertebral bodies are small (76). Mild scoliosis also can occur (129). Children often have recurrent upper respiratory infections. Corneal clouding is present, as are hepatomegaly and splenomegaly. Cardiomegaly also may be present. There is a normal appearance at birth (32). The bone changes of dysostosis multiplex (multiple radiographic skeletal abnormalities) begin by 6 months of age among infants with Hurler syndrome, 1 to 2 years among children with Hurler-Scheie syndrome, and 7 to 10 years among children with Scheie syndrome.

The skeletal changes of Hurler syndrome include severe dysostosis multiplex with gibbus deformity. In Hurler-Scheie syndrome, mild to moderate dysostosis multiplex occurs with no gibbus deformity. In Scheie syndrome, there are mild dysostosis multiplex and no gibbus deformity. Hurler syndrome appears to be associated with an increased incidence of hypoplasia of the odontoid process and the presence of abnormal, excess soft tissue adjacent to the odontoid process (132,136).

J.F. Sarwark and C. DiRaimondo: Division of Orthopedic Surgery, The Children's Memorial Hospital, Chicago, Illinois 60614 and Department of Orthopedic Surgery, Northwestern University, Chicago, Illinois 60611.

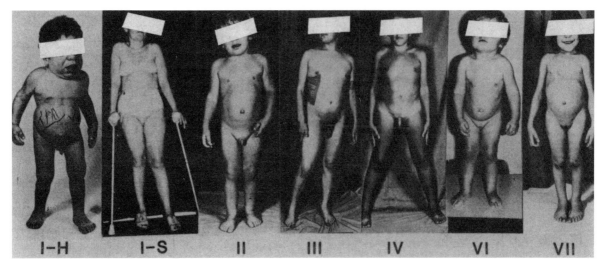

FIGURE 1. Clinical appearance of patients with various types of mucopolysaccharidosis (MPS). *IH*, Eight-year-old patient with Hurler syndrome. *IS*, Adult with Scheie syndrome. *II*, Three-year-old patient with Hunter syndrome. *III*, Eighteen-year-old patient with Sanfilippo A syndrome. *IV*, Twelve-year-old patients with Morquio A syndrome. The patient is standing with spread legs to prevent the femoral heads from slipping out of the acetabular fossae. *VI*, Four-year-old patient with Maroteaux-Lamy syndrome. *VII*, Eight-year-old patient with MPS VII. (From, with permission from ref. 120a.)

TABLE 1. SITES OF SPECIFIC ENZYMATIC DEFECTS IN GLYCOSAMINOGLYCAN CATABOLISM IN MUCOPOLYSACCHARIDOSIS INVOLVING HEPARAN SULFATE AND DERMATAN SULFATE

Heparan sulfate	
–IA–	
1NAcGlc	
4–GA–	
6NAc	
4Glc	
1–IA–	
4NAcGLc–	
SO_4^2	SO_4^3
Dermatan sulfate	
–IA–NAc	
1Gal–GA–	
6NAcGal	
1–IA-NAcGal–	
SO_4^2	SO_4^5

Enzyme	Mucopolysaccharidosis
α-L-iduronidase	I
Sulfoiduronide sulfatase	II
Sulfoglucosamine sulfatase	IIIA
N-acetyl-α-D-glucosaminidase	IIIB
Glucosamine-6-sulfatase	IIID
N-Acetylgalactosamine-6-sulfate	IVA
β-Galactosidase	IVB

Information from Baker E, Guo X, Orsborn AM, et al. (1993): The Morquio syndrome (mucopolysaccharidosis IVA) gene maps to 16q24.3. *Am J Hum Genet* 52:96–98. Kelly TE (1978): The mucopolysaccharidoses and mucolipidoses. *Clin Orthop* 114:116–136. Nakashima Y, Tomatsu S, Hori T, et al. (1994): Mucopolysaccharidosis IVA: molecular cloning of the human *N*-acetylgalactosamin-6-sulfatase gene (GALNS) and analysis of the 5'-flanking region. *Genomics* 20:99–104.

There is a high incidence of airway problems in association with Hurler syndrome. Factors that contribute to airway problems include thickening of the soft tissues of the oropharynx, narrow nasal airway, narrow trachea, short neck and trunk, kyphoscoliosis, and hepatomegaly. Careful preoperative assessment by an experienced anesthesiologist helps to minimize the potential for airway complications (7,102,106,112,143).

The ultimate height in types IH and IH/S MPS is short, but height is normal in type IS MPS. Intelligence is normal in type IS MPS and normal to mildly retarded in MPS IH/S. Fibroblast studies demonstrate deficiency of α-L-iduronidase activity in all forms of type I MPS (37,129).

Radiographic Features and Findings of Other Imaging Studies

The chief radiographic features relating to the spine are hook-shaped vertebrae on the anterior surface; small vertebral bodies, especially at the thoracolumbar region; and thoracolumbar gibbus (23) (Figs. 2, 3). The beaking defect is seen at T12-L2, and the greatest defect is superior and anterior. When C1–2 subluxation occurs, failure of development or hypoplasia of the dens is best seen on lateral radiographs of the cervical spine (25,145).

Calcification of the stylohyoid ligament is frequent among children with Hurler syndrome (150). The ligament is normally calcified to some extent in approximately 25% of all children. When calcification occurs among healthy children, the ossification pattern is a relatively thin configuration. Calcification is a helpful sign in the radiographic examination of children believed to have MPS, but it does not have an appreciable clinical effect (92).

TABLE 2. CHARACTERISTICS OF MUCOPOLYSACCHARIDOSIS

Mucopoly-saccharidosis	Eponym Mucopoly-sacchariduria Abnormality	Enzyme Defect	Inheritance	Chromosomal	Location	Life Expectancy (y)	Intelligence	Spinal
IH	Hurler syndrome	α-L-iduronidase	AR	*4p16.3*	DS, HS	6–10	MR	Thoracolumbar kyphosis, hypoplasia of odontoid process, lumbar gibbus
IS	Scheie syndrome	α-L-iduronidase	AR	—	DS, HS	Normal	Normal	No gibbus
IH/S	Hurler Scheie syndrome	α-L-iduronidase	AR	—	DS, HS	20s	Mild MR	No gibbus
II	Severe Hunter syndrome	L-iduronate sulfatase	XR	*Xq28*	DS, HS	Teens	MR	Thoracolumbar kyphosis
II mild	Hunter syndrome	L-iduronate sulfatase	XR	—	DS, HS	Adulthood–normal	Normal	Thoracolumbar kyphosis
III A	Sanfilippo syndrome	2-deoxyglucoside-2-sulfamate sulfatase	AR	—	HS	Teens–20s	MR	Minimal
III B	Sanfilippo syndrome	α-N-acetyl-glucosaminidase	AR	17	HS	Teens–20s	MR	Minimal
III D	—		—	12q14				
IVA	Morquio syndrome	N-acetylgalactosamine-6-sulfate sulfatase	AR	*16q24.3*	KS	20–40	Normal	Platyspondyly, odontoid dysplasia, C1-2 instability, lumbar gibbus
IVB	Morquio syndrome	β-galactosidase	AR	3p21.33	—	20–50	Normal	Milder, but similar to IVA
V	Formerly Scheie syndrome	—	—	—	—	—	—	—
VI severe	Maroteaux-Lamy syndrome	arylsulfatase B	AR	5q31.3	DS	10–20	Normal	Cervical myeleopathy, lumbar radiculopathy, dural thickening, lumbar gibbus
VI mild	Maroteaux-Lamy syndrome	arylsulfatase B	AR	—	DS	20s–normal	Normal	Milder but similar to VI severe
VII	Sly syndrome	β-Glucuronidase	AR	7q21.11	DS	Restricted (? degree)	MR	Thoracolumbar kyphosis, kyphoscoliosis

AR, autosomal recessive; DS, dermatan sulfate; HS, heparan sulfate; MR, mental retardation; XR, X-linked recessive; KS, keratan sulfate.
Information from Baker E, Guo X, Orsborn AM, et al. (1993): The Morquio syndrome (mucopolysaccharidosis IVA) gene maps to 16q24.3. *Am J Hum Genet* 52:96–98. Dietz FR, Mathews KD (1996): Current concepts review: update on the genetic bases of disorders with orthopaedic manifestations. *J Bone Joint Surg Am* 78:1583–1598. Kelly TE (1978): The mucopolysaccharidoses and mucolipidoses. *Clin Orthop* 114:116–136. Levin TL, Berdon WE, Lachman RS, et al. (1997): Lumbar gibbus deformity in storage diseases and bone dysplasias. *Pediatr Radiol* 27:289–294.

Treatment

Primary therapy for Hurler syndrome is bone marrow transplantation. The greatest benefit is gained when transplantation is performed early (34,93,147).

Course of Disease

The course of type IH MPS is rapid progression to death before 10 years of age. In type IH/S MPS, there is intermediate progression of disease. Slow progression occurs in type IS MPS (129).

Hunter Syndrome

Type II MPS, or Hunter syndrome, is another form of dysostosis multiplex in which the characteristic skeletal changes develop more slowly than they do in type IH MPS, but they can become severe in adolescence (39,122). Hunter syndrome appears to have a wide spectrum of clinical manifestations (82,138). Three forms of Hunter syndrome are generally recognized: type IIAXR MPS, the severe form; type IIBXR MPS, the mild form; and type IIAR MPS, the autosomal recessive form.

Epidemiology and Etiology

Hunter syndrome is rare. One estimate is an incidence of 0.66 cases per 100,000 births (82). This is the only sex-linked recessive lysosomal storage disease. All reported patients have been boys (39,51,91,142). Hunter syndrome is caused by a deficiency of L-iduronate sulfatase. Persons with this syndrome store large

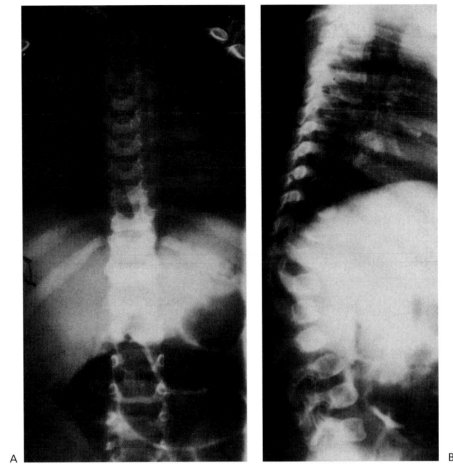

FIGURE 2. A: Hurler-Scheie syndrome. **B:** Hurler-Scheie syndrome with mild thoracolumbar kyphosis and minimal dysplastic changes.

amounts of sulfated acidic glycosaminoglycans (dermatan sulfate and heparan sulfate) in the tissues and excrete them in urine. Inheritance of all the other known MPS syndromes is autosomal recessive.

Clinical Features and Pathologic Anatomy

The clinical phenotype in type II MPS is less severe than in Hurler syndrome (39). Life span is longer, and mental deficiency is not as severe. The mild and severe phenotypes have been reported to occur within the same set of siblings (148). Extensive multisystem involvement occurs, including papilledema, upper airway obstruction, and degenerative changes at the hip (39). Cervical stenosis caused by dural thickening and cervical kyphosis have been reported. A case has been reported of isolated neurogenic bladder as the only initial symptom of cervical stenosis (65,103,141).

Radiographic Features and Findings of Other Imaging Studies

The skeletal changes of dysostosis multiplex are similar to those of Hurler syndrome, but the findings are less severe and develop more slowly (Fig. 4). The skeletal changes may become severe among adolescents. Thoracolumbar kyphosis occurs with development and is associated with a hooklike deformity of the upper lumbar vertebrae on the anterior surface. This may occur among patients as young as 2 years (133). Ventriculomegaly, atrophy of the brain, cystic lesions within the brain stem, periodontoid soft-tissue thickening, and disc dehydration in association with platyspondylisis all have been found at magnetic resonance imaging (MRI) of the brain and spinal cord (Fig. 5) (98,103).

Course of Disease

The life span of patients with Hunter syndrome is longer than that of patients with Hurler syndrome (39). One long-term report discussed the findings for a 31-year-old man. Although he had no signs or symptoms of spine-related problems, life-threatening complications, including laryngeal edema and tracheal narrowing, did occur. The patient also had recurrent episodes of chest infection and painful degenerative arthritis in both hips (149). Treatment options are limited, but there have been reports of successful bone marrow transplantation that eased some of the clinical manifestations of Hunter syndrome (17).

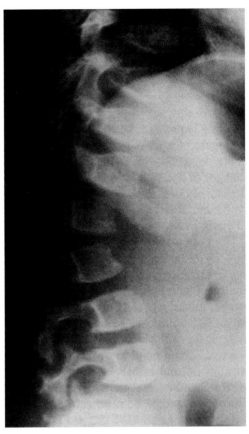

FIGURE 3. Hurler-Scheie syndrome with mild thoracolumbar kyphosis. The hook shape of the anterior surface of the vertebrae is evident.

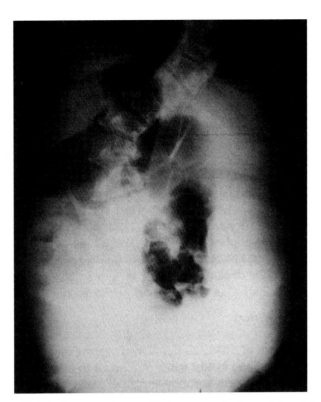

FIGURE 4. Hunter syndrome with less severe findings of dysostosis multiplex. Scoliosis is severe.

Sanfilippo Syndrome

Sanfilippo syndrome (type III MPS with subtypes A, B, C, and D) is a lysosomal storage disease characterized by mental retardation and relatively mild somatic involvement.

Epidemiology and Etiology

It is generally agreed that Sanfilippo syndrome is the most common form of MPS, which is rare in all its forms (3,120,139). A series in the Netherlands had 75 patients, for an incidence of 1:24,000 (139). The enzyme deficiencies of Sanfilippo syndrome are divided into four biochemical types, designated as types A, B, C, and D. The inactive enzymes are 2-deoxyglucoside-2-sulfamate sulfatase in type A; α-*N*-acetylglucosaminidase in type B; acetyl-coenzyme:α-glucosaminide *N*-acetyl-transferase in type C; and *N*-acetylglucosamine-6-sulfate sulfatase in type D (31,56). All diseases are transmitted in an autosomal recessive mode. The enzyme deficiencies impair heparan sulfate metabolism, and this glycosaminoglycan accumulates in many different tissues and organs. Large amounts of heparan sulfate are detected in the urine of patients with Sanfilippo syndrome (31).

Clinical Features and Pathologic Anatomy

Mental retardation with relatively mild somatic involvement characterizes Sanfilippo syndrome. In general, early development

is normal but is followed by progressive, severe deterioration. These children are not strikingly dwarfed, the corneas are not clouded, and joint stiffness is mild (46). Changes of dysostosis multiplex are minimal, and the skeleton may be normal. The enzyme activity in fibroblasts may not be a true reflection of the in vivo activity in the liver, brain, skin, and other tissues. Variability in enzyme activity from organ to organ may explain the differences in progression (56).

Orthopedic problems, including severe kyphoscoliosis, have been reported in a follow-up study of adult patients with MPS III B (107).

Radiographic Features and Findings of Other Imaging Studies

Radiographs show minimal changes of dysostosis multiplex. Results of the skeletal radiographic evaluation may be nearly normal. Thickening of the calvaria occurs. Irregular configuration of the lumbar vertebral bodies and occasionally T11 or T12, including an ovoid shape on the lateral projection in the thoracic and lumbar areas, is reported (31,68). This mild radiographic abnormality has not been associated with gibbus deformity (36). One of the involved vertebrae may be hypoplastic or retroplaced (68). The transverse process may be hypoplastic. One patient in a long-term follow-up study was found to have severe kyphoscoliosis (140). The ribs may be thickened.

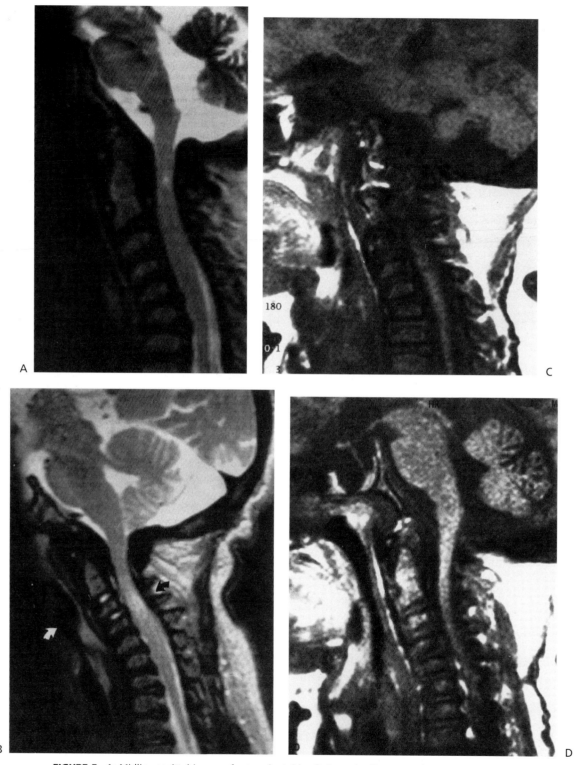

FIGURE 5. A: Midline sagittal image of retroodontoid soft tissue leading to cord compression shows high signal changes in the cord and a giant cisterna magna. **B:** Sagittal image shows high signal changes in the cord (*black arrow*), upper airway narrowing (*white arrow*), and platyspondylysis. **C:** Parasagittal image shows the low signal cystic areas in the thalamus. **D:** Sagittal image shows abnormal ossification of the odontoid peg with thickening of the parapharyngeal soft tissues. (From Parsons VJ, Hughes DG, Wraith JE [1996]: Magnetic resonance imaging of the brain, neck, and cervical spine in mild Hunter syndrome (mucopolysaccharidosis type II). *Clin Radiol* 51:719–723, with permission.)

Course of Disease

Because of the small number of reports of children with Sanfilippo syndrome, it is difficult to make a specific prognosis for duration and quality of life (59). The onset of detectable abnormalities occurs in early childhood. Mental deterioration begins by school age and becomes severe in the teens. Survival past the age of 40 years has been reported among persons with mild Sanfilippo B disease. All patients in that report had severe mentally retardation, as is usually the case. One had severe uncontrolled kyphoscoliosis (59,140).

Morquio Syndrome

Morquio syndrome, or type IV MPS, is synonymous with Morquio-Brailsford disease, Morquio-Ullrich disease, chondroosteodystrophy, osteochondrodystrophy deformans, and eccentro chondroplasia (48,54,95). It is an autosomal recessive lysosomal storage disorder characterized by short-trunk dwarfism and dysostosis multiplex with universal platyspondyly, normal intelligence, and excessive urinary excretion of keratan sulfate (14,48,66,78,109,150). Clinical heterogeneity of the condition is known (90).

Epidemiology and Etiology

Morquio syndrome is rare. Of the 80 cases reported in a literature review in 1964, approximately 41 represented Morquio disease and 39 another condition. An incidence of 1:100,000 births was estimated by Eggli and Dorst (40). This specific mucopolysaccharide storage disease is caused by a deficiency of the enzyme *N*-acetylgalactosamine-6-sulfate sulfatase (8,79,113). This deficiency has been designated type IVA MPS, and a *β*-galactosidase deficiency is designated type IVB MPS (113). The metabolic lesion responsible for this disease is not uniformly expressed in all cell types; thus it appears to be a cell-type-limited mucopolysaccharide storage disease, with excessive mucopolysaccharide accumulation in specific tissues. Whether tissue specificity is caused by unique tissue distribution of the deficient enzymes, unique tissue distribution of mucopolysaccharide substrates, or other factors is unknown (48).

Clinical Features and Pathologic Anatomy

Morquio syndrome is characterized by short-trunk dwarfism, corneal opacities, dental abnormalities, cardiopulmonary complications, normal intelligence, and dysostosis multiplex with universal platyspondylisis, increased thoracic kyphosis, knock knees, lumbar lordosis, and pectus carinatum (43,90,111). Cord compression caused by odontoid dysplasia and thickened retrodental soft tissue is well established in this syndrome (33,79). Excessive urinary excretion of keratan sulfate occurs in type IVA MPS, but type IVB MPS is a non–keratan sulfate–excreting form (48,89).

Abnormalities are not suspected until after the child begins to walk. Acute traumatic quadriparesis, chronic myelopathy of variable rate, and sudden death due to respiratory arrest have been associated with dysplasia caused by abnormal ossification

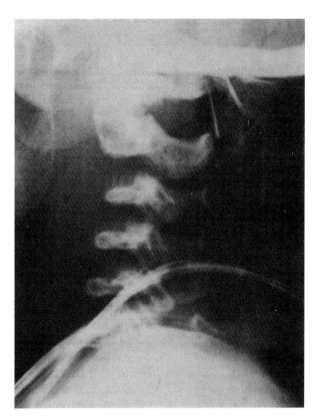

FIGURE 6. Morquio syndrome with C1–2 subluxation after posterior C1–2 fusion with autologous (only) iliac bone graft and halo application.

or complete absence of the odontoid process and the inevitable development of atlantoaxial instability (21,33,79). Ligamentous laxity also plays an important role in the development of C1–2 instability (33). The incidence of cord compression in Morquio syndrome is such that investigators have recommended prophylactic elective posterior cervical fusion in all patients (21,41,69,79).

In a review of 11 selected patients, 6 had neurologic signs and symptoms, and 5 had quadriparesis. The age at onset of the neurologic symptoms ranged from 19 months to 35 years (79). Acute onset of quadriplegia has been reported to occur after atlantoaxial subluxation during general anesthesia (15,62). In addition to subluxation of C1 on C2 in 10 patients, there were abnormally small canals at these vertebral levels (range, 10 to 15 mm) (79).

Radiographic Features and Results of Other Imaging Studies

The dysostosis multiplex is generalized and severe. Universal platyspondylisis is evident. Smallness or disappearance of the odontoid process causes atlantoaxial subluxation and narrowing of the spinal canal at this level (15,21,79,133) (Fig. 6). The margins of the vertebral bodies are irregular. The thoracic vertebrae are oval in infancy; older children have an anterior tongue

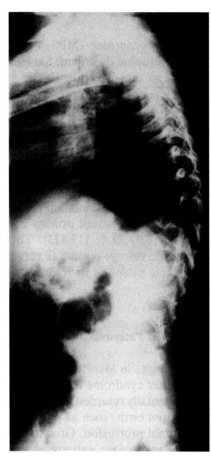

FIGURE 7. Morquio syndrome with severe dysostosis. Anterior tongue from the center of the vertebrae is evident.

from the center of the vertebral body (Fig. 7). The vertebrae are flat and rectangular in adults. Hyperlordosis and kyphoscoliosis have been found in long-term follow-up studies. In Morquio syndrome B, the radiographic skeletal abnormalities are similar to those of Morquio syndrome A but are of a milder nature (133).

Radiographs of the cervical spine should be obtained by the age of 2 years. Patients with symptoms need posterior fusion. For patients who do not have symptoms, the space available for the cord (more than 13 mm observed, less than 13 mm at MRI) can be assessed in flexion and extension to determine whether spinal cord changes are present. When cord changes are evident, posterior spinal fusion should be undertaken (86,107).

Course of Disease

Survival to 67 years of age has been reported. The patient had short-trunk dwarfism, clear corneas at gross examination, scoliosis, and genu valgum. The vertebrae were markedly flattened and osteoporotic. The patient died of unexplained episodic apnea. Postmortem examination showed abnormalities of cartilaginous structures, such as the laryngeal cartilage, sternum, and thoracic vertebrae.

Maroteaux-Lamy Syndrome

Maroteaux-Lamy syndrome (type VI MPS) is synonymous with polydystrophic dwarfism. Skeletal changes may be as severe as those of Hurler syndrome. Mental deficiency does not occur.

Epidemiology and Etiology

Type VI MPS is a cytosomal storage disorder transmitted through autosomal recessive inheritance. It is associated with decreased lysosomal enzymatic activity of arylsulfatase B and increased urinary excretion of dermatan sulfate (19,82,124,130). This form of mucopolysaccharide storage disease is very rare. Few reports are available to define the frequency of occurrence (133). Three forms based on the severity of symptoms have been recognized: infantile, most severe; juvenile, intermediate; and adult, mildest (52).

Clinical Features and Pathologic Anatomy

The skeletal changes of Maroteaux-Lamy syndrome rival those of Hurler syndrome in severity. Children with Maroteaux-Lamy syndrome, however, do not have mentally retarded, and certain physical signs are present from birth, such as prominence of the forehead and sternal protrusion. Growth may be normal to 4 years of age but may cease entirely at 8 years. Hurler-like changes include dysostosis, corneal opacities, and hepatosplenomegaly (130). The bony abnormalities are variable (Fig. 8). The two conditions (type VI MPS and type IH MPS) can be differentiated at radiographic examination. Mucopolysacchariduria occurs with a preponderance of dermatan sulfate (chondroitin sulfate B), and there are abnormal granulations in leukocytes. Cervical and lumbar radiculopathy and cervical myelopathy have been reported (104). Hypoplasia of the odontoid process is associated with cervical myelopathy and narrowing of the spinal canal. Lumbosacral radiculopathy has been associated with spinal stenosis due to dural thickening (104,117).

Radiographic Features and Findings of Other Imaging Studies

The radiographic skeletal changes can be variable in severity and extent. The vertebral bodies are oval or bullet shaped. Kyphosis be present at the lower thoracic or upper lumbar region. A wedge-shaped vertebra may be present at the center of the kyphosis, and there may be posterior displacement. The ribs may be paddle shaped. Narrowing of the cervical spinal canal has been reported to be caused by concentric impingement on the subarachnoid space. Cord compression can be caused by dural thickening in the cervical region, narrowing of the subarachnoid space in the occipitocervical junction, dysplastic arch of C1 protruding dorsally into the foramen magnum, and displacement of the cervical cord (117,133).

Course of Disease

Neurologic deterioration may occur in the form of optic atrophy, progressive hearing loss, or myelopathy. Hydrocephalus may be

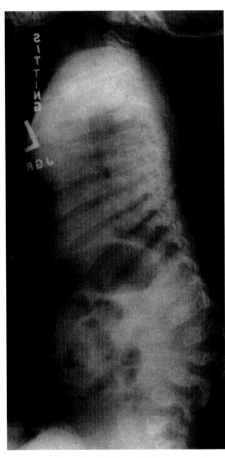

FIGURE 8. Seventeen-month-old boy with Maroteaux-Lamy syndrome. Thoracolumbar kyphosis and vertebral body changes are evident. (Courtesy of F. Deitz, MD.)

present. The myelopathy may manifest as gait abnormality, pain, paresthesia, or urinary or bowel incontinence. The myelopathy is caused by meningeal changes in both the cervical and lumbar regions (117,133). Symptoms may improvement after bone marrow transplantation (67,133). Patients may survive into late childhood or even into adulthood. Persons with milder forms of the disease have survived to their forties (10,124).

Sly Syndrome

Sly syndrome (type VII MPS) is a severe form of dysostosis multiplex.

Epidemiology and Etiology

Sly syndrome is rare. By 1985, only 17 cases had been reported in the literature (71). It is caused by accumulation of chondroitin-4-sulfate and chondroitin-6-sulfate from a deficiency of lysosomal β-glucuronidase activity (114,115). Both the clinical and biochemical manifestations can vary, a deficiency of β-glucuronidase being the only consistent finding. The mode of inheritance is autosomal recessive.

Clinical Features and Pathologic Anatomy

The clinical features of Sly syndrome include short stature, hepatosplenomegaly, progressive skeletal deformities of the thorax and spine, granular leukocytic inclusions, frequent pulmonary infections, and developmental delay (115). Thoracolumbar kyphosis or kyphoscoliosis is common. This disorder occurs among patients whose only clinical finding is kyphosis or scoliosis (71). Laboratory findings include mucopolysacchariduria and the absence of β-glucuronidase in leukocytes and cultured skin fibroblasts.

Atlantoaxial instability has been reported, but in this case report, it may have been a posttraumatic finding (105). The patient died 3 months after cervical fusion, at home in his sleep with no foreshadowing signs or symptoms. For patients with Sly syndrome, detailed preoperative evaluation is recommended, including assessment for cervical instability, chronic hypoventilation, and upper respiratory infections.

Radiographic Features and Findings of Other Imaging Studies

Various degrees of dysostosis multiplex with considerable phenotypic variation occur with Sly syndrome. Platyspondyly is present and is associated with vertebral beaking. Thoracolumbar kyphosis and kyphoscoliosis have been reported (29,40,49,133). The odontoid process is dysplastic (115), and atlantoaxial instability may occur.

Course of Disease

The onset of symptoms is in early infancy and childhood. Severe thoracolumbar kyphosis or kyphoscoliosis may develop. Death in early childhood occurs in the severe form (133).

DiFerrante Syndrome

DiFerrante syndrome (type VIII MPS) is the last of the identifiable and classified disorders of mucopolysaccharide metabolism. The deficient enzyme is glucosamine-6-sulfate sulfatase. Because of the rarity of this syndrome, it is not discussed herein.

MUCOLIPIDOSIS

In 1975, Spranger (120) and others found that other conditions had combined features of MPS and sphingolipidosis and had be classified separately. To delineate these intermediate conditions, the term *mucolipidosis* was coined. The term is a misnomer in the biochemical sense, however. First, a mucolipid is not a known chemical compound; second, in many forms of mucolipidosis, there is no true storage of either mucopolysaccharides or lipids. Children with so-called mucolipidosis excrete excessive amounts of oligosaccharides in the urine (73). The term *oligosaccharidosis* may therefore be more appropriate, but the term *mucolipidosis* remains. Clinically and radiographically, the mucolipidosis resembles the MPS syndromes, but urinary mucopolysaccharide levels are normal. The spectrum of severity in the various forms of mucolipidosis is even wider than in MPS. The severity of dysostosis multiplex is surprisingly variable.

Epidemiology and Etiology

These Hurler variant syndromes are rare. From 1 to approximately 20 cases had been described for each specific enzyme defect, according to the report by Spranger and Wiedemann in 1970 (127). Mucolipidosis is an inherited metabolic disease characterized by accumulation of excessive amounts of mucopolysaccharides and sphingolipids in visceral and mesenchymal cells. The differentiating features of the forms of mucolipidosis, including the enzyme defect and the major storage substance, are as follows.

Mucolipidosis I is a neurodegenerative disorder in which neuraminidase deficiency is the only defect that has been demonstrated (128). Spranger (120) described mucolipidosis I as a nosologic entity that combines clinical and radiographic features of MPS with signs of a neurodegenerative process that affects gray and white matter. To establish the diagnosis, in addition to thin-layer chromatography, urine and fibroblast sialic acid measurements are needed (128).

Mucolipidosis II is an autosomal recessive Hurler-like disorder caused by deficiency of the lysosomal hydrolase glycoprotein *N*-acetylglucosaminylphosphotransferase. This deficiency occurs in cultured skin fibroblasts (97).

Mucolipidosis III is an autosomal recessive inherited disorder, closely related to mucolipidosis II. The specific enzyme deficiency has not been clearly established.

Mucolipidosis IV is a recessively inherited lysosomal disease found in relatively high frequency among Ashkenazi Jews (2,6). The definitive diagnosis is made by means of electron microscopic examination, which reveals storage organelles typical of mucolipidosis (2).

Clinical Features and Pathologic Anatomy

Biochemically mucolipidosis is a lysosomal storage disease with multiple primary defects of lipid, mucopolysaccharide, and glycoprotein metabolism in various combinations (127,137). Noteworthy is the thoracolumbar scoliosis or kyphosis of mucolipidosis I. Thoracolumbar kyphosis occurs in I-cell disease (mucolipidosis II), along with calcification of the intervertebral discs (5,87). Clinically, mucolipidosis resembles the MPS syndromes. Urine mucopolysaccharide levels are normal, however. The spectrum of severity of mucolipidosis is even wider than that of the MPS syndromes.

In mucolipidosis I, the major manifestations are coarse facies, cloudy cornea, hepatosplenomegaly, joint limitation, developmental delay, and dysostosis multiplex (18). Kyphosis is a common finding (42). Mucolipidosis I should be included in the differential diagnosis of disorders that display a Hurler syndrome–like phenotype in infancy (58).

In I-cell disease (mucolipidosis II), the skeletal findings are so severe that they resemble those of Hurler syndrome (20,72,99,100,131). Atlantoaxial subluxation and cervical myelopathy following minor injuries have been reported. A cartilaginous, noncalcified composition of the odontoid process may

contribute to the instability (44). Calcification of the intervertebral disc occurs in I-cell disease and presumably is related to the excessive cartilage degeneration that takes place in this disorder (87). There have been no reports of morbidity associated with this finding. A developmental thoracolumbar gibbus similar to that of Hurler syndrome is common.

Mucolipidosis III, or pseudo-Hurler polydystrophy, is closely related to mucolipidosis II, but onset of signs occurs somewhat later. It is characterized by growth retardation, severe dysostosis multiplex, joint stiffness, tight indurated skin, swollen eyelids, late-onset hepatosplenomegaly, corneal opacities, and only slight impairment of mental and neurologic development (47). Thoracolumbar kyphosis is a common finding.

The clinical manifestations of mucolipidosis IV include profound psychomotor retardation and visual impairment in the first year of life. In type I or generalized gangliosidosis, the dysostosis may be identical to that of Hurler syndrome. The dysostosis multiplex is milder in most of the other types of mucolipidosis, such as type II gangliosidosis, fucosidosis, mannosidosis, juvenile sulfatidosis (Austin type), Farber disease, and mucolipidosis I.

Radiographic Features and Findings of Other Imaging Studies

Mucolipidosis I is a neurodegenerative disorder similar in clinical presentation to Hurler syndrome in infancy. Thoracolumbar gibbus may manifest in late infancy, and mild to moderate thoracolumbar kyphoscoliosis may be seen in early childhood (42,58,123,128). In mucolipidosis II (I-cell disease), radiographic features include ovoid vertebral bodies, narrowing of the interpediculate distance in the lower thoracic vertebrae, and intervertebral disc calcification (87) (Fig. 9). In early childhood, the thoracolumbar vertebrae have a short anteroposterior diameter, there is inferior beaking of the vertebral bodies at T12 through L3, and the occurrence of thoracolumbar kyphosis and scoliosis is variable (13,64,74,97,133,134,146).

In mucolipidosis III (pseudo-Hurler polydystrophy), radiographic changes are similar to the dysostosis changes of the Hurler and Hunter syndromes. In the spine, these include beaking of upper lumbar vertebrae with mild thoracolumbar kyphosis, varying degrees of platyspondylisis, and absence of hypoplasia of the dens (4,47,60,61,85,94,145). Mucolipidosis IV is characterized by psychomotor retardation and ophthalmologic abnormalities but not by skeletal deformities (2).

Course of Disease

Patients with mucolipidosis I have a variable course of progressive neurologic deterioration. Cardiomegaly and hepatomegaly may predominate and contribute to early death. Although kyphosis is known to occur, serious morbidity related to the deformity of developmental thoracolumbar kyphosis or kyphoscoliosis has not been reported (58).

Children with I-cell disease (mucolipidosis II) have extreme psychomotor delay and failure to thrive. Death has been reported to occur as early as 2 weeks of age and as late as 8 years (74,146). Significant morbidity relating to C1–2 instability has been re-

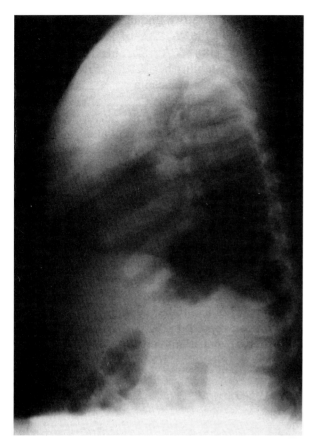

FIGURE 9. I-cell disease with mild thoracolumbar kyphosis. The vertebrae are ovoid.

ported (44), but serious morbidity associated with the thoracolumbar gibbus has not. The latter has not been studied with advanced imaging studies such as MRI. The use of MRI as a noninvasive diagnostic tool may lead to more specific treatment recommendations.

The course of mucolipidosis III has been described in one of a pair of dizygotic twin girls. The odontoid process was short in the affected child, but no neurologic deficits occurred. Growth deficiency and moderate mental deficiency did occur. When the girl was 10 years of age, the chronic course of the disease continued (75).

The course of mucolipidosis IV among 20 patients between the ages of 2 and 17 years has been described (2). The highest developmental level was 12 to 15 months in language and motor function. The disease may be slow and protracted, however, with little deterioration despite the infantile onset (2). Substantial musculoskeletal involvement has not been reported.

HOMOCYSTINURIA

Homocystinuria is an autosomal recessive disease caused by an inborn error of methionine metabolism. In its most common

form, homocystinuria is caused by a deficiency of cystathionine β-synthase activity (22,26). In classic homocystinuria, methionine and homocysteine accumulate in tissues and blood and are excreted in large amounts in the urine; cysteine levels are low. The clinical signs and symptoms are heterogeneous (12,22).

Epidemiology and Etiology

The incidence of homocystinuria has been estimated to be about 1:24,000 to 1:200,000 (22,135). The cause of homocystinuria in its most common form is clearly defined as an inborn error of methionine metabolism due to a deficiency of cystathionine β-synthase activity. This enzyme sulfurates homocysteine—the metabolite of the essential amino acid methionine—to cystathionine, which is converted to cysteine. Homocystinuria as an end pathway is a feature in two other extremely rare inherited metabolic defects—Imerslund-Grasbeck syndrome and a deficiency of 5-methyltetrahydrofolate-homocysteine methyltransferase (22,88). In defects of amino acid metabolism, it appears to rank second in frequency to phenylketonuria. The causative gene is located on chromosome 5p15.2–15.3.17 (70).

Clinical Features and Pathologic Anatomy

The most frequent clinical signs of homocystinuria are dislocated lens (ectopia lentis), premature arteriosclerosis and serious thromboembolic complications, osteoporosis, scoliosis and kyphoscoliosis, arachnodactyly, pectus excavatum or carinatum, mental retardation, and neurologic and psychiatric disorders.

The clinical resemblance of homocystinuria to Marfan syndrome often leads to misdiagnosis. Although the two diseases are similar, differences have emerged. Florid arachnodactyly and scoliosis are more common in Marfan syndrome. Patients with homocystinuria have osteoporosis at a young age and a high incidence of vertebral involvement, including biconcavity and flattening. The osteoporosis associated with homocystinuria is caused by a dearth cross-links in type I collagen (80). Patients with Marfan syndrome do not have osteoporosis and may have excessively tall vertebrae. Mental retardation and thrombosis are common in homocystinuria but not in Marfan syndrome (22,24). The therapeutic relevance of misdiagnosis is that the patient with homocystinuria is deprived of treatment with pyridoxine, folic acid, and methionine restriction, which has a favorable clinical effect in most instances (22).

Children with homocystinuria are considered to be healthy at birth. Motor and speech development may be slow by 1 year of age. Gait may be clumsy or awkward, and a regression in motor and speech skills may occur. With growth, the extremities appear long but not well muscled. The characteristic facial feature is malar flush. The hair is thin and often slightly curled and blond or light brown (12,28).

The most life-threatening components of the disease are venous and arterial thrombosis. Early death of myocardial infarction, pulmonary embolism, mesenteric thrombosis, and cerebral vascular accident has been reported. Venous thrombosis has occurred frequently enough after surgery or illness that a surgeon may be reluctant to perform an elective surgical procedure (12,27,63).

The skeletal manifestations of homocystinuria include long thin extremities, scoliosis, chest deformity, genu valgum, cubitus valgus, and cavus or flat feet. Pectus carinatum or excavatum may be present in the absence of scoliosis. The most common pattern of scoliosis are right thoracic and left lumbar, the left lumbar curve being greater. Osteoporosis also usually occurs (12).

Radiographic Features and Findings of Other Imaging Studies

Marked generalized osteoporosis is the radiographic feature that differentiates homocystinuria from Marfan syndrome. There are no characteristic radiographic abnormalities at birth (116). Other radiographic features described include coxa valga, slender and possibly bowed bones, biconcave (codfish) vertebrae, scoliosis and kyphoscoliosis, retarded bone age, hyperaeration of the sinuses, and enlarged carpal bones (12,81,82) (Fig. 10).

Course of Disease

More than one third of patients with homocystinuria have skeletal deformities. Of 26 patients in one series, 14 died of arterial

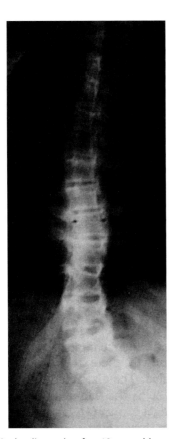

FIGURE 10. Spinal radiographs of an 18-year-old man with homocystinuria, moderate scoliosis, and osteoporosis.

or venous thrombosis (135). Survival rate appears to be highly variable and related to the absence of major complications such as thrombosis.

TREATMENT RECOMMENDATIONS FOR PATIENTS WITH MUCOPOLYSACCHARIDOSIS AND MUCOLIPIDOSIS

Nonsurgical

Enzyme replacement therapy is not yet available as a primary therapy for the enzyme deficiencies in these lysosomal storage diseases. Therefore, all treatments are secondary and consist of management of the phenotypic expressions of the diseases. The effect of multiple transfusions on a patient with Hunter syndrome was studied. For this patient, who also had Cooley anemia, the usual clinical manifestations of Hunter syndrome were fully developed and did not appear to be ameliorated by the transfusions (11).

Bone marrow transplantation has been used to manage Maroteaux-Lamy syndrome (67). Full engraftment occurred, and arylsulfatase B activity, which was previously deficient, increased to normal levels in peripheral lymphocytes and granulocytes. Hepatosplenomegaly was substantially decreased, and cardiopulmonary function was normal. Bone marrow transplantation provided a source of enzymatically normal cells, which altered the metabolic and clinical course of the disease (67).

Subluxation of C1 on C2 occurs in Hurler syndrome (136) and in Morquio syndrome. This may or may not be associated with quadriparesis. Immobilization in traction is recommended until definitive posterior cervical fusion is performed with postoperative immobilization in a halo vest.

Atlantoaxial instability and myelopathy following minor injuries occur among children with I-cell disease (mucolipidosis II). It is reported that the atlantoaxial joint is unstable because the transverse ligament is incompetent and there is infiltration by storage cells. A cartilaginous rather than calcified composition of the odontoid process may contribute to the instability (44). Posterior cervical fusion with halo-vest immobilization is recommended for demonstrated or suspected instabilities. Temporary immobilization of the cervical spine is used until the operation is performed.

Dysplasia of the odontoid process and subsequent atlantoaxial instability with or without quadriparesis occur at such an alarming rate in Morquio syndrome that cervical fusion has been recommended for all patients with Morquio syndrome (79,119). Cervical cord signs become evident during the first two decades of life. Spinal cord compression has been documented in two patients with Morquio syndrome at the level of thoracolumbar kyphosis. In one, the patient had labored walking and corticospinal tract signs at 36 years of age. Myelographic findings confirmed cord compression at the level of the gibbus. The other patient also had onset of symptoms during the fourth decade of life (21). Preventive measures against the development of thoracolumbar kyphosis, such as the use of a thoracolumbosacral orthosis (TLSO) or cervical-TLSO, have been reported and are being used. The experience with prophylactic bracing is not extensive enough to allow conclusions regarding effectiveness.

Management of the thoracolumbar kyphosis associated with many of these disorders is not well studied or well documented. Whether the course of kyphosis can be modified or reversed is not known. It remains debatable whether bracing should be considered. On the one hand, there is little or no documentation of any neurologic deterioration, such as paraparesis or cauda equina syndrome, that may be associated with this deformity (except in Morquio syndrome). On the other hand, as the prospect improves for primary enzyme replacement therapy, prevention of progressive spinal deformity and neurologic deficit may become imperative. As long as immobilization in a custom TLSO does not impair pulmonary status and does not contribute to the development of atelectasis, pneumonia, or upper airway obstruction, it is reasonable to recommend bracing for management of thoracolumbar kyphosis associated with these diseases when the child begins an upright posture.

Surgical

Posterior cervical fusion is recommended for demonstrated atlantoaxial instabilities. Fusion of C1–2 is recommended for all patients with Morquio syndrome (21,41,69,79). The suggested technique is a posterior muscle-splitting midline procedure performed after application of a halo and the anterior portion of the vest. The halo-vest application allows for initial stabilization of the cervical spine after induction of anesthesia and appropriate airway management. Preoperative planning must include assessment for cord compression due to either displacement and relative fixation of C1 in relation to C2 or stenosis associated with dural abnormalities (107,117). If cord compression is found, stabilization and fusion alone may not resolve signs of cord compression. Adjunctive posterior decompression of C1 or C2 and possible durotomy and grafting of dural defects may be needed. When cervical fusion is performed for Morquio syndrome, bone for the graft is best obtained from the proximal tibial metaphysis, because the iliac crest is a poor source of graft bone in this disease (1).

Posterior spinal fusion, with or without anterior fusion and possible anterior decompression, is recommended for progressive thoracolumbar kyphosis. Few or no reports are available in the literature on the results of surgical management of this spinal deformity in these rare lysosomal storage disorders. It is recommended that in the event of cord or cauda equina compression, anterior decompression of the ventrally compressed cord be performed. Adequate decompression can be achieved by means of removal of the middle column portion of the involved vertebrae and discs with preservation of the anterior column.

Anterior discectomy and fusion of the kyphotic region and posterior fusion in situ of the kyphotic region with postoperative casting would appear appropriate for preadolescent, juvenile, and infant patients. The addition of instrumentation in the treatment of adolescents and adults is recommended, because there is no narrowing of anteroposterior diameter of the intraspinal canal. In the absence of substantial deformity, reduction should be judiciously evaluated.

TREATMENT RECOMMENDATIONS FOR HOMOCYSTINURIA

Nonsurgical

Management of homocystinuria with pyridoxine, folic acid, and methionine restriction has a favorable biochemical response and clinical effect (22). Few reports are available on the nonoperative management of scoliosis and kyphoscoliosis in this rare disorder. Clinical indications used in the management of idiopathic scoliosis can be applied to the care of children with homocystinuria, scoliosis, and kyphoscoliosis.

Surgical

Life-threatening thromboembolic complications, including myocardial infarction, are associated with illness of and surgical procedures on patients with homocystinuria. Appropriate and in-depth consultation with a hematologist experienced in treating patients with this rare disorder is recommended before an operation is scheduled. Surgical plans and techniques used to manage idiopathic scoliosis can be applied to the care of patients with homocystinuria. The principles include posterior fusion with instrumentation, anterior fusion with instrumentation for thoracolumbar curves, and staged anterior spinal release or fusion and posterior fusion with instrumentation.

ACKNOWLEDGMENTS

The assistance of Robyn Mann in the preparation of this chapter and of Andrew Poznanski, MD, in the preparation of the references and radiographic illustrations is gratefully acknowledged.

REFERENCES

1. American Academy of Orthopaedic Surgeons (1987): *Orthopaedic knowledge update 2: home study syllabus.* Chicago: American Academy of Orthopaedic Surgeons.
2. Amir N, Ziotogora J, Bach G (1987): Mucolipidosis type IV: clinical spectrum and natural history. *Pediatrics* 79:953–959.
3. Arviddsson J, Chester MA, Hecht H (1983): The first case of the Sanfilippo type C syndrome in Scandinavia. *Acta Paediatr Scand* 72: 313–316.
4. Aviad I, Stein H, Zilberman Y (1974): Roentgen findings of pseudo-Hurler polydystrophy in the adult, with a note on cephalo-metric changes. *Spine* 122:56–66.
5. Babcock DS, Bove KE, Hug G, et al. (1986): Fetal mucolipidosis II (I-cell disease): radiologic and pathologic correlation. *Pediatr Radiol* 16:32–39.
6. Bach G (1979): Mucolipidosis type IV. In: Goodman RM, Motulsky A, eds. *Genetic diseases among Ashkenazi Jews.* New York: Raven Press, pp. 187–193.
7. Baines D, Keneally J (1983): Anaesthetic implications of the mucopolysaccharidoses: a fifteen-year experience in a children's hospital. *Anaesth Intensive Care* 11:198–202.
8. Baker E, Guo X, Orsborn AM, et al. (1993): The Morquio syndrome (Mucopolysaccharidosis IVA) gene maps to 16q24.3. *Am J Hum Genet* 52:96–98.
9. Barton RW, Neufeld EF (1971): The Hurler corrective factor. *J Biol Chem* 246:7773.

10. Barton RW, Neufeld EF (1972): A distinct biochemical deficit in the Maroteaux-Lamy syndrome (mucopolysaccharidosis VI). *J Pediatr* 80.

11. Bartsocas CS, Papasotiriou N, Karageorga M, et al. (1973): Hunter's syndrome and Cooley's anaemia in the same patient. *Acta Paediatr Scand* 62:66–68.

12. Beals RK (1969): Homocystinuria. *J Bone Joint Surg Am* 51: 1564–1572.

13. Beck M, Barone R, Hoffman R, et al. (1995): Inter and intrafamilial variability in mucolipidoses II (I-cell disease). *Clin Genet* 47:191–199.

14. Beck M, Glossl J, Grubisic A, et al. (1986): Heterogeneity of Morquio disease. *Clin Genet* 29:325–331.

15. Beighton P, Craig J (1973): Atlanto-axial subluxation in the Morquio syndrome. *J Bone Joint Surg Br* 55.

16. Belcher RW (1972): Ultrastructure of the skin in the genetic mucopolysaccharidoses. *Arch Pathol* 94.

17. Bergstrom SK, Quinn JJ, Greenstein R, et al. (1994): Long-term follow-up of a patient transplanted for Hunter's disease type IIB: a case report and literature review. *Bone Marrow Transplant* 14:653–658.

18. Berman ER, Livni N, Shapira E, et al. (1974): Congenital corneal clouding with abnormal systemic storage bodies: a new variant of mucolipidosis. *J Pediatr* 84:519–526.

19. Black SH, Pelias MZ, Miller JB, et al. (1986): Maroteaux-Lamy syndrome in a large consanguineous kindred: biochemical and immunological studies. *Am J Med Genet* 25:273–279.

20. Blank E, Linder D (1974): I-cell disease (mucolipidosis II): a lysosomopathy. *Pediatrics* 54:797–805.

21. Blaw ME, Langer LO (1969): Spinal cord compression in Morquio-Brailsford's disease. *J Pediatr* 74:593–600.

22. Boers GHJ, Polder TW, Cruysberg JRM, et al. (1984): Homocystinuria versus Marfan's syndrome: the therapeutic relevance of the differential diagnosis. *Neth J Med* 27:206–212.

23. Brandner ME, Maroteaux P, Rampini S, et al. (1971): Differentiation of different types of mucopolysaccharidosis by vertebral body and intervertebral disk indices. *Ann Radiol* 14:321–328.

24. Brenton DP, Dow CJ, James J (1972): Homocystinuria and Marfan's syndrome. *J Bone Joint Surg Br* 54:277–298.

25. Brill CB, Rose JS, Godmillow L, et al. (1978): Spastic quadriparesis due to C1–C2 subluxation in Hurler syndrome. *J Pediatr* 92.

26. Brill PW, Mitty HA, Gaull GE (1974): Homocystinuria due to cystathionine synthase deficiency: clinical-roentgenologic correlations. *Am J Roentgenol Radium Ther Nucl Med* 121.

27. Carson NAJ, Dent CE, Field CMB, et al. (1965): Homocystinuria: clinical and pathological review of ten cases. *J Pediatr* 66:565–583.

28. Carson NAJ, Neill DW (1962): Metabolic abnormalities detected in a survey of mentally backward individuals in Northern Ireland. *Arch Dis Child* 37:505–513.

29. Chapman S, Gray RGF, Constable TJ, et al. (1989): Atypical radiological features of β-glucoronidase deficiency (mucopolysaccharidosis VII) occurring in an elderly patient from an inbred kindred. *Br J Radiol* 62:491–494.

30. Clausen J, Dyggve HV, Melchior JC (1963): Mucopolysaccharidosis. *Arch Dis Child* 38:364–374.

31. Coppa GV, Giorgi PL, Felici L, et al. (1983): Clinical heterogeneity in Sanfilippo disease (mucopolysaccharidosis III) type D: presentation of two new cases. *Eur J Pediatr* 140:130–133.

32. Crawford MA, Dean MF, Hunt DM, et al. (1973): Early prenatal diagnosis of Hurler's syndrome with termination of pregnancy and confirmatory findings on the fetus. *J Med Genet* 10:144.

33. Crockard HA, Stevens JM (1995): Craniovertebral junction anomalies in inherited disorders: part of the syndrome or caused by the disorder? *Eur J Pediatr* 154:504–512.

34. Crocker AC (1968): Therapeutic trials in the inborn errors: an attempt to modify Hurler's syndrome. *Pediatrics* 42:887–888.

35. Danes BS (1977): Variant of iduronidase deficient mucopolysaccharidoses. *J Med Genet* 14:346–351.

36. Danks DM, Campbell PE, Cartwright E, et al. (1972): The Sanfilippo syndrome: clinical, biochemical, radiological, haematological and pathological features of nine cases. *Aust Paediatr J* 8:174–186.

37. DeJong BP, Van B, Robertson W, et al. (1968): Failure to induce scurvy by ascorbic acid depletion in a patient with Hurler's syndrome. *Pediatrics* 42:889–903.

38. Dietz FR, Mathews KD (1996): Current concepts review: update on the genetic bases of disorders with orthopaedic manifestations. *J Bone Joint Surg Am* 78:1583–1598.

39. Dorst JP (1974): Mucopolysaccharidosis II. In: Kaufman HJ, ed. *Progress in pediatric radiology*, vol 4. Basel: Karger.

40. Eggli KD, Dorst JP (1988): The mucopolysaccharidoses and related conditions. *Semin Roentgenol* 8:275–294.

41. Einhorn NH, Moore JR, Rowntree LG (1946): Osteochondrodystrophia deformans (Morquio's disease): observations at autopsy in one case. *Am J Dis Child* 72:536–544.

42. Feingold M (1983): Mucolipidosis I. *Am J Dis Child* 137:907–908.

43. Gardner DG (1975): The dental manifestations of the Morquio syndrome (mucopolysaccharidosis type IV). *Am J Dis Child* 129: 1445–1449.

44. Goodman ML, Pang D (1988): Spinal cord injury in I-cell disease. *Pediatr Neurosci* 14:315–318.

45. Gwinn JL, Barnes GR (1968): Radiological case of the month. *Am J Dis Child* 15:347–348.

46. Harper PS, Laurence KM, Parkes A, et al. (1974): Sanfilippo A disease in the fetus. *J Med Genet* 11:123–132.

47. Herd JK, Dvorak AD, Wiltse HE, et al. (1978): Mucolipidosis type III. *Am J Dis Child* 132:1181–1186.

48. Hollister DW, Cohen AH, Rimoin DL, et al. (1975): The Morquio syndrome (mucopolysaccharidosis IV): morphologic and biochemical studies. *Johns Hopkins Med J* 137:176–183.

49. Hoyme HE, et al. (1981): Presentation of mucopolysaccharidosis VII (β-glucoronidase deficiency) in infancy. *J Med Genet* 18:237–239.

50. Humbel R, Marchal C, Fall M (1972): Diagnosis of Morquio's disease: a simple chromatographic method for the identification of keratosulfate in urine. *J Pediatr* 81:107–108.

51. Hunter C (1917): Hunter: a rare disease in two brothers. *Proc R Soc Med* 10:104–116.

52. Isbrandt D, Arlt G, Brooks DA, et al. (1994): Mucopolysaccharidosis VI (Maroteaux-Lamy Syndrome): six unique arylsulfatase B gene alleles causing variable disease phenotypes. *Am J Hum Genet* 54: 454–463.

53. Jackson WPU, Hanelin J, Albright F (1954): Metaphyseal dysplasia, epiphyseal dysplasia, diaphyseal dysplasia and related conditions. *Arch Intern Med* 94:898–899.

54. Jenkins P, Davies GR, Harper PS (1973): Morquio-Brailsford disease. *Br J Radiol* 46:668–675.

55. Kaplan D, McKusick V, Trebach S, et al. (1968): Keratosulfate-chondroitin sulfate peptide from normal urine and from urine of patients with Morquio syndrome (mucopolysaccharidosis IV). *J Lab Clin Med* 71:48–55.

56. Kaplan P, Wolfe LS (1987): Sanfilippo syndrome type D. *J Pediatr* 110:267–271.

57. Kelly TE (1978): The mucopolysaccharidoses and mucolipidoses. *Clin Orthop* 114:116–136.

58. Kelly TE, Bartoshesky L, Harris DJ, et al. (1981): Mucolipidosis I (acid neuraminidase deficiency). *Am J Dis Child* 135:703–708.

59. Kelly TE, Graetz G (1977): Isolated acid neuraminidase deficiency: A distinct lysosomal storage disease. *Am J Med Genet* 1:31–46.

60. Kelly TE, Thomas GH, Taylor HA, et al. (1975): Mucolipidosis III (pseudo–Hurler polydystrophy): clinical and laboratory studies in a series of 12 patients. *Johns Hopkins Med J* 137:156–175.

61. Kelly TE, Thomas GH, Taylor HA, et al. (1978): Mucolipidosis III: Clinical and laboratory findings. *Birth Defects* 11:295–299.

62. Kempthorne PM, Brown TCK (1983): Anaesthesia and the mucopolysaccharidoses: a survey of problems and problems. *Anaesth Intensive Care* 11:203–207.

63. Kombower GM, Wilson VK (1963): Homocystinuria. *Proc R Soc Med* 56:996–997.

64. Kousseff BG, Beratis NG, Strauss L, et al. (1976): Fucosidosis type 2. *Pediatrics* 57:205–213.

65. Koyama k, Moda Y, Sone A, et al. (1994): Neurogenic bladder in Hunter's syndrome. *J Med Genet* 31:257–258.

66. Kozlowski K, Bartkowiak K, Chmeilowa M (1971): Mucopolysac-

charidosis IV (Morquio's disease) in a twenty-month-old child. *Australas Radiol* 15:362–366.

67. Krivit W, Pierpont ME, Ayaz K, et al. (1984): Bone-marrow transplantation in the Maroteaux-Lamy syndrome (mucopolysaccharidosis type VI). *N Engl J Med* 311:1606–1611.

68. Langer LO (1964): The radiographic manifestations of the HS-mucopolysaccharidosis of Sanfilippo with discussion of this condition in relation to the other mucopolysaccharidoses and a classification of these fundamentally similar entities. *Ann Radiol* (Paris) 10:315–325.

69. Langer LO, Carey LS (1966): The roentgenographic features of the KS mucopolysaccharidosis of Morquio (Morquio-Brailsford's disease). *Am J Roentgenol Radium Ther Nucl Med* 97.

70. Leclerc D, Wilson A, Dumas R, et al. (1998): Cloning and mapping of cDNA for methionine synthase reductase, a flavoprotein defective in patients with homocystinuria. *Genetics* 95:3059–3064.

71. Lee JES, Falk RE, Ng WG, et al. (1985): Beta-glucuronidase deficiency. *Am J Dis Child* 139:57–59.

72. Lemaitre L, Remy J, Farriaux JP, et al. (1978): Radiological signs of mucolipidosis II or I-cell disease. *Pediatr Radiol* 7:97–105.

73. Leroy JG (1982): The oligosaccharidoses: proposal of a new name and a new classification for the mucolipidoses. *Birth Defects* 18:3–12.

74. Leroy JG, Spranger JW, Feingold M, et al. (1971): I-cell disease: a clinical picture. *J Pediatr* 79:360–365.

75. Leroy JG, Van Elsen AF (1975): Natural history of a mucolipidosis: twin girls discordant for ML III. *Birth Defects* 11:325–334.

76. Levin TL, Berdon WE, Lachman RS, et al. (1997): Lumbar gibbus deformity in storage diseases and bone dysplasias. *Pediatr Radiol* 27:289–294.

77. Lichtenstein JR, Bilbray GL, McKusick VA (1972): Clinical and probable genetic heterogeneity within mucopolysaccharidosis II: report of a family with a mild form. *Johns Hopkins Med J* 131:425–435.

78. Linker A, Evans LR, Langer LO (1970): Morquio's disease and mucopolysaccharide excretion. *J Pediatr* 77:1039–1047.

79. Lipson SJ (1977): Dysplasia of the odontoid process in Morquio's syndrome causing quadriparesis. *J Bone Joint Surg Am* 59:340–344.

80. Lubec B, Fang-Kircher S, Lubec T, et al. (1996): Evidence for McKusick's hypothesis of deficient collagen cross-linking in patients with homocystinuria. *Biochim Biophys Acta* 1315:159–162.

81. MacCarthy JMT, Carey MC (1968): Bone changes in homocystinuria. *Clin Radiol* 19:128–134.

82. McKusick VA (1972): Non-keratan-sulfate-excreting Morquio syndrome. In: *Heritable disorders of connective tissue*. St. Louis: CV Mosby, pp. 600–604.

83. McKusick VA (1988): *Mendelian inheritance in man*. Baltimore: Johns Hopkins University Press.

84. McKusick VA (1965): The genetic mucopolysaccharidoses. *Circulation* 31:1–4.

85. Melhem R, Dorst JP, Scott CI, et al. (1973): Roentgen findings in mucolipidosis III (pseudo-Hurler polydystrophy). *Radiology* 106:153–160.

86. Mikles M, Stanton RP (1997): A review of Morquio syndrome. *Am J Orthop* 26:533–540.

87. Mogle P, Amitai Y, Rotenberg M, et al. (1986): Calcification of intervertebral disks in I-cell disease. *Eur J Pediatr* 145:226–227.

88. Mudd SH, Levy HL (1982): Disorders of transsulphuration. In: Stanbury JB, Wyngaarden JB, Frederickson DS, eds. *The metabolic bases of inherited diseases*. New York: McGraw-Hill, pp. 522–559.

89. Nakashima Y, Tomatsu S, Hori T, et al. (1994): Mucopolysaccharidosis IVA: molecular cloning of the human *N*-acetylgalactosamin-6-sulfatase gene (GALNS) and analysis of the 5′-flanking region. *Genomics* 20:99–104.

90. Nelson J, Broadhead D, Mossman J (1988): Clinical findings in 12 patients with MPS IV A (Morquio's disease). *Clin Genet* 33:111–120.

91. Neufeld EF, Liebaers I, Epstein CJ, et al. (1977): The Hunter syndrome in females: is there an autosomal recessive form of iduronate sulfatase deficiency. *Am J Hum Genet* 29:455–461.

92. Neuhauser EBD, Griscom NT, Gilles FH, et al. (1968): Arachnoid cyst in the Hurler-Hunter syndrome. *Ann Radiol* 11:453–469.

93. Nishioka J, Mizushima T, Ono K (1979): Treatment of mucopolysaccharidosis. *Clin Orthop* 140:194–203.

94. Nolte K, Spranger J (1975): Early skeletal changes in mucolipidosis III. *Eur Soc Pediatr Radiol* 19:151–159.

95. Norman ME, Pischnotte WO (1972): Morquio's disease. *Am J Dis Child* 124:719–722.

96. O'Brien JS, Nyhan WL, Shear C, et al. (1976): Clinical and biochemical expression of a unique mucopolysaccharidosis. *Clin Genet* 9:399–411.

97. Okada S, Kato T, Oshima T, et al. (1983): Heterogeneity in mucolipidosis II (I-cell disease) *Clin Genet* 23:155–159.

98. Parsons VJ, Hughes DG, Wraith JE (1996): Magnetic resonance imaging of the brain, neck, and cervical spine in mild Hunter's syndrome (mucopolysaccharidosis type II). *Clin Radiol* 51:719–723.

99. Patriquin HB, Kaplan P, Kind HP, et al. (1977): Neonatal mucolipidosis II (I-cell disease): clinical and radiologic features in three cases. *Am J Roentgenol* 129:37–43.

100. Pazzaglia UE, Beluffi G, Danesino C, et al. (1989): Neonatal mucolipidosis 2: the spontaneous evolution of early bone lesions and the effect of vitamin D treatment. *Pediatr Radiol* 20:80–84.

101. Pedrini V, Lennzi L, Zambotti V (1962): Isolation and identification of keratosulphate in urine of patients affected by Morquio-Ullrich disease. *Proc Soc Exp Biol Med* 110:847–849.

102. Peters ME, Langer LO (1985): The narrow tracheae in the mucopolysaccharidoses. *Pediatr Radiol* 15:225–228.

103. Piccirilli CB, Chadduck WM (1996): Cervical kyphotic myelopathy in a child with Morquio syndrome. *Childs Nerv Syst* 12:114–116.

104. Pilz H, von Figura K, Goebel HH (1979): Deficiency of arylsulfatase B in 2 brothers age 40 and 48 years (Maroteaux-Lamy syndrome, type B). *Ann Neurol* 6:315–325.

105. Pizzutillo PD, Osterkamp JA, Scott CI, et al. (1989): Atlantoaxial instability in mucopolysaccharidosis type VII. *J Pediatr Orthop* 9:76–78.

106. Pritzker MR, King RA, Kronenberg RS (1980): Upper airway obstruction during head flexion in Morquio's disease. *Am J Med* 69:467–470.

107. Ransford AO, Crockard HA, Stevens JM, et al. (1996): Occipito-atlanto-axial fusion in Morquio-Brailsford syndrome. *J Bone Joint Surg Br* 78:307–313.

108. Rezvani I, Collipp PJ, DeGeorge AM (1973): Evaluation of screening tests for urinary mucopolysaccharides. *Pediatrics* 52:64–68.

109. Schenk EA, Haggerty J (1964): Morquio's disease. A radiologic and morphologic study. *Pediatrics* 34:839–850.

110. Scott HS, Bunge S, Gal A, et al. (1995): Molecular genetics of mucopolysaccharidosis type I: diagnostic, clinical, and biological implications. *Hum Mutat* 6:288–302.

111. Sela M, Eidelman E, Yatzim S (1975): Oral manifestations of Morquio's syndrome. *Oral Surg Oral Med Oral Pathol* 39.

112. Shapiro J, Strome M, Crocker AC (1985): Airway obstruction and sleep apnea in Hurler and Hunter syndromes. *Ann Otol Rhinol Laryngol* 94:458–461.

113. Singh J, DiFerrante NM, Niebes P, et al. (1976): *N*-acetylgalactosamine-6-sulfate sulfatase in man: absence of the enzyme in Morquio's disease. *J Clin Invest* 57:1036–1040.

114. Sly WS, Brot FE, Glaser JH, et al. (1974): β-Glucoronidase deficiency mucopolysaccharidosis. *Birth Defects* 10:239–245.

115. Sly WS, Quinton BA, McAlister WH, et al. (1973): Beta glucuronidase deficiency: report of clinical, radiologic, and biochemical features of a new mucopolysaccharidosis. *J Pediatr* 82:249–257.

116. Smith SW (1967): Roentgen findings in homocystinuria. *Am J Roentgenol Radium Ther Nucl Med* 100:147–154.

117. Sostrin RD, Hasso AN, Peterson DL, et al. (1977): Myelographic features of mucopolysaccharidoses: a new sign. *Radiology* 125:421–424.

118. Spranger J (1969): The genetic mucopolysaccharidoses. *Birth Defects* 5:145–156.

119. Spranger J (1972): The systemic mucopolysaccharidoses. *Ergeb Inn Med Kinderheilkd* 32:165–265.

120. Spranger J (1975): The genetic mucolipidoses: definition and classification. *Birth Defects* 11:279–282.

121. Spranger J (1987): Mini review: inborn errors of complex carbohydrate metabolism. *Am J Med Genet* 28:489–499.

122. Spranger J, Cantz M, Gehler J, et al. (1978): Mucopolysaccharidosis II (Hunter disease) with corneal opacities. *Eur J Pediatr* 129:11–16.

123. Spranger J, Gehler J, Cantz M (1977): Mucolipidosis I-a sialidosis. *Am J Med Genet* 1.

124. Spranger JW, Koch F, McKusick VA, et al. (1970): Mucopolysaccharidosis VI: Maroteaux-Lamy's disease. *Helv Paediatr Acta* 25:337–362.

125. Spranger JW, Langer LO, Wiedemann HR (1974): *Bone dysplasias: an atlas of constitutional disorders of skeletal development*, Philadelphia: WB Saunders.

126. Spranger J, Schuster W (1969): Classifiable and non-classifiable mucopolysaccharidoses. *Ann Radiol* 12:365–375.

127. Spranger JW, Wiedemann HR (1970): The genetic mucolipidoses diagnosis and differential diagnosis. *Humangenetik* 9:113–139.

128. Staalman CR, Bakker HD (1984): Mucolipidosis I. *Skeletal Radiol* : 153–161.

129. Stevenson RE, Howell RR, McKusick VA, et al. (1976): The iduronidase-deficient mucopolysaccharidoses: clinical and roentgenographic features. *Pediatrics* 57:111–122.

130. Stumpf DA, Austin JH, Crocker AC, et al. (1973): Mucopolysaccharidosis type VI (Maroteaux-Lamy syndrome). *Am J Dis Child* 126: 747–755.

131. Taber P, Gyepes MT, Philippart M, et al. (1973): Roentgenographic manifestations of Leroy's I-cell disease. *Am J Roentgenol Radium Ther Nucl Med* 118:213–221.

132. Tandon V, Williamson JB, Cowie RA, et al. (1996): Spinal problems in mucopolysaccharidosis I (Hurler syndrome). *J Bone Joint Surg Br* 78:938–944.

133. Taybi H, Lachman RS (1990): *Radiology of syndromes, metabolic disorders, and skeletal dysplasias*. Chicago: Year Book Medical Publishers.

134. Terashima Y, Tsuda K, Isomura S, et al. (1975): I-cell disease. *Am J Dis Child* 129:1083–1090.

135. Thomas PS, Carson NAJ (1978): Homocystinuria: the evolution of skeletal changes in relation to treatment. *Ann Radiol (Paris)* 21: 95–104.

136. Thomas SL, Childress MH, Quinton B (1985): Hypoplasia of the odontoid with atlanto-axial subluxation in Hurler's syndrome. *Pediatr Radiol* 15:353–354.

137. Tondeur M, Vamos-Hurwitz E, Mockel-Pohl S, et al. (1971): Clinical, biochemical and ultrastructural studies in a case of chondrodystrophy presenting the I-cell phenotype in tissue culture. *J Pediatr* 79: 366–378.

138. Tsuzaki S, Matsuo N, Nagai T, et al. (1987): An unusually mild variant of Hunter's syndrome in a 14-year-old boy. *Acta Paediatr Scand* 76:844–846.

139. van de Kamp JJP (1979): *The Sanfilippo syndrome: a clinical and genetical study of 75 patients in the Netherlands* [thesis] Gravenhage: JH Pasmans.

140. van Schrojenstein-de Valk HMJ, van de Kamp JJP (1987): Follow-up on seven adult patients with mild Sanfilippo B-disease. *Am J Med Genet* 28:125–129.

141. Vinchon M, Cotton A, Clarisse J, et al. (1995): Cervical myelopathy secondary to Hunter syndrome in an adult. *Am J Neuroradiol* 16: 1402–1403.

142. Wakai S, Minami R, Kameda K, et al. (1988): Skeletal muscle involvement in mucopolysaccharidosis type IIA: severe type of Hunter syndrome. *Pediatr Neurol* 4.

143. Walker RWM, Darowski M, Morris P, et al. (1994): Anaesthesia and mucopolysaccharidoses: a review of airway problems in children. *Anaesthesia* 49:1078–1084.

144. Wassman ER, Johnson K, Shapiro LJ, et al. (1982): Postmortem findings in the Hurler-Scheie syndrome (mucopolysaccharidosis I-H/S). *Birth Defects* 18:13–18.

145. Watts RWE, Spellacy E, Kendall BE, et al. (1981): Computed tomography studies on patients with mucopolysaccharidoses. *Neuroradiology* 21:9–23.

146. Whelan DT, Chang PL, Cockshott PW (1983): Mucolipidosis II: the clinical, radiological and biochemical features in three cases. *Clin Genet* 24:90–96.

147. Whitley CB, Belani KG, Chang P, et al. (1993): Long-term outcome of Hurler syndrome following bone marrow transplantation. *Am J Med Genet* 46:209–218.

148. Yatzin S, Erickson RP, Epstein CJ (1977): Mild and severe Hunter syndrome (MPS II) within the same sibships. *Clin Genet* 11:319–326.

149. Young ID, Harper PS (1979): Long-term complications in Hunter's syndrome. *Clin Genet* 16:125–132.

150. Zellweger H, Ponseti IV, Pedrini V, et al. (1961): Morquio-Ullrich's disease. *J Pediatr* 59:549–561.

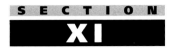

NEUROMUSCULAR DISEASE

NEUROMUSCULAR SPINAL DEFORMITIES

JOHN E. LONSTEIN

This chapter reviews the general principles of neuromuscular spinal deformities as a basis for discussion of each etiologic subgroup.

ETIOLOGY

Neuromuscular spinal deformities form a diverse group of diseases and conditions that have involvement of the neuromuscular system in common (4,11–13) and share principles in course of disease, evaluation, and management. These deformities have been classified by the Scoliosis Research Society into neuropathic and myopathic conditions. The neuropathic conditions have been subdivided into upper and lower motor neuron lesions. The upper motor neuron group includes diseases such as cerebral palsy, syringomyelia, and spinal cord trauma; the lower motor neuron group includes poliomyelitis and spinal muscular atrophy. Certain conditions such as myelodysplasia and spinal trauma have both upper and lower motor neuron involvement. The myopathic conditions include arthrogryposis, Duchenne muscular dystrophy, and other forms of myopathy. The prevalence of spinal deformity in these conditions is much higher than that in idiopathic scoliosis, varying from 25% to 100% (Table 1). In general, the greater the neuromuscular involvement, the greater are the likelihood and severity of scoliosis.

Although the foregoing conditions vary greatly in causation, they share many features. Many are genetic in origin, and they all involve more than one systems, necessitating evaluation by a multidisciplinary team. Whereas idiopathic scoliosis is only a spinal deformity, patients with neuromuscular disorders have many possible attendant problems, such as contractures, dislocated hips, seizures, mental retardation, insensate skin, and pressure sores. Thus the evaluation of these patients cannot be confined to the spine alone; it must encompass all these areas.

At first glance, it may be easy to assume that scoliosis in these conditions is caused by muscle weakness. But this conclusion is difficult to support, because some conditions are accompanied by spasticity and others by flaccidity. No consistent pattern of scoliosis is associated with a particular pattern of weakness or side of weakness. Real understanding comes with an appreciation of spinal muscle control and control of spinal balance by the central pathways.

CURVE PATTERNS

Because spinal surgeons typically see more cases of idiopathic scoliosis, and therefore base their principles of evaluation and treatment on that condition, the neuromuscular deformities need to be contrasted to idiopathic scoliosis. The curve patterns in idiopathic scoliosis are well recognized and constant, the thoracic deformity being lordoscoliosis. The curve patterns in neuromuscular conditions are varied; some resemble idiopathic scoliosis patterns, and others are long C curves that collapse into scoliosis or kyphosis. A common curve pattern is a thoracolumbar curve that extends to the pelvis, the sacrum being a part of the curve.

Kyphosis is important in neuromuscular deformities, and it has two possible causes. The kyphosis can be caused by true posterior angulation of the vertebrae, as in collapsing kyphosis or in myelodysplasia developmental kyphosis. The second cause of what appears clinically to be kyphosis is vertebral rotation—what Stagnara (15) called *kyphosing scoliosis.* Because of vertebral rotation at the apex of the curve, the deformity appears as posterior spinal angulation (kyphosis) rather than as lateral deformity (scoliosis). The apical vertebra, when rotated 90 degrees, continues to deviate laterally in relation to itself, but because of the rotation, this appears as kyphosis related to the torso as a whole.

COURSE OF DISEASE

When considering the course of neuromuscular disease, there are two aspects to consider. The first is the course of the underlying disease: Is it progressive, as in Duchenne muscular dystrophy, or nonprogressive, as in cerebral palsy? The answer may affect decision making and definitely affects discussions with the family. Certain conditions are not progressive but cause progressive weakness with growth, such as spinal muscular atrophy. As the

J.E. Lonstein: Department of Orthopedics, University of Minnesota, Twin Cities Spine Center, Minneapolis, Minnesota 55317.

TABLE 1. PREVALENCE OF SPINAL DEFORMITIES IN DIFFERENT NEUROMUSCULAR DISEASES

Disease	Percentage
Cerebral palsy	25
Myelodysplasia	60
Spinal muscle atrophy	67
Friedreich ataxia	80
Duchenne muscular dystrophy	90
Traumatic paralysis (before 10 y of age)	100

body or extremities grow, the weak muscles cannot control the increased length or weight of the body or extremity; thus the weakness "progresses" while the underlying disease is unchanged. The second aspect of the course of disease is progression of the spinal deformity. In neuromuscular spinal deformities, progression occurs much more frequently than in idiopathic scoliosis. In addition, progression often continues into adulthood.

The long-term effects of the spinal deformity in these neuromuscular conditions are more disabling to the patient than are those of idiopathic scoliosis. There is a loss of sitting ability with an accompanying loss of functional ability, especially loss of hand use. In addition, there is a marked effect on pulmonary function. In idiopathic scoliosis, the effect of a 70- or 80-degree curve on pulmonary function is minimal. In neuromuscular scoliosis, the effect of this curve added to the pulmonary compromise caused by weak intercostal muscles can be devastating.

PATIENT EVALUATION

The evaluation of a patient with neuromuscular scoliosis involves more than assessment of the spinal deformity. Accurate diagnosis of the underlying disease entity is essential and often entails muscle biopsy. The patient and family should be counseled in every case. Counseling should include information about the inheritance and course of the disease and the spinal deformity.

A full family history should be obtained. The physical examination should cover the underlying disease, all aspects of involvement in all the systems, and the spinal deformity. Of special importance is assessment of nutrition and feeding and of pulmonary function. Regarding idiopathic scoliosis, all such information is obtained from the patient and family. Regarding neuromuscular problems, however, additional information is sought from the child's caregivers, attendants, teachers, and physical therapists. In no area is this information of more use than in an appreciation of the patient's functional level. How does the patient move around? Is assistance necessary? Does the patient use a wheelchair? What is the sitting ability? What is the hand use? Has this functional level changed? For example, has there been a loss of sitting ability, loss of hand use, increased weakness, or a change in respiratory function with increased frequency of pneumonia? In assessing a change in functional level, one must ascertain whether it is caused by increasing spinal deformity or progression of the underlying neuromuscular disease. Questions

are asked to evaluate the growth pattern and, in the second decade, to determine whether the child is in the growth spurt.

The physical examination is divided into three areas: general patient evaluation, orthopaedic evaluation, and evaluation of the spinal deformity. The patient's overall size, height, weight, and nutritional status are documented. Signs of puberty, such as development of breasts and pubic hair are documented and graded according to the Tanner system (17). Members of the multidisciplinary team evaluate intelligence, hearing, and vision. The orthopedic examination includes assessment of all extremities and joints for contractures and an evaluation of hand function. If the patient can cooperate, the muscle strength of each muscle group is tested. The spinal deformity, decompensation, and shoulder balance are documented.

Ambulatory status is evaluated, and patients are classified as walkers, sitters, or nonsitters. Further subdivision is based on whether the activity (walking or sitting) depends on assistance. For sitters, the amount of help necessary to achieve a balanced upright posture is assessed. The flexibility of the scoliosis is evaluated clinically with a supine assessment and by means of passive side bending of the patient to judge the rigidity of each curve. Is there any pelvic obliquity? If there is obliquity, which side is high? Can the pelvis be leveled in the supine and sitting positions (10)?

The entire musculoskeletal system is evaluated for contractures and the range of motion of each joint (3). The status of the hips is important among these patients. There may be contractures or dislocation, or the hips may be windswept, which is adduction contracture of one side combined with an abduction contracture of the opposite side, the hip on the adducted side usually being dislocated or subluxed. Areas of pressure breakdown on the sacrum or greater trochanter must also be sought. Whenever possible, full muscle testing and an evaluation of sensation in the upper and lower extremities is performed.

A general medical evaluation is performed with emphasis on nutrition (7). This includes the nutritional history, feeding history, and a battery of blood tests when necessary to evaluate current nutritional status. These include hemoglobin, total lymphocyte count, red blood cell mean corpuscular volume, total protein, albumin, electrolytes, serum blood urea nitrogen, creatinine, and transferrin (18). Other areas of involvement are evaluated depending on the specific neuromuscular disease. These include, when necessary, hearing, vision, intelligence, communication, and hand function, as well as assessment of any seizures and their control.

RADIOLOGIC EVALUATION

An accurate, consistent radiologic examination is essential. For very young patients and those who do not sit, a supine anteroposterior spinal radiograph is obtained. For all other patients, upright radiographs are obtained—standing for patients who can stand, sitting for the others. The posteroanterior position is used for those able to stand, and the anteroposterior position for sitters. All these upright radiographs are obtained with minimal support. Standing patients do not support themselves with crutches, and the sitters use no hand support. This gives an accurate appreciation of the true magnitude of the spinal deformity under the effect of gravity and of pelvic obliquity and spinal balance. Clinically spinal balance is the relation of the head and torso to the pelvis; radiographically, it is the relation of the torso to the pelvis and of the spinous process of C7 to the midsacral line—a vertical drawn from the middle of the sacrum (the spinous process of S1).

All curves are identified and measured. To evaluate the flexibility of the curves (either scoliosis or kyphosis), a traction radiograph is obtained. This can be done in the radiology department with manual distraction with a head halter and leg traction. This is not very effective if the patient has spasticity or hip flexion contracture, as in cerebral palsy. For these patients a better method is to obtain a traction radiograph on a Risser-Cotrel frame.

TREATMENT

The treatment options are the same as those for any spinal deformity—observation, nonoperative, and operative. The choice depends on the initial problem, such as curvature, loss of sitting or function, or pressure sores, and the child's age and maturity.

Observation

Observation plays an important role in the management of spinal deformities in neuromuscular diseases. Because of the high prevalence of spinal deformities, routine clinical or radiologic evaluation should be performed regularly. This means yearly examination in the multidisciplinary or neurology clinic with a spinal examination or radiography. When a curve is present, it is followed by the clinic, or the patient is referred for appropriate spinal care—continued observation or nonoperative or operative treatment.

Nonoperative Treatment

Nonoperative treatment of patients with neuromuscular spinal deformities is directed at two areas: seating and curve treatment. The curves of these patients are either postural—the spine collapses in the upright sitting or standing position because of a lack of muscle control—or structural in nature. Seating systems are used for patients who are unable to sit without support. For curve control, orthoses are used—either a Milwaukee brace or a thoracolumbosacral orthosis (TLSO).

Seating Support

If the patient is unable to walk, seating support is necessary. There are many choices, and the appropriate type of seating support depends on the patient's sitting balance. Sitting balance is evaluated by means of seating the patient on the side of the examining table to see whether he or she can sit unaided. When the patient cannot sit unaided, support is given in a progressive way until the patient can sit upright. First the pelvis is supported, then the lateral and anterior thorax, then the head. The seating support needed for each child is determined in this evaluation.

Firm Seat and Back

When minimal or no support is needed, a firm seat and firm back are adequate to supply a stable pelvis. This can be accomplished with the addition of a padded wooden or plastic seat and back to the wheelchair, or the sling seat and back can be pulled taut to supply the required support.

Upholstered Sitting Support

When pelvic support and some lateral thoracic support are needed, an upholstered sitting system is best (Fig. 1). This can be made of wood or molded thermoplastic. Gillette Children's Hospital developed a molded thermoplastic seating system that comes in a number of sizes. Upholstered pads can be added to hold the pelvis, and lateral thoracic supports can be used where necessary. A thoracic vest can be added if anterior support is needed. The advantage of this system is that it can be tailored to the individual support needs of the patient, and it can be adjusted for growth by varying the thickness of the lateral pelvic pads.

Molded Sitting Support

When more support is necessary because of the lack of sitting balance or the size of the patient, the Gillette sitting support orthosis has proved ideal (Fig. 2). This is a molded polypropylene shell made from a positive mold of the patient. It is a total-contact orthosis. Support is provided from the distal posterior thighs to the shoulders or occiput. This orthosis gives excellent pelvic and thoracic control, and because of the total-contact concept, skin problems are few. A thoracic vest is added to give anterior thoracic support; a head support is added when neces-

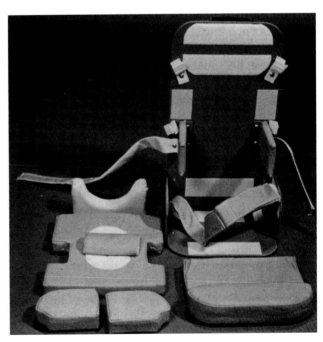

FIGURE 1. Upholstered sitting support orthosis consists of a molded plastic frame that has back, seat, and side support. There are covered foam inserts for the seat, back, and sides of the pelvis. The latter inserts can be made in varying thicknesses to accommodate the child's growth.

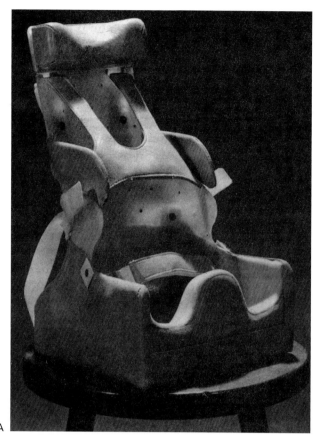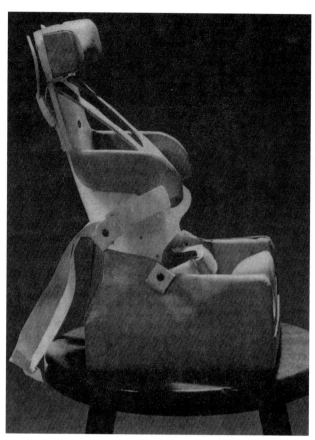

FIGURE 2. Gillette molded sitting support orthosis. The orthosis is made from a positive mold of the child. There is total contact from the back of the thighs to the head, with lateral pelvic and thoracic support. A lap belt and thoracic vest are added to keep the child positioned in the orthosis. The orthosis is shown in oblique front **(A)** and side **(B)** views. The orthosis is tilted back to aid in head control.

sary. When it is necessary to control the tendency of the head to flex, head control can be aided by means of reclining the entire seating system.

All these sitting systems have to support the pelvis and posterior thighs, the latter being essential to distribute the pressures in sitting. The feet have to be placed on footrests to prevent too much popliteal pressure. In all sitting supports, a lap belt is mandatory to hold the pelvis in the support and to prevent the pelvis from sliding forward. When these supports are placed in a wheelchair, they must be held there with a seat belt.

Commercial Sitting Supports

There are a variety of commercially available supports to aid these patients with sitting. For a very young or small child, a car seat can provide support. For these children, a system of plastic molded supports—Tumbleform seats—also is available. These seats come in a number of sizes and can support very flexible curves, but they place the child in a reclined position, which is not conducive to interaction on the child's level. A large number of commercial chairs (e.g., Mullholland, Orthokinetic) usually have some type of pelvic and thoracic support. These are effective for very flexible spines, but they do not work well for larger children or in cases of severe spasticity. It is essential

to assess the effect of the support on the spine with radiographs. With the straps and supports in place, it is impossible to assess curve control clinically.

These sitting supports also help control the collapsing postural curve—scoliosis or kyphosis—by holding the patient in an upright, balanced posture. If a structural curve is present, the sitting support helps sitting balance without controlling the curve. When the child is small, it is easy to support the spine and control postural curves. With growth the spine becomes longer, the child becomes heavier, and the postural curves become more difficult—and at times impossible—to control.

Curve Control

In idiopathic scoliosis, the aim of bracing is to control the curve and prevent the need for surgical intervention. In neuromuscular deformities, the aim of bracing is to control the curve during the period of growth and delay the need for surgical stabilization. For most of these patients, this control is possible in the juvenile years. With the onset of the pubertal growth spurt, however, control is lost, and surgical stabilization is necessary. It is foolhardy to delay fusion until the end of growth. At the onset of puberty, approximately 85% to 90% of spinal growth has already occurred. In addition, during puberty there is usually rapid deterioration in the curve with a marked increase in curve magnitude and structurality. Any additional growth will produce a spine that is not longer but is more curved, stiffer, and shorter overall.

Orthotic management of neuromuscular scoliosis is more demanding than that of idiopathic scoliosis. The duration of bracing is longer, there are more skin problems because of the prevalence of insensate skin among these patients, and full-time bracing is not always necessary. In cases of very flexible curves that are well controlled in an orthosis, bracing is necessary only when the patient is upright under the effect of gravity. At night during sleep, bracing is not necessary, because gravity is not loading the spine and causing the curve to collapse.

Operative Treatment

The operative management of neuromuscular scoliosis differs markedly from that of idiopathic scoliosis. Traction rarely is necessary in idiopathic scoliosis, but it plays a role in the care of paralyzed patients either to improve preoperative pulmonary status or to aid in postoperative care by providing upright support.

The preoperative evaluation differs in that many more areas have to be evaluated for patients with neuromuscular scoliosis. Pulmonary status is important, but in many cases pulmonary function testing is impossible because of lack of patient cooperation or because of paralysis of the intercostal muscles. In such cases, the test results are inaccurate and give a false impression of the pulmonary function of these patients. A good assessment of pulmonary function can be obtained with the history of upper respiratory infection or pneumonia. A good nutritional assessment is important, especially for patients with swallowing or feeding problems.

Overall ambulatory function is assessed, as is the functional level of the patient. Sitting ability, hand use, mental ability, presence of seizures, vision, and functioning in activities of daily living are documented. These areas are critical and can be adversely affected by an increase in spinal deformity. It must be remembered, however, that in many cases the underlying neuromuscular disease is not static and that a change in the patient's examination or functional status may be caused by progression of the disease rather than the spinal deformity. In the patient assessment, information from the patient's family, caregivers, school staff, and physical therapist is invaluable.

The surgical principles in the management of neuromuscular scoliosis differ from those in idiopathic scoliosis. Fusion is necessary at a younger age, and the fusions are longer. Fusion to the sacrum is fairly common, because many of these children do not have sitting balance or there is pelvic obliquity. With idiopathic scoliosis in an adolescent, fusion to the sacrum is never needed. Combined anterior and posterior fusion is common in the treatment of patients with neuromuscular scoliosis either because posterior elements are absent, as in myelodysplasia, or because it is necessary to gain correction in a rigid lumbar or thoracolumbar curve and achieve a spine fused in balance over a level pelvis. Vertebral bone is osteopenic, so segmental fixation with the Luque system is preferred. Autogenous bone graft usually is in-

sufficient because the small pelvic size or the need to fuse to the sacrum with the use of the Galveston technique or iliac screws. Blood loss is greater because the bone is osteopenic, the muscles are poor, and the procedures take a long time. In assessing blood loss, the absolute volume lost is of less importance than the proportion of blood lost from the patient's circulating blood volume. Intraoperative blood salvage with a cell saver is fairly routine in these procedures.

Anterior fusion and instrumentation alone play no role in the management of neuromuscular deformities. Combined anterior and posterior fusion and posterior fusion alone are used in neuromuscular spinal fusion. Combined fusion is used when there are no posterior elements (myelodysplasia) or when there are large, stiff curves and an anterior release and fusion is necessary to achieve a balanced spine over a level pelvis. Achieving a level pelvis is essential in the management of a sitter with neuromuscular spinal deformity and insensate skin. Pelvic obliquity among these patients causes unequal pressure distribution and pressure sores. Combined fusion usually is performed sequentially under the same anesthesia rather than as a staged procedure (9).

The child is positioned on the spinal frame (Hall-Relton or similar design) for the posterior fusion. Positioning often is difficult when hip flexion contractures are present (Fig. 3). In these cases, the pelvic positioning blocks are placed at the lower end of the holding board to allow the hips to be flexed to the required degree. When the contractures are great (more than 60 to 70 degrees), it is necessary to raise the lower end of the board on a sandbag so that the hips can be adequately flexed. Hip flexion after positioning has to be such that when the hips are extended, there is no pelvic tilt and induction of more lumbar lordosis. Sufficient padding is placed under the knees, which are flexed with pillows or rolls. As the board and patient are tilted with the head down, the operating table is tilted in a reverse manner to place the back horizontal.

The extent of posterior fusion depends on the curve pattern and the ambulatory status of the patient. For patients with neuromuscular spinal deformities who can walk, the guidelines for the selection of the fusion area follow those of idiopathic scoliosis. For patients who cannot walk and have pelvic obliquity, fusion extends to the sacrum and cranially to the upper thoracic area (T2 or T3). For patients who cannot walk who have a level pelvis, I fuse to the sacrum, but some surgeons fuse to the lower lumbar spine (16). The instrumentation used is segmental with either (a) a multiple hook-rod system with or without addition of sublaminar wires or (b) a Luque rod and sublaminar wires or a Unit Rod device (5). When fusion to the sacrum is necessary, it can be performed with the Luque-Galveston technique or with iliac screws (2,8,14).

Blood loss is monitored during the procedure by means of weighing the sponges and measuring the cell-saver return. In operations on children with neuromuscular deformities, it is important to relate any calculation of blood loss and replacement to a percentage of the calculated circulating blood volume, not to the volume of loss alone. The use of intraoperative blood salvage techniques is common in these spinal fusions. It is not unusual for these small children to have loss that equals or exceeds a circulating volume. It is imperative in cases of extensive

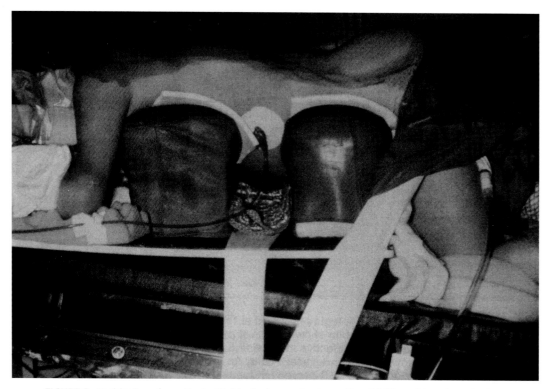

FIGURE 3. Positioning of a patient with hip flexion contractures. The child is positioned on the four-poster frame with the lower posts at the edge of the wooden board. The lower edge of the board is elevated with a sandbag to allow accommodation of full hip flexion. Padding is placed under the knees, which are flexed with a pillow. The operating table is tilted head up until the patient's back is horizontal.

blood loss to replace clotting factors with fresh frozen plasma and platelets with the addition of calcium.

Because in many of these operations inadequate iliac autograft is available, either because a small iliac crest or because of the use of iliac fixation, there is a need for graft augmentation with allograft or a bone graft substitute. Unlike operations on adults, spinal fusion with allograft use in the treatment of children is successful with good incorporation and a low pseudarthrosis rate. Crushed cancellous allograft is the easiest to use and has an excellent success rate (19).

Postoperative care of these patients is demanding. Attention has to be paid to pulmonary support, fluid status, and nutrition in addition to routine postoperative monitoring. The patients are mobilized as rapidly as possible for a return to preoperative ambulatory and functional status. Because of the secure fixation afforded by segmental fixation systems (multiple hook-rod or Luque segmental wiring) and the lower functional demands of these patients, postoperative immobilization is rarely needed.

Postoperative Complications

Postoperative complications among patients with neuromuscular spinal deformities are the same as those that affect any children undergoing spinal fusion. Because of the multitude of other problems these patients have, the complication rate after surgery is high, especially the rate of pulmonary, fluid balance, and skin

problems. Some complications, however, are more common or important than others. These include respiratory problems, ileus, nutritional problems, hip problems, and crankshaft phenomenon.

Respiratory Problems

A child with neuromuscular disease may have intercostal paralysis and a poor cough reflex. As a result, the incidence of postoperative respiratory complications (atelectasis or pneumonia) is high. To minimize or prevent this problem, attention to postoperative respiratory care is essential. It is common to leave the endotracheal tube in place for 1 or 2 days after the operation and to use ventilator assistance. When prolonged support is anticipated, the tube is placed through the nasotracheal route. Secretions are handled with repeated suctioning, which is continued after tube removal. Any cough reflex present will be stimulated by suctioning. Postural drainage and chest percussion are also used to manage atelectasis.

Ileus

Ileus is common among these children after the retroperitoneal approach is used. It also occurs after the posterior approach is used because narcotics are used for pain control. Intestinal hypomotility may persist, necessitating prolonged parenteral support. Because many of these children have nutritional problems before the operation, this inability to resume oral or gastrostomy feeding is important. In these cases, hyperalimentation by the central intravenous route is necessary until adequate gastrointestinal feeding can be resumed. When there is postoperative return of intestinal motility but the child cannot tolerate oral feedings, a small feeding tube can be passed into the stomach or duodenum to allow nutritional support until oral feeding is tolerated.

Hip Problems

Hip problems—subluxation, dislocation, and contracture—are frequent among patients who do not walk. Their hips must be assessed preoperatively, and the parents and caretakers must be told that the hip position may appear worse after the operation when contractures are present. When there are postoperative hip contractures and the child is supine, the legs need to be supported on pillows with 90 degrees of hip and knee flexion. This prevents windswept abduction and adduction contractures from worsening. The forces on the pelvis are reduced, protecting the Galveston pelvic fixation.

The question arises as to when hip range of motion and stretching of contractures can be resumed after fusion to the sacrum. The danger in these cases is torque on the pelvis, which puts sacral and pelvic fixation in jeopardy. Gentle range of motion, short of the extremes, is advised in the healing phase, and stretching is not allowed. These restrictions are in effect until the fusion is solid, which usually takes 4 to 6 months. At that time, the full preoperative hip program of range of motion and stretching can be resumed.

Fusion Too Short

Incorrect selection of the fusion area can cause problems. Failure to fuse to the sacrum, when indicated, leads to a lack of sitting balance and a tilted torso. Failure to include the entire thoracic kyphosis in the fusion area increases the kyphosis immediately above the fusion as the spine falls forward over the top of the fusion.

Crankshaft Phenomenon

Because a large percentage of these children need fusion at a young age, continued anterior growth in the presence of a solid posterior fusion can occur (crankshaft phenomenon) (6). This can increase rotational deformity and even cause torquing of the fusion. Crankshaft phenomenon can be prevented with anterior fusion, which eliminates the anterior growth potential. In these children, the crankshaft phenomenon is a change in appearance only and has not been shown to have any functional effect. The decision to perform anterior fusion to prevent this phenomenon should be seriously considered in light of the added operative time, blood loss, and complications of additional surgery, especially because the functional benefits of the anterior approach

in these cases have not been shown. The prospect of adding an anterior approach to an operation on a patient with respiratory compromise must be considered.

SUMMARY

Spinal deformities are an important problem among children with neuromuscular diseases. These children can have spasticity or flaccidity. Multisystem involvement includes contractures, insensate skin, mental retardation, and respiratory problems. A detailed evaluation of all these areas and of the child's nutritional status and functional ambulatory level is essential. Nonoperative treatment plays a role in following scoliosis for progression. Active treatment involves the use of sitting supports to improve sitting function. Use of an orthosis (TLSO) plays a small role in the treatment of these children.

The two main indications for surgery are curve progression and deterioration in sitting function. A traction radiograph is the best radiographic determination of the flexibility of the spinal deformity. Leveling of the pelvis and the balance of the torso over the pelvis also are evaluated on this traction radiograph. A posterior approach alone is used for "idiopathic like" curves and for curves that balance over a level pelvis on a traction radiograph. Most fusions are long (T2 to the sacrum), the Luque-Galveston technique being the instrumentation of choice. For curves that do not balance or show pelvic obliquity on a traction radiograph, combined anterior and posterior fusion is indicated. This approach also is indicated in the care of patients with myelodysplasia when there are no posterior elements.

Postoperative care is concentrated on the respiratory system and on early implementation of nutritional support. With care in surgical technique and adequate postoperative care, complications can be minimized. The child can be returned to preoperative functional level with a successful surgical result—a solidly fused spine in balance in the coronal and sagittal planes over a level pelvis.

REFERENCES

1. Arlet V, Aebi M (2001): Anterior and posterior cervical spine fusion and instrumentation. In: Weinstein SL, ed. *The pediatric spine: surgery.* Philadelphia: Lippincott Williams & Wilkins, 2001, pp. 000–000.
2. Asher MA (2001): Isola spinal implant system updat: emphasizing application during the first two decades of life. In: Weinstein SL, ed. *The pediatric spine: surgery.* Philadelphia: Lippincott Williams & Wilkins, 2001, pp. 000–000.
3. Bleck E (1987): *Orthopedic management in cerebral palsy.* Philadelphia: JB Lippincott.
4. Bradford D, Hu S (1995): Neuromuscular spinal deformities. In: Lonstein JE BD, Winter RB, Ogilvie JW, eds. *Moe's textbook of scoliosis and other spinal deformities,* 3rd ed. Philadelphia: WB Saunders, p. 295.
5. Bulman W, Dormans J, Ecker M, et al. (1996): Posterior spinal fusion for scoliosis in patients with cerebral palsy: a comparison of Luque rod and unit rod instrumentation. *J Pediatr Orthop* 16:314–323.
6. Dubousset J, Herring J, Shufflebarger H (1989): The crankshaft phenomenon. J Pediatr Orthop 9:541.
7. Dvarik D, Roberts J, Burke S (1986): Gastroesophageal evaluation in totally involved cerebral palsy patients. Presented at AAOS meeting.
8. Ferguson RL (2001): Luque rod instrumentation. In: Weinstein SL,

ed. *The pediatric spine: surgery.* Philadelphia: Lippincott Williams & Wilkins, 2001, pp. 000–000.

9. Ferguson R, Hansen M, Nicholas D, et al. (1996): Same-day versus staged anterior-posterior spinal surgery in a neuromuscular scoliosis population: the evaluation of medical complications. *J Pediatr Orthop* 16:293–303.

10. Haas S (1942): Spastic scoliosis and obliquity of the pelvis. *J Bone Joint Surg* 24:775.

11. Lonstein J, Renshaw T (1987): Neuromuscular spine deformity: *Instr Course Lect* :285.

12. Shapiro F, Bresnan M (1982): Orthopedic management of childhood neuromuscular disease. *J Bone Joint Surg Am* 64:785–789.

13. Shapiro F, Bresnan M (1982): Orthopedic management of childhood neuromuscular disease. *J Bone Joint Surg Am* 64:949–953.

14. Shufflebarger HL (2001): Moss Miami spinal instrumentation. In:

15. Weinstein SL, ed. *The pediatric spine: surgery.* Philadelphia: Lippincott Williams & Wilkins, 2001, pp. 000–000.

15. Stagnara P (1974): Deviations laterales du rachis: scoliosis. In: *Encyclopedie mediocochirurgicale.* Paris: Appareil Locomoteur.

16. Sussman M, Little D, Alley R, et al. (1996): Posterior instrumentation and fusion of the thoracolumbar spine for the treatment of neuromuscular scoliosis. *J Pediatr Orthop* 16:304–313.

17. Tanner J (1975): Growth and endocrinology of the adolescent. In: Gardner L, ed. *Endocrine and genetic disease of childhood.* Philadelphia: WB Saunders, p. 14.

18. Winter S (1994): Preoperative assessment of the child with neuromuscular scoliosis. *Orthop Clin North Am* 25:239–245.

19. Yazici M, Asher M (1997): Freeze-dried allograft for posterior spinal fusion in patients with neuromuscular spinal deformities. *Spine* 22:1467–1471.

SPINE DEFORMITIES DUE TO CEREBRAL PALSY

JOHN E. LONSTEIN

The term *cerebral palsy* originally referred to birth anoxia or trauma that caused cerebral dysfunction and spasticity. Today it is more of an all-inclusive term for static encephalopathy whether it is caused prenatally, perinatally, or postnatally (23). It includes all the nonprogressive brain disorders such as genetic demyelination, intrauterine cerebral infection (toxoplasmosis), perinatal anoxia, cerebral trauma or hemorrhage, and postnatal trauma, hemorrhage, or infection.

Because of the generalized brain involvement, all cerebral functions are affected, and there are many associated features—mental retardation, seizures, delayed motor and mental development, and vision and hearing problems (2,3). Mental retardation occurs with motor involvement in 71% of cases, but it can also occur alone. It was present among 29% of patients in a recent surgical series (16). Associated with the motor involvement is the development of contractures, hip dislocation, spinal deformities, pelvic obliquity, and ischial, sacral, and trochanteric pressure sores. Patients with cerebral palsy motor involvement can be divided into groups depending on muscle tone—flaccid, spastic, athetoid, or mixed—the most common problem being spasticity. In addition, the involvement can be symmetric or asymmetric, ranging from spastic monoplegia to spastic quadriplegia with lack of head control—what some have called *spastic pentaplegia* or *total body involvement*. It is important to realize that the motor and intellectual involvement can be independent. There can be major motor involvement with spastic quadriplegia but normal intelligence. The latter is difficult to recognize and appreciate, however, because of the presence of expressive aphasia.

SPINAL DEFORMITIES

The spinal deformities of these patients can be divided into postural curves (caused by lack of sitting balance) and structural curves. The curves of cerebral palsy can be scoliosis, kyphosis, or lordosis. Kyphosis alone occurs fairly commonly among patients who lack sitting balance and is managed nonoperatively, as dis-

cussed later. Lordosis is rare and occurs among patients who can walk and have hip flexion contractures. Lordosis also occurs among patients with severe extensor muscle overactivity, which is an unusual spinal problem. Scoliosis is the most common spinal deformity among patients with cerebral palsy.

At first glance, the cause of the structural scoliosis appears to be easy to explain on the basis of muscle imbalance on the two sides of the body and an overall incidence of spinal deformity in cerebral palsy of 20% to 25%. There is, however, a low incidence of scoliosis (5%) in spastic diplegia and a high incidence (65% to 70%) in spastic quadriplegia. Other factors that have been correlated with the incidence of scoliosis, including degree of spasticity, ambulatory status, home or institutional setting, and other system involvement. There also are other factors, some of which may be related to the brain stem and balance.

COURSE OF DISEASE

In considering the course of the spinal deformities of cerebral palsy, one must ask two questions: What are the effects of the disease if uncontrolled? How commonly does curve progression occur? In cerebral palsy, a progressive or large curve that is uncontrolled affects the patient's functional abilities and pulmonary function. Because scoliosis is more common among patient who cannot walk, the effects are more marked in this group. The scoliosis affects sitting ability, necessitating constant repositioning by the patient, parent, or caregivers. A high incidence of pressure sores on the ischium, sacrum, or trochanter accompanies this loss of sitting ability. Eventually sitting becomes difficult and limited, and the patient loses all sitting ability. Patients with severe cerebral palsy have frequent respiratory infections because they have difficulty clearing oral secretions and have problems swallowing. When scoliosis is added to this, especially accompanied by reduced pulmonary space and a raised diaphragm, pulmonary infection and pneumonia become more common.

Progression of scoliosis in a person with cerebral palsy differs from that in a person with idiopathic scoliosis. Among persons with idiopathic scoliosis, puberty occurs predictably at the age of 10 to 14 years among girls and 12 to 16 years among boys. Progression of scoliosis, when it occurs, is mainly during the

J.E. Lonstein: Department of Orthopedics, University of Minnesota, Twin Cities Spine Center, Minneapolis, Minnesota 55317.

rapid growth spurt of puberty. Among persons with cerebral palsy, the onset of puberty is variable and can occur as early as 8 years of age or as late as the early twenties. Progression continues into adulthood in a high percentage of cases (15,20,21,29). This means that the patient must be kept under observation for a long time, well into adulthood.

PATIENT EVALUATION

The history obtained for a patient with cerebral palsy is extensive. It covers not only the spinal deformity but also the mother's pregnancy, the delivery, and the growth and development of the patient. This background provides the cause of cerebral palsy and elucidates the child's neurodevelopmental status. The effect of the spinal deformity on the child's function is evaluated with information from the child whenever possible aided by information from parents, attendants, teachers, and therapists. Has there been any change in the back? What changes have been noticed in ability to get around—walking or sitting? What associated problems are present—seizures, contractures, hearing or visual difficulties, pressure sores? Information is sought regarding feeding, nutrition, drooling, and previous respiratory infections. Inquiries are directed at the child's growth and maturity. Questions are asked to evaluate the growth pattern and, in the second decade of life, to determine whether the child is in the growth spurt.

The physical examination is divided into the three areas described in Chapter 44: general patient evaluation, orthopaedic evaluation, and evaluation of the spinal deformity. The patient's overall size, height, weight, and nutritional status are documented. Because of the delayed development that accompanies severe cerebral palsy, patients often are below the twenty-fifth or even the fifth percentile for age. Signs of puberty, such as development of breasts or pubic hair, are documents and graded with the Tanner system (28). It is important to remember that among these children puberty can be premature or delayed. The general evaluation must include hearing, vision, intelligence, communication, and hand function, as well as assessment of any seizures and their control. The orthopaedic examination emphasizes assessment of all extremities and joints for contractures with emphasis on the hips for dislocation, contractures, and windswept status. Ambulatory status is documented and classified (see Chapter 44). The spinal deformity is documented, as are decompensation and shoulder balance. The flexibility of the scoliosis is evaluated clinically with supine assessment and passive side bending of the patient to judge the rigidity of each curve. Is there any pelvic obliquity? If there is obliquity, which side is high? Can the pelvis be leveled in the supine and sitting positions (14)?

A general medical evaluation is performed with emphasis on nutrition and swallowing (9). A history of feeding is obtained. Does the child feed him or herself, or must the child be fed? How long does it take to feed the child, and is positioning or food consistency a factor? What does the diet consist of? What is the child's height to weight ratio? Swallowing is assessed with the feeding history, history of drooling, and history of episodes of aspiration pneumonia. For a complete assessment, swallowing studies are performed to assess the child's ability to handle foods of different consistencies. A full assessment of nutritional status is necessary for surgical patients. This includes nutritional history, feeding history, and a battery of blood tests to evaluate current nutritional status. These include hemoglobin, total lymphocyte count, red blood cell mean corpuscular volume, total protein, albumin, electrolytes, serum blood urea nitrogen, creatinine, and transferrin (30).

RADIOGRAPHIC EVALUATION

Upright frontal and lateral views, either standing or sitting, form the basis of the radiographic evaluation of the spine. The radiographs are obtained with minimal or no support, so that a true appreciation of the spinal deformity under the effect of gravity can be obtained. The posteroanterior position is used for patients who can stand, and the anteroposterior position is used for those sitters. All the curves present are identified and measured. To evaluate the flexibility of the curves (scoliosis or kyphosis), a traction radiograph is obtained. This can be done in the radiology department with manual distraction with a head halter and leg traction, but it is not very effective in cerebral palsy because of spasticity and spastic reflexes and the presence of hip flexion contractures. A better method is to obtain a traction radiograph on a Risser-Cotrel frame. The patient is positioned on the frame with the hips flexed if there are flexion contractures. Traction is applied with a head halter and pelvic straps. Every effort is made to level the pelvis; gradual forces are used so that there is minimal stimulation of any spastic reflexes. A Cotrel side strap can be applied to the convexity of the scoliosis. Anteroposterior and lateral radiographs are obtained so that the flexibility of the curves can be evaluated.

An anteroposterior hip radiograph is routinely obtained to show the status of the hips. Additional radiographs sometimes are necessary to evaluate the lumbosacral area. Spot radiographs are obtained if there is a congenital spinal abnormality.

TREATMENT

The treatment options are the same as those for patients with any spinal deformity—observation, nonoperative, and operative. The choice depends on the problem (curvature, loss of sitting or function, pressure sores) and the child's age and maturity.

Observation

Observation alone plays a small role in the treatment of patients with cerebral palsy. When the curve causes no loss of function and there is no documented progression, the patient is observed. The magnitude of the curve is not a factor; even large curves in patients with severe spastic quadriplegic need not be managed if there is no definite evidence of progression and no change in sitting ability. The exception is a curve greater than 25 to 30 degrees in an immature, still growing child who can walk. Such a patient would be treated for the curve. Depending on the age and maturity of the patient, the examination and radiographic evaluation are repeated in 4 to 12 months. In all cases that are followed for progression, the current radiograph is always compared with the previous and with the initial radiographs.

Nonoperative Treatment

There are two roles of nonoperative treatment: seating support and curve control.

Seating Support

Because a large percentage of patients with cerebral palsy cannot walk, the use of seating supports is important. There are many choices, and the appropriate type of seating support depends on the patient's sitting balance. Sitting balance is evaluated by means of seating the patient on the side of the examining table to see whether he or she can sit unaided. When this not possible, support is given in a progressive way until the patient can sit upright. First the pelvis is supported, then the lateral and anterior thorax, and then the head. The seating support needed for each child is determined in this evaluation. The seating supports available are a firm seat and back, upholstered sitting supports, molded sitting supports, and commercial seating systems (see Chapter 44).

Some experts have questioned the benefits of sitting to patients with severe spastic quadriplegic cerebral palsy. They state that there is no benefit in sitting someone who has no ability to respond to the environment and that the results are not worth the time, cost, and effort involved. A study conducted at Gillette Children's Hospital on the effect of the molded sitting support orthosis showed that these supports did not control curves, but they improved hand function among those able to use their hands. For the others, the greatest effect was in nursing care. Patients in sitting supports needed less repositioning. This left more time for other children in a family setting or more time for other duties in an institutional setting. Transportation was facilitated, and feeding time decreased.

Curve Control

A thoracolumbosacral orthosis (TLSO), either back opening or bivalved, is used to control scoliosis during the growing years. In most instances, this control is temporary. Curve control is achieved during the juvenile years, but the curve progresses during the adolescent growth spurt (32). One small study, however, found that bracing did not help these patients (22). Most of these children do not walk. They have long, flexible curves that are not controlled by means of sitting support alone. They need a TLSO for curve control and a sitting support for sitting balance. Among my patients with more structural curves, a TLSO has not been able to control the curve. The TLSO has proved to be effective in the management of curves (scoliosis or kyphosis) in patients with cerebral palsy who can walk. The scoliosis in these cases has the same curve patterns and response to bracing as idiopathic scoliosis. In these cases, nonoperative treatment is successful in controlling the curves during adolescence, and surgery rarely is necessary.

Operative Treatment

The indication for surgery in the treatment of patients with cerebral palsy who have nearly normal intelligence is generally not difficult. In these cases, surgery is indicated for curves greater than 45 to 50 degrees in a growing child or when there is documented progression of the curve. The role of surgery in the treatment of patients with severe disabilities and spastic quadriplegia, however, is controversial (16). These patients should be given every opportunity and not be pushed into a corner and ignored. The two main indications for surgery are documented progression of the curve and deterioration in function. An increase of a minimum of 10 degrees is considered progression, because achieving a comparable and repeatable position for radiographs is difficult. This is a more liberal definition of progression. In most other causes of scoliosis, in which dependable and reproducible radiographic positioning is possible, a 5-degree increase constitutes progression.

The other indication for surgery is a change in functional level due to the curve. This is usually a loss of or change in sitting ability. The child's caregivers (parents, attendants) report more difficulty in positioning and that constant repositioning is necessary. In addition, the child becomes fussy and may even have pressure areas over the sacrum, ischium, or greater trochanter. Information from all caregivers (parents, attendants, teachers, and therapists) is necessary to gain a full appreciation of changes in the child's functional level.

In the preoperative assessment, evaluation of the child's health is important. The two areas of greatest importance are the respiratory assessment and an evaluation of nutritional status (see Chapter). When the nutritional status is not optimal, a feeding gastrostomy tube often is placed and surgery postponed until nutrition is improved.

Once a decision has been made that surgery is indicated, the next decision concerns the extent of fusion (19). Which curve or curves should be fused? What vertebrae form the fusion limits? The curve patterns in cerebral palsy have been divided into two patterns: group I and group II curves (16) (Fig. 1). Group I curves are single or double curves that resemble the patterns of idiopathic scoliosis with a level pelvis. They occur most often among children who can walk. Group II curves occur among children who cannot walk and are long thoracolumbar or lumbar curves with pelvic obliquity. The high side of the pelvis is on the side of the concavity of the curve. There are two subgroups of this pattern. In type IIA, the curve continues into the sacrum, which thus forms the caudal extent of the curve. In type IIB, there is a short fractional curve in the lumbosacral area, and the sacral vertebrae are not part of the thoracolumbar or lumbar curve.

For group I curves among children who can walk, the fusion-level criteria are the same as those for idiopathic scoliosis (Fig. 2). In group II curves, the fusion should extend to the sacrum, because this forms part of the curve, although some surgeons prefer to stop at L5 (26). This places the fusion on a solid base and helps achieve the surgical objective in these cases—a solidly fused spine in balance over a level pelvis. The head and thorax must be balanced over the pelvis in the sagittal and coronal planes with normal thoracic kyphosis and lumbar lordosis.

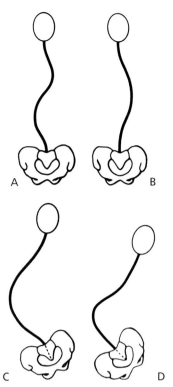

FIGURE 1. Curve patterns in cerebral palsy scoliosis. Group I curves are double curves with thoracic and lumbar components. There is little pelvic obliquity; the child may be well balanced **(A)** or, if the thoracic curve is more extensive, there may be some imbalance **(B)**. Group II curves are large lumbar or thoracolumbar curves with marked pelvic obliquity. There may be a short fractional curve between the end of the curve and the sacrum **(C)**, or the curve may continue into the sacrum, the sacral vertebrae forming part of the curve **(D)**.

Questions often arise about the cranial extent of the fusion. The upper extent of the main thoracolumbar or lumbar curve usually is in the midthoracic area with perhaps a small compensatory curve above, but the latter curve often is absent among patients who have very poor sitting balance. If the fusion stops in the midthoracic area in these cases, there is a tendency for the spine to bend over the top of the fusion, and the result is thoracic hyperkyphosis. Therefore the fusion should extend to the upper thoracic level. Thus the general fusion level for group II curves is from T2 to the sacrum.

What is the management of a group I curve in a child who cannot walk but has a level pelvis and good sitting balance? The first inclination is to fuse to L4 or L5 and not fuse to the sacrum, but I have found that this usually fails. During the growth spurt, a curve develops below the fusion. The result is pelvic obliquity and a subsequent loss of sitting balance. Because of this, I recommend fusing to the sacrum for all sitters regardless of the curve pattern.

The next question is whether to perform posterior fusion alone or combined anterior and posterior fusion. For group I curves, posterior fusion alone is performed. The question of approach generally applies to group II curves, and this decision is made with the use of a traction radiograph. Evaluation of the flexibility of the curve is performed with a Risser-Cotrel casting frame. The child is placed on the frame, and traction is applied with a head halter and muslin waist straps. More tension is placed on the high hip when pelvic obliquity is present. This maneuver is an attempt to achieve maximum correction of the pelvic obliquity. A Cotrel side strap is added over the convexity of the curve to maximally correct the scoliosis. With hip flexion contractures, the hips are placed in flexion on the leg frame on the table. Traction is gradually applied so that any spastic response is minimized. Anteroposterior and, when necessary, lateral radiographs are obtained with a long film (36 inches [90 cm]) so that the entire spine and pelvis can be included on one radiograph. The anteroposterior radiograph shows the flexibility of the scoliosis, the correction of the pelvic obliquity, and the balance of the thorax over the pelvis. A balanced thorax is a nontilted thoracic cage positioned over the pelvis. When this traction radiograph shows a level pelvis and the thorax in balance over the level pelvis, a posterior fusion alone achieves the surgical aim—a solidly fused, balanced spine (the thorax balanced in the coronal and sagittal planes over a level pelvis) (Fig. 3). When the traction radiograph shows pelvic obliquity or an unbalanced thorax (tilted or not positioned over the pelvis), anterior and posterior fusion is necessary to achieve the surgical aim (Fig. 4). No imbalance can be accepted on the traction radiograph, but a minimal amount of pelvic obliquity (less than 10 degrees) is permissible. The other indication for combined anterior and posterior fusion is the rare case that balances on the traction radiograph but still has a large lumbar or thoracolumbar curve.

Posterior Fusion

A posterior fusion alone is performed for group I curves (Fig. 2) and for the group II curves that balance on a traction radiograph (Fig. 3). For patient who can walk, the principles of treatment—selection of fusion levels, use of autograft, and selection of instrumentation—are the same as for idiopathic scoliosis (Fig. 2). When there is osteopenic bone, the Luque system with sublaminar wiring has proved to be effective and secure, because it distributes the forces over all the laminae.

Group II curves, which occur among patients who do not walk, are markedly different from idiopathic scoliosis. The fusions are long, extending on average from T2 to the sacrum. There is greater blood loss, and the bone is extremely osteopenic and soft. The pelvis is small and is used for fixation, so it is not a source of autograft. The surgical technique and planning address these issues. Intraoperative cell salvage is performed with a cell saver. The instrumentation of choice in these cases is a Luque rod with sublaminar wires and Galveston pelvic fixation technique or with iliac screws (1,4,5,7,8,12,13,16–18,24, 25,27). I prefer 16-gauge wire (0.048 mm) with a double strand around each rod at each level. Thick wire is less likely to cut through the lamina. Whenever possible a ¼-inch (6.4 mm) Luque rod is used. A ³⁄₁₆-inch (4.8 mm) rod is used when the pelvis is thin and cannot accept a larger rod. For the fusion, all the local bone from the spinous processes and laminae is placed in the lumbosacral area, and allograft cancellous cubes are added for the rest of the fusion (31).

The child is positioned on a spinal frame (Hall-Relton or similar design) as described in Chapter 44. The techniques of

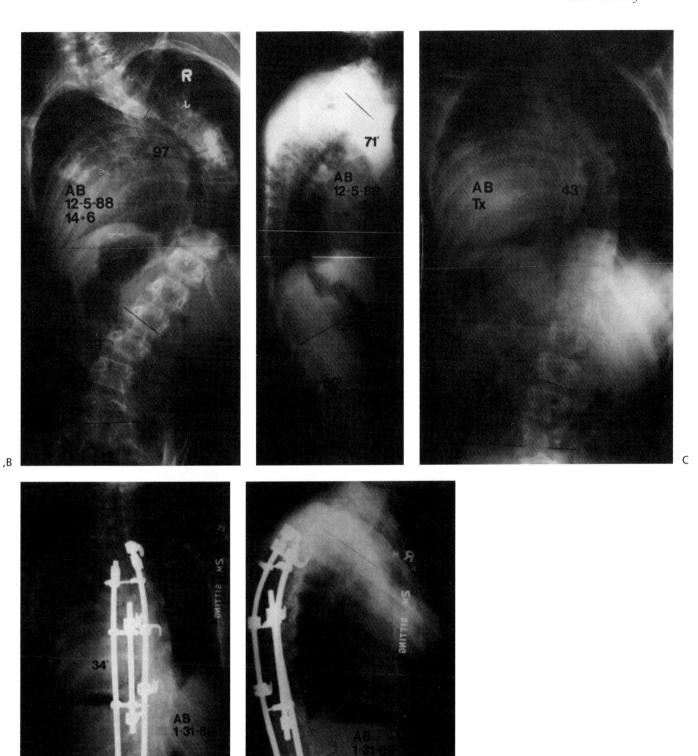

,B

C

,E

FIGURE 2. Images of a patient first evaluated at the age of 14 years 6 months with cerebral palsy, spastic quadriplegia, a right thoracic curve of 97 degrees **(A)**, and thoracic kyphosis of 71 degrees **(B)**. He could walk with hand holding and had marked visual impairment. The curve was flexible. **C:** Traction radiograph shows the curve corrected to 43 degrees. The patient underwent a posterior spinal fusion from T3 to L4 with Cotrel-Dubousset instrumentation and the three-rod technique. Postoperatively there was correction of the scoliosis to 34 degrees **(D)** and of the kyphosis to 56 degrees **(E)**.

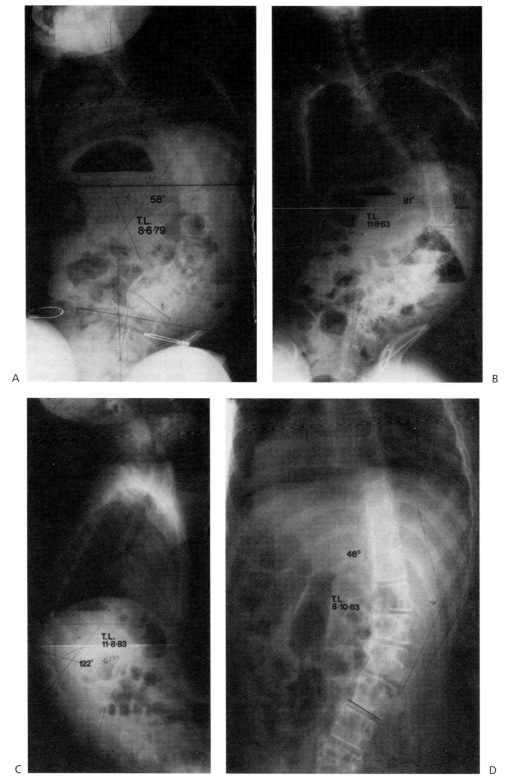

FIGURE 3. A: A 12-year-old girl with cerebral palsy and spastic quadriplegia had a 58-degree long C curve and difficulty sitting. She was placed in a molded sitting support orthosis. The curve progressed. **B:** Unsupported sitting radiograph obtained 4 years after **A** shows a level pelvis and a compensatory curve below the 81-degree thoracolumbar curve. **C:** Lateral radiograph shows a 122-degree thoracolumbar rotatory kyphosis. **D:** Traction radiograph obtained on a Risser-Cotrel frame shows a balanced torso over a level pelvis and correction of the scoliosis to 46 degrees and of the kyphosis to 40 degrees. *(Figure continues.)*

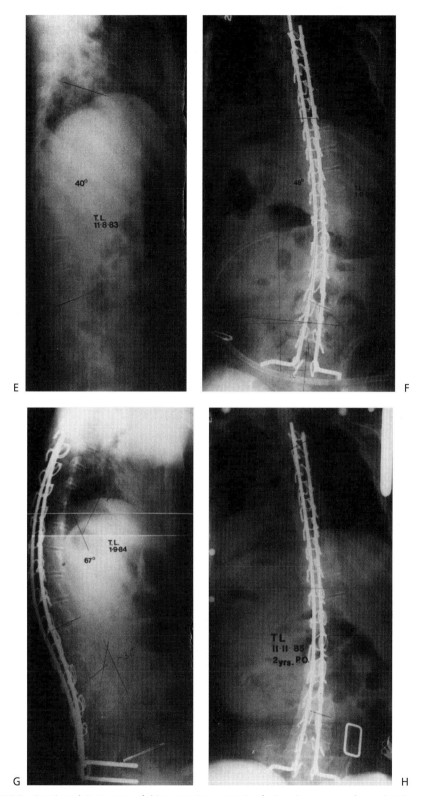

FIGURE 3. *Continued.* **E:** Because of this correction, posterior fusion alone was performed with Luque-Galveston instrumentation. **F:** Postoperative radiograph shows correction of the scoliosis to 48 degrees. **G:** Lateral postoperative radiograph shows restoration of thoracic kyphosis and lumbar lordosis. Evident are the balanced torso and the smaller ³⁄₁₆-inch (4.8 mm) rods used because of the thinness of the pelvis. Two years later the fusion was solid with no change. **H:** Sitting posteroanterior radiograph shows excellent lumbar fusion mass.

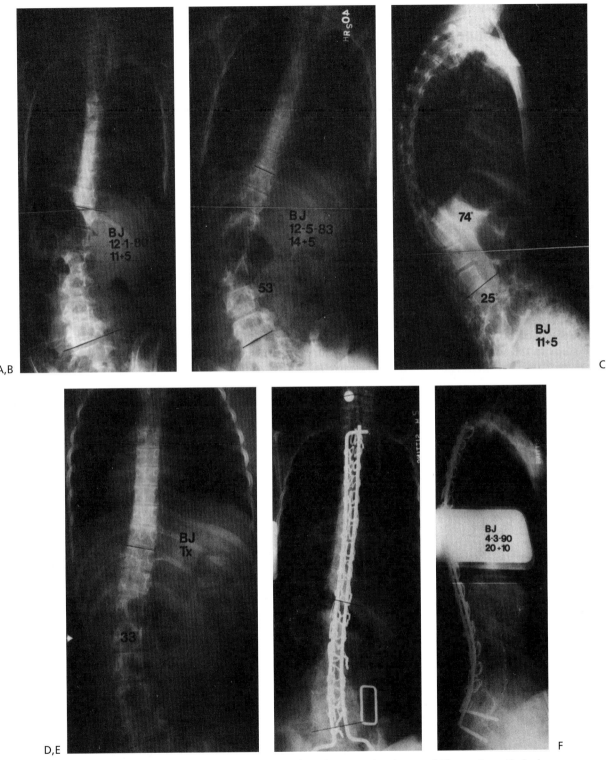

FIGURE 4. Girl with spastic quadriplegia first evaluated presented at the age of 11 years 5 months had difficulty sitting. **A:** Unsupported sitting radiograph shows level pelvis and a small left lumbar curve. A molded sitting support orthosis was fitted and was effective in providing sitting support until the beginning of puberty and the adolescent growth spurt 3 years later. **B:** Unsupported anteroposterior radiograph obtained 3 years after **A** shows pelvic obliquity and a 53-degree left lumbar curve, the sacrum forming part of the curve. **C:** Lateral view shows 74-degree thoracic kyphosis and loss of lumbar lordosis. **D:** Traction radiograph shows curve correction to 33 degrees, but the pelvis did not become level and the torso was not in balance. The patient underwent anterior fusion from T12 to S1 and posterior fusion from T2 to the sacrum with Luque-Galveston instrumentation. Six years after the operation the fusion was solid, the pelvis level, the torso balanced, and sagittal contours restored. Posteroanterior **(E)** and lateral **(F)** views show excellent fusion mass in the lumbar areas.

posterior instrumentation using multiple hook-rod system (1a,15a,23a,23b), Luque rod and sublaminar wiring (9a), Luque-Galveston pelvic fixation (9a), and insertion of iliac screws (1a) are described elsewhere. The steps in the surgical procedure differ from surgeon to surgeon. I use the following steps: (a) exposure of the spine, (b) exposure of the iliac crests, (c) facet excision and flavectomy, (d) drilling of the iliac crest, (e) rod bending, (f) passage of the sublaminar wires on the concavity of the curve, (g) insertion of the rod on the concavity of the curve, (h) passage of the wires on the convexity of the curve, (i) insertion of the rod on the convexity of the curve, (j) decortication and bone grafting, (k) closure.

Blood loss is monitored during the procedure by means of weighing the sponges and measuring the cell saver return. In operations on children with cerebral palsy, it is important to relate any calculation of blood loss and replacement to a percentage of the calculated circulating blood volume, not to the volume of loss alone. It is not unusual for these small children to have a loss that equals or exceeds circulating volume. It is imperative in cases of large blood loss to replace clotting factors with fresh frozen plasma and platelets with the addition of calcium.

Postoperative care is concentrated on fluid balance, blood replacement, and pulmonary care. Operations on these children differ from other pediatric procedures in that children with cerebral palsy do not have a well-developed cough reflex. Postoperative suctioning is necessary to stimulate any cough reflex and to control oral and respiratory secretions. For pulmonary care it often is useful to leave the endotracheal tube in place for the first night after the operation and to use a respirator to aid pulmonary function in the immediately postoperative period. Because of the excellent fixation afforded by the Luque system, no postoperative immobilization is needed. The child should be returned to the preoperative sitting position as soon as possible, and appropriate adjustments should be made to sitting support.

When hip flexion contractures are present, careful positioning is necessary in the postoperative period. The legs are supported on pillows when the child is supine, and the hip and knees are placed in flexion. Any hip flexion or hip windswept deformity appears worse after surgery, because the possible compensation by pelvic flexion or rotation is eliminated with the fixation of the pelvis in the Galveston technique. It is important to be aware of this possible side effect of spinal fusion and to warn family and caregivers of this before surgery. The question always arises whether the hips should be operated on before the spinal fusion. It is easier, however, to perform spinal fusion first and then to assess the hips. Because most of these children are sitters, hip surgery is indicated only when an extremely windswept position or painful dislocation interferes with sitting. Once the child is returned to preoperative ambulatory status, a decision regarding the need for hip surgery can be made.

Anterior and Posterior Fusion

Combined anterior and posterior fusion is indicated when the traction radiograph does not show a level pelvis and balanced spine. The imbalance can be caused by a tilt of the thorax in relation to the pelvis or lack of balance of the thorax over the pelvis. When the curve is large, even with a balanced spine on a traction radiograph, combined fusion gives a better result than posterior fusion alone. Because it shortens the convexity of the curve, the anterior release corrects the thoracolumbar or lumbar curve and helps balance the spine (6,8,10). The technique of anterior discectomy and fusion is described by Herring (14a).

After the anterior procedure is concluded, the patient's condition is assessed and the timing of the posterior fusion is discussed with the anesthesiologist. In most instances, both procedures are performed under the same anesthesia. That is, when the patient's condition is stable, blood loss minimal, and the anterior procedure not prolonged, posterior fusion is performed immediately (11). After anterior fusion, the patient is turned prone and positioned on the spinal frame, and the posterior procedure is performed. In cases of large blood loss, a long anterior procedure, or suboptimal patient status, posterior fusion is delayed for 7 to 10 days to allow the patient to recover from the anterior procedure before the second-stage posterior fusion is performed. During this time, nutrition is of utmost importance. A central intravenous catheter is inserted at the conclusion of the anterior procedure and used for hyperalimentation between the two stages.

If fusion is staged, the question of traction between the stages arises. It has been found that any improvement—either improved correction or improved thoracopelvic balance—is due to the anterior release and not to any traction used. Anterior release allows additional curve correction by making the spine more flexible. Traction provides no additional correction or flexibility. If the patient is uncooperative, halo traction can be used between the stages to help control the patient, but this situation is rare.

After anterior fusion with either a concurrent or staged posterior procedure, the most important part of postoperative care is focused on the respiratory system. After thoracotomy, hypoventilation and atelectasis are common, often making respiratory support necessary in the immediately postoperative period. Bronchial secretions are handled with repeated suctioning, which also has the benefit of stimulating any cough reflex that is present. This helps minimize or prevent atelectasis and thus reduce the likelihood of superimposed pneumonia. Routine care of the chest tube is performed with daily chest radiographs to monitor the presence of air or fluid in the pleural space. The tube is removed when the drainage is minimal, usually on the third or fourth postoperative day.

After posterior fusion, whether performed on the same day or as a second stage, the aftercare regarding positioning and return to the upright preoperative ambulatory status is the same as described earlier. When the procedures are performed on the same day, postoperative recovery is a day or two longer.

Postoperative Complications

Postoperative complications among patients with cerebral palsy are the same as those for any child undergoing spinal fusion for neuromuscular spinal deformities. There are, however, specific complications that are more common or important for children with cerebral palsy. These include respiratory problems, nutritional problems, hip problems, and pseudarthrosis.

Respiratory Problems

Children with cerebral palsy have a poor cough reflex and difficulty swallowing, the latter causing inability to handle normal salivary secretions. As a result, the incidence of postoperative respiratory complications (atelectasis and pneumonia) is high. To minimize or prevent this problem, attention to postoperative respiratory care is essential (see Chapter 44).

Nutritional Problems

Nutrition is important among children with cerebral palsy undergoing surgery. A good preoperative nutritional assessment is essential, and preoperative nutritional counseling and a feeding gastrostomy are provided when necessary. Whenever surgery is performed in two stages 7 to 10 days apart, parenteral hyperalimentation is essential, regardless of how well the child tolerates the first stage. The hyperalimentation should be planned at the time of the first anesthesia, and an appropriate central line is inserted so that a portal for nutritional support is available. When posterior fusion is performed alone or in combination under one anesthesia, nutritional support sometimes is necessary. This may be accomplished through the parenteral route in the case of prolonged ileus or with a feeding tube when intestinal motility has returned but the child does not tolerate oral feedings.

Hip Problems

Hip problems—subluxation, dislocation, and contractures—are frequent among patients who do not walk. Their hips must be assessed preoperatively, and the parents and caregivers must be told that postoperatively the hip position may appear worse when contractures are present. When there are hip contractures and the child is supine, the legs need to be supported postoperatively on pillows with 90 degrees of hip and knee flexion. This prevents the windswept abduction and adduction contractures from worsening. In addition, the forces on the pelvis are reduced to protect the Galveston pelvic fixation.

Question arises about when hip range of motion and stretching of contractures can be resumed when fusion has been performed to the sacrum. The danger in these cases is torque on the pelvis, which puts the sacral and pelvic fixation in jeopardy. Gentle range of motion, short of the extremes, is advised in the healing phase, and stretching is not allowed. These restrictions are in effect until the fusion is solid, which usually takes 4 to 6 months. At that time, the full preoperative hip program of range of motion and stretching can be resumed.

Another important question concerns the need for and timing of hip surgery in relation to spinal fusion. Assessment of the need for release of hip contractures is best made after the spinal fusion, when the pelvis is fixed in position and no spinal compensation for the contracture can take place. Only if the hip contractures prevent standing (ambulators) or sitting (nonambu-lators) is release indicated. This is rare, because flexion contracture of the hips up to 90 degrees does not interfere with sitting. In this case, good leg support is essential when the child is supine. Alteration of the child's position in the chair often is necessary. Placing the seating support at a slight angle to the chair may give a better-appearing seated position. If hip surgery is planned, usually for dislocation or subluxation, the operation should be performed after spinal fusion. The pelvis is fixed in the final position to allow better assessment of hip position.

Pseudarthrosis

Pseudarthrosis is an important complication of operations on the spines of patients with cerebral palsy. It is related to the type of curve and the fusion technique. In a review of mainly Harrington instrumentation, the overall rate of pseudarthrosis was 17% to 25% with a posterior approach and 4% with a combined approach (16). With the introduction of Luque instrumentation with more secure internal fixation, the pseudarthrosis rate for posterior fusion has fallen dramatically. The pseudarthrosis rate for group I curves has fallen from 20% to near zero. The rate for group II curves and for combined fusions has not changed greatly. The most common sites of pseudarthrosis are the lumbosacral and thoracolumbar areas.

The fusion is evaluated with supine oblique radiographs, and defects are identified if present. Nine to 12 months after surgery, the fusion is more mature and the defects are more easily identified, often on anteroposterior or lateral radiographs. In some cases the instrumentation can fracture, and correction can be lost. It must be remembered that the defect can be difficult to identify, and the rods may remain intact and fracture many years after the original fusion procedure. There also can be associated pain, but this is rare and difficult to identify.

The need for reoperation is rare, even when a pseudarthrosis is present. Only with loss of correction and definite pain is pseudarthrosis repair indicated. Thus most pseudarthroses in these children are radiographic defects that do not necessitate surgical repair.

SUMMARY

Spinal deformities are important orthopaedic problems among children with cerebral palsy. As with all neuromuscular diseases, multisystem involvement includes spasticity, contractures, hip dislocation and subluxation, seizures, mental retardation, vision and hearing deficits, and respiratory and feeding problems. A detailed evaluation of all these areas when the patient first arrives for treatment is essential, as is evaluation of the nutritional status and functional ambulatory level. Nonoperative treatment plays a role in following scoliosis for progression. Active treatment involves the use of sitting supports to improve sitting function. Orthoses (TLSO) play a small role in the treatment of these children.

Surgical treatment of patients with cerebral palsy, especially patients with spastic quadriplegia, is controversial in both indications and approach. The two main indications for surgery are curve progression and deterioration in sitting function. Findings on a traction radiograph are the best radiographic determinants of the flexibility of the spinal deformity. Leveling of the pelvis and balance of the torso over the pelvis also are evaluated on a traction radiograph. A posterior approach alone is used for "idiopathic-like" curves and for curves that balance over a level pelvis on a traction radiograph. Most fusions are long (T2 to the sacrum). The Luque-Galveston technique is the instrumentation of choice. For curves that do not balance or show pelvic obliquity on a traction radiograph, combined anterior and posterior fusion is indicated.

Postoperative care is concentrated on the respiratory system and early implementation of nutritional support. With care in surgical technique and adequate postoperative care, complications can be minimized. The child can be returned to the preoperative functional level with a successful surgical result—a solidly fused spine in balance in the coronal and sagittal planes over a level pelvis.

REFERENCES

1. Allen BJ, Ferguson R (1982): L-rod instrumentation for scoliosis in cerebral palsy. *J Pediatr Orthop* 2:87–96.
1a. Asher MA (2001): Insola spinal implant system update: emphasizing application during the first two decades of life. In: Weinstein SL, ed. *Pediatric spine: surgery.* Philadelphia: Lippincott Williams & Wilkins, pp. 437–470.
2. Balmer G, MacEwen G (1968): The incidence and treatment of scoliosis in cerebral palsy. *Dev Med Child Neurol* 10:447.
3. Bleck E (1987): *Orthopedic management in cerebral palsy.* Philadelphia: JB Lippincott.
4. Boachie-Adjei O, Lonstein J, Winter R, et al. (1989): Management of neuromuscular spine deformities with Luque segmental instrumentation. *J Bone Joint Surg Am* 78:548–562.
5. Broom M, Banta J, Renshaw T (1989): Spinal fusion augmented by L-rod segmental instrumentation for neuromuscular scoliosis. *J Bone Joint Surg Am* 71:32.
6. Brown J, Swank S, Specht L (1982): Combined anterior and posterior fusion in cerebral palsy. *Spine* 7:570–573.
7. Bulman W, Dormans J, Ecker M, et al. (1996): Posterior spinal fusion for scoliosis in patients with cerebral palsy: a comparison of Luque rod and Unit Rod instrumentation. *J Pediatr Orthop* 16:314–323.
8. Cohen D, Swank S, Branon J (1988): Spine fusion in cerebral palsy with L-rod segmental spinal instrumentation and analysis of single and two stage combined approach. Presented at the Annual Meeting of the Scoliosis Research Society. Baltimore.
9. Dvarik D, Roberts J, Burke S (1986): Gastroesophageal evaluation in totally involved cerebral palsy patients. Presented at AAOS meeting.
9a. Ferguson RL (2001): Luque rod instrumentation. In: Weinstein SL, ed. *Pediatric spine: surgery.* Philadelphia: Lippincott Williams & Wilkins, pp. 471–491.
10. Ferguson R, Allen BJ (1983): Staged correction of neuromuscular scoliosis. *J Pediatr Orthop* 3:555–562.
11. Ferguson R, Hansen M, Nicholas D, et al. (1996): Same-day versus staged anterior-posterior spinal surgery in a neuromuscular scoliosis population: the evaluation of medical complications. *J Pediatr Orthop* 16:293–303.
12. Gau Y, Lonstein J, Winter R, et al. (1991): Luque-Galveston procedure for correction and stabilization of neuromuscular scoliosis and pelvic obliquity: a review of 68 patients. *J Spinal Disord* 4:399–410.
13. Gersoff W, Renshaw T (1988): The treatment of scoliosis in cerebral palsy by posterior spinal fusion with Luque-rod segmental instrumentation. *J Bone Joint Surg* 70A:41–44.
14. Haas S (1942): Spastic scoliosis and obliquity of the pelvis. *J Bone Joint Surg* 24:775.
14a. Herring JA (2001): Anterior spinal surgery. In: Weinstein SL, ed. *Pediatric spine: surgery.* Philadelphia: Lippincott Williams & Wilkins, pp. 239–255.
15. Horstman H, Boyer B (1984): Progression of scoliosis in cerebral palsy patients after skeletal maturity. *Dev Med Child Neurol* 26:261.
15a. Lenke LG (2001): Cotrel-Dubousset spinal instrumentation. In: Weinstein SL, ed. *Pediatric spine: surgery.* Philadelphia: Lippincott Williams & Wilkins, pp. 367–416.
16. Lonstein J, Akbarnia B (1983): Operative treatment of spinal deformities in patients with cerebral palsy or mental retardation. *J Bone Joint Surg Am* 65:43–55.
17. Luque E (1982): Segmental spinal instrumentation or correction of scoliosis. *Clin Orthop* 163:192–198.
18. Luque E (1988): The treatment of neuromuscular patients with SSI. Presented at the Annual Meeting of the Scoliosis Research Society. Baltimore.
19. MacEwen G (1972): Operative treatment of scoliosis in cerebral palsy. *Reconstr Surg Traumatol* 13:58.
20. Madigan R, Wallace S (1981): Scoliosis in the institutionalized cerebral palsy population. *Spine* 6:583–590.
21. Majd M, Muldowny D, Holt R (1997): Natural history of scoliosis in the institutionalized adult cerebral palsy population. *Spine* 22:1461–1466.
22. Miller A, Temple T, Miller F (1996): Impact of orthoses on the rate of scoliosis progression in children with cerebral palsy. *J Pediatr Orthop* 16:332–335.
23. Samilson R, Bechard R (1973): Scoliosis in cerebral palsy: incidence, distribution of curve patterns and natural history. *Curr Pract Orthop Surg* 5:183.
23a. Shufflebarger HL (2001): Moss Miami spinal instrumentation. In: Weinstein SL, ed. *Pediatric spine: surgery.* Philadelphia: Lippincott Williams & Wilkins, pp. 351–366.
23b. Shufflebarger HL (2001): Theory and mechanisms of posterior multiple hook, screw, rod devices. In: Weinstein SL, ed. *Pediatric spine: surgery.* Philadelphia: Lippincott Williams & Wilkins, pp. 417–435.
24. Stanitski C, Micheli L, Hall J, et al. (1982): Surgical correction of spinal deformity in cerebral palsy. *Spine* 7:563–569.
25. Sullivan J, Conner S (1982): Comparison of Harrington instrumentation and segmental spinal instrumentation in the treatment of neuromuscular spinal deformity. *Spine* 7:299.
26. Sussman M, Little D, Alley R, et al. (1996): Posterior instrumentation and fusion of the thoracolumbar spine for the treatment of neuromuscular scoliosis. *J Pediatr Orthop* 16:304–313.
27. Taddonio R (1982): Segmental spinal instrumentation in the management of neuromuscular spinal deformity. *Spine* 7:305–311.
28. Tanner J (1975): Growth and endocrinology of the adolescent. In: Gardner L, ed. *Endocrine and genetic disease of childhood.* Philadelphia: WB Saunders, p. 14.
29. Thometz J, Simon S (1988): Progression of scoliosis after skeletal maturity in institutionalized adults who have cerebral palsy. *J Bone Joint Surg Am* 70:1290–1296.
30. Winter S (1994): Preoperative assessment of the child with neuromuscular scoliosis. *Orthop Clin North Am* 25:239–245.
31. Yazici M, Asher M (1997): Freeze-dried allograft for posterior spinal fusion in patients with neuromuscular spinal deformities. *Spine* 22:1467–1471.
32. Zimbler S, Craig C, Harris J (1985): Orthotic management of severe scoliosis in severe neuromuscular disease: results of treatment. *Orthop Trans* 9:78.

46

SPINAL DEFORMITIES IN FRIEDREICH'S ATAXIA

HUBERT LABELLE

Nicolaus Friedreich was born on July 31, 1825, in Wurtzburg, a small city in Germany. He studied biology and medicine in his hometown. At the age of 32 years, Friedreich accepted the directorship of the medical clinic and the chair of internal medicine at the nearby University of Heidelberg, where he worked for the next 25 years (4). Few eponyms in neurology are as closely identified with a specific condition as the one Friedreich described in a series of five papers published between 1863 and 1877 (4,18). The term *maladie de Friedreich*, or Friedreich's ataxia, was coined by the French School of Neurology in 1882, the year of Friedreich's death (4). Friedreich's original clinical and pathologic observations and ideas are still up to date and were the basis for all subsequent knowledge of hereditary spinocerebellar degeneration.

DEFINITION AND CLASSIFICATION

Friedreich's ataxia is the most common hereditary and progressive spinocerebellar degenerative disease characterized by ataxia. To date, more than 57 hereditary ataxic syndromes have been identified. To facilitate differentiation of these various syndromes, Barbeau et al. (9) proposed a clinical classification that is user-friendly, flexible, and based on the natural order of questions asked by a clinician (Table 1). First, the genetic mode is established. Is the pattern observed in the family autosomal dominant, autosomal recessive, or sex-linked recessive? Second, the pattern of progression is obtained from the history—nonprogressive, intermittent, or progressive ataxia. Age at onset of the first symptom further divides the syndrome into infantile (onset birth to 2 years), early (onset 2 to 25 years of age), or adult (onset after 25 years of age). Next, the state of deep tendon reflexes is recorded as either hyperactive or normoactive (positive reflexes, recorded with +) or hypoactive or areflexic (negative reflexes, recorded with a −). Finally, the type of ataxia present is recorded as either "pure ataxia" (predominant spinocerebellar or cerebellar incoordination) or "ataxia plus" (spinocerebellar or cerebellar incoordination with other central nervous system involvement).

According to this classification, Friedreich's ataxia is defined as an autosomal recessive ataxia of a progressive nature, of early onset, with weak or absent reflexes, and with predominant spinocerebellar incoordination.

EPIDEMIOLOGY

The prevalence of Friedreich's ataxia is approximately 1:100,000 population (38,40). The incidence has been reported to be between 1:25,000 and 1:50,000 with a heterozygote frequency of 1:110 (38,41). The sexes are equally affected. Although it is rare, the syndrome appears to have a worldwide geographic distribution. Most series described have been in Europe and North America (8,13,17,19,22,35,38).

ETIOLOGY

Since Friedreich's original description (18), it has been known that the disease is genetic in origin and inherited as an autosomal recessive trait, but it was only in 1988 that Chamberlain et al. (15) mapped the gene on chromosome 9 by means of genetic linkage. Since then, with linkage mapping techniques, the classic form of Friedreich's ataxia has been localized to 9q13-q21, a region on the long arm of chromosome 9, and the interval for the defective gene has been narrowed to a few hundred thousand base pairs (24,25,34). It is likely that the Friedreich's ataxia gene will be cloned soon. This confirms the suspicion that there is no evidence of genetic heterogeneity, despite the clinical variations encountered in the syndrome. These variations are probably caused by mutations at the same locus (25).

Extensive genealogic studies have been performed in the province of Québec, which is ideal for such investigations because most of its inhabitants (5 million of 6.5 million total) are of French extraction, originating from a pool of 70,000 immigrants who crossed the Atlantic before 1760. Most of these immigrants are known, and their descendants can easily be traced through church or civil records. Barbeau et al. (8) traced most cases of Friedreich disease in French Canada to one common ancestral couple arriving in New France (Québec) in 1634: Jean Guyon, a mason, and his wife, Mathurine Robin, both born in Perche

H. Labelle: Department of Orthopaedic Surgery, Sainte-Justine Mother-Child University Hospital, University of Montreal, Quebec, H3T 1C5 Canada.

TABLE 1. CLASSIFICATION OF HEREDITARY ATAXIA

Heredity	Progression	Onset	Reflexes		Ataxia		Entity
1.0 Dominant	1.1 Nonprogressive	1.1.1 Infantile					
		1.1.2 Early					
		1.1.3 Adult					
	1.2 Intermittent	1.2.1 Infantile					
		1.2.2 Early					
		1.2.3 Adult					
	1.3 Progressive	1.3.1 Infantile					
		1.3.2 Early	1.3.3.1 + Reflexes	1.3.2.1.1	Pure ataxia		Dominant spastic ataxia
		1.3.3 Adult	1.3.3.2 − Reflexes	1.3.2.1.2	Ataxia plus		
2.0 Recessive	2.1 Nonprogressive	2.1.1 Infantile					
		2.1.2 Early					
		2.1.3 Adult					
	2.2 Intermittent	2.2.1 Infantile					
		2.2.2 Early					
		2.2.3 Adult					
	2.3 Progressive	2.3.1 Infantile					
		2.3.2 Early	2.3.2.1 + Reflexes	2.3.2.2.1	Pure ataxia		Friedreich ataxia
		2.3.3 Adult	2.3.2.2 − Reflexes	2.3.2.2.2	Ataxia plus		
3.0 X-linked	3.1 Nonprogressive	3.1.1 Infantile					
		3.1.2 Early					
		3.1.3 Adult					
	3.2 Intermittent	3.2.1 Infantile					
		3.2.2 Early					
		3.2.3 Adult					
	3.3 Progressive	3.3.1 Infantile					
		3.3.2 Early					
		3.3.3 Adult					

Overall scheme of classification (9). The coding procedure is subdivided progressively from left to right as heredity, progression, onset, reflexes, and ataxia are determined. To date, more than 57 syndromes have been identified, but for clarity, only two examples are shown: dominant spastic ataxia coded 1.3.2.1.1 and Friedreich ataxia coded 2.3.2.2.1, which translates into autosomal recessive ataxia of a progressive nature, early onset, diminished or absent knee jerks, and without major involvement of other systems within the brain.

(northwest of France). It is probable that these ancestors are also responsible for cases reported among the Cajuns of Louisiana (25). The Cajuns' ancestors came from the French colony of Acadia, which includes the territory of Canada now known as Nova Scotia and New Brunswick. The area was first colonized in 1604 by fishermen from the northern coastal regions of France.

Unfortunately, the biochemical abnormality underlying the disorder has not yet been identified. Four areas of metabolic disturbances have been investigated: a taurine retention defect, abnormality in the pyruvate dehydrogenase complex, defective incorporation of linoleic acid in fatty acids, and disturbance of pyruvate-malate metabolism (6,7).

DIAGNOSIS

Because of the large number of ataxic syndromes identified, it is of utmost importance to establish a clear diagnosis for every patient believed to have Friedreich's ataxia. Geoffroy et al. (19) proposed the following classification system, later modified by Harding (20), which is now universally accepted:

Group I: Typical Friedreich's ataxia
Group Ia: Complete picture
Group Ib: Incomplete picture

Group IIa: Atypical Friedreich's ataxia
Group IIb: Not Friedreich's ataxia

Typical Friedreich's ataxia (groups Ia and Ib) can be characterized by a number of primary, constant symptoms and signs that are present in all cases and are essential for diagnosis. There also are secondary signs that are present in more than 90% of cases. Finally, there are a large number of accessory symptoms and signs that cannot be used to establish a diagnosis. Patients with group Ib Friedreich's ataxia are identical to those with group Ia ataxia except that they lack any evidence of pes cavus. Patients with group IIa ataxia differ from those in group I mainly through lack of progression of the ataxia and a very mild degree of scoliosis. Group IIb is heterogeneous; specifically, dysarthria, posterior column signs, and muscle weakness are lacking.

The primary symptoms and signs needed for diagnosis of Friedreich's ataxia are onset of symptoms before 25 years of age, progressive ataxia of limbs and of gait, absent knee and ankle jerks, extensor plantar responses, decreased motor nerve conduction velocity in upper limbs with small or absent sensory action potentials, and dysarthria. The secondary symptoms and signs are present in most cases but are not essential for diagnosis. These are scoliosis, pyramidal weakness in lower limbs, absent reflexes in upper limbs, distal loss of joint position and vibration sense in lower limbs, and abnormal electrocardiographic findings. Finally, the accessory symptoms and signs present in less than 50% of cases are optic atrophy, nystagmus, distal weakness and wasting, partial deafness, pes cavus, and diabetes.

PATHOLOGIC ANATOMY

The anatomic lesions of the peripheral and central nervous system found at autopsy or biopsy of persons with typical Friedreich's ataxia are remarkably similar among published reports (23,32,33). There is moderate to marked loss of large myelinated fibers and limited loss of small fibers in the peripheral nerves. Degeneration does not affect unmyelinated fibers, and there is limited evidence of myelin breakdown at the periphery. There is extensive degeneration of large neuron cell bodies in the posterior root ganglia with segmental demyelination and remyelination. This suggests dying-back axonopathy whereby axonal degeneration slowly progresses from the distal portion of the fiber toward the cell body.

In the spinal cord, anterior horns and cranial motor nerves appear normal, but there is marked loss of large myelinated fibers in the posterior columns. In the cerebellum, the most striking alterations are moderate to marked loss of dentate neurons and myelinated fibers in the dentate nucleus. Pathologic changes in the brain stem are variable, and the cerebral cortex and white matter are normal.

LABORATORY STUDIES

Nerve conduction studies (14,36) reveal markedly decreased or absent sensory action potentials in the digital and sural nerves. Conduction velocity along the motor and sensory fibers of the median and tibial nerves is moderately slowed. Somatosensory evoked potentials (35) show a marked reduction in amplitude along all registration levels and a prolonged latency of the first cortical event. At electromyography, most patients have a moderate to severe loss of motor units, an increase in mean duration of motor unit potentials, and an increase in incidence of polyphasic potentials (14,36).

Pulmonary function studies show evidence of restrictive lung disease that is proportional to the severity of scoliosis (12). These findings are comparable with the alterations found in adolescent idiopathic scoliosis. Electrocardiography, echocardiography, angiography, and cardiac catheterization all reveal findings consistent with progressive hypertrophic cardiomyopathy but without any clear correlation between the degree of abnormal findings and the severity of neurologic impairment (16). All results of routine hematologic and biochemical laboratory tests are normal except for an increased prevalence of clinical and chemical diabetes (around 40%) with an abnormal glucose tolerance test result and hyperinsulinemia (7).

COURSE OF SCOLIOSIS

Since the original description in 1863, very little has been published on the behavior of the scoliosis that is so intimately associ-

ated with Friedreich's ataxia. Earlier reports (21) were mostly anecdotal and based on the personal experience of the authors, who had treated a limited number of patients. Furthermore, many unrelated ataxia syndromes probably were mistaken for typical Friedreich's ataxia before Geoffroy's classification was accepted. This may explain why scoliosis in Friedreich's ataxia was previously considered a neuromuscular curve pattern similar to the curve of muscular dystrophy or spinal muscular atrophy, characterized by a relentlessly progressive, predominantly *C*-shaped thoracolumbar pattern associated with pelvic obliquity and severe muscle weakness.

More recent evidence based on larger retrospective series of 42 patients (13), 19 patients (17), and a pool of 56 patients with typical Friedreich's ataxia observed for an average of 9 years (1–3,29,31) does not support many previous beliefs. The results of these studies suggest that scoliotic deformities in this disease follow a distinct pattern of behavior that is important to understand to plan treatment.

The prevalence of scoliotic deformities is close to 100% (13,31). This figure is higher than that generally reported in the orthopaedic literature, which probably reflects exclusion of other closely related syndromes through strict adherence to the criteria of typical Friedreich's ataxia. Scoliosis appears to be a constant finding, although it is not always present at the time of diagnosis.

The sexes are equally affected, and left-sided curves are as frequent as right-sided curves, as is the case in many neuromuscular deformities. The curve pattern, however, is more closely related to that of idiopathic scoliosis with a clear predominance of double structural thoracic and lumbar curves (57% of cases at my institution [1–3,29,31]) followed by single thoracic or lumbar curves. The classic *C*-shaped thoracolumbar curve pattern occurred in only 18% of cases in Cady and Bobechko's (13) series, 25% of cases reported by Daher et al. (17) series, and 14% of cases at my institution (1–3,29,31) (Fig. 1). In a comparison between subjects with cerebral palsy, Friedreich's ataxia, and adolescent idiopathic scoliosis, Aronsson et al. (5) found that the scoliosis curve patterns among children with Friedreich's ataxia and adolescent idiopathic scoliosis were similar. In contrast, the curve pattern among children with cerebral palsy was distinctly different. The cerebral palsy pattern had more rotation of the apical vertebrae into the convexity of the scoliosis curve (transverse plane deformity) in relation to the amount of lateral deviation of the apical vertebrae from the spinal axis (coronal plane deformity).

Nonstructural curves with a Cobb angle less than 20 degrees and little or no vertebral body rotation are frequent among immature patients and are a reflection of the postural abnormality caused by ataxia. These curves are highly variable and can change dramatically between follow-up visits. Eventually a more definite structural curve pattern with vertebral body rotation is established as the syndrome progresses (Fig. 2).

My colleagues and I (31) studied progression of structural curves by assigning patients to one of three groups according to behavior of scoliosis during a follow-up period. Group I, comprising approximately one third of the patients, included those with clearly progressive curves and Cobb angles greater than 60 degrees. Group II, comprising one third of patients,

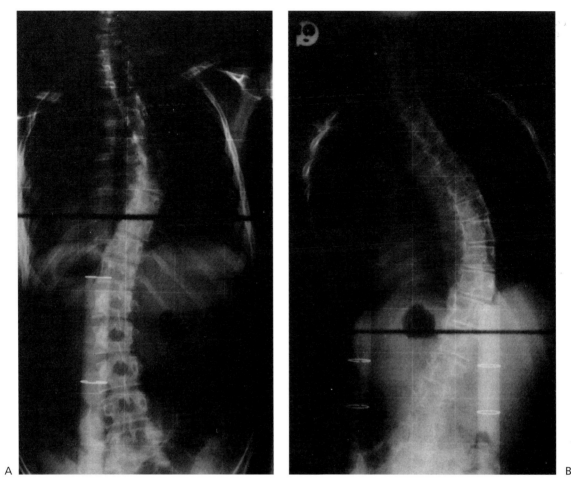

FIGURE 1. Structural scoliotic curve patterns. **A:** Double structural thoracic and lumbar curve pattern that occurs among most patients. **B:** C-shaped thoracolumbar curve pattern with pelvic obliquity that occurs among approximately 20% of the population.

included those with nonprogressive curves and Cobb angles less than 40 degrees at skeletal maturity after more than 10 years of follow-up evaluation. Group III comprised the last one third of patients, among whom the presence or absence of progression could not be established because of insufficient follow-up evaluation.

It thus appears reasonable to state that scoliotic deformities are not always relentlessly progressive and that at least one third of the population does not need treatment. Because patients with Friedreich's ataxia die, on average, early in the third decade of life (22), many do not live long enough to experience scoliosis progression that necessitates treatment. It is also clear that many patients have curves that deteriorate rapidly and necessitate some form of treatment.

Early recognition of these two distinct patterns of progression is important. Although a pathognomonic sign has yet to be identified, many risk factors have been studied (31). Age, sex, type of curve, pelvic obliquity, trunk alignment, and duration of disease are similar for both groups and do not appear to influence the prognosis. There is, however, a statistically significant correlation between progression of the scoliosis and age at onset of disease or age at recognition of scoliosis.

The maximum growth spurt of patients with Friedreich's ataxia occurs between 10 and 15 years of age for girls and between 12 and 17 years for boys (1). For most patients with a progressive curve pattern, onset of the disease or recognition of scoliosis occurs before this growth spurt. Progression of the curve is more severe while the growth spurt continues, suggesting that skeletal immaturity is a key factor in development of the deformity. Few patients with late-onset disease have severe scoliosis.

My colleagues and I have studied muscle weakness as a possible prognostic factor (10,26,29,31). No significant correlation was established between overall muscle weakness and curve progression, as would be expected in neuromuscular scoliosis such as muscular dystrophy or spinal muscular atrophy. The muscle weakness is symmetric, slowly progressive in the first decades of the disease, and rapidly progressive when functional walking is lost. First and mainly, it involves the proximal rather than distal lower limb muscles, whereas the upper limbs and trunk remain relatively spared. There is no apparent correlation between extent of muscle weakness and level of functional walking, suggesting that muscle weakness is not the primary cause of gait deterioration (10).

Although not proved beyond doubt, it is probable that ataxia

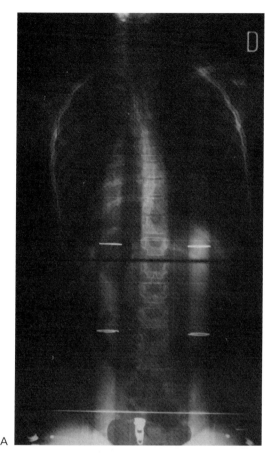

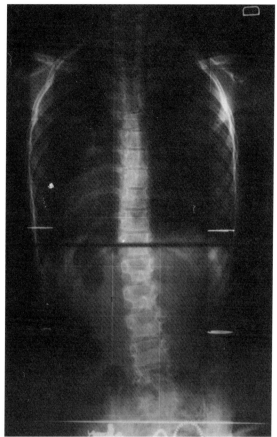

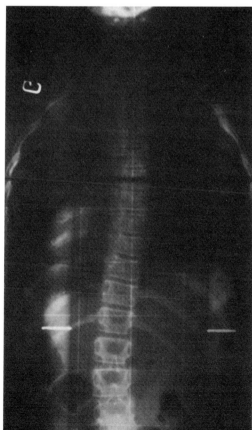

FIGURE 2. Nonstructural scoliotic curve patterns. **A:** Small, nonstructural right thoracic curve with little or no vertebral body rotation in a 10-year-old boy. **B:** Same patient 6 months later. The curve pattern has changed to a left thoracolumbar curve. **C:** Same patient 1 year later. There is now a right thoracic and left lumbar curve. Small nonstructural curves are highly variable among young patients and probably reflect the postural abnormality present before a definite structural curve is established.

is the other prime determinant of curve progression, just as severity of ataxia and not muscle weakness is primarily responsible for gradual loss of the ability to walk during the second decade of life. It is tempting to postulate that the pathogenesis of scoliotic deformities in this disorder is mainly ataxia, which causes a disturbance of equilibrium and postural reflexes—a disturbance that more and more investigators are suggesting is operative in idiopathic scoliosis. The effect of early-onset ataxia coupled with an immature and rapidly developing spine might explain the progressive curves.

In summary, scoliosis among patients with Friedreich's ataxia usually does not have the typical pattern of neuromuscular scoliosis. It appears to behave as an idiopathic curve in the following respects. The curve patterns are similar, many curves are not progressive or slowly progressive, there is no relation to muscle weakness, and early onset of the disease and the presence of a scoliosis before puberty are major factors of progression.

SAGITTAL PLANE ABNORMALITIES

Clinical studies (13,17,29,31) have shown a 40% to 66% incidence of increased thoracic kyphosis and a frequent decrease in lumbar lordosis during clinical and radiologic evaluation of patients with Friedreich's ataxia. The decrease in lumbar lordosis is easily explained by the sitting position of patients who cannot walk. The increased thoracic kyphosis, however, is somewhat controversial, because it implies that a kyphoscoliotic deformity is present. This would be an argument against the statement that the course of these deformities tends to resemble, in some respects, that of idiopathic scoliosis. It is now well recognized that idiopathic curves are lordoscoliotic and not kyphoscoliotic.

Investigations by our research group (1,28,30) using three-dimensional reconstructions of thoracic and thoracolumbar scoliosis deformities in Friedreich's ataxia have shed some light on this apparent contradiction. These studies demonstrated that both kyphotic and lordotic segments can coexist in the same person (Fig. 3). The thoracic or thoracolumbar scoliotic segment is most frequently associated with hypokyphosis or even lordosis as in idiopathic scoliosis. Many kyphotic segments seen on lateral radiographs are really pseudokyphotic from vertebral body rotation. Stagnara calls this kyphosis due to vertebral rotation *kyphosing scoliosis* (see Chapter 44).

True kyphotic segments do occur, but they are usually located above the scoliotic segment in the upper thoracic area or sometimes at the thoracolumbar junction between two curves. Ky-

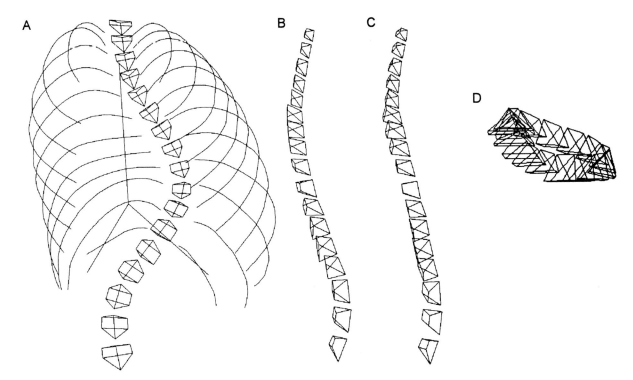

FIGURE 3. Example of a three-dimensional computer-generated graphic representation of a scoliotic deformity reconstructed from standardized anteroposterior and lateral radiographs of a patient with Friedreich's ataxia (27,28,30). **A:** Posteroanterior view of the spine from T1 to L5 shows a right thoracic curve pattern. **B:** Lateral view of the same deformity shows thoracic kyphosis, but it is located mostly above the scoliotic segment between T1 and T5. The thoracic scoliotic segment between T6 and L1 is not visible in a true lateral view because of the associated vertebral body rotation. **C:** True lateral view of the thoracic scoliotic segment. The same model has been rotated en bloc to show the lateral aspect of the thoracic scoliosis centered on T10. The scoliotic segment between T6 and L1 is clearly hypokyphotic. **D:** Apical view of the same spinal deformity shows high thoracic kyphosis from T1 to T5. The rest of the spine is straight or lordotic.

photic deformities tend to appear later in the course of the disease, many years after the appearance of a scoliotic deformity. These deformities often are supple, compensated for by an upper cervical lordosis, and tend to progress when the patient uses a wheelchair full-time and has acquired considerable muscle weakness.

TREATMENT

The earlier discussion of the course of this condition shows that although scoliosis in Friedreich's ataxia can certainly be classified as neuromuscular scoliosis, it should be considered more "neurologic" than "muscular." This implies that the scoliotic deformity is not a collapsing spinal disorder such as that of Duchenne muscular dystrophy or poliomyelitis. Except for true thoracic kyphotic deformities that appear later in the course of the disease and are somewhat related to muscle weakness, the behavior of the scoliotic deformity has many similarities to adolescent idiopathic scoliosis. Treatment principles should take these facts into consideration.

Nonoperative treatment has generally been unsuccessful and is not recommended (13,17,21,31). In particular, attempts at holding curves with various types of bracing have repeatedly been shown to be of limited value. Bracing often is poorly tolerated and may impair walking ability at a time when patients are struggling to continue walking. Bracing may be indicated for

skeletally immature patients with progressive curves to delay surgery and allow maximal growth of the spine. Electrospinal instrumentation has been tried in the treatment of a limited number of patients and has failed in every case (13).

There are no data on the efficiency of physical therapy, but it probably does not alter the natural course of the deformity. Similarly, among patients who use a wheelchair full-time, various positioning devices are routinely prescribed, but it is doubtful that they have any solid effect in preventing curve progression. They are, however, useful for improving sitting ability and correcting flexible scoliotic or kyphotic deformities.

Surgery is the only treatment that can clearly alter the prognosis by providing curve correction and stabilization of a progressive curve (13,17,31,39). An adequate preoperative investigation is important. Careful evaluation should be conducted for cardiomyopathy. Pulmonary function tests are mandatory. Because muscle weakness usually is not severe when a surgical procedure is performed in the adolescent period (10), respiratory complications are less likely than with other neuromuscular disorders. Screening for diabetes also should be routine. During anesthesia, careful monitoring of cardiopulmonary function should be instituted, because Friedreich's ataxia has been reported to cause marked sensitivity to nondepolarizing muscle relaxants and to cause hyperkalemia, with resulting cardiac arrhythmias after administration of succinylcholine (suxamethonium) (11). Because somatosensory evoked potentials are markedly reduced or absent, spinal cord monitoring should be done

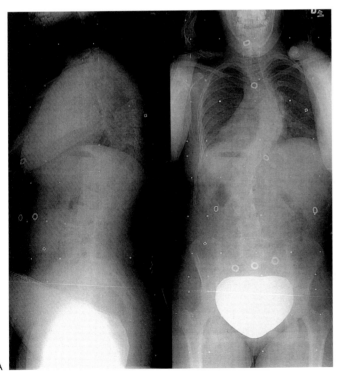
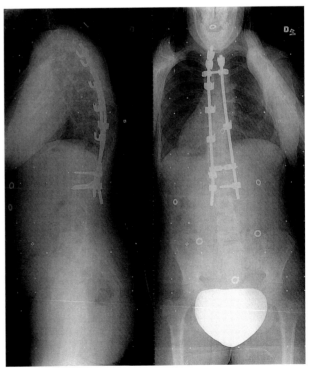

A

B

FIGURE 4. Preoperative and postoperative posteroanterior and lateral digital radiographs of a 12-year-old girl with Friedreich ataxia. **A:** Fusion and instrumentation were done with combined anterior thoracic release and posterior instrumentation and fusion with a multiple-rod, hook and screw system. **B:** The instrumentation was extended high in the thoracic area to include the upper thoracic kyphotic segment.

with motor evoked potentials (37) and the Stagnara wake-up test.

The indications for surgery are similar to those for adolescent idiopathic scoliosis and include all scoliotic deformities with a clearly progressive curve and a Cobb angle greater than 40 degrees in the frontal plane. On the basis of the data available in the literature, the following treatment protocol is recommended. Curves less than 40 degrees should be followed, curves more than 60 degrees should be managed surgically, and curves between 40 and 60 degrees can be either followed or managed surgically. In the latter case, treatment decisions are based primarily on the patient's age at onset of the disease, age when the scoliosis is first recognized, and evidence of curve progression. A 50-degree thoracic curve with no further evidence of progression in a young adult probably does not necessitate treatment, whereas a 45-degree curve in a skeletally immature patient with early-onset disease should be managed by means of surgical stabilization and fusion.

Most series dealing with treatment have reported good results of spinal fusion with Harrington, Harrington-Luque, or Luque instrumentation (13,17,21,39). Because of the ataxia and the balance problems associated with the disease, postoperative bracing with a thoracolumbosacral orthosis (TLSO) may be useful for a few months after the operation to decrease the risk of early implant failure, particularly among patients who walk. Although there are no reports in the literature, the use of the newer-generation of multiple rod, hook and screw systems that allow improved three-dimensional correction of scoliotic curves appears logical and is recommended (Fig. 4).

It is not necessary to extend fusion and instrumentation to the sacrum except for C-shaped thoracolumbar curves with associated pelvic obliquity. In all other curves, the lower level of instrumentation should be selected with the same criteria as for idiopathic scoliosis. On the other hand, fusion and instrumentation should be extended high (T2 or T3) in the thoracic area to prevent the development or deterioration of kyphosis above the scoliotic segment (Fig. 5). Anterior surgical release with or without instrumentation, usually followed by posterior instrumentation, should be limited to rigid curves greater than 60 degrees associated with poor sitting balance.

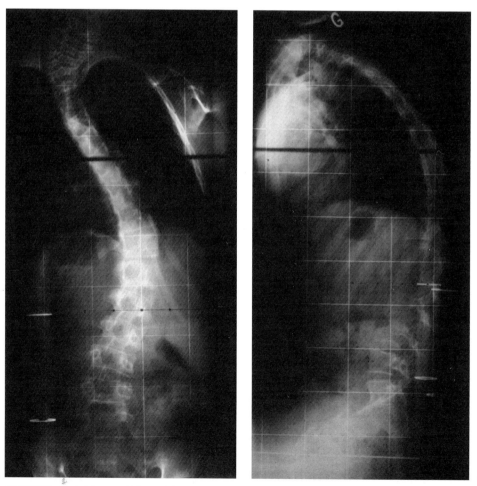

FIGURE 5. A: A 10-year-old boy with a progressive neuromuscular-like thoracolumbar curve pattern. In this case, progression of the disease was rapid, with early loss of ambulation and severe muscle weakness. **B:** Lateral radiograph of same patient as **A** in the sitting position. Associated high thoracic kyphosis is evident. When present, such kyphosis should always be considered in surgical planning. *(Figure continues.)*

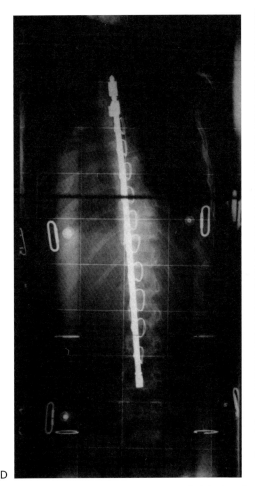
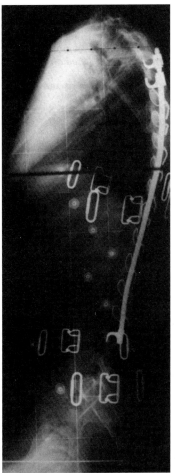
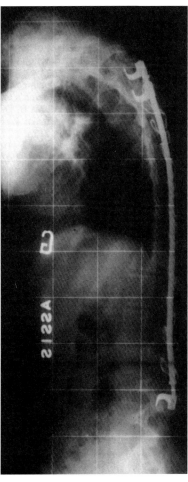

C,D

E

FIGURE 5. *Continued.* **C, D:** Results soon after Harrington-Luque instrumentation and fusion. A lightweight bivalved orthosis has been added for further protection during walking because of the severe ataxia and frequent falls. Fusion to the sacrum was not done, because there was no associated pelvic obliquity. **E:** Late postoperative result at 17 years of age. There has been recurrence and deterioration of the kyphosis above the instrumentation. In retrospect, instrumentation and fusion should have been extended higher in the thoracic area, as suggested by the preoperative lateral radiograph.

SUMMARY

Friedreich's ataxia is a relatively rare disorder, but it is by far the most frequent ataxic syndrome and deserves particular attention, because a scoliotic deformity is nearly always associated. The course of scoliosis in this disorder is different from that of other types of neuromuscular scoliosis and tends to behave as idiopathic scoliosis in many respects. The curve patterns are similar, many curves are nonprogressive, there is no relation between muscle weakness and the scoliotic deformity, and onset of the scoliosis before puberty is a major factor in progression. In most cases, the scoliotic segment is associated with hypokyphosis or lordosis, but kyphotic deformities frequently occur in the high thoracic area above the scoliotic segment.

So far, nonoperative treatment has been unsuccessful in preventing curve progression. Surgical stabilization with fusion is the only treatment that can clearly alter the prognosis of progressive curves. The following treatment protocol is recommended. Curves less than 40 degrees should be followed; curves more than 60 degrees should be managed surgically; and curves between 40 and 60 degrees should be either followed or managed surgically. Treatment decisions should be based primarily on the patient's age at disease onset, the age when the scoliosis was first recognized, and evidence of curve progression.

REFERENCES

1. Allard P, Dansereau J, Duhaime M, et al. (1984): Scoliosis assessment in Friedreich's ataxia by means of intrinsic parameters. *Can J Neurol Sci* 11:582–587.
2. Allard P, Dansereau J, Thiry PS, et al. (1982): Scoliosis in Friedreich's ataxia. *Can J Neurol Sci* 9:105–111.
3. Allard P, Duhaime M, Raso JV, et al. (1980): Pathomechanics and management of scoliosis in Friedreich's ataxia patients. *Can J Neurol Sci* 7:383–388.
4. Andermann F (1976): Nicolaus Friedreich and degenerative atrophy of the posterior columns of the spinal cord. *Can J Neurol Sci* 3:275–277.
5. Aronsson DD, Stokes IAF, Ronchetti PJ, et al. (1994): Comparison of curve shape between children with cerebral palsy, Friedreich's ataxia, and adolescent idiopathic scoliosis. *Dev Med Child Neurol* 36:412–418.

6. Barbeau A (1982): Friedreich's disease 1982: Etiologic hypothesis: a personal analysis. *Can J Neurol Sci* 9:243–263.

7. Barbeau A (1984): The Quebec cooperative study of Friedreich's ataxia: 1974–1984—ten years of research. *Can J Neurol Sci* 11:646–660.

8. Barbeau A, Sadibelouiz M, Roy M, et al. (1984): Origin of Friedreich's disease in Quebec. *Can J Neurol Sci* 11:506–509.

9. Barbeau A, Sadibelouiz M, Sadibelouiz A, et al. (1984): A clinical classification of hereditary ataxias. *Can J Neurol Sci* 11:501–505.

10. Beauchamp M, Labelle H, Duhaime M, et al. (1995): Natural history of muscle weakness in Friedreich's ataxia and its relation to loss of ambulation. *Clin Orthop* 311:270–275.

11. Bell CF, Kelly M, Jones RS (1986): Anesthesia for Friedreich's ataxia. *Anaesthesia* 41:296–301.

12. Bureau MA, Ngassam P, Lemieux B, et al. (1976): Pulmonary function studies in Friedreich's ataxia. *Can J Neurol Sci* 3:343–346.

13. Cady RB, Bobechko WP (1984): Incidence, natural history, and treatment of scoliosis in Friedreich's ataxia. *J Pediatr Orthop* 4:673–676.

14. Caruso G, Santoro L, Perretti A, et al. (1983): Friedreich's ataxia: electrophysiological and histological findings. *Acta Neurol Scand* 67: 26–40.

15. Chamberlain S, Shaw J, Rowland A, et al. (1988): Mapping of mutation causing Friedreich's ataxia to human chromosome 9. *Nature* 334: 248–250.

16. Côté M, Davignon A, Elias G, et al. (1976): Hemodynamic findings in Friedreich's ataxia. *Can J Neurol Sci* 3:333–337.

17. Daher YH, Lonstein JE, Winter RB, et al. (1985): Spinal deformities in patients with Friedreich's ataxia: a review of 19 patients. *J Pediatr Orthop* 5:553–557.

18. Friedreich N (1863): Ueber degenerative atrophie der spinalen Hinterstrange. *Virchows Arch Pathol Anat* 26:391–419.

19. Geoffroy G, Barbeau A, Breton G, et al. (1976): Clinical description and roentgenologic evaluation of patients with Friedreich'sataxia. *Can J Neurol Sci* 3:279–286.

20. Harding AE (1981): Friedreich's ataxia: a clinical and genetic study of 90 families with an analysis of early diagnosis criteria and intrafamilial clustering of clinical features. *Brain* 104:589–620.

21. Hensinger RN, MacEwen GD (1976): Spinal deformities associated with heritable neurological conditions. *J Bone Joint Surg Am* 58:13–23.

22. Hewer RL (1968): Study of fatal cases of Friedreich's ataxia. *Br Med J* 3:649–652.

23. Hughes JT, Brownell B, Hewer RL (1968): The peripheral sensory pathway in Friedreich's ataxia. *Brain* 91:803–820.

24. Johnson WG (1995): Friedreich ataxia. *Clin Neurosci* 3:33–38.

25. Keats B, Ward L, Shaw J, et al. (1989): "Acadian" and "classical" forms of Friedreich's ataxia are most probably caused by mutations at the same locus. *Am J Med Genet* 33:266–268.

26. Labelle H, Beauchamp M, Lapierre L, et al. (1987): Pattern of muscle weakness and its relation to loss of ambulatory function in Friedreich's ataxia. *J Pediatr Orthop* 7:496.

27. Labelle H, Dansereau J, Bellefleur C, et al. (1995): Variability of geometric measurements from 3-D reconstructions of scoliotic spines and rib cages. *Eur Spine J* 4:88–94.

28. Labelle H, Duhaime M, Allard P (1987): Kyphosis and scoliosis in 3-D in Friedreich's ataxia. *Orthop Trans* 11:214.

29. Labelle H, Fassier F (1991): Maladie de Friedreich et scoliose: mise à jour. *Rachis* 3:423–426.

30. Labelle H, Poitras B, Duhaime M, et al. (1990): Scoliosis in Friedreich's ataxia: kyphoscoliosis or lordoscoliosis? *Orthop Trans* 14:789,812.

31. Labelle H, Tohmé S, Duhaime M, et al. (1986): The natural history of scoliosis in Friedreich's ataxia. *J Bone Joint Surg Am* 68:564–572.

32. Lamarche JB, Lemieux B, Lieu HB (1984): The neuropathology of "typical" Friedreich's ataxia in Quebec. *Can J Neurol Sci* 11:592–600.

33. Oppenheimer DR (1979): Brain lesions in Friedreich's ataxia. *Can J Neurol Sci* 6:173–176.

34. Pandolfo M, Sirugo G, Antonelli A, et al. (1990): Friedreich's ataxia in Italian families: genetic homogeneity and linkage disequilibrium with the marker loci D9S5 and D9S15. *Am J Hum Genet* 47:228–235.

35. Pelosi L, Fels A, Petrillo A, et al. (1984): Friedreich's ataxia: Clinical involvement and evoked potentials. *Acta Neurol Scand* 70:360–368.

36. Peyronnard JM, Lapointe L, Bouchard JP, et al. (1976): Nerve conduction studies and electromyography in Friedreich's ataxia. *Can J Neurol Sci* 3:313–317.

37. Phillipps LH, Blanco JS, Sussman MD (1995): Direct spinal stimulation for intraoperative monitoring during scoliosis surgery. *Muscle Nerve* 18: 1214–1215.

38. Romeo G, Menozzi P, Ferlini A, et al. (1983): Incidence of Friedreich's ataxia in Italy estimated from consanguineous marriages. *Am J Hum Genet* 35:523–529.

39. Rivard CH, Duhaime M, Poitras B, et al. (1984): Spinal segmental instrumentation for the treatment of all types of paralytic scoliosis. *J Bone Joint Surg Br* 366:299.

40. Sjogren T (1943): Klinische und erbbiologische Unsersuchungen uber die Heredoataxien. *Acta Psychiatr Neurol Scand Suppl* 27:1–200.

41. Winter RM, Harding AE, Baraitser M, et al. (1981): Intrafamilial correlation in Friedreich's ataxia. *Clin Genet* 20:419–427.

47

MUSCULAR DYSTROPHY

GREGORY V. HAHN
SCOTT J. MUBARAK

DUCHENNE AND BECKER MUSCULAR DYSTROPHY

For many years, the Duchenne and Becker forms of muscular dystrophy were described as two distinct diseases. They are now considered to be mild and severe forms of the same disease. They occur mainly among boys, are characterized by proximal muscle weakness, and have an X-linked recessive inheritance pattern (women are carriers). Children with Duchenne muscular dystrophy have more severe clinical manifestations than do those with Becker muscular dystrophy.

The gene defect has been isolated to the Xp21 locus of the X chromosome. The protein product, dystrophin, is a large (427 kd), intracellular, structural component of the plasma-membrane system in normal muscle fibers (17,54). It is also found in the neural tissues of the cerebrum, cerebellum, and peripheral axons. The exact biologic function of dystrophin remains unknown. At the genetic level, both forms of muscular dystrophy are caused by mutations of the X-linked gene encoding dystrophin. However, at the biochemical level, Duchenne muscular dystrophy is caused by a deficiency of dystrophin, and the Becker form occurs when dystrophin is present but is abnormal in either amount or molecular structure (54).

Portions of the coding sequences of the gene (c-DNA) have been used to produce polyclonal antiserum directed against the protein product of the normal gene. The polyclonal antibodies have been used to assess the quantity and quality of dystrophin in muscle biopsy specimens from patients believed to have Duchenne or Becker muscular dystrophy. According to the dystrophin level in the muscle biopsy specimen, clinical categories are defined as follows: Duchenne dystrophy, less than 3% of normal; severe Becker dystrophy, 3% to 10% of normal; and moderate to mild Becker dystrophy, 20% or more of normal dystrophin levels. Most patients with Duchenne dystrophy have undetectable levels of dystrophin, and most of those with Becker dystrophy have nearly normal levels of an altered form of dystrophin (54).

The diagnosis of Duchenne muscular dystrophy usually is made between the ages of 3 and 5 years. Motor milestones may be delayed by a few months but tend to occur within the normal range. Running is found to be awkward by the age of 18 months to 2 years, although often only in retrospect. Stair climbing becomes progressively more difficult. Some children are seen first by an orthopaedic surgeon with a main symptom of toe-walking or flat-feet. Other clinical findings of the condition that usually are apparent by 3 years of age include enlarged calf muscles, mild iliotibial band and Achilles tendon contractures, proximal weakness, and a positive Gowers sign, which indicates gluteus maximus and quadriceps weakness (Fig. 1). Later, a wide-based, lordotic stance and waddling Trendelenburg gait become apparent.

The diagnosis has traditionally been confirmed with the laboratory finding of a massively elevated level of creatinine phosphokinase (50 to 100 times normal), an electromyogram showing myopathy, and a muscle biopsy characterized by variations of fiber size in internal nuclei, split fibers, degenerating or regenerating fibers, and fibrous tissue deposition (17). Often a family history of muscular dystrophy can be elicited. Diagnostic evaluation includes DNA analysis to identify the specific mutation and protein analysis to determine the quantity and quality of dystrophin in the muscle tissue. This allows for quick and accurate differentiation between Duchenne and Becker muscular dystrophy.

Many advances have been made in prenatal testing. Reliable prenatal diagnosis can be made with chorionic villus biopsy, although this procedure carries some inherent risk. Other options include immunologic analysis of dystrophin expression obtained from fetal amniocytes or fibroblasts. Noninvasive prenatal DNA diagnosis of fetal cells in maternal blood is being studied but is not yet clinically available (47).

Clinical Course

After 5 years of age, walking gradually becomes more labored for patients with Duchenne muscular dystrophy. A typical preadolescent patient stands with anterior pelvic tilt and increased lordosis. Gluteus maximus and quadriceps weakness makes independent walking precarious generally by 8 to 10 years of age. As a result of increasing muscle weakness and decreasing activity level, children have hip and knee flexion contractures and equi-

G.V. Hahn: Department of Orthopaedic Surgery, All Children's Hospital St. Petersburg, Florida 33701.
S.J. Mubarak: Departments of Orthopedic Surgery, University of California San Diego, and Pediatric Orthopedics, Children's Hospital San Diego, San Diego, California 92123.

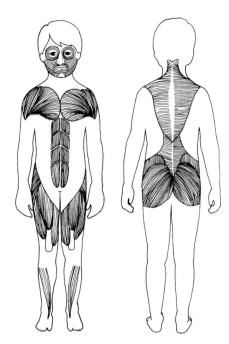

FIGURE 1. Patients with Duchenne muscular dystrophy have a characteristic, symmetric pattern of muscle weakness that involves the facial muscles, shoulder and pelvic girdles, spinal extensors and abdominals, and tibialis anterior.

novarus deformities of the feet. At this stage, patients are treated with iliotibial band release and Achilles tendon lengthening coupled with anterior transfer of the posterior tibialis muscle and the introduction of knee-ankle-foot orthoses. This combined surgical and orthotic approach prolongs walking for about 1.5 years for most patients. The patients typically stand in lordosis, which protects them from kyphoscoliosis until early in the second decade, when standing with orthoses becomes limited. These patients generally begin using a wheelchair full-time by 11 to 13 years of age and then have progressive thoracolumbar scoliosis. Other clinical findings include cardiomyopathy and decreased mental capacity. A relentless progression of spinal deformity and associated decline in pulmonary function contribute directly to early death. Death usually occurs in the late teens or early twenties as a result of cardiopulmonary failure and respiratory infections.

Becker muscular dystrophy has symptoms similar to those of Duchenne muscular dystrophy. The onset of symptoms occurs later, however, and the condition is less severe, so ability to walk often persists into the twenties and beyond. In the past, the most dependable differentiation between the Duchenne and Becker types was the clinical course. In the Becker variant, similar electromyographic and creatinine phosphokinase abnormalities are seen, and only subtle distinctions may be evident in a biopsy specimen. Cardiac involvement and mental retardation are much less frequent in Becker muscular dystrophy. Most patients do not need surgical intervention to maintain ambulation until the adolescent years. The clinical presentation of Becker dystrophy tends to overlap with that of other non–sex-linked neuromuscular disorders, such as limb-girdle dystrophy and some metabolic and mitochondrial forms of myopathy.

Course of Spinal Deformities in Duchenne Muscular Dystrophy

Wilkins and Gibson (53) theorized two pathways of spinal deformity in Duchenne muscular dystrophy—a stable pathway characterized by a position of extension and an unstable pathway exhibiting progressive thoracolumbar kyphosis and scoliosis. A prophylactic electric wheelchair spinal support system was proposed to guide the early straight spine into a stable extended posture, thereby averting the need for operative intervention (13). Although there is a relation between extension of the lumbar spine and severity of scoliosis at the time of final follow-up examination, maintenance of lumbar lordosis is difficult and rarely prevents development of severe scoliosis even when support systems and braces are used (18,43,51).

The incidence of progressive scoliosis is about 95% among patients with Duchenne muscular dystrophy (8,32). The course of these curves is progression to more than 100 degrees. This usually occurs within 5 years of the beginning of full-time use of a wheelchair and greatly interferes with sitting comfort and proper positioning in the wheelchair, upper-extremity function, caloric ingestion, respiratory function, and appearance.

Smith et al. (43) reviewed the clinical charts and spinal radiographs of 51 boys who had Duchenne muscular dystrophy, no surgical management of the spinal deformity, and follow-up evaluation until death. All had scoliosis. However, the rate of progression of the curve was a determinant of the magnitude of the final curve ($P < .001$). The age at death correlated inversely with the rate of progression of the curve ($P < .01$). None of the following were useful factors in predicting which curves would become severe: age when walking began, age when walking ceased, age at onset of spinal collapse, surgical release of the iliotibial bands, or age at death. The authors found that when a curve exceeded 35 degrees, vital capacity usually was less than 40% of the predicted normal value. Hsu (18) found that the curve progressed 0.3 to 4.5 degrees each month in all eight of his patients, who were between the ages of 13 and 22 years at the time of follow-up evaluation.

In a study performed at Children's Hospital San Diego, investigators found an average 10-degree increase in thoracic scoliosis for each year of life once the child began using a wheelchair full-time (26). Cambridge and Drennan (8) found that in 95% of patients, some of whom were observed until death, the curve had progressed to an average of 75 degrees at the last examination. Curve progression was found even in the 32 boys with curves of more than 30 degrees who wore braces.

Oda et al. (37) classified the course of spinal deformity into three types: unremitting progression of scoliosis with kyphosis (type I), transition from kyphosis to lordosis before 15 years of age (type II), and mild deformity without prominent longitudinal changes (type III). The authors found that all patients with type I deformities had a Cobb angle greater than 30 degrees by 15 years of age and that the deformity progressed to a condition of "a collapsing spine." Patients with type II deformities had a less predictable progression of scoliosis, especially those with double curves. Patients with Type III deformities had a more benign course that was associated with improvement in pulmonary function. In the series of 46 patients, 21 (46%) were classified as having type I deformity, 18 (39%) as having type II, and only seven (15%) as having type III deformity. The authors recommended surgical intervention for all patients with type I deformities and selected patients with type II deformities.

Pulmonary Function in Duchenne Muscular Dystrophy

Duchenne muscular dystrophy produces a restrictive pulmonary disease pattern, but the mechanics that cause this restriction are not well defined. Muscle weakness, muscle contractures, and severe spinal deformities that affect respiratory mechanics are important factors. A decline in respiratory function with increasing age in association with Duchenne muscular dystrophy is well recognized (7,15,19,21,22,38,39,48). Decreased respiratory function leads to pulmonary infection and respiratory failure. The forced vital capacity is the best prognostic factor in evaluating pulmonary function (26). Monitoring the rate of decline of forced vital capacity is necessary to ensure that the patient has sufficient pulmonary reserve to safely undergo spinal stabilization.

In idiopathic scoliosis, the degree of scoliosis shows a strong linear correlation with a decline in percentage of predicted forced vital capacity and total lung capacity (23,50,52). There is general agreement that the degree of thoracic scoliosis is the most important causative factor in declining pulmonary function in idiopathic scoliosis. In contrast, among patients with paralytic scoliosis there is a multifactorial influence on declining pulmonary function, increasing scoliotic deformity being only one of these factors (22).

Although numerous studies had described the pulmonary function abnormality among patients with Duchenne muscular dystrophy, none had showed a correlation with scoliosis until 1983, when investigators at our center conducted a study with 25 patients with this condition (26). We found that forced vital capacity peaked at approximately the age when standing ceased then declined rapidly. Percentage of forced vital capacity was found to be the measure of pulmonary function most strongly correlated with age and thoracic scoliosis measurements. Age and thoracic scoliosis together were better predictors of forced vital capacity than either one alone. Once patients were using a wheelchair full-time, each year of age had approximately the same negative influence on percentage of forced vital capacity as each additional 10 degrees of thoracic scoliosis; both decreased forced vital capacity approximately 4%. A regression equation for percentage of forced vital capacity was used to develop the theory that a patient with scoliosis, the progression of which is halted by spinal instrumentation and fusion, would after the surgery show a slower rate of decline in percentage of forced vital capacity and that this rate is quantifiable and predictable and depends solely on the patient's advancing age.

Our conclusions were supported by Galasko et al. (11), who reported results of the treatment of 55 patients with Duchenne muscular dystrophy observed for scoliosis and pulmonary function. All patients were offered surgical stabilization when the scoliosis measured 20 degrees. Thirty-two accepted, and the 23 who refused were used as the control group. The investigators found that in the group that underwent surgical treatment, forced vital capacity remained static during the first 36 months after the operation and then decreased slightly. In the group that did not undergo surgical treatment, forced vital capacity progressively diminished. Peak expiratory flow rate increased considerably among the group that underwent surgical treatment but remained the same among the controls. The survival data showed a significantly higher mortality among those who declined surgical treatment, indicating that spinal stabilization can improve survival for several years after the operation, provided the procedure is performed promptly before marked progression occurs.

Results of several other studies have contradicted these observations. Miller et al. (32), from the Hospital for Sick Children, Toronto, found that patients who underwent spinal fusion and instrumentation had the same decline in respiratory function postoperatively as the untreated group. Miller et al. (33), of Children's Hospital, San Francisco, described patients with Duchenne muscular dystrophy. These investigators also found no significant difference between the group that underwent surgical treatment and the group that did not in terms of declining respiratory function. Kennedy et al. (24), in Australia, compared pulmonary function and survival rates for 38 patients with Duchenne muscular dystrophy, 17 of whom underwent surgical stabilization of the spine and 21 of whom were treated nonoperatively. These authors also found no difference in pulmonary function or survival among the two groups and reported the decline in forced vital capacity to be 3% to 5% per year. All of these studies, however, were comparisons of patients who underwent surgical stabilization at a relatively advanced stage. The surgical group in all three studies had a mean preoperative Cobb angle greater than 50 degrees. Pulmonary function may be too poor at this stage to benefit from surgical correction. In addition, when patients with larger curves undergo instrumentation full postoperative correction often is not achieved. The residual curve may further compromise pulmonary function.

In summary, percentage of forced vital capacity remains the best test for monitoring the pulmonary function of patients with Duchenne muscular dystrophy. This percentage begins to decline rapidly (approximately 4% a year) once patients begin to use a wheelchair full-time and stabilizes at approximately 25% of normal until death (24,26). The benefit of early surgical correction of scoliosis in regard to pulmonary function remains unclear. It appears that once the curve reaches 40 degrees, surgical correction does not influence pulmonary function. Tracheostomy and mechanical ventilation are treatment options to be considered in the more advanced stages of the disease.

Options in the Management of Scoliosis

Nonsurgical

Scoliosis and kyphosis rarely develop while a patient with Duchenne or Becker muscular dystrophy is able to walk. During the later stages of walking, marked lordosis develops, but it is rarely fixed. This is a functional position to compensate for weakness of the gluteus maximus muscle and the subsequent anterior pelvic tilt. It should not be considered a spinal deformity (40). If scoliosis does develop while the child is still able to walk, bracing will be ineffective and will probably end the ability to walk.

Among most patients who have Duchenne or Becker muscular dystrophy, severe spinal deformity develops once the patient begins using a wheelchair full-time. Patients with the Becker type have fewer problems, because the scoliosis usually develops after maturity. Severe scoliosis makes comfortable sitting difficult; even frequent and elaborate position adjustments often cannot prevent pressure sores and pain. Thus some patients become bedridden years before they die, even if prophylactic bracing or positioning in a spinal support system has been used. Braces and spinal support systems may slow the rate of progression of the curve but do not halt it (8,18,45,51).

Gibson et al. (13) initially reported good control of scoliosis with their wheelchair spinal support system. Among 17 patients observed an average of 27.5 months, the average rate of curve progression was held to 0.7 degree per month, or 8.4 degrees a year. Gibson et al. also found that if the curve progressed to 20 to 30 degrees, an anterior-opening spinal orthosis or an anteroposterior bivalved body jacket could be used. For curves greater than 60 degrees, the pressure of the brace was uncomfortable, and effective correction could not be obtained. Further follow-up information from this center showed that the spinal support system only delays the progression of scoliosis; it does not prevent it (51).

It is now generally believed that orthotic management is inappropriate because curve progression is only slowed. The systemic manifestations of the disease continue and cause further deterioration in cardiac and pulmonary function. The braced spinal deformity eventually progresses rapidly. By this time, the patient's may be too debilitated by decreases in pulmonary function to withstand surgery. All these patients should use well-fitting wheelchairs with solid, cushioned seat, back, and lateral trunk supports until spinal fusion is indicated. Patients with power-driven wheelchairs should use a midline control.

Surgical

Posterior spinal instrumentation with fusion is the therapy of choice for scoliosis among patients with Duchenne muscular dystrophy once they are no longer able to walk. This treatment is indicated to improve quality of life and upright wheelchair positioning.

In 1982, Luque (29) revolutionized the surgical management of paralytic scoliosis when he introduced his segmental spinal instrumentation. This procedure eliminated the need for prolonged postoperative immobilization, which is characteristic of Harrington instrumentation. Segmental instrumentation has the

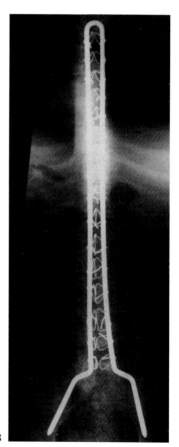 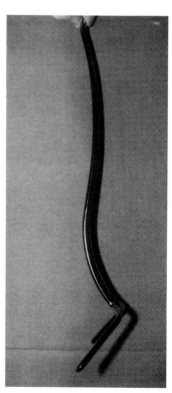 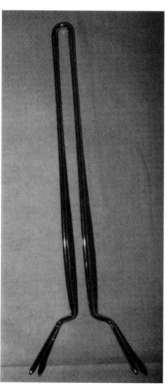

A,B   C

FIGURE 2. A 13-year-old boy with Duchenne muscular dystrophy and progressive scoliosis underwent posterior spinal fusion and instrumentation with a unit rod and sublaminar wires. **A:** Anteroposterior radiograph 2 months after the operation. **B:** Prebent sagittal plane contours of the Unit Rod. **C:** Unit Rod. (Courtesy of Stuart L. Weinstein, M.D.)

advantage of allowing immediately postoperative mobilization without a Risser cast or spinal orthosis. Later, the addition of the Galveston technique of pelvic instrumentation allowed stable spinal instrumentation to the pelvis to manage paralytic scoliosis (1). An additional modification in instrumentation is the unit II rod described by Moseley et al. (34), which allows improved control over pelvic obliquity and tilt to prevent relative translation and rotation (Fig. 2).

It is generally agreed that fusion must be extended into the upper thoracic area to avoid cephalic progression of the curve due to progressive trunk and neck muscle weakness. However, the caudal extent of the fusion continues to be debated. It is essential to center the patient's head over the midpelvis in both the coronal and sagittal planes to prevent the upper body weight from acting as a pendulum, which could lead to loss of head control and cephalic extension of the curve. Because of these concerns, it was initially recommended that instrumentation and fusion be performed to the sacrum to prevent or correct pelvic obliquity (27). However, as Allen and Ferguson (1) pointed out, pelvic fixation is technically demanding, increases operative time, and poses increased risk of complications. In 1984, Sussman (45) suggested that fusion and fixation to the level of L5 may be sufficient for Duchenne muscular dystrophy, but the follow-up period of the study was limited.

To better define this issue, Mubarak et al. (35) conducted a prospective study with two groups of patients: 12 undergoing instrumentation and fusion to the sacrum and ten undergoing to L5 only. For all patients, instrumentation and fusion were performed cephalad to the high thoracic level, generally T2–3. The average follow-up period was 7 years. The minimum was 5 years for all living patients. There were no significant differences in estimated blood loss or length of stay in the intensive care unit and hospital between the two groups. The operative time was approximately 30 minutes longer among patients who underwent fusion to the sacrum. Review of the patients' sitting balance and pelvic obliquity revealed only minor differences between the two groups (Figs. 3, 4). Only one patient (with a preoperative curve of 50 degrees) had marked preoperative pelvic obliquity that was not fully corrected at surgery (Fig. 5). No other patients had substantial pelvic obliquity, and all maintained an upright or only slightly shifted sitting position postoperatively (Fig. 6). It was concluded that instrumentation to L5 is sufficient if treatment is initiated early.

Alman and Kim (2) reported a similar comparison of 48 patients with Duchenne muscular dystrophy. Ten patients underwent fusion and instrumentation to the pelvis, and 38 patients underwent fusion and instrumentation to L5. The authors reported an increase in pelvic obliquity in 32 of the 38 patients

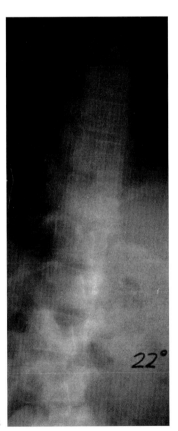
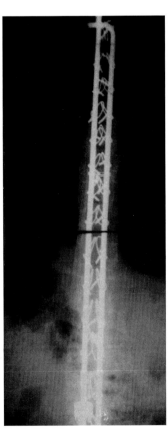
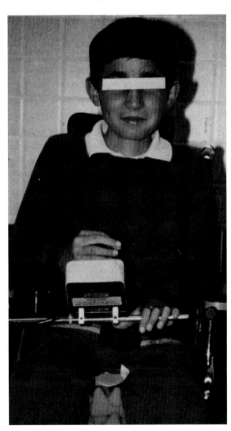

A,B   C

FIGURE 3. A 13-year-old boy with Duchenne muscular dystrophy had 15-degree right thoracic, 22-degree left lumbar scoliosis **(A)**. **B:** Five years after Luque segmental instrumentation to L5, the spine is straight with no substantial residual lumbar curve or pelvic obliquity. **C:** Clinical appearance 5 years after the operation.

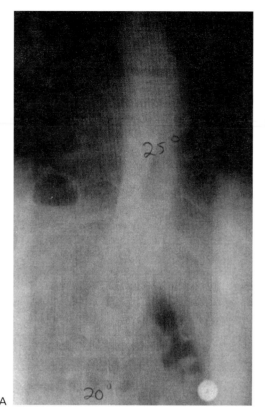

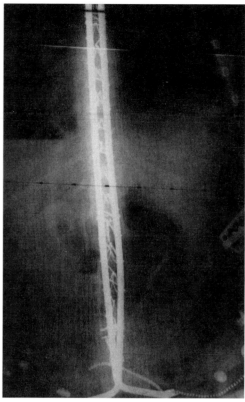

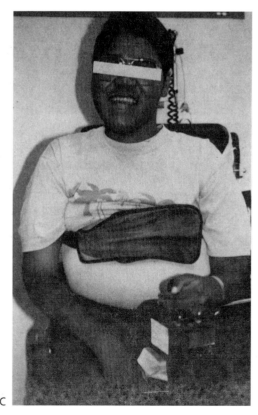

FIGURE 4. A 14-year-old boy with Duchenne muscular dystrophy. **A:** A 25-degree right thoracic, 20-degree left lumbar curve was managed with spinal instrumentation and fusion. **B:** Seven years after Luque segmental instrumentation and fusion from T2 to the pelvis, there is no substantial scoliosis or pelvic obliquity. **C:** The patient sits in a shifted position.

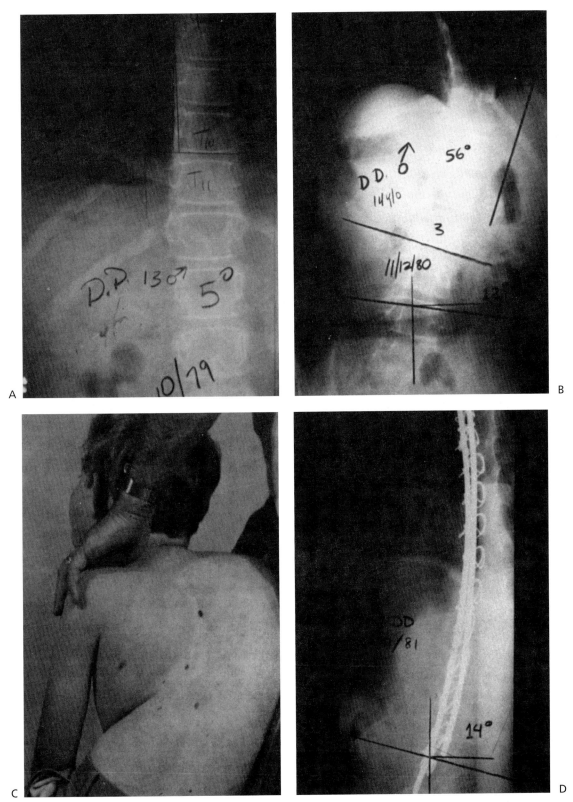

FIGURE 5. A 13-year-old boy with Duchenne muscular dystrophy. **A:** First spinal radiograph shows a 5-degree left lumbar curve. **B:** One year after **A,** a 56-degree right thoracolumbar C-shaped curve necessitates segmental spinal instrumentation and fusion. **C:** Preoperative appearance. **D:** Appearance 10 months after fusion from T3 to L5. The rods shifted, and the patient maintained pelvic obliquity with residual curve of 30 degrees and obliquity of 14 degrees. He was the only patient in either group with marked residual pelvic obliquity.

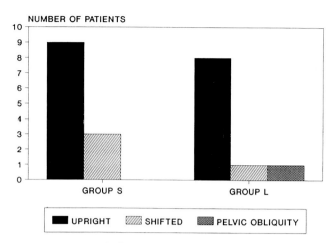

NUMBER OF PATIENTS

UPRIGHT   SHIFTED   PELVIC OBLIQUITY

FIGURE 6. Bar graph shows clinical and radiographic categories for each of the two groups of patients. Among the 12 patients who underwent fusion to the sacrum (*group S*), nine were upright, and three had shifting. Among the ten patients who underwent fusion to L5 (*group L*), eight were upright, one had shifting, and one had pelvic obliquity (35).

who underwent fusion to L5 and in two of the ten patients who underwent fusion to the sacrum. They found substantial increases only when the apex of the preoperative curve was below L1. They therefore recommended fusion to the sacrum for all curves with an apex below L1.

In a series described by Brook et al. (5), results for ten patients who underwent fusion above the pelvis were compared with those for seven patients who underwent Luque-Galveston fixation to the pelvis. The authors found marked sitting imbalance or progression of scoliosis among six of the ten patients who underwent fusion above the pelvis and recommended fusion to the pelvis in all cases. However, three of the ten patients underwent fusion only to L4, and 1 patient underwent fusion to L3. The preoperative curves of eight of the ten patients exceeded 40 degrees, and preoperative pelvic obliquity was not recorded for any of the 10 patients who underwent fusion above the pelvis. We agree that marked preoperative pelvic obliquity or a curve greater than 40 degrees necessitates fusion to the sacrum and pelvis.

We have found the following surgical treatment plan to be successful for patients with Duchenne muscular dystrophy and for those with Becker muscular dystrophy who need surgery. Spinal fusion is performed when the curve reaches 20 degrees, and forced vital capacity is still greater than 40% (Fig. 7). For patients with curves greater than 40 degrees, an operation usually can be performed without difficulty if the vital capacity is more than 35%. For patients with a smaller vital capacity, complications increase, and postoperative tracheostomy may be needed. We generally decline to operate on patients with vital capacities less than 30% because of the high incidence of pulmonary complications. At some centers, however, such patients do undergo surgery (24).

The recommended surgical technique is Luque segmental instrumentation and posterior fusion from the high thoracic level (T2 or T3) down to L5. If the preoperative pelvic obliquity is greater than 10 degrees or the scoliosis curve is greater than 40 degrees, one should consider instrumentation to the pelvis to correct this obliquity and ensure a level pelvis (Fig. 8). Texas

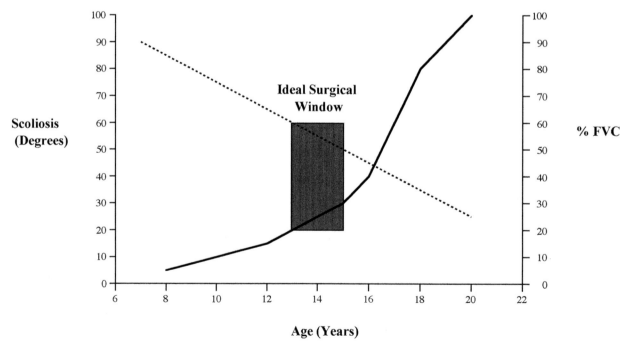

FIGURE 7. Line graph shows the natural progression of scoliosis (*solid line*) plotted against age and declining pulmonary function (*dotted line*) measured as percentage forced vital capacity (*%FVC*) plotted against age. The *shaded area* represents the ideal surgical window for correction of scoliosis—the curve measures between 20 and 30 degrees and the %FVC is greater than 40%.

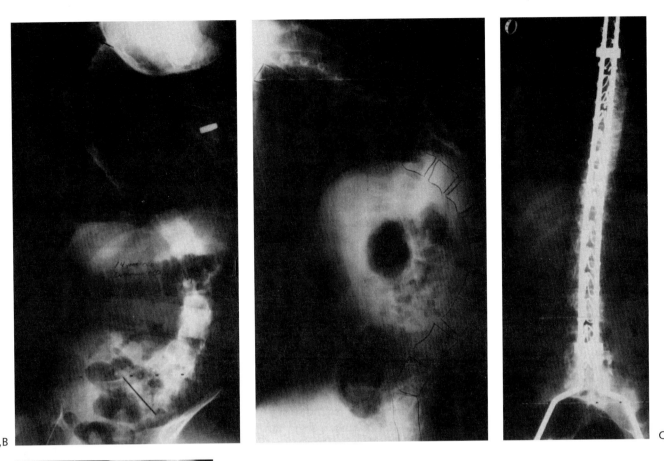

A,B

C

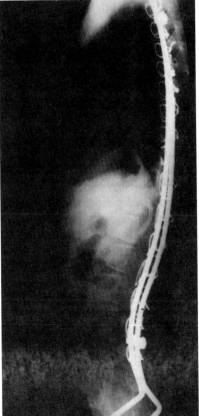

D

FIGURE 8. A 14-year-old boy with Duchenne muscular dystrophy had a 75-degree scoliosis with pelvic obliquity and a severe kyphotic deformity. The patient was successfully treated by means of posterior spinal fusion from T2 to the sacrum with Luque-Galveston instrumentation and Texas Scottish Rite Hospital cross-links. Preoperative sitting anteroposterior **(A)** and lateral **(B)** radiographs. Anteroposterior **(C)** and lateral **(D)** radiographs 6 months after the operation (Courtesy of Stuart L. Weinstein, M.D.)

Scottish Rite Hospital cross-links also can be used for additional stability between the two Luque rods. The intensive care unit stay usually is 2 days, and the average hospital stay is about 7 days. Use of a lightweight Orthoplast body jacket for 6 months is recommended for both comfort and safety when the patient is upright or being transferred.

A recent modification of the original Luque technique was described by Marchesi et al. (31). Two sacral screws are used to supplement the pelvic fixation. They found no instrumentation failure or loss of correction greater than 3 degrees among 25 patients (mean follow-up period 36 months). Intraoperative anaphylaxis to an antibiotic was the only complication recorded. This appears to a reasonable surgical alternative.

The goal in the management of spinal deformity in Duchenne muscular dystrophy is maintenance of upright sitting posture and maximal pain-free function. Many of our patients who have undergone surgical treatment are now older than 20 years, have an upright posture, can operate a power-driven wheelchair, have minimal positioning difficulties, and have an improved quality of life.

FACIOSCAPULOHUMERAL DYSTROPHY

Facioscapulohumeral dystrophy (Landouzy-Dejerines disease) is a more mild form of muscular dystrophy involving the shoulder girdle and facial muscles to varying degrees. The molecular defect has been localized on chromosome 4, but the gene has not yet been identified. The disease is transmitted in an autosomal dominant pattern with variable expression, and the prevalence is estimated at five cases per 100,000 persons (46). In most cases of facioscapulohumeral dystrophy, the onset of symptoms occurs in late childhood or adolescence. Clinical signs generally develop slowly and progressively, often with periods of arrest. Functional disability may not occur until late in the course of the disease.

In some instances the disease course is severe and rapidly progressive, symptoms beginning in infancy or early childhood. This presentation is associated with greater morbidity and higher mortality at a younger age and until recently was believed to be a distinct genetic defect (3,16,46). The parents of children with facioscapulohumeral dystrophy may have no symptoms or have minimal clinical evidence of the disease.

In all cases of facioscapulohumeral dystrophy, facial weakness occurs early in the disease course. Patients have a characteristic stare and may lack the ability to whistle, blow out the cheeks, or completely close the eyes. The usual facial creases may be absent. Weakness of the muscles of the shoulder girdle develops bilaterally, and, as is not true of any other form of muscular dystrophy, the weakness may be asymmetric. Involvement of the trapezius, serratus anterior, and rhomboid muscles is characteristic, and there is later and more variable involvement of the latissimus dorsi and pectoralis major and minor muscles (Fig. 9). Glenohumeral motion is initially preserved, and the deltoid muscle is spared until late in the disease.

With this typical pattern of muscle involvement, patients lose the ability to stabilize the scapula against the thorax and thus

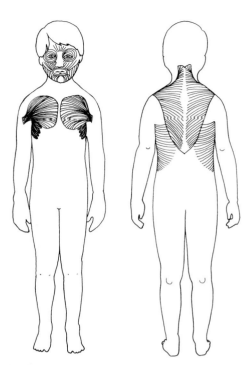

FIGURE 9. Diagram shows initial muscle involvement in facioscapulohumeral dystrophy.

cannot fully abduct or flex the shoulder. Without a stable fulcrum, attempts at shoulder abduction generate scapulothoracic, rather than glenohumeral, motion. Activation of the deltoid causes winging of the scapula as it rotates superiorly and internally unrestrained.

Ketenjian (25), Copeland and Howard (9), and Letournel et al. (28) described methods of scapulothoracic stabilization to improve the upper-extremity function of patients with facioscapulohumeral dystrophy. Ketenjian (25) described a method of scapulocostal fasciodesis. With fascia lata, polyester mesh (Mersilene), or polyester (Dacron) strips, the scapula is secured to the underlying ribs in a position of 20 degrees of external rotation. Five shoulders evaluated over an average of 34 months had improved appearance and an average increase of 33 degrees (37%) in active shoulder abduction. Critics of such procedures, which rely on soft-tissue stabilization, claim that the improvement in active shoulder abduction gradually deteriorates (28). Letournel et al. (28) described an alternative method of stabilization consisting of arthrodesis with a wire-plate construct. Among nine patients who underwent 16 arthrodesis procedures, the authors found a mean increase in shoulder abduction of 25 degrees. With an average follow-up period of 5.7 years, they found substantial and enduring improvement in ability to perform activities of daily living. Patients with facioscapulohumeral dystrophy also may have pelvic girdle weakness as the disease progresses. Weakness of the hip extensors contributes to an increase in lumbar lordosis, which may become severe and symptomatic among

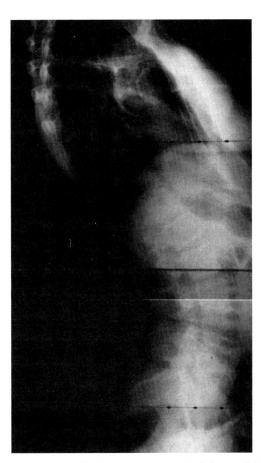

FIGURE 10. Radiograph shows a patient with facioscapulohumeral dystrophy and characteristic increase in lumbar lordosis.

lature. Both autosomal dominant and recessive forms are described, and at least six distinct chromosomal abnormalities have been identified (16,30). Symptoms of limb-girdle dystrophy are similar to those of facioscapulohumeral dystrophy except that the facial muscles are not involved. The symptoms may follow one of several patterns of muscular involvement, shoulder girdle muscles affected first followed by pelvic girdle weakness, or vice versa. In the scapulohumeral type (49), the muscles of the shoulder girdle constitute the primary area of involvement (Fig. 11). Symmetric weakness of the trapezius, serratus anterior, rhomboids, latissimus, and pectoralis major develops with variable subsequent involvement of the fingers and wrists. The deltoid muscle usually is spared early in the course of the disease. Patients with the pelvifemoral type (Leyden-Möbius) have hip extensor and abductor weakness, which increases in lumbar lordosis, gait abnormalities, and hip instability (Fig. 12). The distal musculature eventually is affected, specifically the tibialis anterior and peroneal muscles. The gastrocnemius and soleus muscles are not affected until late in the course of disease.

The onset of symptoms in limb-girdle dystrophy is variable, ranging from the first through fourth decades of life, but symptoms usually occur in mid to late adolescence. Symptoms progress slowly and symmetrically, but marked disability usually is present 20 years after onset. Significant structural scoliosis rarely develops in limb-girdle dystrophy because the onset of disease usually occurs during adolescence, and progression is slow and symmetric. When it is present, scoliosis usually occurs after completion of growth and is rarely severe enough to necessitate treatment (10,42).

some adults (Fig. 10). It may necessitates bracing, hip flexor release, or spinal fusion if the lordosis impairs the ability to walk (6).

Scoliosis is rare in facioscapulohumeral dystrophy because growth usually is nearly complete at the onset of disease (10,12,41). Among 16 adult patients with facioscapulohumeral dystrophy, Siegel (41) found no structural scoliosis. Patients with earlier onset of facioscapulohumeral dystrophy, however, may have marked structural scoliosis. Among these children, asymmetric muscle involvement contributes to curve progression. These patients usually respond well to bracing and surgery. Segmental instrumentation and fusion as described for Duchenne muscular dystrophy are used. The intelligence and life span of patients with facioscapulohumeral dystrophy are normal.

LIMB-GIRDLE MUSCULAR DYSTROPHY

Limb-girdle muscular dystrophy represents a group of autosomal disorders characterized by proximal muscle weakness with predominant involvement of the pelvic and shoulder girdle muscu-

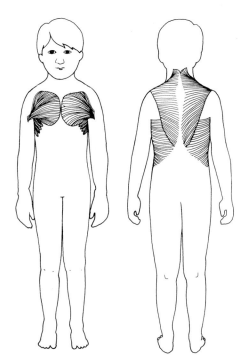

FIGURE 11. Diagram shows muscle involvement in scapulohumeral type of limb-girdle muscular dystrophy.

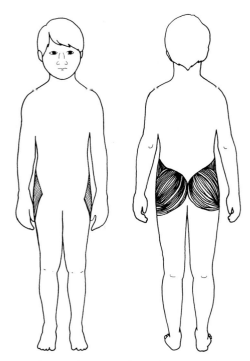

FIGURE 12. Diagram shows muscle involvement in the pelvifemoral type of limb-girdle muscular dystrophy (Leyden-Möbius).

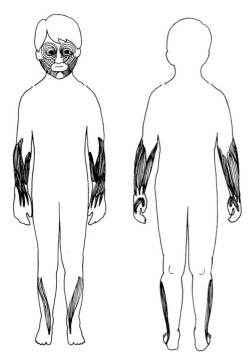

FIGURE 13. Diagram shows muscle involvement in myotonic dystrophy.

MYOTONIC MUSCULAR DYSTROPHY

Myotonic muscular dystrophy (dystrophia myotonica, Steinert disease) is characterized by myotonia and progressive muscular weakness. It is the most common form of muscular dystrophy among adult, affecting one in 7,000 to 8,000 persons. Myotonic dystrophy is transmitted in an autosomal dominant pattern with variable penetrance through a defective gene segment on chromosome 19 (16,44). Myotonic dystrophy causes progressive weakness in an initially distal distribution (Fig. 13). Symptoms may be apparent in early childhood, but the classic form manifests in late adolescence or early adulthood.

The disease is characterized by facial weakness with ptosis and the inability to whistle or close the eyes. Patients may have myopathic facies—a long, narrow face lacks expression. Speech and swallowing may be affected. Unlike the pattern of proximal limb weakness in facioscapulohumeral and limb-girdle muscular dystrophy, muscle involvement in myotonic dystrophy is in the distal limbs. In the upper extremities, intrinsic hand function and wrist and forearm strength are affected early. In the lower extremities, tibialis anterior and peroneal weakness occurs, leading to progressive footdrop deformities in adults. In addition to muscle weakness, myotonia occurs early in the disease course. Persistent involuntary muscle contraction occurs when a patient is unable to release a grasp.

In the congenital form of myotonic dystrophy, patients are not myotonic at birth but are hypotonic. They display the classic facial diplegia with a dull, expressionless face. Fifty percent have rigid equinovarus deformities similar to those of arthrogryposis (4). The clubfoot deformities initially respond well to serial cast-ing but eventually recur and necessitate soft-tissue release in later childhood or triple arthrodesis at skeletal maturity. Congenital myotonic dystrophy often is associated with respiratory and feeding problems at birth and with psychomotor retardation. Patients with congenital and childhood forms of myotonic dystrophy also may have cardiac problems, cataracts, frontal balding, and testicular atrophy (4,36). Because the axial and proximal limb muscles are spared until late in the disease, scoliosis rarely develops in myotonic dystrophy (41,42). Myotonic dystrophy is a progressive disorder that usually causes marked disability within 20 years of onset and often diminishes life span. Subsequent generations may be more severely affected.

MALIGNANT HYPERTHERMIA

Malignant hyperthermia is a potentially catastrophic series of events associated with general anesthesia and, on occasion, with local anesthesia or even stress unrelated to surgery (14,20). It tends to occur among otherwise healthy persons, but there is an increased incidence among persons with myopathy. The condition is genetic, but both recessive and dominant patterns with variable penetrance have been reported. It is thought to be associated with a defect in skeletal muscle that allows a marked rise in intracellular calcium levels. The syndrome results in a rapid increase in temperature (above 105°F [40.6°C]), tachycardia, muscle rigidity, especially of the masseter muscle, but often becoming generalized, hypoxemia, acidosis, hyperkalemia, and rhabdomyolysis. If not reversed, this syndrome is fatal. The mortality rate has been estimated to be 28%. Malignant hyperthermia occurs soon after induction of general anesthesia; succinylcholine and halothane are the anesthetic agents usually implicated. Once recognized, prompt intervention is required: immediate discontinuation of anesthesia and surgery, administration of oxygen, body cooling for patients with temperatures greater than 40.6°C, administration of sodium bicarbonate, frequent monitoring of acid-base and arterial blood gas values, and administration of dantrolene, which is thought to be specific for reversing the effects of malignant hyperthermia.

If malignant hyperthermia occurs, a neuromuscular evaluation should be performed that includes a detailed family history of response to surgery and anesthetic agents. Creatine kinase levels should be determined. A muscle biopsy sample can be assessed for excess reactivity to halothane, caffeine, or both. If a personal or family history of malignant hyperthermia is established, safe anesthetic agents for susceptible patients are nitrous oxide, opiates, thiopental, and pancuronium. Patients with known or suspected malignant hyperthermia also can be treated with dantrolene before undergoing required surgery (35a).

REFERENCES

1. Allen BL, Ferguson RL (1984): The Galveston technique of pelvic fixation with L-rod instrumentation of the spine. *Spine* 9:388–394.
2. Alman BA, Kim H (1998): Pelvic obliquity after fusion of the spine to L5 in Duchenne muscular dystrophy. Presented at the Annual Meeting of the Pediatric Orthopaedic Society of North America, Cleveland.
3. Bailey RO, Marzulo DC, Hans MB (1986): Infantile facioscapulohumeral muscular dystrophy: new observations. *Acta Neurol Scand* 74: 51–58.
4. Bowen RS Jr, Marks HG (1984): Foot deformity in myotonic dystrophy. *Foot Ankle* 5:125–130.
5. Brook PD, Kennedy JD, Stern LM, et al. (1996): Spinal fusion in Duchenne's muscular dystrophy. *J Pediatr Orthop* 16:324–331.
6. Bunch WH (1974): Muscular dystrophy. In: Hardy JH, ed. *Spinal deformity in neurological and muscular disorders.* St. Louis: Mosby, pp. 92–110.
7. Burke S, Grove N, Houser C, et al. (1971): Respiratory aspects of pseudohypertrophic muscular dystrophy. *Am J Dis Child* 121: 230–234.
8. Cambridge W, Drennan JC (1987): Scoliosis associated with Duchenne muscular dystrophy. *J Pediatr Orthop,* 7:436–440.
9. Copeland SA, Howard RC (1978): Thoracoscapular fusion for facioscapulohumeral dystrophy. *J Bone Joint Surg Br* 60:547–551.
10. Daher YH, Lonstein JE, Winter RB, et al. (1985): Spinal deformities in patients with muscular dystrophy other than Duchenne: a review of 11 patients having surgical treatment. *Spine* 10:614–617.
11. Galasko CSB, Delaney C, Morris P (1992): Spinal stabilization in Duchenne muscular dystrophy. *J Bone Joint Surg Br* 74:210–214.
12. Garfin SR, Leach J, Mubarak SJ, et al. (1988): Experiential approach—and literature review—of spinal care in adults with a neuromuscular disorder. *J Spinal Disord* 1:202–205.
13. Gibson D, Koreska J, Robertson D, et al. (1978): The management of spinal deformity in Duchenne's muscular dystrophy. *Orthop Clin North Am* 9:437–450.
14. Grohert GA (1980): Malignant hyperthermia. *Anesthesiology* 53:395.
15. Hapke E, Meek J, Jacobs J (1972): Pulmonary function in progressive muscular dystrophy. *Chest* 61:41–47.
16. Harper PS (1995): Myotonic dystrophy and other autosomal muscular dystrophies. In: Sciver CR, et al., eds. *The metabolic and molecular bases of inherited disease,* 7th ed. New York: McGraw-Hill, pp. 4227–4246.
17. Hoffman EP, Fischbeck KH, Brown RH, et al. (1988): Characterization of dystrophin in muscle biopsy specimens from patients with Duchenne's or Becker's muscular dystrophy. *N Engl J Med* 318:1363.
18. Hsu JD (1983): The natural history of spine curvature progression in the non-ambulatory Duchenne muscular dystrophy patient. *Spine* 8: 771–775.
19. Inkley S, Oldenburg F, Vignos P (1974): Pulmonary function in Duchenne muscular dystrophy related to stage of disease. *Am J Med* 56: 297.
20. Jarden OM, Wingard DW, Barak AJ, et al. (1979; Malignant hyperthermia: a potentially fatal syndrome in orthopaedic patients. *J Bone Joint Surg Am* 61:1064–1070.
21. Jenkins J, Bohn D, Edmonds J, et al. (1982): Evaluation of pulmonary function in muscular dystrophy patients requiring spinal surgery. *Crit Care Med* 10:645.
22. Kafer E (1974): Respiratory function in paralytic scoliosis. *Am Rev Respir Dis* 110:450.
23. Kafer E (1975): Idiopathic scoliosis; mechanical properties of the respiratory system and the ventilatory response to carbon dioxide. *J Clin Invest* 55:1153.
24. Kennedy JD, Staples AJ, Brook PD, et al. (1995): Effect of spine surgery on lung function in Duchenne muscular dystrophy. *Thorax* 50: 1173–1178.
25. Ketenjian AY (1978): Scapulocostal stabilization for scapular winging in facioscapulohumeral muscular dystrophy. *J Bone Joint Surg Am* 60: 476–480.
26. Kurz LT, Mubarak SJ, Schultz P, et al. (1983): Correlation of scoliosis and pulmonary function in Duchenne muscular dystrophy. *J Pediatr Orthop* 3:347–353.
27. LaPrade RF, Rowe DE (1992): The operative treatment of scoliosis in Duchenne muscular dystrophy. *Orthop Rev* 21:39–45.
28. Letournel E, Fardeau M, Lytle JO, et al. (1990): Scapulothoracic arthrodesis for patients who have facioscapulohumeral muscular dystrophy. *J Bone Joint Surg Am* 72:78–84.
29. Luque E (1982): The anatomic basis and development of segmental spinal instrumentation. *Spine* 7:256.
30. Mahjneh I, Bushby K, Pizzi A, et al. (1996): Limb-girdle muscular dystrophy: a follow-up study of 79 patients. *Acta Neurol Scand* 94: 177–189.
31. Marchesi D, Arlet V, Stricker U, et al. (1997): Modification of the original Luque technique in the treatment of Duchenne's neuromuscular scoliosis. *J Pediatr Orthop* 17:743–749.
32. Miller F, Moseley CF, Koreska P, et al. (1988): Pulmonary function and scoliosis in Duchenne dystrophy. *J Pediatr Orthop* 8:133–137.
33. Miller RG, Chalmers AC, Dao H, et al. (1991): The effect of spine fusion on respiratory function in Duchenne muscular dystrophy. *Neurology* 41:38–40.
34. Moseley CF, Musca V, Laden L, et al. (1985): Improved stability in segmental instrumentation of neuromuscular scoliosis. Presented at the Annual Meeting of the Pediatric Orthopaedic Society of North America, San Antonio, Texas.
35. Mubarak S, Morin W, Leach J (1993): Spinal fusion in Duchenne muscular dystrophy: fixation and fusion to the sacropelvis? *J Pediatr Orthop* 13:752–757.
35a. Murray DJ, Forbes RB (2001): Anesthetic considerations. In: Weinstein SL, ed. Pediatric spine surgery. Philadelphia: Lippincott Williams & Wilkins, pp. 3–32.
36. O'Brien TA, Harper PS (1984): Course, prognosis and complications of childhood-onset myotonic dystrophy. *Dev Med Child Neurol* 26: 62–67.
37. Oda T, Shimizu N, Yonenobu K, et al. (1993): Longitudinal study of spinal deformity in Duchenne muscular dystrophy. *J Pediatr Orthop* 13:478–488.
38. Rideau Y (1979): Profils evolutifs de la dystrophie musculaire de Duchenne en l'absence de traitement. *Union Med Can* 108:61.
39. Rideau Y, Janowski L, Grellet J (1981): Respiratory function in the muscular dystrophies. *Muscle Nerve* 4:155.
40. Shapiro F, Bresnan MJ (1982): Orthopedic management of childhood neuromuscular disease, III: diseases of the muscle. *J Bone Joint Surg Am* 64:1102–1107.
41. Siegel IM (1973): Scoliosis in muscular dystrophy: some comments about diagnosis, observations on prognosis, and suggestions for therapy. *Clin Orthop* 93:235–238.

42. Siegel IM (1977): Orthopedic correction of musculoskeletal deformity in muscular dystrophy. *Adv Neurol* 17:343–364.

43. Smith AD, Koreska P, Moseley CF (1989): Progression of scoliosis in Duchenne muscular dystrophy. *J Bone Joint Surg Am* 71A:1066–1074.

44. Stirpe NS, ed. (1992): *MDA reports.* Muscular Dystrophy Association, pp. 1–7.

45. Sussman MD (1984): Advantage of early spinal stabilization and fusion in patients with Duchenne muscular dystrophy. *J Pediatr Orthop* 4: 532–537.

46. Tawil R, Figlewicz DA, Griggs RC, et al. (1998): Facioscapulohumeral dystrophy: a distinct regional myopathy with a novel pathogenesis. *Ann Neurol* 43:279–282.

47. Van Essen AJ, Kneppers ALJ, van der Hout AH, et al. (1997): The clinical and molecular genetic approach to Duchenne and Becker muscular dystrophy: an updated protocol. *J Med Genet* 34:805–812.

48. Vignos P (1977): Respiratory function and pulmonary infection in Duchenne muscular dystrophy. *Isr J Med Sci* 13:207.

49. Walton JN, Nattrass FJ (1954): On the classification, natural history, and treatment of the myopathies. *Brain* 77:169–231.

50. Weber B, Smith J, Briscoe W, et al. (1975): Pulmonary function in asymptomatic adolescents with idiopathic scoliosis. *Am Rev Respir Dis* 111:389.

51. Weimann RL, Gibson DA, Moseley CF, et al. (1983): Surgical stabilization of the spine in Duchenne muscular dystrophy. *Spine* 8:776–780.

52. Weinstein S, Zavala D, Ponseti I (1981): Idiopathic scoliosis. Long-term follow-up and prognosis in untreated patients. *J Bone Joint Surg Am* 63:702–712.

53. Wilkins KE, Gibson DA (1976): The patterns of spinal deformity in Duchenne muscular dystrophy. *J Bone Joint Surg Am* 58:24–32.

54. Worton RG, Brooks MH (1995): The X-linked muscular dystrophies. In: Sciver CR, et al., eds. *The metabolic and molecular bases of inherited disease,* 7th ed. New York: McGraw-Hill, pp. 4195–4218.

48

SPINAL MUSCULAR ATROPHY

J. RICHARD BOWEN
GLENN E. LIPTON

Spinal muscular atrophy is a rare autosomal recessive disorder in which the anterior horn cells of the spinal cord and the neurons of the lower bulbar nuclei undergo degeneration. Clinically common to all variants of the disease is symmetric limb and trunk weakness and muscular atrophy that affects the lower extremities more than the upper extremities and the proximal muscles more than the distal muscles. Muscle fasciculation is common in the tongue and deltoid muscles, and trembling of the hands also occurs (20,49). Sensibility is not affected, and pyramidal long-tract signs are absent. Intelligence usually is normal (39). Scoliosis, contractures, and hip dislocation are the most common orthopaedic conditions associated with this disease.

EPIDEMIOLOGY

Spinal muscular atrophy is a common group of fatal recessive diseases and is one of the most frequently occurring neurodegenerative diseases (25,27,53). The incidence is 1 in 15,000 livebirths, and 1 in 40 to 80 persons is a carrier of a gene for spinal muscular atrophy (53). It was initially reported that women have less severe disease, and this has been refuted by other investigators. More recent studies, however, suggest that women do have a less severe disease course (20,38,50,53).

Scoliosis is the most common spinal deformity among patients with spinal muscular atrophy, yet the reported incidence varies. Benady (3) found that 31 of 54 (57%) patients with spinal muscular atrophy had scoliosis. In that report, however, only one of the patients who did not have scoliosis had reached skeletal maturity. The mean age of the skeletally immature patients without scoliosis was 6.3 years (3). Phillips et al. (57) reported that 34 of 57 (60%) patients had scoliosis diagnosed at an average age of 9 months and had an average follow-up period after diagnosis of 8.8 years. Schwentker and Gibson (66) studied the records of 50 patients with an average age of 11.5 years (range 2 to 29 years). They found 35 (70%) patients had

scoliosis. In a long-term study by Evans et al. (29), 45 of 49 patients had scoliosis. All four patients without scoliosis had better motor function than those with scoliosis. Russman et al. (63) found that 48 of 48 patients had scoliosis greater than 15 degrees; only 50% were observed for more than 10 years. In all these studies many of the patients were not observed to skeletal maturity or the usual maximum age for the onset of scoliosis. Most patients with spinal muscle atrophy who survive into adulthood eventually have scoliosis.

ETIOLOGY

Spinal muscular atrophy among children is an autosomal recessive disorder. Genetic mapping has shown that the chronic childhood onset of spinal muscular atrophy is linked to a region of chromosome 5 (ql2-ql4) and that the acute childhood onset form of the disease is linked to the same or lower region of the chromosome at the 5q position (8,43). Results of some studies suggest that different clinical presentations are allelic and caused by different mutations of the same gene (75,77). Other studies, however, have shown that this condition may be heterogeneous. They challenge the character of autosomal recessive inheritance, which does not explain atypical families and the male predominance without additional hypotheses, such as the Becker allelic model, incomplete penetrance of the gene, or X-linked inheritance (35,40,77,78). A group with autosomal dominant inheritance has been reported but is still under discussion (40,52,76).

Results of current studies suggest reduced levels or mutations in the survival of motor neurons protein has been implicated as the cause of the Werdnig-Hoffman form of the disease (spinal muscular atrophy type I). In 98% of the patients with the Werdnig-Hoffman form of the disease, the gene (5q13) for the survival of motor neurons protein was deleted or mutated. The gene product usually is present in nucleus and cytoplasm of cells from all tissues; especially high levels are present in motor neurons. In patients with the Werdnig-Hoffman form of the disease, the gene product has been found at barely detectable levels (12,43,44,56).

PATHOGENESIS

The pathogenesis of spinal muscular atrophy is largely unknown. Insidious glial proliferation in motor roots of the brain stem and

J.R. Bowen: Department of Orthopaedics, Alfred I. duPont Institute, Wilmington, Delaware 19899, and Department of Orthopaedic Surgery, Jefferson Medical College of Thomas Jefferson University, Philadelphia, Pennsylvania 19107–5083.
G.E. Lipton: Temple University School of Medicine, Philadelphia, Pennsylvania 19140.

spinal cord and deficiency of vitamin E in the plasma have been reported among infants with Werdnig-Hoffmann disease (11,67). The spinal deformity of spinal muscular atrophy develops because of muscle weakness. Severe and diffuse weakness frequently causes collapse of the spine and a progressive deformity that may involve the entire spine and pelvis. The deformity usually is progressive and is independent of the patient's remaining growth in that the curve may progress despite skeletal maturity. In a less severely compromised patient, the deformity can start in a limited area and involve only part of the spine. However, many of these patients eventually have more extensive and severe involvement of the spine. The presence of contractures in the pelvis and lower limbs, hip subluxation or dislocation, and the lack of equilibrium may contribute to progression of the spinal deformity. Shapiro and Bresnan (68) and Eng et al. (28) suggest that dislocation of the hip causes a pelvic tilt, which complicates the developing scoliosis.

PATHOLOGIC ANATOMY

In most cases of spinal muscular atrophy, the cranial nerves are involved. Cranial nerves V, VI, and VII may be affected without clinical manifestations. Cranial nerves IX, X, and XI may be affected with clear neuronal loss. Cranial nerve XII also may be affected. The range of degeneration of the lesions can include central chromatolysis, neuronophagia, nerve cell loss, and gliosis. The process is always symmetric. Reports have shown abnormalities of the cerebrum and cerebellum, marked hypoplasia, a decrease in the number of astrocytes and microglia in the cortex, and cell loss. The Betz cells at area 4 are normal (32).

Examination of the spinal cord shows anterior horn cell loss. The injury is found in the large anterior cells, markedly in the ventromedian group. Besides diminution in the number of cells, pyknotic and neuronophagia cells are found (71,72). Secondary changes occur in the roots and nerves with wallerian degeneration. Although clinical sensory involvement is not detected, microscopic studies developed by Carpenter et al. (10) and Marshall and Duchen (46) show alteration of the posterior columns. There is loss of myelin, especially at nerve fibers from the lumbar area, and involvement of sensory lumbar ganglia.

The muscles that usually are spared are the diaphragm, sternothyroid, sternohyoid, and the involuntary muscles of the intestine, bladder, heart, and sphincters (53). Microscopic examination shows normal groups of muscles mixed with groups showing denervation atrophy. The affected fibers are smaller in diameter, and there is more adipose and fibrous tissue between the fiber bundles than normal.

CLINICAL FEATURES

Spinal muscular atrophy is a spectrum of disorders. The characteristics common to all types of spinal muscular atrophy are symmetric muscular atrophy and weakness, predominance in the lower limbs, and greater involvement in the proximal muscles than in the distal. Fasciculation of the muscles, especially the tongue, and trembling of the hands are common. Most persons

with this disorder have no trembling during relaxation or sleep. Fatigue and stress may cause trembling to increase. Deep tendon reflexes usually are decreased or absent. Although both sensibility and intelligence are unaffected in most patients, the pyramidal long tract is not involved.

Because of the wide range of the clinical course, the most practical method for consideration of treatment is to divide patients into two groups: those with the acute infantile form (acute Werdnig-Hoffmann disease or spinal muscular atrophy type I) and those with the chronic childhood forms of disease. The chronic forms of disease are further divided into chronic Werdnig-Hoffmann disease (spinal muscular atrophy type II) and Kugelberg-Welander disease (mild spinal muscular atrophy type III).

Type I: Acute Infantile, Acute Werdnig-Hoffmann Disease

Patients come to medical attention with severe involvement of the disease. The onset is noticed within the first 2 months of life. Pearn (53) pointed out that 30% of cases have a prenatal onset. The mother often recalls lack of movement of the fetus, and after birth, the cry is of low volume and not sustained. The infant manifests severe, generalized weakness. This patient never walks, turns over, or sits alone, and there usually is lack of head control and bulbar paralysis. The only spontaneous movement of the extremities may be of the fingers and toes. Areflexia is universal. There is intercostal weakness with severe collapse of the ribs and a bell-shaped lower chest. Respiratory movements are paradoxic, and respiratory insufficiency can lead to pneumonia and atelectasis (26). Nasogastric tubes may be needed for feeding. Involvement of the cranial nerves is present but not easily detected clinically. Bland facial expressions and a striking facial resemblance are noticed because of facial weakness. Dysphagia, aphonia, and stridor also may be present (16,21,23,37,55).

Almost all patients have a spinal deformity, and many lie in a characteristic posture with the hips flexed, abducted, and externally rotated; the shoulder abducted and externally rotated; and the hands elevated to the level of the head. The knees and elbows are flexed, and the forearms are pronated. The posture is flaccid, and the child can be moved easily. With rare exception, these children do not survive beyond the age of 3 years. Therefore orthopaedic intervention is rarely warranted (22,73).

Some patients who appear to have the acute infantile of spinal muscular atrophy variety can have a more benign course. In such cases, the disease is not rapidly progressive, and the clinical behavior is similar to that of the chronic disease.

Type II: Chronic Childhood, Chronic Werdnig-Hoffmann Disease

In spinal muscular atrophy type II, chronic Werdnig-Hoffmann disease, the onset of symptoms occurs between 2 months and 2 years of age. These children have less disease involvement than do patients with spinal muscular atrophy type I; however, they are never able to walk independently. Weakness is not generalized at first. It starts in the legs more often than the arms, and the proximal muscles such as the gluteals and quadriceps are affected initially. Fine tremor in the hands and fasciculations of the tongue can occur but do so less frequently than in the acute form. Fasciculation of the eyelids also can occur (69). Chest collapse is uncommon, and respiratory impairment develops after a variable initial asymptomatic period (21,27,55).

Some patients can sit if placed in position, and some can walk. These patients have a waddling gait, lumbar lordosis, genu recurvatum, a protuberant abdomen, and scoliosis. Their walking becomes progressively impaired until they have to use a wheelchair full-time, usually by the second decade of life. Life expectancy also varies widely, ranging from 18 months to adulthood. Most patients live longer than 10 years and may live up to the fifth decade. The principal cause of death is pulmonary compromise (24).

Type III: Chronic Childhood, Kugelberg-Welander Disease

In spinal muscular atrophy type III, Kugelberg-Welander disease, the onset of symptoms occurs after 2 years of age but usually manifests itself before the age of 10 years. The patient has normal or slightly delayed motor milestones (42,74) and usually can walk, run, or climb stairs. These patients usually are able to walk independently until late childhood and sometimes into early adolescence. However, motor capability decreases. A positive Gower sign occurs in which the patient has difficulty in rising from the floor because of weakness in the pelvic girdle. There is atrophy in the lower limbs, and pseudohypertrophy of the calf develops because of sparing of the gastrocnemius muscle. Hypotonia is present, and the reflexes are hypoactive or absent. Muscles innervated by the cranial nerves usually are not affected. The capability to walk can be present for at least 8 years after the diagnosis is made and usually continues until the third decade. Life expectancy can reach the fifth decade.

FUNCTIONAL CLASSIFICATION

A functional classification relating progression of deformities to prognosis is based on the maximum physical function achieved by an individual patient (29,47,61,63,66). The classification divides the patients into the four following groups:

Group I: Patients never have the strength to sit independently, even when placed in optimal position. Head control is poor. They have early and progressive scoliosis.

Group II: Patients have head control and can sit but cannot stand or walk.

Group III: Patients can stand by themselves and have a limited walking ability.

Group IV: Patients can walk, run, or climb stairs. The mean age at diagnosis of scoliosis in this group is 8 years.

DIAGNOSIS

The diagnosis of spinal muscular atrophy is based on the clinical features and genetic evidence in the family. Diagnostic studies include electromyography, conduction velocity, muscle biopsy, and nerve biopsy.

The electromyographic signs of spinal muscular atrophy increase in frequency incidence and magnitude in relation to the duration of the disease. Fibrillation potentials associated with denervation are the best diagnostic sign. Regular spontaneous motor-unit activity occurs frequently and is specific for this disease. This occurs at all ages (9). Conduction velocity in motor fibers usually is normal with a slight decrease among severely affected children and a faster than expected velocity among less severely affected children (17,49,59). Findings of a muscle tremor defect may be present on an electrocardiogram (62).

Muscle biopsy should be performed on only moderately affected muscle. Compromised areas of musculotendinous junctions, scars or sites of recent trauma, injections, or electromyographic needle insertion must be avoided. The vastus lateralis portion of the quadriceps usually is the best muscle for biopsy. Open biopsy is preferable for correct quantity and orientation of muscle fibers. Local anesthesia should not penetrate the muscle, and atraumatic technique should be used. The specimen is maintained in the lengthened position for histologic tests and the contracted position for electron microscopic evaluation. Part of the specimen must be rapidly frozen to preserve the enzymes and prevent artifacts for histochemical evaluation (6). Histologic findings include loss and atrophy of fibers within normal groups of fiber bundles and no evidence of primary myopathy. Proliferation of perimysial connective tissue and groups of giant fibers (usually type 1) also are present. Among neonates, the only finding is perimysial fibrosis and nonspecific variation in muscle-fiber diameter. At a few months of age, the characteristic findings are present. The same pattern is maintained in adulthood, yet there is a progressive recent denervation and necrosis of fibers within the groups of hypertrophic fibers (48,64).

Differential diagnosis should include all conditions that characterize a floppy baby. Congenital myopathy manifesting as an autosomal dominant pattern should be considered. Dislocation of the hip and torticollis are common, and electromyographic studies show myopathic findings. Patients with infantile myasthenia gravis may recover within 12 weeks without relapse. Cerebral palsy can manifest as a stage of hypotonia and flaccid paralysis. Congenital muscular dystrophy is rare but has signs and symptoms similar to those of spinal muscular atrophy. Further, chronic disease should be differentiated from Duchenne muscular dystrophy.

SPINAL DEFORMITY

In the forms of spinal muscular atrophy in which survival into adolescence is anticipated, the occurrence of spinal deformity should be expected. Scoliosis occurs among almost 100% of the patients with type II spinal muscular atrophy and among most patients with type III spinal muscular atrophy (7,29,34,57, 61,66). Scoliosis is the most common and severe orthopaedic problem among children with spinal muscular atrophy and usually appears before 10 years of age. The deformity usually is a progressive *C*-shaped right-sided thoracolumbar paralytic curve. In almost all investigations, scoliosis is the principal spinal deformity, and its association with kyphosis is reported in about one third of cases (34,60). In addition several cases of a solitary kyphotic deformity have been reported. Some authors suggest the kyphosis appears earlier than the scoliosis, collapsing kyphosis occurring among patients younger than 3 years (60). The pulmonary function of patients with spinal muscle atrophy often decreases, and the decrease is attributed to the primary muscle weakness and the developing scoliosis and kyphosis. Some authors have reported pulmonary function less than 50% of normal among patients with moderate to severe scoliosis (26,61).

Factors Affecting Deformity

The age at onset and the severity of spinal deformity have been the subject of many studies, and there appears to be a relation between maximal motor function obtained and scoliosis. Russman et al. (63) found that the mean age at diagnosis of spinal deformity ranged from 6 years for patients with severe deformity to 18 years for patients who could run before the onset of the disease. Benady (3) reported that, the diagnosis of scoliosis was made after 1 year of age, most cases being diagnosed before the patients were 4 years of age. Other authors (2,13,60) have reported a mean age at diagnosis of 6 to 8 years, curve progression occurring in most patients. Kyphosis develops in 20% to 30% of the patients. In a study conducted at the Rizzoli Institute, all 13 patients with mild spinal muscular atrophy (type III) who had stopped walking had scoliosis that ranged from 30 degrees to 153 degrees (34).

The strongest factor related to the occurrence and severity of scoliosis seems to be the retained level of motor function (29,47,61,63,66). Factors related to the severity and progression of the disease, such as age at onset, type of spinal muscular atrophy, and presence of familial cases, also can be associated with spinal deformity. Controversy exists regarding the relation between motor development and age at onset and severity of the scoliosis. Aprin et al. (2) conducted a study with 22 patients who underwent spinal fusion. The investigators found no differences in the age at onset of scoliosis between the group of patients who could walk and the group who could not. In contrast, Schwentker and Gibson (66) found that seven of 15 patients able to walk had scoliosis and that only one patient had a curve greater than 60 degrees. Evans et al. (29) reported the existence of a direct relation between motor function development and age at onset and severity of the spinal deformity. Patients with more severe muscle weakness had a deformity as early as 2 years of age, whereas patients with less involvement had deformities at a mean age of 8.4 years (range 4 to 14 years). Only in the group who could walk or run were there patients with no spinal deformity. However, even in this group, seven of the 11 patients had spinal deformity. In the other three groups, spinal deformity developed in all patients. The results of these studies (29,34) show that patients who retain the ability to walk are unlikely to have early and severe scoliosis, whereas patients who have more severe involvement have early and more progressive scoliosis.

Radiographic Features

Even for patients who can stand, we suggest that radiographic studies be performed with the patient in the seated position.

This avoids compensation to keep the patient standing and eliminates the decrease in the real value of the deformity when the patient is supine. Posteroanterior and lateral radiographs should include the entire spine from the occiput to the pelvis. This allows analysis of pelvic obliquity and alignment of the head over the pelvis.

Type and Localization of Curves

The pattern of scoliosis is similar to that in most cases of neuromuscular scoliosis: a single, large, collapsing C-shaped curve involving the thoracolumbar spine. Usually at least six segments are involved and more frequently between eight and ten segments are involved. The area involved ranges from the low or midthoracic region to the low lumbar region and often produces pelvic obliquity.

Approximately 90% of patients have single curves, and more than 60% have thoracolumbar curves. Eighteen percent of curves are reported as thoracic curves, lumbar curves alone and double curves being less frequent (2,13,58,66). Single thoracic curves usually are right-sided. In the small number of patients who lose the ability to walk, double curves are common, usually with a right thoracic and left lumbar pattern. Among patients with severe asymmetric involvement, no relation between the direction of the convexity of the curve and the side of greater muscle weakness has been shown (66). The curve in patients with spinal muscular atrophy tends to remain more flexible than comparable idiopathic curves; however, rigidity and structural changes may eventually occur. As these curves progress, more segments become involved and pelvic obliquity occurs, the process being hastened among patients who do not walk.

Kyphosis of varying degrees of severity can be associated with the scoliosis. The kyphotic curve usually compromises the upper thoracic to lower lumbar area. In most instances the kyphotic component is not severe. However, in one study, among 18 patients observed without treatment, five had severe kyphosis associated with the scoliosis with four patients had a kyphotic deformity greater than 100 degrees (60).

TREATMENT

Orthotic Treatment

We believe orthotic treatment will not stop development or progression of the deformity but may lend support to the spines of select patients who need the support to perform activities of daily living. Careful attention must be paid to brace tolerance and respiratory function. If vital capacity decreases markedly or if the brace is poorly tolerated, orthotic treatment should be discontinued. Orthotic treatment may be prescribed with the objective of reducing the rate of progression of the spinal deformity or of helping to maintain the sitting posture. Among adult patients with severe deformity, orthotic treatment can be used to avoid painful impingement of the lower ribs on the iliac crest (29).

Studies have shown the use of a brace does not halt the progression or prevent the development of scoliosis among patients who used a brace before scoliosis developed (66). Most reports state that an orthosis can decrease the rate of progression of scoliosis. In the study of Aprin et al. (2), 15 patients received conservative treatment before spinal fusion. Most of the patients had the orthosis applied after the curve reached 40 degrees. Five patients had this treatment discontinued because respiratory difficulty was caused by the lateral pressure of the brace. The rate of progression in the other ten patients was not reported, except to state that the deformities soon progressed and necessitated spinal fusion. Shapiro and Bresnan (68) suggested a brace be prescribed when a curve reaches 15 or 20 degrees to minimize the rate of progression of the scoliosis. They reported the brace was uncomfortable for patients who walked because of the force of the brace against the patient's thighs and torso. Savini et al. (65) found that an orthosis had an effect in preventing scoliosis among patients who could stand or walk, but they did not mention the patients' comfort level. Riddick et al. (60) reported on 20 patients who received conservative treatment. Although half of the patients were observed 2 years or less, the data suggested the use of a brace was effective in slowing curve progression.

In one series (29), the success of orthotic treatment was related to physical function of the patient. Patients who could stand or walk benefited more from brace use. Patients with severe weakness tolerated the brace poorly, and it did not avoid progression of the deformity. Bracing was recommended for use in the care of young children when the deformity reached 20 degrees to decrease the rate of progression. This treatment allows delay of spinal fusion until the child is 10 years or older. Granata et al. (34) did not find braces useful in preventing progression of scoliosis, but the orthosis was believed to improve the functional performance of all children.

A review of the aforementioned studies reveals more opinions and impressions regarding orthotic treatment than it does conclusive data. The different forms of presentation and severity, the relatively small number of patients treated with braces, the absence of description of the course of disease and the characteristics of progression, and the lack of control groups in the studies make it difficult to assess the effectiveness of orthoses in the management of scoliosis in spinal muscular atrophy.

For young children with severe involvement and poor control of the neck, a sitting-support orthosis is used. A molded plastic posterior shell with control from the head to the pelvis is useful and can have a separate removable anterior shell or straps (17,19). The purpose is to support the spine to provide sitting ability. Walking may be promoted by early fitting of lower-limb orthoses (33).

For a child, a lightweight three-point pressure brace can be used. For most patients, the thoracolumbosacral orthosis (TLSO) is a good option. The Wilmington and Boston braces are recommended for their ease of application and light weight. The Milwaukee brace is not recommended because of its heaviness and poor tolerance by children with spinal muscular atrophy. The cervical ring of the Milwaukee brace causes problems for a child with poor neck control, and the chin pad may cause severe dental deformities (29). The Milwaukee brace also may decrease pulmonary function and respiratory difficulty owing to lateral pressure to the thoracic cage.

Orthotic management of scoliosis is indicated to help maintain posture or to slow curve progression among children younger than 9 years with a deformity between 20 and 40 degrees. If the deformity progresses to more than approximately 50 degrees, conservative treatment should be discontinued, and spinal fusion should be considered. Orthotic treatment may be attempted in the care of a child younger than 9 years with a curve greater than 40 degrees if the deformity remains flexible. If the curve becomes rigid or progresses 15 degrees or more, operative treatment should be considered.

Spinal Fusion

The indications for operative treatment are based on the following considerations: (a) in most cases spinal deformity develops and progresses independently of conservative treatment; (b) severe scoliosis causes poor sitting posture, which diminishes the patient's functional and pulmonary capacities; and (c) deterioration of pulmonary function proceeds with increasing curve magnitude and disease progression, which may lead to death. The goal of operative treatment is to have a normally positioned, fused spine over a level pelvis (36,66,68,70).

With these considerations, posterior spinal fusion should be performed before the deformity becomes severe and pulmonary function becomes compromised. At this stage, the operation should not require anterior release or traction. In addition, better correction may be achieved and less postoperative complications occur if the spine is fused before a large-magnitude curve develops that necessitates a more aggressive procedure. With severe deformity, the rate of complications increases with the severity of the curve. The goal of achieving a stabilized spine centered over the pelvis in a severe deformity must be assessed with consideration of the risks involved. Attention should be given to the increased muscular weakness, decreased vital capacity, and the need for anterior release (60).

Most authors recommend posterior spinal fusion at moderate deformity after 10 years of age. Some authors recommended operative intervention when the curve is between 40 and 60 degrees and anterior release if the curve is greater than 100 degrees (18,29,68). Others recommend earlier fusion for curves of approximately 35 degrees or greater (8,57). Still other authors suggest the operation not be performed on a routine basis or for preventive reasons but should be performed only after the development of a severe curve of approximately 85 degrees (47). In consideration of the risk versus the benefits, we recommend posterior spinal fusion for patients with moderate deformity of approximately 50 degrees. If possible, arthrodesis should be performed after the age of 10 years for the benefit of growth. Fusion should not be delayed if delay necessitates anterior release or will cause substantial increase in risk.

Patients scheduled for an operation benefit from a comprehensive evaluation by a pulmonologist, a neurologist, an anesthesiologist, and a physical therapist. Evaluation of pulmonary function a few weeks before the operation provides a useful and relatively simple baseline of preoperative condition. In a study conducted at the Alfred I. du Pont Institute involving patients who underwent posterior spinal fusion for neuromuscular scoliosis, it was found that patients with a vital capacity of 50% or less of predicted value were at risk of development of pulmonary edema or atelectasis. Patients with a vital capacity of more than

60% did not have pulmonary complications after the operation (51). Patients with a vital capacity of less than 25% are at severe risk of pulmonary complications and need extensive therapy (30).

The use of preoperative halo-dependent traction in an attempt to improve pulmonary function is controversial. Although it has some reported benefit, this treatment is not routine, and the limited effect on the pulmonary function should be counterbalanced with the inconvenience and complications for the patient, family, and medical team. In reviewing the records of our patients who underwent halo-dependent traction before surgery, we found a small increase in vital capacity (in most less than 10%). Although physical and respiratory therapy techniques have improved in the last few years, no reports have shown data about improvement in the preoperative pulmonary condition.

Spinal Instrumentation

In spinal muscular atrophy, as in the many other forms of neuromuscular scoliosis, the function of instrumentation is to produce safe correction of the deformity, allow fixation from the upper thoracic spine to the pelvis, and provide rigid fixation that eliminates the need for postoperative casting or traction.

Use of the Harrington system to manage scoliosis in spinal muscular atrophy has been reported (2,5,41,53,66). This system has an increased risk of failure, because it fixes the spine at only two points and fails to restore normal alignment of the spine in the sagittal plane. In addition, cast immobilization is needed after the operation. This is detrimental to children with spinal muscular atrophy. There is greater loss of correction with the use of the Harrington system of fixation (7,13).

Segmental fixation with Luque rods or a Unit Rod is the current standard in the management of neuromuscular scoliosis (Fig. 1). These systems provide good rigid fixation and usually do not necessitate postoperative external immobilization. Correction of pelvic obliquity and decompensation of the torso are controlled through the intrailiac fixation (1,15). This is important because pelvic obliquity places excessive force on a single ischium, and the ability to sit for long periods becomes limited. Physiologic realignment in the sagittal plane is another advantage provided by these systems. When a single Unit Rod (Fig. 1) cannot be used, a connection link between rods, such as the device for transverse traction or the Texas Scottish Rite Hospital cross-link, provides better rigidity in the Luque system. No major neurologic deficits have been related to the correction or to the use of sublaminar wires. However, high blood loss often occurs (5,15).

We recommend spinal fusion from T1 or T2 to the sacrum using a Unit Rod for fixation of the spine. The Unit Rod provides the best correction, stability, and sitting balance with fusion to the pelvis. In addition postsurgical care is easier, and no immobilization is needed. This facilitates early and complete physical therapy. Luque rods may be used in place of a Unit Rod, but the two Luque rods should be connected as previously mentioned to provide better stability and decrease the likelihood of occurrence of the "windshield wiper" effect (Fig. 2).

Anterior Spinal Fusion

The usual indication for an anterior procedure to manage neuromuscular scoliosis is a severe and rigid curve with a pelvis that cannot be leveled or a torso that cannot be placed in balance over the pelvis with external maneuvers (5,15). In the care of children with spinal muscular atrophy, other factors should be considered. Because of weakness of the muscles in the neck and thorax, these children are more dependent on the diaphragm and abdominal muscles for breathing. An anterior approach and fusion, especially through a thoracoabdominal approach, decreases the respiratory and coughing capacities of these patients and increases the risk of pulmonary complications. At our institution, such complications occurred among five of six patients who underwent anterior spinal fusion. Three patients needed endotracheal intubation and ventilatory assistance for an average of 5 days. Other reports have shown similar data. Patients who need an anterior procedure have more severe imbalance and more pulmonary constriction preoperatively, which makes them more likely to have complications. Anterior release combined with posterior fusion and instrumentation may be performed only if there is a severe fixed lumbar curve with pelvic obliquity. The disadvantage of restricting pulmonary function among these patients should be carefully considered in decision making.

Bone Grafting

The generous use of crushed allograft, approximately 100 to 120 g, is recommended in the treatment of patients with spinal muscular atrophy undergoing spinal fusion. Autograft of iliac bone is not recommended to not disturb or weaken the site of intrailiac fixation. The iliac wing often is osteopenic and provides an inadequate quantity of graft.

Postoperative Care and Results

With arthrodesis from T1 or T2 to the sacrum and the use of segmental fixation with allograft bone, postoperative immobilization usually is not necessary. A TLSO can be applied for comfort.

The most important postoperative concern is respiratory care. Coughing capacity decreases after the operative procedure, especially after an anterior procedure with involvement of the diaphragm. This, along with restriction of the patient's mobility, increases the incidence of pneumonitis and atelectasis. Patients with severe involvement (vital capacity 30% or less) may need endotracheal intubation and ventilatory assistance for several days after the operation. Pulmonary therapy with respiratory and postural exercises and mobilization of the patient are fundamental to minimize respiratory complications (14). In extreme conditions, tracheostomy can be performed to maintain respiratory support for a longer time.

No significant functional gain should be expected after spinal fusion. One team of investigators (2) found no difference in the ability to perform tasks of daily hygiene and self-feeding. Eighty-six percent of the patients were happy with the results, although only three patients had improvement in the performance of daily activities. The main reason for increased patient satisfaction was

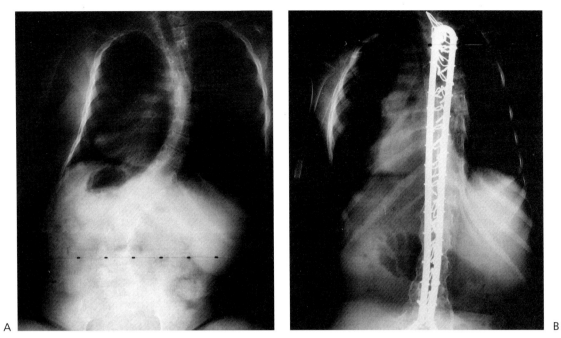

FIGURE 1. **A:** Patient with spinal muscle atrophy had 78-degree neuromuscular scoliosis that was fused and instrumented with a Unit Rod. **B:** Two and one-half years after the operation the correction is maintained at 22 degrees with good balance.

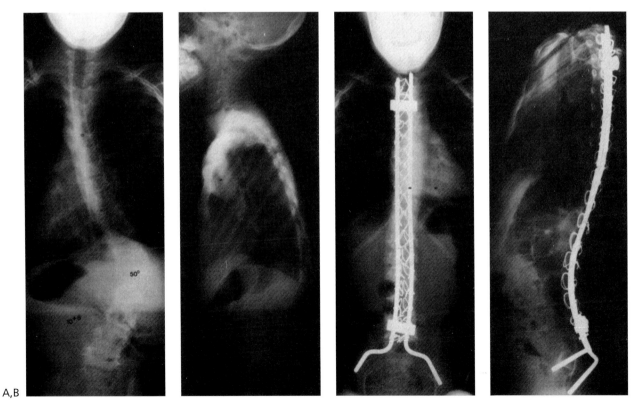

FIGURE 2. A boy 10 years 6 months with spinal muscular atrophy and progressive scoliosis measuring 50 degrees was treated surgically. **A:** Sitting anteroposterior preoperative radiograph. **B:** Sitting lateral preoperative radiograph. **C:** Sitting anteroposterior radiograph 10 months after insertion of Luque rod from T1 to the sacrum by means of the Luque-Galveston technique. **D:** Sitting lateral radiograph 10 months after the operation. (Courtesy of Stuart L. Weinstein, M.D.)

that patients no longer needed to use their arms to support their trunks and could therefore sit better. Other investigators have reported improvement in function after spinal arthrodesis (41,58,60). In contrast are reports (7,31) of a decline in motor activity, including bathing, toileting, transferring, feeding, and self-feeding, after the operation. Additional mobile arm supports, lapboards, and reachers were necessary after the operation. The upper-extremity activities of these patients had declined at the 2-year follow-up evaluation but had improved slightly 5 years after the operation. However, the patients never reached preoperative levels of function. Physical therapy should begin as soon as possible after the operation to maintain the maximum amount of motor function possible (28).

The fusion mass should be evaluated with periodic postoperative radiographs. If back pain develops several months after the operation, loss of internal fixation occurs, or the the deformity progresses, investigation with radiographs and bone scintigraphy should be performed to localize a possible pseudarthrosis.

Postoperative Complications

Complications occur among approximately 40% of patients who undergo surgery, especially older patients and those with severe curves (57). Respiratory insufficiency and atelectasis are the most common postoperative complications. Patients with severe complications may need endotracheal intubation and ventilatory support for several days or, in rare cases, a tracheostomy if the respiratory insufficiency is prolonged. Brown et al. (7) reported that tracheostomy was needed by 30% of their patients. The need for tracheostomy has been related to use of the anterior approach (2). Patients with a preoperative vital capacity less than 50% are at risk of pulmonary complications, but patients with vital capacities as low as 25% of normal can tolerate the procedure (58). Postoperative pneumonia, rupture of the diaphragm with severe loss of pulmonary function, pulmonary embolism, and acute gastric volvulus and late narrowing of the diameter of the chest have been reported after spinal arthrodesis and instrumentation (2,45,58,60).

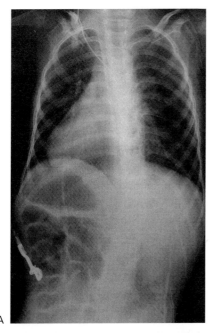
A

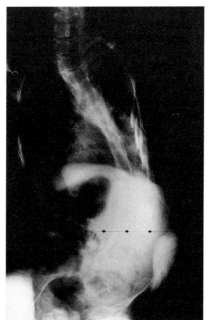
C

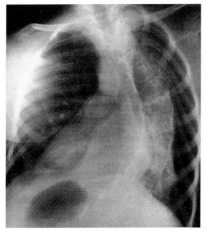
B

FIGURE 3. A: A patient with spinal muscle atrophy had a preoperative deformity of 64 degrees. The curve was initially instrumented with a Unit Rod. During the operation, the sublaminar wires pulled through the lamina, necessitating removal of the rod for loss of fixation. The patient underwent fusion in situ with 6 months of immobilization. **B:** Pseudarthrosis developed, and an operation was performed to repair the pseudarthrosis and to bone graft the nonfused mass. **C:** Postoperative radiograph shows a poor result due to uncontrolled crankshaft deformity.

Complications with the use of spinal instrumentation have been reported. Luque instrumentation for neuromuscular scoliosis has been associated with an index of complications as high as 15% (4). Complications of spinal fusion among patients with spinal muscle atrophy include rod breakage, pull-out of the sublaminar wires, dislocation of the sacral hooks, and painful prominence of the Luque rod (Fig. 3) (2,57,60). Manifestations of pseudarthrosis are pain, progression of the deformity, and breakage of the instruments, although results of some studies suggest that pseudoarthrosis can be asymptomatic (29). The reported incidence of pseudarthrosis after spinal fusion for all kinds of neuromuscular scoliosis ranges from 6.5% to 27% (4,5,60).

Other complications include wound infection and postoperative urinary tract infection (58). Weakness of the neck muscles associated with traction or cast immobilization also occurs. Support with a soft collar and neck-muscle exercises gradually improve the strength of the neck muscles. Narrowing of the chest diameter as a major late complication has been attributed to postoperative cast immobilization (2).

Regression of the functional status of the patient can be considered a complication of operative treatment. This complication may be associated with the use of postoperative traction or a cast. Another cause of regression of the functional status of the patient may be neurologic complications. In the study by Boachie-Adjei et al. (4), this complication was verified for 6.5% of patients with all forms of neuromuscular scoliosis who underwent Luque instrumentation. No studies involving patients with spinal muscular atrophy have addressed this issue. It is important to observe for manifestations that can be caused by neurologic complications after spinal fusion. These include such as paresthesia, progressive weakness, deterioration of pulmonary function, and autonomous dysreflexia.

SUMMARY

Posterior spinal arthrodesis of T1 or T2 to the sacrum is indicated in the care of patients with spinal muscular atrophy with a curve greater than approximately 50 degrees, regardless of age. At this stage, the deformity usually is quite flexible, and pulmonary function is relatively preserved. Therefore, excellent correction and results are expected with a low incidence of complications. For patients with a more severe curve, posterior fusion is still the best option until the curve reaches approximately 80 degrees. For curves greater than 80 degrees, careful evaluation is performed to determine the most appropriate treatment. If the curve is flexible and can be corrected to give relatively good balance with the spine over a level pelvis and a pelvic obliquity of 25 degrees or less, posterior fusion with a Unit Rod is the procedure of choice. Combined procedures with both anterior and posterior fusion are indicated for severe cases of spinal muscular dystrophy with a rigid curve in which a balanced spine is not possible or when the torso cannot be placed over the pelvis. Total correction of pelvic obliquity is not always necessary; however, some correction is preferred.

In the care of patients who are candidates for spinal fusion, pulmonary function is the principal issue. Vital capacity is a guideline for the preoperative condition. If vital capacity is greater than 25%, the planned operation may proceed. However, respiratory therapy rehabilitation should be performed to minimize the risk of pulmonary complications. The therapy should include passive and assisted cough techniques, breathing exercises, postural drainage, and vibration. Patients should be taught to perform breathing exercises that maintain chest-cage expansion and ventilatory capacity, but excessive exercise that causes fatigue should be avoided (28,30).

Posterior spinal fusion with segmental spinal instrumentation should include the entire spine from T1 to the sacrum. The Luque rod or Unit Rod technique is suggested. We believe the Unit Rod system yields superior correction and maintenance of the correction. Blood loss usually is substantial, even when the operation is performed by an experienced surgeon. Most patients have a blood loss of 1,000 mL or more. Respiratory and positional exercises are started immediately after the operation.

REFERENCES

1. Allen BL, Ferguson RL (1982): The Galveston technique for L-rod instrumentation of the scoliotic spine. *Spine* 7:276–284.
2. Aprin H, Bowen JR, MacEwen GD, et al. (1982): Spine fusion in patients with spinal muscular atrophy. *J Bone Joint Surg Am* 64: 1179–1187.
3. Benady SG (1978): Spinal muscular atrophy in childhood: review of 50 cases. *Dev Med Child Neurol* 20:746–757.
4. Boachie-Adjei O, Lonstein JE, Winter RB, et al. (1989): Management of neuromuscular spinal deformities with Luque segmental instrumentation. *J Bone Joint Surg Am* 71:548–562.
5. Bonnett C, Brown JC, Perry J, et al. (1975): Evaluation of treatment of paralytic scoliosis at Ranchos Los Amigos Hospital. *J Bone Joint Surg Am* 57:206–215.
6. Bowen JR, MacEwen GD (1992): Muscle and nerve disorders. In: Chapman MW, ed. *Operative orthopaedics*, 2nd ed. Philadelphia: JB Lippincott, 3277–3313.
7. Brown JC, Zeller JL, Swank SM, et al. (1989): Surgical and functional results of spine fusion in spinal muscular atrophy. *Spine* 14:763–770.
8. Brzustowicz LM, Lehner T, Castilla LH, et al. (1990): Genetic mapping of chronic childhood onset spinal muscular atrophy to chromosome 5q11.2–13.3. *Nature* 344:540–541.
9. Buchthal F, Olsen PZ (1970): Electromyography and muscle biopsy in infantile spinal muscular atrophy. *Brain* 93:15–30.
10. Carpenter S, Karpati G, Rothman S, et al. (1978): Pathological involvement of primary sensory neurons in Werdnig-Hoffmann disease. *Acta Neuropathol* 42:91–97.
11. Chou SM, Nomaka J (1978): Werdnig-Hoffmann disease: proposal of a pathogenetic mechanism. *Acta Neuropathol (Berl)* 41:45–54.
12. Coovert D, Le TT, McAndrew PE, Strasswimmer J, et al. (1997): The survival motor neuron protein in spinal muscular atrophy. *Hum Mol Genet* 6:1205–1214.
13. Daher YH, Lonstein JE, Winter RB, et al. (1985): Spinal surgery in spinal muscular atrophy. *J Pediatr Orthop* 5:391–395.
14. Delmas MC, Berard C (1990): Global management of infantile spinal muscular atrophy: practical guide for medical staff. *Pediatrie* 45: 457–464.
15. Dias RC, Miller F, Dabney KW, et al. (1996): Surgical correction of spinal deformity using a unit rod in children with cerebral palsy. *J Pediatr Orthop* 16:734–740.
16. Dorr JR, Brown JC, Perry J (1973): Results of posterior fusion in patients with spinal muscular atrophy: a review of 25 cases. *J Bone Joint Surg Am* 55:436–437.
17. Drennan JC (1978): Skeletal deformities in spinal muscular atrophy. *Clin Orthop* 133(Abst):266–267.
18. Drennan JC (1983): *Orthopaedic management of neuromuscular disorders.* Philadelphia: JB Lippincott, pp. 137–154.
19. Drennan JC, Renshaw TS, Curtis BH (1979): The thoracic suspension orthosis. *Clin Orthop* 139:33–39.

20. Dubowitz V (1964): Infantile muscular atrophy: a prospective study with particular reference to a slowly progressive variety. *Brain* 87:707–718.

21. Dubowitz V (1969): *The floppy infant.* London: William Heineman.

22. Dubowitz V (1974): Benign infantile spinal muscular atrophy. *Dev Med Child Neurol* 16:672–675.

23. Dubowitz V (1978): *Muscle disorders in childhood.* Philadelphia: WB Saunders, pp. 146–178.

24. Duval-Beaupere G, Barois A, Quinet I, et al. (1985): Respiratory, spinal and thoracic problems in children with prolonged spinal muscular atrophy. *Arch Fr Pediatr* 42:625.

25. Dyken P, Krawiecki N (1983): Neurodegenerative diseases of infancy and childhood. *Ann Neurol* 13:351–364.

26. Echenne B, Georgesco M, Dapres G (1984): Motor nerve conduction velocities in spinal muscular atrophy: diagnosis problems. *Rev Electroencephalogr Neurophysiol Clin* 13:329–335.

27. Emery AEH, Hausmanowa-Petrusewicz I, Davie AM, et al. (1976): International collaborative study of the spinal muscular atrophies, 1: analysis of clinical and laboratory data. *J Neurol Sci* 29:83–94.

28. Eng GD, Binder H, Koch B (1984): Spinal muscular atrophy: experience in diagnosis and rehabilitation management of 60 patients. *Arch Phys Med Rehabil* 65:549–553.

29. Evans GA, Drennan JC, Russman BS (1981): Functional classification and orthopaedic management of spinal muscular atrophy. *J Bone Joint Surg Br* 63:516–522.

30. Frownfelter DL (1987): *Chest physical therapy and pulmonary rehabilitation. An interdisciplinary approach,* 2nd ed. Chicago: Year Book.

31. Furumasu J, Swank SM, Brown JC, et al. (1989): Functional activities in spinal muscular atrophy patients after spinal fusion. *Spine* 14:771–775.

32. Goutieres F, Aicardi J, Farkas EV (1977): Anterior horn cell disease associated with ponte cerebellar hypoplasia in infants. *J Neurol Neurosurg Psychiatry* 40:370–378.

33. Granata C, Cornelio F, Bonfiglioli S, et al. (1987): Promotion of ambulation of patients with spinal muscular atrophy by early fitting of knee-ankle-foot orthoses. *Dev Med Child Neurol* 29:221–224.

34. Granata C, Merlini L, Magni E, et al. (1989): Spinal muscular atrophy: natural history and orthopaedic treatment of scoliosis. *Spine* 14:760–762.

35. Greenberg F, Feuolia KR, Hetmancik JF, et al. (1988): X-linked infantile spinal muscular atrophy. *Am J Dis Child* 142:217.

36. Gui L, Savini R, Merlini L, et al. (1984): Il trattamento chirurgico delia scoliosi nella atrofia muscolare spinale: primi risultati. *Arch Ortop Reum* 97:21.

37. Hausmanova-Petrusewicz I (1978): *Spinal muscular atrophy: infantile or juvenile type.* Warsaw: National Center for Scientific, Technical and Economic Information, p. III.

38. Hausmanowa-Petrusewicz I, Borkowska J, et al. (1982): Juvenile motor neuron diseases: the sex influence in benign juvenile pseudodystrophic spinal muscular atrophy. *Adv Neurol* 36:131.

39. Hausmanowa-Petrusewicz I, Zaremba J, Borkowska J, et al. (1984): Chronic proximal spinal muscular atrophy of childhood and adolescence: sex influence. *J Med Genet* 21:447.

40. Hausmanowa-Petrusewicz I, Zaremba J, Borkowska J (1985): Chronic proximal spinal muscular atrophy of childhood and adolescence: problems of classification and genetic counselling. *J Med Genet* 22:350–353.

41. Hensinger RN, MacEwen GD (1976): Spinal deformity associated with heritable neurological conditions: spinal muscular atrophy, Friedreich's ataxia, familial dysautonomia, and Charcot-Marie-Tooth disease. *J Bone Joint Surg Am* 58:13–23.

42. Kugelberg E, Welander L (1956): Heredofamilial juvenile muscular atrophy simulating muscular dystrophy. *Arch Neurol Psychiatry* 75:500.

43. Lefebvre S, Burglen L, Reboullet S, et al. (1995): Identification and characterization of a spinal muscular atrophy–determining gene. *Cell* 80:155–165.

44. Lefebvre S, Burlet P, Liu Q, et al. (1997): Correlation between severity and SMN protein level in spinal muscular atrophy. *Nature Genet* 16:265–269.

45. Linson M, Bresnan M, Eraklis A, et al. (1981): Acute gastric volvulus following Harrington rod instrumentation in a patient with Werdnig-Hoffmann disease. *Spine* 6:522–523.

46. Marshall A, Duchen LW (1975): Sensory system involvement in infantile spinal muscular atrophy. *J Neurol Sci* 26:349.

47. Merlini L, Granata C, Bonfiglioli S, et al. (1989): Scoliosis in spinal muscular atrophy: natural history and management. *Dev Med Child Neurol* 31:501–508.

48. Mike T, Tamari H, Ohtani Y, et al. (1983): A fluorescent microscopy study of biopsied muscles from infantile neuromuscular disorders. *Acta Neuropathol* 59:48.

49. Moosa A, Dubowitz V (1973): Spinal muscular atrophy in childhood: two clues to clinical diagnosis. *Arch Dis Child* 48.386–388.

50. Munsat TL, Woods R, Fowler W, et al. (1969): Neurogenic muscular atrophy of infancy with prolonged survival: the variable course of Werdnig-Hoffmann disease. *Brain* 92:9–24.

51. Padman R, McNamara R (1990): Postoperative pulmonary complications in children with neuromuscular scoliosis who underwent posterior spinal fusion. *Del Med J* 62:999–1003.

52. Peam J (1978): Autosomal dominant spinal muscular atrophy: a clinical and genetic study. *J Neurol Sci* 38:263–275.

53. Peam J (1980): Classification of spinal muscular atrophies. *Lancet* 1:919–922.

54. Peam JH, Gardner-Medwin D, Wilson J (1978): A clinical study of chronic childhood spinal muscular atrophy: a review of 141 cases. *J Neurol Sci* 38:23–37.

55. Peam JH, Hudgson P, Walton JN (1978): A clinical and genetic study of spinal muscular atrophy of adult onset. *Brain* 101:591.

56. Pellizzoni L, Kataoka N, Charroux B, et al. (1998): A novel function for smn, the spinal muscular atrophy disease gene product, in pre-mRNA splicing. *Cell* 95:615–624.

57. Phillips DP, Roye DP Jr, Farcy JPC, et al. (1990): Surgical treatment of scoliosis in a spinal muscular atrophy population. *Spine* 9:942–945.

58. Piasecki JO, Mahinpour S, Levine DB (1986): Long-term followup of spinal fusion in spinal muscular atrophy. *Clin Orthop* 207:44–54.

59. Renault F, Raimbault J, Praud JP, et al. (1983): Etude electromyographique de 50 cas de maladie de Werdnig-Hoffmann. *Rev Electroencephalogr Neurophysiol Clin* 13:301–305.

60. Riddick MF, Winter RB, Lutter LD (1982): Spinal deformities in patients with spinal muscle atrophy: A review of 36 patients. *Spine* 7:476–483.

61. Rodillo E, Marini ML, Heckmatt JZ, et al. (1989): Scoliosis in spinal muscular atrophy: review of 63 cases. *J Child Neurol* 4:118–123.

62. Russman BS, Fredericks EJ (1979): Use of the ECG in the diagnosis of childhood spinal muscular atrophy. *Arch Neurol* 36:317–318.

63. Russman BS, Melchreit R, Drennan JC (1983): Spinal muscular atrophy: The natural course of disease. *Muscle Nerve* 6:179–181.

64. Sarnat HB (1983): *Muscle pathology and histochemistry.* Chicago: American Society of Clinical Pathologists Press.

65. Savini R, Cervellati S, Granata C, et al. (1980): La scoliosi nelle atrofie muscolari prossimaii infantile. In: Grupo Italiano di Studio della Scoliosi, ed. *Progressi in patologia vertebrate.* Bologna: Editore Aulo Gaggi.

66. Schwentker EP, Gibson DA (1976): The orthopaedic aspects of spinal muscular atrophy. *J Bone Joint Surg Am* 58:32–38.

67. Shapira Y, Amit R, Rachmilewitz E (1981): Vitamin E deficiency in Werdnig-Hoffmann disease. *Ann Neurol* 10:266–268.

68. Shapiro F, Bresnan MJ (1982): Orthopaedic management of childhood neuromuscular disease, 1: spinal muscular atrophy. *J Bone Joint Surg Am* 64:785–789.

69. Skouteli H, Dubowitz V (1984): Fasciculation of the eyelids: an additional clue to clinical diagnosis in spinal muscular atrophy. *Neuropediatrics* 15:145.

70. Taddonio RF (1982): Segmental spinal instrumentation in the management of neuromuscular spinal deformity. *Spine* 7:305–311.

71. Thieffry S, Arthus M, Bargeton E (1955): Quarante cas de maladie de Werdnig-Hoffman avec onje examens anatomiques. *Rev Neurol* 93:621–644.

72. Towfighi J, Young RSK, Ward RM (1985): Is Werdnig-Hoffmann disease a pure lower motor neuron disorder? *Acta Neuropathol* 65:270.

73. Van Wijngaarden GK, Bethlem J (1973): Benign infantile spinal muscular atrophy: a prospective study. *Brain* 96:163–170.

74. Welander L (1951): Myopathia distalis tarda hereditaria. *Acta Med Scand (Suppl)* 265:1.

75. Winson EJ, Murphy EG, Thompson MW, et al. (1971): Genetics of childhood spinal muscular atrophy. *J Med Genet* 8:143.

76. Zellweger H, Simpson J, McCormick WF, et al. (1972): Spinal muscular atrophy with autosomal dominant inheritance. *Neurology* 22: 957.

77. Zerres K, Rudnik-Schoneborn S, Rietschel M (1990): Heterogeneity in proximal spinal muscular atrophy. *Lancet* 336:749–750.

78. Zerres K, Stephen M, Kehreu U (1987): Becker's alielic model to explain unusual pedigrees with spinal muscular atrophy. *Clin Genet* 31: 276.

MYELOMENINGOCELE SPINE

RICHARD E. LINDSETH

Spinal deformity is so common in myelomeningocele that it should be considered part of the disease complex. It is rare for a child with myelomeningocele to reach adulthood without undergoing some treatment of the spine (30). The spinal deformities are usually progressive and may cause severe disability, interfere with rehabilitation, and negate previous treatment to maintain ambulation. They may also resemble other, more common congenital and developmental spinal deformities, with angulation and displacement of the vertebral column in the sagittal, coronal, and transverse planes. However, spinal deformities in myelomeningocele exhibit unique characteristics that must be considered during treatment if the results are to be satisfactory.

The most obvious and consistent abnormality that sets myelomeningocele spinal deformity apart from other spinal deformities is the incomplete posterior arch in the lumbar spine. This abnormality affects many aspects of treatment for scoliosis and kyphosis. Other congenital malformations may also be present (5). Hemivertebrae, diastematomyelia, or unsegmented bars may occur at any level along the spine. Unsegmented bars are particularly difficult to identify and evaluate if they occur in the area of the spina bifida where the facet joints, laminae, and spinous processes are difficult to identify on standard radiographs.

Another consistent problem is the abnormal nervous system. In addition to paralysis, which may be asymmetric, the central nervous system may show abnormalities of the upper spinal cord and brain stem, producing spasticity or increased muscle tone. The central nervous system abnormalities are often the cause of the scoliosis and must be dealt with before or at least concurrent with any orthopaedic treatment of the scoliosis (6,16,17).

The spinal curvature often appears at a younger age than is typical for most developmental abnormalities. It may be present by 2 to 3 years of age, becoming severe by 7 years of age. Because of the early onset of the deformity, treatment plans need to anticipate growth of the spine. However, the projections for growth in children with myelomeningocele are different from those for children with normal growth potential. Children with myelomeningocele have slow growth because of growth hormone deficiency, and they mature earlier than usual, often by 9 to 10 years of age in girls and 11 to 12 years of age in boys.

Another factor that needs to be considered in the surgical

treatment of these patients is the high infection rate (9,23,41,48). These patients are subject to septicemia from urinary tract infections and skin ulcerations. Also, the skin in the area of the meningocele repair is often of poor quality and gives minimal coverage to the instrumentation.

These children also have deformities of the pelvis and hips that affect spine balance. For example, asymmetric hip contractures may cause lumbar scoliosis, pelvic obliquity, and abnormal lordosis in the standing or sitting position. Likewise, correction of the spine in the treatment of scoliosis can position the legs in such a way as to prevent functional sitting, standing, or walking.

As with all children with spinal deformities, the goals of treatment are the prevention of further deformity and the creation of a stable, balanced spine. Children with myelomeningocele, however, require more precise correction of their deformities; because of their paralysis, they are unable to compensate for any residual deformity, which may prevent them from sitting or from standing and walking. Pressure sores are likely to develop if pelvic obliquity remains, and their sagittal plane alignment must allow them to perform intermittent self-catheterization.

Three types of spinal deformity occur with myelomeningocele: scoliosis, usually associated with severe lordosis; congenital malformation of the spine secondary to lack of segmentation or formation; and kyphosis, which is usually congenital in nature and centered in the upper lumbar spine. The sagittal plane deformities are often of greater significance than the coronal plane deformities.

SCOLIOSIS AND LORDOSIS

Scoliosis is common, particularly in the higher levels of paraplegia (3,13,24). Almost 100% of patients with thoracic-level paraplegia develop scoliosis (37), and 85% of these curves are greater than 45 degrees. As the paralysis level lowers, so does the incidence of scoliosis. At the fourth lumbar level of paraplegia, the incidence of curvature decreases to about 60%, with only 40% requiring surgical intervention (37). Lordosis without concurrent scoliosis is rare and is usually caused by hip flexion contractures. Historically, it has been seen after spinal-peritoneal shunting for hydrocephalus. However, this procedure is rarely performed today.

Several causes have been identified for the scoliosis. A *C-*

R. E. Lindseth: School of Medicine, Indiana University, Indianapolis, Indiana 46202.

shaped scoliosis is usually caused by muscle weakness associated with high-level paraplegia. It may also be associated with asymmetric levels of paralysis or a spastic hemiplegia due to the hydrocephalus. This type of scoliosis may be associated with kyphosis rather than lordosis. Typically, this curve pattern occurs at a young age, often in infancy, and it is almost always progressive.

Hydromyelia or hydrosyringomyelia associated with uncompensated hydrocephalus can cause scoliosis (15–17,25). The scoliosis is usually in the thoracic or the thoracolumbar region. It is typically *S* shaped and resembles idiopathic scoliosis. Because of stiffness in the area of the myelomeningocele in the lumbar spine, the compensation for the major curve may be incomplete and associated with pelvic obliquity. Scoliosis may be the only clinical sign of shunt malfunction or progressive hydromyelia and may occur at any age, even early in childhood. Headache, nausea, vomiting, and vision changes—the usual signs of hydrocephalus—may be absent. Other symptoms of hydromyelia are back pain, weakness of the upper extremities, and increasing paralysis of the legs (25). It has been shown that reinserting a functional shunt may decrease the scoliosis if it is less than 50 degrees (17).

Another cause of scoliosis is the tethered cord syndrome (6,12,45). This abnormality is caused by attachment of the spinal cord to the area of the myelomeningocele, preventing its upward migration with growth. This syndrome may be associated with other intraspinal pathology such as dermoid tumors, lipomas, or diastematomyelia. In my experience, the tethered cord usually causes a dorsolumbar or lumbar scoliosis with a marked increase in lumbar lordosis. Other associated symptoms are increased spasticity in the legs, increasing level of paralysis, and back or leg pain. Results of releasing the tethered cord are variable, but in 75% of cases, curve progression stopped or improved 10 degrees at 1 year (45). If the curve is more than 50 degrees, the scoliosis should be corrected and stabilized with spinal fusion at the time of the tethered cord release or shortly thereafter.

Spasticity is another cause of scoliosis that interferes with attempts at nonoperative and operative treatment. If the spasticity is not caused by hydromyelia or a tethered cord, intraspinal rhizotomy and cordectomy may be necessary (35).

Congenital malformations, including the lack of formation and the lack of segmentation (5,51), may exist in combination with hydromyelia, tethered cord, or muscle paralysis. When evaluating a child with scoliosis, the physician must consider each component of the scoliosis in the treatment program. It may be necessary to reinsert the shunt, detether the spinal cord, and treat the congenital scoliosis, if all are present.

Diagnostic Studies

The spine should be evaluated by physical examination each time the patient is seen—from newborn to adult. Note should be made of the coronal and sagittal plane alignment. The examination should be carried out with the child seated without support of the arms. Because of weakness of the legs, standing without the use of arm support is difficult and gives inaccurate results. This eliminates the problems related to hip flexion contracture and asymmetric abduction and adduction. In the coronal plane,

balance is the most important consideration. The occiput should lie over the midsacrum, and the pelvis should be level (41). In the sagittal alignment, particular attention should be paid to increased lumbar lordosis and to the appearance of kyphosis at the thoracolumbar junction. In an ambulatory child, any changes in the lumbar lordosis between sitting and standing should be noted.

Hip range of motion should be carefully documented. Particular note should be made of hip flexion contractures and of asymmetry between abduction and adduction.

A thorough neurologic examination of muscle strength, levels of sensation, and reflex activity of the upper and lower extremities should be carefully documented. If scoliosis is developing, the documented changes in neurologic function are of major diagnostic importance regarding the etiology of the scoliosis.

An assessment of the overall growth of the child should be made. If the child is dropping below the fifth percentile in length, the child is probably suffering from growth hormone deficiency. Note should be made of this for future assessment of anticipated skeletal growth. Likewise, evaluation of the relative maturity of the child should be made. Early onset of puberty is common and decreases the overall length of the spine.

Radiographic evaluation should be carried out annually from the age of 1 year. These radiographs should be taken while the child is sitting as soon as the child is able to do so. If there is documented progressive scoliosis, additional radiographic examination is indicated. Magnetic resonance imaging (MRI) probably gives the most information without requiring invasive studies. MRI of the head and cervical spine evaluates the hydrocephalus and the degree of Arnold-Chiari malformation. The cervical, thoracic, and lumbar spine should also be scanned. The cervical spine and thoracic spine are evaluated for the appearance of syrinx or hydromyelia. The scan of the lumbar spine provides information on the posterior displacement of the conus and the presence of intraspinal tumors, such as lipoma or dermoid cysts. The MRI studies must be interpreted in association with the clinical findings to determine the cause of the scoliosis. The presence of a tethered cord is common, and it alone may not be the cause of the deformity.

Computed tomography (CT) can also be used. To achieve the maximal benefit from the study, however, contrast material is usually necessary for evaluation of the spinal cord. Both MRI and CT usually require sedation or anesthesia in young children.

Treatment

The treatment of each child is individualized and depends on the level and type of curve, the level of paralysis, the age of the patient, and the patient's ambulatory status. The first step is to determine whether there are neurologic causes for the scoliosis. Fortunately, it is often possible to treat the etiology of the scoliosis rather than the curve itself. A prompt referral to a neurosurgeon should be made at the first sign of scoliosis, before the curve becomes severe. Minor curves may correct spontaneously without orthopaedic treatment.

Orthoses

If the scoliosis continues to progress after neurologic problems have been corrected, orthopaedic treatment is indicated. If the

spine is balanced and the curve is 30 degrees or less, observation is probably indicated. If the curve is unbalanced or greater than 30 degrees, however, the spine will be unstable, and progression of the deformity is almost assured. A trial of bracing is indicated in children younger than 7 years of age if the curve is supple and can be corrected easily. Because bracing in paralytic scoliosis is passive, however, the brace has a tendency to deform the rib cage and produce pressure sores in the area of insensate skin. In infants, special care is needed to avoid abdominal compression, which may make it difficult for the child to breathe and eat. Although the use of a brace is only temporary, it may delay the need for surgery until the child is 8 or 9 years of age, when many of these children are beginning adolescence and a satisfactory surgical correction can be made (4,5).

The most effective spinal orthosis is a two-piece, polypropylene, bivalved, molded body jacket. This design allows the brace to be expanded or contracted throughout the day to permit eating and also allows some adjustability for growth. With a body jacket, meticulous skin care is required because pressure sores are common; after pressure sores develop, it is almost impossible to continue using the brace for control of the curve. Therefore, prevention is the rule. In general, the child begins orthosis wear slowly, starting at 1-hour intervals, after which the skin should be inspected. If any redness does not disappear within 4 hours, the orthosis must be modified. The time in the brace is gradually increased over a period of 2 to 3 weeks until the child is wearing it throughout the day except for naps and at night. If the family or caregivers are unable to provide this degree of care, an orthosis is probably not indicated.

Spinal Fusion

Most of these children require surgical correction and spinal fusion. Levels of fusion depend on the age of the child, location of the curve, level of paralysis, and ambulatory status. Generally, the same guidelines for instrumentation and fusion of idiopathic scoliosis are applicable to the myelomeningocele spine. The fusion should go from neutral vertebra to neutral vertebra, and the end vertebra should be located within the stable zone. This holds true for thoracic and thoracolumbar curves. In double curves, uncompensated curves, or primary lumbar curves, however, the decision becomes more difficult. Here, the guidelines for fusion and instrumentation differ from those for idiopathic scoliosis. In general, it is a mistake to fuse short; if there is any question, fuse long. This is particularly true in compensatory thoracic curves, in which reoperation is most common because of progression of the compensatory curve in the thoracic spine (26). In general, a compensatory thoracic curve should be fused for its entire length.

The selection of the level at the distal end is usually complicated by the open vertebral arch, which prevents attachment of the instrumentation to the end vertebra. There is a decreased stability in the vertebral column if the spinal fusion ends in the middle of the spina bifida. Lumbar hyperlordosis is usually present, compounding the problem of deciding on the distal level of fusion. In the past, the instrumentation was extended to the pelvis because of the difficulty of getting a firm attachment to the lower lumbar vertebra (1). With the newer methods of pedicle fixation, it may be possible to control some curves without fusing the lumbosacral joint. At the present, the indications for extending the fusion mass to the sacrum are not well established. Lumbosacral arthrodesis is difficult to obtain because of the lack of posterior vertebral arch to fuse to. Consequently, pseudarthroses and instrumentation failures are common (48). Attempts to correct these problems require repeated surgical procedures and have an uncertain outcome. If a successful fusion to the sacrum is obtained, it may deprive ambulatory patients of the ability to walk (39). For this reason, extending the fusion to the pelvis in an ambulatory child should be avoided, if possible. Even in wheelchair-bound patients, a lumbosacral fusion may cause difficulty as a result of increased occurrence of pressure sores, if the residual pelvic obliquity is 15 degrees or greater. Movement in the lumbosacral spine absorbs much of the angular and rotational movements of the trunk during wheelchair activities. If the lumbosacral spine is fused, these torsional movements are transmitted to the pelvis, creating increased shear between the pelvis, skin, and wheelchair seat. Unless the lumbar scoliosis can be corrected to less than 20 degrees and the pelvic obliquity to less than 15 degrees, however, the scoliosis will continue to progress if the lumbosacral spine is not fused (26). Therefore, it is important to treat the scoliosis while the curve is small and can be corrected to less than a 40-degree lumbar curve and a 15-degree pelvic obliquity, whether or not fusion to the sacrum is planned. Delaying surgical correction of the scoliosis to allow the spine to grow may lead to an unsatisfactory correction. After spinal correction, residual pelvic obliquity greater than 15 degrees can be corrected by a bilateral posterior iliac osteotomy with transfer of a wedge of bone from the long side to the short side (27) (Fig. 1).

The sagittal deformity must also be evaluated because increased lumbar lordosis is a common deformity. Assessment of sitting, supine, and standing posture must be made before correcting the lumbar lordosis. These children often require a greater degree of lordosis than normal. Bringing the lumbar lordosis back to the normal range may uncover a hip flexion contracture and prevent the child from standing or walking. If too much lordosis is fused into the lumbar spine of a female patient, she may not be able to carry out intermittent self-catheterization. The degree of lordosis left in the spine after fusion needs to be individually tailored to each patient. In general, it is best to treat the hip contractures before correcting the spine. It is difficult to maintain the correction of the hip when there is an uncorrected spinal deformity. If the hip deformity is not corrected first, however, positioning of the spine on the operating table will be difficult and will torque the spine postoperatively, leading to instrument failure and pseudarthrosis.

Ischial pressure sores should also be treated before spinal fusion to lessen the chance of infection. This is often difficult to do because the pelvic obliquity is a major cause of the ulceration, and unless it is corrected, pressure cannot be relieved from the ulcer. In this circumstance, a gluteus maximus myocutaneous flap can be used to promote primary healing. The patient is maintained on an air-mattress bed until the spinal correction can be performed. This may seem extreme, but it is much less of a problem than an infected spinal fusion that requires instrument removal.

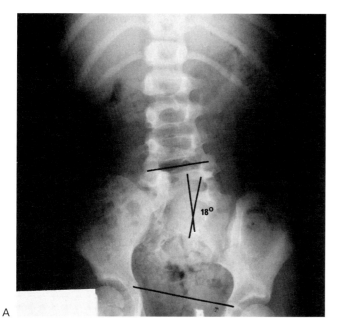

A

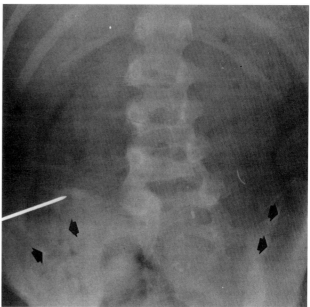

B

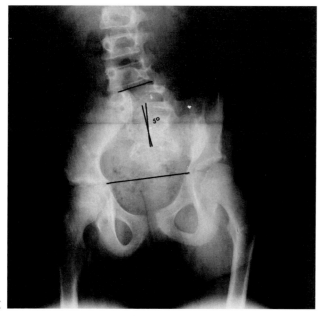

C

FIGURE 1. Eleven-year-old girl who has 18 degrees of pelvic obliquity because of congenital malformation of the lumbosacral spine. This deformity was stable without progression for 5 years. Her level of paralysis was L4 on the right and S1 on the left. **A:** Anteroposterior radiographs show the 18-degree pelvic obliquity. **B:** Postoperative radiographs show the wedge of bone that has been transferred from the long side to the short side. The graft is shown by the opposing *arrows*; the donor site by the *parallel arrows*. **C:** Follow-up radiographs show correction of the pelvic obliquity to 5 degrees.

The age of the child at the time of surgery is an important consideration. If the child has not yet reached adolescence, there is an almost 100% assurance that the curve will continue to progress despite posterior fusion unless the anterior spine is fused to the same level (10). The lumbar spine will almost always be fused anteriorly as well as posteriorly because of the deficient posterior vertebral arch, but if the posterior fusion extends up into the thoracic spine, it must be fused anteriorly as well.

In a child with a progressive curve that cannot be controlled by a brace who is too young to have the entire thoracolumbar spine fused, the preferred treatment is extraperiosteal segmental Luque instrumentation without spinal fusion (Fig. 2). Postoper-

ative brace treatment is still indicated, and complications from this approach include rod breakage, wire breakage, and spontaneous fusion. To provide a definitive solution, reoperation is often necessary when the child reaches maturity. In the interim, however, valuable spine growth often occurs.

There is a growing belief that before surgical correction of the scoliosis, the tethered spinal cord should be surgically released. As yet, there are no control studies to support or contradict this belief. Certainly, the correction of the scoliosis lengthens the posterior column of the spine and puts stretch on the cord. Whether this causes changes in neurologic function is unproved and probably varies on an individual basis. My

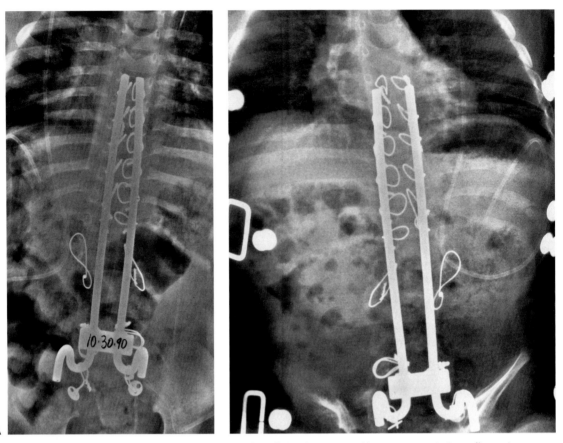

A   B

FIGURE 2. Segmental fixation of a spine without fusion in a 2-year-old. **A:** Anteroposterior radiograph after surgery showing the relationship of the sacral wrap rod to the sacrum. A spinous process wire is used to prevent upper migration of the rod. **B:** Radiograph 1 year later showing growth along the rod. (Courtesy of James Aronson, M.D., Arkansas Children's Hospital, Little Rock, Arkansas.)

approach is to have the child evaluated by neurosurgeons and abide by their recommendation. If a release is to be done, I prefer that it is performed before the spine surgery as a separate procedure.

Instrumentation

Spinal fusion is still the most important part of the surgical treatment of scoliosis despite the recent advances in spinal instrumentation. The role of the instrumentation is to improve spinal alignment, improve the fusion rate, and reduce the need for recumbency or postoperative immobilization. Regardless of the instrumentation used, the degree of correctability of the curve is limited. It is, therefore, important to carry out an early fusion when the deformity is still manageable. The amount of correction that is possible is probably limited to about 60 degrees, regardless of the size of the curve. Occasionally, it is possible to produce truly amazing degrees of correction, but this is not the rule. It is better to correct a 60-degree curve completely than to correct a 120-degree curve to 60 degrees.

It is generally agreed that anterior and posterior fusion is necessary in the area of the lumbar spine (36,37,39,41). There is no agreement, however, about whether the anterior spine

needs to be instrumented. In general, the more severe the deformity to be corrected, the greater the indication for using anterior instrumentation. Anterior instrumentation has recently gone through considerable development. Dwyer and Zielke instrumentation corrected frontal plane deformity but had little control of the sagittal deformity. They usually required external support until healing, a problem in asensate skin. Recent instrumentation using thicker rods up to $\frac{1}{4}$ inch appear able to control the spine in frontal and sagittal planes (21). Experience is still too short, however, to determine whehter the results are lasting. Instrumentation to the sacrum is difficult, and fusion of L5 to S1 anteriorly should not be attempted unless posterior instrumentation is to be used. Normally, this is a stable joint, and adequate posterior fusion can be obtained by grafting from the lamina and transverse process of L5 to the sacral ala. When the anterior longitudinal ligament is destroyed along with the annulus fibrosus, however, instability and severe deformity of this joint may occur if the child develops a pseudarthrosis of the lumbosacral joint. Because repair of this deformity and pseudarthrosis can be exceedingly difficult, it is preferable to end the anterior instrumentation at L4 in those patients who have a dorsolumbar curve that ends or is stable at L3 to L4. If it is necessary to extend the fusion down to the pelvis, perform an

anterior fusion only down to L5 and do not use anterior instrumentation. If the primary curve is less than 60 degrees, use only posterior instrumentation; if the primary curve is more than 60 degrees, instrument anteriorly to L4 and posteriorly to the pelvis.

Posterior instrumentation has evolved considerably. Initially, Harrington instrumentation was used, but because of the lack of posterior vertebral arch, distal fixation of the fusion was difficult unless the instrumentation was extended down to the sacral ala. The alar hooks frequently became displaced, and the pseudarthrosis and complication rates were unacceptably high (40,41). The child also required postoperative immobilization, which increased the occurrence of pressure sores.

Luque instrumentation has probably become the standard instrumentation for these children (1). Because of the segmental fixation to each vertebra, there is much better control over the spine, and postoperative immobilization is not required. However, it does not fix to the length of the spine as a rod with hooks does; therefore, the spine may settle or collapse along the rod, with loss of some of the correction in the immediate postoperative period. If the rod is contoured to maintain a normal sagittal alignment, there is a tendency for the rod to twist into the coronal plane deformity, with loss of correction. This is lessened somewhat by the use of the unit rod or multiple transverse rod connectors. Fixation to the open posterior spine in the lumbar area is weak, and extension of the instrumentation to the ilium is usually necessary. Even this distal attachment of the Luque rods is weak because there may be significant osteoporosis of the pelvis. Loosening of the instrumentation and pseudarthrosis of the lumbosacral joint are common.

The development of instrumentation that allows segmental fixation, distraction, and compression on the same rod along with the use of pedicle screws may solve many of the problems of instrumentation of the distal spine. The pedicle screws allow the end vertebra to be positioned in three planes and provide stable segmental instrumentation. This instrumentation may lessen the desirability of anterior instrumentation. Long-term studies have not yet been performed, but early reports indicate that satisfactory results can be obtained.

Whatever the instrumentation used posteriorly, it should be low profile in design. In the area of the meningocele sac, there is poor skin and soft tissue coverage. Prominence of hardware will invariably lead to ulceration over the hardware, eventual infection, and the need to remove the instrumentation.

Surgical Techniques

Luque Instrumentation Without Fusion

A midline incision is made from the midsacrum to the upper dorsal spine. The upper level of instrumentation should include the compensatory curve. Cephalad to the meningocele, the incision is carried down to the fascia. In the area of the meningocele, the skin and subcutaneous tissues that may be present are carefully dissected off the dural sac laterally until a strip of lumbar dorsal fascia 1 inch wide is exposed. Between the upper level of instrumentation and the first open spinal arch, the spine is

approached by carefully dissecting the paraspinous muscles off the periosteum of the spinous process. Bleeding vessels must be carefully coagulated. Injury to and elevation of the periosteum are to be avoided. In the area of the myelomeningocele, the dura is carefully dissected away from the periosteum and ligamenta flava on the inside of the open canal. On the outside of the canal, the paraspinous muscles are carefully dissected extraperiosteally down to the transverse process. At each interspace along the length of instrumented spine, the interspinous ligament and the ligamenta flava are carefully removed with a narrow rongeur to expose the epidural space. Care is taken to avoid removing any bone from the spinous processes. It may be necessary to place a small towel clip in the spinous processes above and below the area of dissection; this can be used to spread the spinous processes to provide sufficient space so that the ligament can be removed without damaging periosteum or bone. A small angled rongeur may be necessary to remove enough ligamenta flava to permit sublaminar wire passage. In the area of the meningocele, wires can be looped around the pedicle or lamina.

The distal fixation point for the rod can be determined in two ways. If the child has intact neurologic function at the lower lumbar and upper sacral levels, an *S*-shaped rod can be looped around the sacral ala (Fig. 2). To keep the rod from displacing

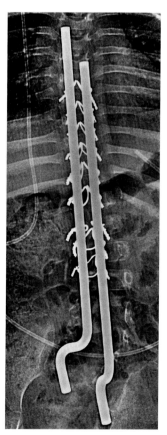

FIGURE 3. Luque rods that were bent to insert into the first sacral foramen. A transverse rod-connecting device was not used, resulting in shift of the rods and recurrence of the pelvic obliquity.

proximally and losing control over the sacrum, it is necessary to wire the rod to the sacrum with a sublaminar or spinous process wire. Bone should be grafted between the L5 transverse process and the ala. The rod should be relatively straight, with no contouring, and should be as large as possible. Unless the child is very small, ¼-inch rods are preferable. If possible, the two rods should be connected at the sacrum with some type of transverse rod-connecting device. This anchors the pelvis and prevents the occurrence of pelvic obliquity in relationship to the rods (Fig. 3). The rods should be as long as possible to allow for growth. It is common for these children to grow at least 6 cm after the rod has been inserted, and they will probably grow off the end of the rod. If this becomes a major problem, a longer rod may need to be inserted at a later date.

If the child has an upper lumbar level of paraplegia, an alternative method of fixation to the sacrum is possible, making use of the L5 to S1 or S1 foramen for the point of fixation (50). The distal end of the Luque rod is bent in two angles. The first, about 1 inch from the end, is bent at an angle of about 120 degrees. About half an inch proximal to this bend is a right-angle bend going in the opposite direction (Fig. 4). The segmental nerve and vessel are ligated and divided at the selected foramen anchor site. With blunt dissection, the foramen is freed of

soft tissue, and the rod is inserted. Even in a 3- or 4-year-old child, a ¼-inch rod fits nicely into this foramen. A transverse rod-connecting device should be used to secure the rod in relationship to the pelvis (see Fig. 4C, D). If this rod system is used, care must be taken to bend a slight outward bow in the rod to follow the contour of the meningocele and then back to midline, as the intact spine is approached. This prevents undue pressure on the dural sac. Lordosis should also be bent into the rod so that the end of the rod is against the anterior surface of the sacrum.

With the Galveston technique, it may be extremely difficult to anchor the distal rod to the pelvis. The pelvis in an infant or small child is small and osteoporotic and provides an inadequate anchor site. Loss of fixation and eventual protrusion of the rods through the skin have been common.

Postoperatively, the patient is placed in a body jacket for day activities; night protection is not necessary.

Anterior Instrumentation and Fusion

If only thoracolumbar fusion is necessary, a standard thoracolumbar approach removing the tenth rib is appropriate. The diaphragm is usually detached about 1 inch from its lateral bor-

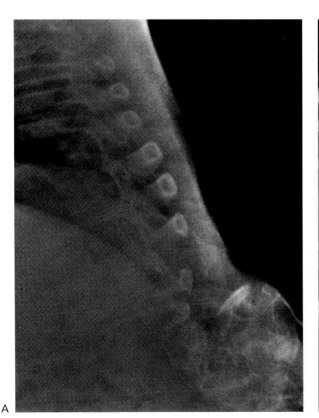 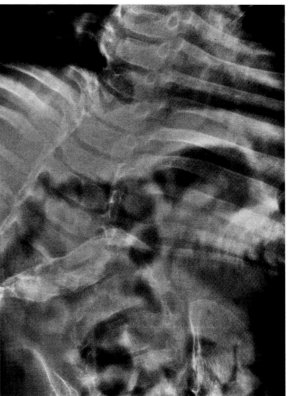

A   B

FIGURE 4. A 2-year-old T12-level paraplegic child with a form of medial spinal aplasia and severe kyphosis. **A:** Lateral radiograph showing severe kyphosis that is unmeasurable because of the disorganized anatomy. The proximal lordosis is also severe and rigid. The deformity resembles the more common S-shaped kyphosis. Treatment consists of excision of the vertebrae between the thoracic lordosis and the apex of the lumbar kyphosis. **B:** Anteroposterior radiograph showing the presence of scoliosis as well as the absence of several lumbar vertebrae. *(Figure continues.)*

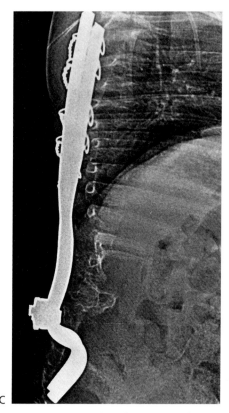 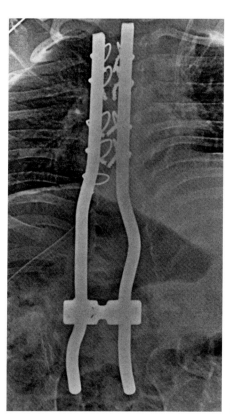

C   D

FIGURE 4. *Continued.* **C:** After excision of two vertebrae in the lordotic segment, satisfactory reduction of the deformity was achieved. This lateral radiograph shows lordosis of the remaining lumbar spine. The Luque rods are bent to enter the L5 to S1 foramen and lie along the anterior border of the sacrum. **D:** Anteroposterior radiograph showing correction of the scoliosis. A transverse rod-connecting device is maintaining the relationship of the rods. The bend in the rod is to avoid compression of the dural sac.

der, and a retroperitoneal approach is made to the lumbar spine. If anterior discectomy and fusion without instrumentation are anticipated, it is possible to retract the soft tissues carefully around the disc space so that the disc can be removed and bone graft inserted into the disc space without ligation of the segmental vessels. If instrumentation is required, the segmental vessels are ligated and retracted, exposing the lateral vertebral body. The vertebral screws should be placed as far posteriorly as possible to avoid producing kyphosis in the lumbar spine. A ¼-inch rod is able to correct the frontal and sagittal deformities (Fig. 5).

Anterior spinal fusions that extend proximal to T10 require more than one rib excision. The spine is approached from the direction of the major deformity, particularly if instrumentation is anticipated. The compensatory curve can be approached from the concave side using this approach. The skin incision extends along the proximal rib to be excised from the posterior rib angle to the costochondral junction, where it then curves distally along the lateral border of the rectus abdominal muscle. The incision is carried down through the subcutaneous tissue, exposing the chest musculature. The skin and subcutaneous tissue are carefully removed by sharp dissection from the chest musculature distally to the tenth rib and proximally to the upper rib to be excised. The incision in the latissimus dorsi is made at the level

of the tenth rib. The latissimus dorsi is detached along its anterior border from the chest wall along with the origin of the serratus anterior, preserving the nerve supply. This flap is elevated to expose the entire rib cage from T4 down to T10. Any rib, typically the tenth, may be removed at this point to allow access to the spine. The rib at the uppermost level of the fusion or instrumentation is also removed.

At the termination of the procedure, the wound is closed in layers. The latissimus dorsi can easily be brought down and repaired, and the origin of the serratus can be reattached.

Posterior Fusion and Instrumentation

A standard midline approach can be used, with a subperiosteal approach to the spine. The skin is carefully removed from the dural sac. If a tethered cord is present and there is any function in the lumbar cord, the tether should be released at the time of spinal fusion. Otherwise, there may be a change in nerve function, including bowel and bladder control. If the skin over the meningocele is poor and scarred to the dural sac and the neurosurgeon is not performing a simultaneous tethered cord release, an inverted *Y* incision is made (38). Segmental instrumentation is preferred—either a Luque rod or one of the newer types (e.g.,

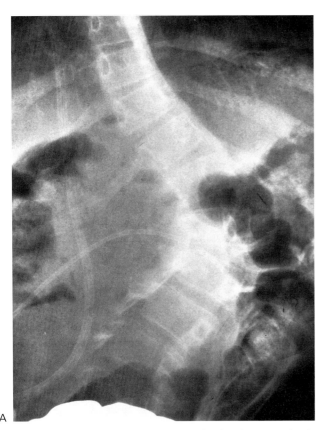 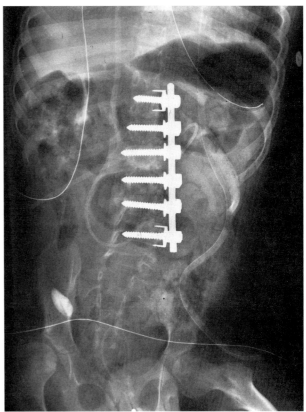

A   B

FIGURE 5. A 12-year-old girl with a motor level paralysis at L4. **A:** 80-degree scoliosis. **B:** Correction to 10 degrees with anterior instrumentation from T11 to L4. The ¼-inch rod also controls sagittal alignment.

TSRH, Moss-Miami) of instrumentation. If the compensatory curves are fused, they must not be overcorrected and must provide a balanced spine. The rods are bent to provide sagittal alignment of the spine, with special care given to the lumbar lordosis.

Segmental fixation of the rods to the dorsal spine usually presents little difficulty because of adequate anchor sites for hooks or wires, but rod fixation in the lumbar spine may be quite difficult. If the distal end of the fusion ends in an area of an intact posterior arch, only routine hook, wire, or screw fixation is necessary. This is not usually the case, however, and the fusion usually ends in the area of the meningocele. If the spine has been instrumented anteriorly, wire fixation to the pedicle is sufficient, but if anterior instrumentation has not been used, pedicle screws in the end vertebra are probably the best choice (Fig. 6). However, care must be taken when attempting to use pedicle screws. Although the pedicle is easily identifiable under direct vision after retracting the dural sac, it is occasionally too small in diameter to accept even a 5.5-mm screw. If adequate fixation cannot be obtained in the area of the meningocele, the fusion should be extended to the sacrum. The instrumentation is carried down and fixed to the ilium using the Galveston technique. Additional fixation at L5 with pedicle screws attached to the rod gives additional fixation to the sacrum and the lower lumbar spine (Fig. 7).

A meticulous lateral mass fusion from the lumbar vertebrae is essential. This must be performed with the same care as one would use for a lumbosacral fusion for spondylolisthesis. The bone graft is then placed along the lamina and transverse process. Care must be taken to curet and bone graft the facet joints in the lumbar vertebrae, which is somewhat difficult because of their abnormal orientation.

Postoperatively, the patient is mobilized as soon as possible to prevent problems with osteoporosis and pressure sores. If the neurosurgeon has performed a tethered cord release, mobilization depends on the adequacy of the dural repair and the possibility of dural leak. Activities are restricted for the first 3 months. If the child is ambulatory and the fusion ended at L3, resumption of ambulation with assistance and the use of crutches or a walker is allowed after 2 or 3 weeks. If the child is a thoracic-level paraplegic and the fusion included the sacrum, activity is limited for at least 3 months. These children are not allowed to transfer themselves without assistance or to participate in activities that would torque the pelvis in relationship to the spine. They must not be transferred to the bathtub (necessitating sponge baths), and they must have assistance getting on and off the toilet and with their intermittent catheterization. They are allowed to wheel their wheelchairs by themselves. After the spine has shown evidence of fusion, usually at 3 months, activities are gradually

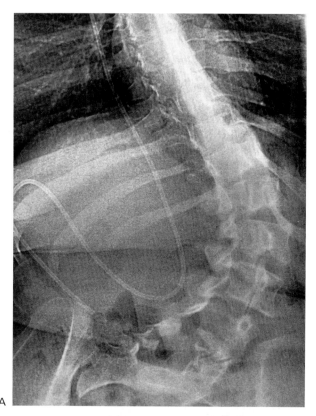

A

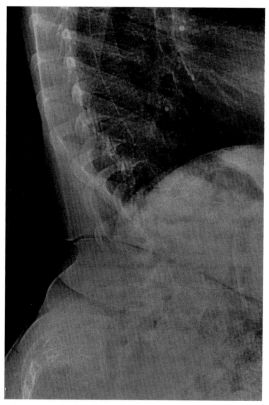

B

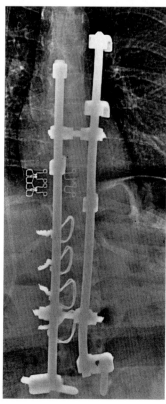

C

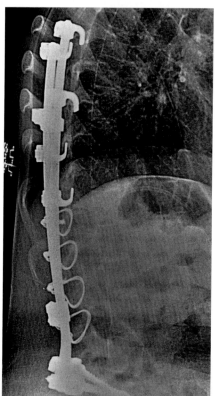

D

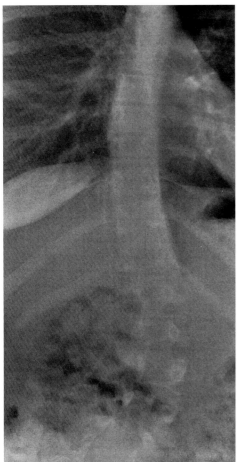
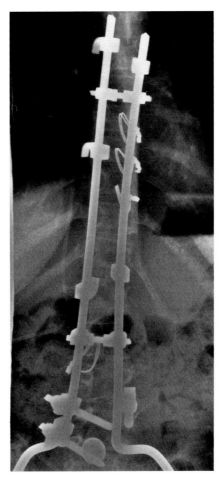
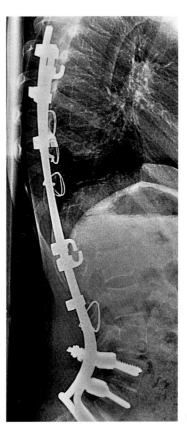

A,B

C

FIGURE 7. A 13-year-old girl who has an L3-level paraplegia but is not ambulatory. She is obese and has a progressive lumbar scoliosis and increase in pelvic obliquity. A tethered spinal cord was released previously. **A:** Anteroposterior radiograph showing a 50-degree uncompensated lumbar scoliosis resulting in 35 degrees of pelvic obliquity. There is also excessive lumbar lordosis. **B:** Postoperative anteroposterior radiograph showing complete correction of the scoliosis. The fusion included the sacrum because the lumbar scoliosis included the first sacral vertebra and the child was not ambulatory. Pedicle screws were used to secure the segmental instrumentation to L4 and L5. Anterior interbody fusion was performed from T10 to the sacrum. **C:** Postoperative lateral radiograph showing restoration of normal sagittal alignment. Lumbar lordosis now measures 55 degrees. She has full extension of her hips and is able to perform intermittent self-catheterization.

FIGURE 6. A mature 12-year-old girl with progressive lumbar scoliosis. She has an L4 level of paraplegia and is a community walker with ankle-foot orthoses and crutches. Neurologic evaluation showed a functional ventriculoperitoneal shunt and the presence of a tethered spinal cord. **A:** Anteroposterior radiograph showing a 55-degree lumbar scoliosis from T9 to L3. There is a 20-degree compensatory curve from L4 to the sacrum, but because this is insufficient, there is a residual 30-degree pelvic obliquity. The last intact vertebral arch is L2. **B:** Lateral radiograph showing a severe 120-degree lordosis, which is typical of the deformity associated with a tethered cord. **C:** Anteroposterior radiograph showing correction of the scoliosis and pelvic obliquity. Pedicle screws are used to fix the distal end vertebra at L5. The lumbosacral joint was left unfused to allow the patient enough pelvic mobility to continue walking. A release of the tethered cord was performed at the same time as the spinal fusion. An anterior interbody fusion was also performed from T9 to L5. **D:** Lateral radiograph showing correction of the lordosis to 45 degrees and the achievement of a normal sagittal alignment.

increased. Unrestricted activities are not allowed for at least 6 to 9 months.

CONGENITAL SCOLIOSIS

Congenital scoliosis may occur anywhere along the spine, including the cervical, thoracic, and lumbosacral spine. Congenital malformations may be caused by the lack of formation, the lack of segmentation, or a combination of the two. If the malformation occurs in the lumbosacral area, the progression of deformity is usually rapid and uncompensated, causing severe pelvic obliquity. Nonoperative methods of treatment do not correct congenital scoliosis or prevent it from worsening. Because of their neurologic abnormalities, these children are unable to tolerate an unbalanced spine. Therefore, it is important that treatment be carried out in infancy when the deformity is small rather than waiting until the child is older and heroic measures are needed to obtain satisfactory alignment.

Posterior fusion of the malformation is rarely successful in preventing progression (49). This is particularly so in the lumbar spine, where there is an incomplete posterior arch. Anterior and posterior fusion appears to be the procedure of choice, and it should be performed as soon as a diagnosis of progressive scoliosis is made, usually at about 1 year of age. An alternative to approaching the spine in staged or separate procedures, the anterior and posterior interbody fusions may be performed through a posterior approach, using the pedicle as the access conduit to the anterior spine (18,28). This is especially true when the malformation is in the upper thoracic spine, where the anterior approach is very difficult. If the lumbar curve is already so severe that the pelvic obliquity is greater than 15 degrees, an osteotomy of the spine to correct the deformity should be considered. Another possibility in a child older than 10 years of age is to perform a bilateral posterior iliac osteotomy to balance the pelvis after the spine has been fused (28).

Surgical Techniques

Anteroposterior Spinal Fusion: Posterior Approach

Preoperative evaluation includes tomograms to identify correctly the anatomy of the vertebral abnormality. Occasionally, a CT evaluation is also indicated to look at cartilaginous abnormalities that may not be visible on conventional radiographs. If there is a suspicion of a diastematomyelia in association with the congenital malformation, an MRI is useful to look at the dural contents. If a diastematomyelia is present, it should be addressed at the same time as the fusion. Pulmonary function tests are indicated if the congenital curve involves the thoracic spine and a thoracotomy is anticipated to perform the anteroposterior fusion.

The child is placed in the prone position on an operating table that allows either radiographic or fluoroscopic examination to be performed during the surgical procedure. The longitudinal incision is centered over the congenital malformation. A subperiosteal dissection is made of the abnormal vertebrae, including the vertebrae above and below the anticipated level of fusion. Only the convex side of the spine is exposed. Minimal exposure is made above and below the intended fusion site to prevent spontaneous fusion from occurring as a result of dissection in areas where fusion is not wanted.

After the spinous process, lamina, and transverse process have been dissected free, the area of the pedicle is identified and confirmed by radiograph. The posterior cortical bone is removed from the lamina overlying the pedicle. It may be necessary to remove part of the inferior facet joint from the vertebra above. Using a small 3-0 or 4-0 straight curet, the cancellous bone is removed from the pedicle (Fig. 8). It is important to use a tog-

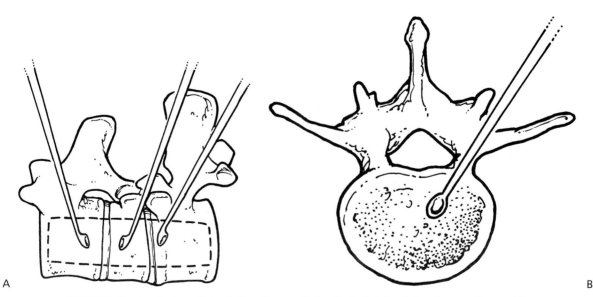

A

B

FIGURE 8. Transpedicular anterior fusion of congenital scoliosis. **A:** Lateral view showing the curet in the pedicles clearing out a trough of the vertebrae that cross the disc space. **B:** Transverse view showing the position of the curet in the pedicle and the vertebral body.

gling motion rather than a pushing motion to identify the canal of the pedicle. Some resistance may be met in the area of the pedicle physis. However, with care, this area can be traversed without breaching the cortical margins of the pedicle. After this resistance has been overcome, the curet will pass easily into the vertebral body. Again, it is important not to push, but rather to use a toggling motion to allow the curet to advance. A tapping motion can be used to confirm that the curet has not perforated the cortex of the vertebral body. With an ever-expanding toggle to the curet, most of the cancellous bone can be removed from the convex half of the vertebral body. Care is taken not to penetrate cortical bone. If bleeding is encountered, small patties can be packed into the pedicle for a few minutes and then removed. An angled 3-0 curet is then used to continue the removal of the cancellous bone up to and including the subchondral bony plate of the vertebral end plate. A similar procedure is performed at each vertebra for the length of the intended fusion (Fig. 9). This includes the abnormal vertebrae plus the vertebrae above and below. Using angled curets, one from above and one from below, the disc can be penetrated and carefully removed. When dissecting posteriorly, it is important not to penetrate the annulus, which would injure the segmental nerve and vessel. The dissec-

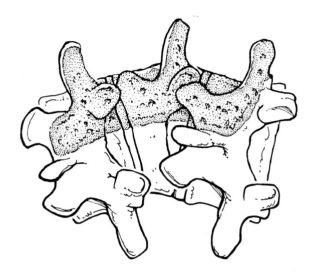

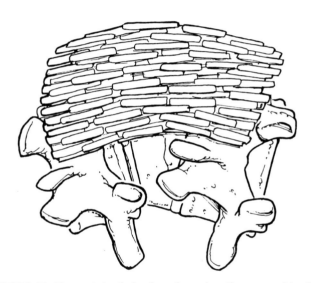

FIGURE 10. The posterior fusion is performed on the convex side of the scoliosis.

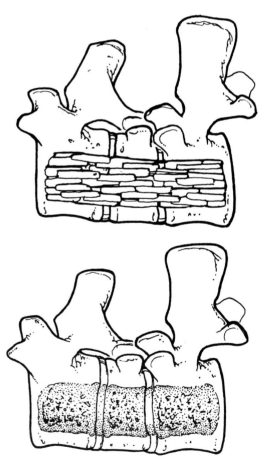

FIGURE 9. *Bottom:* The anterior trough has been completed along the length of the congenital curve. *Top:* Bone graft has been inserted through the pedicles into the trough to promote the anterior spinal fusion.

tion should be checked at frequent intervals using radiographic control.

After a satisfactory trough has been created in the lateral vertebra from the top to the bottom of the fusion mass, small strips of cortical cancellous autogenous graft are removed from the ilium. They are fitted through the pedicle into the anterior trough in the vertebra. The entire trough is packed with bone extending from one vertebra to the next (Fig. 9). The facet joints and the laminae are then decorticated along the convex side of the curve, and additional bone graft is added posteriorly (Fig. 10). Wound closure is carried out in layers.

Rarely, a pedicle is too small to accept a curet. In this situation, a posterior fusion is performed. The child is then rolled into the lateral position, a standard anterior approach to the vertebra is made, and an anterior interbody fusion is performed.

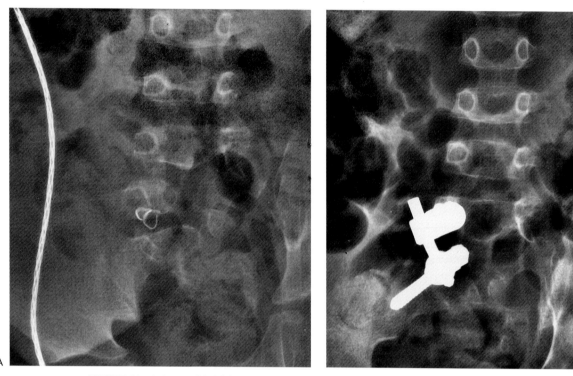

FIGURE 11. A 6-year-old child with severe congenital scoliosis due to hemivertebra. **A:** Radiograph shows the hemivertebra at L5 and an unsegmented bar on the concave side. **B:** Postoperative radiograph shows excision of the hemivertebra and osteotomy of the unsegmented bar. The vertebrae on each side of the hemivertebra were opposed by means of a pedicle screw and a connecting rod. This technique was used instead of a wire because of her age.

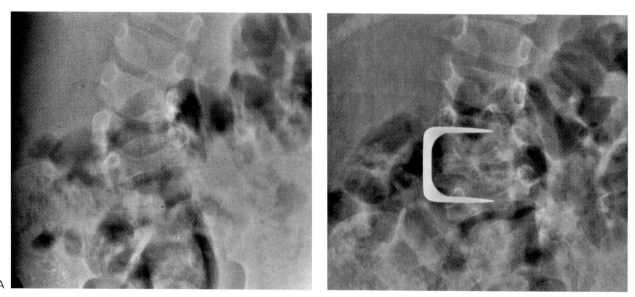

FIGURE 12. A 3-year-old child with congenital scoliosis due to hemivertebra at L4. Posterior excision of the posterior arch of L4 was followed by an anterior excision of the hemivertebra and fixation with a staple. A staged procedure was used because the neurologic level was below S1. **A:** Preoperative radiograph showing the hemivertebra. **B:** Postoperative radiograph shows correction of the deformity.

Typical blood loss from the anteroposterior fusion is about 100 to 150 mL. Operative time averages about 3 hours, which is considerably less than the traditional separate anterior and posterior fusions.

Postoperatively, the child is allowed to resume preoperative activities without restrictions. No brace or cast is used.

Excision of Hemivertebra in the Lumbar Spine: Posterior Approach

This procedure is limited to the lumbar spine in the area of the spina bifida or where neurologic function is intact at the level of the deformity (Fig. 11). It is not appropriate for the dorsal spine, where a more traditional anterior and posterior excision of the hemivertebra in a staged procedure is appropriate.

A longitudinal incision is made in the lumbar spine. Skin and subcutaneous tissue are carefully dissected off the dural sac and lateral to the paraspinous muscles. The dural sac is carefully freed extraperiosteally from the convex side of the curve. The paraspinous muscles are stripped subperiosteally from the convex side of the curve to the transverse process. The hemivertebra is then exposed by a dural retractor retracting the dural sac medially. The spinous process, lamina, and transverse process are removed with a rongeur, exposing the pedicle. Using a small curet, the cancellous bone is removed from the hemivertebra. The cortical bone can then be removed laterally and posteriorly, exposing the anterior cortex. Under direct vision, it is also removed. The disc space and subchondral bone are removed with a curet and rongeur superiorly and inferiorly to the hemivertebra. The deformity can then be reduced by bringing the opposing surfaces together. Bone from the removed hemivertebra can be used for bone graft. Reduction is held by a wire around the pedicle of the vertebra above and below the excised hemivertebra or by pedicle screws and rod. Postoperatively, the patient is placed in a pantaloon cast for 3 months (Fig. 12).

KYPHOSIS

Lumbar kyphosis is a major deformity that occurs in 8% to 15% of patients with myelomeningocele (8,12,22,29,43,46,47). It often measures 80 degrees or more at birth and usually progresses with growth. Children with extensive kyphosis have difficulty wearing braces and sitting in a wheelchair and often have ulcerations over the prominent kyphos. Progression of the kyphosis may lead to breathing difficulty because the abdominal contents are crowded into the chest cavity by increasing upward pressure on the diaphragm. These children also have difficulty eating because of loss of abdominal size, which results in a failure to thrive. They are underweight and short in stature. The increased flexion of the trunk may also interfere with drainage of urine and cause technical difficulties with urethrostomy, vesicotomy, or ileostomy.

Kyphosis is almost always progressive, and attempts to delay definitive treatment until the child is older lead to a more severe deformity (2). Unfortunately, the aorta and vena cava do not follow the anterior border of the spine across the kyphosis (32); they take the short route like a bowstring. Therefore, the amount

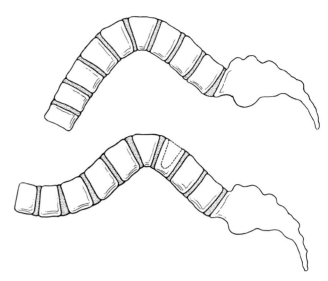

FIGURE 13. Two types of lumbar kyphosis: the *C*-shaped collapsing curve (*top*) and the *S*-shaped curve (*bottom*).

of surgical correctability is limited. For this reason, it is important to carry out treatment early, even though it may be only a temporizing procedure. A more definitive procedure can be performed later.

The goal of treatment is to increase abdominal height to allow more room for the abdominal contents and relieve pressure on the diaphragm and the lungs. In addition, the kyphosis must be minimized to lessen the incidence of pressure sores, and the center of gravity must be moved posteriorly to center it over the ischium. This improves the child's ability to sit without using the arms for support.

The kyphosis deformity can be divided into three types (Fig. 13). The first type is a collapsing kyphosis; it is often *C*-shaped and supple, at least during the initial stages. The apex may occur anywhere from the lower dorsal spine to the lumbosacral joint. The second is a rigid *S*-shaped lumbar kyphosis with a proximal dorsal lordosis. The kyphosis is usually centered at L2 and the proximal rigid lordosis at about T10. This is the most common variety of congenital kyphosis in the older child. Some children progress from the *C* type to the *S* type as they grow. The third type of kyphosis is rare and is associated with partial aplasia of the lumbar spine (7) (Fig. 4). It can exist in either the proximal or distal portion of the lumbar spine and is distinguished from sacral agenesis by the presence of a sacrum. Because the treatment of this type is similar to that used for the rigid *S*-shaped deformity, they are discussed together.

Collapsing Kyphosis

Conservative treatment, which consists of observation, is usually futile. The curve progresses rapidly, and it is not unusual to see a 2- or 3-year-old child with a kyphosis greater than 100 degrees. In those few instances in which the collapsing curve does not progress rapidly and is less than 20 to 30 degrees, an initial period of observation may be worthwhile. At the first sign of progression, however, treatment is indicated. If the curve is very small and the skin is in excellent condition, a brace can be used. However, because any orthotic device must push over the apical vertebra posteriorly and against the protuberant abdomen anteriorly, this leads to pressure sores over the gibbus and increased pressure on the abdominal contents. This pressure decreases the child's appetite and pulmonary reserve, jeopardizing survival. The kyphosis almost always requires surgical correction; this should not be delayed if brace treatment is unsatisfactory.

Collapsing scoliosis in an immature child is difficult to treat. Posterior spinal fusion without instrumentation usually fails because of tension forces in the fusion mass. When instrumentation is used, instrument failure is common. Attempts to provide stability by anterior strut fusion with a strut graft also tend to fail in young patients. The fusion creates an anterior unsegmented bar, with growth potential remaining posteriorly. As the child grows, the kyphosis increases. If the surgeon waits until the child is older to carry out anteroposterior fusion with instrumentation along the dorsolumbar spine, the curve is often so severe that satisfactory correction is difficult, if not impossible, to obtain. If the anteroposterior fusion is carried out in infancy, the result-

ing spine is too short to allow sufficient room for abdominal volume and respiratory sufficiency.

Satisfactory treatment of this deformity requires that the spine be brought into normal sagittal alignment. McCarthy (34) has developed a technique of incising the disc space anteriorly and laterally using a posterior approach (Fig. 14). This is performed at about five levels centered at the apex of the curve. A catheter is placed in one of the foot arteries and hooked to a monitor to watch for a pressure wave as the spine is gradually corrected by pressure over the apical vertebra. Steinmann pins are drilled crosswise through the vertebral body to act as a fixation point for specially contoured Luque rods, which maintain the reduction. In 14 patients, McCarthy has had no vascular compromise (32).

Most authors, however, found that the anterior structures, including the abdominal wall, aorta, and vena cava, are of insufficient length to allow correction to occur without shortening the spine to remove tension from these structures (32). Many different procedures have been described to shorten the posterior spine to allow it to be straightened and put into more normal sagittal alignment. Most of these techniques require fusion of

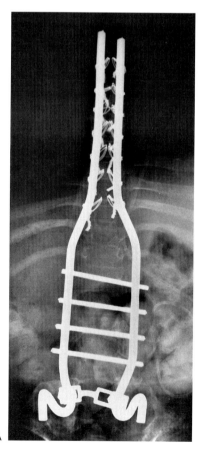 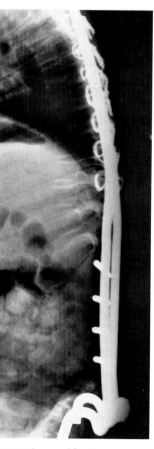

FIGURE 14. Postoperative radiograph showing the instrumentation used for the procedure performed by McCarthy (34). **A:** Anteroposterior radiograph showing the bend of the rod around the dural sac. The pins through the vertebrae are present in the area of the kyphosis. **B:** Lateral radiograph shows a good alignment of the trunk, with the dorsal spine over the sacrum despite a residual kyphosis of 70 degrees. The flexion of the pelvis remains despite the sacral wrap rod. (Courtesy of R. E. McCarthy, M.D., Arkansas Spine Center, Little Rock.)

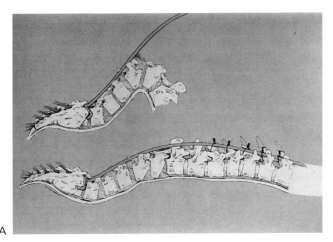

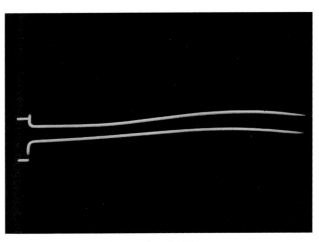

A

B

FIGURE 15. Correction of the spine using multiple disc excision and a rod fixation described by Dunn (11). **A:** Lateral diagram showing the rod attachment to the sacrum and thoracic spine. **B:** The rod is bent with three right-angle bends so that it can pass through the L5 foramen and into the sacral ala. (Courtesy of H. K. Dunn, M.D., University of Utah Medical Center, Salt Lake City, Utah.)

the spine to maintain correction and should therefore be performed only in a mature child; otherwise, the spine will be too short. The most common technique uses an excision of the apical vertebra and a variable amount of the neighboring vertebrae. However, because the deformity usually extends over three or more vertebrae, it is difficult to obtain satisfactory correction; recurrence of the deformity and failure of instrumentation are common.

The procedure described by Dunn (11) has been successful in obtaining satisfactory correction. In this procedure, the disc space and end plate are removed from each vertebral space over the entire length of the deformity. This gives sufficient mobility of the spine to correct most deformities. If additional shortening is needed, bone can be removed from each interspace as well. This procedure destroys all stability of the spine, and rigid segmental fixation is needed until the fusion is complete. Dunn (11) uses a specially contoured Luque rod (Fig. 15). Because the

procedure requires transection of the segmental nerves and vessels at each level and elevation of the spinal cord, it can be used only in patients with thoracic-level paraplegia.

Another method used to shorten the spine is to remove the ossific nuclei from the vertebrae above and below the apical vertebra, which is left intact (Fig. 16A, B). The pedicle and posterior arch are, likewise, removed from these two vertebrae. The apical vertebra is pushed forward, correcting the kyphosis (Fig. 16C). Segmental wiring is used to create a tension band between the pedicles of the apical vertebra and the vertebrae above and below the osteotomy in the newborn child. In a child older than 1 year of age, rods without fusion maintain the correction (Fig. 4). Because the vertebral body growth centers are left intact, the growth of the spine continues, often producing a gradual increase in the lordosis. The spine is not fused; hence, the procedure can be performed at any age, even in newborns (Figs. 17 and 18). It is also possible to perform this surgery

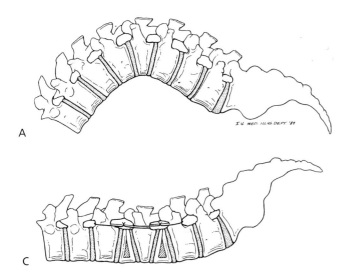

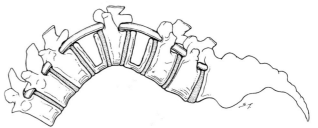

A

B

C

FIGURE 16. Correction of the C-shaped curve by removing the ossific nuclei of the vertebrae above and below the apical vertebra. **A:** The C-shaped kyphosis before removal of the ossific nuclei from the vertebrae. **B:** Spinous processes, laminae, pedicles, and ossific nuclei have been removed from the vertebrae above and below the apical vertebra. The growth plate disc and anterior cortex are left intact. **C:** The deformity is reduced by pushing the apical vertebra forward. Tension band wiring around the pedicles maintains the reduction. (From Lindseth RE [1991]: Spine deformity in myelomeningocele. *Instr Course Lect* 40:276, with permission.)

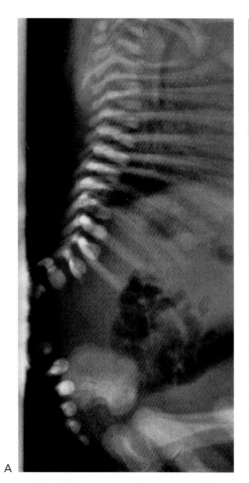

A

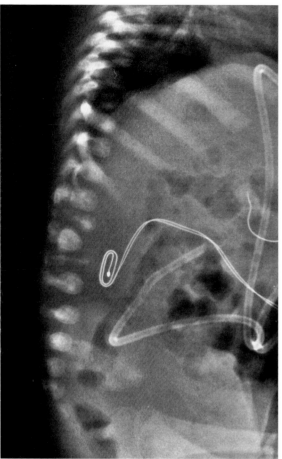

B

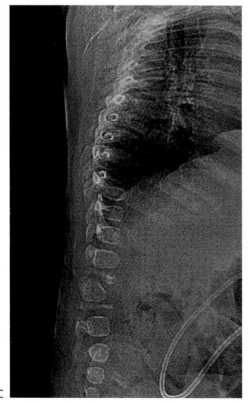

C

FIGURE 17. Newborn infant with severe kyphosis and my-elomeningocele that extends from T12 to the sacrum. Correction was obtained at birth at the same time as the meningocele closure. **A:** Lateral radiograph showing a 100-degree kyphosis. Although there was a proximal lordosis of the distal thoracic spine, it appeared to be supple upon examination, and the decision was made to treat this as a C-shaped curve. **B:** Postoperative radiograph showing that the kyphosis has been reduced to 10 degrees. Nonabsorbable suture was used instead of wire to hold the correction because of the weakness of the infantile bone. After reduction of the kyphosis, the paravertebral muscles could be closed behind the dural sac. Also, the skin was closed primarily without the need for skin flaps. The resected vertebrae are visible as narrow bands of bone on each side of the apical vertebrae. **C:** One-year postoperative lateral radiograph shows further correction of the kyphosis to 2 degrees. Reformation of the excised vertebrae is beginning, as shown by the increased width of the bone above and below the apical vertebrae.

child, a $^3/_{16}$-inch rod is probably satisfactory; in an older child, a $^1/_4$-inch rod often fits into this foramen. The $^1/_4$-inch rod should be used if possible. The $^3/_{16}$-inch rod usually breaks after several years and needs to be replaced. The rod is bent, with the first bend of about 135 degrees being made 1 inch from the end. Half an inch proximal to this, a right-angle bend is made in the opposite direction. The prebent rod is available commonly from AcroMed (325 Paramount Drive, Raynham, MA 02767-0350). The rods are then inserted carefully into the foramen and should be positioned so that they are tight up against the anterior surface of the sacrum. If possible, a transverse loading device should be used to hold the rods separated at the sacrum. The rods are bent to allow a place for the spinal cord as the rods pass through the midline and for the sublaminar wiring proximally. If the spinal cord is pinched between the rods, a spinal cord reflex may develop. Sublaminar wires are then placed in the proximal vertebrae that have already been prepared for their passage. At least three wires are needed for each rod proximally. The sublaminar wires are tightened, correcting the deformity. Because of the bend in the rod at the sacrum, there is usually about 40 degrees of lordosis at the lumbosacral joint. This establishes normal sagittal alignment in this area. The paraspinous muscles are then closed over the rod, and the subcutaneous skin is closed in the routine manner. The rod is cut about 2 inches above the most proximal wire to allow for growth.

Postoperatively, no splint or body cast is needed. The child is allowed to sit after 1 week. When the child is ready to resume physical therapy and standing, a two-piece body jacket may be worn for protection during periods of increased activity.

If the child has intact nerve function, the ossific nuclei of the vertebrae are approached as in the newborn procedure, with care taken to avoid injury to the spinal cord and the segmental nerves. Tension band wiring similar to that in the newborn is used. Because the wiring is of insufficient strength for an older child, however, and the tension band wires will cut through the pedicle when the child begins to sit, the osteotomy must be protected with instrumentation. The distal instrumentation to the pelvis or sacrum is performed as described previously with sacrifice of the S1 nerve root so that the rod can be inserted in the S1 foramen. The sacral wrap rods, similar to the McCarthy (34) and Dunn (11) techniques, may allow the pelvis to tip forward, causing kyphosis at the lumbosacral joint (Fig. 14). The Galveston technique has been unsuccessful in obtaining satisfactory control of the spine for the treatment of kyphosis. The direction of the rods makes it difficult for them to resist the forward flexion that occurs in the treatment of kyphosis.

In children who have reached adolescence, the procedure is further modified by performing a spinal fusion that is instrumented for the entire length of the spine.

Rigid *S*-Shaped Kyphosis

Treatment of the rigid form of upper lumbar kyphosis is difficult and controversial. Conservative nonoperative treatment invariably leads to an increased deformity and difficulty in later correction. In 1968, Sharrard (44) first described resection of the apical vertebral body for the treatment of kyphosis; since then, most authors have recommended vertebral excision as part of the oper-

ative treatment (20). Most of these reports also showed that excision of the apical vertebra may lead to initial correction of the deformity. However, the deformity has a tendency to recur, often to a worse degree than the initial kyphosis (28), leading to feelings of futility and frustration.

Treatment of the rigid form of kyphosis requires a different approach. Because both the kyphosis and the proximal lordosis are rigid, it is necessary to correct both deformities at the same time. This can be accomplished by excising the vertebrae (usually two) between the kyphosis and lordosis (14,29) (Fig. 19) and fusing the apical vertebra to the distal end of the thoracic spine at the level of the resection. In a young child, this is the only area fused, and the osteotomy is held in position by tension band wiring around the pedicle above and below the resected vertebrae (29) (Fig. 18). It is important that the paraspinous muscles be sutured behind the area of the spine to add a corrective force, decreasing the likelihood of recurrence of the deformity (Fig. 18).

An evaluation of 39 patients who underwent this resection of the lordotic segment proximal to the apical vertebra, with a mean follow-up of 11 years, showed that most patients maintained at least 50% of the correction demonstrated on the postoperative radiographs (31). Even though this long-term follow up showed satisfactory outcome, I now use the S1 sacral spinal rod described in the collapsing kyphosis in all patients older than 1 year of age.

Occasionally, there is an associated congenital scoliosis in the same area of the congenital kyphosis. In most instances, resection of the two vertebrae proximal to the apical vertebra allows correction of both the scoliosis and the kyphosis. There is also an increased incidence of diastematomyelia at the proximal end of

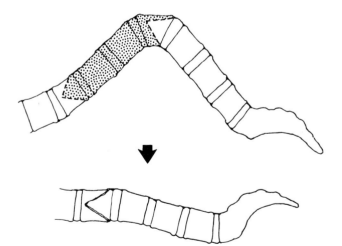

FIGURE 19. Stippled area shows the bone removed for correction of a rigid *S*-shaped lumbar kyphosis. It usually includes one or two vertebrae proximal to the apical vertebra in the area of the fixed lordosis. The vertebrae proximal to the resection and the apical vertebra are shaped to receive each other in a tongue-and-groove joint to provide stability until bony union is achieved. (From La Marca F, Herman M, Grant JA, et al. [1997]: Presentation and management of hydromyelia in children with Chiari type-II malformation. *Pediatr Neurosurg* 26(2):57–67, with permission).

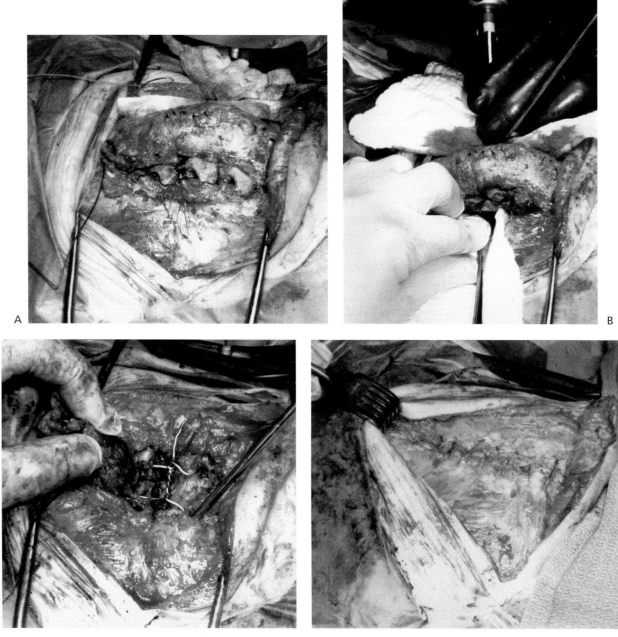

FIGURE 20. Operative photographs of resection of the proximal vertebrae in an *S*-shaped kyphosis. **A:** The head of the child is at the left. A transverse skin incision has been used. The dural sac can be seen posterior to the spine. The paraspinous muscles have been stripped from the spinous process and the lamina. This shows the anatomy of the turned-out lamina and spinous process. The paraspinous muscles are anterior to the spine. **B:** The segmental vessels and nerves have been divided. Soft tissues are stripped from the front of the spine from each side. A lap sponge is used to protect the soft tissues from the periosteal elevators. **C:** Two vertebrae (T12 and L1) have been removed above the apical (L2) vertebra. The apical vertebra has been pushed down to the proximal vertebra (T11). The reduction is held by two stainless-steel wires around the pedicle of T11 and L3. These wires are visible in place. The spine now lies anterior to the paraspinous muscles. **D:** The paraspinous muscles have been closed behind the dural sac and the spine.

the myelomeningocele. This should also be addressed at the time of the vertebral excision.

Surgical Technique

Newborn

A technique similar to the procedure described for a collapsing kyphosis in newborns should be performed. In most cases, the proximal lordosis is not rigid in newborns, and satisfactory alignment can be obtained (Fig. 17). If the proximal lordosis is rigid, correction of the kyphosis should be delayed until the child is at least 1 year of age.

One Year or Older

If the kyphosis is not corrected at the time of the sac closure in the newborn period, the procedure should be delayed until the child is at least the size of a 1-year-old, although the child may be considerably older than 1 year chronologically. A midline incision is made from at least three vertebrae proximal to the last complete neural arch to the midsacrum.

The dissection is started proximally three levels above the last intact vertebral arch and carried distally along the everted spinous process and lamina. The incision is made in the periosteum overlying the posterior surface of these vertebrae and by extraperiosteal dissection. The paraspinous muscles are removed from the undersurface of the spinous process, lamina, and transverse process (Fig. 18). This dissection extends from the last intact arch to the sacrum. The dural sac is freed from the lamina and the inner border of the pedicle, exposing the segmental nerves and vessels. The segmental nerves and vessels are ligated and divided, starting distal to the apical vertebra and extending a distance of at least two segments above the apical vertebra.

The everted spinous process, lamina, and transverse process of the apical vertebra and the two more proximal vertebrae are removed by rongeur. Using careful dissection with a Cobb periosteal elevator, the surgeon dissects the front part of the vertebra free of soft tissue attachments (Fig. 18). The anterior abdominal structures are protected by a sponge during the dissection, which is carried out from both sides. After dissection is complete, a malleable retractor is passed anterior to the vertebral bodies, protecting the soft tissues from injury. The neurotube is divided at one segment level distal to the apical vertebra, and the distal segment is oversewn for hemostasis. The proximal end is opened, and the neuroplate is dissected free of the dura and allowed to fall back into the sac. The sac is closed with a watertight closure with 6-0 silk dural suture. The surgeon then elevates the dural sac, cauterizing bleeding vessels, and retracts it proximally to expose the apical vertebra and the vertebra just proximal to the apex. The disc space between these vertebrae is incised with a scalpel. The anterior soft tissues are protected by the previously inserted malleable retractor. The disc space proximal to this vertebra is incised with a scalpel, and the entire vertebra is removed. This provides considerable relaxation to the spine and allows for additional exposure. The next most proximal vertebral end plate can then be seen. With careful dissection, it is possible to free this proximal vertebra circumferentially and excise it through the proximal disc space. Rarely are more than two vertebrae excised. The end plate of the proximal vertebra is denuded of

disc and growth plate, and a transverse groove is cut into the vertebral body about 1 cm deep and 1 cm high. The apical vertebra is shaped into a wedge by removing the disc and subchondral bone from its undersurface. This wedge-shaped vertebra fits into the groove of the proximal vertebra (Fig. 19) and is held in position by tension band wiring looped around the pedicle of the proximal vertebra and around the pedicle of the vertebra just distal to the apical vertebra (Fig. 20). Bone graft obtained from the excised vertebrae is placed around the osteotomy site. The dura is allowed to fall back into its normal position.

The S1 nerve root and artery are ligated and divided. The prebent sacral rod is carefully inserted through the S1 foramen, similar to the procedure described previously for a collapsing *C*-shaped kyphosis. Proximally, the rod is held by at least three sublaminar wires and the rod cut 2 inches longer than the most proximal wire. In a child older than 10 years of age, a fusion is performed along the instrumented spine.

Paraspinous muscles are freed of attachments to the quadratus lumborum and, if necessary, from the lateral abdominal musculature. The paraspinous muscles are closed over the dural sac posterior to the vertebrae (Fig. 20) to the level of about L3 to L4, where they begin to attach to the ilium. A hemovac drain is placed for drainage, and the skin is closed.

Typical blood loss during this procedure is 50% or more of blood volume (28). It is therefore necessary to perform blood replacement and to maintain blood volume during the procedure.

Postoperatively, the child is kept flat for 24 hours to avoid cerebrospinal fluid leakage. Thereafter, the child may sit up and move with assistance to wheelchair. No cast or brace is used. Activities are limited to avoid bending, twisting, reaching, or lifting for a period of 3 months. The child may then begin his or her usual activities.

Revision Surgery

Occasionally, the deformity recurs as the child matures. This does not represent a failure of the initial surgery. In most instances, growth has occurred, increasing the length of the spine, and the deformity is still less than it would have been without treatment. If it becomes necessary to reoperate, a procedure similar to that described for a collapsing kyphosis can be performed. The instrumentation is anchored to the pelvis in the same fashion, and a fusion is carried out throughout the length of the instrumented spine. The area of increase in the kyphosis is usually distal to the previous osteotomy and fusion, forming a collapsing *C*-shaped type of curve (Fig. 18).

REFERENCES

1. Allen BL Jr. (1979): The operative treatment of myelomeningocele spinal deformity. *Orthop Clin North Am* 10:845.
2. Banta JV, Hamanda JS (1976): Natural history of the kyphotic deformity in myelomeningocele. *J Bone Joint Surg Am* 58:279.
3. Banta JV, Whiteman S, Dyck RM, et al. (1976): Fifteen year review of myelodysplasia. *J Bone Joint Surg Am* 58:726.
5. Bunch WH (1975): The Milwaukee brace in paralytic scoliosis. *Clin Orthop* 110:63.
4. Bunch WH (1976): Treatment of the myelomeningocele spine. *Instr Course Lect* 25:93.

6. Bunch WH, Scarff TB, Dvonch VM (1983): Progressive loss in myelomeningocele patients. *Orthop Trans* 7:185.

7. Carstens C, Schneider E (1989): Zur Kenntnis der partiellen Wirbelsäulenaplasie. *Z Orthop* 127:569–574.

8. Drennan JC (1970): The role of muscles in the development of human lumbar kyphosis. *Dev Med Child Neurol* 12:33.

9. Drummond DS, Moreau M, Cruess RL (1980): The results and complications of surgery for the paralytic hip and spine in myelomeningocele. *J Bone Joint Surg Br* 62:49.

10. Dubousset J, Herring JA, Shufflebarger H (1989): The crankshaft phenomenon. *J Pediatr Orthop* 9:541–550.

11. Dunn HK (1983): Kyphosis of myelodysplasia: operative treatment based on pathophysiology. *Orthop Trans* 7:19.

12. Eyring EJ, Wanken JJ, Sayers MP (1972): Spinal osteotomy for kyphosis in myelomeningocele. *Clin Orthop* 88:24.

13. Hall JE, Martin R (1970): *The natural history of spine deformity in myelomeningocele: a study of 130 patients.* Presented at the Canadian Orthopaedic Association meeting, Bermuda, June.

14. Hall JE, Poitra B: The management of kyphosis in patients with myelomeningocele. *Clin Orthop* 128:33.

15. Hall PV, Campbell RH, Kalsbeck JE (1975): Myelomeningocele and progressive hydromyelia: Progressive paresis in myelodysplasia. *J Neurosurg* 43:457.

16. Hall PV, Lindseth RE, Campbell RL, et al. (1976): Myelodysplasia and developmental scoliosis. *Spine* 1:48.

17. Hall PV, Lindseth RE, Campbell RL, et al. (1979): Scoliosis and hydrocephalus in myelocele patients: the effect of ventricular shunting. *J Neurosurg* 50:174.

18. Heinig CF, Boyd BM Jr (1985): One stage vertebrectomy or eggshell procedure. *Orthop Trans* 9:130–131.

19. Heinz ER, Rosenbaum AE, Scarff TB, et al. (1979): Tethered spinal cord following myelomeningocele repair. *Radiology* 131:153.

20. Heydemann JS, Gillespie R (1987): Management of myelomeningocele kyphosis in the older child by kyphectomy and segmental spinal instrumentation. *Spine* 12:37–41.

21. Hopf CG, Eysel P, Dubousset J (1997): Operative treatment of scoliosis with Cotrel-Dubousset-Hopf instrumentation: new anterior spinal device. *Spine* 26(6):618–627.

22. Hoppenfeld S (1967): Congenital kyphosis in myelomeningocele. *J Bone Joint Surg Br* 49:276.

23. Hull WJ, Moe JH, Lai C, et al. (1974): The surgical treatment of spinal deformities in myelomeningocele. *J Bone Joint Surg Am* 57:1767.

24. Hull WJ, Moe JN, Winter RB (1974): Spinal deformity in myelomeningocele: natural history, evaluation, and treatment. *J Bone Joint Surg Am* 56:1767.

25. La Marca F, Herman M, Grant JA, et al. (1997): Presentation and management of hydromyelia in children with Chiari type-II malformation. *Pediatr Neurosurg* 26(2):57–67.

26. Lindseth RE (1990): Myelomeningocele. In: Morrissy RT, ed. *Lovell and Winters' pediatric orthopaedics,* 3rd ed. Philadelphia: JB Lippincott, p. 552.

27. Lindseth RE (1978): Posterior osteotomy for fixed pelvic obliquity. *J Bone Joint Surg Am* 60:17.

28. Lindseth RE, Graziano GP (1988): One stage anterior transpedicular and unilateral fusion for congenital scoliosis. *Orthop Trans* 12:184.

29. Lindseth RE, Slezer L (1979): Vertebral excision for kyphosis in children with myelomeningocele. *J Bone Joint Surg Am* 61:699.

30. Lindseth RE (1991): Spine deformity in myelomeningocele. *Instr Course Lect* 40:276.

31. Lintner SA, Lindseth RE (1994): The long-term follow-up after proximal vertebral resection in children with myelomeningocele and a kyphos deformity. *J Bone Joint Surg Am* 76:1301–1307.

32. Loder RT, Shapiro P, Towbin R, et al. (1991): Aortic anatomy in children with myelomeningocele and congenital lumbar kyphosis. *J Pediatr Orthop* 11:31–35.

33. Lubicky JP, Fredrickson BE (1985): The combined use of kyphectomy, spinal cord resection, Luque instrumentation, and myocutaneous flaps for severe kyphosis in the myelomeningocele. *Orthop Trans* 9:495.

34. McCarthy RE (1991): Personal communication.

35. McLaughlin TP, Banta JV, Gahm NH, et al (1986): Intraspinal rhizotomy and distal cordectomy in patients with myelomeningocele. *J Bone Joint Surg Am* 68:88.

36. McMaster MJ (1987): Anterior and posterior instrumentation and fusion of thoracolumbar scoliosis due to myelomeningocele. *J Bone Joint Surg Br* 69:20.

37. Mackel JL, Lindseth RE (1975): Scoliosis in myelodysplasia. *J Bone Joint Surg Am* 57:1031.

38. Mayfield JK (1981): Severe spine deformity in myelodysplasia and sacral agenesis: an aggressive surgical approach. *Spine* 6:498.

39. Mazur J, Menelaus MB, Dicksen DR, et al. (1986): Efficacy of surgical management for scoliosis in myelomeningocele: correction of deformity and alteration of functional status. *J Pediatr Orthop* 6:568.

40. Moe JK, Winter RB, Bradford DS, et al. (1987): *Scoliosis and other spinal deformities.* Philadelphia: WB Saunders.

41. Osebold WR, Mayfield JK, Winter RB, et al. (1982): Surgical treatment of the paralytic scoliosis associated with myelomeningocele. *J Bone Joint Surg Am* 64:841.

42. Pontari MA, Bauer SB, Hall JE, et al. (1998): Adverse urologic consequence of spinal cord resection at the time of kyphectomy: value of preoperative urodynamic evaluation. *J Pediatr Orthop* 18:820–823.

43. Raycroft JE, Curtis BH (1972): *Spinal curvature in myelomeningocele: natural history and etiology.* St. Louis: CV Mosby.

44. Sharrard WJW (1968): Spinal osteotomy for congenital kyphosis in myelomeningocele. *J Bone Joint Surg Br* 50:466.

45. Sarwark JF, Weber DT, Gabrieli AP, et al. (1996): Tethered cord syndrome in low motor level children with myelomeningocele. *Pediatr Neurosurg* 25(6):295–301.

46. Sharrard WJW (1972): *The kyphotic and lordotic spine in myelomeningocele.* St. Louis: CV Mosby.

47. Shurleff DB, Bourney R, Gordon LH, et al. (1976): Myelodysplasia: the natural history of kyphosis and scoliosis. A preliminary report. *Dev Med Child Neurol* 18[Suppl 37]:126.

48. Sriram K, Bobrtchko WT, Hall JE (1972): Surgical management of spinal deformities in spina bifida. *J Bone Joint Surg Br* 54:666.

49. Terek RM, Wehner J, Lubicky JP (1991): The crankshaft phenomenon in congenital scoliosis. *Orthop Trans* 15:26–27.

50. Warner WC, Vander Woude L, Fackler CD (1990): Comparison of two instrumentation techniques in treatment of lumbar kyphosis in myelodysplasia. *Orthop Trans* 14:768.

51. Winter RB, Moe JN, Eilers VE (1968): Congenital scoliosis: a study of 234 patients treated and untreated. Part I. Natural history. Part II. Treatment. *J Bone Joint Surg Am* 50:1.

POLIOMYELITIS SCOLIOSIS

PO-QUANG CHEN
YOUNG-SHUNG SHEN

Acute poliomyelitis is an infectious disease caused by one of the three polioviruses known as Leon (type 3), Lansing (type 2), and Brunhilde (type 1). Humans and monkeys are the only hosts for polioviruses. In humans, these viruses have a specific affinity for nervous tissue and, in particular, for the large motor neurons of the anterior horn of the brain stem and spinal cord. Most poliovirus infections have a benign course, with no or only mild gastrointestinal symptoms. Less than 1% develop into the severe paralytic form.

Poliomyelitis was recognized as a clinical entity in the first half of the nineteenth century. Large epidemics occurred in Europe and North America until the first half of the twentieth century. There have been no large-scale epidemics since the immunization programs using both the Salk and the Sabin vaccines (57,58), but endemic outbreaks are still reported in third-world countries, where sanitary conditions are poor and large-scale immunization has not been accomplished. In 1988, the World Health Assembly adopted the goal of worldwide poliomyelitis eradication by the year 2000. Despite substantial progress in that direction, there remain multitudes of postpolio patients in need of scoliosis surgery. In China alone, about 60,000 of these patients need scoliosis surgery (71).

Poliomyelitis is primarily an intestinal infection. The virus gains entrance by way of the oropharynx and can be isolated from the pharynx and feces in both the preparetic and postparetic stages. The virus can be discovered from the blood of abortive cases of poliomyelitis and from chimpanzees after oral feedings (2). However, once the central nervous system is invaded, the motor neuron cells of the anterior horns of the spinal cord and brain stem are destroyed or temporarily lose the ability to function. This loss of function in the motor neuron may be either reversible or irreversible, which is reflected clinically by the recovery of some muscle power in certain patients.

The true incidence of scoliosis in poliomyelitic patients cannot be determined precisely. Colonna and Vom Saal (11) found that of 600 patients with poliomyelitis, 150 developed scoliosis. An island-wide survey of 840 polio victims was conducted during 1986 and 1987 in Taiwan. Scoliosis with Cobb angle larger than 10 degrees was found in 144 children (17.14%) (65). Kuo

and colleagues (31) stated that in a long-term follow-up of 118 adult polio victims in southern Taiwan, the most common deformity was scoliosis (67.8%), followed by limb length inequality (54.1%) and foot deformity (51.7%).

CURVE PATTERNS IN POLIOSCOLIOSIS

The type and severity of the scoliotic curvature depends on the level of involvement of the spinal cord, extent and residual power of the involved trunk muscles, and pelvic obliquity (20,24, 36,41,42). Thus, the curve may be in the high thoracic, thoracolumbar, or lumbar area, depending on which groups of muscles are paralyzed.

Roaf (56) classified the curve patterns into four types:

1. The thoracolumbar C-shaped curve is supposed to occur in patients with relatively slight paralysis and who have been allowed to get up too early. The deformity becomes more evident on standing.
2. The general "collapse" type, or combined thoracic and lumbar curve, is usually caused by extensive spinal weakness. The curves are mobile, and head suspension usually produces marked correction. Rotational deformity is moderate.
3. The primary lumbar curve is caused by a combination of pelvic obliquity resulting from limb length inequality and imbalance of the trunk muscles. Compensatory thoracic curves of less magnitude are often noted. This is the common type.
4. The primary thoracic curve is often associated with weakness of the scapular muscles, and there are secondary compensatory curves above and below.

In a series of 144 children among the 840 polio victims, as surveyed by the Cheng Hsin Rehabilitation Center, lumbar scoliosis was found in 71 patients (49.31%), followed by thoracolumbar curve in 34 patients (23.61%), double major thoracic and lumbar curve in 26 (18.06%), and thoracic curve in 13 (9.03%) patients (65). Mayer and associates (43), in a study of 118 cases of polioscoliosis, found that the most common deformity was the double major thoracic and lumbar curve (92 cases), followed by the thoracic, or thoracolumbar curve (20 cases). Long C-shaped curves were infrequent. From 1977 to 1988, 404 patients with polioscoliosis were operated on to correct the spinal deformity at Pingtung Christian Hospital. The curve pat-

P-Q Chen: Department of Orthopedic Surgery, College of Medicine, National Taiwan University, Taipei, Taiwan.

Y-S Shen: Po-Cheng Orthopedic Institute, Kaohsiung, Taiwan.

terns were classified as double major thoracic and lumbar, 223 cases (55.2%); thoracolumbar (C type), 95 cases (23.5%); lumbar, 68 cases (16.8%); thoracic, 17 cases (4.2%); and double thoracic, 1 case (0.3%). Pelvic obliquity was noted in 339 patients, with 207 patients having a pelvic tilt angle of more than 30 degrees.

Because of severe rotation of the spine, kyphosis in the lumbar spine and lordosis in the thoracic spine are frequently noted in these patients. Rotation of the thoracic spine also produces a prominent rib hump and significant thoracic cage deformity. For these reasons, surgical exposure of the spine and implant placement is difficult. If the spine is left untreated, the disc spaces become narrow, the vertebral bodies and the laminae become hypoplastic and osteoporotic, and adjacent spinal segments on the concave side may coalesce. Therefore, the corrective spinal surgery is more difficult in polio patients than in patients with idiopathic scoliosis.

PATIENT EVALUATION FOR SCOLIOSIS

The principles of evaluation of scoliosis secondary to polio are basically the same as those for idiopathic scoliosis or scoliosis of other etiologies. Unfortunately, polio patients often present for surgical correction of the spine when curves are severe and progressing. Because the natural history of polioscoliosis is not as clear as that of idiopathic scoliosis, it is difficult to predict outcome and eventual severity of the curve. Fortunately, most scoliosis secondary to polio appears be mild and nonprogressive.

Patients must be followed annually with a careful examination and the orthopedic conditions recorded in detail. The extent of muscle involvement, degree of motor power, and any deformity, joint contracture, or limb length inequality must be measured and recorded. The presence of pelvic obliquity and the ambulatory status of the patient (independent walking, crutch-assisted walking, or wheelchair use) are significant for determining the optimal methods and time of treatment of the joint and spine problems. The degree of limb length inequality and the presence of pelvic obliquity accentuate the deformity in the lumbar region. Pavon and Manning (53) noted that leg length inequality was present in about half of their patients with pelvic obliquity.

The severity and location of the spinal deformity in three dimensions may modify the treatment plan. The age of the patient and growth potential at the onset of scoliosis are also important factors in determining management and predicting the outcome of treatment. In young patients, in whom the spine is relatively flexible, surgical correction may be easier. In more mature patients in their late 20s to early 30s with severe curves, the bone stock may be very porotic, and the spine may be severely rotated. Disc spaces become narrow, and the facet joints fuse together; these may render the spinal segments more rigid. Serial casting, brace application, and surface electrical muscular stimulation are ineffective in controlling or correcting spinal deformity in this group of patients. Physiotherapy or muscle training also fails to reduce or even maintain curve magnitude (5,48,55). Braces can be used in young children with collapsing spines, but it is not effective in the long-term (13).

CORRECTION OF LIMB DEFORMITIES

Perry and coauthors (54) considered the postpolio syndrome to be the result of overuse of muscles in adulthood. Modification of lifestyle and use of orthosis or other passive devices are important for these patients. Surgical procedures to correct and stabilize deformities are often necessary.

Irwin (28) believed that abduction contracture of one side hip was a major etiologic factor in producing an oblique pelvis and secondary scoliosis. In teenagers, hip or knee contracture may cause difficulty in ambulation. A soft tissue procedure, such as the Campbell (6) or Wilson (69) procedure, can easily release the deformities caused by such contracture. Hip dislocation may occur if pelvic tilting becomes severe. Complete release of abduction contracture of the hip (18) or pelvic osteotomy and muscle transfer (32) is helpful in stabilizing the hip joint. Lee and associates (33) classified two types of pelvic obliquity resulting from poliomyelitis, according to the level of the pelvis relative to the short leg. In the subtype D, in which moderate to severe paralytic scoliosis was noted, appropriate spinal fusion was usually necessary. Lumbar lordosis and anterior tilt of the pelvis may aggravate flexion contracture of the hip (18). In this circumstance, unless the flexion contracture is severe enough to interfere with the spinal approach, the spinal deformity should be corrected first; otherwise, further release may be necessary.

Foot deformities are corrected by various procedures, such as Achilles tendon lengthening for the equinus deformity and tendon transfer for varus or valgus deformities of the foot. Bony procedures are reserved for patients older than 12 years of age and when soft tissue procedures are not sufficient to maintain stability or provide good function. Osteotomy of the lower femur or upper tibia can be done to correct the valgus or varus deformity of the knee. Triple arthrodesis is often necessary for the correction of foot deformities. Limb length inequality can also be corrected with modern leg lengthening devices. A balanced and stable trunk is crucial for performing daily activities.

PULMONARY FUNCTION

Nickel and colleagues (46) demonstrated that respiratory paralysis due to poliomyelitis results from severe involvement of the muscles in the trunk and extremities; however, the breathing ability of these patients does not dictate their ability to tolerate surgery. It merely indicates their relative need for mechanical respiratory assistance during and immediately after surgery.

Werner and coauthors (68) found that vital capacity was significantly restricted in some patients with extensive respiratory muscle paralysis. Mackley and associates (39) studied pulmonary function in both paralytic and nonparalytic groups and found that pulmonary function was significantly impaired if the Cobb angle was greater than 66 degrees in the thoracic spine. Preliminary cast correction of the curvature reduced vital capacity, whereas halo traction had no influence on it. There was also no significant improvement of pulmonary function after spinal fusion. Swank and associates (63) reported a series of 20 severe scoliosis patients (curves ranging from 90 to 200 degrees) who had overt cor pulmonale. The results of preoperative halo traction showed that, in polioscoliosis patients, there was an average increase of vital capacity and PaO_2, whereas $PaCO_2$ was reduced. Bradford (4) recommended preliminary halo traction to facilitate the evaluation of the reversibility of pulmonary dysfunction and to improve the patient's general cardiopulmonary status before surgery.

In our experience of 38 adult patients with severe polioscoliosis, 35 were found to have impaired pulmonary function. Single-staged or multiple-staged surgery did not result in exacerbation of the patients' cardiopulmonary status. However, the patients were taught to perform pulmonary exercise long before surgery. On admission, patients should be taught to use the respirator; this will reduce the morbidity if overt respiratory insufficiency occurs immediately after surgery.

Modern anesthetic techniques and improved monitoring devices, such as right heart catheterization, continuous arterial monitoring, and serial blood gas studies, enable the detection of subtle changes in cardiopulmonary status and allow early correction. Tracheotomy is rarely needed either before or after surgery.

INDICATIONS FOR SURGICAL CORRECTION

Curve Progression

Curve progression is the main reason patients seek treatment. In progressive thoracic curvatures, the deformity can be severe. The thoracic cage becomes prominent, with secondary pulmonary function impairment. In patients with lumbar scoliosis, pelvic tilting can be relentless, causing severe trunk deviation and unilateral ischial sitting. The goal of treatment of spinal deformity is to obtain a vertical torso centered over a level pelvis. This permits stable sitting on level buttocks and helps prevent ischial pressure callosities and paralytic dislocation of the hip on the high side of the pelvis. The patient does not have to use the arms for support and is able to use both hands freely to perform other activities. When the spinal curvature is severe or is collapsing, the lower costal margin sometimes impinges against the upper margin of the iliac crest, causing pain. Respiratory capacity and ambulation are also hampered. In this situation, a straight and stable spine can relieve symptoms and facilitate walking. Back pain may be a major problem in adult polioscoliosis patients.

Curve Magnitude

Surgery should be considered only when the Cobb angle is larger than 40 degrees or when the spine is collapsing. The indications for posterior instrumentation only are thoracic and long *C*-shaped curves with minimal pelvic obliquity or thoracolumbar or lumbar curves of less than 60 degrees. If the curvature is larger than 60 degrees, whether flexible or rigid, or pelvic obliquity is severe, a two-staged anterior and posterior surgery should be recommended because this results in better correction of the deformity and less pseudarthrosis (8,34,43). This combined approach may be performed in single or separate occasions.

PROCEDURES FOR SURGICAL CORRECTION OF SCOLIOSIS

Application of Halo Traction

The halo was developed by Nickel and colleagues (47). DeWald and Ray (12) and O'Brien and associates in Hong Kong (52) popularized the application of halo-pelvis traction in ambulatory patients, such as polioscoliosis and the spinal deformity caused by spinal tuberculosis. The apparatus is mounted on patients with severe scoliotic curves or kyphoscoliotic deformity before definitive surgery. Clark and coauthors (10) found that the maximal effect was achieved about 1 week after initiation and that a 2-week period was usually sufficient to release the viscoelastic properties of muscular and ligamentous tension. The advantage of the apparatus is that it provides effective, controlled distraction of the spine.

Because of possible neurologic and pelvic pin complications (16,30,35,66) and inconvenience of ambulation after femoral pin insertion, halo gravity traction is now used when traction is deemed necessary (Fig. 1). Traction can be exerted anytime to the halo, with the patient either lying in bed, sitting on the bed or on a wheelchair, or even walking with the imposed weight attached to the wheelchair. Preliminary traction is used when the scoliotic spine in a child is stiff and severe or the Cobb angle is greater than 100 degrees (57,58). However, the use of preliminary halo traction has been challenged. Flierl and Carstens (19) claimed that halo gravity traction only accounted for 16.9% improvement in six patients with severe polioscoliosis. This method can also be used between staged surgery to reduce the severe curvature, when no implant is added after the completion of anterior spinal release. This is our preferred method. If an anterior implant is placed, halo traction becomes superfluous. The maximal load should be about one third of the body weight. The load should be determined by the patient's tolerance. Daily evaluation of the pin tightness and pin care are mandatory. Repeated neurologic evaluations are also mandatory.

Posterior Instrumentation of the Spine

Bunch (5) considered orthotics to be effective in preventing curve progression in young children with paralytic scoliosis. The number of patients under study was small, however, and the follow-up period was only 2 years. Present concepts exclude the use of orthosis in polio scoliosis (13).

The introduction of Harrington instrumentation in the early 1960s revolutionized the treatment of scoliosis (25–27). The experience of Rancho Los Amigos Hospital using halo-femoral traction and posterior Harrington instrumentation showed that the best result for paralytic scoliosis was a 57% correction; the pseudarthrosis rate was 27% (3). Gui and colleagues (23), using Harrington instrumentation, showed that the curve correction rate was 37% for thoracic scoliosis, 40% for lumbar scoliosis, and 28% for double scoliosis. Loss of correction is generally a result of hardware loosening or bending before fusion. After solid fusion, it does not progress.

The segmental spinal instrumentation system devised by Luque (38) is a powerful implant for the correction and stabilization of spinal deformities. Basically, it consists of two smooth, round, L-shaped rods on both sides of the spinous

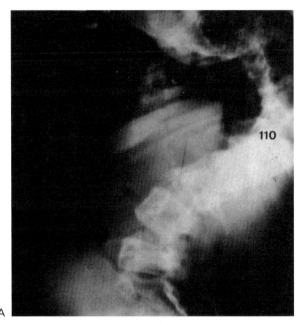

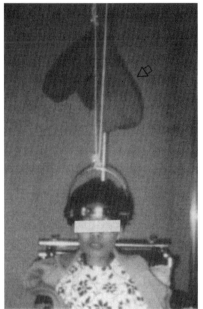

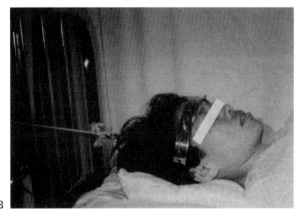

FIGURE 1. A 30-year-old woman with rigid kyphoscoliosis. She underwent two-staged surgery. A halo was also mounted between the operations. **A:** Radiograph reveals 110-degree thoracic scoliosis and 99-degree kyphosis. **B:** The patient under traction while lying in bed. **C:** The patient under halo gravity traction while sitting in a wheelchair. The traction apparatus was connected high on the wheelchair; the *arrow* denotes the sandbags. In this manner, the patient can achieve continuous traction in different positions during the entire day.

processes. Correction of scoliosis is accomplished by twisting stainless steel sublaminar wires to the precontoured rods at each level of lamina. By sequential twisting of the wires, the rods and laminae are approximated, and the deformed segments of the spine are gradually straightened. Bone chips are placed in the excised facet joints and the exposed bony parts of the spine (Fig. 2). This instrumentation is strong enough to resist torsional and compressive stresses (9,29,44,67). Luque instrumentation is suitable for the correction of small-angle curvatures, but the instrumented segments should be long enough to avoid junctional kyphosis. Instrumentation should not end at the apex of a curve in any plane.

Cardoso (7), Sullivan and Conner (62), and Taddonio (64) reported that the use of Luque rods for neuromuscular scoliosis resulted in a balanced spine because of better correction in the coronal and sagittal planes. In nearly all patients operated on, external support became unnecessary; pulmonary function also improved. If fusion and correction to the pelvis are necessary, lower Harrington hooks can be placed at the sacral rim (Fig. 3). The Galveston technique, by contouring the lower end of the rods to enter iliac wings, is favorable (1,21).

Arthrodesis of the spine in a young child results in growth retardation of the spine (22,45). Luque and Cardoso (37) reported that segmental spinal fixation of the involved spine without bone grafting could be a good alternative in a growing child. The advantages include good control of the curve, expected continuous spinal growth, and elimination of the need for bracing. Eberle (17) reported a series of 16 patients with severe paralytic polioscoliosis who were between 5 and 12 years old. In 15 of the 16 patients, the segmental spinal implants failed to control the deformity. In these patients, however, the Cobb angle was the same before and after correction. Spontaneous fusion of the instrumented portion of the spine was also noted in some cases. Implant complications were noted, including rod breakage, longitudinal shifting, and rotation of the short limb of the rod out of the pelvis, which perforated the skin and resulted in infection.

In older children with paralytic scoliosis due to poliomyelitis, Harrington rods with segmental wiring or the combination of Harrington and Luque rods is preferable to Harrington rods alone (Fig. 4). A Harrington square-ended rod is placed on the concave side of the curve and inserted into the squared hole of the hooks, whereas a Luque rod is placed on the convex side.

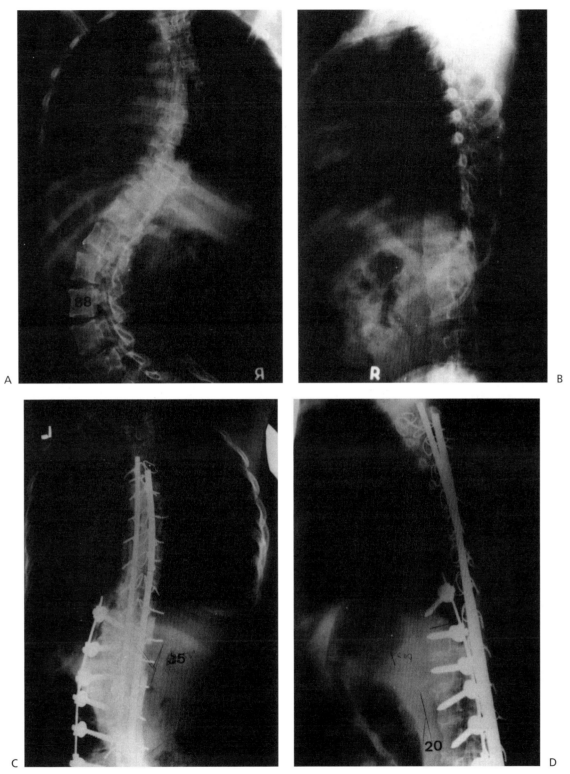

FIGURE 2. This 18-year-old girl needed crutches and pelvic shift for walking. Anterior Zielke VDS and subsequent Luque rods were implanted. **A, B:** Radiographs reveal 88-degree lumbar scoliosis and 5-degree lordosis. **C, D:** Radiographs show the spinal contour 2 years after surgery.

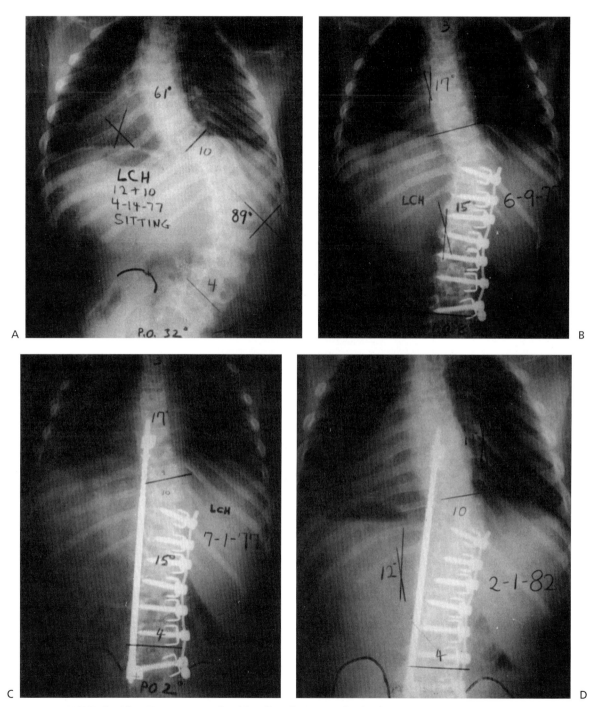

FIGURE 3. A boy 12 years 10 months with polioscoliosis. He walked with crutches. **A:** Radiograph reveals scoliosis with a 61-degree Cobb angle from T2 to T9 and an 89-degree Cobb angle from T10 to L4. Pelvic obliquity is 32 degrees. **B:** After Dwyer instrumentation, the scoliosis is reduced to 15 degrees at the lower curvature. Pelvic obliquity is now less than 8 degrees. **C, D:** The spine after Harrington instrumentation and at 56 months' follow-up. The coronal balance was well corrected and maintained. Note that the lower Harrington hook was anchored at the sacral rim.

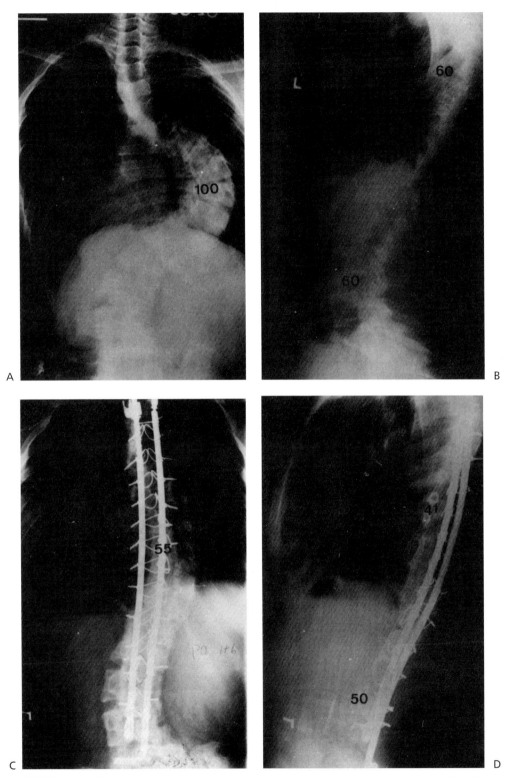

FIGURE 4. This 20-year-old woman underwent anterior release and rib grafting. Two weeks later, combined posterior Harrington-Luque instrumentation and fusion were performed. **A, B:** Lower thoracic scoliosis with a Cobb angle of 100 degrees and thoracic kyphosis of 60 degrees. **C, D:** Spinal contour 18 months after correction. Both coronal and sagittal planes were much improved.

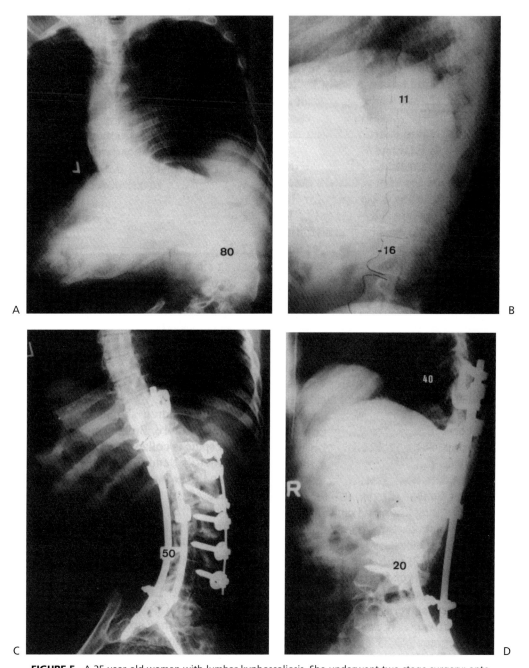

FIGURE 5. A 25-year-old woman with lumbar kyphoscoliosis. She underwent two-stage surgery: anterior Zielke VDS and posterior Cotrel-Dubousset instrumentation from T9 to S1. She had no external support after the second instrumentation. **A, B:** Lumbar scoliosis was 80 degrees, and lordosis was 16 degrees. **C, D:** The spine 3 years after surgery.

Both rods can be bent according to the magnitude and contour of the deformity. With proper distraction of the Harrington rod and segmental wiring of both rods, this combined method is useful for the correction of cases with large Cobb angles. Both these implants should be available as a correcting device in countries where resources are still inadequate. If pelvic obliquity is to be corrected simultaneously, fixation and fusion to the pelvic region can be helpful. In the severe and rigid curves, anterior release and instrumentation are usually necessary. Many new

implants have been developed, such as Cotrel-Dubousset instrumentation (Fig. 5), Isola, TSRH, or Moss-Miami. Using these modern implants, the deformity can be corrected without the need for external support.

Anterior Surgery on the Spine

Dwyer (14,15) introduced a cable and screw system for correction and stabilization of the spine. O'Brien and colleagues

(49–51) adopted it to correct scoliosis due to poliomyelitis. They recommended combined, staged anterior and posterior correction and fusion using Dwyer-Harrington instrumentation. Preliminary halo-femoral traction was preferred for cases with pelvic obliquity or rigid and severe curves. In a study of 110 patients from Hong Kong, Leong and associates (34) demonstrated that combined anterior Dwyer instrumentation and fusion and posterior Harrington instrumentation and fusion resulted in excellent correction. In the lumbar region, the correction rate was 79% for moderate curves and 64% for severe, major curves. Pelvic obliquity was also corrected. For rigid thoracic and long *C*-shaped curves, the combined procedure also gave better correction, but with higher morbidity in the former group. Preoperative traction was found to be useful only in rigid curves and in those with a Cobb angle larger than 80 degrees. The pseudarthrosis rate was 12.5% for long *C*-shaped curves, 7% for lumbar curves, and 0% for thoracic curves, This was in contrast to a 25% pseudarthrosis rate for patients having posterior fusion alone.

The experience in Taiwan (43) with 54 patients who had traction and combined Dwyer-Harrington procedures was also reported. The preoperative Cobb angle for the upper and lower curves averaged 79 degrees and 115 degrees, respectively. After surgery, these were reduced to 52 degrees (40.73%) in the upper curve and 60 degrees (56.2%) in the lower curve. In 20 patients operated on using only Harrington instrumentation and fusion, the correction was 43.2% in the upper curve and 44% in the lower curve. The correction of pelvic obliquity was 43.6% after the posterior fusion only procedure and 68.4% after the combined procedure. In a further study of 290 patients with double major thoracolumbar and lumbar polioscoliosis, pelvic obliquity was reduced from 35.5 degrees to 14.2 degrees (59.9%) (59).

Zielke and coauthors (70) reported the experience of anterior ventrale derotations-spondylodese (VDS) instrumentation to correct scoliosis in the thoracolumbar and lumbar regions. More recently, the more rigid implants, such as Webb-Morley, Moss-Miami, and so forth, have replaced the previously mentioned systems.

If anterior instrumentation is not used after anterior release, or if the patient has a double major curve, halo gravity traction can be applied during the waiting period for posterior surgery. In adult scoliosis, the patients usually present with a very rigid and severely rotated large curve, and the spine becomes osteoporotic and hypoplastic, the disc spaces are narrow, and the bony parts become adhered. Therefore, two- or three-staged surgery is mandatory. This generally consists of initial anterior release and fusion using rib or pelvic bone grafts, followed by posterior release, long instrumentation, and bony fusion. In some patients, the posterior bony elements are fused, necessitating release of the fused bony segments as the first procedure. Halo gravity traction can be applied between the periods of a staged operation.

TREATMENT RECOMMENDATIONS

Young children should be carefully evaluated for spinal curvature. Bracing may be necessary, especially if the spine is collapsing. If curve progression is noted, Marchetti's "end-fusion" technique may be helpful in saving the growth potential of the vertebra (40). The chance of rod breakage in this technique is so high, however, that repeated surgery is inevitable.

For adolescents, when the spine is still supple and the curve is less than 60 degrees, there are several treatment alternatives. If the deformity is in the thoracic spine or is the collapsing long C type, we recommend double Luque rods or the Harrington-Luque combination. Both rods must be bent to conform to the contour of the spine; in the sagittal plane, thoracic kyphosis and lumbar lordosis are reconstituted, and the coronal plane deformity is also corrected. This greatly facilitates the patient's ambulation. The instrumentation and fusion segments should be long enough to avoid junctional kyphosis.

Harrington-Luque combination has both mechanical and clinical advantages. It allows both axial distraction and transverse correction. The rods can be contoured according to the shape of the spinal curvature. Using a curved pusher to approximate the rod to laminae, allowing close tightening of the wire loops during manual correction can further minimize the curvature. The final step is the application of wires to link the two rods at several levels to stabilize the whole construct. The square-ended Harrington rod is superior for the segmental correction of scoliosis because it prevents rotation of the rod during wiring. In most circumstances, external support after surgery is not necessary.

In countries in which economic conditions allow, Cotrel-Dubousset instrumentation or the newer implants, such as Isola, TSRH, or Moss-Miami, are preferred (Fig. 6). Better curve correction and increased stability have been noted. These implants have been widely adopted in the surgery of scoliosis. In choosing these implants, the size of the implant parts should be considered because many of these patients are very thin.

After the hooks and the pedicle screws are placed or inserted in the proper segments of the spine, the rod is carefully mounted over the heads of the hooks and screws. The parts are distracted or compressed along the rods, as needed, to minimize the curve and obtain the normal contour of the spine. Manual rotation of the rods is not an important procedure in the polio cases, however, because the aim of surgery is to achieve truncal stability and balance. At the end of instrumentation, the lumbar spine should be corrected to be in the form of lordosis to avoid the flat-back syndrome. This is important, especially in the lumbar scoliosis with kyphotic deformity.

Bone grafting technique must be carried out meticulously; the ligaments, tendons, and capsules must be removed completely. The facets must be excised and exposed completely. Bone chips are placed in the facet regions and are extended laterally to the transverse processes in the lumbar spine and the costotransverse processes in the thoracic spine.

For rigid curves and those larger than 60 degrees, or sometimes 80 degrees, or in the presence of obvious pelvic tilting, two-stage surgery is suggested. These patients usually have large lumbar curves. The Zielke VDS system or the newer anterior implant can be used anteriorly, and bone chips are placed in the released disc spaces as the first stage in the lumbar or thoracolumbar region. This results in better balance and stability of the trunk and correction of pelvic obliquity. The lower screws placed down to L5 are sufficient. In these cases, preliminary halo traction is not necessary. If anterior release is performed without

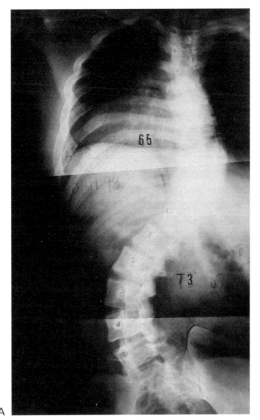

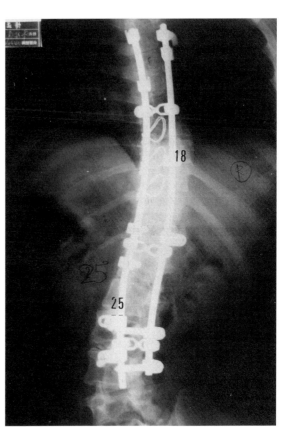

A

B

FIGURE 6. A 16½-year-old boy with double thoracic and lumbar scoliosis. He underwent two-staged surgery: anterior release of the lumbar spine from T12 to L4, followed by posterior Isola instrumentation extending from T4 to L4. **A:** The spine before surgery. The Cobb angle at the thoracic spine was 65 degrees and at the lumbar spine, 73 degrees. **B:** After Isola instrumentation, the Cobb angle in the thoracic spine was reduced to 18 degree; in the lumbar spine, it became 25 degrees.

instrumentation, halo traction is preferably used. The time between the two operations is about 10 days to 3 weeks, depending on the curve magnitude and the effect of traction. At the second stage, posterior instrumentation and spinal fusion are performed. This combined approach is advantageous in that the spinal construct can be more rigid, bony fusion rates are higher, and correction is better. If the deformity is in the thoracic region, anterior release and rib grafting, followed by posterior Luque or Harrington-Luque instrumentation, are sufficient.

Many polio victims present as adults with curve progression despite previous attempts at fusion or with a synostosis of the posterior bony elements. In these situations, posterior osteotomies should be considered. This is followed by traction, and possibly, further anterior release, if the disc spaces are still wide. The final stage is posterior instrumentation and fusion.

In selecting the fusion level, we should consider the conditions of the upper extremities. If the upper extremities are flaccid, fusion of both the thoracic and lumbar spine is necessary. This reflects the weakness of the upper trunk musculature. If the child had lumbar scoliosis without the presence of flaccid upper extremities, fusion of the lumbar curve down to fifth lumbar segment is enough. However, if both the thoracic and lumbar spine are deformed, fusion level depends on the magnitude of the thoracic curve. When the Cobb angle of the thoracic spine

is greater than 40 degrees, both segments should be fused; otherwise, fusion of only the lumbar segment is sufficient. In any case, it is desirable to achieve lumbar lordosis by using modern instrumentation, especially in adults.

Fusion down to sacrum should be carefully considered. If a patient needs pelvic swing to facilitate ambulation, fixation at the lumbosacral region will greatly impair ambulatory activity. Thus, if pelvic tilting is not severe, lumbosacral fusion should be avoided, in cases in which fusion to sacrum is desirable, instrumentation by the Luque-Galveston technique or by double sets of sacral screws offers better stability. Fusion to the sacrum is often necessary to provide truncal balance and to correct pelvic obliquity.

External support is not used in most cases. During hospitalization, patients are encouraged to exercise to maintain their strength, prevent osteoporosis, and avoid prolonged convalescence.

Long-segment fusion for polioscoliosis is usually the rule. This necessitates large amounts of bone chips. In idiopathic scoliosis, autogenous bone taken from one ilium or both ilia is enough. But many polio patients present with a hypoplastic pelvis, making the use of bone grafts from this area impractical. Allograft is often used alone or mixed with autograft. Because anterior fusion requires less bone graft, the resected rib, the iliac bone, or both are usually sufficient. Bony fusion is dependent on providing a large amount of exposed bony areas, performing meticulous facet joint excision, selecting suitable implants, and avoiding excessive loading.

POSTOPERATIVE CARE

Immediately after surgery, the neurologic status of the lower limbs must be checked. Adequate fluid replacement should be administered. Patients should be carefully monitored for respiratory status and cardiac function. Patients with obvious respiratory insufficiency should be monitored in the intensive care unit and given respiratory assistance as needed. Blood gas studies and chest radiographs must be obtained as a treatment guide. Abdominal distention can be annoying, but it is usually not too severe. Menthol packing of the abdominal wall or a rectal suppository to stimulate bowel peristalsis is usually adequate. Gastric tube decompression may be necessary if the abdominal distention is significant. Sphincter training is started soon after the surgery. Patients are allowed to sit 3 or 4 days after posterior instrumentation. A well-molded plastic jacket (TLSO), if needed, should be worn before the patient is allowed to walk.

PATIENT SATISFACTION

Some patients may have higher than reasonable expectations of the results of surgery. A thorough examination of the patient's musculoskeletal function and an understanding of his or her expectations are mandatory. Good communication between the surgeon, patient, and family must be obtained before surgery.

Shen and Cheung (60) studied patient satisfaction after combined anterior and posterior surgery in 148 polio cases. After an average of 4.7 years of follow-up, 117 patients (79.6%) were satisfied with the operative results. 53% of the patients still complained of low back pain after sitting or standing for long periods, but only three patients needed analgesics for relief; the remainder required only rest. Nearly half of the patients (49.7%) could walk more steadily and for a longer distance, but 17% of patients felt that they had more difficulty walking after spinal fusion. Daily activities were improved in 63.3% of the patients; however, 17.7% complained that after fusion their spines became stiffer, hampering their daily functions. The most gratifying result may be that patients have better sitting balance. Eighty-eight patients had to sit on one hip before the operation. At final follow-up study, 48% of the patients had achieved balanced ischial sitting, which greatly facilitates free motion of the upper extremities.

A 15-year or longer follow-up of 88 patients among this same group of patients was carried out (61). The most rewarding result was that after surgery, patients could sit on a stool without using their hands or any other support. This was noted in 54 (61.4%) cases, whereas only 12.9% of the patients could do this before surgery. Relief of back pain was also noted. At follow-up, only 19.3% complained of pain, whereas before surgery, 64% had this complaint. Interestingly, whether patients had fusion down to L5 or to the sacrum, there was no difference in terms of ambulation, daily activities, sitting balance, or back pain.

The management of spinal deformities is difficult in poliomyelitis and requires a thorough understanding of the condition, its natural history, and the alternatives of management. Realistic expectation and meticulous attention to surgical detail can lead to gratifying results.

ACKNOWLEDGMENTS

We appreciate the financial assistance from the Taiwan Spine Research Foundation and the National Science Council, ROC. Thanks are also extended to Dr. S. L. Weinstein for his kind suggestions.

REFERENCES

1. Allen BL Jr, Ferguson RL (1982): The Galveston technique for L-rod instrumentation of the scoliotic spine. *Spine* 7:119–127.
2. Bodian D (1952): Reconsideration of pathogenesis of poliomyelitis. *Am J Hygiene* 55:414–438.
3. Bonnett C, Brown JC, Perry J, et al. (1975): Evolution of treatment of paralytic scoliosis at Rancho Los Amigos Hospital. *J Bone Joint Surg Am* 57:206–215.
4. Bradford DS (1987): Neuromuscular spinal deformity. In: Bradford DS, ed. *Moe's textbook of scoliosis and other spinal deformities.* Philadelphia: WB Saunders, pp. 271–305.
5. Bunch W (1975): The Milwaukee brace in paralytic scoliosis. *Clin Orthop* 110:63–68.
6. Campbell WC (1923): Transference of the crest of the ilium for flexion contraction of the hip. *South Med J* 16:289.
7. Cardoso JJ (1984): Paralytic scoliosis. In: Luque ER, ed. *Segmental spinal instrumentation.* Thorofare, NJ: Slack, pp. 119–145.
8. Chen PQ (1990): *Surgical treatment of adult scoliosis.* Presented at the International Conference on Spinal Surgery; April 13; Taipei.
9. Chen PQ, Shi CM, Cheng CK, et al. (1990): Biomechanical studies of posterior spinal instrumentation system for scoliosis: an intact porcine spine model. *J Orthop Assoc ROC* 7:1–12.
10. Clark JA, Hsu LCS, Yau ACMC (1975): Viscoelastic behaviour of deformed spines under correction with halo-pelvic distraction. *Clin Orthop* 110:90–111.
11. Colonna PC, Vom Saal F (1941): A study of paralytic scoliosis based on 500 cases of poliomyelitis. *J Bone Joint Surg* 23:335–353.
12. DeWald RL, Ray RD (1970): Skeletal traction for the treatment of severe scoliosis. *J Bone Joint Surg Am* 52:233–237.
13. Dickson RA, Weinstein SL (1999): Bracing (and screening): yes or no? *J Bone Joint Surg Br* 81:193–198.
14. Dwyer AF, Newton NC, Sherwood AA (1969): An anterior approach in scoliosis: a preliminary approach in scoliosis. A preliminary report. *Clin Orthop* 62:182–202.
15. Dwyer AF (1972): Experience of anterior correction of scoliosis. *Clin Orthop* 93:191–206.
16. Dove J, Hsu LCS, Yau ACMC (1980): The cervical spine after halo-pelvic traction: an analysis of complications in 83 patients. *J Bone Joint Surg Br* 62:158–161.
17. Eberle CF (1988): Failure of fixation after segmental spinal instrumentation without arthrodesis in the management of paralytic scoliosis. *J Bone Joint Surg Am* 70:696–703.
18. Eberle CF (1982): Pelvic obliquity and the unstable hip after poliomyelitis. *J Bone Joint Surg Br* 64:300–304.
19. Flierl S, Carstens C (1997): Der Effekt der Halo-Schwerkraft-Traktion bei der praoperativen Behandlung der neuromuskularen Skoliose. *Z Orthopaedie Grenzgebiete* 135(2):162–170.
20. Garrett AL, Perry J, Nickel VL (1961): Stabilization of the collapsing spine. *J Bone Joint Surg Am* 43:474–484.

21. Gau YL, Lonstein JE, Winter RB, et al. (1991): Luque-Galveston procedure for correction and stabilization of neuromuscular scoliosis and pelvic obliquity: a review of 68 patients. *J Spinal Disord* 4:399–410.

22. Gillespie R, O'Brien J (1981): Harrington instrumentation without fusion. In: Proceedings of the Canadian Orthopedic Association. *J Bone Joint Surg Br* 63:461.

23. Gui L, Savini R, Vicenzi G, et al. (1964): Surgical treatment of poliomyelitic scoliosis. *Ital J Orthop Traumatol* 2:191–205.

24. Hamel AL, Moe J (1964): The collapsing spine. *Surgery* 56:364–373.

25. Hall JE, Spira IS (1973): Harrington instrumentation in the management of paralytic scoliosis. *J Bone Joint Surg Am* 55:437.

26. Harrington PR (1962): Treatment of scoliosis: correction and internal fixation by spinal instrumentation. *J Bone Joint Surg Am* 44:591–610.

27. Harrington P, Dickson JH (1973): An eleven year clinical investigation of Harrington instrumentation. *Clin Orthop* 93:113–130.

28. Irwin CE (1973): The iliotibial band: its role in producing deformity in poliomyelitis. *J Bone Joint Surg Am* 31:141–146.

29. Johnston CE II, Ashman RB, Sherman MC, et al. (1987): Mechanical consequences of rod contouring and residual scoliosis in sublaminar segmental instrumentation. *J Orthop Res* 5:206–216.

30. Kalamchi A, Yau ACMC, O'Brien JP, et al. (1976): Halo-pelvic distraction apparatus. *J Bone Joint Surg Am* 58:1119–1125.

31. Kuo SH, Lin MD, Chen YY, et al. (1991): *A preliminary study of the post-poliosyndrome in Taiwan.* Presented at annual meeting of the Rehabilitation Association ROC; May 27; Taipei.

32. Lau JHK, Parker JC, Hsu LCS, et al. (1986): Paralytic hip instability in poliomyelitis. *J Bone Joint Surg Br* 68:528–533.

33. Lee DY, Choi IH, Chung CY, et al. (1997): Fixed pelvic obliquity after poliomyelitis: classification and management. *J Bone Joint Surg Br* 79(2):190–196.

34. Leong JCY, Wilding K, Mok CD, et al. (1981): Surgical treatment of scoliosis following poliomyelitis: a review of 110 cases. *J Bone Joint Surg Am* 63:726–740.

35. Letto R, Palkar G, Bobechko W (1975): Preoperative skeletal traction in scoliosis. *J Bone Joint Surg Am* 57:616–619.

36. Lowman CL (1932): The relation of the abdominal muscles to paralytic scoliosis. *J Bone Joint Surg Am* 14:763–772.

37. Luque ER, Cardoso A (1977): Treatment of scoliosis without arthrodesis or external support: preliminary report. *Orthop Trans* 1:37–38.

38. Luque ER (1980): Segmental spinal instrumentation for correction of scoliosis. *Clin Orthop* 163:192–198.

39. Mackley JT, Herndon CH, Inkley S, et al. (1968): Pulmonary function in paralytic and non-paralytic scoliosis before and after treatment. *J Bone Joint Surg Am* 50:1379–1399.

40. Marchetti P (1978): End fusions in the treatment of some progressing or severe scoliosis in childhood or early adolescence. *Orthop Trans* 2:271.

41. Mayer L (1931): Fixed paralytic obliquity pelvis. *J Bone Joint Surg* 13:1–15.

42. Mayer L (1936): Further studies of fixed paralytic pelvis obliquity. *J Bone Joint Surg* 18:87–100.

43. Mayer PJ, Dove J, Ditmanson M, et al. (1981): Post-poliomyelitis paralytic scoliosis: a review of curve patterns and results of surgical treatment in 118 consecutive patients. *Spine* 6:573–582.

44. McAfee PC, Lubicky JP, Werner FW (1983): The use of segmental spinal instrumentation to preserve longitudinal spinal growth. An experimental study. *J Bone Joint Surg Am* 65:935–942.

45. Moe JH (1977): Harrington instrumentation without fusion combined with the Milwaukee brace for difficult scoliosis problems in young children. *Orthop Trans* 1:111.

46. Nickel VL, Perry J, Affeldt JE, et al. (1957): Elective surgery on patients with respiratory paralysis. *J Bone Joint Surg Am* 39:989–1001.

47. Nickel VL, Perry J, Garret A, et al. (1960): Application of the halo. *Orthop Pros App J* 14:31–35.

48. Nash CL (1980): Current concept review: scoliosis bracing. *J Bone Joint Surg Am* 62:848–852.

49. O'Brien JP, Dwyer AP, Hodgson AR (1975): Paralytic pelvic obliquity: its prognosis and management and the development of a technique for full correction of the deformity. *J Bone Joint Surg Am* 57:626–631.

50. O'Brien JP, Yau ACMC (1972): Anterior and posterior correction and fusion for paralytic scoliosis. *Clin Orthop* 86:151–153.

51. O'Brien JP, Yau ACMC, Gertzbein S, et al. (1975): Combined staged anterior and posterior correction and fusion of the spine in scoliosis following poliomyelitis. *Clin Orthop* 110:81–89.

52. O'Brien JP, Yau ACMC, Hodgson AR (1973): Halo-pelvic traction: a technique for severe spinal deformities. *Clin Orthop* 93:179–190.

53. Pavon SJ, Manning C (1970): Posterior spinal fusion for scoliosis due to anterior poliomyelitis. *J Bone Joint Surg Br* 52:420–431.

54. Perry J, Barnes G, Gronley J (1988): The postpolio syndrome: an overuse phenomenon. *Clin Orthop* 233:145–162.

55. Risser JC (1955): Scoliosis: the application of body casts for the correction of scoliosis. *Instr Course Lect* 12:255–259.

56. Roaf R (1956): Paralytic scoliosis. *J Bone Joint Surg Br* 38:640–659.

57. Sabin AB (1985): Oral poliovirus vaccine: history of its development and use and current challenge to eliminate poliomyelitis from the world. *J Infect Dis* 151:420–436.

58. Salk D (1980): Eradication of poliomyelitis in the United States. *Rev Infect Dis* 2:228–242.

59. Shen YS, Cheung CW, Shannon R (1987): "End-fusion" in the treatment of severe scoliosis in childhood. *Spine Deformity* 2:83–100.

60. Shen YS, Cheung CW (1985): Evaluation of polioscoliosis after spinal fusion. *J Rehabil Med ROC* 12:1–4 (in Chinese).

61. Shen WJ, Shen YS (1997): Spinal fusion for post-poliomyelitis scoliosis: minimum 15 year follow-up of 88 patients. *Orthop Trans* 21:45.

62. Sullivan JA, Conner SB (1982): Comparison of Harrington instrumentation and segmental spinal instrumentation in the management of neuromuscular spinal deformity. *Spine* 7:299–304.

63. Swank SM, Winter RB, Moe JH (1982): Scoliosis and cor pulmonale. *Spine* 7:343–349.

64. Taddonio RF (1982): Segmental spinal instrumentation in the management of neuromuscular spinal deformity. *Spine* 7:305–311.

65. Teng SW, Chao SL, Chu SH, et al. (1989): *Follow-up study and rehabilitation of children with poliomyelitis in Taiwan area: report of its therapeutic results.* Taipei, Taiwan: Cheng Hsin Rehabilitation Center, 1989.

66. Tredwell SJ, O'Brien JP (1975): Avascular necrosis of the proximal end of the dens: a complication of halo-pelvic distraction. *J Bone Joint Surg Am* 57:332–336.

67. Wenger DR, Carollo JJ, Wilkerson JA, et al. (1982): Laboratory testing of segmental spinal instrumentation versus traditional Harrington instrumentation for scoliosis treatment. *Spine* 7:265–269.

68. Werner AY, Zumeta GR, Newman RW, et al. (1951): Comparison of vital capacity in normal and poliomyelitic subjects. *J Bone Joint Surg Am* 33:628–635.

69. Wilson PD (1929): Posterior capsuloplasty in certain flexion contractures of the knee. *J Bone Joint Surg* 11:40.

70. Zielke K, Stunkat R, Beaujean FR (1976): Ventrale Derotations-spondylodese. Vorlaeufiger Ergebnisbericht ueber 26 operierte Faelle. *Arch Orthop Unfall-Chirurgie* 85:257–277.

71. Wu HB (1998): Personal communication.

51

OTHER NEUROMUSCULAR DEFORMITIES

MICHAEL J. BARNES

This chapter discusses a miscellaneous group of neuromuscular disorders that share a propensity to produce spinal deformity. The etiologies are diverse, and it is imperative to diagnose the underlying conditions accurately and to make attempts to predict the natural course not only of the condition itself but also of any associated spinal deformities. This allows prediction of the likely effects of the deformity on the patient, which helps to guide treatment recommendations. Even so, the disorders discussed in this chapter are generally uncommon or rare, and guidelines from the literature consequently are often either lacking or taken from a historical era. Frequently, therefore, the surgeon charged with treating these patients needs to revert to the principles outlined in Chapter 46. Many of these conditions are associated with a severe and rigid spinal deformity at a relatively early stage in spinal maturation. This dictates that the surgeon possess a thorough understanding of normal growth and maturation of the spine (see Chap. 1, Appendix B) and the effect of evolving deformity on pulmonary parameters (see Chap. 17) and that the surgeon apply this knowledge in recommending observation, orthotic treatment, or surgical treatment.

RETT SYNDROME

Rett syndrome is a progressive neurologic disorder affecting females almost exclusively (11). It is not excessively rare, with a prevalence between 0.1 and 0.15 per 1000 population (27). Rett syndrome now appears to be a developmental rather than a degenerative disorder (57). It is not, in most cases, an inherited condition, even though the overwhelming female preponderance suggests a genetic origin (1,64,87). Patients with Rett syndrome develop a characteristic cluster of clinical manifestations, including early psychomotor regression with autistic features, loss of purposeful use of the hands that is replaced by stereotypical activity, ataxia and apraxia of gait, and acquired microcephaly (27).

Rett syndrome is remarkable for a period of apparently normal initial development, although affected girls may be somewhat hypotonic from birth (46). The onset of clinical manifesta-

tions is between 6 months and 3 years of age, and affected patients progress at variable rates through four recognizable neurobiologic stages (84). Stage I (early-onset stagnation) occurs between 6 and 18 months of age. Stage II (rapid developmental regression) occurs between 1 and 3 years of age. Stereotypical hand movements develop in this stage, language is lost, and autistic manifestations appear. Stage III (pseudostationary period) follows, persists for years, and is marked by resolution of some of the autistic features but is followed inevitably by stage IV (late motor deterioration). Most patients develop seizures. Only one fourth to one third ever acquire independent ambulation; this is generally lost in stage IV, at which time muscle wasting, spasticity, and contractures become more marked (28).

The syndrome was first described by Rett in 1966 and came to clinical prominence after Hagberg's description in 1980 (26). Even so, it is only recently that most patients have been correctly diagnosed and surviving patients followed into their fourth of fifth decade. The diagnosis of Rett syndrome received attention in the orthopaedic literature in the late 1980s when reports appeared documenting the musculoskeletal manifestations. Foremost among these, and most likely to necessitate intervention, is spinal deformity, although lower limb contractures, acquired hip instability, and foot deformities (equinovarus or planovalgus) also occur (24,29,36,48,70,71). Because of the relatively recent recognition of this disorder, natural history data are still emerging. It is becoming apparent that most patients followed through stage IV develop a spinal deformity (7,14,35,36,39,47,48). Age of onset is variable and correlates more closely with neurobiologic stage than chronologic age (47). The incidence of spinal deformity, therefore, increases with age and is well established in many patients by 8 or 9 years of age. Patients who are hypotonic at birth may develop significant deformity during the infantile period (47). Most curves progress (39,47), and progression accelerates during stage III and especially stage IV. A moderate curve may quickly become severe at this time (7,33,47,48).

In general, these patients develop long C-shaped curves, and pelvic obliquity is frequently seen in association with larger curves. Single thoracic and double curve patterns are also seen (7,33,47,48). Often, the curve has a major kyphotic component, although a thoracic hypokyphosis is sometimes observed, particularly in association with smaller curves (48). Also apparent radiographically is the markedly diminished spine bone mineral density (34).

M. J. Barnes: Starship Children's Hospital, Auckland, New Zealand

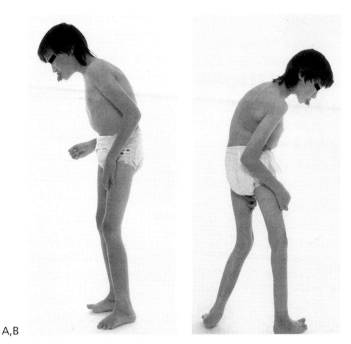

A,B

FIGURE 1. A, B: Stage III Rett syndrome in a 9-year-old demonstrating truncal imbalance disproportionate to the structural scoliosis.

Although curve progression accelerates in stage IV, moderate to severe curves are observed in ambulatory patients. In these patients, a severe truncal imbalance may be noted out of proportion to the structural component of the curve (Fig. 1).

There is no definite evidence that bracing alters the natural progression of spinal deformity in Rett syndrome or prevents a severe deformity ultimately developing (33,39,40,41). It is possible, however, that the use of a TLSO will delay curve progression and allow trunk lengthening through spinal growth before definitive spinal fusion. The best indication for the use of an orthosis, and the situation in which it is most likely to be accepted, is as a temporizing measure when it is found that standing or seated balance is improved with the brace in situ.

As with other, more common neuromuscular conditions (see Chap. 46), surgical treatment of spinal deformity now appears to be an accepted modality in Rett syndrome and holds benefits for both patients and their families. Unfortunately, there is a paucity of published data to allow firm conclusions regarding timing of surgery, posterior only versus anterior and posterior surgery, and fusion levels, particularly with regard to the necessity to fuse to the sacrum. For many curves in the 60- to 70-degree range, segmental posterior instrumentation can effect a correction of about 50 degrees (36). Only one author (33) has reported anterior fusion in addition to posterior instrumentation and fusion, suggesting that this will only be necessary for severe,

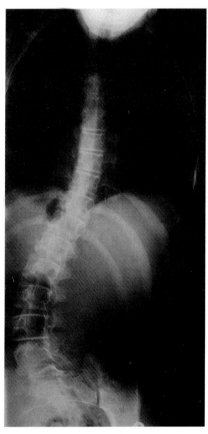

A

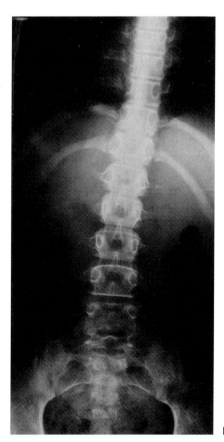

B

FIGURE 2. Rett syndrome in a 12-year-old ambulator. **A:** Standing radiographs demonstrate a moderate but severely unbalanced curve. **B:** Supine radiographs demonstrate the curve to be almost completely postural.

rigid, or neglected curves or in older patients. Because these patients display what could be termed a cerebral imbalance, and ultimately become nonambulators, crankshaft is not really an issue (Fig. 2). Several authors report an improvement in gait after spinal surgery in patients with Rett syndrome (33,39). Loss of ambulatory function as a result of spinal fusion has not been described.

As in other neuromuscular conditions, the timing of surgery is a product of curve magnitude, stiffness, and spinal growth. As with bracing, the primary aim of surgery is to achieve truncal balance, and surgical recommendations are not dictated by Cobb angle alone. For example, a severely unbalanced 40-degree curve in an ambulatory patient may merit spinal fusion, whereas in other patients, a partially compensated and flexible curve may safely be able to progress to 60 or 70 degrees before surgery. It seems that in Rett syndrome, surgery can usually be delayed past 10 years of age and that posterior procedures alone often suffice in ambulatory patients. Because of severe truncal ataxia and imbalance, frequently associated sagittal plane deformity, and the fact that these patients ultimately become spastic, fusion for thoracolumbar or lumbar curves generally commences at T2 and extends to the sacrum (Fig. 3). Patients are certainly encountered in whom, by virtue of spinal flexibility or a fractional compensatory lower lumbar curve, it is possible to end the fusion caudally at L4 or L5 and achieve static spinal balance. However, the risks for decompensation due to truncal ataxia or late pelvic obliquity due to evolution of deformity in unfused lower lumbar segments make it prudent to fuse to the sacrum in most cases. When it is anticipated that posterior segmental instrumentation does not

effect sufficient correction to restore balance, it should be preceded by anterior discectomy and, if necessary, instrumentation. In the absence of data to the contrary, perioperative management should mirror that of scoliosis surgery in cerebral palsy (see Chap. 45).

ARTHROGRYPOSIS

Arthrogryposis translated literally means "curved joint" and is a purely descriptive term. It was expanded to "arthrogryposis multiplex congenita" by Stern in 1923 (80) to denote a syndrome present at birth involving multiple joints. Currently, arthrogryposis is defined as a congenital, generally nonprogressive limitation of movement of two or more joints in different body regions (79). The estimated incidence is 1 per 3000 live births (79).

Animal studies support the concept that joint contractures are a direct result of fetal akinesia (55,82). This failure of normal in utero joint movement may be due to intrinsic causes, namely abnormal formation or function of striated muscle (myopathic origin), a neurologic process (neuropathic origin), or an abnormality of connective tissue (fibropathic origin) (6). Less commonly, it is due to extrinsic causes, including oligohydramnios, structural uterine abnormalities, or various maternal illnesses (76,79).

Under the descriptive umbrella of multiple congenital joint contractures, as many as 150 clinical or genetic entities have been delineated. Many specific types of arthrogryposis have now been mapped to loci on the human chromosomes (31,32). In any one child, it is clearly important to make a precise diagnosis if possible. The sparse orthopaedic and spinal deformity arthrogryposis literature largely predates these diagnostic distinctions. This literature has tended to focus on the common clinical and treatment-related features, specifically the unyielding soft tissues and osteopenia that are the hallmarks of this condition. Historically, the causative distinctions have been considered more important by other specialists, such as clinical geneticists and neurologists.

The term *amyoplasia* (77), itself descriptive and nonetiologic, has been used to denote the classic, extensive arthrogrypotic syndrome seen in orthopaedic services. It is predominantly these patients who form the basis of published spinal deformity series. This subgroup occurs sporadically with an incidence of 1 per 10,000 live births. Other distinct but orthopaedically recognizable syndromes include the various distal arthrogryposes, contractural arachnodactyly or Beals syndrome, the multiple pterygium syndromes, the popliteal pterygium syndromes, and the Freeman-Sheldon syndromes. According to Sarwark and colleagues (74), it is only occasionally difficult to distinguish patients with amyoplasia from those with other specific arthrogrypotic syndromes.

Patients with amyoplasia most typically display symmetric positioning of the limbs with severe equinovarus feet, deformities of all major joints, absent muscle tissue with fibrotic or fatty replacement, midfacial hemangioma, and normal intelligence. The absence of normal functioning muscle mass creates smooth,

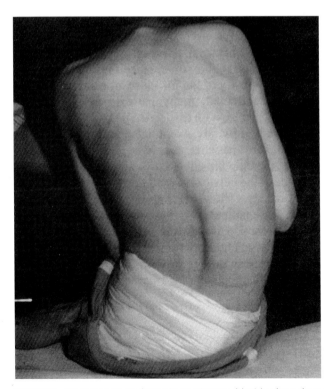

FIGURE 3. Stage IV Rett syndrome in an 18-year-old with a long thoracolumbar, "paralytic" curve pattern and associated pelvic obliquity.

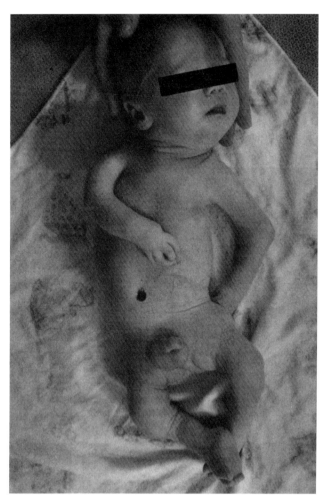

FIGURE 4. Arthrogryposis in a 4-week-old neonate. Classic features of amyoplasia congenita are present and a scoliosis already evident. (Courtesy of the Alfred I. du Pont Institute, Wilmington, DE.)

note congenital vertebral anomalies in other contractural syndromes (74). Other authors make no mention of vertebral anomalies (10,13), with the exception of Drummond and Mackenzie (15), whose seven patients with congenital anomalies probably represented other diagnostic subgroups of arthrogryposis.

Excluding curves with congenital vertebral anomalies, characteristic curve patterns have been noted. Lumbar and thoracolumbar curve patterns predominate (10,12,38,73), frequently associated with increased lordosis and pelvic obliquity. Double (thoracic and lumbar) and single thoracic curves are also seen. Available data do not allow comment on the contribution of the ambulatory status or hip position to the development of spinal deformity, which occurs in all categories. A significant proportion (8% to 38%) of patients with scoliosis exhibit curvatures at birth. By 5 years of age, it is present in 63% of patients who will ultimately develop scoliosis. The remaining curves develop in the juvenile and adolescent periods (Fig. 5) such that the average age a curve is noted is 5 years (12,38,73).

Natural history data are limited. Herron and coauthors (38) noted curve progression in six of seven untreated immature patients, averaging seven degrees per year. No useful data exist on these patients after maturity. Progressive curves do not necessarily become severe by skeletal maturity. As might be expected, the earlier the onset of curvature, the more likely it is to become severe. Authors almost invariably comment on the inflexible, rigid nature of the curves.

fusiform limbs (Fig. 4). The skin is glossy and atrophic, creaseless, and often dimpled over bony prominences. Most patients have all four limbs involved. Hip contractures (50%) and dislocation of one or both hips (33%) are common (79).

Ten percent of patients with amyoplasia are said to have abdominal structural anomalies, which may be a major factor in the genesis of early-onset scoliosis. The reported incidence of scoliosis in arthrogryposis multiplex congenita is 10% to 30% (30,73,79). The variance is accounted for by etiologic heterogeneity and patient selection under study. In amyoplasia, it is about 35% (73).

It is generally considered that patients with amyoplasia and scoliosis do not have congenital vertebral anomalies (73). In a radiographic study of 14 patients with arthrogryposis multiplex congenita and scoliosis, Poznanski and associates (66) found no congenitally anomalous vertebrae. In clinically based studies of spinal deformity in arthrogryposis multiplex congenita, the findings are similar. Herron and coauthors (38) found no such anomalies in 16 patients. Sarwark and associates (73) found no anomalies in 23 patients with scoliosis and amyoplasia but did

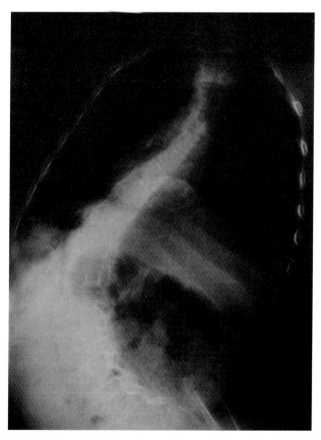

FIGURE 5. Amyoplasia in an 8-year-old nonambulator. A severe, rigid scoliosis is already present.

Nonsurgical treatment modalities consist of passive trunk stretching and orthoses. Sarwark and colleagues (73) stated that trunk contractures present at birth respond to passive stretching. Various authors document orthotic treatment with TLSOs or Milwaukee braces. No attempt was made to assess curve correction after initial brace application. Herron and associates (38) were not able to demonstrate a significant reduction in rate of curve progression over natural history in five patients braced. None of the authors reported successful bracing based on currently accepted stringent criteria.

No series documents surgical outcomes with segmental instrumentation. The available literature documents seven cases only that underwent an instrumented correction. Harrington rods were used in all cases, and treatment included preoperative halo-femoral traction in some patients. The average preoperative curve magnitude was 60 degrees, and the average curve magnitude at follow up was 48 degrees, giving a correction of only 20%. This is consistent with the impression that these are indeed relatively rigid curves.

In view of the paucity of published data, it is necessary to invoke the basic neuromuscular deformity principles when treating these patients. Hip dislocation and deformity should be treated at an early age on their own merits, although it is doubtful that this will materially alter the development or progression of any spinal deformities. Bracing is indicated for the occasional patient with a relatively small flexible curve in the 20- to 40-degree range; however, such a patient is seldom encountered. Because of the tendency for these curves to progress and become rigid at an early age, surgery is often required in the juvenile period. In determining the ideal timing of surgery, it should be recognized that, even with aggressive modern surgical techniques, correction is likely to be much less than that obtained in other neuromuscular conditions as a result of the malignant combination of soft tissue rigidity and osteopenia. Surgery should therefore be recommended before curves become severe and before substantial pelvic obliquity develops. If pelvic obliquity is present, fusion to the sacrum is generally necessary. As always, fusion to the sacrum should be recommended cautiously in ambulatory patients but probably carries little penalty in patients with stiff lumbar or thoracolumbar curves. Provided that pulmonary function is adequate, posterior segmental instrumentation and fusion frequently need to be preceded by anterior disc excision to enhance curve mobility and prevent crankshaft.

At the time of surgery, peripheral venous access is frequently limited or absent. Care should be taken in positioning the patient for surgery because the combination of stiff, deformed joints and osteopenia predisposes to pathologic fractures. Finally, difficulty in establishing a subperiosteal plane because of deficient muscle and soft tissue adherence as well as osteopenia may predispose to moderate or excessive blood loss (12).

HEREDITARY MOTOR AND SENSORY NEUROPATHIES

The current classification of hereditary motor and sensory neuropathies (HMSN) is based in part on the pathology (axonal or myelinic); their electroclinical manifestations, especially the motor and sensory conduction velocities; and their mode of inheritance. Classifications are rapidly changing as a result of progression in molecular genetics (1).

For example, the term *peroneal muscular atrophy* or *Charcot-Marie-Tooth disease* was originally believed to be specific for one disorder. Dyck and Lambert (16,17) in 1968 were the first to suggest that peroneal muscular atrophy occurs in several inherited muscular disorders. They distinguished between the hypertrophic neuropathy variety now commonly known as HMSN type I, and the neuronal variety, or HMSN type II.

HMSN I, also referred to as Charcot-Marie-Tooth disease type I, is genetically heterogenous and has been further subdivided. According to Dyck (19), perhaps less than 10% of patients affected with HMSN I have sought medical consultation. This conclusion comes from examination of relatives of probands diagnosed with HMSN. The clinical manifestation of HMSN II are similar but with a later onset and even slower course (1).

In contrast, HMSN III, also known as *hypertrophic neuropathy of infancy* or *Déjérine-Sottas syndrome*, has a course that is more often severe, and loss of independent walking before adolescence may occur. Déjérine and Sottas' original description (cited by Dyck) pertained to two siblings with this disorder, whose clinical manifestations included kyphoscoliosis. Ouvrier and colleagues (60) noted kyphoscoliosis in two of six patients with this disorder.

HMSN IV, alternatively known as *hypertrophic neuropathy* or *Refsum's disease*, which is associated with phytanic acid excess, is rare, and although skeletal abnormalities are common in this disorder, spinal deformity has only been sporadically recorded. HMSN V is spastic paraplegia, and types VI and VII have features of HMSN I in addition to ocular manifestations. Scoliosis has not yet been described in association with these variants.

Onset of HMSN I is usually within the first decade of life, and it occasionally occurs in the neonatal period or the first year of life. Foot deformity and gait disturbance are the usual presenting manifestations. Examination reveals symmetric atrophy of the peroneal muscles, later involving the calves and eventually the distal thighs, although about half of affected children and adolescents do not display wasting (1). In the upper extremities, atrophy of the small muscles of the hand may occur, although this is usually a later manifestation. Deep tendon reflexes are often lost early. Sensory abnormalities are mild and may be difficult to evidence.

HMSN II has a later onset, during the second or third decade of life, and a slower course. Absent reflexes and foot deformities are less common. Differentiation from type I is by electrophysiologic parameters. Even in HMSN I, most patients remain active indefinitely, but some severe cases exist. The prevalence of HMSN I and II is about 40 per 100,000 population, with the disorder remaining undiagnosed in perhaps most cases (18).

Orthopaedic considerations relate to instability and deformity of the foot and ankle, occult hip dysplasia (44,61), and spinal deformities. Because affected patients with HMSN I and II do not always come to medical attention, the proportion of affected individuals with scoliosis is uncertain. Hensinger and MacEwen (37) noted kyphoscoliosis in 7 of 69 patients with Charcot-Marie-Tooth disease. This report appears to form the basis of the statement that scoliosis is seen in about 10% of patients with HMSN, which is widely quoted in the orthopaedic literature (76). However, Ouvrier and colleagues (60) found evidence of spinal deformity in 3 of 10 patients with HMSN I, Nukada and associates (58) in three of four patients with HMSN II, and recently Walker and colleagues (85) noted scoliosis greater than 10 degrees in 34 of 89 children examined with HMSN I and II and followed to or close to skeletal maturity. Many of these curves exhibited a kyphotic component, and pure kyphosis (greater than 40 degrees) was seen in a further three children. Spinal deformity was found in 84% of children with HMSN I and in only 19% with HMSN II. Of the 34 patients with scoliosis, single thoracic curves, more often left sided, predominated, although all curve patterns were seen (Fig. 6). Daher and coauthors (13) also noted an associated kyphosis in six of 12 patients with Charcot-Marie-Tooth disease and scoliosis. In the pediatric and adolescent group of Walker and colleagues (85), most scoliotic curves were less than 20 degrees, and only two were greater than 40 degrees. Six patients, however, had a kyphotic component of greater than 60 degrees. Similarly, Daher and coauthors (13) found an average scoliotic curve of 19 degrees only. The average ages at diagnosis of spinal deformity in these two series were 10 years and 13 years, 10 months, respectively (13,85).

The literature reports few orthotically and surgically treated patients, probably reflecting and confirming the relatively nonprogressive nature of the deformity in most cases. Hensinger and

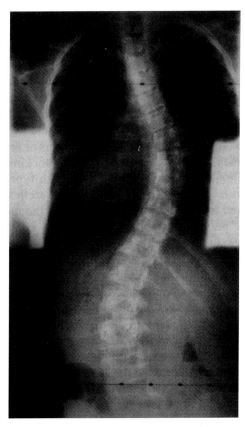

FIGURE 6. Charcot-Marie-Tooth disease in a 13-year-old. The right thoracic, left lumbar curve pattern is similar to that seen in adolescent idiopathic scoliosis.

MacEwen (37) reported that a Milwaukee brace was successful in three of six patients, with the remainder coming to surgery. Likewise, bracing controlled progression in one of Daher's (13) two patients and in one of Walker's (85) three patients so treated. The two patients in Walker's (85) series who underwent spinal fusion had no complications, whereas two of Daher's (13) four patients, who had Harrington instrumentation, developed a pseudarthrosis.

Hensinger and MacEwen (37) believed that spinal deformity in Charcot-Marie-Tooth disease may be managed by the same techniques used for idiopathic scoliosis, including the effective use of a Milwaukee brace. Currently, it would be reasonable to apply bracing criteria and indications developed for adolescent idiopathic scoliosis, using an underarm TLSO when applicable. Because the disorder is slowly progressive and rarely leads to severe disability, adult progression would be predicted to occur only in larger curves by extrapolation from adolescent idiopathic scoliosis data. On the other hand, the occasional patient may develop late curve progression as a result of a neuropathic spinal arthropathy, as recently reported by Anand and coauthors (3) in a 45-year-old man who had been managed as a teenager in a Milwaukee brace.

Even fewer patients require surgical treatment. This most often involves a posterior spinal fusion with segmental instrumentation. The pattern of hook placement and the length of fusion should take account of the frequently associated sagittal plane deformity and the neuromuscular etiology. The occasional patient with a large, stiff curve or a major kyphotic component may require a preliminary anterior disc excision. Anterior and posterior surgery is required if there are any neuropathic features on radiograph, although these are unlikely to be present before maturity (14). As noted recently by Krishna and colleagues (43), surgeons should anticipate failure of conventional somatosensory evoked potential monitoring in these patients.

HEREDITARY SENSORY AND AUTONOMIC NEUROPATHIES

Inherited peripheral sensory neuropathies are rare, and their definitive diagnosis is difficult. Relative insensitivity to pain is common to all and underpins many of the clinical features. Surgeons treating patients with spinal deformity need to be cognizant of the existence of the Riley-Day syndrome or familial dysautonomia (HSAN III). Although the most common of the hereditary sensory and autonomic neuropathies, HSAN III is only rarely encountered outside Israel in several centers in the United States. Nevertheless, the disorder's protean clinical manifestations and the numerous dangers associated with surgical and anesthetic management of these patients are likely to leave an unforgettable clinical impression out of proportion to the condition's prevalence (81). Rarely, patients with other hereditary sensory and autonomic neuropathies are encountered in scoliosis clinics (Fig. 7). Their recognition may result from identification of characteristic clinical features, including anhidrosis, recurrent fractures, Charcot joints, osteomyelitis, acral and oral mutilation, autoamputation, deafness, and behavioral problems or mental retardation (1,19,25). These patients rarely present for spinal surgery as a result of deformity or neurologic compromise associated

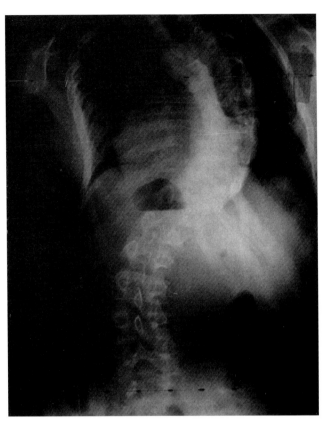

FIGURE 7. Congenital insensitivity to pain (HSAN II) in a 15-year-old demonstrating a severe thoracic scoliosis. (Courtesy of the Alfred I. du Pont Institute Wilmington, DE.)

with the development of Charcot arthropathy of the spine (9,35,65) (Fig. 8).

Five types of hereditary sensory and autonomic neuropathies have been categorized. With the exception of HSAN III, in which scoliosis is almost invariable and its management well documented, reports of patients with spinal deformity are sporadic (20) and do not generally distinguish between the various HSAN subtypes.

The hereditary sensory and autonomic neuropathies are, as the name implies, inherited and are characterized by the fact that primary sensory and autonomic neurons either undergo atrophy and degeneration (HSAN I) or fail to develop (HSAN II to IV). HSAN type I typically has a symptomatic onset during late childhood or adolescence, affects predominately the lower limbs, and is slowly progressive. HSAN types II to V are congenital, the disorder is more generalized (upper limbs, trunk, and face are variably affected), and clinically the disorders are static. However, the present classification is assumed to be temporary and imperfect, and rarer forms exist (19).

Reports of HSAN in the orthopaedic literature either predate the currently accepted classification (50,63) or, with rare exceptions, (7,59) fail to take cognizance of it. Although reports of small numbers of patients exist in both the older and more recent orthopaedic literature (7,20,23,42,45), only three such reports (7,20,23) specifically describe scoliosis in patients other than

those with HSAN III. These various reports highlight the particular difficulties in management of joint instability (both congenital and acquired), fractures, bone and joint infections, acral mutilation, and other orthopaedic problems imposed by the underlying sensory and autonomic neuropathies.

HSAN type III is a recessively inherited disorder seen predominantly but not exclusively in Jewish people. Although there is an overlap of symptoms and signs in this disorder with those of other varieties of HSAN, HSAN III can be distinguished by the predominance of autonomic symptoms (defective lacrimation, defective temperature control, skin blotching, extensive perspiration, hypertension, postural hypotension), absence of fungiform papillae, and occurrence particularly among the Ashkenazi Jews (18). The initial account of the disorder was published by Riley, Day, and coworkers in New York in 1949 (68). The disease has an incidence among Ashkenazi Jews of between 0.5 and 1 per 10,000 live births (51).

The presence of the disorder may be apparent soon after birth or during infancy as a result of hypotonia, poor sucking, vomiting, failure to thrive, unexplained fever, and repeated episodes of pneumonia. Presenting symptoms at an older age may include developmental delay, growth impairment, corneal abrasions, excessive sweating, blotching of the skin with emotion, emotional lability, clumsiness, decreased pain sensation, and spinal deformity (18).

The disorder affects peripheral autonomic, sensory and motor neurons, and possibly other classes of central nervous system neurons (18). Autonomic and spinal ganglia are markedly diminished in number, and significantly reduced numbers of unmyelinated fibers are found in cutaneous nerve biopsies (18,68). The sensory deficit is variable and increases progressively with age (4). Deep tendon reflexes tend to be lost early in the disease, ataxia develops in some patients, and mental retardation may be observed, although more often intelligence is normal. Additional diagnostic criteria include lack of an axon flare after intradermal histamine injection and a hypersensitivity to parasympathetic drugs.

The course of HSAN III is severe. Whereas in the 1960s, only 20% of patients survived to adulthood, improvements in management have seen that proportion rise to 50% (5). From an orthopaedic standpoint, acral mutilation is not a feature, and although Charcot joints do occur, spinal deformity is the leading musculoskeletal abnormality and develops in most patients. The reported frequency of either scoliosis or kyphosis ranges from 60% to 96% (72,86), depending obviously on the age of patients under study and selection criteria. Much of the natural history data derive from patients registered with the Familial Dysautonomia Center of New York University, and it is likely that many patients are common to chronologically successive studies (22,52,72,86). Additional treatment-related data come from Toronto (2) and Israel (71). Scoliosis is the most common deformity, with perhaps one half of these patients also having significantly increased kyphosis (22,52) and with pure kyphosis also occurring occasionally (71). Single thoracic curve patterns predominate, often left sided, although double curve patterns are not infrequent (22,72). The apex of the scoliotic curve is often several vertebrae cephalad to that seen in idiopathic scoliosis (86). The apex of the kyphosis may also be high, and the thoracic

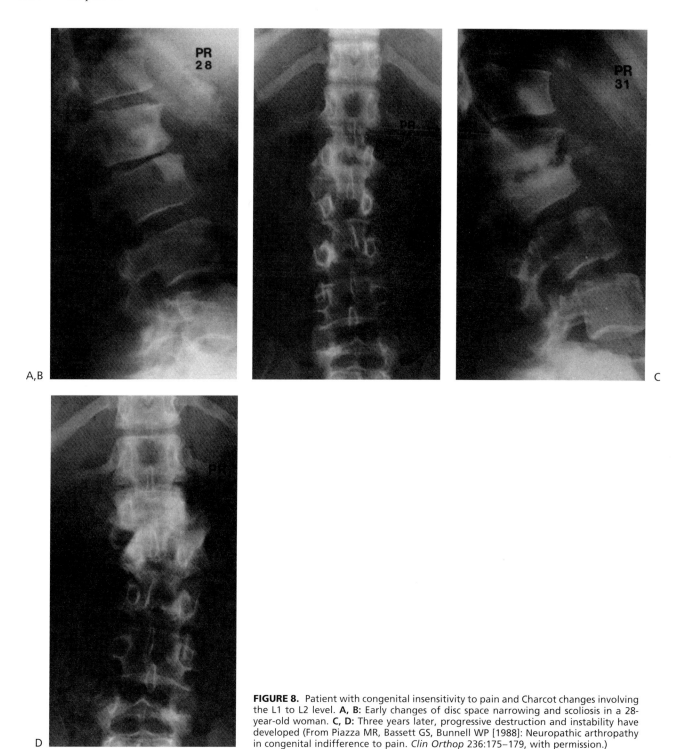

FIGURE 8. Patient with congenital insensitivity to pain and Charcot changes involving the L1 to L2 level. **A, B:** Early changes of disc space narrowing and scoliosis in a 28-year-old woman. **C, D:** Three years later, progressive destruction and instability have developed (From Piazza MR, Bassett GS, Bunnell WP [1988]: Neuropathic arthropathy in congenital indifference to pain. *Clin Orthop* 236:175–179, with permission.)

kyphosis may extend to the caudad portion of the cervical spine, where it may meet a rigid cervical lordosis (72).

Onset of spinal deformity is usually noted between 5 and 10 years of age and is progressive in most patients; frequently, moderately severe or severe curves that tend to be rigid are thought to contribute to cardiopulmonary morbidity and mortality (71,86).

Treatment of spinal deformity is discussed in depth by three authors (2,71,72), with by far the most comprehensive report provided by Rubery and colleagues (72). They considered that failure of bracing to prevent progression of kyphoscoliosis to 45 degrees was an indication for operative treatment. The other authors report limited success with bracing, either Milwaukee or TLSO. Brace efficacy is compromised by the high and rigid curves and the tendency to repeated pneumonia, impaired thermoregulation and hence pressure sores, gastrostomy feeding tubes, and emotional lability. Nevertheless, bracing should probably be attempted for smaller, supple curves in immature patients using modern bracing principles and techniques.

This is particularly so because surgical treatment is likewise often associated with complications of both a medical and surgical nature. Rubery and colleagues (72) reported operative treatment of 22 patients with a mean preoperative scoliosis of 70 degrees and kyphosis of 68 degrees. All patients underwent posterior spinal fusion using Harrington instrumentation with the exception of three patients treated with Cotrel-Dubousset instrumentation. Two patients had an additional anterior fusion. At the most recent follow-up, modest improvements in the scoliosis were noted, with no significant improvement in the kyphosis. Cut out of the upper hook occurred in four patients, one patient required reoperation for pseudarthrosis, and one patient died from paraplegia associated with deep infection. Severe medical complications, including pneumonia and gastrointestinal hemorrhage, were more common early in the series.

Despite these many difficulties, surgery is indicated for scoliotic curves that progress beyond 45 degrees. Fusion length may often be dictated by the extent of the frequently associated kyphosis, and preoperative planning should take into account sagittal plane deformity in cervical, thoracic, and lumbar segments to maximize sagittal balance postoperatively. Segmental instrumentation should reduce the incidence of implant failure, and combined anterior and posterior procedures should be considered for large, rigid curves, especially if there is a major kyphotic component. Unless perioperative medical, anesthetic, and intensive care management is ideal, however, complications will occur with unacceptable frequency. Preoperatively, adequate hydration and avoidance of atropine should reduce the incidence of inspissation of secretions plugging endotracheal tubes (72). Intraoperatively, the surgical practice of infiltration with epinephrine solution should be avoided (2), and blood pressure should be controlled with sedatives rather than antihypertensive medications (72). Postoperatively, cardiovascular, pulmonary, and gastrointestinal symptoms should be adequately supported and monitored.

CONGENITAL MYOPATHIES

The congenital myopathies constitute a group of disorders characterized clinically by hypotonia and weakness from birth and pathologically by distinctive histologic and electron microscopic findings, an absence of dystrophic features, and a normal or only mildly elevated serum creatine kinase (1,75). The current classification is based on histopathologic findings rather than genetic or clinical characterizations. Consequently, there is considerable clinical overlap between the various pathologic entities as well as marked variability in clinical severity within the spectrum of each pathologic class.

Central core disease was the first congenital myopathy to be described and is a rare disease with autosomal dominant inheritance as well as sporadic occurrence. The responsible gene appears to be allelic with the gene that has been implicated in malignant

hyperthermia, and the two conditions frequently coexist, although they may occur discordantly (21,56,78). Histologically, the muscle fibers contain central areas that are devoid of the normal histochemical reactions for oxidative enzymes, myophosphorylase, and glycogen and that ultrastructurally consist of closely packed myofibrils that lack mitochondria, cytoplasmic reticulum, and glycogen.

Nemaline myopathy is predominantly an autosomal recessive trait, although rarely it has an autosomal dominant transmittance. Histologically, multiple small, rodlike particles, thought to represent Z-band proteins, are present within most muscle fibers. There are several patterns of clinical presentation, including a severe, usually fatal, neonatal form; a milder congenital form; and an adult-onset form (53).

The term *congenital fiber-type disproportion myopathy* is applied when biopsy samples demonstrate a disparity between type I and type II fibers in the absence of other histologic abnormalities. *Myotubular myopathy* (or *centronuclear myopathy*) produces a histologic picture of type I fiber predominance and centrally located nuclei, with or without fiber hypertrophy. Variability of both clinical severity and genetic transmittance are also hallmarks of these remaining two categories, and a large number of even rarer categories exist.

Spinal deformity has been described in patients with each of these major divisions of congenital myopathy, as have other musculoskeletal abnormalities, including congenital hip instability, various foot deformities (cavovarus, equinovarus), and contractures (75). The spinal deformity is often rigid but may, less commonly, at least in the early stages, be flexible. Double curve patterns and typical long, thoracolumbar "paralytic" curves are encountered. Within each diagnostic category, phenotypic variability may range from a severe or even fatal neonatal or infantile form to a barely detectable adult picture with little or no clinical impact. There are even cases in which an improvement in strength is noted after the end of infancy. Consequently, treatment must be individualized, but if possible, the underlying condition should be accurately diagnosed and its natural course defined.

An evolving scoliosis can add significantly to the burden of respiratory muscle weakness in these children. In the more severe forms, bracing may be contraindicated, either by virtue of the presence of a severe rigid curve or because of marginal respiratory reserves. However, patients should be kept under regular review. Occasionally a patient is encountered in the infantile period who appears to be untreatable with a grave prognosis, is oxygen dependent, and already has a well-established scoliotic or kyphoscoliotic curve. Surprisingly, at subsequent follow-up, such a child is sometimes seen to be much more robust and perhaps even a candidate for surgery.

Provided that respiration is adequate, attempts should be made to control smaller, flexible curves with an orthosis. Failing this, definitive fusion should be recommended to control progressive curves and should be applied at an age that is calculated to maximize ultimate trunk length and lung capacity and at the same time minimize deformities. This calculation should take account of thoracic vertebral rotation and lordosis, which can severely limit thoracic volume in these patients (see Chap. 46). The possibility of malignant hyperthermia must be investigated if surgery is planned in these patients. Congenital myopathy is probably one of the few diagnostic categories in which the occasional patient may warrant consideration of a growth-preserving surgical approach (49,54,62,69,83). Such a patient would generally be encountered in the infantile or early juvenile period and have a long, flexible, thoracolumbar curve that is too large or too rotated to allow bracing or for which bracing without internal fixation has already failed.

ACKNOWLEDGMENTS

The author gratefully acknowledges the able assistance rendered by Christine Ganly, research assistant, Starship Children's Hospital Orthopaedic Department, in researching and preparing this manuscript.

REFERENCES

1. Aircardi J (1998): *Diseases of the nervous system in childhood*, 2nd ed. London: Mac Keith Press.
2. Albanese S, Bobechko W (1987): Spine deformity in familial dysautonomia (Riley-Day syndrome). *J Pediatr* 7:179–183.
3. Anand N, Levine DB, Burke S, et al. (1997): Neuropathic spinal arthropathy in Charcot-Marie-Tooth disease: a case report. *J Bone Joint Surg Am* 79:1235–1239.
4. Axelrod FB, Iyer K, Fish I, et al. (1997): Progressive sensory loss in familial dysautonomia. *Pediatrics* 67:517–522.
5. Axelrod FB, Abularrage JJ (1982): Familial dysautonomia: a prospective study of survival. *J Pediatr* 101:234–236.
6. Banker B (1985): Neuropathologic aspects of arthrogryposis multiplex congenita. *Clin Orthop* 194:30–43.
7. Bassett GS, Bunnell WP, Bowen JR, et al. (1987): Spinal deformity in congenital indifference to pain. *Orthop Trans* 11:120.
8. Bassett GS, Tolo VT (1990): The incidence and natural history of scoliosis in Rett syndrome. *Dev Med Child Neurol* 32:963–966.
9. Brown CW, Jones B, Donaldson DH, et al. (1992): Neuropathic (Charcot) arthropathy of the spine after traumatic spinal paraplegia. *Spine* 17:S103–108.
10. Carlson WO, Speck GJ, Vicari V, et al. (1985): Arthrogryposis multiplex congenita: a long-term follow-up study. *Clin Orthop* 194: 115–123.
11. Coleman M (1990): Is classical Rett syndrome ever present in males? *Brain Dev* 12:31–32.
12. Daher YH, Lonstein JE, Winter RB (1985): Spinal deformities in patients with arthrogryposis: a review of 16 patients. *Spine* 10:609–613.
13. Daher YH, Lonstein JE, Winter RB, et al. (1986): Spinal deformities in patients with Charcot-Marie-Tooth disease. *Clin Orthop* 202: 219–222.
14. Devlin VJ, Ogilvie JW, Transfeldt EE, et al. (1991): Surgical treatment of neuropathic spinal arthropathy. *J Spinal Disord* 4:319–328.
15. Drummond DS, Mackenzie DA (1978): Scoliosis in arthrogryposis multiplex congenita. *Spine* 3:146–151.
16. Dyck PJ, Lambert EH (1968): Lower motor and primary sensory neuron disease with peroneal muscle atrophy. Part I. Neurologic, genetic, and electrophysiological findings in hereditary polyneuropathies. *Arch Neurol* 18:603–618.
17. Dyck PJ, Lambert EH (1968): Lower motor and primary sensory neuron disease with peroneal muscle atrophy. Part II. Neurologic, genetic, and electrophysiological findings in various neuronal degenerations. *Arch Neurol* 18:619–625.
18. Dyck P (1993): Neuronal atrophy and degeneration predominantly affecting peripheral sensory and autonomic neurons. In: Dyck P, Thomas P, Lambert E, et al., eds. *Peripheral neuropathy*, vol. 2. Philadelphia: WB Saunders, pp. 1065–1093.
19. Dyck P (1993): Hereditary motor and sensory neuropathies. In: Dyck P, Thomas P, Lambert E, et al., eds. *Peripheral neuropathy*, vol. 2. Philadelphia: WB Saunders, pp. 1600–1655.
20. Fath M, Hassanein MR, James JIP (1983): Congenital absence of pain: a family study. *J Bone Joint Surg Br* 65:186–188.
21. Gamble JG, Lawrence RL, Lee JH (1988): Orthopaedic aspects of central core disease. *J Bone Joint Surg Am* 70:1061–1066.
22. Ganz SB, Kahanovitz N, Levine DB, et al. (1982): Comprehensive rehabilitation of the patient with dysautonomia. *Orthop Trans* 6:116.
23. Guidera KJ, Multhopp H, Ganey T, et al. (1990):. Orthopaedic manifestations in congenitally insensate patients. *J Pediatr Orthop* 10: 514–521.
24. Guidera KJ, Borrelli J, Raney E, et al. (1991): Orthopaedic manifestations of Rett syndrome. *J Pediatr Orthop* 11:204–208.
25. Guille JT, Forlin E, Bowen JR (1992): Charcot joint disease of the shoulders in a patient who had familial sensory neuropathy with anhidrosis: a case report. *J Bone Joint Surg Am* 74:1415–1417.
26. Hagberg B (1980): *Infantile autistic dementia and loss of hand use: a report of 16 Swedish girl patients*. Presented at the research session of the European Federation of Child Neurology Societies, Manchester, England.
27. Hagberg B, Aircardi J, Dias K, Ovidio R (1983): A progressive syndrome of autism, dementia, ataxia, and loss of purposeful hand use in girls. Rett's syndrome: report of 35 cases. *Ann Neurol* 14:471–479.
28. Hagberg B (1989): Rett syndrome: clinical peculiarities, diagnostic approach, and possible cause. *Pediatr Neurol* 5:75–83.
29. Hagberg B (1993): Rett syndrome: Clinical and biological aspects. Clinics in developmental medicine. London, MacKeith Press.
30. Hall JG, Reed SD, Driscoll EP (1983): Part 1. Amyoplasia: a common, sporadic condition with congenital contractures. *Am J Med Genet* 15: 571–590.
31. Hall JG (1985): Genetic aspects of arthrogryposis. *Clin Orthop* 194: 44–53.
32. Hall JG (1997): Arthrogryposis multiplex congenita: etiology, genetics, classification, diagnostic approach, and general aspects. Part B. *J Pediatr Orthop* 6:159–166.
33. Harrison DJ, Webb PJ (1990): Scoliosis in the Rett syndrome: natural history and treatment. *Brain Dev* 12:154–156.
34. Hass RH, Dixon SD, Sartoris DJ, et al. (1997): Osteopenia in Rett syndrome. *J Pediatr* 131:771–774.
35. Heggeness MH (1994): Charcot arthropathy of the spine with resulting paraparesis developing during pregnancy in a patient with congenital insensitivity to pain: a case report. *Spine* 19:95–98.
36. Hennessy MJ, Haas RH (1988): The orthopaedic management of Rett syndrome. *J Child Neurol* 3:S43–S47.
37. Hensinger RN, MacEwen GD (1976): Spinal deformity associated with heritable neurological conditions: spinal muscular atrophy, Friedreich's ataxia, familial dysautonomia, and Charcot-Marie-Tooth disease. *J Bone Joint Surg Am* 58:13–24.
38. Herron LD, Westin GW, Dawson EG (1978): Scoliosis in arthrogryposis multiplex congenita. *J Bone Joint Surg Am* 60:293–299.
39. Holm VA, King HA (1990): Scoliosis in the Rett syndrome. *Brain Dev* 12:151–153.
40. Huang TJ, Lubickey JP, Hammerberg KW (1994): Scoliosis in Rett syndrome. *Orthop Rev* 23:931–937.
41. Keret D, Bassett GS, Bunnell WP, et al. (1988): Scoliosis in Rett syndrome. *J Pediatr Orthop* 8:138–142.
42. Koster G, von Knoch M, Willert HG (1999): Unsuccessful surgical treatment of hip dislocation in congenital sensory neuropathy with anhidrosis: a case report. *J Bone Joint Surg Br* 81:102–105.
43. Krishna M, Taylor JF, Brown MC, et al. (1991): Failure of Somatosensory-evoked-potential monitoring in sensorimotor neuropathy. *Spine* 16:479.
44. Kumar S, Marks HG, Bowen JR, et al. (1985): Hip dysplasia associated with Charcot-Marie-Tooth disease in the older child and adolescent. *J Pediatr Orthop* 5:511–514.
45. Kuo RS, Macnicol MF (1996): Congenital insensitivity to pain: orthopaedic implications. *J Pediatr Orthop* 5:292–295.
46. Leonard H, Bower C (1998): Is the girl with Rett syndrome normal at birth? *Dev Med Child Neurol* 40:115–121.

47. Lidstrom J, Stokland E, Hagberg B (1994): Scoliosis in Rett syndrome: clinical and biological aspects. *Spine* 19:1632–1635.
48. Loder RT, Lee CL, Richards BS (1989): Orthopaedic aspects of Rett syndrome: a multicenter review. *J Pediatr Orthop* 9:557–562.
49. Luque ER (1982): Paralytic scoliosis in growing children. *Clin Orthop* March, 163:202–209.
50. MacEwen GD, Floyd GC (1970): Congenital insensitivity to pain and its orthopedic implications. *Clin Orthop* 68:100–107.
51. McKusick VA, Norum RA, Farkas HJ, et al. (1967): The Riley-Day syndrome: observations on genetics and survivorship. An interim report. *Isr J Med Sci* 3:372–379.
52. McMillan RD Levine DB, Axelrod F, et al. (1980): Spinal surgery in familial dysautonomia. *Orthop Trans* 3:34.
53. Martinez BA, Lake BD (1987): Childhood nemaline myopathy: a review of clinical presentation in relation to prognosis. *Dev Med Child Neurol* 29:815–820.
54. Moe JH, Kharrat K, Winter RB, et al. (1984): Harrington instrumentation without fusion plus external orthotic support for the treatment of difficult curvature problems in young children. *Clin Orthop* 185: 35–45.
55. Moessinger AC (1983): Fetal akinesia deformation sequence: an animal model. *Pediatrics* 72:857–863.
56. Mulley JC, Kozman HM, Phillips HA, et al. (1993): Refined genetic localization for central core disease. *Am J Hum Genet* 52:398–405.
57. Naidu S (1997): Rett syndrome: natural history and underlying disease mechanisms. *Eur Child Adolesc Psychiatry* 6:S14–S17.
58. Nukada H, Pollock M, Haas LF (1982): The clinical spectrum and morphology of type II hereditary sensory neuropathy. *Brain* 105: 647–665.
59. Okuno T, Inoue A, Izumo S (1990): Congenital insensitivity to pain with anhidrosis: a case report. *J Bone Joint Surg Am* 72:279–282.
60. Ouvrier RA, McLeod JG, Conchin TE (1987): The hypertrophic forms of hereditary motor and sensory neuropathy: a study of hypertrophic Charcot-Marie-Tooth disease (HMSN type I) and Dejerine-Sottas disease (HMSN type III) in childhood. *Brain* 110:121–148.
61. Pailthorpe CA, Benson MK (1992): Hip dysplasia in hereditary motor and sensory neuropathies. *J Bone Joint Surg Br* 74:538–540.
62. Patterson JF, Webb JK, Burwell RG (1990): The operative treatment of progressive early onset scoliosis: a preliminary report. *Spine* 15: 809–815.
63. Petrie JG (1953): A case of progressive joint disorders caused by insensitivity to pain. *J Bone Joint Surg Br* 35:399–401.
64. Philippart M (1990): The Rett syndrome in males. *Brain Dev* 12: 33–36.
65. Piazza MR, Bassett GS, Bunnell WP (1988): Neuropathic arthropathy in congenital indifference to pain. *Clin Orthop* 236:175–179.
66. Poznanski AK, La Rowe PC (1970): Radiographic manifestations of the arthrogryposis syndrome. *Radiology* 95:353–358.
67. Rett A (1966): Uber ein eigenartiges hirnatrophisches syndrom bei hyperammonaemie in kindersaler. *Wien Med Wochenschr* 116: 723–726.
68. Riley CM, Day RL, Greeley DMcL, et al. (1949): Central autonomic dysfunction with defective lacrimation: report of five cases. *Pediatrics* 3:468–478.
69. Rinsky LA, Gamble JG, Bleck EE (1985): Segmental instrumentation without fusion in children with progressive scoliosis. *J Pediatr Orthop* 5:687–690.
70. Roberts AP, Conner AN (1988): Orthopaedic aspects of Rett's syndrome: brief report. *J Bone Joint Surg Br* 70:674.
71. Robin GC (1984): Scoliosis in familial dysautonomia. *Bull Hosp Joint Dis Orthop Inst* 44:16–26.
72. Rubery PT, Speilman JH, Hester P, et al. (1995): Scoliosis in familial dysautonomia: operative treatment. *J Bone Joint Surg Am* 77: 1362–1369.
73. Sarwark JF, MacEwen GD, Scott CI (1986): Scoliosis in amyoplasia congenita (classic arthrogryposis). *Orthop Trans* 10:19.
74. Sarwark J, MacEwen GD, Scott CI (1990): Current concepts review: amyoplasia (a common form of arthrogryposis). *J Bone Joint Surg Am* 72:465–469.
75. Shapiro F, Specht L (1993): The diagnosis and orthopaedic treatment of inherited muscular diseases of childhood. *J Bone Joint Surg Am* 75: 439–454.
76. Shapiro F, Specht L (1993): The diagnosis and orthopaedic treatment of childhood spinal muscular atrophy, peripheral neuropathy, Friedreich ataxia, and arthrogryposis. *J Bone Joint Surg Am* 75: 1699–1714.
77. Sheldon W (1932): Amyoplasia congenita. *Gen Dis Child* 7:117–136.
78. Shuaib A, Paasuke RT, Brownell KW (1987): Central core disease: clinical features in 13 patients. *Medicine* (Baltimore) 66:389–396.
79. Staheli LT, Hall JG, Jaffe KM, et al. (1998): Arthrogryposis: a text atlas. Cambridge, UK: Cambridge University Press.
80. Stern WG (1923): Arthrogryposis multiplex congenita. *JAMA* 81: 1507–1510
81. Sweeney BP, Jones S, Langford RM (1985): Anaesthesia in dysautonomia: further complications. *Anaesthesia* 40:783–786.
82. Swinyard CA, Bleck EE (1985): The etiology of arthrogryposis (multiple congenital contracture). *Clin Orthop* 194:15–29.
83. Tello CA (1994): Harrington instrumentation without arthrodesis and consecutive distraction program for young children with severe spinal deformities: experience and technical details. *Orthop Clin North Am* 25:333–351.
84. Trevathan E, Naidu S (1988): The clinical recognition and differential diagnosis of Rett syndrome. *J Child Neurol* 3:S6–16.
85. Walker JL, Nelson KR, Stevens DB, et al (1994): Spinal deformity in Charcot-Marie-Tooth disease. *Spine* 1(19):1044–1047.
86. Yoslow W, Becker MH, Bartels J, et al. (1971): Orthopaedic defects in familial dysautonomia: a review of sixty-five cases. *J Bone Joint Surg Am* 53:1541–1550.
87. Zoghbi H (1988): Genetic aspects of Rett syndrome. *Child Neurol* 3: S76–S77.

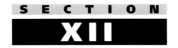

ORTHOTICS

ORTHOTIC TREATMENT FOR SPINAL DISORDERS

THOMAS M. GAVIN
WILTON H. BUNCH
AVINASH G. PATWARDHAN
KEVIN P. MEADE
AND DONALD G. SHURR

The history of mechanical devices to support or correct deformities of the spine in children is long and respectable (2,14). Galen (131–201), Ambroise Paré (1510–1590), and Nicolas Andry (1658–1742) (4) all used and wrote about orthotic devices. Throughout the nineteenth century, the Europeans developed a large number of devices fashioned from steel, leather, and plaster, designed to correct deformities of the spine.

The modern era of orthotic treatment for spinal deformities began with the development of the Milwaukee brace (cervicothoracolumbosacral orthosis, CTLSO) by Blount and Schmidt (9) in the late 1940s. The Milwaukee brace was first used as a postoperative device to replace plaster casts, but in the 1960s it became the mainstay of nonoperative management of spinal deformities due to the leadership of John Moe (8). The 1970s heralded a better understanding of the biomechanical function of spinal orthoses and resulted in the design of low-profile orthoses (thoracolumbosacral orthosis, TLSO), which were used on the more caudal curves and functioned through the mechanism of transverse loading.

But the 1970s and 1980s were also a time of misgivings and even nihilism concerning the efficacy of orthotic treatment. Part-time regimens, electrical stimulation, and observation until the time of surgery all had their advocates. The uncertainty about natural history and the role of orthoses is now relegated to the past, and the value of orthotic treatment has been convincingly demonstrated.

Modern orthotic treatment decision making for pediatric patients requires knowledge of biomechanical mechanisms of action combined with sound clinical procedures, adequate follow-up, proper patient instruction, and physical therapy to ensure the best result. This chapter discusses state-of-the-art biomechanics,

technical parameters, indications for treatment, and treatment outcomes for orthotic treatment of the pediatric spine.

SPINAL DEFORMITY

Biomechanics of Orthotic Treatment

To understand the biomechanical principles of orthotic treatment for idiopathic scoliosis it is necessary to first understand why curves progress. Only when we understand the concepts of why and when curves progress will we understand why and how our clinical treatments will best arrest curve progression and yield a stable spine after skeletal maturity. Long-term clinical studies of children with idiopathic scoliosis have yielded a general understanding of who is at risk of progressing and when we should treat curves, and gives us expectations for the outcome of treatment (51,53,60,76). Understanding the conceptual framework for progression permits formulation of individually tailored clinical treatment plans to fulfill the specific requirements of each patient.

Curve Progression

Curve progression in idiopathic scoliosis may be explained theoretically by using Euler's theory of elastic buckling of a slender column (80). For a flexible column fixed at the base, free at the upper end, and subjected to an axial compressive force (Fig. 1A), there is an upper limit on the magnitude of this force at which point the column will buckle. The buckling load of a column is a function of its flexibility, length, and end support (boundary) conditions (80). For the column shown in Fig. 1A, the relationship is given by:

$$Pe = \pi^2 EI/4L^2$$

where Pe is the buckling load, EI is the flexural rigidity (resistance to bending), and L is the length.

This is an excellent analogy to show the relationship between patient growth and curve progression. In a child at a given age, the weight of the upper torso and arms may not exceed the buckling load of the spinal column. Therefore, an existing scoliotic curve may not progress. However, with height increase and

---

T. M. Gavin: Department of Orthopaedic Surgery and Rehabilitation, Loyola University Medical Center, Maywood, Illinois 60143.
W. H. Bunch: St. Alban's Episcopal Church, St. Pete Beach, Florida 33706–1546.
A. G. Patwardhan: Department of Orthopaedic Surgery and Rehabilitation, Loyola University Medical Center, Maywood, Illinois 60143.
K. P. Meade: Department of Mechanical, Materials and Aerospace Engineering, Illinois Institute of Technology, Chicago, Illinois 60616.
D. G. Shurr: Programs in Physical Therapy, University of Iowa, and American Prosthetics, Inc., Iowa City, Iowa 52240.

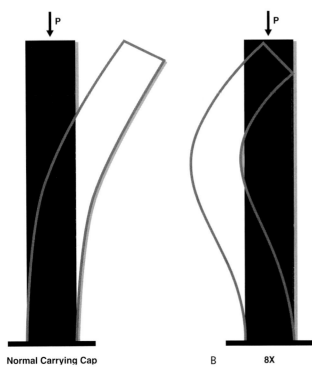

A **Normal Carrying Cap**   B   **8X**

FIGURE 1. A: Flexible column fixed at the base, free at the upper end under an axial load. (Redrawn from Gavin TM, Patwardhan AG, Bunch WH, et al. [1997]: Principles and components of spinal orthoses. In: American Academy of Orthopaedic Surgeons, ed. *Atlas of orthoses and assistive devices,* 3rd ed. St. Louis: Mosby–Year Book Publishers, pp. 155–194.) **B:** Stabilizing the superior end of a flexible column by means of a "pin." (Redrawn from Gavin TM, Patwardhan AG, Bunch WH, et al. [1997]: Principles and components of spinal orthoses. In: American Academy of Orthopedic Surgeons, ed. *Atlas of orthoses and assistive devices,* 3rd ed. St. Louis: Mosby–Year Book Publishers, pp. 155–194.)

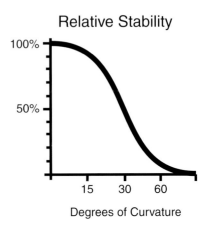

Relative Stability

FIGURE 2. The effect of curve magnitude or degree on the stability of a spinal curve. (Redrawn from Bunch WH, Patwardhan AG [1989]: Biomechanics of orthoses. In: Bunch WH, Patwardhan AG. *Scoliosis: making clinical decisions.* St. Louis: CV Mosby, pp. 204–215.)

with a larger curve, for any given maturity state, is more likely to experience progression than one with a smaller curve (12,53). With plastic deformation, the axial load may be removed *without* the spine returning to the original shape, thus yielding a permanent, or plastic, deformation.

Curve Magnitude Effect

The effect of curve magnitude or degree on the stability of a spinal curve, as reported by Bunch and Patwardhan (11), is shown in Figure 2. This graph shows that larger curves have low critical load values and are usually progressive. However, smaller curves have much higher critical load values and therefore are usually stable, requiring observation alone. The moderate curve range has a rapidly decreasing critical load value for increasing curve magnitude. This explains why these curves are sensitive to small changes in height and weight. Moderate curves are usually the ones wherein orthotic treatment is initiated. Curves of 60 degrees or greater are severely reduced in their critical load value and are unstable. That is why orthoses usually fail to stabilize these curves and why such curves often progress after skeletal maturity.

Biomechanics of Orthoses for Spinal Deformities

Mechanism of Action

Early attempts at correcting curves with external devices led to the development of orthoses that functioned by pure distraction (2,8). Andry reported on "depressing bony protuberances" (4), which may have implied the use of a transverse directed force. The controversy of using distractive versus transverse force may be best explained by White and Panjabi (85), who showed that curves less than 53 degrees respond better to transverse force, whereas curves greater than 53 degrees respond better to axial

weight gain of the upper trunk and arms, this relation may help explain progression of the curve. The formula for the buckling load indicates that an increase in the child's height greatly affects the capacity of the spinal column to support axial load. This formula implies that a 10% increase in height would result in about a 20% decrease in the buckling load. As a patient's height and weight increase, these two factors act together and may explain progression seen during the preadolescent growth spurt.

Curve progression seen in idiopathic scoliosis is not truly *elastic* buckling, which implies a *sudden* departure from the straight configuration of the column followed by total collapse (74). In idiopathic scoliosis, curve progression is a *gradual* deviation from the normal configuration of the spine over an extended period. Furthermore, in elastic buckling the critical load remains the same regardless of the magnitude of curvature.

Progression of a spinal curvature is actually a *plastic* (permanent) deformation. For plastic deformation of the spine, the upper limit of axial load that the spine can withstand without undergoing a permanent increase in curvature is termed "critical load" (74). There is a direct relationship between the magnitude of deformation and critical load. Clinical observations clearly document a strong relationship between the risk of progression and curve magnitude as the literature clearly shows that a patient

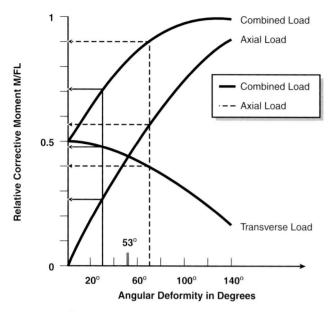

FIGURE 3. Effect of axial distractive loads and transverse loads on the curved spinal column. (From White AA, Panjabi MM [1978]: *Clinical biomechanics of the spine.* Philadelphia: JB Lippincott, p. 105.)

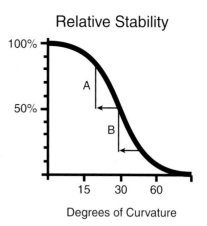

FIGURE 4. Stabilizing effect of curve correction yielded by an orthosis. (Redrawn from Bunch WH, Patwardhan AG [1978]: Biomechanics of orthoses. In: Bunch WH, Patwardhan AG. *Scoliosis: making clinical decisions.* St. Louis: CV Mosby, pp. 204–215.)

distraction (Fig. 3). This has resulted in the development of the current era of orthoses wherein the mechanism of distraction has yielded to the use of orthoses that only utilize transverse forces.

The clinical expectation of scoliosis orthosis is that it will prevent progression of an existing spinal curve and stabilize it until skeletal maturity. Three primary mechanisms of action are utilized to achieve this goal and are considered as separate but interactive effects (11). These are end point control, curve correction, and transverse loading.

End Point Control

End point control is the column sway resistance provided by the mechanical constraints of a spinal orthosis. For example, the neck ring of the Milwaukee brace reduces the sway in all directions by keeping the head and neck centered over the pelvis. Also, to provide a stable base of support from which pad loads may be applied, the pelvic interface fixes the orthosis rigidly to the base of the spine.

End point control alone provides an initial increase in the critical load of a curved spine (11). Stabilizing the superior end of the spine by means of a hinge (Fig. 1B) results in a theoretical critical load value that is eight times that for the column shown in Figure 1A.

The mechanical analogy shown in Figure 1B is an approximation of the constraints imposed by an orthosis on the end points of the scoliotic curve. For example, even though the neck ring of the Milwaukee brace limits the lateral sway, the superior end point of the scoliotic curve (usually T5) is caudal to the neck ring and does not provide the same kinematic constraint as the Euler model (Fig. 1B). Thus, the actual beneficial effect of the neck ring on the stability of a scoliotic curve may be much

smaller than that predicted by this analogy. However, this illustration of the concept clearly emphasizes the value of end point control in orthotic treatment for idiopathic scoliosis.

Curve Correction

Curve correction produced by an orthosis has the single greatest effect on increasing the overall critical load of the spinal column. Reducing a curve of 30 degrees to 20 degrees in the orthosis, which is considered a suboptimal clinical result by today's standards, will increase the stability of the curve from 50% to about 80% of normal. This is shown in Figure 4 by the vertical bar on the left.

This effect is also significant for larger curves. A curve of 45 degrees has a critical load of about 20% of normal. If the curve can be reduced to 30 degrees, the critical load increases to about 50% of normal. This is shown in Figure 4 as the vertical bar on the right.

Transverse Load

The defining characteristic of scoliosis orthoses is some form of a transversely directed load to the curvature of the scoliotic spine, usually through accessories known as pads. A transverse load alone directed at the apex of the curve increases the critical load that the spine can carry. In Figure 5 the lower line represents the critical load for an unsupported spine of increasing degree of curvature while the upper line indicates the critical load of the spine with a transverse support applied at the apex of the curve. For curves of 25 to 30 degrees, the transverse support increases the critical load from approximately 50% to 70% of normal.

This increase is shown in Figure 5 as the left vertical bar. It may be enough to prevent the curve from progressing; however, transverse support without curve correction will usually yield a clinically suboptimal result. Orthotic treatment may only keep the curve unchanged through the growth phase while the ortho-

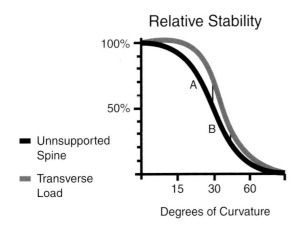

FIGURE 5. Stabilizing effect of transverse load directed at the apex of the curve. (Redrawn from Bunch WH, Patwardhan AG [1989]: Biomechanics of orthoses. In: Bunch WH, Patwardhan AG, eds. *Scoliosis: making clinical decisions*. St. Louis: CV Mosby, pp. 204–215.)

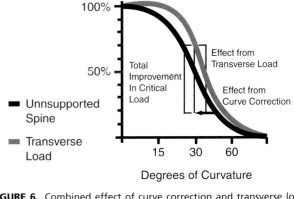

FIGURE 6. Combined effect of curve correction and transverse load. (From Bunch WH, Patwardhan AG [1989]: Biomechanics of Orthoses. In: Bunch WH, Patwardhan AG, eds. *Scoliosis: making clinical decisions*. St. Louis: CV Mosby, pp. 204–215.)

sis is donned. For curves of small magnitudes, maintenance of the status quo is satisfactory but should be considered a clinically suboptimal result.

However, for curves of progressively larger magnitudes, the effect of transverse support is reduced. In contrast to the smaller curves, a curve of 45 degrees would have its critical load increased from about 20% of normal to about 30%. This is shown in Figure 5 as the right vertical bar. The resultant stability may not be enough to stabilize the curve, and progression could be expected despite the use of an orthosis. This analysis suggests that orthoses that do not produce much correction should not be used on curves larger than 25 to 30 degrees.

A comparison of results shown in Figures 4 and 5 illustrates that for any given curvature, reduction of curve magnitude improves the critical load of the spine far more than transverse support alone.

Combined Effect

The effects of curve correction and continued transverse support are additive as shown in Figure 6. Once a curve of 45 degrees is reduced in the orthosis to 30 degrees, the corrective pads of an orthosis can be tightened maximally to provide continued lateral support (transverse load) to the corrected curve to further increase the critical load. This cumulative orthosis adjustment, which usually is done three times over the first 9 months of orthosis wearing, has the potential of increasing the critical load value of 20% to approximately 70% of normal (Fig. 6). Thus, with initial response from pad tightness and subsequent pad tightening, significant curve correction in the orthosis and continued transverse load must be obtained to optimize the results of orthotic treatment.

The Milwaukee Brace

The Milwaukee brace (Fig. 7) was developed in the late 1940s as a substitute for postoperative casting (9). It was subsequently

used for nonoperative treatment, and its traditional design was improved and refined (8). Several authors (3,8,11,51,59, 74,72,70) have reported the clinical and biomechanical mechanisms of action of the Milwaukee brace for stabilizing curves. In some studies, the magnitudes of forces generated by the various components of the orthosis were measured experimentally (29,59). In the standing position, the average distractive force was about 10 to 20 N and the lateral pad forces were about 20 to 40 N. Removal of the thoracic pad substantially increased

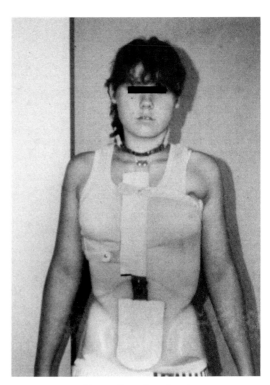

FIGURE 7. The Milwaukee brace.

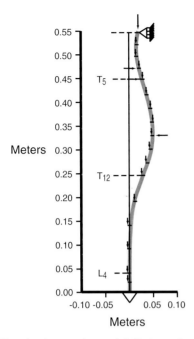

FIGURE 8. Milwaukee brace-spine model. (Redrawn from Patwardhan AG, Gavin TM, Bunch WH, et al. [1996]: A biomechanical comparison of the Milwaukee brace and TLSO. *J Prosth Orth* 8(4):115–122.)

the distractive forces, implying that the thoracic pad plays a primary role in providing curve stability.

Andriacchi et al. (3) used a mathematical model of the spine to analyze curve correction achieved by various components of the Milwaukee brace. In moderate curves of 40 to 45 degrees, the lateral pad load was the predominant corrective component as compared to the distractive force due to the superstructure of the orthosis (29,59).

Given the spine model described above, it is possible to think theoretically about the Milwaukee brace (Fig. 8). The sacrum was first fixed in all degrees to simulate the pelvic interface (70). To simulate the neck ring, the lateral displacement of the first thoracic vertebra was constrained to prevent sway. Transverse loads were then applied at the apex of the curve and were subsequently varied to vertebra above and below the apex.

For primary right thoracic curves with T5 cephalic end point and T8 apex, axillary pad resistive forces were applied in addition to thoracic and lumbar pads to complete the force triangulation. This resists having the neck ring be pulled into the neck on the side contralateral to the thoracic pad, in response to thoracic pad force (neck ring reaction). The axillary sling force was set to minimize or eliminate the neck ring reaction (relative to the magnitude of thoracic pad force) and was placed at the most common superior end point of an idiopathic curve with a T8–9 apex (T4 and T5). The force was directed onto the concave side of the curve.

The magnitude of the axillary sling forces was found to be in the range 15 to 34 N for various combinations of the pad placements and a maximum thoracic pad load of 50 N. Addition of a lumbar pad decreased the magnitude of shoulder sling force needed to minimize the neck ring reaction.

In these simulations, as well as in the simulations of the TLSO, the stabilizing effect of the pad forces was evaluated in a two-stage manner corresponding directly to the clinical procedure used in fitting a patient with an orthosis. The loads were applied and the corrections produced were calculated. The spine was initially loaded to simulate axial load after orthosis pad loads were applied (19). Then additional force was applied to the corrected curve to simulate pad adjustments done by the orthotist during follow-up visits to regain lateral support in the orthosis that was lost when the curve responded to the initial force and was reduced. The stability of the curve was measured by calculating the critical load under these different conditions.

Primary Thoracic

This model supports much of the trial-and-error–generated clinical knowledge gained from experience. The best correction and maximum stability of the primary thoracic curve can be achieved by applying the thoracic pad load at its apex. However, incorrect placement of the thoracic pad cephalad to the apex reduces the stability of the thoracic curve and might suggest a strong sensitivity to pad placement. This reinforces the need of frequent clinical follow-ups to adjust the pads for growth, thus ensuring continual optimum thoracic pad placement. Placement of the thoracic pad two levels caudad to the apex reduces the stability achieved by the correctly placed thoracic pad by 16% (Fig. 9).

Although necessary for double curves, the lumbar pad at the apex of the lumbar compensatory curve tends to decrease the correction of the primary thoracic curve and the stability achieved by a correctly placed thoracic pad. A lumbar pad one level too cephalad causes a further reduction in the correction of the thoracic primary curve, with an even greater loss in the stability gained by the use of the thoracic pad. This is shown in Figure 9. The loss of stability caused by having the lumbar pad one level too cephalad is about equal to that of having the thoracic pad two levels too caudad.

In midthoracic curves, placement of a thoracic pad at the apex of the curve produced maximum correction. Correction of the midthoracic curve decreased when the thoracic pad was placed two levels caudad to the apex and also with the addition of a lumbar pad. When treating primary thoracic curves, a single thoracic pad without a lumbar pad on the compensatory curve provides the maximum critical load of the curve and therefore the maximum stability. This may help us to understand why double curves with both thoracic and lumbar pads are usually less responsive to orthotic force than single thoracic curves and therefore correct less in an orthosis.

Primary Lumbar

Primary lumbar curves, which are usually not treated with a Milwaukee brace, were modeled to better understand the effect of pad forces and to be able to compare the Milwaukee brace to the TLSO (70).

The best correction and maximum stability for a primary lumbar curve treated with a Milwaukee brace can be achieved by placement of a lumbar pad on the apex of the primary curve and a thoracic pad counterforce of a sufficient magnitude to

Primary Thoracic Curve

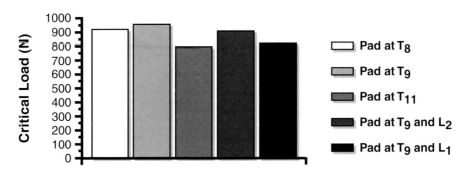

FIGURE 9. Stability yielded by thoracic and lumbar pads in the Milwaukee brace for thoracic primary curves. (Redrawn from Patwardhan AG, Gavin TM, Bunch WH, et al. [1996]: A biomechanical comparison of the Milwaukee brace and TLSO. *J Prosth Orth* 8(4):115–122.)

minimize the neck ring reaction. A lumbar pad alone at the apex of the primary curve without a thoracic counterforce results in about the same amount of curve correction, although the resultant critical load is nearly 25% less than that achieved when a thoracic apical counterforce is used, and therefore it is not as effective in *stabilizing* the primary lumbar curve (Fig. 10). Incorrect placement of the lumbar pad one level too cephalad reduces its stabilizing effect by about 12%. This suggests that a three-point orthosis for lumbar primary curves (1, pelvic constraint; 2, lumbar apical load; 3, thoracic apex) is clearly more optimal than a two-point orthosis (1, pelvic constraint; 2, lumbar apical load; 3, righting reflex) and should be used to optimize results when treating these curves.

Correct placement of the pads is of great importance. In the thoracic area, misplacement of a pad one level too high or too low greatly reduces the stabilizing effect of the thoracic pad. This effect is even more significant in the lumbar area. Placing a lumbar pad one level too high effectively eliminates any benefit

of the pad. Therefore, the sensitivity of pad placement for primary lumbar curves is similar to the sensitivity for the primary thoracic curves. Thus, follow-up growth adjustments to reposition the pads are essential for optimal outcome of treatment.

The Thoracolumbosacral Orthosis

The same type of modeling has been done for the TLSO (70). The sacrum was fixed to simulate the stabilizing effect of the pelvic section. The lateral walls of the orthoses and the trim line (concave side superior endpoint counterforce) were simulated by linear springs at the appropriate vertebral levels. The springs denote the equivalent resistance of the ribs to deformation along the medial-lateral direction. As before, the procedure was to apply a load and calculate the correction. Then additional force was applied to this corrected configuration to simulate the maintenance of lateral support in the orthosis.

Primary Lumbar Curve

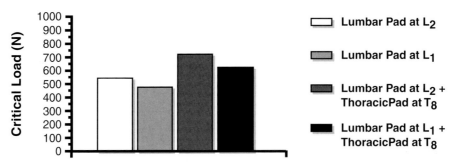

FIGURE 10. Stability yielded by thoracic and lumbar pads in the Milwaukee brace for lumbar primary curves. (Redrawn from Patwardhan AG, Gavin TM, Bunch WH, et al. [1996]: A biomechanical comparison of the Milwaukee brace and TLSO. *J Prosth Orth* 8(4):115–122.)

Primary Thoracic Curve

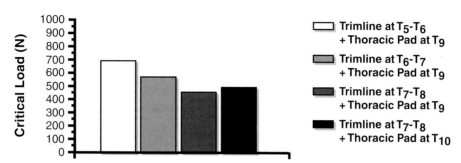

FIGURE 11. Stability yielded by thoracic and lumbar pads in the thoracolumbosacral orthosis for thoracic primary curves. (Redrawn from Patwardhan AG, Gavin TM, Bunch WH, et al. [1996]: A biomechanical comparison of the Milwaukee brace and TLSO. *J Prosth Orth* 8(4):115–122.)

Primary Thoracic

For primary thoracic curves, with T5 as the cephalic end and a T8 apex, maximum stability and curve correction are achieved with the trim line at T5–6 and a pad at the apex to the thoracic curve (Fig. 11). As the trim line of the TLSO moves caudal relative to the superior end point of the curve, curve correction decreases and there is a loss of stability of nearly 18% to 20% with each level.

With the counterforce trim line set at T5–6, moving the thoracic pad one level cephalad to the apex decreases the curve correction and causes a 13% loss in stability. Placement of the thoracic pad up to two levels caudad to the apex has no appreciable effect on the curve correction and stability. Although necessary for double curves, adding a lumbar pad at the apex of the compensatory curve decreases the effectiveness of correctly placed thoracic pad because the critical load value decreases by nearly 15%. A lumbar pad one level too cephalad further decreases the correction of the primary curve and causes a 20%

decrease in stability as compared to that achieved by a correctly placed thoracic pad alone. This is consistent with the behavior of the lumbar pad noted for the Milwaukee brace treatment of primary thoracic curves.

Primary Lumbar

In primary lumbar curves, the optimum result with a TLSO is achieved with the trim line at the apical level of the compensatory thoracic curve and a pad at the apex of the primary lumbar curve. Moving the trim line caudad toward the end point of the primary lumbar curve results in progressively greater loss of stability with each lower level (Fig. 12).

Comparison of the Milwaukee Brace and TLSO

Because we consider the Milwaukee brace the historical gold standard against which other orthoses should be measured, it is

Primary Lumbar Curve

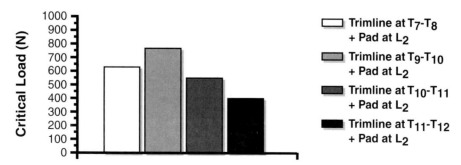

FIGURE 12. Stability yielded by thoracic and lumbar pads in the thoracolumbosacral orthosis for lumbar primary curves. (Redrawn from Patwardhan AG, Gavin TM, Bunch WH, et al. [1996]: A biomechanical comparison of the Milwaukee brace and TLSO. *J Prosth Orth* 8(4):115–122.)

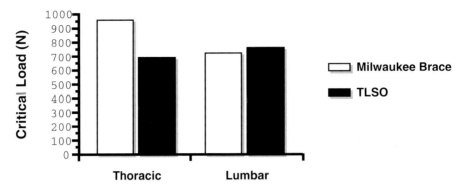

FIGURE 13. Comparison of stability yielded by Milwaukee brace and thoracolumbosacral orthosis for thoracic and lumbar primary curves. (Redrawn from Patwardhan AG, Gavin TM, Bunch WH, et al. [1996]: A biomechanical comparison of the Milwaukee brace and TLSO. *J Prosth Orth* 8(4):115–122.)

important to compare the stability of a TLSO with that of the Milwaukee brace (70). These comparisons are shown in Figure 13. For primary thoracic curves, the stability gained with a TLSO is approximately 25% less than that obtained with the Milwaukee brace.

This suggests that thoracic curves of larger magnitudes that are not well corrected may respond better with a Milwaukee brace than a TLSO. For primary lumbar curves, a properly fitted TLSO appears to be as effective as the Milwaukee brace in stabilizing the curve. This is consistent with clinical experience because the current use of a Milwaukee brace is usually for a thoracic primary curve whereas the TLSO is the exclusive orthosis for lumbar primary curves.

Decompensation

When most people stand, the head in the frontal plane is centered directly over the sacrum or is "compensated." This is also true of patients with scoliosis. However, such individuals develop secondary curves or half-curves to keep the head centered while accommodating the primary curve. This secondary accommodation maintains a compensated posture.

For double curves in which the caudal lumbar end point is rotated counterclockwise, the tendency is to shift to the left of the center sacral line (CSL) or in the direction of the tilt of the lowest vertebra in the lowest curve (30). When patients are placed in orthoses for double curves, this shift, known as *decompensation,* is frequently increased. In a geometrical modeling study, Gavin et al. (30) showed that for double curves corrected in orthoses (with the upper thoracic curve geometry fixed), if there is a greater than 2:1 ratio of either thoracic to lumbar or lumbar to thoracic curve magnitudes, the patient will always decompensate to the left (Fig. 14). With the initial tendency to lean left, care must be taken to counter this to yield a balanced spine in the orthosis. Because patients will be leaning to one side or another due to the position of the orthosis and the confinement, it is important to counteract the decompensation tendency caused from the curve pattern (toward the tilt of the lowest vertebra in the curves).

Effect of Decompensation on Spinal Stability

As shown in Figure 15, decompensation is directly related to progressive decrease in the stability of the spine (11). Correctly placed pads will increase the stability by about the same percentage as for compensated curves. However, as the initial stability was lower due to decompensation, the end result of an orthosis in which the patient is not compensated is a lower critical load of the spine. These results should encourage orthopaedists and orthotists to check brace alignment frequently and with great care in order to avoid decompensation and to make the proper timely adjustments to the orthosis to counteract the tendency to decompensate.

Pad Loading

The modeling studies described above showed that for optimal stability resultant pad forces should be directed at curve apices. Also, counterforces should be directed at the pelvis and cephalad curve end points. This leaves the question: "How should we load the curves to optimize results?"

The traditional three-point loading system for single thoracic, lumbar, or thoracolumbar curves, as reported by Gavin (34), in which a "translatory" or trunk-shifting load is applied at and inferior to the apex of the curve on the convex side, shifting against a concave side counterforce on the superior end of the curve and against an inferior, concave side counterforce on the pelvis, is ideal for single curves. This three-point system will reduce the tilt of the most inferior vertebra in the curve as well as reduce the Cobb magnitude.

However, when we consider right thoracic, left lumbar double-curve patterns in which the thoracic curve is primary, traditional experience would have us placing pads at the thoracic and lumbar apices, with the greatest magnitude of pad pressure directed at and below the primary curve apex (translatory load, or TL). The lumbar pad would be of a lesser load magnitude (constraining load, or CL), placed over the deformity of the lumbar curve, and would increase its load magnitude from the synergy of tightening the thoracic pad (Fig. 16).

Counterforces would then be applied at the pelvis opposite the lumbar pad and the axilla opposite the thoracic pad. This has

Thoracic Cobb

Lumbar Cobb	5	10	15	20	25
5	-25 mm -10 mm Compensated 10 mm	-25 mm -10 mm Compensated	-25 mm		
10	-25 mm -10 mm Compensated	-25 mm -10 mm Compensated 10 mm 25 mm	-25 mm -10 mm Compensated 10 mm	-25 mm -10 mm Compensated	
15	-25 mm -10 mm	-25 mm -10 mm Compensated 10 mm	-25 mm -10 mm Compensated 10 mm 25 mm	-25 mm -10 mm Compensated 10 mm 25 mm	-10 mm Compensated 10 mm
20	-25 mm	-25 mm -10 mm Compensated 10 mm	-25 mm -10 mm Compensated 10 mm 25 mm	-25 mm -10 mm Compensated 10 mm 25 mm	-25 mm -10 mm Compensated 10 mm 25 mm
25	-25 mm -10 mm Compensated 10 mm 25 mm	-25 mm -10 mm	-25 mm -10 mm Compensated 10 mm 25 mm	-25 mm -10 mm Compensated 10 mm 25 mm	-25 mm -10 mm Compensated 10 mm 25 mm
30	-25 mm -10 mm Compensated 10 mm 25 mm	-25 mm	-25 mm -10 mm Compensated 10 mm	-25 mm -10 mm Compensated 10 mm 25 mm	-25 mm -10 mm Compensated 10 mm 25 mm

Coronal Balance Possible for Given Thoracic/Lumbar Angle Combinations

FIGURE 14. Table of possible compensation/decompensation values (-25 mm, -10 mm, 0 mm, 10 mm, 25 mm) for a combination of 30 thoracic/lumbar curve magnitudes with a fixed upper thoracic geometry.

been called the four-point pressure system, which is a synergistic system that utilizes two 3-point force systems: one 3-point system on the thoracic curve and one 3-point system on the lumbar curve. This yields two triangulation of force on the two curves (Fig. 16). Tightening of the thoracic pad results in the increase in force from all four points. The result is a trunk shift from right (convex side of thoracic curve) to left (concave side of thoracic curve). Therefore, the only shifting or translatory load is at the thoracic apex as depicted in Fig. 16A as TL, and the axilla, lumbar apex, and opposite pelvis becomes counterforces or "constraining" loads as depicted in Fig. 16A as CL.

This traditional four-point loading mechanism has an inherent flaw. The translatory force creates a trunk shift to the left of CSL, toward the direction the spinal column, which already displays a tendency to decompensate (32). This may or may not increase decompensation, but it moves the entire column in the area of the curve farther left from center sacral line (CSL) and may resist correction in the orthosis.

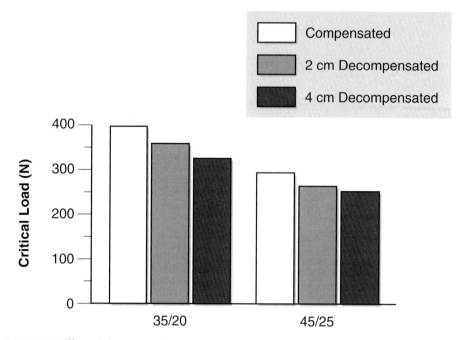

FIGURE 15. Effect of decompensation on curve stability. (From Bunch WH, Patwardhan AG [1989]: Biomechanics of orthoses. In: Bunch WH, Patwardhan AG. *Scoliosis: making clinical decisions*. St. Louis: CV Mosby, pp. 204–215.)

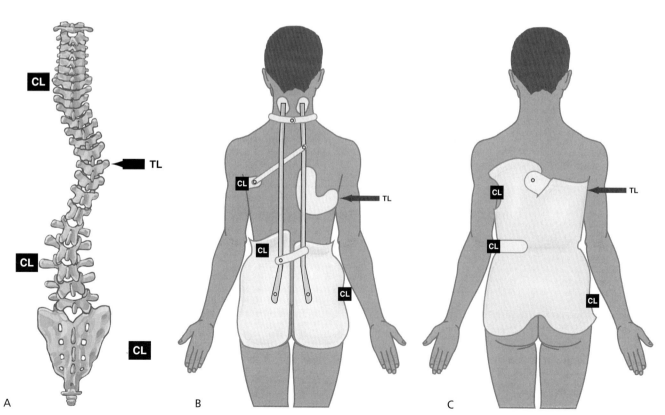

FIGURE 16. **A:** Traditional four-point orthotic curve loading system on a right thoracic, left lumbar curve. **B:** On the Milwaukee brace. **C:** On a thoracolumbosacral orthosis (Rosenberger).

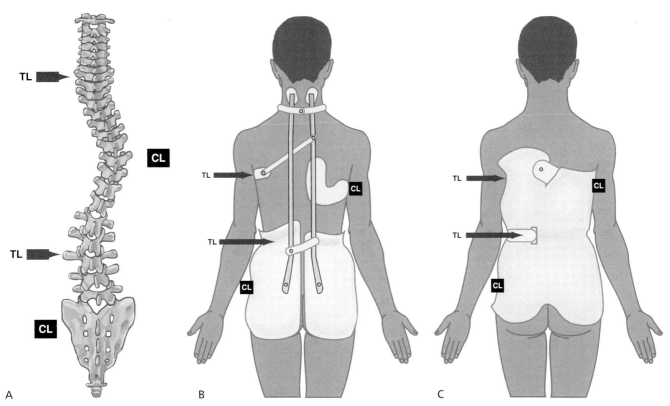

FIGURE 17. A: New four-point curve loading system on a right thoracic, left lumbar curve. **B:** On the Milwaukee brace. **C:** On a thoracolumbosacral orthosis (Rosenberger).

We have reported a four-point force system in which the axilla and lumbar points become translatory loads and shift the torso from left to right, against the thoracic pad, thus loading these three points with a resultant overall shift of the spinal column toward CSL (32) (Fig. 17). Because of the greater magnitude of the axilla load, the orthosis tends to become unstable and rotate counterclockwise (away from the axilla), necessitating a stabilizing force at the pelvis *on the same side as the axilla and lumbar loads.* Thus, the axilla counterforce and lumbar pad become *translatory* force (TL), whereas the pelvis and thoracic sling become *constraining* forces (CL), as depicted in Fig. 17A.

This force system has only one synergistic triangulation of force that is on the primary curve only and a stabilizing force on the pelvis. Therefore, the system yields three points of force on the left side and one point on the right. The tendency of the spinal column to move left is countered first, and then the curves are corrected. This method first reduces the tilt of the lowest vertebra in the lumbar curve and then reduces the Cobb magnitude.

Natural History

Originally, the diagnosis of scoliosis was an indication for treatment. Small curves of 15 and 20 degrees, as well as larger curves of up to 60 degrees, were treated without consideration of the degree of skeletal maturity or documented progression. Studies on prevalence and natural history to provide a rationale for treatment were needed.

Lonstein and Carlson (53) provided this needed natural history and showed the relationship of age and curve magnitude to risk of progression. They found that children first seen at the age of 10 years (or younger) with curve magnitude of 5 to 19 degrees had a 45% risk of progression, whereas those with curves between 20 and 29 degrees had a 100% risk. In children 11 to 12 years of age, the risk of progression in the 5- to 19-degree range was 23%, whereas in the 20- to 29-degree range it was 61%. For children 15 years and older, the 5- to 19-degree group reduced to a 4% risk factor and the 20- to 29-degree group reduced to a 16% risk factor.

Fernandez-Feliberti et al. (26) later confirmed these findings. In their study, 33% of the patients aged 13 or younger and with a curve of less that 29 degrees progressed. However, if the curve of these patients was 30 degrees or greater, 66% progressed. Of the children older than 13 years and with a curve of less than 29 degrees, fewer than 10% needed surgery. If the curve of this group was greater than 30 degrees, 14% needed surgery. This is illustrated in Table 1.

Long-term progression has been studied by Weinstein et al. (82,83). With an average follow-up of 40 years, it was found that 68% of the curves had progressed 5 degrees or more. Although some of this progression probably occurred in late adolescence, 37% had progressed in the last 10 years an average of 13 degrees. As in childhood progression, the degree of curve and the degree of progression were linked. The thoracic curves under 30 degrees did not progress, whereas those between 30 and 50

TABLE 1. RISK OF PROGRESSION[a]

Age	Curve (Degrees)	
	<30	>30
<13	38%	66%
>13	10%	14%

[a] The prediction of curve progression in untreated idiopathic scoliosis during growth. Based on data presented in Brill PW, Mitty HA, Guall GE (1974): Homocystinuria and Marfan's syndrome *J Bone Joint Surg Br* 54: 277–298.

degrees progressed an average of 10 degrees, and curves of 50 to 75 degrees progressed an average of 29 degrees. This study showed that progression was not linear throughout follow-up. Curve progression was greater during the time from skeletal maturity to 30-year follow-up than from 30 to 40 years after diagnosis.

These studies of the nature of curve progression and the relationships of age and curve magnitude lead directly to orthotic treatment indications and expectations.

Indications for Orthotic Treatment

Orthotic treatment is generally indicated for skeletally immature patients with curves between 20 and 40 degrees. There is no indication for treatment of curves under 20 degrees. Orthotic treatment should be started immediately for curves of 20 to 30 degrees if 2 or 3 years of growth remains (i.e., a Risser sign of 0–1 and premenarchal). Those with Risser signs of 2 or 3 with demonstrated progression in this range should also be treated.

Children with curves of 30 to 40 degrees should be treated at the first visit if they have growth remaining. A more mature adolescent with a Risser sign of 4 or 5 and who is 1.5 years post menarche should not need treatment.

There is no convincing evidence that the type of orthosis is critical as long as it is designed for the specific curve problem and corrects the curve in the brace. For optimal results in avoiding surgery, the larger curves must be reduced by at least 50% in the orthosis and maintained throughout the duration of wear (51). With the newer designs, this threshold can and should be reached for all patients.

We believe that the treatment course for all but the Charleston bending brace should be full time until growth is completed followed by a gradual weaning period. Green (37) reported that part-time orthotic treatment can yield good results and that the protocol of full-time treatment is not necessary. However, Edmonsson and Morris (22) found that patients who were not compliant with full-time wearing did not do as well as the full-time wearers. The difference was 25% correction for the full-time wearers and only 14% for the partially compliant. In the meta-analysis to be discussed below, 8 and 16 hours of wearing time were not as effective as full-time protocols. The weight of the evidence is on the side of full-time wearing until growth is completed.

The Charleston bending brace (Fig. 18A) can only be used at night. The principle is demonstrated in Figure 18B and C. Acceptable results have been reported using this orthosis (75). However, it must be noted that in the meta-analysis (76) re-

ported below and in a comparison with the Boston brace (44), the Charleston brace did not give as good a result as others. Because it is only worn at night, the effect of part-time treatment cannot be definitively separated from the effect of brace type.

Studies of Results

Many studies have been carried out to investigate clinical outcome of patients with idiopathic scoliosis treated in the Milwaukee brace (12,17,22,46,51,56,57). However, many of these studies included patients that would not be considered for treatment today because of small curve magnitude, stage of maturity, or lack of documented progression. These inadequacies have been largely overcome in two large-scale studies of patients treated with a Milwaukee brace and one prospective study.

The first is the report by Lonstein and Winter (51) in which 1,020 patients with adolescent idiopathic scoliosis were treated with the Milwaukee brace between 1954 and 1979. Average follow-up was 6.2 years, with all greater than 2 years. Failure was defined as the need for surgery. Overall, 22% of the patients required surgery.

Curve Pattern

Persons with single right thoracic curves needed surgery only 19% of the time. Approximately 27% of patients with lumbar, thoracolumbar, or double thoracic curves required surgery.

Curve Magnitude

Six percent of patients with curves under 19 degrees needed surgery. In the 20- to 29-degree range, 7% required surgery. For curves of 30 to 39 degrees, the rate of surgery increased to 23%; for 40 to 49 degrees, 33%; and for curves greater than 60 degrees at the start of orthotic treatment, 84% of patients required surgery. This trend was constant for all curve patterns (Fig. 19).

Maturity of the Patient

The surgery rate on patients who initiated treatment at Risser 0–1 with curves of 20 to 29 degrees was 32% and for curves 30 to 39 degrees 45%. Both of these were below natural history predictions of 68% for curves over 20 degrees and Risser sign 0–1. For more mature patients with a Risser sign of 2, the comparative figures were 12% and 18%, respectively. This study showed that the incidence of surgery was lower for the more mature patient and that orthotic treatment affects the natural history of progression.

There were two findings that are important in the thinking about treatment course. First, the average time in brace was 3 years 10 months. Good results are not possible when the orthosis wear is terminated after correction is achieved but growth is incomplete. Second, all patients lost a few degrees of correction when the brace was discontinued. This implies that the best possible correction should be obtained and maintained during treatment.

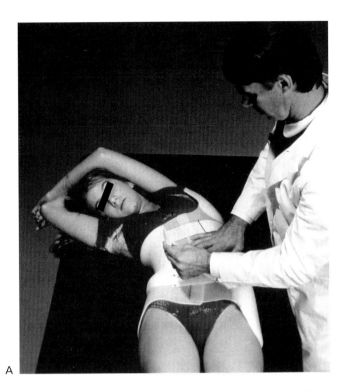

FIGURE 18. **A:** The Charleston bending brace. Note side-bending contour of orthosis. (Courtesy of Ralph Hooper, C.P.O., Charleston Bending Brace Foundation.) **B, C:** The curve unbending principles of the Charleston bending brace.

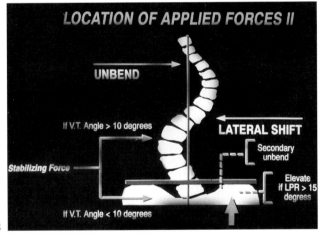

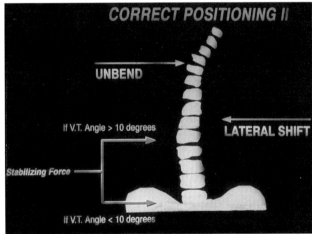

The second large-scale study is a meta-analysis by Rowe et al. (76). Meta-analysis is a statistical method of pooling and analyzing data from a number of reports. Its purpose is to increase the statistical power and resolve uncertainty when the results disagree. There are several objections that can be raised to the use of meta-analysis but none apply to this paper. The application of this technique to scoliosis was long overdue (6).

The report included 1,910 patients from 22 different studies of whom 1,459 had been treated with an orthosis. (The Lonstein and Winter study was not included in this meta-analysis, so that there is no overlap between the two reports.) The authors of this study found that the use of an orthosis, particularly the Milwaukee brace, for 23 hours per day effectively halted progression of the curve. Treatment programs for 8 or 16 hours a day were significantly less effective. Electrical stimulation was completely ineffective.

Although these two papers have large numbers and convincing results, neither is a prospective controlled study. The Scoliosis Research Society, under the leadership of Alf Nachemson, designed such a study (60). This could not be randomized for a number of practical reasons but consisted of each center treating the patient as they believed best. Patients were treated with observation only (129 patients), bracing (111 patients), and electrical stimulation (46 patients). There was a 74% success rate for those treated with an orthosis; observation only and electrical stimulation had only a 33% success rate. Criteria for inclusion and for failure were standardized across all treatment centers.

There are few large long-term studies involving patients treated with TLSOs. However, many reports suggest that excellent results can be obtained. Emans (23) reported on 295 patients with idiopathic scoliosis treated with the Boston brace. Of the patients treated with curves 30 to 40 degrees, only 16%

FIGURE 19. Orthotic failure

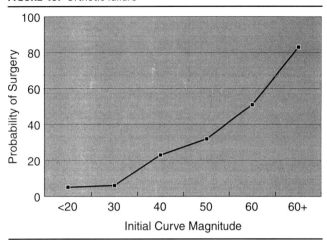

This shows the percentage of orthotic failures as a function of initial curve magnitude. It is clear that orthotic treatment is very effective for curves of 40 degrees or less. Based on data presented in reference 51.

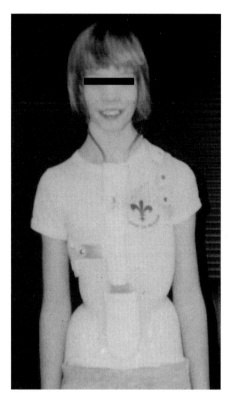

FIGURE 20. Current Milwaukee brace.

required surgery by the time of follow-up, whereas for curves greater than 40 degrees, 32% required surgery. McCollough et al. (55) reported results of a study on 100 patients treated with the Miami orthosis in which 6% of patients required surgery at the time of follow-up. Allington and Bowen (1) showed the surgery rate on a series of patients treated with the Wilmington jacket also to be 6%.

The authors are confident that these studies have convincingly demonstrated the value of orthotic treatment for scoliosis. However, doubters remain (68,78). In some cases the problem has been the lack of correction obtained in the orthosis. If the curve is not corrected in the orthosis, good results cannot be expected.

Some who are opposed to orthotic treatment suggest that psychological damage is a significant risk. Although there are some suggestions of this in the literature, the broad stream of reports from the 1970s (86) to the most recent (67) have indicated that psychological effects, if any, are usually mild and transient.

Idiopathic Scoliosis

The Milwaukee Brace

Contemporary nonoperative treatment of idiopathic scoliosis originated with Blount and Moe (8) in the 1950s. They designed a device fabricated from steel and leather extending from the pelvis to the mandible and occiput (to provide longitudinal distraction) along with a lateral pad against the most displaced ribs on the convex side of the deformity (to control scoliosis in children without resorting to surgery). In its present form, the neck ring does not provide distraction and the superstructure of the Milwaukee brace is a structure to which lateral pads are attached. The neck ring provides resistance to the sway of the vertebral column and functions as a mechanical "pin," keeping the upper thoracic spine constrained over the sacrum (34). Thermoplastics

are used for the pelvic interface, replacing leather and steel in an effort to reduce weight and improve hygiene (Fig. 20).

The TLSO

Low-profile or underarm-type orthoses, more commonly known as TLSOs, are not a modern concept. Crude underarm trunk supports fashioned from tree bark were found in the cave dwellings of pre-Columbian Indians (2). Modern TLSO usage for the nonoperative treatment of scoliosis began with the Boston brace (Fig. 21). The concept began as a method of treating curves with apices at and caudad to T10 with the pelvic aspect of a CTLSO, thus eliminating the superstructure (39). The Boston brace has evolved into a system of prefabricated TLSO modules, custom-fitted for specific patient needs, and is currently used to treat all curves with apices as cephalad as T8. It is the most widely known TLSO for scoliosis treatment.

Unlike the Milwaukee brace, which is still the only CTLSO for treatment of spinal deformity, several different TLSOs have been developed throughout the 1970s and 1980s. The Lyon orthosis was developed in France with modifications used in the United States (Fig. 22). The Lyon was developed for the treatment of more caudal lumbar and thoracolumbar curves (16). The Miami orthosis (55) is an orthosis similar to the Boston brace in many regards, including usage parameters with variations in trim line, and is custom-molded. The Wilmington orthosis (15) (Fig. 23) is a custom-molded TLSO fabricated from a Risser frame plaster impression taken in curve correction. The Rosenberger orthosis (35) (Fig. 24) is a custom-molded TLSO

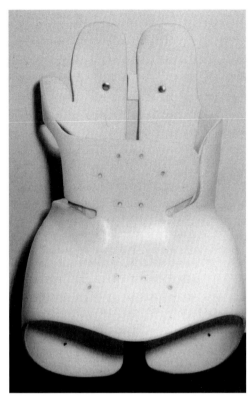

FIGURE 21. The Boston thoracolumbosacral orthosis.

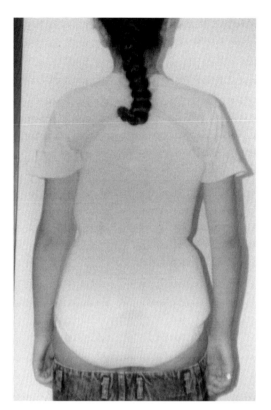

FIGURE 23. The Wilmington thoracolumbosacral orthosis.

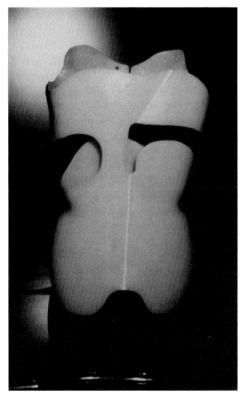

FIGURE 22. The Lyon thoracolumbosacral orthosis. (Photograph courtesy of L. Dreher Jouett, C.P.O. Chicago, IL.)

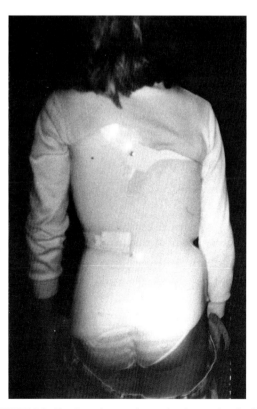

FIGURE 24. The Rosenberger thoracolumbosacral orthosis.

fabricated from a plaster impression taken with curvature correction and uses a Dacron thoracic sling to load thoracic curves.

Description of Thoracolumbosacral Orthoses

The Boston brace is a one-piece, posterior-opening TLSO fabricated from polypropylene that extends anteriorly from the xyphoid process to the symphysis pubis, with posterior and lateral trim lines varied for each curve pattern. This orthosis is modular and does not require a plaster impression. However, it must be custom-fitted for individual size and curve pattern. On the convex side of the curve, the Boston brace is trimmed one level superior to the apex of the curve to provide a wall to function as a thoracic or lumbar pad mount. On the concave side of the curve, an opening is cut opposite the pad to allow an open area for the concave side trunk shift on the level of the primary curve. Above the cutout a band of plastic is left intact to provide concave side superior end-point counterforce to function in the same manner as the axillary sling of the Milwaukee brace (Fig. 20).

The Lyon Orthosis

The Lyon orthosis is a one-piece, anterior-opening orthosis custom-fabricated from a plaster impression and fashioned from polypropylene. This orthosis extends anteriorly from the sternal notch to the symphysis pubis and has lateral trim lines, openings, and counterforce parameters that function similar to the Boston brace. Original fabrication utilized two lateral shells of custom-molded plastic joined posteriorly by a longitudinal aluminum bar, and steel hinges allowing for function as an anterior-opening orthosis. Recent modifications have changed this to a one-piece molded, with a posterior seam used for hinge function, which eliminates the metal structure and lightens the orthosis as seen in Figure 21.

The Miami Orthosis

The Miami orthosis is a one-piece, posterior-opening polypropylene TLSO, custom-molded from a plaster impression. This orthosis has many of the advantages of the Boston brace, yet, unlike the Boston brace, is custom-molded and trimmed short enough to allow forward bending of the patient. Lateral trim line heights and concave side cutout areas for trunk shift are similar to the Boston and Lyon orthoses, as they are all varied according to curve pattern.

The Wilmington Jacket

The Wilmington jacket is unique in that it is casted molding the plaster impression from the Risser frame. This impression is designed to be similar to the localizer cast, as the curves are to be reduced and analyzed by radiograph before proceeding with fabrication. This orthosis was originally designed to be molded with a low-temperature orthoplast. However, many have adopted the high-temperature, vacuum-formed, low-density

polyethylene, as shown in Figure 22, as it will provide greater longevity without material degradation. This is a one-piece, anterior-opening orthosis with anterior trim line from symphysis pubis to sternal notch and bilateral heights to axilla. It does not have concave side cutouts, varied trim lines, or wall-mounted pads, as all loads, counterforces, and concave side area for trunk shift are fabricated into the orthosis.

The Rosenberger Orthosis

The Rosenberger orthosis is a custom-molded, low-density polyethylene, anterior-opening TLSO. It is fabricated from a bivalved plaster impression made on an examination table with corrective forces done in the impression. Although the impression is bivalved and does not require a Risser frame, the procedure is similar to that for the Wilmington jacket. This orthosis extends anteriorly from the pubis to the xyphoid process. The convex side trim line is one rib level superior to the apical height, similar to the Boston or Miami orthosis. However, the concave side is similar to the Wilmington jacket in that there is no cutout for trunk shift because the shift is built into the orthosis. The concave side trim line terminates at the superior end point of the superior curve being treated. This orthosis is unique in that it uses adjustable floating slings for curve loading, as is seen in Figure 23, so that loading can exceed what is achieved by the corrected walls of the orthosis.

The Charleston Orthosis

The Charleston orthosis is unique in that it is prescribed for sleeping hours only. It is a custom-molded, one-piece, anterior-opening TLSO fabricated in a maximal side-bending position to "unbend" the primary curve. This concept is important because it is based on the concept of overcorrection during sleep. Because side bending decompensates the spine, this orthosis is not recommended for standing. Trunk shift is allowed for in the walls of the orthosis similar to the Rosenberger orthosis, and the side-bending correction is built into the orthosis walls similar to the Wilmington orthosis (Fig. 17A).

Neuromuscular Scoliosis

Orthotic treatment for neuromuscular scoliosis has traditionally been a treatment method to delay spinal fusion. Because of the pelvic obliquity and decompensation from neuromuscular scoliosis common to the nonambulatory child, seating balance is a major concern. A properly fitted orthosis will also assist this type of patient with seating balance to reduce fatigue and allow for longer periods of upper limb function. Custom-molded seating orthoses attached to the wheelchair are presently state of the art for this condition. However, these devices frequently do not incorporate continuous circumferential support and may not provide optimal function for curve reduction and maintenance of curves post reduction.

We have developed an orthotic approach to the correction of neuromuscular spinal deformity for the long *C*-shaped curves

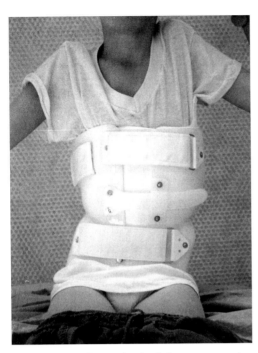

FIGURE 25. Thoracolumbosacral orthosis for neuromuscular scoliosis.

that eliminates the usage of three-point corrective forces. This replaces the three-point approach to curve correction with lateral bending toward the convexity of the curve. The primary focus of this "illiotibial band stretching" mechanism of action is to lengthen the pelvic origin and spinal insertion points of the psoas major muscle. This is coupled with a derotation force at the apex of the curve to lessen the rotational deformity. The result is greater correction of spinal deformity, resistance of deformity progression, and seating balance in the orthosis (31) (Fig. 25).

The ambulatory neuromuscular patient who frequently presents with compensatory curves benefits from the adjustability of three-point orthoses for idiopathic scoliosis, as described earlier in this chapter. Decision making for these patients must be based on primary orthotic goals. If seating stability is primary, then the patient will benefit from custom-molded seating. If, however, curve reduction and delay of fusion is primary, then the TLSO will yield the optimal result (31).

Although Bunch (13) successfully used the Milwaukee brace for paralytic scoliosis, current state of the art for the neuromuscular patient is the custom-molded, total-contact TLSO. Although some are pessimistic about the use of orthoses for neuromuscular scoliosis, the purpose of orthotic treatment is to reduce and maintain the curve until the patient is mature enough for fusion. Even though current treatment protocols call for operating on these patients at a younger age, many neuromuscular patients are either juvenile or infantile at the onset of progressive curvature and will benefit from the use of an orthosis (40). This will allow for trunk growth, which is important because the organs of the thorax and abdomen will continue to grow even if the spine does not.

Congenital Scoliosis

The patient with congenital scoliosis challenges the orthotic creativity of the clinical team. Goals for orthotic treatment of congenital scoliosis are to reduce compensatory curves and to maintain a compensated alignment of the spine during growth. Changing the segmental angulation of the congenital anomaly is not possible using orthoses; any attempt will lead to discomfort and skin breakdown.

The decision for proper choice of orthosis should include clinical requirements as well as mechanism of action. As most of these patients begin treatment at an early age and usually require surgery during the clinical course, they will require several orthoses during treatment. For families with financial difficulties the Milwaukee brace is the orthosis of choice because it is the only orthosis that has longitudinal adjustability, allows for partial refabrication, and is easily converted for postoperative use (34). The TLSO is the orthosis of choice for reasons of cosmesis.

Reduction or control of compensatory curves, compensation of the spine, and correction of any secondary deformity are the goals of orthotic treatment for the congenital patient.

Kyphosis

The sagittal plane deformity of kyphosis has many causes, such as Scheuermann disease, postural round back, neuromuscular disorders, and congenital dysplasia. The most common form to be treated with an orthosis is Scheuermann kyphosis, which manifests radiographically as anterior wedging of several consecutive vertebrae. The orthosis of choice is the Milwaukee brace because the apices of these curves are usually more cephalad than a TLSO can control. The pelvic interface and neck ring provides constraints in space that yield the counterforce to the kyphosis pads (Fig. 26). These pads are usually rectangular and are placed at and inferior to the apex of the curve, mounted on the paraspinal bars. They produce an anteriorly directed force that reduces the curvature, thus opening the wedges and allowing bony remodeling.

As the nature of kyphosis is two-dimensional in comparison with the three-dimensional aspects of scoliosis, reduction of these curves is usually an easy task. Early in the treatment course there is a tendency on the part of the patient to lean on the throat mold because of the force generated by the kyphosis pads. Physical therapy plays a role in teaching these patients thoracic hyperextension exercises so that they can retract from the neck ring, thus providing an active counterforce to the kyphosis pads (33).

For the more caudal thoracic and thoracolumbar curves, a TLSO may gain the desired result because the apex is low and the sternum is cephalad enough to be used as a counterforce without being in opposition to the kyphosis pads (52).

The goal when treating Scheuermann kyphosis is bony remodeling of the wedged vertebrae and overall reduction of the curvature. Sachs et al. (77) reviewed 75 patients who had completed an average of 34 months in the Milwaukee brace and had vertebral wedging corrected to a mean of 5 degrees. At long-term follow-up, there was an average of only 6 degrees loss of

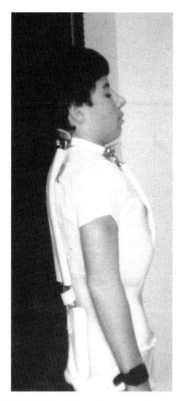

FIGURE 26. The Milwaukee brace for kyphosis.

overall correction. In contrast, Montgomery and Erwin (58) reported poor results for a group of patients who were weaned from orthoses 4 to 6 months after overall correction of the ky-phosis. They showed a 15-degree average loss of correction at follow-up. Because bony remodeling is the goal of orthotic treatment, weaning from the orthosis is recommended only after measurable changes have occurred in the vertebral wedging. Once again, proper follow-up for growth adjustment and increases in pad pressure along with adherence to sound clinical parameters of treatment yield the best possible result.

SPINAL INJURY

Thoracolumbar Injuries

To classify acute thoracolumbar fractures, Denis (20) proposed that the spine is composed of three load-bearing columns. The anterior longitudinal ligament, anterior annulus fibrosis, and anterior part of the vertebral body form the anterior column. The posterior longitudinal ligament, posterior annulus fibrosis, and posterior wall of the vertebral body form the middle column. The posterior arch, supraspinous ligament, interspinous ligament, capsule, and ligamentum flavum form the posterior column. Compression fracture involves failure of the anterior column, with the middle column being totally intact. The burst fracture involves failure of both the anterior and middle columns. Seat belt-type injuries represent failure of the middle and posterior columns. Finally, the fracture dislocation injury represents failure of all three columns.

The stability of the injured spine, measured by its ability to withstand loads without causing the progression of a deformity at the injury site, is a primary biomechanical concern in the treatment of thoracolumbar injuries. The stability of a segment defined by its load displacement behavior is affected by an injury, and the extent of such effect is a function of the type of injury, that is, the anatomical components disrupted by the injury and the severity of the damage.

The axial load carrying capacity of the thoracolumbar spine as a function of injury to the three columns of the spine was studied by Haher et al. (38). Disruption of the anterior column reduced the load carrying capacity (LCC) of the spine by 20%. The reduction in the LCC of the spine was 80%, with disruption of both the anterior and middle columns of the spine. Disruption of the posterior column reduced the LCC by 35%, whereas the reduction in LCC was 60% with disruption of both the posterior and the middle columns. Ferguson et al. (25) found that a two-column injury involving disruption of the anterior and posterior columns caused a 78% loss in flexion stiffness of the T11–L1 segment as compared with the intact value. Thus, disruption of two of the three load-bearing columns led to substantial instability, whereas the three-column injury rendered the segment completely unstable.

Slosar et al. (79) investigated the three-dimensional instability patterns of L1 burst fractures. Analysis of the burst fracture in flexion and lateral bending showed stiffness losses of 71% and 75%, respectively, at low-moment load (up to 3 Nm) applications. Subsequent loss of stiffness through higher moment loads (3 to 10 Nm) showed only a 5% stiffness change in flexion and 25% stiffness loss in lateral bending when comparing intact with burst fracture. Postinjury stiffness losses for rotation were 92% and 67% for low-moment load and high-moment load applications. After the burst fracture, loss of stiffness was much larger at low-moment loads than the subsequent loss of stiffness at high-moment loads.

It may be postulated that the initial instability represents a structural collapse through the fracture itself. Once the collapse is complete, the apposition of the involved cortices limits further significant displacement. With the fracture now maximally collapsed and cortices apposed, the behavior of the injured spine is similar to that of the intact spine. The severe loss of stiffness found through both the low- and high-moment load applications in rotation may indicate that to the unprotected injured spine, rotation is potentially the most destabilizing motion. The authors also determined that posterior column involvement in the form of an isolated lamina fracture did not alter the behavior of a two-column (anterior plus middle) burst fracture. Burst fractures with extensive third-column injuries in the form of facet joint disruptions or bilateral lamina fractures were less stable than two-column injuries.

Biomechanics of Orthoses for Spinal Injuries

Orthoses for spinal injury are designed to protect the spinal column from loads and stresses that cause progression of the angular and translational deformity from the injury (71,84). Orthoses for thoracolumbar injuries have two primary classifications: nonoperative and postoperative. Although there is no agreement on the mechanisms of action, orthoses primarily function to provide biomechanical stability.

Nonoperative Treatment

Mild injuries, such as those that affect only a single level and a single column and are at low risk of progression, require minimally immobilizing orthoses. The more severe two-level and two-column injuries that have only marginal stability but do not require surgery need orthoses that offer maximal stabilization and resistance to further progression of the deformity.

The primary mechanism of action is that of limiting gross trunk motion. Gross trunk motion is the movement and sway of the vertebral column during activities of normal daily living. Orthoses that primarily restrict gross trunk motion provide protection to the vertebral column by minimizing bending moments. Buchalter et al. (10) and Lantz and Schultz (49) studied the effectiveness of spinal orthoses in limiting gross trunk motion in flexion-extension, lateral bending, and axial rotation. The TLSO resulted in the most motion restriction in all three planes, whereas the corset provided the least restriction of gross upper body movement.

Another mechanism of orthotic stabilization is the reduction of intersegmental motion. Orthoses that reduce intersegmental motion may be assumed to also reduce gross motion. Many investigators (27,54,65,69) have studied the effect of orthoses in segmental immobilization. The three-point hyperextension orthosis was fair in limiting flexion-extension motion but had little effect on the motion in lateral bending or axial rotation. The Taylor-Knight orthosis was effective in lateral bending, fair in flexion-extension, but had little effect on limiting axial rotation. The body cast performed satisfactorily in limiting motion in all three modes. In general, the orthoses were more effective in reducing motion at the upper lumbar levels than at lower levels. The canvas corset was found to reduce the segmental motion by one third. The Raney jacket and the Baycast spica reduced the segmental motion by about two thirds at the mid-lumbar levels, and the Baycast spica was the only orthosis that was effective in limiting motion at the lower lumbar levels.

The effects of gross motion limitation on the spine are assumed to affect all vertebrae equally. However, the studies of orthoses for reducing intersegmental motion show that the effect of motion reduction is nonlinear and affects different motion segments differently. Orthoses are less effective in reducing intersegmental motion the more caudal the motion segment is in the lumbar spine.

The third mechanism, limited to the nonoperative treatment, is "three-point" sagittal plane hyperextension. This mechanism was first reported by Chance in 1948 (18). Patwardhan et al. (73) used a finite element model to investigate the effect of the Jewett hyperextension orthosis on single- and two-level injuries. They reported that for single-level injuries that cause up to 50% loss of segmental stiffness, the Jewett orthosis can restore stability under normal gravitational as well as large flexion loads. In severe two-level injuries with loss of stiffness between 50% and 85% of normal, the orthosis can restore stability with restricted patient activity level in the brace. Beyond 85% loss in segmental stiff-

ness, such as three-column injuries, the orthosis alone appears to be ineffective in preventing progression of deformity.

The effects of orthoses on trunk myoelectric activity, abdominal cavity pressures, and intradiscal pressures have also been investigated, but results have been inconsistent (36,47,50,64, 62,81).

The nonoperative treatment of single- and two-column injuries must encompass the known mechanisms of action: three-point hyperextension, gross motion reduction, and intersegmental motion reduction. There is some speculation as to the possibility of load sharing as a viable mechanism of action for some spinal orthoses. This may be unique to molded TLSOs in three-point hyperextension as they increase the Cobb angle of lumbar lordosis as well as increase the height of many patients. If load sharing is a reality with these orthoses, this could indeed be the most significant mechanism of action. Further investigation is necessary to prove this theory.

The state of the art in nonoperative management of spinal injuries is the custom-molded TLSO. Figure 27A depicts a girl with a Chance-type flexion distraction injury. Figure 27B shows the patient in her first orthosis (custom-molded, bivalved TLSO in hyperextension) with only a minimal change in the segmental angle at the fracture. Figure 27C shows the patient after 10 days of gradual hyperextension in her first TLSO with the addition of hyperextension pads upon being refitted into a new TLSO in even more hyperextension. Note the decrease in segmental angle after gradual hyperextension over time. Figure 27D was taken nearly 4 months later when the patient was being weaned from the orthosis.

Postoperative Orthoses

The goal of orthotic stabilization of a thoracolumbar injury that has been surgically reduced and instrumented is to protect the surgical construct from large loads created from torso motion until solid biologic fusion occurs. Nachemson and Elfstrom (63) studied the effect of the Milwaukee brace and body cast on the loads acting on spinal instrumentation in patients with idiopathic scoliosis. Both the Milwaukee brace and the body cast reduced the axial force in the Harrington rod during standing and walking. There exist no objective data regarding reduction of stresses that an orthosis may provide for other, more modern implants.

A postoperative orthosis should protect the surgical construct from the planes of motion in which the construct is vulnerable to failure. For most surgical constructs, these motions are *flexion* and *torsion.* The Harrington distraction rod can carry the axial load in the physiologic range. However, it is vulnerable to forward flexion and rotation. Postoperative orthoses that restrict these motions will minimize the chances of hook dislodgement or fracture. Segmental fixation of the Harrington rods using wires improves the failure strength and rigidity of the construct in flexion and rotation because segmental fixation distributes the load over multiple fixation points. The Luque system benefits from this principle, but it is notably weak in axial loading. The Cotrel-Dubousset system combines the axial load carrying ability of the Harrington rods with improved torsional rigidity of segmental fixation.

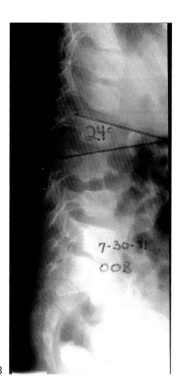
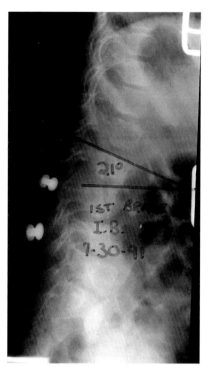

A,B

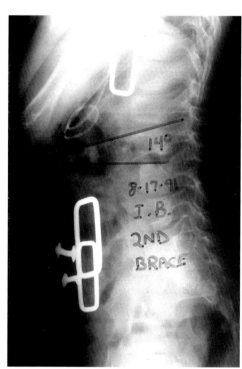

C

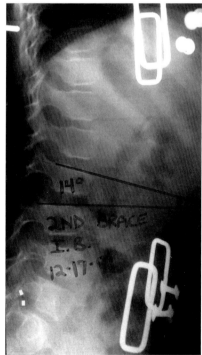

D

FIGURE 27. Orthotic treatment of chance fracture. **A:** Preorthosis radiograph of a girl with a Chance fracture. **B:** With the patient in her first thoracolumbosacral brace, the reduction of the segmental angle was only to 21 degrees despite hyperextension fabricated into the orthosis. **C:** After a gradual increase in extension and refabrication of orthosis, reduction was to 14 degrees. **D:** After 4 months in the orthosis, the patient maintained 14-degree angulation. (From Patwardhan AG, Gavin TM, Slosar P, et al. [1993]: Biomechanics of implants and orthoses for thoracolumbar injuries. In: Lorenz MA, Akbarnia B, eds. *Spine: state of the art reviews*, Vol. 7. Philadelphia: Hanley and Belfus, pp. 261–280.)

The fixation devices utilizing intrapeduncular screw fixation to the spine result in the most stable construct in all modes of loading and therefore can potentially stabilize injury to all three load-bearing columns. The improved rigidity of these constructs is derived from the fixation of screws in the pedicles, which provides a greater control on the three-dimensional motion of the vertebral body. However, it should be noted that both the strength and rigidity of these constructs would be adversely affected by a loss of bone mineral density such as in osteoporotic bone.

The role of a postoperative orthosis is to protect the implant from undue loads during the process of fusion. The segmental motion limiting requirements of a postoperative orthosis are not as stringent as in the case of nonoperative treatment because the orthosis is only being used as an adjunct to protect the implant from loads, moments, and stresses.

A postoperative TLSO should have enough anterior height to resist forward bending at the sternum. However, care must be taken that it does not induce hyperextension, as this will additionally stress the implant.

When spinal fusion is performed across the lumbosacral joint, a thigh extension must be applied to the TLSO to reduce lumbosacral motion in the orthosis. A TLSO without thigh extension has been shown either to have no effect or to actually increase lumbosacral motion (54,69). Despite patient preferences, an orthosis must not interfere with the surgical construct.

Cervical Orthoses

Much of the motion of the upper spine is determined by the structure of the anatomy. An example is the rotation that occurs at the C1 and C2 level. White and Panjabi (84) state that the occipitoatlantoaxial complex is the most complicated series of articulations in the human body. They further state that it supports the head, allows for necessary motion of the head on the spine, and protects the spinal cord from damage. In summary, there is little or no axial rotation at the occipito-C1 joint, but much that occurs is at the C1–2 joint.

Pure flexion of the cervical spine occurs at many levels. It is generally thought that the greatest amount of flexion-extension occurs at C5–6, followed by C4–5 and C6–7. Few studies of cervical spine orthoses for the pediatric patient exist. There are only a small number of studies dealing with cervical orthoses in adults and these are reviewed here.

Nachemson (61) draws a distinction between two groups of cervical orthoses: the cervical orthosis, dealing with C1 and C2; and the cervicothoracic orthosis, dealing with C3–T1. Nachemson classifies cervical orthotics as soft, reinforced, and rigid. Most of these orthoses are prefabricated and are available in pediatric sizes.

A foam collar is an example of a soft collar. It is usually encased in a knitted material and closes in back using velcro. These collars provide very little support or control and are usually used for the mildest of conditions. Beavis (7) measured a 39% reduction in cervical flexion using a soft collar. Beavis also measured a warming effect from the collar, but it was no more than a plain wool scarf.

The Philadelphia collar is the best known example of a reinforced collar. It is made of plastazote reinforced with plastic anteriorly and posteriorly. It is available in 12 sizes, depending on the neck measurement and the distance between the chin and chest. The greater the distance, the more cervical extension given. The pediatric collar has a tracheotomy opening, which allows room for respiratory apparatus if necessary.

Beavis (7) measured a 73% reduction in flexion and a 58% reduction in extension compared to no collar. Lateral flexion was reduced by 35% and rotation reduced by 63%. Interestingly, the study concluded that the custom-fitted plastazote collars were more comfortable to wear, an important concern given the high rejection rate of patients wearing collars. Kaufman et al. (45) found that the plastazote collar immobilized better than the foam but did not control axial rotation as well.

Fisher (28) reported that because most patients loosen the cervical orthoses from the initial adjustment, the effectiveness of the orthosis is much diminished. This report suggests that there is an important fitting component as well as a compliance factor if the orthoses are to be worn effectively.

Most cervical orthoses used for long-term stability rely on fixation on the mandible and therefore cause problems in eating or opening the mouth. One that does not is the frontooccipitozygomatic orthosis (FOZY) (Fig. 28). Developed in Japan, it uses pressure on the frontal bones of the face and leaves the mandible free to move. It purportedly controls all motions of the cervical spine, including rotation. The connecting parts of the orthosis are made of aluminum and thus can be adjusted as the need arises. It weighs only 1 lb (66).

Lango et al. (48) reported success using a custom-fabricated low-temperature plastic orthosis in the treatment of the congenital torticollis patient. It was formed directly on the patient and in the opposite directions of the deformity. By incorporating a thoracic component, the necessary forces were developed from the thorax to control the head.

A second example of the reinforced type of orthosis is the sternooccipitomandibular orthosis (SOMI) (Fig. 29). The SOMI consists of three components: the sternal yoke, the occipital component, and the mandibular component. These are easily fitted and available in pediatric sizes. Johnson reported a mean percentage of normal flexion-extension restriction of 32% to 61% per level from C1–2 to C7–T1. It remains the orthosis of choice in levels C4 and above, where flexion control is critical.

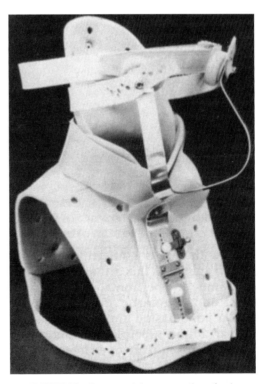

FIGURE 28. Frontooccipitozygomatic orthosis.

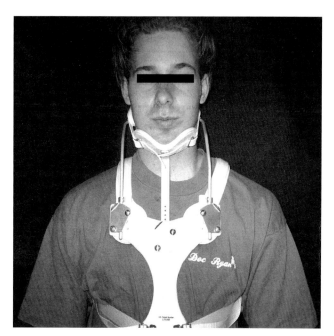

FIGURE 29. Sternooccipitomandibular orthosis.

Below C4, the orthosis of choice is a cervicothoracic orthosis (Fig. 30) when the extra lever is needed (41,42).

Evans and Bethem (24) reported on 24 cases of pediatric cervical spine injuries and their treatment. They concluded that the injury is very rare (only 1.2 cases per year), but that these

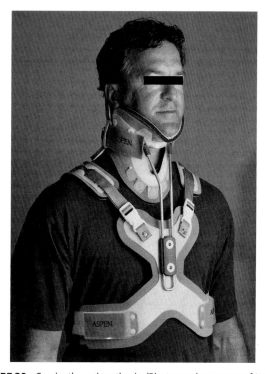

FIGURE 30. Cervicothoracic orthosis. (Photograph courtesy of International Healthcare Devices.)

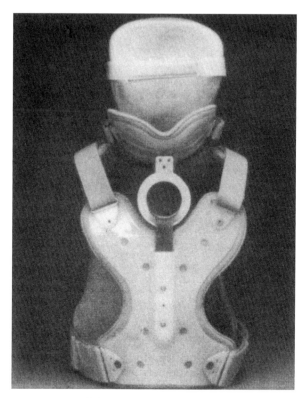

FIGURE 31. Minerva orthosis.

injuries frequently have many other associated injuries and the patients are often treated nonoperatively. Nonoperative treatment was successful 95% of the time, with 14% developing late kyphosis. Since C1 or C2 was involved only 29% of the time, there were many Minerva-type orthotic fittings (Fig. 31). Flexion injuries were recommended for surgical fixation, with postoperative use of orthoses.

Ducker (21) reported on motion allowed using five collars, including the Miami J. Results indicated that the Miami J collar restrained all but 15% of flexion, 25% of extension, 37% of lateral flexion, and 24% of rotation.

Askins and Eismont (5) compared motion restriction in several prefabricated cervical orthoses and determined that the NecLoc and Miami J collars restricted motion better than the other collars tested.

International Healthcare Devices manufactures a pediatric version of their Aspen collar (Fig. 32). This collar is not a scaled down version of an adult collar but rather is designed to fit the different occipital and mandibular shape of the pediatric patient. Most of the other pediatric collars available are shaped much like a small version of an adult collar and do not conform well to the pediatric mandible. This makes immobilization unreliable and creates discomfort in wearing. Many of the newer collars, such as the Aspen, also are made from materials that keep moisture on the skin to a minimum.

An example of a rigid orthosis is the halo (Fig. 33). This provides the best control and support of any cervical orthosis and comes in pediatric sizes. However, often a vest must be customized for a small patient or for one of nonstandard size or

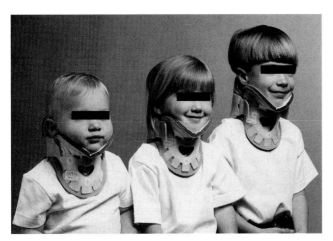

FIGURE 32. Pediatric cervical collars (Aspen). (Photograph courtesy of International Healthcare Devices.)

shape. White and Panjabi (85) refer to the "low stiff viscoelastic transmitter" when describing the medium between the orthosis and the skeletal structures of the spine.

Two inherent flaws in the testing methodology are that the amount of exertion against these collars was not measured and controlled and that some prehospitalization collars that are considered too uncomfortable to wear long term were compared with the more comfortable long-term collars. More reliable testing parameters and better controls for cervical orthoses are

needed to ascertain which collars and related devices have greatest efficacy.

Custom-Molded Cervical Orthoses

As a result of the problems associated with adaptability, deformity control, and patient tolerance, Jurgutis et al. (43) described a custom-designed multiadjustable cervical orthosis. Used for the treatment of torticollis, the posterior device of a thoracic and cranial component is connected with ball-jointed steel rods, allowing adaptability and contouring. Like the FOZY, this orthosis draws purchase on the frontal bones of the face to control and derotate, as well as maintains the position of the head and neck.

CLINICAL TEAM APPROACH

Whereas spinal orthoses are considered to be an off-the-shelf product by some, when used properly they are much more than that. Without careful attention to detail in the design, fitting, and follow-up of spinal orthoses, the results can be disastrous. To maximize the benefit of a spinal orthosis, a well-trained spinal orthotist must communicate with the physician, the patient, the patient support group, and other health care professionals. In the current era, when large clinics with a multitude of health care specialists in attendance are becoming increasingly rare, communication among health care professionals has become more difficult. If the physician is not clear in communicating the desired mechanism of action to the orthotist, the likelihood of achieving maximal result with the least amount of orthosis decreases.

The last decade has seen a sharp decrease in the level of spinal orthotic training of physicians. Therefore, greater reliance on the knowledge and skill of the orthotist has resulted. All too often an orthosis is ordered based on nomenclature or acronym and not on mechanism of action; this frequently results in a breakdown of the clinical treatment. Also, because the increasingly limited knowledge about orthotic treatment on the part of physicians limits orthosis usage to diagnoses commonly treated with orthoses, patients with more sophisticated needs are overlooked for this treatment modality.

The increasing number of poorly trained or untrained individuals attempting to provide orthotic treatment has compounded this problem. The attitude of "if it can't be fitted off the shelf, it can't be fitted" does great disservice to patients who require a customized approach to maximize the effect of the orthosis. However, many such providers do not have the training or access to utilize the laboratory bench science of orthotics and are self-limited to the off-the-shelf modality. Also, as the manufacturing of spinal orthoses is unregulated, the off-the-shelf approach to orthotic treatment leads to a "one size fits all" attitude, which may result in poor in-brace curve reduction for scoliosis, fractures that require hyperextension being fitted in flexion, and cervical orthoses that do not immobilize properly.

The best orthosis is well fitted and delivers the desired mechanism of action to achieve an optimal treatment result with the least amount of structure, the most comfort possible, and at the lowest cost. Any deviation from this is suboptimal and may lead to failure to reach the treatment objective. The physician needs

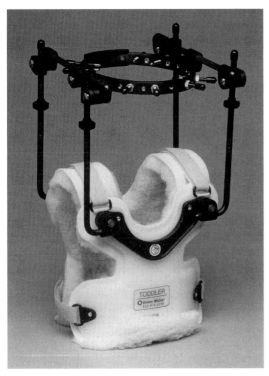

FIGURE 33. Ambulatory halo orthosis.

more than a cursory knowledge of spinal orthotics to be successful with their use. Also, the orthotist needs advanced training in the area of spine and must have the experience and laboratory access necessary to custom-fabricate orthoses. The clinical team approach is still the best model to ensure that one of the oldest known treatment methods for spinal maladies is carried out for the optimal benefit of the patient.

REFERENCES

1. Allington NJ, Bowen JR (1996): Adolescent idiopathic scoliosis: treatment with the Wilmington brace. *J Bone Joint Surg Am* 78(7): 1056–1062.
2. American Academy of Orthopaedic Surgeons (1952): *Atlas of orthopaedic appliances.* Ann Arbor, MI: Edwards, pp. 180–187.
3. Andriacchi TP, Schultz AB, Belytschko TB, et al. (1976): Milwaukee brace correction of idiopathic scoliosis. *J Bone Joint Surg Am* 58:806.
4. Andry N (1961): *Orthopaedia.* Philadelphia: JB Lippincott, Philadelphia. (Facsimile reproduction of the first edition in English, London, 1743).
5. Askins V, Eismont FJ (1997): Efficacy of five cervical orthoses in restricting cervical motion. A comparison study. *Spine* 22(11): 1193–1198.
6. Bailar JC III (1995): The practice of meta-analysis. *J Clin Epidemiol* 48:149–157.
7. Beavis A (1989): Cervical orthoses. Prosth Orthot Int 13:6–13.
8. Blount WP, Moe JH (1973): *The Milwaukee brace.* Baltimore: Williams & Wilkins.
9. Blount WP, Schmidt AC, Keever ED, et al. (1958): Milwaukee brace in the operative treatment of scoliosis. *J Bone Joint Surg Am* 40:511–525.
10. Buchalter D, Kahanovitz N, Viola K, et al. (1988): Three-dimensional spinal motion measurements. Part 2: A non-invasive assessment of lumbar brace immobilization of the spine. *J Spinal Disord* 1(4):284–286.
11. Bunch WH, Patwardhan AG (1989): Biomechanics of orthoses. In: Bunch WH, Patwardhan AG. *Scoliosis: making clinical decisions.* St. Louis: CV Mosby, pp. 204–215.
12. Bunch WH, Patwardhan A (1989): Clinical experience in orthotic treatment. In: Bunch WH, Patwardhan AG. *Scoliosis: making clinical decisions.* St. Louis: CV Mosby, pp. 237–255.
13. Bunch WH (1975): The Milwaukee brace in paralytic scoliosis. *Clin Orthop* 110:63–68.
14. Bunch WH, Keagy R (1975): *Principles of orthotic treatment.* St. Louis: CV Mosby.
15. Bunnell WP, MacEwen GD, Jayakumar S (1980): The use of plastic jackets in the nonoperative treatment of idiopathic scoliosis. *J Bone Joint Surg Am* 62:31–38.
16. Caton J, Michel CR, Fiquet A, et al. (1987): Orthopedic treatment of lumbar and thoracolumbar scolioses using a 3-valve spinal orthosis. Experience covering 17 years and more than 800 orthoses. *Rev Chir Orthop* 73(Suppl 2):138–142.
17. Carr WA, Moe JH, Winter RB, et al. (1980): Treatment of idiopathic scoliosis in the Milwaukee brace: long-term results. *J Bone Joint Surg Am* 62:599.
18. Chance GQ (1948): Note on a type of flexion fracture of the spine. *Br J Radiol* 21:452.
19. Cramer HJ, Liu YK, Von Rosenberg DU (1976): A distributed parameter model of the inertially loaded human spine. *J Biomech* 9:115–130.
20. Denis F (1983): The three-column spine and its significance in the classification of acute thoracolumbar spinal injuries. *Spine* 8:817.
21. Ducker TB (1990): Restriction of cervical spine motion by cervical collars. Scientific Exhibit of the American Association of Neurologic Surgeons, Nashville, TN.
22. Edmonsson A, Morris J (1977): Follow-up study of Milwaukee brace treatment in patients with idiopathic scoliosis. *Clin Orthop* 126:58–61.
23. Emans J (1986): The Boston bracing system for idiopathic scoliosis: follow-up results in 295 patients. *Spine* 11:792–801.
24. Evans DL, Bethem D (1989): Cervical spine injuries in children. *J Pediatr Orthop* 9:563–568.

25. Ferguson RL, Tencer AF, Woodard P, et al. (1988): Biomechanical comparisons of spinal fracture models and the stabilizing effects of posterior instrumentations. *Spine* 13:453–460.
26. Fernandez-Feliberti R, Flynn J, Ramirez N, et al. (1995): Effectiveness of TLSO bracing in the conservative treatment of idiopathic scoliosis. *J Pediatr Orthop* 15:176–181.
27. Fidler MW, Plasmans CMT (1983): The effect of four types of support on the segmental mobility of the lumbosacral spine. *J Bone Joint Surg Am* 65:943–947.
28. Fisher SV (1978): Proper fitting of the cervical orthosis. *Arch Phys Med Rehab* 59:505–507.
29. Galante J, Schultz AB, DeWald RL, et al. (1970): Forces acting in the Milwaukee brace on patients undergoing treatment for idiopathic scoliosis. *J Bone Joint Surg Am* 52:498.
30. Gavin TM, Patwardhan AG, Meade KP (1999): Preventing coronal decompensation in idiopathic scoliosis: a geometric analysis of orthotic correction of right thoracic, left lumbar curves. In: *Proceedings of the American Society of Mechanical Engineers,* 1999 Summer Bioengineering Conference, Big Sky, Montana.
31. Gavin TM, Gavin DQ (1998): Orthotic treatment for neuromuscular scoliosis. Thranhardt Series Lecture of the American Orthotic and Prosthetic Association. Chicago, IL.
32. Gavin TM, Patwardhan AG, Meade KP, et al. (1998): Biomechanical principles of orthoses for adolescent idiopathic scoliosis. In: Rowe DE, ed. *Scoliosis Research Society bracing manual,* Scoliosis Research Society. pp. 1–24.
33. Gavin TM, Patwardhan AG, Bunch WH, et al. (1997): Principles and components of spinal orthoses. In: American Academy of Orthopaedic Surgeons, ed. *Atlas of orthoses and assistive devices,* 3rd ed. St. Louis: Mosby–Year Book, pp. 155–194.
34. Gavin TM (1989): Fabrication and fitting of orthoses. In: Bunch WH, Patwardhan AG, eds. *Scoliosis: making clinical decisions.* St. Louis: CV Mosby, pp. 216–236.
35. Gavin TM, Bunch WH, Dvonch VM (1986): The Rosenberger scoliosis orthosis. *J Assoc Child Prosthet Orthot Clin* 21:35–38.
36. Gilbertson LG, Goel VK, Patwardhan AG, et al. (1991): The biomechanical function of three-point hyperextension orthoses. In: Vanderby R Jr., ed., *Proceedings of the American Society of Mechanical Engineers 112th Annual Meeting,* Atlanta, Georgia, December 1–6, 1991.
37. Green NE (1981): Part-time bracing of idiopathic scoliosis, *Orthop Trans* 5:22.
38. Haher TR, Tozzi JM, Lospinuso MF, et al. (1989): The contribution of the three columns of the spine to spinal stability: a biomechanical model. *Paraplegia* 27(6):432–439.
39. Jodoin A, Hall JE, Watts HG, et al. (1981): Treatment of idiopathic scoliosis by the Boston brace system: early results. *Orthop Trans* 5:22.
40. Johnston CE 2nd, Hakala MW, Rosenberger R (1982): Paralytic spinal deformity: orthotic treatment in spinal discontinuity syndromes. *J Pediatr Orthop* 2(3):233–241.
41. Johnson RM, Owen JR, Hart DC, et al. (1981): Cervical orthoses: a guide to their selection and use. *Clin Orthop* 154:34–35.
42. Johnson RM, Hart DL, Simmons EF, et al. (1977): Cervical orthoses: a study comparing their effectiveness in restricting cervical motion in normal subjects. *J Bone Joint Surg Am* 59:332–339.
43. Jurgutis J, et al. (1984): A multi-adjustable cervical orthosis for use in the treatment of torticollis: a case study. *Orthot Prosthet* 38:51–54.
44. Katz DE, Richards S, Browne RH, et al. (1997): A comparison between the Boston brace and the Charleston bending brace in adolescent idiopathic scoliosis. *Spine* 22:1302–1312.
45. Kaufman W, Lunsford T, Lunsford B, et al. (1986): Comparison of three prefabricated cervical collars. *Orthot Prosthet* 39:21–28.
46. Keiser RP, Shufflebarger HL (1976): The Milwaukee brace in idiopathic scoliosis: evaluation of 123 completed cases. *Clin Orthop* 118: 19–24.
47. Krag MH, Byrne KB, Pope MH, et al. (1986): The effect of back braces on the relationship between intra-abdominal pressure and spinal loads. *Adv Bioeng* 22–23.
48. Lango S, Schwentker E, Sweigart J (1977): Orthotic treatment for muscular torticollis. *Int Clin Info Bull* 16:13–15.

49. Lantz SA, Schultz AB (1986): Lumbar spine orthosis wearing. I. Restriction of gross body motions. *Spine* 11:834–837.

50. Lantz SA, Schultz AB (1986): Lumbar spine orthosis wearing. II. Effect on trunk muscle myoelectric activity. *Spine* 11:838–842.

51. Lonstein JE, Winter RL (1994): Milwaukee brace treatment of adolescent idiopathic scoliosis; review of 1020 patients. *J Bone Joint Surg Am* 76(8):1207–1221.

52. Lonstein JE (1985): Orthotic treatment of spinal deformities. In: American Academy of Orthopaedic Surgeons, ed. *Atlas of orthotics.* St. Louis: CV Mosby, pp. 371–385.

53. Lonstein JE, Carlson JM (1984): The prediction of curve progression in untreated idiopathic scoliosis during growth. *J Bone Joint Surg Am* 66:1061.

54. Lumsden RM, Morris JM (1968): An in vivo study of axial rotation and immobilization at the lumbosacral joint. *J Bone Joint Surg Am* 50: 1591.

55. McCollough NC, Schultz M, Javeck N, et al. (1981): Miami TLSO in the management of scoliosis: preliminary results in 100 cases. *J Pediatr Orthop* 1:141.

56. Mellencamp D, Blount W, Anderson A (1977): Milwaukee brace treatment of idiopathic scoliosis. *Clin Orthop* 126:47–57.

57. Moe JH, Kettleson DN (1970): Idiopathic scoliosis: analysis of curve patterns and the preliminary results of Milwaukee brace treatment in one hundred sixty-nine patients. *J Bone Joint Surg Am* 52:1509.

58. Montgomery SP, Erwin WE (1981): Scheuermann's kyphosis: long-term results of Milwaukee brace treatment. *Spine* 6:5–8.

59. Mulcahy T, Galante J, DeWald RL, et al. (1973): A follow-up study of forces acting in the Milwaukee brace on patients undergoing treatment for idiopathic scoliosis. *Clin Orthop* 93:53.

60. Nachemson AL, Peterson LE. (1995) Effectiveness of treatment with a brace in girls who have adolescent idiopathic scoliosis. *J Bone Joint Surg Am* 77(6):815–822.

61. Nachemson AL (1987): Orthotic treatment for injuries and diseases of the spinal column. *Phys Med Rehab* 1:22–24.

62. Nachemson A, Schultz AB, Andersson GBJ (1983): Mechanical effectiveness studies of lumbar spine orthoses. *Scand J Rehab Med* Suppl. 9.

63. Nachemson A, Elfstrom G (1971): In vivo wireless telemetry of axial forces in Harrington distraction rods in patients with idiopathic scoliosis. *J Bone Joint Surg Am* 53:445–465.

64. Nachemson A, Morris JM (1964): In vivo measurements of intradiscal pressure. *J Bone Joint Surg Am* 46:1077–1092.

65. Nagel DA, Koogle TA, Piziali RL, et al. (1981): Stability of the upper lumbar spine following progressive disruptions and the application of individual internal and external fixation devices. *J Bone Joint Surg Am* 63:62–70.

66. Nakamura T, Oh-Hama M, Shingu H (1984): A new orthosis for fixation of the cervical spine: fronto-occipito-zygomatic orthosis. *Orthot Prosthet* 38:41–45.

67. Noonan KJ, Dolan LA, Jacobson WC, Weinstein SL (1997): Long-term psychosocial characteristics of patients treated for idiopathic scoliosis. *J Pediatr Orthop* 17:712–717.

68. Noonan KJ, Weinstein SL, Jacobson WC, et al. (1996): Use of the Milwaukee brace for progressive idiopathic scoliosis. *J Bone Joint Surg Am* 78(4):557–567.

69. Norton PL, Brown T (1957): The immobilizing efficiency of the back braces: their effect on the posture and motion of the lumbosacral spine. *J Bone Joint Surg Am* 39:111–139.

70. Patwardhan AG, Gavin TM, Bunch WH, et al. (1996): A biomechanical comparison of the Milwaukee brace and TLSO. *J Prosthet Orthot* 8(4):115–122.

71. Patwardhan AG, Gavin TM, Slosar P, et al. (1993): Biomechanics of implants and orthoses for thoracolumbar injuries. In: Lorenz MA, Akbarnia B, eds. *Spine: state of the art reviews*, Vol. 7. Philadelphia: Hanley and Belfus pp. 261–280.

72. Patwardhan AG, Bunch WH, Dvonch VM, et al. (1990): Biomechanics of adolescent idiopathic scoliosis: natural history and treatment. In: Goel VK, Weinstein JN, eds. *Biomechanics of the spine: clinical and surgical perspective.* Boca Raton, FL: CRC Press, pp. 251–285.

73. Patwardhan AG, Li S, Gavin TM, et al. (1990): Orthotic stabilization of thoracolumbar injuries: a biomechanical analysis of the Jewett hyperextension orthosis. *Spine* 15:654–661.

74. Patwardhan AG, Bunch WH, Meade KP, et al. (1986): A biomechanical analog of curve progression and orthotic stabilization in idiopathic scoliosis. *J Biomech* 19:103.

75. Price CT, Scott DS, Reed FR, et al. (1997): Nighttime Bracing for Adolescent Idiopathic Scoliosis with the Charleston Bending Brace: Long-Term Follow-up. *J Pediatr Orthop* 17:703–707.

76. Rowe DE, Bernstein SM, Riddick MF, et al. (1997): A meta-analysis of the efficancy of nonoperative treatment for idiopathic scoliosis. *J Bone Joint Surg Am* 79(5):664–674.

77. Sachs B, Bradford DS, Winter RB, et al. (1987): Scheuermann's kyphosis: follow-up of Milwaukee brace treatment. *J Bone Joint Surg Am* 69: 50–57.

78. Skaggs DL (1996): Letter to the Editor. *J Bone Joint Surg Am* 78(1): 151.

79. Slosar PJ Jr, Patwardhan AG, Lorenz M, et al. (1992): Instability of the lumbar burst fracture and limitations of transpedicular instrumentation. *Spine* 20(13):1452–1461.

80. Timoshenko S, Gere J (1961): *Theory of elastic stability*, 2nd ed. New York: McGraw-Hill, pp. 46–50.

81. Waters RL, Morris JM (1970): Effects of spinal supports on the electrical activity of muscles of the trunk. *J Bone Joint Surg Am* 52:51–60.

82. Weinstein SL, Ponseti IV (1983): Curve progression in idiopathic scoliosis. *J Bone Joint Surg Am* 65:447–455.

83. Weinstein SL, Zavala DC, Ponseti IV (1981): Idiopathic scoliosis: long-term follow-up and prognosis in untreated patients. *J Bone Joint Surg Am* 63:702–712.

84. White A, Panjabi M (1990): *Clinical biomechanics of the spine*, 2nd ed. Philadelphia: JB Lippincott.

85. White A, Panjabi M (1978): *Clinical biomechanics of the spine.* Philadelphia: JB Lippincott.

86. Wickers FC, Bunch WH, Barnett PM (1977): Psychological factors in failure to wear the Milwaukee brace for treatment of idiopathic scoliosis. *Clin Orthop* 126:62–66.

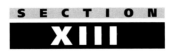

APPENDICES

TERMINOLOGY AND DEFINITIONS

AURELIO G. MARTINEZ-LOZANO

It was the editor's intention that this text would provide the reader with the majority of information related to the pediatric spine, spinal cord and their diseases and disorders in a single location. This appendix is intended to compliment the text chapters and subject areas and to serve as a supplemental reference source for information on terminology and nomenclature, embryology, growth and maturation, laboratory data, radiographic measurements and classifications referable to the pediatric spine and spinal cord. When charts, graphs, or line drawings were available, these were reprinted; when permissions to reprint were not granted, appropriate references were instead provided to enable the reader to know where to look for this information. Each topic area in the appendix is accompanied by additional references related to measurement values and classifications for supplemental reading. The editor and the author hope that you will find the supplemental information included in this appendix helpful.

GLOSSARY

Adolescent scoliosis: Spinal curvature presenting at or about the onset of puberty and before maturity.

Adult scoliosis: Spinal curvature existing after skeletal maturity.

Angle of thoracic inclination: With the trunk flexed 90 degrees at the hips, the angle between horizontal and a plane across the posterior rib cage at the greatest prominence of a rib hump.

Apical vertebra: The most rotated vertebra in a curve; the most deviated vertebra from the vertical axis of the patient.

Body alignment, balance, compensation: 1. The alignment of the midpoint of the occiput over the sacrum in the same vertical plane as the shoulders over hips. 2. Roentgenology: When the sum of the angular deviations of the spine in one direction is equal to that in the opposite direction.

Café au lait spots: Light brown irregular areas of skin pigmentation. If they are sufficient in number and with smooth margins, they suggest neurofibromatosis.

Cervical curve: Spinal curvature that has its apex from C1 to C6.

Cervicothoracic curve: Spinal curvature that has its apex at C7 or T1.

Compensation: Accurate alignment of the midline of the skull over the midline of the sacrum.

Compensatory curve: A curve, which can be structural, above or below a major curve that tends to maintain normal body alignment.

Congenital scoliosis: Scoliosis due to congenitally anomalous vertebral development.

Curve measurement: *Cobb method:* Select the upper and lower end vertebrae. Erect perpendiculars to their transverse axes. They intersect to form the angle of the curve. If the vertebral end plates are poorly visualized, a line through the bottom or top of the pedicles may be used. *Ferguson method:* The angle of a curve is formed by the intersection of two lines drawn from the center of the superior and inferior end vertebral bodies to the center of the apical vertebral body.

Double structural curve: Double major scoliosis: A scoliosis with two structural curves. Two structural curves in the same spine, one balancing the other.

Double thoracic curve (scoliosis): A scoliosis with a structural upper thoracic curve; a larger, more deforming lower thoracic curve; and a relatively nonstructural lumbar curve.

End vertebra: The most cephalad vertebra of a curve whose superior surface, or the most caudad vertebra of a curve whose inferior surface tilts maximally toward the concavity of the curve.

Fractional curve: A compensatory curve that is incomplete because it returns to the erect. Its only horizontal vertebra is caudad or cephalad.

Full curve: A curve in which the only horizontal vertebra is at the apex.

Functional curve, Nonstructural curve: A curve that has no structural component and that corrects or overcorrects on recumbent side-bending radiographic views.

Genetic scoliosis: A structural spinal curvature inherited according to a genetic pattern.

Gibbus: A sharply angular kyphos.

A. G. Martinez-Lozano: Universidad Autónoma De Nuevo León, Monterey, Mexico.

Hysterical scoliosis: A nonstructural deformity of the spine that develops as a manifestation of a conversion reaction.

Idiopathic scoliosis: A structural spinal curvature for which no cause is established.

Iliac epiphysis, Iliac apophysis: The epiphysis along the wing of the ilium.

Iliac epiphysis sign, Iliac apophysis sign: In the anteroposterior radiograhic view of the spine, when the excursion of ossification in the iliac epiphysis (apophysis) reaches its ultimate medial migration, vertebral growth may be complete.

Inclinometer: An instrument used to measure the angle of thoracic inclination or rib hump.

Infantile scoliosis: Spinal curvature that develops during the first 3 years of life.

Juvenile scoliosis: Spinal curvature that develops between the skeletal age of 3 years and the onset of puberty.

Kyphos: A change in the alignment of a segment of the spine in the sagittal plane that increases the posterior convex angulation.

Kyphoscoliosis: Lateral curvature of the spine associated with either increased posterior or decreased anterior angulation in the sagittal plane in excess of the accepted norm for that region. In the thoracic region, 20 to 40 degrees of kyphosis is considered normal.

Lordoscoliosis: Lateral curvature of the spine associated with an increase in anterior curvature or a decrease in posterior angulation thoracic spine where posterior angulation is normally present, less than 20 degrees would constitute lordoscoliosis.

Lumbar curve: Spinal curvature that has its apex from L1 to L4.

Lumbosacral curve: Spinal curvature that has its apex at L5 or below.

Major curve: Term used to designate the larger (largest) curve or curves, usually structural.

Minor curve: Term used to refer to the smaller (smallest) curve or curves.

Myogenic scoliosis: Spinal curvature due to disease or anomalies of the musculature.

Neurogenic scoliosis: Spinal curvature due to disease or anomalies of nerve tissue.

Osteogenic scoliosis: Spinal curvature due to abnormality of the vertebral elements or adjacent ribs, either acquired or congenital.

Pelvic obliquity: Deviation of the pelvis from the horizontal in the frontal plane. Fixed pelvic obliquities can be attributable to contractures either above or below the pelvis.

Primary curve: The first or earliest of several curves to appear, if identifiable.

Rib hump: The prominence of the ribs on the convexity of a spinal curvature, usually due to vertebral rotation best exhibited on forward bending.

Skeletal age, Bone age: The age obtained by comparing an anteroposterior radiographic view of the left hand and wrist with the standards of the Greulich and Pyle Atlas.

Structural curve: A segment of the spine with a fixed lateral curvature. Radiographically, it is identified in supine lateral side-bending views by the failure to correct. They may be multiple.

Thoracic curve: Scoliosis in which the apex of the curvature is between T2 and T11.

Thoracogenic scoliosis: Spinal curvature attributable to disease or operative trauma in or on the thoracic cage.

Thoracolumbar curve: Spinal curvature that has its apex at T12 or L1.

Transitional vertebra: Vertebra that is neutral in relation to rotation usually at the end of a curve.

Vertebral endplates: The superior and inferior plates of cortical bone of the vertebral body adjacent to the intervertebral disc.

Vertebral growth plate: The cartilaginous surface covering the top and bottom of a vertebral body that is responsible for the linear growth of the vertebra.

Vertebral ring apophyses: The most reliable index of vertebral immaturity seen best in the lateral radiographs or in the lumbar region in side-bending anteroposterior views.

BIBLIOGRAPHY

Goldstein LA, Waugh TR (1973): Classification and terminology of scoliosis. *Clin Orthop* 93:10–22.

McAlister WH, Schackelford GD (1975): Classification of spinal curvatures. *Radiol Clin North Am* 13:93–121.

The Terminology Committee of the Scoliosis Research Society. (1976): A glossary of scoliosis terms. *Spine* 1:57–58.

The Pediatric Spine: Principles and Practice, 2nd ed., edited by Stuart L. Weinstein. Lippincott Williams & Wilkins, Philadelphia © 2001.

B

EMBRYOLOGY, GROWTH AND MATURATION

AURELIO G. MARTINEZ-LOZANO

A. SPINE DEVELOPMENT (PRENATAL)

1. Neural Tube Development in Human Embryos

Lemire RJ (1969): Variation in development of the caudal neural tube in human embryos (horizons XIV–XXI). *Teratology* 2:361–70.

2. Spinal Cord Formation

The cephalic and caudal portions of the spinal cord are formed by distinctly different mechanisms and are, therefore, heir to distinctly different types of malformation. The cephalic, or majority, portion of the spinal cord forms by an orderly sequence of (a) creation of neural folds, (b) flexion of neural folds, and (c) closure of the folds into a neural tube. This process is designated neurulation. The caudal, or minority, portion of the cord forms by far less well-organized mechanisms of (a) agglomeration of cells, (b) canalization of the cell mass, and (c) involution of unused portions of the distal cord. This process is designated canalization and retrogressive differentiation (Fig. 1).

Lemire RJ, Loeser JD, Leech RW, et al. (1975): *Normal and abnormal development of the human nervous system.* Hagerstown, MD: Harper & Row.

3. Vertebrae and Disc Development (Fig. 2)

Rothman RH, Simeone FA (1982): *The spine.*

4. Ascent of the Cord

In the early embryo, the spinal cord extends to the distal end of the tail. By approximately 3 months postpartum, the tip of the conus medullaris lies at approximately the L1–2 interspace, this ascent results from two processes: (a) retrogressive differentiation and (b) disproportionately more rapid growth of the vertebral column (Fig. 3).

5. Normal Curvatures of the Spine: Termination of the Spinal Cord (Fig. 4)

It is generally stated that the thoracic and sacral curvatures are primary curves and that the cervical and lumbar curvatures are secondary curves, developing after birth. However, it is likely that the cervical curvature begins to form prenatally. Although the vertebral column and neural tube at first grow synchronously, a difference develops in the fetal period so that the cord ends successively at the sacral and lumbar levels. The level at birth is generally the third lumbar vertebra, and that in the adult is most commonly the first or second lumbar vertebra. The "adult" level is reached at about 2 months after birth so that the vertebral column and spinal cord grow at an equal rate during childhood (Fig.4).

Bagnall KM, Harris, PF, Jones, PRM (1977): A radiographic study of the human fetal spine. I. The development of the secondary cervical curvature. *J Anat* 777–782.

A. G. Martinez-Lozano: Universidad Autónoma De Nuevo León, Monterrey, Mexico.

Barry A (1956): A quantitative study of the prenatal changes in angulation of the spinal nerves. *Anat Rec* 126:970–110.

Barson AJ (1970): The vertebral level of termination of the spinal cord during normal and abnormal development. *J Anat* 106:489–497.

O'Rahilly R, Muller F, Meyer DB (1980): The human vertebral column at the end of the embryonic period proper: the column as a whole. *J Anat* 136: 181–195.

6. Vertebral Ossification Centers in Human Embryos (Tables 1–4)

Mall FP (1906): On ossification centers in human embryos less than 100 days old. *Am J Anat* 5:433–458.

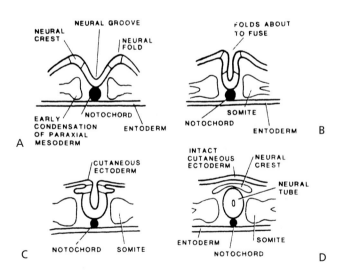
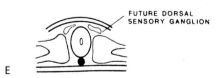

FIGURE 1. Embryonic stages 8 to 12 (18 to 27 days) in cross section showing the process of neurulation, which transforms the neural plate into the neural tube buried beneath a continuous layer of cutaneous ectoderm **(A–E)**. The paraxial mesoderm condenses to form paired segmental blocks, called comites, from which the vertebral bodies will form. If the embryo were sectioned along its length in the early stages of neurulation, all these steps would be seen, with the advanced step **(E)** in the cervicomedullary area. (From French BN [1990]: Midline fusion defects and defects of formation. In: *Youman's neurological surgery,* 3rd ed. Philadelphia: WB Saunders, with permission.)

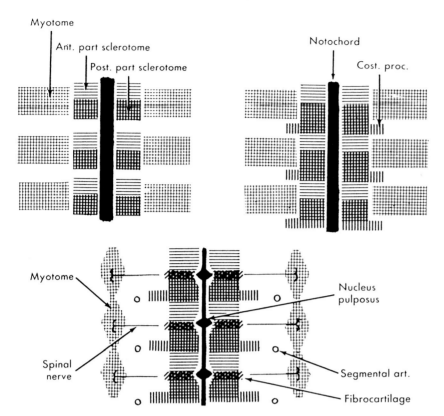

FIGURE 2. Schematic representation of development of vertebrae and discs. (From Rothman RH, Simeone FA [1982]: *The Spine,* vol 1. Philadelphia: WB Saunders).

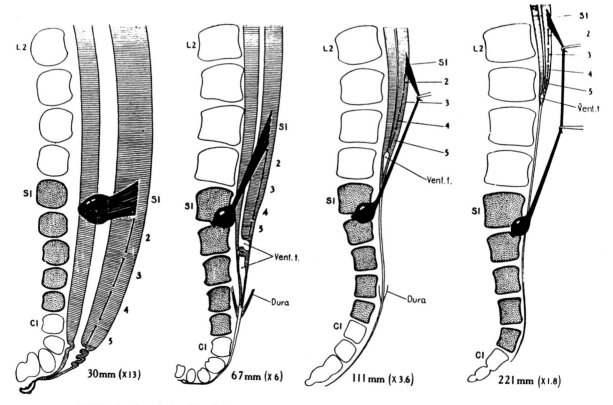

FIGURE 3. The relationship of the caudal end of the developing spinal cord to the vertebral column during the fetal period from the 8th to the 25th week. The increase in length of the S1 nerve root and the filum terminale reflects the "ascension" of the conus medullaris by a combination of regression and disproportionate elongation of the vertebral column. (From Streeter GL [1919]: Factors involved in the formation of the filum terminale. *Am J Anat* 25:1–12, with permission.)

TABLE 1. TIME OF OSSIFICATION OF THE VERTEBRAL ARCHES

Embryo No.	202	274	263,b2	266	263,b1 right	263,b1 left	272	J	I	282	K	284	288b	M	N	300	O	S	306c	Q	306a	306b	P	R
Crown-rump Length (mm)	30	31	32	33	34	34	34	36	41	42	53	54	57	69	70	73	73	75	75	81	100	105	105	110
Probable Age of Embryo (days)	55	56	56	57	58	58	58	60	64	65	72	73	75	83	83	85	85	87	87	90	100	105	105	110
Arches of the vertebrae																								
1					*	*	*	*	*	*	*	*	*	*	*	*	*	*	*	*	*	*	*	*
2				*	*	*	*	*	*	*	*	*	*	*	*	*	*	*	*	*	*	*	*	*
3						*	*	*	*	*	*	*	*	*	*	*	*	*	*	*	*	*	*	*
4							*	*	*	*	*	*	*	*	*	*	*	*	*	*	*	*	*	*
5							*	*	*	*	*	*	*	*	*	*	*	*	*	*	*	*	*	*
6							*	*	*	*	*	*	*	*	*	*	*	*	*	*	*	*	*	*
7					*		*	*	*	*	*	*	*	*	*	*	*	*	*	*	*	*	*	*
8				*	*	*	*	*	*	*	*	*	*	*	*	*	*	*	*	*	*	*	*	*
9					*	*	*	*	*	*	*	*	*	*	*	*	*	*	*	*	*	*	*	*
10						*	*	*	*	*	*	*	*	*	*	*	*	*	*	*	*	*	*	*
11						*	*	*	*	*	*	*	*	*	*	*	*	*	*	*	*	*	*	*
12							*	*	*	*	*	*	*	*	*	*	*	*	*	*	*	*	*	*
13							*	*	*	*	*	*	*	*	*	*	*	*	*	*	*	*	*	*
14							*	*	*		*	*	*	*	*	*	*	*	*	*	*	*	*	*
15							*	*	*		*	*	*	*	*	*	*	*	*	*	*	*	*	*
16							*	*	*		*	*	*	*	*	*	*	*	*	*	*	*	*	*
17							*	*	*		*	*	*	*	*	*	*	*	*	*	*	*	*	*
18							*	*	*		*	*	*	*	*	*	*	*	*	*	*	*	*	*
19							*	*	*		*	*	*	*	*	*	*	*	*	*	*	*	*	*
20									*		*	*	*	*	*	*	*	*	*	*	*	*	*	*
21									*	*	*	*	*	*	*	*	*	*	*	*	*	*	*	*
22									*	*	*	*	*	*	*	*	*	*	*	*	*	*	*	*
23											*	*		*	*	*	*	*	*	*	*	*	*	*
24											*			*	*					*	*	*	*	*
25											*				*							*	*	*
26											*				*								*	*
27											*												*	*
28																								?

From Mall FP (1906): On ossification centers in human embryos less than 100 days old. *Am J Anat* 5:433–58, with permission.
Asterisks indicate that the bone listed in the first column is ossified.

TABLE 2. TIME OF OSSIFICATION OF THE VERTEBRAL BODIES

Embryo No.	202	274	263,b,2	266	263,b,1	272	282	284	288,b	M	N	300	O	S	306,c	Q	306,a	306,b	P	R
Crown-rump Length (mm)	30	31	32	33	34	34	42	54	57	69	70	73	73	75	75	81	100	105	105	110
Probable Age of Embryo (days)	55	56	56	57	58	58	65	73	75	83	83	85	85	87	87	90	100	105	105	110
Bodies of the vertebrae																				
1																				
2											*		0			*			*	*
3											*		0	*		*		*	*	*
4										*	*		0	*	*	*	*	*	*	*
5										*	*	*	0	*	*	*	*	*	*	*
6									*	*	*	*	0	*	*	*	*	*	*	*
7									*	*	*	*	0	*	*	*	*	*	*	*
8								*	*	*	*	*	0	*	*	*	*	*	*	*
9								*	*	*	*	*	0	*	*	*	*	*	*	*
10						*	*	*	*	*	*	*	0	*	*	*	*	*	*	*
11						*	*	*	*	*	*	*	0	*	*	*	*	*	*	*
12						*	*	*	*	*	*	*	0	*	*	*	*	*	*	*
13						*	*	*	*	*	*	*	0	*	*	*	*	*	*	*
14						*	*	*	*	*	*	*	0	*	*	*	*	*	*	*
15						*	*	*	*	*	*	*	0	*	*	*	*	*	*	*
16						*	*	*	*	*	*	*	0	*	*	*	*	*	*	*
17						*	*	*	*	*	*	*	0	*	*	*	*	*	*	*
18						*	*	*	*	*	*	*	*	*	*	*	*	*	*	*
19						*	*	*	*	*	*	*	*	*	*	*	*	*	*	*
20						*	*	*	*	*	*	*	*	*	*	*	*	*	*	*
21						*	*	*	*	*	*	*	*	*	*	*	*	*	*	*
22						*	*	*	*	*	*	*	*	*	*	*	*	*	*	*
23						*	*	*	*	*	*	*	*	*	*	*	*	*	*	*
24						*	*	*	*	*	*	*	*	*	*	*	*	*	*	*
25						*	*	*	*	*	*	*	*	*	*	*	*	*	*	*
26								*	*	*	*	*	*	*	*	*	*	*	*	*
27									*	*	*	*	*	*	*		*	*	?	*
28										*	*							*		*
29											*							*		

From Mall FP (1906): On ossification centers in human embryos less than 100 days old. *Am J Anat* 5:433–58, with permission.
Asterisks indicate that the bone listed in the first column is ossified.

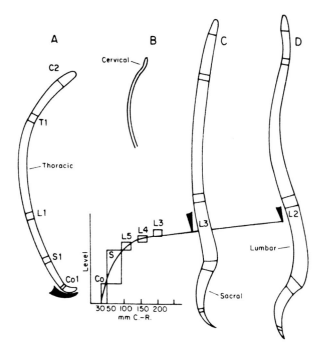

FIGURE 4. The curvatures of the vertebral column and the termination of the spinal cord. **A:** At the end of the embryonic period proper (stage 23), based on O'Rahilly and coworkers. The thoracic curvature is evident. The neural tube *(solid black)* reaches to the end of the column. **B:** An indication of a cervical curvature at the beginning of the fetal period, as illustrated by Bagnall and associates. The graph shows the level of termination of the spinal cord plotted against fetal length, as found by Barry. **C:** Newborn showing the sacral curvature. The cord ends at the third lumbar vertebra. **D:** Adult, showing all four curvatures. The spinal cord generally ends at the level of the first or second lumbar vertebra. (From O'Rahilly R, Benson DR [1985]: The development of the vertebral column. In: Bradford DS, Hensinger RN, eds. *The pediatric spine*, Stuttgart: Georg Thieme, Verlag, with permission.)

TABLE 3. TIME OF OSSIFICATION CENTERS OF THE VERTEBRAL NEURAL ARCHES[a]

1	2	3	4	5
Centers	Smallest Specimen(s) With Center Present (mm CR)	Specimen(s) of a CR Length After Which Center Always Observed	Specimens Between Those Listed in Columns 2 and 3 With the Bone Ossified	Data in Literature in mm CR
Cervical 1	45 (1,2,4)	49	48 (1)	34 (M), 50–60 (T)
2	40 (3)	45 (1,2,4)	44 (1,2)	33 (M), 51–60 (T)
3–7	38 (4)	45 (1,2,4)	40 (3), 44	34 (M), 51–60 (T)
Thoracic 1	38 (4)	45 (1,2,4)	40 (3,4), 44 (2)	33 (M), 51–60 (T)
2	38 (4)	45 (1,2,4)	40 (3), 44 (2)	34 (M), 51–60 (T)
3	40 (3)	52	44 (2), 45 (1,2,4), 48 (1,2), 49	34 (M), 51–60 (T)
4–5	40 (3)	60 (1,2)	44 (2), 45 (1,2,4), 48 (1,2), 49, 52, 53, 54, 56 (1,2), 57	34 (M), 51–60 (T)
6	40 (3)	60 (1,2)	44 (2), 45 (1,4), 48 (1,2), 49, 52, 53, 54, 56 (1,2), 57	34 (M), 51–60 (T)
7	45 (1,4)	60 (1,2)	48 (1,2), 49, 52, 53, 54, 56 (1,2), 57	34 (M), 51–60 (T)
8	45 (1,4)	60 (1,2)	48 (1), 52, 53, 54, 56 (1,2), 57	34 (M), 51–60 (T)
9	45 (1,2,4)	60 (1,2)	48 (1), 52, 53, 56 (1,2), 57	34 (M), 51–60 (T)
10	45 (1,2,4)	60 (1,2)	48 (1), 52, 53, 56 (1,2)	34 (M), 51–60 (T)
11	45 (1,4)	60 (1,2)	48 (1), 52, 53, 56 (1,2)	34 (M), 51–60 (T)
12	45 (1,4)	60 (1,2)	48 (1), 52, 53, 56 (1,2)	34 (M), 52–60 (T)
Lumbar 1	45 (1,4)	60 (1,2)	48 (1), 52, 53, 54, 56 (1,2)	41–53 (M), 51–60 (T)
2	45 (1)	60 (1,2)	48 (1), 56 (1,2)	41–53 (M), 51–85 (T)
3	45 (1)	68 (2)	56 (1,2), 60 (1,2), 61 (1), 62, 65 (1,2,3), 67	41–53 (M), 55–91 (T)
4	45 (1)	68 (2)	60 (1,2), 61 (1), 62, 65 (1,3), 67	53–69 (M), 58–91 (T)
5	60 (1,2)	69 (1,2)	61 (1), 62, 65 (1,3), 67, 68 (2)	53–69 (M), 60–93 (T)
Sacral 1	65 (3)	76	68 (2), 69 (1,2), 71	53–81 (M), 75–110 (T), 65–120 (O), 65–128 (Ad)
2	102 (1,2)	127 (2)	108, 110, 112, 113 (2), 115 (1,2), 116 (1,2), 120 (1,2,3), 124 (2), [69 (1,2)][a]	53–110 (M), 80–139 (T), 115–155 (O), 65–150 (Ad)
3	102 (2)	161	110, 116 (2), 120 (2,3), 127 (2), 134, 135, 139 (1,2), 140, 141, 143, 147 (1,2), 148	53–110 (M), 135–170 (T), 127–155 (O), 100–170 (Ad)
4	135	161	139, 147 (2), 148 (1)	139–205 (T), 127–220 (O), 130–170 (Ad)
5	163 (2)	173		170–350 (T), 190–newborn (O)

From Noback CR, Robertson GG (1951): Sequence of appearance of ossification centers in the human skeleton during the first five prenatal months. *Am J Anat* 89:1–27, with permission.
[a] 136 human embryos ranging in crown-rump (CR) length from 14 to 235 mm were cleared with potassium hydroxide and their bones stained with alizarin red.
Numbers in parentheses refer to specimens in which that specific center apparently appears precociously.
Letters in parentheses refer to previously published reports: (Ad) Adair FL (1918): The ossification centers of the fetal pelvis. *Am J Obstet Dis Women Child* 78:175–99; (M) Mall FP (1906): On ossification centers in human embryos less than 100 days old. *Am J Anat* 5:433–58; (O) Obata R (1912): Die Knochenderene des fetalen menschlichen Beckens. *Z. Begurtsch Bynakol* 22: 533–74; (T) Tessandler J (1944): *L'Ossification des cotes et de la colonne vertebrate chez le foetus human* [Dissertation]. Paris: Faculte de Medicine.

TABLE 4. TIME OF APPEARANCE OF THE PRIMARY OSSIFICATION CENTERS OF THE VERTEBRAL BODY[a]

1 Centers	2 Smallest Specimen(s) With Center Present (mm CR)	3 Specimen(s) of a CR Length After Which Center Always Observed	4 Specimens Between Those Listed in Columns 2 and 3 With The Bone Ossified	5 Data in Literature In mm CR
Cervical 1	135	161		165–195 (T)
2	69 (1)	120 (2,3)	76, 83 (1), 85, 86, 91, 94, 97 (2), 102 (1,2), 104, 108, 110, 112, 113 (1,3), 115 (1,2), 116 (1)	70–105 (M), 75–130 (T)
3	69 (1)	102 (1,2)	76, 83 (1,2), 84 (1), 85, 86, 88, 91, 94, 95, 97 (1,2)	70–105 (M), 75–105 (T)
4	57	85	69 (2,3), 76, 78, 83 (1,2), 84 (1)	69–75 (M), 75–105 (T)
5	57	71	61 (1), 65 (1), 67, 69 (1,3)	69 (M), 65–91 (T)
6	52	71	57, 60 (1), 61 (1), 65 (1), 67, 68 (1,2), 69 (1,2,3)	57 (M), 65–80 (T)
7	52	68 (1)	58 (1), 57, 60 (2), 61 (1), 65 (1,2,3), 67	57 (M), 60–80 (T)
Thoracic 1	52	69 (1,2,3)	54, 56 (1), 57, 60 (1,2), 61 (1,2), 65 (1,2,3), 67, 68 (2)	54 (M), 57–72 (T)
2	52	57	54, 56 (1)	54 (M), 57–65 (T)
3	48 (1)	57	52, 54, 56 (1)	34 (M), 54–60 (T)
4	48 (1)	57	52, 54, 56 (1)	34 (M), 51–60 (T)
5–7	40 (3)	52	45 (4), 48 (1)	34 (M), 51–60 (T)
8	40 (3)	52	45 (4), 48 (1), 49	34 (M), 51–60 (T)
9	40 (3)	52	45 (1,4), 48 (1), 49, 50	34 (M), 51–60 (T)
10–12	40 (3)	52	44 (2), 45 (1,4), 48 (1), 49, 50	34 (M), 43–60 (T)
Lumbar 1	40 (3)	52	44 (2), 45 (1,4), 48 (1), 49, 50	34 (M), 43–55 (T)
2	45 (1,4)	52	48 (1), 49, 50	34 (M), 43–55 (T)
3	45 (1,4)	52	49, 50	34 (M), 51–56 (T)
4	45 (1,4)	54	52	34 (M), 51–56 (T)
5	45 (1)	57	52, 54, 56 (1)	34 (M), 51–65 (T)
Sacral 1	52	65 (1,2,3)	56, 57, 60 (1,2), 61, 62	34 (M), 57–85 (T), 50 (O), 51–60 (Ad)
2	60 (1,2)	68 (2)	61, 62, 65 (1,2), 67	54 (M), 59–93 (T), 65 (O), 60–65 (Ad)
3	60 (1,2)	97 (3)	61 (1), 62, 65 (3), 67, 68 (2), 69 (1,2,3), 71, 72, 76, 78, 83, 84 (1,2), 85, 86, 88, 91, 94, 95	54 (M), 59–93 (T), 66–120 (O), 65–128 (Ad)
4	84	143	88, 95, 97 (3), 102 (1,2), 108, 110, 113 (1,2), 115 (1), 116 (1,2), 120 (1,2,3), 127, 133, 134, 135, 139 (1,2), 140, [62, 69 (1)][a]	57–110 (M), 82–170 (T), 102–165 (O), 77–170 (Ad)
5	135	after 175	148, 163 (2), 236 [62]	70–after 110 (M), 107–350 (T), 155–230 (O)

From Noback CR, Robertson GG (1951): Sequence of appearance of ossification centers in the human skeleton during the first five prenatal months. *Am J Anat* 89:1–27, with permission.
[a] 136 human embryos ranging in crown-rump (CR) length from 14 to 235 mm were cleared with potassium hydroxide and their bones stained with allzerin red.
Numbers in parentheses refer to specimens in which that specific center apparently appears precociously.
Letters in parentheses refer to previously published reports: (Ad) Adair FL (1918): The ossification centers of the fetal pelvis. *Am J Obstet Dis Women Child* 78:175–99; (M) Mall FP (1906): On ossification centers in human embryos less than 100 days old. *Am J Anat* 5:433–58; (O) Obata R (1912): Die Knochenderene des fetalen menschlichen Beckens. *Z. Beguirtsch Bynakol* 22: 533–74; (T) Tessandier J (1944): *L'Ossification des cotes et de la colonne vertebrale chez le foetus human* [Dissertation]. Paris: Faculte de Medicine.

Noback CR, Robertson GG (1951): Sequences of appearance of ossification centers in the human skeleton during the first five prenatal months. *Am J Anat* 89:1–27.

B. SPINE DEVELOPMENT (POSTNATAL)

1. Spine Ossification Centers (Fig. 5)

2. Normal Variations in Shape of Vertebral Bodies According to Age (Fig. 6)

3. Cervical Spine Development (Figs. 7–9)

4. Vertebral Growth (Figs. 10–13)

According to Winter (1977), the average growth of each vertebral segment is 0.07 cm per year. The most caudal vertebral have been reported (Schmorl) to show more growth than those more cephalic. Therefore, the midportion of the column in the newborn lies at the level of T7 and in the adult at T9.

Dimeglio A (1993): Growth of the spine before 5 years. *J Pediatr Orthop* 1-B:102.

Dubousset J, Katti E, Seringe R (1993): Epiphysiodesis of the spine in young children for congenital spinal deformations. *J Pediatr Orthop* 13:123.

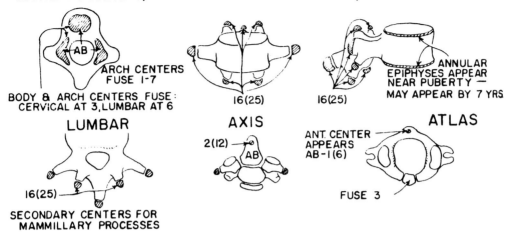

VERTEBRA

OSSIFY FROM 3 PRIMARY CENTERS AND 9 SECONDARY CENTERS – ANY OF THESE SECONDARY CENTERS, EXCEPT FOR ANNULAR EPIPHYSES, MAY FAIL TO FUSE.

ARCH CENTERS FUSE 1-7

BODY & ARCH CENTERS FUSE: CERVICAL AT 3, LUMBAR AT 6

16(25)

16(25)

ANNULAR EPIPHYSES APPEAR NEAR PUBERTY — MAY APPEAR BY 7 YRS

LUMBAR

AXIS

ATLAS

2(12)

ANT. CENTER APPEARS AB-1(6)

16(25)

FUSE 3

SECONDARY CENTERS FOR MAMMILLARY PROCESSES

FIGURE 5. Time of appearance of ossification centers according to Girdany and Golden. The figures indicate the range from the 10th to the 90th percentile in appearance time of centers of ossification. Obtained from data available in 1950. (From Girdan BR, Golden R [1952]: Centers of ossification of the skeleton. *Am J Roentgenol* 69:922–924.)

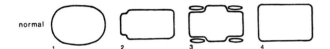

normal

1 2 3 4

FIGURE 6. Normal and abnormal variations in shape of vertebral bodies. Sagittal views. *1*, Newborn; *2*, at 6 to 8 years, with anterior steplike recesses; *3*, partial calcification of ring apophysis; *4*, mature vertebra. (From Kricun ME [1988]: Conventional radiography. In: *Imaging modalities in spinal disorders.* Philadelphia: WB Saunders, with permission.)

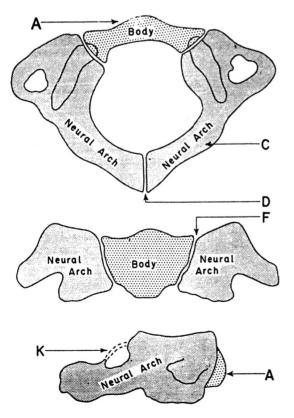

A — Body

Neural Arch   Neural Arch

C

D

F

Neural Arch   Body   Neural Arch

K   Neural Arch   A

FIGURE 7. Diagram of first cervical vertebra (atlas). *A*, Body: not ossified at birth; center (occasionally two centers) appears during first year after birth; body may fail to develop and forward extension of neural arches may take its place. *C*, Neural arches: appear bilaterally about seventh fetal week; most anterior portion of superior articulating surface is usually formed by the body. *D*, Synchrondrosis of spinal processes: unite by 3rd year; union may rarely be preceded by the appearance of a secondary center within the synchondrosis. *F*, Neurocentral synchondrosis: fuses about the 7th year. *K*, Ligament surrounding the superior vertebral notch: may ossify, especially later in life. (From Bailed D [1952]: The normal cervical spine in infants and children. *Radiology* 59:712–719, with permission.)

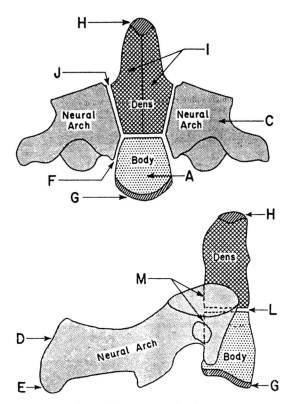

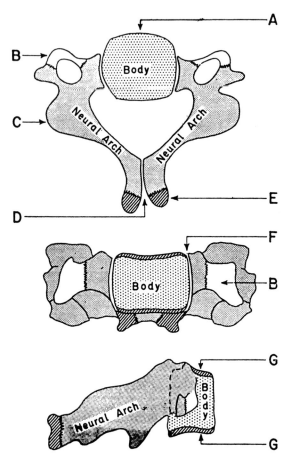

FIG. 8. Diagram of second cervical vertebra (axis or epistropheus). *A*, Body: one center (occasionally two) appears by the fifth fetal month. *C*, Neural arches: appears bilaterally by the seventh fetal month. *D*, Neural arches fuse posteriorly by second or third years. *E*, Bifid tip of spinous process (occasionally a secondary center is present in each tip). *F*, Neurocentral synchondrosis: fuses at 3 to 6 years. *G*, Inferior epiphyseal ring: appears at puberty and fuses at about 25 years. *H*, "Summit" ossification center for odontoid: appears at 3 to 6 years, and fuses with odontoid by 12 years. *I*, Odontoid (dens): two separate centers appear by the fifth fetal month and fuse with each other by seventh fetal month. *J*, Synchondrosis between odontoid and neural arch: fuses at 3 to 6 years. *L*, Synchondrosis between odontoid and body: fuses at 3 to 6 years. *M*, Posterior surface of body and odontoid. (From Bailed D [1952]: The normal cervical spine in infants and children. *Radiology* 59: 712–719, with permission.)

FIGURE 9. Diagram of typical cervical vertebrae C3–7. *A*, Body: appears by fifth fetal month. *B*, Anterior (costal) portion of transverse process: may develop from a separate center that appears by the sixth fetal month and joins the arch by the sixth year. *C*, Neural arches: appears by seventh to ninth fetal week. *D*, Synchondrosis between spinous processes: usually unites by second or third year. *E*, Secondary centers for bifid spine: appears at puberty and unites with spinous process at 25 years. *F*, Neurocentral synchondrosis: fuses at 3 to 6 years. *G*, Superior and inferior epiphyseal rings: appears at puberty and unites with body at about 25 years. The seventh cervical vertebra differs slightly because of a long powerful nonbifid spinous process. (Based on the study of radiographs of the cervical spine from approximately 100 normal children ranging from newborn to 14 years of age.) (From Bailey DK [1952]: The normal cervical spine in infants and children. *Radiology* 59: 712–719, with permission.)

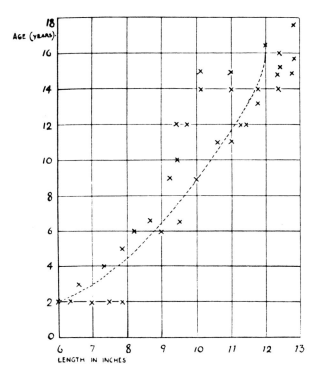

FIGURE 10. Normal growth curve for the thoracic spine. Measurements were made on radiographs obtained with standard technique. The authors did not include the relative height of the patient or the degree of kyphosis or lordosis. (From Roaf R [1960]: Vertebral growth and its mechanical control. *J Bone Joint Surg [Br]* 42:40–59, with permission.)

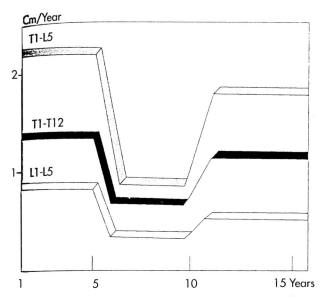

FIGURE 12. Growth velocity of T1–L5 segment, thoracic segment T1–12, and lumbar segment L1–5. (From Dimeglio A [1993]: Growth of the spine before 5 years. *J Pediatr Orthop* 1-B:102.)

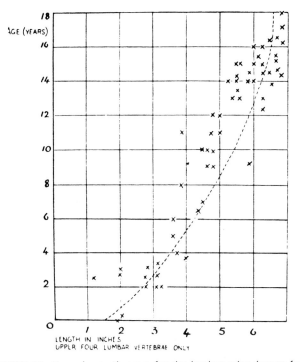

FIGURE 11. Normal growth curve for the lumbar spine (upper four lumbar vertebrae only). (From Roaf R [1960]: Vertebral growth and its mechanical control. *J Bone Joint Surg [Br]* 42:40–59, with permission.)

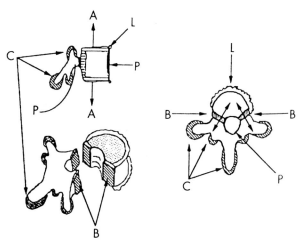

FIGURE 13. Vertebral growth. *A*, Body end plates (superior and inferior). *B*, Neurocentral cartilage (bipolar) fusion at age 7 or 8 years. *C*, Posterior elements cartilage. *P*, Periosteum. *L*, ring apophysis (begins age 7 to 9 years, closed at age 14 to 24 years) (From Dubousset J, Katti E, Seringe R [1993]: Epiphysiodesis of the spine in young children for congenital spinal deformations. *J Pediatr Orthop* 13:123.)

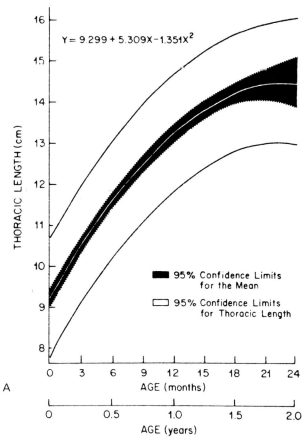

$$Y = 9.299 + 5.309X - 1.351X^2$$

■ 95% Confidence Limits
for the Mean

□ 95% Confidence Limits
for Thoracic Length

A

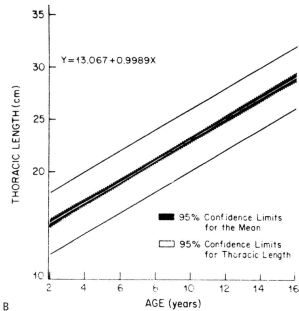

$$Y = 13.067 + 0.9989X$$

■ 95% Confidence Limits
for the Mean

□ 95% Confidence Limits
for Thoracic Length

B

FIGURE 14. Results of statistical analysis in children from birth to 2 years and children from 2 to 16 years. The predicted values for the mean are indicated by the center curve, and the 95% confidence limits for the mean by the shaded area. The boundaries of the unshaded area (outside curves) denote the calculated 95% confidence limits for thoracic length for an individual child. In the equations shown in these figures, Y is the thoracic length in centimeters and X is the age in years. (From Currarino G, Williams B, Reisch JS [1986]: Linear growth of the thoracic spine in chest roentgenograms from birth to 16 years. *Skelet Radiol* 15:628–630, with permission.)

Schmorl G, Junghanns H (1971): The human spine in health and disease, 2nd ed. New York: Grune & Stratton.

Winter RB (1977): Scoliosis and spinal growth. *Orthop Rev* 6:17–20.

5. Thoracic Spine Length from Birth to 16 Years (Fig. 14)

Kuhns LR, Holt JF (1975): Measurement of thoracic spine length on chest radiographs of newborn infants. *Radiology* 116:395–397.

C. NEUROLOGIC MATURATION

1. Primitive Reflexes (Table 5)

2. Reflex Maturation (Fig. 15)

3. Reflexes of Neurophysiologic Maturation (Table 6)

4. Developmental Milestones

Capute AJ, Biehl RF (1973): Functional developmental evaluation. *Pediatr Clin North Am* 20:3–26.

Capute AJ, Palmer FB, Shapiro BK, et al. (1986): Clinical linguistic and auditory milestone scale: prediction of cognition in infancy. *Dev Med Child Neurol* 28:762–771.

Greene MG (1991): *The Harriet Lane handbook,* 12th ed. St. Louis: Mosby–Year Book.

5. Motor Development Evaluation (Tables 7, 8)

Zausmer E (1953): Evaluation of strength and motor development in infants. *Phys Ther Rev* 33:575–581.

Zausmer E (1964): The evaluation of motor development in children. *Phys Ther Rev* 44:247–250.

Zausmer E, Tower G (1966): A quotient for the evaluation of motor development. *Phys Ther Rev* 46:725–727.

6. Motor Maturity Tests (Tables 9, 10)

TABLE 5. PRIMITIVE REFLEXES

Reflex	Present by (months)	Gone by (months)
Intrauterine—birth reflexes		
Palmar grasp	Birth	4
Plantar grasp	Birth	9
Automatic stepping	Birth	2
Crossed extension	Birth	2
Galant	Birth	2
Moro	Birth	3–6
Tonic neck		4
Asymmetric	Birth	8
Symmetric	5	
Lower extremity placing	0.03 (1 day)	—
Upper extremity placing	3	—
Downward thrust	3	—
Late infant reflexes		
Landau (head, trunk and leg extension while prone)	3	12–24
Derotational righting	4	—
Other postural reflexes		
Anterior propping	6	—
Lateral propping	8	—
Posterior propping	10	—

TABLE 6. REFLEXES OF NEUROPHYSIOLOGIC MATURATION

Reflex	Test position	Stimulus	Response	Appears	Disappears	Significance of Absence	Significance of Abnormal Persistence
Palmar (hand) grasp (Fig. 1–35)	Supine; head must be midline	Introduction of a pencil or rod into palm from ulnar side; object pulled on after grasp	Finger will flex and grasp object Thumb will not oppose but will flex if extended If response is marked, infant can be suspended by object he is holding	Birth	2–4 mo	Flaccid paralysis	Flexor hypertonicity as in spastic cerebral palsy Asymmetric in hemiplegia
Plantar (foot) grasp (Fig. 1–36)	Supine	Light digital pressure on planter aspect of foot	Tonic flexion and abduction of toes	Birth	9–12 mo	Flaccid paralysis	Spasticity of leg and foot muscles
Moro's (Fig. 1–37)	Supine with both upper and lower limbs in natural extension	Sudden extension of neck by raising the head off the table, supporting head on palm of hand, then suddenly dropping hand Raising the infant by holding the hands and then rapidly releasing Sharp bang on table or sudden tap on abdomen	*First phase:* adduction and extension of all four limbs and extension of spine; extension and fanning of digits; followed by: *Second phase:* adduction and flexion of all four limbs as if embracing	Birth	3–6 mo	In flaccid paralysis, may be asymmetric in obstetric brachial plexus paralysis In generalized hypotonia or weakness of muscles, amyotonia congenita In severe hypertonicity increased flexor muscle tone prevents extension of limbs	After 6 months, delayed maturation of central nervous system as in cerebral palsy
Startle	Supine with all four limbs in natural extension	Sudden loud noise Tapping sternum	Flexion of elbows and knees, hands closed	Birth	Present through life	Severe hypotonia Asymmetric obstetric brachial plexus paralysis	—
Placing reaction Lower limb (Fig. 1–38)	Vertical suspension by holding at waist	Touching anterior aspect of legs and dorsum of feet on edge of table	Foot placed on table spontaneous flexion of hip and knee and dorsiflexion of ankle	Birth	2–4 mo and may persist	Brain damage if absent at birth	—
Upper limb (Fig. 1–39)	Vertical suspension (feet down) by holding at waist	Bringing dorsum of ulna against edge of table	Hand placed on table by flexion of elbow	Birth	1–2, and may persist	Brain damage if absent at birth	—

(continued)

TABLE 6. *Continued.*

Reflex	Test position	Stimulus	Response	Appears	Disappears	Significance of Absence	Significance of Abnormal Persistence
Walking or stepping (Fig. 1–40)	Upright; hold supporting trunk	Pressing (touching) soles of feet on hard surface and gently inclining and moving child forward	Alternating flexion and extension of lower limbs simulating walking (rhythmical, coordinated, needs only forward movement, no propulsion)	Birth	1–2 mo	Flaccid paralysis if absent at birth	Brain damage persists after 3–4 months
Crossed extension (Phillippson's reflex) (Fig. 1–41)	Supine, lower limbs in midline and extended at hip and knee	Firm pressure to sole of one foot by rubbing or stroking Strong pressure in inguinal region	Opposite free lower limb flexes, adducts, then extends	Birth	1–2 mo	Flaccid paralysis if absent at birth	Partial or incomplete cord lesions Brain damage
Withdrawal	Supine, lower limbs in midline and natural extended posture	Pinprick to sole	Dorsiflexion of ankle, flexion of hip and knee (withdraws limb from noxious stimulus)	Birth	1–2 mo	Flaccid paralysis as in myelomeningocele or intraspinal lesions	Spasticity of lower limbs as in cerebral palsy
Positive support or leg straightening	Upright, supported under axillae and around chest	Press soles of feet to the ground or table several times	Lower limbs and trunk go into extension, serving as strong pillars for weight bearing	Birth	4 mo	—	Reciprocal leg movements cannot appear; infant cannot walk
Extensor thrust	Lower limbs held in flexed position	Apply pressure to the sole of foot	Sudden—extension of entire lower limb (sometimes followed by flexion)	Birth	2 mo	Flaccid paralysis	Brain damage and delayed maturation of central nervous system
Trunk incurvation (Galant's reflex) (Fig. 1–42)	Prone	Strike lumbar region of back with index finger—10th rib to iliac crest—in the paravertebral area about 3 cm from midline Alternate method: prick outer side of gluteal area	Lateral flexion (incurvation) of trunk toward side of stimulus	Birth	2–2¹/₂ mo	?	May cause scoliosis if dominant unilaterally

Reflex	Position	Stimulus	Response	Appears	Disappears	Flaccid paralysis/hypotonia	Severe brain damage
Tonic neck Asymmetric (Fig. 1-43)	Supine with head in midline	Rotate head to one side (without flexion of neck) to the count of 10 seconds, then rotate to the opposite side	Limbs on *chin* side—become rigid and elbow and knee go into extension. Limbs on *occiput* side—elbow and knee become flexed	Birth	4–6 mo	Flaccid paralysis Severe hypotonia	Severe brain damage as in cerebral palsy
Symmetric (Fig. 1-44)	Quadriped position	Extend head-neck Flex head-neck	Upper limbs extend and lower limbs go into flexion. Upper limbs flex and lower limbs extend	5–8 mo	No absolute time (1 year)	Cannot assume "four-point" kneeling position	Prevents reciprocal lower limb motion, hinders ambulation. Prevents crawling. Causes adduction, medial rotation flexion gait pattern
Landau's	Prone, supported under abdomen and lower thorax	First passively flex and then extend the neck-head	On flexion of neck-head, the trunk and lower and upper limbs go into flexion. On extension of head-neck, the limbs and trunk extend	6 mo	24–30 mo	Motor weakness	Delayed reflex maturation, usually breaks up predominant flexion pattern
Parachute (protective extension of arms) Forward (Fig. 1-45)	Prone, suspended in the air by waist	Move head suddenly toward floor by tipping or plunging downward	Sudden extension of arms and wrists to protect head	6 mo	Present through life	Brain damage Delayed maturation	—
Backward	Sitting or standing in neutral position	Sudden tip or push backward with enough force to offset balance	Backward extension of both upper limbs; fingers extended and abducted, weight is born on hands	9 mo	Present through life	Delayed maturation	—
Tilting Prone and supine	Prone (or supine) on tilt table (flat board with all four limbs in neutral extension)	Tilt table slowly to one side	Lateral flexion of trunk with concavity upward. The arm and leg on upper side go into abduction and extension. Arm and leg on lower side go into protection	6 mo	Present through life	—	—

(continued)

TABLE 6. *Continued.*

Reflex	Test position	Stimulus	Response	Appears	Disappears	Significance of Absence	Significance of Abnormal Persistence
Prone and supine cont'd On all fours	Placed on all fours on tilt table	Tilt to either side	As above	12 mo	Present through life	—	
Standing	Supported from waist, standing on tilt board	Movement first to either side and then forward and backward	As above				
Righting Neck	Supine, head in midline and all four limbs fully extended	Flexion and rotation of head to one side, maintaining position to count of 10	Body rotates as *a whole* in same direction as head	Birth	6 mo	Delayed maturation	Brain damage
Body	As for neck righting	Rotation of shoulder to one side, maintaining position to count of 10	Sequential rotation of trunk	6 mo	5 yr to life	—	—
Labyrinthine Prone	Blindfolded to rule out optical righting reflexes)	Posture in space	Extension of neck, bringing face horizontal to floor	1–2 mo	Present through life	Delayed maturation	—
	Suspended prone in space by support to abdomen		Flexion of head-neck, bringing face horizontal to floor	6 mo	Present through life	Delayed maturation	—
Supine	Same as prone but *supine*	Posture in space	Head will automatically right to vertical position with the mouth horizontal	6–8 mo	Present through life	Delayed maturation	—
Upright	Blindfolded, held at pelvis and suspended vertically in space	Tilt to either side	Same as above	6–8 mo	Present through life	Delayed maturation	—
Optical (Fig. 1–46)	Same as labyrinthine but eye open	Same as labyrinthine					

From Tachdjian MO (1990): *Pediatric orthopaedics*, 2nd ed. Philadelphia: WB Saunders, with permission.
Figures cited are in the above reference.

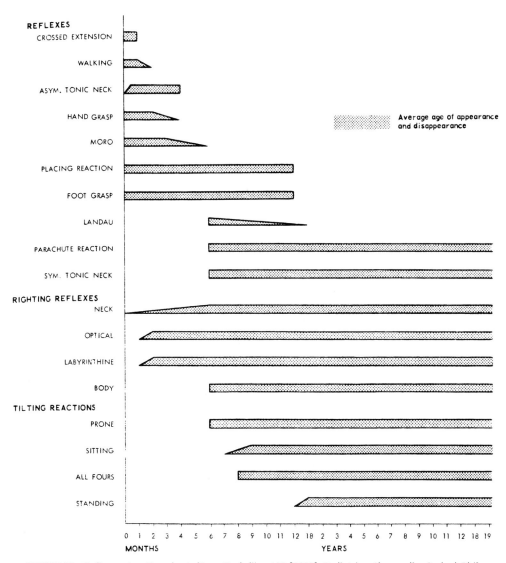

FIGURE 15. Reflex maturation chart. (From Tachdjian MO [1990]: *Pediatric orthopaedics,* 2nd ed. Philadelphia: WB Saunders, with permission.)

TABLE 7. LOCOMOTION DEVELOPMENT

Age	Skill	Age	Skill
3 mo	Lifts head up when prone	18 mo	Ascends stairs with two-hand support
6 mo	Head held steady when sitting Turns head side to side No head lag when pulled to sitting Rolls over	2 yr	Ascends stairs with no support, one foot at a time Runs forward Kicks ball forward
9 mo	Sits without support, legs extended Sits "tailor fashion"–external rotation Sits with legs in internal rotation Pulls self to stand Stand with two-hand support	3 yr	Ascends stairs without support, foot over foot Descends stairs with support, one foot at a time Jumps in place Pedals tricycle
12 mo	Leans and recovers balance when sitting Walks with one-hand support	4 yr	Descends stairs without support, foot over foot Beginning to balance on one foot
14 mo	Stands without support Walks forward without support Stoops and recovers balance	5 yr	Hops on one foot without support Heel-toe walk
		6 yr	Skips one foot at a time Backward heel-toe walk Throws ball up and catches it with one hand Hits small target from 12-in. distance

TABLE 8. MANIPULATION, UPPER EXTREMITY FUNCTION, AND LANGUAGE DEVELOPMENT

3 mo	Hand skills	Symmetric head and arm posture (supine)	2½ yr	Dressing	Unlaces and removes shoes
		Active arm motion on sight of toys			Takes off pants
	Feeding	Lip pressure		Writing	Holds crayon with fingers
		Coordination of sucking and swallowing	3 yr	Hand skills	Creases paper neatly
	Language	Vocalizes without crying			Nine-block tower
6 mo	Hand skills	Purposefully reaches out and touches object			Rides tricycle
		Palmar grasp of rattle		Feeding	Feeds self with fork
		Involuntary release of rattle		Dressing	Dresses self with supervision
	Feeding	Hand to mouth			Learning to lace shoes
	Language	Laughs and smiles			Puts on shoes, not necessarily on correct foot
9 mo	Hand skills	Transfers object both ways			Tries to wash and dry hands
		Extended reach and grasp		Language	Knows whether boy or girl
		Uses finger and thumb to grasp object		Writing	Copies circles, cannot copy cross
		Releases object with flexed wrist			Tries to use scissors, but cannot follow line
	Feeding	Can protrude tongue	4 yr	Hand skills	Overhand throw of ball
		Feeds self cookies		Feeding	Drinks through straw without mashing it
	Language	Da-da, ma-ma (nonspecific)	4 yr	Dressing	Puts on shoes on correct feet
1 yr	Hand skills	Attempts to stack one block on another (brings over and drops)			Laces shoes, but does not tie bow
		Hits two objects together			Dresses, knows back and front of clothes
		Voluntary release of object			Washes and dries face
		Rolls ball imitatively			Brushes or combs hair
		Puts round ball into round hole			Brushes teeth
		Puts cube into container			Manages buttons on self
		Can hold crayon and imitate scribbling		Language	Counts three objects correctly
	Feeding	Picks spoon up from table		Writing	Copies cross
		Chews cookies or toast	5 yr	Hand skills	Bounces ball and catches it
		Drooling controlled at all times			Performs three simple directions in sequence
		Drinks milk from cup, if held		Dressing	Dresses self completely except for back fasteners
	Dressing	Cooperates (extends arm for sleeve)		Language	Names four colors
	Language	Two or more words (other than ma-ma or da-da)			Names penny, nickel, dime
18 mo	Hand skills	Builds three-block tower (1-in cube)			Counts 10 objects correctly
		Turns pages (two or three at a time)		Writing	Draws a recognizable man
		Puts pegs into hole (1-in diameter)			Colors within 1-in area
		Pounds			Uses scissors, follows line
		Hurls ball	6 yr	Feeding	Cuts with knife and fork
		Points to nose, eyes, ears		Dressing	Buttons small buttons on shirt
	Feeding	Drinks from cup (one- or two-handed)			Ties bows on shoes
		Feeds self with spoon, but messy			Combs and brushes hair
	Dressing	Removes socks, shoes		Writing	Copies printing (A, B, C)
	Language	Vocabulary of 10 words, including names			
2 yr	Hand skills	Six-block tower			
		Turns pages one at a time			
		Throws bean bags			
		Strings beads (1-in)			
		Throws 3-in ball, but inaccurately			
	Feeding	Feeds self semisolid food with spoon			
		Drinks from cup or glass (one-handed)			
		Drinks from straw			
	Language	Three-word sentences			
	Writing	Imitates vertical, horizontal, and circular strokes; cannot initiate himself			
		Matches colors			

From Tachdjian MO (1999): *Pediatric orthopaedics*, 2nd ed. Philadelphia: WB Saunders, with permission.
Development is rated according to the Zausmer scale: O, no attempt made; T, attempt made but fails; P, poor or partial completion; F, fair performance, fluctuates; G, good, attaining speed; N, normal skill and speed; NT, not tested.

D. GROWTH CHARTS

1. Recumbent Length Percentiles From Birth to 36 Months (Figs. 16, 17)

2. Weight Percentiles From Birth to 36 Months (Figs. 18, 19)

3. Head Circumference Percentiles From Birth to 36 Months/Weight by Length Percentiles From Birth to 36 Months (Figs. 20, 21)

4. Stature Percentiles From 2 to 18 Years (Figs. 22, 23)

5. Weight Percentiles From 2 to 18 Years (Figs. 24, 25)

6. Weight by Stature Percentiles for Prepubescent Children (Figs. 26, 27)

7. Sitting Height (Fig. 28, Table 11)

8. Upper-Lower Segment Ratio

TABLE 9. BASIC MOTOR MATURITY TESTS PERFORMED AT 3 TO 10 MONTHS

Age (mo)	Supine	Prone	Pull to Sit
3	Limb posture is flexion Limb and trunk postures becoming symmetric	Holds chin and shoulders off table, weight on forearms Pelvis is flat when plane of face is 45 to 90 degrees to table	Head lag in beginning of movement, then keeps head in line with trunk Head will bob forward when sit is completed Lower limbs are flexed
4	Bilateral activities at midline (Resting) legs are in flexion, abduction, and outward rotation (Active) able to flex hips and extend legs, lifting them an inch	Head in midline Prone swimming, jerky movements	Slight head lag in beginning of movement, then keeps head in line with trunk (lower limbs flexed)
5	Back arches and child raises hips (bridges, no progression)	Arms forward, fully extended for support Arms retracted and flexed (hands off support) Support on one forearm and reaches for toys Free kicking of legs	Assists and brings head forward, no head lag (lower limbs flexed)
6	Rolls supine to prone Reaches forward with extended arms to be picked up Lifts legs and plays with feet	Rolls prone to supine (purposeful)	Spontaneous lifting of head Pulls him/herself to sitting Raises extended leg (hips are flexed, knees are extended)
7	Lifts head off table	Commando-crawls Assumes quadruped position	
8	Does not like supine position	Pivots	
9		Goes from prone to sitting	
10		Creeps on hands and knees	

From Bleck EE (1979): *Orthopaedic management of cerebral palsy.* Philadelphia: WB Saunders, with permission.

TABLE 10. BASIC MOTOR MATURITY TESTS PERFORMED AT 3 TO 15 MONTHS

Age (mo)	Sitting	Standing
3	Back somewhat rounded Head mostly held up	Does not accept weight
4	Holds head steady, but set forward Head wobbles when child is swayed Back shows only a lumbar curvature (slight rounding)	Accepts some weight
5	No arm support, arms retracted at shoulders with elbows flexed Child tends to fall backwards (does not push back) Head stable when body is mildly rocked by examiner	Takes almost full weight
6	May sit alone unsupported briefly when placed Arm support forward Sits well when propped	Bounces
8	Sits unsupported, without hand support for 1 min Sits erect Has arm support sideways	Readily bears whole weight when supported (not rigid)
9	Adjusts posture to reach Good sitting balance, sits 10 min	Pulls self to standing
10	Pivots to pick up objects Arm support backward Leans forward and recovers Can lean over sideways and recover Goes forward from sitting to prone	Stands holding on and lifts one foot Lowers self to floor by holding on Collapses if not holding on
11		Walks holding on to furniture
12		Walks with one hand held; attempts to stand alone
13		Stands alone well; walks alone
14		Gets to standing unsupported
15		Stoops and recovers

From Bleck EE (1979): *Orthopaedic management of cerebral palsy.* Philadelphia: WB Saunders, with permission.

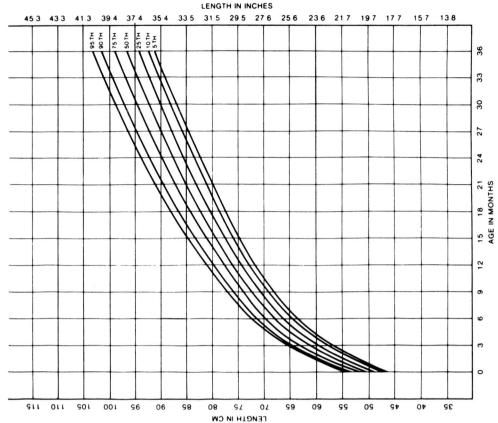

FIGURE 17. Recumbent length by age percentiles for boys aged birth to 36 months. (From Hamill PVV, Drizd PA, Johnson CL, et al. [1977]: Physical growth: national center for health statistics percentiles. *Am J Clin Nutr* 32:607–629, with permission.)

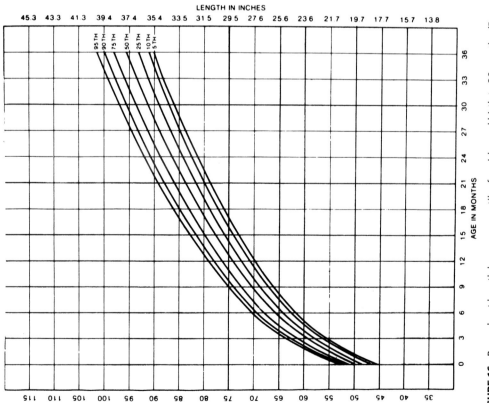

FIGURE 16. Recumbent length by age percentiles for girls aged birth to 36 months. (From Hamill PVV, Drizd PA, Johnson CL, et al. [1977]: Physical growth: national center for health statistics percentiles. *Am J Clin Nutr* 32:607–629 with permission.)

942

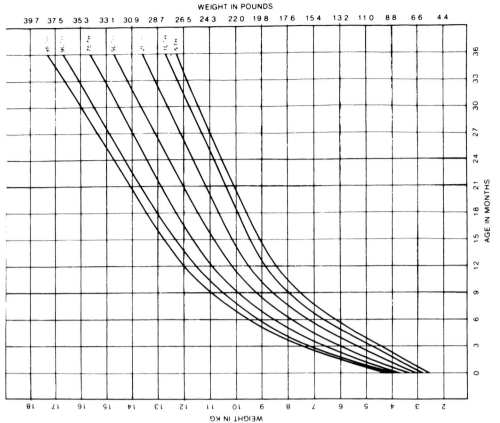
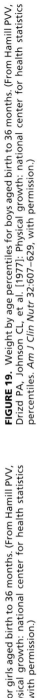

FIGURE 19. Weight by age percentiles for boys aged birth to 36 months. (From Hamill PVV, Drizd PA, Johnson CL, et al. [1977]: Physical growth: national center for health statistics percentiles. *Am J Clin Nutr* 32:607–629, with permission.)

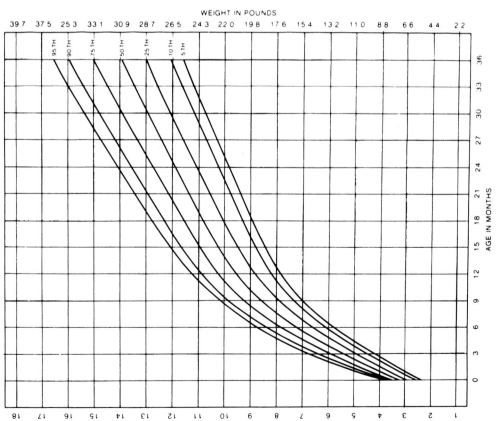

FIGURE 18. Weight by age percentiles for girls aged birth to 36 months. (From Hamill PVV, Drizd PA, Johnson CL, et al. [1977]: Physical growth: national center for health statistics percentiles. *Am J Clin Nutr* 32:607–629, with permission.)

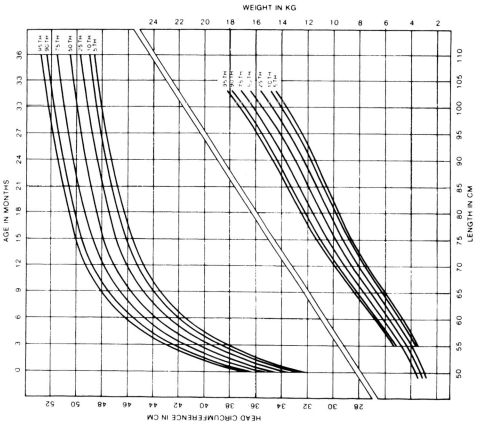

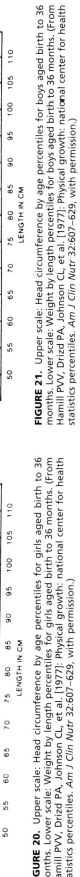

FIGURE 21. Upper scale: Head circumference by age percentiles for boys aged birth to 36 months. Lower scale: Weight by length percentiles for boys aged birth to 36 months. (From Hamill PVV, Drizd PA, Johnson CL, et al. [1977]: Physical growth: national center for health statistics percentiles. *Am J Clin Nutr* 32:607–629, with permission.)

FIGURE 20. Upper scale: Head circumference by age percentiles for girls aged birth to 36 months. Lower scale: Weight by length percentiles for girls aged birth to 36 months. (From Hamill PVV, Drizd PA, Johnson CL, et al. [1977]: Physical growth: national center for health statistics percentiles. *Am J Clin Nutr* 32:607–629, with permission.)

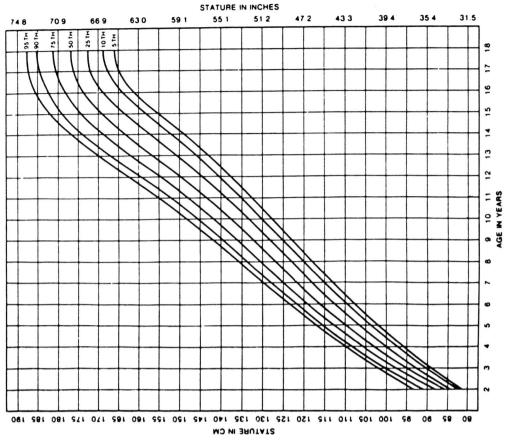

FIGURE 23. Stature by age percentiles for boys aged 2 to 18 years. (From Hamill PVV, Drizd PA, Johnson CL, et al. [1977]: Physical growth: national center for health statistics percentiles. *Am J Clin Nutr* 32:607–629, with permission.)

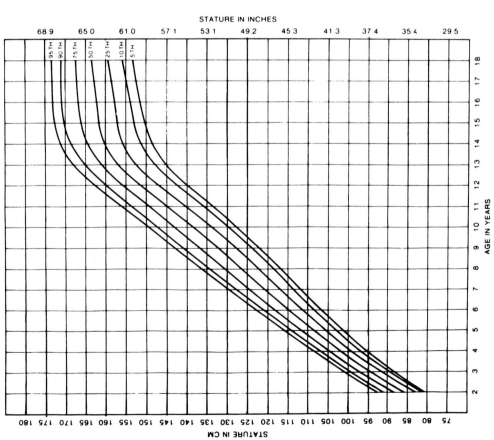

FIGURE 22. Stature by age percentiles for girls aged 2 to 18 years. (From Hamill PVV, Drizd PA, Johnson CL, et al. [1977]: Physical growth: national center for health statistics percentiles. *Am J Clin Nutr* 32:607–629, with permission.)

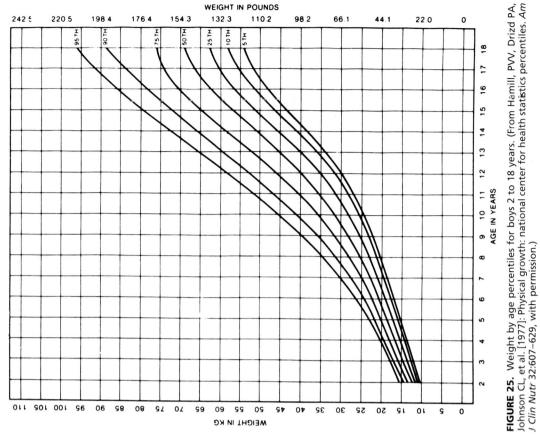

FIGURE 25. Weight by age percentiles for boys 2 to 18 years. (From Hamill, PVV, Drizd PA, Johnson CL, et al. [1977]: Physical growth: national center for health statistics percentiles. *Am J Clin Nutr* 32:607–629, with permission.)

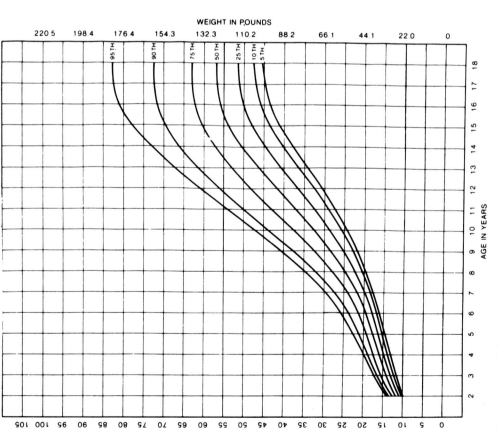

FIGURE 24. Weight by age percentiles for girls aged 2 to 18 years. (From Hamill PVV, Drizd PA, Johnson CL, et al. [1977]: Physical growth: national center for health statistics percentiles. *Am J Clin Nutr* 32:607–629, with permission.)

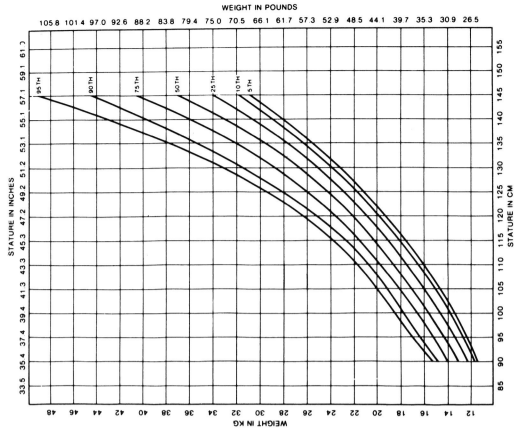

FIGURE 27. Weight by stature percentiles for prepubescent boys. (From Hamill PVV, Drizd PA, Johnson CL, et al. [1977]: Physical growth: national center for health statistics percentiles. *Am J Clin Nutr* 32:607–629, with permission.)

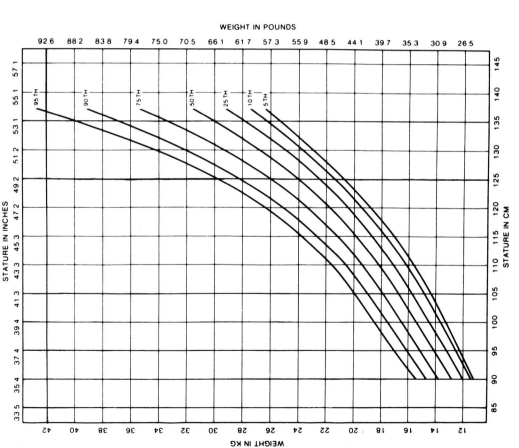

FIGURE 26. Weight by stature percentiles for prepubescent girls. (From Hamill PVV, Drizd PA, Johnson CL, et al. [1977]: Physical growth: national center for health statistics percentiles. *Am J Clin Nutr* 32:607–629, with permission.)

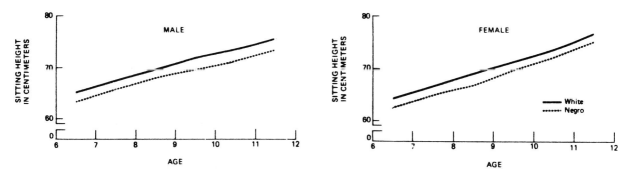

FIGURE 28. Mean sitting height of white and black children by sex and age. (From Hamill PVV, Drizd PA, Johnson CL, et al. [1977]: Physical growth: national center for health statistics percentiles. *Am J Clin Nutr* 32:607–629, with permission.)

TABLE 11. SITTING HEIGHT OF CHILDREN BY RACE, SEX, AND AGE AT LAST BIRTHDAY[a]

Race, Sex, and Age	n	N	$\overline{X}$	s	$s_{\overline{x}}$	Percentile (in cm)						
						5th	10th	25th	50th	75th	90th	95th
White												
Boys												
6	489	1,787	65.0	2.68	0.13	60.4	61.4	63.2	65.1	66.7	68.5	69.7
7	551	1,781	67.2	2.74	0.15	63.0	64.0	65.4	67.2	68.9	70.8	71.8
8	537	1,739	69.5	2.94	0.12	65.1	65.7	67.6	69.6	71.5	73.3	74.3
9	525	1,730	71.6	3.15	0.19	66.4	67.4	69.6	71.6	73.7	75.6	76.7
10	509	1,692	73.3	3.07	0.20	68.3	69.5	71.4	73.3	75.4	77.3	78.7
11	542	1,662	75.6	3.10	0.13	70.6	71.5	73.5	75.5	77.7	79.6	80.7
Girls												
6	461	1,722	64.2	3.00	0.18	59.2	60.4	62.3	64.3	66.1	68.2	69.1
7	512	1,716	66.4	2.99	0.12	61.5	62.6	64.3	66.5	68.4	70.4	71.4
8	498	1,674	68.8	2.89	0.13	63.7	64.8	67.1	68.9	70.8	72.4	73.3
9	494	1,663	71.1	3.19	0.17	65.8	67.1	68.9	71.1	73.4	75.3	76.3
10	505	1,632	73.5	3.39	0.14	68.2	69.2	71.1	73.5	75.7	77.6	79.1
11	477	1,605	76.5	3.96	0.15	70.4	72.0	74.2	76.2	78.8	81.6	83.7
Black												
Boys												
6	84	289	63.2	2.48	0.35	59.2	59.7	61.4	63.2	64.8	66.5	68.1
7	79	286	65.6	2.58	0.29	61.6	62.3	63.5	65.6	67.5	69.1	70.1
8	79	279	67.8	2.81	0.29	63.5	64.3	66.2	67.5	69.4	71.8	72.7
9	74	269	69.3	3.69	0.40	63.7	64.5	66.7	68.6	71.7	74.5	75.8
10	65	264	70.9	3.54	0.33	64.8	66.1	68.3	70.6	73.2	75.4	77.5
11	83	255	73.4	3.36	0.37	67.8	68.7	71.4	73.6	74.8	77.5	79.3
Girls												
6	72	281	62.3	2.78	0.35	57.4	58.8	60.4	62.3	64.5	66.2	66.6
7	93	284	64.9	3.05	0.40	60.0	61.2	62.7	64.7	67.0	69.3	70.5
8	113	281	66.6	3.50	0.26	61.5	62.4	64.5	66.3	68.6	71.5	73.4
9	84	265	69.6	3.43	0.44	64.2	65.4	67.4	69.5	71.6	74.4	75.5
10	77	266	71.9	3.77	0.48	66.3	67.6	69.3	71.5	74.4	76.8	78.9
11	84	253	75.1	4.08	0.38	68.3	69.3	72.5	75.3	78.4	80.3	81.4

From Hamill PVV, Drizd PA, Johnson CL, Reed RB, Roche AF (1977): Physical growth; national center for health statistics percentiles. *Am J Clin Nutr* 32:607–629, with permission.
[a] These are the data from which the growth chart in Figure 28 was constructed.
n, sample size: *N*, estimated number of children in population in thousands; $\overline{X}$, mean; *s*, standard deviation; $s_{\overline{x}}$, standard error of the mean.

Hamill PV, Johnston FE, Gram W (1977): *Height and weight of children, United States: height and weight measurements by age, sex, race, geographic region of children 6 to 11 years of age, United States 1963–1965.* National Center for Health Statistics, Series II, No. 104; Public Health Service Publication No. 1011, No. 104 Washington, D.C.: U.S. Government Printing Office.

9. Height Velocity Standards (Figs. 29, 30)

10. Weight Velocity Standards (Figs. 31, 32)

11. Standard Growth Curves for Achondroplasia (Figs. 33, 34)

12. Mean Heights and Growth Curves for Height in Children With Skeletal Dysplasias

Mean heights and growth curves for diastrophic dysplasia, spondyloepiphyseal dysplasia, and pseudoachondroplasia are given by Horton and colleagues. Only the mean heights at different ages are presented here (Table 12).

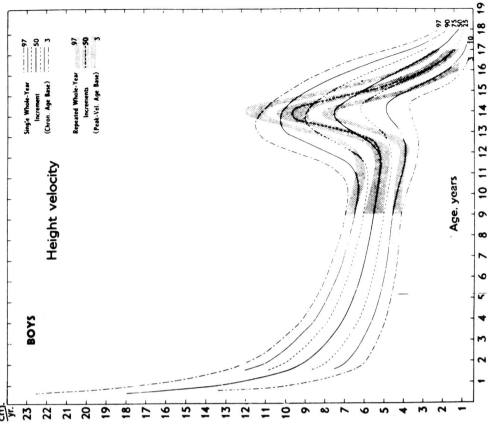

FIGURE 30. Peak height velocity for boys. (From Tanner JM, Whitehouse RH, Takaishi M [1966]: Standards from birth to maturity for height, weight, height velocity and weight velocity: British children Parts I and II. *Arch Dis Child* 41:454–471, 613–635, with permission.)

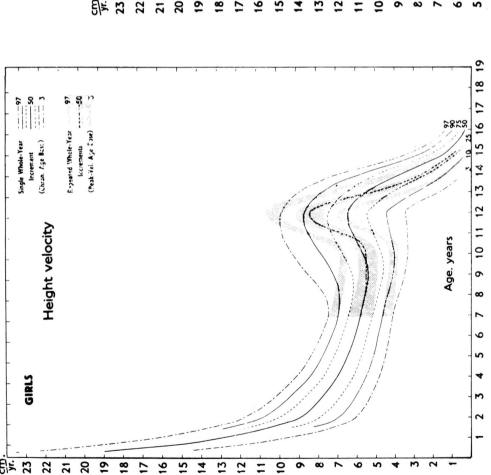

FIGURE 29. Peak height velocity for girls, the graph is composed of single whole-year increments with a chronologic age base displayed in a conventional manner by means of a continuous line indicating the 50th percentile, and broken lines indicating the 3rd and 97th percentiles. These are the standards used before and during adolescence if no data on developmental ages are available. Repeated whole-year increments (peak velocity age base) are plotted as shaded bands with a dashed line for 50th percentile. This individual curve represents the velocity taken at each successive year by an individual who has her peak at the average age and an average velocity through adolescence. The shaded curves represent the shape of the individual child's growth spurt at adolescence better than the increment line. (From Tanner JM, Whitehouse RH, Takaishi M [1966]: Standards from birth to maturity for height, weight, height velocity and weight velocity: British children Parts I and II. *Arch Dis Child* 41:454–471, 613–635, with permission.)

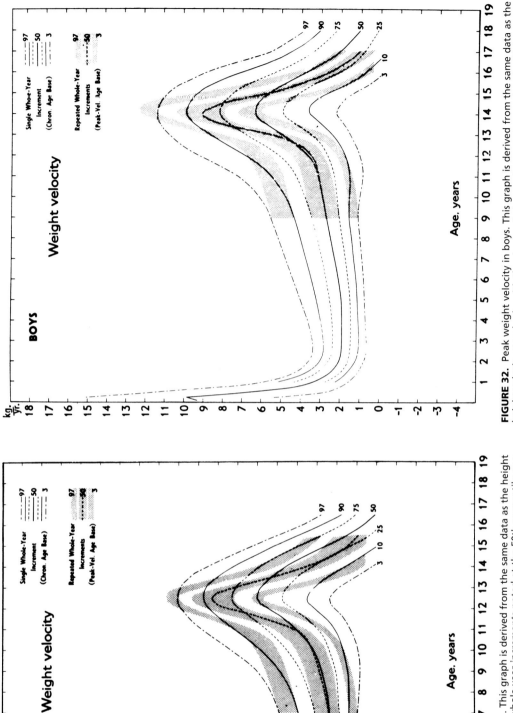

FIGURE 31. Weight velocity in girls. This graph is derived from the same data as the height velocity standards, with the single whole year increments noted at the 50th percentile as a smooth line and the 97th percentile and 3rd percentiles as dotted lines; from birth to adolescence, the peak velocity–centered curves and whole-year increments are presented by the dotted 50th percentile and shaded areas. (From Tanner JM, Whitehouse RH, Takaishi M [1966]: Standards from birth to maturity for height, weight, height velocity and weight velocity: British children Parts I and II. *Arch Dis Child* 41:454–471, 613–635, with permission.)

FIGURE 32. Peak weight velocity in boys. This graph is derived from the same data as the height velocity standards, with the single whole-year increments noted at the 50th percentile as a smooth line and the 97th and 3rd percentiles as dotted lines; from birth to adolescence, the peak velocity–centered curves whole-year peak increments are represented by the dotted 50th percentile and shaded areas. (From Tanner JM, Whitehouse RH, Takaishi M [1966]: Standards from birth to maturity for height, weight, height velocity and weight velocity: British children Parts I and II. *Arch Dis Child* 41:454–471, 613–635, with permission.)

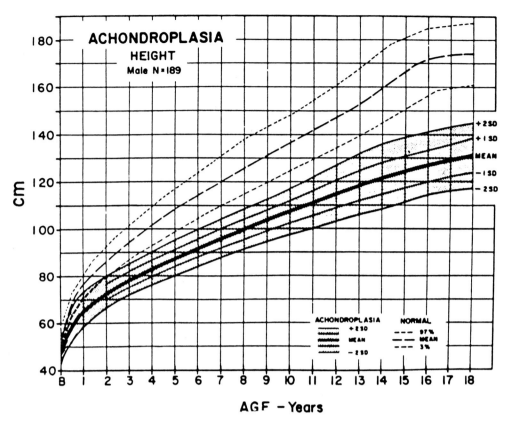

FIGURE 33. Height of men with achondroplasia (*stippled area*) compared with normal male standard height curve (3rd, 50th, and 97th percentiles). (From Horton WA, Rotter JI, Rimoin DL, Scott CI [1978]: Standard growth curves for achondroplasia. *J Pediatr* 93:435–438, with permission.)

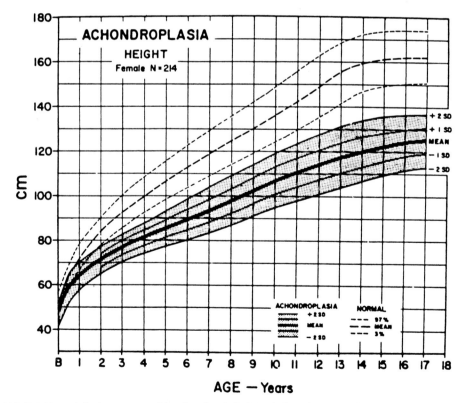

FIGURE 34. Height for women with achondroplasia (*stippled area*) compared to normal female standard height curve. (From Horton WA, Rotter JI, Rimoin DL, Scott CI [1978]: Standard growth curves for achondroplasia. *J Pediatr* 93:435–438, with permission.)

TABLE 12. MEAN HEIGHTS IN DIASTROPHIC DYSPLASIA, SPONDYLOEPIPHYSEAL DYSPLASIA, AND PSEUDOACHONDROPLASIA

	Diastrophic Dysplasia (n = 72)			Spondyloepiphyseal Dysplasia (n = 62)			Pseudoachondroplasia (n = 61)		
	No. of OBS,	Height, cm		No. of OBS,	Height, cm		No. of OBS,	Height, cm	
Age	M + F	Mean	SD	M + F	Mean	SD	M + F	Mean	SD
Birth	12 + 12	41.67	4.69	9 + 5	42.14	2.66	8 + 10	49.39	1.97
6 mo	3 + 0	56.33	1.15	3 + 2	48.00	3.03	2 + 4	63.17	2.86
1	3 + 2	63.40	5.94	2 + 1	58.67	4.04	0 + 6	71.17	1.47
2	3 + 3	70.00	5.51	8 + 5	68.23	4.94	2 + 7	80.22	3.07
4	6 + 7	82.69	6.25	12 + 5	80.00	8.24	4 + 7	88.73	3.07
6	8 + 7	90.87	7.81	8 + 5	88.38	7.01	5 + 6	94.55	3.86
8	5 + 10	100.27	8.50	6 + 7	94.23	11.53	4 + 4	98.13	5.69
10	4 + 5	103.89	9.99	7 + 7	99.43	11.10	2 + 8	106.80	6.41
12	7 + 3	102.90	10.95	7 + 0	106.57	14.73	2 + 5	111.14	9.96
14	7 + 1	104.88	9.93	6 + 3	114.56	19.79	1 + 2	124.00	2.00
16	2 + 1	112.67	13.43	3 + 0	120.33	15.82	0 + 2	120.50	14.85
18	12 + 9	118.33	12.03	9 + 9	115.50	14.88	11 + 19	118.83	12.22

From Horton WA, Hall JG, Scott CI, Pyeritz RE, Rimoln DL (1982): Growth curves for height for diastrophic dysplasia, spondyloepiphyseal dysplasia, congenita, and pseudoachondroplasia. *Am J Dis Child* 136:316–319, with permission.
SD, standard deviation.

E. PUBERTAL EVENTS

1. Pubertal Events in Boys and Girls

Greene MG (1991): *The Harriet Lane handbook,* 12th ed. St. Louis: Mosby—Year Book.
Lee PA (1980): *J Adolesc Health Care* 1:26–32.

2. Pubertal Stages in Girls and Boys (Table 13)

Marshall WA, Tanner JM (1969): Variations in pattern of pubertal changes in girls. *Arch Dis Child* 44:291–303.
Marshall WA, Tanner JM (1970): Variations in the pattern of pubertal changes in boys. *Arch Dis Child* 45:13–23.

F. ASSESSMENT OF SKELETAL MATURATION

1. Bone Age (Greulich-Pyle)

Pyle, Waterhouse, and Greulich have published a new radiographic reference standard for the assessment of skeletal age from hand-wrist film of children and youths. Studies of skeletal age assessments by research workers using left hand-wrist film and the bone-specific Greulich and Pyle method have shown intraobserver differences.
Gruelich WW, Pyle SI (1959): *Radiographic atlas of skeletal development of the hand and wrist,* 2nd ed. Palo Alto, CA: Stanford University Press.
Keats TE (1990): Skeletal maturation. In: *Atlas of roentgenographic measurement.* St. Louis: Mosby—Year Book.

TABLE 13. PUBERTAL STAGES IN GIRLS AND BOYS

Pubertal Stages in Girls	Pubertal Stages in Boys
Breast Staging	**Genitalia Ratings**
Stage 1. Preadolescent; elevation of papilla only	Stage 1. Preadolescent; testes, scrotum, and penis are of about the same size and proportion as in early childhood
Stage 2. Breast bud stage; elevation of breast and papilla as a small mound, enlargement of areola diameter	Stage 2. Scrotum and testes are enlarged with change in texture of the scrotal skin with slight reddening of the skin
Stage 3. Further enlargement of breast and areola, with no separation of their contours	Stage 3. Increase in size of the penis, in length mainly, but also in breadth, with continued growth of the testes and scrotum
Stage 4. Projection of areola and papilla to form a secondary mound above the level of the breast	Stage 4. Further enlargement of the testes, scrotum, and penis with development of the glans and darkening of the scrotal skin
Stage 5. Mature stage; projection of papilla only, due to recession of the areola to the general contour of the breast	Stage 5. Genitalia adult in size and shape
Pubic Hair Stages	**Pubic Hair Stages**
Stage 1. Preadolescent; no pubic hair	Stage 1. Preadolescent; no pubic hair
Stage 2. Slight growth of long, slightly pigmented, downy hair appearing chiefly along the labia	Stage 2. Slight growth of long, slightly pigmented, downy hair, appearing chiefly at the base of the penis
Stage 3. Darker, coarser hair that is more curled and spread sparsely over the junction of the pubes	Stage 3. Darker, coarser hair that is more curled and spread over the junction of the pubes
Stage 4. Hair is adult in type with no spread to medial surface of the thigh	Stage 4. Hair is adult in type with no spread to medial surface of the thigh
Stage 5. Adult in quantity and quality with no inverse triangle distribution and spread to the medial thighs	Stage 5. Adult in quantity and quality with no inverse triangle distribution and spread to the medial thighs

From Tanner JM (1975): Growth and endocrinology of the adolescent. In: Gardner L, ed. *Endocrine and genetic diseases of childhood.* Philadelphia: WB Saunders, with permission.

Pyle SE, Waterhouse AM, Greulich WW (1971): *A radiographic standard of reference for the growing hand and wrist.* Cleveland: The Press of Case Western Reserve University.

Roche AF, Rohmann CG, French Y (1970): Effect of training on replicability of assessment of skeletal maturity. *Am J Roentgenol* 108:511–515.

2. Method of Graham (Table 14)

3. The Oxford Method of Assessing Skeletal Maturity

Standards are presented for the assessment of skeletal maturity based on radiographs of the pelvis and hip. A point is assigned for each maturity indicator, and a total maturity score is developed. The original text should be consulted for more detailed discussion. (Figs. 35, 36)

4. Skeletal Ossification Centers

Figures 37 and 38 indicate the range from 10th to the 90th percentiles in appearance time of centers of ossification. Numbers followed by m indicate months, otherwise all numbers indicate years. Where two sets of numbers are given for one center of ossification, the upper boldface numbers refer to men and the lower numbers refer to women. A single set of numbers applies to both sexes. AB indicates that the ossification center is visible at birth. Numbers in parentheses give approximate time of fusion.

5. Risser Sign (Fig. 39)

Risser JC (1958): The iliac apophysis: an invaluable sign in the management of scoliosis. *Clin Orthop* 11:111–120.

6. Vertebral Ring Apophysis (Fig. 40)

TABLE 14. AGE AT APPEARANCE (YEARS–MONTHS) PERCENTILES FOR SELECTED OSSIFICATION CENTERS[a]

	Percentiles					
	Boys			Girls		
Centers	5th	50th	95th	5th	50th	95th
1. Humerus, head	—	0–0	0–4	—	0–0	0–4
2. Tibia, proximal	—	0–0	0–1	—	0–0	0–0
3. Coracoid process of scapula	—	0–0	0–4	—	0–0	0–5
4. Cuboid	—	0–1	0–4	—	0–1	0–2
5. Capitate	—	0–3	0–7	—	0–2	0–7
6. Hamate	0–0	0–4	0–10	—	0–2	0–7
7. Capitellum of humerus	0–1	0–4	1–1	0–1	0–3	0–9
8. Femur, head	0–1	0–4	0–8	0–0	0–4	0–7
9. Cuneiform 3	0–1	0–6	1–7	—	0–3	1–3
10. Humerus, greater tuberosity	0–3	0–10	2–4	0–2	0–6	1–2
11. Toe phalanx 5M	—	1–0	3–10	—	0–9	2–1
12. Radius, distal	0–6	1–1	2–4	0–5	0–10	1–8
13. Toe phalanx 1 D	0–9	1–3	2–1	0–5	0–9	1–8
14. Toe phalanx 4 M	0–5	1–3	2–11	0–5	0–11	3–0
15. Finger phalanx 3 P	0–9	1–4	2–2	0–5	0–10	1–7
16. Toe phalanx 3 M	0–5	1–5	4–3	0–3	1–0	2–6
17. Finger phalanx 2 P	0–9	1–5	2–2	0–5	0–10	1–8
18. Finger phalanx 4 P	0–10	1–6	2–5	0–5	0–11	1–8
19. Finger phalanx 1 D	0–9	1–6	2–8	0–5	1–0	1–9
20. Toe phalanx 3 P	0–11	1–7	2–6	0–6	1–1	1–11
21. Metacarpal 2	0–11	1–7	2–10	0–8	1–1	1–8
22. Toe phalanx 4 P	0–11	1–8	2–8	0–7	1–3	2–1
23. Toe phalanx 2 P	1–0	1–9	2–8	0–8	1–2	2–1
24. Metacarpal 3	0–11	1–9	3–0	0–8	1–2	1–11
25. Finger phalanx 5 P	1–0	1–10	2–10	0–8	1–2	2–1
26. Finger phalanx 3 M	1–0	2–0	3–4	0–8	1–3	2–4
27. Metacarpal 4	1–1	2–0	3–7	0–9	1–3	2–2
28. Toe phalanx 2 M	0–11	2–0	4–1	0–6	1–2	2–3
29. Finger phalanx 4 M	1–0	2–1	3–3	0–8	1–3	2–5
30. Metacarpal 5	1–3	2–2	3–10	0–10	1–4	2–4
31. Cuneiform 1	0–11	2–2	3–9	0–6	1–5	2–10
32. Metatarsal 1	1–5	2–2	3–1	1–0	1–7	2–3
33. Finger phalanx 2 M	1–4	2–2	3–4	0–8	1–4	2–6
34. Toe phalanx 1 P	1–5	2–4	3–4	0–11	1–7	2–6
35. Finger phalanx 3 D	1–4	2–5	3–9	0–9	1–6	2–8
36. Triquetrum	0–6	2–5	5–6	0–3	1–8	3–9
37. Finger phalanx 4 D	1–4	2–5	3–9	0–9	1–6	2–10
38. Toe phalanx 5 P	1–6	2–5	3–8	1–0	1–9	2–8
39. Metacarpal 1	1–5	2–7	4–4	0–11	1–7	2–8
40. Cuneiform 2	1–2	2–8	4–3	0–10	1–10	3–0
41. Metatarsal 2	1–11	2–10	4–4	1–3	2–2	3–5
42. Femur, greater trochanter	1–11	3–0	4–4	1–0	1–10	3–0
43. Finger phalanx 1 P	1–10	3–0	4–7	0–11	1–9	2–10
44. Navicular of foot	1–1	3–0	5–5	0–9	1–11	3–7

(continued)

TABLE 14. *Continued.*

Centers	Boys			Girls		
	5th	**50th**	**95th**	**5th**	**50th**	**95th**
45. Finger phalanx 2 D	1–10	3–2	5–0	1–1	2–6	3–3
46. Finger phalanx 5 D	2–1	3–3	5–0	1–0	2–0	3–5
47. Finger phalanx 5 M	1–11	3–5	5–10	0–11	2–0	3–6
48. Fibula, proximal	1–10	3–6	5–3	1–4	2–7	3–11
49. Metatarsal 3	2–4	3–6	5–0	1–5	2–6	3–8
50. Toe phalanx 5 D	2–4	3–11	6–4	1–2	2–4	4–1
51. Patella	2–7	4–0	6–0	1–6	2–6	4–0
52. Metatarsal 4	2–11	4–0	5–9	1–9	2–10	4–1
53. Lunate	1–6	4–1	6–9	1–1	2–7	5–8
54. Toe phalanx 3 D	3–0	4–4	6–2	1–4	2–9	4–1
55. Metatarsal 5	3–1	4–4	6–4	2–1	3–3	4–11
56. Toe phalanx 4 D	2–11	4–5	6–5	1–4	2–7	4–1
57. Toe phalanx 2 D	3–3	4–8	6–9	1–6	2–11	4–6
58. Radius, head	3–0	5–3	8–0	2–3	3–10	6–3
59. Navicular of wrist	3–7	5–8	7–10	2–4	4–1	6–0
60. Greater multangular	3–6	5–10	9–0	1–11	4–1	6–4
61. Lesser multangular	3–1	6–3	8–6	2–5	4–2	6–0
62. Medial epicondyle of humerus	4–3	6–3	8–5	2–1	3–5	5–1
63. Ulna, distal	5–3	7–1	9–1	3–3	5–4	7–8
64. Calcaneal apophysis	5–2	7–7	9–7	3–6	5–4	7–4
65. Olecranon of ulna	7–9	9–8	11–11	5–7	8–0	9–11
66. Lateral epicondyle of humerus	9–3	11–3	13–8	7–2	9–3	11–3
67. Tibial tubercle	9–11	11–10	13–5	7–11	10–3	11–10
68. Adductor sesamoid of thumb	11–0	12–9	14–7	8–8	10–9	12–8
69. Os acetabulum	11–11	13–6	15–4	9–7	11–6	13–5
70. Acromion	12–2	13–9	15–6	10–4	11–11	13–9
71. Iliac crest	12–0	14–0	15–11	10–10	12–9	15–4
72. Coracoid apophysis	12–9	14–4	16–4	10–4	12–3	14–4
73. Ischial tuberosity	13–7	15–3	17–1	11–9	13–11	16–0

From Graham BC (1976): Assessment of bone maturation: methods and pitfalls. *Clin North Am* 10:186–202, with permission.
[a] Based on a study of 143 healthy, middle-class Ohio-born children of northwestern European ancestry.
P, proximal; M, middle; D, distal.

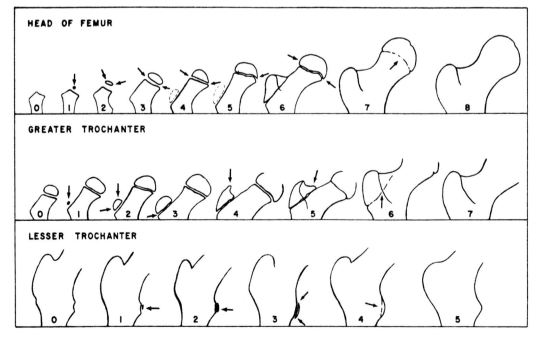

FIGURE 35. Maturity indicators at the proximal end of the femur. Head of the femur, greater trochanter, and lesser trochanter. (From Acheson RM [1957]: The Oxford method of assessing skeletal maturity. *Clin Orthop* 10:19–39, with permission.)

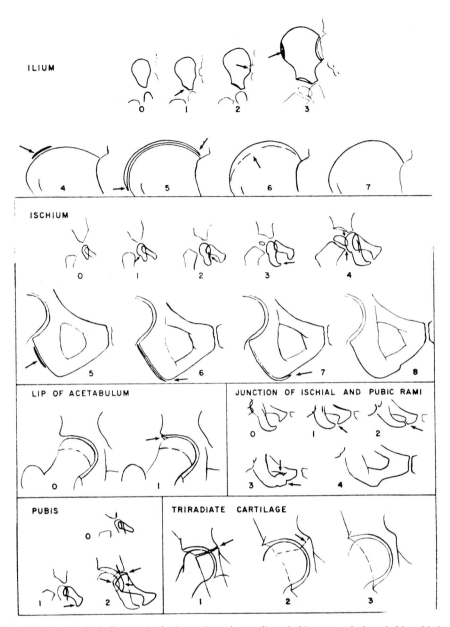

FIGURE 36. Maturity indicators in the innominate bone. Ilium, ischium, acetabulum, ischiopubic junction, pubis, and triradiate cartilage. (From Acheson RM [1957]: The Oxford method of assessing skeletal maturity. *Clin Orthop* 10:19–39, with permission.)

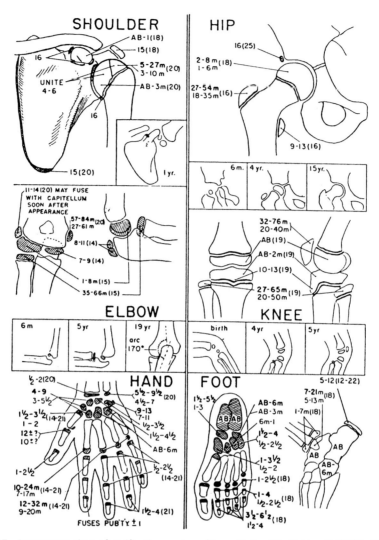

FIGURE 37. Appearance time of ossification centers. (From Girdan BR, Golden R [1952]: Centers of ossification of the skeleton. *Am J Roentgenol* 68:922–924, with permission.)

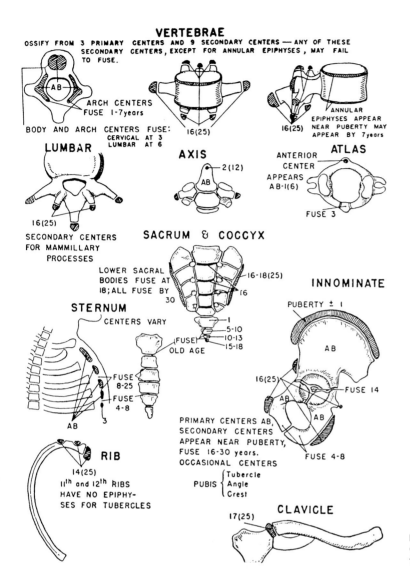

FIGURE 38. Appearance time of ossification centers. (From Girdan BR, Golden R [1952]: Centers of ossification of the skeleton. *Am J Roentgenol* 68:922–924, with permission.)

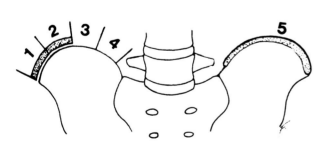

FIGURE 39. Risser sign. Ossification of the iliac apophysis as a method to assess maturation of the vertebral column. The ossification begins at the anterior superior iliac spine. After completion of its excursion, the ossified iliac apophysis fuses to the body of the ilium. *1:* Risser 1: 25% excursion. *2:* Risser 2: 50% excursion. *3:* Risser 3: 75% excursion. *4:* Risser 4: complete excursion. *5:* Risser 5: iliac crest fuses to the ilium. (From Lonstein JE [1987]: Patient evaluation. In: Bradford DS, et al., eds. *Moe's textbook of scoliosis and other spinal deformities.* Philadelphia: WB Saunders, with permission.)

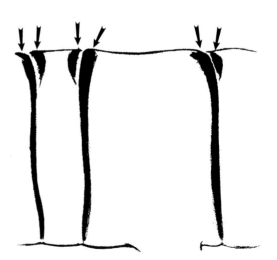

FIGURE 40. Ossification of the vertebral ring apophysis. The arrows indicate the apophyseal areas.

Garn SM, Silverman SN, Rohmann CG (1962): A rational approach to the assessment of skeletal maturation. *Ann Radiol* 7:297–307.

Hansman CF (1962): Appearance and fusion of ossification centers in the human skeleton. *Am J Roentgenol* 88:476–482.

Sontag LW, Snell D, Anderson M (1939): Rate of appearance of ossification centers from birth to the age of five years. *Am J Dis Child* 58:949–956.

Tanner JM, Whitehouse RH, et al. (1975): *Assessment of skeletal maturity and prediction of adult height (TW2 method)*. London: Academic Press.

Tanner JM (1975): *Growth and endocrinology of the adolescent in Gardner endocrine and genetic diseases of childhood and adolescence*. Philadelphia: WB Saunders.

G. NEUROLOGIC EXAMINATION

1. Cranial Nerves (Table 15)

2. Dermatome Patterns (Fig. 41)

3. Motor Scale: Manual Testing

The definitions recommended by the American Spinal Injury Association (ASIA) in the booklet Standards for Neurological Classifications of Spinal Injury Patients adapted from Austin, provide an accurate method of communicating information on the extent of neurologic injury. Manual muscle testing is performed using the standard six-grade scale:

Absent = 0
Trace = 1 Visible of palpable contraction
Poor = 2 Active movement through range of motion with gravity eliminated

TABLE 15. CRANIAL NERVES

I	(Olfactory)	Smell
II	(Optic)	Acuity, fields, fundi
III	(Oculomotor)	Extraocular muscle, pupillary reaction, eyelid opening
IV	(Trochlear)	Extraocular muscle (superior oblique muscle)
V	(Trigeminal)	Facial sensation, corneal reflex (sensory component), muscles of mastication
VI	(Abducens)	Extraocular muscle (lateral rectus muscle)
VII	(Facial)	Facial movement (motor component), taste (anterior 2/3 of tongue), salivation, tearing, hyperacusis (stapedius)
VIII	(Acoustic)	Hearing, balance
IX	(Glossopharyngeal)	Gag, taste (posterior 1/3 of tongue)
X	(Vagus)	Gag, taste, visceral parasympathetics, larynx
XI	(Accessory)	Trapezius and sternocleidomastoid muscles
XII	(Hypoglossal)	Tongue strength

Fair = 3 Active movement through range of motion against gravity
Good = 4 Active movement through range of motion against resistance
Normal = 5

American Spinal Injury Association (1989): *Standards for neurological classification of spinal injury patients.*

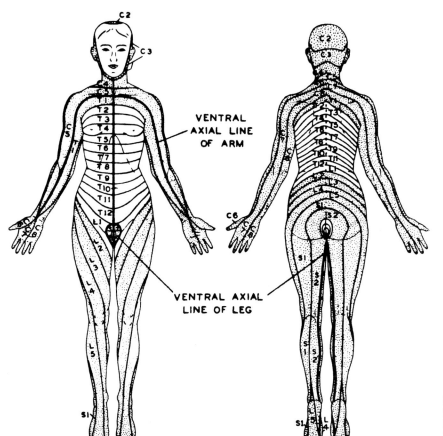

FIGURE 41. Anterior and posterior views of the dermatome patterns. (From Keegan JJ, Garett FD [1948]: The segmental distribution of the cutaneous nerves in the limbs of man. *Anat Rec* 102: 409–437, with permission.)

TABLE 16. INNERVATION OF MUSCLES RESPONSIBLE FOR MOVEMENTS OF THE SHOULDER GIRDLE AND UPPER EXTREMITY

Muscle	Segmental Innervation	Peripheral Nerve
Trapezius	Cranial XI: C(2)3–C4	Spinal accessory nerve
Levator anguli scapulae	C3–C4	Nerves to levator anguli scapulae
	C4–C5	Dorsal scapular nerve
Rhomboideus major	C4–C5	Dorsal scapular nerve
Rhomboideus minor	C4–C5	Dorsal scapular nerve
Serratus anterior	C5–C7	Long thoracic nerve
Deltoid	C5–C6	Axillary nerve
Teres minor	C5–C6	Axillary nerve
Supraspinatus	C(4)5–C6	Suprascapular nerve
Infraspinatus	C(4)5–C6	Suprascapular nerve
Latissimus dorsi	C6–C8	Thoracodorsal nerve (long subscapular)
Pectoralis major	C5–T1	Lateral and medial anterior thoracic
Pectoralis minor	C7–T1	Medial anterior thoracic
Subscapularis	C5–C7	Subscapular nerves
Teres major	C5–C7	Lower subscapular nerve
Subclavius	C5–C6	Nerve to subclavius
Coracobrachialis	C6–C7	Musculocutaneous nerve
Biceps brachia	C5–C6	Musculocutaneous nerve
Brachialis	C5–C6	Musculocutaneous nerve
Brachioradialis	C5–C6	Radial nerve
Triceps brachii	C6–C8 (T1)	Radial nerve
Anoconeus	C7–C8	Radial nerve
Supinator brevis	C5–C7	Radial nerve
Extensor carpi radialis longus	C(5)6–C7(8)	Radial nerve
Extensor carpi radialis brevis	C(5)6–C7(8)	Radial nerve
Extensor carpi ulnaris	C6–C8	Radial nerve
Extensor digitorum communis	C6–C8	Radial nerve
Extensor indicis proplus	C6–C8	Radial nerve
Extensor digiti minimi proprius	C6–C8	Radial nerve
Extensor pollicis longus	C6–C8	Radial nerve
Extensor pollicis brevis	C6–C8	Radial nerve
Abductor pollicis longus	C6–C8	Radial nerve
Pronator teres	C6–C7	Median nerve
Flexor carpi radialis	C6–C7(8)	Median nerve
Pronator quadratus	C7–T1	Median nerve
Palmaris longus	C7–T1	Median nerve
Flexor digitorum sublimis	C7–T1	Median nerve
Flexor digitorum profundus (radial half)	C7–T1	Median nerve
Lumbricales 1 and 2	C7–T1	Median nerve
Flexor pollicis longus	C8–T1	Median nerve
Flexor policis brevis (lateral head)	C8–T1	Median nerve
Abductor pollicis brevis	C8–T1	Median nerve
Opponens pollicis	C8–T1	Median nerve
Flexor carpi ulnaris	C7–T1	Ulnar nerve
Flexor digitorum profundus (ulnar half)	C7–T1	Ulnar nerve
Interossei	C8–T1	Ulnar nerve
Lumbricales 3 and 4	C8–T1	Ulnar nerve
Flexor pollicis brevis (medial head)	C8–T1	Ulnar nerve
Flexor digiti minimi brevis	C8–T1	Ulnar nerve
Abductor digiti minimi	C8–T1	Ulnar nerve
Opponenens digiti minimi	C8–T1	Ulnar nerve
Palmaris brevis	C8–T1	Ulnar nerve
Abductor pollicis	C8–T1	Ulnar nerve

Austin GM (1972): *The spinal cord: basic aspects and surgical considerations,* 2nd ed. Springfield IL: Charles C Thomas.

4. Muscle Innervation (Tables 16, 17)

5. Spinal Pathways (Long Tracts) (Fig. 42)

6. Deep Reflexes (Level, Muscle) (Table 18)

7. Glasgow Coma Scale (Table 19)

James HE (1986): Neurologic evaluation and support in the child with an acute brain insult. *Pediatr Ann* 15:16–22.

Jennet B, Teasedale G (1977): Aspects of coma after severe head injury. *Lancet* 1:878–881.

H. BODY SURFACE AREA NOMOGRAM (Fig. 43)

I. VITAL SIGNS (FOR DIFFERENT AGES) (Tables 20–22, Fig. 44)

TABLE 17. INNERVATION OF MUSCLES RESPONSIBLE FOR MOVEMENTS OF THE LOWER EXTREMITIES

Muscle	Segmental Innervation	Peripheral Nerve
Psoas major	L(1)2–L4	Nerve to psoas major
Psoas minor	L1–L2	Nerve to psoas minor
Iliacus	L2–L4	Femoral nerve
Quadriceps femoris	L2–L4	Femoral nerve
Sartorius	L2–L4	Femoral nerve
Pectineus	L2–L4	Femoral nerve
Gluteus maximus	L5–S2	Inferior gluteal nerve
Gluteus medius	L4–S1	Superior gluteal nerve
Tensor fasciae latae	L4–S1	Superior gluteal nerve
Piriformis	S1–L2	Nerve to piriformis
Adductor longus	L2–L4	Obturator nerve
Adductor brevis	L2–L4	Obturator nerve
Adductor magnus	L2–L4	Obturator nerve
	L4–L5	Sciatic nerve
Gracilis	L2–L4	Obturator nerve
Obturator externus	L2–L4	Obturator nerve
Obturator internus	L5–S3	Nerve to obturator internus
Gemellus superior	L5–S3	Nerve to obturator internus
Gemellus inferior	L4–S1	Nerve to quadratus femoris
Quadratus femoris	L4–S1	Nerve to quadratus femoris
Biceps femoris (long head)	L5–S1	Tibial nerve
Semimembranosus	L4–S1	Tibial nerve
Semitendinosus	L5–S2	Tibial nerve
Popliteus	L5–S1	Tibial nerve
Gastrocnemius	L5–S2	Tibial nerve
Soleus	L5–S2	Tibial nerve
Plantaris	L5–S1	Tibial nerve
Tibialis posterior	L5–S1	Tibial nerve
Flexor digitorum longus	L5–S1	Tibial nerve
Flexor hallucis longus	L5–S1	Tibial nerve
Biceps femoris (short head)	L5–S2	Common peroneal nerve
Tibialis anterior	L4–S1	Deep peroneal nerve
Peroneus tertius	L4–S1	Deep peroneal nerve
Extensor digitorum longus	L4–S1	Deep peroneal nerve
Extensor hallucis longus	L4–S1	Deep peroneal nerve
Extensor digitorum brevis	L4–S1	Deep peroneal nerve
Extensor hallucis brevis	L4–S1	Deep peroneal nerve
Peroneus longus	L4–S1	Superficial peroneal nerve
Peroneus brevis	L4–S1	Superficial peroneal nerve
Flexor digitorum brevis	L4–S1	Medial plantar nerve
Flexor hallucis brevis	L5–S1	Medial plantar nerve
Abductor hallucis	L4–S1	Medial plantar nerve
Lumbricales (medial 1 or 2)	L4–S1	Medial plantar nerve
Quadratus plantae	S1–S2	Lateral plantar nerve
Adductor hallucis	L5–S2	Lateral plantar nerve
Abductor digiti quinti	S1–S2	Lateral plantar nerve
Flexor digiti quinti brevis	S1–S2	Lateral plantar nerve
Lumbricales (lateral 2 or 3)	S1–S2	Lateral plantar nerve
Interossei	S1–S2	Lateral plantar nerve

TABLE 18. DEEP TENDON REFLEXES

Neurologic Level	Reflex
C5	Biceps
C6	Brachioradialis
C7	Triceps
L4	Knee jerk (quadriceps)
S1	Ankle jerk (gastrocnemius)

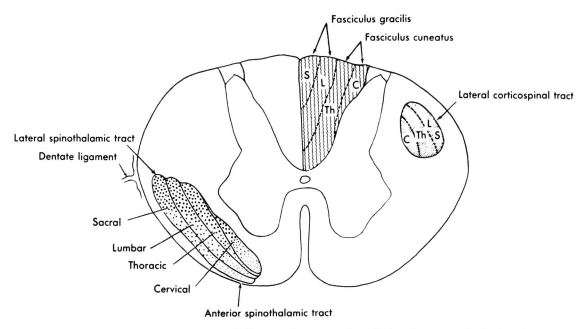

FIGURE 42. Laminar arrangement of the axons from successive spinal cord segments in the lateral spinothalamic tract *(left)*. Laminar separation of the fibers mediating temperature *(large dots)*, pain *(medium dots)*, and light touch *(small dots)* within the tract is also illustrated. Similar laminations for the ascending proprioceptive (posterior column) and descending lateral corticospinal tract are shown on the right.

TABLE 19. GLASGOW COMA SCALE AND MODIFIED COMA SCALE FOR INFANTS

Modified Coma Score for Infants			Glasgow Coma Score		
Activity	Best Response	Score	Activity	Best Response	Score
Eye opening	Spontaneous	4	Eye opening	Spontaneous	4
	To speech	3		To verbal stimuli	3
	To pain	2		To pain	2
	None	1		None	1
Verbal	Coos, babbles	5	Verbal	Oriented	5
	Irritable cries	4		Confused	4
	Cries to pain	3		Inappropriate words	3
	Moans to pain	2		Nonspecific sounds	2
	None	1		None	1
Motor	Normal spontaneous movements	6	Motor	Follows commands	6
	Withdraws to touch	5		Localizes pain	5
	Withdraws to pain	4		Withdraws in response to pain	4
	Abnormal flexion	3		Flexion in response to pain	3
	Abnormal extension	2		Extension in response to pain	2
	None	1		None	1

From James HE (1986): Neurologic evaluation and support in the child with an acute brain insult. *Pediatr Ann* 15:16–22.

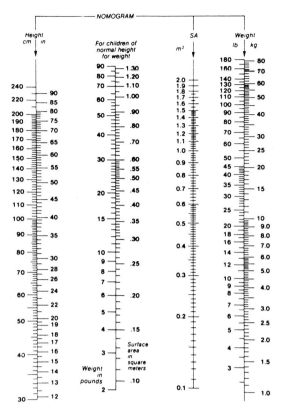

FIGURE 43. Nomogram for calculation of body surface area from height and weight. (From Herndon DN, Thompson PB, Desai, MH, Van Osten TJ [1985]: Treatment of burns in children. *Pediatr Clin North Am* 32:1311–1332, with permission.)

TABLE 20. NORMAL RESPIRATORY RATES

Age (y)	Boys	Girls	Age (y)	Boys	Girls
0–1	31 + 8	30 + 6	9–10	19 + 2	19 + 2
1–2	26 + 4	27 + 4	10–11	19 + 2	19 + 2
2–3	25 + 4	25 + 3	11–12	19 + 3	19 + 3
3–4	24 + 3	24 + 3	12–13	19 + 3	19 + 2
4–5	23 + 2	22 + 2	13–14	19 + 2	18 + 2
5–6	22 + 2	21 + 2	14–15	18 + 2	18 + 3
6–7	21 + 3	21 + 3	15–16	17 + 3	18 + 3
7–8	20 + 3	20 + 2	16–17	17 + 2	17 + 3
8–9	20 + 2	20 + 2	17–18	16 + 3	17 + 3

From Iliff A, Lee V (1952): Pulse rate, respiratory rate, and body temperature of children between two months and eighteen years of age. *Child Dev* 23:240–245 with permission.
Mean ± 1 SD.

TABLE 21. AGE-SPECIFIC HEART RATES (BEATS/MINUTE)

Age	2%	Mean	98%
<1	93	123	154
1–2 d	91	123	159
3–6 d	91	129	166
1–3 w	107	148	182
1–2 m	121	149	179
3–5 m	106	141	186
6–11 m	109	134	169
1–2 y	89	119	151
3–4 y	73	108	137
5–7 y	65	100	133
8–11 y	62	91	130
12–15 y	60	85	119

TABLE 22. CLASSIFICATION OF HYPERTENSION BY AGE GROUP

Age Group (y)	Significant Hypertension (mm Hg)	Severe Hypertension (mm Hg)
Newborn	Systolic BP ≥96	Systolic BP ≥106
7 days	Systolic BP ≥104	Systolic BP ≥110
8–30 days		
Infant (<2)	Systolic BP ≥112	Systolic BP ≥118
	Diastolic BP ≥74	Diastolic BP ≥82
Children (3–5)	Systolic BP ≥116	Systolic BP ≥124
	Diastolic BP ≥76	Diastolic BP ≥84
Children (6–9)	Systolic BP ≥122	Systolic BP ≥130
	Diastolic BP ≥78	Diastolic BP ≥86
Children (10–12)	Systolic BP ≥126	Systolic BP ≥134
	Diastolic BP ≥82	Diastolic BP ≥90
Adolescents (13–15)	Systolic BP ≥136	Systolic BP ≥144
	Diastolic BP ≥86	Diastolic BP ≥92
Adolescents (16–18)	Systolic BP ≥142	Systolic BP ≥150
	Diastolic BP ≥92	Diastolic BP ≥98

From Report of the second task force on blood pressure control in children (1957): *Pediatrics* 79:1–25, with permission.
BP, blood pressure.

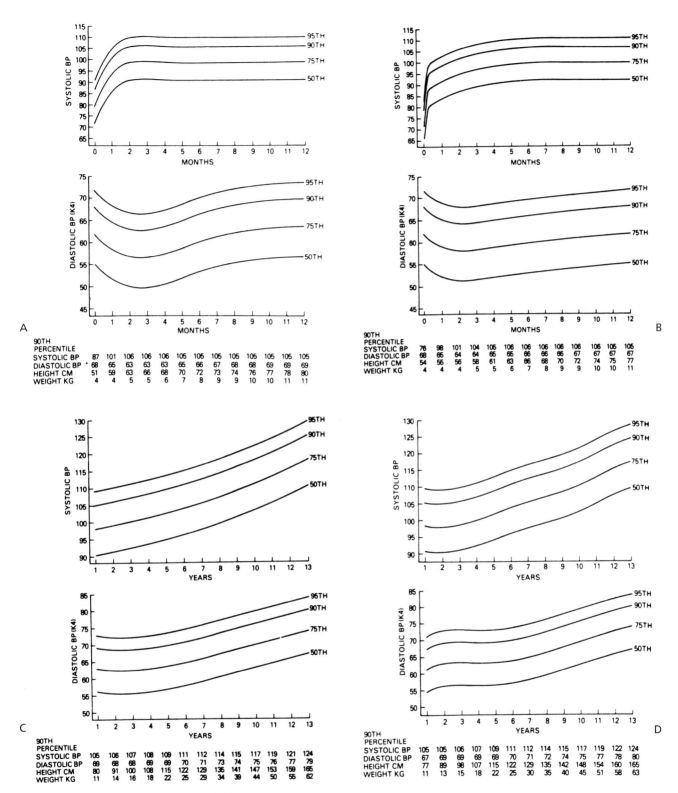

FIGURE 44. **A:** Arterial blood pressure. Ages 0 to 12 months, boys. **B:** Arterial blood pressure. Ages 0 to 12 months, girls. **C:** Arterial blood pressure. Ages 1 to 13 years, boys. **D:** Arterial blood pressure. Ages 1 to 13 years, girls. *(Figure continues.)*

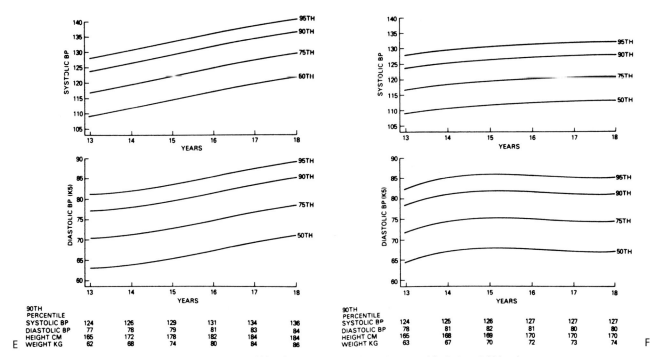

90TH PERCENTILE						
SYSTOLIC BP	124	126	129	131	134	136
DIASTOLIC BP	77	78	79	81	83	84
HEIGHT CM	165	172	178	182	184	184
WEIGHT KG	62	68	74	80	84	86

E

90TH PERCENTILE						
SYSTOLIC BP	124	125	126	127	127	127
DIASTOLIC BP	78	81	82	81	80	80
HEIGHT CM	165	168	169	170	170	170
WEIGHT KG	63	67	70	72	73	74

F

FIGURE 44. *Continued.* **E:** Arterial blood pressure. Age 13 to 18 years, girls. **F:** Arterial blood pressure. Age 13–18 years, boys. (From Report on the second task force on blood pressure control in children [1987]: *Pediatrics* 79:1–25, with permission.)

RADIOGRAPHIC MEASUREMENTS

AURELIO G. MARTINEZ-LOZANO

A. RADIOGRAPHIC MAGNIFICATION

The relative positions of the radiographic source, the spine, and the film are the factors that affect the magnification (Fig. 1).

The most commonly used value for the distance D1 (source-to-film distance) is 1.83 m (72 in); the magnification factors for different D2 (object-to-film distance) can be calculated (Table 1).

To avoid variations in the magnification, standardized distances have been suggested to facilitate comparisons of radiographs of the same patient, taken at different times. This approach also avoids the need for repeated computations to determine magnification for different patients. White and Panjabi have suggested the following standard distances:

ML > Radiographic source-to-film distance D1 = 1.83 m (72 in)

Spine to film distance D2 = 0.36 m (14 in)

These two distances give a linear magnification of 24%: M = 24%.

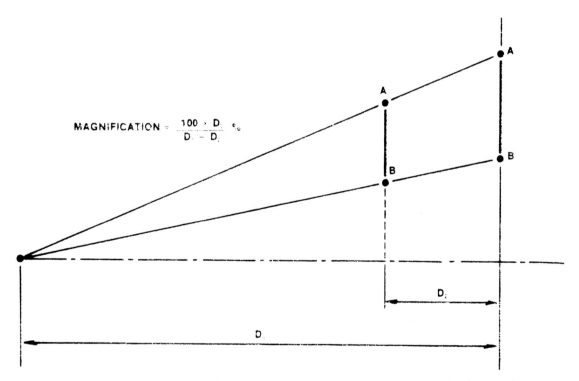

$$\text{MAGNIFICATION} = \frac{100 \cdot D_2}{D_1 - D_2} \%$$

FIGURE 1. On a radiograph, the image is always bigger than the object: A'B' is greater than AB. The magnification depends on the source-to-film and object-to-film distances, D1 and D2, respectively. D2 is the distance that is the more sensitive in regard to magnification. (From White AA, Panjabi MM [1990]: The problem of clinical instability in the human spine. A systematic approach. In: *Clinical biomechanics of the spine.* Philadelphia: WB Saunders, with permission.)

A. B. Martinez-Lozano: Universidad Autónoma De Nuevo León, Monterrey, Mexico.

965

TABLE 1. PERCENTAGE MAGNIFICATION OF IMAGE ASSOCIATED WITH DIFFERENT SPINE-TO-FILM DISTANCES

Spine-to-film Distance m (in.)	Magnification %
0.15 (6.0)	9
0.20 (8.0)	12.5
0.25 (10.0)	16
0.30 (12.0)	20
0.36 (14.0)	24

Source-to-film distance = 1.83 m (72 in.).
From White AA, Panjabi MM (1990): The problem of clinical instability in the human spine: a systematic approach. In: *Clinical biomechanics of the spine.* Philadelphia: WB Saunders, with permission.

B. MAGNIFICATION: GEOMETRIC DISTORTION OF THE ROENTGEN IMAGE AND ITS CORRECTION

A number of devices have been constructed that give a fully compensated value of a given object dimension. These devices have usually been made for use in pelvicephalometry. A nomogram (Fig. 2) may be used for finding corrected dimensions.

C. RADIATION EXPOSURE

Compared with other conventional radiographic procedures, the radiographic examination of the lumbosacral spine delivers one of the highest doses of radiation to the skin, bone marrow, and gonads. The mean value of radiation to the gonads from a lumbosacral examination is exceeded only by urography and colon examinations. For women, the radiation dose to the gonads is higher than that for men during the lumbosacral examination. The current dose can be 1.5 to 4 times lower if newer film-screen combinations are used. Gonadal doses are higher when there is poor centering, poor coning, or poor calibration of radiographic equipment, or when repeated films are taken. Unfortunately, radiographs frequently ordered to evaluate acute low back pain ("strain") in young adults deliver a high direct gonadal dose of radiation in this self-limiting disorder. Because of the high radiation dose of the lumbosacral examination, various authors have stressed the need for eliminating unnecessary radiographic examinations and limiting the number of views per radiographic study. Among those suggestions are the following: a single, well-centered lateral spine radiograph to replace the combination of lateral and cone lateral views; obtaining only anteroposterior and lateral views; and eliminating oblique views.

In patients with scoliosis who receive repeated follow-up examinations, there is also increased radiation to the gonads, thyroid gland, and breast (in girls). However, proper selection of screen-film-grid combinations, collimation of x-ray beam, proper technical factors, and proper shielding reduce the radiation burden. Using posteroanterior exposure reduces the radiation to the breast but increases the absorbed dose to bone marrow.

Kricun ME (1988): Conventional radiography. In: Kricun ME. *Imaging modalities in spinal disorders.* Philadelphia: WB Saunders.

Waggener RG, Kereiakes JG, Shalek, RJ (1984): *CRC handbook of medical physics,* Vol. 2. Boca Raton, Fla: CRC Press, Inc.

Webster EW, Merrill OE (1957): Radiation hazards. II. Measurements of gonadal dose in radiographic examinations. *N Engl J Med* 257:811–819.

D. RELATIVE COMPLICATIONS OF RADIOTHERAPY

Radiation, either from external or internal sources, may lead to alterations in the axial skeleton. The effects of radiation depend on the dose absorbed by bone, duration of radiation, quality of radiation, area of the spine irradiated, age of the patient when irradiated, and whether irradiation occurred to abnormal bone. As a general rule the greater the treatment dose and the younger the child at the time of radiotherapy, the greater the radiographic alterations. Children who receive less than 1000 cGy by orthovoltage therapy do not develop gross, permanent spinal abnormalities (although growth retardation can occur with 800 cGy); however, those who receive 1000 to 2000 cGy may develop minor changes of growth arrest. Those who receive over 2000 cGy will probably experience growth disturbance. Patients who receive less than 2600 cGy from megavoltage therapy do not develop spinal deformities, whereas those who receive more than 3070 cGy develop spinal deformities. The skeletal changes observed with megavoltage therapy occur as frequently but are not as pronounced as those following orthovoltage therapy (Table 2).

Riseborough EJ, Grabias SL, Burton RJ, et al. (1976): Skeletal alterations following irradiation for Wilms' tumor: with particular reference to scoliosis and kyphosis. *J Bone Joint Surg [Am]* 58:526–536.

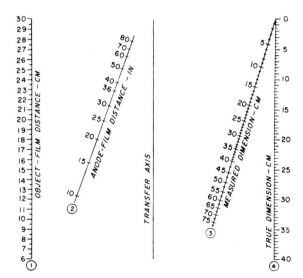

FIGURE 2. Nomogram (designed by Holmquist) for securing corrected dimension. 1. Draw a straight line from the object-film distance (a) through the anode-film distance (b) to the transfer axis. 2. Draw a second line from this point on the transfer axis through the measured dimension (c) to the true dimension (d). (From Holmquest HJ [1938]: Nomogram for roentgenographic mensuration. *Radiology* 31:198–205, with permission.)

TABLE 2. RELATIVE COMPLICATIONS OF RADIOTHERAPY

	Orthovoltage	Megavoltage
Growth recovery lines	28%	45%
Endplate irregularity	83%	70%
Anterior beak	20%	25%
Decreased vertebral height	83%	Data not available
Vertebral asymmetry	75%	45%
Decreased vertebral development	100%	Data not available
Scoliosis	70%–81%	80%–100%
Degree of curve	20% >20°	100% <20°
	61% <25°	
	2% <5°	69% <5°
Kyphosis	26%–30%	45%–56%
Degree of curve (average)	21°	14°
Degree of curve (range)	7°–57°	<10°–25°

From Kricun ME (1988): Conventional radiography. In: *Imaging modalities in spinal disorders.* Philadelphia: WB Saunders, with permission.

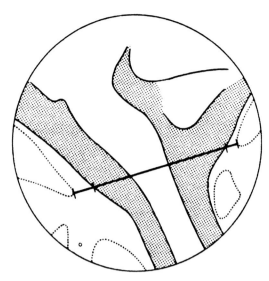

FIGURE 3. On a midsagittal pneumotomogram, the landmarks used for the measurement of the bony canal and the subarachnoidal canal at the level of the foramen magnum are indicated. (From Schmeltzer A, Babin E, Wenger JJ [1971]: Foramen magnum in children: measurement of the anteroposterior diameter on midsagittal pneumotomograms. *Neuroradiology* 2:162–163, with permission.)

E. CRANIOVERTEBRAL JUNCTION

1. Measurement of the Foramen Magnum in Children and Adults

Measurements made on a line drawn between the lower margin of the occipital bone and the basion (anterior margin of foramen magnum) are shown in Figure 3. During growth, the average anteroposterior diameter of the foramen increases from 30 to 35 mm and the average anteroposterior diameter of the subarachnoidal canal increases from 24 to 28 mm (Fig. 4).

2. Basilar Impression

a. *Lateral Craniometry*

Deformity of the bones of the base of the skull at the margin of the foramen magnum, where the base of the skull appears to be indented by the upper cervical spine. There are two types of basilar impression. Primary basilar impression is

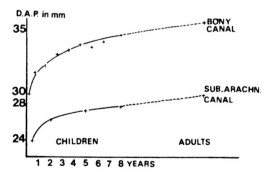

FIGURE 4. Diagram showing the anteroposterior diameter of the bony canal and subarachnoidal canal at the foramen magnum according to age: Normal measurements have been corrected for magnification. Based on measurement of 200 children and 100 adults. (From Schmeltzer A, Babin E, Wenger JJ [1971]: Foramen magnum in children: measurement of the anteroposterior diameter on midsagittal pneumotomograms. *Neuroradiology* 2:162–163, with permission.)

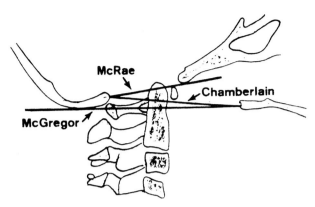

FIGURE 5. Lateral craniometry showing the three most commonly used lines to determine basilar impression. Chamberlain, McGregor, and McRae lines. McGregor's line is the best method for routine screening because the bony landmarks can be defined clearly at all ages on a routine lateral radiographic view. (From Hensinger RH [1986]: Osseous anomalies of the craniovertebral junction. *Spine* 11:323–333, with permission.)

a congenital anomaly that is often associated with other vertebral defects. Secondary basilar impression is a developmental condition usually attributed to softening of the osseous structures of the base of the skull. It is difficult to assess radiographically, and many measurement schemes have been proposed. The most commonly used are the Chamberlain, McGregor, and McRae lines.

1. *Chamberlain's Line.* Chamberlain's line is drawn from the posterior margin of the hard palate to the posterior margin of the foramen magnum (opisthion). According to Poppel, the odontoid process should not project above this line in the normal case (SD 3.3 mm). In any individual case, an odontoid process 6.6 mm (2 SD) or more above the line should be considered strongly indicative of basilar impression, based on his study of 102 normal skull radiographs (Fig. 5)

Line	No. of cases	Mean position of tip of odontoid in relation to Chamberlain's line (mm)	Standard deviation (mm)
Saunders	100	−1	3.6
McGregor (Bantu)	203	−1.32	2.62
Poppel	102	+0.06	3.3

2. *McGregor's Line.* McGregor's line is drawn from the posterosuperior margin of the hard palate to the lower-most point on the midline occipital curve. It is the best method for routine screening because the bony landmarks can be defined clearly at all ages on a routine lateral radiographic view. The position of the tip of the odontoid is measured in relation to this baseline; a distance of 4.5 mm above McGregor's line is considered to be on the extreme edge of normality. However, Hinck and associates demonstrated a wide range of normal as well as differences between men and women (Table 3, Fig. 5).

3. *McRae's Line (Foramen Magnum Line).* McRae's line is drawn from the anterior margin of the foramen magnum (basion) to the posterior border (opisthion). The tip of the odontoid should lie below this line (Fig. 5).

4. *Bull's Method.* Bull's method is a line drawn along the plane of hard palate that intersects a line drawn along the plane of the atlas. If the angle formed by the intersection of these two lines is greater than 13, the position of the odontoid process is abnormal. This angle has been shown to vary significantly with flexion and extension (Fig. 6).

5. *Ranawat's Method.* Ranawat's method is useful when the hard palate is not visualized in the film. The distance between the center of the pedicle of C2 and the line drawn in the coronal axis of C1 is measured. In men, this distance averages 17 mm, with a SD of 2 mm. In women, it measured 15 mm, with a SD of 2 mm. Superior migration of the odontoid has occurred in the cases in which this distance is decreased based on radiographs of 26 normal individuals and 33 patients with rheumatoid arthritis (Fig. 7).

TABLE 3. MEASSUREMENT OF THE BASE OF THE SKULL FOR BASILAR INVAGINATION[a]

Children: Both Sexes (mm)		
Age	Mean Baseline	90% Tolerance Range
3	1.94	− 0.8 to 4.7
4	2.07	− 0.7 to 4.8
5	2.17	− 0.6 to 4.9
6	2.24	− 0.5 to 5.0
7	2.29	− 0.4 to 5.1
8	2.31	− 0.4 to 5.1
9	2.30	− 0.4 to 5.1
10	2.27	− 0.5 to 5.0
11	2.21	− 0.5 to 5.0
12	2.13	− 0.6 to 4.9
13	2.01	− 0.7 to 4.8
14	1.88	− 0.9 to 4.6
15	1.71	− 1.0 to 4.5
16	1.52	− 1.2 to 4.3
17	1.31	− 1.4 to 4.1
18	1.07	− 1.7 to 3.8

Adults mm			
Sex	Mean	SD	90% Tolerance Range for Normal
Male subjects	0.33	3.81	− 7.4 to + 8.0 mm
Female subjects	3.67	1.69	− 2.4 to + 9.7 mm
M–F average difference	− 3.06	—	—

From Hinck VC, Hopkins CE, Savara BS (1961): Diagnostic criteria of basilar impression. *Radiology* 76:572–85, with permission.
[a] McGregor's line: *Children:* mean baseline and 90% tolarance range for both sexes at different ages. *Adults:* mean, SD, and 90% tolerance range for both sexes. Based on radiographs of 66 normal adults and a series of 258 films taken at yearly intervals in 43 normal children aged 3–18 years.

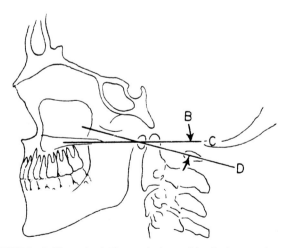

FIGURE 6. Bull's method. The angle formed by the intersection of a line drawn along the plane of the hard palate and a line drawn along the plane of the atlas should be normally less than 13 degrees. Based on roentgenograms of 120 normal skulls. (From Hinck VC, Hopkins CE, Savara BS [1961]: Diagnostic criteria of basilar impression. *Radiology* 76:572–585, with permission.)

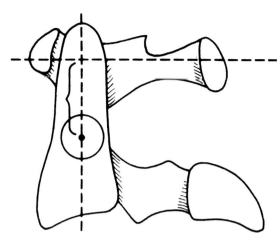

FIGURE 7. A line is drawn connecting the center of the anterior arch of the first cervical vertebra with its posterior ring. The center of the sclerotic ring of the second cervical vertebra, presenting the pedicle is marked. The distance between the center of the pedicle of C2 and the line drawn in the coronal axis of C1 is measured. (From Ranawat CS, O'Leary P, Pellicci P [1979]: Cervical spine fusion in rheumatoid arthritis. *J Bone Joint Surgery [Am]* 61:1003–1010, with permission.)

6. *Redlund-Johnell Method.* Redlund-Johnell and Petterson described a method of measurement that uses McGregor's line, the apex of the dens, and the lower plate of C2. They measured the distance between the apex of the dens and McGregor's line, and the distance between the lower plate of C2 and McGregor's line in 200 normal adults (100 men and 100 women), and compared them with measurements in 61 patients with rheumatoid arthritis (10 men and 51 women). The distance between McGregor's line and the lower plate end of the body of C2 in normal men was 41.6 4.0 mm, in normal women it was 37.1 4.3 mm; in patients with rheumatoid arthritis: for men, 32.3 4.9 mm and women 28.7 4.3 mm. Values under 34 mm in men and 29 mm in women indicate cranial settling. The distance from McGregor's line to the apex of the dens was for normal subjects: men, 2.4 3.2 mm; women 2.5 3.3 mm; for patients with rheumatoid arthritis: men 10.2 3.3 mm; women 9.3 3.7 mm. All the differences between normal (control) patients and patients with rheumatoid arthritis were statistically significant. (Fig. 8).

7. *Station of the Atlas.* The station of the atlas is the simplest way to quickly screen for the possibility of cranial settline (Fig. 9)

b. Anterior Craniometry

1. *Bimastoid Line.* Line drawn between the tips of the mastoid processes is the bimastoid line. Normally it should cross the atlanto-occipital joints. This

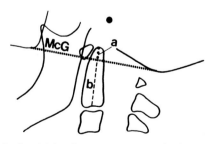

FIGURE 8. Redlund-Johnell measurement method. *McG,* the palato-occipital line, or McGregor's line. *a,* The distance between the apex of the dens and McG. If the apex is situated below this line, the value will be negative. *b,* The distance between the lower end plate of the C2 and McG. (From Redlund-Johnell I, Petterson H [1984]: Radiographic measurements of the craniovertebral region. *Acta Radiol Diagn* 25: 23–28, with permission.)

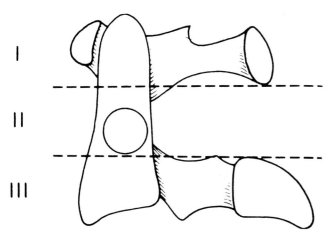

FIGURE. 9. The station of the atlas is determined by dividing the odontoid process into thirds in the sagittal plane. Normally, the anterior ring of the atlas should be adjacent to the cephalad third of the axis *(station I)*. If the ring of the atlas is adjacent to the middle third of the axis, mild cranial settling is indicated *(station II)*. If the anterior ring of the atlas is adjacent to the base of the axis, it is considered evidence of severe cranial settline *(station III)*. (From Clark CC, Goetz DD, Menezes AH [1989]: Arthrodesis of the cervical spine in rheumatoid arthritis. *J Bone Joint Surg [Am]* 71:381–392, with permission.)

line has been supplanted by the digastric line. Because the mastoid process varies considerably in length from one individual to another, the normal position of a reference line based on these structures is therefore quite variable. According to Fischgold, the odontoid apex should lie an average of 2 mm above this line, with a range between 3 mm below and 10 mm above (Fig. 10)

2. *Digastric Line.* The digastric line is between the two digastric grooves that lie just medial to the bases of the mastoid processes. According to Fischgold, the distance measured from this line to the middle of the atlanto-occipital joints is normally about 10 mm. The distance in millimeters between this line and the apex of the dens and the atlanto-occipital joint is shown in Table 4.

3. *Temporomandibular Line.* The distance of the temporomandibular line

TABLE 4. MEASUREMENT OF THE BASE OF THE SKULL FOR BASILAR INVAGINATION[a]

Sex	Mean	SD	90% Tolerance Range for Normals
Measured on laminagrams to atlanto-occipital joint (mm)			
M or F	11.66	4.04	3.8–19.5
Measured on laminagrams to apex of dens (mm)			
M or F	10.70	5.06	1.0–20.4

From Hinck VC, Hopkins CE, Savara BS (1961): Diagnostic criteria of basilar impression. *Radiology* 76:572–85, with permission.
[a] Mean, SD, and 90% tolerance range based on skull laminagrams of 68 normal adults.

is measured between two parallel lines, one (TM) at the level of the temporomandibular joints and one (AA) at the superior margin of the anterior arch of the atlas. Either an anteroposterior or lateral projection may be used. These lines are usually about 30 mm apart, with a range from 22 to 39 mm. The distance is diminished in basilar impression (Fig. 11).

c. Summary of Measurements for Basilar Impression

A summary of the most widely used lines and their points of reference, normal values, and their implications has recently been presented by Menezes and VanGilder (Figs. 12, 13; Tables 5, 6).

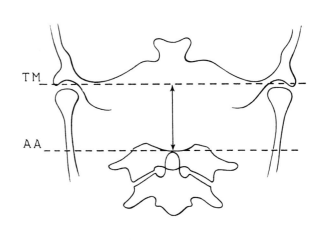

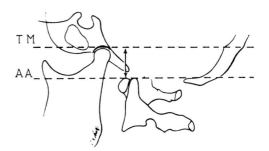

FIGURE 11. Temporomandibular line. The distance is measured between two parallel lines, one (TM) at the level of the temporomandibular joint and one (AA) at the superior margin of the anterior arch of the atlas. Either an anteroposterior or lateral projection may be used. (From Hinck VC, Hopkins CE, Savara BS [1961]: Diagnostic criteria of basilar impression. *Radiology* 76:572–585, with permission.)

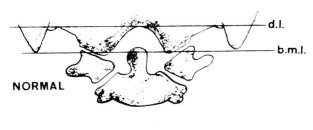

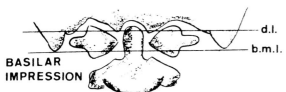

FIGURE 10. Anterior craniometry. Fischgold and Metzger noted that in the normal skull, a line joining the lower poles of the mastoid processes *(bml)* passes through the tip of the odontoid. Owing to the variability in the size of mastoid processes, this was further refined to a line drawn between the digastric grooves *(dl)*. These lines are best visualized on an anteroposterior transoral tomogram. Although this is the most accurate method for assessing basilar impression, routine use of this method is impractical. (From Hensinger RN [1986]: Osseous anomalies of the craniovertebral junction. *Spine* 11:323–333, with permission.)

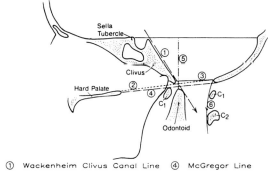

① Wackenheim Clivus Canal Line   ④ McGregor Line
② Chamberlain Line   ⑤ Height Index of Klaus
③ McRae Line   ⑥ Spinous Interlaminar Line
                                   (Posterior Canal Line)

FIGURE 12. Lateral craniometry with points of reference. (From Menezes AH, VanGilder JC [1990]: Anomalies of the craniovertebral junction. In: *Youman's neurological surgery*, 3rd ed. Philadelphia: WB Saunders, with permission.)

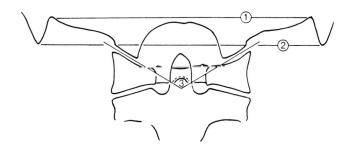

① Fishgold Diagastric Line
② Fishgold Bimastoid Line
③ Schmidt—Fischer Angle
     (angle of axes of Atlanto—occipital joints)

FIGURE 13. Craniometry lines and angles in anteroposterior view. (From Menezes AM, VanGilder JC [1990]: Anomalies of the craniovertebral junction. In: *Youman's neurological surgery*, 3rd Ed. Philadelphia: WB Saunders, with permission.)

TABLE 5. CRANIOMETRIC LINES IN LATERAL VIEWS

Synonyms	Definition	Normal Measurements	Implications
Wackenheim's line (clivus canal line)	Line drawn along clivus into cervical canal	Odontoid tip is ventral and tangential to this line	Odontoid process transects the line in basilar invagination or forward position of skull
Chamberiain's line (palato-occipital line)	Joins posterior pole of hard palate to opisthion	Tip of dens 1 mm + 3.6 mm below this line	Odontoid process bisects the line in basilar invagination
McRae's line (foramen magnum line)	Joins anterior and posterior edges of foramen magnum (basion to opisthion)	Tip of dens does not exceed this line	When effective sagittal canal diameter is less than 20 mm, neurological symptoms occur
McGregor's line (basal line)	Hard palate to lowest point of occipital bone	Tip of dens should not exceed 5 mm above the line	Line position varies with flexion-extension—hence not important
Height-index of Klaus	Distance between tip of dens and tuberculum-cruciate line	40–41 mm	<30 mm seen in basilar invagination
Spinolamellar line (spinous interlaminar line)	Line drawn from interoccipital ridge above and down along the fused spinous process of C2 and C3	Should intersect posterior arch of atlas	If atlas is fused, posterior arch is anterior to the line; posterior compression of spinal cord may occur

From Menezes AM, VanGilder JC (1990): Anomalies of the craniovertebral junction. In: *Youman's neurological surgery*, 3rd ed. Philadelphia: WB Saunders, with permission.

TABLE 6. CRANIOMETRIC LINES AND ANGLES IN ANTEROPOSTERIOR VIEW

Synonyms	Definition	Normal Measurements	Implications
Fishgold's diagastric line (biventer line)	Joins the fossae for diagastric muscles on undersurface of skull just medial to mastoid process	Dens tip should not project above this line; central axis of dens should be perpendicular to the line	Corresponds to McRae's line on lateral view; may be oblique in unilateral condylar hypoplasia; oblique odontoid suggests paramedian abnormality
Fishgold's bimastoid line	Line connecting tips of mastoid process	Runs across atlanto-occipital joints; line is 10 mm below diagastric line	Odontoid tip may be 10 mm above the line
Schmidt–Fischer angle (angle of axes of atlanto-occipital joints)	Angle of axes of atlanto-occipital joints	124–127 degrees; should be measured in plane of dens on tomograms	Angle is wider in condylar hypoplasia

From Menezes AM, VanGilder JC (1990): Anomalies of the craniovertebral junction. In: *Youman's neurological surgery*, 3rd ed. Philadelphia: WB Saunders, with permission.

Bull JWD, Nixon WLB, Pratt RTC (1955): The radiological criteria and familial occurrence of primary basilar impression. *Brain* 78:229–247.

Chamberlain WE (1939): Basilar impression (platybasia). *Yale J Biol Med* 11:487–496.

Clark CC, Goetz DD, Menezes AH (1989): Arthrodesis of the cerivcal spine in rheumatoid arthritis. *J Bone Joint Surg [Am]* 71:381–392.

Fischgold H, Metzger J (1952): Etude radiographique de l'impression basilaire. *Rev Rheum* 19:261–264.

Hensinger RN (1986): Osseous anomalies of the craniovertebral junction. *Spine* 11:323–333.

Hinck VC, Hopkins CE, Savara BS (1961): Diagnostic criteria of basilar impression. *Radiology* 76:572–585.

McGregor M (1948): The significance of certain measurements of the skull in the diagnosis of basilar impression. *Br J Radiol* 21:171–181.

McRae DL, Barnum AS (1953): Occipitalization of the atlas. *Am J Roentgenol* 70:23–46.

Menezes AH, VanGilder JC (1990): Anomalies of the craniovertebral junction. In: *Youman's neurological surgery,* 3rd ed. Philadelphia: WB Saunders.

Poppel MH, Jacobson HG, Duff BK, Gottlieb C (1953): Basilar impression and platybasia in Paget's disease. *Am J Roentgenol* 61:639–644.

Ranawat CS, O'Leary P, Pellicci P, et al. (1979): Cervical spine fusion in rheumatoid arthritis. *J Bone Joint Surg [Am]* 61:1003–1010.

Redlund-Johnell I, Petterson H (1943): Radiographic measurements of the craniovertebral region. *Acta Radiol Diagn* 25:23–28.

Saunders WW (1943): Basilar impression: the position of the normal odontoid. *Radiology* 41:589–590.

Platybasia

Platybasia denotes flattening of the angle formed by the intersection of the plane of the anterior fossa with the plane of the clivus. It does not have clinical significance and it is merely an anthropologic term. The basal angle is the angle formed by a line drawn from the nasion to the center of the seila turcica, and a line drawn from the center of the sella turcica to the anterior margin of the foramen magnum (Fig. 14).

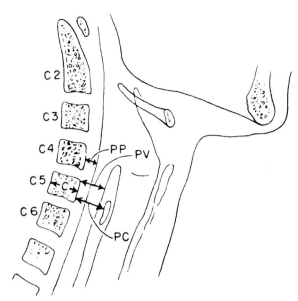

FIGURE 15. Measures of the soft tissues of the neck. *PV,* Postventricular soft tissues for use in children in which the cricoid cartilage is not visible. The distance is measured between the posterior commisure of the larynx and the nearest portion of the cervical spine. *PP,* Postpharyngeal soft tissue, measured at a point where the soft tissues run parallel to the vertebra. *PC,* Postcricoid soft tissue, measured between the posterior surface of the cricoid cartilage and the anterior surface of the adjacent cervical vertebra. *C,* Anteroposterior dimension of C5 vertebral body at its middle. (From Templeton PA, et al. The value of retropharyngeal soft tissue measurements in trauma of the adult cervical spine. *Skeletal Radiol* 16:98–104, with permission.)

F. CERVICAL SPINE

1. Measurement of the Soft Tissues of the Neck in Children

In children, the thickness of the soft tissue between the pharyngeal lumen and the vertebrae should be about three fourths the diameter of the adjacent vertebra. According to Templeton, in films made in the lateral projection using 40-in focus film distance, values between 7 and 10 mm at C2, C3, or C4 should suggest possible abnormality. Values of 10 mm or more definitely indicate the need for additional investigation. He found considerable overlap in the retropharyngeal soft tissue space of normal and abnormal patients. (Fig. 15).

Adran GM, Kemp FH (1968): The mechanism of changes in form of the cervical airway in infancy. *Med Radiogr Photogr* 44:26–54.

TABLE 7. NORMAL VALUES IN MILLIMETERS FOR PREVERTEBRAL SOFT TISSUE SPACE AT DIFFERENT LEVELS[a]

| Level | Average Width (range) in mm | | |
	Flexion	Midposition	Extension
C1	5.6 (2–11)	4.6 (1–10)	3.6 (1–8)
C2	4.1 (2–6)	3.2 (1–5)	3.8 (2–6)
C3	4.2 (3–7)	3.4 (2–7)	4.1 (3–6)
C4	5.8 (4–7)	5.1 (2–7)	6.1 (4–8)
C5	17.1 (11–22)	14.9 (8–20)	15.2 (10–20)
C6	16.3 (12–20)	15.1 (11–20)	13.9 (7–19)
C7	14.7 (9–20)	13.9 (9–20)	11.9 (7–21)

From Penning L (1981): Prevertebral hematoma in cervical spine injury: incidence and etiologic significance. *Am J Roentgenol* 136:553–61, with permission.
[a] Sites of measurements shown in Figure 15. Based on 50 non-injured adults. Flexion and extension films were made on 20 adults.

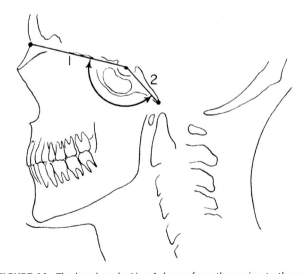

FIGURE 14. The basal angle. Line 1 drawn from the nasion to the center of the sella turcica. Line 2 drawn from the center of the sella turcica to the anterior margin of the foramen magnum. (From Poppel MH, Jacobson HG, Duff BK, Gottlieb C [1953]: Basilar impression and platybasia in Paget's disease. *Am J Roentgenol* 61:639–644, with permission.)

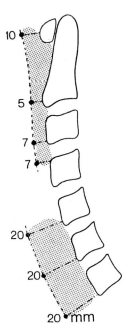

FIGURE 16. Upper limits of width of the normal prevertebral space in adults. (From Penning L [1981]: Prevertebral hematoma in cervical spine injury: incidence and etiologic significance. *Am J Roentgenol* 136: 553–561, with permission.)

Hay PD (1939): *In annals of roentgenogenology,* Vol. 9. New York: Paul B. Hoeber.

Keats TE (1990): The neck. In: *Atlas of roentgenographic measurements,* 6th ed.

2. Normal Cervical Spine Prevertebral Space in Adults

Measurements made a line describing the shortest distance between (a) the anterior arch of the atlas and the anterosuperior and anteroinferior edges of the vertebral bodies of C2 and C7 and (b) the air shadows of the pharynx and trachea. (Fig. 16, Table 7).

Wholey MH, Brewer AJ, Baker HL Jr (1958): Lateral roentgenograms of the neck with comments on atlanto-odontoid-basion relationship. *Radiology* 71: 350–356.

3. Atlantodens Interval in Children

Measurement of the atlantodens interval is made between the posteroinferior margin of the anterior arch of the atlas and the anterior surface of the odontoid process (Fig. 17).

Average normal distance is 2.0 mm; 99% of patients will be between 1 and 4 mm. Maximum distance found in a patient was 5 mm (Fig. 18). Less than 4 mm is considered normal in children.

4. Atlantodens Interval in Adults

The average normal atlantodens interval in adults is as follows:

Female (age 20 to 80): .238 − (0.0074 × age in years) 0.90 mm
Male (age 30 to 80): 2.052 − (0.0192 × age in years) 1.00 mm

About 95% of normal adults will have an atlas-odontoid distance in flexion between 0.3 and 1.8 mm, in neutral position between 0.4 mm and 2.0 mm, and in extension between 0.3 and 2.2 mm, based on studies of 25 men and 25 women. Less than 3 mm is considered normal. Values of 5 mm or more usually indicate rupture of the transverse ligament.

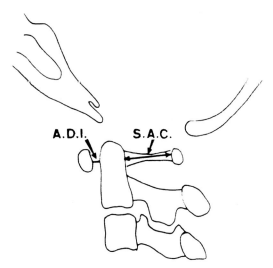

FIGURE 17. Atlantoaxial joint demonstrating the normal atlas-dens interval *(ADI)* and the normal space available for the spinal cord *(SAC),* the distance between the posterior aspect of the odontoid and the nearest posterior structure. (From Hensinger RN [1986]: Osseous anomalies of the craniovertebral junction. *Spine* 11:323–333, with permission.)

Hinck VC, Hopkins CE (1960): Measurement of the atlantodental interval in the adult. *Am J Roentgenol* 84:945–951.

Fielding JW, Cochran GV, Lawsing JF, Hohl M (1974): Tears of the transverse ligament of the atlas. *J Bone Joint Surgery [Am]* 56:1683–1691.

5. Space Available for the Spinal Cord

The atlantodens interval is of limited value in evaluating chronic atlantoaxial instability. In this condition, the odontoid is frequently found to be hypermobile with a widened atlantodens interval, particularly in flexion (Fig. 19). In this situation, attention should be directed to the amount of space available for the spinal cord. This is accomplished by measuring the distance from the posterior aspect of the odontoid or axis to the nearest posterior structure (foramen magnum or posterior margin of the atlas). This measurement is particularly helpful when evaluating a patient with nonunion of the odontoid or os odontoideum because in both conditions the atlantodens interval may be normal, yet in flexion or extension there may be considerable reduction in the space available for the spinal cord (Fig. 20). Steel defined the "rule of thirds," in that the area of the vertebral canal at the first cervical vertebra can be divided into one-third cord, one-third cervical vertebra, and one-third "space." The one-third "space" represents a safe zone in which displacement can occur without neurologic impingement. It is generally agreed that a reduction of the lumen of the spinal canal to 13 mm or less may be associated with neurologic problems (Fig. 21).

Fielding JW, Hawkins RJ, Ratzan SA (1976): Spine fusion for atlanto-axial instability. *J Bone Joint Surg [Am]* 58:400–407.

Spierlings ELH, Braakman R (1982): Os odontoideum: analysis of 37 cases. *J Bone Joint Surg [Br]* 64:422–48.

Steel HH (1968): Anatomical and mechanical considerations of the atlantoaxial articulation. *J Bone Joint Surg [Am]* 50:1481–1482.

6. Normal and Abnormal Relationships Between the Occiput and Atlas: Detection of Anterior Atlanto-occipital Dislocation.

The ratio BC/OA is used to determine anterior atlanto-occipital dislocation (Fig. 22). BC/OA is equal to or greater than 1 in all cases of atlanto-occipital dislocation. Ratios less than 1 are normal. This relationship is valid only in the absence of associated fractures of the atlas. Data are from 100 normal adults and 50 normal children, and four cases of dislocation.

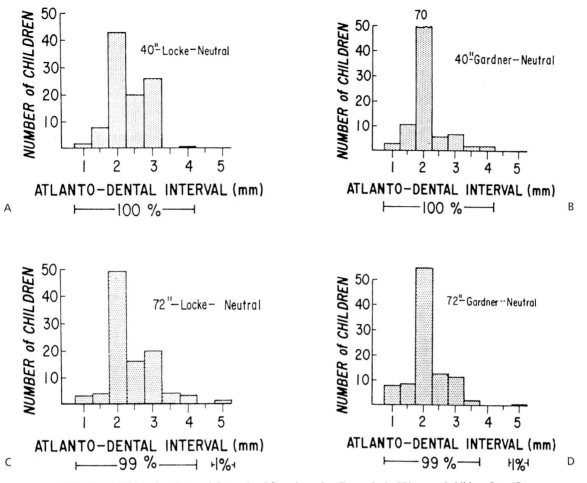

FIGURE 18. Atlantodens interval determined from lateral radiographs in 200 normal children 3 to 15 years of age. The lower limit of 3 years was selected because of the summit of the epiphysis of the odontoid process is not present earlier, and adequate radiographs are more dificult to obtain in the younger children. In the upright position, 100 studies were done using a 72-in tube-to-film distance and were interpreted by one examiner **(A, B)**. Another 100 studies were shot at 40-in tube-to-film distance with the patient supine and the film exposed with the horizontal beam and again read by one examiner **(C, D)**. These positions were selected because supine studies are usually used in trauma investigations, whereas children with inflammatory disease are examined upright. (From Locke GR, Gardner JL, Van Epps EF [1966]: Atlas-dens interval (ADI) in children: survey based on 200 normal cervical spines. *Am J Roentgenol* 97:135–140, with permission.)

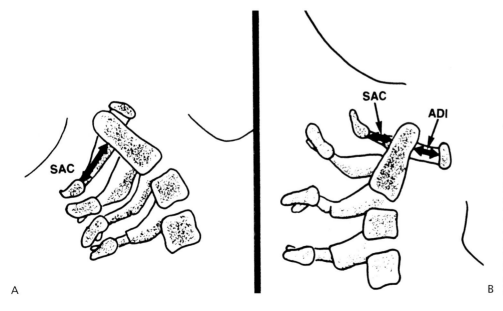

FIGURE 19. Atlantoaxial instability with intact odontoid. **A:** Extension: The atlas-dens interval (ADI) and space available for the spinal cord (SAC) are normal because the intact odontoid provides a bony block to subluxation in hyperextension. **B:** Flexion: Forward sliding of the atlas with an increased ADI and decreased SAC. (From Hensinger RN [1986]: Osseous anomalies of the craniovertebral junction. *Spine* 11: 323–333, with permission.)

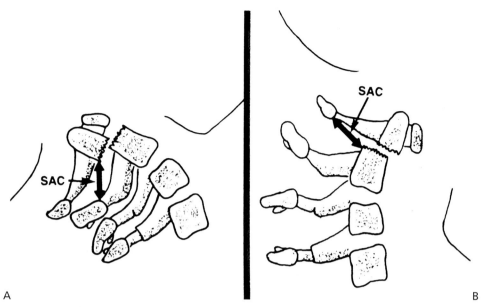

A

B

FIGURE 20. Atlantoaxial instability with os odontoideum, absent odontoid, or traumatic nonunion. **A:** Extension: Posterior subluxation with reduction in SAC and no change in the ADI. **B:** Flexion: Forward sliding of the atlas with reduction of the SAC. (From Hensinger RN [1986]: Osseous anomalies of the craniovertebral junction. *Spine* 11:323–333, with permission.)

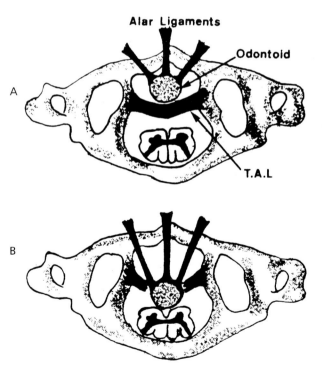

FIGURE 21. Atlantoaxial joint as viewed from above. **A:** Normal. **B:** Disruption of the transverse atlantal ligament (TAL); odontoid occupies the "safe zone of Steel." The intact alar ligaments (second line of defense) prevent spinal cord compression. (From Hensinger RN [1986]: Osseous anomalies of the craniovertebral junction. *Spine* 11:323–333, with permission.)

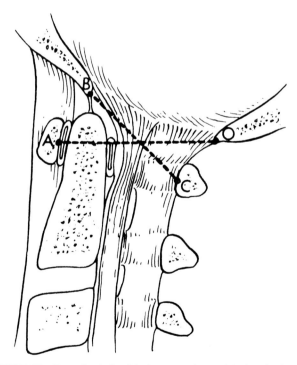

FIGURE 22. Normal relationship between the occipital and atlas. *A,* Anterior arch of the atlas; *B,* basion; *C,* Posterior arch of the atlas; *O,* Opisthion of the occipital bone. (From Powers B, Miller MD, Kramer RS, et al. [1979]: Traumatic anterior atlanto-occipital dislocation. *Neurosurgery* 4:12–17, with permission.)

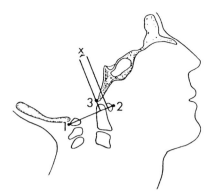

FIGURE 23. Method of measuring atlanto-occipital instability according to Wiesel and Rothman. These lines are drawn on flexion and extension lateral roentgenograms, and the translation should be no more than 1 mm. (From Gabriel KR, Mason DE, Carango P [1990]: Occipitoatlantal translation in Down's syndrome. *Spine* 15:997).

The method of Weisel and Rothman of measuring atlanto-occipital instability. Lines are drawn on a lateral cervical spine x-ray as shown in Figure 23, on flexion and extension, and the translation should be no more than 1 mm.

7. Anterior Displacement of C2 in Children. C2–3 Pseudo subluxation (Fig. 24).

8. Measurement of the Interspinous Distance for the Detection of Anterior Cervical Dislocation in the Supine Frontal Projection

A widened interspinous distance (ISD), which measures more than 1.5 times the ISD above and more than 1.5 times the ISD below, indicates the presence of an anterior cervical dislocation at the level of the abnormal widening based on a study of 500 patients with normal cervical spine and 14 patients with documented anterior cervical dislocations.

Naidich JB, et al. (1977): The widened interspinous distance: a useful sign of anterior cervical dislocation in the supine frontal projection. *Radiology* 123: 113–116.

Vertebral level	Mean diameter in mm
C2	12.5
C3	11.5
C4	11.5
C5	12.2
C6	12.6
C7	12.1

9. Measurement of the Sagittal Diameter of the Cervical Spinal Canal in Infants

Standard deviation is 0.7 mm (Fig. 25).

10. Sagittal Diameter of the Cervical Spine Canal in Children (Figs. 26–28; Tables 8, 9)

Hinck VC, Hopkins CE, Savara BS (1962): Sagittal diameter of the cervical spinal canal in children. *Radiology* 79:97–108.

Yousefzadeh DK, El-Khoury GY, Smith WL (1982): Normal sagittal diameter and variation in the pediatric cervical spine. *Pediatr Radiol* 144:319–325.

11. Sagittal Diameter of the Bony Cervical Spinal Canal in Adults (Fig. 29).

Esimont FJ, Clifford S, Goldverg M, Green B (1984): Cervical sagittal spinal canal size in spine injury. *Spine* 9:663–670.

Edwards WC, LaRocca H (1983): The developmental segmental sagittal diameter of the cervical spine in patients with cervical spindylosis. *Spine* 8: 20–27.

12. Cervical Spine Stenosis: Spinal Canal Vertebral Body Ratio

A ratio of 1.00 or more is considered normal. A ratio of 0.8 to less is considered to indicate significant spinal stenosis (Torg-Pavlov ratio) (Fig. 30).

Pavlov H, Torg JS, Robie B, Jahre C (1987): Cervical spinal stenosis: determination with vertebral ratio method. *Radiology* 164:771–775.

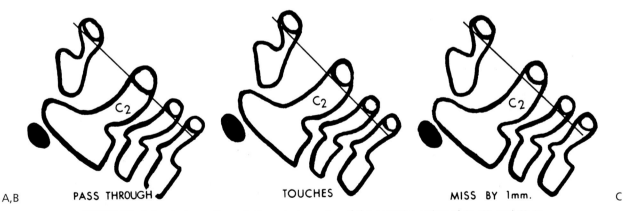

FIGURE 24. A line is drawn through the anterior cortex of the posterior arches of C1, C2, and C3. In the normal situation or in pseudosubluxation, the line is normal if it *(A)* passes through or just behind the anterior cortex of the posterior arch of C2, *(B)* touches the anterior aspect of the cortex of C2, or *(C)* comes within 1 mm of the cortex of C2. In pathologic dislocation of C2 or C3, the posterior cervical line misses the posterior arch of C2 by 2 mm or more. If the line misses the arch by 1.5 mm, one should be suspicious, but if the distance is 2 mm or more, true dislocation should be assumed unless further tests show that there is no dislocation. Based on a study of 500 children up to the age of 14 years. (From Swischuk LE [1977]: Anterior displacement of C2 in children: physiologic or pathologic? *Radiology* 122: 759–763, with permission.)

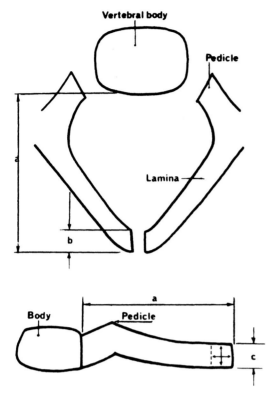

FIGURE 25. Method of measuring the sagittal diameter. *A,* The distance from posterior border of vertebral body to the tip of the spinous process; *B,* the thickness of the spinous process; and *C,* the height (on lateral radiograph) of the spinal process. At this age, b = c, and the sagittal diameter in the radiographs is equal to a minusc. Measured in 25 normal spines in infants younger than 12 months of age studied postmortem. (From Naik DR [1970]: Cervical spinal canal in normal infants. *Clin Radiol* 21:323–326, with permission.)

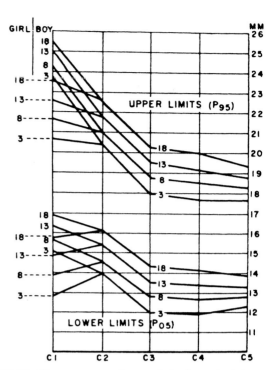

FIGURE 27. Ninety percent tolerance limits for sagittal diameters in C1–C5. In boys and girls 3 to 18 years of age: 90% tolerance limits for sagittal diameters in C1–C5. Measurements were made on 333 films, on 48 white children aged 3 to 18 years, at annual intervals. (From Markuske H [1977]: Sagittal diameter measurements of the bony cervical spinal canal in children. *Pediatr Radiol* 6:129–131, with permission.)

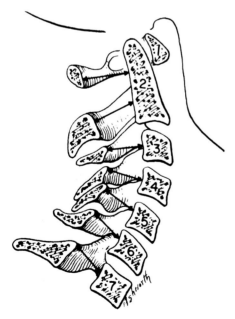

FIGURE 26. The sagittal diameter was measured from the middle of the posterior surface of the vertebral body to the nearest point on the ventral line of the cortex seen at the junction of spinous processes and laminae *(arrows).* Measurements were made on 333 films, on 48 white children aged 3 to 18 years, at annual intervals. (From Markuske H [1977]: Sagittal diameter measurements of the bony cervical spinal canal in children. *Pediatr Radiol* 6:129–131, with permission.)

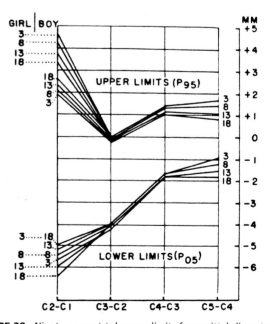

FIGURE 28. Ninety percent tolerance limits for sagittal diameter differences between adjacent vertebrae, C1–C5, in boys and girls from 3 to 18 years of age. Measurements were made on 333 films, on 48 white children aged 3 to 18 years, at annual intervals. (From Markuske H [1977]: Sagittal diameter measurements of the bony cervical spinal canal in children. *Pediatr Radiol* 6:129–131, with permission.)

TABLE 8. SAGITTAL DIAMETER OF THE BONY CERVICAL SPINAL CANAL IN 120 NORMAL CHILDREN: RELATION TO AGE[a]

	3–6 years			7–10 years			11–14 years		
	Boys (20)[b] Mean mm	Girls (20) Mean mm	Total (40) Mean/SD mm	Boys (20) Mean mm	Girls (20) Mean mm	Total (40) Mean/SD mm	Boys (20) Mean mm	Girls (20) Mean mm	Total (40) Mean/SD mm
C1	20.2	19.6	19.9 ± 1.3	20.5	20.6	20.6 ± 1.3	21.2	21.4	21.3 ± 1.4
C2	18.2	17.6	17.9 ± 1.3	18.8	18.9	18.8 ± 1.0	19.3	19.5	19.4 ± 1.1
C3	16.3	15.8	16.0 ± 1.3	17.3	17.2	17.2 ± 1.0	17.8	17.7	17.8 ± 1.0
C4	16.0	15.6	15.8 ± 1.3	17.0	16.9	16.9 ± 0.9	17.3	17.2	17.3 ± 0.9
C5	15.9	15.5	15.7 ± 1.3	16.7	16.6	16.7 ± 0.9	17.1	16.9	17.0 ± 0.9
C6	15.8	15.3	15.6 ± 1.2	16.5	16.3	16.4 ± 0.9	16.8	16.6	16.7 ± 0.9
C7	15.6	15.0	15.3 ± 1.1	16.1	15.9	16.0 ± 0.9	16.3	16.2	16.2 ± 0.9

From Markuske H (1977): Sagittal diameter measurements of the bony cervical spinal canal in children. *Pediatr Radiol* 6: 129–31, with permission.
[a] Based on lateral radiographic views of the cervical spine in 120 normal children between 3 and 14 years of age.
[b] Number in parentheses indicate number of subjects.

TABLE 9. SAGITTAL DIAMETER OF THE BONY CERVICAL SPINAL CANAL IN 120 NORMAL CHILDREN: RELATION TO HEIGHT[a]

Height (cm)	Age (years)	No. of boys and girls	C1 Mean mm	C2 Mean mm	C3 Mean mm	C4 Mean mm	C5 Mean mm	C6 Mean mm	C7 Mean mm
91–100	2.84–4.41	12	19.0	17.2	15.3	15.0	14.9	14.8	14.6
101–110	3.13–5.78	13	19.9	17.7	15.9	15.6	15.5	15.4	15.3
111–120	4.04–7.48	16	20.6	18.5	16.8	16.5	16.4	16.1	15.7
121–130	5.44–10.50	20	20.5	18.8	17.2	16.9	16.6	16.4	16.0
131–140	7.79–11.51	18	20.7	18.9	17.3	17.0	16.7	16.4	16.1
141–150	8.83–13.50	19	21.2	19.2	17.6	17.2	16.9	16.6	16.0
151–160	11.22–14.39	14	21.3	19.5	17.8	17.2	17.1	16.8	16.5
161–170	13.09–14.48	8	21.4	19.6	17.9	17.5	17.2	16.9	16.4

From Markuske H (1977): Sagittal diameter measurements of the bony cervical spinal canal in children. *Pediatr Radiol* 6: 129–131, with permission.
[a] Based on lateral radiographic views of the cervical spine in 120 normal children between 3 and 14 years of age.

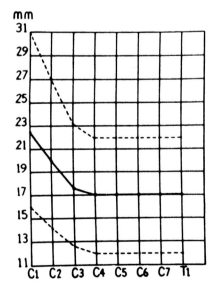

FIGURE 29. Curves for average, maximal, and minimal sagittal measurements of cervical spinal canal in adults. Plotted values are uncorrected measurements from lateral neck films taken at 72-in target-table top distance. Truce measurements are 1.5 mm less than those shown. Based on measurements made on 200 adults with no known neurologic disturbances and showing no obvious bone or joint changes on the films. (From Wolf BS, Khilnani M, Malis L [1956]: The sagittal diameter of the bony cervical spinal canal and its significance in cervical spondylosis. *J Mount Sinai Hosp* 23:283–292, with permission.)

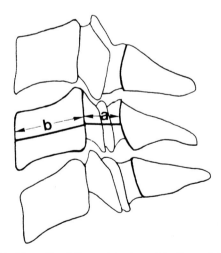

FIGURE 30. The ratio of the vertebral canal to the vertebral body is the distance from the midpoint of the posterior aspect of the vertebral body to the nearest point on the corresponding spinolaminar line *(a)* divided by the anteroposterior width of the vertebral body *(b)*. Based on measurements made at the level of the third to the sixth vertebral body on a routine lateral view of the cervical spine on 24 patients and 49 normal adults. (From Torg JS, Pavlov H, Genuario SE, et al. [1986]: Neuropraxia of the cervical spinal cord with transient quadriplegia. *J Bone Joint Surg [Am]* 68:1354–1370, with permission.)

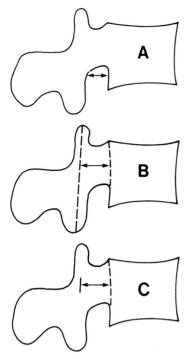

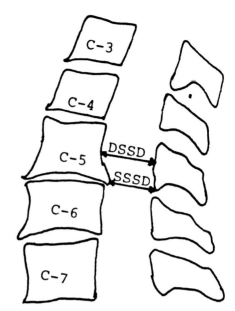

FIGURE 32. The developmental segmental sagittal diameter (DSSD) is determined at the level of the pedicle. A perpendicular line is drawn to the posterior margin of the spinal canal as determined by the most anterior bony landmark for the segment. A second perpendicular line is drawn at the level of the disc indicating the spondylotic segmental sagittal diameter (SSSD). The difference between these two measurements is the spondylosis index (SI) and represents the amount of narrowing of the spinal canal due to the disease process. (From Edwards WC, LaRocca H [1983]: The developmental segmental sagittal diameter of the cervical spinal canal in patients with cervical spondylosis. *Spine* 20–27, with permission.)

FIGURE 31. Three different methods recommended for measuring the sagittal diameter of the spinal canal. *A,* In Epstein's method, measurements are made from the uppermost level of the intervertebral foramen to the nearest point on the dorsal surface of the centrum. *B,* In Einstein's method, the sagittal diameter is measured from a line drawn from the midheight of posterior vertebral border to the nearest point of the interfacet line. The latter joints the apex of the superior articular facet to the inverted apex of the inferior facet. *C,* In Hinck's method, the sagittal diameter is the shortest perpendicular distance between the vertebral body and the inner surface of the neural arch. (From Omojola MF, Vas W, Banna M [1981]: Plain film assessment of spinal canal stenosis. *J Can Assoc Radiol* 32:95–96, with permission.)

15. Cervical Spine Lordosis (Table 10)

16. Radiographic Measurements of the Normal Cervical and Thoracic Spinal Cord in Childhood (Figs. 33, 34)

17. Normal Cord (Cervical, Thoracic, and Conus) in Infants and Children Examined with Computed Tomographic Metrizamide Myelography (Fig. 35 and Table 11).

18. Measurement of the Width of the Cervical Spinal Cord in Adults

Measurements were made at the level of the fourth and sixth cervical vertebrae when possible. Average width = 1.4 cm; minimum width = 1.0 cm; maximum width = 1.7 cm. The distance between the "inner" shadow of the

13. Other Methods of Assessing Spinal Canal Stenosis on Plain Films

Methods of assessing spinal canal stenosis based on plain films have been criticized because significant discrepancy exists between them. Three-dimensional assessment by computed tomography has been recommended (Fig. 31).

Einstein S (1977): The morphometry and pathological anatomy of the lumbar spine in South African negroes and caucasoids with specific reference to spinal stenosis. *J Bone Joint Surg [Br]* 59:173–180.

Epstein BS, Epstein JA, Lavine L (1964): The effect of anatomic variations in the lumbar vertebrae and spinal canal on cauda equina and nerve root syndromes. *Am J Roentgenol* 91:1055–1063.

Hinc VC Hopkins CE, Clark WM (1965): Sagittal diameter of the lumbar spinal canal in children and adults. *Radiology* 85:929–937.

14. Developmental Segmental Sagittal Diameter, Spondylotic Segmental Sagittal Diameter, and Spondylosis Index

Normally, the spinal canal is oval shaped in the midcervical region, and there is a sagittal diameter of 17 mm. The cervical cord diameter varies little from C1 to C7 and averages 10 mm. The diameter of the spinal canal increases with flexion and decreases with extension. The spinal cord moves as much as 3 mm at C7 during flexion and extension, and results in angulation of the nerve roots at their foramina (Fig. 32).

Burrows EH (1963): The sagittal diameter of the spinal canal in cervical spondylosis. *Clin Radiol* 14:77–86.

TABLE 10. CERVICAL SPINE LORDOSIS[a]

| Age in Years | Angle in Degrees | |
	Men	Women
20–25	16 ± 16	15 ± 10
30–35	21 ± 14	16 ± 16
40–45	27 ± 14	23 ± 17
50–55	22 ± 15	25 ± 11
60–65	22 ± 13	25 ± 16

From Gore DR, Sepic SB, Gardner GM (1986): Roentgenographic findings of the cervical spine in asymptomatic people. *Spine* 11:521–524, with permission.
[a] Mean (±1 standard deviation). Based on radiographs of 200 asymptomatic adults.

TABLE 11. RANGE OF CORD MEASUREMENTS BY AGE GROUP[a]

Age	Cervical		Midthoracic		Conus	
	Sagittal Diameter	Transverse Diameter	Sagittal Diameter	Transverse Diameter	Sagittal Diameter	Transverse Diameter
0–3 mo	4.5–5	4.5–7	2.5–5	3–4	4	5
3–18 mo	5–7	7–12	4.5–6	5–7.5	5.5–7	6.5–7
1½–6 y	7–7.5	10.5–12	5–6.5	6–7	6.5–7	6.5–9
Older than 6 y	7.5–9	10–14	5–6.5	7–8.5	6.5–9	8–11

From Resjo IM. Harwood-Nash DC, Fitz CR, Chuang S (1979): Normal cord in infants and children examined with computed tomographic metrizamide myelography. *Radiology* 130:691–6, with permission.
[a] Measurements taken from normal cords in 24 infants and children. Data in millimeters.

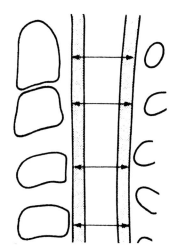

FIGURE 33. Measurement of the sagittal width of the subarachnoid space. The spinal cord and the subarachnoid space are measured in the sagittal diameter of the midvertebral level, at right angles to the long axis of the cord, and in the transverse diameter at the interpedicular level. The cord/subarachnoid space (cord/SAS) ratio is calculated. Normal values are given in Figure 32. (From Boltshauser E, Hoare RD [1976]: Radiographic measurements of the normal spinal cord in childhood. *Neuroradiology* 10:235–237, with permission.)

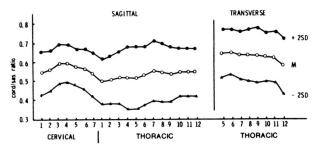

FIGURE 34. Mean and two standard deviations of cord subarachnoid space ratio in the sagittal and transverse plane. Data from 100 normal air myelograms in children aged 1 month to 15 years. (From Boltshauser E, Hoare RD [1976]: Radiographic measurements of the normal spinal cord in childhood. *Neuroradiology* 10:235–237, with permission.)

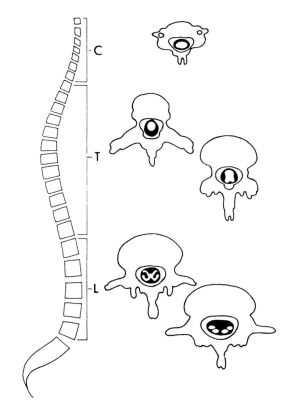

FIGURE 35. Diagram of the spinal cord at different levels in children older than 6 months. (From Resjo IM, Harwood-Nash DC, Fitz CR, Chuang S [1979]: Normal cord in infants and children examined with computed tomographic metrizamide myelography. *Radiology* 130: 691–696, with permission.)

true cord was measured rather than the entire central shadow, which includes the nerve roots. Measurements were taken from 20 patients undergoing lumbar myelography because of suspected herniated disc. There was no clinical suspicion of cervical pathology.

Devkota J, El Gammal T, Lucke JF (1982): Measurement of the normal cervical cord by metrizamide myelography. *South Med J* 75:1363–1365.

Gellad F, et al. (1983): Measurement of normal thoracic spinal cord and subarachnoid space in adults by CT metrizamide myelography. *Am J Neuroradiol* 4:614–618.

Jirout J (1966): Pneumographische Diagnostik der Ruckenmarksatrophie. *Geb Roentgenstr* 104:89–96.

Porter EC (1956): Measurement of the cervical spine cord in pantopaque myelography. *Am J Roentgenol* 76:270–272.

Thijssen HOM, Keyser A, Horstink MWM, Meijer E (1979): Normal frontal and sagittal diameter of the cervical spine on computer myelography. *Neuroradiology* 18:57–62.

19. Normal Interpediculate Distances in Children and Adults: Cervical, Thoracic, Lumbar (Tables 12–15)

TABLE 12. MEAN INTERPEDICULATE DISTANCE OF EACH VERTEBRA BY AGE: MALES[a]

	Age							
Vertebra	3, 4, 5 (4.0)	6, 7, 8 (7.0)	9, 10 (9.4)	11, 12 (11.6)	13, 14 (13.5)	15, 16 (15.6)	17, 18 (17.4)	Adult (>18)
C3	24.3	26.3	26.9	26.0	26.9	27.9	28.6	28.6
4	25.5	27.4	27.3	27.8	28.0	28.8	29.5	29.5
5	26.1	27.8	27.5	27.0	28.4	29.3	29.9	30.3
6	25.8	28.2	27.3	27.2	28.4	29.2	30.1	30.2
7	24.8	27.1	26.2	26.0	27.3	28.0	28.8	29.3
T1	22.5	22.7	23.8	23.8	24.2	25.2	24.5	25.1
2	19.4	19.7	20.4	20.6	20.6	21.7	21.2	21.4
3	17.9	18.1	19.0	18.8	19.1	19.2	19.4	19.6
4	16.9	17.6	18.2	17.6	18.3	18.0	18.7	18.8
5	16.4	17.3	17.4	17.4	18.3	17.7	18.4	18.2
6	16.5	17.3	18.8	17.4	18.3	17.3	18.2	17.8
7	16.7	17.5	16.5	17.4	18.5	17.6	17.9	17.8
8	17.0	18.1	16.7	17.6	18.9	18.3	18.4	18.0
9	17.0	18.5	17.0	17.8	19.3	18.6	18.7	18.6
10	16.9	18.8	17.3	18.1	19.5	18.1	18.9	19.1
11	18.2	20.1	18.8	19.2	20.9	19.8	20.2	20.4
12	20.4	22.5	21.3	21.8	23.5	23.2	23.4	23.5
L1	20.7	22.5	23.3	23.9	23.8	24.5	25.1	25.9
2	20.7	22.4	23.5	24.2	23.3	24.6	24.8	26.5
3	21.2	23.0	24.1	24.6	23.6	25.1	25.2	26.8
4	21.9	23.6	24.8	23.6	24.7	26.0	26.6	27.6
5	24.7	26.9	28.4	28.9	28.0	30.1	29.9	30.7

From Hinck VC, Clark WM, Hopkins CE (1966): Normal interpediculate distances (minimum and maximum) in children and adults. *Am J Roentgenol* 97:141–53, with permission.
[a] Data are given in millimeters.

TABLE 13. MEAN INTERPEDICULATE DISTANCE OF EACH VERTEBRA BY AGE: FEMALES[a]

	Age							
Vertebra	3, 4, 5 (4.2)	6, 7, 8 (7.2)	9, 10 (9.6)	11, 12 (11.6)	13, 14 (13.7)	15, 16 (15.5)	17, 18 (17.8)	Adult (>18)
C3	22.1	25.5	24.8	26.6	27.5	26.6	26.5	27.4
4	22.2	26.0	25.6	27.4	28.4	27.7	27.5	28.2
5	22.3	26.4	25.9	28.0	28.7	28.1	27.9	28.7
6	23.6	26.7	26.0	27.3	28.6	27.5	28.0	28.6
7	24.0	25.5	26.3	25.8	27.1	26.1	26.1	27.1
T1	19.8	22.1	23.1	23.0	22.6	22.3	22.4	23.1
2	16.6	18.2	19.7	18.8	19.6	18.9	19.1	19.8
3	15.2	17.0	17.9	17.5	18.3	17.6	17.9	18.2
4	14.6	16.3	17.1	16.6	17.8	16.9	17.4	17.4
5	14.6	16.3	16.6	16.0	17.2	16.8	17.1	17.1
6	14.5	16.1	16.3	15.9	17.4	16.5	16.9	16.9
7	14.7	16.3	16.5	16.1	17.8	16.6	17.4	17.0
8	15.0	16.9	16.6	16.4	18.0	16.8	17.8	17.4
9	15.1	17.1	16.9	16.8	18.1	17.3	18.2	17.9
10	15.4	17.3	17.1	17.1	18.2	17.7	18.7	18.4
11	16.5	18.0	18.2	18.4	19.8	19.2	19.9	20.0
12	19.1	20.2	21.1	20.9	22.8	21.7	22.5	22.9
L1	20.1	21.0	22.5	22.2	23.7	23.6	24.1	24.3
2	20.0	21.1	22.6	22.3	23.6	23.6	24.2	24.9
3	20.2	21.7	23.2	22.8	24.6	24.4	24.5	25.4
4	21.1	23.0	24.7	24.2	26.9	25.4	25.8	26.4
5	23.9	26.1	28.2	28.5	30.4	28.6	29.5	29.0

From Hinck VC, Clark WM, Hopkins CE (1966): Normal interpediculate distances (minimum and maximum) in children and adults. *Am J Roentgenol* 97:141–153, with permission.
[a] Data are given in millimeters.

TABLE 14. MEAN INTERPEDICULATE DISTANCE OF EACH VERTEBRA BY AGE: MALES AND FEMALES COMBINED[a]

Vertebra	3, 4, 5 (4.1)	6, 7, 8 (7.1)	9, 10 (9.4)	11, 12 (11.6)	13, 14 (13.6)	15, 16 (15.6)	17, 18 (17.5)	Adult (>18)
C3	23.9	26.0	26.4	26.2	27.2	27.1	27.7	28.0
4	24.9	26.8	26.9	27.0	28.3	28.2	28.7	28.8
5	25.3	27.2	27.1	27.4	28.6	28.6	29.1	29.4
6	25.3	27.6	27.0	27.3	28.5	28.2	29.1	29.3
7	24.4	26.4	26.2	25.9	27.2	26.9	27.6	28.0
T1	21.4	22.4	23.4	23.5	23.4	23.5	23.1	24.0
2	18.2	18.9	20.0	19.8	20.1	19.9	19.8	20.5
3	16.9	17.6	18.4	18.1	18.7	18.1	18.4	18.8
4	16.0	17.0	17.6	17.2	18.1	17.3	17.8	18.1
5	15.8	16.8	16.9	16.8	17.7	17.1	17.5	17.6
6	15.8	16.7	16.5	16.8	17.8	16.7	17.3	17.3
7	16.0	16.9	16.5	16.8	18.2	16.9	17.5	17.4
8	16.3	17.6	16.7	17.1	18.4	17.3	18.0	17.7
9	16.4	17.8	17.0	17.4	18.7	17.7	18.3	18.2
10	16.4	18.1	17.2	17.7	18.8	17.8	18.8	18.7
11	17.6	19.2	18.5	18.9	20.3	19.5	20.0	20.2
12	19.9	21.2	21.2	21.4	23.1	22.3	22.8	23.2
L1	20.5	21.8	23.0	23.0	23.7	23.9	24.5	25.0
2	20.4	21.9	23.2	23.1	23.4	23.9	24.4	25.5
3	20.8	22.4	23.8	23.6	24.0	24.6	24.8	26.0
4	21.7	23.3	24.8	24.9	25.7	25.6	26.1	26.9
5	24.5	26.5	28.3	28.7	29.1	29.1	29.6	29.7

From Hinck VC, Clark WM, Hopkins CE (1966): Normal interpediculate distances (minimum and maximum) in children and adults. *Am J Roentgenol* 97:141–153, with permission.
[a] Data are given in millimeters.

TABLE 15. TOLERANCE RANGE (90%) OF INTERPEDICULATE DISTANCE OF EACH VERTEBRA BY AGE: MALES AND FEMALES COMBINED[a]

Vertebra	3, 4, 5	6, 7, 8	9, 10	11, 12	13, 14	15, 16	17, 18	Adult
C3	18–29	22–30	21–32	20–32	24–31	23–31	23–32	25–31
4	19–30	23–31	21–32	21–33	25–32	24–32	24–33	26–32
5	20–31	23–31	22–32	21–33	25–32	25–32	25–34	26–33
6	20–31	24–31	22–32	21–33	25–32	24–33	25–34	26–33
7	19–30	23–31	21–32	20–32	24–31	21–32	23–32	24–32
T1	17–26	19–26	20–27	20–27	19–28	18–29	20–26	20–28
2	14–22	15–22	17–24	16–24	16–24	14–25	17–23	17–24
3	13–21	14–21	15–21	14–22	15–23	15–22	15–21	16–22
4	12–20	14–21	15–21	14–21	14–22	14–20	15–21	15–21
5	12–20	13–20	14–20	13–21	14–22	14–21	15–21	14–21
6	12–20	13–20	14–20	13–20	14–22	13–20	14–20	14–20
7	12–20	13–21	14–20	13–20	14–22	13–21	15–21	14–20
8	12–21	14–21	14–20	13–21	14–23	14–21	15–21	15–21
9	12–21	14–21	13–21	14–21	15–23	14–22	15–21	15–21
10	12–21	15–22	13–21	14–21	15–23	14–22	16–22	16–22
11	13–22	16–23	14–23	15–22	16–25	16–23	17–23	17–24
12	16–24	18–25	17–25	18–25	19–27	18–26	20–26	19–27
L1	17–24	17–27	19–28	19–27	20–27	20–28	20–29	21–29
2	17–24	17–27	19–28	19–27	20–27	20–28	20–29	21–30
3	17–24	17–27	19–28	20–27	21–28	21–29	20–29	21–31
4	18–25	18–28	20–29	20–28	19–33	21–30	19–33	21–33
5	21–28	22–32	24–33	24–34	22–36	23–35	23–37	23–37

From Hinck VC, Clark WM, Hopkins CE (1966): Normal interpediculate distances (minimum and maximum) in children and adults. *Am J Roentgenol* 97:141–153, with permission.
[a] Data are given in millimeters.

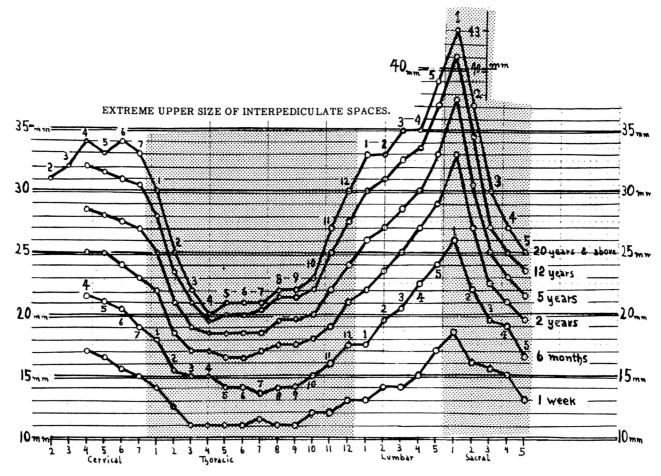

FIGURE 36. Extreme upper limits of interpediculate spaces. All curves delineate the maximum measurement observed for a given vertebra at the age designated. For ease of orientation, the thoracic segment and the sacrum are shaded. Based on findings from 200 patients. (From Schwarz GS [1956]: The width of the spinal canal in the growing vertebra, with special reference to the sacrum. Maximum interpediculate distances in adults and children. *Am J Roentgenol* 76:476–481, with permission.)

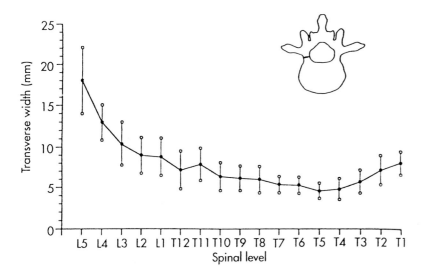

FIGURE 37. Transverse pedicle isthmus widths. (From Zindrick MR, Wiltse LL, Doornik A, et al. [1987]: Analysis of the morpholometric characteristics of the thoracic and lumbar pedicles. *Spine* 12:160–166, with permission.)

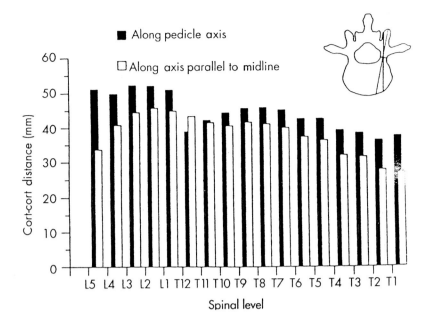

FIGURE 38. Distance to anterior cortex through pedicle angle axis versus through line parallel to midline axis of vertebra widths. (From Zindrick MR, Wiltse LL, Doornik A, et al. [1987]: Analysis of the morphometric characteristics of the thoracic and lumbar pedicles. *Spine* 12:160, with permission.)

Abnormal Interpedicular Distances

Wide: Intraspinal tumor, dural ectasia, dysraphism

Narrow: Achondroplasia, diastrophic dwarfism, thanatophoric dwarfism. Interpediculate distance is the shortest distance between the medial surfaces of the pedicles of a given vertebra.

20. Maximum Interpediculate Distances in Adults and Children: Cervical, Thoracic Lumbar (Fig. 36)

Halworth JB, Keillor B (1962): Use of transparencies in evaluating the width of the spinal canal in infants, children and adults. *Radiology* 79:109–114.

Hinck VC, Hopkins CE, Clark WM (1965): Sagittal diameter of the lumbar spinal canal in children and adults. *Radiology* 85:929–937.

Ulrich CG, Binet EF, Sanecki MG, Kieffer SA (1980): Quantitative assessment of the lumbar spinal canal by computed tomography. *Radiology* 134:137–143.

Wynne-Davies R, Walsh WK, Gormley J (1981): Achondroplasia and hypochondroplasia. Clinical variation and spinal stenosis. *J Bone Joint Surg [Br]* 63:508–515.

21. Transverse Pedicle Isthmus Widths (Fig. 37)

22. Distance to Anterior Cortex Through Pedicle Angle Axis Versus Through Line Parallel to Midline Axis of Vertebra (Fig. 38)

Zindrick MR, Wiltse LL, Doornik A, et al. (1987): Analysis of the morphometric characteristics of the thoracic and lumbar pedicles. *Spine* 12:160.

Zindrich MR (1992): Clinical pedicle anatomy, Spine. *State of the Art Reviews* 6:11.

F. THORACOLUMBAR SPINE

1. Measurement of Thoracic Spine Length (Fig. 39)

Kuhns LR, Holt JF (1975): Measurement of thoracic spine length on chest radiographs of newborn infants. *Radiology* 116:395–397.

2. Vertebral Body and Intervertebral Disc Index T12–L3 in Children (Fig. 40; Tables 16–18)

Brander ME (1972): Normal values of the vertebral body and intervertebral disc index in adults. *Am J Roentgenol* 114:411–414.

Farfan HF, Huberdeau RM, Dubow HI (1972): Lumbar intervertebral disc degeneration. *J Bone Jone Surg [Am]* 54:492–510.

Nicholson AA, Roberts GM, Williams LA (1988): The measured height of the lumbosacral disc in patients with and without transitional vertebrae. *Br J Radiol* 61:454–455.

3. Measurement of the Normal Wedging of the Dorsolumbar Vertebrae

The degree of anterior wedging was measured as the ratio between the heights of the anterior (A) and the posterior (P) aspects of the vertebral bodies at a distance of 2 mm from the vertebral margins to avoid the edges, which are difficult to define. The mean A/P ratios were calculated and are shown in Table 18.

4. Scoliosis (See also under classifications)

a. Radiographic Measurements

Posteroanterior and lateral views of the entire spine are the basic films used for evaluation of any type of scoliosis. They should show the entire spine from the occiput to the coccyx on a single film. Appropriate filters can help render all parts of the spine almost equally visible, despite different tissue densities. The basic films can be taken in the supine position (gravity eliminated) or in the upright position, either sitting or standing. Standing films are the standard technique. Sitting films show the spine under the influence of gravity but eliminate the effect of leg length discrepancies and hip contractures on the spine. Supine films are recommended in patients who had just begun to walk (younger than the age of 2 or 3 years). For valid comparisons to be made on sequential radiographic examinations, it is important to use the same technique.

(1) *Methods of Determining Magnitude.* The most commonly used method is that described by Cobb (Fig. 41). The Ferguson method is employed when the end plates of the vertebral bodies are difficult to determine (as in congenital scoliosis with multiple anomalies) (Fig. 42).

Cobb JR (1948): Outline for the study of scoliosis. *AAOS Instr Course Lect* 5:261–275.

Ferguson AB (1945): Roentgen diagnosis in the extremities and spine. *AAOS Instr Course Lect* 2:214–224.

Ferguson AB (1949): *Roentgen diagnosis of the extremities and spine,* 2nd ed. New York: Paul B. Hoeber.

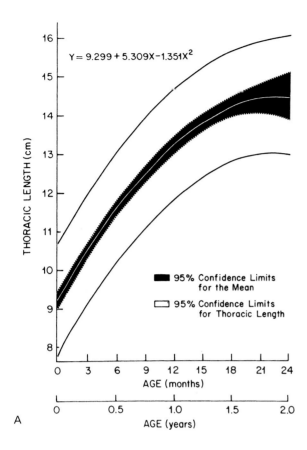

A

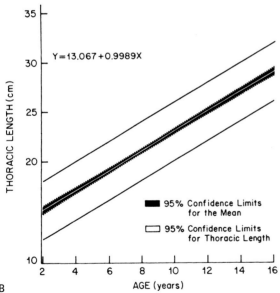

B

FIGURE 39. Results of statistical analysis in children from birth to 2 years **(A)** and children from 2 to 16 years **(B)**. The predicted values for the mean are indicated by the center curve, and the 95% confidence limits for the mean by the shaded area. The boundaries of the unshaded area *(outside curves)* denote the calculated 95% confidence limits for thoracic length for an individual child. In the equations shown in these figures, Y is the thoracic length in centimeters and X is the age in years. (From Currarino G, Williams B, Reisch JS [1966]: Linear growth of the thoracic spine in chest roentgenograms from birth to 16 years. *Skeletal Radiol* 15:628–630, with permission.)

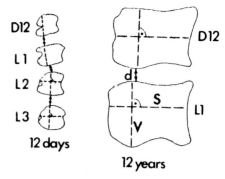

FIGURE 40. Method of measuring vertebral bodies and disc spaces. Only dotted lines were measurable. This is the method used to form the indices. *Ivb,* Vertebral body index; *v/s,* Height of vertebral body/sagittal diameter of vertebral body; *id,* intervertebral disc index; *d/v,* intervertebral disc thickness/height of vertebral body. Upper disc and lower vertebral body are compared.

TABLE 16. VERTEBRAL BODY INDEX AT DIFFERENT AGES AND LEVELS

Vertebral Body	Age (Sex)	N	Mean *v/s*
D12	0–1 m	13	0.81
	2–18 m	26	0.91
	19–36 m	22	0.86
	4–12 y (F)	18	0.86
	4–12 y (M)	35	0.78
	≥13 y (F)	7	0.93
	≥13 y (M)	20	0.84
L1	0–1 m	16	0.87
	2–18 m (F)	11	1.02
	2–18 m (M)	16	0.96
	2–18 m (M & F)	27	0.98
	19–36 m	23	0.89
	4–12 y (F)	20	0.87
	4–12 y (M)	40	0.80
	≥13 y (F)	19	1.03
	≥13 y (M)	27	0.87
L2	0–1 m	10	0.92
	2–18 m	21	1.01
	19–36 m	20	0.91
	4–12 y	49	0.82
	≥13 y (F)	15	1.03
	≥13 y (M)	25	0.88
L3	0–1 m	11	0.95
	2–18 m	17	0.98
	19–36 m	16	0.88
	4–12 y	35	0.79
	≥13 y (F)	11	1.00
	≥13 y (M)	17	0.87

N, number of subjects; F, female; M, male; m, months; y, years.

TABLE 17. INTERVERTEBRAL DISC INDEX AT DIFFERENT AGES AND LEVELS[a]

Vertebral Segment	Age Group	N	Mean d/v
D11–D12	0–1 m	12	0.37
	2–18 m	26	0.30
	19–36 m	19	0.25
	4–12 y	49	0.24
	≥13 y	21	0.18
D12–L1	0–1 m	17	0.35
	2–18 m	27	0.28
	19–36 m	20	0.26
	4–12 y	53	0.25
	≥13 y	37	0.19
L1–L2	0–1 m	15	0.35
	2–18 m	26	0.26
	9–36 m	19	0.27
	4–12 y	44	0.28
	≥13 y	37	0.20
L2–L3	0–1 m	9	0.38
	2–18 m	18	0.28
	19–36 m	15	0.30
	4–12 y	32	0.30
	≥13 y	22	0.21

From Brander ME (1970): Normal values of the vertebral body and intervertebral disc index during growth. *Am J Roentgenol* 110:618–27, with permission.
N, number of subjects; m, months; y, years.
[a] The average intervertebral disc is only one-third to one-fourth the height of the adjacent vertebral body. Based on 187 radiographs of dorsal and lumbar spines from newborns to adolescents. (Note: Additional work by Brander based on a study of adults indicates that the intervertebral disc index d/v in adults is comparable to the results obtained in children.)

TABLE 18. DEGREE OF VERTEBRAL WEDGING IN THE MALE AND FEMALE GROUPS

	Confidence Limits				
Vertebrae	80%	90%	95%	97.5%	Total
Males					
T8	0.81	0.77	0.75	0.72	62
T9	0.84	0.81	0.78	0.76	67
T10	0.86	0.83	0.80	0.78	67
T11	0.85	0.81	0.79	0.76	66
T12	0.84	0.81	0.79	0.77	63
L1	0.86	0.84	0.82	0.80	68
L2	0.90	0.88	0.86	0.84	68
L3	0.95	0.92	0.90	0.88	67
Females					
T8	0.86	0.84	0.82	0.80	94
T9	0.90	0.88	0.85	0.84	95
T10	0.91	0.89	0.87	0.85	95
T11	0.87	0.85	0.82	0.80	94
T12	0.89	0.87	0.85	0.84	96
L1	0.90	0.88	0.86	0.84	95
L2	0.94	0.92	0.90	0.89	95
L3	0.96	0.94	0.92	0.90	95

From Lauridsen KN, DeCarvalho A, Andersen AH (1991): Degree of vertebral wedging of the dorsolumbar spine. *Acta Radiol Diagn* 25:29–32, with permission.
[a] Data based on a study of 164 persons: 96 women aged 25 to 59 years and 68 men aged 17 to 59 years. Subjects selected at random, and those with fractures were excluded.

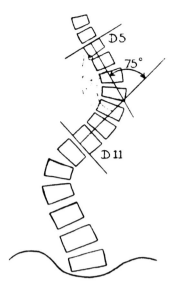

FIGURE 41. Cobb method. First, determine the end vertebrae. The top vertebra of the curve is the highest one whose superior surface tilts to the side of the concavity of the curve. The bottom vertebra is the lowest one whose inferior surface tilts to the side of the concavity of the curve. Draw intersecting perpendicular lines from the superior surface of the top and the inferior surface of the bottom vertebrae of the curve. The angle formed by these lines is "the angle of the curve."

(2) *Method of Determining Rotation.* In the Cobb method, the relationship of the spinous process to the center of the vertebral body is noted in the antero-posterior radiograph (Fig. 43). The Nash and Moe method is probably the most commonly used method of measuring vertebral rotation. It is based on the rotation of the pedicles (Figs. 44–46, Table 19).

(a) *Other methods of measuring curve rotation have been described.*

Benson DR, Schultz AB, Dewald RL (1976): Roentgenographic evaluation of vertebral rotation. *J Bone Joint Surg [Am]* 58:1125–1129.

Bunnell WP (1985): Vertebral rotation: a simple method of measurement in routine radiographs. *Orthop Trans* 9:114.

Coetsier M, Vercauteren M, Moerman P (1977): A new radiographic method for measuring vertebral rotation in scoliosis. *Acta Orthop Belg* 43: 598–605.

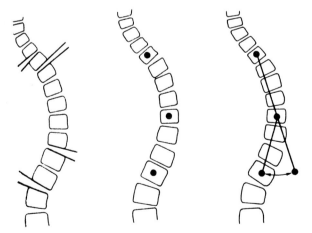

FIGURE 42. Ferguson method. The center of the shadow of the vertebral body is marked at the most unrotated vertebra at the ends of the curve and at the most rotated vertebra at the apex of the curve. Lines are drawn from the apical to the end marks and the deviation of these lines from 180 degrees is the angle of the curve.

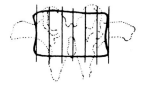
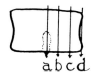

NORMAL VERTEBRA
NO ROTATION

Spinous process is in center of body.
Divide width of vertebra in sixths.

ROTATION

If spinous process
is at b = + rotation
is at c = ++ rotation
is at d = +++ rotation
beyond d = ++++ rotation

FIGURE 43. Cobb method of determining degree of rotation.

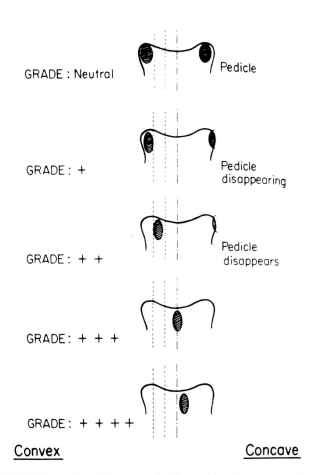

FIGURE 44. Nash and Moe method of determining degree of rotation.

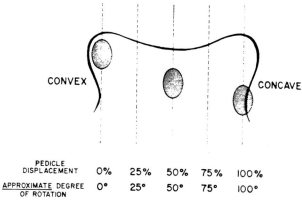

| | PEDICLE DISPLACEMENT | 0% | 25% | 50% | 75% | 100% |
| APPROXIMATE DEGREE OF ROTATION | 0° | 25° | 50° | 75° | 100° |

FIGURE 45. A simplified technique of describing vertebral rotation and estimating the degrees of rotation present. (From Nash C, Moe J [1969]: A study of vertebral rotation. *J Bone Joint Surg [Am]* 51: 223–229, with permission.)

TABLE 19. SUMMARY OF THE RESULTS COMPARING THE AMOUNT OF ROTATION OF THE COBB METHOD (SPINOUS PROCESS) AND THE METHOD USED BY NASH AND MOE (PEDICLES)

| Location | Technique | Degrees | | | |
		+	++	+++	++++
Upper thoracic (T2–T5)	Pedicle	5–15	20–35	40	>50
	Cobb	5	10	15–20	>25
Thoracic (T7–T10)	Pedicle	5–10	15–30	35–40	>50
	Cobb	5	10–15	20–25	>30
Lumbar (L2–L4)	Pedicle	5–15	20–35	40–50	>60
	Cobb	5–10	15–20	25–35	>40

From Nash C, Moe J (1969): A study of vertebral rotation. *J Bone Joint Surg [Am]* 51:223–229, with permission.

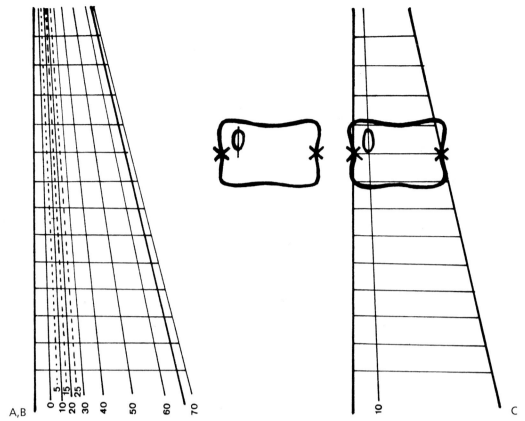

FIGURE 46. The measurement of rotation is performed using a torsiometer. **A:** The measurement is made from the pedicle situated at the convexity of the apical vertebra under consideration. **B:** Mark the greatest diameter of the pedicle. Mark a reference *(x)* at the waist of each lateral border of the vertebra. **C:** Superimpose the torsiometer on the vertebra at the edges of the rule at the sides of the vertebral body. The amount of rotation of the vertebral body is read from the rotation scale (10 degrees in this example). (From Pedriolle R [1979]: *La scoliose.* In: Maloine SA, ed. Paris: Masson, with permission.)

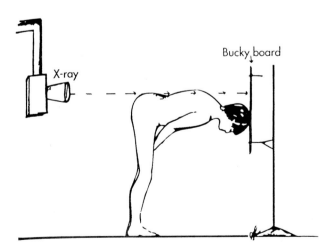

FIGURE 47. Patient positioning for tangential roentgenographic rib view. (Redrawn from Harvey CJ, Betz RR, Clements DH, et al. [1993]: Are there indications for partial rib resection in patients with adolescent idiopathic scoliosis treated with Cotrel-Dubousset instrumentation? *Spine* 18:1593, with permission.)

Drerup B (1984): Principles of measurement vertebral rotation from frontal projections of the pedicles. *J Biomech* 17:923–935.

Fait M, Janovec M (1970): Establishing of the rotation angle in the vertebra. *Scripta Medica* 43:207–215.

Harvey CJ, Betz, RR, Clements DH, et al. (1993): Tangential rib view. *Spine* 18:1593.

Mehta MH (1973): Radiographic estimation of vertebral rotation in scoliosis. *J Bone Joint Surg (Br)* 55:513–520.

(3) *Metha's Rib Vertebral Angle.* The value of Metha's rib vertebral angle is in the prediction of whether infantile scoliosis is of the resolving or progressive type. According to Metha, if the angle difference is greater than 20, there is an 80% chance that the scoliosis is progressive (Figs. 48, 49)

(4) *Torso Balance.* Measured on a posteroanterior film of the entire spine, a plumb line dropped from C7 should fall on the midline of the sacrum.

Stage I:	1.5 cm off center	One-half vertebral body
Stage II:	3 cm	One vertebral body
Stage III:	5 cm	One and one-half vertebral bodies
Stage IV:	Over 5 cm	

Goldstein LA, Waugh TR (1973): Classification and terminology of scoliosis. *Clin Orthop* 93:10–22.

(5) *Moire Screen Method (Fig. 50).* The Moire technique is adapted from the field of engineering and allows three-dimensional measurements of the spine. Moire fringe topography has been accepted optical engineering practice since it was first described by Rayleigh in 1974. Its reintroduction into the medical field has come through the work of Takasaki (1970, 1973). Takasaki's work showed

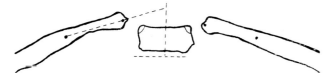

FIGURE 48. Method of measurement of Metha's rib vertebral angle (RVA). A perpendicular is drawn to the middle of either the upper or lower border of a selected thoracic vertebra (in a scoliotic curve, the apical vertebra). Another line is drawn from the midpoint of the head of the rib to the midpoint of the neck of the rib, just medial to the region where the neck widens into the shaft of the rib. The rib line is extended medially to intersect the vertebral line to make the RVA. (From Metha MH [1972]: The rib-vertebral angle in the early diagnosis between resolving and progressive infantile scoliosis. *J Bone Joint Surg [Br]* 54:230–243, with permission.)

the feasibility of using the shadow Moire fringe method to get accurate and reproducible contour lines on the suface of the back. Using the shadow Moire technique, three-dimensional evaluations have been carried out for a variety of disorders of the spine.

Moreland and colleagues (1981) defined fringe patterns for normal spines, kyphosis, and different types of scoliosis (Fig. 46). They based the pattern classification on the form of the contour lines formed by the Moire fringe. They described the following patterns: (a) Upper M (M1), (b) 0 (01), (c) W, (d) V, (e) Lower M (M2), and (f) Gluteal (02).

The M1 pattern is formed in the upper thoracic region, as the height descends cephalad from the elevated scapular regions toward the base of the neck, the contour lines become discontinuous laterally at the shoulder region to form an upper M pattern (M1). Because the contour lines formed by the Moire fringe represent lines of uniform height, they tend to be continuous around the elevated, and usually steeper areas of each scapula and the gluteal region form 0 patterns, designed 01 for the scapula and 02 for the gluteal region. Beginning at the scapula region, there is usually a descending pattern of contour lines proceeding caudally, becoming discontinuous laterally in the axillary region and forming a

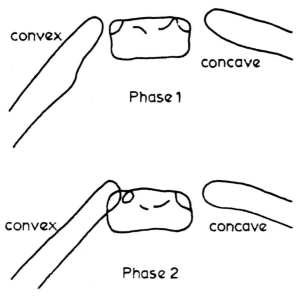

FIGURE 49. The two phases in progression of infantile scoliosis as described by Metha. Phase I (early stage): The rib head on the convex side of the curve does not overlap (is separated from) the vertebral body. Phase II: With progression of the curve, the rib head overlaps the vertebral body. According to Metha, the transition from Phase I to Phase II indicates a progressive curve. (From Metha MH [1972]: The rib-vertebral angle in the early diagnosis between resolving and progressive infantile scoliosis. *J Bone Joint Surg Br* 54:230–243, with permission.)

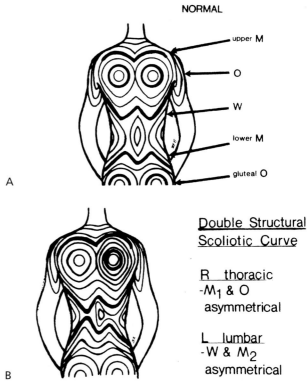

FIGURE 50. Moire fringe patterns. **A:** Normal patterns with symmetric right and left sides of the back. **B:** Deformed back surface patterns in a patient with right thoracic, left lumbar scoliosis. (From Moreland MD, Bigalow LC, Stokes IAF [1986]: Concordance of back surface rotation and scoliosis. In: Harriw JD, Turner-Smith AR, eds. *Surface topography and spinal deformity.* Proceedings of the 3rd international symposium. Stuttgart: Gustav Fischer, with permission.)

W pattern. The lower base points of the W descend along the paravertebral thoracolumbar ridges into the upper lumbar region, where they are replaced by vertically oriented contour levels descending on either side of the waist, designed lateral V left and right. The pattern of the upper back begins to repeat itself, proceeding caudally in the lumbar region, with the lower O (02) invariably representing the gluteal region and which evidences this rising slope through the lumbar region, creating the lower M (M2) pattern. The upper tips of the M represent extensions of the lumbar paravertebral ridges broadening into the gluteal mass.

Willner has devised a method of assessing the amount of asymmetry of the Moire fringe patterns. He described the use of an opalescent ruler consisting of horizontal and vertical lines. The thick mean vertical line is positioned between the vertebral prominence of C7 and the crena ani. One of the horizontal lines is placed over the lower point of the most asymmetric contour line at the convex side. A symmetric point on the same horizontal line (at the same distance of the vertical line, but on the opposite side) is found. These two points should, in a symmetric spine, be found on the same contour line. In structural scoliosis, these two points will be on different shadow lines. By recording the number of lines that differentiate these points, the difference in distance to the grid between these points can be calculated. He found a statistical significant correlation between the deviation of the Moire fringe shadows and the radiographic magnitude of the lateral deviation.

Takasaki H (1970): Moire topography. *Appl Opt* 9:1467.
Takasaki H (1973): Moire topography. *Appl Opt* 12:845.
(6) *Integrated Shape Investigation System (Figs. 51, 52).*

5. Prediction of Curve Progression

a. Progression in Untreated Congenital Scoliosis (Fig. 53)

b. Prediction of Curve Progression in Idiopathic Scoliosis (Fig. 54)

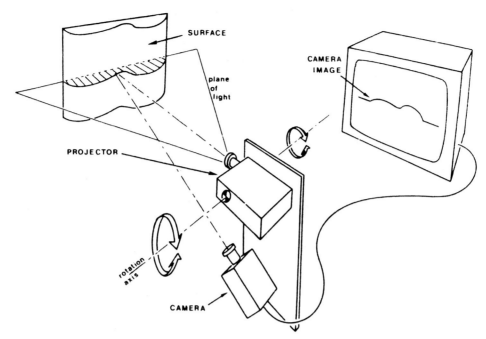

FIGURE 51. Principle of the integrated shape investigation system (ISIS). ISIS is a structured light technique in which a plane of light is cast across the patient by an ordinary 35-mm projector. This line is viewed from below the projector by a television camera mounted on a unit with the projector. The camera does not see a straight line but a curved line, the curvature being the result of the prospective view of the line as it falls on a curved three-dimensional surface. The shape of the line is recorded by a television computer system, while the projector and camera unit is scanned over the patient's back by a speed-controlled motor. The sequence of 50 to 100 television pictures is processed to convert the two dimensional television information and a record of the angle of the projector camera unit to three-dimensional real world coordinates. (From Turner-Smith AR, Harris D [1986]: ISIS: An automated shape measurement and analysis system. In: Harris JD, Turner-Smith AR, eds. *Surface topography and spinal deformity,* with permission.)

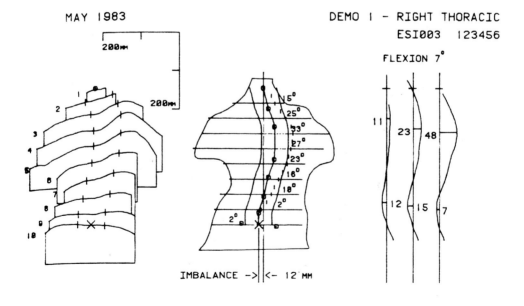

FIGURE 52. Example of the images obtained by ISIS. (From Turner-Smith AR, Harris D [1986]: ISIS: An automated shape measurement and analysis system. In: Harris JD, Turner-Smith AR, ed. *Surface topography and spinal deformity,* with permission.)

Site of curvature	Type of congenital anomaly					
	Block vertebra	Wedged vertebra	Hemivertebrae: Single	Hemivertebrae: Double	Unilateral unsegmented bar	Unilateral unsegmented bar and contralateral hemivertebrae
Upper thoracic	< 1° – 1°	★ – 2°	1° – 2°	2° – 2.5°	2° – 4°	5° – 6°
Lower thoracic	< 1° – 1°	1° – 2°	2° – 2.5°	2° – 3°	5° – 6.5°	6° – 7°
Thoracolumbar	< 1° – 1°	1.5° – 2°	2° – 3.5°	5° – ★	6° – 9°	> 10° – ★
Lumbar	< 1° – ★	< 1° – ★	< 1° – 1°	★	> 5° – ★	★
Lumbosacral	★	★	< 1° – 1.5°	★	★	★

No treatment required — May require spinal fusion — Require spinal fusion

★ Too few or no curves

FIGURE 53. Median yearly rate of deterioration without treatment for each type of single congenital scoliosis in each region of spine. Numbers on the left in each column refer to patients seen while they were younger than 10 years of age; numbers on right refer to patients seen at age 10 years or older. (From McMaster MJ, Ohtsuka K [1982]: The natural history of congenital scoliosis. *J Bone Joint Surg* 64-A:1128.)

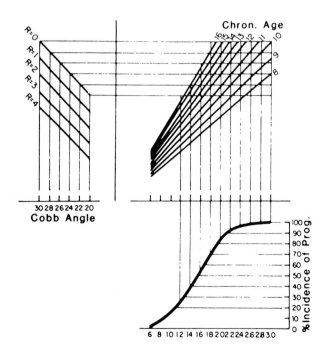

Nomogram devised using the formula:

$$\text{progression factor} = \frac{\text{Cobb angle} - 3 \times \text{Risser sign}}{\text{chronological age}}$$

FIGURE 54. Knowing the Cobb angle of the major curve, the Risser grade (0 to 5) of the iliac crest apophysis, and the patient's age permits the likelihood of progression to be estimated for curves between 20 and 29 degrees. To use the nomogram, start with the Cobb angle and follow the corresponding line vertically until the oblique line corresponding to the appropriate Risser value is encountered. Turn horizontally until the chronologic age line is met, then turn directly vertically downward until the curved line is encountered, then horizontally to the right to read the approximate percentage incidence of progression. (Reproduced from Lonstein JE, Carlson JM [1984]: The prediction of curve progression in untreated idiopathic scoliosis during growth. *J Bone Joint Surg* 66A:1061–1071).

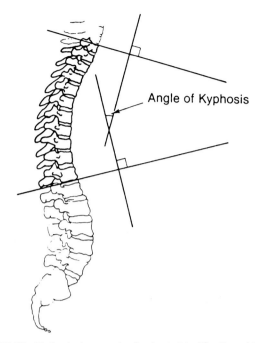

FIGURE 55. Method of measuring kyphosis. Modification of the Cobb method of measuring scoliosis. First, determine the end vertebrae, which are the last ones tilted to the convexity of the curve. Second, draw perpendicular lines to the inferior and superior vertebral end plates. The angle formed between these two lines is the degree of kyphosis (positive value) or lordosis (negative value). (From Fon GT, Pitt MJ, Thies AC Jr [1980]: Thoracic kyphosis: range in normal subjects. *Am J Roentgenol* 134:979–983, with permission.)

Knowing the Cobb angle of the major curve, the Risser grade (0 to 5) of the iliac crest apophysis and the patient's age permits the likelihood of progression to be estimated for curves between 20 and 29 degrees. To use the nomogram, start with the Cobb angle and follow the corresponding line vertically until the oblique line corresponding to the appropriate Risser value is encountered. Turn horizontally until the chronologic age line is met, then turn directly vertically downward until the curved line is encountered, then horizontally to the right to read the approximate percentage incidence of progression.

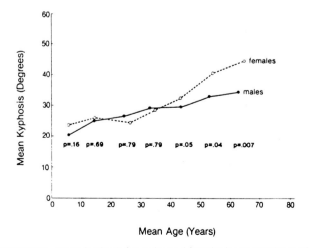

FIGURE 56. Mean kyphosis for males and females by 10-year intervals. (From Fon GT, Pitt MJ, Thies AC Jr [1980]: Thoracic kyphosis: range in normal subjects. *Am J Roentgenol* 134:979–983, with permission.)

TABLE 20. DEGREE OF KYPHOSIS IN MALES BY AGE

Age (Years)	No. Cases	Kyphosis (°)			
		Mean	SD	Minimum	Maximum
2–9	26	20.88	7.85	5	40
10–19	28	25.11	8.16	8	39
20–29	37	26.27	8.12	13	48
30–39	26	29.04	7.93	13	49
40–49	20	29.75	6.93	17	44
50–59	10	33.00	6.46	25	45
60–69	9	34.67	5.12	25	62
70–79	3	40.67	7.57	32	66

From Fon GT, Pitt MJ, Thies AC Jr (1980): Thoracic kyphosis: range in normal subjects. *Am J Roentgenol* 134:979–983, with permission.

6. Thoracic Kyphosis: Range in Normal Subjects (Fig. 55, 56; Tables 20, 21)

7. Radiographic Determination of Lordosis and Kyphosis and Lumbosacral Angle in Normal and Scoliotic Children

Lordosis was defined in this study as the angle formed by perpendicular lines drawn from the superior end plate of L1 and the inferior endplate of L5 on the lateral radiograph. Kyphosis was measured similarly from T5 to T12. The lumbosacral angle was measured as the angle formed by lines drawn on the lower endplate of L5 and the top of the sacrum (Table 22).

8. Sagittal Profiles of the Spine: Kyphosis, Lordosis, Sacral Inclination

The study was based on 670 normal subjects; lateral standing radiographs of the spine, with the arms supported and flexed about 50 to 60 degrees. Thoracic kyphosis between 20 and 50 degrees and lumbar lordosis between 20 and 70 degrees are considered normal (Table 23).

Farfan HF, Huberdeau RM, Dubow HI (1972): Lumbar intervertebral disc degeneration. *J Bone Joint Surg [Am]* 54:492–510.

Stagnara P, et al. Reciprocal angulation of vertebral bodies in a sagittal plane: approach to references in the evaluation of kyphosis and lordosis. *Spine* 7:335–342.

9. Sagittal Contour (Figs. 57, 58)

10. Measurement of the Lumbosacral Angle

According to Hellems, the mean lumbosacral angle is 41.1 degrees and the standard deviation is 7.7 degrees. Ninety-five percent of all values will lie between 25.7 and 56.5 degrees. The angle was formed by the intersection of two lines. Line 1 is the plane of the top of the sacrum, and line 2 is a horizontal line

TABLE 21. DEGREE OF KYPHOSIS IN FEMALES BY AGE

Age (Years)	No. Cases	Kyphosis (°)			
		Mean	SD	Minimum	Maximum
2–9	23	23.87	6.67	8	36
10–19	22	26.00	7.43	11	41
20–29	24	26.83	7.98	7	40
30–39	26	28.42	8.63	10	42
40–49	32	32.66	6.72	21	50
50–59	17	40.71	9.88	22	53
60–69	7	44.86	7.80	34	54
70–79	6	41.67	9.00	30	56

From Fon GT, Pitt MJ, Thies AC Jr (1980): Thoracic kyphosis: range in normal subjects. *Am J Roentgenol* 134:979–983, with permission.

TABLE 22. SUMMARY OF DISTRIBUTION OF LORDOSIS, KYPHOSIS, AND L5–S1 ANGLE[a]

| | Lordosis | | Kyphosis | | L_3–S_1 Angle | |
	Normal	Scoliotic	Normal	Scoliotic	Normal	Scoliotic
Median	40	48.5	27	28	12	10.5
25–75%	31–49.5	40–55	21–33	16.5–36	9–16	6–14.5
10–90%	22.5–54	33.5–61.5	11.5–39.5	9–53	5–21	4–18

From Propst-Proctor SL, Bleck EE (1983): Radiographic determination of lordosis and kyphosis in normal and scollotic children. *J Pediatr Orthop* 3:344–346, with permission.
Data are in degrees.
[a] Based on a total of 218 lateral standing radiographic views, 104 normal and 114 scoliotic patients.

TABLE 23. MEAN VALUES AND STANDARD DEVIATIONS (SD) FOR COBB MEASUREMENTS OF SAGITTAL CURVATURES BY AGE-GENDER GROUPS

| | | 5–9 Years | | | 10–14 Years | | | 15–20 Years | | |
		M + F	M	F	M + F	M	F	M + F	M	F
Thoracic kyphosis	Mean	36.7	35.8	37.4	37.5	37.6	37.5	38.5	39.4	37.9
	SD	6.9	6.4	7.1	8.0	7.7	8.2	8.1	8.8	7.6
Lumbosacral lordosis	Mean	52.2	49.1	54.1	56.1	55.0	56.6	56.6	57.4	56.1
	SD	10.0	9.7	9.7	8.7	8.3	8.9	9.1	8.6	9.4
Sacral inclination	Mean	51.7	48.7	53.6	56.6	56.4	56.7	56.5	58.2	55.3
	SD	9.7	10.5	8.6	7.7	7.7	7.6	9.3	9.3	9.2

From Voutsinas SA, MacEwen GD (1986): Sagittal profiles of the spine. *Clin Orthop* 210:235–242, with permission.

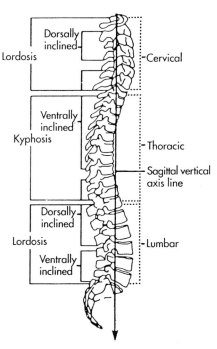

FIGURE 57. Balance of sagittal contour depends on sagittal vertical axis. Each vertebra has unique orientation and spatial relationship to apical vertebra. (From Hammerberg KW [1991]: Kyphosis. In: Bridwell KH, De Wald RL, eds. *The textbook of spinal surgery.* Philadelphia: JB Lippincott.)

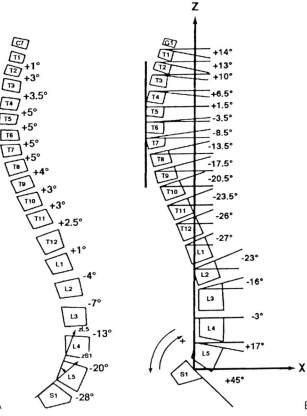

FIGURE 58. Normal local **(A)** and global **(B)** standing (assuming normal sagittal plane sacral angulation of +45 degrees) segmental angular position. Maximal sagittal plane displacement occurs dorsally at T5–T6 and ventrally at L4. (**A** adapted from Bernhardt M, Bridwell HK (1989): Segmented analysis of the sagittal plane alignment of the normal thoracic and lumbar spines and thoracolumnar junction. *Spine* 14:717; **B** adapted from Asher MA: *Isula Spine Implant System: Principles and Practice.* Cleveland: Acromed.)

drawn parallel to the bottom margin of the film. This was measured on a standing spot lateral radiographic view of L5–S1.

Hellems HK, Keats TE (1971): Measurement of the normal lumbosacral angle. *Am J Roentgenol* 113:642–645.

11. L4–5 Seating: Intercrestal Line

Based on the study of various skeletal configurations on the lumbar spine, MacGibbon and Farfan concluded (Fig. 59):

a. Criteria for probable L4–5 degeneration

(1) A high intercrestal line passing through the upper half of L4
(2) Long transverse processes on L5
(3) Rudimentary rib
(4) Transitional vertebra

b. Criteria for probable L5–S1 degeneration

(1) An intercrestal line passing through the body of L5
(2) Short transverse processes on L5
(3) No rudimentary ribs
(4) No transitional vertebra

12. Spondylolisthesis (Also see under classifications)

Measurements: Many different methods for measurement of spondylolisthesis have been used. The most comonly used are presented:

a. Anterior Displacement: Meyerding (Fig. 60)

b. Anterior Displacement: Taillard (Fig. 61)

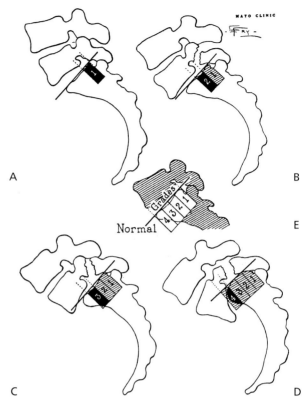

FIGURE 60. **A:** *Grade I,* The anterior displacement is 25% or less, that is, the posteroinferior angle of the displaced vertebra lies within the first segment. **B:** *Grade II,* The displacement is between 25% and 50%. **C:** *Grade III,* The displacement is between 50% and 75%. **D:** *Grade IV,* The displacement is greater than 75%. **E:** *Normal,* The superior border of the anteroposterior diameter of the anteroposterior diameter of the subjacent vertebra is divided into four equal parts. Displacement greater than 100% (spondyloptosis) may be classified as type V. (From Meyerdin HW [1932]: Spondylolisthesis. *Surg Gynecol Obstet* 54: 371–377, with permission.)

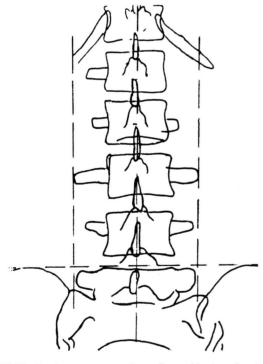

FIGURE 59. Tracing anteroposterior radiographic view showing construction lines for comparing transverse process length and height of the intercrestal line. (From MacGibbon B, Farfan HF [1979]: A radiologic survey of various configurations of the lumbar spine. *Spine* 4:258–266, with permission.)

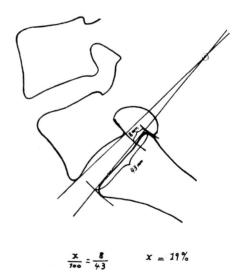

$$\frac{x}{100} = \frac{8}{43} \qquad x = 19\%$$

FIGURE 61. The anterior displacement is expressed as a percentage obtained by dividing the amount of displacement (determined by the relationship of the posterior part of the cortex of the fifth lumbar vertebral to the posterior part of the cortex of the first sacral vertebra) by the maximum anteroposterior diameter of the first sacral vertebra, and multiplying by 100. (From Taillard W [1964]: Le spondylolisthesis chez l'enfant et l'adolescent: etude de 50 cas. *Acta Orthop Scand* 24: 115–144, with permission.)

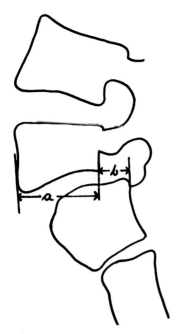

FIGURE 62. The amount of slipping is calculated by measuring the distance from a line parallel to the posterior portion of the first sacral vertebral body to a line drawn parallel to the posterior portion of the body of the fifth lumbar vertebra. The anteroposterior dimension of the fifth lumbar vertebra inferiorly is used to calculate the percentage of slipping. Taillard used the anteroposterior dimension of the first sacral vertebra. Because of the erosion of the first sacral vertebra, Boxall and coworkers proposed using the fifth lumbar vertebra (as described by Laurent and Einola) as a more accurate method. (From Laurent LE, Einola S [1961]: Spondylolisthesis in children and adolescents. *Acta Orthop Scand* 31:45–64, with permission.)

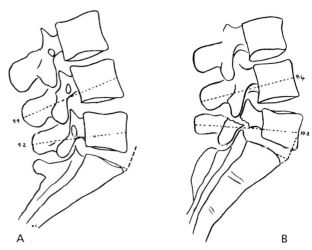

FIGURE 63. Displacement is measured by comparison of anteroposterior diameters of the spondylolytic vertebra and the normal vertebra above it. Ullmann's sign is demonstrated by drawing a line at right angles to the upper border of the sacrum at its anterior edge. Note that in the normal spine **(A)**, the fifth lumbar vertebra lies entirely behind this line, whereas in spondylolisthesis **(B)**, the perpendicular line is intersected by the slipped vertebral body. Garland and Thomas also reported on the value of Ullmann's line. (From Capener N [1931]: Spondylolisthesis. *Br J Surg* 19:374–386, with permission.)

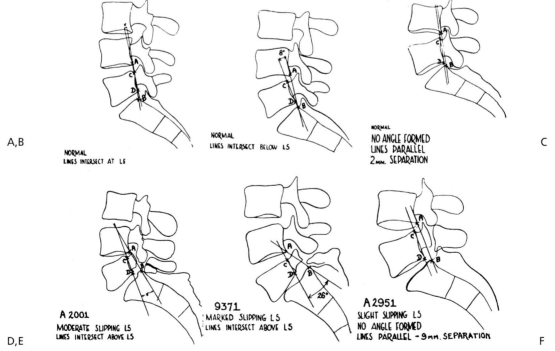

FIGURE 64. Two lines are drawn. The first line (A–B) extends between the posterior lower lip of the vertebra above and the posterior upper lip of the vertebra below. The second line (C–D) is drawn between the posterior upper and lower lips of the slipped vertebra. The lines are extended: If they are not parallel, they will meet and form an angle. When the angle is as much as 10 degrees, the spondylolisthesis can be called slight; 11 to 20 degrees, moderate; and greater than 20 degrees, severe. If the lines are parallel, a distance of more than 3 mm is abnormal. (From Mescham I [1945]: Spondylolisthesis. *Am J Roentgenol* 53:230–243, with permission.)

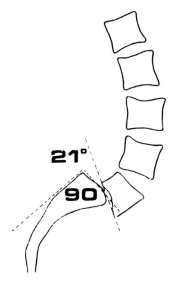

FIGURE 65. The angle of slipping measures the degree of forward tilting of the fifth lumbar vertebral body over the first sacral vertebral body, or the gibbus at the level of the slipping. The slip angle is formed by a line drawn parallel to the inferior aspect of the fifth lumbar vertebral body and a line drawn perpendicular to the posterior aspect of the body of the first sacral vertebra. (From Boxall D, Bradford DS, Winter RB, Moe JH [1979]: Management of severe spondylolisthesis in children and adolescents. *J Bone Joint Surg [Am]* 61:479–495, with permission.)

c. Anterior Displacement: Laurent-Einola and Boxall-Bradford Modification of Taillard Method (Fig. 62)

Boxall D, Bradford DS, Winter RB, Moe JH (1979): Management of severe spondylolisthesis in children and adolescents. *J Bone Joint Surg [Am]* 61: 479–495.

d. Anterior Displacement: Capener and Ullman Sign (Fig. 63)

Garland LH, Thomas SF (1946): Spondylolisthesis: criteria for more accurate diagnosis of true anterior slip of the involved vertebral segment. *Am J Roentgenol* 55:275–291.

Ullman HJ (1924): Diagnostic line for determining subluxation of the fifth lumbar vertebra. *Radiology* 2:305–306.

e. Anterior Displacement: Mescham (Fig. 64)

f. Slip Angle (Fig. 65)

g. Lumbosacral Kyphosis (Fig. 66)

h. Sacral Inclination (Fig. 67)

i. Sagittal Rotation (Fig. 68)

j. Slip Degree (Fig. 69)

k. Rounding of the Sacrum (Fig. 70)

An alternative method of measuring was proposed by Boxall and colleagues. The convexity of the proximal portion of the body of the first sacral vertebra is graded zero, I, II, or III depending on whether none, none to one third, one third to two thirds, or more than two thirds of it is rounded on the lateral radiographic views. This represents the amount of anterior and posterior erosion of the first sacral vertebral body.

Boxall D, Bradford DS, Winter RB, Moe JH (1979): Management of severe spondylolisthesis in children and adolescents. *J Bone Joint Surg [Am]* 61: 479–495.

l. Lumbar Lordosis (Fig. 71)

m. Ferguson's Lumbosacral Angle: Wiltse's Sacrohorizontal Angle (Fig. 72)

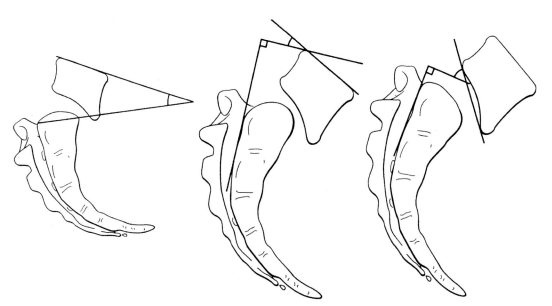

FIGURE 66. *Left,* Lumbosacral kyphosis is represented by the angle between the superior end plate of L5 and the superior end plate of S1. *Center,* it is difficult to establish a reference line for the superior end plate of a dome-shaped sacrum. The end plate can be approximated by a line drawn orthogonal to the posterior cortex of the sacrum. *Right,* The inferior end plate of L5 undergoes remodeling changes during slip progression and is not a reliable reference point. The superior end plate of L5 does not undergo these changes and should be used to measure the lumbosacral kyphosis. (Reproduced from Burkus JK, Lonstein JE, Winter RB, et al. [1992]: Long term evaluation of adolescents treated operatively for spondylolisthesis. *J Bone Joint Surg* 74A:693–704.)

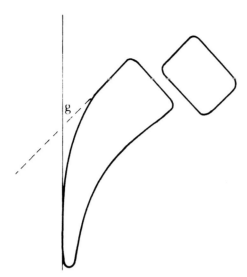

FIGURE 67. The sacral inclination angle is determined by drawing a line along the posterior border of the first sacral vertebra and measuring the angle created by this line intersecting a true vertical line. (From Wiltse L, Winter RB [1983]: Terminology and measurement of spondylolisthesis. *J Bone Joint Surg [Am]* 65:768–772, with permission.)

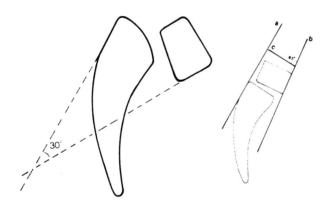

FIGURE 68. Sagittal rotation is the term used to express the angular relationship between the fifth lumbar and first sacral vertebrae. It is determined by extending a line along the anterior border of the body of the fifth lumbar vertebra until it intersects a line drawn along the posterior border of the body of the first sacral vertebra. The drawing on the right shows an alternative method of measuring sagittal rotation, which is to be used when the degree of olisthesis is small and lines *a* and *b* do not intersect. A third line, *c*, is added perpendicular to line *a*. Lines *c* and *b* intersect to form the angle of sagittal rotation. (From Wiltse L, Winter RB [1983]: Terminology and measurement of spondylolisthesis. *J Bone Joint Surg [Am]* 65:768–772, with permission.)

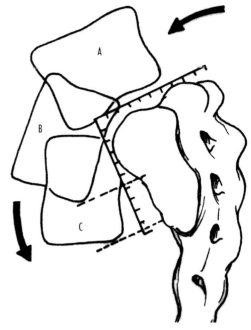

FIGURE 69. Forward displacement develops into lumbosacral kyphosis. Modified Newman spondylolisthesis grading system. The degree of slip is measured using two numbers: the first along the sacral end plate, and the second along the anterior portion of the sacrum. A = 3 + 0; B = 8 + 6; C = 10 + 10. (Reproduced from DeWald RL [1977]: Spondylolisthesis. In: Bridwell KU, DeWald RL, eds. *Textbook of Spinal Surgery,* 2nd ed. Philadelphia: Lippincott-Raven, p. 1207.)

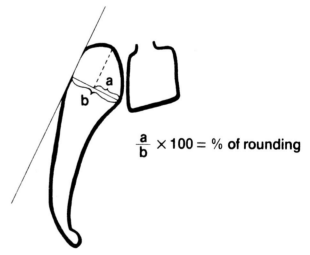

$$\frac{a}{b} \times 100 = \% \text{ of rounding}$$

FIGURE 70. Rounding of the top of the centrum of the first sacral vertebra is expressed as the relationship between lines *a* and *b,* drawn as shown. The result, when multiplied by 100, gives the percentage of rounding of the first sacral vertebra. (From Wiltse L, Winter RB [1983]: Terminology and measurement of spondylolisthesis. *J Bone Joint Surg [Am]* 65:768–772, with permission.)

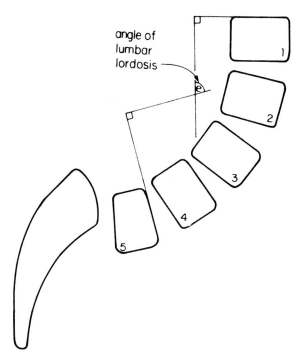

FIGURE 71. The degree of lumbar lordosis is defined as angle *e*, as shown. With significant sagittal rotation of the fifth lumbar vertebra, there may be lordosis extending well up into the thoracic spine, in which case "total spinal lordosis" should be distinguished from "lumbar lordosis." (From Wiltse L, Winter RB [1983]: Terminology and measurement of spondylolisthesis. *J Bone Joint Surg [Am]* 65:768–72, with permission.)

This angle was first described by Ferguson in 1934 as the lumbosacral angle. In Wiltse's paper, it is denominated sacrohorizontal angle. According to Hellems and Keats, the mean value is 41.1 degrees and the standard deviation is 7.7 degrees. Ninety-five percent of all values will lie between 25.7 and 56.5 degrees.

Ferguson AB (1934): Clinical and roentgen interpretation of the lumbosacral spine. *Radiology* 22:348–358.

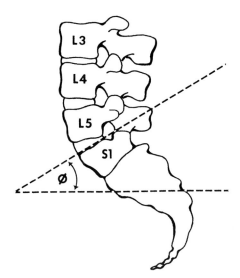

FIGURE 72. The sacrohorizontal angle is the angle between a line drawn across the cranial border of the body of the first sacral vertebra and the horizontal. (From Hellems KH, Keats TE [1971]: Measurement of the normal lumbosacral angle. *Am J Roentgenol* 113:542–645, with permission.)

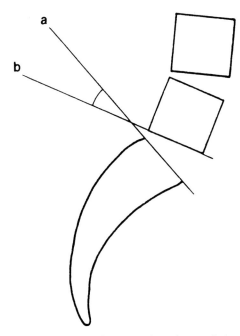

FIGURE 73. The lumbosacral joint angle is that angle between the longitudinal axes of the bodies of the fifth lumbar and first sacral vertebrae. In the normal spine, one can use lines across the caudal and cranial borders of the center of these vertebrae. The angle between these two lines is the lumbosacral joint angle. (From Wiltse L, Winter RB [1983]: Terminology and measurement of spondylolisthesis. *J Bone Joint Surg [Am]* 65:768–772, with permission.)

Wiltse L, Winter RB (1983): Terminology and measurement of spondylolisthesis. *J Bone Joint Surg [Am]* 65:768–772.

n. Lumbosacral Joint Angle as Defined by Wiltse (Fig. 73)

o. Lumbar Index: Wedging of the Olisthetic Vertebra (Fig. 74)

p. Composite Drawing of Various Angles in the Normal Lumbosacral Spine (Fig. 75)

Dandy DJ, Shannon MJ (1971): Lumbosacral subluxation. *J Bone Joint Surg [Br]* 53:578–595.

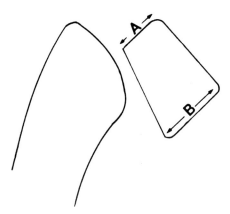

FIGURE 74. Wedging of the olisthetic vertebra is expressed as a percentage determined by dividing line *A* by line *B*, drawn as shown, and mutiplying by 100. (From Wiltse L, Winter RB [1983]: Terminology and measurement of spondylolisthesis. *J Bone Joint Surg [Am]* 65:768–772, with permission.)

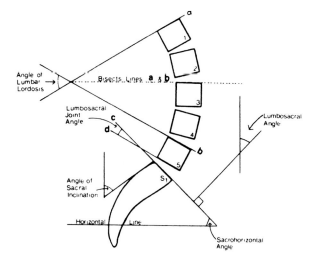

FIGURE 75. Composite drawing of various angles in the normal lumbo-sacral spine. (From Wiltse L, Winter RB [1983]: Terminology and measurement of spondylolisthesis. *J Bone Joint Surg [Am]* 65:768–772, with permission.)

Ferguson AB (1949): Roentgen diagnosis of the extremities and spine, 2nd ed. New York: Paul B. Hoeber.

Laurent LE, Einola S (1961): Spondylolisthesis in children and adolescents. *Acta Orthop Scand* 31:45–64.

Newman PH (1965): A clinical syndrome associated with severe lumbosacral subluxation. *J Bone Joint Surg [Br]* 47:39–53.

Vallois HV, Lozarthes G (1942): Indices lombaires et indice lombaire totale. *Bull Soc Antropol* 3:117.

Wiltse LL, Newmann PH, MacNab I (1976): Classification of spondylolisis and Spondylolisthesis. *Clin Orthop* 117:23–29.

11. Spine Motion (Table 24, Fig. 76)

12. Facet Orientation at Different Spine Levels (Fig. 77)

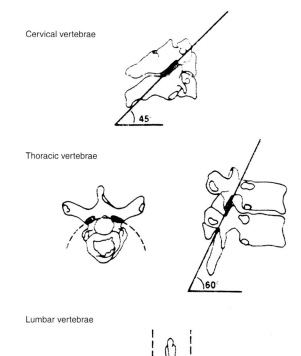

FIGURE 77. Characteristic facet orientation in the cervical, thoracic, and lumbar regions. The spatial alignment of the facet joints determines, to a large extent, although not completely, the characteristic kinematics of different regions of the spine. (From White AA, Panjabi MM [1990]: *Clinical biomechanics of the spine,* 2nd ed. Philadelphia: JB Lippincott, with permission.)

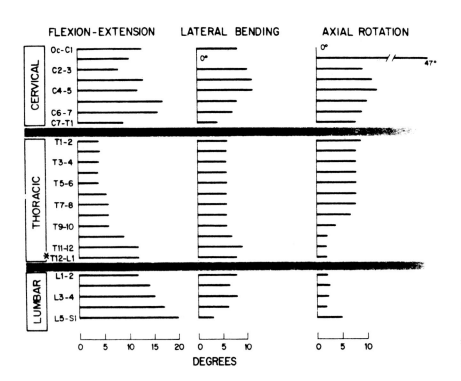

FIGURE 76. Spine motion. Composite of rotation in the traditional modalities and traditional planes of movement for the different regions of the spine. (From White AA, Panjabi MM [1978]: The basic kinematics of the human spine. *Spine* 3: 12–20, with permission.)

TABLE 24. SPINE MOTION AT DIFFERENT LEVELS ACCORDING TO WHITE AND PANJABI

Area of Spine	Flexion-Extension, *x*-Axis Rotation		Lateral Bending, *z*-Axis Rotation		Axial Rotation, *y*-Axis Rotation	
	Compiled Rotary Range (Degrees)	Representative Angle (Degrees)	Compiled Rotary Range (Degrees)	Representative Angle (Degrees)	Compiled Rotary Range (Degrees)	Representative Angle (Degrees)
Occiput–C1	4–33	13	4–14	8	0	0
C1–C2	2–21	10	0	0	22–58	47
C2–C3	5–23	8	11–20	10	6–28	9
C3–C4	7–38	13	9–15	11	10–28	11
C4–C5	8–39	12	0–16	11	10–26	12
C5–C6	4–34	17	0–16	8	8–34	10
C6–C7	1–29	16	0–17	7	6–15	9
C7–T1	4–17	9	0–17	4	5–13	8
T1–T2	3–5	4	6	6	14	9
T2–T3	3–5	4	5–7	6	4–12	8
T3–T4	2–5	4	3–7	6	5–11	8
T4–T5	2–5	4	5–6	6	4–11	8
T5–T6	3–5	4	5–6	6	5–11	8
T6–T7	2–7	5	6	6	4–11	8
T7–T8	3–8	6	3–8	6	4–11	8
T8–T9	3–8	6	4–7	6	6–7	7
T9–T10	3–8	6	4–7	6	3–5	4
T10–T11	4–14	9	3–10	7	2–3	2
T11–T12	6–20	12	4–13	9	2–3	2
T12–L1	6–20	12	5–10	8	2–3	2
L1–L2	9–16	12	3–8	6	<3	2
L2–L3	11–18	14	3–9	6	<3	2
L3–L4	12–18	16	5–10	8	<3	2
L4–L5	14–21	17	5–7	8	<3	2
L5–S1	18–22	20	2–3	3	<3	5

From White AA, Panjabi MM (1978): The basic kinematics of the human spine. *Spine* 3:12–20, with permission.

D

CLASSIFICATIONS

AURELIO G. MARTINEZ-LOZANO

1. CONGENITAL ANOMALIES OF THE ODONTOID (Fig. 1)

Fielding JW, Hensinger RN, Hawkins RJ (1980): Os odontoideum. *J Bone Joint Surg [Am]* 62:376–383.

2. TORTICOLLIS (Table 1)

3. ATLANTOAXIAL ROTATORY FIXATION (ROTATORY SUBLUXATION) (Fig. 2)

Goddard NJ, Stabler J, Albert JS (1990): Atlanto-axial rotatory fixation and fracture of the clavicle: an association and a classification. *J Bone Joint Surg [Br]* 72:72–75.

Wortzman G, Dewar FP (1967): Rotary fixation of the atlantoaxial joint: rotational atlantoaxial subluxation. *Radiology* 90:479–487.

4. KLIPPEL-FEIL SYNDROME

Type I: Extensive cervical and upper thoracic spine fusion
Type II: One or two interspace fusions, often associated with hemivertebrae and occipitoatlantal fusion
Type III: Combination of cervical and lower thoracic or lumbar fusion

Pizzutillo and colleagues proposed the following classification based on clinical and radiographic findings on 111 patients flexion-extension lateral radiographs of the cervical spine.

Class I: Normal range of motion in flexion and extension with no instability
Class II: Excessive range of motion or instability of the upper cervical segment, or the presence of basilar impression or iniencephaly
Class III: Hypermobility, instability, or degenerative changes of the lower cervical segment
Class IV: Combination of the findings as defined by Class II and Class III

Based on this study, they suggested that neurologic compromise is to be suspected in patients with hypermobility of the upper cervical segment or in the presence of iniencephaly (iniencephaly is an unusual disorder of the cervical spine consisting of congenital cervical synostoses, fixed retroflexion of the head, severe cervical lordosis, and varying degrees of incomplete posterior closure.) Degenerative changes of the cervical spine may be expected to develop when hypermobility of the lower cervical segment exists.

Nagib and colleagues suggested a classification for patients at neurologic risk.

Group I: Patients with an unstable fusion pattern
Group II: Patients with craniocervical abnormalities
Group III: Patients with fusions associated with spinal stenosis

Hensinger and colleagues have pointed out the high incidence of associated conditions in patients with Klippel-Feil syndrome:

A. G. Martinez-Lozano: Universidad Autónoma De Nuevo León, Monterrey, Mexico.

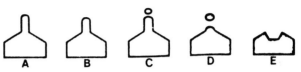

FIGURE 1. Gradations for odontoid anomalies. **A:** Normal odontoid. **B:** Hypoplastic odontoid. **C:** Ossiculum terminale. **D:** Os odontoideum. **E:** Aplastic odontoid. (From Hensinger RN, Fielding JW [1990]: The cervical spine. In: *Lovell and Winter's pediatric orthopedics*, 3rd ed. Philadelphia: JB Lippincott, with permission.)

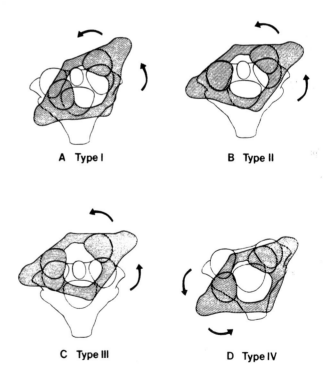

FIGURE 2. The four types of rotatory fixation. **A:** *Type 1*—Rotatory fixation with no anterior displacement and the odontoid acting as the pivot. **B:** *Type II*—Rotatory fixation with anterior displacement of 3 to 5 mm, one lateral articular process acting as the pivot. **C:** *Type III*—Rotatory fixation with anterior displacement of more than 5 mm. **D:** *Type IV*—Rotatory fixation with posterior displacement. (From Fielding JW, Hawkins RJ [1990]: Atlanto-axial rotatory fixation (fixed rotatory subluxation of the atlanto-axial joint). *J Bone Joint Surg [Am]* 59:37–44, with permission.)

TABLE 1. DIFFERENTIAL DIAGNOSIS OF CONGENITAL MUSCULAR TORTICOLLIS

Congenital anomalies
Occipitocervical anomalies
Klippel-Feil syndrome
Atlantooccipital synostosis
Basilar impression
Odontoid anomalies (aplasia, hypoplasia, os odontoideum)
Occipital vertebra
Asymmetry of occipital condyles (hypoplasia)
Absent C1 facet (unilateral)
Hemivertebra, cervical-superior dorsal spine
Unilateral congenital absence of sternocleidomastoid muscle
Pterygium colli (skin web)
Congenital muscular torticollis

Trauma, particularly C1–C2
Subluxation
Fracture
Dislocations

Inflammatory
Cervical lymphadenitis
Tuberculosis
Spontaneous hyperemic subluxation of the atlas
Rheumatoid arthritis

Neurologic disorders
Visual disturbances
Syringomyella
Cervical spinal cord tumor
Cerebellar tumor, posterior fossa
Bulbar palsies

Idiopathic disorders
Atlantoaxial rotary displacement
Subluxation
Fixation
Sandfidar syndrome
Acute calcification of cervical disc

From Hensinger RN, Fielding JW (1990): The cervical spine. In: *Lovell and Winter's pediatric orthopedics*, 3rd ed. Philadelphia: JB Lippincott, with permission.

Scoliosis, 60%
Renal abnormalities, 35%
Sprengel's deformity, 30%
Deafness, 30%
Synkinesis (involuntary paired movements of the hands and occasionally of the arms), 20%
Congenital heart disease, 14%

Feil A (1919): *L'absence et la diminution des vertèbres cervicales; le syndrome de reduction numberique cervicale*. Thèses de Paris.

Hensinger RN, Lang JE, MacEwen GD (1974): Klippel-Feil syndrome: a constellation of associated anomalies. *J Bone Joint Surg [Am]* 56:1246–1251.

Nagib MG, Maxwell RE, Chou SN (1984): Identification and management of high risk patients with Klippel-Feil syndrome. *J Neurosurg* 61:525–530.

Pizzutillo PD, Woods MW, Nicholson L (1987): Risk factors in Klippel-Feil syndrome. *Orthop Trans* 11:473.

5. BONY ABNORMALITIES OF THE CRANIOCERVICAL JUNCTION (Table 2; Fig. 3)

6. ARNOLD-CHIARI MALFORMATION (Fig. 4)

Type I: The cerebellar tonsils are elongated, flattened, and atrophic. They are stretched downward through the foramen magnum to the level of the first cervical vertebra.

Type II: Not only is there downward displacement of the inferior portion of the cerebellar vermis and hemispheres but the medulla and fourth ventricle are also herniated into the upper reaches of the cervical canal.

TABLE 2. CLASSIFICATION OF CRANIOVERTEBRAL JUNCTION ABNORMALITIES

I. Congenital anomalies and malformations
  A. Malformations of the occipital bone
    1. Manifestations of occipital vertebrae
      a. Clivus segmentation
      b. Remnants around foramen magnum
      c. Variants at atlas
      d. Dens segmentation anomalies
    2. Basilar invagination
    3. Condylar hypoplasia
    4. Assimilation of atlas
  B. Malformations of atlas
    1. Assimilation of atlas
    2. Atlantoaxial fusion
    3. Aplasia of atlas arches
  C. Malformations of axis
    1. Irregular atlantoaxial segmentation
    2. Dens dysplasias
      a. Ossiculum terminale persistens
      b. Os odontoideum
      c. Hypoplasia-aplasia
    3. Segmentation failure of C2–C3

II. Development and acquired abnormalities
  A. Abnormalities at the foramen magnum
    1. Secondary basilar invagination, e.g., Paget's disease, osteomalacia, rheumatoid cranial settling
    2. Foraminal stenosis, e.g., achondroplasia
  B. Atlantoaxial instability
    1. Errors of metabolism, e.g., Morquio syndrome
    2. Down syndrome
    3. Infections, e.g., Grisel syndrome
    4. Inflammatory, e.g., rheumatoid arthritis
    5. Traumatic occipitoatlantal and atlantoaxial dislocations, os odontoideum
    6. Tumors, e.g., neurofibromatosis, syringomyella
    7. Miscellaneous, e.g., fetal warfarin syndrome, Conradi syndrome

From Menezes AH, Van Gilder JC (1990): Anomalies of the craniovertebral junction. In: *Youman's neurological surgery*, 3rd ed. Phildelphia: WB Saunders, with permission.

Type III: Similar to type I, but associated with a meningocele at the craniocervical junction into which the prolapsed cerebellar tissue has descended.

Type IV: Hypoplasia of the cerebellar hemisphere with an enlarged fourth ventricle. This is not considered a type of dysraphism.

Type I is not necessarily associated with hydrocephalus, and symptoms, if they occur at all, are due to impaction and embarrassment of the brainstem at the foramen magnum. It is one of the conditions associated with a communicating syringomyelia. *Type II* is the most common of these abnormalities. It is usually associated with spina bifida. Obstruction to the outflow of cerebrospinal fluid (CSF) from the fourth ventricle leads to hydrocephalus, while compression of the brainstem can result in abnormalities affecting all the functions contained within it. One further syndrome may occur. With the obliteration of the outlets of the fourth ventricle, CSF is now pumped downward from the fourth ventricle into the central canal of the spinal cord, which may in turn become dilated causing the clinical complex known as syringomyelia.

Arnold J (1894): Myelocyste, transposition von Gewebskeimen und Sympodie. *Beihr Pathol Anat* 16:1–28.

Carmel PW, Markesbery WR (1972): Early descriptions of the Arnold-Chiari malformation: the contribution of John Cleland. *J Neurosurg* 37: 543–547.

Chiari H (1896): Über Verandeningen des Kleinhirns infolge von Hydrocephalie des Grosshirns. *Dtsch Med Wochenschr* 17:1172.

Chiari H (1896): Über Verandeningen des Kleinhirns, des Pons und der Medulla oblongata in Folge von congenitaler Hydrocephalie des Grosshirns. *Denschr Akad Wiss Wien* 63:71.

7. SPINAL ARTERIOVENOUS MALFORMATIONS (Figs. 5–9)

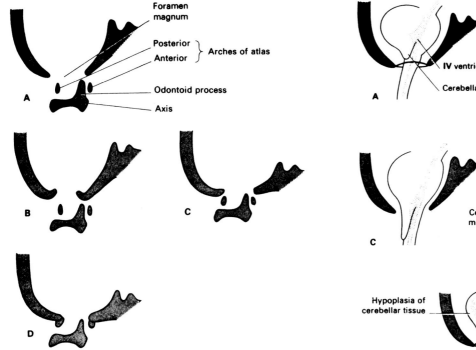

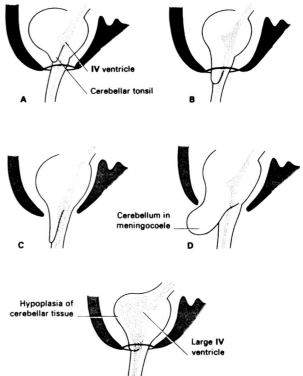

FIGURE 3. Schematic representation of a lateral view of the craniocervical junction. **A:** Normal. **B:** Basilar invagination or impression. **C:** Platybasia. Flattening of the skull base with a small posterior fossa, short clivus, and high odontoid. **D:** Platybasia and fusion of the atlas to the skull base. (From Hayward R [1980]: Skull and brain abnormalities. In: Essentials in neurosurgery. London: Blackwell, 1980, with permission.)

FIGURE 4. The Chiari malformations. **A:** Normal. **B:** Chiari type I. **C:** Chiari type II (Arnold-Chiari). **D:** Chiari type III. **E:** Chiari type IV. (From Hayward R [1980]: Skull and brain abnormalities. In *Essentials of neurosurgery.* London: Blackwell, with permission.)

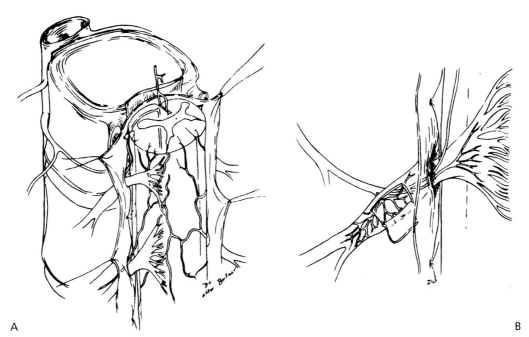

FIGURE 5. Normal vasculature of the spinal cord. **A:** The spinal ramus of each intercostal artery divides after entering the intervertebral foramen and penetrating the surface of the dura, into dural arteries, which supply the root sleeve and spinal dura, and radicular arteries, which supply the anterior and posterior nerve roots. In addition, the spinal ramus of the intercostal artery also is the origin of a medullary artery in a sporadic fashion. **B:** This vessel enters the dura adjacent to the nerve root ganglion, after which it ascends and joins an anterior or posterolateral spinal artery to supply the spinal parenchyma. The spinal cord is drained by radial veins, which carry blood to the coronal venous plexus, which is, in turn, drained by medullary veins, which pierce the dura adjacent to the nerve roots.

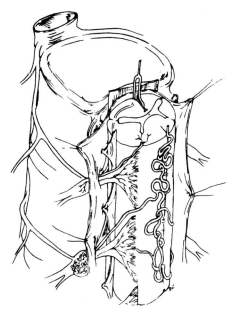

FIGURE 6. Dural arteriovenous (AV) fistula. The dural AV fistula is supplied by a dural artery and is drained by a medullary vein, which carries blood retrograde to the normal direction of venous drainage to the coronal venous plexus. The coronal plexus becomes elongated, tortuous, thickened, and dilated by the increased venous pressure, which is, in turn, transmitted to the cord tissue and causes myelopathy.

A. Dural Arteriovenous Fistulas (Type I)

B. Intradural Arteriovenous Malformations (AVMs)

- Glomus AVMs (Type II)
- Juvenile AVMs (Type III)
- Direct arteriovenous fistulas (Type IV)

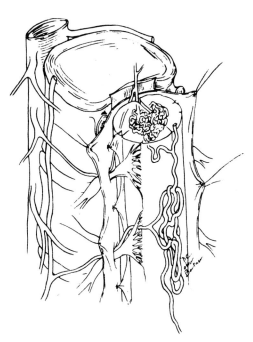

FIGURE 7. Glomus arteriovenous malformations (AVMs). The nidus of the glomus type of intramedullary AVM is a tightly packed congeries of blood vessels confined to a short segment of the spinal cord. It receives its blood supply from spinal medullary arteries.

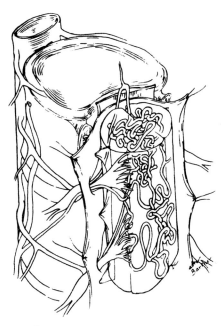

FIGURE 8. Juvenile arteriovenous malformations (AVMs). The juvenile type of intramedullary AVM is fed by medullary arteries through the anterior and posterolateral spinal arteries. The nidus of the AVM is large, often fills the spinal canal, and contains cord tissue within the interstices of the vessels of the AVM.

C. Extradural Venous Varices (Type V)

D. Associated Conditions With Intradural Spinal AVMs

- Other arteriovenous malformations
- Cerebral aneurysms
- Vascular agenesis/hypoplasia
- Rendu-Osler-Weber syndrome
- Klippel-Trenaunay-Weber syndrome

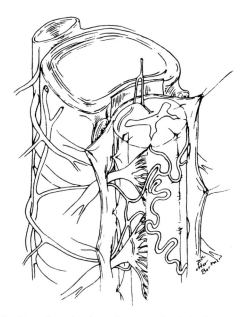

FIGURE 9. Direct intradural arteriovenous fistula in the pia. Medullary arteries provide the arterial supply.

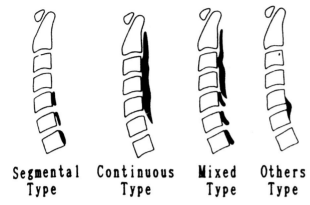

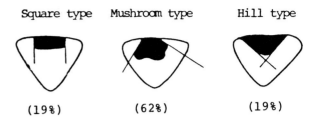

FIGURE 11. Classification of ossification of the posterior longitudinal ligament (OPLL) as seen on computed tomography (CT) scan. CT is particularly helpful in determining the existence of OPLL as well as its thickness, lateral extension, shape, and the extent of narrowing of the spinal canal. (From Hirabayashi K, Satomi K, Sasaki T [1989]: Ossification of the posterior longitudinal ligament in the cervical spine. In The Cervical Spine Research Society, ed. *The cervical spine.* Phildelphia: JB Lippincott, 1989, with permission.)

FIGURE 10. Classification of ossification of the posterior longitudinal ligament as seen on lateral radiographic views: *segmental type,* in which ossification is observed behind individual vertebral bodies; *continuous type,* in which ossification is observed through several vertebrae; *mixed type,* which is a combination of segmental and mixed; and other types, in which ossification is observed over the intervertebral disc space. (From Hirabayashi K, Miyakawa J, Satomi K, et al. [1981]: Operative results and postoperative progression of ossifications among patients with ossification of cervical posterior longitudinal ligament. *Spine* 6:354–364, with permission.)

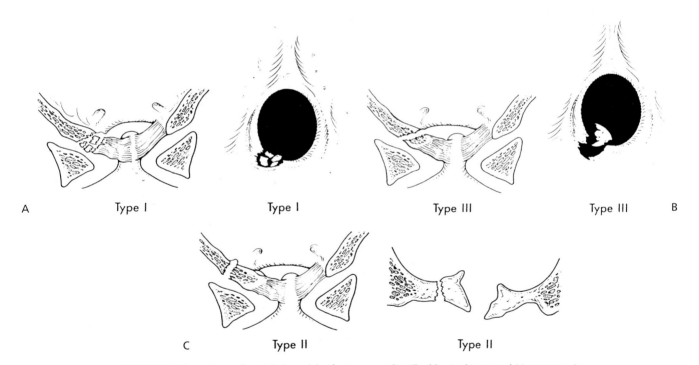

FIGURE 12. Three types of occipital condylar fractures, as described by Anderson and Montesano. **A:** *Type I:* Impacted fracture. **B:** *Type II:* Basilar skull fracture. **C:** *Type III:* Avulsion fracture (Redrawn from Anderson PA, Montesano PX [1988]: Morphology and treatment of occipital condyle fractures. *Spine* 13:731.)

8. OSSIFICATION OF THE POSTERIOR LONGITUDINAL LIGAMENT IN THE CERVICAL SPINE (Figs. 10, 11)

9. FRACTURES OF THE OCCIPITAL CONDYLES (Fig. 12)

10. CRANIOCERVICAL TRAUMA WITH INJURIES AROUND THE C1–C2 COMPLEX (Figs. 13, 14)

A. Jefferson's Fracture

Jefferson's fracture is a bursting of the ring of C1 as a result of axial loading. An anteroposterior view generally shows widening of the distance between the odontoid and lateral masses of C1. Spence's rule is that the overhang from the lateral masses of C1 on each side should not be more than 6.9 mm. Fractures are classified as stable if the transverse ligament is intact and unstable when it is ruptured. (Fig. 13)

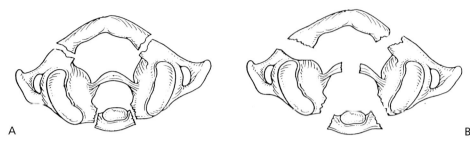

FIGURE 13. **A:** Drawing indicating axial view of stable Jefferson's fracture (transverse ligament intact). **B:** Drawing indicating axial view of unstable Jefferson's fracture (transverse ligament ruptured). (Redrawn from Schlicke LH, Callahan R [1981]: A rational approach to burst fractures of the atlas. *Clin Orthop* 154:18).

FIGURE 14. Craniocervical trauma with injuries around the C1–C2 complex. In injuries high in the cervical spine, there is a series of fractures that occur depending on the major vector of the traumatic force. As represented in this clock of injuries, the vector of force at 12 o'clock is distraction, at 3 o'clock is forced extension, at 6 o'clock is compression, and at 9 o'clock is forced flexion. When these vectors cause trauma at the C1–C2 complex, including the cranial junction, there are known injury patterns. If the resultant injury is severe with marked malalignment, the majority of the patients are killed instantaneously or die soon afterward for lack of respiration and cardiovascular support. Such injuries, which cause complete cord damage, give not only paralysis but also give a complete sympathectomy and destroy all drive for respiration, including the phrenic nerve function. However, many injuries through this area give an incomplete cord injury or do hardly any damage to the nervous system at all. Each of these injuries is discussed separately in this chapter.

At *12 o'clock,* there is primarily a distraction injury wherein the condyles of the occiput are pulled from the C1–C2 complex. This particular injury is more likely to be seen on the lateral skull radiograph as opposed to a lateral cervical spine radiograph. Also, it can occur in young children, in whom the head is much bigger in proportion to the body. It is also commonly reported in those patients sustaining an injury who are killed in the accident wherein there is no other obvious reason for death.

At *2 o'clock,* the extension injury may cause a high fracture of the odontoid process itself. There is usually retrolisthesis of the C1 complex on the C2 vertebral body and its surrounding lamina and spinous process.

At *3 o'clock,* the extension injury often causes fractures through the lamina of C1 and C2. If the fracture through C2 comes more anteriorly, then it will cause traumatic spondylolosis. Even on rare occasions, the odontoid may be fractured as well.

At *4 o'clock,* one sees a typical hangman's fracture with a traumatic spondylolosis between the facet area of C2 and the major body of C2. The line of trauma will separate the body of C2 with all of C1, leaving behind the C2 lamina and spinous process, which are in turn attached to the C3 vertebra. The hangman's fracture can truly occur with hangings, but one will rarely see that clinically. More commonly, it is associated with a vehicular accident in which there is forced extension of the head and upper part of the spine on the mid and lower part of the cervical spine.

At *5 o'clock,* one is more likely to see a compression fracture into the body of C2. This may be a form of the type III odontoid fracture, where there is a burst in the body.

At *6 o'clock,* there tends to be two types of fractures. When the C1 vertebra alone is involved, some form of a Jefferson ring fracture is apparent. Or, in some lesions, the ring of C1 will be maintained and there will be a burst fracture of C2. Admittedly, the latter is rare but has been documented. This would be marked as a very severe type III odontoid fracture in select cases, but there is bursting of the body below.

At *7 o'clock,* there are various types of type II and type II odontoid fractures. If the force is considerably anterior as well as compressed, there will be a form of the type III fracture. However, as the force becomes more pure flexion, more likely the patient will suffer a type I fracture. On rare occasions, one can see the trauma as depicted at *8 o'clock,* usually with a devastating outcome to the patient. There is marked displacement on a type II fracture with disruption of the anterior ligaments.

At *9 o'clock,* one typically sees the type II dens fracture with displacement of the C1 vertebra along with the dens of C2 anteriorly.

At 10 o'clock, there can be disruption of the ligaments from the C1 vertebral body, which holds the peg of the C2 dens in alignment. This rupture of the cruciate ligament can lead to anterior displacement of C1 with all the bony elements of C2 being maintained.

At *11 o'clock,* there is the rare type I dens fracture. This is an avulsion fracture. It is rarely documented.

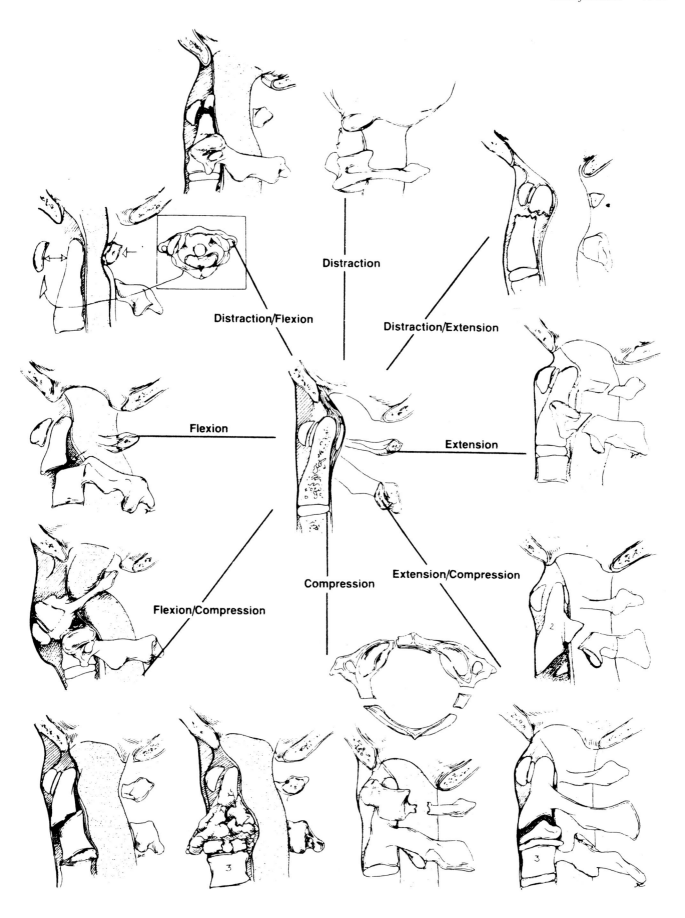

Distraction

Distraction/Flexion

Distraction/Extension

Flexion

Extension

Flexion/Compression

Compression

Extension/Compression

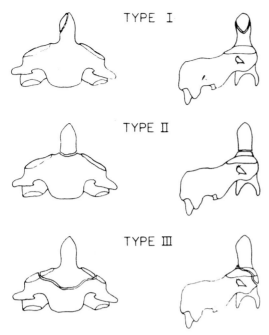

TYPE I

TYPE II

TYPE III

FIGURE 15. Three types of odontoid fractures as seen in the anteroposterior and lateral planes: *Type I* is an oblique fracture through the upper part of the odontoid process itself. *Type II* is a fracture at the junction of the odontoid process with the vertebral body of the second cervical vertebra. *Type III* is really a fracture through the body of the axis. (From Anderson LD, D'Alonzo RT [1974]: Fractures of the odontoid process of the axis. *J Bone Joint Surg [Am]* 56:1663–1674, with permission.)

B. Fractures of the Odontoid Process of the Axis (Odontoid Fractures as Classified by Anderson and D'Alonzo) (Fig. 15)

Clark CR, White AA (1985): Fractures of the dens: a multicenter study. *J Bone Joint Surg [Am]* 67:1340–1348.

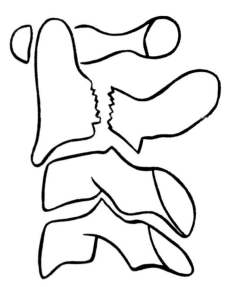

FIGURE 17. *Type II:* Fractures with both significant angulation and significant displacement. (From Levine AM, Edwards CC [1985]: The management of traumatic spondylolisthesis of the axis. *J Bone Joint Surg [Am]* 67:217–226, with permission.)

C. Traumatic Spondylolisthesis of the Axis (Hangman's Fracture) (Figs. 16–21)

11. FRACTURES AND DISLOCATIONS OF THE LOWER CERVICAL SPINE (Fig. 22)

A. Fractures and Dislocations of the Lower Cervical Spine (Fig. 23)

McAfee PC (1991): Cervical spine trauma. In: Frymoyer JW, ed. *The adult spine: principles and practice.* New York: Raven Press.

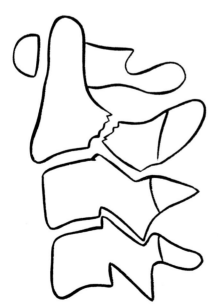

FIGURE 16. *Type I:* Fracture through the neural arch with no angulation and as much as 3 mm of displacement. (From Levine AM, Edwards CC [1985]: The management of traumatic spondylolisthesis of the axis. *J Bone Joint Surg [Am]* 67:217–226, with permission.)

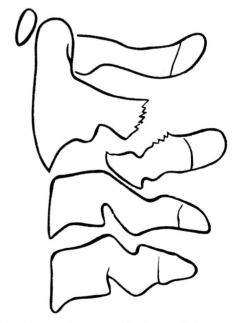

FIGURE 18. *Type IIA:* Fractures with minimal displacement but with severe angulation, apparently hinging from the anterior longitudinal ligament. (From Levine AM, Edwards CC [1985]: The management of traumatic spondylolisthesis of the axis. *J Bone Joint Surg [Am]* 67: 217–226, with permission.)

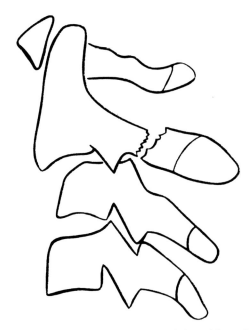

FIGURE 19. *Type III:* Fractures that combine bilateral facet dislocation between the second and third cervical vertebrae with a fracture of the neural arch. (From Levine AM, Edwards CC [1985]: The management of traumatic spondylolisthesis of the axis. *J Bone Joint Surg [Am]* 67: 217–226, with permission.)

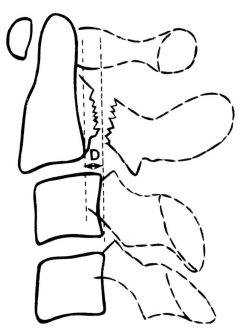

FIGURE 21. Anterior translation is measured as the distance between a line drawn parallel to the posterior margin of the body of the third cervical vertebra and the posterior margin of the second cervical vertebra at the level of the disc space between the second and the third cervical vertebrae. (From Levine AM, Edwards CC [1985]: The management of traumatic spondylolisthesis of the axis. *J Bone Joint Surg [Am]* 67:217–226, with permission.)

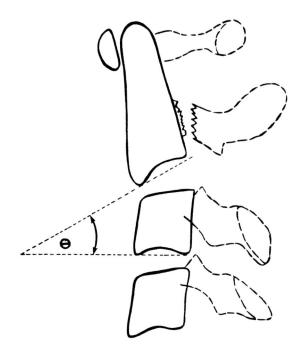

FIGURE 20. Angulation is calculated as the angle between the inferior end plate of the second cervical vertebra and the inferior end plate of the third cervical vertebra. (From Levine AM, Edwards CC [1985]: The management of traumatic spondylolisthesis of the axis. *J Bone Joint Surg [Am]* 67:217–226, with permission.)

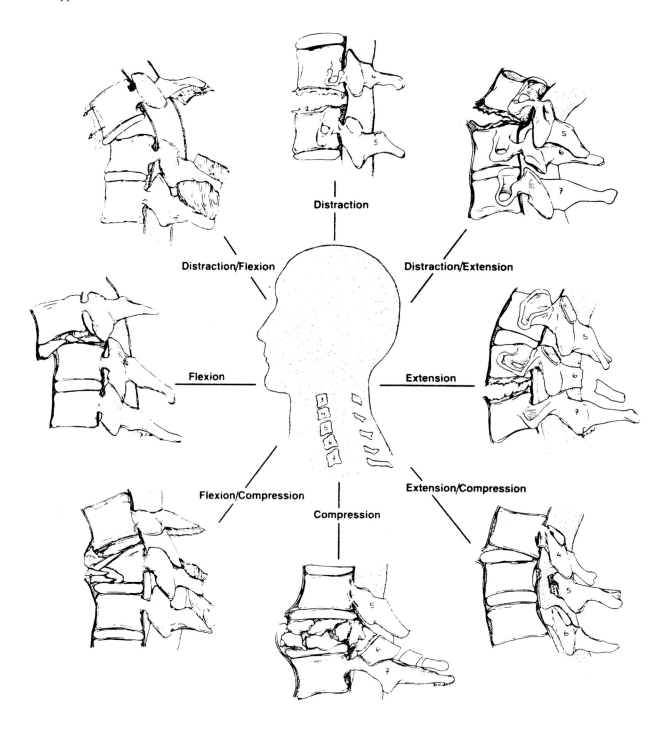

Distraction

Distraction/Flexion

Distraction/Extension

Flexion

Extension

Flexion/Compression

Compression

Extension/Compression

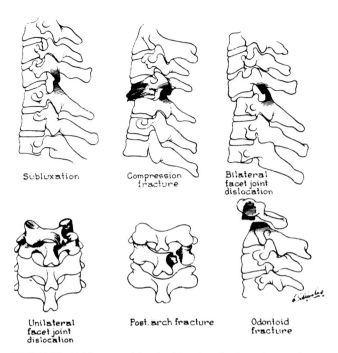

Subluxation   Compression fracture   Bilateral facet joint dislocation

Unilateral facet joint dislocation   Post. arch fracture   Odontoid fracture

FIGURE 23. Robinson and Southwick's classification of cervical spine injuries.

Robinson RA, Southwick WO (1960): Surgical approaches to the cervical spine. *AAOS Instr Course Lect* 17:299–330.

B. Mechanistic Classification of Fractures and Dislocations of the Lower Cervical Spine (Figs. 24–29)

Compression flexion: five stages
Vertical compression: three stages
Distractive flexion: four stages
Compressive extension: five stages
Distractive extension: two stages
Lateral flexion: two stages

The hypotheses on which this classification is based are as follows:

- The forces producing either fracture or dislocation of the cervical spine can be considered as major and minor injury vectors.
- The injury vectors can be deduced from the radiographic examination of the cervical spine.
- The magnitude of the vectors determines the severity of an injury.
- Similar injuries result from similar injury vectors.
- Within a given injury mechanism, there is a spectrum of injury, a phylogeny, which ranges from trivial to severe.

Allen BL Jr, Ferguson RL, Lehmann TR, O'Brien RP (1982): A mechanistic classification of closed, indirect fractures and dislocations of the lower cervical spine. *Spine* 7:1–27.

Rizzolo SJ, Cotler JM (1993): Unstable cervical spine injuries: specific treatment approaches. *J Am Acad Orthop Surg* 1:57–66.

FIGURE 22. Mid and lower cervical spinal fractures involve the vertebrae 3 through 7 and do follow a common pattern. This clock of injuries (see also Figure 12) again shows 12 o'clock with distraction, 3 o'clock with extension, 6 o'clock with compression, and 9 o'clock with flexion injuries.

At *1* or *2 o'clock,* extension injuries in the midcervical spine can cause disruption of the anterior longitudinal ligament with some posterior displacement of the superior or cephalad vertebrae on the more caudal vertebrae. When there is some forced extension, as in the *3 o'clock* injury, there may be fracture of the spinous process, and even the lamina. This is to be differentiated from a stress fracture, referred to as clay shoveler's fracture, which occurs on the C7 spinous process.

A *4 o'clock* injury represents a forced extension injury, wherein there is some form of fracture through the facet area, like an incomplete spondylolosis, which is seen in the lumbar spine or seen at C2. All of the injuries at 2 o'clock, at 3 o'clock, and at 4 o'clock can occur in the elderly population in whom there is preexisting cervical spondylytic stenosis. When the injuries occur in the elderly patient, there is buckling of the disc and joint space anteriorly into the canal, and buckling of the inner spinous ligament and the ligamentum flavum posteriorly to squeeze the spinal canal and squeeze the spinal cord to give the central cord syndrome.

With further compression injuries, as seen at *6 o'clock,* the patient typically suffers a burst fracture. If there is a strong vector posteriorly, the bones may be displaced posteriorly. If there is a strong vector more anteriorly, the bones can be displaced and malaligned anteriorly. With the bursting of the fracture, the bone segments are in many pieces. Typically, bone is fractured back into the spinal canal to compress the spinal cord.

At *7* and *8 o'clock,* there is a combination of flexion and compression. The vertebral body anteriorly will fracture. There is permanent compression anteriorly. There may be posterior disruption of the inner spinous ligaments. If these injuries are mild, the neurologic deficit is not great, and the disc material may not be ruptured back into the canal, although that can occur.

At *9 o'clock,* the flexion injury causes either a unilateral or bilateral facet dislocation. There may be various fractures of the facet. In these injuries, the disc material is often disrupted. There is always a fear that the disc may be dislodged back in the canal with alignment.

At *10* and *11 o'clock,* there may be forced distraction injuries in which the posterior elements are torn and the vertebral bodies themselves are intact, along with the disc space. In some of these patients, the muscle spasm will cause the spine to realign, yet the neurologic injury may be quite devastating. In other cases, the muscle spasms will cause the spine to malalign with either a unilateral or bilateral facet dislocation. In these patients, the neurologic deficit is often severe and often will ascend above the level of the trauma.

Finally, the *12 o'clock* injuries, which are seen when there are separations of C4–5, are usually only documented after a forced flexion injury with traction maintained at a joint where there was complete ligamentous disruption. Obviously these lesions are very unstable. More likely, the distraction injuries will occur higher in the cervical spine.

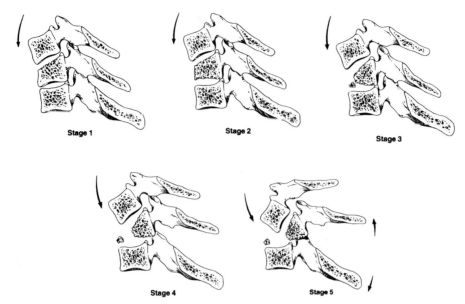

FIGURE 24. Allen and Ferguson classification of traumatic cervical spine injuries. Compression flexion injury. *Stage 1:* Blunting and rounding off of anterosuperior vertebral margin. *Stage 2:* Loss of anterior height and beaklike appearance anteroinferiorly. *Stage 3:* Fracture line from anterior surface of vertebral body extending obliquely through the subcondral plate (a fractured beak). *Stage 4:* Some displacement (< 3 mm) of the posteroinferior vertebral margin into the neural canal. *Stage 5:* Displacement (> 3 mm) of the posterior part of vertebral body. Although vertebral arch is intact, entire posterior ligamentous complex is ruptured (From Rizzolo SJ, Cotler JM [1993]: Unstable cervical spine injuries: specific treatment approaches. *J Am Acad Orthop Surg* 1:57–66.)

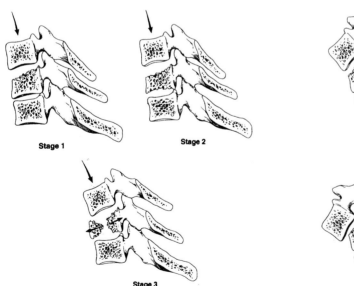

FIGURE 25. Allen and Ferguson classification of traumatic cervical spine injuries. Vertical compression injuries. *Stage 1:* Central cupping fracture of superior or inferior end plate. *Stage 2:* Similar to stage 1, but fracture of both end plates; any fracture of the centrum is minimal. *Stage 3:* Fragmentation and displacement of vertebral body. (From Rizzolo SJ, Cotler JM [1993]: Unstable cervical spine injuries: specific treatment approaches. *J Am Acad Orthop Surg* 1:57–66.)

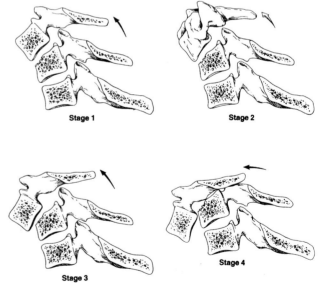

FIGURE 26. Allen and Ferguson classification of traumatic cervical spine injuries. Distraction flexion injury. *Stage 1:* Facet subluxation in flexion and divergence of spinous processes (flexion sprain); some blunting of anterosuperior vertebral margin as in a stage 1 compression flexion injury. *Stage 2:* Unilateral facet dislocation; there may be some rotary spondylolisthesis. *Stage 3:* Bilateral facet dislocation with about 50% anterior vertebral body displacement. Facets may have completely leap frogged over those below or may be "perched." *Stage 4:* Full width vertebral body displacement or completely unstable motion segment. (From Rizzolo SJ, Cotler JM [1993]: Unstable cervical spine injuries: specific treatment approaches. *J Am Acad Orthop Surg* 1:57–66.)

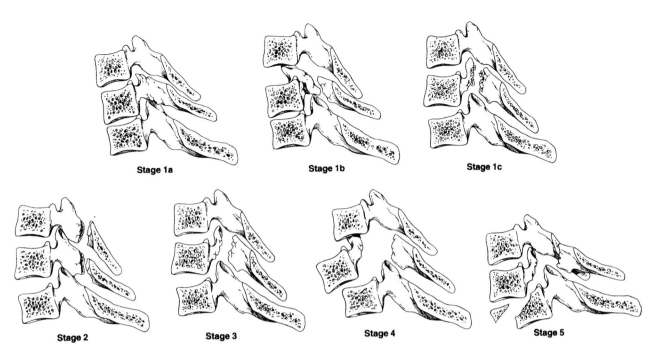

FIGURE 27. Allen and Ferguson classification of traumatic cervical spine injuries. Compression extension injury. *Stage 1:* Unilateral vertebral arch fracture; may be through articular process (stage 1a), pedicle (stage 1b), or lamina (stage 1c); there may be rotary spondylolisthesis of centrum. *Stage 2:* Bilaminar fracture, which may be at multiple contiguous levels. *Stage 3:* Hypothetical modes not seen clinically by authors of classification, characterized by bilateral fractures of vertebral arch (articular processes, pedicles, or laminae) and partial-width anterior vertebral body displacement. *Stage 4:* Partial-width anterior vertebral body displacement. *Stage 5:* Full-width anterior vertebral body displacement. (From Rizzolo SJ, Cotler JM [1993]: Unstable cervical spine injuries: specific treatment approaches. *J Am Acad Orthop Surg* 1:57–66.)

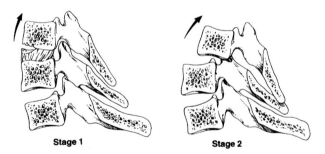

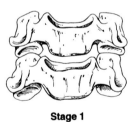 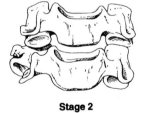

FIGURE 28. Allen and Ferguson classification of traumatic cervical spine injuries. Distractive extension injury. *Stage 1:* Failure of anterior ligamentous complex. Injury may be a nondeforming transverse fracture through the centrum or widening of disk space. *Stage 2:* Injury may be anterior marginal avulsion fracture of centrum. Some posterior ligamentous complex failure may be revealed by posterior displacement of upper vertebra. Fracture reduces in flexion. (From Rizzolo SJ, Cotler JM [1993]: Unstable cervical spine injuries: specific treatment approaches. *J Am Acad Orthop Surg* 1:57–66.)

FIGURE 29. Allen and Ferguson classification of traumatic cervical spine injuries. Lateral flexion injury. *Stage 1:* Asymmetric compression fracture of centrum with associated vertebral arch fracture ipsilaterally; anteroposterior film shows no displacement. *Stage 2:* Displacement of ipsilateral arch fracture seen on anteroposterior view. There also may be ligamentous tension failure on contralateral side with facet separation. (From Rizzolo SJ, Cotler JM [1993]: Unstable cervical spine injuries: specific treatment approaches. *J Am Acad Orthop Surg* 1:57–66.)

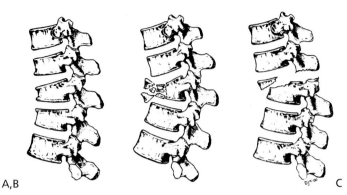

A,B   C

FIGURE 30. A: Simple wedge fracture. **B:** Comminuted fracture. **C:** Fracture-dislocation.

12. THORACOLUMBAR SPINE FRACTURES

A. Watson-Jones Classification

According to Watson-Jones, three types of vertebral body fractures are to be distinguished (Fig. 30).

Watson-Jones R (1938): The results of postural reduction of fractures of the spine. *J Bone Joint Surg [Am]* 20:567–586.

B. Nicoll Classification (1949)

Nicoll classified thoracolumbar fractures into four main types:

1. Anterior wedge fracture
2. Lateral wedge fracture
3. Fracture-dislocation
4. Isolated fractures of the neural arch

Nicoll considered stable fractures to be all anterior and lateral wedge fractures and all laminar fractures above the fourth lumbar level. Unstable fractures included fracture-dislocations and all laminar fractures at the level of the fourth and fifth lumbar level.

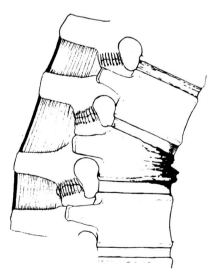

FIGURE 31. Diagram of a wedge compression fracture of the vertebral body. The posterior ligament complex is intact. (From Holdsworth FW [1963]: Fractures, dislocations and fracture-dislocations of the spine. *J Bone Joint Surg [Br]* 45:6–20, with permission.)

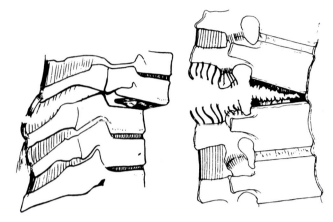

FIGURE 32. Diagrams of dislocations of the cervical and of the lumbar spine. The posterior ligament complex is ruptured in each case. More flexion is necessary to dislocate the lumbar spine than to dislocate the cervical spine. (From Holdsworth FW [1963]: Fractures, dislocations and fracture-dislocations of the spine. *J Bone Joint Surg [Br]* 45:6–20, with permission.)

Nicoll EA (1949): Fractures of the dorso-lumbar spine. *J Bone Joint Surg [Br]* 31:376–394.

C. Holdsworth Classification (1963)

According to Holdsworth, the spine may be subjected to four types of violence: flexion, flexion and rotation, extension, and compression. The type of fracture, dislocation, or fracture-dislocation that results from each of these types of violence will depend on whether or not the posterior ligament complex is ruptured and on the part of the spine involved. This classification is based on a two-column subdivision of the spine.

Compression fractures result from pure *flexion*. Most common in the thoracic and lumbar spine, these are stable injuries (Fig. 31).

With *flexion-rotation* violence the posterior ligament ruptures and a pure dislocation results. Pure dislocations are unstable (Fig. 32). Rotation or flexion-rotation may result in fracture-dislocation in the lumbar spine. These are generally very unstable injuries (Fig. 33).

In pure *extension,* either the posterior elements (lamina and pedicles) fracture or an extension dislocation occurs. This is common in the cervical spine as a result of "whiplash" injuries (Fig. 34) *Compression* leads to the comminuted "burst fracture" (Fig. 35).

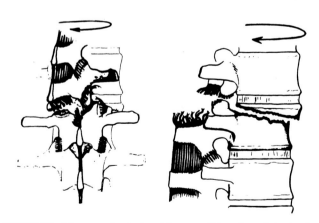

FIGURE 33. Diagram of rotational fracture-dislocation of the lumbar spine. The posterior ligament complex is ruptured, and the vertebral body is fractured. This is a very unstable injury. (From Holdsworth FW [1963]: Fractures, dislocations and fracture-dislocations of the spine. *J Bone Joint Surg [Br]* 45:6–20, with permission.)

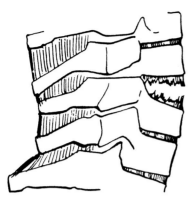

FIGURE 34. Diagram of extension injury. The anterior common ligament is ruptured. The posterior complex is intact. (From Holdsworth FW [1963]: Fractures, dislocations and fracture-dislocations of the spine. *J Bone Joint Surg [Br]* 45:6–20, with permission.)

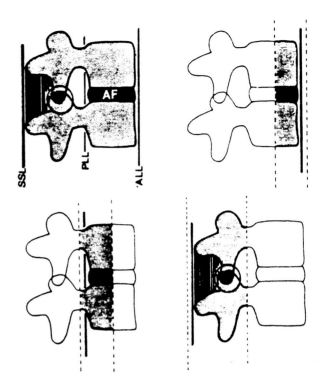

FIGURE 36. The three-column spine. The anterior column is formed by the anterior longitudinal ligament, the anterior annulus fibrosus, and the anterior part of the vertebral body. The middle column is formed by the posterior longitudinal ligament, the posterior annulus fibrosus, and the posterior wall of the vertebral body. The posterior column is formed by the posterior bony complex (posterior arch), alternating with the posterior ligamentous complex (supraspinous ligament, interspinous ligament, capsule, and ligamentum flavum). (From Denis F [1983]: The three-column spine and its significance in the classification of acute thoracolumbar spinal injuries. *Spine* 8:817–831, with permission.)

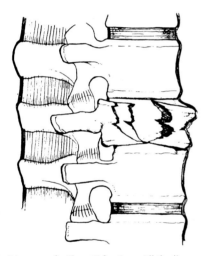

FIGURE 35. Diagram of a "burst" fracture. All the ligaments are intact. (From Holdsworth FW [1963]: Fractures, dislocations and fracture-dislocations of the spine. *J Bone Joint Surg [Br]* 45:6–20, with permission.)

Holdsworth FW (1970): Fractures, dislocations and fracture-dislocations of the spine. *J Bone Joint Surg [Br]* 52:1534–1551.

D. Denis Classification

Denis popularized the concept of the *three-column theory* (Fig. 36; Table 3). Denis classified spinal fractures into major and minor injuries. He identified four major types of spinal injuries: compression fractures, burst fractures, seatbelt injuries, and fracture-dislocations. The key in distinguishing among these injuries is the middle column's mode of failure.

TABLE 3. BASIC MODES OF FAILURE OF THE THREE COLUMNS IN THE FOUR MAJOR TYPES OF SPINAL INJURIES

	Column		
Type	Anterior	Middle	Posterior
Compression	Compression	None	None or distraction (severe)
Burst	Compression	Compression	None or splaying of pedicles
Flexion-distraction	None or distraction	Distraction	Distraction
Fracture/dislocation	Compression	Distraction	Distraction
	Rotation	Rotation	Rotation
	Shear	Shear	Shear

From Denis F (1985): The three-column spine and its significance in the classification of acute thoracolumbar spinal injuries. *Spine* 8:817–831, with permission.
In seat belt-type injuries, the component of compression failure on the anterior column is either absent or minimal and takes place in the anterior part of the vertebral body (collapse of about 10% to 20% of the anterior height).

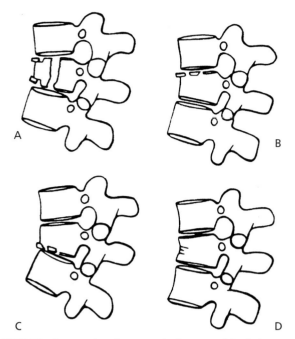

FIGURE 37. Compression fractures. **A:** Fracture of both lower and upper end plates. **B:** Isolated fracture of the upper end plate. **C:** Lower end plate fracture. **D:** Lateral compression (this is best identified in the frontal plane, anteroposterior radiographic view). (From Denis F [1983]: The three-column spine and its significance in the classification of acute thoracolumbar spinal injuries. *Spine* 8:817–831, with permission.)

In compression fractures, the middle column is not injured and the fracture is stable. In burst fractures, the middle column fails in compression and the injury is most likely unstable. In shearing injuries, such as the seat-belt–related fractures, the middle column fails in distraction, whereas in fracture-dislocations, the middle column fails in rotation or shear. In addition to the injury to individual motion segments of the spine, stability relates to the presence or absence of neurologic injury.

(1) Compression Fractures

Compression fractures result from an axial load combined with flexion or lateral bend (Fig. 37). They are the most common injury, comprising 89% of Denis' series. If the loss of vertebral body height is less than 50% (40% according to some authors) or the angled deformity is less than 20°, the fractures have been considered stable. In instances in which compression injuries are contiguous, the angulatory and compression deformities are summated. The two subtypes of compression fractures are anterior and lateral. The most frequent type of compression fracture involves fracture of the upper end plate of the vertebra in its anterior portion; however, other types occur.

(2) Burst Fractures

The burst fracture results from failure of the vertebral body under axial load (Fig. 38). The essential feature of the burst injury is disruption of the middle column with varying degrees of retropulsion into the neural canal, best identified on CT scans. Involvement of the posterior elements is common. When the posterior elements are involved, neurologic injury is present in 50% of the cases. The neural injury may be the result of neural element entrapment in laminal fractures. Dural laceration is to be anticipated. Five subtypes have been identified by Denis, based on which end plate is involved and on the rotational or lateral flexion component.

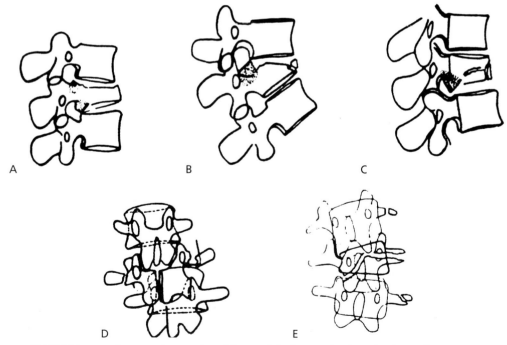

FIGURE 38. Burst fractures. Types A, B, and C are mainly diagnosed on lateral radiographic views: *Type A:* Fracture of both endplates, seen in the low lumbar region. Its mechanism is pure axial load. *Type B:* Fracture of the superior end plate. This is the most frequent burst fracture. It is seen at the thoracolumbar junction. The mechanism of injury is axial load and flexion. *Type C:* Fracture of the inferior end plate. This fracture is rare. The mechanism of injury also appears to be axial load and flexion. *Type D:* Burst rotation. This is typically a midlumbar fracture, which could be misdiagnosed as a fracture-dislocation. The mechanism of injury is axial load and rotation. *Type E:* Burst lateral flexion. This fracture results from axial load and lateral flexion. It differs from the lateral compression fracture in that the posterior wall of the vertebral body fractures, allowing retropulsion of bone back into the canal. (From Denis F [1983]: The three-column spine and its significance in the classification of acute thoracolumbar spinal injuries. *Spine* 8:817–831, with permission.)

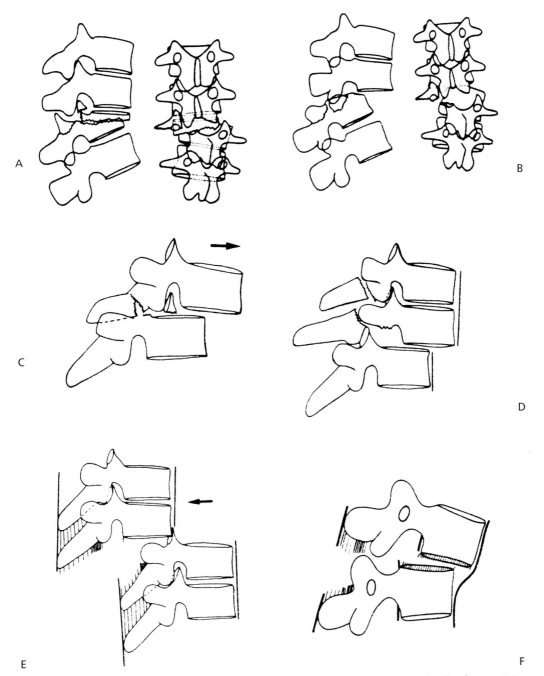

FIGURE 39. Fracture-dislocations. **A:** Flexion rotation through the vertebral body "slice fracture." **B:** Flexion rotation through the disc. It is accompanied by unilateral fracture of the superior articular process. **C:** Posteroanterior shear injury. Intact anterior vertebral bodies and fracture of the superior articular facet, which has been sheared off by the anterior. The spinous process or entire posterior arch may be fractured by the same mechanism. **D:** Posteroanterior shear injury in which a large part of the posterior arch may be left behind (floating lamina). **E:** Anteroposterior shear injury. The posterior arches and anterior vertebral bodies may be entirely intact, but the three ligamentous columns are disrupted. **F:** Flexion distraction. The posterior, middle, and anterior ligamentous columns are disrupted but for the anterior longitudinal ligament, which strips off the vertebral body below. (From Denis F [1983]: The three-column spine and its significance in the classification of acute thoracolumbar spinal injuries. *Spine* 8:817–831, with permission.)

(3) Fracture-Dislocations

Fracture-dislocation injuries are unstable because all three columns have failed (Fig. 39). Multiple forces are involved, including rotation, distraction, compression, and shear. In general, these injuries are divided into

I: Flexion rotation
II: Shear
III: Flexion-distraction

Gertzbein and Eismont have added a fourth category: the combined dislocation-burst injury.

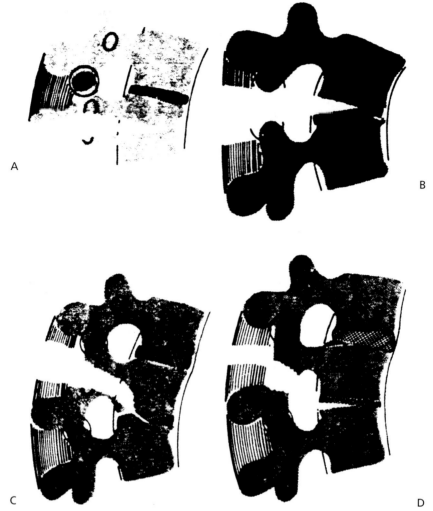

FIGURE 40. Seat-belt–type injuries: flexion distraction injuries. **A:** One-level, through bone (Chance fracture). **B:** One-level, through the ligaments. **C:** Two-level, through bone at the level of the middle column. **D:** Two-level, through ligaments at the level of the middle column. (From Denis F [1983]: The three-column spine and its significance in the classification of acute thoracolumbar spinal injuries. *Spine* 8:817–831, with permission.)

(4) Seat-Belt Injuries

(a) *Seat-Belt–Type Spinal Injuries (Flexion Distraction Injuries) in Adults*

The seat-belt–type of injury represents failure of both the posterior and middle columns under tension forces generated by flexion and sometimes by superadded distraction (Fig. 40)

(b) *Seat-Belt Fractures in Children (Fig. 41)*

(5) Fractures (Slipping of the Vertebral apophysis) (Fig. 42)

Slipping of the apophysis can be classified into three types according to radiographic appearance:

Type I: Separation of the posterior rim of the involved vertebra. A calcified arc is seen on CT scan with no evidence of associated large bony fracture. This type is most common in children aged 11 to 13.

Type II: Avulsion fracture of part of the vertebral body, annular rim, and cartilage. This type is most common in adolescents and young adults aged 13 to 18 years.

Type III: More localized injury that includes smaller posterior irregularities of the cartilaginous end plate. This is most common in young adults older than age 18 years.

Type IV: Spans the entire length and breadth of the posterior vertebral margin between end plates.

Epstein NE, Epstein JA (1991): Limbus lumbar vertebral fractures in 27 adolescents and adults. *Spine* 16:962–966.

Epstein NE, Epstein JA, Mauri T (1989): Treatment of fractures of the vertebral limbus and spinal stenosis in five adolescents and five adults. *Neurosurgery* 24:595–604.

(6) Isolated Injuries of the Posterior Elements (Minor Injuries)

Transverse process fractures are the result of blunt trauma or violent contracture of the spinal musculature. When multiple fractures are present, or particularly when the L5 transverse process is fractured, there is a significant association with intraabdominal (renal) injuries and pelvic disruption. Occasionally, neuropraxias results, most typically involving the L3 and L4 nerve roots.

Spinous process avulsions are fairly rare in the lumbar spine and are usually the result of direct trauma.

Isolated facet fractures (articular process fractures) are uncommon but may occur in patients with prior laminectomies, most commonly by a fatigue, rather than an acute injury mechanism.

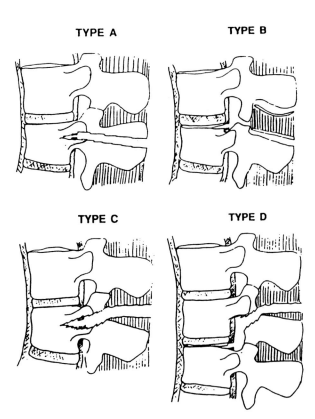

TYPE A   **TYPE B**

TYPE C   **TYPE D**

FIGURE 41. Seat-belt fracture patterns in skeletally immature children. *Type A* is a bony disruption of the posterior column extending just into the middle column. *Type B* is an avulsion of the posterior elements with facet joint disruption or fracture and extension into the apophysis of the vertebral body. *Type C* is a posterior ligamentous disruption with a fracture line entering the vertebra close to the pars interarticularis and extending into the middle column. *Type D* is a posterior ligamentous disruption with a fracture line traversing the lamina and extending into the apophysis of the adjacent vertebral body. (From Rumball K, Jarvis J [1992]: Seat-belt injuries of the spine in young children. *J Bone Joint Surg* 74B:571–574, with permission.)

Traumatic spondylolisthesis (pars interarticularis fracture) is rare compared with the far more common isthmic defect.

E. Flexion-Distraction Injuries (Gertzbein and Court-Brown)

Court-Brown and Gertzbein have further subdivided flexion-distraction injuries into three categories related to the posterior element fracture, the anterior column fracture, and the state of the vertebral body (Fig. 43).

F. Magerl Classification (1989)

Magerl and associates have proposed a classification based on morphologic injury patterns. Three basic forces (compression, distraction, rotation) produce main injury types. These types have been applied to all levels of the spine and are divided into A, B, and C with subcategories (A1, A2, A3, and so on), with the further subdivisions of 1, 2, and 3 indicating severity.

> *Type A:* Compression lesions (loss of vertebral body height)
>   *Type A1:* Body impaction
>   *Type A2:* Splitting
>   *Type A3:* Burst
> *Type B:* Distraction injuries
>   *Types B1 and B2:* Increased distance between posterior elements
>   *Type B3:* Increased distance between the anterior structures
> *Type C:* Torsional injuries, which are the most unstable injuries and are a combination of types A and B with rotation; there is anteroposterior element destruction with torsion

Magerl F, Harms H, Gertzbein S, Aebi M (1989): Classification of spinal fractures. Presented at a meeting of the American Academy of Orthopaedic Surgeons, Vail, Colorado, 1989.

13. SACRAL FRACTURES

Denis and Comfort have classified sacral fractures based on direction, location, and level of fracture (Fig. 44).

Zone I, the region of the ala, was occasionally associated with partial damage to the fifth lumbar root.

Zone II, the region of the sacral foramina, is frequently associated with sciatica but rarely with bladder dysfunction.

Zone III, the region of the central sacral canal, is frequently associated with saddle anesthesia and loss of sphincter function.

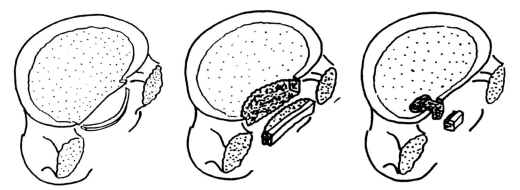

FIGURE 42. Schematic representation of the three types of avulsion fractures. In type I *(left),* an arcuate fragment is found, but no osseous defect is seen at the posterior rim of the vertebral body. Type II *(middle)* is an avulsion fracture of the posterior rim of the vertebral body that includes a rim of bone. The fragment is not arcuate, and it is thicker than in type I. The sharply avulsed osseous edge is recognized on computed tomograms. Type III *(right)* is a localized fracture posterior to an irregularity of the cartilage end plate. The osseous defect anterior to the fragment, as depicted on computed tomograms, is larger than the fragment. (From Tarr RW, et al. [1987]: Imaging of recent spinal trauma. *J Comput Assist Tomogr* 11:412–417.)

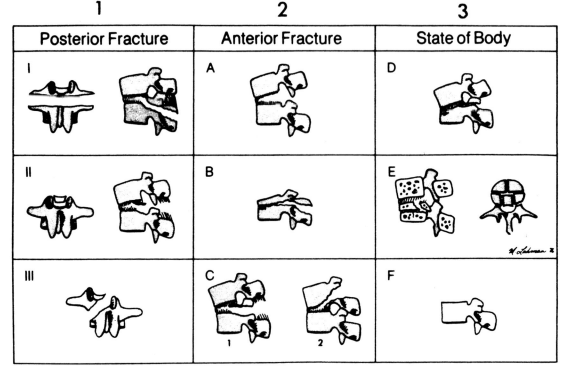

1	**2**	**3**
Posterior Fracture	Anterior Fracture	State of Body

FIGURE 43. Flexion-distraction injuries. *Posterior fractures:* In type I, the fracture line enters the spinous process and passes symmetrically through the laminae, transverse processes, and pedicles to enter the vertebral body. Type II is similarly symmetric, but the fracture line enters at the base of the spinous process. Type III enters obliquely, involving more of the posterior elements on one side than the other. *Anterior fractures:* There are three constant locations of the exiting anterior fracture in the vertebral body. Group A: The injury exits through the disc; Group B: the fracture passes through the vertebral body; Group C: extension occurs through the superior end plate (Subgroup 1) or the inferior end plate (Subgroup 2). State of the vertebral body: Group D: the injury may affect the vertebral body by a wedge compression fracture, or Group E: a burst injury, or Group F: the vertebral body may be intact. (From Gertzbein SD, Court-Brown CM [1988]: Flexion-distraction injuries of the lumbar spine. *Clin Orthop* 227: 52–60, with permission.)

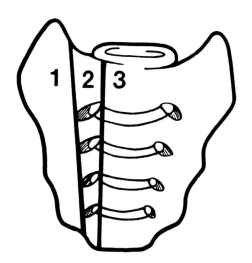

FIGURE 44. Denis classification of sacral fractures: *Zone I*—the region of the ala; *Zone II*—the region of the foramina; and *Zone III*—the region of the central canal. (From Denis F, Davis S, Comfort T [1988]: Sacral fractures: an important problem. *Clin Orthop* 227:67–81, with permission.)

Routine pelvic radiographs were almost useless in identifying the pathologic process in sacral injuries with neurologic symptoms. Computed tomography is recommended.

14. POSTTRAUMATIC NEUROLOGIC DEFICIT

A. Definitions

The definitions recommended by the American Spinal Injury Association (ASIA) in the booklet Standards for Neurological Classifications of Spinal Injury Patients, adapted from Austin, provide an accurate method of communicating information on the extent of neurologic injury.

(1) Manual Muscle Testing

Manual muscle testing is performed using the standard six-grade scale:

Absent = 0
Trace = 1, visible or palpable contraction
Poor = 2, active movement through range of motion with gravity eliminated
Fair = 3, active movement through range of motion against gravity
Good = 4, active movement through range of motion against resistance
Normal = 5

(2) Neurologic Level of Injury

The most caudal segment that tests as intact for both sensory and motor functions on both sides of the body is the neurological level of injury. If a muscle has at least a grade of "Fair," it is considered intact.

(3) Motor Level

The motor level is the level of the lowest key muscle having a grade of at least "Fair." All levels above the neurologic level of injury or motor level must be intact.

(4) Incomplete Spinal Cord Injury

When the preservation of sensory or motor function exists more than three neural segments below the neurologic level of injury, the spinal cord injury is incomplete. These patients have a good potential for progressive recovery of neurologic function. There are three basic syndromes that can be identified, each with its own specific physical findings and prognostic implications (Fig. 45).

(5) Complete Spinal Cord Injury

Complete spinal cord injury (SCI) means no preservation of motor and sensory function exists more than three segments below the neurologic level of injury. If the patient has no active muscle control or sensibility below the zone of injury, specifically with no retained perianal sensation or sphincter, one may diagnose a "presumed" complete lesion. The patient may be in spinal shock, however, which is a short period of paralysis, insensitivity, and absence of reflex activity following any severe traumatic injury to the spinal cord. This period rarely lasts more than several hours. The end of spinal shock is heralded by the presence of the bulbocavernosus reflex. Therefore, if the patient has no active muscle power and has no sensibility below the level of the injury, and the

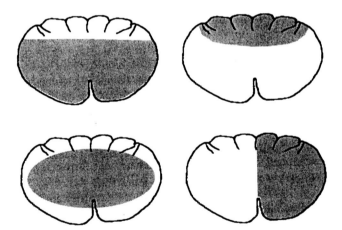

FIGURE 45. Incomplete spinal cord injury syndromes. Anterior cord syndrome: Only deep pressure sensitivity is retained, no evidence of sharp or dull discrimination or voluntary muscle control. These patients have only a 10% to 20% chance of any functional recovery. There is virtually no chance of full recovery. Posterior cord syndrome is rare. There is preservation of motor function with loss of sensory function below the level of injury. Central cord syndrome: The patient has severe quadriparesis but has "sacral sparing." This means sharp or dull discrimination is present around the perineum. The prognosis is good for functional recovery in 50% to 70% of the patients. Approximately 5% may have full recovery. Brown-Séquard syndrome: The patient has voluntary function and sensibility below the zone of injury, and the muscle weakness is greater on one side and the loss of sensibility is greater on the opposite side. The prognosis for progressive recovery is excellent. (From Kasser JR, ed [1996]: *Orthopaedic knowledge update 5.* Rosemont, IL, American Academy of Orthopaedic Surgeons, p 576, with permission.)

bulbocavernosis reflex is present, the patient has a "confirmed" complete spinal cord lesion. The relevance of this finding is that the patient will make no significant functional recovery.

(a) *Zone of Injury*

In patients with complete SCI, the zone of injury is defined as up to three neural segments below the level of injury having partial motor and sensory function. Because the most caudal normal sensory segment may not be the same as the most caudal normal motor segment, and the motor and sensory levels may not be the same on the right and left sides, it is possible to express the differences individually in a given patient.

(b) *Vertebral Level of Injury*

The vertebral level of injury is the highest spinal level with radiographic evidence of vertebral injury.

(c) *Respirator-Dependent Quadriplegia*

If the patient has a functional level above C4, he will be respirator dependent. These patients usually die at the scene of the accident owing to respiratory paralysis. These patients have control only of their face, head, and mouth muscles.

(d) *Pentaplegia*

If the patient has an injury of C1 or C2, which produces a complete spinal cord injury, the patient is not only respirator-dependent but has lost the use of the head and neck muscles, and only has sensation over the face with no voluntary control of the head other than facial muscles.

American Spinal Injury Association (1989): *Standards for neurological classification of spinal injury patients.* pp 1–21.

Austin GM (1972): The spinal cord: basic aspects and surgical considerations, 2nd ed. Springfield, IL: Charles C Thomas.

15. NEUROLOGIC GRADING SCALES

The classifications are designed to monitor the extent of the initial neurologic injury and its progression, as well as to provide a method for assessing treatment efficacy by different methods.

The Frankel scale is well known and widely used. Its disadvantage is that it does not include complete assessment of rectal or bladder function, nor is it sensitive to significant neurologic improvement in those patients classified as grade D. An additional problem is that the lesion level is not indicated, so that a paraplegic falls into the same category as a quadriplegic.

The Sunnybrook cord injury scale consists of 10 neurologic grades. It differs from the Frankel system in that sensory loss can be classified as complete or incomplete. There is also a coding system to assess change in neurologic status. Unfortunately, motor grades 6 to 8 comprise a large and heterogeneous group. Bladder and bowel function are not assessed. It is not easy to commit to memory and thus has diminished bedside utility, particularly in acute management.

The motor index of Lucas and Ducker has been modified by the American Spinal Injury Association into a motor index score in which 100 represents the perfect score. Its deficiency is that bowel and bladder function are not evaluated.

The classification of Lucas and Duckworth has two subdivisions:

1. The level of vertebral trauma documented by radiographic examination
2. The resulting motor examination

The level of vertebral trauma was subdivided into single sites, multiple sites, and no evidence of vertebral trauma. The motor function was assessed by testing different muscle groups and grading them on a scale of 0 to 5. Certain patterns of motor dysfunction below the level of injury were found and used to classify patients into five different motor patterns—two complete and three partial lesions.

Complete at bony level (CBL): complete loss of motor function within two cord segments below the site of vertebral trauma

Graded complete (GC): complete motor loss that occurs two to four cord segments below the site of vertebral trauma

Partial with secondary caudal loss (PCL): partial loss may be secondary or complete; by definition, approaches zero function at least four segments below the level of bony trauma

Partial with caudal gain or caudal sparing (PCS)

Uniform partial lesions (PLU)

The classification of Bracken and colleagues has many of the features of the Sunnybrook cord injury system and, like it, is difficult to memorize and apply at the bedside. It also makes no specific mention of bowel or bladder function.

TABLE 4. SUNNYBROOK CORD INJURY SCALE

Grade	Description	Corresponding Frankel Scale
1	Complete motor and sensory loss	A
2	Complete motor loss; incomplete sensory loss	B
3	Incomplete motor but unclear	C
4	Incomplete motor loss; incomplete sensory loss	C
5	Incomplete motor but useless; normal sensory	C
6	Incomplete motor; complete sensory	D
7	Incomplete motor; incomplete sensory	D
8	Incomplete motor; normal sensory	D
9	Normal motor; incomplete sensory	D
10	Normal motor; normal sensory	E

Recently, Esses and Botsford described a neurologic grading system, attempting to overcome some of these deficits. The scale includes assessment of motor and sensory function, rectal tone, and bladder control. Motor index is assessed by function.

A. Frankel Classification

Each patient should be classified at the time of injury and again at 1-year follow-up to document improvement.

A *Complete:* The lesion is found to be complete both motor and sensory below the segmental level marked.

B *Incomplete:* Sensory only: There is some sensation present below the level of the lesion, but the motor paralysis is complete below that level.

C *Incomplete:* Motor useless: There is some motor power present below the lesion, but it is of no practical use to the patient.

D *Incomplete:* Motor useful: There is useful motor power below the level of the lesion. Patients in this group can move the lower limbs and many can walk with or without aids.

E *Normal:* Full recovery. The patient is free of neurologic symptoms (i.e., no weakness, no sensory loss, no sphincter disturbance). Abnormal reflexes may be present.

B. Sunnybrook Cord Injury Scale (Table 4)

C. Bracken Classification (Tables 5, 6)

In the Bracken classification, assessment of sensory level was based on the patient's response to five stimuli:

Superficial pain
Light touch
Position sense
Vibratory sense
Deep pain

The patients were then grouped in a Sensory Severity Scale:

1. Normal
2. Some segments decreased
3. Some segments absent
4. Paraparetic
5. Quadriparetic
6. Paraplegic
7. Quadriplegic

The motor level of function was assessed by a 0 to 5 scale, and the patients were then grouped in a five-category Motor Severity Scale.

TABLE 5. CRITERIA USED FOR SENSORY SEVERITY SCALE

Sensory Severity Scale	Description	Pain (pinprick)				
		Higher Level			Lower Level	
		Normal	Decreased	Absent	Decreased	Normal
7	Quadraplegic	Yes	Yes	C1 to T1	No	No
6	Paraplegic	Yes	Yes	T2 to S5	No	No
5	Quadraparetic	Yes	C1 to T1	No	Yes	No
4	Paraparetic	Yes	T2 to S5	No	Yes	No
3	Some segments absent	Yes	Yes	Any level	Yes	Yes
2	Some segments decreased	Yes	Any level	No	No	Yes
1	Normal	Yes	No	No	No	Yes

From Bracken MB, Wabb SB, Wagner FC (1978): Classification of the severity of acute spinal cord injury: Implications for management. *Paraplegia* 15:319–26, with permission.

TABLE 6. CRITERIA USED FOR MOTOR SEVERITY SCALE

Motor Severity Scale	Higher Level			Lower Level	
	Active Antigravity Against Resistance	Flicker, Trace Active Antigravity	No Contraction	Flicker, Trace Active Antigravity	Active Antigravity Against Resistance
5	Yes	Yes	C5 → T1	No	No
4	Yes	Yes	L1 → S2	No	No
3	Yes	C5 → T1	No	Yes	No
2	Yes	L1 → S2	No	Yes	No
1	C5 → T1	No	No	No	Yes

From Bracken MB, Webb SB, Wagner FC (1978): Classification of the severity of acute spinal cord injury: implications for management. *Paraplegia* 15:319–326, with permission.

TABLE 7. AMERICAN SPINAL INJURY ASSOCIATION (ASIA) MOTOR SCORE[a]

Grade On Right		Muscle		Grade On Left
0 to 5	C5	Deltoid and/or biceps	C5	0 to 5
0 to 5	C6	Wrist extensors	C6	0 to 5
0 to 5	C7	Triceps	C7	0 to 5
0 to 5	C8	Flexor profundus	C8	0 to 5
0 to 5	T1	Hand intrinsics	T1	0 to 5
0 to 5	L2	Iliopsoas	L2	0 to 5
0 to 5	L3	Quadriceps	L3	0 to 5
0 to 5	L4	Ankle dorsiflexors	L4	0 to 5
0 to 5	L5	Extensor hallucis longus	L5	0 to 5
0 to 5	S1	Gastrocnemius/soleus		0 to 5
0 to 50			S1	0 to 50

[a] Total possible score: 100.

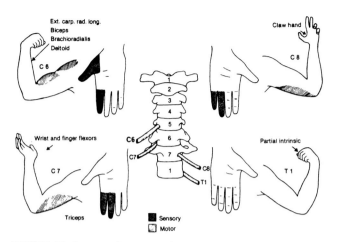

FIGURE 46. Segmental motor and sensory changes, C6 to T1. (From McQueen JD, Khan MI [1989]: Neurologic evaluation. In: The Cervical Spine Research Society, ed. *The cervical spine.* Philadelphia: JB Lippincott, with permission.)

D. ASIA Motor Score

The extent of motor function below the level of injury can be determined numerically by the ASIA motor score (Lucas). The strength of a key muscle at each level from C5 through T1 and from L2 through S1 is determined using the numerical scale for motor strength described above. A total score of 100 is possible (Table 7).

In gunshot injuries, the neurologic level is at least one level higher than the vertebral level in approximately 70% of injuries; in 20%, the neurologic and vertebral level are the same, and in 10%, the vertebral level is two levels lower than the neurologic level. More than half of all gunshot injuries, resulting in spinal cord injury, cause a complete neurologic lesion.

American Spinal Injury Association (1989): *Standards for neurological classification of spinal injury patients.*

Austin GM (1972): The spinal cord: basic aspects and surgical considerations, 2nd ed. Springfield, IL: Charles C Thomas.

Bracken MB, et al (1990): A randomized, controlled trial of methylprednisolone or naloxone in the treatment of acute spinal-cord injury. *N Engl J Med* 322:1405–1411.

Esses S, Botsford D (1990): *Development of a new neural grading scale.* Presented at the annual meeting of the American Spinal Injury Association, Orlando, Florida, 1990.

Frankel H, Hancock D, Hyslop G, et al. (1969): The value of postural reduction in the initial management of closed injuries of the spine with paraplegia and tetraplegia. *Paraplegia* 7:179–192.

Lucas JT, Ducker TB (1979): Motor classification of spinal cord injuries with mobility, morbidity, and recovery indices. *Am Surg* 45:151–158.

Tator CH, Rowed DW, Schwartz ML (1982): Sunnybrook cord injury scales for assessing neurologic injury and neurological recovery. In: Tator CH, ed. *Early management of acute spinal cord injury.* New York: Raven Press.

Waters RL, Hu SS (1991): Penetrating injuries of the spinal cord. In: Frymoyer JW, ed. *The adult spine: principles and practice.* New York: Raven Press.

16. DETERMINATION OF LEVEL OF NEUROLOGIC INJURY

A. Localization of Cervical and Lumbar Root Lesions (Table 8)

B. Segmental Motor and Sensory Changes, C6 to T1 (Fig. 46)

C. Method to Determine Level of Neurologic Injury (Table 9)

17. ASSOCIATION OF NEUROLOGIC PATTERNS AND INJURY MECHANISM IN THE CERVICAL SPINE (Table 10)

18. NEUROLOGIC LOSS IN CERVICAL SPONDYLOTIC MYELOPATHY

Nurick classified cervical spondylotic myelopathy largely on the basis of gait (Table 11).

The Japanese Orthopaedic Association has devised an objective assessment scale to quantitate the degree of involvement secondary to spondylotic myelopathy. The scale involves four categories (Table 12).

19. CLINICAL FEATURES OF INTERMEDULLARY AND EXTRAMEDULLARY LESIONS OF THE CERVICAL SPINE (Table 13)

20. CLINICAL MANIFESTATIONS OF SPINAL CORD, PERIPHERAL NERVE, AND SKELETAL MUSCLE DISEASES (Table 14)

TABLE 8. LOCALIZATION OF CERVICAL AND LUMBAR ROOT LESIONS BY PHYSICAL EXAMINATION

Neurologic Level	Weakness	Reflex Depression	Sensation Decreased
C5	Deltoid and biceps	Biceps	Lateral aspect of upper arm
C6	Biceps flexion and wrist extension	Brachioradialis	Thumb and index finger
C7	Finger and elbow extensions	Triceps	Middle finger
C8	Finger flexions	None	Ulnar aspects of forearm
L4	Anterior tibial, quadriceps	Knee jerk	Medial foot
L5	Extensor hallucis longus	—	Middorsum of foot
S1	Peroneals, calf muscles, hamstrings	Ankle jerk	Lateral foot

From White AA, Panjabi MM (1990): *Clinical biomechanics of the spine*, 2nd ed. Philadelphia: JB Lippincott, with permission.

TABLE 9. METHOD TO DETERMINE LEVEL OF NEUROLOGIC INJURY

Level	Muscle Power	Sensory	Reflexes
T2–T5	Upper extremity intact; intercostals paralyzed; breathing diaphragmatic	T2 axialla lost T5 nipple line	None
T6–T9	Intact Intercostals above level of involvement Supraumbilical segments of rectus abdominus intact, umbilicus moves cephalad with forced respiration	T6 xiphoid T7 costal margins	Abdominals absent
T10	Infraumbilical segments of rectus abdominus intact; umbilicus shifts caudad with forced respiration	Umbilicus	
T12	Abdominal muscles intact	Groin	Abdominals present
L1	No lower extremity	Buttocks	Intact ankle jerk, knee jerk = upper motor neuron paralysis Cremasteric present
L2	Possible iliopsoas	Anterior upper third of the thighs	Cremasteric absent
L3	Hip flexion sartorius and iliopsoas intact	Anterior two-thirds of the thighs	Knee jerk absent
L4	Hip flexion; hip adduction; intact sartorius permits some knee flexion	Anterior thigh, medial leg	Knee jerk present
L5	Ankle dorsiflexion Anterior tibial intact	Medial ankle Dorsum of the foot, great toe absent	
S1	As above	Plantar, lateral border of foot absent	
S2	Plantar flexion, intact	Peripheral sensation intact	Ankle jerk present
S3–S4	Cauda equina-type syndrome, including potential loss of bladder and bowel control with sensory losses confined to the genitalia, perineum, anus, and posterior upper thigh; no peripheral motor loss		

TABLE 10. ASSOCIATION OF NEUROLOGIC PATTERNS AND INJURY MECHANISM IN THE CERVICAL SPINE

	Neurologic Damage	Injury
Group 1	Total motor and sensory loss to all four limbs; total transection of cord; no recovery occurred	Burst fracture or bilateral facet dislocation, flexion injury
Group II	Motor loss of varying degrees, either in all four extremities or in the upper limbs only: sometimes segmental or patchy transient sensory loss was associated (*central spinal cord damage*)	Hyperextension injuries
Group III	Complete motor loss in the extremities, with hypoesthesia and hypalgesia up to the level of the lesion; no loss of position and vibratory sense (*anterior spinal cord damage*)	Vertical compression, bursting injury, "teardrop" fracture-dislocation: possibly some associated flexion or extension
Group IV	Motor power in all four limbs or the upper extremities along with no sensory loss	Unilateral facet dislocation, fractured arch of altas, and a variety of injuries
Group V	Brown-Séquard syndrome	Unilateral facet dislocation or a burst fracture

From Marar BC (1974): The patterns of neurological damage as an aid to the diagnosis of the mechanism in cervical-spine injuries. *J Bone Joint Surg (Am)* 56:1648–1654, with permission.

TABLE 11. NURICK'S CLASSIFICATION OF DISABILITY IN SPONDYLOTIC MYELOPATHY

Grade 0	Root signs and symptoms No evidence of cord involvement
Grade I	Signs of cord involvement Normal gait
Grade II	Mildgait improvement Able to be employed
Grade III	Gait abnormality prevents employment
Grade IV	Able to ambulate only with assistance
Grade V	Chairbound or bedridden

From Nurick S. (1972): The pathogenesis of the spinal cord disorder associated with cervical spondylosis. *Brain* 95:687–100, with permission.

TABLE 12. THE ASSESSMENT SCALE PROPOSED BY THE JAPANESE ORTHOPAEDIC ASSOCIATION

I. Motor dysfunction of the upper extremity *Score*
  0 = Unable to feed oneself
  1 = Unable to handle chopsticks, able to eat with a spoon
  2 = Handle chopsticks with much difficulty
  3 = Handle chopsticks with slight difficulty
  4 = None

II. Motor dysfunction of the lower extremity *Score*
  0 = Unable to work
  1 = Walk on flat floor with walking aid
  2 = Up and/or down stairs with handrail
  3 = Lack of stability and smooth reciprocation
  4 = None

III. Sensory deficit
  A. The upper extremity *Score*
    0 = Severe sensory loss or pain
    1 = Mild sensory loss
    2 = None
  B. The lower extremity, same as A
  C. The trunk, same as A

IV. Sphincter dysfunction *Score*
  0 = Unable to void
  1 = Marked difficulty in micturition (retention, strangury)
  2 = Difficulty in micturition (pollakiuria, hesitation)
  3 = None

From Hirabayashi K, Miyakawa J, Satomi K, et al. (1981): Operative results and postoperative progression of ossification among patients with ossification of cervical posterior longitudinal ligament. *Spine* 6:354–364, with permission.

TABLE 13. CLINICAL FEATURES OF INTRAMEDULLARY AND EXTRAMEDULLARY LESIONS OF THE CERVICAL SPINE

Clinical Features	Intramedullary Lesions	Extramedullary Lesions
Motor disturbances		
Spastic paresis	Late onset, lower limbs	Early onset, more marked distally
Flaccid paresis	Early onset, upper limbs	Often absent, except at segmental level
Atrophy of muscles	Often prominent, upper limbs	Uncommon but may be segmental
Fasciculations	Present	Present
Reflex changes		
Muscle stretch reflex	Depressed early in upper limbs, late hyperactivity in lower limbs	Early hyperactivity with possible segmental depression
Babinski's sign	Late appearance	Early sign
Sensory disturbances		
Root pains	Often absent	Often presenting symptom
Local vertebral pain	Usually absent	Often present
Sensory loss	Dissociated sensory loss, maximal at level of lesion	Usually begins below level of lesion
Others		
Tropic skin changes	Often present	Rare
Bladder function	Early incontinence	Late incontinence

From McQueen JD, Khan MI (1989): Neurologic evaluation. In: The Cervical Spine Research Society, ed. *The cervical spine.* Philadelphia: JB Lippincott, with permission.

TABLE 14. CLINICAL MANIFESTATIONS OF SPINAL CORD, PERIPHERAL NERVE, AND SKELETAL MUSCLE DISEASES

Clinical Manifestations	Spinal Cord Lesions (Myelopathies)	Peripharal Nerve Lesions (Neuropathies)	Muscle Disease (Myopathies)
Motor	Upper or lower motor neuron-type weakness, depending on acuity and "age" of the lesion and its location in relation to cord segments Trunk and limb(s) below the lesion affected Atrophy from disuse only	Lower motor neuron (flaccid) weakness only Predominantly in extremities; tends to involve distal limb segments more than proximal Atrophy early	Flaccid weakness only Tends to involve trunk and proximal limb segments earliest
Sensory	Cutaneous "sensory level" or "suspended level" on trunk Sensory dissociation, if present, usually in terms of cord tracts	Rarely involves trunk; tends to begin distally in limbs and ascend limbs or follows distribution of a peripheral nerve supply Dissociation, if present, may be of any combination of modalities	None
Reflexes	Hyperactive tendon reflexes below lesion except during "spinal shock" with acute lesions At level of lesion, if limb segments are involved, hyporeflexia or areflexia persists or both hyper- and hyporeflexia occur in same limb(s) Pathologic reflexes (Babinski's sign, spontaneous flexor or extensor spasms) below lesion likely Cutaneous reflexes lost below lesion	Hyporeflexia or areflexia found early and persists No pathologic relaxes Cutaneous reflexes spared unless their effecter muscles are completely paralyzed	Tendon reflexes normal early, become progressively hypoactive as disease advances Cutaneous reflexes spared No pathologic reflexes
Sphincters	External urethral and anal sphincters often impaired	Sphincters very rarely involved	No sphincter disturbances

From Talbert OR (1990): General methods of clinical examination. In: *Youman's neurological surgery*, 3rd ed. Philadelphia: WB Saunders, with permission.

TABLE 15. DIFFERENTIAL DIAGNOSIS OF MYELORADICULOPATHY

Degenerative
  Cervical spondylosis
  Intervertebral disc disease

Neoplastic
  Metastatic carcinoma (prostate, lung, breast, colon, myeloma, renal, thyroid)
  Spinal cord tumor (glioma, ependymoma, hemangioblastoma, neurofibroma, maningioma)
  Paraneoplastic (acute necrotic myelopathy secondary to systemic carcinoma)

Infectious
  Epidural abscess
  Transverse myelitis (mumps, rabies, vaccinia, variola, varicella, HTLV)
  Infectious arteritis (chronic meningovascular syphilis)
  Tuberculous osteomyelitis of the spine (Pott's disease)
  Acute disseminated encephalomyelitis

Traumatic
  Blunt
  Penetrating

Neurodegenerative (autoimmune, nutritional)
  Demyelinating disease (Devic's neuromyelitis optica)
  Amyotrophic lateral sclerosis (motor neuron disease)
  Subacute combined degeneration (vitamin B_{12} deficiency)

Developmental
  Syringomyelia
  Arachnoid cyst
  Meningomyelocele
  Spinal arteriovenous malformation
  Intracranial dural arteriovenous fistula

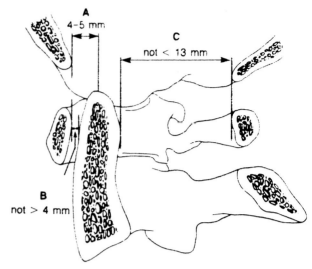

FIGURE 47. C0-1-2 lateral view. **A:** The distance between the basion of the occiput and the top of the dens is 4 to 5 mm. An increase of more than 1 mm in this distance with flexion or extension views is believed to indicate instability of C0-1, if one assumes that the transverse ligament of the atlas is intact. **B:** The distance between the anterior border of the dens and the posterior border of the ring of C1 should not be greater than 4 mm. **C:** There is another important measurement that we must consider. We refer to the distance between the posterior margin of the dens and the anterior cortex of the posterior ring of C1. This distance is of concern should it be less than 13 mm. (From White AA, Panjabi MM (1990): The problem of clinical instability in the human spine: a systematic approach. In *Clinical biomechanics of the spine*, 2nd ed. Philadelphia: JB Lippincott, with permission.)

21. DIFFERENTIAL DIAGNOSIS OF MYELORADICULOPATHY (Table 15)

22. SPINE INSTABILITY

Segmental instability is a loss of spinal motion segment stiffness, such that force application to that motion segment produces greater displacement or displacements than would be seen in a normal structure, resulting in a painful condition, the potential for progressive deformity, and neurologic structures at risk.

A. C0-1-2 Instability (Table 16; Fig. 47)

White AA, Panjabi MM, Posner I, et al. (1981): Spinal stability: evaluation and treatment. *AAOS Inst Course Lect* 30:457–483.

TABLE 16. CRITERIA FOR C0-1-2 INSTABILITY

>8°	Axial rotation C0–1 to one side
>1 mm	C0–1 translation*
>7 mm	Overhang C1–2 (total right and left)
>45°	Axial rotation C1–C2 to one side
>4 mm	C1–2 translation[a]
<13 mm	Posterior body C2-posterior ring C1
Avulsed transverse ligament	

[a] See Figures 37, 38, and 39 for measurement techniques.

TABLE 17. CLINICAL CHECKLIST FOR THE DIAGNOSIS OF CLINICAL INSTABILITY IN THE LOWER CERVICAL SPINE

Element	Point Value
Anterior elements destroyed or unable to function	2
Posterior elements destroyed or unable to function	2
Positive stretch test	2
Radiographic criteria	4
A. Flexion/extension radiographs	
1. Sagittal plane translation >3.5 mm or 20% (2 points)	
2. Sagittal plane rotation >20° (2 points)	
or	
B. Resting radiographs	
1. Sagittal plane displacement >3.5 mm or 20% (2 points)	
2. Relative sagittal plane angulation >11° (2 points)	
Abnormal disc narrowing	1
Developmentally narrow spinal canal	1
1. Sagittal diameter <13 mm	
or	
2. Pavlov's ratio <0.8	
Spinal cord damage	2
Nerve root damage	1
Dangerous loading anticipated	1
Total of 5 or more = unstable	

From White AA, Panjabi MM (1990): The problem of clinical instability in the human spine: a systematic approach. In: *Clinical biomechanics of the spine* 2nd ed. Philadelpha: JB Lippincott, with permission.
See Figures 38 and 39 for information on making radiographic measurements.

B. Lower Cervical Spine

See Table 17 and Figures 48 and 49.

C. Thoracic and Thoracolumbar Spine (Table 18)

See Figures 48 and 49 for information on making radiographic measurements. Measurement techniques are the same as for the cervical spine, except for Pavlov's ratio.

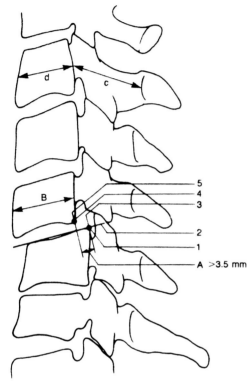

FIGURE 48. The method for measuring translatory displacement is as follows: *1,* A point is marked at the posterosuperior angle of the projected image of the vertebral body below the interspace of the functional spinal unit (FSU) being evaluated. *2,* A line is drawn along the upper vertebral end plate of the vertebra, below the interspace of the FSU under analysis. *3,* At the point where this intersects the mark, at the posterior portion of the end plate, a short perpendicular line is drawn. *4,* Next, a mark is made at the posteroinferior angle of image of the vertebral body above the interspace of the FSU being evaluated. *5,* A short line that goes through the second mark and is perpendicular to the line on the subjacent vertebral end plate is drawn. The linear distance between the two perpendicular lines is measured. This can be called distance *A.* The anteroposterior sagittal plane diameter at the midlevel of the supraadjacent vertebra is measured. This distance is called *B.* If distance *A* is less than 20% of distance *B,* then this is considered evidence of instability and should be so entered on the checklist. An alternative method is simply to measure the linear distance *A,* and if this is greater than 3.5 mm, it is considered to be suggestive of instability, and two points are entered onto the checklist. Pavlov's ratio is a reliable, accurate method for recognizing a developmentally narrow canal without the variables involved in linear measurements. The measurement *c* is the distance between the midlevel of the posterior aspect of the vertebral body and the nearest point on the corresponding spinolaminar line. The measurement *d* is seen on lateral view as the anteroposterior distance from the front to the back of the vertebral body measured at the midlevel. The ratio *c/d* is considered normal if ≥1 and abnormal is <0.80. These measurements are used in conjunction with the checklist. (From White AA, Panjabi MM [1990]: The problem of clinical instability in the human spine: a systematic approach. In *Clinical biomechanics of the spine,* 2nd ed. Philadelphia: JB Lippincott, with permission.)

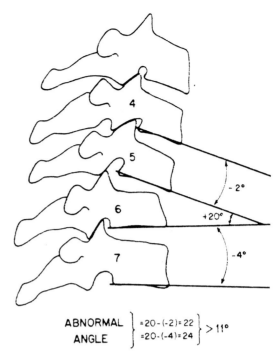

FIGURE 49. Measurement of rotation. The angulation between C5 and C6 is 20°, which is more than 11° greater than at either adjacent interspace. The angle at C4 and C5 measures −20°, and the one at C6 and C7 measures −4. (From White AA, Johnson RM, Panjabi MM, Southwick WO [1975]: Biomechanical analysis of clinical stability in the cervical spine. *Clin Orthop* 109:85–96, with permission.)

D. Lumbar Spine (Table 19; Figs. 50–52)

Posner I, White AA, Edwards WT, et al. (1982): A biomechanical analysis of the clinical stability of the lumbar and lumbosacral spine. *Spine* 7:374–389.

E. Sacroiliac Joint and Pubis (Table 20)

F. Lumbar Segmental Instabilities (Table 21)

G. Degenerative Segmental Instabilities (Table 22)

23. PEDICLE ABNORMALITIES (Tables 23, 24)

TABLE 18. CHECKLIST FOR THE DIAGNOSIS OF CLINICAL INSTABILITY IN THE THORACIC AND THORACOLUMBAR SPINE

Element	Point Value
Anterior elements destroyed or unable to function	2
Posterior elements destroyed or unable to function	2
Disruptions of costovertebral articulations	1
Radiographic criteria[a]	4
1. Sagittal plane displacement >2.5 mm (2 points)	
2. Relative sagittal plane angulation >5° (2 points)	
Spinal cord or cauda equina damage	2
Dangerous loading anticipated	1
Total of 5 or more = unstable	

From White AA, Panjabi MM (1990): The problem of clinical instability in the human spine: a systematic approach. In: *Clinical biomechanics of the spine,* 2nd ed. Philadelphia: JB Lippincott, with permission.
See Figures 42, 43, and 44 for measurement techniques.

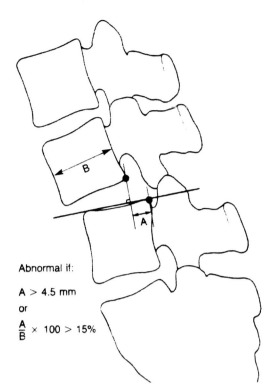

Abnormal if:

A > 4.5 mm

or

$\dfrac{A}{B} \times 100 > 15\%$

FIGURE 50. Measurement to determine vertebral translation or displacement in the lumbar spine. If the translation or displacement is as much as 4.5 mm or 15% of the sagittal diameter of the adjacent vertebra, it is considered to be abnormal. These measurements are to be used in conjunction with the checklist in Table 19. (From White AA, Panjabi MM [1990]: The problem of clinical instability in the human spine: a systematic approach. In *Clinical biomechanics of the spine*, 2nd ed. Philadelphia: JB Lippincott, with permission.)

TABLE 19. CHECKLIST FOR THE DIAGNOSIS OF CLINICAL INSTABILITY IN THE LUMBAR SPINE

Element	Point Value
Anterior elements destroyed or unable to function	2
Posterior elements destroyed or unable to function	2
Radiographic criteria[a]	4
A. Flexion-extension radiographs	
1. Sagittal plane translation >4.5 mm or 15% (2 points)	
2. Sagittal plane rotation	
>15° at L1–L2, L2–L3, and L3–L4 (2 points)	
>20° at L4–L5 (2 points)	
>25° at L5–S1 (2 points)	
or	
B. Resting radiographs	
1. Sagittal plane displacement >4.5 mm or 15% (2 points)	
2. Relative sagittal plane angulation >22° (2 points)	
Cauda equina damage	3
Dangerous loading anticipated	1
Total of 5 or more = unstable	

From White AA, Panjabi MM (1990): The problem of clinical instability in the human spine: a systematic approach. In: *Clinical biomechanics of the spine*, 2nd ed. Philadelphia: JB Lippincott, with permission.
See Figures 41 and 42 for measurement techniques.

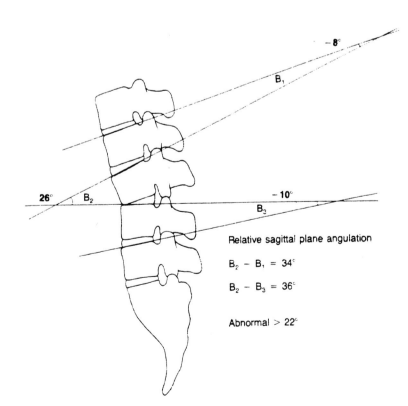

Relative sagittal plane angulation

$B_2 - B_1 = 34°$

$B_2 - B_3 = 36°$

Abnormal > 22°

FIGURE 51. Measurement of relative sagittal plane angulation in the lumbar spine. A method of measuring relative sagittal plane angulation on the L4–5 functional spine unit (FSU) on a static (resting) lateral view radiograph. Relative sagittal plane angulation greater than 22 degrees is abnormal and potentially unstable in the lumbar spine. Note that this means 22 degrees greater than the amount of angulation at the FSU above or below the FSU in question. By convention, negative values denote lordosis, and positive values denote kyphosis. These measurements are to be used in conjunction with the checklist in Table 19.

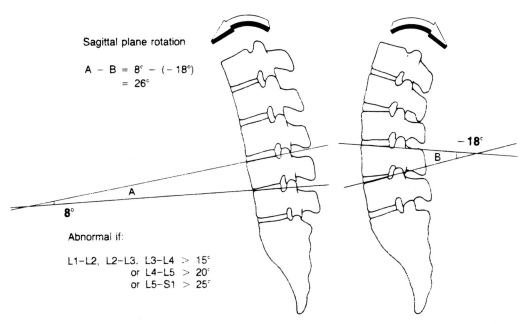

Sagittal plane rotation

$$A - B = 8^c - (-18°)$$
$$= 26^c$$

$8°$

A

B -18^c

Abnormal if:

L1–L2, L2–L3. L3–L4 $> 15^c$
or L4–L5 $> 20^c$
or L5–S1 $> 25^c$

FIGURE 52. Measurement of sagittal plane rotation in the lumbar spine. A method of measuring sagittal plane rotation of the L4–5 functional spinal unit on dynamic (flexion and extension) lateral radiographs. The sagittal plane rotation is the difference between the Cobb measurements taken in flexion (*A*) and extension (*B*). Sagittal plane rotation greater than 15 degrees at L1–2, L2–3, and L3–4, greater than 20 degrees at L4–5, or greater than 258 at L5–S1 is abnormal and potentially unstable. Note that negative values denote lordosis and positive values denote kyphosis. These measurements are to be used in conjunction with the checklist in Table 19.

TABLE 20. CHECKLIST FOR THE DIAGNOSIS OF CLINICAL INSTABILITY OF THE SACROILIAC JOINT AND PUBIS

Element	Point Value
Pain relief with pelvic fixation	3
Abnormal displacement	
>1 cm sacroiliac	2
>2 cm pubic diastasis (horizontal)	1
>1 cm pubic displacement (vertical)	1
Audible click with associated pain	1
Pain with maneuvers to stress pelvic ring	1
Dangerous loads anticipated	1
Total of 5 or more = unstable	

From White AA, Panjabi MM (1990): The problem of clinical instability in the human spine: a systematic approach. In: *Clinical biomechanics of the spine*, 2nd ed. Philadelphia; JB Lippincott, with permission.

TABLE 21. LUMBAR SEGMENTAL INSTABILITIES

I. Fractures and fracture-dislocations

II. Infections involving anterior columns
   A. With progressive loss of vertebral body height and deformity despite treatment with antibiotics
   B. With progressing neurologic symptoms despite treatment with antibiotics (if accompanied by progressive loss of vertebral body height and deformity)

III. Primary and metastatic neoplasms
   A. With progressive loss of vertebral body height and deformity
   B. With progressing neurologic symptoms not resulting from direct tumor involvement of the spinal cord, cauda equina, or nerve roots (e.g., caused by progressive loss of vertebral body height and deformity)
   C. Postsurgical (after resection of neoplasm)

IV. Spondylolisthesis
   A. Isthmic spondylolisthesis
      1. L5–S1 progressive deformity in a child, particularly when accompanied by radiographic risk signs (this lesion is rarely unstable in adults)
      2. L4–L5 deformity (probably unstable in adults)

V. Degenerative instabilities

VI. Scoliosis (any progressive deformity in a child, subclassified by the criteria of the Scoliosis Research Society)

From Hazlett JW, Kinnard P (1982): Lumbar apophyseal process excisions and spinal instability. *Spine* 7:171–178, with permission.

TABLE 22. DEGENERATIVE SEGMENTAL INSTABILITIES

Primary instabilities
Axial rotational instability
Translational instability
Retrolisthetic instability
Progressing degenerative scoliosis
Disc disruption syndrome

Secondary instabilities
Post-disc excision: subclassified according to the pattern of instability as subscribed under primary instabilities
Postdecompressive laminectomy
Accentuation of preexistent deformity
New deformity, i.e., no deformity existed at the time of original decompression: further subclassified as for primary instabilities
Postspinal fusion
Above or below a spinal fusion, subclassified as for primary instabilities
Pseudarthrosis
Postchemonucleolysis

TABLE 23. PEDICLE ABNORMALITIES

Absent
Tumor
Congenital
Histiocytosis
Infection (rare)

Hypoplasis
Neurofibromatosis
Congenital
Renal abnormalities
Following radiation therapy

Narrow
Normal (T spine)
Intraspinal tumor
Dural ectasla
Dysraphism
Scoliosis
Spondylolisthesis

Large
Contralateral abnormalities of vertebral arch
Neurofibromatosis
Paget's disease
Expansile tumors and tumor-like conditions
Infection
Histiocytosis
Normal

From Kricun ME (1988): Conventional rediography. In: *Imaging modalities in spinal disorders*. Philadelphia: WB Saunders, with permission.

TABLE 24. ABNORMAL INTERPEDICULAR DISTANCES

Wide
Intraspinal tumor
Dural ectasia
Dysraphism

Narrow
Achondroplasia
Diastrophic dwarfism
Thanatophoric dwarfism

From Kricun ME (1988): Conventional rediography. In: *Imaging modalities in spinal disorders*. Philadephia: WB Saunders, with permission.

24. SPINAL DEFORMITIES: SCOLIOSIS, KYPHOSIS, LORDOSIS (Table 25)

Goldstein LA, Waugh TR (1973): Classification and terminology of scoliosis. *Clin Orthop* 93:10–22.

McAlister WH, Schackelford GD (1975): Classification of spinal curvaturea. *Radiol Clin North Am* 13:93–112.

White AA, Panjabi MM (1990): Biomechanical classification of scoliosis. In: *Clinical biomechanics of the spine*, 2nd ed. Philadelphia: JP Lippincott.

A. Congenital Scoliosis (Fig. 53)

There are three basic categories, as classified by Winter (based on MacEwen classification): defects of formation, defects of segmentation, and mixed defects.

I. Unclassifiable; usually a collection of defects
II. Fusion of ribs
   A. At a distance from the vertebrae, with little or no significance
   B. Adjacent or continuous with the vertebrae (usually associated with an unsegmented bar) where curve progression is very likely
III. Unilateral, partial failure of formation of a vertebra (wedge or trapezoid vertebra)
IV. Unilateral, complete failure of formation of a vertebra (hemivertebra)
V. Bilateral failure of segmentation (block vertebra)
VI. Unilateral failure of segmentation (unsegmented bar)

B. Congenital Kyphosis (Fig. 54)

In 1973, Winter and associates proposed a three-type classification. This classification was modified in 1977, and it is widely accepted in this form.

Type I: Failure of formation: aplasia or hypoplasia
   Absence of the body
   Absence of the body associated with microspondylia of neighboring body
   Microspondylia of one body
   Microspondylia of two neighboring bodies
Type II: Failure of segmentation
Type III: Mixed

Kostuik JP (1991): Adult kyphosis. In: Frymoyer JW, ed. *The adult spine: principles and practice*. New York: Raven Press.

Winter RB, Moe JH, Wang JF (1973): Congenital kyphosis. Its natural history as observed in a study of one hundred and thirty patients. *J Bone Joint Surg [Am]* 55:223–256.

Winter RB (1977): Congenital kyphosis. *Clin Orthop* 128:26–32.

C. Congenital Spine Deformities (Winter)

In 1983, Winter presented a comprehensive classification of congenital deformities of the spine.

(1) Defects of Segmentation

- Anterior failure of segmentation results in kyphosis. Commonly called *anterior unsegmented bar* (Fig. 55).
- Posterior failure of segmentation results in lordosis; the condition Commonly called *laminar synostosis*. Usually involves the lamina and the facet joints (Fig. 56).
- Lateral failure of segmentation. Commonly called *unilateral unsegmented bar*. Produces a purely lateral curvature without kyphosis or lordosis (Fig. 57).
- Posterolateral failure of segmentation. Because of the continued growth anteriorly and on the opposite side, a *lordoscoliosis* is produced.
- Anterolateral failure of segmentation (very rare). Produces *kyphoscoliosis*.
- Total failure of segmentation. Commonly known as *block vertebra* (Fig. 58).

TABLE 25. CLASSIFICATION ENDORSED BY THE SCOLIOSIS RESEARCH SOCIETY

SCOLIOSIS
Idiopathic
  Infantile (0–3 years)
    Resolving
    Progressive
  Juvenile (4 years to puberty onset)
  Adolescent (puberty onset to epiphyseal closure)
  Adult (epiphyses closed)
Neuromuscular
  Spinal muscular atrophy
  Myelomeningocele (paralytic)
  Dysautonomia (Riley-Day syndrome)
  Other
Myopathic
  Arthrogryposis
  Muscular dystrophy
    Duchenne syndrome (pseudohypertrophic)
    Limb-girdle
    Facioscapulohumeral
  Congenital hypotonia
  Myotonia dystrophica
  Other
Congenital
  Failure of formation
    Partial unilateral (wedge vertebra)
    Complete unilateral (hemivertebra)
      Fully segmented
      Semisegmented
      Nonsegmented
  Failure of segmentation
    Unilateral (unilateral unsegmented bar)
    Bilateral (bloc vertebrae)
  Mixed
    Associated with neural tissue defect
      Myelomeningocele
      Meningocele
      Spinal dysraphism
        Diastematomyelia
        Other
Neurofibromatosis
Mesenchymal
  Marfan syndrome
  Homocystinuria
  Ehlers-Danlos syndrome
  Other
Traumatic
  Fracture or dislocation (nonparalytic)
  Postradlation
  Other

Soft tissue contractures
  Postempyema
  Burns
  Other
Osteochondrodystrophies
  Achondroplasia
  Spondyloepiphyseal dysplasia
  Diastrophic dwarfism
  Mucopolysaccharidoses
  Other
Tumor
  Benign
  Malignant
Rheumatoid disease
Metabolic
  Rickets
  Juvenile osteoporosis
  Osteogenesis imperfecta
Related to lumbosacral area
  Spondylolysis
Neuropathic
  Upper motor neuron lesion
    Cerebral palsy
    Spinocerebeliar degeneration
      Friedreich's disease
      Charcot-Marie-Tooth disease
      Roussy-Levy syndrome
    Syringomyelia
    Spinal cord tumor
    Spinal cord trauma
    Other
  Lower motor neuron lesion
    Poliomyelitis
    Traumatic
  Spondylolisthesis
  Other
Thoracogenic
  Postthoracoplasty
  Postthoracotomy
  Other
Hysterical
Functional
  Postural
  Secondary to short leg
  Due to muscle spasm
  Other

KYPHOSIS
Postural
Scheuermann disease
Congenital
  Defect of segmentation
  Defect of formation
  Mixed
Paralytic
  Poliomyelitis
  Anterior horn cell
  Upper motor neuron
Myelomeningocele
Posttraumatic
  Acute
  Chronic
Inflammatory
  Tuberculosis
  Other infections
  Ankylosing spondylitis
Postsurgical
  Postlaminectomy
  Postexcision (e.g., tumor)
Postradiation
Metabolic
  Osteoporosis
    Senile
    Juvenile
  Osteogenesis imperfecta
  Other
Developmental
  Achondroplasia
  Mucopolysaccharidoses
  Other
Tumor
  Benign
  Malignant
    Primary
    Metastatic

LORDOSIS
Postural
Congenital
Paralytic
  Neuropathic
  Myopathic
Contracture of hip flexors
Secondary to shunts

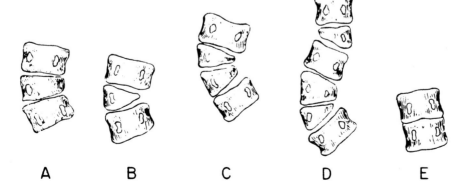

FIGURE 53. Congenital scoliosis. **A:** Unilateral failure of vertebral formation, partial (wedged vertebra). **B:** Unilateral failure of vertebral formation, complete (hemivertebra). **C:** Double hemivertebra, unbalanced. **D:** Double hemivertebra, balanced. **E:** Symmetric failure of segmentation (congenital fusion). *(Figure continues.)*

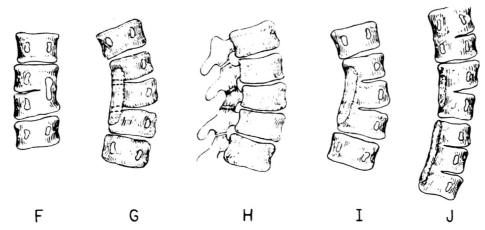

F G H I J

FIGURE 53. *Continued.* **F:** Asymmetric failure of segmentation (unsegmented bar). **G:** Asymmetric failure of segmentation (unsegmented bar involving posterior elements only, anteroposterior view) **H:** Asymmetric failure of segmentation, oblique view showing intact disc space and lack of segmentation confined to the posterior elements (surgically easy to divide). **I:** Unsegmented bar involving both the disc area and posterior elements (a very difficult surgical problem to divide). **J:** Multiple unsegmented bar, unbalanced. (From Winter RB, Moe JH, Eilers VE [1968]: Congenital scoliosis: a study of 234 patients treated and untreated. *J Bone Joint Surg [Am]* 50:1–47, with permission.)

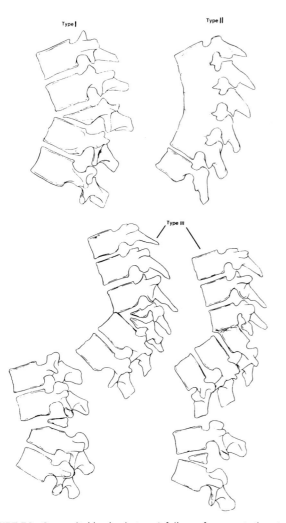

FIGURE 54. Congenital kyphosis *type I:* failure of segmentation; *type II:* failure of formation; *type III:* mixed. (From Winter RB [1983]: Classification and terminology. In: *Congenital deformities of the spine.* New York: Thieme-Stratton, with permission.)

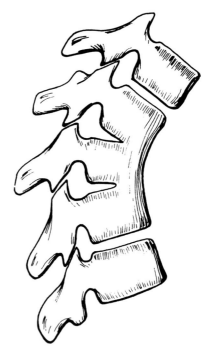

FIGURE 55. Anterior unsegmented bar (congenital kyphosis type I). (From Winter RB [1983]: Classification and terminology. In: *Congenital deformities of the spine.* New York: Thieme-Stratton, with permission.)

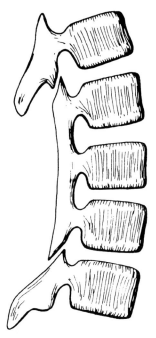

FIGURE 56. Laminar synostosis. (From Winter RB [1983]: Classification and terminology. In *Congenital deformities of the spine.* New York: Thieme-Stratton, with permission.)

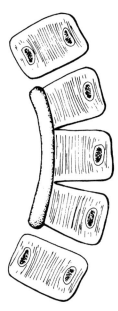

FIGURE 57. Unilateral unsegmented bar. (From Winter RB [1983]: Classification and terminology. In *Congenital deformities of the spine.* New York: Thieme-Stratton, with permission.)

(2) Defects of Formation

- Anterior failure of formation. Results in kyphosis. These defects may range from only a minimal failure to total absence of the bodies of several adjacent vertebrae (Fig. 59).
- Posterior failure of formation (extremely rare). Results in lordosis.
- Lateral failure of formation. This is a very common defect. May vary from a mild wedging for a vertebra to nearly total absence of all, except a pedicle and facet joint on one side. This is commonly called a hemivertebra (Fig. 60).
- Anterolateral defect of formation. This is frequently called a "corner" hemivertebra but is in reality more of a "quarter" vertebra. This defect results in an angular true kyphoscoliosis.
- Anterior central defect of formation. Involves a defect in midline fusion of the lateral halves of the vertebral body. This is commonly called a "butterfly" vertebra. Frequently associated with kyphosis (Fig. 61).

(3) Mixed Failures

- Mixed failure of formation and segmentation in the sagittal plane (mixed congenital kyphosis) (Fig. 62). Mixed failure of segmentation and formation in the frontal plane leads to scoliosis.
- Unilateral unsegmented bar with hemivertebra (Fig. 63).
- Hemivertebra with defects of segmentation (Fig. 64).

D. Hemivertebra

(1) Incarcerated Versus Nonincarcerated Hemivertebrae

An incarcerated hemivertebra is one that is "tucked into" the spine without producing any distortion of the vertebral column. The pedicle line is intact (Fig. 65*A*).

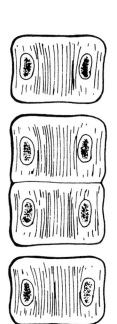

FIGURE 58. Block vertebra. (From Winter RB [1983]: Classification and terminology. In *Congenital deformities of the spine.* New York: Thieme-Stratton, with permission.)

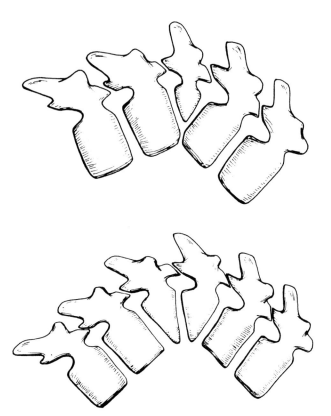

FIGURE 59. Anterior failure of formation (congenital kyphosis type II). (From Winter RB [1983]: Classification and terminology. In *Congenital deformities of the spine.* New York: Thieme-Stratton, with permission.)

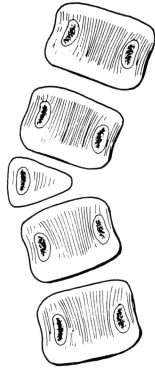

FIGURE 60. Lateral failure of formation. Hemivertebra. (From Winter RB [1983]: Classification and terminology. In *Congenital deformities of the spine.* New York: Thieme-Stratton, with permission.)

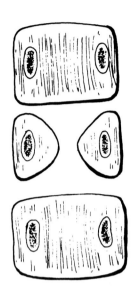

FIGURE 61. Butterfly verte-bra. (From Winter RB [1983]: Classification and terminology. In *Congenital deformities of the spine.* New York: Thieme-Stratton, with permission.)

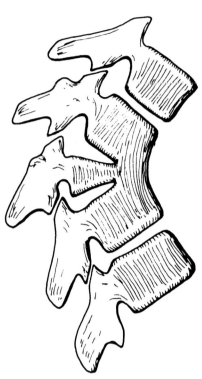

FIGURE 62. Mixed congenital kyphosis (type III congenital kyphosis). (From Winter RB [1983]: Classification and terminology. In *Congenital deformities of the spine.* New York: Thieme-Stratton, with permission.)

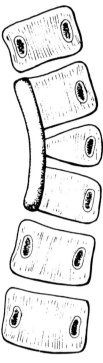

FIGURE 63. Unilateral unseg-mented bar with hemivertebra. (From Winter RB [1983]: Classi-fication and terminology. In *Congenital deformities of the spine.* New York: Thieme-Strat-ton, with permission.)

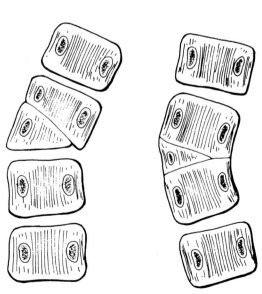

FIGURE 64. Hemivertebra with defects of segmentation. (From Winter RB [1983]: Classification and terminology. In *Congenital deformities of the spine.* New York: Thieme-Stratton, with permission.)

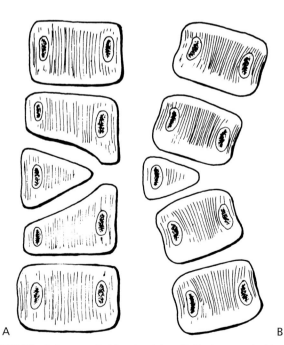

A   B

FIGURE 65. A: Incarcerated hemivertebra. **B:** Nonincarcerated hemiv-ertebra. (From Winter RB [1983]: Classification and terminology. In *Con-genital deformities of the spine.* New York: Thieme-Stratton, with per-mission.)

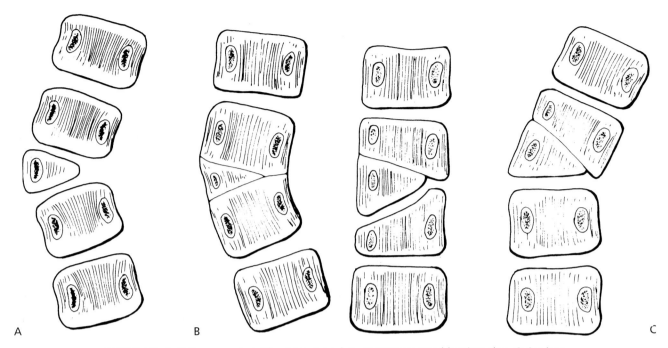

FIGURE 66. A: Fully segmented, "free" hemivertebra. **B:** Nonsegmented hemivertebra. **C:** Semisegmented hemivertebra. (From Winter RB [1983]: Classification and terminology. In *Congenital deformities of the spine.* New York: Thieme-Stratton, with permission.)

A nonincarcerated hemivertebra is one that is lying at the apex of the definite scoliosis. The pedicle line is disturbed, that is, the vertebral column is distorted (Fig. 65B).

(2) Segmented Versus Nonsegmented Hemivertebrae

A fully segmented hemivertebra is one in which there is a normal disc space above and below. It is frequently called a "free" hemivertebra (Fig. 66A).

A nonsegmented hemivertebra is one in which there is a defect of segmentation both above and below (Fig. 66B).

A semisegmented hemivertebra is one in which there is a normal disc space on one side of the hemivertebra, but the other side is nonsegmented from the adjacent vertebra (Fig. 66C).

(3) Hemimetameric Segmental Displacement

Hemimetameric segmental displacement results from a failure of the normal union of hemimetameres across the midline. One or more malunions occur, resulting in two "hemivertebrae," one on each side at the top and bottom of the area of malunion. It is usually called hemimetameric "shift" (Fig. 67).

E. Idiopathic Scoliosis

Approximately 80% of the patients with structural scoliosis have idiopathic scoliosis.

(1) Chronologic Classification

Infantile: From birth to 3 years of age
Juvenile: From 4 years until the onset of puberty
Adolescent: At or about the onset of puberty and before closure of the physes
Adult: After skeletal maturity

(2) Clinical Measurements

Decompensation: Balance of the thorax over the pelvis. A plumb line from C7 should fall in the intergluteal cleft; otherwise describe if it is to the left or right, and measure in centimeters the distance between the plumb line and the cleft.

Shoulder level: Measured from the acromioclavicular joints. The height of the high shoulder is compared with that of the low shoulder measured and recorded.

Trapezius neckline: Record asymmetries.

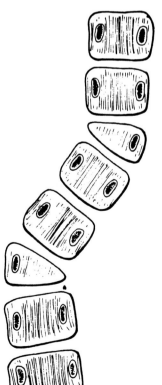

FIGURE 67. Hemimetameric segmental displacement. Hemimetameric shift. (Figures 45–57) (From Winter RB [1983]: Classification and terminology. In *Congenital deformities of the spine.* New York: Thieme-Stratton, with permission.)

Pelvis level: Differences in the levels of the anterosuperior iliac spine are measured in centimeters.

With the patient viewed from the side, the sagittal contours are noted on the forward-bending test (Adams' test):

- Trunk rotation angle (scoliometer)
  —Thoracic rib hump; measurement of the prominence in centimeters
  —Also can be measured in the Tangential Rib View (See Fig. 4/, Appendix C)
- Sagittal alignment (kyphosis, lordosis)
- Determine flexibility by side bending and by head-neck traction
- Moire screen

(3) Curve Patterns

Curves are designated according to the level of the apex of the curvature. Right and left refer to the side of the convexity of the curve (Fig. 68). Ponseti and Friedman in 1950 defined five curve patterns in idiopathic scoliosis:

Curve Type	Apex	End Vertebrae
Cervicothoracic	T3	C7 or T1 to T4 or T5
Thoracic	T8 or T9	T6 to T11
Thoracolumbar	T11 or T12	T6 or T7 to L1 or L2
Lumbar	L1 or L2	T6 or T7 to L1 or L2
Double curve	L1 or L2	T11 to L3

According to the Terminology Committee of the Scoliosis Research Society.

Cervical: When the apex is between C1 and C6
Cervicothoracic: Apex between C7 and T1
Thoracic: Apex between T2 and T11
Thoracolumbar: Apex at T12 and L1

Lumbar: Apex between L2 and L4
Lumbosacral: Apex between L5 and S1

Double structural curves:

A. Double thoracic
B. Combined thoracic and lumbar
C. Combined thoracic and thoracolumbar

Moe JH, Kettleson DN (1970): Idiopathic scoliosis: analysis of curve patterns and the preliminary results of Milwaukee brace treatment in 169 patients. *J Bone Joint Surg [Am]* 52:1509–1533.

Ponseti IV, Friedman B (1950): Prognosis in idiopathic scoliosis. *J Bone Joint Surg [Am]* 32:381–395.

The Terminology Committee of the Scoliosis Research Society (1976): A glossary of scoliosis terms. *Spine* 1:57–58.

(4) Classification of Thoracic Idiopathic Curves (King and Colleagues) (Table 26; Figs. 69–73)

(5) Assessment of Maturity

Bone age (Greulich and Pyle)
Risser Sign
Tanner-Whitehouse
Graham
Oxford
Girdany
Vertebral ring apophysis

(6) Selection of Fusion Levels

A traditional teaching principle has been fusion from T4 to L4 for combined thoracic and lumbar curves. However, fusion in the lumbar spine should be avoided when possible.

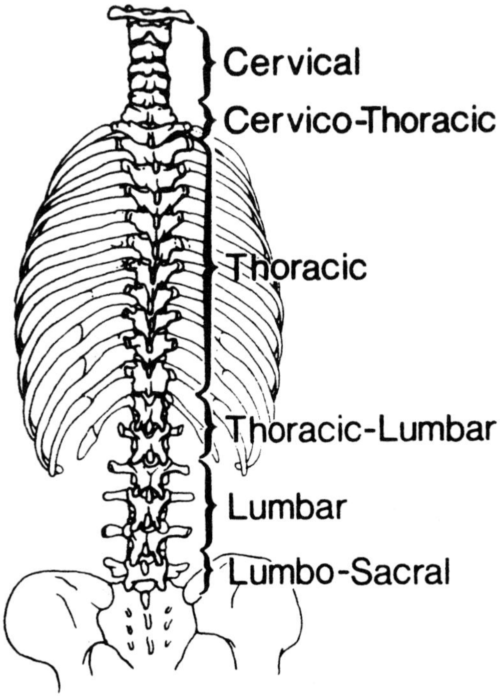

FIGURE 68. Description of the curve based on the apical vertebra (Scoliosis Research Society). (From Morrissy RT [1985]: Clinical and radiologic evaluation of spinal disease. In: Bradford DS, Hensinger RM, eds. *The pediatric spine.* Stuttgart: Georg Thieme, with permission.)

TABLE 26. CURVE PATTERNS

	Criteria	No. of Patients in the Present Series (%)
Type I	S-shaped curve in which both thoracic curve and lumbar curve cross midline Lumbar curve larger than thoracic curve on standing radiograph Flexibility index a negative value (thoracic curve = lumbar curve on standing radiograph, but more flexible on side-bending)	52 (12.9)
Type II	S-shaped curve in which thoracic curve and lumbar curve cross midline Thoracic curve = lumbar curve Flexibility index = 0	132 (32.6)
Type III	Thoracic curve in which lumbar curve does not cross midline (so-called overhang)	133 (32.8)
Type IV	Long thoracic curve in which L5 is centered over sacrum, but L4 tilts into long thoracic curve	37 (9.2)
Type V	Double thoracic curve with T1 tilted into convexity of upper curve Upper curve structural on side-bending	47 (11.6)

From King, HA, Moe JH, Bradford DS, et al. (1983): The selection of fusion levels in thoracic idiopathic scoliosis. *J Bone Joint Surg [Am]* 65: 1302–1313, with permission.

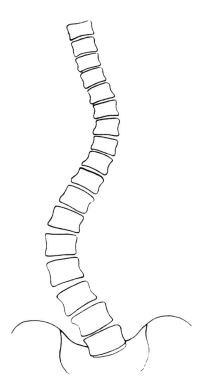

FIGURE 69. Type 1 curve. (From King HA, Moe JH, Bradford DS, Winter RB [1983]: The selection of fusion levels in thoracic idiopathic scoliosis. *J Bone Joint Surg [Am]* 65:1302–1313, with permission.)

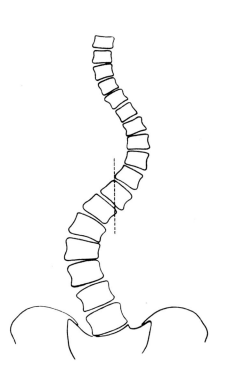

FIGURE 70. Type 2 curve. (From King HA, Moe JH, Bradford DS, Winter RB [1983]: The selection of fusion levels in thoracic idiopathic scoliosis. *J Bone Joint Surg [Am]* 65: 1302–1313, with permission.)

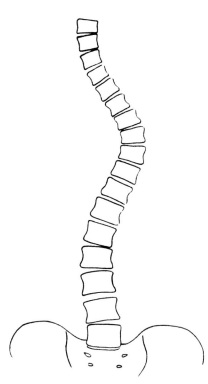

FIGURE 71. Type 3 curve. (From King HA, Moe JH, Bradford DS, Winter RB [1983]: The selection of fusion levels in thoracic idiopathic scoliosis. *J Bone Joint Surg [Am]* 65: 1302–1313, with permission.)

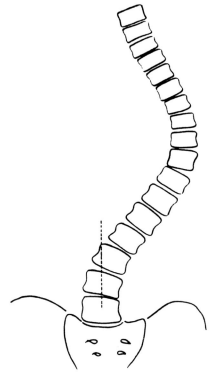

FIGURE 72. Type 4 curve. (From King HA, Moe JH, Bradford DS, Winter RB [1983]: The selection of fusion levels in thoracic idiopathic scoliosis. *J Bone Joint Surg [Am]* 65: 1302–1313, with permission.)

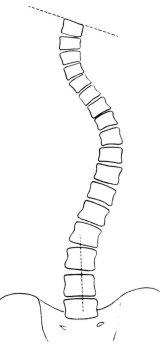

FIGURE 73. Type 5 curve. (From King HA, Moe JH, Bradford DS, Winter RB [1983]: The selection of fusion levels in thoracic idiopathic scoliosis. *J Bone Joint Surg [Am]* 65:1302–1313, with permission.)

Ferguson suggested that the ideal fusion should extend to the vertebrae that have their distant surfaces parallel to each other.

Moe and Goldstein suggested that the levels of fusion should extend from the neutrally rotated vertebra above to the neutrally rotated vertebra below. The neutral vertebra is determined by the criteria established by Nash and Moe. It can be established when both pedicles are symmetric on a posteroanterior radiograph. Moe has also recommended side-bending radiographic views to define curve flexibility. He has advocated selective thoracic fusion in patients with double curves but a flexible lumbar curve.

(a) *Harrington's "Stable Zone"*

Harrington proposed that the lower level of the fusion should lie between two vertical lines drawn through the lumbosacral facets. He recommended that the fusion should be extended one level above and two levels below the measured curve (by the Cobb method) if the end vertebra was in the "stable zone" (Fig. 74).

(b) *King's Center Sacral Line and Stable Vertebra*

King and colleagues have proposed the central sacral line and the concept of the stable vertebra. The fusion should extend to the stable vertebra (Fig. 75).

Ferguson AB (1930): The study and treatment of scoliosis. *South Med J* 23: 116–120.

Ferguson AB (1945): Roentgen diagnosis in the extremities and spine. *AAOS Instr Course Lect* 2:214–24.

Goldstein LH (1966): Surgical management of scoliosis. *J Bone Joint Surg [Am]* 48:167–1696.

Goldstein LH (1971): Surgical management of scoliosis. *Clin Orthop* 77: 32–56.

Harrington PR (1962): Treatment of scoliosis: correction and internal fixation by spine instrumentation. *J Bone Joint Surg [Am]* 44:591–610.

Harvey CJ, Betz RR, Clements DH, et al. (1993): Tangential rib view. *Spine* 18:1593.

King HA, Moe JH, Bradford DS, Winter RB (1983): The selection of fusion levels in thoracic idiopathic scoliosis. *J Bone Joint Surg [Am]* 65:1302–1313.

Moe JH (1972): Methods of correction and surgical techniques in scoliosis. *Orthop Clin North Am* 3:17–48.

Nash CL, Moe JH (1969): Study of vertebral rotation. *J Bone Joint Surg [Am]* 51:223–229.

(7) Special Views

(a) *Supine Films for Detail: Spot Films*

Supine cone-down views or spot films give good detail of specific areas of the spine.

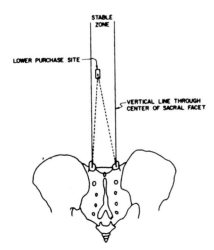

FIGURE 74. The "stable zone" of Harrington, defined by parallel lines drawn through the lumbosacral facets. The vertebral bodies within these lines are in the stable zone. (From Harrington PR [1972]: Technical details in relation to the successful use of instrumentation in scoliosis. *Orthop Clin North Am* 3:49–67, with permission.)

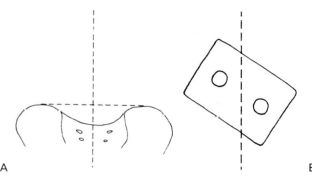

FIGURE 75. A: Center sacral line. The line is drawn through the center of the sacrum perpendicular to the iliac crest. When a limb length discrepancy is present, the pelvis should be leveled with an appropriate lift under the short limb. The central vertical line must always be based on a horizontal pelvis. **B:** The vertebra that is bisected or most closely bisected by this line is determined and is recorded as being the stable vertebra. (From King HA, Moe JH, Bradford DS, Winter RB [1983]: The selection of fusion levels in thoracic idiopathic scoliosis. *J Bone Joint Surg [Am]* 65:1302–1313, with permission.)

(b) *Bending Films*

Bending films are used to evaluate the rigidity or flexibility of a curve. These films should be taken with the patient supine and should use the maximal voluntary cooperation of the patient. For uncooperative or nonunderstanding patients, passive bending films can be obtained.

(c) *Traction Films*

For patients with neuromuscular scoliosis, a good evaluation of the rigidity or flexibility of a curve can be obtained by using traction in the supine position, or vertically by using suspension devices.

(d) *Hyperextension Films*

In hyperextension films, to assess flexibility or rigidity in patients with kyphosis, a lateral view is taken with a firm radiolucent object placed under the apex of the kyphosis and the patient supine.

(e) *Oblique Views*

Oblique views are useful to evaluate the fusion mass. They are also used to evaluate the pars interarticularis in cases where spondylolysis is suspected.

(f) *Ferguson View*

The Ferguson view is taken with the film tilted 30 degrees cephalad in men and 35 degrees in women, or with the patient's hips flexed 90 degrees to eliminate lordosis. This view shows the anatomy of the lumbosacral junction.

(g) *Derotated View (Stagnara)*

The derotated view is useful in large curves (usually around 100 degrees or larger). This view eliminates the kyphosis associated with rotation in large curves. This view should be a true coronal view of the apical vertebra, revealing the true scoliosis.

(h) *Tangential rib view*

Method of assessment of the rib prominence. This view is taken with the patient standing in the Adams maneuver position. (See Fig. 47 in Appendix C.)

25. PELVIC OBLIQUITY (Fig. 76)

26. SCHEUERMANN DISEASE (JUVENILE KYPHOSIS)

Thoracic Scheuermann disease usually affects the T7–9 area, less often the T11–12. There are also cases of "lumbar Scheuermann disease" in which the affection predominantly affects the L1–2 area.

The radiographic diagnosis of Scheuermann kyphosis is made by the presence of irregularities of the vertebral endplates, anterior vertebral wedging, Schmorl's nodes, and decreased intervertebral disc space height. There is some discrepancy in the literature as to the number of consecutive vertebrae that need to be wedged to make the diagnosis of Scheuermann kyphosis. By one criterion

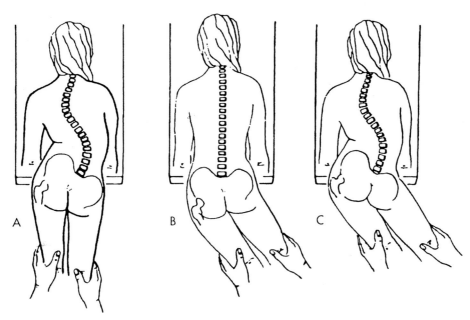

FIGURE 76. A: Pelvic Obliquity. **B:** If pelvic obliquity is eliminated by abduction or adduction of hips, pelvic-femoral muscle contracture is caused. **C:** If obliquity persists despite abducion or adduction of hips, fixed spinal-pelvic deformity exists. (From Shook JE, Lubicky JP [1996]: Paralytic scoliosis. In: Bridwell KH, DeWald RI, eds. *The textbook of spinal surgery*, 2nd ed. Philadelphia: JB Lippincott.)

(Sorensen's criterion) there should be wedging in three or more adjacent vertebrae of more than 5 degrees. In other studies the diagnosis is made by the presence of only wedged vertebrae of more than 5 degrees. Total kyphosis in excess of 50 degrees is considered abnormal.

Sorensen KH (1964): *Scheuermann's juvenile kyphosis.* Copenhagen: Munskgaard.

Bradford DS, Moe JH, Montalvo FJ, Winter RB (1974): Scheuermann's kyphosis and roundback deformity. *J Bone Joint Surg Am* 56:740–758.

27. SPONDYLOLISTHESIS

A. Classification (Figs. 77, 78; Table 27)

Newmann PH (1963): Spondylolisthesis, its course and effect. *Ann R Coll Surg Engl* 16:305–323.

This classification was later modified and it is now the most widely accepted classification (Wiltse et al., 1976).

  I. *Dysplastic.* In this type, congenital abnormalities of the upper sacrum or the arch of L5 permit the listhesis to occur.
  II. *Isthmic.* The lesion is in the pars interarticularis. Three types can be recognized.
    A. Lytic-fatigue fracture of the parts.
    B. Elongated but intact pars.
    C. Acute fracture.
  III. *Degenerative.* Owing to long-standing intersegmental instability.
  IV. *Traumatic.* Owing to fractures in other areas of the bony hook than the pars.
  V. *Pathologic.* There is generalized or localized bone disease (Fig. 67).

Wiltse LL, Newmann PH, Macnab I (1976): Classification of spondylolisis and spondylolisthesis. *Clin Orthop* 117:23–29.

Camins M, O'Leary P (1987): *The Lumbar Spine.* New York: Raven Press.

B. Risk Factors for Progression of Spondylolisthesis

(1) Clinical

Age: Young child, younger than 10 years
Sex: Girls at greater risk
Symptoms: Children with backache have greater likelihood
Excessive ligamentous laxity

TABLE 27. MARCHETTI-BARTOLOZZI CLASSIFICATION

Developmental
High dysplastic
  With lysis
  With elongation
Low dysplastic
  With lysis
  With elongation

Acquired
Traumatic
  Acute fracture
  Stress fracture
Postsurgery
  Direct surgery
  Indirect surgery
Pathologic
  Local pathology
  Systemic pathology
Degenerative
  Primary
  Secondary

Orthopaedic Knowledge Update #6. *American Acad Orthop Surg.* ed: Beaty J 1999:69.

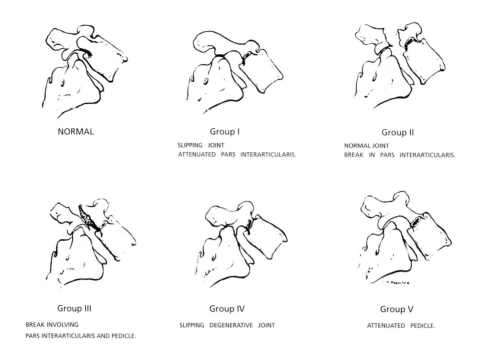

NORMAL

Group I

SLIPPING JOINT
ATTENUATED PARS INTERARTICULARIS.

Group II

NORMAL JOINT
BREAK IN PARS INTERARTICULARIS.

Group III

BREAK INVOLVING
PARS INTERARTICULARIS AND PEDICLE.

Group IV

SLIPPING DEGENERATIVE JOINT

Group V

ATTENUATED PEDICLE.

FIGURE 77. Normal L5–S1 relationship. *Group I:* Congenital (dysplastic). *Group II:* Spondylolitic (isthmic or true spondylolistheses). *Group III:* Traumatic. *Group IV:* Degenerative. *Group V:* Pathologic. Group I and Group IV were also frequent. (From Newman PH [1963]: The etiology of spondylolisthesis. *J Bone Joint Surg [Br]* 45:39–59, with permission.)

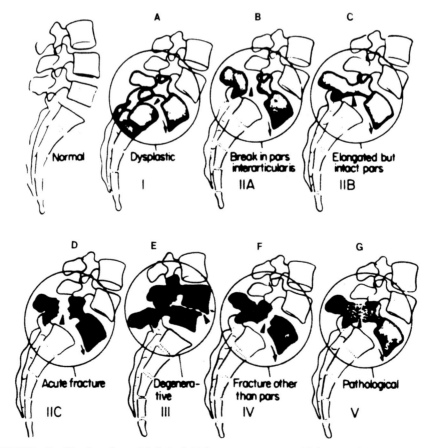

FIGURE 78. Classification of spondylolisthesis (Wiltse, Newmann, McNab). (From Tachdijan MO: Spondylolisthesis. In: *Pediatric orthopedics,* 2nd ed. Philadelphia: WB Saunders, with permission.)

(2) Radiologic

Type of spondylolisthesis
Dysplastic lesions have greater tendency than isthemic defects

(3) Degree of Slips

Mild displacement, minimal chances; 50% and over, greater probability; high slip angle—40 to 50 degrees and over.

(4) Mobility at L5–S1

Mobility at L5–S1 indicates instability and greater probability of progression.

(5) Anatomic Stability

A trapezoid or wedge-shaped fifth lumbar vertebra and a dome-shaped top of the first sacral vertebra means instability and greater likelihood of progression. An anterior slip of the sacrum and narrowed L5–S1 disc interspace indicates stability and minimal chance of further slip.

28. SPINAL STENOSIS

Definition: Any type of narrowing of the spinal canal, nerve root canals (or tunnels), or intervertebral foramina. It may be local, segmental, or generalized. It may be caused by bone or by soft tissue, and the narrowing may involve the bony canal alone, the dural sac, or both. It can be classified according to the Anatomical area of the spine affected and the specific pathologic entity involved (Table 28).

TABLE 28. CLASSIFICATION OF SPINAL STENOSIS

Anatomical Area	Anatomical Region (Local Segment)
ANATOMIC	
Cervical	Central
	Foraminal
Thoracic	Central
Lumbar	Central
	Lateral recess
	Foraminal
	Extraforaminal (far-out)
PATHOLOGIC	
Congenital	
Achondroplastic (dwarfism)	
Congenital forms of spondylolisthesis	
Scoliosis	
Kyphosis	
Idiopathis	
Degenerative and inflammatory	
Osteoarthritis	
Inflammatory arthritis	
Diffuse idiopathic skeletal hyperostosis (DISH)	
Scoliosis	
Kyphosis	
Degenerative forms of spondylolisthesis	
Metabolic	
Paget disease	
Fluorosis	

Wood GW II. In: Camele ST, ed. *Cambell's Operative Orthopaedics,* 9th ed. Mosby, 1998, p. 3143.

TABLE 29. CLASSIFICATION OF SPINAL STENOSIS BASED ON PATHOLOGIC PROCESSES

I. Congenital-development stenosis
  A. Idiopathic
  B. Achondroplastic
II. Acquired stenosis
  A. Degenerative
    1. Central portion of spinal canal
    2. Peripheral portion of canal
      a. Lateral recess
      b. Foraminal
  B. Combined
    1. Any combination of all types
  C. Spondylolisthetic/spondylolytic
    1. May also include lateral recess, foraminal and far-out forms
  D. Iatrogenic
    1. Postlaminectomy
    2. Postfusion (anterior or posterior)
  E. Posttraumatic, late changes
  F. Miscellaneous (metabolic/inflammatory)
    1. Paget disease
    2. Fluorosis
    3. Forestier disease
    4. DISH

Modifiers
I. Segmental disease
II. Generalized disease

Adapted from Arnoldi CC, Brodsky AE, Cauchoix J. et al. (1976): *Clin Orthop* 115:4.

29. LUMBAR SPINAL STENOSIS: Arnoldi proposed a classification scheme for the lumbar spine based on pathologic processes (Fig. 79; Table 29).

Postacchini F (1990): Lumbar spinal stenosis: classification and treatment. In: The International Society for the Study of the Lumbar Spine, ed. *The Lumbar Spine.* pp 594–611.

30. DISC HERNIATION (Fig. 80)

The distortion of the annular contour that occurs because of a disc herniation may be as follows:

Contained: This is a simple disc protrusion in which the annular fibers are intact and contain the protruded nuclear material.
Noncontained: Disc material has ruptured through the annulus and is no longer contained.

The following two varieties occur:

1. Extruded disc material: subligamentous (subannular) or transligamentous
2. Sequestered: free fragment of disc material in the spinal canal

A. Criteria for the Diagnosis of Acute Radicular Syndrome (Sciatica due to a Herniated Nucleus Pulposus) (Table 30)

31. CLASSIFICATION OF NERVE ROOT ANOMALIES (Figs. 81–84)

32. DIFFERENTIAL DIAGNOSIS OF BACK AND LEG PAIN (Table 31)

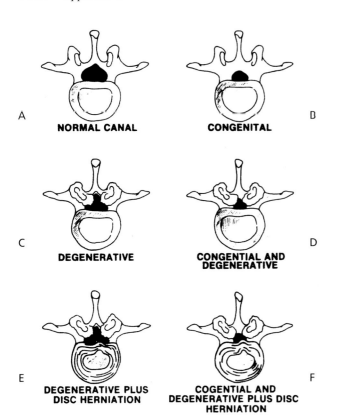

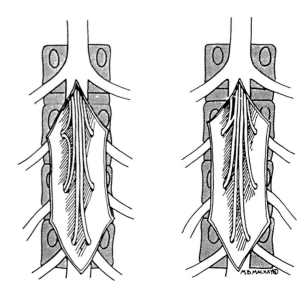

FIGURE 81. Nerve root anomalies. Type I nerve root anomaly: intradural anastomosis. (From Kadish LJ, Simmons EH [1984]: Anomalies of the lumbosacral nerve roots: an anatomical investigation and myelographic study. *J Bone Joint Surg [Br]* 66:411.)

FIGURE 79. Types of lumbar spinal stenosis. **A:** Normal canal. **B:** Congenital and developmental stenosis. **C:** Degenerative stenosis. **D:** Congenital and developmental stenosis with disc herniation. **E:** Degenerative stenosis with disc herniation. **F:** Congenital/developmental stenosis with superimposed degenerative stenosis. (From Arnoldi CC, et al. [1976]: Lumbar spinal stenosis and nerve root entrapment syndromes: definition and classification. *Clin Orthop* 115:4–5, with permission.)

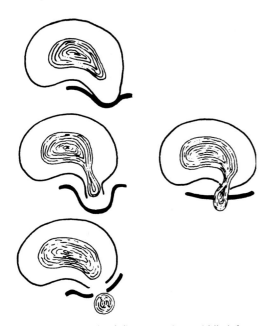

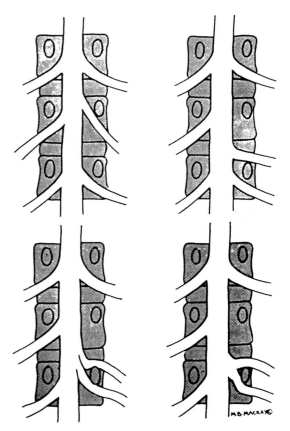

FIGURE 80. *Top,* A contained disc protrusion. *Middle left,* A noncontained subligamentous disc extrusion. *Middle right,* A noncontained transligamentous disc extrusion. *Bottom,* A noncontained disc sequestration. (From McCulloch JA, Inoue S, Moriya H, et al. [1990]: The intervertebral disc: surgical indications and techniques. In: The International Society for the Study of the Lumbar Spine, ed. *The lumbar spine.* Philadelphia: WB Saunders, with permission.)

FIGURE 82. Nerve root anomalies. Type II anomalous origin of nerve roots. **A:** Cranial origin. **B:** Caudal origin. **C:** Closely adjacent nerve roots. **D:** Conjoined nerve roots (From Kadish LJ, Simmons EH [1984]: Anomalies of the lumbosacral nerve roots an anatomical investigation and myelographic study. *J Bone Joint Surg [Br]* 66:411.)

TABLE 30. CRITERIA FOR THE DIAGNOSIS OF ACUTE RADICULAR SYNDROME (SCIATICA DUE TO A HERNIATED NUCLEUS PULPOSUS[a]

1. Leg pain (including buttock) is the dominant complaint, rather than back pain

2. Neurologic symptoms are specific (e.g., paresthesia in a typical dermatomal distribution)

3. Significant straight-leg raising (SLR) changes occur
    SLR less than 50% of normal
    Bowstring discomfort
    Crossover pain (any one or a combination of these)

4. Neurologic signs: 2 out of 4 of weakness, wasting, sensory loss, or reflext alteration

From McCuiloch JA, et al. (1990): The intervertebral disc: surgical indications and techniques. In: The International Society for the Study of the Lumbar Spine, ed. *The lumbar spine*. Philadelphia: WB Saunders, with permission.
[a] Three or four of these criteria must be present, the only exception being the young patients who are very resistant to the effects of nerve root compression and thus may not have neurologic symptoms (criterion 2) or signs (criterion 4).

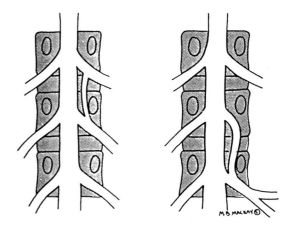

FIGURE 83. Nerve root anomalies. Type III. Extradural anastomosis. (From Kadish LJ, Simmons EH [1984]: Anomalies of the lumbosacral nerve roots an anatomical investigation and myelographic study. *J Bone Joint Surg Br* 66:411.)

TABLE 31. DIFFERENTIAL DIAGNOSIS OF BACK AND LEG PAIN

1. Peripheral nerve problems
    a. Piriformis syndrome
    b. Meralgia paresthetica
    c. Iliohypogastric ilioinguinal, and genitofemoral neuritis
    d. Femoral neuropathy
    e. Obturator neuropathy
    f. Sacral notch or sciatic neuropathy

2. Metabolic and inflammatory diseases
    a. Bony infection of the spine (pyogenic, fungal, parasitic, tuberculosis)
    b. Spinal epidural abscess
    c. Rheumatoid variants: ankylosing spondylitis, psoriatic arthritis, Reiter syndrome, intestinal arthropathies
    d. Paget disease
    e. Gout
    f. Pseudogout
    g. Fibrositis
    h. Ochronosis
    i. Hemochromatosis
    j. Osteogenesis imperfecta
    k. Diabetic amyotrophy
    l. Hyperparathyroidism
    m. Bursitis
    n. Osteoporosis
    o. Osteoarthritis
    p. Diffuse idiopathic skeletal hyperostosis
    q. Adhesive arachnoiditis

3. Psychogenic pain

4. Tumors
    a. Intramedullary
    b. Extradural
    c. Intradural-extramedullary
    d. Metastatic tumors of the spine

    e. Primary benign and malignant tumors to bone
    f. Sacral cysts
    g. Retroperitoneal tumors and fibrosis
5. Referred pain syndrome
    a. Gastrointestinal: peptic ulcer, pancreatic disorders, gallbladder disorders
    b. Vascular: abdominal aortic aneurysm, arterial occlusion or insufficiency, other aneurysms
    c. Renal: nephrolithiasis, infection, prostatitis
    d. Gynecological/obstetrical: pregnancy, pelvic tumors, pelvic inflammatory disorders
    e. Hip disorders
    f. Knee disorders
    g. Sacroiliac disorders
    h. Coccygodynia

6. Mechanical
    a. Segmental instability
    b. Trauma
    c. Spinal deformity
    d. Spinal stenosis
    e. Leg length inequality
    f. Iliac crest syndrome
    g. Facet syndrome
    h. Herniated intervertebral disc

7. Congenital
    a. Ilium—transverse process pseudarthrosis

8. Miscellaneous
    a. Charcot's spine (vertebral osteoarthropathy)
    b. Compartment syndromes (posterior thigh and paraspinal muscles)
    c. Scheuermann disease
    d. Radiation-induced disorders
    e. Spondylosis and spondylolithesis

From Watson T, Benson D (1990): Nondiscogenic back and leg pain. In *Youman's neurological surgery*, 3rd ed. Philadelphia: WB Saunders, with permission.

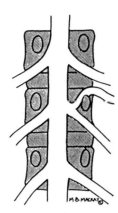

FIGURE 84. Nerve root anomalies. Type IV. Extradural division. (From Kadish LJ, Simmons EH [1984]: Anomalies of the lumbosacral nerve roots an anatomical investigation and myelographic study. *J Bone Joint Surg [Br]* 66:411.)

33. DIFFERENTIAL DIAGNOSIS OF SCIATICA (Table 32)

34. NONORGANIC PHYSICAL SIGNS OF LOW BACK PAIN

Waddell's tests (nonorganic physical signs of low back pain):

Tenderness: This category should be scored positive if light touch or rolling of the skin on the back causes pain, or if deep tenderness is spread over large areas of the body.

Simulation test: This is scored positive if gentle axial rotation of the pelvis and shoulders causes back pain, or if light pressure of 1 to 2 pounds of force applied to the head by the examiner's hand causes back pain.

Distraction test: This is scored positive if the patient's pain, which is presented in some activities, is not present when those same activities occur in a different context, for example, if the straight leg–raising test is present in the supine position but totally absent when sitting. This is considered a positive distraction test.

Regional disturbances: This is positive when the patient demonstrates "cogwheel" weakness ("give-away weakness" followed by increased resistance) or nonneu-

roanatomic numbness, such as stocking-and-glove numbness in the absence of peripheral neuropathy.

Overreaction: A positive score is awarded here when there is excessive body language, grimacing, verbalization, groans, tremors, collapsing, excessive sweating, or stumbling.

Scoring: If three out of the five tests listed are positive, then nonorganic psychological pain behavior is likely.

Wadell G, McCulloch JA, Kummel E, Venner RM (1980): Nonorganic physical signs in low-back pain. *Spine* 5:117–125.

35. MIDLINE DYSRAPHISM (Table 33)

36. CONGENITAL ABSENCE OF THE SACRUM AND LUMBOSACRAL VERTEBRAE (LUMBOSACRAL AGENESIS) (Figs. 85–88)

37. LUMBOSACRAL TRANSITIONAL VERTEBRA

Classification of the different types of lumbosacral transitional vertebra
Type 1: Dysplastic transverse process:
  A. Unilateral
  B. Bilateral

This type presents a large transverse process that is triangular in shape and measures at least 19 mm in width.

Type 2: Incomplete lumbarization and sacralization (i.e., the total number of vertebrae were not determined.)

TABLE 32. DIFFERENTIAL DIAGNOSIS OF SCIATICA

Intraspinal causes
  Proximal to disc
    Conus and cauda equina lesions (e.g., neurofibroma, ependymoma)
  Disc level
    HNP
    Stenosis (canal or recess)
    Infection—osteomyelitis or discitis (with nerve root pressure)
    Inflammation—arachnoiditis
    Neoplasm—benign or malignant with nerve root pressure

Extraspinal causes
  Pelvis
    Cardiovascular conditions (e.g., peripheral vascular disease)
    Gynecologic conditions
    Orthopaedic conditions (e.g., osteoarthritis of hip)
    Sacroiliac joint disease
    Neoplasms (invading or compressing lumbosacral plexus)
  Peripheral nerve lesions
    Neuropathy (diabetic. tumor, alcohol)
    Local sciatic nerve conditions (trauma, tumor),
    Inflammation (herpes zoster)

From McCulloch JA, et al. (1990): *The intervertebral disc.* Philadelphia: WB Saunders, with permission.

TABLE 33. CLASSIFICATION OF CRANIAL AND SPINAL DYSRAPHISM

Spina bifida aperta
  Myeloschisis
  Myelomeningocele
  Hemimyelomeningocele
  Syringomyelomeningocele
  Spinal meningocele

Arnold-Chiari malformation

Dandy-Walker malformation

Cranium bifidum
  Cranial meningocele
  Encephalomeningocele

Occult cranial dysraphism
  Cranial dermal sinus

Occult spinal dysraphism
  Spinal dermal sinus
  Tethered cord syndrome
  Lumbosacral lipoma
  Diastematomyelia
  Neurenteric cyst
  Combined anterior and posterior spina bifida
  Anterior sacral meningocele
  Occult intrasacral meningocele

Nondysraphic malformations
  Perineurial (Tarlov's) cyst
  Spinal extradural cyst
  Nondysraphic spinal meningocele
  Caudal regression syndrome
  Sacrococcygeal teratoma

From French BN (1990): Midline fusion defects and defects of formation. In *Youman's neurological surgery.* 3rd ed. Philadelphia: WB Saunders, with permission.

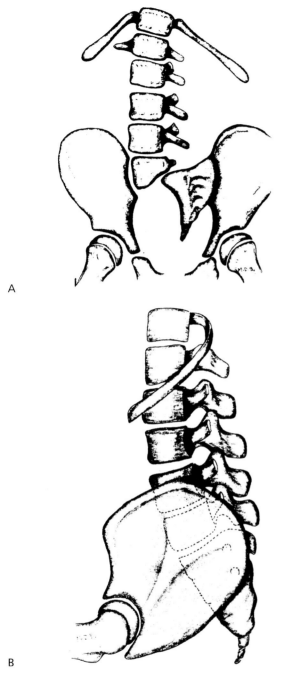

A

B

FIGURE 85. Type I: Total or partial unilateral sacral agenesis. Vertebro-pelvic articulation is usually stable. The unilateral absence of the sacrum results in an oblique lumbosacral joint and lumbosacral scoliosis. **A:** Anteroposterior drawing. **B:** Lateral view diagram.

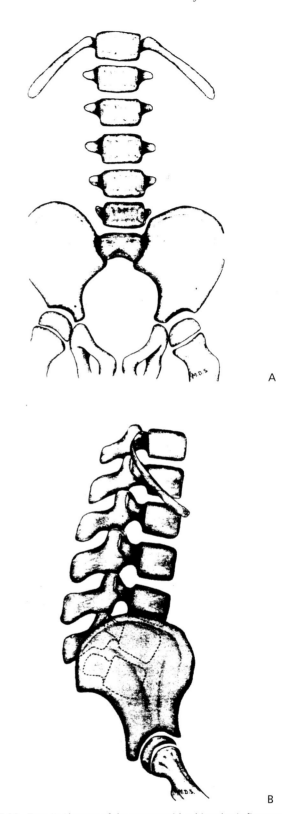

A

B

FIGURE 86. Type II: Absence of the sacrum with a hipoplastic first sacral vertebra providing a lumbopelvic articulation. **A:** Anteroposterior drawing. **B:** Lateral view diagram.

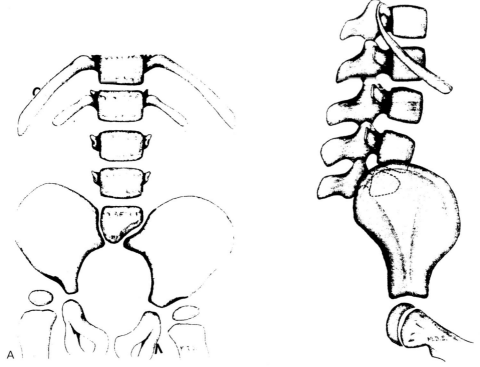

FIGURE 87. Type III: Absent fourth and fifth lumbar vertebrae, sacrum, and coccyx. The sides of the third lumbar vertebra articulate with the ilia. The lumbopelvic junction is relatively stable. **A:** Anteroposterior drawing. **B:** Lateral view diagram.

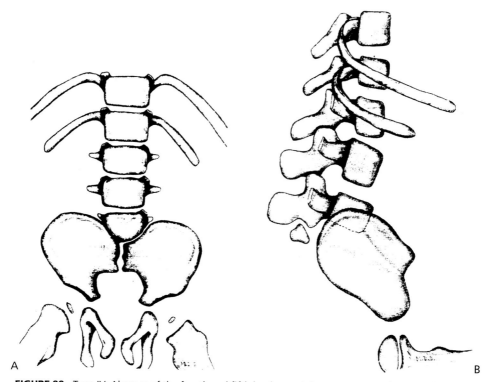

FIGURE 88. Type IV: Absence of the fourth and fifth lumbar vertebrae, sacrum, and coccyx. The caudal end plate of the third lumbar vertebra rests above an iliac amphiarthrosis. The pelvis is very unstable under the spine. **A:** Anteroposterior drawing. **B:** Lateral view diagram. (Figures 85–88 from Renshaw TS [1978]: Sacral agenesis: a classification and review of twenty-three cases. *J Bone Joint Surg. [Am]* 60: 373–380, with permission.)

A. Unilateral
B. Bilateral

This type has a large transverse process, which appears to follow the contour of the sacral ala. They are considered incomplete because there appears to be a diarthrodial joint between the transverse process and the sacrum.

Type 3: Complete lumbarization and sacralization (i.e., the total number of vertebrae were not determined)
A. Unilateral
B. Bilateral

This is similar to type 2 except that instead of a diarthrodial joint between the transverse process and the sacrum, there is a true bony union.

Type 4: Mixed.
The patients who fall in this category exhibit type 2 on one side and type III on the other.

Type 2 presents a high incidence of herniated lumbar disc at the level of transition. It also presents a greater incidence of disc herniations at the level just above the lumbosacral transitional vertebra (Fig. 89).

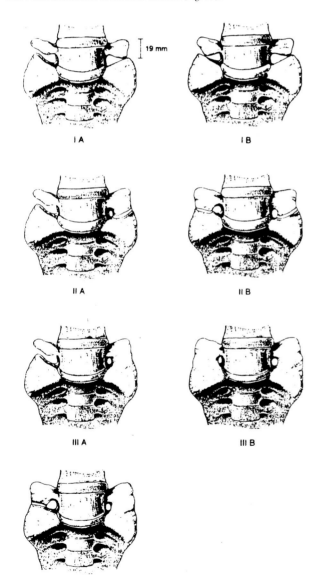

FIGURE 89. Classification of lumbosacral transitional vertebrae according to radiomorphological and clinical relevance with respect to lumbar disc herniation. (From Castelvi AE, Goldstein LA, Chan DPK [1984]: Lumbosacral transitional vertebrae and their relationship with lumbar extradural defects. *Spine* 9:493–495, with permission.)

TABLE 34. VERTEBRAL BEAKING

Inferior	Central
Hurler syndrome	Morqulo syndrome
Cretinism	Achondroplasia
Morquio syndrome	Spondyloepiphyseal dysplasia
Achondroplasia	Normal (6–8 years, mild)
Diastrophic dwarfism	
Trisomy 21	
Phenylketonuria	
Muscle hypotonia	
Trauma	
Normal children—early sitting	

From Kricun ME (1988): Conventional radiography. In: *Imaging modalities in spinal disorders.* Philadelphia: WB Saunders, pp. 75–78, with permission.

TABLE 35. CENTRAL VERTEBRAL DEPRESSION ("H" VERTEBRA)

Sickle cell anemia
Uremic osteopathy (renal osteodystrophy)
Gaucher disease
Homocystinuria
Hereditary spherocytosis (rare)
Thalassemia (rare)
Normal (mild)

From Kricun ME (1988): Conventional radiography. In: *Imaging modalities in spinal disorders.* Philadelphia: WB Saunders, pp. 75–78, with permission.

38. NORMAL AND ABNORMAL VARIATIONS IN VERTEBRAL BODY SHAPE (Fig. 90; Tables 34–38)

Mitchell GE, Lourie H, Berne AS (1967): The various causes of scalloped vertebrae with notes on their pathogenesis. *Radiology* 89:67–74.

39. ABNORMALITIES IN VERTEBRAL BODY DENSITY

The density of the vertebral bodies is best appreciated on the lateral radiograph, and changes in density, either increased (osteoblastic, osteosclerotic) or

TABLE 36. POSTERIOR VERTEBRAL SCALLOPING

Physiologic

Increased intraspinal pressure
    Tumor
    Syringohydromyelia
    Uncontrolled communicating hydrocephalus

Dural actasia
    Neurofibromatosis
    Marfan syndrome
    Ehlers-Danlos syndrome
    Morquio syndrome

Narrow spinal canal
    Achondroplasia

Bone disorders
    Neurofibromatosis
    Hurler syndrome
    Morquio syndrome
    Acromegaly

From Kricun ME (1988): Conventional radiography. In: *Imaging modalities in spinal disorders.* Philadelphia: WB Saunders, pp. 75–78, with permission.

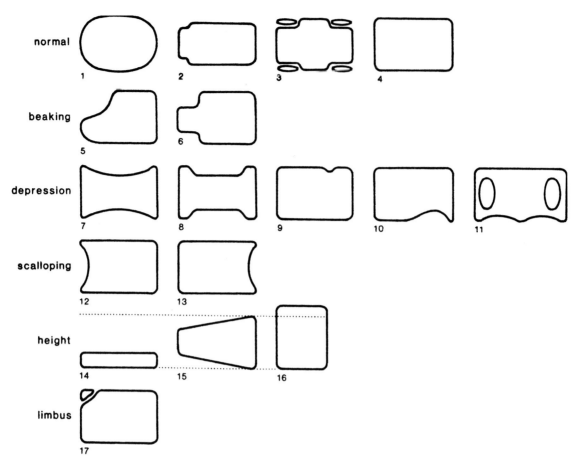

FIGURE 90. Normal variations in shape of vertebral bodies. KEY: 1–10 and 12–17, sagittal view; 11, coronal view; 1–4, normal stages of vertebral development; 1, newborn; 2, 6 to 8 years with anterior steplike recesses; 3, partial calcification of ring apophyses; 4, mature vertebra; 5, inferior beaking; 6, central beaking; 7, biconcavity; 8, "H" or "Lincoln log"; 9, focal indentation—Schmorl's node; 10, posterior concavity; 11, "cupid's bow" configuration; 12, anterior scalloping; 13, posterior scalloping; 14, vertebra plana; 15, anterior wedging; 16, high "canine" vertebra; 17, limbus vertebra. (From Kricun GE [1988]: Conventional radiograph. In: *Imaging modalities in spinal disorders*. Philadelphia: WB Saunders, with permission.)

decreased (osteopenic), may be diffuse or patchy or may involve one vertebral level or part of a vertebral complex.

A. Increased Density (Tables 39–44)

B. Decreased Density (Tables 45, 46)

TABLE 37. ANTERIOR VERTEBRAL SCALLOPING

Thoracic or upper lumbar aneurysm

Tortuous iliac arteries

Paravertebral tumor (metastasis, lymphoma, neurofibroma, and sarcoma)

Abscess

Bony dysplasia of neurofibromatosis

A pseudoscalloping appearance may occur on the lateral radiograph in patients with osteopenia and anterolateral osteophyte formation, or in those with overlying densities

From Kricun ME (1988): Conventional radiography. In: *Imaging modalities in spinal disorders*. Philadelphia: WB Saunders, pp. 75–78, with permission.

40. SPINAL INFECTIONS (Fig. 91)

A. Comparison of Pyogenic and Tuberculous Spinal Infection

The radiographic differentiation of pyogenic and tuberculous infection of the spine may be difficult to establish. There are several features that are more commonly observed in each of the disorders (Table 47)

Kricun ME (1988): Conventional radiography. In: *Imaging modalities in spinal disorders*. Philadelphia: WB Saunders.

TABLE 38. LATERAL SCALLOPING

Tumor (metastasis, lymphoma, neurofibroma, sarcoma)

Abscess

Bony dysplasia of neurofibromatosis

Tortuosity of vertebral arteries in the cervical region and dilated lumbar venous collaterals with or without vena cava obstruction may also cause lateral vertebral scalloping

From Kricun ME (1988): Conventional radiography. In: *Imaging modalities in spinal disorders*. Philadelphia: WB Saunders, pp. 75–78, with permission.

TABLE 39. DIFFUSE INCREASED DENSITY

Metastasis (prostate, breast)
Leukemia
Uremic osteopathy (renal osteodystrophy)
Myelosclerosis
Sickle cell disease in adults
Paget's disease
Osteopetrosis
Pycnodysostosis
Mastocytosis
Fluorosis

From Kricun ME (1988): Conventional radiography. In: *Imaging modalities in spinal disorders*. Philadelphia: WB Saunders, pp. 75–78, with permission.

TABLE 40. PATCHY INCREASE IN DENSITY

Metastasis (prostate, breast)
Lymphoma
Paget disease
Myeloma

From Kricun ME (1988): Conventional radiography. In: *Imaging modalities in spinal disorders*. Philadelphia: WB Saunders, pp. 75–78, with permission.

TABLE 41. IVORY VERTEBRA (EXTENSIVE AND UNIFORM OSTEOSCLEROSIS OF THE ENTIRE VERTEBRAL BODY)

Metastasis
Lymphoma
Paget disease
Osteosarcoma
Chronic osteomyelitis
Melorheostosis
Chordoma (rare)
Myeloma (rare)
Osteoid osteoma (rare)

From Kricun ME (1988): Conventional radiography. In: *Imaging modalities in spinal disorders*. Philadelphia: WB Saunders, pp. 75–78, with permission.

TABLE 42. BANDLIKE INCREASED DENSITY (RUGGER JERSEY SPINE)

Renal osteodystrophy with secondary hyperparathyroidism
Long-term steroid therapy
Cushing disease
Osteopetrosis
Pycnodysostosis
Paget disease

From Kricun ME (1988): Conventional radiography. In: *Imaging modalities in spinal disorders*. Philadelphia: WB Saunders, pp. 75–78, with permission.

TABLE 43. FOCAL OSTEOSCLEROSIS

Metastasis (prostate, breast)
Lymphoma
Bone islands (enostoses)
Degenerative disease (associated to disc space narrowing)
Osteomyelitis

From Kricun ME (1988): Conventional radiography. In: *Imaging modalities in spinal disorders*. Philadelphia: WB Saunders, pp. 75–78, with permission.

TABLE 44. BONE WITHIN BONE (SCLEROTIC OUTLINE OF A SMALLER VERTEBRA WITHIN THE VERTEBRAL BODY)

Normal (50% of infants under two months of age)
Previous severe systemic illness
Chronic intermittent disease
Osteopetrosis
Heavy metal intoxication
Generalized infection
Following radiation therapy
Thorotrast

From Kricun ME (1988): Conventional radiography. In: *Imaging modalities in spinal disorders*. Philadelphia: WB Saunders, pp. 75–78, with permission.

TABLE 45. DIFFUSE DECREASE IN BONY DENSITY

Normal aging
Multiple myeloma
Metastatic disease
Steroids (endogenous or exogenous)
Marrow replacement
Disuse

From Kricun ME (1988): Conventional radiography. In: *Imaging modalities in spinal disorders*. Philadelphia: WB Saunders, pp. 75–78, with permission.

TABLE 46. FOCAL OSTEOPENIA

Tumor
Infection
Histiocytosis
Schmorl's nodes

From Kricun ME (1988): Conventional radiography. In: *Imaging modalities in spinal disorders*. Philadelphia: WB Saunders, pp. 75–78, with permission.

TABLE 47. PYOGENIC SPONDYLITIS VERSUS TUBERCULOUS SPONDYLITIS

	Spondylitis	
	Pyogenic	Tuberculous
Behavior (aggressiveness)	+ + +[a]	+
Bone destruction	+ + +	+ + +
Anterior erosion	+	+ + +
Sclerosis	+ + + (more rapid)	+
Osteophytes	+ + +	+
Vertebral collapse	+ +	+ + +
Osteopenia	+ + +	+
Disc narrowing	+ + +	+ + +
Vertebral fusion	+ + +	+ + (lumbar)
Abscess incidence	+ +	+ + +
Abscess size	+ +	+ + +
Abscess calcification	+	+ + +
Multiple vertebral segments	+	+ + +
Skip lesions	+	+ +
Posterior elements	Rare	Rare
Kyphosis	+	+ + +

From Kricun ME (1988): Conventional radiography. In: *Imaging modalities in spinal disorders*. Philadelphia: WB Saunders, pp. 75–78, with permission.
Key: + + +, frequent; + +, moderately frequent; +, occasional.
[a] Occasionally the behavior is not aggressive.

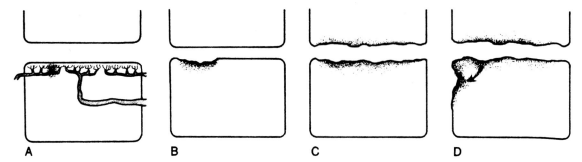

A   **B**   **C**   **D**

FIGURE 91. The formation and spread of infection in the vertebral body, adjacent disc, and prevertebral region. **A:** Infection *(shaded area)* begins in the subchondral region. Disc height is normal. **B:** Further subchondral destruction and extension into the intervertebral disc, causing diminution of disc height. **C:** Extension of infection to involve the opposing vertebral margin. **D:** Infection extends anteriorly into the prevertebral subligamentous region, forming an abscess. (From Kricun ME [1988]: Conventional radiography. In: *Imaging modalities in spinal disorders.* Philadephia: WB Saunders, with permission.)

B. Prediction of final gibbus deformity in Spinal Tuberculosis (Figs. 92, 93)

Rajasekaran and Shanmugasundaram compared the development of kyphosis with the degree of collapse at the time of presentation of tubercular disease and the institution for antibiotic treatment. A formula was developed to predict the degree of final gibbus deformity: x is the initial loss of vertebral body, and a and b are constants 5.5 and 30.5, retropectively. Initial vertebral loss was determined by dividing the vertebra into tenths for each involved vertebra (Figs. 92,

93). This formula may be used to identify patients who are most likely to develop significant kyphosis.

Rajasekaran S, Shanmugasundaram TK (1987): Prediction of the angle of gibbus deformity in tuberculosis of the spine. *J Bone Joint Surg [Am]* 69:503.

41. SPINAL TUMORS (Table 48, adapted from Simeone and Weinstein)

Simeone FA (199)): Spinal cord tumors in adults. In *Youman's neurological surgery,* 3rd ed. Philadelphia: WB Saunders.

Weinstein JN (1991): Differential diagnosis and surgical treatment of primary benign and malignant neoplasms. In: Frymoyer JW, ed. *The adult spine: principles and practice.* New York: Raven Press.

A. Anatomic Extent of Spinal Tumors by Zone (Fig. 94A–D; Table 49)

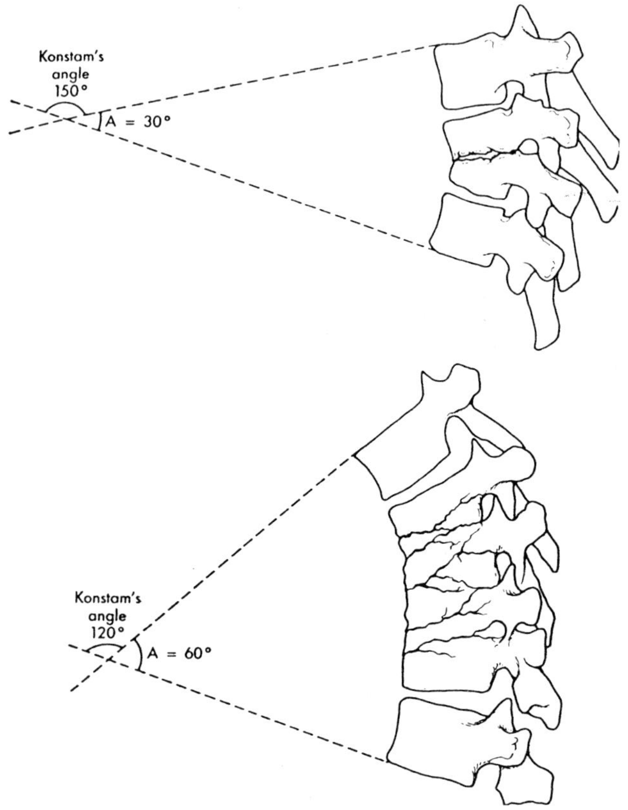

Konstam's angle 150°   A = 30°

Konstam's angle 120°   A = 60°

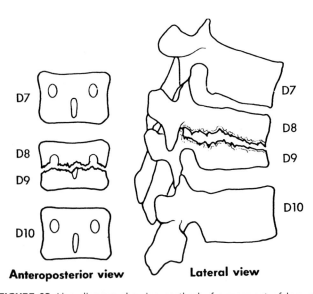

D7   D8   D9   D10

D7   D8   D9   D10

Anteroposterior view   **Lateral view**

FIGURE 92. Line diagrams showing Konstam angle (K) and angle A. (From Rajasekaran S, Shanmugasundaram TK [1987]: Prediction of the angle of gibbus deformity in tuberculosis of the spine. *J Bone Joint Surg [Am]* 69:503.)

FIGURE 93 Line diagram showing method of assessment of loss of vertebral body (From Rajasekaran S, Shanmugasundaram TK [1987]: Prediction of the angle of gibbus deformity in tuberculosis of the spine. *J Bone Joint Surg [Am]* 69:503.)

TABLE 48. MOST COMMON SPINAL TUMORS AND THEIR LOCATION

Intradural

Extramedullary intradural tumors
   Neurofibromas
   Meningiomas
   Exophytic ependymomas
   Sarcomas
   Exophytic astrocytoma
   Vascular tumors
   Epidermoid tumors
   Lipomas

Intramedullary tumors
   Ependymomas
   Astrocytomas
   Lipomas
   Teratomas
   Dermoids
   Meningoblastomas
   Oligodendrogliomas
   Epidermoids

Extradural

Primary malignant tumors
   Chordomas
   Myeloma
   Lymphoma
   Chondrosarcoma
   Osteosarcoma
   Ewing sarcoma
   Fibrosarcoma
   Anglosarcoma
   Giant cell tumor

Primary benign tumors
   Osteochondroma
   Osteoblastoma-osteoid
      osteoma
   Aneurysmal bone cyst
   Hemangioma
   Eosinophilic granuloma
   Giant cell tumors

Metastatic (most common)

TABLE 49. ANATOMIC EXTENT BY ZONE

Zones I to IV	Site A—intraosseous; site B—extraosseous; site C—regional or distant metastasis
Zones IA to IVA	Intraosseous lesions confined within the cortical boundaries
Zones IA	Includes spinous processes to the pars interarticularis and inferior articular processes
Zones IIA	Includes the transverse processes, superior articular processes, and the pedicles to their junction with the vertebral body
Zones IIIA	Anterior three fourths of the vertebral body
Zones IVA	Posterior and medial one fourth of the vertebral body
Zones IB to IVB	Extraosseous extension beyond the cortical boundaries. Lesions having extraosseous extension extend beyond the bony margins of their respective zones.
Zones IC to IVC	Intraosseous or extraosseous lesions associated with regional or distant metastases

Weinstein JN, 1991.

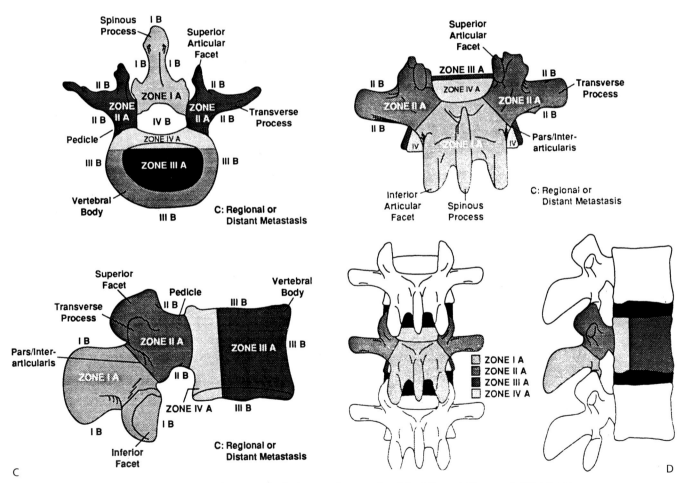

FIGURE 94. **A:** Anatomic extent of spinal tumors by zone *A:* axial cut through L1; *zones I–IVA:* intraosseous lesions are confined within the boundaries of the cortical spine. **B:** Posterior view of L1, *zones I–IVB:* extraosseous extension beyond the boundaries of the cortical spine. **C:** Lateral view of L1. **D:** Posterior view of L1–3.

TABLE 50. DIFFERENTIAL DIAGNOSIS OF PEDIATRIC SPINAL TUMORS

Lesion	History	Physical Examination	Neurodiagnostic Findings	Cerebrospinal Fluid
Syringomyelia/ hydromyelia	Slow onset	Dissociated sensory loss, atrophy	Widened cord, syrinx on magnetic resonance imaging, associated Chiari malformation	Normal
Lipomeningocele	Slow onset, autonomic dysfunction	Lumbosacral soft tissue mass, pes cavus, atrophy	Spina bifida, large subarachnoid space lipoma on magnetic resonance imaging	Normal
Tethered cord	Slow onset, autonomic dysfunction	Pes cavus	Spina bifida; conus below L2–3 thickened or fatty filum on magnetic resonance imaging	Normal
Dermoid/epidermoid	Slow onset, autonomic dysfunction	Dermal sinus, wiry hairs, hemangioma	Spina bifida, intradural extramedullary mass	Normal, unless previous meningitis
Multiple sclerosis	Rapid onset, multiple metachronous lesions	Determined by location of current plaque	Normal, magnetic resonance imaging may show multiple intracranial foci of demyelination	Increased oligoclonal bands; increased IgG index
Vitamin B$_{12}$ deficiency	Insidious onset, motor and sensory deficits start distally	Weakness, loss of proprioception (most marked distally)	Normal	Normal
Landry-Guillain-Barré syndrome	Weakness over days, starts distally	Weakness without sensory loss, loss of tendon reflexes, autonomic function usually preserved	Normal	Increased protein, increased cells
Congenital myopathy	Decreased motor activity from birth, delayed development	Decreased muscle tone, rigidity, diagnosis by muscle biopsy	Normal	Normal
Perinatal ischemic brain injury	Decreased motor activity in one extremity or on one side of the body	Increased tone, weakness, athetosis	Normal spine, infarcts on computed tomography or magnetic resonance imaging scans of brain	Normal
Transverse myelitis	Rapidly progressive painful paraplegia	Motor and sensory level, spinal shock, may have associated blindness (neuromyelitis optica)	Normal	Increased protein

From Raffel C, Edwards MSB (1988): Intraspinal tumors in children. In: *Youman's neurological surgery*, 3rd ed. Philadelphia: WB Saunders, with permission.

B. Differential Diagnosis of Pediatric Spinal Tumors (Table 50)

Weinstein JN, McLain RF (1987): Primary tumors of the spine. *Spine* 12: 843–851.

Weinstein JN (1991): Differential diagnosis and surgical treatment of primary benign and malignant neoplasms. In: Frymoyer JW, ed. *The adult spine: principles and practice.* New York: Raven Press.

C. Classification of Spinal Metastases (Fig. 95)

Harrington has described five classes of tumors. Class I is present without significant bony destruction or canal compromise. Class II bone destruction is present in less than half the vertebral body, without any evidence of fracture or instability, and with no compromise of the spinal canal or neurologic deficit. Class III, spinal compromise due to epidural disease without significant bone involvement. Class IV pathologic fracture with or without spinal deformity but without significant neurologic compromise. Class V pathologic fracture with collapse, instability, and significant neurologic compromise due to either epidural tumor, retropulsed bony debris, or kyphosis.

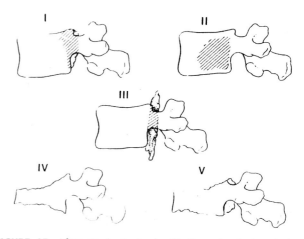

FIGURE 95. After Harrington's classification of spinal metastases. (From Harrington KD [1993]: Metastatic tumors of the spine: diagnosis and treatment. *J Am Acad Orthop Surg* 1:76–86.)

Harrington KD (1993): Metastatic tumors of the spine: Diagnosis and treatment. *J Am Acad Orthop Surg* 1:76–86.

42. NEUROFIBROMATOSIS

Young and associates (1970) classified neurofibromatosis into three hereditary forms:

1. The peripheral form, with café au lait spots and neurofibromas
2. The central form, with multiple tumors in the central nervous system, which are typical of neurofibromatosis
3. A mixed form, with both peripheral signs of neurofibromatosis and tumors in the central nervous system

Most investigators now accept two clinical forms of neurofibromatosis: central and peripheral.

NF-1: Von Recklinhausen's neurofibromatosis; peripheral neurofibromatosis (most common type, autosomal dominant affects about 1 in 4,000 persons)
NF-2: Central neurofibromatosis; bilateral acoustic neurofibromatosis (autosomal dominant, affects about 1 in 50,000 persons)

Central neurofibromatosis may be subdivided in two groups:

A. Isolated bilateral acoustic neuroma
B. Patients with multiple nervous system involvement, such as neuroaxial neoplasia, meningoneuroplasia, and cranial schwannoma

Diagnostic criteria for von Recklinhausen's neurofibromatosis (NF-1 neurofibromatosis or peripheral neurofibromatosis). Two or more of the following criteria must be met:

A. Six or more café au lait macules larger than 5 mm in greatest diameter in prepubertal children and more than 15 mm in greatest diameter in postpubertal persons
B. Two or more neurofibromas of any type or one plexiform neurofibroma
C. Freckling in the axillary or inguinal regions
D. Optical glioma
E. Two or more Lisch nodules (iris hamartomas)
F. A distinctive osseous lesion, such as sphenoid dysplasia or thinning of long bone cortex with or without pseudarthrosis
G. A first-degree relative (parent, sibling, or offspring) with NF-1 by the above-mentioned critera

Diagnostic criteria for central neurofibromatosis (NF-2):

A. Evidence from computed tomography scans or magnetic resonance imaging of bilateral internal auditory canal masses consistent with acoustic neuroma
or
B. A first-degree relative with NF-2 and either
   1. Unilateral acoustic neuroma or
   2. Two of the following:
      Neurofibroma
      Meningioma
      Glioma
      Schwannoma
      Juvenile posterior subcapsular lentricular opacity

Scoliosis is the most common osseous defect associated with neurofibromatosis. Up to 60% of the patients with neurofibromatosis may have some spinal disorder.

There are two patterns of scoliosis found in neurofibromatosis:

Dysplastic: The dysplastic curves are characteristically short-segmented, sharply angled, with severe wedging of the vertebral bodies, strong rotation of the apical vertebra, scalloping of the vertebral bodies, spindling of the transverse processes, foraminal enlargement, and penciling of the apical ribs.
Nondysplastic: These curves resemble idiopathic scoliosis and show no dysplastic changes in the vertebral bodies.

The dysplastic curves usually present in the thoracic area produce a short-segmented, sharply angled curvature involving four to six vertebrae and are usually progressive. Scoliosis is frequently accompanied by severe kyphosis. This has very important implications. Kyphosis produces elongation and deformation of the spinal cord that may lead to paraplegia. Also a high incidence of pseudarthrosis has been reported when dystrophic scoliosis associated with kyphosis in excess of 50 degrees is treated by posterior fusion with or without instrumentation. Combined anterior and posterior fusion is recommended in these cases.

Another common problem is the abnormalities found in the cervical spine in patients with neurofibromatosis. These are more common and more severe in patients with dystrophic scoliosis.

Aoki S, Barkovich Aj, Nishimura K, et al. (1989): Neurofibromatosis types 1 and 2: cranial MR findings. *Radiology* 172:527–534.
Crawford AH, Bagemary N (1986): Osseous manifestations in neurofibromatosis in childhood. *J Pediatr Orthop* 6:72–88.
National Institute of Health (1987): Neurofibromatosis. *Consensus Development Conference Statement* 6:1–7.
Winter RB, Moe JH, Bradford DS, et al. (1979): Spine deformity in neurofibromatosis. *J Bone Joint Surg [Am]* 61:677–694.
Yong-Hing K, Kalamchi A, McEwen GD (1979): Cervical spine abnormalities in neurofibromatosis. *J Bone Joint Surg [Am]* 61:695–699.
Young DF, Eldridge R, Gardner WJ (1970): Bilateral acoustic neuroma in a large kindred. *JAMA* 214:347–353.

43. NEUROMUSCULAR DISORDERS

A. Cerebral Palsy

Most of the classifications used today are modifications of the one presented by Phelps in 1932 (not published). Bleck has proposed the following classifications according to the type of movement disorder and topography (Table 51).
Bleck EE (1987): Classification. In: *Orthopaedic management in cerebral palsy.* London: Mac Keith Press.
Phelps WM (1932): *Cerebral birth injuries: their orthopedic classification and subsequent treatment.* New York: Academy of Medicine.

B. Hereditary Sensory Motor Neuropathies

Hereditary sensory motor neuropathies (HSMNs) are a heterogeneous group of familial distal muscular atrophy and weakness with relatively minor sensory deficit. Dick and Lambert developed a classification of peripheral neuropathies in which intrinsic atrophy and weakness are prominent features early in the course of the disease. These neuropathies are slowly progressive, but life expectancy is normal. Women are more severely affected than men.

Type I: Hypertrophic type of Charcot-Marie-Tooth disease, includes hereditary areflexic dystaxia (Roussy-Levy syndrome), and is inherited as an autosomal dominant disease. Compared with patients affected with type II, these patients have a greater tendency to show weakness of the hands, upper limb tremor and ataxia, generalized tendon areflexia, more distal sensory loss, and more frequent foot and spinal deformities. Clinical presentation is most common during the second decade.
Type II: Represents the neuronal form of Charcot-Marie-Tooth disease and is inherited as an autosomal dominant trait. Onset is delayed until the second decade, with more profound distal lower extremity involvement than in type I. A characteristic "stork leg" appearance is frequently seen caused by atrophy of the distal third of the quadriceps and hamstrings.
Type III: This includes the hypertrophic neuropathy of infancy (Déjérine-Sottas disease) and is an autosomal recessive trait. The disease is first noted in infants or in young children with delayed lower extremity motor milestones. Sensory modalities are lost in a stocking-and-glove type of distribution. Significant spinal deformity develops in most patients, and confinement to a wheelchair occurs during the third or fourth decade of life. The motor nerve conduction velocity is markedly slow. Nerve biopsy shows "onion bulb" formation with frequent segmental demyelination.

TABLE 51. CLASSIFICATION OF MOVEMENT DISORDERS

Type	Major Clinical Findings	Common Etiology
Physiological (according to the movement disorder)		
Spasticity (pyramidal)	Increased stretch reflex in muscles, i.e., hypertonicity of "clasp knife type"	Prematurity
	Hyperreflexia (deep tendon reflexes)	Perinatal hypoxia
	Clonus	Cerebral trauma
	Presence of Babinski sign	Rubella (maternal)
	Esotropia or exotropic	Familial
Athetosis		
Tension type	Tension can be "shaken out" of limb by examiner	Kernicterus due to Rh incompatibility
	Extensor pattern (usually)	
	Normal or depressed reflexes	
	Paralysis of upward gaze	
	Deafness (often)	
Dystonia	Intermittent distorted posturing of limbs, neck, trunk	
	No contractures	
	Full range of joint motion when relaxed	
Chorea	Spontaneous jerking of distal joints (fingers and toes)	Neonatal jaundice
		Hyperbilirubinemia
		Cerebral anoxia
		Encephalitis, meningitis, or both
Ballismus (rotary, flailing)	Uncontrolled involuntary motions of proximal joints (shoulders, elbows, hips, and knees)	
Rigidity	Rigid limbs	
	Lead pipe type—continuous resistance to passive motion	
	Cog-wheel type—discontinuous resistance to passive motion	
Ataxia	Lack of balance	Head injury
	Uncoordinated movement	Cerebral maldevelopment
	Dysmetria	
	Dysarthria	
	Wide-based gait (patient sways when walking)	
	Pes valgus (flexible) common	
Tremor	Rare	
	Intentional or nonintentional	
	Rhythmic or nonrhythmic	
Atonia	Rare	Cerebral anoxia
	Hypotonia of limbs and trunk	
	Often evolves into athetosis as child matures	
Mixed types	Spasticity and athetosis usual	Encephalitis
	Total body involvement used	Cerebral anoxia
		Birth trauma
Topographical		
Monopregia	One limb involved	
	Spasticity (usually)	
	Patient should run to excluda hemiplegic pattern	
Hemiplegia	Spastic upper and lower limb on same side	
Paraplegia	Lower limb involvement only	
	Rare in spastic type of cerebral palsy	
	Common in familial type	
	Spasticity	
Diplegia	Minor involvement of upper limbs (slight incoordination of finger movement)	
	Major involvement of lower limbs	
	Spasticity	
Triplegia	Three limbs involved	
	Spasticity	
Quadriplegia or total body involved	Total body involvement (all four limbs, head, neck, and trunk)	
	Spastic, athetoid, and mixed types	

From Block EE (1979): Definitions. In: *Orthopaedic management of cerebral palsy*. Philadelphia: WB Saunders, with permission.

TABLE 52. MUSCULAR DYSTROPHIES

The Pure Muscular Dystrophies
X-linked recessive
  Duchenne muscular dystrophy—severe
  Backer muscular dystrophy—benign
  Emery-Dreifus dystrophy—benign with early contracture

Autosomal recessive
  Scapulohumeral—"limb girdle," "quadriceps myopathy"
  Early onset in childhood—"Duchenne-like"
  Congenital muscular dystrophies

Autosomal dominant
  Facioscapulohumeral
  Scapuloperoneal
  Late-onset proximal
  Distal (adult onset)
  Distal (infantile onset)
  Ocular
  Oculopharyngeal

Dystrophies with Myotonia
  Myotonia congenita
  Dystrophia myotonica
  Paramyotonia congenita

Type IV: Type IV is Refsum disease. The condition is inherited as a autosomal recessive trait, with onset in childhood or puberty. Initial findings are anosmia, progressive deafness, and night blindness. Hypertrophic neuropathy and areflexia are common. Orthopaedic manifestations include scoliosis, pes cavus, and pes equinus. Motor nerve conduction are slow. Onion bulb formation is noted on nerve biopsy. Serum elevation of phytanic acid levels is pathognomonic.

Dick PJ, Lambert EH (1968): Lower motor and primary sensory neuron disease with peroneal muscle atrophy. Part I. Neurologic genetic and electrophysiologic finding in hereditary polineuropathies. *Arch Neurol* 18:603–628.

C. Progressive Muscular Dystrophy (Table 52)

Walton JN, Gardner-Medwin D (1981): Progressive muscular and myotonic disorders. In: *Disorders of voluntary muscle*, 4th ed. Endinburgh: Churchill-Livingstone.

D. Differential Diagnosis of Muscle Dystrophies (Table 53)

44. SKELETAL DYSPLASIAS (Tables 54–56)

Wynne-Davies R, Hall CM, Graham-Apley A (1985): *Atlas of skeletal dysplasias.* Edinburgh: Churchill Livingstone.

TABLE 53. DIFFERENTIAL DIAGNOSIS OF THE PRINCIPAL TYPES OF MUSCULAR DYSTROPHY

Clinical Features	Duchenne-Type	Limb Girdle	Facioscapulohumeral	Distal	Progressive Dystrophia Ophthalmoplegia	Congenital or Infantile
Incidence	Commonest	Less common, but not infrequent	Not common	Rare	Rare	Rare
Age at onset	Usually prior to 3 y, some between 3 and 8 y	Variable (usually by second decade, occasionally latar)	Variable (usually in second decade)	20–77 y (mean: 47 y)	At any age (infancy to >50 y)	At or soon after birth
Sex preponderance	Male	Either sex	Male and female equally affected	Either sex	Either sex	Not yet determined
Inheritance	Sex-linked recessive, autosomal less than 10%	Autosomal recessive, on rare occasions autosomal dominant	Autosomal dominant usually, autosomal recessive very rarely	Autosomal dominant	Simple dominant or simple recessive	Unknown
Pattern of muscle involvement	Proximal (pelvic and shoulder girdle muscles affected early, spreads to periphery limbs late in course)	Proximal (shoulder and pelvic girdle, spreads to periphery late)	Face and shoulder girdle, later spreads to pelvic girdle)	Distal (hand first, anterior tibial, and calf in leg)	Usuality limited to extend ocular muscles	Generalized
Muscle spared until late	Gastrocnemius, toe flexors posterior tibial, hamstrings, hand muscles, upper trapezius, biceps, triceps, face, jaw, pharyngeal, laryngeal, and ocular	In upper extremity brachioradialis and hand, calf muscles	Back extensors, iliopsoas, hip abductors, quadriceps	Proximal until late	See above	—
Pseudohypertrophy	80% of cases (calf muscles)	Less than 33% of cases	Rare	Not seen	Not seen	Not seen

(continued)

TABLE 53. *Continued.*

Clinical Features	Duchenne-Type	Limb Girdle	Facioscapulohumeral	Distal	Progressive Dystrophia Ophthalmoplegia	Congenital or Infantile
Myotonia	Absent	Absent	Absent	Absent	Absent	Absent
Contractural deformities	Common	Develop late in course, less severe than Duchenne syndrome	Mild, occur late	Mild, late	—	Severe
Scoliosis and kyphoscoliosis	Common in late stage	Mild, in late stage	Mild, occur late	—	—	?
Heart involvement	Hypertrophy and tachycardia common: in late stages widespread degeneration, fibrosis, and fatty infiltration	Very rare	Very rare	Very rare	Not seen	Not observed
Endocrine changes	Not seen	Not seen	Not seen	Not seen	Not seen	?
Intellectual level	Commonly decreased	Normal	Normal	Normal	Normal	?
Course	Steady rapid progression	Slow progression, considerable variation in pace of disease	Progresses insidiously	Comparatively benign	Slow progression	Steady progression

From Tachdjian MO (1990): Progressive muscular dystrophy. In: *Pediatric orthopaedics*. Philadelphia: WB Saunders, with permission.

TABLE 54. DYNAMIC CLASSIFICATION OF BONE DYSPLASIAS

I. Epiphyseal dysplasias
  A. Epiphyseal hypoplasias
    1. Failure of articular cartilage: spondyloepiphyseal dysplasia, congenita, and tarda
    2. Failure of ossification of center: multiple epiphyseal dysplasia, congenita, and tarda
  B. Epiphyseal hyperplasia
    1. Excess of articular cartilage; dysplasia epiphysealis hemimelica

II. Physeal dysplasias
  A. Cartilage hypoplasias
    1. Failure of proliferating cartilage: achondroplasia, congenita, and tarda
    2. Failure of hypertrophic cartilage: metaphyseal dysostosis, congenita, and tarda
  B. Cartilage hyperplasias
    1. Excess of proliferating cartilage: hyperchondroplasia
    2. Excess of hypertrophic cartilage: enchondromatosis

III. Metaphyseal dysplasias
  A. Metaphyseal hypoplasias
    1. Failure to form primary spongiosa: hypophosphatasia, congenita, and tarda
    2. Failure to absorb primary spongiosa: osteopetrosis, congenita, and tarda
    3. Failure to absorb secondary spongiosa: craniometaphyseal dysplasia, congenita, and tarda
  B. Metaphyseal hyperplasias
    1. Excessive spongiosa: multiple exostoses

IV. Diaphyseal dysplasias
  A. Diaphyseal hypoplasias
    1. Failure of periosteal bone formation: osteogenesis imperfecta, congenita, and tarda
    2. Failure of endosteal bone formation: idiopathic osteoporosis, congenita, and tarda
  B. Diaphyseal hyperplasias
    1. Excessive periosteal bone formation: progressive diaphyseal dysplasia
    2. Excessive endosteal bone formation: hyperphosphatasemia

From Rubin P (1964): *Dynamic classification of bone dysplasias*. Chicago: Year Book Medical Publishers, with permission.

TABLE 55. INTERNATIONAL NOMENCLATURE OF CONSTITUTIONAL DISEASE OF BONE

Osteochondrodysplasias
  Abnormalities of cartilage and/or bone growth and development

Defects of Growth of Tubular Bone and/or Spine
A. Identifiable at birth
  1. Achondrogenesis type I, Parenti-Fraccaro
  2. Achondrogenesis type II, Langer-Saldino
  3. Thanatophoric dysplasia
  4. Thanatophoric dysplasia with clover-leaf skull
  5. Short rib-polydactyly syndrome type I, Saldino-Noonas (perhaps several forms)
  6. Short rib-polydactyly syndrome type II, Majewski
  7. Chondryodysplasia punctata
     a. Rhizomelic form
     b. Dominant form
     c. Other forms, excluding symptomatic stippling in other disorders (e.g., Zellweger syndrome, Warfarin embryopathy)
  8. Campomelic dysplasia
  9. Other dysplasias with congenital bowing of long bones (several forms)
  10. Achondroplasia
  11. Diastrophic dysplasia
  12. Metatropic dysplasia (several forms)
  13. Chondroectodermal dysplasia, Ellis Van Creveld
  14. Asphyxiating thoracic dysplasia, Jeune
  15. Spondyloepiphyseal dysplasia congenita
     a. Type Spranger-Wiedemann
     b. Other forms (see B, 11–12)
  16. Kniest dysplasia
  17. Mesomelic dysplasia
     a. Type Nievergelt
     b. Type Langer (probable homozygous dyschondrosteosis)
     c. Type Robinow
     d. Type Rheinhardt
     e. Other forms
  18. Acromesomelic dysplasia
  19. Cleidocranial dysplasia
  20. Larsen syndrome
  21. Otopalatodigital syndrome
B. Identifiable in later life
  1. Hypochondroplasia
  2. Dyschondrosteosis
  3. Metaphyseal chondrodysplasia type Jansen
  4. Metaphyseal chondrodysplasia type Schmid
  5. Metaphyseal chondrodysplasia type McKusick
  6. Metaphyseal chondrodysplasia with exocrine pancreatic insufficiency and cyclic neutropenia
  7. Spondylometaphyseal dysplasia
     a. Type Kozlowski
     b. Other forms
  8. Multiple epiphyseal dysplasia
     a. Type Fairbank
     b. Other forms
  9. Arthro-ophthalmopathy, Stickler
  10. Pseudoachondroplasia
     a. Dominant
     b. Recessive
  11. Spondyloepiphyseal dysplasia tarda
  12. Spondyloepiphyseal dysplasia, other forms (see A, 15–16)
  13. Dyggve-Melchior-Clausen dysplasia
  14. Spondyloepiphyseal dysplasia (several forms)
  15. Myotonic chondrodysplasia, Catel-Schwartz-Jampel
  16. Parastremmatic dysplasia
  17. Trichorhinophalangeal dysplasia
  18. Acrodysplasia with retinitis pigmentosa and nephropathy Saldino-Mainzer

Disorganized Development of Cartilage and Fibrous Components of Skeleton
  1. Dysplasia epiphysealis hemimelica
  2. Multiple cartilaginous exotoses
  3. Acrodysplasia with exotoses Giedion-Langer
  4. Enchondromatosis, Olliar
  5. Enchondromatosis with hemangioma, Maffucci
  6. Metachondromatosis
  7. Fibrous dysplasia, Jaffe-Lichtenstein
  8. Fibrous dysplasia with skin pigmentation and precocious puberty, McCune-Albright
  9. Cherubism (familial fibrous dysplasia of the jaws)
  10. Neurofibromatosis

Abnormalities of Density of Cortical Diaphyseal Structure and/or Metaphyseal Modelling
  1. Osteogenesis imperfecta congenita (several forms)
  2. Osteogenesis imperfecta tarda (several forms)
  3. Juvenile idiopathic osteoporosis
  4. Osteoporosis with pseudoglioma
  5. Osteoporosis with precocious manifestations
  6. Osteopetrosis with delayed manifestations (several forms)
  7. Pycnodysostosis
  8. Osteopoikliosis
  9. Osteopathia striata
  10. Melorheostosis
  11. Diaphyseal dysplasia, Camurati-Engelmann
  12. Craniodiaphyseal dysplasia
  13. Endosteal hyperostosis
     a. Autosomal dominant, Worth
     b. Autosomal recessive, Van Buchem
  14. Tubular stenosis, Kenny-Caffey
  15. Pachydermoperiostosis
  16. Osteodysplasty, Melnick-Needles
  17. Frontometaphyseal dysplasia
  18. Craniometaphyseal dysplasia (several forms)
  19. Metaphyseal dysplasia, Pyle
  20. Sclerosteosis
  21. Dysosteosclerosis
  22. Osteoectasia with hyperphosphatasia

Dysostoses
  Malformation of individual bones singly or in combination.

Dysostoses with Cranial and Facial Involvement
  1. Craniosynostosis (several forms)
  2. Craniofacial dysostosis, Crouzon
  3. Acrocephalosyndactyly, Apert (and others)
  4. Acrocephalopolysyndactyly, Carpenter (and others)
  5. Mandibulofacial dysostosis
     a. Type Treacher Collins, Franceschetti
     b. Other forms
  6. Oculomandibulofacial syndrome, Hallermann-Streiff-Francois
  7. Nevoid basal cell carcinoma syndrome

Dysostoses with Predominant Axial Involvement
  1. Vertebral segmentation defects, including Klippel-Feil
  2. Cervico-oculoacoustic syndrome, Wildervanck
  3. Sprengel anomaly
  4. Spondylocostal dysostosis
     a. Dominant form
     b. Recessive forms
  5. Oculovertebral syndrome, Weyers
  6. Osteo-onychodysostosis
  7. Cerebrocostomandibular syndrome

(continued)

TABLE 55. *Continued.*

Dysostoses with Predominant Involvement of Extremities
  1. Acheiria
  2. Apodia
  3. Ectodactyly syndrome
  4. Aglossia-adactyly syndrome
  5. Congenital bowing of long bones (several forms) (see also osteochondrodysplasias)
  6. Familial radioulnar synostosis
  7. Brachydactyly (several forms)
  8. Symphalangism
  9. Polydactyly (several forms)
  10. Syndactyly (several forms)
  11. Polysyndactyly (several forms)
  12. Camptodactyly
  13. Poland syndrome
  14. Rubenstein-Taybi syndrome
  15. Pancytopenia-dysmelia syndrome, Fanconi
  16. Thrombocytopenia-radialaplasia syndrome
  17. Orodigitofacial syndrome
      a. Type Papillon-Leage
      b. Type Mohr
  18. Cardiomelic syndrome, Holt-Oram (and others)
  19. Femoral facial syndrome
  20. Multiple-synostoses (includes some forms of symphalangism)
  21. Scapuloiliac dysostosis, Kosenow-Sinlos
  22. Hand-foot-genital syndrome
  23. Focal dermal hypoplasia, Goltz

Idiopathic Osteolyses
  1. Phalangeal (several forms)
  2. Tarsocarpal
      a. including Francois form (and others)
      b. With nephropathy
  3. Multicentric
      a. Hajdu-Cheney form
      b. Winchester form
      c. Other forms

Chromosomal Aberrations
  Specific entities not listed

Pulmonary Metabolic Abnormalities

Calcium and/or Phosphorus
  1. Hypophosphatemic rickets

  2. Pseudodeficiency rickets, Prader, Royer
  3. Late rickets, McCance
  4. Idiopathic hypercalcuria
  5. Hypophosphatasia (several forms)
  6. Pseudohypoparathyroidism (normo- and hypocalcaemic forms, include acrodysostosis)

Complex Carbohydrates
  1. Mucopolysaccharidosis, type I (alpha-ι-iduronidase deficiency)
      a. Hurler form
      b. Scheie form
      c. Other forms
  2. Mucopolysaccharidosis, type II, Hunter (sulfolduronate sulfatase deficiency)
  3. Mucopolysaccharidosis, type III San Filippo
      a. Type A (heparin sulfamidase deficiency)
      b. Type B (N-acetyl-alpha-glucosaminidase deficiency)
  4. Mucopolysaccharidosis, type IV, Morquio (N-acetylgalactos-amine-6-sulfate-sulfatase deficiency)
  5. Mucopolysaccharidosis, type VI, Maroteaux-Lamy (aryl sulfate B deficiency)
  6. Mucopolysaccharidosis, type VII (beta-glucuronidase deficiency)
  7. Aspartylglucosaminuria (aspartylglucosaminidase deficiency)
  8. Mannosidosis (alpha-mannosidase deficiency)
  9. Fucosidosis (alpha-fucosidase deficiency)
  10. GMI-gangilosidosis (beta-galatosidase deficiency)
  11. Multiple sulfatase deficiency, Austin, Thieffry
  12. Neuraminidase deficiency (formerly mucolipidosis I)
  13. Mucolipidosis II
  14. Mucolipidosis III

Lipids
  1. Niemann-Pick disease
  2. Gaucher disease

Nuclic Acids
  1. Adneosine-deaminase deficiency and others

Amino Acids
  1. Homocystinuria and others

Metals
  1. Menkes' kinky hair syndrome and others

From Horan F, Beighton P (1982): *Orthopaedic problems in inherited skeletal disorders.* New York: Springer Verlag, with permission.

TABLE 56. CHARACTERISTIC SPINAL PROBLEMS IN SKELETAL DYSPLASIAS

Condition	Deformity	Anomaly	Instability	Stenosis	Special Features
Achondroplasia	T1 kyphosis ages 0–2	0		Foramen magnum; entire spine	Adult weakness due to stenosis
Diastrophic dysplasia	Cervical kyphosis; T1 scoliosis	Cervical spina bifida occulta			Cervical kyphosis may resolve; scoliosis usually rigid
SED congenita	Scoliosis	Odontoid hypoplasia	C1–2		
Morquio syndrome	T1 scoliosis	Odontoid hypoplasia	C1–2		
Hurler syndrome	T1 kyphosis; scoliosis		C1–2		Most live 1–2 decades
Osteogenesis imperfecta	Kyphosis; scoliosis				Scoliosis related to overall severity
Larsen syndrome	Cervical kyphosis	Cervical spondylolisthesis; cervical spina bifida	Midcervical		Kyphosis should be fused posteriorly

Orthopaedic Knowledge Update #6, American Academy of Orthopaedic Surgeons 1999:28.

45. OSTEOGENESIS IMPERFECTA (Table 57)

Sillence D (1981): Osteogenesis imperfecta: an expanding panorama of variants. *Clin Orthop* 159:11–25.

46. MARFAN SYNDROME (Table 58)

47. EHLERS-DANLOS SYNDROME (Cutis hyperelastica) (Table 59)

48. MUCOPOLYSACCHARIDOSIS (Table 60)

49. OSTEOPOROSIS IN CHILDHOOD (Table 61)

50. RHEUMATOID DISORDERS

A. Diagnostic Criteria for Rheumatoid Arthritis (Table 62)

B. Diagnostic Criteria for Ankylosing Spondylitis (Tables 63, 64)

Bennett PH, Burch TA (1968): *Population studies in rheumatic disease.* Amsterdam: Excerpta Medicus.
Katz, JN, Liang MH (1991): Differential diagnosis and conservative treatment of rheumatic disorders. In: Frymoyer JW, ed. *The adult spine: principles and practice.* New York: Raven Press.
Kellgren JH, Jeffrey MR, Ball S (1963): *The epidemiology of chronic rheumatism,* Vol. 1. Oxford: Blackwell, pp. 326–327.

TABLE 57. OSTEOGENESIS IMPERFECTA

Type		Transmission*	Biochemistry	Orthopaedic	Miscellaneous
I	A	AD	Half normal amount of type I collagen	Mild to moderate bone fragility, osteoporosis	Blue sclerae, hearing loss, easy bruising, dentinogenesis imperfecta absent
	B	AD		Short stature	More severe than IA with dentinogenesis imperfecta
II		AD, AR and mosaic	Unstable triple helix	Multiple intrauterine fractures, extreme bone fragility	Usually lethal in perinatal period, delayed ossification of skull, interuterine growth retardation
	A		Long bones broad, crumpled; ribs broad with continuous beading		
	B		Long bones broad, crumpled; ribs discontinuous or no beading		
	C		Long bones thin, fractured; ribs thin, beaded		
	D		Severely osteopenic with generally well-formed skeleton; normally shaped vertebrae and pelvis		
III		AD (new mutation) and AR (rare)	Abnormal type I collagen	Progressive deforming phenotype, severe bone fragility with fractures at birth, scoliosis, severe osteoporosis, extreme short stature	Hearing loss, short stature, blue sclerae becoming less blue with age, shortened life expectancy, dentinogenesis imperfecta, relative macrocephaly with triangular faces
IV	A	AD	Shortened pro alpha, (I) chains	Mild to moderate bone fragility, osteoporosis, bowing of long bones, scoliosis	Light sclerae, normal hearing, normal dentition, dentinogenesis imperfecta absent
	B	AD			Dentinogenesis imperfecta present

* AR, autosomal recessive; AD, autosomal dominant
* Cole WG. The molecular pathology of osteogenesis imperfecta. *Clin Orthop* 1997;343:235–248.

TABLE 58. DIAGNOSTIC CRITERIA FOR MARFAN SYNDROME

System	Major Criteria	Minor Criteria
Musculoskeletal[a]	Pectus carinatum; pectus excovatum requiring surgery; dolichostenomelia, wrist and thumb signs; scoliosis > 20° or spondylolisthesis; reduced elbow extension; pes planus; protrusio acetabulae	Moderately severe pes excovatum; joint hypermobility; highly arched palate with crowding of teeth; focies (dolichocephaly, malar hypoplasia, enophihalmos, retognathio, down-slanting palebral fissures)
Ocular[b]	Ectopia lentis	Abnormally flat comea; increased axial length of globe; hypoplastic iris or hypoplastic ciliary muscle causing decreased miosis
Cardiovascular[c]	Dilatation of ascending aorta ± aortic regurgitation, involving sinuses of Valsalva; or dissection of ascending aorta	Mitrol valve prolapse ± regurgitation; dilatation of main pulmonary artery without valvular or peripheral pulmonic stenosis or obvious cause below 40 years; calcification of mitrol anulus below 40 years; or dilatation or dissection of descending aorta below 50 years

(continued)

TABLE 58. *Continued.*

System	Major Criteria	Minor Criteria
Family/genetic history[d]	Parent, child, or sibling meets diagnostic criteria; mutation in *FBN1* known to cause Marfan syndrome; or inherited haplotype around *FBN1* associated with Marfan syndrome in family	None
Skin and integument**	None	Stretch marks not associated with pregnancy, weight gain, or repetitive stress; or recurrent or incisional hernias
Dural[d]	Lumbosacral dural ectasia	None
Pulmonary**	None	Spontaneous pneumothorax or apical blebs

[a] Two or more major or one major + two minor criteria required for involvement
[b] At least two minor criteria required for involvement
[c] One major or minor criteria required for involvement
[d] One major criteria required for involvement
** One minor criteria required for involvement
Data taken from Paepe A, Deveraux RB, Dietz HC, et al. (1996): Revised diagnostic criteria for the Marfan Syndrome. *Am J Med Genet* 62:417–426.

TABLE 59. EHLERS-DANLOS SYNDROME (CUTIS HYPERELASTICA)

Type	Acronym	Transmission[a]	Clinical Findings	Miscellaneous	Basic Defect
I	Gravis type	AD	Hyperextensible skin, poor wound healing, scoliosis, pes planus; hypermobility of small and large joints; osteoarthritis, clubfoot and hip dislocation in the newborn	Easy bruising, "cigarette paper" scars, varicose veins, miscarriages, prematurity, mitral valve prolapse	COL5A1 mutations
II	Mitis type	AD	Similar to EDS I; joint laxity less severe but remarkable in small joints	Less severe than EDS I, no prematurity	COL5A1 mutations, COL1A2 null alleles
III	Hypermobile type	AD	Early onset osteoarthritis, joint dislocations, marked large and small joint hypermobility	Soft skin, no scarring	Unknown
IV	Vascular type	AR (rare)	Hands and feet appear prematurely aged, thin skin without hyperextensibility, minimal joint hypermobility	Severe vascular fragility; uterine and bowel ruptures; stroke; abnormal facies with large eyes, thin nose, thin lips; short life expectancy	COL3A1 mutations; numerous point mutations and exon skips, rarely deletions
	IVA acrogeric	AD			
	IVB acrogeric	AR			
	IVC ecchymotic	AD			
V	x-linked type	XR	Joint laxity	Very rare; similar to EDS I, II, III	Unknown
VI	Ocular scoliotic VIA decreased lysyl hydroxylase levels, VIA normal levels	AR	Kyphoscoliosis (occasionally intractable), muscle hypotonia, moderate joint laxity, skin hyperextensibility	Easy bruising, arterial rupture, ocular fragility	Lysyl hydroxylase point mutations or exon skips (homozygosity and double heterozygosity)
VII	A and B arthrocholosis multiplex congenita	AD	Multiple joint dislocations, bilateral hip dislocation at birth, increased skin elasticity without fragility; diffuse hypotonia, increased bone fragility	Easy bruising, short stature	A: COL1A1 exon 6 skipping mutations; B: COL1A2 exon B skipping mutations
	C	AR	Soft fragile, bruisable skin; marked joint hypermobility	Blue sclera	C: procollagen peptidase deficiency
VIII	Periodontis type	AD	Joint laxity, increased skin elasticity with fragility	Periodontal disease with early tooth loss, easy bruising	Some are COL3A1, others not
IX[b]	Vacant				
X	Fibronectin abnormality	AR	Mild, similar to EDS II or EDS III without dislocations	Platelet aggregation dysfunction resulting in poor clotting	Defect in fiber section
XI[c]	Vacant				

[a] AD, autosomal dominant; AR, autosomal recessive; XR, x-linked recessive
[b] EDS type IX is no longer part of EDS; it has been reclassified as a disease of copper metabolism
[c] EDS type XI is now reclassified as a disorder of joint instability
Pope FM, Burrow NP: Ehlers-Danlos syndrome has varied molecular mechanisms. *Am J Med Genet* 1997;34:400–410.

TABLE 60. DIFFERENTIAL DIAGNOSIS OF MUCOPOLYSACCHARIDOSIS

Type	Enzyme Defect	Increased Urinary Excretion of Acid Mucopolysaccharide	Inheritance	Age at Which Features Present	Facies	Corneal Clouding
Hurler syndrome MPS 1	Deficient α-L-iduronidase	Dermatan sulfate ++ Heparan sulfate +	Autosomal recessive	First few months; may appear normal at birth	Grotesque Gargoyle	Present
Hunter syndrome MPS II	Low sulfoiduronate sulfatase	Heparan sulfate ++ Dermatan sulfate +	Sex-linked recessive; all patients male	6–12 m	Similar to Hurler syndrome; less severe	Absent
San Filippo syndrome MPS III	Low N-heparan sulfatase or α-acetyl-glucosaminase	Heparan sulfate ++	Autosomal recessive	Early childhood	Not coarse	Absent
Morquio syndrome MPS IV	N-Ac-Gal-8 sulfate sulfatase	Keratin sulfate ++ (diminishes with age)	Autosomal recessive	2–4 y	Not coarse Wide mouth Prominent maxilla	Present; slowly progressive
Scheie syndrome MPS I-S	α-L-iduronidase	Heparan sulfate + Dermatan sulfate ++	Autosomal recessive	Late childhood	Somewhat coarse	Present
Maroteaux-Lamy syndrome MPS VI	N-Ac-Gal-4-sulfate	Dermatan sulfate ++	Autosomal recessive	Early to late childhood	Coarse	Present, poor vision

Deafness	Hepatosplenomegaly	Cardiovascular Abnormalities	Stature	Skeletal Changes	Mental Retardation	Prognosis
Present	Present	Present	Normal at birth; later may be moderately short	Moderate dorsolumbar kyphosis; anterior-inferior beaking of body of L2 or L1	Severe	Progressive disease, usually death by 10 years of age, due to heart disease or respiratory infection
Frequent	Present	Present; pulmonary hypertension	Normal at birth; later may be moderately short	Moderate, absence of lumbar kyphosis	Late in onset, less severe than in Hurler	Survival usually into the third decade of life; eventual death from cardiopulmonary disease
Present	Minimal or moderate	Absent	Normal	Minimal widening of clavicles at medial ends, no kyphosis	Severe	Survival to third or fourth decade
Present	Usually absent	Minimal, if present aortic regurgitation	Markedly short (under 4 ft)	Severe and diffuse platyspondyly with central tongue; capital femoral epiphyses irregular, eventually disappear	Absent	Normal longevity; respiratory failure due to rib cage rigidity
Present	Absent	Present, aortic valve disease	Normal	Small epiphysis on hands	Absent	Normal longevity
Present	Hepatomegaly rather than splenomegaly	Absent	Normal at birth; later markedly short	Severe (same as Hurler syndrome)	Absent	Guarded, death from cardiovascular complications

From Techdijian MO (1990): The mucopolysaccharidosis. In: *Pediatric orthopedics*, 2nd ed. WB Saunders, Philadelphia, with permission.

TABLE 61. CAUSES OF OSTEOPOROSIS IN CHILDHOOD

Endocrine disorders
   Hyperthyroidism
   Hyperparathyrodism
   Hypogonadism
   Glucocorticoid excess—Cushing syndrome, steroid therapy

Metabolic disorders
   Homocystinuria
   Gastrointestinal malabsorption
   Idiopathic hypoproteinemia
   Vitamin C deficiency
   Rickets-osteomalacia
   Liver disease

Renal disease
   Chronic tubular acidosis
   Idiopathic hypercalciuria
   Lowe syndrome
   Uremia and regular hemodialysis

Bone affections
   Osteogenesis imperfecta
   Idiopathic juvenile osteoporosis
   Idiopathic osteolysis
   Turner syndrome (XO chromosome anomaly)

Malignant diseases
   Leukemia
   Lymphoma

Miscellaneous causes
   Disuse osteoporosis of paralyzed limbs as in myelomeningocele
   Generalized osteoporosis of Still disease, especially after steroid therapy
   Heparin therapy
   Anticonvulsant drug therapy

From Tachdijian MO (1990): Idiopathic juvenile osteoporosis. In: *Pediatric orthopedics*. 2nd ed. Philadelphia: WB Saunders, with permission.

TABLE 62. THE 1987 REVISED CRITERIA FOR THE CLASSIFICATION OF RHEUMATOID ARTHRITIS (TRADITIONAL FORMAT)[a]

Criterion	Definition
1. Morning stiffness	Morning stiffness in and around the joints, lasting at least 1 hour before maximal improvement
2. Arthritis of 3 or more joint areas	At least 3 joint areas simultaneously have had soft tissue swelling or fluid (not bony overgrowth alone) observed by a physician. The 14 possible areas are right or left PIP, MCP, wrist, elbow, knee, ankle, and MTP joints
3. Arthritis of hand joints	At least 1 area swollen (as defined above) In a wrist, MCP, or PIP joint
4. Symmetric arthritis	Simultaneous involvement of the same joint areas (as defined in criterion 2) on both sides of the body (bilateral involvement of PIPs, MCPs, or MTPs is acceptable without absolute symmetry)
5. Rheumatoid nodules	Subcutaneous nodules, over bony prominences, or extensor surfaces, or in juxtaarticular regions, observed by a physician
6. Serum rheumatoid factor	Demonstration of abnormal amounts of serum rheumatoid factor by any method for which the result has been positive in <5% of normal control subjects
7. Radiographic changes	Radiographic changes typical of rheumatoid arthritis on posteroanterior hand and wrist radiographs, which must include erosions or unequivocal bony decalcification localized in or most marked adjacent to the involved joints (osteoarthritis changes alone do not qualify)

From Arnett FC, Edworthy SM, Bloch DA, et al. (1988): The American Rheumatism Association 1987 revised criteria for the classification of rheumatoid arthritis. *Arthritis Rheum* 31:315–324, with permission.
[a] For classification purposes, a patient shall be said to have rheumatoid arthritis if he or she has satisfied at least four of these seven criteria. Criteria 1 through 4 must have been present for at least 6 weeks. Patients with two clinical diagnoses are not excluded. Designation as classic, definite, or probable rheumatoid arthritis is not to be made.
PIP, proximal interphalangeal joint; MCP, metacarpophalangeal joint; MTP, metatarsophalangeal joint.

TABLE 63. ROME CRITERIA FOR THE DIAGNOSIS OF ANKYLOSING SPONDYLITIS

1. Low back pain and stiffness for more than 3 months, which is not relieved by rest
2. Pain and stiffness in the thoracic region
3. Limited motion in the lumbar spine
4. Limited chest expansion
5. History or evidence of iritis or its sequelae

Ankylosing spondylitis diagnosed if bilateral sacroiliitis present and associated with any one of the above clinical criteria

TABLE 64. NEW YORK CRITERIA FOR THE DIAGNOSIS OF ANKYLOSING SPONDYLITIS

1. Limitation of motion of the lumbar spine in all three planes (anterior flexion, lateral flexion, and extension)
2. A history of pain or the presence of pain at the dorsolumbar junction or in the lumbar spine
3. Limitation of chest expansion to 1 inch (2.5 cm) or less, measured at the level of the fourth intercostal space

Radiographic sacroiliac changes
0.   Normal
I.   Suspicious
II.   Minimal sacroiliitis
III.   Moderate sacroiliitis
IV.   Ankylosis

Definite ankylosing spondylitis if
   Grade 3–4 bilateral sacroiliitis associated with at least one clinical criterion
   Grade 3–4 unilateral or grade bilateral sacroiliitis associated with clinical criterion 1 or with both clinical criteria 2 and 3
   Probable ankylosing spondylitis if grade 3–4 bilateral sacroiliitis exists without any signs or symptoms satisfying the clinical criteria

INDEX

Page references for figures are in italics and page references for tables are followed by a t.